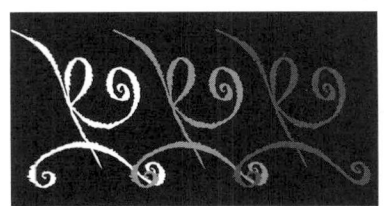

Contents

ALEXANDER'S

CARE OF THE PATIENT IN SURGERY

ALEXANDER'S
CARE OF THE PATIENT IN SURGERY

MARGARET H. MEEKER, RN, BSN, CNOR
Director of Women and Infants Services
Former Director of Perioperative Nursing
The Ohio State University Medical Center
Columbus, Ohio

JANE C. ROTHROCK, RN, DNSc, CNOR
Professor and Program Coordinator
Perioperative Nursing
Delaware County Community College
Media, Pennsylvania

ELEVENTH EDITION

with 1468 illustrations

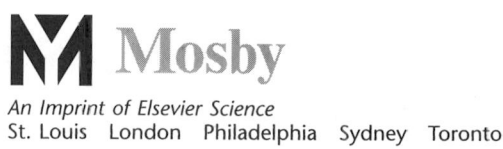 Mosby

An Imprint of Elsevier Science
St. Louis   London   Philadelphia   Sydney   Toronto

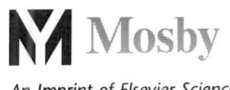

Publisher	Nancy L. Coon
Editor	Michael Ledbetter
Developmental Editor	Nancy L. O'Brien
Project Manager	Dana Peick
Senior Production Editor	Jeffrey Patterson
Designer	Pati Pye
Manufacturing Manager	Betty Mueller

A NOTE TO THE READER:

The author and publisher have made every attempt to check dosages and nursing content for accuracy. Because the science of pharmacology is continually advancing, our knowledge base continues to expand. Therefore we recommend that the reader always check product information for changes in dosage or administration before administering any medication. This is particularly important with new or rarely used drugs.

ELEVENTH EDITION

Copyright © 1999 by Mosby, Inc.

All rights reserved. No part of this publication may be reproduced, stored in a retrieval system, or transmitted in any form or by any means, electronic, mechanical, photocopying, recording, or otherwise, without written permission of the publisher.

Permission to photocopy or reproduce solely for internal or personal use is permitted for libraries or other users registered with the Copyright Clearance Center, provided that the base fee of $4.00 per chapter plus $.10 per page is paid directly to the Copyright Clearance Center, 222 Rosewood Drive, Danvers, MA 01923. This consent does not extend to other kinds of copying, such as copying for general distribution for advertising or promotional purposes, for creating new collected works, or for resale.

Printed in the United States of America

Mosby, Inc.
11830 Westline Industrial Drive
St. Louis, Missouri 63146

Library of Congress Cataloging-in-Publication Data

Alexander's care of the patient in surgery   /   [edited by] Margaret H. Meeker, Jane C.
   Rothrock. — 11th ed.
        p.   cm.
      Includes bibliographical references and index.
      ISBN 0-323-00134-3 (hard cover)
      1. Surgical nursing. 2. Therapeutics, Surgical. I. Alexander, Edythe Louise. II. Meeker, Margaret
   Huth. III. Rothrock, Jane C. IV. Title: Care of the patient in surgery.
      [DNLM: 1. Perioperative Nursing. 2. Nursing Care. WY   161   A3756   1999]
   RD99.M387   1999
   610.73'677—dc21
   DNLM/DLC   98-37345

02 / 9 8 7 6 5 4

Contributors

Kay A. Ball, RN, BSN, MSA, CNOR, FAAN
Perioperative Consultant/Educator
Lewis Center, Ohio
Ch. 3 — Surgical Modalities

Anna H. Burns, RN, BS, CNOR, RNFA
RN First Assistant
White Plains Hospital Center
White Plains, New York
Ch. 16 — Thyroid and Parathyroid Surgery

Brenda S. Gregory Dawes, RN, MSN, CNOR
Editor
AORN Journal
New Port Richey, Florida
Ch. 25 — Thoracic Surgery

Katherine J. Donahoe, RN, CNOR
Perioperative Staff RN
Crozer-Chester Medical Center
Upland, Pennsylvania
Ch. 24 — Plastic and Reconstructive Surgery

Althea R. Dunscombe, RN, PhD, CRNFA
President, RNFA Program Director
Professional Assistants PRN, Inc.
Chair, Postgraduate Perioperative Nursing Education
Southwest Florida College
Naples, Florida
Ch. 6 — Sutures, Needles, and Instruments

Diane L. Fecteau, RN, MSA
Executive Director
Brighton Surgical Center
Portland, Maine
Ch. 2 — Patient and Environmental Safety

Nancye Rue Feistritzer, RN, MSN
Assistant Hospital Director
Perioperative Patient Care Center
Vanderbilt University Hospital
Nashville, Tennessee
Ch. 9 — Mechanics of Wound Healing

Dorothy M. Fogg, RN, BSN, MA
Perioperative Nursing Specialist
Center for Nursing Practice, Policy, and Research
Association of Operating Room Nurses, Inc.
Denver, Colorado
Ch. 4 — Infection Prevention and Control

Vicki J. Fox, RN, MSN, ACNP-CS, CRNFA
Acute Care Nurse Practitioner
Tyler, Texas
Ch. 10 — Patient Education and Discharge Planning

Denise L. Geuder, RN, MS, CNOR
Vice President, Patient Care Services
Saint Francis Hospital
Tulsa, Oklahoma
Ch. 28 — Ambulatory Surgery

Charlotte L. Guglielmi, RN, BSN, CNOR
Clinical Nurse III
Beth Israel Deaconess Medical Center
Carl J. Shapiro Ambulatory Operating Room
Boston, Massachusetts
Ch. 20 — Rhinologic and Sinus Surgery

Pauline Anne Heizenroth, RN, MSN, CNOR
Clinical Nurse Educator, Surgical Services
The Bryn Mawr Hospital
Bryn Mawr, Pennsylvania
Ch. 5 — Positioning the Patient for Surgery

J. Lee Hoffer, MD, PhD
Professor of Anesthesiology
Texas A&M University Health Science Center
Scott & White Memorial Hospital & Clinic;
Professor of Engineering
Texas A&M University College of Engineering
Temple, Texas
Ch. 7 — Anesthesia

Theresa M. Jasset, RN, BSN, CNOR
Clinical Nurse III
Beth Israel Deaconess Medical Center
Carl J. Shapiro Ambulatory Operating Room
Boston, Massachusetts
Ch. 20 — Rhinologic and Sinus Surgery

Antoinette F. Kanne, RN, MS, TNS, CNOR
Trauma Coordinator
St. John's Mercy Medical Center
St. Louis, Missouri
Ch. 31 — Trauma Surgery

Carol Slusarz Ladden, RN, MSN, CNOR, CRNP
Lecturer
University of Pennsylvania
Philadelphia, Pennsylvania
Ch. 1 — Concepts Basic to Perioperative Nursing

Porter C. Layne, RN, BS, CNOR, CRNFA
RN First Assistant
Beacon Orthopaedics and Sports Medicine
Cincinnati, Ohio
Ch. 22 — Orthopedic Surgery

Beth Ann MacVittie, RN, MS, CNOR
Primary Service Nurse, Peripheral Vascular Surgery
Strong Memorial Hospital
University of Rochester
Rochester, New York
Ch. 26 — Vascular Surgery

Susie Maldonado, RN, CNOR, RNFA
Cardiovascular Coordinator
Driscoll's Children Hospital
Corpus Christi, Texas
Ch. 29 — Pediatric Surgery

Maryann Skasko Mawhinney, RN, BSN, MEd, CNOR
Staff Nurse/Preceptor, Surgical Services
Holy Spirit Hospital
Camp Hill, Pennsylvania
Ch. 18 — Ophthalmic Surgery

Patricia Felice Meckes, RN, MN, CNOR
Director of Education
Kaiser Permanente Medical Centers
Bellflower and Baldwin Park, California
Ch. 30 — Geriatric Surgery

Gratia M. Nagle, RN, CNOR, CRNFA, CURN
RN First Assistant
James R. Bollinger, MD, FACS, PC
Surgical and Clinical Urology
Paoli, Pennsylvania
Ch. 15 — Genitourinary Surgery

Gwen Lynn Nelson, RN, MSN, CNOR
Clinical Educator
Valleylab, Inc.
Boulder, Colorado
Ch. 14 — Gynecologic Surgery and Cesarean Birth

Cheryl L. Nygren, RN, BSN, CNOR, CRNFA
Cardiothoracic Operating Room Nurse
Nemours Cardiac Center at A.I. Dupont Hospital for Children
Wilmington, Delaware
Ch. 29 — Pediatric Surgery

Jan Odom, RN, BSN, MS, CPAN, FAAN
Clinical Nurse Specialist, Surgical Services
Forrest General Hospital
Hattiesburg, Mississippi
Ch. 8 — Postoperative Pain Care and Complications

Lynda R. Petty, RN, BSN, CNOR, RNFA
Perioperative Education and Training
The Arthur G. James Cancer Hospital and Research Institute at The Ohio State University
Columbus, Ohio
Ch. 11 — Gastrointestinal Surgery
Ch. 12 — Surgery of the Liver, Biliary Tract, Pancreas, and Spleen

Carol A. Richard, RN, BSN, CNOR
Nurse in Charge, Operating Room
Brigham & Women's Hospital
Boston, Massachusetts
Ch. 19 — Otologic Surgery

Rosemary Ann Roth, RN, MSN, CNOR, CNAA
Director, Surgical Services
The Genesee Hospital
Rochester, New York
Ch. 17 — Breast Surgery

Laurie A. Saletnik, RN, BSN, CNOR
Assistant Director, Department of Surgery
Johns Hopkins Hospital
Baltimore, Maryland
Ch. 21 — Laryngologic and Head and Neck Surgery

Patricia C. Seifert, RN, MSN, CNOR, CRNFA
Manager, Open Heart Surgery
Halifax Medical Center
Daytona Beach, Florida
Ch. 27 — Cardiac Surgery

Dale A. Smith, RN, CNOR, RNFA
RN First Assistant
Brighton Surgical Center
Portland, Maine;
Adjunct Faculty, Perioperative, & RNFA Programs
Delaware County Community College
Media, Pennsylvania
Ch. 13 — Repair of Hernias

Ruth E. Vaiden, RN, CNOR
Director, Surgical Services
HealthSouth Medical Center
Richmond, Virginia
Ch. 23 — Neurosurgery

Donna S. Watson, RN, MSN, CNOR
Staff Nurse
St. Joseph Medical Center Same Day Surgery
Gig Harbor, Washington
Ch. 32 — Contemporary Issues

Clinical Consultants

Emmie Amerine, RN, BS, CURN
Clinical Urology/Urodynamic Specialist
Office of James R. Bollinger, MD, FACS, PC
Paoli, Pennsylvania

Susan D. Bell, RN, MS, CNRN, CNP
Adult Nurse Practitioner
Division of Neurosurgery
Ohio State University Medical Center
Columbus, Ohio

Sally Betz, RN, MS, CEN, CCRN
Trauma Patient Care Resource Manager
Ohio State University Medical Center
Flight Nurse, Med Flight of Ohio
Columbus, Ohio

James R. Bollinger, MD, FACS, PC
Chairman, Department of Urology
Paoli Memorial Hospital;
Co-Chairman, Department of Urology
Chester County Hospital
Paoli, Pennsylvania

Christopher B. Caldwell, MD
Senior Attending Physician
The Genesee Hospital
Rochester, New York

Wayne Dennis, SA
New York Territory Manager
Influence, Inc.
San Francisco, California

Teresa DiMeo, RN, MS, CNOR, CNP
Adult Nurse Practitioner
Division of Neurosurgery
Ohio State University Medical Center
Columbus, Ohio

Marvin P. Fried, MD
Otolaryngologist-in-Chief
Beth Israel Deaconess Medical Center
Brigham and Womens Hospital;
Professor of Otology and Laryngology
Harvard Medical School
Boston, Massachusetts

William P. Homan, MD, PhD
Attending Surgeon
White Plains Hospital Center;
Clinical Assistant Professor of Surgery
New York Medical College
White Plains, New York

Richard C. Lanning, MD, FACS
Retina and Oculoplastic Consultants, PC
Camp Hill, Pennsylvania

Jeffery H. Levine, MD
Associate Director, Trauma Services
St. John's Mercy Medical Center
St. Louis, Missouri

Robert Mackin
Laser Consultant
Mackin Medical Accessories, Inc.
Bryn Mawr, Pennsylvania

Bruce E. Mathern, MD
Assistant Professor, Department of Surgery
Division of Neurosurgery
Medical College of Virginia
Richmond, Virginia

Kim McKenna, RN, BSN, CEN, EMT-P
Coordinator, Paramedic Education
St. John's Mercy Medical Center
St. Louis, Missouri

Terence M. Moore
Regional Sales Manager
Influence, Inc.
San Francisco, California

Robert C. Neilson, DO
General Surgeon
Clinical Faculty
New England College of Osteopathic Medicine
Portland, Maine

Tonie Nichols, BSEE, CRLS
Lithotripsy Unit Manager
Signal Medical Corp.
Farmington, Connecticut

Victoria U. Nugent, RN, MS
Adult Nurse Practitioner
Genesee Surgical Associates
Rochester, New York

Carol Orr, RN, BSN, MHR, CNOR
Clinical Manager, Ambulatory Surgery
Outpatient Admit/Discharge, Endoscopy
University of Tulsa
University of Oklahoma
Tulsa, Oklahoma

Thomas R. Pheasant, MD, FACS
Chief, Department of Ophthalmology
Holy Spirit Hospital
Camp Hill, Pennsylvania

J. G. Prensky, MD, FACS
Retina and Oculoplastic Consultants, P.C.
Camp Hill, Pennsylvania

Jeffery Rosenblum, MD, PC
Adult and Pediatric Urology
Exton, Pennsylvania

Alan L. Schein, MD, FACS
Ophthalmologist
Holy Spirit Hospital
Camp Hill, Pennsylvania

John J. Schietroma, MD, FACS
Retina and Oculoplastic Consultants, P.C.
Camp Hill, Pennsylvania

Virginia Schuster
Implant Consultant
American Medical Systems
Minnetonka, Minnesota

George Skinner, BS
Director of Positioning Products
Allen Medical Systems
Garfield Heights, Ohio

Dale A. Smith, RN, CNOR, RNFA
Registered Nurse First Assistant
Brighton Surgical Center/Maine Medical Center
Portland, Maine

Patricia A. Timmins, AB, RNFA, CNOR
Operating Room Staff Nurse
Pennsylvania Hospital
Philadelphia, Pennsylvania

Mary Ann Toy, RN, CNOR, CRNFA
Staff Nurse
Halifax Medical Center
Open Heart Surgery
Daytona Beach, Florida

Bryan R. Troop, MD, FACS, FCCM
Director, Trauma Services
Director, Surgical Education
Associate Director, Critical Care Medicine
St. John's Mercy Medical Center
St. Louis, Missouri

David E. Tunkel, MD
Associate Professor of Otolaryngology
Head and Neck Surgery and Pediatrics
Johns Hopkins University School of Medicine
Baltimore, Maryland

Debra J. Watson, RN, BSN, MS
Staff Registered Nurse
Bryn Mawr Hospital
Bryn Mawr, Pennsylvania

Richard M. Yelovich, MD
Director, Radiation Oncology
Paoli Cancer Center, Division of Fox-Chase Cancer Center
Paoli, Pennsylvania

Karen Ann Yohn-Williams, RN, MSN
Certified Enterostomal Therapy Nurse
The Bryn Mawr and Lankenau Hospitals
Wynnewood, Pennsylvania

Reviewers

Kim E. Anasoulis, RN, BSN, CNOR
Staff Nurse, Thoracic/Cardiovascular Surgery
The Queen's Medical Center
Honolulu, Hawaii

Sandra L. Beidelschies, RN, MSN, CNOR
Assistant Administrator, Perioperative and Diagnostic
Services
The University Hospital
Cincinnati, Ohio

Nelda D. Britton, RN, MEd, CNOR
Clinical Nurse Specialist, Perioperative Nursing
University of South Alabama Medical Center;
Adjunct Faculty, University of South Alabama College
of Nursing
Educational Consultant and Instructor
Mobile, Alabama

Ellen Carson, RNCS, PhD
Associate Professor, Department of Nursing
Pittsburg State University
Pittsburg, Kansas

**Joanne D. Cimorelli, RN, BS, CNOR,
CRNFA**
RN First Assistant, Presbyterian Medical Center of the
University of Pennsylvania Health System
Philadelphia, Pennsylvania

**Nancy B. Davis, RN, BSN, NP, CRNFA,
CNOR**
Registered Nurse First Assistant
Cardiovascular and Chest Surgical Associates
Boise, Idaho

Lucylle L. Duffy, RN, BSN, MA
Director of Nursing, Surgical Services/MCH
Co-Director, Surgical Development
Holy Name Hospital
Teaneck, New Jersey

**Susan Jane Fetzer, RN, BA, BSN, MSN,
MBA, PhD, CCRN**
Assistant Professor
University of New Hampshire
Durham, New Hampshire

Paul A. Gregor, RN, BSN, CNOR
Staff Nurse, Thoracic/Cardiovascular Surgery
The Queen's Medical Center
Honolulu, Hawaii

Patricia L. Griffith, RN, CNOR, RNFA
Staff Nurse, RN First Assistant
Southampton Hospital
Southampton, New York

Donna N. Hershey, RN, MSN, CNOR
Care and Outcomes Coordinator
Masonic Homes
Elizabethtown, Pennsylvania

Roxanne Huckstep, RN, AA, BS, CNOR
Orthopaedic Specialist
Riverside Regional Medical Center
Newport News, Virginia

Marilyn A. Hunter, RN, PhD, CNOR
Program Director, Surgical Technology
Daytona Beach Community College
Daytona Beach, Florida

Debra A. Johnson, RN, MSN, NP, CNOR
Nurse Practitioner and Manager of Ambulatory
Anesthesia Services
Anesthesia Group of Onondaga, P.C.
Syracuse, New York

Cecil A. King, RN, MS, CNOR
Assistant Nurse Manager
University of Washington Medical Center
Seattle, Washington

Mary JB Larsen, RN, BSN, CNOR, RNFA
Staff Nurse, Operating Room
Wixom, Michigan

Kathleen Kelly Lunday, RN, MSN
Instructor, School of Nursing
Emory University
Atlanta, Georgia

Susan M. McCullough, RN, BSN
Nurse Clinician, Ophthalmology
Cleveland Clinic Eye Institute
Cleveland, Ohio

Donna R. McEwen, RN, BSN, CNOR, CNRN
Nurse Manager, Outpatient Surgery
St. Luke's Baptist Hospital, Baptist Health System
San Antonio, Texas

Ann T. McKennis, RN, CNOR, CORLN
Staff Nurse, Otolaryngology/Head and Neck Surgery
The Methodist Hospital
Houston, Texas

Joseph J. Napolitano, RN, MSN, MPH, CS, CRNP, CCRN
Assistant Nurse Manager, Rhoads 5 SICU
Hospital of the University of Pennsylvania
Philadelphia, Pennsylvania

Elaine K. Neel, RN, BSN, MSN
Instructor, School of Nursing
Methodist Medical Center of Illinois
Peoria, Illinois

Sister Trudy O'Connor, RN, BSN, MEd, MSN, CNOR
Clinical Specialist, Surgery and Anesthesia Services
St. John's Hospital
Springfield, Illinois

Jess Q. Salinas, RN, ADN, BA
Staff Nurse
Children's Hospital Medical Center
Seattle, Washington

Christine E. Smith, RN, MSN, CNOR
Perioperative Clinical Specialist/Educator
Delaware County Community College
Media, Pennsylvania

Judith A. Spraley, RN, BSN, MEd
Nursing and Allied Health
Curriculum Consultant
Cincinnati, Ohio

Katie Steuer, RN, BSN, CNOR
Perioperative RN, Level III
Dartmouth Hitchcock Medical Center
Lebanon, New Hampshire

Vicki Suster, RN, BSN
Operating Room Manager
Mt. Sinai Medical Center
Cleveland, Ohio

Allan R. Thomes, RN, BSN, CNOR, CRNFA
Cardiac and Neurosurgery
Sauk Rapids, Minnesota

Sheri J. Voss, RN, MS, CNOR
Administrative Director, Surgical Services
St. Mary's Hospital
Richmond, Virginia

Jacquelyn Walker, RN, BSN
Registered Nurse
University of Washington Medical Center
Seattle, Washington

Denise L. Witt, RN, BSN, MA, CST, CNOR
Professor, Surgical Technology
Nassau Community College
Garden City, New York

Terri Zimon, RN, BSN, MSN, NP
Nurse Practitioner
Hinsdale Hospital
Hinsdale, Illinois

Just as *Alexander's Care of the Patient in Surgery* has promoted quality care for all patients undergoing surgical interventions for more than 50 years, the Association of Operating Room Nurses (AORN) has helped guide perioperative nursing practice during that same period. Both have been known for their dedication to perioperative nursing education. In recognition of AORN's approaching celebration of one-half century of setting standards and recommended practices for perioperative nurses and serving as a driving force for the improvement of perioperative patient care, this edition is dedicated to AORN, its leaders, and its members. Many patients have benefitted from their efforts, and many nurses, including the editors and authors of *Alexander's*, owe much of the credit for their professional nursing opportunities and accomplishments to this outstanding organization.

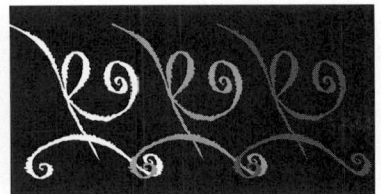

Preface

The eleventh edition of *Alexander's Care of the Patient in Surgery* has been extensively updated to reflect new concepts in perioperative nursing practice and the increased sophistication and complexity of surgical procedures as the new millennium approaches. However, the goal of this text remains essentially the same: to provide a comprehensive basic reference that will assist perioperative personnel with safely, cost-effectively, and efficiently meeting the needs of patients during surgical interventions.

The standard in perioperative nursing for over 50 years, *Alexander's Care of the Patient in Surgery* is written primarily for professional perioperative nurses, but is also useful for nursing students, surgical technologists, healthcare industry representatives, medical students, interns, residents, and government officials concerned with healthcare issues. Practitioners of perioperative nursing, clinical nurse specialists, and educators from many geographic areas of the United States have served as contributors to this text, providing a vast range of perioperative nursing knowledge and procedural information.

This thoroughly revised edition highlights the most current techniques and innovations in surgery. Hundreds of illustrations, including many new photographs and drawings, help familiarize the reader with new procedures, methods, and equipment. Classic illustrations, particularly of surgical anatomy, have been preserved to enhance the text.

A new aspect of this edition is that we have added the opportunity for our readers to use the Internet and computer technology as a learning tool. A special feature at the end of each chapter is the presentation of websites, list servers, or e-mail addresses to assist teachers and learners in accessing some of the most current information via the "information superhighway." Our goal is to move forward in traveling to the new millennium with an Internet Connection that suggests websites related to the focus of each of the chapters in this edition of the text. There are many different types of sites listed as well as e-mail addresses for specialty nursing organizations that did not have website addresses when the text went into production. These websites have not been reviewed for the reader; instead, we invite you to experience the excitement of visiting sites and bookmarking those you find most useful.

Overall, the text imparts state-of-the-art information that reflects quality contemporary practice and promotes the delivery of comprehensive perioperative patient care.

Unit I, Foundations for Practice, provides information on basic principles and patient-care requisites essential to the care of all recipients of perioperative patient care. The nursing process, a model for developing therapeutic nursing interventional knowledge, reflects a six-step process that includes the identification of desired patient outcomes. Interest in patient outcomes and their improvement continues to be an essential element of nursing as reformation of the healthcare delivery system escalates. Realizing that the collection of health data in an expansive information age requires clear identification of contributions to patient outcomes and quantification of these in data-driven improvement of quality patient care, perioperative nurses must continue to link their interventions to clearly identified outcomes. This relationship is presented in Chapter 1 and explicated in each Sample Care Plan throughout the text. Research Highlights continue to be included in every chapter, reflecting the steady increase in the amount and quality of research relevant to perioperative patient care. Because the findings of research are often not effectively used in clinical practice, the editors and authors of *Alexander's* are committed to closing this research-practice gap. The Research Highlights will help perioperative nurses use the findings of research in their practice. Chapter 1 also sets the stage for an emphasis on patient and family education and discharge planning throughout the text, with a subsequent entire chapter dedicated to this important topic. A new component of all chapters in Units II and III addresses specific patient and family education and discharge planning relevant for patients undergoing the respective specialty surgical procedures. As the responsibilities of perioperative nurses become greater with regard to these important care components, it is imperative that we effectively educate patients and families. With the length of stay in healthcare facilities continuing to decrease, patients and families must be informed and prepared to appropriately deal with postoperative needs after discharge. A new chapter in Unit I, Surgical Modalities, provides comprehensive coverage of endoscopic surgery, lasers, electrosurgical modalities, cryosurgery, videoconferencing, and robotics.

The chapters within Unit II, Surgical Interventions, include over 400 contemporary and traditional specialty surgical interventions, as well as numerous minimally invasive surgical procedures that have been developed since the last edition. Each chapter provides a helpful review of pertinent anatomy and details the steps of each procedure. Perioperative nursing considerations are once again presented within the nursing process framework. Current NANDA-approved nursing diagnoses and Sample Care Plans for each surgical specialty are intended to help perioperative nurses plan, implement, and evaluate individualized perioperative patient care. Each of these chapters also provides an example of a clinical pathway (also referred to as a care map) for a select surgical procedure. These tools are increasingly being developed to contain costs, improve outcomes, foster consistency in care delivery, and identify best practice. Typically multidisciplinary in nature, they reflect additional efforts by perioperative practitioners to link research, care processes, and outcome measurement and management.

The unique needs of ambulatory, pediatric, geriatric, and trauma surgery patients are presented in Unit III, Special Considerations. Surgical procedures that are typically performed on pediatric patients have been incorporated within the Pediatric Surgery chapter rather than being interspersed in the respective specialty surgery chapters to provide a more comprehensive resource for perioperative nurses who care for pediatric patients. The chapter on Contemporary Issues has been expanded to include a review of the concept of best practices and benchmarking, healthcare report cards, and the expanded use of unlicensed assistive personnel. A subject of significant interest to all healthcare practitioners, the recommendations of the Pew Health Professions Commission, and associated perioperative implications are succinctly presented to encourage nurses to continuously monitor legislative actions that may ultimately affect their practice.

Many expert perioperative practitioners, RN first assistants, clinical nurse specialists, and educators have contributed to this eleventh edition, and we owe a debt of gratitude to all of them for sharing their expertise in the development of this text. We extend special thanks to Christine E. Smith, RN, MSN, CNOR and Dale A. Smith, RN, CNOR, RNFA for helping us locate websites and check to see that they were up and live! We also acknowledge the valuable assistance of editors, reviewers, photographers, and illustrators who have contributed their time and expertise to the revision of this text.

Alexander's Care of the Patient in Surgery is written by and for perioperative nurses, and is dedicated to excellence in perioperative nursing practice.

MARGARET H. MEEKER
JANE C. ROTHROCK

Contents

UNIT ONE FOUNDATIONS FOR PRACTICE

UNIT TWO   SURGICAL INTERVENTIONS

UNIT THREE   # SPECIAL CONSIDERATIONS

UNIT I

FOUNDATIONS
FOR PRACTICE

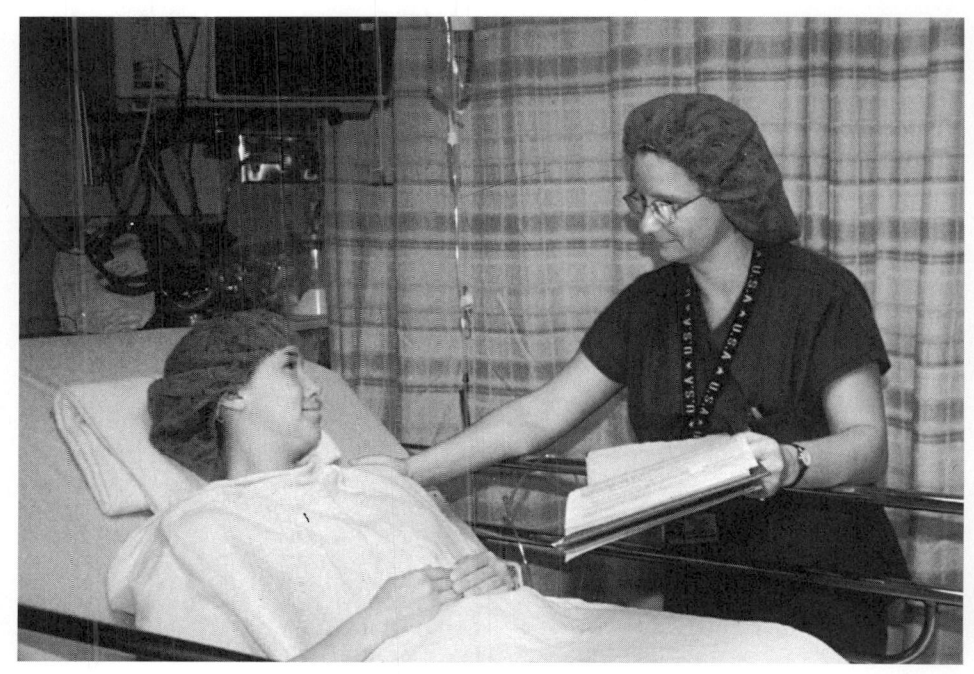

CHAPTER ONE

Concepts Basic to Perioperative Nursing

Carol Slusarz Ladden

THE SPECIALTY OF perioperative nursing has come of age in both image and practice. In the few years since the last edition of this text was published, perioperative nurses have continued to expand their responsibilities and firmly establish perioperative nursing as a professional nursing specialty, all with vibrant enthusiasm for their profession and enduring commitment to the patient.

The term *perioperative nursing* is now used in both nursing and medical circles. Perioperative nursing is recognized and practiced in surgical suites, ambulatory surgery centers, endoscopy suites, laser centers, interventional radiology departments, mobile surgical units, and physician's offices across the United States. Remote surgery and virtual endoscopy are but two of the innovations being developed as part a vast array of futuristic technology.[17] As we approach a new millennium, perioperative patient care is very different than it was in the past.

Historically, the term *operating room (OR) nursing* was used to describe the care of patients in the immediate preoperative, intraoperative, and postoperative phases of the surgical experience (Fig. 1-1). Such a term, however, intimated that nursing care activities were circumscribed to the geographic limits of the surgical suite. The term may have contributed to stereotypic images of an OR nurse who took care of the operating room and had little interface or nursing responsibility for medicated and anesthetized patients in the surgical suite (Research Highlight 1-1). With such a perspective, nursing practitioners outside the operating room had difficulty ascribing important elements of the nursing process and patient care accountability to the nurse who practiced behind the doors of the surgical suite. The current view of perioperative nursing connotes the delivery of patient care in the preoperative, intraoperative, and postoperative periods of the patient's surgical experience through the framework of the nursing process. In such a framework, the perioperative nurse engages in patient assessment, collecting, organizing, and prioritizing patient data; establishes nursing diagnoses; identifies desired patient outcomes; develops and implements a plan of nursing care; and evaluates that care in terms of outcomes achieved by the patient (Fig. 1-2). In these activities the perioperative nurse functions both independently and interdependently. The perioperative nurse collaborates with other health care professionals, makes appropriate nursing referrals, and delegates and supervises nursing care.

When perioperative nursing is practiced in its broadest scope, nursing care may begin in the patient's home, a clinic, a physician's office, the patient care unit, the presurgical care unit, or the holding area (see Research Highlight 1-1). After the surgical intervention, nursing care may continue in the perianesthesia care unit (PACU) or in patient evaluation on the patient care unit, in the physician's office, in the patient's home, in a clinic, or through written or telephone patient surveys.

When perioperative nursing is practiced in the narrower sense, patient care activities may be confined to the common areas of the surgical suite. Assessment and data collection may take place in the holding area; evaluation may take place on discharge from the operating room. Despite the way perioperative nursing is practiced in a health care setting, it is underscored by the nursing process and all the care activities inherent in that process.

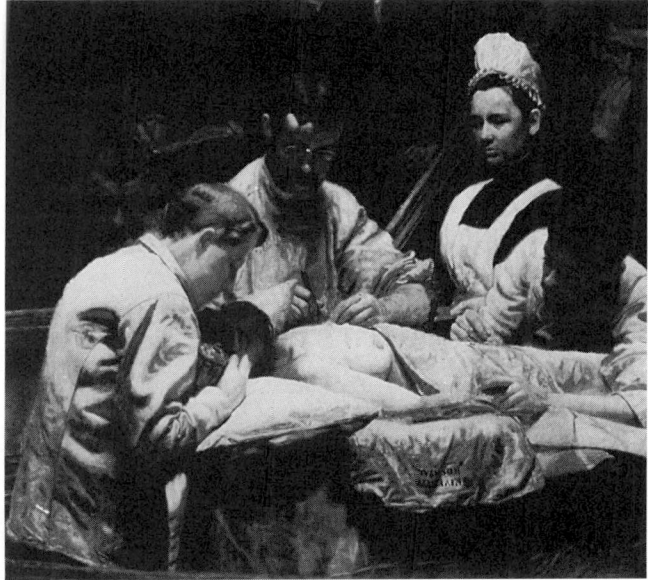

FIGURE 1-1 Thomas Eakins, *The Agnew Clinic*, 1889. In this painting, reforms and advancements in surgical techniques and procedures are apparent. Surgeons wear gowns, instruments are sterilized, ether is used, and the patient is covered. An operating room nurse is a prominent member of the team.

OVERVIEW OF PERIOPERATIVE NURSING PRACTICE

The various perioperative nursing roles all subsume elements of the behaviors and technical practices that characterize professional nursing. Probably no other area of nursing requires the broad knowledge base, the instant recall of nursing science, the need to be intuitively guided by past nursing experience, the diversity of thought and action, the stamina, and the flexibility needed in perioperative nursing endeavors. Whether a generalist or a specialist, the perioperative nurse depends on knowledge of surgical anatomy, physiologic alterations and their consequences for the patient, intraoperative risk factors, potentials for patient injury and the means of preventing them, and psychosocial implications of surgery for the patient and significant others. This knowledge enables the perioperative nurse to anticipate needs of the patient and surgical team and rapidly initiate appropriate nursing interventions. This is part of patient advocacy, of doing for the patient what needs to be done to provide a safe and caring environment.

The size of this mental repertoire is staggering and emphasizes the constant discipline, attention, ongoing education, and presence of mind demanded in perioperative nursing. However, the greater the requirements, the more satisfactory and indelible are the joys that come with practice at this level of excellence. The perioperative nurse is recognized by other members of the health care team as an integral team member, truly an expert!

1-1 RESEARCH HIGHLIGHT

In this historical review four periods were analyzed to identify the changing focus of preoperative patient preparation. From 1900 to 1919 preparation of the patient for surgery took place primarily in the patient's home, where much of surgery was also done. The patient took light, nourishing food; baths; and frequent rest periods to build up the body. The nurse arrived at the home a few hours before surgery, choosing and preparing a room, emptying it of furniture, boiling sheets and instruments, and preventing excitement on the patient's part. The nurse also obtained a personal and family history from the patient, though little patient teaching took place. Between 1920 and 1939, physicians became affiliated with hospitals, and minimum standards of preoperative patient preparation began to evolve. Both physical and mental preparation of the patient was stressed, the concept of patient consent for surgery was initiated, and preparation of the OR and instruments was addressed. Nursing manuals on care of the surgical patient included normal anatomy and physiology, pathophysiology, medical and surgical treatments, and nursing interventions. The years between 1940 and 1959 witnessed enormous scientific medical discoveries; nursing care of surgical patients became more complex to accommodate rapid changes in surgical care. Patient teaching became part of preoperative patient preparation, individual patient needs were emphasized, and the psychologic preparation of the patient was increasingly recognized as important. From 1960 to 1979 nursing research was being conducted and emphasized; early research linked preoperative preparation and postoperative recovery. Patients' emotional needs were recognized as they related to individual patients, and concepts of structured preoperative instruction were introduced and validated by nursing research.

From Oetker-Black, S.L. (1993). Preoperative preparation: historical development. *AORN Journal, 57*(6), 1402-1410.

Perioperative nursing is a purposeful and dynamic process. By planning patient care and identifying required nursing interventions and actions, perioperative nurses assure surgical patients of scientific, professional nursing care. Perioperative nurses historically have assumed responsibility for providing a safe, efficient, and caring environment for surgical patients, one in which the surgical team can function smoothly and efficiently to achieve positive patient outcomes. Such mutuality between nursing and other health care disciplines and the role of patient advocacy continue to be part of the essence of perioperative nursing in the late 1990s and well into the future.

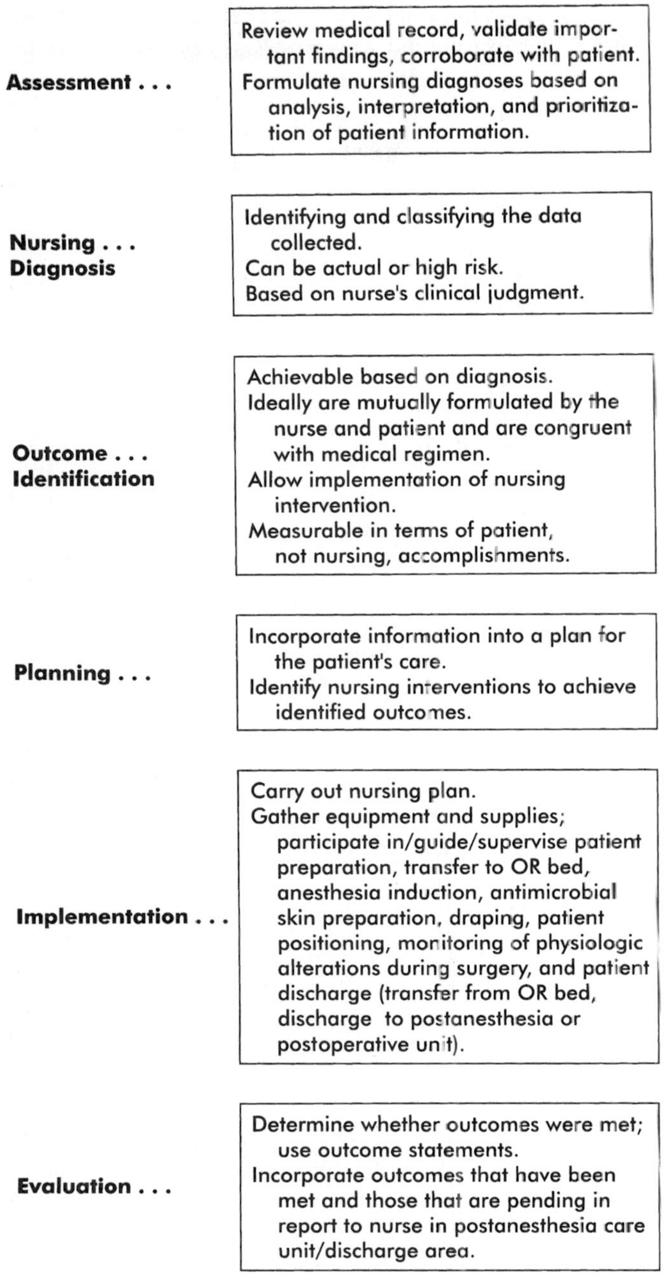

Assessment . . .

> Review medical record, validate important findings, corroborate with patient.
> Formulate nursing diagnoses based on analysis, interpretation, and prioritization of patient information.

Nursing . . . Diagnosis

> Identifying and classifying the data collected.
> Can be actual or high risk.
> Based on nurse's clinical judgment.

Outcome . . . Identification

> Achievable based on diagnosis.
> Ideally are mutually formulated by the nurse and patient and are congruent with medical regimen.
> Allow implementation of nursing intervention.
> Measurable in terms of patient, not nursing, accomplishments.

Planning . . .

> Incorporate information into a plan for the patient's care.
> Identify nursing interventions to achieve identified outcomes.

Implementation . . .

> Carry out nursing plan.
> Gather equipment and supplies; participate in/guide/supervise patient preparation, transfer to OR bed, anesthesia induction, antimicrobial skin preparation, draping, patient positioning, monitoring of physiologic alterations during surgery, and patient discharge (transfer from OR bed, discharge to postanesthesia or postoperative unit).

Evaluation . . .

> Determine whether outcomes were met; use outcome statements.
> Incorporate outcomes that have been met and those that are pending in report to nurse in postanesthesia care unit/discharge area.

FIGURE 1-2 The nursing process is continuous, leading to a higher level of care.

A significant part of perioperative nursing is the delivery of scientifically based care: understanding the necessity for certain techniques of care; knowing how and when to initiate them; being creative in maintaining a technique when the situation calls for flexibility; and evaluating the safety, cost, and outcomes of the care delivered. Knowledge of surgical interventions, instruments, and equipment is essential during the implementation phase of nursing care. Without such knowledge, the perioperative nurse is unable to prepare for or anticipate the steps in the surgical procedure, with their concomitant implications for the patient and for the surgical team.

1-2 RESEARCH HIGHLIGHT

Since Benner's landmark work on the description of differences in nurse performance on a continuum from novice to expert, many nurse researchers have described what nurses do at various stages on the continuum. This study explored how nurses move from novice to expert and differences in patient outcomes based on the expert or nonexpert status of the nurse. Both observation and unstructured interviews were used to capture what was done differently by expert nurses; expert nurses were not identified by years of experience or by educational preparation but by their characteristics (distinct ways of "being with" patients) and their ability to focus on patient outcomes. In general, the expert nurse determines the need to "be with" the patient based on a guided, focused assessment of the patient situation; no previous contact with the patient may be necessary for the expert nurse to sense a patient need. Expert nurses also had decisive action and outcome orientation; they were aware of possibilities, understood the interrelationships of what was "going on," focused on the patient response, and therefore prevented complications while maintaining a humanistic approach to patient care. Nonexpert nurses had a more unfocused assessment and were guided by a strong task orientation.

From Hanneman, S.C. (1996). Advancing nursing practice with a unit-based clinical expert. *Image: Journal of Nursing Scholarship, 28*(4), 331-337.

Scientific nursing interventions and caring, comforting behaviors are at the heart of perioperative nursing. The chapters in Unit Two of this text focus on surgical interventions common to patients in inpatient and ambulatory settings. Each of the chapters on surgical interventions contains a *Sample Care Plan,* and suggested nursing interventions have been integrated as part of the perioperative nurse's plan of care. A fundamental assumption is that perioperative nursing is a blend of the technical and behavioral; it is critical thinking as well as doing and caring for patients.

A model depicting perioperative practice would illustrate a continuum on which the nurse functions from beginning competency to excellence (Research Highlight 1-2). The practice of perioperative nursing encompasses both traditional and expanded nursing activities during intraoperative care, preoperative and postoperative patient education, counseling, assessment, planning, and evaluation functions. Perioperative nursing practice revolves around an individual patient who is undergoing a surgical intervention. The perioperative nurse's activities address the psychologic, social, and physiologic problems that may result. Perioperative nurses scrub, circulate, assist during surgery (registered nurse first assistant [RNFA]), manage, teach, and conduct research. From admission through discharge and home follow-up, the perioperative nurse plays a significant role in managing the patient's care. Research will continue to test and validate the contribution of perioperative nursing to patient care outcomes in all settings where it is practiced.

STANDARDS OF CLINICAL NURSING PRACTICE

Perioperative nursing is a systematic planned process, a series of integrated steps. If viewed only as setting up cases, perioperative nursing becomes nothing more than rote equipment preparation and paper shuffling. When it is viewed as patient care, it becomes a scientific process and stimulates the nurse to perform optimally. For professional nursing, standards set forth the expectations of the full professional role within which the nurse practices. As early as the 1960s, the American Nurses Association (ANA) engaged in standards development. First published in 1973, these standards have helped to shape nursing practice. Specialty nursing organizations such as the Association of Operating Room Nurses (AORN) have worked with the ANA to develop their own standards and guidelines using the ANA framework. This has resulted in the use of common language and a consistent format for the profession. The *Standards of Clinical Nursing Practice* are the standards of care and professional performance. The standards of care are based on the nursing process.

Nursing Process

The nursing process is a way of looking at nursing and bringing it into perspective as methodical critical thinking that guides actions, which contrasts with considering nursing as only a set of cookbook rituals and procedures to be learned. The focus of the nursing process is on the patient, and the nursing interventions prescribed are those that meet patient needs. Because of the setting and the nature of the work, perioperative nursing is particularly vulnerable to being considered only a conglomeration of

mechanical techniques and a carrying out of surgeons' orders. By using the nursing process, perioperative nurses focus on the patient and, at the same time, utilize skills and knowledge in caring for patients and making clinical decisions. Use of the nursing process, nursing care plans, and clinical pathways (discussed later in this chapter) has become an integral part of patient care.

In its simplest form, the nursing process defined by the ANA consists in six steps: assessment, nursing diagnosis, outcome identification, planning, implementation, and evaluation (Fig. 1-3). The process is circular and continuous. In all areas of nursing practice, responsibilities inherent in the nursing process are the provision of culturally and ethnically sensitive care that is also age appropriate, maintenance of a safe environment, education of patients and their families or significant others, assuring continuity and coordination of care through discharge planning and referrals, and communicating information.[2]

Assessment

Assessment is the collection of relevant data about the patient (Box 1-1). Sources of data may be a preoperative interview with the patient and the patient's family by a perioperative or unit nurse; review of the nursing care plans and patient's medical record; examination of the results of presurgical diagnostic studies; and consultation with the surgeon and anesthesia provider, unit nurses, or other personnel.

The format this assessment takes may vary from institution to institution but always includes both the physiologic and the psychosocial aspects of the patient. For a perioperative nurse caring for a healthy patient, assessment may mean a thoughtful, quick scan of the patient and medical record, a review of the surgical procedure, and a mental rehearsal of the resources and knowledge necessary to direct the patient through an operative course. At other times the perioperative nurse must thoroughly assess all aspects of the patient and the patient's condition, along with preoperative and postoperative reviews. Assessment may be performed by a

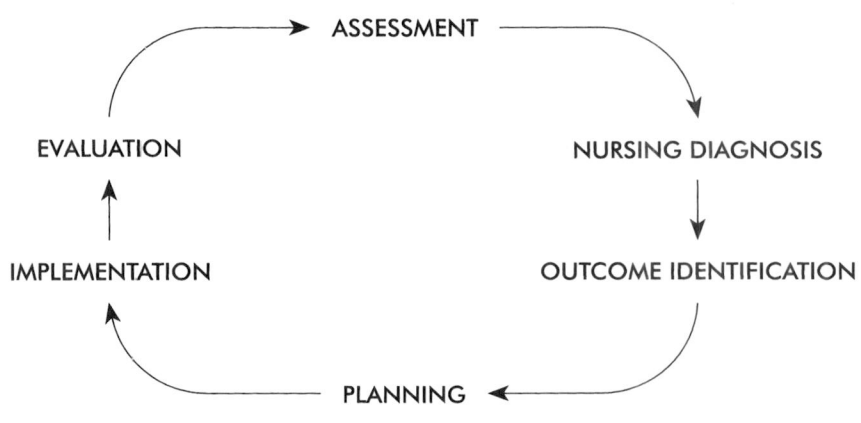

FIGURE 1-3 Six phases of nursing process.

perioperative nurse in the presurgical care unit or by telephone before the day of surgical admission.

When developing guidelines for preoperative assessment, patient and family education, and discharge planning, the perioperative nurse should consider the following: Is relevant, concise patient information already available to the perioperative nursing staff? Is enough information available to allow perioperative nurses to consider patient care needs when setting up the room (special equipment, accessory items, instruments, sutures)? Is sufficient time available to initiate a meaningful perioperative nurse-patient interaction? Are surgical patients satisfied with their perioperative nursing care (do they express feelings of comfort and satisfaction regarding their care in the surgical setting), and do they have knowledge of the perioperative nurse's role? Is there continuity of care between the perioperative unit and other nursing care units?

BOX 1-1 | Standard I: Assessment

The Perioperative Nurse Collects Patient Health Data.

Interpretive Statement

Assessment is the systematic and ongoing collection of data, guided by the application of knowledge of physiological and psychological principles and experience, and is used to make judgments and predictions about a patient's response to illness or changes in life processes. Assessment is essential to establishing a nursing diagnosis and predicting outcomes. Assessment may occur in a variety of settings.

Criteria

1. The priority of data collection is determined by the patient's immediate condition or needs, and the relationship to the proposed intervention. Pertinent data include, but are not limited to,

   - current medical diagnoses and therapies;
   - physical status and physiological responses;
   - psychosocial status of the patient;
   - cultural, spiritual, and lifestyle information;
   - the individual's understanding, perceptions, and expectations of the procedure;
   - previous responses to illness, hospitalizations, and surgical, therapeutic, or diagnostic procedures; and
   - results of diagnostic studies.

2. Pertinent data are collected using appropriate assessment techniques.
3. Data collection involves the patient, significant others, and health care providers when appropriate. It may be accomplished through diverse means, such as interview, review of records, assessment, and/or consultation.
4. Data collection is systematic and ongoing.
5. Relevant data are documented in retrievable form.

Reprinted with permission from AORN *Standards, Recommended Practices, and Guidelines,* 1998, pp. 125-127. Copyright © AORN, Inc., Denver, Colorado.

Being able to exchange information about their patients in face-to-face meetings, by telephone, or by written messages is helpful for unit and perioperative nurses. A thorough assessment, made and recorded by the unit nurses, can accompany inpatients to the operating room and serve as a guide to perioperative nursing personnel. Then the perioperative nurse completes a more focused preoperative patient assessment. With the burgeoning number of ambulatory surgery procedures, preoperative assessment is often integrated in preadmission testing (PAT). In some institutions, group preoperative sessions are held. These not only help nurses get to know the patients but also permit nurses to impart information on common routines, reactions, sensations, and nursing procedures that will take place preoperatively, intraoperatively, and postoperatively. The perioperative setting determines the type of interaction that may occur. The use of preoperative phone calls and questionnaires has gained acceptance. Soliciting information before the patient's arrival in the perioperative setting and this one-on-one contact from the perioperative nurse can affect patient outcomes. The important point is that some form of assessment, patient and family education, and discharge planning should be done. How it is accomplished is up to the particular facility and nursing staff.

Assessment then is knowing and understanding the patient as a feeling, thinking, and responsible person and as a candidate for a surgical procedure (Research Highlight 1-3). Data identified through assessment assists the perioperative nurse in meeting unique patient needs throughout the surgical intervention. Based on the data collected, recorded, and interpreted during patient assessment, nursing diagnoses are formulated.

Nursing diagnosis

Nursing diagnosis is the process of identifying and classifying data collected in the assessment in a way that will yield a focus for the planning of nursing care (Box 1-2). Nursing diagnoses have been evolving since they were first introduced in the 1950s. They have now reached the stage of development of being identified, named, and classified according to human response patterns and functional health patterns. The organization responsible for delineating the accepted list of nursing diagnoses is the North American Nursing Diagnosis Association (NANDA) (Box 1-3). Each NANDA-approved nursing diagnosis has a set of components: definition (meaning of the diagnostic term); defining characteristics (pattern of cues that make the meaning of the diagnosis clear); and related, risk, or contextual factors (patient behaviors and factors in the environment that interact to place the individual at high risk of developing a particular diagnosis).

Not all patient problems encountered in the perioperative setting can be described by the list of accepted nursing diagnoses. Perioperative nurses must participate in the describing and naming new of nursing diagnoses that characterize unique perioperative patient problems. NANDA has established a "to be developed" category to

1-3 RESEARCH HIGHLIGHT

This study was designed to quantify, through description, "good nursing care" by surgical patients undergoing back operations. Structured interviews of 30 patients yielded information about satisfaction with care during preoperative, intraoperative, and postoperative phases of care. Data indicated that patients had a strong need for information regarding the surgery, its risks and prognosis, and anesthesia. The majority of patients preferred this information 1 or 2 days before surgery, and the surgeon was identified as the preferred information giver. For the intraoperative phase, patients identified friendly, competent staff members who provided reassurance and protection for the patient; patients expressed confidence in the perioperative nurse's ability to care for them during anesthesia. Patients had vague recall of PACU care but were able to identify close monitoring by a nurse and pain control as important to satisfaction with care provided. Based on interview results, four areas for nursing research were noted: development and evaluation of perioperative information delivery systems, descriptions of nurse-patient roles and relationships, quantification of ways patients are respected during care episodes, and an analysis of the concept of loneliness during perioperative care phases.

From Leino-Kilpi, H., & Vuorenheimo, J. (1993). Perioperative nursing care quality: patient's opinions. *AORN Journal, 57*(5), 1061-1071.

BOX 1-2 | Standard II: Diagnosis

The Perioperative Nurse Analyzes the Assessment Data in Determining Diagnoses.

Interpretive Statement

The outcome of assessment is the potential for one or more nursing diagnoses. Nursing diagnoses are concise statements about actual, or high risk for, health problems/clinical conditions that are amenable to nursing intervention. Diagnoses result from analysis and interpretation of data about the patient's problems, needs, and health status.

Criteria

1. Diagnoses are consistent with the assessment data.
2. Diagnoses are validated with the patient, significant others, and health care providers, when possible.
3. Diagnoses are documented in a manner that facilitates the determination of outcomes and plan of care.

Reprinted with permission from AORN *Standards, Recommended Practices, and Guidelines*, 1998, pp. 125-127. Copyright © AORN, Inc., Denver, Colorado.

---

designate nursing diagnoses that are partially developed and deemed useful to the nursing profession; perioperative nurses may develop unique diagnostic labels and definitions and then work to further develop and validate them through this process. This becomes even more important as health care moves toward the use of information systems to document nursing practice. The Nursing Information and Data Set Evaluation Center (NIDSEC), established by ANA in 1997, evaluates such systems according to set criteria[26]; these criteria require that codes for clinical data be consistent with accepted nursing nomenclature such as NANDA.[19]

Outcome identification

Outcome identification is a statement that describes the desired or favorable patient condition that can be achieved through nursing interventions (Box 1-4). The study of patient outcomes is not new. Nurse historians attribute the beginnings of outcome measurement to Nightingale, who analyzed health care conditions and patient outcomes during the Crimean War. To be useful for assessing the effectiveness of nursing care, patient outcomes should be "nursing sensitive"; that is, they should be influenced by nursing and describe a patient state that can be measured

and quantified.[16] Nursing-sensitive patient outcomes are derived from nursing diagnoses and direct the interventions to resolve the nursing diagnoses. They are the standards or criteria by which the effectiveness of the interventions is measured. Outcomes should be stated in terms of expected or desired patient behavior and be specific and measurable in time. The appropriate time to measure perioperative nursing-sensitive outcomes varies. Some outcomes result from intraoperative nursing interventions and can be evaluated immediately. Others result over a longer period of time. In this textbook, the use of "the patient will . . ." indicates an outcome that is expected to occur over time. Identification of expected and desired outcomes unique to the surgical patient provides the opportunity to prioritize care, becomes a basis for continuity of care, and directs evaluation (outcomes research). In this type of research, the relationship between the process of care (what the perioperative nurse does, described below in the implementation section) and the outcomes of that care are studied, enhancing the perioperative nurse's ability to improve care.[7] In many instances, outcomes research efforts result in the identification of "best practice" for improving patient care.[9] (See Chapter 32 for more discussion of best practice.)

Planning

Having collected and interpreted patient data, arrived at appropriate nursing diagnoses, and established desired outcomes, the perioperative nurse is prepared to *plan* the nursing care for the patient (Box 1-5). Planning, in part, requires use of nursing knowledge and information about the patient to prepare the surgical environment. Perioperative nurses check equipment, have usual and unusual supplies ready, and use their knowledge of anatomy to have

BOX 1-3	NANDA-Approved Nursing Diagnoses 1997-1998

Activity intolerance

Activity intolerance, risk for

Adaptive capacity, decreased: intracranial

Adjustment, impaired

Airway clearance, ineffective

Anxiety

Aspiration, risk for

Body image disturbance

Body temperature, altered, risk for

Bowel incontinence

Breastfeeding, effective

Breastfeeding, ineffective

Breastfeeding, interrupted

Breathing pattern ineffective

Cardiac output, decreased

Caregiver role strain

Caregiver role strain, risk for

Communication, impaired verbal

Community coping, potential for enhanced

Community coping, ineffective

Confusion, acute

Confusion, chronic

Constipation

Constipation, colonic

Constipation, perceived

Coping, defensive

Coping, family: potential for growth

Coping, ineffective family: compromised

Coping, ineffective family: disabling

Coping, ineffective individual

Decisional conflict (specify)

Denial, ineffective

Diarrhea

Disuse syndrome, risk for

Diversional activity deficit

Dysreflexia

Energy field disturbance

Environmental interpretation syndrome, impaired

Family processes, altered: alcoholism

Family processes, altered

Fatigue

Fear

Fluid volume deficit

Fluid volume deficit, risk for

Fluid volume excess

Gas exchange, impaired

Grieving, anticipatory

Grieving, dysfunctional

Growth and development, altered

Health maintenance, altered

Hopelessness

Hyperthermia

Hypothermia

Incontinence, functional

Incontinence, reflex

Incontinence, stress

Incontinence, total

Incontinence, urge

Infant behavior, disorganized

Infant behavior, disorganized: risk for

Infant behavior, organized: potential for enhanced

Infant feeding pattern, ineffective

Infection, risk for

Injury, perioperative positioning: risk for

Injury, risk for

Knowledge deficit (specify)

Loneliness, risk for

Management of therapeutic regimen, community: ineffective

Management of therapeutic regimen, families: ineffective

Management of therapeutic regimen, individual: effective

Management of therapeutic regimen, individual: ineffective

Memory, impaired

Memory, impaired physical

Mobility, impaired physical

Noncompliance (specify)

Nutrition, altered: less than body requirements

Nutrition, altered: more than body requirements

Nutrition, altered: risk for more than body requirements

Oral mucous membrane, altered

Pain

Pain, chronic

Parent/infant/child attachment, altered: risk for

Parental role conflict

Parenting, altered

Parenting, altered, risk for

Peripheral neurovascular dysfunction, risk for

Personal identity disturbance

Poisoning, risk for

Post-trauma response

Powerlessness

Protection, altered

Rape-trauma syndrome

Rape-trauma syndrome: compound reaction

Rape-trauma syndrome: silent reaction

Relocation stress syndrome

Role performance, altered

Self-care deficit, bathing/hygiene

Self-care deficit, dressing/grooming

Self-care deficit, feeding

Self-care deficit, toileting

Self-esteem disturbance

Self-esteem, chronic low

Self-esteem, situational low

Self-mutilation, risk for

Sensory/perceptual alterations (specify) (visual, auditory, kinesthetic, gustatory, tactile, olfactory)

Sexual dysfunction

Sexuality patterns, altered

Skin integrity, impaired

Skin integrity, impaired, risk for

Sleep pattern disturbance

Social interaction, impaired

Social isolation

Spiritual distress (distress of the human spirit)

Continued

| BOX 1-3 | NANDA-Approved Nursing Diagnoses 1997-1998—cont'd |

Spiritual well-being, potential for enhanced
Suffocation, risk for
Swallowing, impaired
Thermoregulation, ineffective
Thought processes, altered
Tissue integrity, impaired
Tissue perfusion, altered (specify type) (renal, cerebral, cardiopulmonary, gastrointestinal, peripheral)

Trauma, risk for
Unilateral neglect
Urinary elimination, altered
Urinary retention
Ventilation, inability to sustain spontaneous
Ventilatory weaning response, dysfunction (DWR)
Violence, risk for: directed at others

| BOX 1-4 | Standard III: Outcome Identification |

The Perioperative Nurse Identifies Expected Outcomes Unique to the Patient.

Interpretive Statement

Patient outcomes are derived from nursing diagnoses and direct the interventions to correct, alter, or maintain the nursing diagnoses. Areas for the perioperative nurse to consider when formulating outcomes should include, but are not limited to,

- absence of infection;
- maintenance of skin integrity;
- absence of adverse effects through proper use of safety measures related to positioning, extraneous objects, and chemical, physical, and electrical hazards;
- maintenance of fluid and electrolyte balance;
- knowledge of the patient and significant others of the physiological and psychological responses to surgical intervention; and
- participation of the patient and significant others in the rehabilitation process.

Criteria

1. Outcomes are derived from the diagnoses and are mutually formulated with the patient, significant others, and health care providers, when possible.
2. The patient's present and potential physical capabilities and behavioral patterns are congruent with the expected outcomes.
3. Outcomes are attainable with consideration to human and material resources available to the patient.
4. Outcome statements include measurable criteria for determining expected outcomes as a result of nursing interventions.
5. Outcomes include a time estimate for attainment.
6. Outcomes are prioritized.
7. Outcomes are communicated to appropriate people.
8. Outcomes are documented in a retrievable form.
9. Outcomes provide direction for continuity of care.

Reprinted with permission from AORN *Standards, Recommended Practices, and Guidelines*, 1998, pp. 125-127. Copyright © AORN, Inc., Denver, Colorado.

| BOX 1-5 | Standard IV: Planning |

The Perioperative Nurse Develops a Plan of Care That Prescribes Interventions to Attain Expected Outcomes.

Interpretive Statement

The outcome statements become the guide for nursing interventions necessary to achieve the desired results. The individualized plan of care reflects the perioperative assessment and a logical sequence to attain outcomes. Priorities for the provision of nursing care are established by the perioperative nurse in collaboration with the patient, significant others, and health care providers. Examples of interventions performed include, but are not limited to,

- provision of information and supportive perioperative teaching specifically related to the surgical intervention and nursing care,
- identification of the patient,
- verification of the surgical site,
- verification of the operative consent and reports of essential diagnostic procedures,
- positioning according to physiological principles,
- adherence to principles of asepsis,
- provision of appropriate and properly functioning equipment and supplies for the patient,
- provision for comfort measures and supportive care to the patient,
- environmental monitoring and safety,
- evaluation of outcomes in relation to the identified interventions, and
- communication of intraoperative information to significant others and the health care team to provide for continuity of care.

Criteria

1. The plan of care reflects current nursing practice.
2. The plan of care provides for continuity of care.
3. The plan of care specifies nursing diagnoses, interventions necessary to achieve the outcomes, and a logical sequence of interventions.
4. Human and material resources are available to implement the plan of care.
5. The plan of care is communicated to appropriate people.
6. Evidence of a plan of care is retrievable through documented intervention and evaluation of progress toward expected outcome.

Reprinted with permission from AORN *Standards, Recommended Practices, and Guidelines*, 1998, pp. 125-127. Copyright © AORN, Inc., Denver, Colorado.

proper instruments and sutures on hand for the procedure to be performed. They know the sequence of steps in the operative or other invasive procedure and use surgeons' preference cards, nursing care guides, and other resources such as computerized data sheets to ready the room and equipment for the patient.

Planning is preparing ahead of time for what will happen and determining the priorities for care. Planning, based on patient assessment, results in knowing the patient and the patient's unique needs so that alterations in events such as positioning or the surgical process are anticipated and readily accommodated. Planning also requires knowledge of the patient's psychosocial state and feelings about the proposed operation so that an extra, needed explanation, comforting, or emotional support can be provided when patient care is being implemented.

Implementation

Implementation is performing the nursing care interventions that were planned as well as responding to changes in surgical routine, the patient's condition, or emergencies with critical thinking and orderly activities (Box 1-6). It is employing established standards of nursing care, recommended practices, and other guidelines developed and maintained by the nursing profession. During this phase of the nursing process, the perioperative nurse continues to assess the patient to determine the appropriateness of selected interventions and to alter the intervention as necessary to achieve the desired outcomes of care. Bowles and Naylor[4] have described nursing interventions as the "work of nursing." The study of nursing interventions can link nursing diagnoses with interventions and outcomes and lead to the validation of selected interventions or the development of new ones. This enhances clinical practice, decision-making, and research-based practice. It also assists in the delivery of cost-effective care by quantifying resource allocation. Implementation also means being the patient's advocate by recognition and acknowledgment of a patient's concern or unmet need. Advocacy is part of nurse-caring, and it encompasses nursing interventions that promote both emotional and physical comfort. Caring behaviors include establishing a friendly relationship, responding to the individuality of the patient, and meeting the expectations of the patient and family[14] (Research Highlight 1-4). The role of patient advocate is especially important in surgical settings when patients are sedated or unconscious and unable to speak for themselves.

BOX 1-6	**Standard V: Implementation**

The Perioperative Nurse Implements the Interventions Identified in the Plan of Care.

Interpretive Statement

Interventions are consistent with the established plan of care and provide continuity of nursing care in the perioperative period. Interventions are based on expert opinion, scientific principles, and/or consensus. They reflect the rights and desires of the patient and significant others.

Criteria

1. Interventions are consistent with the established plan of care.
2. Implementation of the plan of care is an ongoing process and is based on the patient's response.
3. Interventions reflect the rights and desires of the patient and significant others.
4. Interventions are implemented with safety, skill, and efficiency and are adjusted according to patient responses.
5. Interventions may be assigned or delegated as appropriate.
6. Interventions are documented and communicated verbally as appropriate to promote continuity of care.

Reprinted with permission from AORN *Standards, Recommended Practices, and Guidelines,* 1998, pp. 125-127. Copyright © AORN, Inc., Denver, Colorado.

1-4 RESEARCH HIGHLIGHT

In a managed care environment, patient education assumes importance, both in the philosophy of managed care and in the determination of methods of delivering patient and family education with less time and limited access to patients. In one study by Brumfield, Kee, and Johnson, researchers compared what preoperative teaching content was important to ambulatory surgery patients and what was important to perioperative nurses. For patients, information describing the activities and events that would take place (situational information) was most important. Perioperative nurses, on the other hand, believed that psychosocial support for the patient was most important. When asked about timing of preoperative education, patients expressed the need to have teaching done before they were admitted; perioperative nurses believed that some teaching could be done after admission.

Another study by Lookinland and Pool examined timing of education, along with the effects of structured content on patient satisfaction, postoperative recovery, and return to functional status. Patients in the experimental group received structured education at least 2 or 3 days before admission; the control group received instruction on the day of admission according to what the admitting nurse believed was important and had time for. Results indicated that the group of patients who received structured preoperative education before admission did have higher satisfaction with their care, described a more favorable recovery, and returned sooner to a normal functional status.

From Brumfield, V.C., Kee, C.C., & Johnson, J.Y. (1996). Preoperative patient teaching in ambulatory surgery settings. *AORN Journal, 64*(6), 941-952; Lookinland, S., & Pool, M. (1998). Study of effect of methods of preoperative education in women. *AORN Journal, 67*(1), 203-213.

Delegation

During the implementation of patient care, the perioperative nurse may delegate certain nursing interventions. Perioperative patient care is delivered by a team; there are numerous categories of personnel who assist in various direct and indirect patient care activities. Often referred to as unlicensed assistive personnel (UAP), these health care workers emerged during the nursing shortages of world wars I and II and were part of the team model of delivering patient care. In the 1980s, delivery models shifted the skill mix away from assistive personnel; RNs were the principal caregivers in primary nursing models. However, during the fiscally constrained 1990s, health care facilities began to reintroduce assistive personnel, who are less trained and less expensive. Instead of using UAP in narrowly defined job categories (such as clerical, housekeeping, orderly, and patient transport), the trend in the late 1990s is to create a set of multiskilled UAP who can assist the nurse in various activities, rather than just a single activity.[21]

As the use of UAP quickly burgeoned in the 1990s, questions and concerns arose regarding delegation of activities that were formerly performed by the registered nurse. In many states, the board of nursing defines the scope of practice for registered nurses based on the nursing process. The legal definition of nursing is contained in each state's nurse practice act, a state law that protects the health and safety of the public by establishing legal qualifications for who can practice nursing. Because implementation of the plan of care and the interventions to accomplish it are part of the nursing process, guidelines for delegating some of these interventions were required. The National Council of State Boards of Nursing (NCSBN) defines delegation as a transfer, to a competent person of the authority to perform a selected nursing task in a selected situation[27] according to the five "rights" of delegation (Box 1-7). When the perioperative nurse delegates a task, he or she retains the accountability for delegation. Nursing functions of assessment, evaluation, and nursing judgment cannot be delegated.[10] It is important for perioperative nurses to understand that institutional policy cannot contradict the nurse practice act of their state. Although tasks and procedures may be delegated to UAP, the perioperative nurse is responsible for supervising care; supervision cannot be delegated.[9]

Documenting Interventions

Accurate documentation of nursing care is an integral part of all phases of the nursing process, especially implementation of the plan of care. A description of the patient, the nursing diagnoses and desired patient outcomes, the nursing care given, and the patient's response to care (outcomes) should be included in the patient's record. Documentation of the nursing care given should include more than the technical aspects of care, such as the sponge count or the application of the electrosurgical dispersive pad. Nursing care documentation should be related to

---

| BOX 1-7 | The 5 Rights of Delegation |

1. **The Right task.** The perioperative nurse determines that this task is one that is delegable for a specific patient, taking into consideration such factors as potential for harm, the complexity of the task, necessary problem solving, and the predictability of the outcome.
2. **The Right circumstances.** The perioperative nurse considers the patient care setting, the resources available, and other relevant factors.
3. **The Right person.** The perioperative nurse is the right person to delegate the right task to the right person to be performed on the right patient. The perioperative nurse must be familiar with the job description of the UAP, capabilities, skill level, and learning needs to assure that safe, quality patient care is provided.
4. **The Right communication and direction.** The perioperative nurse provides a clear, concrete, and concise description of the task, with key information relating to its objectives, rationale, limits, and expectations. There should be an opportunity for questions and clarifying instructions. Information the perioperative nurse needs to know from the person performing the task must be identified.
5. **The Right supervision.** The perioperative nurse appropriately monitors the task or person performing it, evaluates the results, intervenes if necessary, and provides feedback. Providing immediate feedback or identifying a problem with performance as it occurs is essential to upholding standards of care and performance expectations.

Perioperative nurses must be actively involved in providing the assessment, evaluation, and judgment needed to coordinate and supervise perioperative patient care. When delegating care activities, the perioperative nurse retains accountability for analyzing and evaluating the outcome of the delegated task. Activities that rely on the nursing process, such as assessment, nursing diagnosis, establishing plans of care, extensive patient and family education, and discharge planning, cannot be delegated.

Adapted from National Council of State Boards of Nursing Response to the PEW Taskforce Principles and Vision for Health Care Workforce Regulation, 1996, Chicago, the Council, pp. 4-5.

---

assessment and nursing diagnoses, with preestablished outcomes against which the appropriateness and effectiveness of care may be judged. The form for this documentation may include standardized protocols and interventions as noted on clinical pathways; space should be provided to write in interventions that are unique to individual patients or to describe variances in care. Documentation should require little time to complete, be specific to the perioperative setting, and provide continuity across the various areas in surgery from presurgery holding areas to the perianesthesia care units.

Evaluation

Evaluation is checking, observing, and appraising the results of what was done (Box 1-8). Although evaluation is traditionally listed as the last phase of the nursing process, it

---

BOX 1-8 | **Standard VI: Evaluation**

The Perioperative Nurse Evaluates the Patient's Progress Toward Attainment of Outcomes.

Interpretive Statement

Evaluation is systematic and ongoing. It is based on observations and patient responses to nursing interventions; the effectiveness of interventions is evaluated in relation to the outcomes. Ongoing assessment data are used to revise diagnoses, the plan of care, and/or outcomes as needed. The patient, significant others, and health care providers are involved in the evaluation process.

Criteria

1. Evaluation of the effectiveness of interventions is systematic and ongoing.
2. The effectiveness of interventions is evaluated in relation to outcomes.
3. Documentation of the patient's progress toward achievable outcomes is retrievable.
4. Ongoing assessment data are used to revise diagnoses, outcomes, and the plan of care, as needed.
5. Revisions in diagnoses, outcomes, and the plan of care are documented.
6. The patient, significant others, and health care providers are involved in the evaluation process when appropriate.

Reprinted with permission from AORN *Standards, Recommended Practices, and Guidelines*, 1998, pp. 125-127. Copyright © AORN, Inc., Denver, Colorado.

---

is an integral, systematic, and ongoing component of providing perioperative patient care. Evaluation is directed toward the patient's progress in attaining identified outcomes. When feasible and appropriate, the patient and family or significant others should be involved in the evaluation process. The attainment of outcomes or the need to revise nursing diagnoses or modify outcomes and the plan of care must be documented. Since perioperative patient care processes and interventions are often multidisciplinary, additional evaluation methods may be used in health care facilities.

Performance assessment and improvement activities, notably monitoring of important aspects of care, problem identification, problem solving, and peer review, may be part of the overall system evaluation. Often referred to as *quality improvement (QI) programs*, multidisciplinary teams address areas for improvement in patient care, identify problems, propose solutions, and monitor and evaluate the effectiveness of the improvements. This is discussed in more detail later in this chapter.

Perioperative Nursing Practice Standards

Perioperative nurses are responsible for identifying, interpreting, and implementing contemporary professional standards. The AORN[3] has established standards for perioperative nursing practice that can serve as guidelines for measuring the quality of patient care. These sound principles are broad in scope, attainable, definitive, and relevant for perioperative nurses. The standards represent a

comprehensive approach to meeting the health care needs of surgical patients. Nursing care standards consist of three elements: structure, process, and outcome. The AORN *Standards of Perioperative Administrative Practice* are *structure* standards, describing organizational characteristics, administrative and fiscal accountabilities, personnel qualifications, and facilities and environmental requirements. These standards provide guidance for evaluating operational systems.

Process standards relate to nursing activities, interventions, and interactions and are used to explicate clinical, professional, and quality objectives in perioperative nursing. Examples of process standards are the AORN *Standards of Perioperative Clinical Practice, Standards of Perioperative Professional Performance, and Quality Improvement Standards for Perioperative Nursing.*

Outcome standards identify desirable and measurable physiologic and psychologic responses of patients to nursing interventions. Patient outcomes are an essential indicator of the quality of care. AORN's *Patient Outcomes: Standards of Perioperative Care* provide outcome statements, interpretations, and criteria guidelines for measuring patient responses. The common goal of standards is quality care for the surgical patient.

Standards of Professional Performance

The pace and complexity of advances in surgical procedures, minimally invasive surgery, newly developed technology with surgical applications, professional nursing issues, ongoing health care reform measures, changes in recommended practices, and the burgeoning body of nursing research and practice guidelines demand constant attention to professional education and development. Perioperative professionals must continue to tenaciously search for new research on patient outcomes, link nursing interventions to outcomes, and seek to determine methods that conserve resources when implementing interventions. Such activity is part of the *Standards of Professional Performance*, part of which is the expectancy for the perioperative nurse to evaluate the effectiveness of nursing practice and the quality of that practice.[2] Professional performance standards also require perioperative nurses to evaluate their own practice in relation to AORN's professional practice standards. Life-long learning and maintaining competency and current knowledge in perioperative nursing are the hallmarks of a professional. Other standards of professional performance address ethics, collaboration, and collegiality.

Patient and family education and discharge planning

As part of the *Standards for Professional Performance*, there is an expectation that the nurse collaborates with the patient and family in formulating goals, the plan of care, decisions regarding care, and delivery of health care services.[2] In a managed care philosophy, there is a strong recognition that emphasizing patient education and prevention is a key to improving outcomes; longitudinal care, prevention of problems, and providing emotional as well as physical support for the patient and family are integral components.[20] As short-stay, same-day admission, and ambulatory surgery continue to grow, patient and family education and discharge planning become crucial perioperative nursing activities (Research Highlight 1-5). Because many procedures once done in an acute care, inpatient setting are now performed on an ambulatory basis, education and discharge planning must also take into consideration the environment to which the patient will be returning (usually the home), resources available, and self-care requisites.

In developing a plan for patient and family education and discharge planning, the perioperative nurse must consider an educational assessment (what the patient needs to know and wants to know and the factors that influence the patient's readiness and ability to learn), an environmental assessment, the level of information provided to the patient and family (materials should be between sixth and eighth grade reading levels), supportive patient education materials (print, video, computer based), and the participation of the family or significant others.[5] Goals of patient education include providing information and support, correcting misconceptions, and assisting the patient in understanding self-care roles and responsibilities.

1-5 RESEARCH HIGHLIGHT

Surgery is usually a source of anxiety to both patients and their families. Perioperative nurses have well-developed interventions to assist patients with anxiety; these interventions can be found in many of the sample care plans in this book. However, perioperative nursing interventions for families are less well defined. This study was designed to answer two questions: What are reported anxiety levels of family members of elective surgery patients? What is the relationship of family member characteristics and length of waiting period to report anxiety levels? Fifty family members of patients undergoing elective surgery that lasted for more than 30 minutes were included in the study. State anxiety levels were measured using a written tool; a portable monitor was used to measure blood pressure and heart rate. Results confirmed findings that family members waiting during elective surgery experience higher mean anxiety levels. Perioperative nurses need not only recognize this anxiety but also develop nursing interventions designed to reduce it in family members during the intraoperative waiting period.

From Lesky, J.S. (1993). Anxiety of elective surgical patient's family members: relationship between anxiety levels, family characteristics. *AORN Journal, 57*(5), 1091-1101.

To be an effective educator, the perioperative nurse should have knowledge of the subject, empathy and caring, unconditional positive regard, good verbal and nonverbal communication skills, and counseling skills.[24] A comprehensive discussion of patient and family education and discharge planning may be found in Chapter 10. In the chapters in Unit Two of this text, there is a section summarizing important features of patient education for selected types of surgical intervention.

Clinical pathways

Another expectation in the *Standards of Professional Performance* is that the nurse utilize the best available evidence, preferably research data, in planning patient care and participate in research activities.[2] Dahl suggests that clinical pathways (also referred to as care maps) will lead to improvement in patient care because they are based on research and outcomes.[6] In general, clinical pathways are multidisciplinary practice guidelines that allow one to recommend key resources and activities with targeted time frames during various phases of a patient's care. Their intent is to improve patient and family satisfaction, reduce or control costs, and improve quality of care.[15]

In 1997, the AORN Project Team on Professional Practice Issues oversaw the development of a perioperative clinical path template (Fig. 1-4). In the chapters on surgical interventions in Unit Two of the text, sample clinical pathways for select surgical interventions are provided to assist the perioperative nurse in using findings of best available evidence and research in planning and delivering perioperative patient care.

Institutional Standards of Care

Perioperative departments have delegated responsibility, through the governing board of the institution, for the development of policies and procedures. Often referred to as *surgical services standards of care*, these serve as the institution's standards for delivering quality care. Policies are written statements that clearly outline responsibilities and appropriate actions for specific circumstances. Falkenhagen suggests that five criteria must be met for an effective policy:[8] the policy must be consistent with both national and state practice standards; it needs to be realistic and achievable; it should be consistently followed, except where prior approval has been obtained; the policy should be based on reasoned and rational thinking; and it should be related to the long-term intent of the surgical services department.

Procedures are the guides to implementing a policy; they set forth the detailed chronologic sequence of activities as they relate to a particular policy. Policies and procedures are usually combined into a manual that is kept readily available as a perioperative care resource in departments where operative or other invasive procedures are performed. Participation of staff members in policy and procedure development increases their knowledge of the

AORN Clinical Pathway Template

1. Focus of Clinical Pathway: _____
2. Timeline: _____

3. Patient Care Problems		Preoperative:	Intraoperative:	Postoperative:
A. B. C. D. E. F.	4. I N T E R V E N T I O N S			
5. E X P E C T E D O U T C O M E S		Immediate:	Discharge:	
6. V A R I A N C E S		For concurrent intervention:	For retrospective analysis:	

FIGURE 1–4 AORN Clinical Pathway Template

subject matter and generates a sense of ownership, resulting in meaningful interpretation of the approved policy or procedure to peers and its successful implementation.

PERFORMANCE ASSESSMENT AND IMPROVEMENT

Trends in health care have mandated increased control of costs, efficient use of resources and supplies, decreased length of stay for surgical patients, and shifting of many surgical procedures from inpatient to ambulatory care settings. Along with this shift has come an increasing awareness of the need for continued quality improvement in the provision of perioperative patient care. The Joint Commission on the Accreditation of Healthcare Organizations (JCAHO) has taken a strong position on the need for continuously monitoring and evaluating the quality and appropriateness of care delivery to resolve any identified problems while striving to constantly improve delivery systems and processes. In 1994 the JCAHO instituted performance assessment, measurement, and improvement as the core of its standards. This represented an evolution from quality assurance, to continuous quality improvement, to performance improvement. Such a transition was underscored by the belief that measuring outcomes and improving care are the essential purposes of health care delivery. Performance improvement efforts encompass improvements in quality and productivity (Box 1-9). Harrington suggests that organizational performance improves under three conditions:[11] when productivity remains constant but quality goes up; when quality remains constant and productivity goes up; or when both quality and productivity go up. However, attempts to improve either quality or productivity must be based on both ethical and economic perspectives.[14]

The surgical services performance assessment and improvement program should be based on established standards of care. The intent of each standard should be reflected in realistic and measurable outcomes. A plan to monitor and improve care should be in place, which includes both the scope of care and the important aspects of care. Specific indicators should be identified that reflect these important aspects of care. Thresholds that identify the level of acceptability of variance for each indicator are then established. Measurement methods include retrospective review, review of incident reports, utilization review, patient surveys and interviews, and peer review. Emphasis has evolved from process auditing to the current emphasis on structure, process, and outcome indicators. In 1995, the ANA worked on developing a report card for acute care. In 1996, the ANA embarked on *Nursing's Safety and Quality Initiative*, part of which was the development and validation of quality indicators. The AORN has also begun work on a perioperative nursing report card. These efforts underscore nursing's commitment to improving processes and outcomes of care.

BOX 1-9	Concepts and Methods of Performance Assessment and Improvement

1. Effective performance assessment and measurement systems should provide accurate, complete, and relevant quality-of-care data that can be used in improvement efforts.
2. Both process and outcome assessment and measurement are essential to performance improvement.
3. Health care professionals and organizations must understand and believe in the benefits of performance assessment and improvement. Potential barriers must be identified and resolved.
4. The organization's performance can be correlated with a variety of attributes such as outcomes of care, cost of care, quality, and patient satisfaction, and perceived value.
5. Performance improvement requires the ability to measure specific functions and dimensions of performance such as appropriateness, availability, continuity, effectiveness, efficacy, efficiency, respect and caring, safety, and timeliness.
6. Organizational functions, structures, and key processes can be elucidated through common quality-improvement tools such as flowcharting, cause-and-effect diagraming, brainstorming, and charting performance to understand and identify common and special cause variations.
7. Steps to establish a performance measurement system include establishing units of measure, developing instruments and tools that can quantify the units of measure, and using these instruments and tools to collect and analyze data for performance improvement.

A process-improvement approach facilitates measurement of perioperative patient care. When processes are understood, they can be improved through a systematic plan of action. Involvement on teams that work on the surgical services performance assessment and improvement plans can strengthen the staff's commitment to meeting standards and enhance program effectiveness (Fig. 1-5).

PERIOPERATIVE NURSING ROLES OF THE FUTURE

The profession of nursing and the culture of health care in the United States continues to undergo rapid transformation. The environment of health care is changing in response to many elements. An aging population, with an anticipated over-65 population expected to top 40 million by the year 2000, will create a significant increase in the demand for health services.[22] New ambulatory settings for delivery of health services, including operative and other invasive procedures, will continue to develop, as will community-based clinics, school-linked clinics, mobile clinics, and drive-by health centers. Health care organizations that are agile and flexible and able to respond to change quickly will have an edge in the health care industry of the future. Perioperative nurses who under-

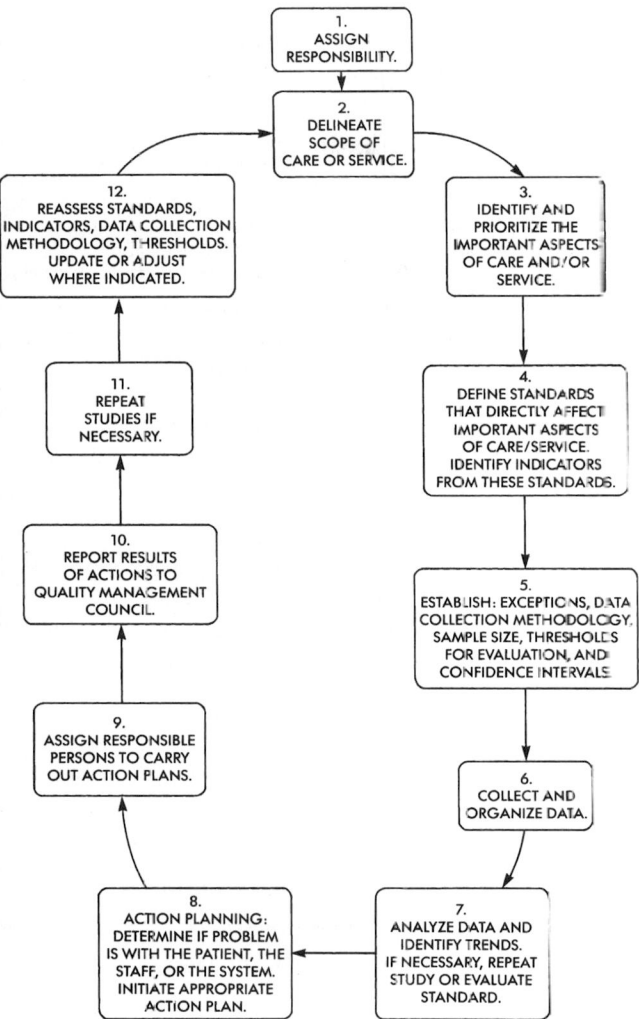

FIGURE 1-5   Team responsibilities in quality improvement.

stand the needs for both clinical and service quality, cost effectiveness, information management, efficiency, and the importance of patient satisfaction will be able to anticipate and position themselves for this future. Roles in nursing research, industry, consulting, informatics, case management, and advanced practice are all possibilities for perioperative nurses. Perioperative nurses need personal strategic plans for enhancing their education, skill sets, and professional goals as they expand their practice horizons and move into some of these roles that directly or indirectly support perioperative patient care. To assist in exploring possible career paths, a few of these roles are described below.

Registered Nurse First Assistant

The role of the perioperative nurse as assistant at surgery is a good example of an evolving new role. In 1984 the AORN approved an official statement on the RNFA; the statement was revised in 1993 and 1998 to reflect changes in role evolution. The RNFA, who must have formal education for role preparation in an academic setting,

works collaboratively with the surgeon (and the patient and surgical team) by handling tissue and instruments, providing exposure and hemostasis, and suturing as components of assisting-at-surgery behaviors. Many experienced perioperative nurses have obtained education to prepare themselves for this role. Performing as an RNFA allows the experienced perioperative nurse to advance in clinical knowledge and skill while still remaining directly involved with the provision of perioperative nursing care. The role of the RNFA has gained wide acceptance and is just one of the ways perioperative nurses are developing themselves to meet the changing needs of health care delivery.

Nursing Informatics Specialist

Pressures for more efficient management of fiscal, material, and human resources have stimulated the development of automated information systems for diverse functions in perioperative patient care settings. Prompt access to accurate data is essential to maintain and improve the management and functioning of a surgical suite. A well-designed management information system can efficiently synthesize large volumes of data into meaningful reports. Ad hoc delivery reporting capabilities are a vital component that can enhance decision making. Although administrative systems were probably the first area of nursing informatics, newer nursing applications include clinical practice, computer-based patient records, patient education, and research. Fueling the need for information systems is managed care, where decisions to "purchase" health care from an institution rely heavily on information that demonstrates cost effectiveness and efficiency of care provided.[13] The field of nursing informatics, defined by Turley as the interaction of cognitive science, computer science, and information science, which rests on a foundation of nursing science, is growing rapidly.[23] Perioperative nurse informatics specialists have the opportunity to develop clinical nursing systems that incorporate care protocols, critical paths, and patient education materials and track patients over time, sharing information across wide networks as patients access health care at different points and times over a continuum of care. The possibilities of interactive computer/television, where perioperative nurses can communicate with their patients over phone or cable lines that allow the perioperative nurse to "view" the patient's wound or "discuss" overall recovery and rehabilitation from surgery, will be available with future technology systems. Many surgical patients themselves are information literate in the age of the Internet, using this technology to search out health care providers, best institutions, and knowledge about their disease process and current, up-to-date results of various treatment protocols. Perioperative nurse informatics specialists can assist in developing information infrastructures that support a broad range of future information technology.

Case Manager

Many perioperative nurses prize their role as practitioner-caregiver and have been reluctant to move away from the "bedside" of the patient. A career path as a perioperative case manager allows the professional nurse to participate indirectly in patient care through coordination, monitoring continuity of care, and managing and scheduling ancillary services.[1] The perioperative case manager is also teacher and patient advocate, educating and counseling patients and their families or significant others, working with discharge planners to assure continuity of care, and following patients after discharge.

Advanced Practice

Advanced nurse practitioners, either nurse practitioner (NP) or Clinical Nurse Specialist (CNS), have become valuable members of health care teams in multiple settings. Traditionally NPs practiced in primary care or outpatient settings, whereas the CNS was employed in acute care settings. However, as residency programs have been downsized and part of the revenue stream for specialty preparation (surgical residents) diverted to primary care medicine, acute care NPs have begun to fill the gap in providing care for patients with increased acuity and complex medical-surgical problems. NPs and CNSs have graduate nursing education and, as a result of the Balanced Budget Act of 1997, receive Medicare reimbursement in a variety of settings. This legislation also provided for Medicare reimbursement of RNFAs when they are an NP or a CNS.[18] The AORN has developed competency statements for the perioperative advanced practice nurse, which include managing health or illness status, competency in helping and healing, in teaching and coaching disease prevention and health promotion, organizational and work role competence, and competence in monitoring and promoting the quality of perioperative practice.[3]

CONCLUSION

The perioperative nurse works in collaboration with surgeons, anesthesia providers, and other health care providers to plan the best course of action for each patient. To ensure the highest quality of care, input from each of the health care disciplines represented in the perioperative practice setting is crucial. Because the education of the professional nurse has more breadth than that of many other health care providers, the nurse is often in the best position to serve in a leadership role in fostering collegiality and collaboration among a variety of disciplines.

Perioperative nurses are accountable to their patients and demonstrate it by using standards, recommended practices, performance assessment and improvement activities and by constantly strengthening their professional skills through education. As the transformation of health care continues, new perioperative nursing roles will emerge, but perioperative nurses in any role will continue to demonstrate humanized care for surgical patients and their families. *Scrubbing* and *circulating* may become obsolete terms; already we know that they define circumscribed functions that are only a part of the perioperative nurse's sphere of responsibility. The future may bring new titles and functions but will never erase the critical function in surgical patient care that every perioperative nurse fulfills. The future of perioperative nursing is directly related to the sophistication of its practitioners. Sophistication means that perioperative nurses must be superior thinkers (knowledge) and doers (clinical skills). Outcomes of surgical interventions are related to the quality of perioperative nursing care provided, which in turn reflects the aptitudes and motivations of perioperative practitioners. With this perspective, the reader should consider the remainder of this book as one part of a perioperative nurse's knowledge bank. The remaining chapters contain vital information related to nursing practices and care processes that are needed to function in perioperative practice settings.

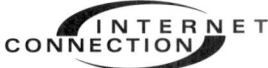

Association of Operating Room Nurses: http://www.aorn.org

American Academy of Ambulatory Care Nursing: http://www.inurse.com/~AAACN

American Academy of Nurse Practitioners: http://www.aanp.org

American Association for the History of Nursing: http://users.aol.com/NsgHistory/AAHN.html

American College of Nurse Practitioners: http://www.nurse.org/acnp

American Nurses Association: http://www.nursingworld.org

Case Management Society of America: http://www.cmsa.org

National Council of State Boards of Nursing: http://www.ncsbn.org

Agency for Health Care Policy and Research: http://www.ahcpr.gov/

Nursing Management: http://www.nursingmanagement.com

Quality Improvement: http://www.ipro.org

Nursing Informatics: http://www.cini.com/cin/

Clinical Pathways: http://www.surgyinfosys.com http://www.cinahl.com/ (search under "Critical Path" or "Critical Path Development")

National Institute of Nursing Research: http://www.nih.gov/ninr/

RN First Assistants: http://www.rnfa-firsthand.com

REFERENCES

1. Adler, S. (1994). The case manager. In Mundinger, M.O (Ed.), *The Pfizer guide: nursing career opportunities*. New York: Merritt Communications, pp. 300-303.
2. *ANA Standards of Clinical Practice*. (1998). Washington, DC: the Association.
3. AORN Standards, Recommended Practices and Guidelines. (1998). Denver: the Association.
4. Bowles, K.H., & Naylor, M.D. (1996). Nursing intervention classification systems. *Image: Journal of Nursing Scholarship, 28*(4), 303-308.
5. Canobbio, M.M. (1996). *Mosby's handbook of patient teaching*. St. Louis: Mosby.
6. Dahl, S. (1998). Navigating clinical pathways. *Surgical Services Management, 4*(1), 10-11.
7. Eisenberg, J.M. (1997). Outcomes research: engine for quality improvement. *Research Activities, 211*, 11-13.
8. Falkenhagen, K. (1993). Policies/procedures. In *Optimizing resources: a manager's guide to success*. Denver: AORN.
9. Fiesta, J. (1996). Legal update—1996, Part 1. *Nursing Management, 28*(4), 28.
10. Fiesta, J. (1997). Delegation, downsizing and liability. *Nursing Management, 28*(12), 14.
11. Harrington, H.J. (1998). Performance improvement: back to basics. *Quality Digest, 18*(2), 19.
12. Jenny, J., & Logan, J. (1996). Caring and comfort metaphors used by patients in critical care. *Image: Journal of Nursing Scholarship, 23*(4), 349-352.
13. Jones, L.D. (1997). Building the information infrastructure required for managed care. *Image: Journal of Nursing Scholarship, 29*(4), 377-382.
14. Larrabee, J.H. (1996). Emerging model of quality. *Image: Journal of Nursing Scholarship, 28*(4), 353-358.
15. Lawson, M.L., Lapinski, B.J., & Velasco, E.C. (1997). Tonsillectomy and adencidectomy pathway plan of care for the pediatric patient in day surgery. *Journal of Perianesthesia Nursing, 12*(6), 387.
16. Maas, M.L., Johnson, M., & Moorhead, S. (1996). Classifying nursing-sensitive patient outcomes. *Image: Journal of Nursing Scholarship, 28*(4), 295-301.
17. Mathias, J.M. (1996). OR of the future: remote surgery and virtual endoscopy on the horizon. *OR Manager, 12*(2), 1, 9-10.
18. Rothrock, J.C. (1997). Medicare reimbursement. *First Hand, 12*(3), 1-2.
19. Simpson, R.L. (1998a). A NIDSEC primer: Part 2. Setting the standards. *Nursing Management, 29*(2), 26-27, 29.
20. Simpson, R.L. (1998b). Take advantage of managed care opportunities. *Nursing Management, 28*(3), 24-25.
21. Speer, A.T., & Ziolkowski, L. (1998). Perioperative assistants are a new resource. *AORN Journal, 67*(2), 420-427.
22. Stilwell, K. (1998). Welcome to 1998 and focus on the future. *American Society for Quality–Health Care Division Newsletter*, Jan, 1998, 1,4.
23. Turley, J.P. (1996). Toward a model for nursing informatics. *Image: Journal of Nursing Scholarship, 28*(4), 309-313.
24. Winthrop, E. (1995). *Mosby's patient teaching tips*. St. Louis: Mosby.
25. Wojner, A.W. (1996). Outcomes management: driving enhancement of interdisciplinary practice with outcomes research. *Seminars in Perioperative Nursing, 5*(1), 3-11.
26. Zielstorff, R.D. (1997). ANA develops nursing data set standards for information systems. *Surgical Services Management, 3*(12), 47-48.
27. Zimmermann, P.G. (1996). Delegating to unlicensed assistive personnel. *Nursing Spectrum, 5*(11), 12-13.

C H A P T E R T W O

Patient and Environmental Safety

Diane Fecteau

THE SAFETY AND welfare of patients during surgical interventions are primary concerns of perioperative nurses. Risk management, a systematic way of detecting potential problems and ensuring safe patient care, has become increasingly important in the health care environment. Patient injuries during operative or other invasive procedures have serious consequences, necessitating a clear understanding of risk management by perioperative nursing personnel. Numerous hazards can be prevented, reduced, or controlled by adherence to sound policies, procedures, and regulations, thereby managing risk. Patients entering perioperative settings are at risk for infection, impaired skin integrity, altered body temperature, fluid volume deficit, and injury related to positioning and chemical, electrical, and physical hazards.

Policies and procedures are designed to ensure the safety of patients and personnel and to provide a setting in which all activities of the surgical team and ancillary personnel fit together, resulting in an efficient course of action for the benefit of each patient.

Regulations are mandated activities with which the institution must comply to meet certain standards set by outside agencies. There are several agencies that regulate the health care environment and affect practice in perioperative settings, including the following:

- The Environmental Protection Agency (EPA), which regulates the use of chemicals for disinfection and sterilization, as well as the disposal of medical wastes.
- The Joint Commission for Accreditation of Healthcare Organizations (JCAHO), which sets standards related to the structure, process, and outcomes of services provided by healthcare facilities. Accreditation is voluntary but recommended for Medicare and Medicaid reimbursement for services.
- The Occupational Safety and Health Administration (OSHA), which regulates safety and health issues in the workplace environment. Its regulations regarding preventing exposure to bloodborne pathogens and permissible levels of exposure to toxic substances in the environment (e.g., ethylene oxide and gluteraldehyde) most directly affect operating room practices.
- The federal Food and Drug Administration (FDA), which regulates implantable medical devices and requires surgical facilities to track them.[25]
- Many state health agencies have strict regulations affecting healthcare facilities and practices in surgical suites, including staffing and sterilization practices. In addition, local fire department regulations often control issues around corridor clearance and the storage of combustible supplies. It is important to become familiar with local and state regulations affecting perioperative practice.

SAFE ENVIRONMENT

Safety Design Features

Designing a safe environment incorporates features that prevent or control the risk of infection, fire, explosion, and chemical and electrical hazards. Well-devised traffic patterns, material-handling systems, disposal systems, positive-pressure and well-dispersed clean ventilation, and high-flow, unidirectional ventilation systems for special applications all contribute to a safe surgical environment. In addition, a reliable and adequate emergency power source must be available for use during electrical interruptions and be tested regularly to ensure working order. Emergency shutoffs for piped medical gases, such as oxygen and nitrous oxide, must be clearly labeled and readily available. Education designed to familiarize staff with all safety and hazard-prevention programs is required by the JCAHO.[15] Flame and explosion hazards have decreased significantly in recent years as a result of the use of nonflammable anesthetics and skin-prepping solutions. Electrical hazards continue to be of concern and are discussed at length later in this chapter.

Physical Plant Design Elements

Surgical suite design should take into consideration the need for adequate space to accommodate technology employed such as video monitors, microscopes, lasers, and cardiopulmonary bypass machines. Operating rooms that are too small compromise the safety of staff as well as the safety of patients. It is difficult to maneuver around equipment and to monitor and maintain the sterile field in a crowded room. Generally, the standard operating room is approximately 400 square feet, with a minimum 20-foot clear dimension between any cabinets and built-in shelves. Specialty operating rooms, such as those used for minimally invasive, orthopedic, neurologic, or cardiac surgery procedures, require at least 600 square feet of floor space, again with at least a 20-foot clear floor space. Specialty rooms designed for endoscopy and cystoscopy may be as small as 350 square feet.[12] Operating rooms designated for ambulatory surgery were once designed at the lower range of square footage; however, as more and more minimally invasive procedures are done on an ambulatory basis, larger surgery rooms have become necessary to accommodate this technology.

Surface materials used in operating rooms must be nonporous, smooth, easy to clean, waterproof, and fire resistant. High-impact vinyl materials and flexible wall coverings, together with new adhesives, permit completely sealed wall, ceiling, and floor joints so that the surfaces may be washed effectively with microbicidal cleaning solutions. The surfaces should be as free as possible of seams, joints, and crevices to prevent the harboring of microorganisms. Tile walls are no longer used in operating rooms because the grout lines are porous and can harbor microorganisms. Bumper guards should be placed on the corridor walls and corners to avoid damage from movement of surgical equipment and stretchers. Damaged walls cannot be cleaned properly and can harbor microorganisms.

Floor coverings should also be nonporous, seamless, and easy to clean. They should be made of slip-proof materials to prevent injuries to personnel. The color of the floor covering should be such that surgical needles are readily visible against its surface should they fall to the floor. The juncture between the floor and the wall should be curved to prevent material from gathering in the floor-to-wall juncture and to facilitate cleaning.

Sliding doors are recommended to eliminate the air turbulence caused by swinging doors. A pronounced increase in microbial counts has been noted when swinging doors are opened or closed. Doors should be made of the surface-sliding type, if possible, to facilitate cleaning of all surfaces.

Supply cabinets inside operating rooms should be enclosed with wire shelving to facilitate cleaning and minimize the collection of dust. Stainless steel cabinets with sliding glass doors are preferred to provide for ease of cleaning and ready visibility of contents to the circulating nurse.

When the supplies for a specific procedure are picked in the central sterile department and sent up to the operating room on an enclosed cart (case cart), the amount of supplies that are stocked in each operating room can be minimized. Fewer supplies in each operating room centralizes and reduces excess inventory for the hospital, allows for greater control, and makes it easier to keep the environment clean and free from dust. Ideally, clean carts with clean and sterile supplies are brought up to the operating room via a clean lift system (elevator, dumbwaiter, or cart lift). At the end of the procedure, contaminated instruments and supplies are placed into the cart and returned via a contaminated lift, where they are reprocessed and the cart is washed. Case carts work well when preference cards, or computerized data sheets, specific to a given procedure and surgeon, are accurate and routinely updated. Communication and collaboration between perioperative staff and central processing staff is critical to the success of a case cart system.

Operating room suite design with a sterile core is the most common design of modern operating rooms. This design eliminates cross traffic of staff and supplies from the contaminated or soiled areas to the clean or sterile areas. If decontamination and clean assembly processes occur outside of the operating room (in a central processing department), design of the suite needs to allow for the flow of items from dirty to clean areas without compromising principles of infection control, standard precautions (see Chapter 4), or aseptic technique.

The design of an operating room suite must be made with consideration for adequate space for storage of supplies and equipment. Storage space is usually underestimated when a new facility is being planned, resulting in clutter and inefficient movement of staff to gather equipment from distant storage spaces. One method to determine the amount of storage space needed in an OR is to add 50% of the total square footage of the surgical suite into the design for storage.[7] Storage space should be planned adjacent to the operating rooms. Several medium-sized storage rooms are preferable to one large room, to avoid the difficulty of retrieving items from the back of a large room.

Traffic Flow

Perioperative patient care requires movement of patients, personnel, and materials within and through the surgical suite. Development and implementation of appropriate traffic patterns, based on the design of the surgical suite, helps contain contamination. According to the Association of Operating Room Nurses (AORN) Recommended Practices for Traffic Patterns in the Surgical Suite, a three-zone designation of areas within the surgical suite facilitates appropriate movement of patients and personnel.[3] *Unrestricted* areas are those in which personnel may wear street clothes, and traffic is not limited. In *semirestricted* areas, such as processing and storage areas for instruments and supplies, as well as corridors leading to the restricted areas of the surgical suite, personnel must wear surgical attire and patients must wear gowns and hair coverings. *Restricted* areas include operating rooms and clean core and scrub sink areas. Surgical attire and masks are required in these areas when there are open sterile supplies or scrubbed persons in the area.

The flow of supplies should be from the clean core area through the operating rooms to the peripheral corridor. Soiled materials should not reenter the clean core area. Soiled linen and trash collection areas should be separated from personnel and patient traffic areas for infection control purposes. If instruments and other supplies are partially or totally reprocessed within the surgical suite, a unidirectional traffic pattern should ensure movement of items from the decontamination area to processing and storage areas. Work areas for each task should be clearly identified to eliminate crossover or mixing of these soiled and cleaned instruments or supplies. These recommended practices decrease the risk of infection by separating the clean from the contaminated.[3]

Ventilation

Appropriate ventilation systems aid in the control of infection by minimizing microbial contamination. Temperatures in an operating room should be maintained between 68° and 73° F (20° to 23° C), with relative humidity of 30% to 60% to reduce bacterial growth and suppress static electricity. Temperatures in that range allow for comfort of the surgical team and are tolerated by most patients. Each operating room should have individual temperature controls to accommodate patient safety, as when increased warmth is required for patients at high risk

for inadvertent hypothermia during operative procedures.

Currently, 15 air exchanges per hour are required in an operating room, at least three of which must be fresh air.[12] Air flow in an operating room is filtered through high-efficiency particulate air (HEPA) filter systems. These can filter 99% of all particles larger than 0.3 micrometers before air enters the operating room. Flow of air is designed so that clean, filtered air enters the operating room through vents located centrally at the ceiling and leaves the room close to the floor through exhaust vents in the walls. There is positive pressure inside the operating room, compared to the substerile rooms, corridors, and scrub areas, preventing potentially contaminated air from entering the operating room through these adjacent areas. To maintain this pressure gradient, doors to the operating room must be kept closed at all times, except when necessary for patient and personnel entry and exit.[10]

Each facility needs to have policies and procedures for the regular maintenance of the air-handling system in the operating room. This includes routine inspection and changing of filters, regular cleaning and inspection of vents and ductwork, and periodic measurement of air flow and air exchanges.

Emergency Signals

Every surgical suite should have an emergency signal system that can be activated inside each operating room. A light should appear outside the door of the room involved, and a buzzer or bell should sound in a central nursing or anesthesia area. The signals should remain on until the alarm is turned off at the source. All personnel should be familiar with the system and should know both how to send a signal and how to respond to it. Such a system, restricted to use in life-threatening emergencies, saves invaluable time in bringing additional personnel and resources for assistance.

STAFF AND PATIENT SAFETY

A safe environment, even in a well-designed facility, is dependent on a safety program with well-defined policies and procedures and a well-trained staff. All staff members, regardless of their position, need to recognize potential hazards in the surgical environment, implement safety practices, and contribute to making the environment safe for themselves, their coworkers, and the patients. The staff should be prepared through education programs (inservice) and practice drills to care for patients in a variety of emergency situations.

Staff Safety

All perioperative personnel should be instructed in the use of good body mechanics to avert common falls and strains when reaching, stretching, lifting, or moving heavy patients or other articles. Where possible, mechanical devices should be used for lifting patients and other heavy objects. Good body mechanics and application of work-simplification principles conserves energy, protects the worker, and thereby promotes good performance. Personnel should also be instructed and supervised in proper use of equipment to prevent injury such as burns from autoclaves and electrical equipment, abrasions from contact with metal accessory levers, injuries from swinging doors, cuts from knife blades, needle sticks, and splash exposures.

Personnel must be cognizant of and use appropriate protective apparel in the surgical suite in accordance with OSHA's final rule on exposure to bloodborne pathogens and the CDC's standard precautions. Eye protection, face masks, head and shoe covers, gowns, gloves, and any other protective wear must be used whenever the potential for blood and body fluid contact exists. Standard precautions are applied to all patients receiving care regardless of their diagnosis or presumed infection states. A blood and body fluid exposure control plan for the institution should be developed, identifying areas of high risk in the perioperative environment.

The exposure control plan for the operating room should be well documented and contain these key elements (see Chapter 4 for a thorough discussion of these elements):

1. A determination of exposure
2. Methods for complying with the OSHA and CDC guidelines
3. A procedure to evaluate exposures when they occur
4. A list of job classifications or tasks that have exposure potential
5. A plan for offering hepatitis vaccine
6. A definition of Standard Precautions, including a clear plan of compliance

The maintenance and cleaning program should be clearly defined and understood by the perioperative staff. Prompt attention to spills, immediate drying of wet floors, use of warning signs in danger areas, and keeping corridors and traffic areas clear of obstacles are important parts of maintaining a safe environment.

Effective disposal procedures for soiled materials and hazardous waste are essential to render the area safe for patients and personnel. AORN has proposed a definition of regulated medical waste (the part of medical waste with the potential to transmit infectious disease) as being one of four categories: sharps, cultures and stocks of infectious waste, animal waste, and selected isolation waste. Also included in regulated medical waste (because of esthetic concerns of the public) are pathologic waste, human blood, blood products, and body fluids. Some method for reducing the microbiological content for items falling in these four categories is recommended.[3] In addition, all surgical procedures are treated as potentially contaminated (Standard Precautions); outmoded "dirty-case" rituals have been eliminated to ensure a safe environment.

The professional nursing staff has a responsibility to work with the designated facility committees in establishing appropriate policies and reporting occurrences. Cleaning, disinfection, and sterilization of equipment, control of contaminants, and application of Standard Precautions and aseptic prectices are basic to an effective infection control program that helps protect patients and staff from the transmission risk of bloodborne and other pathogens.

Staff and Patient Safety Environmental Issues

In most facilities, the maintenance or engineering departments are responsible for regularly scheduled inspection of steam, electrical, vacuum, hydraulic, ventilation, plumbing, and emergency generator systems. It is important to verify that these systems are indeed checked regularly as an important part of maintaining a safe environment for patients and perioperative staff.

Electrical and fire hazards

The types of electrical hazards encountered in the OR environment include electric shock, fire, explosions, and burns. Electric shock results from current flowing through the body and can result from touching a damaged plug or an ungrounded piece of metal equipment. Fires can result from faulty wires, inappropriate use of extension cords, and careless use of electrical equipment, such as lasers and electrosurgical units (ESUs), particularly in the presence of an oxygen-enriched environment or flammable liquids.

The electrical and fire safety plan, identifying policies and procedures pertinent to the operating room, should be approved by the operating room committee and hospital administration. Perioperative nursing management should be delegated the responsibility and authority to see that the plan is put into effect by all staff members. The plan includes the following:

1. Prohibit smoking and the use of any apparatus or device producing an open flame.
2. Evaluate and test all new equipment to ensure optimum safety and performance.
3. Inspect all electrical equipment, regardless of the source, for safety and proper functioning before use, and label with an inspection sticker, according to institutional procedure
4. Have the biomedical technician or electrical safety officer determine whether electrical equipment, cameras, lights, and electrosurgical units are safe for use in a given situation.
5. Establish inventory control, regular inspection, preventive maintenance, and safety approval systems.
6. Instruct personnel in the safe use of all equipment and require a return demonstration of their proficiency.
7. All personnel must be familiar with the procedure for

prompt removal from use and expeditious repair of defective equipment.

8. A qualified electrician should inspect electrical outlets and equipment at designated intervals or as requested and should file written reports with the director of surgical services.

9. A standard procedure for care and use of electrical equipment should include the following:
   a. The plug, cord, and connections of electrical equipment must be checked before each use.
   b. All electrical cords should be of adequate length and flexibility to reach an outlet without stress and without the use of extension cords. Kinks and curls should be removed from electrical cords before the plugs are inserted into wall outlets.
   c. The plug, not the cord, should be handled when electrical cords are plugged into or removed from an outlet. Pulling on the cord may cause it to break at the point where the wire is attached to the plug.
   d. Cords and connections should be handled in accordance with their delicacy. They cannot withstand pulling or rough treatment. Cord breakage is inconvenient and dangerous, and replacing broken cords is extremely expensive.
   e. Cords should not be wrapped tightly around equipment, which causes the protective covering to wear and breaks the wires inside the covering.
   f. Cords should always be removed from traffic pathways before equipment such as a bed or a machine is moved. If the position of electrical equipment necessitates cords lying on the floor where persons will be walking during surgery, the cords should be taped down to prevent tripping.[3]

Isolated power system

An isolated power system, though no longer required by the National Fire Protection Agency in nonflammable anesthetizing locations, is still found in many operating rooms. These systems may reduce the hazard of shock or burn from electrical current flowing through the body to ground by allowing identification of a piece of equipment in the system that is not appropriately grounded. Each isolated power system must have a continually operating line-isolation monitor that indicates possible leakage or fault currents to ground.[3]

Most monitors have a green signal lamp that indicates when the system is isolated from ground. A red signal lamp and an audible warning signal indicate when a ground fault is detected. All perioperative personnel must know the procedure to follow when this occurs:

1. The last electrical device to be plugged in must be shut off and unplugged.
2. If the red signal remains on, each piece of nonessential equipment must be systematically unplugged until the defective device is found.

3. A replacement must be obtained and the defective device removed from service, properly labeled as to the problem, and sent to the appropriate department for inspection and repair.
4. If a defective device cannot be identified and the red lamp remains on, the operating room must be shut down after the completion of that patient's surgery until the situation is corrected.
5. Individuals responsible for ensuring electrical safety must be notified.

Volatile liquids

Flammable liquids, including alcohol, must be properly stored. Volatile liquids such as acetone and aerosol sprays are prohibited for cleaning and incidental use in hazardous locations. Skin-prepping solutions should be applied with care to prevent pooling, which can lead to a chemical burn. Towels should be tucked under the patient along the area to be prepped to catch any dripping solution and removed as soon as the prep is completed. In addition to being a chemical irritant, the prep solution may be ignited by a spark from an active electrode of the ESU or from a charge of static electricity. Ignition of vapors can occur as the solution evaporates. Whenever an ESU is used, all solutions used for skin prepping should be nonflammable.

The Right to Know directive published by OSHA in 1983[22] sets the standard for providing information to employees about hazardous substances encountered in the workplace. Material Safety Data Sheets (MSDSs) are information sheets that are the basis for the standard. Each manufacturer of a chemical or solution is required to provide safety information about their products, and employers are required to have this information available to employees to review at any time. Personnel should be familiar with the MSDSs for chemicals and solutions used in the operating room because they provide valuable patient and personnel safety information.

Electrosurgery

High-frequency current from an ESU is frequently used to cut tissue and to coagulate blood vessels. Advanced technology has dramatically improved electrosurgical capabilities with the development of solid-state generators and isolated systems (Fig. 2-1). Solid-state, isolated units are made to ignore all grounded objects that may come into contact with the patient undergoing surgery, referring current only to the generator. These units significantly decrease the burn potential and the shock hazards that were inherent in the original spark-gap units. In those units current could be split to an alternate pathway if a patient were in contact with a grounded object (i.e., OR bed, ECG electrode). Personnel must receive education and demonstrate competence in the proper use of electrosurgical equipment.

Before each use, the ESU and associated safety features should be inspected for signs of damage and tested to

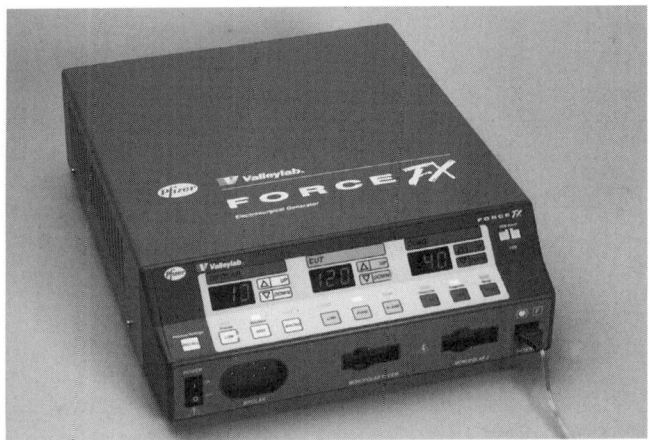

FIGURE 2-1 Computer-controlled Instant Response technology uses Tissue Density Feedback circuitry and computer-controlled output for automatic response to changes in tissue density, reducing the need to adjust power settings for different types of tissue. It also includes the REM Contact Quality Monitoring System, providing safety against electrosurgical burns under the return electrode. Dual, independent, simultaneous, hand- or foot-switching monopolar outputs allow two surgeons or the surgeon and assistant to coagulate simultaneously yet independently from the same unit. Coagulation modes include low, medium, and high; cut modes include low, pure, and blend. Improved performance at lower voltages reduces sparking, neuromuscular stimulation, and RF interference. Bipolar modes include low, medium, and macro. Low cut and low coagulation use lower voltages to reduce risks of laparoscopic electrosurgery. Macrobipolar mode is designed for today's new generation of macrobipolar cutting instruments.

ensure that they are functioning properly. The patient's skin integrity must be assessed before and after ESU use, particularly at positional pressure points and the area under the dispersive pad (inactive electrode, or grounding pad).

After the patient has been positioned, the desired connection between the patient and the ESU is established by placement of the dispersive pad on a nonhairy area of clean, dry skin. The pad should be placed as close to the operative site as possible, on the same side of the patient's body as the operative site, and over a large muscle mass if possible because muscle is a better conductor of electricity than adipose tissue is. Bony prominences, skin over metal prostheses, pressure points, and scar tissue should be avoided because these increase the resistance to the flow of current. Care is taken to be sure to avoid placing the dispersive electrode where blood and body fluids or irrigation solution may pool because the pad could lose contact with the skin. If a dispersive pad requiring gel is used, the pad must be checked before placement to identify any dry spots on its surface. Placement should ensure that the pad's entire surface area maintains uniform body contact, without tenting or gapping.

The ESU power settings should be as low as possible for each procedure. Settings are determined by the surgeon in conjunction with the manufacturer's recommendations and confirmed orally by the circulating nurse before activation. When not in use, the ESU active electrode

should be placed into a clean, well-insulated, safety container (holster) in a visible area to prevent accidental activation and injury.[3]

The current supplied by the ESU is dispersed by the active electrode (electrosurgical pencil) through the body and is directed back to the generator by the dispersive electrode. In a nonisolated system, failure of this electrical pathway can result in current traveling in alternate pathways and causing burns in areas of contact. A faulty return pathway should be suspected if the surgeon requests higher settings because of inadequate cutting or coagulation. The connection from the patient to the generator should be examined immediately. A faulty return pathway may result from (1) inadequate patient contact with the dispersive pad, (2) poor placement of the pad, (3) inadequate connection of the cable to the pad, or (4) inadequate connection at the unit itself.

Electrosurgical burns may result from the unit's action on other electrical equipment. When an ECG monitor is used, the electrodes should be placed on the patient's shoulders and upper chest. The placement of ECG electrodes should always be as far as possible from the operative site. Distant positioning minimizes the alternate flow of electrosurgical current through the electrodes and monitor to ground.

Contemporary ESUs possess a patient return electrode monitoring (REM) system. Current flowing from the active electrode is measured and compared with current returning from the patient return electrode. If the currents are not balanced, the circuit determines that the patient return electrode is not functioning properly, and the unit is deactivated. A significant safety feature is the capability of the REM system to measure the potential current concentration that may result in a burn at the return electrode site, such as inadequate electrode application or reduction of electrode contact area. It also measures the continuity of the entire electrical circuit (patient-pad-cord) for safe current flow. This capability represents a vital patient safety feature. (See Chapter 3 for a thorough discussion of electrosurgical physics, modes, tissue effects, and special considerations during endoscopy.)

Surgical smoke

There has been an increased awareness of the potential harmful effects of surgical smoke in the operating room environment on staff and patients. Surgical smoke is composed of aerosols produced when lasers or ESUs are used and has been found to contain particulate matter, gases, mutagens, carcinogens, and sometimes DNA components. However, whether DNA materials found are infectious has not been established. Because particulate matter such as human papillomavirus (HPV) has been found in both laser and ESU vapors after treatment of warts,[23] the National Institute for Occupational Safety and Health (NIOSH) has issued an alert regarding the "Control of Smoke From Laser/Electric Surgical Procedures."[20]

Operating room air exchanges alone are not effective at clearing surgical smoke because the recommended air exchanges for ORs are 15 per hour, and it takes 20 minutes after the ESU machine is turned off for the smoke to return to the baseline level. Wall suction might be useful for small amounts of smoke but are designed for evacuation of fluids, not gases, and they don't have the power to remove large quantities of smoke. Particles found in surgical smoke are too small to be effectively filtered by a surgical mask.[24]

Smoke evacuators, machines specifically designed to remove surgical smoke from the operating room environment, are increasingly being used. Controversy regarding their use continues, however, because of their cost (estimated between $10,000 and $12,000 per year per OR), noise level, and the lack of conclusive data correlating surgical smoke exposure with actual physical effects. To be effective, filter nozzles from smoke evacuators must be placed within 2 inches of the source of surgical smoke.[9]

Institutions should review the studies concerning hazards of surgical smoke and develop policies for its safe evacuation from the environment. A multidisciplinary team consisting of surgeons; nurses; anesthesia providers; safety, infection control, risk management, and clinical engineering personnel should reach a consensus about which procedures generate the most smoke and have the highest priority for smoke evacuation. The team should then determine what equipment is appropriate for which types of procedures and should evaluate smoke–evacuation devices.

Radiation safety

Radiation presents environmental safety concerns for both patients and staff. Many surgical procedures utilize radiologic studies that are performed immediately before, during, or after surgery, therefore increasing the potential for radiation exposure. X rays of all frequencies can damage tissues and may produce long-term effects. The effects of radiation are dose dependent and cumulative; the larger the dose, or the more frequent the exposure, the greater the risk of the effects of radiation.

Sources of radiation exposure in the OR include ionizing sources: portable radiography (x-ray) machines and portable fluoroscopy units (C-arm), and non-ionizing sources: lasers (see Chapter 3 for a thorough discussion of laser safety). Members of the surgical team should avoid unnecessary exposure to radiation sources and comply with practices that reduce potential for exposure. Personnel present in the operating room must maintain the greatest practical distance from the radiation source when ionizing radiation is used during surgery. Nonessential personnel should leave the room, and members of the scrubbed team should wear protective devices and move as far from the radiation source as is possible, while still adhering to aseptic technique.

When feasible, appropriate devices should be used to hold patients or the x-ray cassettes during radiography procedures to limit exposure of the surgical team. Protective equipment is used to reduce the intensity of radiation exposure. Radiation safety devices include but are not limited to special eyewear, lead gloves, aprons, and thyroid shields. Careful handling and regular examination of leaded garments are important to ensure the integrity of shielding. Staff-development programs on radiation safety should be done periodically to reinforce radiation safety practices as well as to correct misconceptions or unrealistic practices relating to radiation exposure and monitoring.

Radiation-monitoring devices (film badges) are used in accordance with radiation safety standards by personnel who may be exposed to radiation. A film badge comprises the film holder, metal filters (aluminum or copper), and a film packet. The badge should be worn consistently in the same area of the body, attached to the front of clothing either at the chest or waist level. When a protective apron is worn, the film badge should be worn on the collar above the apron. Badges are collected monthly and sent to a monitoring company. A written monthly report provides a permanent record of an individual's occupational exposure.[11]

Patient protection during procedures utilizing radiation is accomplished by shielding and by using machines that limit the size of the beam, thereby reducing the amount of tissue being exposed to direct radiation. Shields should be placed over reproductive organs, where possible. A careful preoperative history is an important part of radiation safety, especially related to a female's reproductive status. If a woman might be pregnant, especially during the first trimester, it is very important to avoid radiation exposure, which might damage the fetus.[16]

Latex allergy

A subject critical to the health and safety of both the patient and the healthcare worker is that of latex allergy. Latex is the material of choice for surgical gloves because it is resealable and flexible, maintaining the wearer's tactile sensitivity. Although natural rubber latex has been a common component in thousands of medical and consumer products for many years, latex sensitivity is a relatively new problem for patients and healthcare personnel. Latex reactions have ranged from mild contact dermatitis to moderately severe symptoms of urticaria, rhinitis, conjunctivitis, and bronchospasm and to severe life-threatening anaphylaxis.[21]

There are two types of reactions: type IV—delayed cell-mediated reaction, including symptoms of contact dermatitis (e.g., pruritus, edema, erythema, vesicles, drying papules, and crusting and thickening of the skin) that spread beyond the areas of contact—and type I—immediate, IgE mediated, and anaphylactic. The onset of an anaphylactic reaction usually occurs within minutes with symptoms of generalized urticaria, wheezing, dyspnea, laryngeal edema, bronchospasm, tachycardia, angioedema, hypotension, and cardiac arrest. Many serious anaphylactic reactions have occurred when there is direct contact with a latex product (e.g., surgical gloves) with mucous membranes during surgical procedures. This situation permits a rapid introduction of latex antigen directly into the vascular circulation.[14]

Individuals at high risk for latex allergy include healthcare workers (prevalence values of 3% to 17%), patients with spina bifida, genitourinary tract anomalies, and who have undergone multiple surgical procedures. People who work in the rubber industry and those who have a hereditary tendency for immediate allergic reactions are also at risk.[18]

Until recently, it was assumed that the sensitization to latex resulted only from cutaneous absorption in healthcare workers or from direct mucosal contact during clinical treatments. Recent studies confirm that latex protein allergens effectively bind to glove powder and, when airborne, can remain suspended for prolonged periods of time. Therefore, inhalant exposure is an additional risk factor for sensitization to latex allergens (Research Highlight 2-1).

Healthcare facilities need to develop policies and procedures for caring for latex-sensitive patients, and all staff members must adhere to these policies.[12] One of the first steps to protect latex-sensitive patients is the replacement of latex-containing devices and products with alternate synthetic materials for surgical procedures. Such efforts are hampered by the difficulties in identifying latex-containing products. For example, the rubber stopper on a medication vial or syringe plunger might release a sufficient amount of protein to trigger the reaction in an extremely sensitive patient.[14]

Latex allergy carts that contain alternate products should be set up, maintained, and used with known allergic or high-risk patients (Table 2-1). If the designation of latex-free rooms is not possible, the access to any latex product in the room needs to be prohibited by means of locking or taping closed cabinet doors that contain these products. It is preferable for patients who are latex sensitive to have their procedures performed in an OR where no latex products have been recently used (such as the first procedure of the day). Prominent signs identifying the risk of latex allergy should be posted at all entrances to an operating room where the latex-allergic patient is having surgery.

In addition, institutions need to develop strategies for limiting healthcare workers' occupational exposure to latex. This includes switching to low-allergen latex gloves

---

2-1 RESEARCH HIGHLIGHT

LATEX ALLERGEN LEVELS IN OPERATING ROOM AIR

This study explored the effect of substituting low-allergen–containing latex gloves for high-allergen–containing latex gloves on operating room (OR) air latex allergen levels. Latex allergen levels in the air on high-allergen glove days were significantly higher than on low-allergen glove days. In a multivariable consideration of four variables (glove type, total number of gloves used, OR time, and operating procedure time), glove type and OR time emerged as independent factors associated with latex allergen air levels. The use of gloves containing low levels of latex allergen was associated with significant reductions in air latex allergen levels (more than a ten-fold reduction) in a typical OR setting. This usage should minimize latex-induced asthma and allergic rhinoconjunctivitis in many latex-sensitized healthcare workers. This is not a substitute for latex-free precautions to prevent cutaneous, mucosal, and serosal contact with rubber in latex-sensitive persons. It does, however, offer a means to reduce sensitizing healthcare workers to latex allergens that is less costly than the complete removal of all latex-containing items in operating rooms.

From Heilman, D.K., Jones, D.T., Swanson, M.C., & Yuninger, J.W. (1996). A prospective, controlled study showing that rubber gloves are the major contributor to latex aeroallergen levels in the operating room, *Journal of Allergy and Clinical Immunology, 98*(2): 324-330.

TABLE 2-1 | Product Identification for Latex Allergy

PRODUCTS WITH LATEX	NONLATEX ALTERNATIVE
Adhesive tape	3M tapes: Durapore, Micropore; J&J Dermicel or Dermiclear
Blood-pressure cuff, or tourniquet cuff tubing	Cover patient's arm, tubes, bulb, with softroll or stockinette
Foley catheters	Silastic, or silicone, elastomer Foley catheters
Intravenous supplies: rubber injection ports on bags	Three-way stopcock on intravenous tubing and other tubing
Latex gloves	Tactylon, vinyl, or Sensicare gloves
Medication vials	Remove rubber stopper, wipe with alcohol, or use glass ampules
Penrose drains	Silicone drains
Pulse oximeter with rubber	Use Tegaderm on finger before applying pulse oximeter
Rubber bands	Vessel loops
Rubber dams	Sterile plastic bowel bags
Rubber shods, suture bolsters	Cut pieces of Silastic catheter
Syringes	Nonlatex brands, or glass

Source: Johns Hopkins Hospital Operating Room latex allergy chart (1996). Baltimore: The Johns Hopkins Hospital.

or nonlatex gloves. The expense of completely eliminating latex gloves is often a barrier for facilities. The next best alternative is low-allergen, powder-free gloves. The cornstarch powder on powdered latex gloves is an efficient allergen carrier and contributes to airborne contamination, especially in ORs where glove use is high. The use of low-allergen, powder-free gloves reduces the airborne latex allergen content (to below detectable levels), thereby reducing occupational exposure.[29]

Patient Safety

Protecting patient's rights

Protection of patients' personal, moral, and legal rights begins at the time of admission. The course of action involves correctly identifying patients, safeguarding their right to privacy and their right to make choices regarding their care, and keeping confidential all records and reports.[15] Conditions of admission to the hospital, consent forms for treatment or surgical procedures, and advance directives are important records that protect both the patient and the personnel who render care to them.

The facility administration provides legally appropriate forms. Personnel who obtain consents or witness them should be aware of the conditions that ensure validity of the consent. A signed consent must also be an informed consent, which implies adequate communication with the patient regarding the procedure or procedures for which the consent is being signed. No surgical procedure should be performed without a signed and witnessed informed consent. The surgeon is ultimately responsible for informing the patient about the proposed operation or other invasive procedure, its inherent risks and complications, and for obtaining consent. Consent forms must be signed before the administration of preoperative medications. On the patient's arrival in the operating room, the circulating nurse and anesthesia provider are responsible for verifying that the consent is on the chart and is correct, properly signed, and witnessed before the administration of anesthesia.

Special permits for anesthesia administration, specific operations, such as sterilization and therapeutic abortion, disposal of severed body parts, organ donation, and autopsy provide additional safeguards for the patient, staff, and institution.

General patient safety measures

Minimizing human error helps eliminate hazardous conditions for the patient undergoing operative or other invasive procedures. In all perioperative settings, where the patient is unable to protect himself or herself, nursing personnel must provide protection for the patient.

Communication of vital medical information to surgical team members is essential to safe patient care. An allergy identification band is used to communicate a patient's allergy to a given medication or substance. This is a safety measure that prevents the administration of drugs

or the use of materials that would evoke an allergic reaction in the patient. Even in the absence of an allergy band, patients should be queried regarding allergies to medications or food products.

All medications must be checked three times before administration: (1) when removed from the drug cabinet, (2) before being drawn up in the syringe, and (3) before being given to the patient.

Patients' hearing tends to become more acute after the administration of the preoperative medication and in the induction stage of anesthesia. A quiet environment is essential for all patients awaiting surgery. Recent studies indicate that some patients' hearing is acute throughout the surgical procedure. Even with the use of amnesia-invoking drugs, a small percentage of the population experience recall of noise and events that occurred during their surgery.[13] In addition, high noise levels interfere with accurate communication among members of the surgical team and may increase the likelihood of error. For both of these reasons, noise in the operating room should be controlled and conversations kept to a minimum.

Stretchers and operating room beds must be stabilized with the wheels locked when a patient is moving from one to another. One person should stabilize the stretcher while another stands on the opposite side of the operating room bed to receive the patient. All safety devices on stretchers and operating room beds must be in proper working order. Locking mechanisms, side rails, restraint straps, intravenous standards, hydraulic controls, armboards, and other protective devices should be used whenever necessary.

Admission of the Patient to the Operating Room

Admission of patients to the operating room is a critical time for the perioperative nurse to gather data to help plan for the patients' care and safety. It is the opportunity to collaborate with the patient by identifying and verifying his or her needs and then planning care to meet those needs. Empathic communication, good listening skills, being alert to nonverbal communication, offering gentle reassurance, providing explanations, and utilizing comforting behaviors are essential attributes of perioperative nurses

Institutional policy and procedure for patient admission should include the following steps:

1. The perioperative nurse verifies the patient's identification orally with the patient (if feasible) and compares the name on the surgical schedule with the name on the patient's armband and medical record. Information on the surgical schedule pertaining to the patient's name, hospital number, date of birth, and physician's name must match the information on the patient's identification band and medical record.
2. The procedure to be performed (including the operative site, side, and surgical approach) is verified by the patient and matched with the surgical posting,

medical record, and consent form. Similar validation is undertaken by the anesthesia provider and the surgeon.

3. The operative consent form, history and physical examination record, laboratory results, and other examination or diagnostic results should be complete before surgery[15] and reviewed by the perioperative nurse as part of patient assessment. Facility policy determines which examinations are mandatory as part of the patient's preoperative preparation. These may include completed records for health history and physical examination, recent determinations of blood and urine testing, and chest x-ray and ECG examinations.

4. Allergies; previous unfavorable reactions to anesthesia or blood transfusions; previous reactions to latex; religious, cultural, spiritual, or ethnic preferences; and any relevant advanced directive must be carefully noted.[30]

5. The patient should be queried about personal effects, including clothing, money, jewelry, wigs, religious symbols, and prostheses such as dentures, lenses, glass eyes, and hearing aids. The nurse is responsible for ensuring the safe handling and proper disposition of patient property and valuables.

6. The perioperative nurse should review the orders and results concerning preoperative skin preparation, medication administration, and elimination, such as enema results and the amount of urine voided or collected through a catheter.

7. It is important to determine whether preoperative dietary and fluid restrictions (NPO status) have been maintained; this is crucial in preventing the aspiration of gastric contents during anesthesia induction. (During induction, additional precautions should be taken to prevent such an occurrence by ensuring that the suctioning apparatus is functional and by having personnel present to assist the anesthesia provider.)

8. The nurse should meticulously document any medications, fluids, blood, or blood products administered as ordered during the immediate preoperative period.

9. The nursing staff should apply siderails, locking devices, and safety straps on stretchers and operating room beds to prevent falls and injury to the patient during transport, transfer, and positioning.

A preoperative checklist, frequently used to prevent oversights, omissions, and sentinel events (Box 2-1), displays critical items to be checked preoperatively. Fig. 2-2 demonstrates a preoperative checklist as an integrated part of the perioperative nursing record.

Clinical Documentation

The JCAHO requires that a record be kept of each operation, including the preoperative diagnosis, the surgery performed, a description of findings, the specimens removed, the postoperative diagnosis, and the names of all persons participating in intraoperative care. This

operative record is a permanent part of the patient's chart. The AORN Recommended Practices for Documentation of Perioperative Nursing Care[3] suggest that the intraoperative patient care record should also include but not be limited to the following:

1. Evidence of a patient assessment upon arrival in the operating room, which includes an assessment of the patient's skin condition immediately before and after the procedure

2. Evidence of a plan of care individualized for the patient

3. Any sensory aids or prosthetic devices worn by the patient on admission to the operating room and their subsequent disposition

4. Patient position, including supports or restraints used

5. Location of dispersive electrode pad placement and identification of ESU and settings used

6. Location of temperature-control device placement, with identification of unit used and recording of time and temperature

7. Placement of monitoring electrodes

Text continued on p. 37

BOX 2-1 | **Sentinel Events**

Perioperative nursing practice has a fundamental goal of protecting patients from injury related to numerous events, equipment and activities such as physical hazards, extraneous objects, chemicals, electrical equipment, positioning, radiation (ionizing and non-ionizing), inadvertent hypothermia, incorrect administration of medications, fluid therapy, and medical devices. In 1997, the Joint Commission defined a *sentinel event* as an "unexpected occurrence involving death or serious physical or psychological injury, or risk thereof." Organizations accredited by the Joint Commission are required to report a sentinel event that has occurred if it *has* resulted in an unanticipated death or major permanent loss of function or is one of the following:

- Infant abduction
- Infant discharge to the wrong family
- Rape (by another patient or staff)
- Hemolytic transfusion reaction
- Surgery on the wrong patient or wrong body part

"Risk thereof" includes any process variation for which a recurrence would carry a significant chance of a serious outcome. When a sentinel event has occurred, the facility must perform a root-cause analysis and submit an action plan to the Joint Commission within 30 days. The analysis must focus on systems and processes, with identification of process improvements that could reduce a similar event from occurring in the future. The Joint Commission then follows up by requiring a written progress report or conducting an on-site visit in 6 months of implementing the system or process improvements identified in the institution's root-cause analysis.

Adapted from Kobs, A. (1998). Sentinel event: a moment in time, a lifetime to forget. *Nursing Management, 29*(2), 1-13.

PREOPERATIVE ASSESSMENT

PLANNED PROCEDURE DATE		Pre-Op Testing: BMC/Other _____	
PROPOSED PROCEDURE			
DIAGNOSIS			

Historian: ☐ Patient ☐ Other _____ ☐ In Person ☐ Telephone

Patient's Chief Complaint: _____
_____

Medications	Dose	Frequency	Patient Med. Knowledge

Are you presently taking ASA or Bloodthinner Y ☐ N ☐ Last Dose _____

ALLERGIES _____

☐ NKDA _____

Latex Allergy ☐ No ☐ Yes

Escort Name _____

Escort Phone _____

Hgt. _____   Wgt. _____

P _____   BP _____

Date:	Previous Hospitalizations/Surgery:	Complications:

Health Problems:

☐ NO ☐ YES Respiratory _____

☐ NO ☐ YES Cardiovascular Disease: (Circle)
MI _____ yr., Angina, Stroke,
Rheumatic Fever, Mitral Valve Prolapse
Hypertension, murmur
_____

☐ NO ☐ YES Implants: i.e. pacemaker, subcutaneous port,
metal hardware: _____

☐ NO ☐ YES Pregnant _____

☐ NO ☐ YES Diabetes _____

☐ NO ☐ YES Hepatitis _____ yr _____

☐ NO ☐ YES Seizures _____

☐ NO ☐ YES Cancer _____

☐ NO ☐ YES Muscular/Skeletal _____

☐ NO ☐ YES Emotional Problems _____

☐ NO ☐ YES Significant health problems _____
_____

Other:

☐ NO ☐ YES Smoking _____ pk/day x _____ yrs.

☐ NO ☐ YES Alcohol/Drug Use (circle): _____

Immunization History:

☐ NO ☐ YES ☐ Unknown Childhood immunizations

☐ NO ☐ YES ☐ Unknown Recent exposure to communicable
disease, i.e. chicken pox, measles, mumps or TB

NSG DX: Potential for Alteration in Self Care

ROLE RELATIONSHIP PATTERN/DISCHARGE PLANNING

Occupation: _____

Financial concerns: ☐ NO ☐ YES

Living conditions: Alone ☐ NO ☐ YES _____
Stairs ☐ NO ☐ YES ☐ N/A

Do you anticipate homecare/equipment needs: ☐ NO ☐ YES

Social Service/discharge planning referral made: ☐ NO ☐ YES

Advance directive: ☐ NO ☐ YES ☐ INFO GIVEN

Patient/Significant other education needs: ☐ NO ☐ YES

GOAL: Patient is able to verbalize the need for home care.
Goal met _____ Goal not met _____ (explain in nurse's notes)

NSG DX: Knowledge deficit R/T upcoming procedure.

PATIENT TEACHING/INSTRUCTIONS Initials _____

☐ Y ☐ N/A NPO after Midnight or _____
☐ Y ☐ N/A Take Preop Meds
☐ Y ☐ N/A Bring Meds
☐ Y ☐ N/A No Make-up, Jewelry, Nail polish, contacts
☐ Y ☐ N/A Wear Appropriate Clothing
☐ Y ☐ N/A Bring Crutches, Walker
☐ Y ☐ N/A Preps, Tests, Treatments
☐ Y ☐ N/A Pain Scale 0-10
☐ Y ☐ N/A Arrival Time

GOAL: Patient verbalizes understanding.
Goal met _____ Goal not met _____ (explain in nurse's notes)

COMMENTS: _____
_____
_____

Date _____ 24-HR Time _____ RN Signature _____

FIGURE 2-2 Perioperative nursing record form. This form incorporates a preoperative checklist and combines documentation from all perioperative areas to avoid duplication of patient history and assessment data.

Continued

PERI

PERIOPERATIVE NURSING RECORD

Date: _____

Arrival 24-HR Time: _____ ☐ Amb.   ☐ W/C   ☐ _____

Emotional Response	Skin/Mucous Membrane
☐ Talkative	☐ Warm/Dry
☐ Quiet/Calm	☐ Moist/Clammy
☐ Crying/tearful	☐ Cyanosis
☐ Anxious	☐ Pink
☐ Agitated	☐ Jaundice
☐ Cooperative	☐ Pale
☐ Uncooperative	☐ Ruddy

NPO Since: _____
Medications Taken Today:

_____
_____
_____
_____

Voided/Time: _____

PATIENT TEACHING DONE

_____Review of day's events
_____Wound Care, Mobility
_____Pain Scale 0 - 10
_____Patient/Responsible Adult verbalizes understanding

INTRAVENOUS RECORD

24-HR Time	IV Solutions	Site	Cath Size	Initials

PROCEDURE	
PHYSICIAN	ROOM

ANESTHESIA TYPE   ☐ LOCAL   IV   IV CONSCIOUS
GEN. ☐   SAB ☐   EPIDURAL ☐   BLOCK ☐   REGIONAL ☐   MAC ☐   SEDATION ☐

CHART READY

_____ Y ☐ N/A   H&P
_____ Y ☐ N/A   Procedure permit complete
_____ Y ☐ N/A   Anesthesia permit complete
_____ Y ☐ N/A   Lab
_____ Y ☐ N/A   EKG
_____ Y ☐ N/A   Pre-op Consults
_____ Y ☐ N/A   CXR and/or PFT results
_____ Y ☐ N/A   BGM or FBS (on all diabetics) _____
_____ Y ☐ N/A   Height & Weight, VS charted
_____ Y ☐ N/A   Allergies Noted

PATIENT READY

_____ Y ☐ N/A   Identification Band
_____ Y ☐ N/A   Dentures Removed/In
_____ Y ☐ N/A   Jewelry Secured
_____ Y ☐ N/A   Glasses/Contacts: Removed/On
_____ Y ☐ N/A   Hearing Aid Removed/On
_____ Y ☐ N/A   Patient seen by Anesthesia

SKIN PREP   ☐ N/A   Initials _____
Area: _____   ☐ Wet/Razor ☐ Clippers

NSG DX: High risk for injury r/t sensory/motor deficits secondary to sedation or anesthesia.

POSITION FOR SURGERY	POSITION DEVICES ☐ N/A
_____ Supine	_____ Shea Head Rest
_____ Prone	_____ Donut Under
_____ Lateral R L	_____ Blanket Roll
_____ Lith L H	_____ Pillow Under
_____ Other_____	
_____ Safety Strap On	**ARMS POSITIONS ☐ N/A**
_____ Side Rails Up	_____ Arm Boards R L

LASER ☐ N/A	_____ Tucked @ Sides R L
_____ CO2 _____ YAG	_____ Across Chest
_____ Eye protection by policy	_____ Under Head

THERMAL ☐ N/A

MACH #	TYPE	TEMP SET

TOURNIQUET #   ☐ N/A

LOCATION	24-HR TIME UP	APPLIED BY
PRESSURE	24-HR TIME DOWN	TESTED

ESU ☐ N/A

MACH #	KLEPS #	BICAP #
CUT	ABC	COAG	BIPOLAR	☐ SNARE ☐ HOT BX
PAD SITE	APPLIED BY	SITE ___ CHECKED

☐ Scope # _____

GOAL: The patient's safety will be maintained.
Goal met _____   Goal not met _____
(explain in nurse's notes)

NSG DX: High risk for infection r/t break in skin integrity.

DRESSINGS ☐ N/A

	PREPS ☐ N/A
_____ Soft Sterile _____ Steri Strips	_____ Beta/Scrub
_____ Band-aids _____ Eye Patch	_____ Dura Prep
_____ Peri-Pad	_____ Beta/Paint
_____ Splint _____ Collodian	_____ Hibiclens
_____ Cast _____ Otomed/Ear	_____ Solo/Gel
_____ Cold Pack _____ Other	_____ Alcohol
	_____ Other

GOAL: The patient will be protected from potential wound infection.
Goal met _____   Goal not met _____   N/A _____
(explain in nurse's notes)

NSG DX: Fluid volume, excess/deficit
r/t physiological response to stress 2° to procedure.

IRRIGATION ☐ N/A

_____ NACL   _____ Epi   _____ Antibiotic
_____ H2O   Dose _____   Dose _____
_____ BBS   _____ LR
_____ Tis-u-sol   _____ Mannitol   Dose_____
_____ Heparin   Intake _____
Dose _____   Output _____

	NA	TYPE	SITE
Drains			
Packs			

URINARY CATH ☐ N/A

FOLEY SIZE	CATH BY	STR. CATH
CAME WITH _____		

GOAL: The patient will maintain fluid volume balance.
Goal met _____   Goal not met _____   N/A _____
(explain in nurse's notes)

SPECIMENS/PERMANENT   ☐ N/A

F/S Site ☐ N/A

CULTURES ☐ N/A

_____ Aerobic Site:
_____

_____ Anaerobic Site:
_____

_____ Gram Stain Site:
_____

OTHER EQUIPMENT ☐ N/A

FIGURE 2-2—cont'd   Perioperative nursing record form.

PERI

PERIOPERATIVE NURSING RECORD

Site	Oxygen	Level of Response
R = Right L = Left	R/A = Room Air	5 = Unresponsive
G = Gluteal	M = Mask	4 = Sedated - Responsive only to tactile stimuli
T = Thigh	N = Nasal	3 = Sedated - Delayed response to stimuli
A = Arm	T = T-Piece	2 = Sedated - Responds readily to verbal stimuli
OP = Op Site	P = Pedicup	1 = Awake and responds appropriately
N/A = Not Applicable		

*Indicates further documents in Patient Care Focus Notes

NSG DX #1: High risk for fluid volume deficit/excess R/T surgery.   **NSG DX #2:** Pain R/T physiological response to surgery

24-HR TIME	TEMP	P	R	BP	MAP	SaO$_2$	O$_2$	LOR	PAIN SCALE	FOCUS PHRASES	INITIAL

INTAKE: TYPE	OR/ENDO	PACU	ASU	TOTAL	OUTPUT: TYPE	OR/ENDO	PACU	ASU	TOTAL

MEDICATION RECORD									
24-HR TIME	MEDICATION - DOSAGE	RT. OF ADM.	SITE	INITIALS	24-HR TIME	MEDICATION - DOSAGE	RT. OF ADM.	SITE	INITIALS

FIGURE 2-2—cont'd   Perioperative nursing record form.   *Continued*

PERI

PERIOPERATIVE NURSING RECORD

		24-HR TIME										

T H E R M O / **R E G U L A T I O N**

NSG DX #3: Ineffective thermoregulation R/T environmental temperatures & effects of sedation.

Skin Status: W/D = Warm & Dry   C/D = Cool & Dry
M/C = Moist, clammy   S = Shivering

Skin Color: P = Pink   PA = Pale   D = Dusky
N = Normal for Race   J = Jaundiced

P S Y C H O / **S O C I A L**

NSG DX #4: Anxiety R/T Post-op status, unfamiliarity with environment, separation from family/significant other.

Emotional Response: C = Calm   CR = Crying   A = Agitated
D = Disoriented   U = Uncooperative   N/A = Not Applicable

N E U R O / **L O G I C A L**

NSG DX #5: High risk for injury R/T sensory/motor deficits 2° to sedation.

Ability to move extremities: C = Complete P = Partial/Weak N = None   UE
R = Right   L = Left   B = Bilat   LE

Dermatone Level:
Full sensation to: K = Knee → A = Ankle → B = Buttock F = Full Sensation N/A ☐

V A S C U L A R

Pulse: Site: _____   N/A ☐
P = Palpable   D = Doppler   U = Unable to assess due to dressing

Circulation: P = Pink   W = Warm   N/A ☐
CL = Cool   D = Dusky

Capillary Filling: N = Normal   SL = Sluggish   A = Absent   N/A ☐

Sensation: F - Full/Normal   P = Partial/Tingling   N = Numbness   N/A ☐

Limb Elevated: Y = Yes   N = No   N/A ☐

W O U N D / **D R E S S I N G**

#1 Location/Type _____   D = Dry & Intact N/A ☐
S = Scant
#2 Location/Type _____   M = Moderate
L = Large
#3 Location/Type _____   Δ = Dressing Change
I = Ice Pack

C A R D I O / **P U L M O N A R Y**

NSG DX #6: High risk for impaired gas exchange R/T ineffective airway clearance.

Breath Sounds: L = Left   R = Right   B = Bilat
C = Clear CO = Coarse CR = Crackles RH = Rhonchi W = Wheeze
I = Inspiratory   E = Expiratory   D = Diminished   N/A = Not Assessed

Respirations: SP = Spontaneous   D = Deep
S = Shallow   L = Labored   U = Unlabored

Cardiac Rhythm: NSR = Normal Sinus Rhythm   ST - Sinus Tach   N/A = Not
SB = Sinus Brady   SA = Sinus Arrhythmia   Assessed
* = Other Write in:

S A F E T Y

NSG DX #7: High risk for impaired mobility R/T procedure and/or pain

Activity: B = Bed   C = Chair   A = Ambulatory   H = Held by Adult

Tolerance: W = Well   F = Fair   P = Poor

(√ if yes)	PACU	ASU	Initial									
Alarms On	☐	☐										
Side Rails ↑	☐	☐	Bed Station PACU _____									
Call Bell		☐	Bed Station ASU _____									
Fall Prevention		☐										

FIGURE 2-2—cont'd Perioperative nursing record form.

PERI

PERIOPERATIVE NURSING RECORD

Date	24-HR Time	Focus	Notes

#146750* 5/96 Page 5

FIGURE 2-2—cont'd Perioperative nursing record form.

Continued

PERI

PERIOPERATIVE NURSING RECORD
PATIENT TRANSFER

24-HR TIME	TRANSFER TO	MODE	REPORT TO	INIT.

KEY W/C = Wheelchair A = Ambulatory
C = Chair S = Stretcher

DISCHARGE SUMMARIES

PACU/ENDO				ASU		
Yes	No	N/A	N/A = NOT APPLICABLE	Yes	No	N/A
			1. Awake and oriented			
			2. Vital signs stable			
			3. Airway patent, gag reflexes present			
			4. Minimal pain or discomfort			
			5. Minimal nausea or emesis			
			6. No unexpected bleeding			
			7. Oxygen saturation > 90% or at Pre-Admission level			
			8. All tubings, catheters & drains patent			
			9. SAB patients meet orthostatic challenge			
			10. Ambulates with minimal assistance			
			11. Voided or absence of bladder distention			
			12. Discharge instructions given and understood			
			13. Adult escort available			

Initials: _____   Initials: _____

GOAL MET	GOAL NOT MET	GOAL SUMMARY	*IF GOAL NOT MET, EXPLAIN IN PATIENT CARE NOTES
		GOAL #1: The patient will be hemodynamically stable.	
		GOAL #2: The patient will achieve an adequate level of comfort.	
		GOAL #3: The patient's temperature will be compatible with pre-op levels.	
		GOAL #4: The patient will communicate verbally/nonverbally reasonable emotional comfort.	
		GOAL #5: The patient's safety will be maintained.	
		GOAL #6: The patient's respiratory status will be maintained with $SaO_2 \geq 90\%$, or Pre-Admission level.	
		GOAL #7: The patient will achieve optimal level of mobility.	

Discharge at: _____ via ☐ W/C ☐ Ambulatory ☐ Stretcher

Accompanied & Driven by: _____

Date: _____
☐ Unable to Reach

PATIENT FOLLOW-UP   PHONE NUMBER:

PATIENT PROBLEMS/CONCERNS: ☐ Yes ☐ No (if yes, √ below)
☐ Pain uncontrolled by medication. ☐ Cephalalgia which ▲ severity with sitting/standing. ☐ Nausea & Vomiting ☐ Other (explain below)

Initials: _____

SIGNATURES	INITIALS	SIGNATURES	INITIALS

#146750* 5/96 Page 6

FIGURE 2-2—cont'd   Perioperative nursing record form.

8. Medications administered or dispensed by the perioperative nurse
9. Presence of catheters, drains, packing, and dressings
10. Location of tourniquet cuff placement, identification of unit, pressure setting, and inflation and deflation times
11. Fluid output, including blood loss estimates, as appropriate
12. Type, size, and appropriate identifying information (such as serial number) of implants
13. Skin-preparation solutions used, areas prepped, and any reactions to prep
14. Known allergies to medications, prep solutions, tape, latex, etc.
15. Sponge, sharp, and instrument counts taken and results obtained
16. Wound classification
17. Time of discharge and disposition of patient from operating room, including mode of transfer and patient status

Perioperative nursing documentation needs to describe the assessment, planning, and implementation of perioperative care that reflects individualization of care, as well as the evaluation of patient outcomes. Careful thought should be given in the design of perioperative nursing documentation tools that include the identified elements in a format that minimizes time needed for the documentation process (such as checklists). Ideally, collaboration with the preoperative, perianesthesia, and postoperative nursing units would produce one documentation tool that is used across the areas, avoiding duplication of patient data by different nursing staff (see Fig. 2-2).

PERIOPERATIVE PATIENT CARE ACTIVITIES

Maintaining Fluid and Electrolyte Balance

Fluid and electrolyte balance within the body is important to the health and safety of the patient in surgery. The body's fluids and electrolytes play a key role in maintaining homeostasis, transporting the necessary oxygen and nourishment to the cells, removing waste products of cellular metabolism, and helping to maintain the temperature of the body. Electrolytes are essential to the processes of transmitting nerve impulses, regulating water distribution, contracting muscles, generating adenosine triphosphate (ATP) (needed for cellular energy), regulating acid-base balance, and clotting blood. The intake, distribution, and output of water and electrolytes, regulated by the renal and pulmonary systems, normally maintains fluid and electrolyte balance.

Fluid and electrolyte imbalances may occur rapidly in the surgical patient, caused by any number of factors, including preoperative fluid and food restrictions, intraoperative fluid loss, or the stress of surgery. The surgical patient is unable to regulate the body's fluid and electrolyte requirements by normal activities of drinking, eating, excreting, and breathing unaided. Therefore it is imperative that the perioperative nurse monitor and collaborate in controlling the fluid and electrolyte status of the patient intraoperatively.

Body fluids

The adult human body is approximately 60% water, although water content varies by age, gender, and body mass. In the elderly, body water content averages 45% to 55% of body weight, whereas it is 70% to 80% in infants. Older adults therefore are at risk because they have less fluid reserve, and the very young are at risk for fluid problems because a greater percentage of their body weight is water. Both age groups have a decreased ability to compensate for fluid loss. Muscular tissue contains more water than the same amount of adipose tissue; therefore men generally have higher water content because they usually have more lean body mass (more muscular tissue) than women.

Body fluids are distributed in two main functional compartments: intracellular and extracellular. Intracellular fluids (ICF) are liquids within cell membranes that contain dissolved substances essential to fluid and electrolyte balance and metabolism. Extracellular fluids (ECF) are those fluids in compartments outside the cells of the body, including plasma, intravascular fluids, fluids in the gastrointestinal (GI) tract, and cerebrospinal fluid. Fluid spacing is a term used to classify the distribution of body water. First spacing is the normal distribution of fluid in both the extracellular and intracellular compartments. Second spacing refers to an excess accumulation of interstitial fluid (edema), and third spacing occurs when fluid accumulates in areas that normally have no fluid or only a minimum amount of fluid. This occurs with burns, ascites, peritonitis, or small bowel obstructions. Third spacing traps fluid away from the normal fluid compartments and results in a deficit in extracellular fluid volume.[17]

Electrolytes

Electrolytes are substances found in intracellular fluids and extracellular fluids that, when dissolved in water, dissociate into ions and are able to carry an electric current. Positively charged ions are cations, and negatively charged ions are anions. The electrolytes found in the ECF and ICF are essentially the same, but the concentration of each electrolyte differs in extracellular and intracellular fluids (Table 2-2). The primary intracellular cation is potassium, and the primary extracellular cation is sodium. The primary intracellular anion is phosphate, and the primary extracellular anion is chloride. Fluids and electrolytes move between the intracellular and extracellular spaces to facilitate body processes, such as acid-base

TABLE 2-2 | Major Electrolyte Composition of the Fluid Compartments

ELECTROLYTE	FLUID COMPARTMENT	CONCENTRATION (mEq/L)
Sodium (cation)	Intravascular compartment	142
	Interstitial fluid	145
	Intracellular fluid	12
Potassium (cation)	Intravascular compartment	4.5
	Interstitial fluid	4.4
	Intracellular fluid	150
Chloride (anion)	Intravascular compartment	104
	Interstitial fluid	117
	Intracellular fluid	4
Bicarbonate (anion)	Intravascular compartment	24
	Interstitial fluid	27
	Intracellular fluid	12
Phosphate (anion)	Intravascular compartment	2
	Interstitial fluid	2.3
	Intracellular fluid	40

Source: Horne, M.M., Heitz, U.E., & Swearingen, P.L. (1997). *Fluid, electrolyte, and acid-base balance*, St. Louis: Mosby.

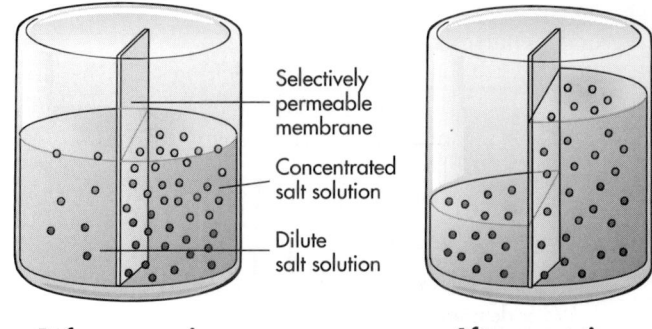

FIGURE 2-3 Osmosis is the movement of solvent molecules across a membrane to an area of higher solute concentration. The solvent moves because the solute cannot pass through the membrane. The result of osmosis is two solutions, separated by a selectively permeable membrane, that are equal in concentration.

balance, tissue oxygenation, response to drug therapies, and response to illness. Diffusion, active transport, and osmosis control this movement.[26]

Diffusion, active transport, osmosis

Diffusion is the movement of molecules from an area of high concentration to one of low concentration across a permeable membrane. Movement continues until there is an equal concentration of molecules on both sides of the membrane.

Active transport is a process where molecules are moved across a cell membrane, against a concentration gradient, with the use of external energy. The sodium and potassium pump moves sodium out of the cell and potassium into the cell to maintain the intracellular and extracellular concentration differences of sodium and potassium. ATP is the energy source for the sodium-potassium pump.

Osmosis is the movement of a fluid through a semipermeable membrane from a solution that has a lower solute concentration to one that has a higher solute concentration (Fig. 2-3). The semipermeable membrane prevents movement of solute particles. The number of particles is measured in a unit called the *osmol*. Osmolality is the term used to express the concentration of a solution in osmoles per kilogram (osm/kg) of water. A solution with the same osmolality as blood plasma is called *isotonic*. Isotonic solutions, such as 0.9% normal saline or lactated Ringer's solution administrated intravenously, prevent the shift of fluid and electrolytes from intracellular compartments. A hypotonic IV solution (0.45% saline or 2.5% dextrose) has a lower concentration of solutes than plasma does and will move water into the cells. Administration of a hypertonic IV solution (5% dextrose in normal saline or 5% dextrose in lactated Ringer's), with a greater concentration of solutes than that of plasma, will move water out of the cells.[18]

Preoperative considerations

A critical part of assisting the surgical patient to maintain fluid and electrolyte balance is preoperative assessment and identification of risk factors for fluid and electrolyte imbalances. Preoperative laboratory analysis of electrolyte levels should be checked, and abnormalities corrected to within normal limits before any surgical procedure, unless the surgery is needed to correct a life-threatening problem. Preexisting conditions, such as diabetes mellitus, liver disease, or renal insufficiency may be aggravated by surgical stress, increasing a patient's risk of fluid and electrolyte imbalances. Diagnostic procedures, such as arteriogram or intravenous pyelogram, require the administration of IV dyes, which may produce osmotic diuresis, with a resulting urinary excretion of water and electrolytes. Preoperative steroids or diuretics affect the excretion of water and electrolytes; diuretics, used in the management of hypertension, cause the loss of potassium. Preoperative surgical regimens, such as administration of enemas or laxatives, may act to increase fluid loss from the GI tract. Medical management of preexisting conditions, such as gastric suction and lavage, can affect fluid and electrolyte balance in the surgical patient, just as preoperative fluid restriction can.

Preoperative fluid restrictions are used to reduce nausea, vomiting, and aspiration risk in the surgical patient. This practice is being modified in ambulatory care settings because newer anesthetic agents cause less nausea and vomiting than in the past. Prolonged fluid restrictions may not be necessary in healthy patients before outpatient surgery; therefore the ingestion of black coffee or pulpfree juice 2 to 3 hours before surgery may be done safely, without an increase in gastric volume.[19]

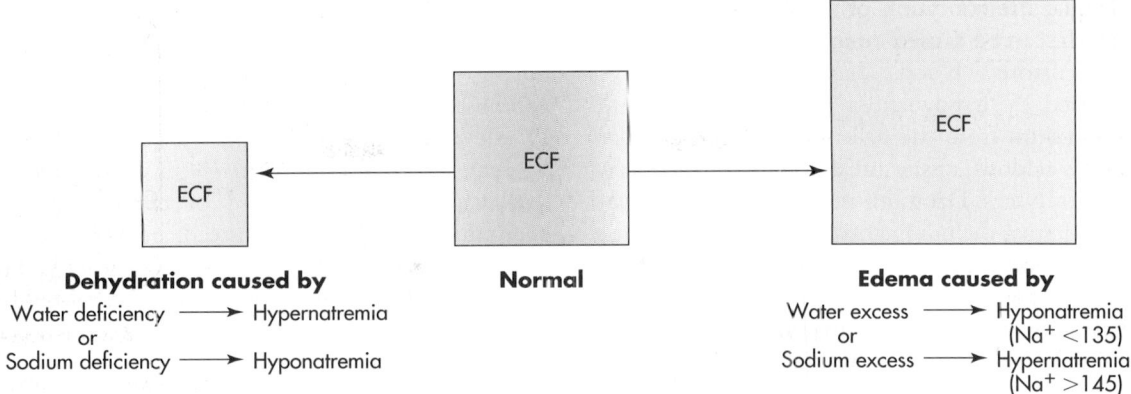

FIGURE 2-4   Changes in extracellular fluid (ECF) volume caused by sodium imbalance.

Fluid volume deficit

The most common patient problems associated with fluid and electrolyte balance during surgery include fluid volume deficit, sodium and water imbalances, and potassium imbalances. Fluid volume deficit is an imbalance in isotonic body fluids related to either abnormal fluid loss or decreased oral intake. Very young and very old surgical patients are affected most rapidly by fluid losses from bleeding; inadequate intake because of previous NPO status; inadequate IV fluid replacement; excessive cutaneous losses from fever and sweating; third-space losses attributable to bowel obstructions, ascites, or peritonitis; excessive GI losses resulting from diarrhea, vomiting, GI suctioning, or fistulas; evaporation of fluid from the exposed peritoneum during abdominal surgery; shifting of intravascular fluid into the surgical site (third-space edema); and inhalation of dry gases. Third-space fluid shift cannot be measured directly, but it can be considerable after extensive dissection of tissue. Intraoperative use of an electrolyte solution, such as lactated Ringer's solution, for fluid replacement can help correct intraoperative third-space fluid losses.[26]

The effect of fluid loss on the surgical patient depends on the amount of fluid lost and the speed at which the fluid is lost. A patient who loses a large amount of fluid (more than 500 ml), or loses fluid rapidly, will exhibit symptoms of shock; fluid replacement therapy will be required. A slow loss of fluid may be compensated for through albumin synthesis and erythropoiesis.

Sodium and water imbalances

Sodium is a cation in extracellular fluid, playing a major role in maintaining the osmolality and water balance of the extracellular fluid (Fig. 2-4). Because cell membranes are permeable to water, it also affects the intracellular fluid volume. Sodium also helps in the maintenance of acid-base balance in the body. The sodium-potassium pump plays a vital role in neuromuscular activity.[17]

Hyponatremia, the condition of a serum sodium level of less than 135 mEq/L, can be caused by increased excretion of sodium with diuretic therapy and the abnormal loss of sodium through nasogastric suctioning and third spacing. Patients undergoing transurethral resection of the prostate (TURP) and uterine endoscopic laser surgery are at risk for dilutional hyponatremia and volume overload, caused by absorption of the irrigation solution used in those procedures. Because saline is a good conductor of electrical current, fluids that contain no electrolytes, such as glycine, sorbitol, and mannitol, must be used to irrigate in the presence of the electrical current used in the dissection during these procedures.[19]

Potassium imbalances

Potassium is the major intracellular cation and is necessary for the contraction of both skeletal muscle and smooth muscle. It is necessary for cardiac contractions and for movements of the GI tract. It plays a role in the transmission of nerve impulses by regulating neuromuscular excitability and in the formation of muscle protein by transporting glucose into the cells with insulin. It is also involved in the maintenance of acid-base balance and intracellular osmotic pressures.[17]

Hypokalemia, the condition of a serum potassium of less than 3.5 mEq/L, can occur intraoperatively because of the suctioning of large amounts of body fluids or the use of diuretic therapy and other drugs (such as mannitol) that cause increased renal flow. Signs and symptoms of hypokalemia include cardiac effects, such as ectopy, dysrhythmias, conduction abnormalities, and altered sensitivity to digitalis. The neuromuscular effects of hypokalemia include muscle weakness; smooth muscle effects include gastric distention, paralytic ileus, and urinary retention.

Treatment of hypokalemia includes IV replacement when the deficit is severe, as in the development of cardiovascular or other serious symptoms. Potassium is very irritating to veins upon infusion; the infusion site should be monitored for redness, heat, swelling, or site pain, all signs of chemical phlebitis. One must take care to avoid overcorrection and subsequent hyperkalemia by monitoring serum potassium levels every 2 to 4 hours.

Hyperkalemia, the condition of a serum potassium of over 5.5 mEq/L, can be caused during surgery by massive transfusions of stored blood, decreased excretion of potassium caused by hypovolemia or renal failure, and shifting of potassium from the cells into the extracellular fluid caused by acidosis, tissue breakdown from surgery, crush injuries, or burns. Drugs infused during surgery can induce hyperkalemia, including anti-inflammatory agents, beta-adrenergic receptor blockers, digitalis, succinylcholine, heparin, and penicillins.

The signs and symptoms of hyperkalemia include neuromuscular symptoms, such as weakness and paresthesias in the arms and legs. Smooth muscle symptoms include diarrhea and abdominal distention. Excess potassium can cause serious cardiac symptoms, including ventricular dysrhythmias, heart block, and asystole. Cardiac side effects of hyperkalemia are treated by calcium gluconate. Sodium bicarbonate or insulin-glucose infusions can be given to cause the serum potassium to move into the cells, thereby reducing the level of potassium in the plasma.[16]

Estimating Blood Loss

Measuring blood loss is a vital procedure in the surgical management of critically ill or elderly patients, patients undergoing complex, extensive surgery, and infants. Weighing sponges provides a reliable means of judging the amount of blood lost and in gauging the need for replacement of fluids and blood products. The weight of the unit of dry sponges and the plastic bag for soiled sponges must be identified and excluded from the weight tally. Grams measured are then converted to milliliters on a one-to-one basis, and blood loss estimates are reported to the anesthesia provider.

Setup

- Blood-loss record
- Gram scale
- Plastic bags and twist ties to hold soiled sponges

Procedure

1. Weigh the unit of dry sponges and the plastic bag, and adjust the scale to register zero.
2. Place bagged sponges on the scale.
3. Record the scale reading: 1 g equals 1 ml of blood loss.
4. Note the blood loss on the record.
5. Add subsequent weight to the preceding weight each time sponges are weighed so that a running total blood loss, calculated from sponges, is available.
6. Measure blood in the suction bottles at regular intervals, subtracting the amount of irrigating solution used.
7. Add the amount of blood loss calculated from suction bottles to the total recorded from sponges to obtain accurate blood loss estimates.

Handling Blood and Blood Products

Maintenance of circulating blood volume is critical during surgical procedures; this is accomplished with administration of whole blood or blood components. Whole blood is rarely administered unless the patient has an acute, massive loss (often empirically determined as a loss that exceeds one third of circulating volume, or approximately 1500 ml). Instead, packed red blood cells (RBCs) to improve oxygen-carrying capacity and oxygen transport to tissues, with or without crystalloid or colloid solutions, are administered to maintain intravascular blood volume.[6] Crystalloid solutions include normal saline and lactated Ringer's solution; colloid solutions include albumin, purified protein factors, dextran, and hydroxyethyl starch (hetastarch). When blood must be given, appropriate precautions are necessary to reduce the hazards of its administration.

Safe administration of blood or blood products begins with the pretransfusion blood sample that is sent for typing and cross matching (compatibility testing). Elective surgery patients have this sample taken no more than 3 to 5 days before surgery to ensure compatibility and to avoid antibodies that may emerge either in response to exposure through blood transfusions, pregnancy, or environmental factors, or resulting from the patient's disease process. Typing refers to the test to determine the ABO and Rh blood type compatibility. Cross matching refers to testing the compatibility of the recipient's serum with the donor's red blood cells. It is crucial to correctly identify the patient before the pretransfusion blood sample is drawn and to ensure that the sample is properly labeled. Improperly identified pretransfusion blood samples can result in acute hemolytic transfusion reactions at the time of transfusion.[4]

A patient having an elective surgical procedure where blood has been requested should not be anesthetized without someone validating that the requested blood products are typed, crossmatched, and available. The appropriate institutional blood requisition form, with complete and accurate patient identification information, should be sent to the blood bank when blood or blood components are being requested. Included on or with this requisition should be the number of units desired. Many institutions have computerized ordering; the same information is required when blood is requested by computer.

If the patient is sent to the operating room directly from the emergency department or trauma admitting area without a chart, all patient identification information must be plainly printed on a piece of paper. The perioperative nurse should contact the blood bank to explain the emergency situation and facilitate release of the needed blood products.

The storage of blood products is important to both the safety of the patient and the avoidance of wasteful discarding of improperly stored blood units. Whole blood, packed RBCs, and thawed fresh frozen plasma (FFP) must be stored between 33.8° and 42.8° F (1.0° and 6.0° C), under continuously monitored conditions, according to the American Association of Blood Banks (AABB) and FDA regulations. Once blood components have been out of monitored refrigeration for more than 30 minutes, they cannot be returned to the blood bank for reissue. The use of ice chests for the temporary storage of refrigerated blood products is used in some institutions. Caution is urged for such a practice because of the difficulty in verifying the appropriate storage of the products in ice chests. To ensure a safe environment, the perioperative nurse must constantly monitor the storage and administration of blood products.

Before the administration of any blood product, the circulating nurse and the anesthesia provider (or a second licensed individual) must confirm the following:

- The number on the unit of blood corresponds with the number on the blood requisition.
- The name and number on the patient's identification band agree with the name and number on the unit of blood.
- The patient's name on the unit of blood corresponds with the name on the requisition.
- The blood group indicated on the unit of blood corresponds with that of the patient.
- The date of expiration has not been reached.
- The blood bag is free of leaks, damage, or signs of possible bacterial contamination, such as the presence of fine gas bubbles, discoloration, clots, or excessive air in the bag.

If there is a discrepancy identified with any of these checks, the blood product must not be infused until the discrepancy is resolved.

When it becomes apparent that more blood will be needed than that originally anticipated, the perioperative nurse should request the blood bank to prepare a specified number of units in advance of the actual need to transfuse. This procedure allows the blood bank time to carefully crossmatch the units without rushing and jeopardizing patient safety. Crossmatch requisitions should be sent for any additional units requested. A new, properly labeled sample with a blood grouping requisition may also need to be sent to have adequate serum for crossmatching or to assure antibody compatibility after a significant amount of transfusion has been required.

The need for rapid blood transfusion necessitates the warming of blood to prevent hypothermia, which may induce cardiac arrest. Blood should be warmed during its passage through the transfusion set. The warming device should incorporate a temperature monitor and, ideally, an audible warning system. Blood should never be warmed above 37° C (98.6° F).[1] The probability of a transfusion reaction increases in direct proportion to the number of units transfused. The circulating nurse

should be alert to any signs of reaction, including the following:

- Increased intraoperative bleeding
- Weak pulse
- Hypotension
- Visible hemoglobinuria
- Vasomotor instability
- Greatly decreased or absent urinary output

If any suspicious reactions occur, the circulating nurse should assist the anesthesia provider to do the following:

1. Stop the transfusion
2. Report the reaction to the surgeon and the blood bank
3. Return the unused portion of the blood, the IV tubing used during transfusion, and a sample of the patient's blood to the blood bank
4. Send a urine sample to the lab as soon as possible
5. Complete an incident report covering the details of the reaction
6. Monitor the patient's reaction carefully

Any unused blood should be returned as soon as the patient leaves the operating room suite. Returned blood can be reissued if it has not been allowed to warm above 10° C. New external blood thermometers (such as a Hemo Temp II), much like a skin contact tape thermometer, are being used on blood bags by many blood banks to quickly identify blood that has exceeded safe storage temperatures.

Autotransfusion—the reinfusion of a patient's own blood—is being used with increasing frequency. In autologous blood donations, the blood is predonated up to 1 month before surgery for use in the patient's own planned surgery. During intraoperative autotransfusion, blood is collected as it is lost during the surgical procedure and reinfused to the patient after it is filtered or washed. This technique can be lifesaving in emergency situations, such as major trauma, or in procedures with major blood loss, as in liver transplantation.

Maintaining Normothermia in the Surgical Patient

An important component of patient safety is the avoidance of hypothermia. The incidence of inadvertent hypothermia (below 36° C, or 96.8° F) in the perioperative patient is estimated at 50% to 90% of all surgical cases. Studies have demonstrated that perioperative hypothermia contributes to increased postoperative discomfort, increased surgical bleeding, incidents of postoperative cardiac events (ischemia and tachycardia), as well as impaired wound healing with susceptibility to wound infection and longer lengths of stay[8] (Research Highlight 2-2).

The temperature and humidity in the OR, the number of room air exchanges occurring per hour, open body

MAINTAINING NORMOTHERMIA IN THE SURGICAL PATIENT

A study of patients with cardiac risk factors undergoing noncardiac surgery was conducted to examine the relationship between body temperature and cardiac morbidity during the perioperative period. Previous studies have identified that when core temperature decreases by approximately $1.0°$ Celsius shivering occurs and total-body oxygen consumption increases, placing increased demands on the cardiovascular system. In this study, high-risk patients were randomly assigned to receive either hypothermic care (IV fluids, blood, and respiratory gases warmed, patient covered by surgical drapes alone) or normothermic care (IV fluids, blood, and respiratory gases warmed, and an upper- or lower-body forced-air warming cover to maintain core temperature at or near $37°$ C) intraoperatively. Postoperatively the hypothermic group had a greater incidence of ECG events (ventricular tachycardia or ischemia), ventricular tachycardia, and morbid cardiac events (unstable angina or ischemia, cardiac arrest, or myocardial infarction), an indication that a certain number of early postoperative cardiac complications can be prevented by maintaining normothermia.*

In other research, a study of patients undergoing colorectal surgery was done to determine the effect of hypothermia on surgical-wound infection rates and length of hospitalization. In this study[†], hypothermic patients, whose final intraoperative core temperature was $34.7 \pm 0.6°$ C, demonstrated a significant increase in surgical wound infections (19% versus 6%) and lengths of stay, with hospital length of stay prolonged by 2.6 days (approximately 20% increase). Maintaining normothermia intraoperatively was determined to decrease the incidence of infectious complications and to shorten patients' hospitalizations.

*From Frank, S.M., Fleisher, L.A., Breslow, M.J., et al. (1997). Perioperative maintenance of normothermia reduces the incidence of morbid cardiac events, *JAMA,* 277(14), 1127-1134.
†From Kurz, A., Sessler, D.I., Lenhardt, R. (1996). Perioperative normothermia to reduce the incidence of surgical-wound infection and shorten hospitalization, *New England Journal of Medicine,* 334(19), 1209-1215.

cavities, the use of anesthetics (all of which impair thermoregulation), and cool air currents contribute to the loss of body heat. Patients at greatest risk include those undergoing complex surgeries lasting long periods of time because body cavities are exposed to cold temperatures for extended times. Other patients at risk include those that are thin (fat acts as insulation to conserve heat), elderly (shivering occurs less in the elderly because the vasoconstrictive response to cold is blunted), and patients whose positioning causes them to have a greater body surface exposed to cool room temperatures.[28]

Nursing interventions to reduce the incidences of inadvertent hypothermia include the following[5]:

1. Identify risk factors for hypothermia.
2. Keep the patient warm preoperatively.
3. Frequently assess the patient's body temperature.
4. Increase the ambient room temperature of the OR.
5. Use a temperature-regulating blanket under the patient, or forced-air warming blankets over the upper or lower body.
6. Apply warm blankets immediately postoperatively.
7. Use warm irrigation fluids.
8. Assist the anesthesia provider to infuse warm IV fluids and use heated humidified gases.

Care and Handling of Specimens

The proper care and handling of specimens is important to the safe outcome of a patient's surgical experience. It is the responsibility of the circulating nurse to identify, document, and properly care for specimens collected in the operating room. Blood, soft tissue, bone, body fluids, and foreign bodies are examples of specimens commonly handled. Complete and accurate identification and labeling of specimens, as well as their timely arrival to the proper laboratory for analysis, is the responsibility of the perioperative nurse. A mislabeled specimen could result in misdiagnosis and subsequent inappropriate treatment of the patient. The circulating nurse must ensure that each specimen is labeled with the proper patient name and specific origin of the specimen (for example, Jane Doe, 100001, right breast biopsy). The surgeon should provide descriptive information about the specimen (for example, suture tag at 6 o'clock). All specimens and their disposition are documented on the operating room record.

Each specimen is cared for according to the specific protocol established by the receiving laboratory. Generally, all tissue should be kept moist and transported to the laboratory as soon as possible.

Formalin, a combination of methanol, water, and formaldehyde, is frequently used to preserve specimens if they will not be taken to the laboratory immediately. Formaldehyde is considered a hazardous substance that can cause watery eyes and respiratory irritation. Care must be taken in handling to avoid exposure to skin and the respiratory tract. Gloves must be worn, and adequate ventilation provided in areas where formaldehyde is handled. Exposure to formaldehyde fumes should be monitored at least quarterly, and an MSDS should be available. Institutional policy should identify procedures to follow in case of formaldehyde spills.

When immediate tissue identification, or the identification of malignancy is needed, specimens are quick-frozen, sliced, stained, and examined in the laboratory under a microscope—a method of tissue examination known as *frozen section*. The results of frozen-section reports are communicated to the surgeon intraoperatively. Specimens for frozen section are placed on a moist towel, on Telfa, or into a dry specimen container. They are **never** placed in saline solution or formalin.

All specimens are considered a potential source of infection. The specimen containers must be placed in an impervious plastic bag and labeled "biohazard" to prevent contamination of the individuals transporting or receiving them. Gloves should always be worn when handling specimens.

Sponge, Sharp, and Instrument Counts

Sponge, sharp, and instrument counts are performed to prevent patient injury from a retained foreign object. They are also an important risk-management activity. Every operating room should have established written policies and procedures for sponge, sharp, and instrument counts that define materials to be counted, the times when counts must be done, and the documentation required.[3]

Certain general guidelines are pertinent to counting all three categories of items. The scrub person and the circulating nurse should count all items in unison and aloud, quietly, as the scrub person touches each item. Counting should not be interrupted. If any uncertainty exists about a count, it should be repeated. The circulating nurse should immediately record the count for each type of item on the count record or worksheet (Fig. 2-5). If additional sponges, instruments, sharps, or other items are dispensed during the procedure, they are similarly counted, and the circulating nurse records and initials the number added. The names of the circulating nurse and the scrub person should be recorded as soon as each count is completed. Additional counts should be performed whenever there is a change in personnel.

Once items are counted, linen or trash bags should not be removed from the operating room until the procedure is completed and the patient has been taken out of the room. Emergency or trauma surgery may sometimes necessitate omission of counts. If this occurs, it should be documented on the operative record, and an x-ray film should be obtained after the procedure to assure that items are not left in the patient.

Sponge counts

All types of sponges should be counted in all procedures. The scrub person and the circulating nurse should count them before the beginning of the operation, before any closure begins, and when skin closure is begun. Additional counts may be indicated according to individual institutional policy and circumstance. Additional counts should always be taken before a cavity within a cavity is closed as when the uterus is closed after a cesarean birth. Types and sizes of sponges used should be kept to a minimum. All soft goods that are used within a wound and are not intended to be left in the wound after closure must contain a radiopaque marker. Radiopacity allows a retained item to be identified or the surgeon to rule out a retained item with an x-ray film taken after an incorrect count. X ray–detectable sponges should never be used for dressings to avoid the appearance of a retained item on postoperative x-ray studies.

Each type and size of sponge should be kept separate from the other types. Sponges must be kept away from other supplies such as towels and drapes to prevent a sponge from being misplaced or carried inadvertently into the wound. To minimize the possibility of an incorrect count, counted sponges should never be taken from the operating room for any reason during surgery.

If an incorrectly numbered package of sponges is dispensed to the field, it should be handed off the field in its entirety, not included in the count, and removed from the room. This practice reduces the potential for error by using only standard multiples of sponges.

During surgery the scrub person should discard soiled sponges into a plastic-lined bucket or receptacle. Throughout the procedure the circulating nurse transfers the discarded sponges from the bucket into impermeable plastic bags or other appropriate containers, according to type and prescribed number. Each time this is done, the sponges are counted by the scrub person. The bag is then closed, secured, and labeled with the type and number of sponges and the initials of the persons who counted them. The bag can be set aside, and unless a discrepancy occurs, the sponges need not be taken out and counted again at the time of the closure sponge counts. Bagging of sponges reduces the possibility of airborne contamination arising from the sponges as they become dry, facilitates weighing of sponges for estimating blood loss, and enables a visual assessment of the patient's blood loss to be made by the anesthesia provider.

The circulating nurse should tally the number of each type of sponge dispensed, as recorded on the count worksheet before the closure counts are taken. As the first layer of closure is begun, the scrub person and the circulating nurse should count all sponges consecutively, proceeding from the sterile field to the back table and off the field. The circulating nurse should inform the surgeon of the results of the count. The procedure should be repeated as skin closure is begun.

Sharp counts

The scrub person and the circulating nurse should count sharps in all procedures at the same time as sponges are counted. In addition to suture needles, sharps may include scalpel and electrosurgical blades, hypodermic needles, and safety pins. When needles are counted before surgery begins, opening every package of suture dispensed onto the field is not necessary. The needles may be counted according to the number indicated on the package. If a package indicates that five needled sutures are

OR5O

Brighton Surgical Center
Surgery

SHARP, SPONGE & INSTRUMENT COUNT

Page 1 of 1

Date ______________ 24-Hour time ______________

Raytec	Laps	Sutures	Blades	Hypos	Bovie Tip	Bovie Scraper	Suture Boots	T & A Bobs	Pea-nuts	Clip Racks	Neuro Patties	Other
Setup												
1st												
2nd												
Final												
Misc												

Instrument Count ☐N/A	Set Up	Add Ons	Final Count
Towel clips			
Mosquitos			
Stats			
Allis			
Babcocks			
Kellys			
Kochers			
Right angles			
Sponge sticks			
Needle holders			
Scissors			
Knife handles			
Skin hooks			
Forceps			
Sarrotts			
Schnidts/bridge			
Retractors			
Balfour retractor			
Gall bladder CDE			
Doyan clamps			
Ligaclip appliers			
Miscellaneous			

Set up Count	1st Closing Count	2nd Closing Count	Final Skin	Misc

Count ☐ Correct ☐ Incorrect

If unresolved, x-rays taken ☐ Yes ☐ No *(If no, explain in Nursing Notes)*

148550* 11/96

SIGNATURE & INITIALS

Init	Signature

FIGURE 2–5 Sharp, sponge, and instrument count sheet.

contained within, five needles should be documented on the worksheet. The scrub person is responsible for verifying the number of needles at the time the package is opened. The scrub person should continually count needles during the procedure and hand them to the surgeon on an exchange basis. Hands-free transfer of sharps by using an emesis basin or magnetic pad is recommended to prevent staff and surgeon needlestick injuries.

Collecting used needles on a needle pad or container facilitates counting and helps to ensure their containment on the table. In procedures that may require use of a high volume of needles, the scrub person can count any filled needle pad with the circulating nurse and hand it off the field. The circulating nurse should then bag it and label it with the number of needles contained and the initials of the individuals who counted them.

Needles broken during the procedure must be accounted for in their entirety. Like sponges, needles should never be taken from the room for any reason during a procedure. Closure counts are conducted in the same format as that for sponges.

Instrument counts

Instrument counts for all procedures are recommended. However, the policy of some institutions specifies that instrument counts be taken only when a major body cavity is entered or when the depth and location of the wound are such that an instrument could inadvertently be left in the patient. Individual facility policy must be followed without deviation. Instrument sets should be standardized for ease in counting, with the minimum number and type of instruments in each set. Instruments should be counted in the instrument room as sets are being assembled, in the operating room by the scrub person and circulating nurse before the beginning of the operation, and before closure begins. Additional counts may be indicated according to facility policy or individual circumstance. Instruments that are broken or disassembled during the procedure must be accounted for in their entirety. No instruments should be taken from the operating room during a procedure. Printed instrument count sheets with the names of all items to be counted help expedite the count procedure.

Incorrect counts

An incorrect count occurs when the number of items on the count record or worksheet does not match the number of items during the actual count. Any incorrect closure count should be repeated immediately, and attempts must be made to resolve the discrepancy. If it remains incorrect, the circulating nurse should notify the surgeon of the incorrect count, and a search should be made for the missing item, including the surgical wound, field, floor, linen, and trash (if they can be searched safely). All personnel should direct their immediate attention to locating the missing item. If it is not found, an x-ray film is taken. If the x-ray study is negative, the count is recorded as incorrect, and the x-ray results are noted on the operating room record. An incident report should be initiated according to institution policy. Accurate counting and recording of sponges, sharps, and instruments are essential for the protection of the patient, personnel, and the institution.

Cardiopulmonary Resuscitation

An important part of a patient safety plan is training staff in cardiopulmonary resuscitation (CPR). CPR is the immediate restoration of circulatory and respiratory functions by means of manual and mechanical methods and the administration of drugs to provide for ventilation and conversion of the heartbeat to normal sinus rhythm. Cardiac arrest, standstill, or fibrillation may occur in patients undergoing surgery because of the hazards of surgery, including blood loss and shock, or because of unfavorable reactions to anesthesia, such as hypoxia and poor ventilation. CPR is vital to the survival of these patients.

All body organs and tissues must receive sufficient oxygen through the circulatory system for life to be sustained. The circulating blood must carry the oxygen supplied by pulmonary ventilation. Ventilation may be reestablished by mouth-to-mouth breathing or by other means of artificial respiration, such as oxygen apparatus, facemask, and intubation (artificial airway and endotracheal tube), with the use of an Ambu-Bag or mechanical ventilator. Cardiac compression is directed toward the reestablishment of circulation.

A well-defined written protocol should be posted in a designated area in each operating room and should be clearly understood by all personnel. Periodic practice sessions for delegated duties should be scheduled as part of the safety program. Basic life-support training should be provided for all perioperative nurses.

Setup

A movable emergency cardiopulmonary arrest cart (crash cart) containing all items that may be needed for CPR should be immediately available. The surgical committee, the perioperative nursing staff, and the anesthesia department should collaboratively determine the equipment needed. It is important to stress the team approach for successful cardiopulmonary resuscitation of the patient in surgery. The following items should be included on or with the emergency cart:

- **Emergency thoracotomy kit**
  - 1 knife handle no. 4 with blade no. 20
  - 1 mallet
  - 1 Lebsche knife
  - 1 rib retractor
  - 1 Finochietto or Harken self-retaining retractor

- **Ventilation and resuscitation equipment**
  - Ambu resuscitator (bag), anesthesia machine, or mechanical ventilator
  - Airways—oral and nasal
  - Endotracheal tubes
  - Laryngoscope and endotracheal forceps or stylets
  - Suctioning devices
  - O_2 tank

- **Syringes (Luer-Lok) and needles**
  - 3 syringes, 3 ml
  - 4 syringes, 5 ml
  - 4 syringes, 10 ml
  - 2 syringes, 20 ml
  - 2 syringes, 50 ml
  - 5 needles, 25 gauge, ⅝ inch
  - 5 needles, 20 gauge, 1½ inches
  - 5 needles, 18 gauge, 1½ inches
  - 2 needles, 20 gauge, 3 inches (intracardiac)

- **Emergency drugs**

  Where available, commercially prefilled syringes should be used
  - Sodium bicarbonate
  - Lidocaine
  - Epinephrine
  - Calcium chloride
  - Dopamine
  - Dobutamine
  - Isoproterenol hydrochloride (Isuprel)
  - Methylprednisolone sodium succinate (Solu-Medrol)
  - Magnesium sulfate
  - Adenosine
  - Atropine
  - Propranolol hydrochloride (Inderal)
  - Levarterenol bitartrate (Levophed)
  - Procainamide (Pronestyl)
  - Cedilanid-D (Deslanoside)
  - Aminophylline
  - Bretylium
  - Naloxone hydrochloride (Narcan)
  - Dextrose 50%
  - Flumazenil (Mazecon)
  - Sodium chloride for injection
  - Water for injection

- **Infusion equipment**
  - Fluids for intravenous infusion
  - Venesection tray
  - Infusion administration sets
  - Cutdown tray and intracatheters
  - Stopcocks
  - Alcohol wipes (sponges)
  - Prep swabs
  - Tourniquets
  - Infusion pump

- Blood sampling kit
- Blood tubes
- Heparinized syringes

- **Cardiac support equipment**
  - Defibrillator
  - External paddles
  - Sterile internal paddles
  - Pediatric paddles, if indicated
  - Cardiac monitoring equipment

- **Cardiac arrest board** (for use if patient is in a bed)

- A **thoracotomy setup** (Chapter 25) should be available in case open-heart massage is attempted. Open-heart massage is rarely performed today unless the chest is already open and a thoracic surgeon is present. Closed-chest massage is considered equally effective with fewer inherent hazards.

Procedure

1. Activate the emergency alarm to alert appropriate surgical and anesthesia personnel. Record the exact time of arrest and obtain additional assistance as required.
2. Nursing personnel responding to the alarm should bring the cardiopulmonary arrest cart to the room. (The circulating nurse should **never leave the room** to get the crash cart because he or she must stay with the patient.)
3. If not already established, an airway should be established and ventilation of the patient begun by means of artificial respiration to restore and maintain oxygenation. Mouth-to-mouth resuscitation is begun if resuscitative equipment is not immediately available.
4. Closed-chest massage is performed to maintain circulation and provision of oxygen to vital tissues.
5. Designate one person to run the arrest (usually the anesthesia provider) and another to record (usually the circulating nurse). The recorder should maintain ongoing documentation of all medications given and procedures performed.
6. Prepare and administer medications as ordered.
7. Procure and prepare infusions or transfusions as ordered.
8. Assist the surgeon and anesthesia provider as needed.
9. Document the event, care given, and outcomes of the patient.
10. Notify appropriate administrative services as the situation requires. This may include a request to the service supplying pastoral care and notification to the proper services of the change in the patient's condition and the need to inform the patient's family.

Successful cardiopulmonary resuscitation of the patient in surgery depends on a coordinated team effort, starting with early recognition of impending danger, and rapid response by all team members.

A separate cart or box for malignant hyperthermia (MH; see Chapter 7) is also recommended to facilitate prompt initiation of treatment protocols for a patient diagnosed with MH. Emergency drugs and equipment include 36 ampules of dantrolene sodium, sterile water (preservative-free) for injection, sodium bicarbonate, furosemide, 50% glucose, and antiarrhythmic agents. Equipment and supplies to cool the patient are typically stocked with the MH cart.[13, 27]

The operating room is a complex environment with many hazardous substances as well as equipment. The perioperative nurse, through the activities described in this chapter, plays a critical role in helping maintain a safe environment for the patient in surgery as well as for other members of the surgical team.

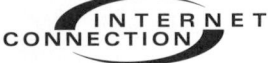

INTERNET CONNECTION

Joint Commission on Accreditation of Healthcare Organizations: http://www.jcaho.org

Health Care Financing Administration: http://www.hcfa.gov

Best Practices Network: http://www.Best4Health.org

Materials Safety Data Sheets (MSDS):
http://www.chem.uky.edu/resources/msds.html

Latex Allergy Sites: http://latex.fdli.org
http://www.cdc.gov/niosh/latexalt.html
http://www.anesth.com/lair/lair.htm

Food and Drug Administration (FDA):
http://www.fda.gov

Occupational Safety and Health Administration (OSHA):
http://www.osha.gov

American Society for Testing and Materials (ASTM):
http://www.astm.org

Association for the Advancement of Medical Instrumentation (AAMI): http://www.aami.org

Emergency Care Research Institute (ECRI): e-mail:
ecri@hslc.org

Radiology Resources:
Radiology Society of North America: http://www.rsna.org/
Society of Nuclear Medicine: http://www.snm.org/
US Nuclear Regulatory Commission: http://www.nrc.gov/
Center for Devices and Radiological Health:
http://www.fda.gov/cdrh/index.html

State and Local Governments:
http://lcweb.loc.gov/global/state/stategov.html

ACLS Algorithms: http://www.cardiac.org/aclsalgr.html#algor

Information About Medications:
http://www.rxlist.com/

http://pharminfo.com
http://www.intmed.mcw.edu/drug.html

Laboratory Values: http://www.ghsl.nwu.edu/Norm.html

On-line Clinical Calculator:
http://www.intmed.mcw.edu/clincalc.html

REFERENCES

1. American Association of Blood Banks (1993). *Standards for blood banks and transfusion services* (ed 14). Arlington, VA: the Association.
2. American Nurses Association (1997). *Position statement on latex allergy*. Washington, DC: the Association.
3. Association of Operating Room Nurses (1998). *AORN standards, recommended practices, and guidelines*. Denver: the Association.
4. Craig, V., Bower, J.O. (1987). Blood administration in perioperative settings. *AORN Journal, 66*(1), 133-143.
5. Dennison, D. (1995). Thermal regulation of patients during the perioperative period. *AORN Journal, 61*(5), 827-831.
6. Dreger, V., Tremback, T. (1998). Blood and blood product use in perioperative patient care. *AORN Journal, 67*(1), 154-190.
7. Fogg, D. (1995). Clinical issues. *AORN Journal, 62*(2), 102-104.
8. Frank, S.M. (1998). *Body temperature and clinical outcome in the perioperative period*. Paper presented at Consensus Conference on Perioperative Thermoregulation, February 7, 1998, Bethesda, MD.
9. Giordano, B. (1996). Don't be a victim of surgical smoke. *AORN Journal, 63*(3):520-522.
10. Groah, L. (1996). *Perioperative nursing* (ed. 3). Stamford, CT: Appleton & Lange.
11. Gruendemann, B., Fernsebner, B. (1995). Comprehensive perioperative nursing, vol.1, *Principles*. Boston: Jones & Bartlett Publishers.
12. *Guidelines for construction and equipment of hospitals and medical facilities*. (1996). Washington, DC: The American Institute of Architects Press.
13. Haas, R.E. (1998) Learning during anesthesia: myth or reality? *Seminars in Perioperative Nursing, 7*(1), 46-53.
14. Jackson, D. (1995). Latex allergy and anaphylaxis—what to do? *Journal of Intravenous Nursing 18*(1), 33-52.
15. Joint Commission on Accreditation of Healthcare Organizations. (1996). *Accreditation manual for hospitals*. Chicago: the Commission.
16. Kneedler, J., Dodge, G. (1994). *Perioperative patient care: the nursing perspective* (ed. 3). Boston: Jones & Bartlett Publishers.
17. Lewis, S.M., Collier, I.C., & Heitkemper, M.M. (1996). *Medical-surgical nursing* (ed. 4). St. Louis: Mosby.
18. Meeropol, E. (1996). Latex allergy update: clinical practice and unresolved issues. *Journal of Wound, Ostomy and Continence Nursing, 23*(4), 193-196.
19. Metheny, N. (1995). *Fluid and electrolyte balance: nursing considerations* (ed. 3). Philadelphia: Lippincott-Raven.
20. National Institute for Occupational Safety and Health. (1996). *Control of smoke from laser/electric surgical procedures*, Pub. No. 96-128. Cincinnati: OSHA (NIOSH). pp 1-2.
21. National Institute for Occupational Safety and Health. (1997). *NIOSH alert: preventing allergic reactions to natural rubber latex in the workplace*, Pub. No. 97-135. Cincinatti: OSHA (NIOSH).
22. Occupational Safety and Health Administration (Nov. 25, 1983). Toxic and hazardous substances, hazard communication standard, *Code of federal regulations*, title 29, chapter xvii, section 1910.7200, 48 FR 53280, Washington, DC: U.S. Government Printing Office.
23. O'Grady, K., & Easty, A.C. (1996). Electrosurgery smoke: hazards and protection. *Journal of Clinical Engineering, 21*(2),149-154.
24. Patterson, P. (1997). Meeting airs differences on need for smoke evacuation. *OR Manager, 13*(4), 1,8, 10, 12-13.
25. Phippin, M., & Wells, M. (1994). *Perioperative nursing practice*. Philadelphia: W.B. Saunders.
26. Potter, P.A., & Perry, A.G. (1996). *Fundamentals of nursing* (ed. 4). St. Louis: Mosby.

27. Stolworthy, C., & Haas, R.E. (1998). Malignant hyperthermia: a potentially fatal complication of anesthesia. *Seminars in Perioperative Nursing,* 7(1), 58-66.

28. Tappen, R, & Andre, S P. (1996). Inadvertent hypothermia in elderly surgical patients. *AORN Journal, 63*(3), 639-643.

29. Tarlo, S.M., Sussman, G., Contala, A., Swanson, M.C. (1994). Control of airborne latex by use of powder-free latex gloves. *Journal of Allergy and Clinical Immunology 93*(6), 985-989.

30. Young, M.A., Meyers, M., & McCulloch, L.D. (1992). Latex allergy: a guideline for perioperative nurses. *AORN Journal, 56*(3), 488.

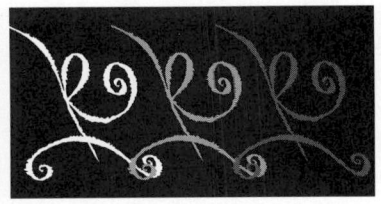

CHAPTER THREE | # Surgical Modalities

Kay A. Ball

SURGERY CONTINUES TO evolve as less invasive procedures and instrumentation are introduced and accepted. A variety of modalities have been developed that have enhanced and advanced surgical procedures. This chapter provides detailed information about the evolution of some of the more popular surgical modalities, including endoscopy, video technology, and energies used during surgical intervention.

ENDOSCOPY

Evolution of Endoscopy

Endoscopy, the examination of body organs or cavities by means of an endoscope, has been practiced for several centuries. Although primitive, the first use of reflected light for inspection of the vagina and uterine cervix is credited to Abul Kasim (936-1013), an Arabian physician.[11] From this new conquest came instrumentation to examine the nasal sinuses and urinary bladder. Of primary concern during this initial era of endoscopy was the thermal tissue injury caused by the intense heat emitted by the light sources utilized. Incandescent lighting was eventually incorporated into the tips of certain endoscopes (such as cystoscopes and ureteroscopes) that could be cooled by continuous irrigation. Modifications allowed for examination of the nasal sinuses, larynx, bronchus, and sigmoid colon. Procedures, however, were restricted to those performed through endoscopic placement in external body orifices.

In 1910 Jacobaeus, a Swedish physician, first reported using a cystoscope to examine the peritoneal cavity.[12] Only the diagnostic capability was realized; pneumoperitoneum (the introduction of a gas into the peritoneum to increase visualization and operative exposure) was yet to be developed. Thus numerous complications were associated with these brave attempts. Commonly reported were injuries to bowel and vascular structures, complications that today, although not unknown, are quite uncommon.

In an attempt to reduce morbidity Decker[4] introduced the cul-de-sac approach to pelvic endoscopy (culdoscopy).

Instead of inserting the scope through the abdomen, he did so through the cul-de-sac. During this era, the importance of introducing air into the abdomen was recognized. Air introduction was enhanced through the use of a syringe and needle. Knee-chest and Trendelenburg's positions were used to facilitate this procedure.

It was not until 1964 that an automatic insufflation device was developed by the German surgeon Kurt Semm.[10] Laparoscopy was still considered to be "blind" surgery and because of this did not gain rapid popularity in either North America or Europe. During this decade, two other developments enhanced the endoscopic revolution. In 1966 the rod-lens system designed by the British optical physicist Hopkins improved brightness and clarity. Fiberoptic (cold) light sources were also introduced, and they even further reduced the risk of visceral and bowel burns.

In the late 1970s to early 1980s endoscopic surgery moved from the category of diagnostic to that of operative. Kurt Semm termed his pioneering work *pelviscopy*. His work led to many technologic advances in instrumentation, equipment, and practice. Diagnostic and operative laparoscopies were becoming the techniques of choice for gynecologists throughout the world. Flexible and rigid endoscopic procedures were also increasing for urologists, internists, and otorhinolaryngologists. In the 1970s orthopedic surgeons began to appreciate the art of arthroscopy.

It was not until the 1980s that the laparoscope was introduced in general surgery. General surgeons were familiar with laparoscopy, since many were consulted to assist gynecologists when evaluating right lower quadrant pain in young female patients. The evolutionary process enabled surgeons to perform their own laparoscopic procedures to diagnose acute appendicitis.

In the late 1980s the "laparoscopy revolution" began in the United States. As surgeons and perioperative nurses were scrambling for knowledge and information, industry was desperately trying to accommodate the rapid change from open surgical procedures to the newer techniques of minimally invasive surgery (Table 3-1). Perioperative nurses experienced an increased opportunity for knowledge growth with new equipment, instrumentation, surgical approaches, and patient education. Professional self-satisfaction resulted despite initial frustration. More rapid changes in surgery to incorporate endoscopic procedures continue to present multiple and complex challenges for the surgical team while offering patients potentially shorter hospital stays, reduced postoperative pain, and faster recuperation (see Research Highlight 3-1).

Endoscopes

An endoscope is a tube that is inserted into a natural body orifice or through a tiny incision to access internal organs or structures.[2] Endoscopes can be flexible, rigid, or semirigid. Flexible endoscopes include but are not limited to angioscopes, bronchoscopes, choledochoscopes (Fig.

3-1), colonoscopes, cystonephroscopes, hysteroscopes, mediastinoscopes, ureteroscopes, and ureteropyeloscopes. Rigid endoscopes include, but are not limited to, cystoscopes, laparoscopes, sinuscopes, arthroscopes, bronchoscopes, laryngoscopes, and hysteroscopes (Fig. 3-2). Some endoscopes may be manufactured in both flexible and rigid forms. A semirigid endoscope, such as the ureteroscope, provides some movement, although it remains fairly rigid (Fig. 3-3).

Endoscopes can be diagnostic or operative. Diagnostic scopes are for observation only and have no operating channels. The system is sealed at both ends. A diagnostic scope can be used, however, when multiple access sites are planned for the introduction of other instrumentation to perform a surgical procedure. Operative endoscopes are channeled for irrigating, suctioning, inserting, and con-

TABLE 3-1	Advantages of Minimally Invasive Surgery Over Open Surgery
MINIMALLY INVASIVE	**OPEN**
Ambulatory or short hospital stay	Hospital admission
Short postoperative recuperation	4- to 6-week recuperation
Reduced postoperative pain; reduced need for pain medications	Postoperative pain related to surgical site; more analgesics
Earlier return to normal life-style	Return to normal life-style varies with recuperation period

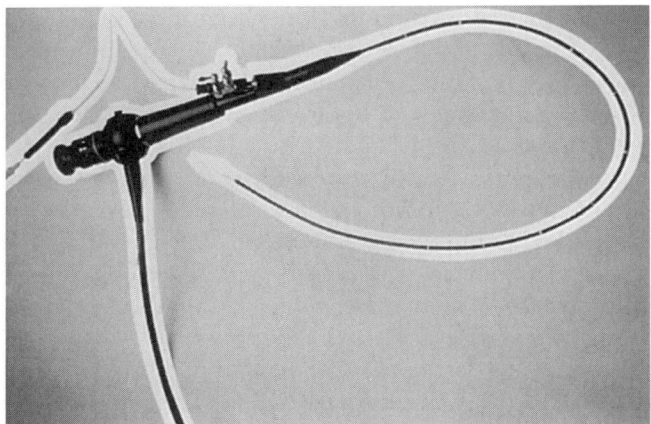

FIGURE 3-1 Flexible translaparoscopic choledochoscope.

3-1 RESEARCH HIGHLIGHT

Many open procedures are being replaced today by endoscopic approaches. Endoscopic techniques are often challenged as physicians and the surgical team members are forced to learn new skills and practices. Research from University Hospital Utrecht in the Netherlands is being called the most definitive evidence supporting laparoscopic hernia repair over the traditional open method. The patient sample for this study totaled 994, which is a very impressive number. Of this patient group, 487 patients underwent laparoscopic extraperitoneal inguinal hernia repair, whereas 507 patients underwent conventional open hernia repair. The laparoscopy patients required an average of 6 days to return to their normal activities, whereas the patients who experienced the open procedure returned to normal activities after 10 days. The laparoscopy patients had a 3% recurrence rate that mostly occurred within the first postoperative year. The conventional surgery patients experienced a 6% recurrence rate with recurrences equally divided between the first and the second postoperative year. The laparoscopic approach added approximately 5 minutes to the procedure length. This study was conducted to determine whether the country's national health service should reimburse for the laparoscopic hernia repair approach. These results indicated that the laparoscopic patients not only experienced a faster recovery but also had fewer recurrences. Other laparoscopic procedures will begin to be accepted by the surgical community and will replace traditional procedures as studies such as this one are published.

From Liem, M.S.L., Van Der Graaf, Y., Van Steensel, C.J., et al. (1997). Comparison of conventional anterior surgery and laparoscopic surgery for inguinal-hernia repair, *New England Journal of Medicine, 336,* 1541-1547.

necting accessory instrumentation (Fig. 3-4). For example, when a neodymium:yttrium–aluminum–garnet (Nd:YAG) laser is used, the laser fiber is inserted into the operating port of the laparoscope.

Endoscopes come in a variety of diameters and lengths depending on access to the area being visualized and the requirements of the procedure. Optical capability through a rigid scope is controlled by the lens system and can be direct (0-degree angle) or angled (30, 70, and 120 degrees) (Fig. 3-5). Flexible scopes by their very nature allow for a more panoramic view.

There are two types of flexible endoscopes—fiberoptic endoscopes and videoscopes. A fiberoptic endoscope has an eyepiece lens for visualization while the image is carried through the endoscope via a bundle of tiny glass fibers. A videoscope has, at the scope's distal end, a video chip that provides an image that is directly viewed on a monitor; therefore a videoscope does not have an eyepiece for direct viewing. Flexible endoscopes have four distinct components:

- Control body (angulation knobs, air-water channels, biopsy port, eyepiece for fiberoptic endoscopes, etc.)
- Insertion tube (a flexible tube containing channels for suction, biopsy, irrigation, air and water, image bundles for the fiberscope, light bundles, etc.)
- Bending section at distal tip (bending rubber, lenses, air-water nozzle, C-cover, CCD chip for video-scopes, etc.)
- Light-guide connector unit (suction, air-water channel, etc.)

Rigid endoscopes also have four distinct components:

- Eyepiece (ocular lenses, etc.)
- Body (light-guide connector, valves, etc.)
- Shaft (rod lenses, spacers, etc.)
- Distal end (objective lens, negative lens, etc.)

Understanding the anatomy of an endoscope can help assess technical problems that can occur during an endoscopic procedure. The internal components are complex, sophisticated, and sometimes delicate (Fig. 3-6); therefore the endoscope must be treated with care.

Light Sources and Fiberoptic Cables

As previously discussed, incandescent light sources were used for early endoscopic procedures. These became very hot and were hazardous to use. With the

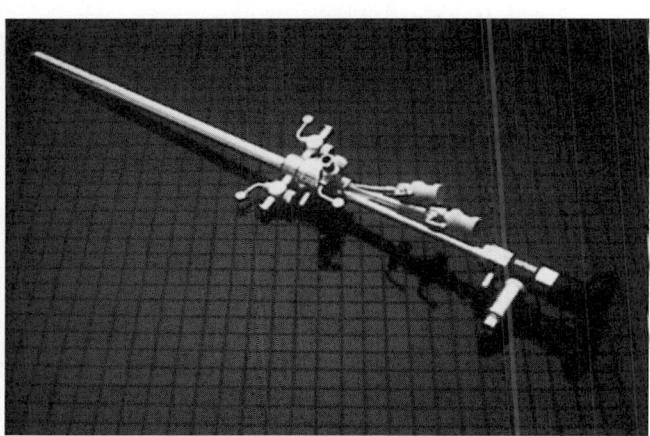

FIGURE 3-2   Rigid endoscope.

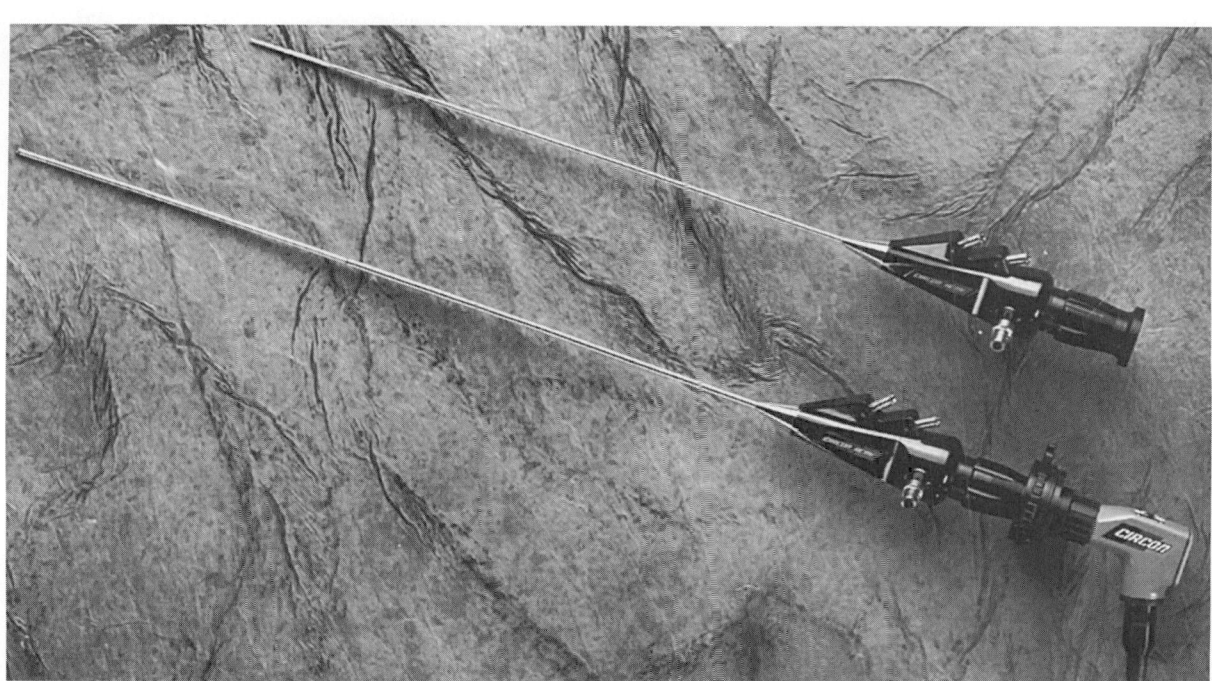

FIGURE 3-3   Semirigid ureteroscope with and without video camera connected.

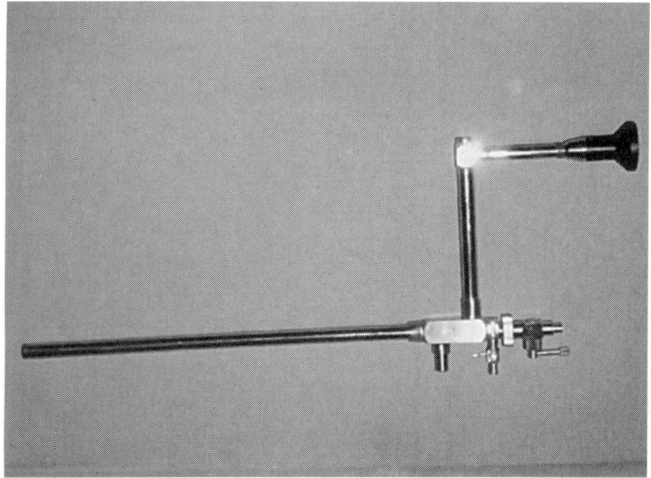

FIGURE 3-4   Operative laparoscope.

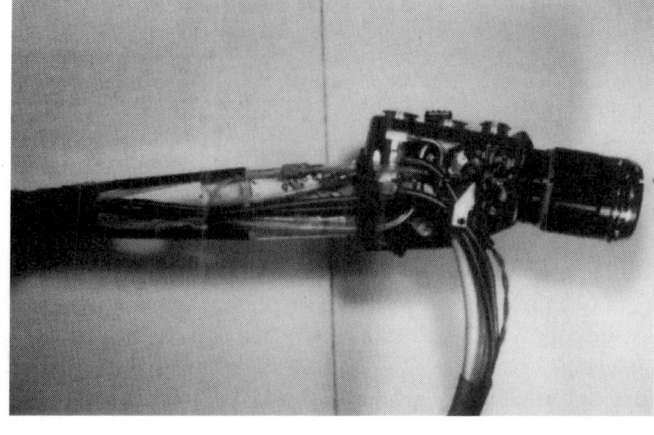

FIGURE 3-6   The dissected flexible endoscope, showing the complexity of the internal structure and design.

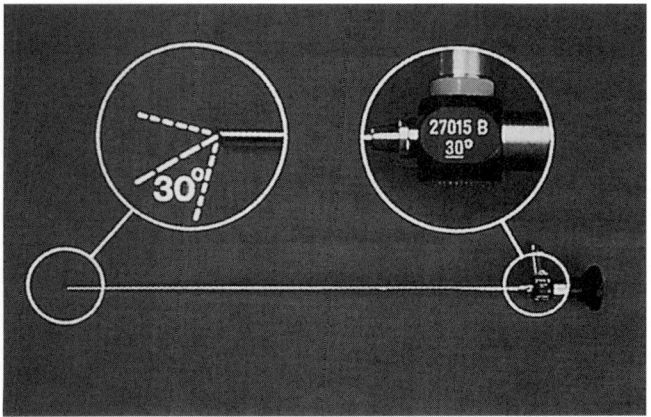

FIGURE 3-5   The lenses inside the endoscope determine the angle of view.

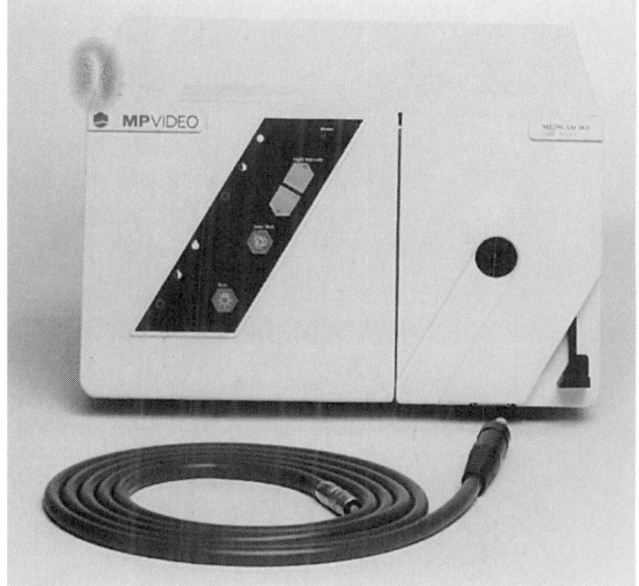

FIGURE 3-7   Light source with universal light cable adapter.

development of fiberoptics an entirely new surgical approach became possible. Fiberoptic design offers increased illumination, cold–light capability, and a control unit where intensity can be adjusted accordingly and from a distance.

Endoscopic light is often referred to as *cold light* meaning that the heat from the light source is not transmitted through the length of the scope; therefore tissue damage from heat at the distal tip is eliminated. The surgical team must be extremely cautious, however, to keep the ends of the fiberoptic cables when disconnected from the scope out of contact with patient and personnel skin or any flammable material. These ends are extremely hot. If the fiberoptic cable is disconnected from the endoscope during surgery, the scrub nurse must ensure that the cable end is held away from drapes or placed on a moist towel to prevent burns and fires. Ideally the light should be turned off whenever disconnected from the endoscope.

Light sources should have adjustable brightness modes,

both manual and automatic. The automatic mode adjusts brightness according to the video image. If set in this mode, it eliminates the need for the circulating nurse to constantly make the adjustments.

When selecting a light source, certain options should be considered. A light source that can adapt to several rigid endoscopic systems is desirable, such as one with a universal light cable adaptor, which enhances flexibility and usage (Fig. 3-7). If a previously purchased unit does not provide this feature, universal light cables with an interchangeable light source as well as endoscope adapters are available (Fig. 3-8). This allows a generic cord to be utilized with most scopes as well as light sources. Light sources also must have connection capability with different camera units.

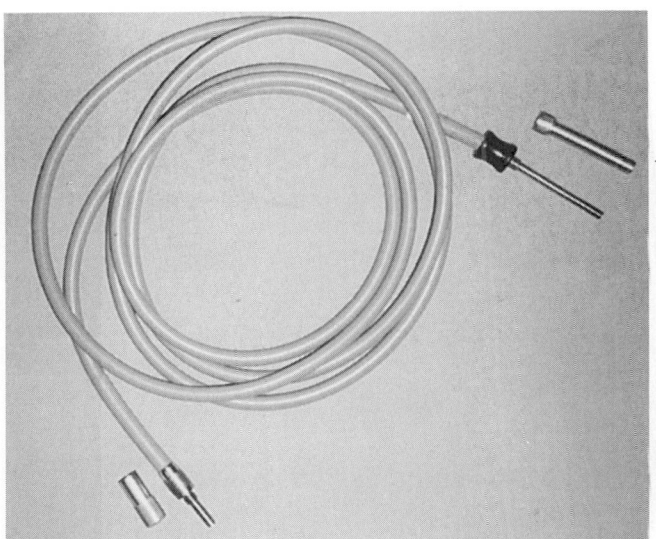

FIGURE 3-8   Universal light cable with interchangeable light source as well as endoscope adapters.

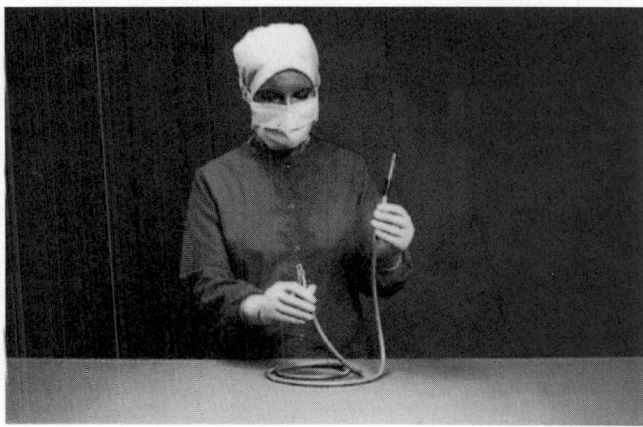

FIGURE 3-10   The light cable can be checked for broken fibers by holding one end toward a bright light while looking at the other end.

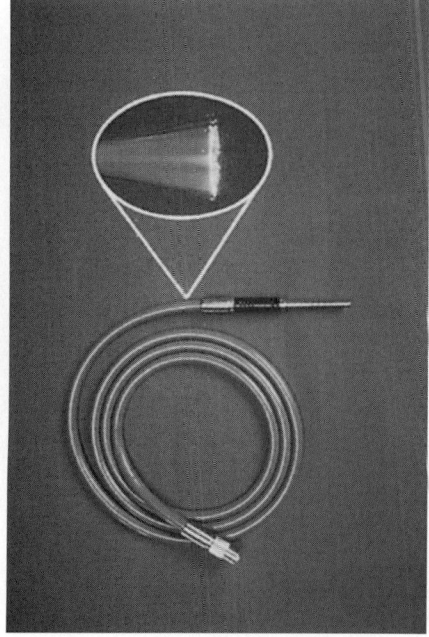

FIGURE 3-9   Inside the light cable are hundreds of glass fibers that transmit light.

Light cables must be handled with extreme care because these fiberoptics consist of hundreds of glass fibers that transmit light (Fig. 3-9). The tiny fibers can be broken if kinked or dropped. Cables should be loosely coiled, not bent, when not in use. After multiple uses, fibers can break. Cables should be checked after each use. To do this, one should hold one end of the cable pointing toward a bright light while the opposite end is observed for light transmission (Fig. 3-10). One should not test the cable by looking into the end while it is attached to the light source. The visible light and ultraviolet light produced by the light

source could be harmful to the eye if directly viewed for extended periods of time. "Peppering" on the light cable end indicates broken fibers. Once 18% to 20% of the fibers are broken, the cable should be replaced because adequate light for visualization will not be transmitted through fractured fibers.

Bulbs within the light source are usually very easy to replace. Most are located in lamp-assembly drawers, which are readily accessible. The bulb itself should not be touched because it may be very hot and the oils on a person's hands and fingers can adhere to the bulb causing the bulb to burn out more quickly. Nonmetal handles are usually built into the light source for bulb removal and replacement when the bulb is hot.

There are three popular types of light sources available today—xenon, metal halide, and halogen. Advantages and disadvantages are associated with each. Xenon bulbs are more expensive but can last longer. A xenon light is better for the smaller-diameter endoscopes (2 mm or less) because the light can focus down to a smaller spot size. Metal halide bulbs have a shorter life span (about 250 hours) and are less expensive. These bulbs are easier than the others to handle and replace and do not require large fans for cooling. Halogen light sources are used for office and hospital applications. They do not offer the light intensity necessary for many endoscopic and video requirements though. Personal preference and conditions for use are the parameters considered to choose an appropriate light source for endoscopy. A light source that incorporates a lamp-life status-testing mode is desirable so that bulb replacement can be anticipated.

Since light sources produce different colors of light, whenever a camera is used, white balancing must be performed during each procedure. White balancing is merely adjusting the camera to all other optical compo-

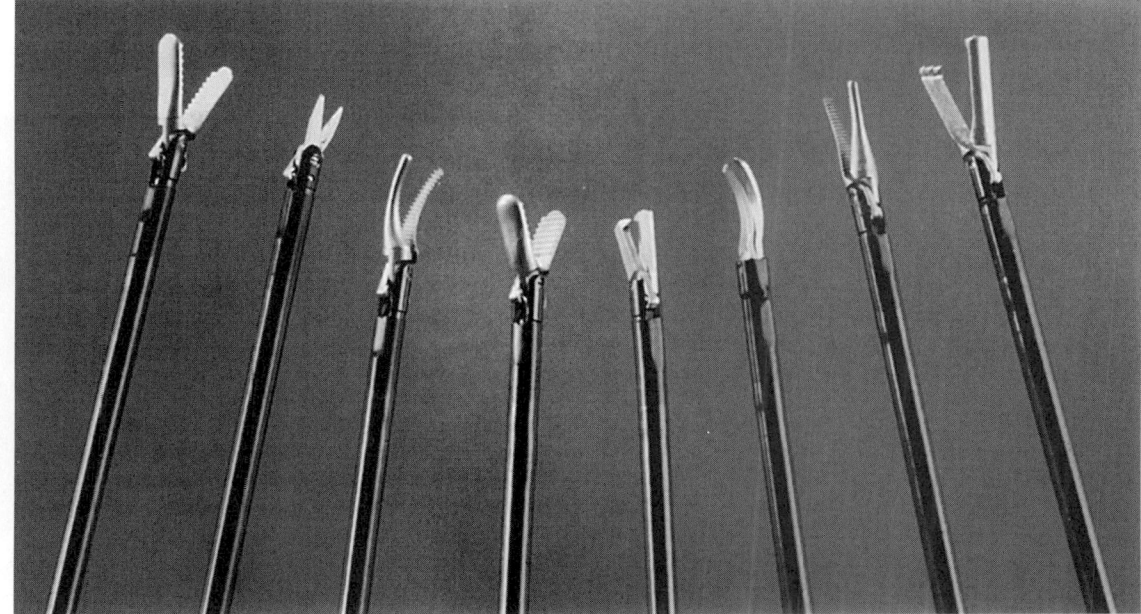

FIGURE 3-11   Disposable endoscopic instruments are designed to meet procedural needs during endoscopic surgery.

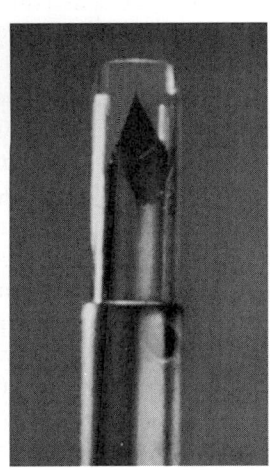

FIGURE 3-12   A close-up view of the trocar safety shield in place.

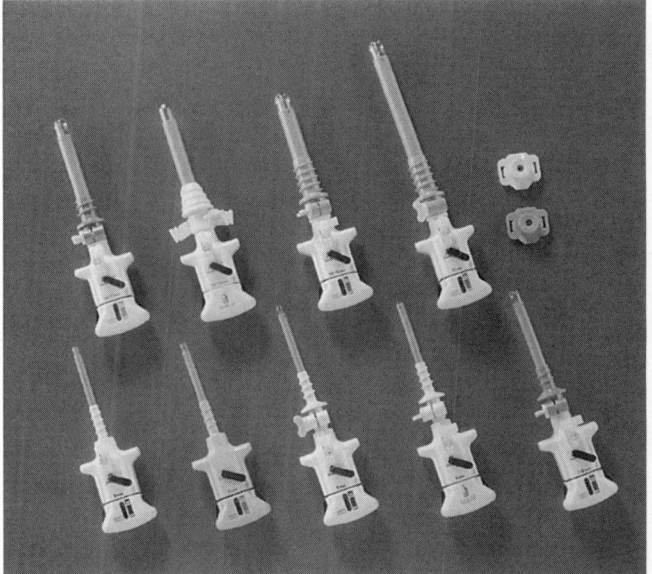

FIGURE 3-13   Disposable trocars and cannulas with grippers. Two converters with reducers are also shown.

nents (endocoupler, light cable, laparoscope). This is a method for the camera to reference white so that it can properly identify all primary colors. White balancing should be performed only when the scope and light cable are connected, the light source is turned on, and the lens is held close to a white gauze or drape.

Endoscopic Instrumentation

Endoscopic instrumentation has been designed to correspond with the surgical site. The length and working end of the device must be adequate to perform surgery at the target site. The hand control is designed for the comfort of the operator. Many times graspers and other instrumentation used by the assistant in surgery are built for a shorter hand span because many women function in this role.

Because endoscopic surgical approaches differ from the traditional open-surgical equivalents, modifications of existing instruments have been made as endoscopic procedures have evolved. Some of the basic patterns have

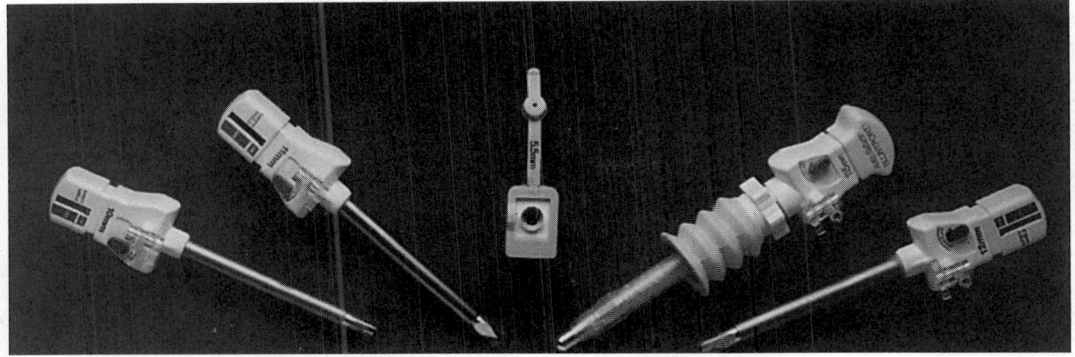

FIGURE 3-14 Blunt port and sheath assembly is often used for open laparoscopies (*second from right*). Sharp trocar and cannula units as well as converter with reducer are also shown.

been used for years and continue to be very popular, whereas others have been designed to accommodate the new endoscopic approaches. The full effect of this new era in surgery has been realized within the last decade, and already instrument designs are in their fourth and fifth generations. As surgery becomes more sophisticated, so do the instruments required for successful less invasive techniques (Fig. 3-11).

Trocars and cannulas

When a natural orifice does not exist for diagnostic or operative procedures, one or several can be created. To do so, a trocar and cannula are necessary. Those used for arthroscopy are very small in comparison to those used to access the chest or abdomen. The basic principle remains the same for all trocars and cannulas. They provide a mechanism for inserting and removing instrumentation while endoscopic surgery is performed. The cannula, or sheath, is inserted to access the operative site by use of a trocar as an obturator. Once the port of entry has been made, the trocar is removed, and the cannula is left in place.

If reusable trocars and cannulas are used, the trocar tip must be sharpened routinely. The stopcock and trumpet valves must be inspected before and after each use to ensure proper functioning. Internal gaskets may need occasional replacement. The trocar and cannula must fit properly and may not always be interchangeable. Component parts must be kept together, but they must be disassembled completely for cleaning and sterilization.

Disposable trocar and cannula units offer several advantages. One of the more popular features is that the trocar is always sharp. When multiple ports of the same size are used, the same trocar can be reused on the same patient. Some manufacturers package one trocar and two or more sheaths of the same size. The same trocar is then used to establish multiple access ports.

Disposable trocar and cannula units also may provide siliconized trocar tips as well as safety features once entry has been made. Systems are available that either engage a safety shield to automatically advance over the trocar tip

once entry is made or provide retractability of the trocar tip once entry is made (Fig. 3-12). No reusable trocar systems currently have built-in automatic safety shields.

Many disposable cannulas have gripping devices that can reduce the risk of accidental cannula removal during repeated advancement and withdrawal of the endoscopic instrumentation (Fig. 3-13). Grippers are incorporated either into the cannula or as separate entities. Grippers can be used with reusable cannulas as long as the fit is appropriate.

Disposable cannulas have a stopcock assembly for the insufflation gas, much the same as the reusable system. One-way flapper valves in disposables provide leak-proof protection and operate automatically for instrument insertion, specimen removal, or rapid desufflation. Since the diameters of instrumentation vary with design and use, various sizes of trocar and cannula units may be required for one procedure. Both reusable and disposable systems come in a variety of diameters and lengths. To increase flexibility, converters and reducers are used to adapt the size of the instrument (see Fig. 3-13). Converters can be separate or built into the cannula as a diaphragm seal. Both systems are designed to reduce the chance of CO_2 leaks.

Radiolucent disposable cannulas offer the ability to visualize tissue and lesions without obstruction. This feature may be critical during an endoscopic cholangiogram so that this instrumentation does not obstruct the view during fluoroscopy. Other times this design may not be necessary. Occasionally a procedure is scheduled as an open laparoscopy. Patients who have had multiple surgeries or have developed adhesions present an added risk. When a surgeon is unsure of underlying structures, the laparoscopy may be done in an open fashion. A small paraumbilical incision is made, and tissues are dissected. Peritoneum is opened and a large blunt-tipped trocar-sheath assembly is inserted (Fig. 3-14). The sheath is designed to fit snugly against the peritoneum from underneath and skin from above. Stay sutures are used to close any excess incision. Wafer seals (much like colostomy wafers) further reduce loss of CO_2 gas. Pneumoperito-

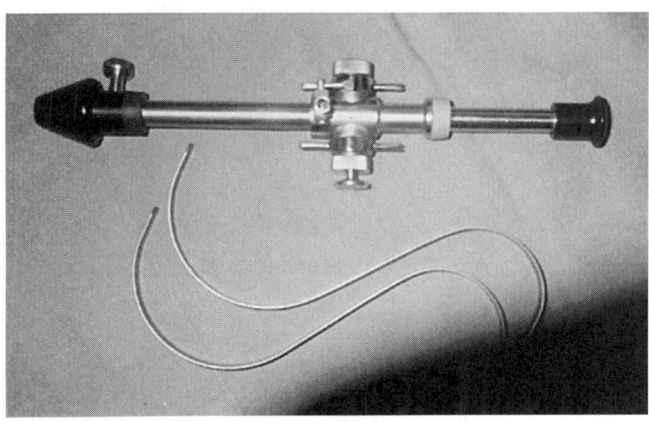

FIGURE 3-15 Reusable blunt-tip Hassan type of trocar and S retractors.

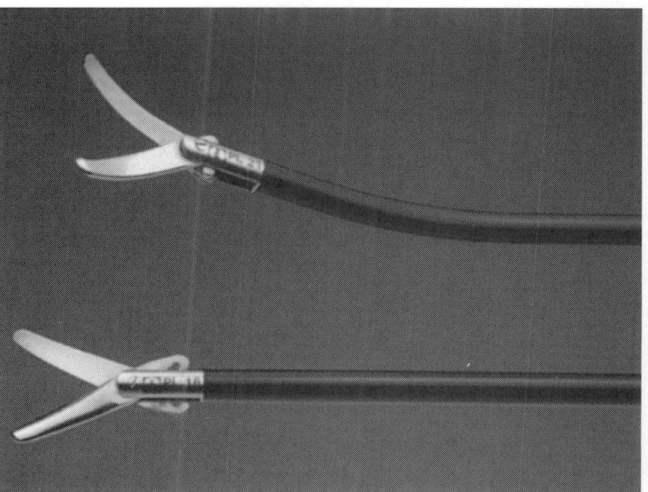

FIGURE 3-17   Straight and curved endoscopic scissors.

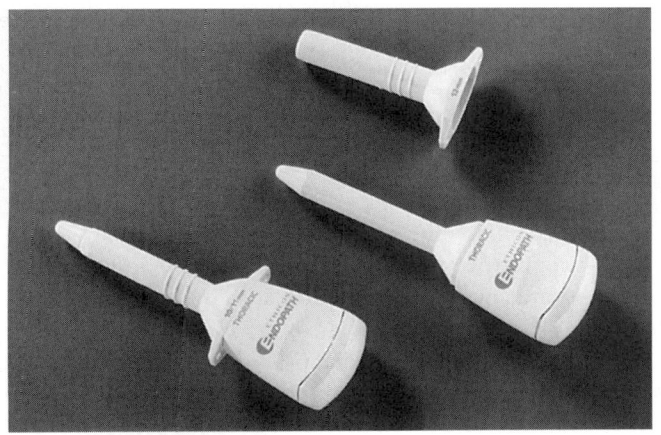

FIGURE 3-16 Thoracic blunt trocar and gripper assembly. Notice absence of stopcock insufflation capability.

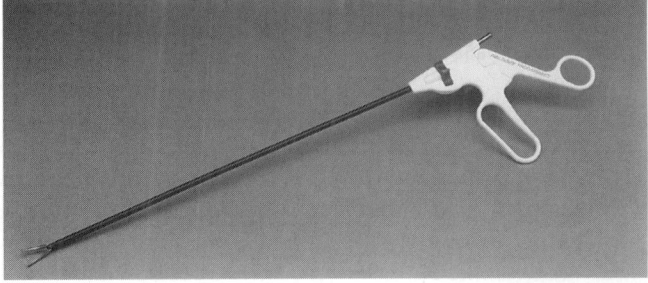

FIGURE 3-18   Disposable dissector with swivel design and monopolar electrosurgical capability.

neum is then created. If a reusable system is used, stay sutures are also used to stabilize the system. S-type retractors are usually needed for both (Fig. 3-15).

When extracorporeal surgery must be performed during laparoscopy (when tissue to be operated on is brought to the outside of the body through a small hole), an even larger diameter port is used. During certain bowel resections, for example, loops of bowel are brought through a larger port to be resected or sutured. When entering the chest, shorter blunt trocars are used with grippers that provide stabilization while in the pleural cavity. This type of trocar does not have insufflation ports (Fig. 3-16). If insufflation is required to assist the anesthesiologist in collapsing the lung, regular ports are used.

Dissecting instruments

Dissecting instruments for endoscopy are used to cut, divide, or separate tissue. Scissors and dissectors that are

very similar to their open–procedure counterparts have been designed for endoscopic use.

Endoscopic scissors are available for blunt or sharp dissection. They can be straight or curved (including hook scissors) depending on the location of the target tissue (Fig. 3-17). Scissors usually have a rounded tip when closed so that they can also be used to manipulate tissue without trauma. When open, both jaws of the scissors should be visualized to prevent inadvertent injury. Some scissors have been designed to be connected to an electrosurgical energy source so that coagulation can be provided during cutting.

Dissectors are used to separate or divide tissue. They come in many different shaped tips for dissecting, spreading, dividing, grasping, retracting, and coagulating structures (Fig. 3-18). Other dissecting instruments, such as balloon dissectors, have been developed for blunt dissection or creation of a space so that surgery can be performed. For example, a balloon dissector is used to

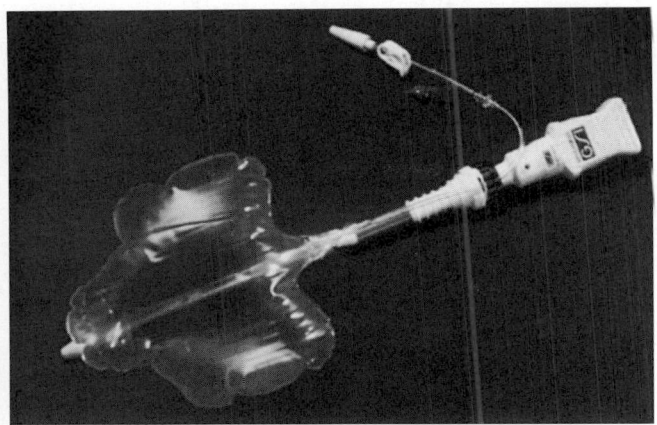

FIGURE 3-19   Balloon dissecting instrument.

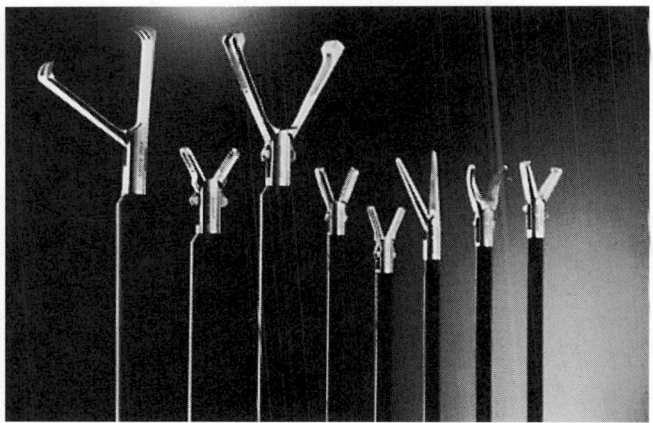

FIGURE 3-20   Endoscopic grasping instruments.

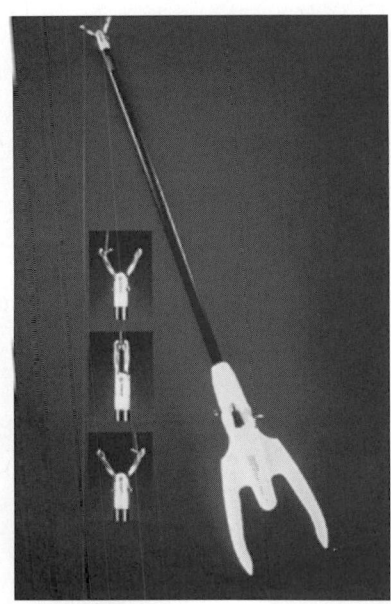

FIGURE 3-21   An endoscopic needle holder that transfers the needle from one prong of the jaw to the other.

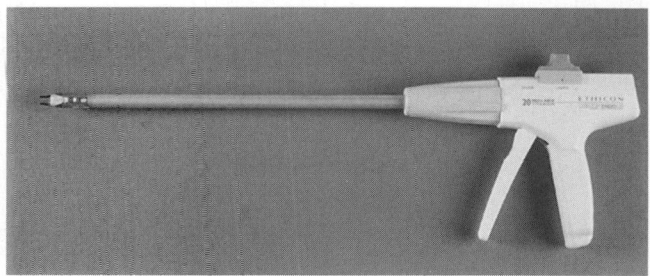

FIGURE 3-22   Disposable endoscopic rotating clip applier.

create a preperitoneal space during laparoscopic herniorrhaphy (Fig. 3-19).

Clamping instruments

Endoscopic clamping instruments are used to grasp and hold tissue or other materials. Ratchets are used in the instrument design to allow the distal tip to be locked onto the tissue or whatever is being grasped. Graspers, forceps, and even biopsy forceps are all classified as clamping instruments.

Graspers and forceps can be traumatic, with sharp teeth, or atraumatic, with a smooth, serrated jaw surface (Fig. 3-20). Traumatic graspers and forceps customarily are used to hold tissue that will be excised, whereas the atraumatic versions are used to gently hold structures, such as the bowel or liver. Some clamping instruments are insulated so that electrosurgical energy can be transmitted to provide coagulation.

Suturing and stapling instruments

Suturing or stapling instruments are used to deliver sutures, staples, or clips to join, hold, and secure tissue.

Needle holders, clip appliers, and staplers are all listed within this category.

Needle holders have been designed to deliver and place sutures within body cavities during endoscopic procedures. Tungsten carbide jaw inserts on the needle holders are often used to prevent rotation of the suture needle. Some needle holders have been designed to transfer the needle from one jaw to the other during suturing (Fig. 3-21). Since endoscopic suturing is so tedious, other instruments have been developed to facilitate this process, including suture passers and curved needle holders.

Another instrument used to provide hemostasis and tissue security is the clip applier. It represents the safest, easiest, and quickest way to occlude small vessels and structures. Reusable appliers exist, but many must be removed from the cannula each time to be reloaded. This adds time, contributes to loss of pneumoperitoneum (if utilized), and causes frustration when the clip is dislodged upon reinsertion. The automatic-feed, reloadable, disposable version remains very popular today (Fig. 3-22).

Endoscopic staplers provide cutting and stapling during endoscopic resections (Figs. 3-23 and 3-24). Certain

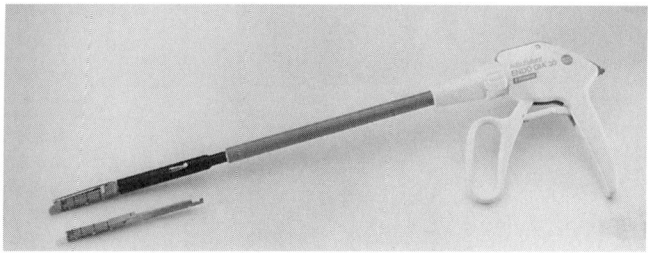

FIGURE 3-23   Disposable endoscopic stapling device (Endo GIA 30 and reloading unit).

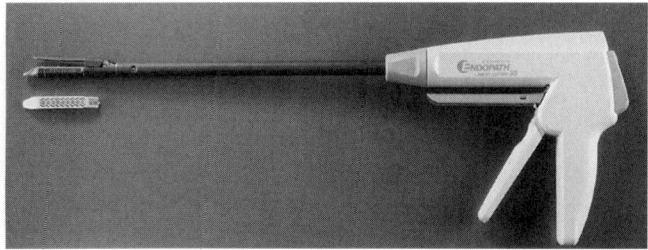

FIGURE 3-24   Disposable linear cutter and reloading unit (Endopath ELC 35).

structures can be easily resected intracorporeally (such as the ovary and appendix). Others may necessitate extracorporeal resection or reanastomosis. If this occurs, traditional stapling devices are used.

The evolution of more complex endoscopic surgical techniques have challenged traditional suturing and ligation methods; therefore, several devices and techniques have been developed for laparoscopic tissue suturing. When surgical clips and staples cannot be used, a laparoscopic suture may have to be substituted. Conditions that preclude the use of clips include large arteries and edematous or inflamed ducts. Most general surgeons prefer to use nonabsorbable sutures and ligation materials to prevent rapid absorption.

The three basic types of laparoscopic suturing materials are loop ligatures, extracorporeal sutures, and intracorporeal sutures.

Loop Ligatures

Preknotted suture loops are used to ligate pedicle tissues. The suture loop is packaged with an introducer sleeve, which can be inserted through one of the trocars. The loop is passed over the targeted tissue or pedicle by means of a grasping forceps to assist. Once the loop is in position the existing suture knot is pushed down the introducer sleeve until it is cinched tightly around the tissue. The suture is then cut with endoscopic scissors (Fig. 3-25).

Extracorporeal Sutures

Tissue can be approximated intraabdominally when the knot is tied extracorporeally (outside the body). To accomplish this, endoscopic swaged sutures are used. The suture is grasped proximally to the needle, and both are inserted through one of the trocars into the abdomen. The needle is then held with the grasper or laparoscopic needle holder and driven through the desired tissue. A second grasper or needle holder inserted through a second trocar is used to assist. The needled end of the suture is pulled through the tissue and out through the trocar. The needle is removed, and a knot is tied extracorporeally. The knot is advanced down the trocar and onto the tissue. The suture is cut by use of laparoscopic scissors (Fig. 3-26). The three types of knots tied extracorporeally are the slip knot, the fisherman's knot, and the surgeon's knot. The surgeon determines which knot is used.

Intracorporeal Sutures

Suture ligature can also be passed through the trocar to be tied while it is inside the body. The tissue is approximated in the same fashion but tied intracorporeally (inside the abdomen) using grasping forceps or laparoscopic needle holders. Some surgeons prefer this simplified technique.

Retractors and accessory instruments

Retractors are used to hold tissue and expose the operative target site (Fig. 3-27). Retractors can be traumatic to some structures, such as the bowel and liver, so they must be used with caution. Miniretractors and balloon retractors have been designed for use on delicate structures.

Other accessory instruments have been designed to enhance the use of basic endoscopic instruments and to facilitate the surgical procedure. Probes that are used to manipulate tissue should be blunt to minimize tissue trauma. Some probes have centimeter gradations to measure structures within the body. Irrigation-aspirator probes are used to enhance visualization of the internal structures, and electrosurgical probes provide hemostasis. Endoscopic specimen bags are available to contain specimens to minimize cross-contamination. Special accessory instruments will continue to be designed to enhance and make possible advanced endoscopic procedures.

Care and handling of endoscopes and instrumentation

Endoscopes and instruments must be clean and free from all bioburden before sterilization or high-level disinfection can be considered. During routine use, bioburden accumulates in channels, ports, crevices, and other movable parts of scopes and instruments. Periodically throughout the procedure, gross blood and bioburden should be removed by flushing of the channels and wiping off of the surfaces with sterile water. Instruments and endoscopes that are kept relatively clean during the procedure helps to prevent debris from drying, thus facilitating the cleaning process.

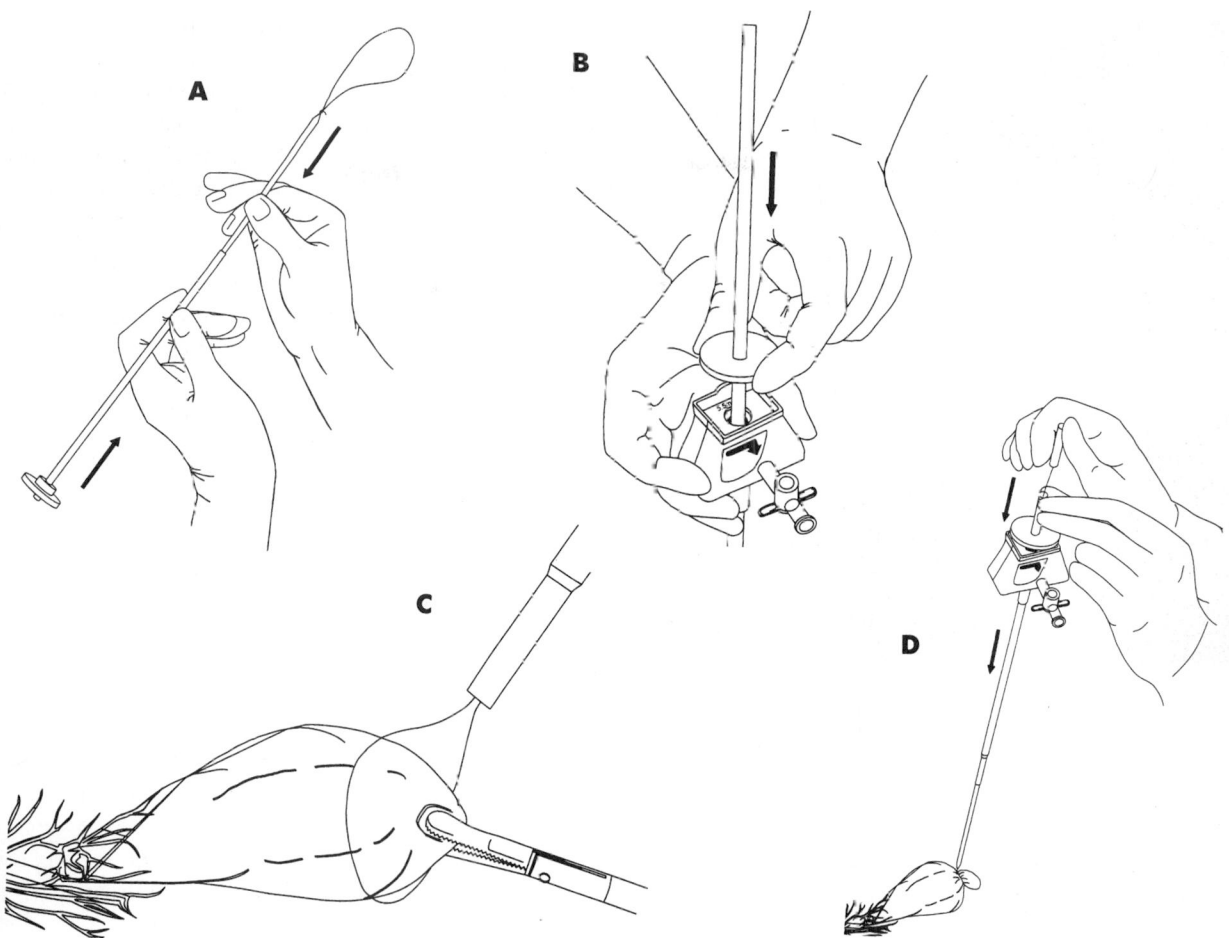

FIGURE 3-25 Surgitie ligating loop. **A,** Back load loop into introducer completely. **B,** Insert introducer into trocar, all the way down. **C,** Push suture loop through introducer. Grasp desired tissue with grasping forceps (passed through another trocar) and maneuver loop over tissue. **D,** Push down knot by advancing nylon carrier all the way until knot is cinched. Cut suture.

After each procedure all instrumentation and devices must be decontaminated thoroughly. Immersible equipment should be cleaned or flushed with an enzymatic or other appropriate detergent solution. This loosens organic material and makes it easier to remove. Instruments that can withstand cavitation or ultrasonic cleaning can be placed in an ultrasonic device. Fiberoptics and endoscopes usually cannot be placed in an ultrasonic machine because the ultrasonic vibration can damage the tiny fiberoptic bundles.

Careful rinsing and flushing with copious amounts of water must follow the cleaning process. Often deionized water is recommended for the final rinse to minimize any mineral buildup from tap water. Manufacturer's written recommendations for cleaning and processing should always be followed. Instruments must be dried before disinfection or sterilization.

Automatic cleaning devices that flush the ports of instruments provide an economical, practical, and effective way to initially clean reusable channeled instruments (Fig. 3-28). Even though instruments have flush ports, debris can become lodged distally. Some automatic

systems provide a means to flush in a retrograde fashion, forcing debris out the larger proximal port. Sealed instruments can also be tested for seal integrity using this type of system. The cleaning and processing of endoscopic instrumentation and equipment have been under scrutiny and heated debate. The need for a dependable method to assess the adequacy of the cleaning process is desperately needed today. Currently many companies are researching cleaning-validation techniques.

Compliance with federal, professional, and regional standards cannot be ignored for reprocessing. High-level (cold-soak) disinfection has been the accepted primary standard for endoscopic instrumentation. Today the concern over viruses and microorganisms such as HIV, hepatitis B and C viruses, *Mycobacterium* (tuberculosis bacteria), and antibiotic-resistant organisms, coupled with the need for comparable levels of patient care, has caused great concern about the adequacy of merely disinfecting devices.

Ideally all instruments and devices coming into contact with sterile tissues and the vascular system should be sterile. Those coming into contact with mucous mem-

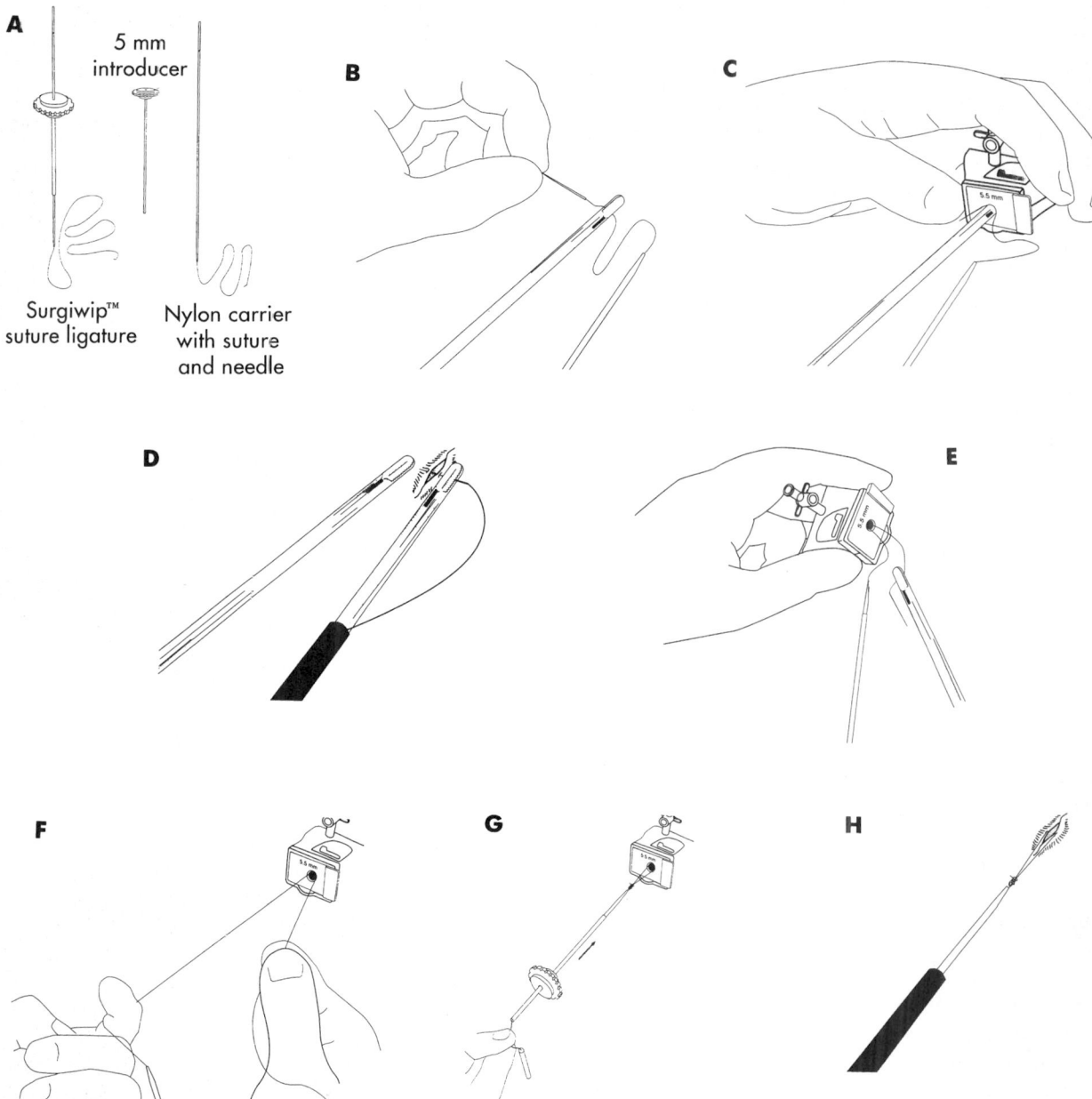

FIGURE 3-26   Surgiwip suture ligature application for approximating tissue intraabdominally by extracorporeal knot tying (outside body). **A,** Component pieces. **B,** Grasp suture behind swage of needle with tissue grasper or needle holder. **C,** Introduce grasper or needle holder and suture through trocar into abdomen. **D,** Drive needle through tissue to be approximated. Place instrument close to center of needle for control. Pull needle through tissue using second grasper (introduced through another trocar). **E,** Regrasp needle behind swage intracorporeally and pull it through and out the same trocar. (Allow for slack of suture to avoid tissue tears.) **F,** Remove needle. Tie fisherman's knot. **G,** Once knot is tied, break end of nylon carrier. **H,** Push knot down with nylon carrier and out onto tissue. Cut suture. For additional suturing, repeat **A** to **H** until tissue is satisfactorily approximated.

branes or nonintact skin can be disinfected at a high level. This means that sterility is required for all laparoscopy, angioscopy, thoracoscopy, and arthroscopy procedures. Cold-soak disinfection may be acceptable for colonoscopy, laryngoscopy, bronchoscopy, cystoscopy, and other diagnostic procedures. However, because more invasive procedures that access the vascular system are being performed

during most of these endoscopy procedures, the adequacy of high-level disinfection is being questioned. Also heartier microorganisms, such as TB spores, are not easily destroyed during high-level disinfection.

The hazards of glutaraldehyde for high-level disinfection are being realized in today's healthcare workplace environment. The maximum recommended exposure

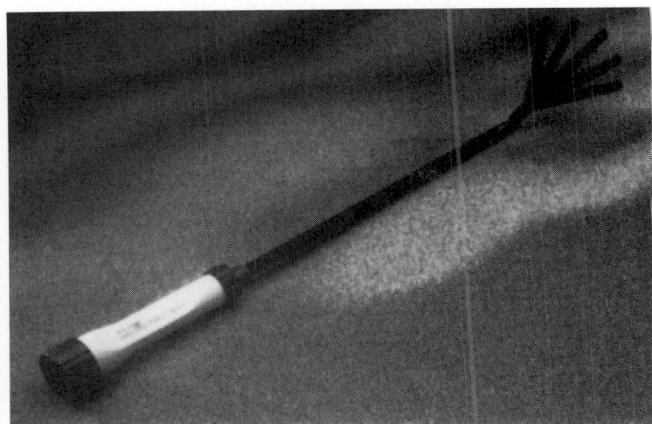

FIGURE 3-27   Endoscopic fan retractor with five fingers.

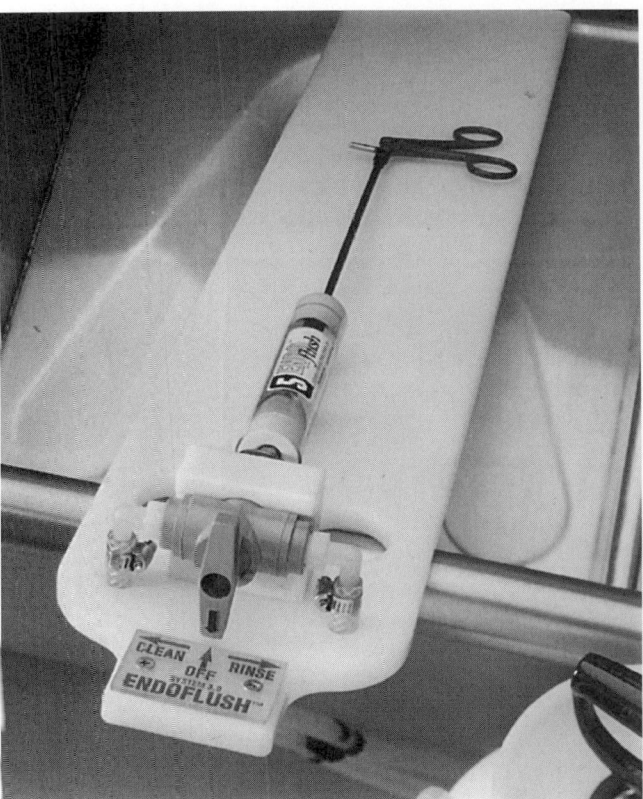

FIGURE 3-28   Endoflush endoscopic instrument cleaner.

level of glutaraldehyde determined by OSHA is 0.2 parts per million (ppm). When solution is being poured after mixing or devices are being submerged, the level rises to approximately 0.4 ppm, which is double the exposure level. The odor of glutaraldehyde becomes an irritant at 0.3 ppm causing tearing, nausea, and other effects.[2] Devices have been designed to absorb the odor and fumes from the glutaraldehyde solution (Fig. 3-29).

Currently much debate is being voiced over the soak times in glutaraldehyde for high-level disinfection to take place. The FDA has stated that items must be soaked for 45 minutes with a solution temperature of 25° C for high-level disinfection to occur. This statement was based on uncleaned instrumentation. Professional organizations, such as the Society of Gastroenterology Nurses and Associates, have supported the 20-minute glutaraldehyde soak at room temperature, on cleaned instrumentation for high-level disinfection.[2]

Institutional policy sets the guidelines from which practitioners will work. Provision of comparable levels of care when there are not equal numbers of instruments to match scheduled procedures takes insight and coordination. If sterile instruments are required for a particular endoscopic procedure, sterile instruments should be used for all patients undergoing that procedure. Enough instrumentation and equipment must be purchased to accommodate the endoscopic patient volume, or other measures must be implemented.

When sterile devices and instrumentation are needed, there are multiple options that provide sterilization today, including steam, ethylene oxide, peracetic acid, and gas-plasma sterilization methods. Many times steam cannot be used on delicate endoscopes, but the endoscopic accessory instrumentation may be able to withstand the heat produced during this type of sterilization.

Ethylene oxide sterilization has been used successfully for many years to sterilize endoscopes and instruments.

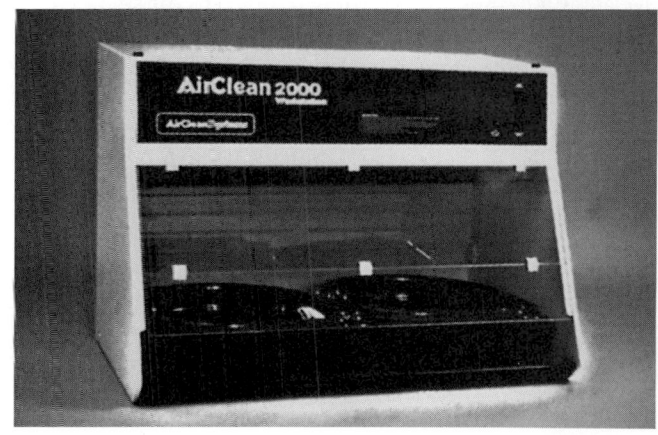

FIGURE 3-29   A covered hood system, which can be used to minimize the glutaraldehyde fumes and odor.

Recent rulings to eliminate the agents that have been combined with the ethylene oxide, such as chlorofluorocarbon (CFC) and halogenated CFC (HCFC), have led to the use of 100% ethylene oxide to provide safe and effective ethylene oxide sterilization.

Peracetic acid sterilization is gaining much popularity for instruments and endoscopes that are immersible but are sensitive to heat. This method provides sterility within 30

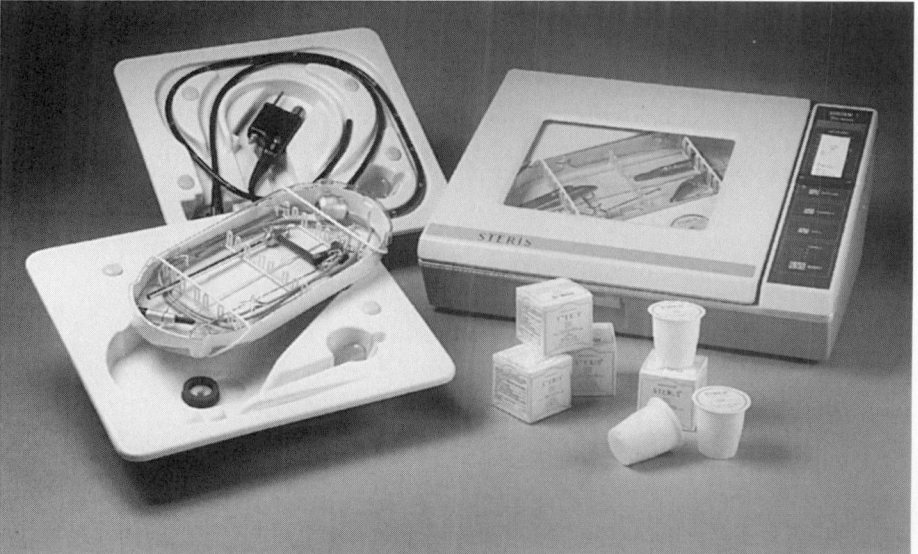

FIGURE 3-30   STERIS System 1.

minutes. Instruments are placed into removable trays where the solution is purged over all surfaces and within all lumens and ports. A four-rinse cycle with sterile water removes all the sterilizing diluent. Devices sterilized in this manner should be used soon after sterilization because this process does not ensure a sterile shelf life for later use (Fig. 3-30).

Plasma sterilization systems have been introduced during this past decade. There are two popular systems today: One uses hydrogen peroxide gas plasma, which sterilizes within 75 minutes, and the other uses peracetic acid vapor and gas plasma, which sterilizes within 3 to 4 hours. Both of these systems use and emit nontoxic and nonflammable gases. Understanding the advantages and limitations of each system is important when determining which system will meet the needs of endoscopic instrumentation sterilization.

Single-use versus reusable instrumentation

The climate surrounding healthcare has become one of uncertainty and ever-present change. With spiraling costs come new opportunities and challenges for the redesign of endoscopic instrumentation. The directive to "do more with less" has become a way of life. Endoscopy has paved the way for surgical and diagnostic procedures to be performed with reduced patient discomfort and earlier discharge (often the same day). Patients are happier because they can go home and return to normal life-styles more quickly.

Case management and clinical pathways are important guides to enable a safe, rapid hospital discharge. Hospital administrators and third-party payers are rapidly turning to the concept of cost per discharge. The endoscopic revolution has indeed reduced a patient's length of stay significantly. Operating room expenditures, on the other hand, have increased. Institutional policy may dictate whether reusable or single-use items are chosen. When analyzing the risk-to-benefit ratio, one should consider several issues.

Many facilities are using a combination of reusable and single-use laparoscopic instruments, which appears to be the most successful practice. Advantages of single-use items include sharpness, reliability related to function, guaranteed sterility, and safety. Indirect advantages include no reprocessing time and effort, no associated repair costs, and the provision of comparable levels of patient care. Upgrade designs are also more easily purchased if they are for single use. Disadvantages may include the need for increased storage space, budgetary implications, and environmental concerns related to disposal and biohazardous waste.

Advantages of reusable instruments include less storage space required, a reduced budgetary effect (except for initial purchase), and minimal waste. With reusables, the decontamination and reprocessing system must be reliable, must be compatible with the devices being processed, and must be monitored for effectiveness. Above all, safe and effective patient outcome should be the criterion against which all else is compared.

The advantages and disadvantages of reusable versus single-use devices must be explored before purchasing decisions can be made. Part of patient advocacy required of a perioperative nurse is to evaluate patient care practices, justify products used, and provide a safe environment for patients and personnel. Being open to suggestions and change is expected in today's healthcare environment. Now is the time for the entire surgical team and industry to form collaborative relationships to enhance practices and patient outcomes. The choice between single-use or reusable instrumentation and equipment must be thoroughly evaluated in each individual practice setting and justified accordingly.

Reprocessing single-use devices

Reprocessing single-use devices is a practice that has evolved recently. Since guidelines are vague about this practice, there is much controversy regarding the appropriateness and effectiveness of reprocessing single-use devices. Reprocessing can take place within a healthcare facility or can be performed by an independent third-party company that is in the business of providing this service. Devices that are reprocessed are usually items that have been opened and not used, items that have an expiration date that has been reached, and items that have been used in surgery but appear not to be damaged. Some items that fall into these categories are endoscopic graspers, scissors, trocars, and other accessory devices.

Liability is the most questioned aspect of reprocessing single-use items. A hospital is liable for this practice if reprocessing is performed within the confines of the facility. If a third-party company provides this service, it is likewise liable and should present documentation of the insurance coverage to the facility contracting for this service. Although the original manufacturer of a device warrants a disposable product for one use, a reprocessing company will also warrant the reprocessed device for one use. Because of the lack of lawsuits involving patients injured by reprocessed single-use devices, a liability precedent has not been set yet.

Another area to explore when determining whether to reprocess single-use items is the actual process involved. Can the disposable device be disassembled for cleaning? Can the device withstand disinfection or sterilization? For example, can the item be adequately aerated if ethylene oxide sterilization is used? No manufacturer of sterilization products will endorse the practice of reprocessing single-use items today. Can the device be tested and checked for proper form and function after cleaning has been completed? Has the device integrity been destroyed during reprocessing? Is there equipment available to test the integrity of the device? For example, how is the integrity of the insulation checked on an electrosurgical probe? Can the device be returned to its original intended use?

If reprocessing is performed within a healthcare facility, determining the integrity of the instrument is often difficult. Appropriate equipment must be available to ensure this process. Customers must ask third-party companies about their reprocessing methods. Usually these companies will have the appropriate equipment to perform comprehensive device testing.

Third-party companies that provide reprocessing services should be registered with the FDA, meaning that they are following good manufacturing practices.[5] For example, reprocessed items are kept in quarantine until the biologic indicators show that the parameters for sterilization have taken place for the reprocessed devices. Many companies are being formed today for the practice of providing this type of reprocessing service. They need to provide documentation of FDA registration and procedures used for reprocessing.

Cost savings is the final criterion that must be explored when determining whether to reprocess single-use devices. Items that are more expensive may be considered appropriate for promoting cost savings, whereas less-expensive items (such as those less than $10) may not show a cost savings benefit. Each single-use item must be evaluated individually when considering this practice. When a significant cost saving is realized, the healthcare facility is ethically responsible for passing this cost saving on to the patient.[9]

Reprocessing single-use devices will continue to be a controversial practice. Healthcare providers and workers as a team must be involved in making the decision to reprocess because this practice can have either very positive financial outcomes or devastating results if not explored and planned carefully.

Complications and Anesthetic Considerations

Although anesthetic technique and delivery are the responsibility of the anesthesia care provider, the perioperative nurse must anticipate and appropriately respond to associated risks during endoscopic intervention. Many open surgical procedures, which require lengthy hospitalization and result in substantial postoperative pain, are now performed endoscopically as ambulatory or short-stay surgeries. Postoperative pain has been minimized for most patients. Because of these changes, anesthetic technique has also changed. Today there is an emphasis on minimal anesthesia during surgery. Short-acting drugs are used so that the patient awakens quickly and experiences as few side effects as possible.

The three major goals of the anesthesia care provider during endoscopic procedures remain the same: respiratory stability, appropriate muscle relaxation, and hemodynamic stability. Additionally, during many laparoscopic and pelviscopic procedures it is necessary to control diaphragmatic excursion.

When Trendelenburg's position is used, there is an increase in intraabdominal pressure, which can result in respiratory complications including hypoxia. CO_2 absorption from the peritoneal cavity can further aggravate this situation. Reverse Trendelenburg's position could result in decreased venous return, cardiac output, and blood pressure. CO_2 insufflation in this position could lead to an increase in total peripheral resistance, especially if intraabdominal pressure is high and the aorta is compressed. The perioperative nurse must be prepared to change the position of the OR bed when necessary and decrease the CO_2 flow rate of the insufflator. The anesthesia care provider may require assistance with medications and extra supplies.

Carbon dioxide, highly soluble in blood, does not

generally become a hazard when used during laparoscopic insufflation because it is rapidly absorbed in the splanchnic vascular region. Excessive intraabdominal pressure or any anesthetic technique that reduces splanchnic blood flow, however, could increase the potential for CO_2 gas emboli. This could lead to circulatory collapse. CO_2 could also advance from the heart to the pulmonary circulation, causing acute pulmonary hypertension with right-sided heart failure. If these effects are undetected and CO_2 insufflation continues, cardiac arrest and death could occur.

Signs of CO_2 embolus include sudden fall in blood pressure, dysrhythmia, heart murmurs, cyanosis, pulmonary edema, and an abrupt increase in end-tidal CO_2. If an embolus is suspected, continuous monitoring of heart sounds, blood pressure, and end-tidal CO_2 can help the anesthesia care provider make a rapid diagnosis. Immediate deflation of pneumoperitoneum is necessary. Treatment may include immediate placement of the patient in a left lateral position and aspiration of the CO_2 gas through a central venous catheter. The perioperative nurse should assist in patient repositioning while maintaining sterility of equipment and the surgical field wherever possible. Assistance may be required during central venous catheter placement. Debilitated patients may require preoperative invasive monitoring.

Hypotension can result from excessive bleeding, excess intraabdominal pressure, and hypoxia. CO_2 insufflation rates may have to be reduced. Extra intravenous fluids may be needed. Hypertension resulting from increased intraabdominal pressure and increased CO_2 gas absorption may also be evidenced. Increased bleeding may result. Again, the perioperative nurse can help by decreasing CO_2 insufflation flow rates; additional hemostatic agents and endoscopic clips may be required.

Gastric reflux is a concern if the patient is obese, a hiatal hernia is present, or excessive pneumoperitoneum occurs. The hiatal hernia could be discovered during the preoperative assessment. A nasogastric or orogastric tube may be inserted after general anesthesia is administered. There will be less postoperative discomfort if an orogastric tube is used. During epidural and regional anesthesia, patients are usually awake, and insertion of a gastric tube may be poorly tolerated. For this reason the tube is not inserted unless gastric distention occurs. The perioperative nurse must be quick to respond if assistance is required during gastric tube insertion. Intercostal nerve blocks offer surgical pain relief and abdominal muscle relaxation when the patient is awake during surgery. This anesthetic technique requires extreme patient cooperation because several injections are necessary. The perioperative nurse's role during intercostal nerve block induction is to remain at the patient's side and help to reduce anxiety. The perioperative nurse's understanding of the potential risks along with appropriate nursing interventions can have a significant effect on the patient's outcome.

VIDEO TECHNOLOGY

Evolution of Video Technology

A basic medical video system includes the scope, light cable, light source, camera head, camera cord, camera-scope coupler, camera control unit, and video monitor. Additional peripheral equipment is also necessary for specific surgical procedures and is discussed later. Since video technology can be so complex, a glossary of terms is included in Box 3-1.

A video system takes light energy from a beginning source and converts it into electrical energy and then back into light energy to provide a picture. The camera head contains a sensor, which is light sensitive. The sensor used today is a solid-state unit, or chip, called a *charged coupled device* (CCD); it produces the unprocessed video signal. The CCD has replaced the outdated vacuum camera tubes and, as a result, offers greater sensitivity and resolution. The CCD is made up of small picture elements called *pixels*, which in the presence of light become conductive and in the absence of light remain nonconductive. Each pixel is capable of sensing either red, blue, or green light. The picture is then transformed into a matrix made up of the conductive and nonconductive pixels. This matrix is usually scanned at a rate of 525 lines per frame, 30 frames per second, generating a signal frequency. The scanning rate is standardized by the National Television Systems Committee (NTSC). The picture is then reproduced at its terminal destination.

The NTSC is the standard video format in the United States, Canada, Japan, and most of South America and Asia. It was established to be used for broadcast purposes. A format is the way electronic camera signals carry brightness and color information. The three most commonly used formats are the composite, the Y/C, and the RGB. The standard format is termed *composite* because it carries both color and brightness on the same signal (Fig. 3-31). The advantage is that it is standard. The disadvantage is that when both color and brightness information are combined on one signal, cross-talk, or interference between the two, can result in increased video noise (disturbance).

Another commonly available signal transmission method is Y/C. Y stands for the brightness signal and C for the color signal. Video information is carried on two different signals and is commonly referred to as *super video home system* (S-VHS) (Fig. 3-32). This transmission method does not have cross-talk problems and produces sharper pictures with higher resolution on both video recorders and hard copy producers. These systems require more expensive monitors and recorders. Another disadvantage is that color and brightness travel at different speeds and, over longer cord distances, may be out of synchronization, requiring extra electronic circuitry.

The third commonly used video format, RGB, also a component system, separates video information into red, green, and blue signals and carries each separately (Fig. 3-33). Brightness is generated as a percentage of the three colors (30% red, 59% green, 11% blue). An advantage of this format is less noise interference, resulting in sharper pictures with distinct color separation. It is the format of choice for computer interfacing, which is rapidly becoming more popular and accepted. Some RGB components are more expensive as compared with the other formats because the three signals must be synchronized.

Several cameras are available with all three formats, which allow for flexibility. One must keep in mind, however, that accompanying equipment must be compatible with the camera's format. For example, for the Y/C or RGB camera format to be advantageous, the monitor utilized must also be capable of handling these formats as well as the composite signals. It becomes apparent that system compatibility is crucial. For this reason the basic composite format is still very desirable.

Visualization Systems

Endoscopes once offered visualization only to the operating physician. The introduction of the teaching arm provided direct visualization not only for the physician but also for the resident, perioperative nurse, or other surgical team members. Often, however, images seen through the teaching arm were not identical to those seen through the primary optics. The inability to effectively interact with the physician and anticipate the surgical needs were frustrating and time consuming.

In the late 1960s and early 1970s medical video and still cameras were being introduced to the marketplace. This allowed for still photography as well as video documentation of select surgical procedures. The tube style of cameras were large, bulky, and heavy, not adequately meeting the video needs of the surgery. Video technology rapidly changed with the introduction of the chip TV camera. Its lightweight, low-profile design triggered the era of video-guided surgery. Cameras that once weighed several pounds now weigh only a few ounces (Fig. 3-34).

The rapid developments in video imaging have also resulted in higher resolution monitors. Together this integrated system provides increased assurance of maintenance of sterility during direct visualization, enhanced participation by assistants, and promotion of accurate assessment and planning by the perioperative nursing staff. Today video technology has evolved to the point of almost being mandatory during endoscopic procedures. All surgical disciplines have been enhanced by the availability and capability of video systems.

Camera, cable, control unit

The video camera represents the optical-electronic interface of the video system. A camera cable transfers the signal frequency to a camera control unit (processor), which modifies the signal and then transmits the image to a video monitor, recorder, or hard copy picture, or all three. The camera is the most important component of the

---

BOX 3-1 | **Video Glossary**

autoexposure An electronic circuit built into cameras to eliminate electronically (within the camera) excess light from the picture; sometimes referred to as *electronic shutter.*

automatic gain control Ability to increase or decrease the video output level depending on the average light level of the viewed object.

blooming A glaring effect on the monitor caused by excessive light.

boost The ability to increase the signal strength of the camera. When used under low light conditions, boost provides increased sensitivity.

chroma Saturation of a color.

chromiance Defines the video camera's ability to handle the color red, the most difficult color to reproduce. The more accurate the color reproduction, the higher is the chromiance.

C-mount Standard thread size and diameter for a standard video camera lens.

color bars A test pattern used to adjust controls on the monitor for color, brightness, and contrast.

color reproduction Ability of an imaging device to reproduce colors exactly as the human eye perceives them.

composite video output (NTSC) The most commonly used video signal; the typical television video signal.

electronic shutter Ability of a camera to freeze image information within fractions of a second ($\frac{1}{60}$, $\frac{1}{125}$, $\frac{1}{1000}$, $\frac{1}{10,000}$).

footcandle Standard measure of luminance; the amount of light emitted by a standard candle at a distance of 1 foot from the frame; 10 luxes equals 1 footcandle. The lower the footcandle or lux number, the more sensitive is the camera.

light gain Another circuit within the camera to electronically amplify the picture to show a brighter image; sometimes referred to as AGC (automatic gain control), or boost circuit.

luminance Intensity or effectiveness of a given light on the eye.

NTSC National Television Standards Committee; type of television signal used in the United States.

orientation A mark or ridge on the camera head to orient the top portion of the video monitor.

pixel A signal-sensor element on a solid-state video chip; most solid-state chips used in medical videography have about 400,000 pixels on their surface. Each pixel is light sensitive and sees its own small part of the total picture.

resolution An optical device's ability to separate fine detail. Usually expressed in TV lines. Traditionally measured by aiming the camera at a target chart with squares of fine lines. The maximum resolution of the optical device is determined at the point where it begins to blur the lines together. If a box showing 400 lines per inch is still clear with spaces between the lines, the optical device has at least 400 lines-per-inch resolution.

sensitivity The response to low light levels by a video system.

S-VHS output A signal from the camera that splits the chroma and luminance, allowing for a richer resolution recording; Super Video Home System (Japan Victor Co.)

white balance Different light sources produce different temperatures of light and therefore different colors of light. White balancing is an adjustment of the camera for various sources of light.

video system. Camera options vary according to available technology, specialty, and personal preference.

Cameras have either one or three CCD chips. Three-chip cameras provide enhanced color and image quality but are somewhat larger, can cost up to three times that of a single-chip camera, and are not as light sensitive as the single-chip type. Color and the resulting image are enhanced because each chip is dedicated to one of the primary colors: red, green, blue. For this reason they are often used with microscopes when higher magnification requires increased resolution.

Newer single-chip cameras are available with digital

-------- COLOR -------- BRIGHTNESS --------

FIGURE 3-31   Standard composite signal format.

-------- COLOR --------

-------- BRIGHTNESS --------

FIGURE 3-32   Component Y/C (S-VHS) signal format.

-------- RED --------

-------- GREEN --------

-------- BLUE --------

FIGURE 3-33   Component RGB signal format. Brightness is generated as percentage of three primary colors.

processing in their control units, which boosts resolution. In essence, this technology incorporates three-chip quality in a single chip. Although the signal processing in the control unit may be digital, the video output from most cameras is an analog signal.

Digital processing refers to the way information is delivered through the various components of the control unit. This processing format allows for image enhancement and manipulation of the video image. It also allows multiple video signals to be shown on one monitor as well as electronic zoom capability. Digital processing also provides the user with freeze-frame capability when using video printers and when using picture-in-picture systems. The disadvantage of complete digital processing of images is the ability to refresh the picture on the monitor in real time. This processing method produces a jumpy, jittery picture. Thus most cameras are currently converting the digital image back to an analog signal before sending it to the video monitor.

Most cameras feature the ability to adjust to changes in light intensity while in use. This is done by an automatic shutter (iris), which measures the availability of light and adjusts accordingly. Automatic shutter activation also helps reduce glare from reflected light off instrumentation and moist viscera. The ability for continuous variable shutter speeds rather than discrete shutter speeds allows for instruments to be brought into the field without glare while still maintaining adequate illumination of background objects. The shutter's response should be rapid and without perceptible stepping of image intensity.

Camera heads now have buttons to control certain functions. Some of these include white balancing, light-sensitivity boosting (ability to provide a brighter picture when the image requires more light, especially

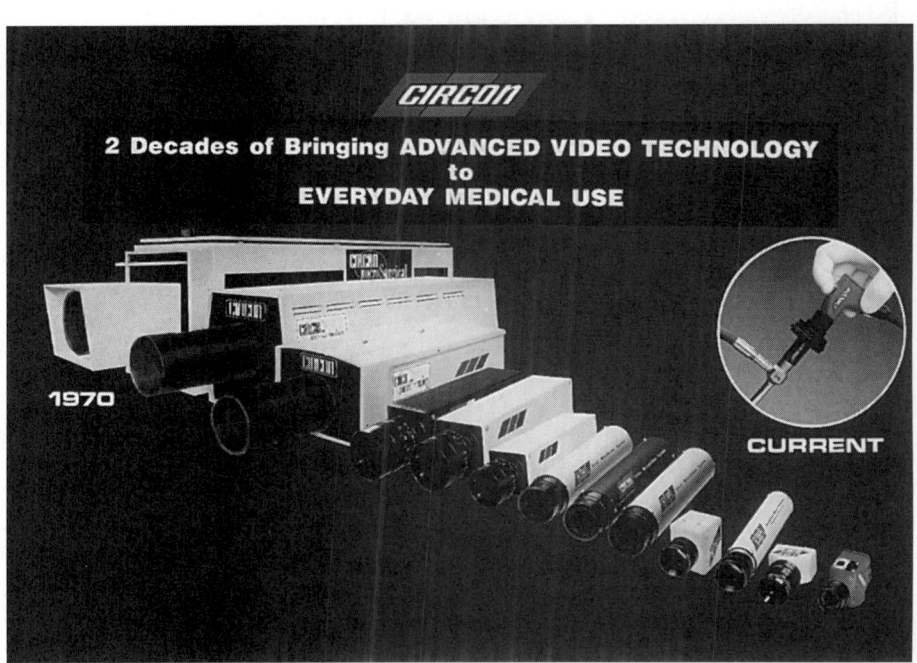

FIGURE 3-34   Evolution of medical video cameras.

when a scope smaller than 3 mm is used during sinuscopy), starting and stopping the VCR, and taking hard copy prints. This gives the surgeon control of these functions instead of requesting the circulating nurse to do so each time. The surgeon also has the ability to capture events exactly when they occur (Fig. 3-35).

Remote-control hand-held devices are also available for additional functions. These mimic the familiar household VCR remote control. As in the home setting, these devices take time to master. If used routinely, they can become the perioperative nurse's best friend (Fig. 3-36).

All cameras have focusing capability at the camera-coupler interface. Some also have zoom capability, allowing for closer visualization of specific structures or pathologic conditions. A camera cable connects the camera head to the camera control unit (Fig. 3-37). Most camera malfunctions are cable, not camera, related. For this reason a system that provides field-replaceable cables is most appealing. Should wires in the cable break, a new cable can be quickly exchanged, reducing downtime from having to ship the camera and cable for repair. Since wires in the flexible cable can break, it must be handled with care. Cables should never be twisted, crimped, or kinked. They should also be long enough to allow sufficient space between the sterile field and the visualization system.

Couplers (adapters)

Endocouplers are optical coupling devices used to connect cameras to various endoscopes. They are usually available in both 28 mm and 35 mm focal lengths and with different optical magnifications.

The specific type of coupler required depends on the type of surgery or diagnostic procedure performed and endoscope to be used. When the surgeon is viewing only on a monitor, a direct link coupler between the telescope and camera head is required (Fig. 3-38). For the surgeon to look directly through the endoscope and also have monitor-viewing capability, a beam-splitter coupler is

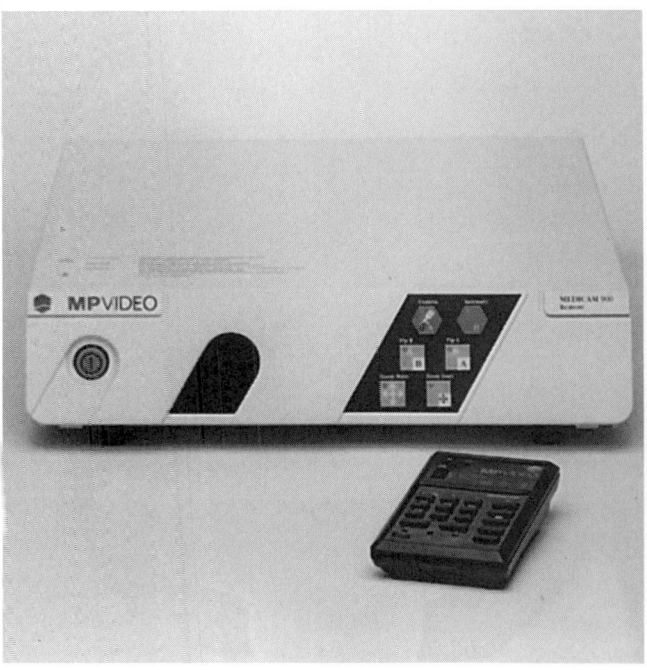

FIGURE 3-36 Camera control unit with remote control.

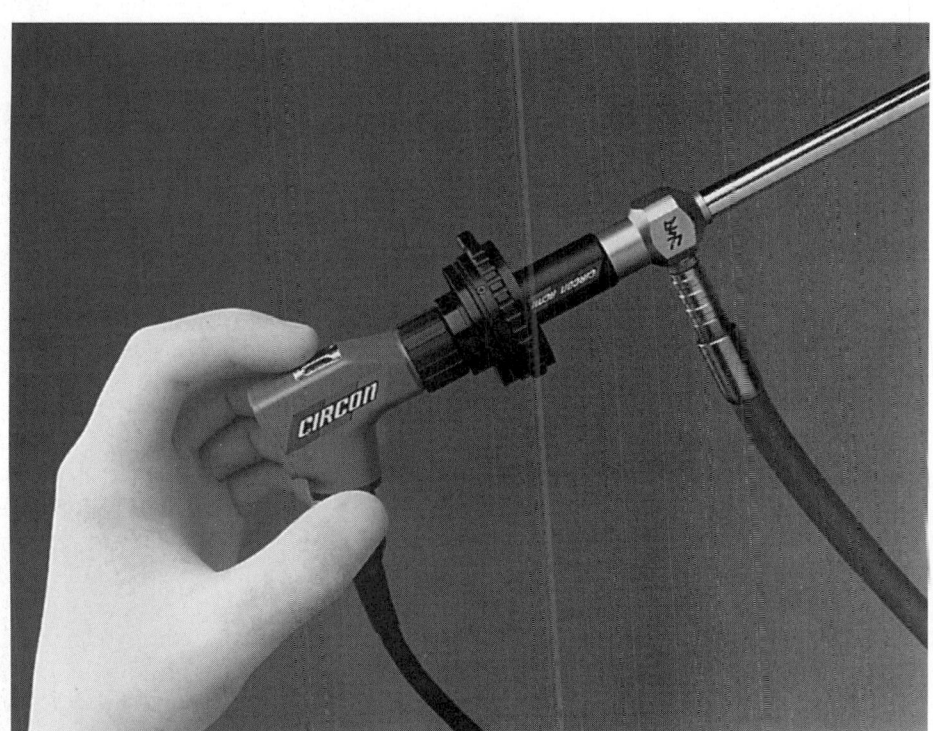

FIGURE 3-35 Microdigital I RGB color video camera with fingertip control.

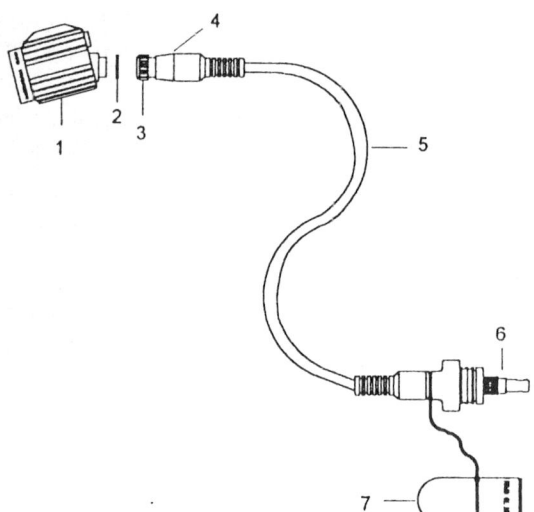

FIGURE 3-37   Camera and field-replaceable cable. *1,* Camera head; *2,* O-ring; *3,* knured ring; *4,* cable connector; *5,* replaceable cable; *6,* camera connector; *7,* soak cap.

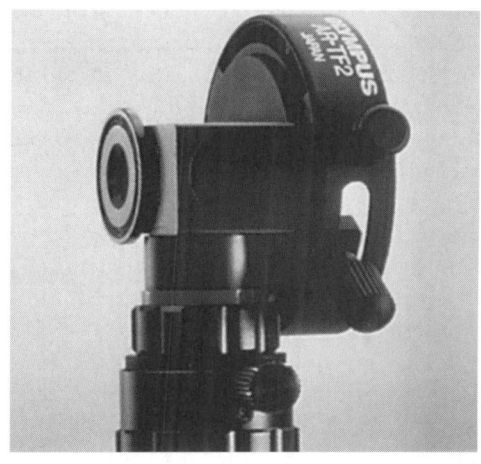

FIGURE 3-39   This camera adapter with a beam splitter allows the physicians to look through the eyepiece while others view the procedure on the monitor.

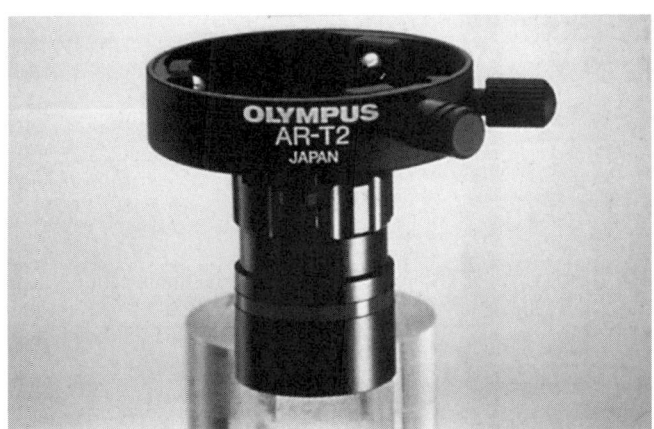

FIGURE 3-38   This camera adapter provides a direct link from the camera to the monitor when eyepiece viewing is not desired.

necessary (Fig. 3-39). Beam splitters are often used with flexible endoscopes. There are rotating beam splitters designed for the surgeon who operates in a sitting position. Zoom couplers provide variable focal lengths, usually from 22.5 to 50 mm.

A videoscope is a new design of camera-to-scope connection without the use of a coupler (Fig. 3-40). Since a coupler adds one more link to the chain, it is an area that can cause loss of light as well as lens fogging. Connecting the camera and scope with a screw-in design instead of the coupler clamp achieves a tighter fit. This design, however, requires that the camera and scope be bought as a unit; thus there is no interchangeability between systems. It also does not allow for sterile bagging of the camera because the camera is part of the endoscope.

Lens fogging can be very frustrating. It occurs because a cool metal scope is introduced into a warm body. Several ways to handle this phenomenon have been developed. The elimination of a coupler has already been discussed. Sterile defogging solutions are available for application to the telescope and coupler lenses (Fig. 3-41). These provide a coating and reduce the incidence of fogging. Other options on the market include O-ring seals at connections, sapphire lenses, and various water seals. Warming of the telescope before insertion may also help reduce fogging. It can be warmed by wrapping the telescope with lap sponges that have been soaked in warm sterile water. Another method is to utilize a CO_2 insufflator, which warms the gas (if used) before it enters the body. It may be sufficient to change the insufflation site to a secondary port, once initial pneumoperitoneum has been achieved. The surgeon may also opt to warm the lens of the telescope by gently touching an intraabdominal structure. This also requires visualization.

Video monitor

High-resolution video monitors represent the end of the chain in endoscopy. They have become the windows of observation during minimally invasive surgery. Monitors should closely match the resolution quality of the camera being used. For example, a high-resolution monitor that meets or exceeds the horizontal resolution specification of the camera used should be purchased. The camera-monitor system will always have the resolution of the least-detailed element. Most monitors outperform the cameras, so discrimination in this purchase is less important. Determining the picture quality of monitors is difficult unless the monitors are side by side. The picture-tube design is the component that alters the monitor's picture quality. Monitors must be able to

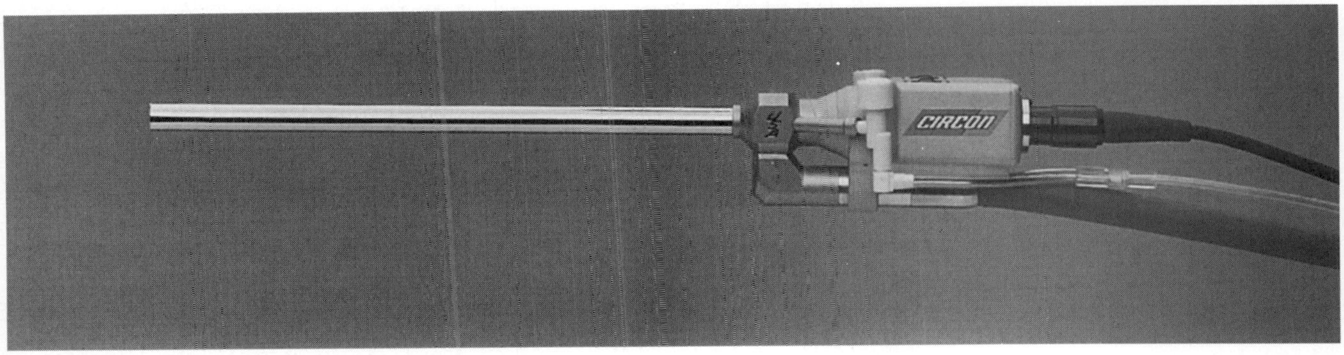

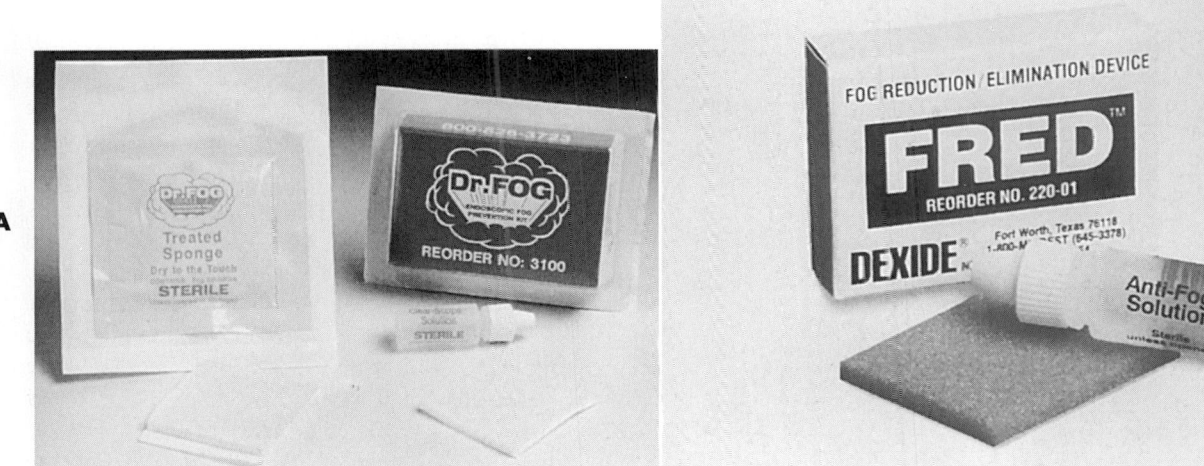

FIGURE 3-40   Videoscope for laparoscopy and thoracoscopy.

A   **B**

FIGURE 3-41   **A,** Dr. FOG sterile endoscopic fog inhibitor. Product is shown in its treated sponge and liquid forms.
B, FRED sterile antifog solution and sponge.

handle the camera/recorder format (composite, Y/C, or RGB).

Some monitors are designed primarily for home viewing. These all have softer colors and less sharpness for a warmer picture. Operating room monitors are designed for sharper imagery, increased edge enhancement, increased contrast, and true color reproduction. Video monitors used for endoscopy differ from televisions in that they are capable only of receiving input through direct cables. They usually cannot receive broadcast signals. Some have the capability of both but are not necessary for the operating room.

Many operative procedures require two video monitors. One is placed on each side of the patient so that both primary surgeon and assistant can view the screen comfortably and simultaneously. The second monitor is called the *slave monitor.* Abdominal and thoracic procedures are performed in this manner. Certain procedures can be accomplished by use of only one monitor. Whenever the monitor can be placed in a position of visibility to both surgeon and assistant comfortably, only one is necessary. This is usually the method of choice for urologists,

endoscopists, gynecologists, and otorhinolaryngologists. Most general surgeons require only one monitor whenever they perform surgery with the endoscope directed toward the patient's feet, (as in endoscopic herniorrhaphy). Of course, monitor selection, as with most equipment, also is based upon personal preference as well as educational training. It is important for the perioperative nurse to be flexible and prepared to help make this purchasing decision.

Monitors should be at least 13 inches (diagonal measurement of screen) for adequate visualization. When the endoscopic revolution began, most institutions purchased 19- or 20-inch main monitors and 13-inch slave monitors. Today many institutions are purchasing only 19- or 20-inch monitors. This size increases flexibility in usage as well as providing excellent visibility from most observational angles and distances.

When one is using only one monitor and a composite signal, the 75-ohm termination on-off switch must be in the on position. When one is using multiple monitors, the switch on the last monitor in line to receive the video signal should be in the on position and all others should be in the off position to enhance picture quality. Some monitors are self-terminating and do not have termination switches (Fig. 3-42).

Recording systems

There are recording devices that allow for archiving the surgical procedure or selected portions of it. The most commonly used is the video printer, or Mavigraph (Fig. 3-43). The video printer is similar to a Polaroid camera in that it takes still photography instantly. The printer stores the selected image and then reprints it onto special paper. Many units can be programed to print one, four, nine, and even 25 pictures on one piece of 5½ 8-inch paper in split-screen fashion. Comparisons can be made as the pathologic condition changes. Information such as patient name, date, time, and operating surgeon usually can also be superimposed on top of the print. These prints can be utilized for teaching purposes or remain as a permanent record on the patient's chart. Some patients are quite interested in seeing prints of "before and after" images of their condition.

Video disk recorders are available when one is considering storage and easy access to information. The disk recorder may very well become the documentation format of the future. To use this format one must also use a video printer because the images are limited to video.

The VCR is used when moving-image documentation is needed. The VCR format usually is required for teaching purposes and is not utilized as often as the printer is. Image quality is not so clear when one is using a commercial VCR. Professional-grade VCRs differ in that they do not have tuners and RF converters. Although rarely used, the best quality recorder available is the ¼-inch U-matic cassette recorder. It provides the best resolution available but also has advantages and disadvantages. It is an expensive piece of equipment, but it has low theft incentive because it cannot be used with standard ½-inch VCR tapes. This feature also becomes a deterrent because videos recorded in surgery are ¾-inch and usually cannot be reviewed in surgeons' offices or at home. If security and quality resolution are both issues, the best VCR is the professional grade ½-inch S-VHS. It costs more but is not subject to theft because it cannot be connected to household televisions. S-VHS recorders have the ability to record in the standard VHS format as well as the S-VHS format. When recorded in the S format, tapes can be played back only on an S-compatible VCR.

Storage systems

Space, storage capability, security, and required components determine the type and size of video storage carts needed. Purchasing a cart that can house multiple

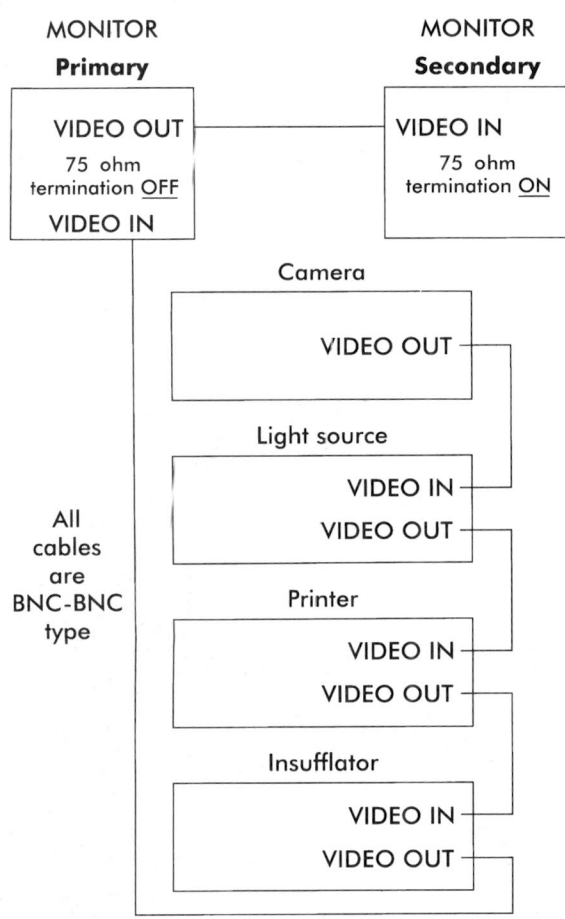

FIGURE 3-42   Basic wiring configuration.

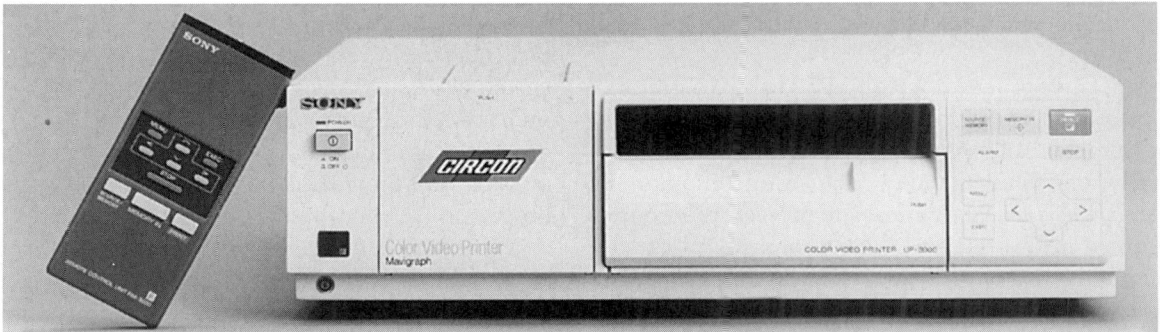

FIGURE 3-43   Video printer with remote control.

components of the video system is beneficial (Fig. 3-44). This eliminates clutter from multiple smaller carts and tables. It also eliminates the number of cord connections to wall outlets because most carts have power strips incorporated in the electrical setup. If the cart has a power strip, there is usually an on-off main switch located near the base. The power switch must be in the on position for the equipment that is plugged into the strip to work. Because of the location of the switch, it can easily be turned off during transport and cleaning. Time and embarrassment can be avoided if this switch position is checked before each use.

Articulating arms can be used as monitor mounts. Surgeon preference and room space determine if this option is necessary. If a surgical or treatment room has been set aside for endoscopy, the monitor can be suspended from the ceiling on a swivel mount. The mount should be placed in a location where the monitor can be easily and comfortably viewed as well as cleaned. Care must be taken to ensure the swivel mount will be able to withstand the weight of the monitor and other equipment.

Carts have either a locked (Fig. 3-45) or open (Fig. 3-46) shelf design. Institutional security will determine this need. Consideration of storage capability, tampering

with equipment, and key availability is important. A locked drawer may be an ideal area to store VCR tapes, printing paper, and the computer disk if these options are available. Carts should also be selected for ease in movement, component accessibility, and cleaning. They should include an optional storage bracket for E-cylinders when insufflation is required. Secondary (slave) monitor carts usually do not contain multiple shelving and cabinet components.

Robotics

Robotic devices to assist with holding and maneuvering a laparoscope have been introduced recently. Robotics were not created to replace surgical staff but to free up team members to perform other roles and attend to other responsibilities. The robotic arm minimizes problems with shaky video images and reduces miscommunication and misunderstanding between the surgeon and the assistant. The robot's movement is directly controlled by foot pedals,

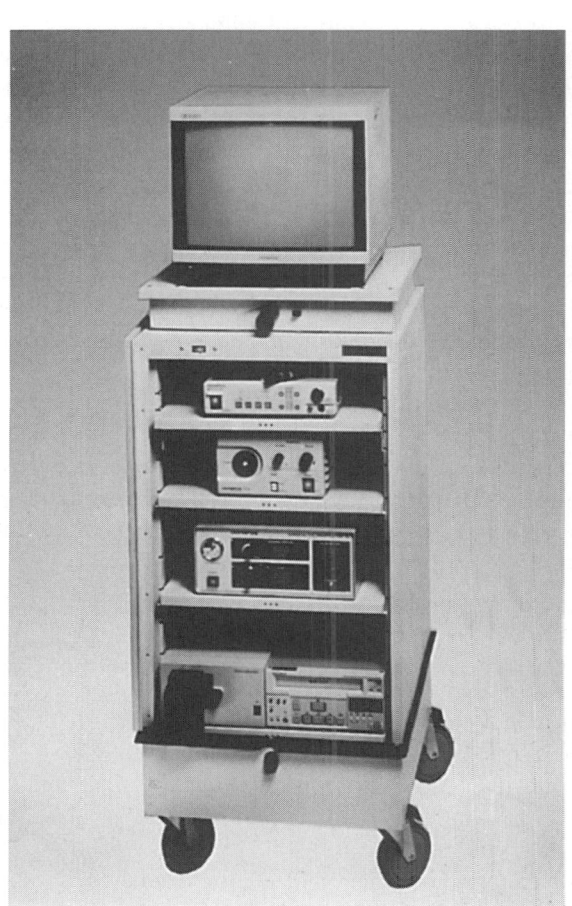

FIGURE 3-44 Video laparoscopy cart.

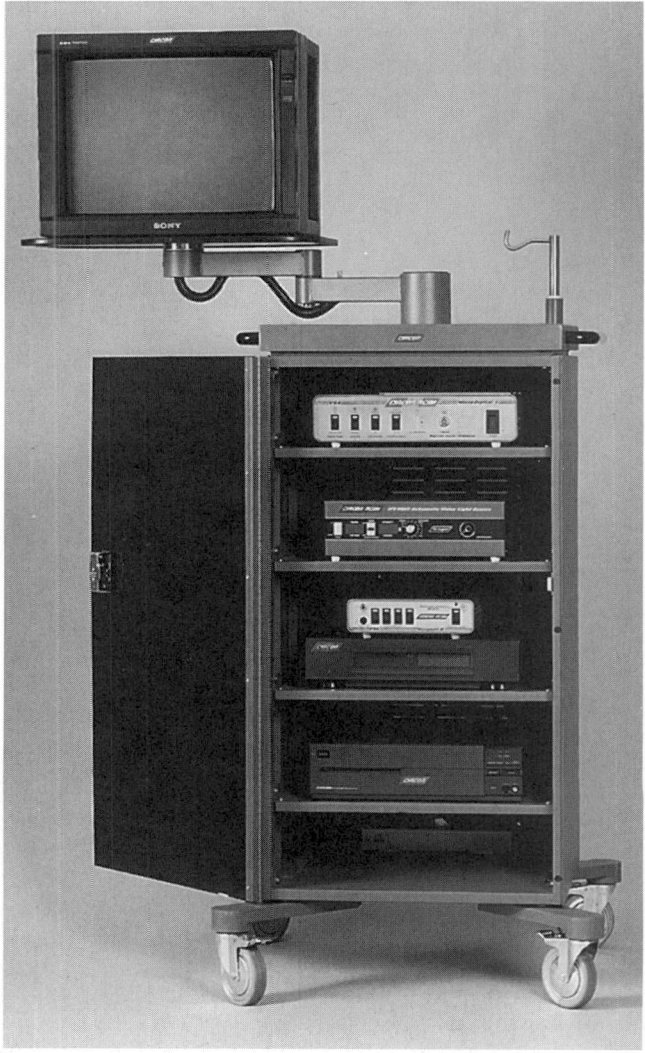

FIGURE 3-45 Video storage cart with swivel monitor arm and lockable door.

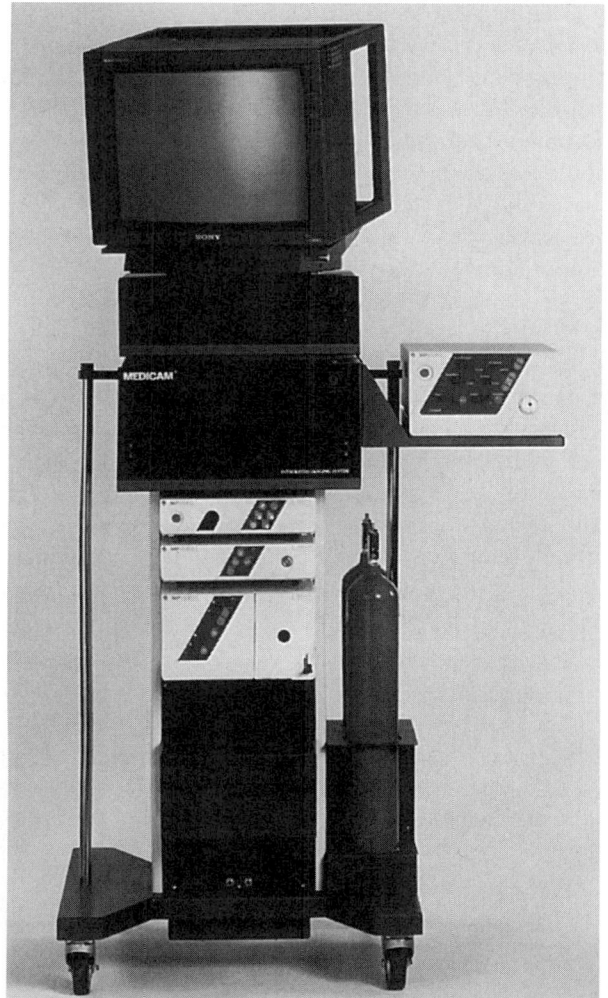

FIGURE 3-46 Combination lockable and open video storage cart. Cart also incorporates shelf for insufflator and bracket for CO_2 cylinder.

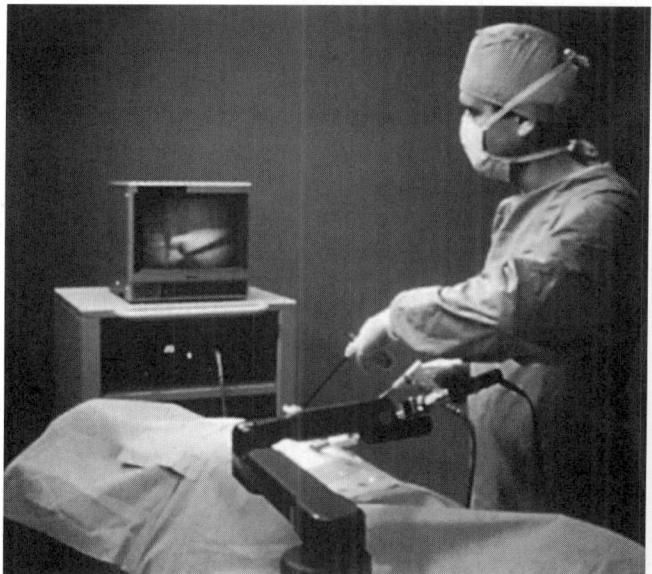

FIGURE 3-47 By being able to command the movement of the robotic arm, the surgeon has complete control over laparoscopic positioning.

- May shorten the procedure time by minimizing scope-positioning time
- Provides a steady image that enhances the video quality
- Ensures the same level of care for every patient (consistent scope positioning and movement) not always possible with different assistants
- Frees the physician's hands to perform other tasks

Videoconferencing

Videoconferencing is a new method to reach distant sites through communication, both audio and visual, occurring in real time. This new technology requires basic telecommunication equipment and a mode to transmit the communication signal to different sites.

The basic equipment pieces needed for most telecommunication that is done today are a monitor, camera, codec, and other various accessory devices. Each site participating in the telecommunication or videoconferencing needs a complete setup to be able to communicate with the people at the other sites.

The high-resolution monitor that is used for viewing endoscopic procedures in surgery or the endoscopy lab also can be used for videoconferencing. Sometimes two monitors are used for videoconferencing, one to view the distant site and one to display the view being sent to the other site. One monitor can be used if it has a picture-in-picture display capability. The main picture is usually of the distant site, whereas the smaller picture is of the near site.

A panoramic camera is needed at each site so that the participants can see each other. The image can be switched to the endoscopic camera so that the surgical target site can be viewed by those at the far end of the transmission.

hand-held control panels, and even voice activation (Fig. 3-47). This advancement in laparoscope stabilization and movement facilitates the procedure, promotes safety, and minimizes the time needed to perform the procedure.[2]

The robotic arm chassis houses the power system and the computerized control unit. An electromechanical positioner bar attaches to the surgical table and connects to the laparoscope with a magnetic coupling device. A sterile drape covers this arm to maintain a sterile field. The robotic arm maintains the laparoscope in proper orientation, a problem experienced with manual scope maneuvering.

Some of the advantages of using a robotic device for laparoscope positioning[2] are as follows:

- Minimizes fatigue associated with endoscope holding and moving
- Returns scope control to the physician
- Can accommodate quick scope movements through a computerized memory

A codec (compressor-decompressor or coder-decoder) at each site is needed to change or compress the analog information of the audio-visual message to a digital signal so that it can be transmitted to the distant site. The codec at the distant end then converts or decompresses the digital signal into analog information so that it can be viewed on the monitor.

Accessory equipment is helpful to enhance the video-conferencing experience. A remote microphone may be placed on the inside of the surgeon's gown so that he or she can narrate what is happening during a procedure. A video slate annotation pad can be used to draw, illustrate, and point out details on freeze-framed images that are transmitted. A document camera, VCR, laser printer, and remote assessment tools (such as stethoscope, otoscope) may also be used.

Connectivity between two sites or among many sites can be achieved through various modes of transmission. Satellite transmission provides a full-motion broadcast-quality picture for the audience but requires an uplink to a satellite and a downlink to the specific locations. This type of transmission can become very expensive, and the satellite time must be scheduled in advance. Satellite transmission is very useful for transmission to and from remote areas where terrestrial transmission is impossible.

Telephone lines also can be used as the mode of transmission for videoconferencing. Videoconferencing requires a bandwidth or carrying capacity measured in thousands of bits per second (kbps). For comparison, a normal telephone call requires 64 kbps. A T-1 telephone line consists of 24 voice channels or lines of 64 kbps each. Connectivity with a full T-1 line provides 1.54 Mbps (million, or mega-, bits per second). A fourth of the T-1 line, or 6 telephone lines (384 kbps), provides adequate bandwidth for many healthcare applications. Generally when a higher bandwidth is used, better image quality and transmission are achieved. When a lower bandwidth or fewer lines are used, visual anomalies may occur, such as motion artifact and unclear images.

Microwaves also provide videoconferencing transmission as the signals are sent from one tower to another. The limitation of this mode is that the towers must be in sight of each other to receive the transmissions. The transmission success is also subject to atmospheric disturbances.

Fiberoptic lines are also being used to provide transmission for videoconferencing. These lines consist of delicate thin glass fibers that transmit the information quickly and with great clarity.

Videoconferencing applications in healthcare include education, remote assessments and consultation, administrative meetings, product development, and other applications.

Since formal education and continuing education are the foundations of quality healthcare, providing education to and from distant sites has gained tremendous popularity during the past decade. Those practicing in remote

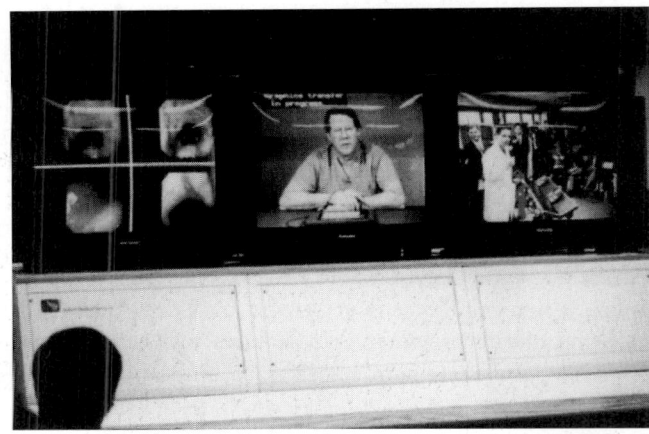

FIGURE 3-48   During a remote consultation, the physician is able to assess the patient's condition and discuss possible treatment options.

areas do not feel so isolated because educational video-conferencing is now available to many of these areas. Distant preceptorships have also been offered as one physician monitors and oversees another physician learning a new surgical technique or using advanced surgical instrumentation.

Remote consultation to evaluate patients at remote sites has been used as assessment technology has been introduced. A physician can assess heart sounds of a patient located at a distant place through the use of a telemedicine stethoscope. The retina of a diabetic patient can be viewed from afar by use of a special remote-assessment otoscope. A nurse practitioner located in a rural area can consult with a specialty physician located in downtown America to ask for advice for the treatment of a patient (Fig. 3-48).

Other videoconferencing applications include conducting administrative and other meetings to minimize travel expenses and time away from work. Product development can also be enhanced through videoconferencing. A company manufacturing surgical devices can communicate on a regular basis with key customers conducting trials of the devices. Device malfunctions and limitations can be assessed easily through real-time audio and video communication.

There are some issues that need to be addressed as videoconferencing becomes accepted universally. Standardization must be accomplished so that videoconferencing equipment can communicate and be compatible with each other. Some governmental and professional organization recommendations and mandates are guiding manufacturers to meet the agreed upon criteria so that this interactivity can be accomplished. Confidentiality is another concern as the popularity of this technology increases. Patient information, assessment data, and treatment results are being shared among providers by means of videoconferencing today. Patient confidentiality and privacy must be maintained. Private networks, advanced coding systems, and other technology can help address this issue. Practicing across state lines also has become a concern as videoconferencing in healthcare evolves. State boards of nursing, medicine, pharmacy, and other professions are currently addressing this situation and are proposing methods to facilitate licensing so that providers can practice across state boundaries. Finally reimbursement for remote consultation and assessment has been under scrutiny by many third-party carriers and reimbursers. Pilot project sites have been established by the Health Care Financing Administration (HCFA) to study this predicament. When reimbursement can be provided, more and more healthcare providers and facilities will get involved with videoconferencing for healthcare applications.

INSUFFLATION

To help in visualization of abdominal structures and safe operative functions during laparoscopic procedures, a pneumoperitoneum is created. To do so, the surgeon makes a paraumbilical incision and inserts an insufflation (Verres) needle into the abdomen (Fig. 3-49). Trendelenburg's position is selected to reduce the risk of visceral perforation. While the surgeon inserts the needle, he or she lifts up the patient's abdomen by grasping a fold of tissue on either side of the umbilicus. Preoperative patient education should include the possibility of finger-pinched bruising at the site where the abdominal tissue is grasped.

The needle safely enters the peritoneum if positioned at a 45-degree angle. Placement is usually confirmed by a negative bowel and blood return on aspiration and by a saline instillation that meets no resistance. This is a relatively blind procedure, since no scope can be introduced until pneumoperitoneum has been established.

Once needle confirmation is established, the insufflation tubing is connected and the process begun. One fills the peritoneal cavity starting at a low flow rate and then increases it to a high flow rate of at least 9 L/min ideally. Flow rate refers only to how quickly a predeter-

mined intraabdominal pressure can be reached. Intraabdominal pressure is the actual parameter that must be closely monitored and should be maintained between 14 and 16 mm Hg. High flow rates are important because during the procedure the insufflation CO_2 gas can escape. The more quickly it can be replaced, the less time will be spent waiting for the abdomen to be redistended.

CO_2 gas normally is used for insufflation. In the past, many gases including air, oxygen, and nitrous oxide have been tried. Air and oxygen have been eliminated as choices because of the risk of air embolism. Additionally, oxygen supports combustion, which could be fatal, since electrosurgery and often laser energy may be employed. Nitrous oxide has also been eliminated because of the potential risk of unpredictable, uncontrollable absorption. CO_2 does not support combustion, can be absorbed at rather large volumes per minute without serious side effects, and is also fairly inexpensive.

Insufflator control panels should monitor and display the following variables:

- Rate of flow
- Volume delivered
- Intraabdominal pressure

Selection of an insufflator that can accommodate a high flow rate is important. In the initial phases of the endoscopic revolution flow rates of 6 L/min were adequate. Today, because of the increased complexity of endoscopic procedures, increased numbers of secondary ports, and longer procedures (attributable to surgical complexity), pneumoperitoneum must be maintained over longer time frames. This requires flow rates of no less than 9 L/min. Those delivering 15 to 20 L/min are much more supportive and effective than those delivering at the slower rate.

Of even greater concern during the insufflator selection process should be the guarantee that an insufflator can and will continuously monitor insufflation pressure, stop the insufflation process once this predetermined set pressure has been reached, and release pressure if there is an inadvertent increase (called "taking a breath"). Intraabdominal pressure can be increased for reasons other than CO_2 insufflation; for example, leaning on the abdomen and additional gas introduction from other sources, such as a CO_2 laser, can inadvertently increase intraabdominal pressure.

Overpressurization can be extremely hazardous to the patient and must be avoided. Excess pressure can force CO_2 to diffuse into the blood, resulting in hypercarbia. End-tidal CO_2 monitoring becomes a critical assessment parameter to detect increased CO_2 absorption. Excess pressure also increases diaphragmatic pressure, which could result in gastric regurgitation and aspiration of stomach contents. It could also reduce intrathoracic space, resulting in decreased respiratory effort and cardiac output. The phrenic nerve innervates the diaphragm and is responsible for some motor activity associated with respiration. CO_2

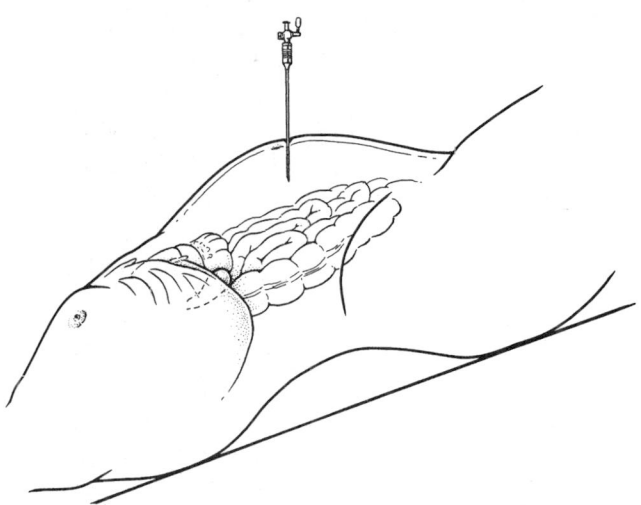

FIGURE 3-49 | Verres needle insertion into abdomen.

gas irritates this nerve, causing postoperative pain in the shoulder and neck. Although a common complaint, excessive pressure could cause tremendous discomfort as well as more severe nerve damage. The surgeon should press on the patient's abdomen to release as much residual CO_2 gas as possible before removal of the last trocar when the procedure is completed. Insufflators that automatically vent excessive CO_2 gas into the air provide assurance that many associated complications can be avoided.

A two-way disposable filter should be incorporated into the insufflation tubing (Fig. 3-50). This is one disposable supply that many institutions choose to purchase because of the time and energy required to reprocess reusable tubing. The filter provides patient protection from harmful gas-tank contamination such as chromium particles.[7] It also provides protection from the colonization of organisms in the insufflator itself. Without a filter, when the insufflator is turned on, organisms such as *Klebsiella*, *Pseudomonas*, and *Staphylococcus aureus* can be blown into the patient. This could jeopardize the patient's welfare and surgical outcome. It could be deadly for a very ill, elderly, or immunocompromised patient. The manufacturer's written instructions must be followed when implementing CO_2 insufflation (Box 3-2).

An insufflator capable of warning the operative team of insufflation parameter problems throughout the procedure is highly desirable. If these parameters are periodically visualized on the monitor, information can be immediately processed and action taken. Alarms that sound when there is an alteration in predetermined parameters also call attention to the need for immediate intervention (Fig. 3-51), such as an alarm ringing and a monitor blinking "Gas supply low." An alarm sounding when overpressurization occurs from a secondary source (such as by leaning on the abdomen) also alerts the team of the need for corrective action.

Insufflators are also available with CO_2 warming devices (Fig. 3-52). Cylinder CO_2 is in liquid form, and as it is released, it expands into a gas. During this conversion from liquid to gas, energy is lost, and the gas becomes colder. The higher the flow, the colder the gas.[8] Some warming does occur as the gas travels through the insufflation tubing. Use of cold CO_2 gas can easily cause a decrease in patient temperature, especially with prolonged laparoscopy. Although there are many factors that contribute to the reduction of body temperature during endoscopic procedures (such as cold irrigation, room temperature, surface exposure, length of the procedure, patient's age and medical history, anesthetic choice), cold CO_2 represents an additional one. The best way to reduce patient heat loss is to address all the variables and intervene wherever possible.

Cold CO_2 gas also contributes to the fogging of telescope lenses. Fogging occurs whenever a cold instrument enters the warm, moist environment of the body. Some methods to reduce this condensation process have

been previously discussed. Moving the insufflation site to a secondary port away from the scope is often sufficient.

ENERGIES USED DURING SURGERY

Laser

One of the healthcare revolutions that has occurred in the last three decades is the birth and evolution of an amazing tool called the laser. The perioperative nurse today must be keenly aware of the expanded responsibilities associated with laser applications. The laser has radically changed surgery by making possible less invasive procedures, thus decreasing inpatient hospitalization, diminishing postoperative complications, and saving healthcare dollars.

Laser biophysics

During the early 1900s Albert Einstein first described the theory that involved the stimulation of matter to cause

BOX 3-2	Steps to Reduce Cross-Contamination of Patient and Insufflator During CO_2 Insufflation Procedures

- Flush insufflator and tubing with CO_2 gas before attaching to patient.
- Use a disposable hydrophobic filter on insufflation tubing. Discard after procedure.
- Disconnect tubing from insufflator *before* turning off, at end of procedure.
- Keep insufflator *elevated* above the patient to prevent fluid backflow.

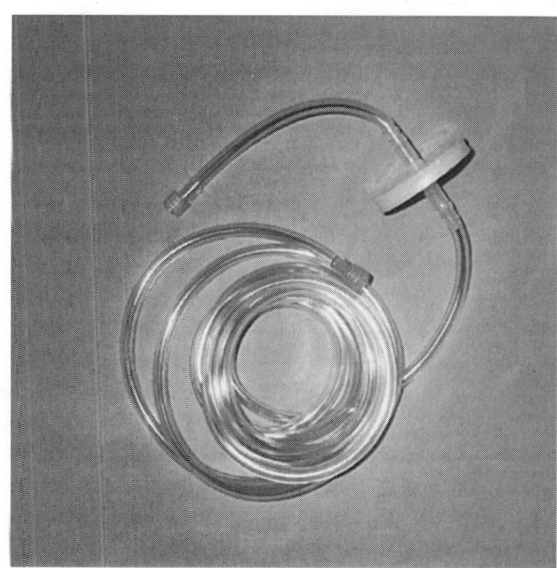

FIGURE 3-50 Disposable insufflation tubing with two-way filter.

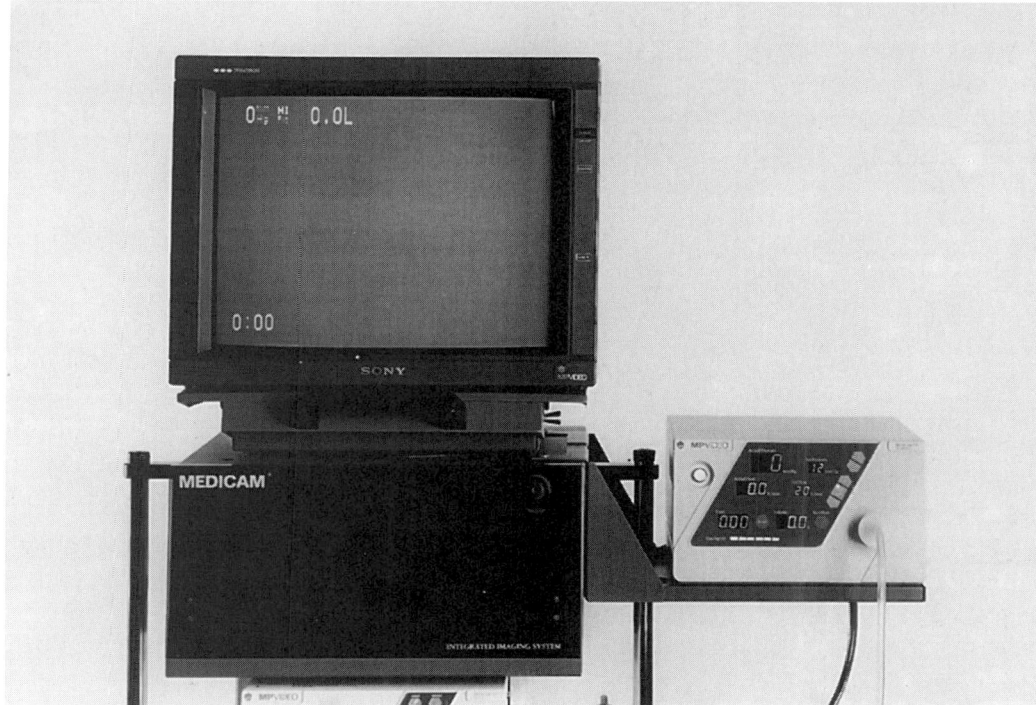

FIGURE 3-51   Insufflation parameters visualized on TV monitor can be immediately processed.

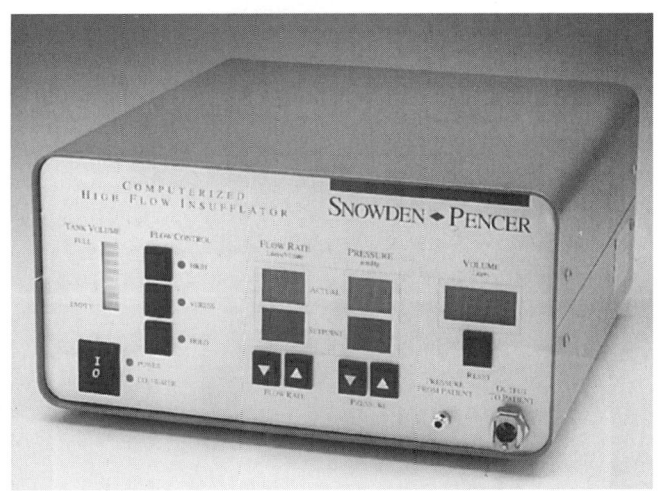

FIGURE 3-52   Computerized high-flow insufflator with CO_2 warmer.

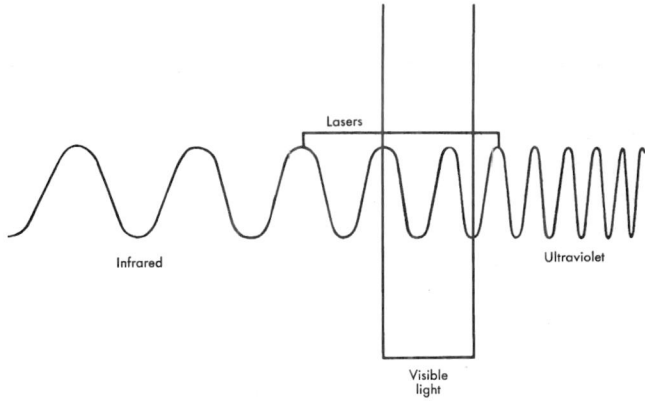

FIGURE 3-53   The electromagnetic spectrum.

the release of energy. In 1958 Schawlow and Townes used this concept of stimulated emission to develop the principle of laser, which is an acronym for light amplification by the stimulated emission of radiation.

In 1962 Theodore Maiman developed the first laser for medicine and surgery using a ruby crystal. The ruby laser was utilized for dermatologic applications and for retinal photocoagulation in patients with diabetic retinopathy. It was not very efficient, however. Other lasers, such as the argon, carbon dioxide, Nd:YAG, holmium, and diode lasers, have been developed and are now being used in many surgical disciplines. Newer lasers, such as the excimer and free-electron lasers, continue to be investigated and refined for clinical use. Advancements in laser technology have provided the physician with a precision tool for cutting, coagulating, vaporizing, and welding tissue during surgical intervention.

Principles of Light

Laser is an acronym that describes a process in which light energy is produced. This term also refers to the device that generates the laser energy.

Light is a form of electromagnetic energy that can be graphically illustrated on a continuum known as the

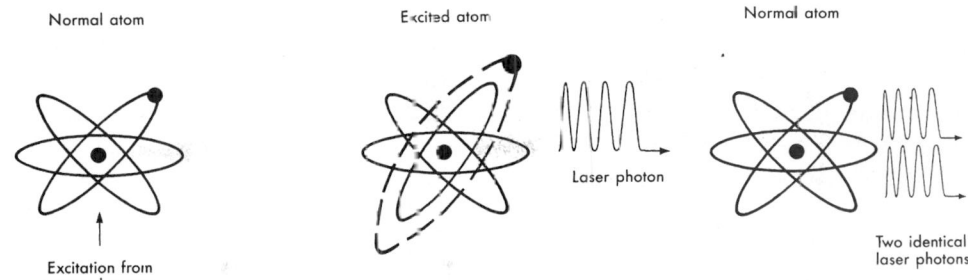

FIGURE 3-54 Laser energy is produced when an external source excites the atom to emit a photon spontaneously. This photon can then "stimulate" the emission of two identical photons.

electromagnetic spectrum (Fig. 3-53). The unit of measurement that delineates the continuum is called a *wavelength*, which is the distance between two successive peaks of a wave. The wavelength determines color and is usually measured in nanometers (10^{-9} m) or micrometers (1000 nm). The various wavelengths of laser energy extend from the shorter waves in the ultraviolet area to the longer waves in the infrared region along this perpetual line. The visible laser wavelengths occupy only a small portion of this continuum. The radiation of laser technology is nonionizing in that it does not present the hazard of cellular DNA disruption through continual tissue exposure. Therefore pregnant women can work with lasers because laser energy does not produce harmful ionizing radiation.

Briefly, the laser functions in the following way. A negatively charged electron orbits a positively charged nucleus while the atom is in its ground or resting state, which is at its lowest possible level of energy. An outside source of energy can excite the atom and cause an electron to jump to a higher, less-stable, orbit. The electron almost immediately returns to its stable orbit, and the atom resumes its normal resting state. As this process occurs, a tiny bundle of surplus energy called a *photon* is spontaneously emitted. If the photon is close to another atom still in the excited state, it then interacts with this atom. The photon triggers the excited second atom to return to its resting state, and in this process another photon of laser light is emitted. These two photons of identical energy then travel together. Thus the process of stimulated emission has occurred, and laser energy has been initially formed (Fig. 3-54).

This activity occurs in the resonating chamber of the laser, where the lasing medium is contained. The name of the laser is usually derived from the actual medium that causes the lasing action. The photons that are generated during the stimulated emission process are reflected back and forth between mirrors at each end of the resonating chamber as the process is amplified, until the number of excited atoms surpasses the number of resting atoms. This is known as *population inversion*. One of the mirrors in the chamber is partially reflective and, when activated, allows a stream of laser photons to escape the unit. These photons

are then introduced to the target area by means of a specific delivery system.

Characteristics of Laser Light

Three distinct characteristics distinguish laser light from ordinary light. Laser light is monochromatic, collimated, and coherent.

Monochromatic light is composed of photons of the same wavelength or color. In contrast, ordinary light consists of many different colors or wavelengths.

A collimated laser beam consists of waves parallel to each other that do not diverge significantly, thus minimizing any loss of power. When a collimated beam is passed through a lens, the light is focused into a tiny spot that tremendously concentrates the energy. In comparison, the light waves from a flashlight are not parallel and lose intensity as they travel away from the source. A lens cannot easily focus these noncollimated waves to concentrate the light into a small area.

Laser light is coherent—all the waves are orderly and in phase with each other as they travel in the same direction. All peaks and troughs of the waves are opposite each other in both time and space. This property provides an additive effect that gives the laser beam power. Ordinary light is incoherent, since the waves radiate away from the source without being in phase or in an orderly pattern.

Laser Power

The power, or energy, of a laser beam is measured in watts. One of the most critical factors in laser application is the concept of power density, or irradiance of the beam. Power density is the amount of power that is concentrated within an area and is described by the following formula:

$$\text{Power density} = \frac{\text{Watts}}{\text{Spot size (cm}^2)}$$

The spot size of the laser beam can be controlled when the beam is passed through a special lens that causes the beam to converge. The focal configuration of the lens determines at what distance from the lens the beam will be most intense; this is called the *focal point*. If the beam is defocused into a larger spot size, the laser energy is spread over a greater area, thus decreasing the intensity or power density of the beam. In contrast, a small spot size of the beam concentrates the power into a smaller area, thus increasing the intensity or power density of the beam. When the power density is increased, the beam has the potential for causing a greater depth of penetration into the tissue.

A joule is the unit of measurement used to describe the total energy used. A joule is expressed by the power multiplied by the time duration of beam exposure. Fluence is a term that involves the power and duration of exposure of the beam and measures the specific amount of energy that is delivered to the tissue. The following equation calculates the fluence:

$$\text{Fluence} = \frac{\text{Watts} \times \text{Duration time}}{\text{Spot size (cm}^2)}$$

The transverse electromagnetic mode (TEM) determines the precision of the beam by the distribution of the power over the spot area. The most precise or fundamental mode, TEM_{00}, evenly distributes the power over an area, with the most concentrated energy in the center and the intensity of the beam decreasing toward the periphery.

Tissue Interaction

When laser energy is delivered to the target area, four different interactions can occur: reflection, scattering, transmission, or absorption (Fig. 3-55). The extent of the reaction of the beam on the target depends on the laser wavelength, power settings, spot size, length of time the beam is in contact with the tissue, and the characteristics of the tissue.

Reflection of the laser beam occurs when the direction of the beam is changed after it contacts an area. Specular reflection occurs when the angle of the incoming light is equal to the angle of the reflected light. Laser light can be intentionally reflected in this manner off a reflective mirror to contact hard-to-reach areas. This type of reflection can also pose safety problems by inadvertently striking untargeted areas if it is not controlled at all times.

Scattering of the laser light occurs when the beam spreads over a large area as the tissue causes the beam to disperse. The intensity of the beam is decreased as the waves travel in different directions. The Nd:YAG laser beam can backscatter up an endoscope and possibly cause damage to the end of the scope, the optics, or the operator's eye.

Transmission of the laser beam occurs when the beam passes through fluids or tissue without thermally affecting the area. For example, the argon beam can be transmitted through the clear fluids and structures of the eye to the retina and cause thermal photocoagulation. The cornea, lens, and vitreous are unaffected by the transmission of the beam.

Absorption of the laser light results when the tissue is altered from the impingement of the beam. This reaction is usually thermal but can sometimes be acoustic. The consistency, color, and water content of the target tissue often determine the rate of absorption of the laser energy. The laser wavelength also affects the absorption of the beam. Certain laser light, such as that from the argon laser, is highly absorbed by pigmented tissues. The CO_2 laser, however, is independent of color-selective absorption. The CO_2 laser light is absorbed superficially by tissue to a shallow depth of approximately 0.1 to 0.2 mm, whereas the holmium laser beam is absorbed to about 0.4 to 0.6 mm. Argon laser light is readily absorbed by pigmented tissue to a depth of approximately 1 to 2 mm, whereas that of the noncontact Nd:YAG laser beam is

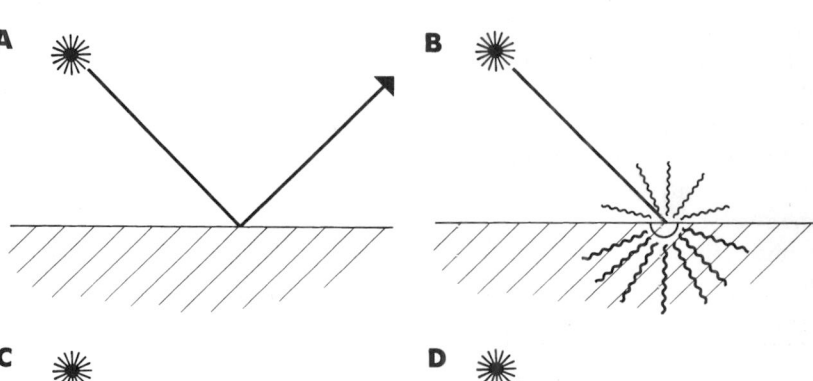
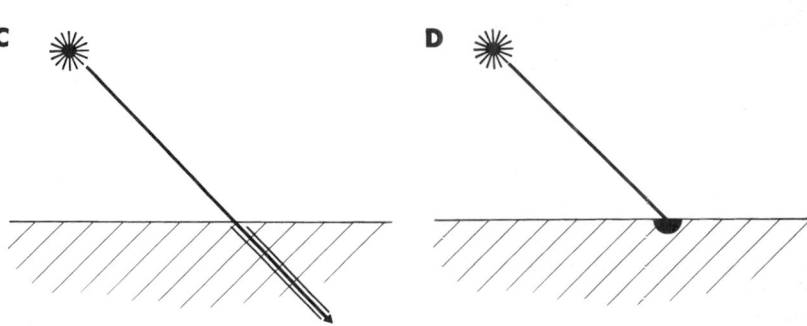

FIGURE 3-55 Laser tissue interaction: **A,** Reflection. **B,** Scattering. **C,** Transmission. **D,** Absorption.

more readily absorbed by darkened tissue to a depth of 3 to 5 mm.

Tissue reaction becomes more pronounced as the temperature of the impingement area increases (Table 3-2). During this thermal reaction the laser energy is absorbed, causing the cellular water to be heated. Intracellular protein is destroyed; as the temperature rises, the water inside the cell turns to steam. Eventually the membrane ruptures from increased pressure, spewing cellular debris and plume (smoke) from the tissue. The surrounding tissue is also heated because it borders the impingement site. The degree of adjacent tissue damage depends on the duration of the laser-beam exposure that causes the thermal injury.

Laser systems

New laser systems are being introduced into healthcare regularly. Constant efforts by researchers and physicians to explore the use of different wavelengths are changing surgical approaches in a variety of specialties. Table 3-3 describes some of the more popular lasers used in medicine and surgery today.

Parts of a Laser System

The five major components of a laser system are the laser head, excitation source, ancillary components, control panel, and delivery system.[3] When a laser malfunctions, an organized investigation of each of these parts (Fig. 3-56) can usually determine the source of the problem.

The laser head, or resonating chamber, is the part where the laser energy is generated and amplified. The laser head contains the active medium or substance that actually produces the photons that generate the laser light. The active medium can be a gas (CO_2 or argon), a solid (Nd:YAG), a liquid (tunable dye), or a semiconductor crystal (diode).

The excitation source supplies the energy to excite the active medium in the laser head. Different sources include flash lamps, electricity, radio waves, battery, chemicals, and other laser systems. For example, the CO_2 laser gas is excited by electrical current or radio waves, and the Nd:YAG laser crystal is excited by flash lamps.

The ancillary components are the other laser parts that are needed to help produce the laser energy. A cooling system maintains the appropriate temperature of the laser head to keep the unit from overheating. Usually lasers are either air cooled or water cooled. A vacuum pump may be required in a CO_2 laser to pull the gas mixture from an external cylinder into the laser head for laser light production.

The control panel consists of the board that regulates the delivery of laser energy. Various power settings, modes, durations, and other parameters can be selected as desired. Many laser panels are now computerized, allowing the laser to be quickly and accurately controlled. Wireless control modules that can be placed into a sterile plastic bag have been developed so that the surgical team can control the laser from the operating field. The laser team should be exceedingly familiar with the operation of the laser control panel or module.

The delivery system of the laser is the device or accessory that actually conducts the laser energy from the laser head to the target area. CO_2 laser energy is usually delivered to the tissue through an articulated arm with a series of special mirrors at each joint. Argon and Nd:YAG lasers deliver energy through a fiber system. Advancements

TABLE 3-3 | **Description of Laser Color and Wavelength**

LASER	COLOR	WAVELENGTH (mm)
Excimer	Ultraviolet	
ArF		193
KrCl		222
KrF		248
XeCl		308
XeF		351
Helium-cadmium		325
Argon	Blue	488
	Green	515
Frequency-doubled YAG (KTP)	Green	532
Krypton	Green	531
	Yellow	568
	Red	647
Dye laser	Variable with dyes	
	Red	632
	Yellow	577-585
Gold vapor	Red	628
Helium neon	Red	632
Ruby	Deep red	694
Nd:YAG	Infrared	1064
		1318
Holmium-YAG	Infrared	2100
Erbium-YAG	Infrared	2900
Carbon dioxide	Infrared	10,600

From Ball, K. (1995). *Lasers: the perioperative challenge* (ed. 2), St. Louis: Mosby.
KTP, Potassium titanyl phosphate crystal.

TABLE 3-2 | **Tissue Changes with Temperature Increases**

TEMPERATURE	VISUAL CHANGE	BIOLOGIC CHANGE
37°-60° C	No visual change	Warming, welding
60°-65° C	Blanching	Coagulation
65°-90° C	White/grey	Protein denaturization
90°-100° C	Puckering	Drying
100° C	Smoke plume	Vaporization, carbonization

From Ball, K. (1995). *Lasers: the perioperative challenge* (ed. 2), St. Louis: Mosby.

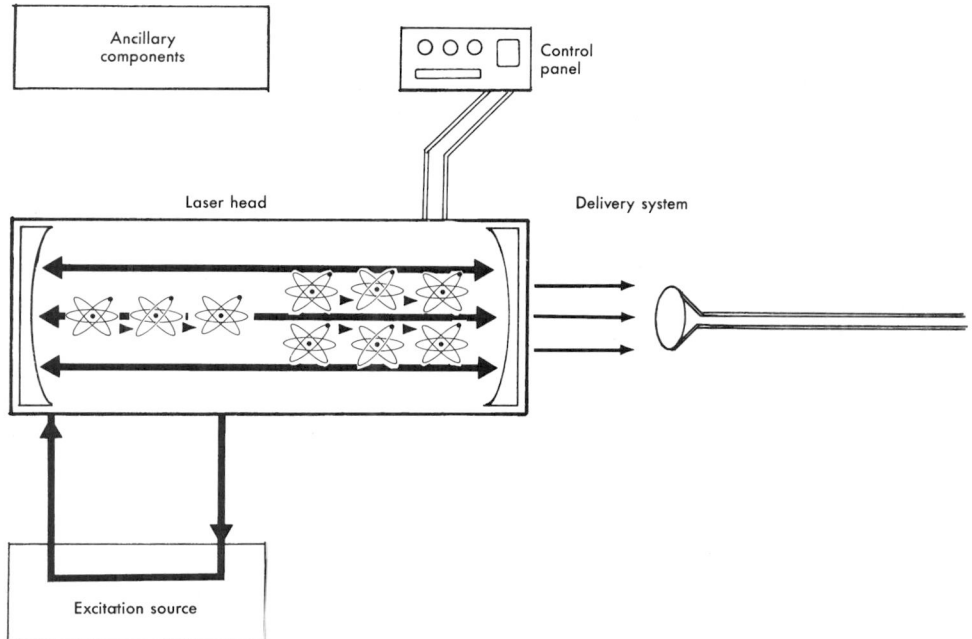

FIGURE 3-56   Parts of a laser system.

in laser technology are refining delivery systems to make them more adaptable, convenient, and user friendly.

CO_2 Laser

The CO_2 laser is versatile and widely used. Its wavelength of 10,600 nm is located in the infrared region of the electromagnetic spectrum. Because this light is invisible, a visible helium-neon laser beam is usually transmitted coaxially with the CO_2 laser energy to serve as an aiming beam.

The CO_2 laser is characterized by its superficial tissue interaction (0.1 to 0.2 mm), since the beam is highly absorbed by water. The degree of tissue response is related to the amount of heat buildup from the absorption. Therefore, the longer the CO_2 beam is in contact with the tissue, as with other laser wavelengths, the more destruction is noted and a greater depth of penetration can be achieved. The tissue reaction is quite visible and has been described as "what you see is what you get." The CO_2 beam is independent of color selectivity, meaning that lighter tissue absorbs the beam as readily as darker tissue.

Currently two types of CO_2 lasers that use electricity or radio waves as the excitation source are available. The free-flowing CO_2 laser system requires an external cylinder of a special laser gas mixture of carbon dioxide, helium, and nitrogen. The concentrations of these gases must be specific to the particular laser unit so that the laser operates properly. The gas is pulled into the laser head by a vacuum pump, laser energy is generated, and then harmless disassociated by-products are discharged from the unit. The laser gas cylinder is replaced when empty.

The other type of CO_2 laser is the sealed-tube system, which contains the special mixture of carbon dioxide, helium, and nitrogen within a tube that is sealed. A catalyst is added to the tube to cause regeneration of the mixture so that lasing action can be produced again. The shelf life (functional period) of this type of tube is usually from 1 to 4 years. At the end of this time the tube can be reprocessed by the manufacturer to replace the special gas and catalyst mixture.

With both types of CO_2 lasers the laser beam is delivered to the target area through a hollow tube called an *articulated arm*. Mirrors are positioned within the arm to reflect the laser energy forward. Because the helium-neon aiming beam runs coaxially with the CO_2 beam, care must be taken when moving the laser so that the mirrors are not jarred out of alignment.

The articulated arm can be attached to a microscope or a special handpiece. A lens system within these attachments causes the beam to converge at the focal point. A special coating on the lens maintains the beam's integrity and intensity and must be cared for carefully so that the coating is not disrupted. The manufacturer's instructions that provide information on the appropriate lens care must be followed closely. The beam is most intense at the focal point because all the energy is concentrated into a very small spot. The size of the spot can be changed by focusing or defocusing of the lens to allow the spot to become larger or smaller. Sometimes tubing is connected to the handpiece or microscope adapter to conduct a purge gas or compressed air that blows the laser smoke away, thus keeping the lens cool and free from debris.

The CO_2 laser beam can also be conducted through a hollow flexible tube that allows the energy to "wiggle" down its path by being reflected off the surface of the inner lumen. Because of this reflection, some of the power of the beam is lost as it leaves this delivery device. Solid fibers that will conduct the CO_2 wavelength to the target site are currently being developed.

The CO_2 laser energy can be delivered to tissue in a variety of modes. The continuous mode allows the laser energy to be delivered continuously as long as the foot pedal is depressed. The timed mode delivers the energy either one pulse at a time or in a repeat manner that specifically controls the duration of exposure. The superpulse mode delivers the energy in an extremely quick sequence of interrupted pulses that may appear to be a continuous mode. The energy may peak from 5 to 10 times higher than the desired wattage, but the duration of exposure is extremely limited, thus providing great precision. This type of interaction allows the adjacent tissue to cool so that tissue destruction is minimized.

Argon Laser

The argon laser is another popular laser system. This laser produces an intense, visible blue-green light of approximately 488 and 515 nm respectively. In clinical applications this combination of light wavelengths allows more complete tissue absorption. The depth of penetration is usually 1 to 2 mm. The aiming system is low-power argon-laser energy because the beam is visible.

The argon energy is highly absorbed by hemoglobin, melanin, and other similar pigmentation and is less absorbed by lighter tissue. The absorbed laser energy is then converted to heat to cause coagulation or vaporization. Because of the high color selectivity of the beam, adjacent tissue injury is reduced significantly when the laser is being used on a localized pigmented area.

The argon wavelength is transmitted through clear fluids and structures. The argon laser energy is delivered to the target area through a fiber system. The fiber can be attached to a slit lamp, microscope, or handpiece, depending on the surgical approach. Because the argon light diverges 10 to 14 degrees when leaving the fiber, the size of the spot can be altered by changing the distance of the fiber tip to the tissue. Special handpieces that contain an internal lens can be adjusted to change the spot size of the beam.

Nd:YAG Laser

The neodymium:yttrium-aluminum-garnet (Nd:YAG) laser wavelength is in the infrared region of the electromagnetic spectrum at approximately 1064 nm. This invisible wave is usually accompanied by a visible helium-neon beam or other colored light, such as white light, to provide an aiming source. The Nd:YAG laser has a solid crystal of yttrium-aluminum-garnet that is doped with neodymium, which produces the lasing energy when exposed to bright flash lamps.

The Nd:YAG wavelength, like the argon wavelength, is transmitted through clear fluids and structures and is more highly absorbed by darker tissue. This laser light tends to scatter within the tissue and cause thermal damage to approximately 5 mm. Tissue absorption produces a homogeneous coagulative effect as tissue is heated to the point of coagulation without vaporization occurring. The Nd:YAG beam can easily backscatter, posing an eye-safety concern when used through an endoscope.

The Nd:YAG energy is delivered to the tissue through a fiber system. The core fiber, usually made of quartz, is surrounded by a Teflon silicone coating or cladding that keeps the light in. This is known as a bare fiber. If the bare fiber is encased by a catheter sheath, a purge gas, air, or fluid can be conducted down the length of the fiber. This purge is used to cool the fiber tip and keep debris from accumulating.

The Nd:YAG laser wavelength can be delivered to the tissue in a noncontact mode, meaning that the fiber does not touch the tissue.

Nd:YAG laser energy can also be delivered to the tissue using the contact method. A synthetic sapphire contact probe or scalpel can be attached to the end of a fiber with a special connector to deliver the Nd:YAG energy directly to the tissue in a more concentrated manner. The depth of penetration then is limited to less than 1 mm.[6] These contact tips are available in a variety of configurations. Depending on the desired tissue effects, the appropriate contact tip is chosen. A scalpel is used to cut, and a rounded probe is used to vaporize. A flat probe may be used to coagulate tissue. The end of the quartz fiber may also be sculpted into a configuration that can be used in direct contact with the tissue. Contact technology provides precision, since the power output of the beam is confined to a very small area. It causes less thermal buildup, so adjacent tissue is relatively unaffected. The beam does not scatter as readily as the free Nd:YAG energy, and less plume is generated.

Another Nd:YAG wavelength being investigated is in the 1318 nm range. This laser causes minimal heat dissipation and allows greater cutting precision than the 1064 nm one does.

Besides the continuous-mode Nd:YAG laser, a special pulsed-mode Nd:YAG laser for ophthalmologic applications delivers the energy to the tissue in extremely short pulsations of nanoseconds. This laser works with an acoustic effect instead of a thermal effect. For example, a clouded membrane behind an artificial lens implant can be ruptured quickly and painlessly with this Nd:YAG laser beam through the production of an acoustic effect at the target site.

The frequency-doubled YAG laser is also popular in healthcare today. An Nd:YAG beam of 1064 nm is passed through a potassium titanyl phosphate (KTP) crystal to produce an intense green laser light of 532 nm. This process of delivering the Nd:YAG incident beam of 1064 nm through the KTP crystal shortens the wavelength in half, to 532 nm, while doubling the beam's frequency. The emergent beam then is visible. If the original Nd:YAG beam is once again desired, the crystal is rotated out of the way when a button is pressed on the control panel.

The 532 nm wavelength responds to tissue in the same manner as the argon beam. It is very color selective and is highly absorbed by hemoglobin, melanin, and other similar pigmentations. The beam is conducted to tissue through a fiber, and this wavelength can also be transmitted through clear solutions and structures. The depth of penetration is approximately 1 to 2 mm.

Holmium:YAG Laser

Another YAG laser that has been widely accepted into the surgical arena today is the holmium:YAG laser. The YAG crystal is doped with holmium, which is a rare earth element. This laser produces a wavelength of 2100 nm and is delivered to the tissue in a quick pulsed mode. The holmium wavelength is absorbed intensely by water, so the depth of penetration is limited to approximately 0.4 to 0.6 mm. It has many of the same benefits of CO_2 laser technology in that it can ablate tissue very precisely but it can also be conducted to the target through a flexible fiber. This wavelength can be delivered to tissues in a fluid environment, since it produces a vapor bubble that transmits the laser energy. If the fiber is held almost in contact or directly in contact with the tissue, cutting occurs. If sculpting or ablating is needed, the fiber is held at a distance of approximately 2 mm from the target. Adjacent tissue is left significantly unharmed, thus enhancing the precision of this wavelength.

Other Laser Systems

The tunable dye laser allows the operator to dial in the desired wavelength within a limited range, such as 400 to 1000 nm. By changing dyes or other certain parameters, one can change the wavelength. Tunable dye lasers produce a range of colors by exposing a liquid dye to an intense light source, such as an argon laser beam. The dye then absorbs the laser light and fluoresces over a broad spectrum of colors. By using special crystal prisms, diffraction gratings, or birefringent filters within the laser, a specific wavelength can be produced.

This laser has become very popular in treating pigmented dermatologic conditions. A yellow laser beam can be generated at 585 nm, which is readily absorbed by hemoglobin and less absorbed by the epidermal melanin, thus resulting in less scarring. The tunable dye lasers have been refined to provide very quick pulsations in milliseconds that allow increased power to be used. Less adjacent tissue damage is realized with the shorter durations of exposure, and greater tissue response occurs through the increased wattage used. Advancements to produce an array of different wavelengths with a variety of pulsation modes are continually being developed to successfully treat dermatologic conditions.

The excimer laser derives its name through the use of an active medium that is an excited dimer. This laser is also known as a rare gas-*n*-halide laser in that it combines a rare gas with a halide, usually a halide-oxide or a halide-halide dimer. The dimeric media are excited to emit the laser energy. Depending on the chemical composition of the active medium, a variety of the shorter ultraviolet wavelengths can be produced. Four of the most popular wavelengths are argon fluoride (ArF) at 193 nm, krypton fluoride (KrF) at 248 nm, xenon chloride (XeCl) at 308 nm, and xenon fluoride (XeF) at 351 nm. One of the hazards of the excimer laser is that these gases are extremely toxic; therefore appropriate laser housings and exhausts must be employed. Some excimer lasers are quite large, so more floor space should be planned for.

Excimer lasers are popular for their significant ablative capabilities. The beam penetrates less than 1 mm into the tissue and disassociates the molecular bonds of the cells. There is no significant damage to the adjacent tissue because the beam provides a sharp, clean cutting action at the target site without any thermal damage. Therefore this laser has been used very successfully to sculpt corneas for refractive purposes and to ablate plaque in arteries. Other applications continue to be developed and researched for FDA approval.

Diode lasers, since they are extremely compact and reliable, are being used in some consumer products, such as video disk players and computers. This technology is now being used for surgical lasers with approximately 30 watts of output in the 750 to 950 nm range. With the efficiency, small size, and reliability of these systems, increasing medical applications can be anticipated in the near future. With the advent of the high-power semiconductor diode lasers in the gallium arsenide family (840 to 910 nm), smaller laser photocoagulators for ophthalmic, urologic, and other applications have been developed. This laser energy can be delivered directly to the tissue through a fiber or can be attached to an existing slit lamp microscope for ophthalmic applications. Other clinical applications that allow this type of laser to be used in place of other wavelengths, such as the Nd:YAG laser, are being introduced.

As technology continues to advance, laser wavelengths are being combined into one unit so that a selection of wavelengths, such as the Nd:YAG or holmium:YAG, can easily be used during a procedure. The delivery systems must be compatible for this type of setup. A variety of wavelengths is being developed as other active media are being explored. New delivery systems are being perfected as different material combinations that will more efficiently conduct the laser energy to the tissue are being discovered.

Benefits of laser technology

Laser technology continues to evolve as more surgical applications are developed. Once controversial the laser has now become a respected and valued medical device that is revolutionizing surgery. As physicians become more adept in laser applications, utilization continues to grow. The laser has fostered the development of new minimally invasive procedures and endoscopic techniques. The true potential of the laser has yet to be realized as healthcare practitioners explore different applications of laser technology. The following list describes some of the advantages that have been associated with laser technology, depending on the procedure performed.

- Seals small blood vessels (less intraoperative and postoperative blood loss)
- Seals lymphatics (decreases postoperative edema and the chance of spread of malignant cells in the lymphatic system)
- Seals nerve endings (on selective procedures, to decrease postoperative pain)
- Sterilizes tissue (from the heat generated at the laser tissue impingement site)
- Decreases postoperative stenosis (by decreasing the amount of scarring that could lead to stenosis)
- Produces minimal tissue damage (from precision of the laser beam).
- Reduces operative and anesthesia time
- Allows shift to more ambulatory surgery procedures
- Allows more use of local anesthesia instead of general anesthesia
- Provides quicker recovery and return to daily activities

As new laser technology is introduced and refined, perioperative nurses have the responsibility of expanding their knowledge base by keeping current with the safety requirements and operation of these systems. Laser technology is a challenge to the perioperative nurse's professional growth. It offers the opportunity to develop creative methods of perioperative nursing practice to deliver high-quality patient care during laser procedures. The full potential of laser use is still being realized, and the perioperative nurse continues to have an instrumental role in the development of this technology.

Laser safety

Because laser systems are capable of concentrating high amounts of energy within very small areas, they present hazards. Safe and appropriate use of the laser during surgical intervention is the responsibility of the entire healthcare team. Each member must be acutely aware of the many controls needed to prevent accidental injury. Often the laser team member is given the responsibility and authority to shut down the laser system if safety policies are not being followed.

The laser is a class III medical device that is subdivided into four subclasses. The lasers designated as subclass 3 and 4 have the potential to cause injury. Some of the ophthalmic Nd:YAG lasers that cause an acoustic instead of a thermal reaction are classified in the subclass 3 category and can cause injury with sustained interaction.

Most of the lasers used in surgical applications today are known as subclass 4 lasers and can cause thermal reactions that can lead to fire, skin burns, and optical damage by either direct or scattered radiation. Specific safety precautions must be followed to prevent injury from these laser systems.

Many agencies are beginning to address the regulation of laser safety. Healthcare facilities must develop safety protocols in anticipation of mandates by these regulatory agencies as the technology advances and grows.

The American National Standards Institute (ANSI), a nongovernmental organization of experts, published the ANSI Z136.1 standards in 1973 as safety guidelines for laser use in warfare, industry, and health care. In 1988 ANSI Z136.3 standards were established to provide specific recommendations for laser use in healthcare environments. The appendix of ANSI Z136.3 discusses a consensus on laser safety in each of the special areas of medicine and surgery. These standards are reviewed periodically and revised as surgical trends continue to change. The latest revision for Z136.3 was published in 1995.[1] It is recommended that both ANSI standards be acquired for reference, since the Z136.3 document often refers to the Z136.1 publication.

Other guidelines have been suggested by the Center for Devices and Radiological Health (CDRH), Association of Operating Room Nurses (AORN), American Society for Laser Medicine and Surgery (ASLMS), Laser Institute of America (LIA), Food and Drug Administration (FDA), Occupational Safety and Health Administration (OSHA), and individual state and local regulatory bodies.

Hospitals and other healthcare delivery facilities need to formulate laser-safety policies and procedures using these groups of experts as resources. In the development of safety guidelines for a facility, protocols should individually address situations without being too general or too specific. A policy or procedure must be general enough to address the need but not so detailed that the surgical team cannot follow it. Facilities must realize that they can be held liable for following their own safety policies and procedures. Therefore basic inservice education on the written laser policies and procedures for all personnel in the surgical environment (including orderlies, aides, and housekeeping personnel) should be mandatory within the healthcare facility.

Eye Protection

Because the eye is extremely sensitive to laser radiation, great care must be taken to protect the eyes during laser intervention. Even low levels of laser radiation can lead to permanent optical damage. The area of possible ophthalmologic injury depends on the type of wavelength. The CO_2 laser can damage the cornea because this beam is readily absorbed by the surface cells. Immediate pain is associated with this injury. The argon and Nd:YAG laser beams, in contrast, are transmitted through the clear

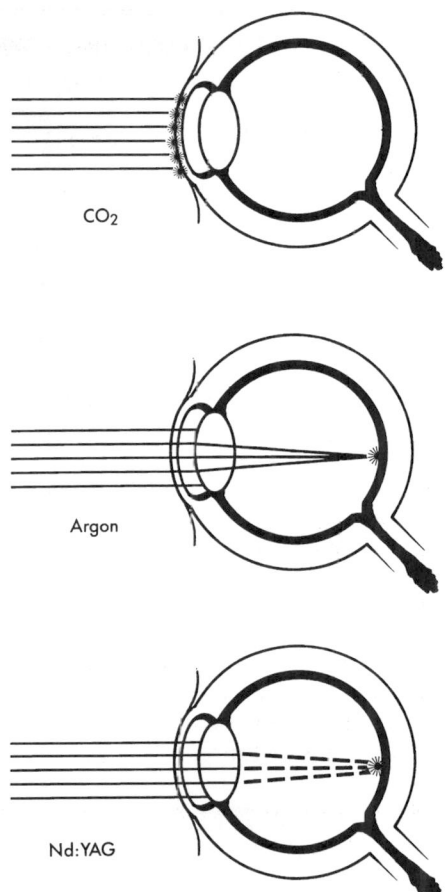

FIGURE 3-57   The CO_2 laser beam can damage the cornea; the argon and Nd:YAG beams can injure the retina.

optical structures and fluids and can be refocused by the lens of the eye. The intensity of the beam after refocusing can permanently damage the retina. Sometimes pain is not even felt during this destruction (Fig. 3-57).

Adequate eye protection requires understanding the two concepts of maximum permissible exposure (MPE) and nominal hazard zone (NHZ). According to the ANSI Z136.3 standards the MPE is the level of laser radiation to which a person may be exposed without hazardous effects to the eye or skin. The MPE levels are determined through consideration of the laser wavelength, power, exposure time, and pulse repetition.

The NHZ is the space where the level of the direct, reflected, or scattered radiation during normal laser operation exceeds the MPE; therefore eye, skin, and fire safety precautions must be followed while one is working within this hazard zone. The NHZ can be calculated mathematically to determine the distance from the laser beam emission in which the beam can cause skin and eye damage. Since the power, operating modes, and other parameters are changed frequently during a procedure, this calculation would also change. Therefore the area inside

the surgical room is usually considered to be within the NHZ so that consistency and simplicity can be maintained when lasers are used in healthcare.

Recommendations suggest that protective goggles, glasses, and endoscope lens covers should be inscribed with the appropriate filtering capabilities and adequate optical densities for the specific wavelength being used. For example, a pair of Nd:YAG goggles may be inscribed "1064 nm, optical density 4." The optical density of the lens is the capability of the lens material to absorb a specific wavelength. The darker lens shades do not necessarily have higher optical density or give more protection than the lighter ones do. Technology has introduced lighter lens shades with high optical densities that provide adequate safety. The perioperative nurse must ensure that eyewear is properly labeled, handled, and stored so that hazards are minimized and scratching and damage are avoided.

During surgical procedures using multiple wavelengths, protective eyewear must be changed as the wavelengths are changed. There are some types of eyewear that protect against a limited range of wavelengths. If the range is expanded to block a greater variety of wavelengths, the eyewear is more difficult to see through.

Controversy exists as to the appropriateness of using one's own prescription glasses to serve as CO_2 laser eye protection when the wearer is not in the immediate vicinity of the laser beam emission (such as the circulating nurse). Prescription eyeglasses do not have the wavelength protection inscribed on them and have not been tested to note the protective ability of the lens; therefore adequate protection cannot be guaranteed. Opponents state that the NHZ is so limited when the CO_2 beam is passed through the focusing lens that those persons who are not close to the laser emission port are not at a high risk for eye damage. Facilities must address this controversial issue and develop a policy for the surgical team to follow. Contact lenses and half glasses definitely do not offer adequate protection against CO_2 laser energy.

During a microscopic procedure the optics of the microscope provide eye protection against CO_2 laser energy. But when other wavelengths are used, such as argon or Nd:YAG, an automatic lens shutter can be connected to the microscope head. During the laser activation the shutter allows a lens filter to drop into place to provide a shield from any laser backscatter. When this device is attached to the microscope head, any observer tube being used must also be placed above the filter so that all portal optics have protection provided.

A lens filter can be placed over the eyepiece of a rigid or flexible endoscope. The lens must offer the appropriate protection for the specific laser being used. Guidelines suggest that the other surgical team members also wear eye protection, even though the laser energy appears to be confined within an enclosed cavity. Optical injury is always possible if a fiber or articulated arm becomes separated from the endoscope while the laser is being activated or if a fiber is fractured and the beam escapes at that fracture site.

The ANSI standards recommend that a baseline eye examination, with visual acuity and retinal health being monitored, be performed on those healthcare professionals who routinely work with laser systems. Another eye examination can be performed after any ophthalmic accident or upon termination of employment. The baseline exam then provides a foundation for comparison with abnormal findings from subsequent examinations. This preventive procedure protects the facility from a potential worker's compensation claim for retinal damage from incidental beam reflection, should the problem occur. Some facilities have opted not to follow this rather expensive and difficult-to-monitor guideline because they strictly enforce their eye-safety policy, thus minimizing the chance of any ophthalmic accidents.

The patient's eyes must be protected during laser intervention. When general anesthesia is used, patients should have their eyes covered with wet gauze, eye pads, or a towel; the eyes should be taped closed. If awake or under local anesthesia, the patient should wear appropriate eye protection. Explanations regarding this safety action should be provided to the patient. If the laser is to be used in the immediate vicinity of the eye, such as to lighten a port-wine stain on the eyelid, a special laser eye shield can be placed on the surface of the eye after instillation of a drop of an ophthalmic local anesthetic. Box 3-3 summarizes actions to promote eye safety during laser surgery.

Controlled Access

Inadvertent access to rooms where laser treatments are being performed should be prevented. Laser warning signs must be placed at all entrances to the treatment area so that access is granted only to those individuals who have been appropriately educated in laser safety. The word "Danger" and the universally accepted laser symbol should be present on any laser warning sign to indicate the possibility of hazards. Laser signs should be removed when the procedure has been completed.

Windows and ports into rooms where lasers are utilized must be covered with appropriate protection for the specific laser being used. The CO_2 laser beam is stopped by clear glass or Plexiglas panels, but the argon and Nd:YAG laser wavelengths can be transmitted through this glass. Therefore the windows and ports must be covered with a blocking barrier that stops the transmission of specific wavelengths.

The laser key must not be left in the laser during storage. The key should be available only to authorized personnel who have the appropriate education and training to operate the laser. Laser keys can be stored in the narcotics cabinet or in a special key lockbox to control access. Box 3-4 summarizes actions that should be initiated to control access to laser rooms.

BOX 3-3 | Guide to Eye Safety during Laser Surgery

- Ensure that everyone in the laser room is wearing the appropriate eye protection before activating the laser. The eyewear should have the laser wavelength protection and optical density of the lens material inscribed on it.
- A special lens cover can be placed over the eyepiece of an endoscope to protect the physician's eye from laser backscatter. Remember that the physician's other eye will be unprotected.
- Everyone in the laser room should wear eye protection during laser endoscopic procedures.
- An automatic lens shutter can be connected to a microscope head to provide eye protection for persons viewing the procedure through the microscope.
- When general anesthesia is used, cover the patient's closed eyes with moistened gauze pads. When the patient is awake, place the appropriate glasses or goggles on the patient. Explain the need for eye protection to the patient.
- During laser surgery near the eye, a special laser eye shield may be placed directly on the anesthetized eye surface.
- Ensure that the appropriate protective eyewear is available at all entrances to the laser room for anyone entering the area.
- When storing protective eyewear, guard against scratches and mishandling. Scratches on the lenses may decrease their effectiveness.

BOX 3-4 | Guide to Controlled Access during Laser Surgery

- Hang laser warning signs at all entrances to the laser room to prevent unauthorized persons from entering.
- The warning sign should include *Danger* and the universal laser symbol.
- Cover windows or ports with the appropriate protection for the specific laser wavelength being used.
- Do not store the laser key in the laser. The laser key must be available only to authorized persons.

Fire Safety

An awareness of laser biophysics and tissue interaction is necessary to understand the actions needed to prevent laser fires. A fire can be started by a reflected beam as easily as from a direct impact. The laser team must be able to respond quickly if a fire occurs. Immediate action is the key to minimize injury to the patient and the surgical team. Box 3-5 summarizes important measures to support fire safety during laser surgery.

Sterile water or saline solution should be readily available to douse a small fire. A halon fire extinguisher should be available to control a fire within the laser system. This fire extinguisher contains halogenated hydrocarbons (halon) that do not produce a residue that could harm the

---

| BOX 3-5 | Guide to Fire Safety during Laser Surgery |

- Sterile water or saline should be immediately available to douse a small fire near or on the patient.
- A halon fire extinguisher should be available in the department in case the laser catches on fire.
- Do not place fluids or solutions on the laser unit. Protect the laser system from spillage or splatter, which could cause short-circuiting and fire.
- Do not place dry combustibles in the vicinity of the laser impact site. Use wet towels, nonflammable drapes, or special laser-retardant materials near the laser target area. Moisten dry drapes and sponges with sterile saline or water to prevent ignition. Constantly monitor the moisture level throughout the procedure.
- Do not use flammable materials near the laser impact site.
- Utilize nonreflective instrumentation in or near the laser tissue impact site to decrease accidental direct reflection of the laser beam. Cover larger instruments, such as retractors, with wet sponges or towels to protect against reflection.
- Do not prep with flammable skin preparations, such as alcohol.
- A wet pack may be inserted into the rectum as a tamponade to prevent methane gas from escaping into the surgical area. A cleansing bowel prep before surgery will also decrease this risk.
- Use a specially prepared or a commercially manufactured laser endotracheal tube or wrap during laser procedures of the oropharynx. An unprotected PVC endotracheal tube can readily be ignited from an inadvertent laser beam impact. Inflate the endotracheal tube cuff with a solution to provide a heat sink if the cuff is penetrated by the laser beam. Protect the endotracheal tube cuff with wet gauze sponges.
- Place the laser in the standby mode when not in use.
- Identify the laser foot pedal to avoid accidental activation.

---

internal delicate components of the laser. Halon is known to destroy the ozone layer, so its use has become controversial. In contrast, a CO_2 fire extinguisher can cause thermal damage to the laser components from the extremely cold temperature of the residue that is emitted. A dry chemical fire extinguisher is not appropriate because it discharges a fine dust that damages the optics and circuitry of the laser system, and this dust is difficult to remove from the surgical environment.

During the surgical intervention, combustibles, such as sponges or towels, near the laser tissue impact site should be kept wet to prevent ignition. The surgical team should constantly monitor the moisture level of the sponges and other materials to prevent drying, which could eventually support a fire.

Flammable draping material can be easily ignited by a laser beam. Some water-repellent drapes and other laser-safe materials are able to withstand laser impact, and thus the flammability of the material is decreased. If the restrictions of draping material or any other supplies are questionable, the item can be tested for flammability in the manufacturer's or researcher's laboratory. The laser beam can be directed to the item using different power settings to determine any limitations before clinical use. Water should be immediately available during these experiments.

Instrumentation used in the immediate vicinity of the laser tissue impact site should be nonreflective to decrease the chance of the laser beam bouncing off the surface and accidentally impinging on another area. The laser beam can easily be reflected off shiny instrument surfaces and can cause skin or eye injury or ignite flammable materials. An instrument may be ebonized by coating the instrument with a special substance (usually black) to decrease reflectivity. Many companies offer this service at a low cost. The instrument should be inspected regularly to ensure the integrity of the coating. Any scratched surface or area where the ebonization has worn off should be recoated as necessary.

An instrument may also be anodized or surfaced with a matte finish to decrease reflectivity. Other coatings and surfaces that cause the laser light to scatter and diffuse upon impingment are being introduced. Larger retractors can be covered with wet sponges or towels so that the laser beam cannot accidentally be reflected off the shiny surface.

Other instrumentation may be used to provide a backstop for the laser energy to decrease adjacent tissue damage and the chance of fire. Titanium rods are effective backstops and can be reprocessed easily. Quartz rods are often used as backstops for the CO_2 laser beam, but the argon and Nd:YAG beams may be transmitted through them. Glass rods must never be used with a CO_2 laser because the glass material heats and shatters after continuous impingement by the laser beam. Teflon backstops should not be used because they can melt when heated and produce toxic fumes. Wet sponges can also be used as backstop material.

Special laser mirrors that directly reflect the beam onto a hard-to-reach area have been introduced. Mirrors may be made of rhodium or stainless steel. Glass-surface mirrors do not withstand laser impact and will heat and shatter instead. Using a laser mirror requires skill, since the beam must be focused on the target area and not on the mirror to deliver the full impact of the laser energy. A laser beam that is misdirected off a mirror can easily cause a fire.

Flammable skin preparations should not be used for laser procedures. During skin cleansing the prep solution can pool underneath a patient, and ethanol vapors from alcohol-based preparations can become trapped beneath the drapes. The volatility of these vapors increases the risk of a surgical drape fire. Iodophor or any other tinted prep solution should be rinsed before argon or Nd:YAG lasers are used, since the tint may unexpectedly increase laser absorption.

When a laser is used in the rectal area, a wet pack may be used to tampon the methane gas, which could enter the surgical area and cause an explosion. The wet sponges used for the pack must be counted so that the packing is not inadvertently left in place after the surgery is completed. A cleansing bowel preparation before surgery also helps to decrease this potential hazard.

Airway explosion caused by the laser beam igniting the endotracheal tube can cause a potentially lethal accident for the patient. A polyvinyl chloride (PVC) endotracheal tube is highly flammable, especially when a high concentration of oxygen flows through it during anesthesia administration. Specific laser-retardant endotracheal tubes, special endotracheal tube–protective wraps, or foil-wrapped red rubber endotracheal tubes should be used during oral, tracheal, or esophageal laser procedures that require general anesthesia (Research Highlight 3-2). The laser power limitations of a commercially prepared endotracheal tube or wrap must be followed closely to ensure proper performance of the protective material. The cuff of the endotracheal tube should be inflated with sterile saline to provide a heat sink and retard a fire if it is perforated by the laser beam. Saline may be tinted with methylene blue to immediately note cuff rupture. A protocol should be developed to describe the emergency procedure needed to control an endotracheal fire. Immediate considerations include the following:

- Remove the flaming endotracheal tube and instruments. Stop the flow of oxygen by pinching the oxygen tube or shutting off the supply valve. Reintubate immediately to prevent laryngospasm.
- Inspect the mouth, oral cavity, and bronchial tree.
- Jet ventilation may also be used during a laser microlaryngoscopy. A jet ventilator is a mechanical ventilation unit that delivers the anesthetic gases through a small metal needle used with a rigid laryngoscope. Under pressurization the jet ventilator is set to deliver a determined amount of anesthesia gas while setting the rate, pressure (in pounds per square inch [psi]), and percentage of inspiratory time. The needle is positioned between the vocal cords on the side opposite the lesion. The needle extends into the trachea so that the proper amount of anesthesia gas can be delivered easily. After the surgery, the patient may be intubated to maintain an open airway if postoperative edema or tracheal spasm is anticipated.

Endoscope Safety

Special precautions should be followed when using the laser during an endoscopic procedure. When a laser fiber is introduced through the biopsy port of a flexible or rigid endoscope, the operator must view the tip of the fiber before activating the laser. If the end of the fiber is still within the sheath of the endoscope and the laser is fired, the heat from the laser energy will quickly damage the optics and channel of the endoscope.

When a "bare" fiber is placed down the biopsy channel of a flexible endoscope, the sharp tip can possibly tear the inside lumen of the channel. A length of medical-grade

3-2 RESEARCH HIGHLIGHT

Since airway fires during laser surgery presents such a devastating hazard, special considerations must be made to provide and improve patient safety. Recommendations have been made to inflate the endotracheal cuff with saline solution, which will provide a heat sink if the cuff is accidentally penetrated by a laser beam. But this tube must also be removed immediately. A research study was conducted to determine the time it takes to remove a red rubber (RR) endotracheal tube versus a polyvinyl chloride (PVC) tube from a model airway after rapid deflation of the cuffs (cutting the pilot tube, removing a pilot tube clamp, or aspirating the pilot tube to deflate the cuff). The pilot tubes used to inflate the cuff of the RR endotracheal tubes were clamped. The pilot tubes of the PVC endotracheal tubes were clamped or left attached to the 10 ml syringe used to fill the cuff. The times involved to unclamp the RR endotracheal tube port and extubate, cut the PVC endotracheal tube port and extubate, and aspirate the cuff with a syringe on the PVC endotracheal tube and extubate were recorded. Results noted that deflating the PVC cuff by aspiration with a 10 ml syringe is faster than cutting the pilot tube. Unclamping the pilot tube on the RR endotracheal tube resulted in the quickest time for endotracheal extubation.

From Sosis, M.B., Braverman, B. (1996). Advantage of rubber over plastic endotracheal tubes for rapid extubation in a laser fire, *Journal of Clinical Laser Medicine and Surgery, 14*(2), 93.

tubing can be placed over the fiber with the tip recessed within the sheath. The entire unit is then passed through the endoscope. Once the end of the tubing is observed, the medical-grade tubing is withdrawn sufficiently to expose the end of the fiber. This procedure effectively protects the inside lumen of the endoscope channel during fiber insertion.

Smoke Evacuation

Smoke evacuation and odor control must be adequate whenever a plume is generated whether it is from the laser, electrosurgical unit, or other surgical devices being used. Research has conclusively determined that the size of the particulate matter in surgical smoke is extremely small and that this plume could coat lung alveoli if inhaled over time, leading to respiratory conditions and complications. Controversy exists today as to the viability of any organism in the surgical plume, and more research is needed to conclusively prove the potential of transmitting infectious diseases through inhalation of the smoke.

A surgical plume contains carbonized particles, water, cellular debris, trace amounts of acrolein, benzene, formaldehyde, and other elements, causing an offensive

| BOX 3-6 | Guide to Smoke Evacuation during Laser Surgery |

- Use the appropriate smoke evacuation system for the amount of plume generated. Never use a nonfiltered in-line suction system to remove surgical smoke.
- Change the smoke evacuation filter or filters as often as recommended.
- Maintain the smoke tube or evacuation device as close as possible to the laser-tissue impact site.
- Wear high-filtration surgical masks that provide adequate filtration (capable of filtering 0.3 or 0.1 μm particular matter) when a surgical plume is generated.

odor; therefore adequate smoke evacuation is necessary to remove these contaminants from the air. Some of the toxins that cause the odor are known carcinogens and must be evacuated to minimize staff exposure.

Small amounts of generated plume can be evacuated through a special in-line suction filter positioned between the wall outlet and the suction canister. If the amount of plume is greater, an individual smoke evacuation unit that can filter particulate matter as small as 0.1 mm should be used. Smoke evacuator filters should be changed regularly as specified by the manufacturer.

Contamination by the surgical plume and tissue splatter is also decreased when the surgical team wears gloves, gowns, and masks. High-filtration masks that filter particulate matter of at least 0.3 mm should be used. A standard surgical mask usually filters particulate matter that is 5 mm.

The key to adequate smoke evacuation and elimination of inhalation hazards is to evacuate the plume at the laser-tissue impact site. Constant vigilance is mandatory to ensure that the smoke evacuation wand or suction device is very close to the laser target. Research continues in this area to develop devices to control the plume so that the surgical team and the patient are not subjected to inhalation contaminants and offensive odors. Box 3-6 summarizes important measures for smoke evacuation during laser surgery.

Other Safety Measures

Foot pedals can also present safety problems if mistakenly activated. Technology has given the physician more pedals to control devices and instrumentation in today's surgical environment. The number of foot pedals placed on the floor for the physician can often be confusing and can easily lead to accidents. The laser pedal should be clearly identified for the physician and should be used by only the physician who is actually delivering the laser energy to the target area.

Laser team members should appreciate the potential for electrical hazards because the laser, like the electrosurgical unit, is a high-voltage piece of equipment. Water and other solutions should not be placed on the laser unit, and the components of the laser should be protected against spillage or splatter, which could cause short-circuiting. The outside housing of the laser should never be removed by unauthorized personnel, since the potential for electrical shock or electrocution is high.

Transportation hazards are always a threat because some of the laser systems are quite heavy. When these units need to be moved from one area to another, proper body mechanics must be employed to prevent injury to the transporter. The laser should never be bumped against a wall because the internal components can be damaged or thrown out of alignment.

Documentation

Complete and accurate documentation that notes the safety parameters followed during a laser procedure is critical. Documenting laser safety is important for medicolegal reasons, as for any hazardous piece of equipment. Documentation can be done on a laser log form or as part of the existing intraoperative nursing notes. Either record should be placed on the patient's chart so that safety activities that were performed can be recorded.

A special laser log can be designed to be a permanent part of the patient's record and could include information such as the laser used, power, pulse duration, and other laser parameters. The use of smoke evacuation, fibers, and contact tips should also be documented, especially if specific charges for these items are made. Sometimes the reimburser will challenge the payment of an item if its use is not documented on the patient's record. A sample laser log is shown in Box 3-7.

Role of the Laser Team Member

As the popularity of laser technology continues to grow, the role of the laser team member becomes increasingly important. The backbone of a progressive and successful laser program is the enthusiastic and dedicated laser team. Expanded responsibilities are being assumed by the laser team member to provide consistency and promote a safe environment for the patient and the surgical team. Some of the roles of the laser team member may include becoming the laser safety officer, serving on the laser committee, becoming actively involved with laser procurement, and promoting the laser program through marketing.

According to ANSI Z136.3 standards the laser safety officer (LSO) is the individual who has the responsibility to determine laser hazards and monitor and enforce laser safety. This person is usually a nurse but can be a technologist, physician, or researcher. The LSO promotes laser safety, investigates laser accidents, and reports safety infractions to the laser committee for evaluation and resolution.

Interpretations of the ANSI Z136.3 standards defining the role of the LSO indicate that each healthcare facility should designate one individual to assume these responsibilities. Other laser team members are guided by the LSO to ensure that consistency and safe laser practices are being maintained within the laser program.

The LSO is also responsible to ensure that the other laser team members have received adequate and appropriate laser education and practical experience. Laser training for the LSO and the laser team member involves attendance at an educational offering that focuses on laser physics, tissue interaction, safety, and clinical application. The laser team member is the generalist who must understand laser applications in all specialty areas. Unlike physicians who focus on their own specialty, the laser team member must be able to provide support during all types of laser procedures. This expertise level is achieved by constant review of the literature to understand new techniques and developments.

The LSO oversees and coordinates the responsibilities of the other laser team members. Consistency within the laser program to provide cohesiveness among the team is critical to ensure satisfaction and success. Some of the expanded responsibilities that the LSO may authorize the laser team member to fulfill are listed below:

- Set up and test fire the laser system.
- Operate the laser control panel.
- Place the laser on standby when it is not actually being used to prevent accidental and uncontrolled laser firing.
- Perform preventive maintenance and minor troubleshooting on the laser.
- Monitor and enforce laser safety according to written policies and procedures.
- Participate in quality management activities.
- Report to the LSO any infractions of the written policies.
- Document the laser procedure, laser charges, and laser service.
- Inventory and maintain laser supplies and accessories.
- Attend laser committee meetings when requested.
- Assist with patient education.
- Help monitor physician credentialing.
- Stay abreast of laser technology by attending continuing education conferences or reading laser publications.
- Actively assist with laser system evaluations when a new laser is needed.
- Act as the laser resource person for the surgical team.
- Make suggestions to enhance the laser program.
- Assist with a laser marketing program to increase visibility and utilization.

Perioperative nurses who are part of the laser team are often involved with patient education. The perioperative nurse reinforces what the physician has described to the patient before the laser procedure. When told that surgery is needed, the patient is often anxious because of the unknown. When it is mentioned that laser surgery is needed, the anxiety may be compounded because the patient is confronted with two alarming unknowns. Many

BOX 3-7 | Sample Laser Log

Date _____ O.R. Room No. _____

Patient Information

Name _____ Patient ID No. _____

Zip Code _____ Sex: M F Age _____

Status: IP OP

Insurance _____

Surgery Information

Physician _____ Anesthesia: General Local

Procedure _____

Laser Information

Laser _____ Wavelength _____

Power _____ Duration _____

Total spots _____ Total energy _____

Laser time on _____ Laser time off _____
Total laser time _____

Laser fiber _____

Contact tip _____

Smoke evacuation _____

Comments: _____
_____
_____
_____

Laser team member _____

patients develop an uneasiness about laser procedures based on information from science-fiction movies, talk shows, and other such sources. The patient should always have the opportunity to discuss the laser procedure to allay any worries. After the physician has explained the procedure and has had the surgical consent form signed, the perioperative nurse may provide additional information if the patient has any further questions about laser technology. Ideally the consent form should reflect that the laser will be used during the surgical experience. Some physicians have noted that the laser is merely a tool used during the surgical intervention and do not feel the need to list the laser use on the consent form.

An adequate amount of time should be allotted for patient questions before the procedure. If local anesthesia is used, the patient should understand what to anticipate during the surgery, what sounds or odors will be present, why eye protection is needed, and what the patient's role is during the procedure. If the patient understands the application, the role of the laser, and his or her responsibility during and after the procedure, the perioperative nurse can expect better compliance and diminished anxiety in the patient.

Discharge instructions are required for any ambulatory procedure; therefore laser discharge instructions may be preprinted for each surgical application. These written instructions should be reviewed and given to the patient upon discharge. A follow-up phone call helps the perioperative nurse evaluate the care delivered during the laser intervention and the patient's compliance with the postoperative instructions.

Sometimes the perioperative nurse is placed in a compromising position by being expected to circulate during the surgical procedure and also operate the laser. This nurse then has the tremendous responsibility of being accountable for two critical roles in the operating room; thus the risk of a laser incident may be increased. In the traditional setting one nurse circulates while another nurse or a technologist, who is part of the laser team, operates the laser. The health care facility must determine what procedures require more staffing to handle each perioperative nursing role.

Electrosurgery

History of electrosurgery

Electrosurgical devices have been very popular for many years to cut and coagulate tissue, but also this energy has been associated with many patient injuries and accidents. Many surgical team members never have attended a formal education session to learn how to prevent and minimize the hazards of electrosurgery. Education is vital to ensure the safe use of electrosurgery by understanding the principles and actions of this surgical energy.

Around 1926, Dr. Harvey Cushing, a neurosurgeon, and Dr. William T. Bovie, a biophysical engineer, combined their talents and knowledge to develop electrosurgical technology for use during neurosurgical procedures. This primitive electrosurgical tool provided hemostasis for surgery in highly vascular areas. The first commercial electrosurgical unit (ESU) was produced in the early 1930s.[2] It stood chest high, weighed about 300 pounds, and was set in a beautifully crafted wooden cabinet. Electrosurgery began to gain acceptance as the benefits of tissue coagulation producing a drier surgical field become recognized by many surgical disciplines.

Physics of electrosurgery

The basic principles of electricity must be understood to comprehend how an ESU works. Electrons orbit the nucleus of an atom. As electrons jump from one atom to the orbit of another, an electric current is generated. Three terms help to describe the properties of electricity—current, voltage, and resistance. Current is the flow of electrons measured in amperes. Voltage is the force or push that moves the electrons from one atom to another and is measured in volts. Resistance is the impedance that obstructs the flow of electrons and is measured in ohms. As electrons encounter resistance, heat is produced and a tissue effect is observed.

An interesting characteristic of electricity is that it must have a complete circuit or pathway so that the electrons can flow. That is, if an electrical current originates from earth, the electricity must be returned to ground to complete the circuit.[2] Two forms of electrical current are used today—direct current (DC) and alternating current (AC). With DC the electrons flow only in one direction, whereas with AC the electrons flow back and forth as the polarity changes. During electrosurgery, the AC actually enters the patient's body causing the patient to become part of the circuit as the energy is returned to anything grounded.

Electrocautery is often misused as a reference for electrosurgery. Electrocautery devices use DC as electrons flow in one direction through a wire. The wire causes resistance, thus heating up. As the hot wire is held in contact with tissue, coagulation results. Electrocautery units are often battery operated, such as the small disposable units used during cataract extraction to coagulate small blood vessels.

Frequency is the number of waves passing through a given point over a specified period of time. This is measured in hertz (Hz). Electrosurgical systems operate at frequencies well over 100,000 Hz (100k Hz). In comparison, the electrical current in a normal household wall outlet alternates at 60 cycles per second, or 60 Hz.

Electrosurgical modes

Two popular modes used today for electrosurgery are monopolar and bipolar. Electrosurgical instruments provide cutting and coagulating abilities by using monopolar or bipolar modes.

In a monopolar electrosurgery system the electrical energy flows from the generator through an active electrode to the patient (Fig. 3-58). Since the energy is concentrated in a small area and the tissue provides increased resistance, controlled heat is generated and cutting or coagulation is achieved. The electrical energy passes through the patient to a dispersive or return electrode pad placed on the patient's body. The dispersive pad surface area is larger so that the energy is not concentrated enough to generate significant heat. The energy is then returned to the generator as the circuit is completed. If the dispersive pad is tented or only a small part of the pad is in contact with the patient's body, the electrical energy becomes concentrated and a burn can result. In summary, monopolar electrosurgery includes the patient to complete the electrical circuit.

In a bipolar system, a dispersive pad is not needed because the electrical energy flows from one tine or prong of the bipolar instrument to be received by the other tine

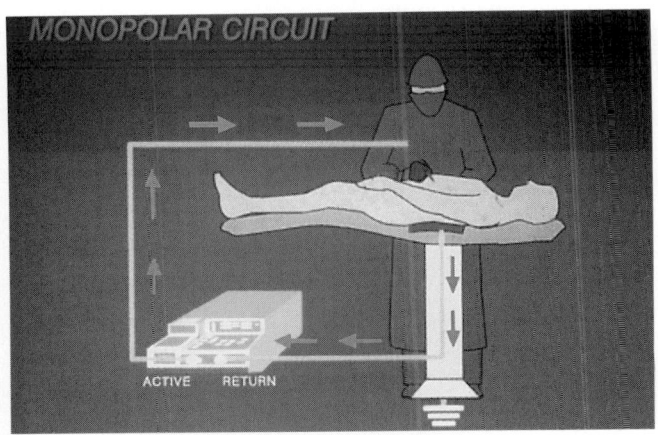

FIGURE 3-58   Monopolar electrosurgery.

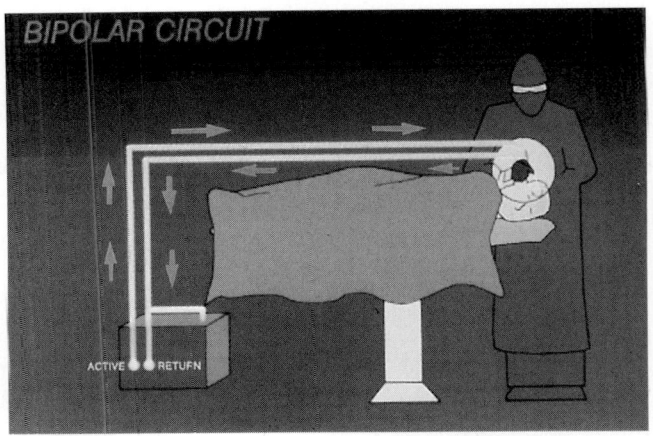

FIGURE 3-59   Bipolar electrosurgery.

as it passes through the tissue located between these tines (Fig. 3-59). The energy is then directly returned to the generator to complete the circuit, thus eliminating the flow of current through the patient's body. During bipolar electrosurgery, the flow of electricity is stopped if a certain impedance level is reached. This is usually 100 ohms. Even though the ESU appears to be activated because an audible sound is heard while the pedal is depressed, the flow of current is actually stopped when the specified resistance is met. Impedance meters are available today to alert the physicians when tissue desiccation is occurring or when complete desiccation has been achieved.

Tissue effects

As electrosurgery variables change, different tissue effects can be achieved. Those variables include:

- Waveform
- Power setting
- Length of exposure
- Active electrode size
- Type of tissue
- Eschar presence

As the waveform changes, so does the tissue effect. Waveforms can range from pure cut to pure coagulation. To produce a pure-cut mode, the generator must be on a 100% duty cycle, meaning that the electrical flow is continually being applied and heat is quickly being generated for cutting and tissue vaporization. The frequency is high, but the voltage is low. Because less force is being used to push the current, the cut mode becomes safer than the other modes. As the cut mode produces a constant bombardment of electrons on the tissue, heat is produced, cells are ruptured, and the tissue is cut. For maximum activity, the active electrode used to deliver the current should be held slightly above the tissue so that the electrons have to jump through the impedance of the air to reach the target site. This generates even more heat. Since this heat is produced so quickly, most of it dissipates as steam and plume as tissue is cut.

In a pure coagulation mode, the frequency is lowered, but the voltage is increased. The duty cycle is on only about 6% of the time leaving 94% of the time with no flow of electrons to the surgical site. To compensate for this duty cycle, the voltage, or force of the push, must be increased making a more hazardous condition. During coagulation, this intermittent delivery of electrons causes the cells to heat up and then cool, producing a coagulative effect. Higher voltage settings allows for the active electrode to be held over the area while a spraying effect delivers the electrical energy to coagulate a larger area. The tissue effect is superficial, collapsing the cells and producing a coagulum (Fig. 3-60).

Most ESUs today have a blend mode that allows the operator to dial in the desired combinations of cut and coagulation modes. If a higher voltage is used, a coagulative effect is achieved, whereas a lower voltage will provide cutting capabilities.

The power setting also determines the tissue effect. Obviously higher power settings produce more observable tissue effects. The longer the exposure of the electrical current, the greater the tissue response. Thermal energy can spread from the target site causing damage to adjacent tissue. Smaller active electrodes will concentrate the electrical energy causing an increased tissue effect; larger electrodes will dispense the electrical energy causing less distinct tissue effects, but more power is needed for the larger electrodes.

Tissue type also influences the tissue reaction. Tissue, such as adipose tissue, that is not well vascularized and is less dense will offer more resistance. As a result electrical energy is not conducted well, and higher power settings will be needed. Muscle tissue is more dense and well vascularized and will require less power to achieve a tissue effect. Eschar is less dense, so it impedes the flow of electrons causing more power to be used to achieve the desired tissue effect. Therefore, electrosurgical tips on the active electrode must be kept clean and free from debris for proper working. Nonstick surfaces minimize this tissue buildup.

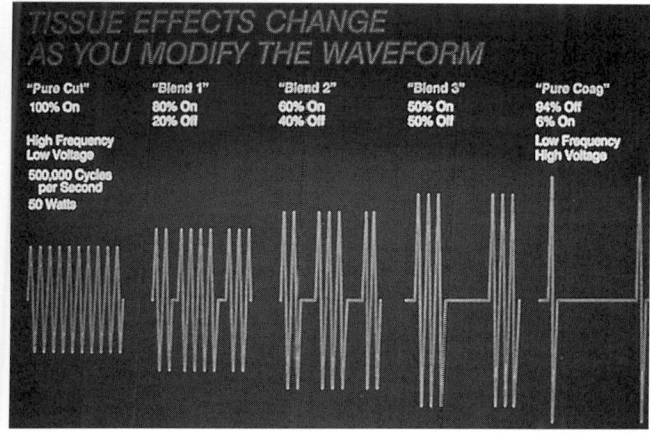

FIGURE 3-60   Cut versus coagulation waveforms.

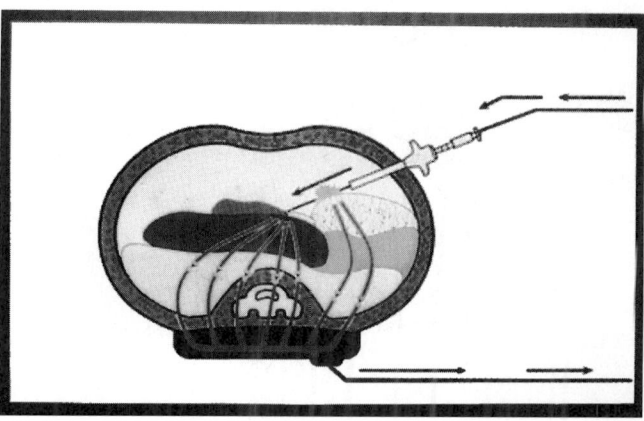

FIGURE 3-61   Insulation failure during laparoscopy.

Electrosurgical units

There are three basic types of ESUs used today: grounded, isolated, and return-electrode monitoring (REM) systems.

Grounded ESU

The grounded ESU delivers the electrical energy from the generator to the patient and returns the energy to the generator. Since electricity takes the path of least resistance, the current can flow through any grounded alternative paths, such as an ECG pad, in its flow to a grounded site. Patients have sustained burns at these alternative path sites as the electricity searches for a path to return to ground or to the generator.

Isolated ESU

An isolated ESU has a transformer that causes the current to return only to the generator and not return to anything grounded. Therefore the current flows through the patient's body and must return to the generator. If this is not possible, the generator will shut down, adding to the safety of this type of unit. An isolated ESU prevents alternative site burns but not dispersive electrode pad burns. For example, if the pad is tented, the electrical current will jump from the patient's skin to the pad to complete the circuit. Passing through the air will increase the impedance and will produce heat causing a burn at this site.

REM System

The REM system protects the patient from dispersive pad site burns. The system continually monitors the impedance or heat buildup under the pad as it is positioned on the patient's skin. The system deactivates the current flow when significant heat is present, thus preventing a burn.

Dispersive pad placement is extremely important to prevent patient injuries. The pad should be placed over an area that is well vascularized, such as a muscle mass. Sites with excessive hair, bony prominences, excessively dry skin, or excessive adipose tissue should be avoided. When a patient is being repositioned after the pad has been placed, the pad site must be inspected to ensure proper adherence.

Special electrosurgery considerations during endoscopy

Three unique problems can occur during endoscopic procedures involving electrosurgery including insulation failure, direct coupling, and capacitive coupling.[2]

Insulation Failure

Insulation failure can occur when the coating or special surface of an endoscopic instrument has been compromised. If there is a crack or break in the insulation along the shaft of the instrument, the electrical energy can escape at the point of defect and burn untargeted tissue (Fig. 3-61). The insulation must be inspected every time a reusable endoscopic electrosurgical tool is used. Even an area of insulation that is weakened may be penetrated by the electrical flow if a high voltage, or pure coagulation mode, is being used. Since the force of the push of the electrons is greater with coagulation, a weakened area may become an actual break along the insulation. The resulting tissue burn may not even be observed or realized by the operating physician.

Direct Coupling

Direct coupling occurs as electrical energy flows from the active electrode to a noninsulated metal instrument that is near or touching. Direct coupling can also occur with metal clips. Therefore the electrosurgical energy should not be activated when the active electrode is near or touching a metal object.

Capacitive Coupling

Capacitive coupling occurs when radio frequency energy (electrosurgical energy) is transferred through

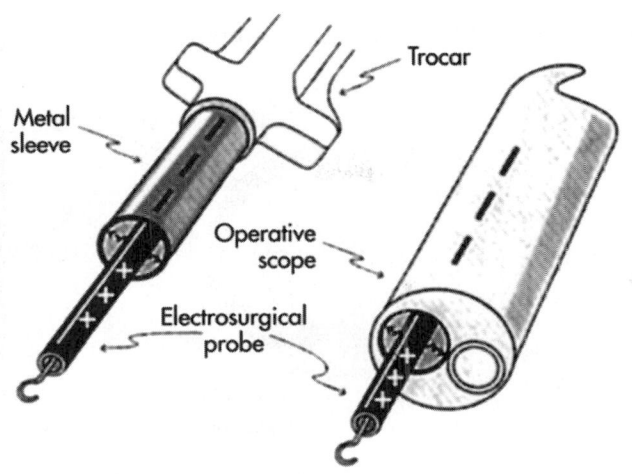

FIGURE 3-62 Capacitive coupling occurs when electrical energy flowing from an instrument charges a nearby metal trocar sheath or laparoscope.

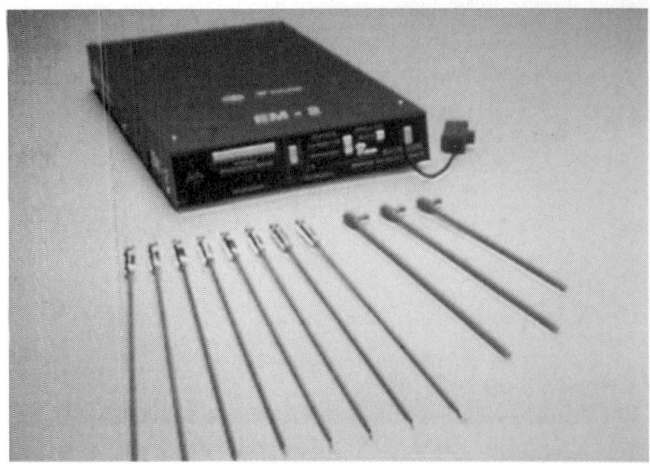

FIGURE 3-63 Protective shields or individual active electrodes are available to prevent patient injury resulting from stray electrical current.

intact insulation into nearby conductive materials (Fig. 3-62). A common example is when an electrode is activated within a suction irrigator. Induced current on the suction irrigator can cause bowel burns. The use of monopolar electrosurgical instrumentation through metal suction irrigators increases the risk of visceral burns through capacitive thermal energy. The laparoscope can also cause alternate-site burns if the electrosurgical electrode is used through the scope. Instruments that are long and narrow with thin insulation combined with high voltage increases the incidence of capacitive coupling. The electrical charge stays in the second metal instrument until a path to the patient dispersive pad is found to complete the circuit. Usually this energy can be safely dispersed through the large surface of the abdominal wall to the dispersive pad. But if a nonconductive device such as a plastic stability collar is in this path, the energy cannot be discharged and will burn any tissue touched by the metal instrument. These burns often go undetected by the operating physician, and the problem is not diagnosed until the patient presents with complications after the surgery. Therefore the use of hybrid instruments (combination of plastics and metals) during laparoscopy are avoided to minimize the problem of capacitive coupling. Special instruments are also available to capture energy that is transferred from one conductive device to another to eliminate the hazard of capacitive coupling (Fig. 3-63).

Argon-enhanced electrosurgery

An argon-enhanced electrosurgical device combines argon gas with electrosurgical energy to improve the effectiveness of the electrosurgical current. Since argon gas is heavier than air, inert, and noncombustible, it creates an efficient pathway for the electrosurgical energy from the electrode to the target tissue. The flow of argon gas also clears the surgical site of fluids and plume thus increasing visibility so that coagulation can be achieved.

The most popular benefits of argon-enhanced electrosurgery include the following:

- Rapid coagulation with reduced blood loss
- Reduced risk of rebleeding
- No need for direct contact with the tissue for coagulation
- Less surgical plume
- Less depth of penetration by the electrical energy, thus less adjacent tissue damage

When the argon-enhanced electrosurgical device is used during laparoscopic procedures, care must be taken not to overinsufflate or overpressurize the abdomen because there is a constant flow of argon gas that could cause the formation of a gas embolism. Often another port is left open during activation of the argon-enhanced electrosurgical device to allow any excess gas to escape. An insufflator with an audible alarm indicating overpressurization should be used. The patient should also be closely monitored so that any early symptoms of an embolism can be detected and treated.

Ultrasonic Device Surgery

Vibrating energy devices have been developed to provide a safe option for cutting and coagulation. High-frequency sound waves are propagated to a blade tip to produce ultrasonic energy. These ultrasonic waves have a frequency of over 20,000 Hz and cannot be sensed by the human ear.

The production of ultrasonic energy begins with an electrical current that generates an electrical signal sent through a coaxial cable to a transducer in a handpiece. The transducer converts the electrical energy to mechanical motion through the contraction and expansion of ceramic elements. A longitudinal vibratory response that moves the tip at the end of the handpiece from 23,000 to more than 55,000 Hz is produced (Fig. 3-64). As the power is

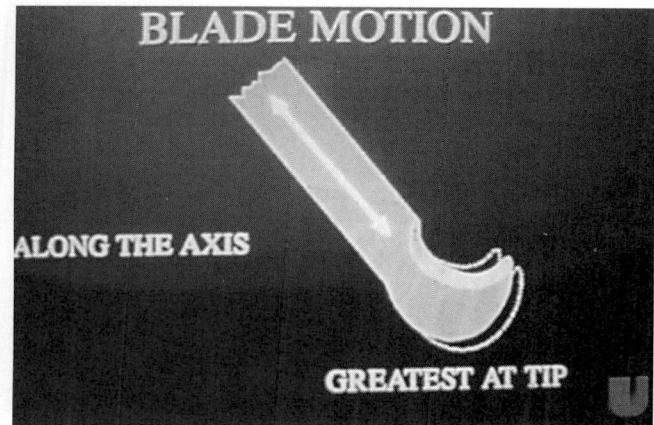

FIGURE 3-64   An ultrasonic blade may move longitudinally more than 55,000 times per second.

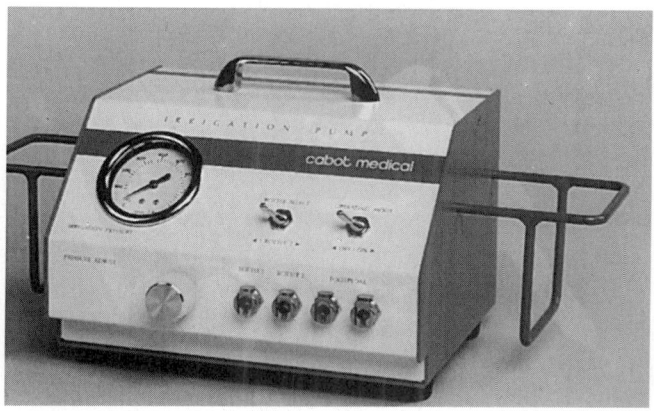

FIGURE 3-65   Irrigation pump used for endoscopic surgery. CO_2 gas is used to force fluid throughout system. Side brackets hold sterile irrigation bottles.

increased, the frequency remains the same, but the longitudinal excursion of the tip becomes longer.

As the tip is in contact with tissue, the mechanical motion causes the tissue protein to become denatured as the hydrogen bonds are broken. This action causes the protein molecules to become disorganized and a sticky coagulum forms and welds and coagulates the smaller bleeding vessels. No tissue plume is generated during the cellular destruction, but a small amount of water vapor is produced and dissipates quickly. Since such a small amount of thermal energy is produced, the adjacent tissue damage is minimal.

Different tip configurations are available, including a blade, ball, or hook. To obtain optimal tissue response, countertraction must be applied to the structure being treated. A shear-grasper to hold the tissue between a blade and tissue pad can be used to eliminate the need for countertraction.

The advantages of using an ultrasonic device for cutting and coagulation include the following[2]:

- No surgical plume or odor is generated.
- Less adjacent tissue is damaged as compared to the laser and electrosurgical device.
- Tactile feedback is provided.
- No nerve or muscle stimulation is present because no electrical current is delivered to the target area.
- No stray electrical or laser energy is produced.
- Precise cutting and control are offered.

Hydrodissection and Irrigation

Irrigation is essential during most open and endoscopic procedures. This is accomplished through irrigation probes for open procedures, through irrigating channels built into endoscopes, or by irrigating systems inserted through an operating port, cannula, or operative endoscope.

Irrigating fluid can be manually introduced through an endoscope by a syringe and stopcock attached to irrigation tubing on one end and an irrigation bag and tubing assembly on the other (the original IV pole, Y tubing, and irrigation system). Fluid flows by gravity and is manually forced through the distal tubing. A pressure bag can be used to increase flow, if desired. Irrigation through a flexible endoscope can also be delivered directly by a syringe attached to the irrigation port. Fluid travels through a specific channel built into the scope. Rigid scopes such as ureteroscopes, cystoscopes, and hysteroscopes also have this capability, just as operative laparoscopes do.

Pumps are available when large quantities of fluid are used and manual operation is cumbersome and time consuming. Pumps are beneficial when irrigation is used for aquadissection because more fluid can be introduced to the surgical site under pressurization. More force can be exerted over longer periods, and the pressure is adjustable (Fig. 3-65).

A common pump irrigation system includes the irrigation pump (CO_2 or electric), irrigation bottle caps, irrigation probe with dual trumpet valves, and Y-tubing irrigation set. When a CO_2-controlled system is in use, an E-cylinder of CO_2 gas must be attached by means of a tank yoke and input hose. A wrench should always be available to turn off the tank when not in use. It is important to check tank pressure before and after each use. The pump usually has an adjustable pressure on-off capability and dual irrigation bottle selection. As one bottle is emptied, a flip of the switch redirects CO_2 flow to the second bottle. Bottles can be replaced as needed. The system operates by the displacement of water or saline with CO_2 gas.

When an electric setup is used, a carrier bag with an inflatable bladder surrounds the solution bag (Fig. 3-66). When the bladder is inflated, an adequate pressure can be achieved and controlled to provide irrigation and hydrodissection.

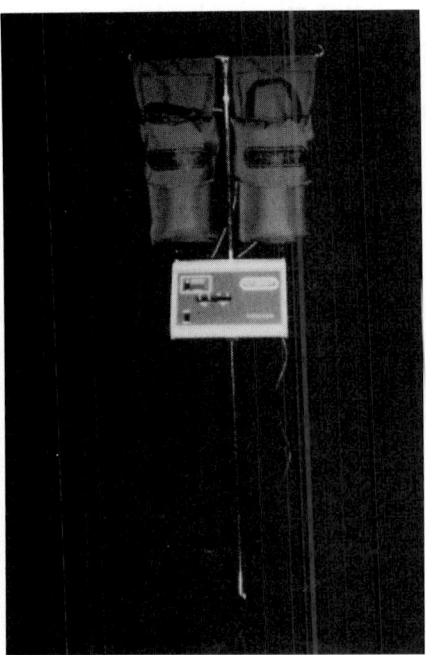

FIGURE 3-66   Hydrodissection system.

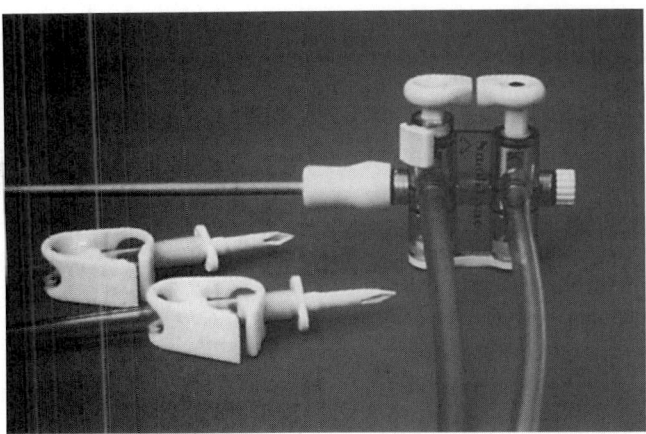

FIGURE 3-67   A trumpet valve controls the flow of irrigant and suction.

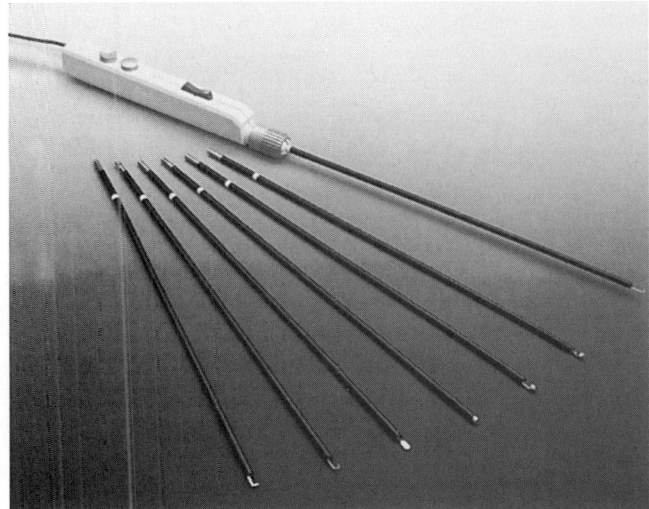

FIGURE 3-68   Disposable laparoscopic system with irrigation, suction, and monopolar electrosurgical capability. Electrosurgical probes are available in a variety of tips.

The distal tubing attaches directly to an irrigation probe. The time and amount of irrigation are controlled by a trumpet valve (Fig. 3-67). Probes are available as reusable, disposable, or a combination of both. All three types incorporate a second trumpet valve for suctioning purposes.

If reusable probes are used, they must be completely disassembled for cleaning and sterilization or disinfection. Each trumpet valve has a spring mechanism (almost like a ballpoint pen). The springs are under pressure when the trumpet valve is inserted. During disassembly it is important to hold one's hand over the valve so that the spring does not become ejected and lost or cause eye injury. Protective eyewear should be worn during this process. Extra springs should be available.

Completely disposable units are also available. Some systems incorporate disposable with reusable. Tubing and pistol-grip handles containing the trumpet valves are disposable, and the suction and irrigation probes are reusable. The disposable and disposable-reusable units also may incorporate electrosurgical capability into the system (Fig. 3-68). This allows the device to be used for three separate functions.

Irrigation fluid depends on surgeon preference. Traditionally, normal saline has been used. Because saline is a conductive fluid, there is concern when monopolar electrosurgery is used. The disadvantage rests with the risk from the transfer of heat and current to adjacent tissues. Because of this, sterile water or other nonconductive solutions should be considered to prevent electrosurgical energy from being transferred to alternative sites whenever excessive monopolar electrosurgery is anticipated. Sorbi-

tol, which is also used as an irrigation medium during hysteroscopy, can be rapidly absorbed into the vascular system, especially during excessive venous bleeding. The patient must be carefully monitored because of the potential for congestive heart failure.

Cryosurgery

Cryosurgery has been used in healthcare for many years, even though it may appear to be a space-age surgical technique. In fact, archeological evidence indicates that even as early as 2500 B.C. freezing tissue was probably employed as an anesthetic. In the early 1800s, cancer was treated using different freezing techniques. Today cryosurgery systems are being used successfully to destroy small quantities of unwanted tissue, such as unwanted skin tumors, and are also being perfected to ablate larger tissue targets, such as liver tumors, prostatic cancer, and cervical dysplasia.

To properly freeze tissue, a cooling device or cryosurgical probe must produce an iceball capable of destroying tissue at approximately -50° C and colder. Some systems produce freezing effects down to -240° C (-400° F). The cooling source of the system is usually gaseous nitrogen or supercooled liquid nitrogen systems.

For external tumors, the liquid nitrogen is applied directly to the dysplastic tissue with a cotton swab or through a spraying device. For internal tumors, liquid nitrogen is circulated through the length of a cryoprobe with an insulated shaft to confine the freezing to the distal tip. Ultrasound imaging is often used to guide the cryoprobe and to monitor the freezing of the cells. By localization of the freezing effects, nearby healthy tissue is spared. Smaller cryoprobes that can be inserted through small trocar sites are being perfected.

The effects produced by cryosurgery cause tumor death by freezing it. When internal tumors (such as liver cancer) are treated, the dead tumor cells are eventually absorbed into the surrounding tissue. Cryosurgery often involves cycles or steps during the treatment as a tumor is frozen, allowed to thaw, and then frozen again. Research continues to validate the effectiveness of this technology.

Cryosurgery has been used successfully to treat early-stage skin cancers (both basal cell and squamous cell carcinomas) and retinoblastoma (a childhood cancer that attacks the retina of the eye). Precancerous lesions, such as actinic keratosis and cervical intraepithelial neoplasia, have also been treated effectively with this technologic method. Cryosurgery has been explored to treat a variety of cancers, including prostate, liver, bone, brain, spinal, lung, and tracheal. It is also being used in combination with other cancer treatments, such as radiation, hormone therapy, chemotherapy, and surgery.

The primary advantage of cryosurgery for cancer treatment over other therapies is that it is less invasive because only a small incision is needed to introduce the cryoprobe through the skin; therefore less bleeding, pain, and other complications are experienced. Cryosurgery is less expensive when compared to other treatments and often requires shorter hospital stays and recovery time. The main disadvantage of cryosurgery is the uncertainty of its long-term effectiveness because microscopic cancer cells can easily spread if these cells are missed during the freezing application. Cryosurgery is an evolving technique that will continue to be explored for treatment cures and palliative therapy.

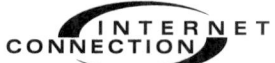

INTERNET CONNECTION

Centers for Disease Control and Prevention (CDC):
http://www.cdc.gov

Occupational Health and Safety Administration:
http://www.osha.gov

American Society for Gastrointestinal Endoscopy (ASGE):
http://www.asge.org

Association for Professionals in Infection Control and Epidemiology (APIC): e-mail: apicinfo@aspic.org

Society of Gastroenterology Nurses and Associates (SGNA): http://www.sgna.org

American Society for Laser Medicine and Surgery:
www.aslms.org

Birthmarks AKA Port Wine Stains:
http://www.fc.net/~msteffan/birthmark.htm

American Society for Testing and Materials (ASTM):
http://www.astm.org

Association for the Advancement of Medical Instrumentation (AAMI): http://www.aami.org

Emergency Care Research Institute (ECRI): e-mail:
ecri@hslc.org

REFERENCES

1. American National Standards Institute, Inc. (1995). American national standard for the safe use of lasers in health care facilities, ANSI Z136.3. New York: the Institute.
2. Ball, K.A. (1997). *Endoscopic surgery.* St. Louis: Mosby.
3. Ball, K.A. (1995). *Lasers: the perioperative challenge* (ed. 2). St. Louis: Mosby.
4. Decker, A. (1946). Pelvic culdoscopy. In Meigs, J., & Sturgis, S. (Eds.), *Progress in gynecology.* New York: Grune & Stratton.
5. English, N. (1996). Reprocessing disposables: one strategy to balance cost reduction and quality patient care. *Today's Surgical Nurse, 18*(4), 23-26.
6. Fuller, T.A. (1993). *Thermal surgical lasers, a technical monograph.* Oaks, PA: Surgical Laser Technologies.
7. Mackin, P. (1991). Laparoscopy risks are focus of research. *Laser Nursing, 6*(3), 74-75.
8. Ott, D. (1991). Correction of laparoscopic insufflation hypothermia. *Journal of Laparoendoscopic Surgery, 1*(4), 183-186.
9. Parsons, M. (1997). The dilemma over the reuse of single-use medical devices—a risk manager's perspective, *Today's Surgical Nurse, 19*(3), 17-21.
10. Semm, K. (1982). Advances in pelviscopic surgery, *Progress in Clinical and Biological Research, 112*, Pt B, 127-129.
11. White R.A., & Klein S.R. (1991). *Endoscopic surgery.* St. Louis: Mosby.
12. Zucker, K.A. (1991). *Surgical laparoscopy.* St. Louis: Quality Medical Publishing.

| # Infection Control

Dorothy Fogg

THE KNOWLEDGE THAT bacteria could cause disease and were transmissible agents was not acquired until the nineteenth century; however, the concept that there were tiny creatures that could cause disease had existed for thousands of years. In the first century B.C. it was believed that swampy land contained minute animals not visible to the naked eye that became airborne, entered humans through the mouth, and caused disease. During the Middle Ages it was the practice to segregate lepers, avoid areas of pestilence, and isolate the severely ill, indicating an awareness that diseases were transmissible. As early as the sixteenth century, Thomas Moffett identified and described lice, fleas, and mites. During the seventeenth century Antony van Leeuwenhoek, inventor of the microscope, discovered previously unseen creatures in his microscopic observations. In the eighteenth century Angostino Bassi linked a disease of the silkworm with a fungal parasite. Bassi went on to suggest that many contagious diseases such as smallpox, typhus, and cholera were the result of live organisms. The first studies of the pathogenic nature of bacteria occurred in the midnineteenth century when Casimir Davaine and Pierre Rayer studied the anthrax bacillus.[47]

Although various forms of surgery were practiced throughout the centuries, the first period of surgical prominence occurred during the 1500s, when Ambroise Paré, a French military surgeon, used ligatures to control bleeding when amputations were done. In that same era, Fracastorius, the world's first epidemiologist, proclaimed that diseases were spread in three ways: by direct contact, by handling articles that infected people had handled previously, and by transmission from a distance. The seventeenth century brought advances in anatomy, physiology, and medical instrumentation. The most momentous advance was the discovery and fundamental understanding of the anatomy and physiology of human circulation. The invention of the microscope by van Leeuwenhoek also contributed to the evolution of surgery.[63] The seventeenth century was a time of specialized anatomical research and a movement from unsubstantiated theory to more scientific thinking. During the eighteenth century the close relationship between surgeons and anatomic research continued. The entire profession of medicine became more organized and more scientific. The first tentative movement toward public health, surgical cleanliness, and surgical statistics occurred during this period. Surgery came to be associated more closely with the field of military medicine.[63]

In the midnineteenth century a new era began, greatly expanding the horizons of surgery. Anesthesia became a beneficial tool of the surgeon, permitting pain-free operations and decreasing the need for speed during surgery. Interest in surgical techniques and the development of new operations flourished. The preservation of life, however, was still not being fulfilled. Wound infections were so common that they were considered normal. When pus appeared in the incision, it was believed to be a healthy sign, signaling the beginning of clinical improvement. *Hospitalism* was a term coined by Sir James Simpson to describe the array of infections that developed among hospitalized patients. Today these are referred to as *nosocomial infections*.[43]

The principles of asepsis as we know them today did not begin until the midnineteenth century. The rudiments of aseptic technique and infection control were described as early as 450 B.C. Hippocrates, the father of surgery, used wine or boiled water to irrigate wounds. Galen, a Roman who lived during the second century A.D., is reported to have boiled his instruments before use.

In the 1850s Louis Pasteur, founder of the science of microbiology, theorized that fermentation was caused by particles of living matter so small that they could not be seen but could be carried freely in the air. He referred to these microorganisms as *germs* and found that heat killed them. The relationship between the fermentation process and the putrefaction of tissue was not understood at that time. In 1860 Joseph Lister learned about Pasteur's work, recognized the analogous relationship between the two processes, and set out to investigate the relationship of the germ theory to the process of infection. By 1867 Lister was advocating carbolic acid soaks and sprays for hands, wounds, dressings, sutures, and the operating room itself. Even though Lister's antiseptic methods and principles were crude and undeveloped, their use resulted in a drop in surgical mortality from 45% to 15%. The antiseptic era and the modern age of surgery had begun.[47,63]

During the mid-1800s three individuals developed concepts of hygiene and antisepsis within the healthcare community but apparently independently of each other. Ignaz Semmelweis made a simple but momentous contribution to infection control by advocating that hands be washed between examinations of patients and that a clean gown be worn for each patient. Joseph Lister was applying principles of antisepsis to wound care in an effort to make surgery a safe practice. The third individual, Florence Nightingale, was instigating radical changes in sanitation, resulting in reductions in mortality from contagious diseases. The interventions of these leaders provided the structure of infection control practice today.[43]

CAUSES OF INFECTION

Asepsis

The term "asepsis" means the absence of infectious organisms. Asepsis is directed at cleanliness and the elimination of all infectious agents. With the knowledge that bacteria could be destroyed by heat, it was but a short intellectual jump from the antiseptic practice of Lister to current aseptic practice. In 1889 Halstead at the Johns Hopkins Hospital asked the Goodyear Rubber Company to make rubber gloves for his operating room scrub nurse because she was allergic to the corrosive hand rinse being used. Gradually the idea of wearing gloves to protect the patient emerged. The usual morning coat worn by surgeons was replaced by white aprons and gowns. Later the color was changed to green for eye comfort. Masks were added as microbiologists measured the microbial soilage that occurred during conversation. Before the use of masks, many procedures were performed in total silence to decrease the probability of surgical wound infection. Sterilizers completed the transition to a truly aseptic approach to surgery, with all items coming into contact with the patient being sterile. By 1910 use of sterile instruments, gowns, masks, and gloves was standard practice in large university hospitals.[41]

Surgical asepsis is designed to exclude all microbes, whereas medical asepsis is designed to exclude microbes associated with communicable diseases. Practices that restrict microorganisms in the environment and on equipment and supplies and that prevent normal body flora from contaminating the surgical wound are termed *aseptic techniques*. The goal of each aseptic practice is to optimize primary wound healing, prevent surgical infection, and minimize the length of recovery from surgery. For perioperative practitioners aseptic principles and practices are the foundation for infection control efforts in the perioperative arena.

The human body has three lines of defense to combat infection. The first line of defense consists of external barriers such as the skin and mucous membranes, which are usually impervious to most pathogenic organisms. The second line of defense is the inflammatory response, which prevents an invading pathogen from reproducing and possibly involving other tissue. The third line of defense, the immune response, is triggered after the inflammatory response. When there is a break in this defense mechanism, the possibility for infection increases. See Box 4-1 for definitions of terms.

Microorganisms that Cause Infection

Microorganisms are living organisms that are too small to be seen with the naked eye. These organisms include bacteria, fungi, protozoa, algae, and viruses. Microorganisms are classified to determine appropriate treatment for an infection. Each organism is assigned two names: genus is the first name, and the specific epithet (species) is the second. Scientific names can be assigned to organisms in various ways. For example, *Staphylococcus aureus* is a microorganism commonly found on the skin. *Staphylo-* describes the clustered arrangement of the cells; *coccus-* (Greek *kokkus* 'berry') indicates that they are shaped like spheres. The species *aureus* is Latin for 'golden,' the color of the colonies of the bacterium.

Gram staining is one method used in identification of bacteria. Gram-positive bacteria have a thicker cell wall, whereas gram-negative bacteria have a thinner cell wall. The Gram stain of bacteria is necessary to determine which drug will be most effective against the disease. Gram-positive bacteria can usually be eliminated with penicillin and sulfonamide drugs. Gram-negative bacteria are resistant to penicillin but sensitive to streptomycin, chloramphenicol, and tetracycline.

Most surgical site infections (SSIs) are caused by bacteria. Those most commonly found in postoperative SSIs include staphylococcal, enterococcal, pseudomonal, and streptococcal species. *Staphylococcus aureus* is by far the most frequently identified organism. Gram-positive cocci, as a group, are the most common cause of SSIs. Although rare, fungal infections can also be serious and difficult to

---

BOX 4-1 | **Definition of Terms**

aerobes Microorganisms unable to live and reproduce without access to free atmospheric oxygen, such as *Mycobacterium tuberculosis*.

anaerobes Bacteria able to survive only in the absence of molecular oxygen, such as *Clostridium perfringens*.

carrier Person who harbors one or more specific pathogens in the absence of discernible clinical disease.

contamination Presence of pathogenic microorganisms on or in animate or inanimate objects. This term generally is used in reference to a specific object, substance, or tissue that contains microorganisms, especially disease-producing microorganisms.

deep incisional SSI Infection involving deep soft tissue, fascia, and muscle.

facultative bacteria Bacteria with enzyme systems that permit them to live and reproduce with or without free oxygen.

infection Invasion and multiplication of microorganisms in body tissues causing cellular injury attributable to competitive metabolism, toxins, intracellular replication or antigen-antibody response.

infectious agent Parasite (bacterium, spirochete, fungus, virus, or any other type of organism) that is capable of producing infection.

nosocomial infections Infections acquired by patients during hospitalization, with confirmation of diagnosis by clinical or laboratory evidence. The infective agents may originate from endogenous sources, as from one tissue to another within the patient (self-infection), or from exogenous sources, as acquired from objects or other patients within the hospital (cross-infection). Nosocomial infections, which are often referred to as *hospital-acquired infections*, may not become apparent until after the patient has left the hospital.

opportunists Microorganisms of low virulence and requiring large numbers to produce infection.

organ or space SSI Infection involving any part of the anatomy other than the incision.

parasites Microorganisms that reside on or within the bodies of living organisms called *hosts* to find the environment and food they require for life and reproduction. Some microorganisms are obligatory parasites, meaning that they depend on their hosts for survival and reproduction. Other microorganisms are facultative parasites, meaning that they normally reside on dead matter but may receive nourishment from living matter. All disease-producing microorganisms are parasites; however, not all parasites are disease producing.

pathogen Any disease-producing agent or microorganism.

primary pathogens Highly virulent organisms that are capable of producing disease in low numbers.

resident microorganisms Organisms that habitually live in the epidermis, deep in the crevices and folds of the skin.

source Object, substance, or individual from which an infectious agent passes to a host. In some cases transfer is direct from the reservoir, or source, to the host.

superficial SSI Infection involving skin and subcutaneous tissue as opposed to deep tissue.

surgical-site (incisional) infection (SSI) Infections involving body wall layers that have been incised.

transient microorganisms Organisms with a very short life span, such as the normal flora present on the skin surface of humans. Gram-negative bacteria are transient on the hands of hospital personnel and account for 60% of infections.

Sources: Horan, T.C., Gaynes, R.P., Martone, W.J., & Emori, T.G. (1992). CDC definitions of nosocomial surgical site infections, 1992; a modification of CDC definitions of nosocomial surgical site infections. *American Journal of Infection Control, 20*(5), 271-274; O'Toole, M.T., (Ed.), (1997). *Miller-Keane encyclopedia and dictionary of medicine, nursing, and allied health* (ed. 6). Philadelphia: W.B. Saunders Co; Stedman, T.L. (1995). *Stedman's medical dictionary* (ed. 26). Baltimore: Williams & Wilkins; CDC. (June 17, 1998). Draft guidelines for surgical site infections, Notice. *Federal Register*, 3168233187.

---

treat. Fungi most often isolated from SSIs are *Candida albicans* and *Rhizopus rhizopodiformis*.[41]

Staphylococci

Staphylococci are gram-positive cocci. They are facultative anaerobes but grow best under aerobic conditions. Staphylococci can be found in the indigenous flora of the skin and mucous membranes of the nasopharynx, urethra, and vagina. They are very resistant to drying, heat, and high salt concentrations. These organisms act as opportunists, usually as a result of trauma or foreign bodies.

There are two recognized species of staphylococci: *Staphylococcus aureus* and *Staphylococcus epidermidis*. Staphylococci are called *coagulase positive* when they are capable of clotting plasma, and *coagulase negative* when they are clumped by the plasma. Coagulase-positive staphylococci are more virulent or pathogenic than coagulase-negative staphylococci are. *Staphylococcus aureus* is hemolytic, parasitic, pathogenic, and coagulase positive. *Staphylococcus epidermidis* is parasitic, less pathogenic, and coagulase negative. *Staphylococcus aureus* is a long-recognized cause of surgical site infections. More recently, *Staphylococcus epidermidis* has been implicated in infections of prosthetic devices, including heart valves.[30]

The skin surface is the most common site of *Staphylococcus epidermidis*. Between 30% and 70% of people carry staphylococci on their skin. This can lead to contamination of clothing and dispersal of the microorganisms. For no known reason, people who are skin carriers of staphylococci differ in their ability to shed the microorganisms. There is no obvious difference in hygiene and skin condition between light and heavy shedders, and no other contributing factor is apparent. Heavy shedders appear to be in normal good health.

Human nasal and throat cavities are the most important reservoirs that continually replenish the external environment. *Staphylococcus aureus* has been found in the nasal passages of 30% to 50% of the adult population.[48] Among operating suite personnel, *Staphylococcus aureus* has been found in the respiratory passages 21% of the time.[35] The potential for patient infection increases greatly as the personnel carrier rate increases. Nasal carriers may also be skin carriers. Carriers usually harbor either coagulase-positive (pathogenic) or coagulase-negative (nonpathogenic) staphylococci—seldom both types—and rarely more than one strain. Because an individual may be a carrier of staphylococci one day and a noncarrier the next, frequent swab testing of the nose as a check to the spread of the microorganisms is impractical. Staphylococci survive for long periods in the air, dust, debris, bedding, and clothing. Pathogenic staphylococci grow in the sweat, urine, and tissue and on the skin of humans. They are more difficult to destroy than many other non–spore-forming organisms. Cleanliness of the environment, proper handling and sterilization of linens and equipment, and adherence to adequate handwashing techniques are important controls to prevent transmission of infection.

Enterococci

Enterococci are gram-positive organisms that are found in the normal flora of the gastrointestinal and female genital tracts. These organisms are responsible for many serious nosocomial infections including surgical site infections, bacterial endocarditis, septicemia, and urinary tract infections (UTIs).[30] In older males having undergone urinary tract instrumentation, 40% of UTIs are the result of enterococci. This organism has also been implicated in polymicrobial wound infections.[31] Enterococcal infections are most often nosocomial. They are usually seen in patients with co-morbid conditions.

Pseudomonas

The best-known pathogenic, aerobic species of *Pseudomonas* for humans is *Pseudomonas aeruginosa*. It thrives in moist environments and is frequently found in soil, water, sewage, debris, and air. It can also be found in the normal flora of the skin and intestines. Until recently it was considered a microorganism of slight pathogenic power. More recently it has been found growing in intravenous fluids and soap solutions. Aqueous solutions such as benzalkonium chloride support the growth of *Pseudomonas*. It is now known to be associated with a great many suppurative infections in humans, including surgical site infections. *Pseudomonas aeruginosa* appears to be pathogenic only when it is introduced into areas where normal defenses are absent, when it is superimposed on staphylococcal infection, or when it is present in a mixed infection. It may attack a debilitated patient who has extensive burns or major trauma. The organism is often seen in critical care and burn units. *Pseudomonas aeruginosa* is resistant to most antimicrobial agents. Other species of *Pseudomonas* have been associated with intravascular cannula infections as with the use of pressure transducers. Environmental sanitation and strict adherence to aseptic techniques are important preventive measures.

Streptococci

Most streptococci are gram-positive, non–spore-forming, facultative microorganisms. They are normally found in the indigenous flora of the upper respiratory, genitourinary, and gastrointestinal tracts. Streptococci are classified as alpha, beta, or gamma according to chemical factors, biochemical tests, and their action on red blood cells.

Group A streptococci account for most streptococcal infections in humans. Known as the *flesh-eating bacteria* because of their ability to cause necrotizing fasciitis, group A streptococci are of concern because of the sporadic and deadly outbreaks of both community-acquired and nosocomial infection.[2] An example is *Streptococcus pyogenes*, which is responsible for most soft tissue infections, otitis media, pharyngitis, impetigo, septicemia, and surgical site infections. Virulent streptococci are more serious invaders than staphylococci are because streptococci tend to involve wide areas of tissue and cause necrosis without localization. However, this tendency is partially counterbalanced by the fact that, whereas these virulent streptococci are usually sensitive to penicillin, staphylococci may not be. Streptococci also occur in mixed infections with other pathogens.

In surgical wounds a streptococcal infection can be introduced into the incision and spread by way of the lymph vessels and nodes. This can result in inflammation, cellulitis, and sometimes suppuration. Transmission of streptococci from the infected person to the susceptible host is accomplished by droplet transmission and by contamination of the environment. Direct contact may occur by inhalation of infectious droplets expelled from the nose and mouth. Indirect contact is by means of infected air and dust in the environment. Group A streptococcus can be carried in the nasal passages, anus, or vagina. The upper respiratory tract is not a significant reservoir for microorganisms that cause surgical site infections except in the presence of an acute upper respiratory infection. Most bacteria in the operating room environment are shed from the skin of personnel.[50] In a randomized, controlled study, Tunevall found the surgical wound infection rate to be unaffected by the use or nonuse of surgical masks by noninfected persons during the operative procedure.[72] However, wearing masks during operative procedures continues to be strongly recommended in the prevention of SSIs.

Mycobacterium tuberculosis

Mycobacterium tuberculosis is a non–spore-forming, non-motile, aerobic bacillus. Disease is produced by establishment and proliferation of virulent microorganisms within the host. Tubercle bacilli spread in the host through the lymphatic channels and bloodstream and by way of the alveoli and gastrointestinal tract. These bacilli can infect almost any tissue including skin, bones, kidney, lymph nodes, intestinal tract, and fallopian tubes.

Tubercle bacilli are transmitted directly by means of discharge from the respiratory tract, by inhalation of droplets expelled during coughing, by kissing, and, less frequently, through the digestive tract. They are transmitted indirectly by means of contaminated articles and dust floating through the air. *Mycobacterium tuberculosis* is carried by way of airborne droplet nuclei when infected persons sneeze, cough, or speak. These nuclei particles are less than 5 μm in size, allowing them to be kept airborne for a prolonged period of time.[27] Infection occurs when persons inhale these infected droplet nuclei. The droplet nuclei travel through the nasal passages, upper respiratory tract, and bronchi to reach the lung alveoli where they are spread throughout the body.

Mycobacterium tuberculosis can be manifested in two ways. Tuberculosis *infection* is the presence of the mycobacteria in the tissue of a host without clinical symptoms. Tuberculosis *disease* is a pathologic manifestation indicating destructive activity by mycobacteria in the host tissue. The probability that a person who is exposed to *Mycobacterium tuberculosis* will become *infected* depends on the concentration of infectious droplet nuclei and the duration of exposure.[24]

Viruses

Viruses are classified as small particles, rather than living cells, because viruses have no metabolic activity and must receive all sustenance for survival from a host cell. Viral pathogens are transmitted via the oral and respiratory tracts (such as poxvirus and rhinovirus), the intestinal and urinary tracts (such as poliovirus and hepatitis A virus [HAV]), the genital tract (such as herpes simplex 2 and human immunodeficiency virus [HIV]), and through blood and some blood products (such as HIV, hepatitis B virus [HBV], and hepatitis C virus, formerly designated non-A, non-B hepatitis virus [NANB]). Some viruses have multiple routes of transmission.

Once a virus invades a host cell, it combines with the host cell's nucleic acid (DNA or RNA) and reprograms the host cell metabolism to accommodate virus replication. If the host cell dies, all the viruses are released; if the host cell lives, one virus at a time is released. This process approximates the latent stage of infection. Virus replication stimulates antibody defense in the host. The presence of viruses may be detected by identification of the virus-specific antibodies that are produced by the infected person's immune system, by detection of the antigens elaborated by the virus and present in the blood, or by growing of a culture of the virus itself. Detection of virus-specific antibodies or antigens is termed *seropositivity*, or *seroconversion*. Viruses are susceptible to destruction by high-level disinfection, a process that destroys most disease-producing microorganisms.

Viral hepatitis is one of the most frequently reported infectious diseases in the United States, evolving from hepatitis A to six identified strains (A to F). Hepatitis A is the causative agent of infectious hepatitis. There is no specific treatment for the disease, but the incidence can be decreased by passive immunization. Persons at high risk can receive immunoglobulin (HBIG), which provides protection for several months. Hepatitis B is the causative agent for serum hepatitis. Some health care workers whose jobs place them at risk for exposure to blood or body fluids become infected with HBV each year. Hepatitis B can be transmitted by virus-carrying blood or any infective body fluid, such as serum, saliva, semen, and vaginal fluids. Hepatitis B is a slow virus with an incubation period of 6 weeks to 4 months. The onset of symptoms is insidious and gradual. Symptoms include anorexia, fatigue, nausea, vomiting, and jaundice. Hepatitis can lead to progressive liver disease.[74] Hepatitis B vaccine is recommended for healthcare workers regularly exposed to blood and body fluids. Postexposure prophylaxis for either percutaneous or permucosal exposure to HBV depends on the vaccination status of the healthcare worker.

Hepatitis C virus (HCV) transmission is most often associated with direct percutaneous exposure to blood. Its presence is often undetected because the patient may be asymptomatic. Currently there is no postexposure treatment plan for healthcare workers after exposure to HCV. It is therefore crucial that education of perioperative personnel about the risk for and prevention of all blood-borne infections, including HCV, be conducted routinely and updated for accuracy of information.

HIV is the causative agent for acquired immunodeficiency syndrome (AIDS). HIV is a latent virus which attacks the immune system by destroying T_{helper} lymphocytes (helper T lymphocytes). The period from HIV exposure to actual disease may be greater than 12 years. During this time, the person is a carrier of the virus.[74] HIV has been isolated from blood, semen, vaginal secretions, saliva, tears, breast milk, cerebrospinal fluid, amniotic fluid, and urine of infected persons. Transmission of HIV can occur by percutaneous or permucosal exposure to blood or other body fluids. The Centers for Disease Control and Prevention (CDC) estimate that at least 5000 needlestick exposures to HIV occur annually in the Untied States.[36] If an exposure incident occurs, the source patient should be informed of the incident. Serology testing should be done after the patient's consent has been obtained. Policies should be established for instances in which consent cannot be obtained. The healthcare worker should be counseled about the risk of infection, and he or she should be evaluated clinically and serologically for evidence of HIV infection as soon as possible after exposure. The healthcare worker should be advised to seek medical evaluation for any acute febrile illness that occurs within 12 weeks of the exposure. Seronegative healthcare workers should be retested after exposure at 6 weeks and then periodically, such as at 12 weeks and 6 months. Serologic testing should be available to all healthcare workers with concern of HIV exposure.

Drug-Resistant Bacteria: Emerging and Resurging Organisms

Historical perspective

In 1935 sulfonamides were introduced, resulting in a cure for staphylococcal and streptococcal infections. After World War II the introduction of penicillin was even more dramatic.[41] This was followed by the discovery of streptomycin in the middle to late 1940s.[30] When the concept of using antibiotics prophylactically before surgery to prevent infection after surgery was introduced, the practice of surgery flourished with "miracle" drugs to prevent septicemia and cure infections.[41]

As early as the mid-1940s strains of previously susceptible microorganisms began showing resistance to penicillin. In the 1950s severe epidemics of staphylococcal infections in pediatric and surgical units occurred in both Europe and the United States.[41] Strains of *Staphylococcus aureus* that were resistant to penicillin, tetracycline, streptomycin, and erythromycin were isolated. At the same time, resistant strains of gram-negative bacteria such as *Klebsiella*, *Proteus*, and *Pseudomonas* emerged as leading causes of nosocomial infections.[30]

During the 1960s, cephalosporin and semisynthetic penicillins were developed, and it was believed that the problem of nosocomial infections was solved. Many of the gram-negative bacteria were found to be susceptible to these new drugs. But by the latter part of the 1970s, strains of *Staphylococcus aureus* resistant to penicillin, methicillin, cephalosporins, aminoglycosides, clindamycin, erythromycin, and other antibiotics were isolated in hospital outbreaks of infection. This led to the development of new antibiotics such as carbapenems, cephamycins, and fluoroquinolones. These broad-spectrum antimicrobials were bactericidal at low concentrations and led to a false sense of euphoria during the 1980s when it was believed that, at last, resistance to these antimicrobials would be impossible.[30]

In the 1990s, it became evident that the potential for resistance to any and all antimicrobials existed, as nosocomial outbreaks of multidrug-resistant tuberculosis (MDR-TB) began to occur. Significant outbreaks of methicillin-resistant *Staphylococcus aureus* (MRSA) and vancomycin-resistant *Enterococcus faecalis* (VRE) also occurred in the 1990s. In some cases organisms seem to acquire resistance almost immediately upon exposure to the particular antibiotic. As fewer new antimicrobial drugs are being developed by the pharmaceutical industry, many consider the 1990s to be the beginning of the postantibiotic era—a frightening prospect.[30]

Mechanisms of resistance

Like their unwilling human hosts, pathogenic bacteria have an instinct to survive. When faced with an antimicrobial attack, they assemble their defensive resources. They have the remarkable capability to incapacitate the threatening antibiotic and to mutate and outwit the most lethal clinical weapons. While carrying only a single chromosome, bacteria by nature have extra mini-chromosomes called *plasmids*. These plasmids are hearty, and some may survive even the most aggressive antibiotic attack. Those surviving are resistant and will reproduce in kind, thus creating dominant organisms within the host. Additionally, infections incompletely or ineffectively treated create the potential for reinfection with resistant organisms.[2]

Microbial resistance can be divided into three categories: presence of a naturally resistant strain of an organism before any drugs are administered, acquisition of a drug-resistant strain from an external source, and drug-resistance from treatment-related causes.

Occurrence of naturally resistant strains of organisms sans drug administration can occur by intrinsic resistance, genetic mutation, or transfer of genetic material. Some microorganisms possess genes that make them resistant to an antibiotic. These genes may always be present in the microorganism but remain in an inactive stage until challenged by an antibiotic. Genetic mutation can occur spontaneously in the course of rapid multiplication of the microbe. These antibiotic-resistant mutants then reproduce within the host. New genetic material can also be transferred into bacteria by means of free DNA that contains resistant genes.[30]

Introduction of drug-resistant microorganisms can occur through a person or an inanimate object. Bacteria become mobile and accessible to humans on the hands or clothing of care providers, through instruments and procedures, or through food. Resistant microorganisms may travel from distant lands by means of infected travelers. Surgical instruments that have been ineffectively cleaned and processed can contribute to the spread of resistant organisms. Use of antibiotics in agriculture in animal feed products has also contributed to the development of resistant organisms. When the food is ingested, resistant genes may be spread to humans.[30]

Drug resistance from treatment-related causes is often the result of either incorrect use, overuse, or underuse of antibiotics. As much as 50% of all antibiotic use in the United States is believed to be misused in one form or another. It is estimated that half of all prescriptions written are not needed.[2,45] During antibiotic therapy the patient may have had a small number of resistant organisms. By natural selection, that is, as the susceptible organisms are killed, the resistant organisms multiply and become predominant. Inadequate drug therapy may contribute to the phenomenon and may be the fault of the patient, the provider, or both. Failure to perform sensitivity testing and prescription of an inappropriate drug can be a contributing factor. Inappropriate dosing can also contribute to resistance. If the patient is noncompliant with the prescribed regime or discontinues the drug prematurely, he or she may be contributing to drug resistance.[30,45]

Perioperative considerations
Methicillin-Resistant *Staphylococcus aureus* (MRSA)

Methicillin-resistant *Staphyloccus aureus* (MRSA) infections have become an increasingly serious problem in the United States since the mid-1970s. Most MRSA infections occur in surgical patients, with the incisional site being the greatest source of MRSA. Other sites in which MRSA can be found include burn wounds, chest tubes, intravenous catheter tips, and intraabdominal abscesses. *Staphylococcus aureus* is the most frequently isolated organism in postoperative surgical site infections. MRSA infections occur most commonly in surgical patients in hospitals where high-risk patients with underlying disease have a prolonged hospitalization, have had previous antimicrobial therapy, receive care in an intensive care unit, or have been in proximity to another patient colonized with MRSA.[21] MRSA is also found among care providers who carry the organism either in their nose or on their skin. Some patients have been colonized or infected by personnel who are carriers of the organism. The ambient environment is rarely a source of MRSA, except for some burn units.[50]

The primary mode of transmission for MRSA is most likely contact transmission by the hands of personnel. The organism has been recovered from the hands of personnel after they touched contaminated material and before they washed their hands. It has also been shown that MRSA carried in the nares of personnel can be transferred to patients by hand contact.[50] Because MRSA is transmitted by contact, perioperative protocols to be used when caring for these patients should include the following:

1. Segregate the patient using contact transmission–based or barrier precaution guidelines.
2. Wear gown and gloves when in contact with contaminated materials.
3. Implement strict handwashing practices.
4. Limit patient transportation to essential movement only.
5. Clean and disinfect patient-care equipment.[26]

Vancomycin-Resistant Enterococci (VRE)

Enterococci are intrinsically resistant to cephalosporins, semisynthetic penicillins, and clindamycin. There are also strains having acquired resistance to erythromycin, chloramphenicol, tetracycline, the fluoroquinolones, and vancomycin.[2] In recent years, there has been a rapid increase in the incidence of vancomycin-resistant enterococci (VRE) infections in the United States. Patient characteristics associated with this increased infection rate include critical illness, intraabdominal or cardiothoracic surgical procedures, presence of central venous catheters, presence of urinary catheters, extended hospital stays, multiple antimicrobial therapies, and proximity to infected persons. Because the enterococcal plasmid carrying the resistant gene can be transferred to organisms such as *Staphylococcus aureus*, VRE infections are of serious concern.[30]

The CDC has issued recommendations regarding vancomycin use. These recommendations include identification of situations in which vancomycin should and should not be used, the need for education programs for practitioners, susceptibility testing, isolation procedures and dedication of equipment and devices, verification of procedures for cleaning and disinfecting the environment, and minimizing movement of personnel between patients with and without VRE.[25]

VRE can be transmitted either directly from patient to patient or indirectly through the hands of care providers or by contact with contaminated environmental surfaces and equipment used for patient care.[73] As with MRSA, contact precautions should be followed when caring for patients infected with VRE. Perioperative protocols are similar to those for MRSA patients and should include the following:

1. Segregate patients using contact transmission–based or barrier precaution guidelines.
2. Wear gown and gloves when in contact with contaminated materials.
3. Implement strict handwashing practices.
4. Limit patient transportation to essential movement only.
5. Clean and disinfect patient-care equipment.[26]

Germicides commonly used for cleaning and disinfecting in hospitals are effective against VRE (Research Highlight 4-1). Isopropyl alcohol and sodium hypochlorite (bleach) are highly effective. With a 10-minute exposure time, some phenolic and some quaternary ammonium compounds are also effective. These are less effective at shorter exposure times. Hydrogen peroxide has been found to be ineffective.[64] There does not appear to be a relationship between microbial resistance to antibiotics and increased resistance to germicides.[4]

Vancomycin-Intermediate Resistant *Staphylococcus aureus* (VISA)

In 1996 the first known incidence of VISA occurred in Japan when the organism was isolated from a surgical site infection and undrained abscess. Treatment with vancomycin for 29 days left the condition unchanged. Further treatment with other antibiotic agents and abscess drainage led to patient recovery.[60] In 1997, the first occurrence of the organism was seen in the United States. A patient having been treated with vancomycin for multiple episodes of peritoneal MRSA developed bacterial strains moderately resistant to vancomycin, the treatment of choice for MRSA. Although the organism demonstrated only intermediate levels of resistance, the CDC views this occurrence as an early warning that strains of *Staphylococcus aureus* with full resistance to vancomycin may emerge.[27]

4-1 RESEARCH HIGHLIGHT

Vancomycin-resistant enterococci (VRE) cause serious nosocomial infections and their incidence has risen considerably in recent years. Environmental cultures and epidemiologic studies have shown antibiotic-resistant enterococci to remain viable on inanimate surfaces. These surfaces can act as reservoirs for drug-resistant organisms and can contribute to the transmission of infection. This study determined and compared the survival rates of VRE and vancomycin-sensitive enterococci (VSE) after exposure to various dilutions of four hospital-grade environmental surface disinfectants.

Four strains of *Enterococcus faecium* were used for this study: two strains of highly resistant organisms and two strains of susceptible organisms. All strains were recovered from blood and wound cultures of infected surgical patients. A series of preparation steps provided inocula for the study. The hospital-grade, commercial disinfectants studied were Hi-Tor and Hi-Tor Plus (quaternary ammonium compounds); Vesphene Ilse (a phenolic); and Wescodyne (an iodophor). All disinfectants were challenged at dilutions recommended by the manufacturer and at extended dilutions.

A disinfectant suspension test was used to determine inocula survival rates for the challenge inocula. Neither VRE nor VSE were recoverable after a 15-second exposure of the inocula to the recommended dilutions of all disinfectants tested. At extended dilutions both VRE and VSE showed similar survival curves with longer periods of time required to achieve a nonsurvival state as the concentration of active ingredient in each disinfectant was increasingly diluted.

The increased incidence of VRE infections and the isolation of the organism from inanimate surfaces has led to the belief that VRE are less susceptible to commonly used hospital disinfectants. This and other studies demonstrate no identifiable link between microbial resistance to antibiotics and resistance to disinfectants. Other studies have shown antibiotic-resistant organisms such as *Klebsiella pneumoniae, Escherichia coli, Staphylococcus aureus,* and *Staphylococcus epidermidis* to be similarly susceptible to commonly used disinfectants.

Authors of this study conclude that routine disinfection and housekeeping protocols need not be changed but rather that stricter adherence to these protocols will decrease the reservoir of VRE and other organisms in healthcare facilities.

From Anderson, R., Carr, J., Bond, W., & Favaro, M. (1997, March). Susceptibility of vancomycin-resistant enterococci to environmental disinfectants. *Infection Control and Hospital Epidemiology,* 195-199.

Multidrug-Resistant *Mycobacterium tuberculosis* (MDR-TB)

Outbreaks of tuberculosis (TB) have heightened concern about nosocomial transmission of this disease. The incidence of multidrug-resistant tuberculosis (MDR-TB) is rising in this country. Transmission is most likely to occur from patients with unrecognized pulmonary or laryngeal tuberculosis. Populations at greatest risk of developing TB or MDR-TB are the elderly, indigent, minorities; immigrants from countries where TB and MDR-TB are prevalent; and HIV-infected persons.[33] Transmission also occurs as a result of procedures such as bronchoscopy, endotracheal intubation, endotracheal suctioning, and open abscess irrigation.

In 1994 the CDC[24] issued *Guidelines for Preventing the Transmission of Mycobacterium tuberculosis in Health-Care Facilities.* These guidelines emphasize the following:

- Importance of control measures including engineering controls and personal respiratory protection, including fit-tested, personal respirators when indicated
- Use of risk assessment to develop a tuberculosis-control plan
- Early detection and treatment of those having tuberculosis
- Screening programs for healthcare workers
- Training and education for healthcare workers
- Evaluation of the tuberculosis control program

Creutzfeldt-Jakob Disease

Creutzfeldt-Jakob Disease (CJD) is an infectious, degenerative neurologic disorder. Depending on the area of the brain infected, the disease is characterized by progressive dementia, cerebellar ataxia, and myoclonic jerking with rapid progression to coma and death. Physiologically the infection produces no inflammatory process but results in neuronal loss.[28] Diagnosis is by means of an abnormal but characteristic electroencephalogram or by isolation of the infectious agent known as a *prion* by means of brain biopsy. The disease is always fatal. Brain tissue examined post mortem resembles that of other spongiform encephalopathies seen in humans and other species.[70]

The incidence of CJD is approximately one case per million persons. Little is known about the natural transmission of CJD, but iatrogenic cases have occurred as a result of brain tissue transplants, injection of contaminated human pituitary–derived growth hormone, and contaminated surgical items, such as neurosurgical instruments, cortical electrodes, corneal transplants, and dura mater grafts.[28] A serious infection control concern is how to destroy the infectious prions, which are extremely hardy and resistant to heat, formaldehyde, glutaraldehyde, ionizing radiation, freezing, drying, and organic detergents.[70] Sodium hydroxide has been found to be the most effective agent in decreasing or eliminating the infectivity of the CJD prion. Other agents are either ineffective or only partially effective. Steam sterilization in a gravity-displacement sterilizer for 60 minutes at 132° C (270° F) after a 60-minute exposure to sodium hydroxide has been shown effective. If a prevacuum sterilizer is used after the 60-minute exposure to sodium hydroxide, the item or items should be sterilized for 18 minutes at 134° C (274° C). Sterilization of tissue that is first fixed with formaldehyde is virtually impossible.[70]

CONTROLLING INFECTION IN THE PERIOPERATIVE ARENA

Infection control practices should focus on prevention. Transmission of infection involves a chain of events, including presence of a pathogenic agent, reservoir, portal of exit, transmission, portal of entry, and host susceptibility. Prevention occurs when there is a break in the chain of transmission. Infection control practices involve both personal and administrative measures. Personal measures include fitness for work and application of aseptic principles. Administrative measures include provision of adequate physical facilities, appropriate surgical supplies, and operational controls.

Universal, Standard, and Transmission-Based Precautions
Universal precautions

In 1985, in response to the growing number of persons testing positive for HIV, the CDC published recommendations for the use of Universal Precautions.[23] Reports of hospital personnel becoming infected with HIV after a needlestick or skin exposure to a patient's blood created an urgent need for new and better measures to protect personnel from patient transmission of infection. With knowledge that many patients with blood-borne infections are undiagnosed, Universal Precautions, for the first time, placed emphasis on applying Blood and Body Fluid Precautions (one of the categories in the 1993 *Guidelines for Isolation Precautions in Hospitals*) universally to all persons regardless of their presumed infection status.[26] Universal Precautions expanded the Blood and Body Fluid Precautions by recommending masks and eye protection to prevent mucous membrane exposures in addition to the routine use of barrier protection such as gowns and gloves. Universal Precautions also emphasized the prevention of needlestick injuries and the use of ventilation devices when resuscitation was done. The CDC continued to recommend the use of Universal Precautions until 1987 when a new system of isolation called Body Substance Isolation (BSI) was proposed. BSI directed isolation of *all* moist and potentially infectious body substances (such as blood, feces, urine, sputum, saliva, wound drainage, and other body fluids) for all persons regardless of their infection status. This was accomplished primarily with the use of gowns and gloves. Because of the similarities yet differences between Universal Precautions and BSI, confusion reigned.

In 1991, the Occupational Safety and Health Administration (OSHA) issued a rule for Occupational Exposure to Bloodborne Pathogens.[55] This document was based on the concept of Universal Precautions. The following is a summary of the requirements of the Final Rule: Occupational Exposure to Bloodborne Pathogens:

1. Each facility must develop and implement an exposure control plan that defines exposure and implements the requirements of the final rule. This plan is to be reviewed and revised annually with information provided to all employees.
2. Engineering and work practice controls must be used to eliminate or minimize employee exposure. Examples follow:
   a. The employer must provide everything necessary for proper handwashing.
   b. Contaminated needles shall not be recapped or removed unless such action is required by a specific medical procedure. Such recapping or removal must be accomplished by the use of a mechanical device or one-handed technique.
   c. A clamp or other mechanical device should be used to disassemble a knife blade and handle.
   d. Sharps are to be placed in labeled or color-coded, puncture-resistant, leakproof containers for disposal.
   e. Specimens of blood or body fluids must be placed in containers that prevent leakage and are labeled or color coded. Warning labels shall be affixed to containers of regulated waste, refrigerators and freezers containing blood or potentially infectious material, and other containers used to transport blood or potentially infectious material (Fig. 4-1). The labels shall be fluorescent orange or orange-red.
   f. Food and drink are not to be kept in the same storage area where blood or other potential infectious materials are present.
   g. Personal protective equipment (PPE) must be provided by the employer at no cost to the employee. Appropriate equipment shall include but is not limited to gloves, gowns, masks, face shields or masks, and eye protection. Protective eyewear must have solid side shields. Gloves are to be worn when contact with blood or body fluids is anticipated. Single-use gloves are to be replaced as soon as possible after contamination occurs. Disposable gloves are not to be washed or decontaminated for reuse. Some facilities may have educational signs posted to assist employees in recognition of appropriate PPE (Fig. 4-2).
   h. Signs must to be posted at the entrance to work areas of potential contamination. These signs are to bear the biohazard legend with the following informa-

tion: name of infectious agent; special requirements for entering the area; and name and telephone number of the responsible person.

i. Housekeeping provisions are to ensure that the workplace is maintained in a clean and sanitary condition. A written schedule for cleaning and a method of decontamination shall be established. All equipment and working surfaces shall be cleaned and decontaminated after contact with blood or other potentially infectious materials.

j. Contaminated laundry must be placed in a labeled or color-coded container that is recognized by all employees.

k. All employees are to receive education and training about safe handling of hazardous substances and materials. Information must be provided to all occupationally exposed employees at no cost to them. Individuals must receive training at the time of employment and annually thereafter. Individual employee training records are to be maintained by the employer for the duration of employment plus 30 years. The health care worker is highly encouraged to receive the hepatitis B vaccine after receiving the required information about the risk of exposure and about the vaccine. If the employee chooses not to accept the vaccination, the employer must have the employee sign a declination statement.

l. Employees are to report all exposures to blood and body fluids for postexposure evaluation.[22,55]

The blood-borne pathogen regulation is enforceable by the Federal and State Occupational Safety and Health Administration. This regulation is based on the concept of Universal Precautions to serve and protect the healthcare provider and to minimize cross-infection of pathogens between patients. Surveyors for OSHA may engage in on-site visits to healthcare facilities. Unannounced visits may occur at any site where an employee exposure occurs. The visit may be a result of a voiced employee concern, referral from another regulatory agency, or random inspections of facilities.

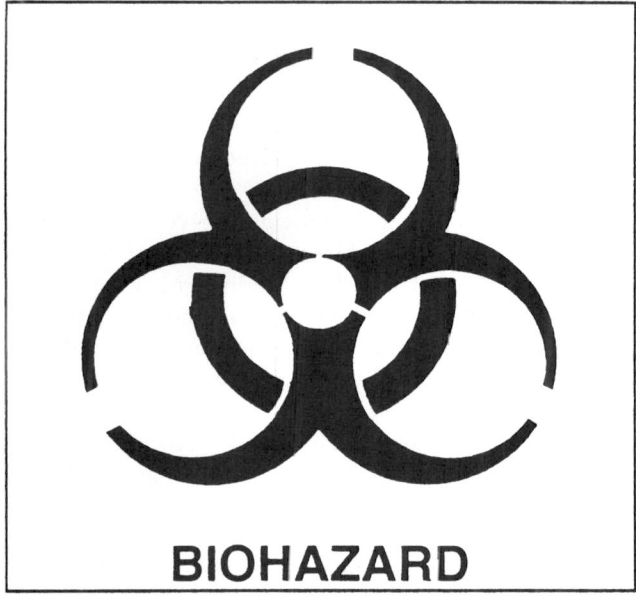

FIGURE 4-1 Biohazard label.

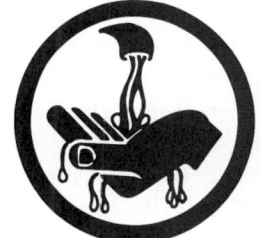   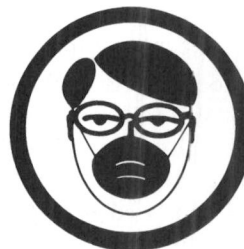 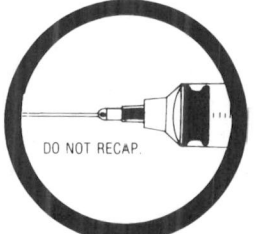

FIGURE 4-2 Example of universal symbols for blood and body fluid protection.

Standard precautions

By the early 1990s the controversy regarding Universal Precautions and Body Substance Isolation had escalated. There was considerable confusion about which body fluids required special care under either Universal Precautions or Body Substance Isolation. There were also concerns about the need for additional precautions to prevent airborne, droplet, and contact transmission of other infectious agents. With this in mind, the CDC developed a single set of precautions incorporating the major features of both Universal Precautions and Body Substance Isolation.[26] These precautions are called Standard Precautions, and they are designed to reduce the transmission risk of blood-borne and other pathogens. Additional precautions based on routes of transmission for patients known or suspected to be infected or colonized with highly transmissible or epidemiologically significant pathogens are included in the document. These are known as Transmission-Based Precautions. They are designed to reduce the risk of airborne, droplet, and contact transmission of organisms

Standard Precautions are intended to reduce the transmission risk for blood-borne pathogens and the risk of transmission of all pathogens from moist body substances. Standard Precautions should be applied to all patients receiving care regardless of their diagnosis or presumed infection status.

Standard Precautions apply to (1) blood, (2) all body fluids, and (3) secretions and excretions (except sweat) regardless of whether they contain visible blood. Standard Precautions also apply to nonintact skin and mucous membranes and include the following:

1. *Handwashing.* Handwashing is the single most important factor in preventing the spread of infection. Hands are to be washed after handling any contaminated item, upon glove removal, and between patient contacts. A plain nonantimicrobial soap may be used unless special circumstances such as hyperendemic conditions dictate the use of an antimicrobial or a waterless antiseptic agent.
2. *Gloves.* Gloves are to be worn when touching blood, body fluids, secretions, excretions, and contaminated items. Freshly donned gloves should be worn when touching mucous membranes and nonintact skin. Gloves should be changed between tasks and after contact with material that may contain high concentrations of organisms. Gloves should be removed immediately after use and hands washed before engaging in another task or administering to another patient.
3. *Masks, eye protection, face shields.* Masks, eye protection, or a face shield are to be worn at any time patient care activities are likely to generate sprays or splashes of blood or body fluids, secretions, and excretions. These protective devices help protect the mucous membranes of the nose, mouth, and eyes.
4. *Gowns.* Gowns are to be worn at any time patient care activities are likely to generate sprays or splashes of blood or body fluids, secretions, and excretions. Gowns help protect the skin and prevent soiling of clothing. The activity to be performed and the amount and type of fluid likely to be encountered will dictate the degree of protective barrier necessary in the gown. Gowns should be removed immediately after use and hands washed before engaging in other activities or administering to other patients.
5. *Sharps.* Needles, scalpels, and other sharps are to be handled in a manner to avoid injury. Needles should never be recapped using any technique that directs the point of the needle toward any body part. If recapping is necessary, it should be done using a mechanical device or a one-handed scoop technique. Used needles should not be removed from disposable syringes nor should they be bent, broken, or otherwise manipulated by hand. Used disposable sharps should be placed in puncture-resistant containers located as close as possible to the point-of-sharps use. Reusable sharps should be contained in a puncture-resistant container for transport to the point of decontamination.
6. *Patient-care equipment.* Single-use items are to be discarded after use. Reusable equipment must be cleaned and reprocessed to ensure safe use for another patient. Equipment soiled with blood, body fluids, secretions, and excretions should be carefully handled to prevent exposure of skin and mucous membrane, clothing contamination, and transfer of organisms to patients, personnel, and the environment.
7. *Linens.* Linens soiled with blood, body fluids, secretions, or excretions should be handled in a manner to avoid skin and mucous membrane exposure, clothing contamination, and transfer of microorganisms to other patients, personnel, and the environment.
8. *Environmental control.* Adequate procedures for routine care and cleaning of environmental surfaces, beds, and associated equipment are to be developed, and the use of these procedures is monitored on a regular basis.
9. *Patient placement.* Patients who contaminate the environment or who are unable to maintain appropriate hygiene or environmental control are to be housed in a private room with appropriate air handling and ventilation. If a private room is not available, the infection-control professional may determine a method for cohorting patients with similar infectious organisms.[26]

Transmission-based precautions

Transmission-Based Precautions are to be used for patients known or suspected of being infected with highly transmissible or epidemiologically important pathogens for which additional precautions are needed beyond the basic Standard Precautions. There are three types of Transmission-Based Precautions: Airborne Precautions, Droplet Precautions, and Contact Precautions. In some cases these precautions may be combined as when a disease has multiple routes of transmission. Transmission-Based Precautions are to be used in addition to Standard Precautions.

Airborne Precautions

Airborne transmission occurs by dissemination of droplet nuclei from evaporated droplets that can remain suspended in the air for long periods of time or by dissemination of dust particles that contain the infectious agent. Droplet nuclei are particles 5 μm or smaller in size. Airborne microorganisms can be dispersed widely depending on air currents and can be inhaled by or deposited on a susceptible host. In addition to Standard Precautions, Airborne Precautions include the following:

1. Patients are to be placed in private, negative-pressure rooms. The air exchange should be at a rate of 6 to 12 exchanges per hour with air discharged to the outdoors or circulated through high-efficiency filters before being circulated to other areas of the facility.
2. Care givers should wear respiratory protection when caring for patients with known or suspected tuberculosis. If susceptible personnel care for patients with rubeola (measles) or varicella (chickenpox), respiratory protection should be worn. If the care giver is immune to rubeola and varicella, respiratory protection is not necessary.
3. All precautions for preventing transmission of tuberculosis should be implemented if the patient is known or suspected to have tuberculosis.[24,26]
4. A surgical mask should be placed over the patient's face if he or she must be transported from one location to another. Patient transport should be limited to essential purposes only.

Droplet Precautions

Droplet Precautions are used for patients known or suspected of being infected with microorganisms that are transmitted by large droplets greater than 5 μm in size. These droplets can be generated when the patient sneezes, coughs, or simply talks. Droplet Precautions are used in addition to Standard Precautions. Droplet Precautions[26] include the following:

1. Patients are to be placed in private rooms when available. If this is not possible, the patient should be placed in a room with another patient who is infected with the same organism and with no other infection. If this is not possible, a three-foot spatial separation should be maintained between the infected patient and other patients in the same room. For Droplet Precau-

tions, no special air-handling is required and doors may remain open.
2. Care givers should wear a mask when working within 3 feet of the patient.
3. Patients should be transported only for essential purposes. When transport is necessary, a mask should be placed over the patient's nose and mouth to minimize dispersal of droplets.

Contact Precautions

In addition to Standard Precautions, Contact Precautions should be used for patients known or suspected to be infected or colonized with epidemiologically important organisms that can be transmitted by direct contact as occur when the care giver touches the patient's skin, or by indirect contact as in touching patient care equipment or environmental surfaces in the patient's room. Contact Precautions include the following:

1. Patients should be placed in a private room. If this is not possible, the patient should be placed in a room with another patient who is infected with the same organism and with no other infection. If this is not possible, patient placement must be determined on an individual basis, depending on the organism involved.
2. Gloves should be worn upon entering the patient's room. These gloves should be changed after handling infective material that might contain a high concentration of microorganisms. When care-giving activities have been completed, gloves should be removed before leaving the patient's room. Hands should be washed with an antimicrobial agent or a waterless antiseptic hand-cleansing agent. To avoid transfer of microorganisms to others, care should be taken to not touch any environmental surfaces in the patient's environment after the hands have been washed.
3. Gowns should be worn upon entering the patient's room if there is a probability that the care giver's clothing will be in contact with the patient or the environmental surfaces, or if the patient is incontinent, has diarrhea, or has an ileostomy or colostomy. The gown should be removed before leaving the patient's room and care exercised to avoid contact with environmental surfaces.
4. Patient transportation should be limited to essential transport only, and Contact Precautions maintained to avoid contamination of personnel, visitors, or the environment.
5. Patient-care equipment should be dedicated to a single patient and not be shared between patients. If this is not possible, equipment must be thoroughly cleaned and disinfected before being used for another patient.

Perioperative staff members historically have relied on Universal Precautions to protect themselves and others from blood-borne pathogens. Little attention has been given in the perioperative setting to routinely protecting healthcare personnel or patients from infectious diseases caused by pathogens other than HIV. Perioperative personnel should be knowledgeable about and practice both Standard Precautions and Transmission-Based Precautions.[34] Implementing these precautions in surgical settings requires perioperative nursing judgment. These precautions serve to protect the healthcare provider and to minimize cross-infection of pathogens between patients.

Engineering Practices to Control Infection

Environment of care

The surgical suite should be designed in such a way as to minimize and control the spread of infectious organisms. Either a central-core or a single-corridor design may be used. With the central-core design, sterile equipment and supplies should be contained within the central-core area, which is surrounded by operating rooms and a peripheral corridor. The single corridor design places the operating rooms on either side of a single corridor, with separate storage rooms along the corridor to house sterile equipment and supplies. If a single-corridor design is used, sterile and contaminated items must be separated by either space or time. That is, sterile, wrapped, or containerized items can pass contaminated items in the corridor when the contaminated items are covered or otherwise contained.

Floors in the operating rooms should be hard, seamless, easily cleaned, and contiguous with the walls. This design eliminates the sharp angle where the floor and walls meet and where bacteria can become lodged and proliferate. If floors must be seamed, all seams should be heat sealed. Walls may be constructed of any hard surface that is easily cleaned and hard enough to withstand the impact of surgical equipment that may accidentally be pushed into the wall during transport. If ceramic tile is used, smooth-surface grouting mortar should be used. This grout provides a surface nearly as smooth as the tile itself, thus eliminating concerns that surface roughness may attract and retain bacteria. Painted walls are less desirable because the paint flakes and peels, particularly in areas of higher humidity. If a hard-finish, epoxy paint is used, it will be only as good as the surface beneath it. Equipment banged into a wall may cause damage and exposure of construction materials into the environment. A soft-colored, matte-finished wall may be preferred to reduce reflectance and glare.[44]

Doors in the operating rooms may swing or slide. If sliding doors are used, they should not recess into the wall but should slide over the adjoining wall to facilitate housekeeping.[44] Cabinets should be recessed into the wall if at all possible. This configuration allows for maximum use of open floor space in operating rooms. Size and configuration of operating rooms are discussed in detail by the American Institute of Architects Academy of Architecture for Health.[3] Stainless-steel cabinets are preferred because the surfaces remain smooth and are easily cleaned. Wooden cabinets become quickly damaged with cracks and crevices where bacteria can collect and proliferate. Wooden cabinets are difficult to clean and disinfect and should be avoided in the operating rooms. Cabinet doors may be of either the swinging or the sliding type. A cleaning protocol should be established for the tracts if sliding doors are used. For noncabinet shelving, open wire shelves are preferred because dust and bacteria do not accumulate and air can circulate freely around shelf contents.[44]

Scrub sinks should be located adjacent to each operating room with a single area serving two operating rooms if possible. Ideally, scrub sinks are located in a room or alcove adjacent to the peripheral or single corridor of the operating room. Scrub sinks should not be within the central core area because aerosolization and splashing may occur where sterile items are stored.

Each surgical suite must contain an enclosed soiled workroom exclusive for its own use. The workroom should contain a flushing hopper, receptacles for waste and soiled linen, a handwashing sink, and a work counter. If the area is used as a holding area as part of a larger system for collection and disposal of soiled materials, the flushing hopper can be eliminated.[3]

Heating ventilation air conditioning (HVAC)

To control bioparticulate matter in the operating room environment, ventilating air should be delivered to the room from ceiling vents or vents located high on the walls of the room. Air should be exhausted from outlets located near the floor and on opposite walls to those containing inlet vents. Airflow should be unidirectional, moving down and through the location, with a minimum of draft, to the floor and exhaust portals.[44]

Air pressure in the operating room should be greater than that in the surrounding corridor. This will help maintain the unidirectional airflow in the room and minimize the amount of corridor air entering the operating room. Each operating room should have a minimum of 15 total air exchanges per hour, with the equivalent of at least three replacements being of outside air to satisfy exhaust needs of the system. No recirculating devices such as cooling fans or room humidifiers or dehumidifiers are to be used. These units create a turbulent airflow and may recirculate settled bacteria. To minimize static electricity and to reduce the potential for bacterial growth, relative humidity in the operating room should be maintained between 30% and 60%. A lower relative humidity may support accumulation of static electricity, whereas a higher humidity rate may result in condensation of ambient moisture, which may result in damp materials and supplies. This dampness will support bacterial growth. In concert with the prescribed humidity range, temperatures in the operating rooms should be maintained at a range of 68° to 73° F.[3]

Work Practices to Control Infection
Sterilization

Sterilization is defined as the complete elimination or destruction of all forms of microbial life. The concept of what constitutes "sterile" is measured as the *probability* of sterility for each item to be sterilized. This probability is known as the *sterility assurance level* (SAL). For terminal steam sterilization processes, 10^{-6} is the recommended probability of survival for microorganisms on a sterilized device.[75] A probability of microorganism survival of 10^{-6} means that there is less than or equal to 1 chance in 1 million that an item is contaminated or unsterile. The SAL of 10^{-6} is considered appropriate for items that will be used on tissue that has lost the integrity of the natural body barriers. For items not intended to come into contact with compromised tissue, the recognized SAL is 10^{-3}, or a 1 in 1000 chance of a surviving microorganism.[7]

Steam Sterilization

Steam sterilization is the oldest, safest, most economical, and best-understood method of sterilization available in healthcare. It is the preferred method of sterilization for those items that can withstand heat and moisture. The efficacy of steam sterilization depends on lowering and limiting the bioburden on the item or items to be sterilized, using effective sterilization cycles, and preventing recontamination of sterile items before delivery to the point of use.[6]

Theory of microbial destruction

Microorganisms are believed to be destroyed by moist heat through a process of denaturation and coagulation of the enzyme-protein system within the bacterial cell. Microorganisms are killed at a lower temperature when moist heat is used as opposed to when dry heat is used. This fact is based on the theory that all chemical reactions, including coagulation of proteins, are catalyzed by the presence of water.

Principles and mechanisms

At standard atmospheric pressure (sea level) when water is heated, the water temperature rises as heat energy is added. After the boiling point of 100° C (212° F) is reached, additional heat energy evaporates the water to form steam. At this point the steam and the water are at the same temperature, but the steam has more energy than the water. This difference in energy is known as the *latent heat of vaporization*. When a cold item is introduced into the steam, some of the steam gives up its latent energy to the object and changes back to liquid water. This phenomenon allows items to be heated much more rapidly in steam than in dry heat. The phenomenon of steam changing to liquid water is called *condensation* and both the steam and the liquid water are at a temperature of 212° F when this occurs. At this point, the steam is said to be saturated. However, this 212° F temperature is insufficient to kill microorganisms. To achieve a saturation temperature sufficient to kill microorganisms (250° F), it is necessary to have a sealed container. When water is boiled in a vessel from which the steam cannot escape, a higher temperature is reached. As more steam is generated with no escape route, pressure in the vessel increases. The higher the steam pressure, the higher the temperature. The steam is the sterilizing agent. Any compressed air remaining in the vessel will mix with the steam and lower the steam temperature. This reduced-temperature steam will be incapable of sterilization. Thus, air acts as a barrier to steam sterilization.[75]

Steam entering the sterilizer chamber should contain little or no entrapped liquid water. The term "steam quality" is used to describe the amount of steam vapor and liquid water in the mixture. A steam quality of 100% indicates that no liquid water is present in the steam. A steam quality of 97% or greater (that is, less than 3% of the mixture is liquid water) is recommended to achieve an efficient sterilization process. Causes of low steam quality include improper boiler operation and inadequate or poorly maintained steam distribution lines to the sterilizer.[75]

Presterilization preparation

Efficacy of the sterilization process will depend in part on lowering or limiting of the amount of bioburden present on the item to be sterilized. Items to be sterilized should be precleaned to lower the bioburden to the lowest possible level.

To prevent infection, all items that come into contact with the patient or sterile field should be systematically decontaminated after a surgical procedure. Handling, transport, and cleaning methods must be selected to prevent cross-contamination to other patients, exposure of personnel to blood-borne pathogens, and damage to instruments. The cleaning and decontamination methods chosen should be economical and of demonstrated effectiveness. Items may be cleaned by hand, by mechanical means, or a combination of the two.[6] Increased productivity, greater cleaning effectiveness, and increased employee safety may result from use of mechanical cleaning methods. Some mechanical cleaning equipment is designed to remove microorganisms through a cleaning and rinsing action, whereas others destroy specific types of microorganisms by thermal or chemical means. Types of mechanical cleaning equipment include washer-sterilizers, washer-disinfectors, or washer-sanitizers, ultrasonic cleaners, utensil washers, and cart washers.

All workers handling soiled surgical instruments, whether in the operating room, substerile room, or a central decontamination area, must wear personal protective attire sufficient to prevent contact with any blood or other body fluid. This generally means scrub attire covered with a liquid-proof gown, coverall, or sleeved apron; hair covering; surgical face mask and eye protection; rubber or latex gloves suitable to the task; and, if fluids may pool on the floor, liquid-proof boots or shoe covers.

Because debris contains microorganisms (bioburden), instruments should be kept as free from body substances and other debris as possible during the surgical procedure. Instruments should be wiped with a sterile, water-moistened sponge as frequently as required. Sterile water is selected as opposed to saline solution because saline causes corrosion of the instrument surfaces. When the surgical procedure is completed, initial decontamination should begin immediately.[10] All instruments that can be immersed are disassembled, or box locks are opened to allow solution contact with all soiled surfaces. These instruments should be placed in a basin, solid-bottom container system, or bin with lid. Scissors and light-weight instruments should be placed on top. Heavy retractors should be placed in a separate tray. Instruments may be covered with a water-moistened surgical towel to prevent drying of any lingering debris.

Some instruments have sharp or pointed edges, such as scissors, forceps with teeth, perforating towel clamps, curettes, and rongeurs. These items can penetrate the gloves and skin, creating a portal of entry for infectious organisms. A different process is used for these instruments. They must not be placed in a basin or tray in such a way that a worker would have to reach into the container to retrieve the instrument, thus risking injury. Instead, they can be placed with points down in a basin small enough that the handles are outside the basin, thus allowing individual instruments to be grasped. An alternative to this is to place all instruments together and not handle them until after they have been through a mechanical cleaning process.

All soiled instruments should be transported from the operating room for cleaning and decontamination. They should be contained in leakproof containers or trays inside plastic bags. If sharps are being transported, the container should be puncture resistant. Means of containing instruments include plastic, rubber, or metal bins with lids, solid-bottom sterilization container systems with the lids in place and filters in place, or simply placement of the instrument tray in a plastic bag. All soiled containment packages should be labeled with the biohazard symbol to warn handlers as to the nature of the contents. Transporting instruments while they are soaking in water is discouraged because of the possibility of a liquid spill with the associated clean-up problems and the difficulty of safely disposing of the contaminated liquid unless a flushing hopper is available.

In the decontamination area, an initial cold water rinse with tap water or a soak in cool water with a protein and blood-dissolving enzyme will help remove blood, tissue, and gross debris from device lumens, joints, and serrations.[6] After this pretreatment, the instruments may then be processed mechanically or washed by hand.

When manual cleaning is done, instruments should be submerged in warm water with an appropriate detergent and cleaned and rinsed while submerged. Cleaning in this manner helps protect personnel from aerosolization or splashing of infectious material and from injury by sharp objects. Harsh abrasives should not be used for manual cleaning because they will damage the protective surfaces of instruments, contribute to corrosion, and impede sterilization.[10]

Mechanical cleaning is the preferred method of processing most instruments. For immersible instruments, washer-sterilizers offer an excellent option. If a washer-sterilizer is to be used, gross debris should be removed with a cold water rinse before the instruments are placed in the washer-sterilizer, with care used to minimize splashing during rinsing. Instruments are placed in perforated or mesh bottom trays or baskets and positioned so that the cleaning portion of the washer-sterilizer cycle can reach all parts of the instrument.

There are two types of washer-sterilizers: those configured like a tunnel, with doors at each end and rotating spray arms on the sides, top, and bottom of the chamber, and those that cover the instruments with water and then blow steam and air through the water to cause agitation that produces the cleaning effect (Fig. 4-3). The former machines are generally found in central decontamination areas and may be connected to an automatic or manual conveyer. The second type of machine is generally small (about 16 to 20 inches in diameter) and located in the substerile room or instrument-processing room of the surgery suite.

After cleaning the instruments with detergent and water and then rinsing them, the washer-sterilizer begins a steam sterilization cycle. The exposure time for this cycle depends on the temperature at which the cycle is run. Some washer-sterilizers of the tunnel type operate at 285° F for less than 1 minute. Others, including all of the second type of washer-sterilizers, operate at 270° F for 10 minutes. All rely on gravity displacement to remove air from the chamber. Instruments processed through a single cycle of a washer-sterilizer are safe to handle and may indeed be sterile, depending on presterilization bioburden. They are not suitable for immediate use in another surgical procedure. They must be inspected, arranged in a manner convenient for the surgical team to use, and steam sterilized again. Debris remaining on the instruments because of possible inefficiencies of the cleaning process will be baked on by the sterilization portion of the process and may be difficult to remove.

In recent years, different types of mechanical instrument washers, washer-sanitizers, and washer-decontaminators have been introduced. In some facilities they have

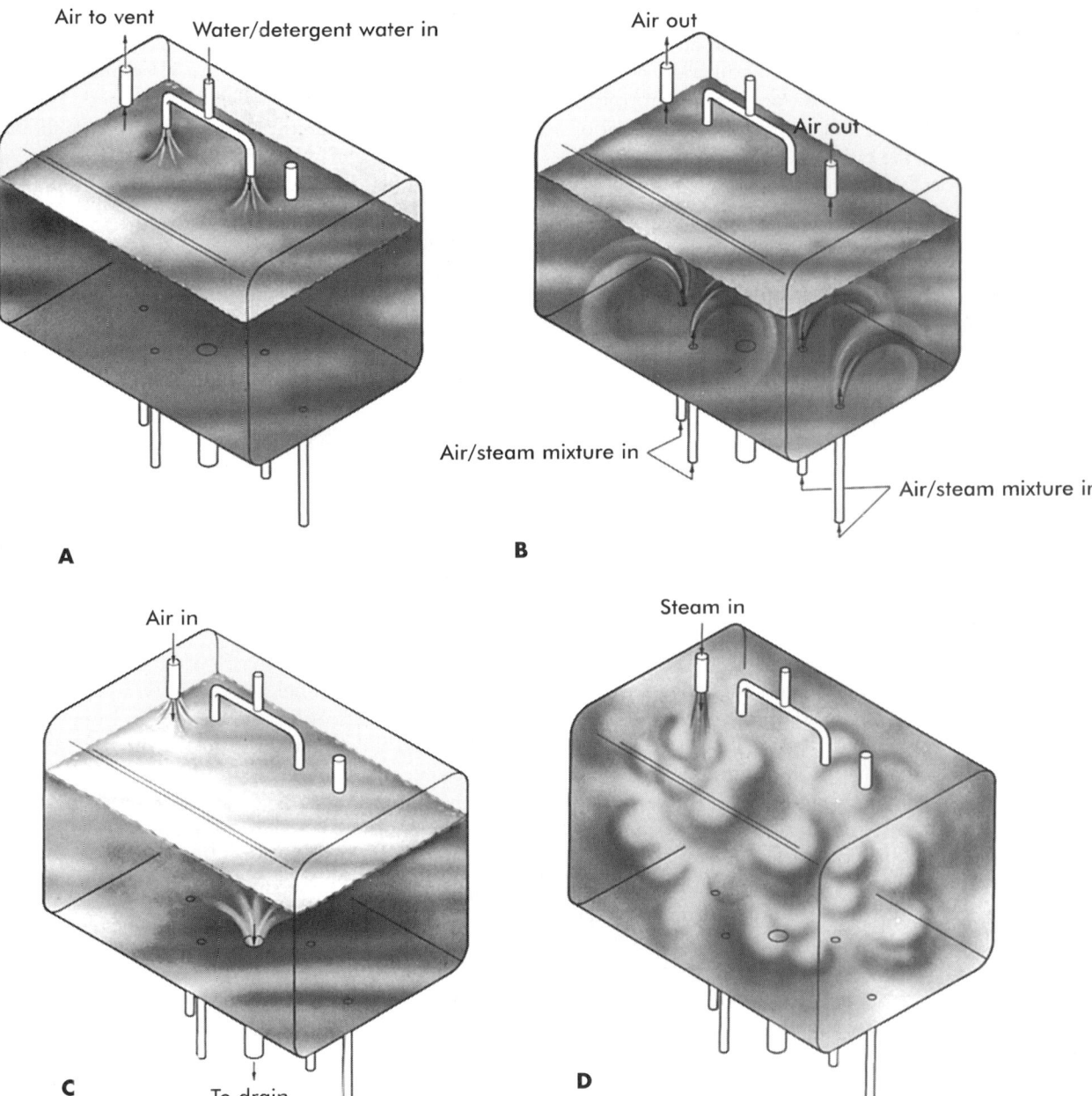

FIGURE 4-3 Automatic washer-sterilizer. **A,** The cycle in this machine begins with a cold water rinse entering through the top of the chamber to loosen and remove gross soil such as blood and tissue without coagulating proteinaceous material, which would cause it to adhere to instruments. Then warm water and detergent enter the chamber to a level to cover the instruments. **B,** Next, jets of steam and air are injected into the filled chamber through ports in the floor of the chamber. Violent turbulence in the detergent-water solution removes any debris remaining on the instruments after the initial rinse. **C,** At the conclusion of the wash time the water drains out of the chamber. Newer model washer-sterilizers may have microprocessor controls that allow the user to set the duration of wash time based on the nature of soil on the instruments. A final rinse coming in through the top of the chamber carries any detergent residues and soil away from the instruments and out the drain. **D,** Finally, saturated steam begins to fill the chamber. Air in the chamber and load is heavier than the steam and, because of gravity, is displaced downward and out the drain. As pressure builds in the chamber from the incoming steam, the temperature rises to 132° C (270° F), the chamber drain closes, and that temperature is held for the duration of the sterilization exposure time selected by the user. Then steam is exhausted through the automatic condenser exhaust. Some machines have the capability of selecting drying times for the instruments. At the conclusion of the cycle, an audible signal indicates that the unit is ready for unloading. Instruments and the inside of the sterilizer are very hot, and, if no dry time was used, the instruments and trays are also wet. Use extreme caution in handling.

replaced both handwashing of instruments and the use of washer-sterilizers. These units may have a single chamber where several phases of a rinsing, cleaning, rinsing, and drying process occur. Or they may have multiple chambers, each specialized for a specific function in the cleaning process, including initial cool-water rinse to remove protein debris, enzymatic-solution soak, washing with detergent, ultrasonic cleaning, sustained hot-water (80° to 95° C) rinse, perhaps a liquid chemical germicide rinse (such as sodium hypochlorite solution), and drying. Soiled utensils such as basins and trays should pass through a utensil washer, washer-disinfector-sanitizer, or a washer-sterilizer.[6]

Not all instrumentation will tolerate this process and not all hospitals have access to mechanical washers that incorporate hot water or chemical decontamination as part of the cleaning cycle. Some instrumentation will not tolerate immersion in water or cannot take the heat or pressures involved in mechanical processes. These items must be hand washed using an appropriate detergent for the type of material and the type of soil on the item. If protein or other organic soil is present, the detergent should have an alkaline pH (greater than 7). If inorganic soil is present, the detergent should have an acid pH (less than 7). The degree of alkalinity or acidity should be selected so that the instrument or item itself will not be damaged in the cleaning process. For example, stainless-steel instrumentation with organic soil is best cleaned by alkaline detergents with a pH range of 7.0 to 10.0, according to most United States surgical instrument manufacturers. Using acidic or harshly alkaline solutions can remove the protective passivation layer from the instrument and allow pitting and other corrosive activity, which cannot be repaired. This advice regarding detergent selection applies to mechanical washing also. The instrument manufacturer should be consulted to determine appropriate cleaning products and procedures.

Items that were soiled with blood or body fluids and that have been cleaned only may not have been sufficiently decontaminated to allow handling by workers not wearing protective attire. If such an item will tolerate steam sterilization, it can be further decontaminated by processing through an unwrapped steam-sterilization cycle (flash sterilized). It is then safe to handle. The item can also be soaked in a liquid chemical germicide such as 2% alkaline glutaraldehyde for 20 minutes to disinfect it. If none of these methods is suitable for the item, either because of damage to the item, cost, or unavailability, workers in the preparation area should wear protective gloves when handling, inspecting, assembling, and packaging these items for sterilization.

The ultrasonic cleaning process is designed to remove fine soil from crevices and box-lock areas of instrumentation. It should be used only after instruments have had gross debris removed. Ultrasonic energy occurs in wave form and is generated by transducers on the sides or bottom of a specially constructed chamber that is filled with water or a water and detergent solution. The ultrasonic waves pass through the water, creating tiny bubbles that then collapse or implode. This creates a negative pressure, which pulls debris away from surfaces. This process is known as *cavitation*. Once the cleaning process is accomplished, the instruments should be rinsed to remove the loose debris. Some ultrasonic consoles have chambers for rinsing and drying instruments.

Effective ultrasonic cleaning requires that most of the dissolved gases be removed from the water in the chamber before cleaning begins. Otherwise, the bubbles formed are too large to produce effective cavitation. Degassing should be done each time the chamber is refilled with clean solution. This can be done by running the ultrasonic machine without a load in the chamber for 5 to 10 minutes, as directed by the manufacturer.

The ultrasonic cleaner should always be used with the lid down. The fine aerosols created by the process can spread over greater distances than large water splashes can. Also, personnel working in the area of the ultrasonic machine should be wearing a surgical face mask and eye protection to protect the mucous membranes. The ultrasonic cleaner can be used in the cleaning process any time after gross debris is removed from the instruments. It is most effective if used before fine debris is baked on, as in the steam-sterilization process. The ultrasonic machine should be placed in the soiled or decontamination area, not in the clean area, regardless of what stage it is used in the process. Previous recommendations for using the ultrasonic machine only after cleaning and sterilization of instruments resulted from concerns over the fine aerosols created by the process and arose in a time when personal protective attire was neither routinely worn nor required by federal regulation.

Not all items will tolerate the energy waves of the ultrasonic process. Chromium-plated instruments should not be cleaned ultrasonically because the energy waves can loosen the chromium from the base metal underneath. Dissimilar metals such as stainless steel, titanium, copper, and lead should not be ultrasonically processed at the same time. The energy waves, combined with the heat and detergent solution, can cause electrolysis to occur, plating one metal onto others, potentially ruining the instruments. Some manufacturers recommend that microsurgery instruments not be placed in the ultrasonic cleaner, both because of their delicate design and the fact that they may contain several types of metal. The detergent or enzyme cleaner used in the ultrasonic machine should be very carefully selected. The corrosiveness and overall effectiveness of some solutions can be dramatically affected by the combination of heat and ultrasonic energy in such a machine.

The final step before sterilization for reuse includes instrument preparation and packaging. These activities occur in a clean area, separate from the area where decontamination occurred. Instruments are carefully inspected for cleanliness and functionality. Soiled instruments are returned for further cleaning. Instruments with movable parts are treated with a water-soluble lubricant solution that contains an antimicrobial agent to retard growth in the lubricant solution. Broken or worn instruments are set aside for repair. Instruments are assembled into sets according to set content lists prepared by perioperative nursing staff.

Packaging and sterilizer loading

Packaging of surgical supplies and their arrangement in loads in the sterilizer are factors that govern the effectiveness of steam sterilization. The prime function of a package containing a surgical item is to permit sterilization of the contents and to ensure the sterility of the contents up to the time the package is opened.[9, 10] Provision must be made for the contents to be removed without contamination. Effective packaging material should have the following characteristics:

1. Allows for adequate air removal and steam penetration
2. Provides an adequate microbial barrier
3. Resists tearing or punctures
4. Has proved seal integrity (does not delaminate when opened and will not allow a reseal after opening)
5. Allows for aseptic delivery of package contents
6. Is free of toxic ingredients and nonfast dyes
7. Is low linting
8. Is cost effective by value analysis

Sterilization-container systems are one way of packaging instruments. As rigid packaging systems that can be sterilized, stacked, and stored, they offer a simple yet effective method. Because they are rigid, they cannot be punctured, abraded, or easily contaminated by environmental microbes. Studies have indicated that, properly initiated, container systems are a cost-effective packaging method. Recommendations for sterilizing containers in various sterilizers should be obtained from the manufacturer. Performance testing should be carried out in the sterile processing department of the healthcare facility to ensure that all conditions essential for both sterilization and drying are effectively achieved. Before opening a container, the perioperative nurse should check for evidence of integrity and sterility. The lid should be removed with care. The scrub person should maintain a margin of safety between himself or herself and the unsterile outer container when removing the inner basket.

If textile wrappers are used, they must be laundered between sterilization exposures to ensure sufficient moisture content of the fibers. This prevents superheating and absorption of the sterilizing agent. Rehydrated materials also deteriorate at a slower rate. All wrappers must be checked for holes or tears before use. Many in-hospital packaging materials—woven and nonwoven, reusable and disposable—are marketed today. Materials should be carefully evaluated before a product is chosen.

The size and density of woven textile packs must be restricted to ensure uniform steam penetration. The pack should not exceed $12 \times 12 \times 20$ inches ($30 \times 30 \times 50$ cm) and should not weigh more than 12 pounds (5.4 kg). When the items in the pack are being assembled, the lighter materials should be placed near the center of the pack. Each succeeding layer of dry goods should be placed crosswise on the layer below to promote free circulation of steam and removal of air. Pack density should not exceed 7.2 pounds per cubic foot. A chemical indicator that accurately reflects one or more of the physical parameters of sterilization should be inserted into the center of each pack. These parameters are time, temperature, and steam saturation and purity.

The pack should be wrapped sequentially in two barrier type of wrappers, which may be disposable or reusable. A single textile reusable wrapper is defined as one layer of 270- to 280-thread-count woven fabric. Cross-stitching and raw edges are not acceptable. Sequential double wrapping creates a package within a package, providing for ease in presenting the wrapped item to the sterile field. Wrappers are made in suitable dimensions for the various items that must be packaged. The familiar envelope wrap is made by placement of the article diagonally in the center of the wrapper. The near corner, which should point toward the worker, is brought over the item, and the triangular tip is folded back to form a cuff. The two side flaps are folded to the center in like manner. The far corner of the wrapper is then folded on top of the other three. The process is repeated with the second wrapper, and the package is secured with autoclave indicator tape.

When the pack is opened for use, the flaps at the corners are used to form a protective cuff over the nurse's hands during dispensing of the sterile contents. When the items are wrapped, the wrappers should be folded securely about the contents. The package should be firm and sealed securely to prevent contamination in handling and storage. Single, disposable, nonwoven wrappers made up of fused material layers are available in the marketplace. When these single wrappers provide a bacterial barrier at least equivalent to the sequential double wrap and allow for safe and easy presentation of the package contents to the sterile field, they may provide an alternative to the sequential double-wrapping procedure. Careful wrapping to prevent tenting and gapping of the package is essential.

Sterilization process (chemical) indicator tape should be used to hold wrappers in place on packages and to indicate that the packages have been exposed to the physical conditions of a sterilization cycle. When packages are opened, these tapes should be removed from reusable wrappers because they create laundry problems, such as occluding screens and filters. In some cases the tapes leave a dye on the wrappers that may cause deterioration of the material. Tapes may also leave an adhesive residue that can interfere with future sterilizations of the fabric.

Every package intended for sterile use should be imprinted or labeled with a load-control number that identifies the date of sterilization, the sterilizer used, and the cycle or load number. Load-control numbers facilitate identification and retrieval of supplies, inventory control, and appropriate rotation to ensure that older packages are used first.

Some instruments or packaging systems may present challenges to the sterilization process. Special preparation or loading procedures may be necessary to meet these challenges. Hinged instruments must be arranged so that the steam can contact all surfaces of the instrument, including the tips, hinged surfaces, and ratchets. To accomplish this, these instruments must be sterilized in the open position. If the instruments have ringed handles for the fingers, the instruments may be placed on a "stringer," which is a U-shaped metal rod made especially for this purpose. Tubular instruments with lumens can trap air, which interferes with the sterilization process. To avoid this problem, lumens should be moistened with water immediately before sterilization. As the instrument is heated, the water turns to steam and forces the air out of the lumen. Instruments with concave or other surfaces that can hold water must be carefully placed on edge to facilitate removal of air, which may get trapped in the concave surface. Placing the instrument on edge will also facilitate drainage of condensate. Items such as basins, which may be stacked for sterilization, should be stacked with sufficient space between all surfaces so that steam can contact all surfaces.[66]

When packaging is complete and the sterilizer chamber is loaded, the bundles and packages should be arranged to minimize resistance to steam, which must pass through the load from the top of the chamber toward the bottom of the sterilizer. All packages should be placed on a vertical edge in the sterilizer in a loose-contact position. This allows free circulation and penetration of steam, enhances air elimination, prevents entrapment of air or water, and precludes excessive condensation. A second or upper layer may be placed crosswise on the first or lower layer. All jars, tubes, canisters, and other nonporous objects should be arranged on their sides with their covers or lids removed to provide a horizontal path for the escape of air and the free flow of steam and heat. To guard against superheating, surgical packs and supplies should not be subjected to preheating in the sterilizer with steam in the jacket before sterilization.

Rigid container systems should be placed flat on the sterilizer shelf. These containers should not be stacked during sterilization unless the manufacturer specifically indicates that this is safe practice. Containers should be stacked only in the manner recommended by the manufacturer. Stacking may interfere with air removal and steam penetration. Additionally, condensation from upper containers may drip down and contaminate lower containers when the sterilizer door is opened and the cooler room air contacts the containers.[66]

Sterilizing

When steam enters the autoclave, it is at the same pressure as the atmosphere. As the valves and doors to the outside close, steam pressure rises inside the chamber, thereby increasing the temperature of the steam. Evacuation of air from the sterilizer is necessary to permit proper permeation of steam. If a sterilizer is improperly loaded, mixing of air with steam acts as a barrier to steam penetration and prevents attainment of the sterilization temperature. (See *Principles and mechanisms* section on p. 110.)

The three factors necessary to achieve steam sterilization are time, temperature, and moisture. The microbial destruction period is based on the known time-temperature cycle necessary to accomplish sterilization in saturated steam. Authorities have shown that the order of death in a given bacterial population subjected to a sterilizing process is determined by definite laws. If the temperature is increased, the time may be decreased. The minimum time-temperature relationships for sterilizing efficiency are shown in Table 4-1.

To provide a safety margin, the minimum estimated exposure is extended to cover the lag between the attainment of the selected temperature in the chamber and the temperature of the load. The length of exposure varies with the type of sterilizer, cycle design, altitude, bioburden, packaging, and size and composition of items to be sterilized. Written instructions for sterilization parameters should be obtained from the sterilizer manufacturer. If a closed-container system is used as packaging for items to be sterilized, the container manufacturer's written instructions for exposure times should be consulted and reconciled with those of the sterilizer manufacturer.[6]

Sterilizers vary in design and performance characteristics. Use of rigid container systems may alter the come-up and exposure times in steam sterilizers. The configuration of some instruments or medical devices may hinder air removal and steam penetration, making sterilization more difficult. In such circumstances the device manufacturer

TABLE 4-1	Minimum Time-Temperature Relationships for Sterilizing Efficiency
TEMPERATURE, IN °C (°F)	**TIME, IN MINUTES**
132 (270)	2
125 (257)	8
118 (245)	18

TABLE 4-2 | **Common Time-Temperature Parameters for Steam Sterilization**

TYPE OF STERILIZER	LOAD CONFIGURATION	TEMPERATURE, IN °C (°F)	TIME, IN MINUTES
Gravity-displacement	Porous or nonporous	121-123 (250-254)	15-30
		132-135 (270-275)	10-25
Prevacuum	Porous or nonporous	132-135 (270-275)	3-4
Steam-flush/pressure pulse	Porous or nonporous	121-123 (250-254)	20
		132-135 (270-275)	3-4

must be able to specify the necessary parameters to achieve steam sterilization. The most common time and temperature parameters are provided in Table 4-2.

The recording thermometer, not the pressure gauge, is the important guide to the sterilizing phase. The recording clock on the sterilizer gives information about the run of the load and to what temperature the goods were exposed. The temperature inside the chamber must be maintained throughout the determined time of exposure.[6]

Drying, cooling, and storing

Upon completion of the sterilization cycle the steam inside the chamber is removed immediately so that it will not condense and wet the packs. To assist in the drying process, the jacket pressure should be maintained to keep the walls of the chamber hot as the steam from the chamber is exhausted. When the chamber pressure has been exhausted, the door may be opened slightly to permit vapor to escape. Another method is to introduce clean, filtered air by means of a vacuum dryer (ejector) device in conjunction with the operating valve on the sterilizer. The minimum drying time for all methods is approximately 15 to 20 minutes.

After removal from the sterilizer, freshly sterilized packs should be left untouched on the loading carriage until they have cooled to room temperature. This is usually accomplished in 30 to 60 minutes, depending on the load contents. If freshly sterilized packages are placed on cool surfaces such as metal table tops, vapor still inside the essentially dry package may condense to water. This water may dampen the package from the inside to the outside. Once the outside is wet, bacteria may follow the moist tract into the contents of the package. Because bacteria are capable of passing through layers of wet material, any packages that are wet must be considered unsterile.

A written record of existing conditions during each sterilization cycle should be maintained. It should include the sterilizer number, the cycle or load number, the time and temperature of the cycle, the date of sterilization, the contents of the load, and the initials of the operator. These records should be retained for the length of time designated by the statute of limitations in each state.

Sterile packages must be handled with care and only as necessary. They should be stored in clean, dry, limited-access areas that are well ventilated and have controlled temperature and humidity. Closed cabinets are preferred to open shelves for sterile storage. If open shelves must be used, the lowest shelf should be 8 to 10 inches from the floor to avoid floor contamination. The highest shelf should be at least 18 inches from the ceiling to allow for circulation around the stored items. All shelves should be at least 2 inches from outside walls to facilitate air circulation and avoid any condensation that might accumulate on the walls during periods of severe temperature change. Shelving should be smooth and well spaced, with no projections or sharp corners that might damage the wrappers. Sterilized packs should never be stacked in close contact with each other. Their arrangement on the shelves should provide for air circulation on all sides of each package. Excessive handling, crowding, dropping, and stacking of sterile packs tend to force particles through the mesh or matrix of the wrapping material, which might contaminate the contents. Sterile items should not be stored near or under sinks or in any area where they can become wet. Storage on window sills, nondesignated shelving, counters, or carts should be avoided.

Shelf life refers to the length of time a pack may be considered sterile. Loss of package sterility is event related as opposed to time related; that is, what happens to the package after sterilization determines its continued sterility, not the length of time the package remains on the shelf ready for use. Variables that must be considered in determining shelf life are the type and number of layers of packaging material used, the presence or absence of impervious protective covers, the number of times a package is handled before use, and the conditions of storage. Impervious protective covers known as *dust covers* may extend shelf life by protecting the sterile package from a contaminating event. When used to protect sterilized items, impervious covers should be designated as such to prevent their being mistaken for a sterile wrap. They should be applied only to thoroughly cooled, dry packs at the time of removal from the sterilizer cart, after the required cooling period.

Supply standards should be planned to maintain adequate stock with prompt turnover. Appropriate volume and proper rotation of supplies reduce the need for concern about shelf life. The longer an item is stored, the greater the chances of contamination. For proper rotation, the most recently dated sterile packages should be placed behind those already on the shelves.

Quality control

All mechanical parts of sterilizers, including gauges, steam lines, and drains, should be periodically checked by a competent engineer. Reports of these inspections should be kept by the person responsible for the sterilizers. Temperature, humidity, and vacuum should be measured with control equipment, independently of the fixed gauges. There are several methods of keeping a constant check on the proper functioning of a sterilizer and ensuring the efficiency of the sterilizing process. Mechanical, chemical, and biological controls assist in identifying and preventing sterilizer malfunction and operational errors made by personnel. Automatic controls are a type of mechanical control that, by a predetermined program, control all phases of the sterilizing process. The controls allow the steam to enter, time the sterilizing cycle, exhaust the steam, and initiate drying. Some lock the door so that it cannot be opened until the cycle is complete.

Recording thermometers are another type of mechanical control that indicate and record the temperature throughout the sterilizing cycle on a dial on the front of the sterilizer. In some cases, the sterilizer may provide a digital readout as opposed to a graphic depicter of the sterilizing cycle. In either case, a drop in temperature is recorded when and if it occurs. This can act as a warning of sterilizer failure. The recording thermometer records the time the sterilizer reaches the desired temperature and the duration of each exposure. The recording thermometer can be helpful if several individuals are using the sterilizer or if the operator should forget to time the load. Its recordings are proof that the exposure time of loads has been correct and proper temperature limits have been maintained. The daily record should show the number of the sterilizer, the number of cycles run, the time, and the date. Mechanical monitoring devices provide real-time assessment of sterilizer-cycle conditions and permanent records by means of either the chart recording or computer printouts.[6] This evidence can be used for detection of malfunctions as soon as possible so that alternative procedures can be implemented while the cause of the malfunction is identified and corrective action is taken. Recording thermometers cannot detect air pockets within the load or pack. Air is a poor conductor of heat; therefore it is one of the most common causes, other than human error, of sterilization failure.

Chemical controls, also commonly known as chemical indicators or integrators, include devices such as pellet-containing, sealed, glass tubes; sterilizer indicator tapes; and color-change cards or strips, which may or may not provide a line of demarcation to indicate use or nonuse of the sterilizer load. These chemical indicators are used to detect failures in packaging, loading, or sterilizer function such as presence of cool air pockets inside the sterilizing chamber. The sealed, glass tube that contains a pellet that melts when favorable time and temperature conditions for sterilization are achieved can be placed in the center of linen packs before sterilization. Chemical indicator cards or strips that are impregnated with a material that changes color or moves up a gauge when steam initiates a chemical reaction can also be used to monitor conditions within linen packs. These indicators or integrators are often used in instrument trays or other packages. There is no chemical monitor that verifies that an item is actually sterile.[6]

An external chemical indicator should be used on all packages to be sterilized except for those that allow direct visualization into the package, where an internal indicator is used (such as paper or plastic pouches). The primary purpose of the external indicator is to differentiate between processed and nonprocessed packages. This indicator should be checked after the sterilization process and before a package is opened for use to determine that the package has been exposed to a sterilization process.

An internal chemical indicator should be placed within each package to be sterilized in the in the area of the package believed to be the least accessible to steam penetration. This indicator should be located and interpreted by the user at the time the package is opened and the contents used.[6,14]

A biological indicator is the most accurate method of checking sterilization effectiveness. Commercially prepared biological indicators (manufactured in accordance with minimum performance criteria of the *United States Pharmacopeia*) should be stored and used according to the manufacturer's written instructions. They contain a known population of *Bacillus stearothermophilus*, a highly heat-resistant, spore-forming microorganism that does not produce toxins and is nonpathogenic.

Biologic testing should be done after initial installation of steam sterilizers, after any major repair of the sterilizer, and with all loads of implantable devices. Whenever possible, implantable devices should be quarantined until the results of the biological testing are available. Rapid-action biological indicators are available commercially for certain types of sterilizers. These indicators provide a preliminary readout of biological kill in 1 to 3 hours, depending on the type of sterilizer and cycle used (Research Highlight 4-2).

Biologic testing for steam sterilizer loads should be conducted at least weekly and preferably daily on the first run of the day. The biological indicator should be placed in a test pack that is positioned on edge in the front, bottom section of a routinely loaded steam sterilizer. This area of the sterilizer will most challenge all sterilization parameters. The Association for the Advancement of Medical Instrumentation (AAMI) has defined the challenge test pack composition, configuration, and use.[6] Commercially prepared test packs are available in the marketplace.

After the sterilization cycle the biological indicators are removed from the pack and incubated according to the manufacturer's instructions. Negative reports (failure to recover any spores from the indicators in the test pack) indicate that the sterilizer is functioning properly. Results

4-2 RESEARCH HIGHLIGHT

Biologic indicators are considered to be the monitors closest to ideal for sterilization processes. They measure the sterilization process directly by using highly resistant bacterial spores. This study compared a rapid-readout indicator designed for a 3-hour incubation period with four, self-contained biologic indicators designed for a 24- to 48-hour incubation period. These biologic indicators were also compared to five chemical indicators to determine whether chemical-indicator results parallel those of biologic indicators.

Biologic indicators used in this test were Attest 1262, Proof Plus, Assert, and Biosign. Chemical indicators tested were Comply 1250, Propper, Chemdi, Sterigage, and Thermalog-S. All indicators were commercially available at the time of testing. An AMSCO Eagle model gravity-displacement sterilizer was used for the test with a temperature setting of 121° C (± 1 degree). Experimental cycle times of 5, 10, and 15 minutes were used.

After a 5-minute exposure time, all biologic indicators, including the test indicator, were positive, demonstrating spore growth at 48 hours. Readings taken at 24 hours were predictors of readings at 48 hours 97% of the time. After a 10-minute exposure time, indicators showed either no growth or infrequent growth after 48 hours of incubation. Again the 24-hour data were a 97% predictor of the 48-hour results. With a 10-minute cycle, the test indicator demonstrated spore growth (measured by florescence) of 27% at 1-hour incubation, 64% at 2-hour incubation, and 72% after 3-hour incubation. After a 15-minute sterilization cycle, all biologic indicators including the test indicator were negative for spore growth.

A comparison with chemical indicators tested in the same sterilizer runs demonstrated that three of the five indicators indicated "successful processing" after a 10-minute cycle. The two indicators indicating "unsuccessful processing" at 10 minutes continued to demonstrate "unsuccessful processing" even after the 15-minute cycle. Such results would normally dictate removal of the sterilizer from use pending further investigation and reprocessing of the sterilizer load, an expensive and time-consuming process.

The authors of this study conclude that the rapid-readout biologic indicator, when read at 3-hour incubation, is an accurate and sensitive indicator of sterilization failure. It is equal to or surpasses other indicators designed for 48-hour incubation. Additionally, the authors conclude that chemical indicators are less reliable measures and should not replace biologic indicators.

From Rutala, W., Jones, S., & Weber, D. (1996, July). Comparison of a rapid readout biological indicator for steam sterilization with four conventional biological indicators and five chemical indicators. *Infection Control and Hospital Epidemiology,* 423-428.

of these tests should be filed as a permanent record. A positive report does not necessarily indicate sterilizer failure because false-positive results sometimes occur. However, the sterilizer should immediately be retested and taken out of service until it is operationally inspected and the results of retesting are negative. If a sterilizer malfunction is found, all items prepared in the suspect load should be considered unsterile. They should be retrieved if possible and washed, repackaged, and resterilized in another sterilizer.

When a prevacuum sterilizer is used (see discussion of the prevacuum sterilizer below), a test designed to detect residual air in the chamber should be run daily. The test, generally known as a *Bowie-Dick test*, is run with an otherwise empty chamber so that residual air is not forced into other packs or materials, thus degrading the test results. The Bowie-Dick test pack and procedure have been described by AAMI.[6] The Bowie-Dick determines the efficacy of the vacuum system of the prevacuum sterilizer. The Bowie-Dick is **not** a sterility-assurance test.

Types of Steam Sterilizers
Gravity-displacement sterilizer

For sterilization to occur, steam must contact all surfaces of the item to be sterilized. To accomplish this, the air in the sterilizer chamber must be evacuated. The terms *gravity displacement* and *prevacuum* describe the methods by which air leaves the sterilizer chamber.

At the beginning of the cycle in a gravity sterilizer, steam begins to enter the chamber after the door is closed and locked (Figs. 4-4 and 4-5). An initial burst of steam enters the chamber and forces out much of the free air in the chamber. Air is heavier than steam, and the two do not mix well. As more steam enters the chamber, the air that is held by gravity at the bottom of the chamber exits down the drain, which is at the bottom of the sterilizer, hence the name *gravity sterilizer.*[66]

Pulsing gravity sterilizer

The pulsing gravity sterilizer introduces pulses of steam to assist with air removal. However, no ejector or vacuum pump is used to facilitate the steam and air removal at the end of each pulse. This type of cycle is less efficient in removing air and aiding steam penetration than a prevacuum cycle but more efficient than a regular gravity cycle.

Prevacuum sterilizer

In a prevacuum cycle, rather than passive air removal as is the case with the gravity sterilizer, air is actively removed from the sterilizer (Fig. 4-6). When the cycle is initiated, steam is injected with force into the chamber. At the same time, the drain at the bottom of the chamber is automatically closed. As more steam enters the chamber, pressure increases and the steam and air form a turbulent mixture. When a specific pressure is reached, the drain opens, and the pressurized steam and air rush from the

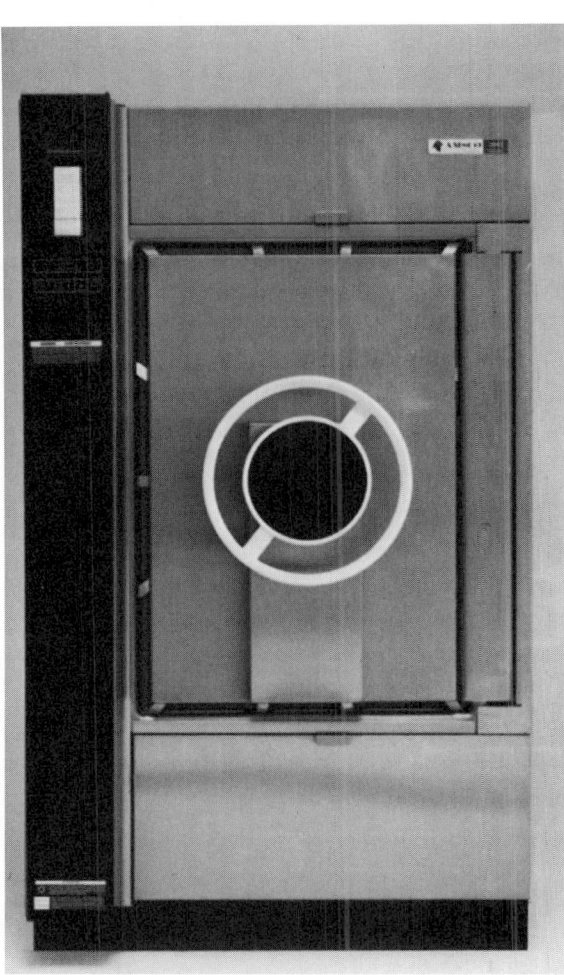

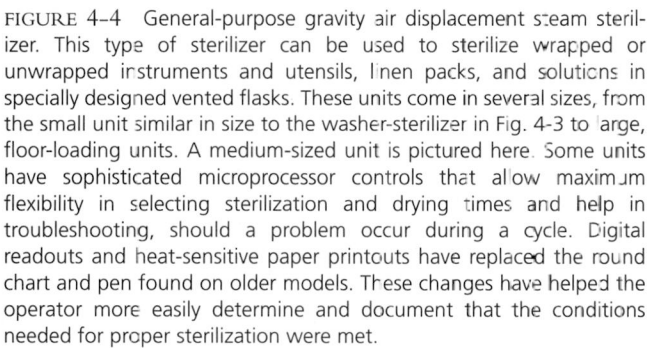

FIGURE 4-4 General-purpose gravity air displacement steam sterilizer. This type of sterilizer can be used to sterilize wrapped or unwrapped instruments and utensils, linen packs, and solutions in specially designed vented flasks. These units come in several sizes, from the small unit similar in size to the washer-sterilizer in Fig. 4-3 to large, floor-loading units. A medium-sized unit is pictured here. Some units have sophisticated microprocessor controls that allow maximum flexibility in selecting sterilization and drying times and help in troubleshooting, should a problem occur during a cycle. Digital readouts and heat-sensitive paper printouts have replaced the round chart and pen found on older models. These changes have helped the operator more easily determine and document that the conditions needed for proper sterilization were met.

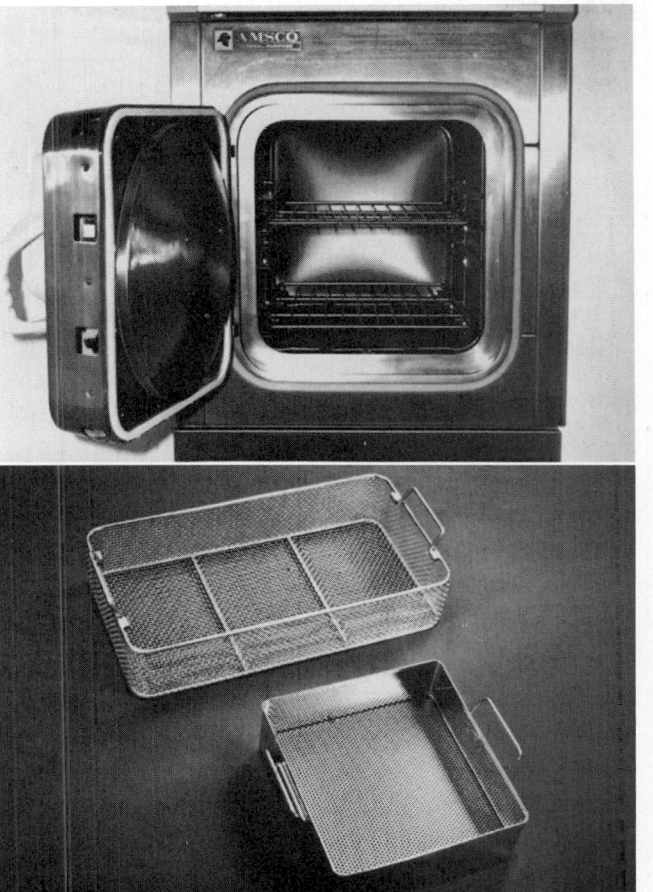

FIGURE 4-5 **A,** Adjustable racks are designed to permit maximum loading efficiency. **B,** Instrument baskets or trays should have either wire-meshed bottoms or a sufficient number of perforations in the sheet metal to allow for air removal and drainage of condensate during the sterilization cycle.

chamber, aided by a water ejector or a vacuum pump. This sudden rush of gas from the chamber creates a vacuum within the chamber. This is the basis for the name *prevacuum sterilizer*. The sterilizer repeats this injection and vacuum process four times in succession in an effort to evacuate all air from the chamber.[66]

Abbreviated prevacuum cycle

Some prevacuum sterilizers have the capability of providing an abbreviated cycle. In this cycle, there are two rather than four pulses of the steam injection–vacuum process. This cycle may be used only for simple metal or glass instruments. No instruments with a lumen should be sterilized using this cycle.[65]

High-speed (flash) sterilizer

The high-speed, steam sterilizer, commonly referred to as a *flash sterilizer*, can be adjusted to operate at 132° C (270° F) and 27 pounds per square inch (psi) of pressure for shortened cycles with no accompanying drying cycle. This sterilizer is most frequently used in the operating room for sterilizing urgently needed unwrapped instruments. This method of sterilization is intended for use with unwrapped items or those sterilizing pans or container systems developed specifically for the flash cycle. Flashed items are to be used immediately after sterilization; they may not be stored for future use. Flash sterilization should be used only in situations when time does not permit processing by the preferred, wrapped, presterilization.[14] Implantable devices should not be flash sterilized because the cycle margin of safety for sterilization is reduced as a result of the speed of the cycle. However, the exposure phase of the cycle has just as much lethality as a routine cycle. If in an emergent situation, an implantable must be flash sterilized, a biological indicator should be included in the tray and the item quarantined until, at a minimum, a preliminary result from

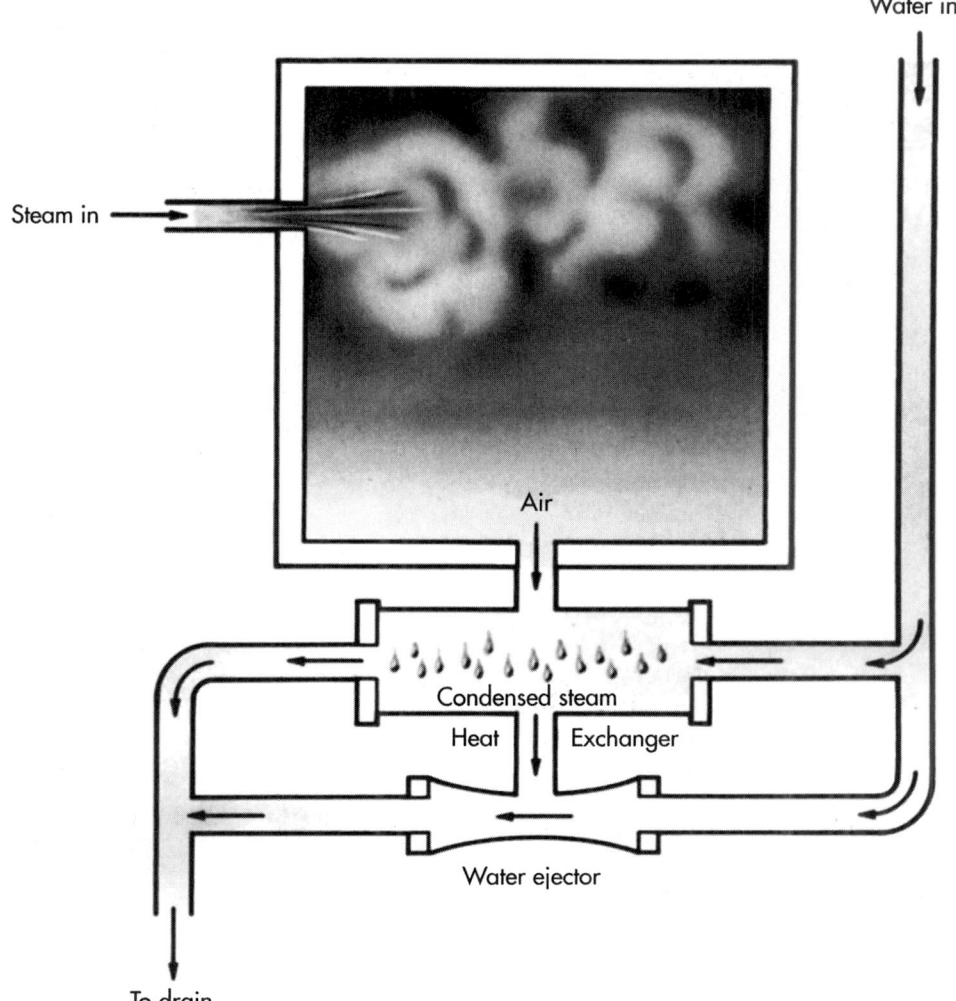

FIGURE 4-6 Prevacuum steam sterilizer. This type of sterilizer features active, aggressive removal of air, rather than relying on the passive action of gravity. When the cycle is initiated, steam is injected with force into the chamber. At the same time, the drain at the bottom of the chamber is automatically closed. As more steam enters the chamber, pressure increases and the steam and air form a turbulent mixture. When a specific pressure is reached, the drain opens, and the pressurized steam and air rush from the chamber, aided by a water ejector or a vacuum pump. This sudden rush of gas from the chamber creates a vacuum within the chamber. This process is repeated several times and deepens the level of vacuum drawn with each pulse. The effect of this pulsing cycle is to displace any air in the load and rapidly increase the chamber and load temperatures. At the conclusion of this conditioning phase, steam flows into the chamber and raises the temperature to sterilization levels, usually 132° C (270° F). The temperature is maintained for at least 3 minutes for unwrapped, nonporous materials and 4 minutes for wrapped or porous items. Steam is then removed from the chamber to draw a partial vacuum once again. Heated, filtered air is introduced into the chamber to dry the load. Drying times are selected and set by the user, depending on the nature of the load. Some units have a special cycle designed for rapid sterilization of an instrument tray in a single wrapper. This express cycle has fewer conditioning pulses, a 4-minute exposure time, and 1 or 2 minutes of dry time, for a total cycle time of approximately 12 minutes. Although the wrapper feels warm and dry to the touch, the contents may not be totally dry. Thus this package should be handled by persons wearing sterile gloves and using sterile towels for protection from burns. The instruments sterilized in this express cycle must be used immediately. Because the contents are not dry, the package is not suitable for any length of storage.

a rapid-indicator system is available. Flash sterilization can be accomplished in either gravity-displacement or prevacuum sterilizers designed with "flash" capabilities. Although flashing is considered a rapid method of sterilization for unwrapped items, both the pulsing gravity and the abbreviated prevacuum cycles have been designed with a brief drying cycle, intended to dry the single wrapper, which may be used to cover the tray holding instruments being sterilized. However, even with the brief drying cycle, the tray itself and its contents may still be wet. The tray should be transported to its point of use only by persons wearing sterile gloves. The tray should be placed

TABLE 4-3 | Time-Temperature Parameters for Flash Steam Sterilization

TYPE OF STERILIZER	LOAD CONFIGURATION	TEMPERATURE, IN °C (°F)	TIME, IN MINUTES
Gravity-displacement	Metal or nonporous items only (no lumens)	132-135 (270-275)	3
	Metal items with lumens and porous items (such as rubber, plastic) sterilized together	132-135 (270-275)	10
Prevacuum	Metal or nonporous items only (no lumens)	132-135 (270-275)	3
	Metal items with lumens and porous items sterilized together	132-135 (270-275)	4
Pulsing gravity	Nonporous, nonlumened instruments only	Manufacturer instructions	
Abbreviated prevacuum	Nonporous, nonlumened instruments only	Manufacturer instructions	

on a sterile impervious drape that will not melt with the heat of the tray. The wrapper should be removed by the person handling the tray so that the scrubbed person can remove the tray contents in an aseptic manner.[65] Routine cycle parameters for flash sterilization are shown in Table 4-3.[8,65]

Chemical Sterilization

New materials that cannot be heat sterilized are continually being introduced for use in healthcare. These materials require the use of other methods of sterilization. Chemical agents provide an effective alternative to steam sterilization. Chemical sterilization is frequently referred to as *cold sterilization*. This term refers to the maximum temperature of 54° to 60° C (130° to 140° F) of gaseous sterilization as compared with the 121° to 132° C (250° F to 270° F) temperatures of steam sterilization.

Sterilization can be achieved by many agents when only vegetative cells are present. If the microbial population is unknown, however, a sporicidal agent must be employed to ensure sterilization. An antimicrobial agent must exhibit a wide microbiological spectrum and sporicidal activity to qualify as a chemosterilant.

Ethylene oxide

In recent years gaseous chemical sterilization has had considerable application for heat-labile and moisture-sensitive items, such as intricate, delicate surgical instruments; large pieces of equipment used in the hospital; plastic and porous materials; and electrical instruments, all of which are difficult to steam sterilize without deterioration and damage. Ethylene oxide (EO) is the gas most frequently used for this purpose. It is colorless at ordinary temperatures, has an odor similar to that of ether, and has an inhalation toxicity similar to that of ammonia gas. EO gas is an effective sterilant but must be used with care because of its toxicity. It is easily stored as a liquid that will boil at 10.73° C (51.3° F) and freeze at -111.3° C (-168.3° F). It is highly explosive and very flammable in the presence of air. These hazards are greatly reduced by dilution of the EO with inert gases such as carbon dioxide and fluorinated hydrocarbons (Freon). Neither of these two inert gases appears to affect the bactericidal activity of

the EO but serves only as an inert diluent that reduces the flammability hazard.

Several theories on how EO kills bacteria have been proposed. The killing rate of bacteria is generally believed to be relative to the rate of diffusion of the gas through their cell walls and the availability or accessibility of one of the chemical groups in the bacterial cell walls to react with the EO. The killing rate also depends on whether the bacterial cell is in a vegetative or spore state. Destruction takes place by alkylation through chemical interference and probably inactivation of the reproductive process of the cell. In the process of alkylation, a hydrogen atom within the microbial cell is replaced with a portion of the EO molecule (such as an alkyl group). This process alters the structure of the microbial molecule and renders it nonfunctional. When sufficient molecules within the microbial cell are subjected to this process, the microbial cell is rendered unable to metabolize or produce infection.

Items to be sterilized must be thoroughly cleaned and towel or air dried so that no visible droplets remain. Drying inhibits the formation of ethylene glycol during the sterilization cycle. Lumens of tubing, needles, and the like should be dry and open at both ends. Caps, plugs, valves, and stylettes should be removed from instruments or equipment to permit the gas to circulate through the items. The packaging material used should possess the characteristics described previously in this chapter.

Items to be sterilized should be placed in a loose configuration within the confines of metal baskets or sterilizer carts. Packages should not touch the chamber walls when loaded into the sterilizer. An excessively large load or a load that is tightly packed will interfere with proper air removal, load humidification, sterilant penetration, and sterilant evacuation at the conclusion of the cycle. Penetration of gas throughout the load is essential. Compression of packages prevents penetration of the gas. If packages are wrapped in plastic, compression hinders evacuation of air and causes packages to open during the decrease in chamber pressure when a vacuum is drawn. Proper loading is essential so that sterilized items do not fall from the container or cart after sterilization, thus requiring personnel to handle them before aeration. Because metal baskets or carts do not absorb EO, they can be handled before aeration. An EO–sensitive chemical indicator should be used with each package to indicate that the package was exposed to the gas. The chemical indicator does not indicate achievement of sterility.[5,76]

Factors affecting sterilization with EO are time of exposure, gas concentration, temperature, humidity, and penetration. The time exposure required depends on temperature, humidity, gas concentration, the ease of penetrating articles to be sterilized, and the type of microorganisms to be destroyed. Gas concentration is affected by the temperature and humidity inside the sterilizing chamber. If the concentration of gas is doubled, the exposure time may be shortened. Temperature and humidity have a pronounced influence on the destruction of microorganisms. They are important in gaseous sterilization with EO because they affect penetration of the gas through bacterial cell walls as well as through wrapping and packaging material. Dry spores are the most difficult to kill, but when such spores are moistened, their resistance to gas penetration is lowered. Dehydration makes some microorganisms nearly immune to EO sterilization, whereas droplets of moisture can inhibit the action of the gas by protecting the organism. EO sterilizers with automatic controls provide for moisture injection to raise the relative humidity within the chamber. Manufacturers of gas sterilizers have developed recommended exposure periods for various EO concentrations in relation to the material to be sterilized. Exposure time is set for absolute destruction of the most resistant microorganisms, which is a very slow process.

The adequacy of every EO cycle should be verified by the use of biological monitors that contain *Bacillus subtilis* var. *niger*. Where feasible, implantable or intravascular items should not be used until the results of the test are known. The AAMI has defined two standard test packs for use in monitoring the EO sterilization cycle.[5] The sterilizer manufacturer's instructions regarding cycle parameters should be followed. In general, the most common parameter ranges are shown in Table 4-4.[5]

EO-sterilized items must be aerated to make them safe for personnel handling and patient use. At the conclusion of the sterilization cycle, items may be safely removed from the chamber to a separate aerator. Certain model sterilizers may have an internal aeration cycle. The sterilizer manufacturer's recommendations relating to opening the sterilizer door after completion of the sterilization cycle

and subsequent transferring of items to the aerator must be closely followed. Excessive exposure to EO represents a health hazard to personnel, since it has been linked to cancer, reproductive problems, and other disorders in animals. Therefore inhalation of EO should be avoided or minimized, and direct contact with items sterilized by EO should be avoided during transfer to the aerator. Various safety features such as a purge system, an audible alarm at the end of the sterilization cycle, and automatic door locking and sealing mechanisms are used on EO sterilizers to protect personnel. Opening the sterilizer door within the capture zone of the scavenging hood for a period of 5 to 10 minutes can reduce operator exposure to the sterilizing gas. If the sterilizer contents are not removed at that time, they will begin to "outgas," resulting in increased EO concentration within the chamber.

Aeration may be accomplished in a mechanical aerator or in the ambient environment. Length of aeration for each item should be based on the manufacturer's instruction. Typical aeration times when a mechanical aerator is used are 8 to 12 hours at 50° to 55° C or 12 to 16 hours at 38° C. Aeration in the ambient environment should be for 7 days. Ambient aeration should be carried out in a limited access, well-ventilated room with controlled temperature between 18° and 22° C (65° and 72° F) and vented to the outside. Intravenous or irrigation fluids packaged in plastic bags should not be stored in this area. When moving items from the sterilizer to the aerator, items should be handled as little as possible. Personnel should not breathe the air that passes over baskets or carts containing EO–sterilized items. To avoid breathing this air, carts should always be pulled as opposed to pushed. Depending on the sterilization-cycle temperature used, items may be warm to the touch at the end of the cycle. Butyl rubber gloves are recommended to protect personnel from contact with liquid EO and from thermal injury.[14]

Smoking is prohibited in the sterilizer and aerator area. Because EO is highly explosive and flammable, the sterilizer and aerator should be installed in a well-ventilated room and should be vented to the outside atmosphere as recommended by the manufacturer and required by the National Institute for Occupational Safety and Health (NIOSH).

Because of EO's suspected carcinogenicity and its potential as a reproductive hazard, OSHA has issued standards regulating personnel exposure to EO. These standards set the permissible exposure level (PEL, the amount of EO in the air) at one part per million (ppm) and the action level (AL, monitored value at which corrective action should occur) at 0.5 ppm. These are calculated as time-weighted averages (TWA) over an 8-hour period. OSHA requires that monitoring and surveillance be performed to ensure that exposure levels do not exceed 1 ppm over an 8-hour period.[53] Additionally, occupational exposure level to EO may not exceed 15 ppm in any

TABLE 4-4	Common Parameters for Ethylene Oxide Sterilization			
TIME	TEMPERATURE, IN °C (°F)	HUMIDITY, %	GAS CONCENTRATION, MG/L	
105-300 minutes	37-63 (99-145)	45-75	450-1200	

15-minute period. This is known as the *excursion level* (EL).[54] EO–monitoring badges are available. Adherence to these guidelines will help protect patients and personnel from problems associated with EO sterilization.

In general, EO sterilization should be used only if the materials are heat sensitive and unable to withstand sterilization by saturated steam under pressure. Any item that can be steam sterilized should never be gas sterilized. EO's advantages are that it is easily available; is effective against all types of microorganisms; easily penetrates through masses of dry material; does not require high temperatures, humidity, or pressure; and is noncorrosive and nondamaging to items. Sterilization with EO also has numerous disadvantages. The long exposure and aeration periods make it a lengthy process. When compared with steam sterilization, EO sterilization is expensive. Liquid EO may produce serious burns on exposed skin if not immediately removed; insufficiently aerated materials can cause skin irritation, burns of body tissue, and hemolysis of blood; and diluents used with EO cause damage to some plastics. Human error and mechanical breakdown can enhance these disadvantages.

Aqueous glutaraldehyde

When used properly, liquid chemosterilants can destroy all forms of microbial life, including bacterial and fungal spores, tubercle bacilli, and viruses. Although formaldehyde is one of the oldest chemosterilants known to destroy spores, it is rarely used because it takes from 12 to 24 hours to be effective, its pungent odor is objectionable, and controversy regarding its potential carcinogenic effect is ongoing. Glutaraldehyde is more rapid and less irritating than formaldehyde solutions.

Activated aqueous glutaraldehyde 2% is recognized as an effective liquid chemosterilant. It is most useful in the disinfection of lensed instruments such as cystoscopes and bronchoscopes because it has minimal deleterious effects on the lens cement and is noncorrosive. Its low surface tension permits easy penetration and rinsing.

Instruments must be free from bioburden and completely immersed in activated aqueous glutaraldehyde solution for 10 hours to achieve sterilization. Any period of immersion less than 10 hours will not kill spores that may be present and must be considered as only a disinfection procedure. During immersion, all surfaces of the instrument must be contacted by the liquid chemosterilant. After immersion, instruments must be rinsed thoroughly with sterile distilled water before being used.

Peracetic acid

Liquid paroxyacetic (peracetic) acid is a biocidal oxidizer that maintains its efficacy in the presence of high levels of organic soil. The mechanism of action of peracetic acid is not well understood. Because peracetic acid is highly corrosive to instruments, it must be used in combination with anticorrosive additives.[71] Commercially available sterilization systems using peracetic acid have found increasing use in recent years because of their relatively short cycles and subsequent ability to quickly ready items for use. These systems should be maintained and used according to the manufacturer's instructions. Although peracetic acid does not leave toxic residues on items that have been adequately rinsed, the agent may cause serious injury if not handled, neutralized, and rinsed properly. Items processed in peracetic acid systems should be used immediately after processing because the item containers are wet and are not sealed from the environment.[14] Some controversy regarding internal-process monitors has existed with peracetic acid sterilization systems. Manufacturer recommendations should be sought and carefully followed.

Gas plasma sterilization

Plasma is the fourth state of matter, the sequence being solid, liquid, gas, and plasma. Gas plasmas are highly ionized gases composed of ions, electrons, and neutral particles. To create gas plasma for sterilization, a precursor solution such as hydrogen peroxide or peracetic acid is introduced into a closed area in the sterilizer under very low vacuum conditions. This precursor is vaporized and either remains within the sterilization chamber or is injected into the chamber via an injection/flow mechanism. Microwave or radiofrequency energy is used to create an electromagnetic field to excite either the precursor vapor or another gas or vapor, creating a variety of charged and uncharged, excited species with biocidal properties. These excited species may be either within the sterilizer chamber or contained within an outer shell, which has an electrode barrier that allows only neutral species to enter the chamber. These highly excited species diffuse through packaging materials to sterilize the package contents of items having been placed within the sterilizer chamber.[42,46,51]

Plasma sterilization has the potential of displacing ethylene oxide sterilization for many but not all applications. It is designed to provide nontoxic, dry, low-temperature sterilization in a shorter turnaround time than that of ethylene oxide. The hydrogen peroxide gas plasma process rapidly destroys a broad spectrum of microorganisms, including gram-negative and gram-positive vegetative bacteria, mycobacteria, yeasts, fungi, lipophilic and hydrophilic viruses, as well as highly resistant aerobic and anaerobic bacterial spores.[38,39] Cycle times for gas plasma sterilization may range from 75 minutes to five hours. For processing endoscopes, longer cycles are required to allow penetration of the devices. At the completion of the sterilization process, no toxic residues remain on the sterilized items. No aeration is needed, making it a safe process for both patients and health care workers. Preparation of instrumentation for sterilization includes cleaning and decontaminating procedures, reassembly, and wrapping with nonwoven polypropylene wraps or Tyvek-mylar

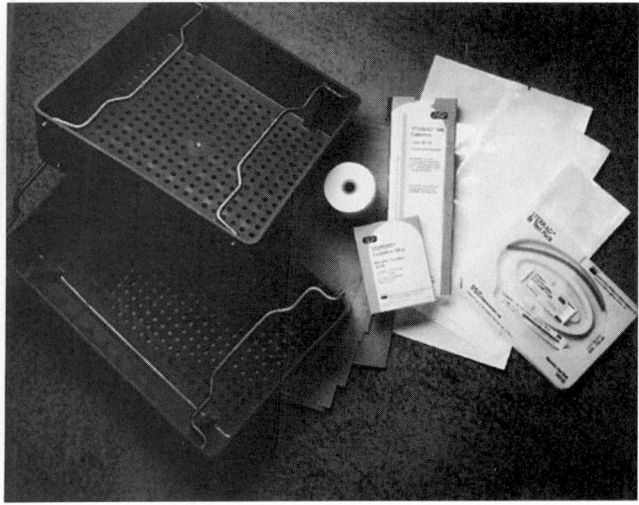

FIGURE 4-7 Supplies for use in low-temperature, gas-plasma, sterilization systems include trays, Tyvek pouches, and biological and chemical indicators for process validation. Cellulosic materials such as paper and linen are not recommended for use with plasma systems because they tend to absorb the precursor vapor and cause the sterilization cycle to abort.

TABLE 4-5	Time-Temperature Parameters for Dry Heat (Hot Air) Sterilization
TEMPERATURE, IN °C (°F)	**TIME**
180 (356)	30 minutes
170 (340)	1 hour
160 (320)	2 hours
150 (300)	2.5 hours
140 (285)	3 hours
121 (250)	6 hours (preferably overnight)

pouches (Fig. 4-7). Cellulosic-based products like paper and linen are not recommended for use with plasma systems because they tend to absorb the precursor vapor and cause the sterilization cycle to abort. Systems that use peractic acid should not be used to sterilize instruments that contain copper, brass, or zinc; toxic salts may form, resulting in patient injury.

Biologic and chemical indicators for process verification are used in the same manner as those for steam and ethylene oxide sterilization procedures. Plasma sterilization processes should be tested with biologic indicators at intervals similar to those used for steam and ethylene oxide sterilization. Manufacturer recommendations should be followed in determining the specific monitor to be used. For some plasma sterilization systems, *Bacillus stearothermophilus* spores demonstrate the greatest resistance to kill. Other systems use *Bacillus circulans* as the challenge organism. Still others use *Bacillus subtilis* var. *niger* spores to be the most resistant to the particular sterilization process. The importance of consulting the system manufacturer for specific instructions cannot be overemphasized.[42,46,51]

Dry Heat Sterilization

Dry heat sterilization should be used only for materials that cannot be sterilized by other methods, when the moisture of other processes would either damage the materials or they would be impermeable to it.[40,58] These materials include grease, anhydrous oils, powders, and some glassware. Dry heat can also be used for delicate sharp instruments that would be substantially dulled by sterilizing with other processes. Dry heat is not a suitable sterilization method for fabrics and rubber goods because the high temperatures necessary for sterilization will cause deterioration of these materials.

There are two kinds of dry heat (also known as hot air) sterilizers—the gravity convection type and the mechanical convection type. Both heat by electricity to achieve accurate and dependable temperature control.

In the *gravity convection sterilizer*, convection is created by the temperature differences within the sterilizing chamber. The heating apparatus present in the bottom of the chamber warms the air within the chamber. The warmed air rises, contacting the items in the chamber to be sterilized. At contact, heat is transferred from the air to the items. With this loss of heat, the cooled air descends toward the bottom of the chamber where it again is warmed by the heating coils.

In the *mechanical convection sterilizer*, the heating apparatus is outside the chamber, in a compartment separated from the chamber by a diffusing wall placed in front of a motor-driven turbine blower. Through an internal process, air is heated and forced into a chamber on the opposite wall. From this chamber the air is discharged into the chamber uniformly over the vertical plane of the chamber.[58] This system provides for uniform delivery of heated air and equal transfer of heat to all regions of the chamber.[58] This system offers the maximum in functional efficiency at a minimum cost and is the system most often used in hospitals.

Because of the variation in items to be sterilized and packaging methods and materials, parameters for dry heat sterilization will vary. Temperature parameters refer to the temperature of the load, not sterilizer chamber temperature. When sterilizing by the dry heat method, the parameters provided in Table 4-5 are believed to be adequate.[58]

Spore tests may be used with dry heat sterilization. *Bacillus subtilis* var. *niger* is the most commonly used challenge microorganism. The sterilizer manufacturer's instructions should be carefully followed for sterilizer monitoring. Steam sterilizers should not be used for dry heat sterilization. Although jacket pressure can heat sterilizer walls to 250° F, absence of monitoring devices within the chamber preclude its use for dry heat sterilization.[58]

Disinfection

Disinfection is defined as the process of eliminating many or all pathogenic organisms except bacterial spores from inanimate objects.[62] In healthcare facilities, equipment is usually soaked in liquid chemicals for a specified period of time to achieve disinfection of the equipment or item. The disinfection process may destroy tubercle bacilli and inactivate hepatitis viruses and enteroviruses but usually does not kill resistant bacterial spores. The term *disinfection* may also refer to treatment of body surfaces that have been contaminated with infectious material. Chemicals used to disinfect inanimate objects are referred to as *disinfectants*. Chemicals used for body surfaces are known as *antiseptics*. The term *germicide* refers to any solution that will destroy microorganisms. Some germicides are both disinfectants and antiseptics.

Disinfectants are categorized as either high level, intermediate level, or low level depending on their disinfecting capability.[62] High-level disinfectants kill all microorganisms except high numbers of bacterial spores. Intermediate-level disinfectants may kill tubercle bacilli, vegetative bacteria, and most viruses and fungi but not bacterial spores. Low-level disinfectants kill most vegetative bacteria and some viruses and fungi.

Just as with sterilization, an item must first be cleaned before it can be disinfected. Proper cleaning removes all foreign substances such as soil or organic material from an object. This is usually accomplished by the use of soap and water or an enzymatic detergent. The term *decontamination* refers to the removal of pathogenic organisms from an object, making the object safe to handle.

Items to be sterilized or disinfected have been classified as critical, semicritical, and noncritical based on the risk of infection for the patient. This classification system, known as the *Spaulding classification system* and named for its developer, Earle Spaulding, was developed many years ago. It has withstood the passage of time and continues to be used today to determine the correct processing method for preparing instruments and other items for patient use. According to the Spaulding system, the level of disinfection required is based on the nature of the item and the manner in which it is to be used.

Critical items are those that enter sterile tissue or the vascular system. These items should be subjected to a sterilization process and be sterile at the time of use. Many critical items are purchased from the manufacturer as sterile. Unsterile critical items should be steam autoclaved if they are heat and moisture stable. If the items cannot withstand heat or moisture, they may be sterilized by one of the other methods as noted in the sterilization section of this chapter. Examples of critical items include surgical instruments, needles, implants, and certain types of catheters.

Semicritical items are those that contact mucous membranes and nonintact skin but do not ordinarily penetrate the blood barrier. Examples of semicritical items include anesthesia breathing circuits, fiberoptic endoscopes, and laryngoscopes. Semicritical instruments require high-level disinfection. That is, these items must be free of microorganisms other than bacterial spores. Because

intact skin and mucous membranes are generally resistant to infection by common bacterial spores but are susceptible to other organisms such as tubercle bacilli and viruses, high-level disinfection is required. Examples of high-level disinfecting agents include glutaraldehyde, stabilized hydrogen peroxide, peracetic acid, and chlorine or chlorine compounds.[62]

Noncritical items are those that come into contact with intact skin but not with mucous membranes. Because skin is an effective barrier to most microorganisms, most noncritical, reusable items can be cleaned at the point of use. Low-level disinfectants may be used to process noncritical items. Examples of noncritical items include blood pressure cuffs, bedpans, linens, utensils, furniture, and floors. Although it is unlikely that infection will be transmitted to patients with intact skin by means of noncritical items, noncritical items can contaminate the hands of healthcare workers or medical equipment that will be used on other patients who may be at greater risk for infection. Examples of low-level disinfectants include alcohols, sodium hypochlorite, phenolic solutions, iodophor solutions, and quaternary ammonium solutions.[62]

Types of Disinfectants
Alcohols

For disinfection in healthcare, alcohol refers to either 70% or 90% isopropyl alcohol. Both of these compounds are water soluble and have a high degree of antimicrobial activity. They are bactericidal as opposed to bacteriostatic against vegetative forms of bacteria. They are also tuberculocidal, fungicidal, and virucidal. Both isopropyl alcohol (isopropanol) and ethyl alcohol (ethanol) are effective against HBV and HIV. The alcohols do not destroy spores or kill certain hydrophilic viruses, such as echovirus and coxsackievirus. Alcohols are flammable and so must be stored in a well-ventilated area. Because they evaporate rapidly, extended contact time is difficult to achieve unless items are immersed. Alcohols lack residual effect and are easily inactivated by protein material. Alcohols tend to damage the shellac on lensed instruments and may cause hardening of certain rubber and plastic tubing after repeated exposure to the compound. Alcohols are considered intermediate-level disinfectants. They are often used to disinfect thermometers and rubber stoppers on medication vials. Alcohol is also used in processing flexible endoscopes. After high-level disinfection with glutaraldehyde and a tap-water rinse, alcohol is effective in inactivating water contaminants. Its speed of evaporation also assists in rapid drying of the endoscope channels.[61,67]

Chlorine compounds

In healthcare facilities, hypochlorites are the most widely used of the chlorine compounds. Hypochlorites are available in a liquid form (sodium hypochlorite [liquid household bleach]) and in a solid form (calcium hypochlorite). Hypochlorites have a broad-spectrum antimicrobial activity. They are inexpensive and fast acting. Low concentrations of free chlorine (50 ppm) are effective against vegetative bacteria and *Mycobacterium tuberculosis*. Free chlorine at 50 ppm will inactivate HIV, whereas a 500 ppm concentration is needed to inactivate HBV. Concentrations as high as 1000 ppm are recommended for inactivation of bacterial spores. Household bleach contains 5.25 % sodium hypochlorite. A dilution of 1:1000 provides 50 ppm of available chlorine. A dilution of 1:50 provides 1000 ppm of available chlorine, which is considered adequate to achieve high-level disinfection. The CDC recommend a 1:10 solution, which provides 5000 ppm of availabke chlorine. Hypochlorite solutions are stable for up to 30 days in opaque containers. Beyond that time, a new solution should be prepared. Hypochlorites are inactivated in the presence of organic matter. Therefore all organic material should be removed before application of the disinfecting solution. Hypochlorites are used sparingly on instruments because of the corrosive action of the compound. Hypochlorites are most often used for counter tops, floors, and other surfaces to be disinfected. Other chlorine compounds that may be used include chlorine dioxide and chloramine-T. Chlorine compounds are the preferred disinfectant in water treatment.[61,67]

Glutaraldehyde

Glutaraldehyde is a saturated dialdehyde that has gained prominence as the best overall disinfecting agent for high-level disinfection. Aqueous solutions of glutaraldehyde are acidic and as such are not sporicidal. The solution is said to be "activated" when alkalinating agents are added to make the solution alkaline. In this state the solution, 2% glutaraldehyde, is sporicidal. Glutaraldehyde has a broad antimicrobial range, being effective against vegetative bacteria, *Mycobacterium tuberculosis*, fungi, and viruses. Although glutaraldehyde is effective against most bacteria in 10 minutes, some species of mycobacteria require a longer exposure time. To achieve high-level disinfection, a minimum exposure time of 20 to 30 minutes is recommended.[67] Glutaraldehyde is noncorrosive to endoscopic equipment, thermometers, and rubber and plastic goods. Glutaraldehyde phenate is a related compound that has been shown to lose efficacy against certain organisms in the recommended dilution. This compound also is not sporicidal and should not be used to achieve high-level disinfection. Another compound, glutaraldehyde with *ortho*-phenylphenol and *para-tertiary* amylphenol, provides a wide range of antimicrobial activity similar to 2% glutaraldehyde. The compound is odorless and minimizes irritation and allergic reactions in users.[61,67]

Hydrogen peroxide

Unstable and low concentrations of hydrogen peroxide (<3% solution) may be used as low-level disinfectant for work-surface cleaning and disinfection. More concentrated (6%) and stable solutions of hydrogen peroxide demonstrate an antimicrobial effect against some bacteria, fungi, and viruses. Stabilized 6% hydrogen peroxide is sporicidal and can be used as a liquid sterilant with sufficient exposure time. However, the solution is corrosive to copper, zinc, and brass. It can also damage rubber and plastic goods. Hydrogen peroxide does not enjoy widespread use as a disinfectant in today's healthcare environment.

Iodine and iodophors

Historically, iodine solutions known as *tinctures* were used in healthcare. Tincture of iodine is a 2% solution of iodine in 50% alcohol. This tincture was been used primarily as a disinfectant on skin and tissue. An iodophor is a water-soluble combination of iodine and a solubilizing agent or carrier that allows for a slow but continuous release of free iodine over time. Iodophors may be used as either disinfectants or antiseptics depending on the concentration of free iodine. Antiseptic formulations contain less free iodine than disinfectant formulations do. The most popular and most often used iodophor is povidone-iodine, a complex of polyvinylpyrrolidone (PVP) and iodine. Interestingly, dilutions of iodophors demonstrate more rapid bactericidal action than a full-strength povidone-iodine. It is believed that dilution of the iodophor weakens the linkage of the iodine to the carrier with an accompanying release of free iodine in solution. As disinfectants, iodophors have the advantage of having the germicidal efficacy of iodine absent the disadvantages of toxicity and surface irritation. Iodophors are usually nonstaining and retain their efficacy in the presence of protein material. Iodophors are effective against vegetative bacteria, *Mycobacterium tuberculosis*, and most viruses and fungi. Iodophors are not considered suitable for high-level disinfection because they have no sporicidal capability.[61,67]

Phenolics

Phenol (carbolic acid) was first used by Joseph Lister in the mid-1800s. Since that time, many phenol derivatives (phenolics) have been developed. These recent formulations are much more effective than the carbolic acid used by Lister. Phenolics are assimilated by porous material, making their removal most difficult. Residual disinfectant can cause tissue irritation. There are few data regarding the antimicrobial properties of phenolics. Most phenolic formulations are tuberculocidal, bactericidal, and fungicidal. Certain viruses including echovirus and coxsackievirus are resistant to the phenolics. Phenolics are not sporicidal nor are they considered effective as high-level disinfectants. They are used primarily as intermediate and low-level disinfectants. Phenolics are most often used for environmental disinfection. Phenolics are known to have toxic effects. Their use has been associated with depigmentation and with hyperbilirubinemia in newborns. Because of this, phenolics are not recommended for cleaning incubators or infant bassinets.

Quaternary ammonium compounds

Quaternary ammonium compounds (Quats) have been used for many years, having enjoyed a reputation for microbicidal activity, good detergent action, and low-level toxicity. In more recent times, it has been noted that environmental factors such as hard water, soap residues, and protein soils reduce or nullify the efficacy of the Quats. Quats are ineffective against *Mycobacterium tuberculosis* and the lipophilic viruses. Quats are not sporicidal. They are not recommended for either high-, intermediate-, or low-level disinfection. They are good cleaning agents and are most often used for noncritical surfaces such as floors, walls, and furniture.[61,67]

Disinfection of Endoscopes

In today's technologically advanced environment, flexible, fiberoptic endoscopes and their associated instrumentation allow for myriad minimally invasive surgical procedures. The list of these procedures grows almost daily. Current technology allows not only for direct visualization of internal sites, but also for diagnostic biopsies and therapeutic procedures to be performed with reduced pain and shorter recovery time for patients. Along with advances in technology, complications have also occurred. Some complications such as bleeding or tissue perforation are immediately obvious. Infectious complications may be more difficult to identify.

Infections related to endoscopic procedures can be caused by both endogenous and exogenous microorganisms. When an infection occurs from endogenous sources, organisms normally present in the procedure area gain access to the bloodstream. Examples of endogenous infections resulting from endoscopy include cholangiitis, pneumonia, endocarditis, brain abscess, and subdural empyema. Infections can also be caused by organisms introduced into the patient via the endoscope (exogenous organisms). Organisms commonly associated with exogenous infection include *Pseudomonas*, *Klebsiella*, *Enterobacter*, *Salmonella*, and *Mycobacterium tuberculosis*. Because the hepatitis A, B, and C viruses and the HIV are inactivated by commonly used chemical germicides, documented endoscopic transmission of these viruses is uncommon. Hepatitis B transmission via the endoscope has been reported[49] as has the transmission of tuberculosis via a contaminated bronchoscope.[1]

For an endoscope to be thoroughly disinfected, the disinfecting agent must contact all surfaces of the endoscope, both internal and external, for the prescribed length of time. Organic soil, such as blood, feces, or respiratory secretions, harbors embedded microorganisms and prevents penetration of the disinfecting agent. Some disinfectants are inactivated by organic material. Rigorous mechanical cleaning is essential to remove soil and debris from the outside of the scope and from the lumens of all accessible channels.[20,57]

Endoscopes and their accessories should be cleaned immediately after use to prevent drying of secretions or other organic soil. They should be cleaned with a nonabrasive enzymatic detergent as recommended by the endoscope manufacturer.[18,49] If a powdered detergent is used, all granules must be completely dissolved before washing begins. Undissolved granules can block the internal channels of the instrument. To soften, moisten, and dilute organic debris, endoscope channels should be flushed with copious amounts of water and detergent. The external surfaces of the endoscope should be washed with a detergent solution and rinsed. Internal channels should be brushed to loosen and remove organic matter. The detergent solution should be suctioned or pumped through all channels to remove loosened debris. Special attention should be given to convoluted areas and crevices where contaminated organic material may lodge. The tip of the endoscope should be gently wiped or brushed to remove any debris or tissue that may be lodged around the air and water outlets. Brushes used for cleaning should be disposable or be thoroughly cleaned and sterilized daily. Detachable parts of the endoscope, such as hoods and suction valves, should be removed and soaked in a detergent solution. They should be thoroughly cleaned with a detergent, using a brush to remove any organic material.[49]

Before immersion in any liquid, endoscopes should be pressure (leak) tested to determine integrity of seals and minimize the potential for damage to the head of the scope. If damage is detected, the scope should not be immersed or reused. The endoscope should be removed from service and returned to the manufacturer for repair. An endoscope sent for repair is considered a contaminated item and must be labeled as such for shipping.

Immediately after decontamination and cleaning, endoscopes should be rinsed of residual debris and cleaning agent. After a tap-water rinse, endoscopes should be rinsed with 70% or 90% alcohol and forced-air dried. Alcohol inactivates organisms normally found in tap water and helps dry the internal channels of the scope. After being cleaned, endoscopes and accessories should be sterilized or high-level disinfected before being stored. Care must be taken to dry internal channels of the scopes after being processed and before being stored. Endoscopes should be stored in a vertical position in an area in which recontamination is unlikely. Ideally, endoscopes should be processed immediately before patient use to avoid any possibility of recontamination. Endoscopes should be sterilized or high-level disinfected depending on their intended use (see *Spaulding classification system* on p. 125). Because of pressure and heat sensitivity, the sterilization method of choice for endoscopes has been EO for many years. More recently liquid peracetic acid with anticorrosive buffers has also been used to process endoscopes. As endoscopic surgery grows and the need for sterile endoscopes increases, additional processing methodologies are expected in the marketplace.

Activated glutaraldehyde is the agent of choice for high-level disinfection of endoscopes. Either a manual or an automated system may be used. When using a manual system, the precleaned endoscope is immersed in a solution of 2% glutaraldehyde for a minimum of 20 minutes at room temperature. The endoscope is then rinsed in three separate sterile water baths to thoroughly rinse all residual agent from the scope. With each processing, the first rinse solution is discarded and solutions number 2 and 3 are moved into the number 1 and 2 positions. The third rinse is always a new bath so that the final rinse of the scope is in an unused sterile water bath. Several automated processors for disinfection are available in the marketplace. They vary in the degree to which all channels are effectively irrigated, whether fluids are reused in the system, and whether cycle times can be adjusted. Rinsing and drying are part of the automated cycle. Regardless of whether a manual or automated system is used, meticulous manual cleaning must precede the disinfection process.[49]

Pasteurization

Pasteurization is a process that uses hot water at temperatures below 100° C to achieve disinfection. The most commonly used time and temperature parameters are use of 75° C water for 30 minutes. This is believed to destroy all microorganisms except for bacterial spores. Advantages of pasteurization include absence of toxic residues and the associated need for postprocess rinsing. Disadvantages of pasteurization include the lack of sporicidal activity and the potential for splash burns to personnel involved with the process.[67]

ASEPTIC PRACTICES TO CONTROL INFECTION

Surgical Aseptic Principles

Asepsis had been defined as the absence of infectious organisms. Surgical aseptic practices are based on the premise that most infections are caused by organisms exogenous to the surgical patient's body. To avoid infection, surgical procedures must be done in a manner that minimizes or eliminates the patient's exposure to exogenous organisms. Using sterile drapes to create a sterile field around the incision site, using sterile instruments for the surgical procedure, and placing the operative team in sterile attire after their hands and arms have been cleansed of surface bacteria aid in avoiding infection.

Aseptic technique stems from the principles of asepsis derived over time from microbiologil and epidemiologic concepts. Although some may believe that current aseptic practices and techniques have become too ritualistic or lack scientific research to support their use, present-day infection-control statistics support the application of aseptic principles for safe perioperative nursing practice.

Until empirical research demonstrates that a technique is unnecessary or ineffective, the basic aseptic principles should be followed. These principles follow:

1. *Only sterile items are used within the sterile field.* The inadvertent use of unsterile items may introduce contaminants into the surgical site. Persons dispensing sterile items to the sterile field must look at the sterilization indicator on or visible in the package, check for package integrity, and check for package expiration date (or appropriate marking for event-related shelf life) before dispensing the item to the field.
2. *Items of doubtful sterility must be considered unsterile.* Some examples of such items include sterile items found in unsterile work areas, sterilized packages wrapped in pervious materials that have become wet, and sterilized packages wrapped in pervious materials that are dropped. If a package wrapped in an impervious material is dropped and the area of contact is dry, the package may be opened and the contents used. However, the package should not be returned to sterile storage for future use.
3. *Whenever a sterile barrier is permeated, it must be considered contaminated.* This principle applies to packaging materials as well as to draping and gowning materials. Obvious contamination occurs from direct contact between sterile and unsterile objects. Other less apparent modes of contamination are the filtration of airborne microorganisms through materials, passage of liquids through materials, and undetected perforations in materials. Moisture soaking through a drape, gown, or package is considered a strikethrough, and the item must be considered contaminated.
4. *Sterile gowns are considered sterile in front from shoulder to level of the sterile field and at the sleeves from 2 inches above the elbow to the cuff.* The cuff should be considered unsterile because it tends to collect moisture and is not an effective bacterial barrier. Therefore the sleeve cuffs should always be covered by sterile gloves. Other areas of the gown that must be considered unsterile are the neckline, shoulders, areas under the arms, and back. These areas may become contaminated by perspiration or by collar and shoulder surfaces rubbing together during head and neck movements. Wraparound gowns that completely cover the back may be sterile when first put on. The back of the gown, however, must not be considered sterile because it cannot be observed by the scrubbed person and protected from contamination. The sterile area of the front of the gown extends to the level of the sterile field because most scrubbed personnel work adjacent to a sterile table. For this reason the scrubbed person should avoid changing levels, as would occur while moving from footstool to floor. To maintain sterility, scrubbed persons should not allow their hands or any sterile item to fall below the level of the sterile field. Scrubbed persons should

neither sit nor lean against unsterile surfaces because the threat of contamination is great. The only time scrubbed persons may be seated is when the entire surgical procedure will be performed at that level. Self-gowning and gloving should be done from a sterile surface separate from the sterile field. This method eliminates the potential for water to be dripped on sterile items or on any part of the sterile field. Once prepared, the scrubbed person's hands should be kept in sight at or above waist level. Elbows should be kept close to the body and the hands kept away from the face. Hands should not be folded under the arms because axillary perspiration may permeate the bacterial barrier of the gown.

5. *Tables are sterile only at table level.* Sterile drapes are used to create a sterile field. Only the top surface of a draped table is considered sterile. Although the drape extends over the sides of a table, the sides cannot be considered sterile. Any portion of the drape that falls below the top edge of the table cannot be brought back up to the table level. Once placed, a drape should not be shifted or moved. Items should be dispensed to a sterile field by methods that preserve the sterility of the items and the integrity of the sterile field. Good judgment must be used when dispensing items either by presenting them to the scrubbed person or by placing them securely on the sterile field. A sterile field should be created as close as possible to the time of use. If a sterile field must be covered because of unavoidable case delay, the cover should be placed in such a manner that it can be removed without contamination. Using a wide cuff on the cover and draping only the top of the table allows for aseptic removal of the cover. In some instances, two covers may be needed to cover all sterile items on the table top. Sterile drapes also are used to create a sterile field when placed over the patient and operative bed. Any item that extends beyond the sterile boundary is considered contaminated and cannot be brought back onto the sterile field. A contaminated item must be lifted clear of the operative field without contacting the sterile surface and must be dropped with minimum handling to an unscrubbed surgical team member, an unsterile area, or a designated receptacle. Interpretation of sterile areas versus unsterile areas on a draped patient requires astute observation and use of good judgment.

6. *The edges of a sterile enclosure are considered unsterile.* Items should be dispensed to the field in a manner that preserves the sterility of the item and the integrity of the sterile field. After a sterile package or container is opened, the edges are considered unsterile. Sterile and unsterile boundaries are often intangible. A 1-inch safety margin is usually considered standard on package wrappers, whereas the sterile boundary on a wrapper used to drape a table is at the table edge. When opening a sterile wrapper, the top flap is first opened away from

the operator. The side flaps follow. The inside or proximal flap is opened last. All flaps are secured in the hand by the operator, so as not to dangle and contaminate other items. When removing items from a sterile package, the scrubbed person should lift it straight up from the package. On peel-pack pouches, the inner edge of the heat seal is the line of demarcation. Peel-pack edges should be pulled back as opposed to being torn. The contents of the package should be flipped by the unscrubbed person or lifted directly upward by the scrubbed person. Its contents should not be allowed to slide over the side of the package. Interpreting sterile boundaries requires good judgment based on an understanding of aseptic principles.

7. *Sterile persons touch only sterile items or areas; unsterile persons touch only unsterile items or areas.* All members of the surgical team must understand which areas are considered sterile and which are considered unsterile. All must maintain a continual awareness of these areas. Scrubbed persons must guard the sterile field to prevent any unsterile item from contaminating the field or the persons themselves. Unsterile persons must not touch or reach over a sterile field or allow any unsterile item to contaminate the field. When a circulating nurse opens a package, hand and arm motions are always from unsterile to unsterile objects. The circulating nurse avoids contact with the sterile area by placing the hands under the cuff to provide a protected wide margin of safety between the inside of the pack (sterile) and the hands (unsterile) (Fig. 4-8). As the unsterile circulating nurse opens a sterile article that is wrapped sequentially in two wrappers with the corners folded toward the center of the article, the corner farthest from the body is opened first, and the corner nearest the body last. When a scrubbed person opens a sterile wrapper, the side nearest the body is opened first. This portion of the wrapper then protects the gown and enables the individual to move closer to the table to open the opposite side (Fig. 4-9). If a solution must be poured into a sterile receptacle on a sterile table, the scrub person holds the receptacle away from the table or sets it near the edge of a waterproof-draped table (Fig. 4-10). This procedure eliminates the need for the unsterile circulating nurse to reach over the sterile field. Maintaining a safe margin of space can reduce accidental contamination when items are passed between sterile and unsterile fields. An instrument may be used as an extension of a team member's hands to ensure a safe margin between fields. The use of transfer forceps, however, is unacceptable. Maintaining the sterility of these forceps is questionable because of many variables, such as sterilization method, type of container, and type and amount of soaking solution used. Incorrect handling of soaked forceps results in contamination. The preferred procedure is for single use of a

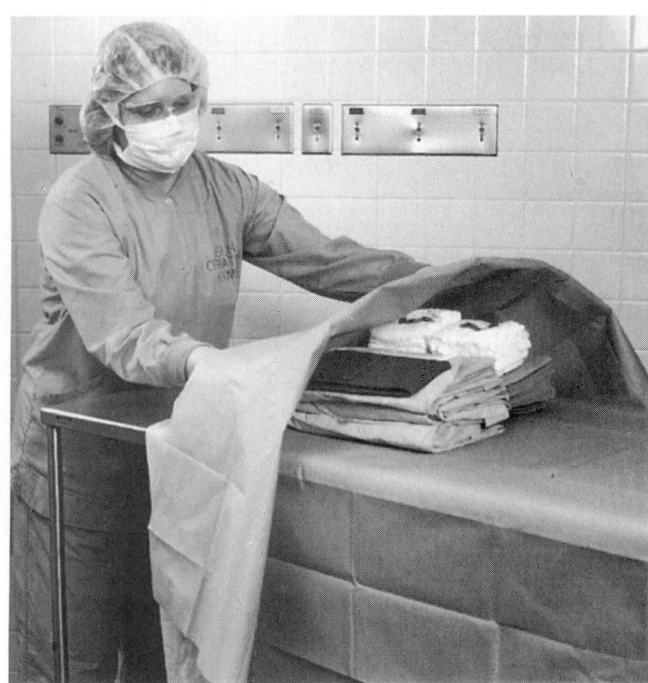

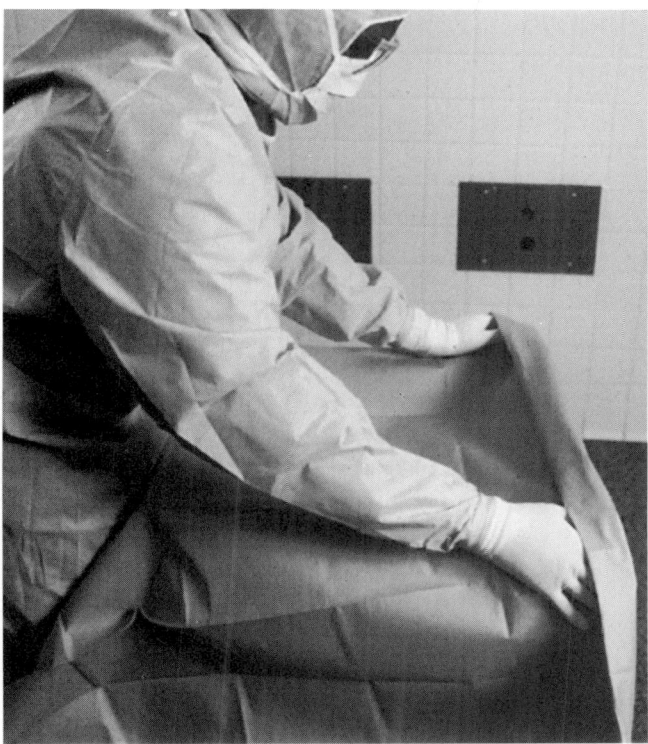

FIGURE 4-8 Circulating nurse is shown opening cover of pack containing sterile drapes for surgery. Cover is cuffed to provide protection for sterile contents. Circulating nurse avoids contact with sterile area by keeping all fingers under cuff as cover is drawn back over table to expose the pack contents.

FIGURE 4-9 Scrub person opens near side of wrapper first, providing protection for the sterile gown. Scrub person protects gloves with cuff of drape as drape is opened to provide sterile table cover.

packaged, sterile ring forceps, which is then discarded into a container for reprocessing.

8. *Movement within or around a sterile field must not contaminate the field.* The patient is the center of the sterile field during an operative procedure; additional sterile areas are grouped around the patient. If contamination is to be prevented, patterns of movement within or around this sterile grouping must be established and rigidly practiced. Scrubbed persons stay close to the sterile field. If they change positions, they turn face to face or back to back with another person while maintaining a safe distance between themselves and other objects. Accidental contamination is a threat to any scrubbed person who wanders into a traffic pathway or out of the clean area of the operating room. Circulating nurses approach sterile areas facing them and never walk between two sterile fields. Keeping sterile areas in view during movement around the area and maintaining a safe distance from sterile fields helps prevent accidental contamination. Bacterial fallout from the body or clothing is a source of contamination when an unsterile person leans over a sterile field. All perioperative personnel must maintain a vigilant watch over sterile areas and point out any contamination immediately. Movement within and around a sterile area should be kept to a minimum to avoid contamina-

tion of the field or the sterile members of the surgical team.

Close adherence to principles of asepsis and consistent observance of the boundaries established in the principles provide protection against infection. Application of the basic principles of aseptic technique depends primarily on the individual's understanding and conscience. Every person on the surgical team must share the responsibility for monitoring aseptic practice and initiating corrective action when a sterile field is compromised.

Traffic Control

The surgical suite should be designed to minimize the spread of infectious organisms and to facilitate movement of patients and personnel within that framework.[17] Ideally the suite is divided into three areas, each defined by the activities occurring within the area. The *unrestricted* area includes areas outside of the surgical suite as well as a control point to monitor the entrance of patients, personnel, and materials. Street clothes are appropriate attire in this area, and traffic is not limited. The *semirestricted* area comprises the peripheral support areas within the surgical suite. These may include storage areas, work areas, and corridors leading to restricted areas of the surgical suite. Traffic in the semirestricted area is limited to

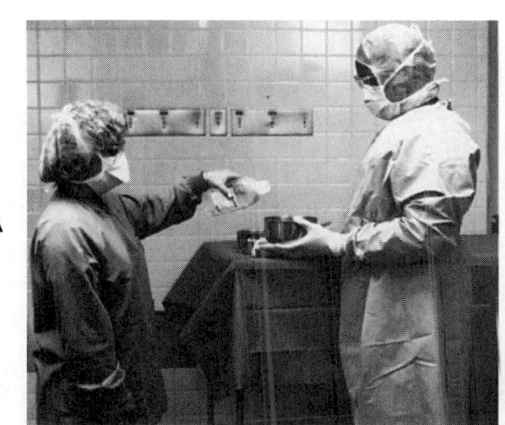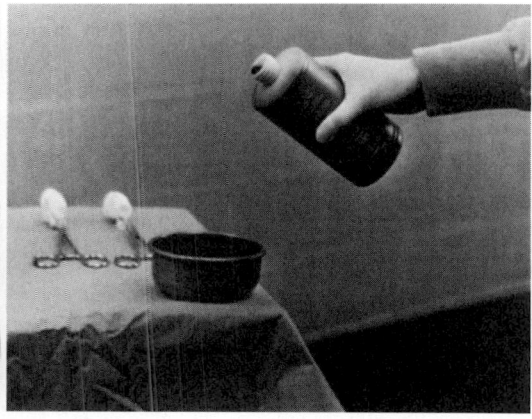

FIGURE 4-10 **A,** When pouring solution into receptacle held by scrub person, circulating nurse maintains safe margin of space to avoid contamination of sterile surfaces. **B,** Care must be used when pouring solution into receptacle on sterile field to avoid splashing fluids onto sterile field. Placement of receptacle near edge of table permits circulating nurse to pour solution without reaching over any portion of sterile field.

appropriately attired personnel and patients. Personnel must wear surgical attire and cover all head and facial hair when in this area. Patients should have their hair covered, wear clean hospital attire, and be covered with clean hospital linens. The *restricted* area includes the operating rooms, procedure rooms (if any), the central core, and the scrub sink area. Personnel must wear surgical attire including hair coverings when in the restricted area. Masks are worn where open sterile supplies or scrubbed persons may be present. Patients should wear hospital attire as above. Masks are not required for patients because a mask could hinder access to the patient's face and airway and cause additional patient anxiety.

Personnel entering semirestricted or restricted areas of the surgical suite should do so through prescribed routes. These routes contain vestibular areas, which serve as transition zones between the outside and inside of the suite. Offices, holding rooms, and locker rooms act as transition zones. Personnel entering the operating rooms should access the locker room via the unrestricted area. After donning clean, hospital-laundered surgical attire, personnel should exit directly into the operating room suite without retracing steps through the unrestricted area.

Air is a potential source of microorganisms that can result in a surgical site infection. Airborne contamination increases with movement of the surgical team. Therefore this movement should be kept to a minimum during operative procedures. Each operating room door should remain closed except during movement of patients, personnel, supplies, and equipment. The positive-pressure gradient of air in the operating room is disrupted if the door remains open. Further, the turbulent flow occurring as the pressure equalizes can increase airborne contamination.

Surgical equipment and supplies also are potential sources of contamination. Clean and sterile supplies should be separated from contaminated items by space, time, or traffic patterns. Clean and sterile items delivered to the surgical suite should be transported in a manner that preserves package integrity and protects the packaged items from contamination along the travel route. Because external shipping containers may collect dust, debris, and insects during shipment, these containers should be removed in the unrestricted area before supplies are brought into the surgical suite. Within the suite, supplies should move from the clean core or storage area through the operating room to the peripheral or semirestricted corridor. Soiled instruments, supplies, and equipment should not reenter the clean core. Instead, soiled items should be covered or contained in closed carts or containers and transported to an area designated for decontamination. This decontamination area should be separate from personnel and patient traffic areas, as should be the soiled linen and trash collection areas.

Surgical Attire

Every surgical department should have a written policy and procedure regarding proper attire in the surgical suite. PPE, which includes protective eyewear, gloves, and fluid-resistant gowns, aprons, and shoe covers, should be included as part of the surgical attire regulations as advocated by OSHA regulations.[22,55]

People are a major source of bacteria in the surgical setting. To reduce bacterial shedding and promote environmental control, all persons entering the semirestricted and restricted areas of the surgical suite should wear clean, hospital-laundered, surgical attire made of multiuse fabric or limited use nonwoven material.[15] Surgical attire, also known as scrub attire, should consist of a two-piece pantsuit, a head cover, mask, and shoe covers, which may be optional depending on the type of surgery being performed, hospital policy, and OSHA regulations (Fig. 4-11). The top of the pant suit should fit close to the body, secured at the waist, or tucked into the trousers. Care

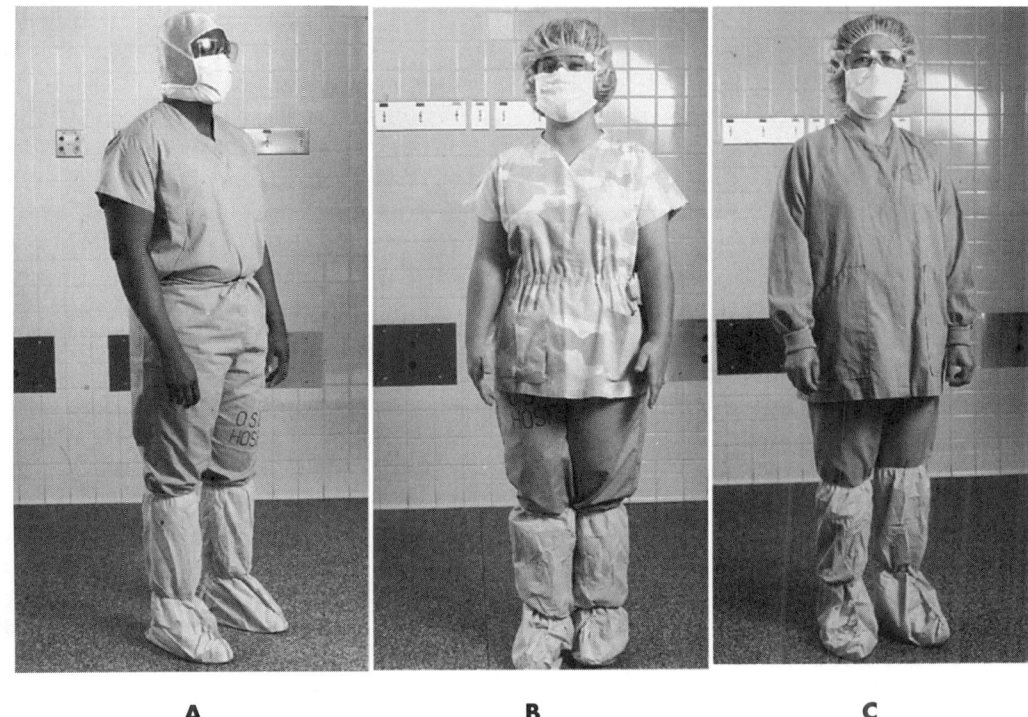

A   **B**   **C**

FIGURE 4-11 Proper surgical attire consists of a two-piece pant suit or a one-piece coverall suit. Shoe covers should be worn when it is reasonably anticipated that spills or splashes will occur. If worn, they should be changed whenever they become wet, torn, or soiled. All head and facial hair should be covered in the semirestricted and restricted areas. In the restricted area, all personnel should wear masks. Jewelry should be removed or totally confined. Artificial nails should not be worn. **A,** When a two-piece scrub suit is worn, loose-fitting scrub tops should be tucked into pants. **B,** Tunic tops that fit close to the body may be worn outside of pants. **C,** Nonscrubbed personnel should wear long-sleeved jackets that are buttoned or snapped closed.

must be taken when donning scrub pants to avoid dragging the pant legs on the floor. To protect both the patient and the healthcare worker, surgical attire should be changed at any time it becomes soiled or wet with blood, any body fluid including perspiration, or food. Nonscrubbed personnel should wear long-sleeved jackets that are buttoned or snapped closed during wear. These jackets will help decrease bacterial shedding from bare arms. Closing the jackets helps prevent inadvertent contamination, which can occur if the loose fabric brushes against a sterile area.

Before scrub attire is donned, a clean, lint-free surgical hat or hood that completely covers all head and facial hair should be donned. This head cover eliminates the possibility of hair or dandruff being shed on the scrub suit. The design and composition of the hat or hood should minimize dispersal of bacteria and be comfortable to wear. All hair must be confined as well as covered. Bouffant and hood types of head covers are preferred. Skullcaps that fail to cover the side hair above the ears and hair at the nape of the neck should not be worn in the operating room. Net caps should not be used because they do not provide a barrier to dandruff and hair fallout. Hair acts as a filter when left uncovered and collects bacteria which are released into the air during activity. Hair attracts, harbors, and sheds bacteria in proportion to its length, curliness,

and oiliness. If reusable hats or hoods are worn, they should be laundered after each use. Disposable head covers should be discarded in a designated receptacle immediately after use. Head covers should always be worn in areas where equipment and supplies are processed and stored.

Shoe covers may be worn by personnel entering the semirestricted or restricted areas of the surgical suite. The primary reason for the use of shoe covers is sanitation. Shoe covers help keep shoes clean and also decrease the amount of soil and bacterial tracking throughout the suite if they are changed when soiled or wet. It is far easier to change a shoe cover than to stop to clean or change a shoe that has become soiled. For personnel safety, shoes that provide protection should be worn. Cloth shoes provide little protection against spilled liquids or sharp items that may be accidentally dropped to the floor. Shoes with enclosed toes and heels help minimize injury. Shoe covers should be kept in an area adjacent to the semirestricted area entrance. They should be removed on leaving the semirestricted area, and clean shoe covers should be put on when returning to that area. Shoe covers are required as part of one's personal protective attire if it is reasonably expected that the feet may become contaminated with blood or body fluids.

A surgical mask should be worn to reduce the dispersal

of microbial droplets expelled from the mouth and nasopharynx of personnel. Masks also help protect healthcare workers from aerosolized pathogenic organisms and aerosol particles from the high-technology surgical environment. Masks should be worn in operating rooms and other designated areas where open sterile supplies or scrubbed persons may be located. It is best to wear a single, high-filtration surgical mask as opposed to wearing a mask over a mask (double masking). A single mask provides a filter; double masking creates a barrier, thereby causing the exhaled air to be expelled through tents and gaps around the mask. Some studies indicate that oral bacteria expelled by personnel in the operating room are of no threat to the surgical patient and that surgical masks for nonscrubbed personnel in the operating room may not be necessary.[52,72] Further research is needed to determine the value of masks in preventing patient infection. State, OSHA regulations, and CDC guidelines should be considered when facility policy related to masks in operating rooms is being developed.

Cloth or gauze masks are not acceptable for use in surgical settings. They have a very low filtration efficiency and may become ineffective as a bacterial barrier within 30 minutes of wear. The wearer who breathes through a face mask that is thickly inoculated with expired bacteria may expel a higher number of microorganisms into the atmosphere than does the person who breathes normally and quietly without a mask. Forceful expulsion of the breath during talking, laughing, or sneezing propels large concentrations of microorganisms into the air. When a mask is being chosen, one with a microbial filtration efficiency of 95% or above should be selected. Aerosol particles generated by the surgical team, sometimes visible to the naked eye, are most likely 10 μm or larger. The plume of lasers or the electrosurgical unit has been found to contain particles with a mass of 0.31 μm, smaller than that expelled by the surgical staff. Therefore the filtration efficiency of masks should ensure protection against aerosol particles as small as 0.1 μm.[29] However, the most effective filter mask is relatively useless if worn incorrectly and can be dangerous if handled improperly. Fig. 4-12 illustrates the proper application and removal of a surgical mask.

The mask must cover the mouth and nose entirely, have facial compliance, and be tied securely to prevent venting. The strings should not be crossed when tied because the sides of the mask will gap and permit nonfiltered air to escape through venting. A pliable metal strip in the top hem of most masks provides a firm, contoured fit over the bridge of the nose. This strip also helps prevent fogging of eyeglasses. Air should pass only through the filtering system of the mask. Masks should be either on (properly) or off. They should not be saved from one operation to the next by being left hanging around the neck or being tucked into a pocket. Bacteria that have been filtered by the mask will become dry and airborne if the mask is worn

necklace fashion. Touching only the strings during removal of the mask reduces contamination of the hands. Masks should be changed between procedures and sometimes during a procedure, depending on the length of the operation and the amount of talking done by the team. The facepiece, which is highly contaminated with droplet nuclei, should not come into contact with the hands of personnel. Immediately after removal, masks should be discarded directly into a designated, covered waste receptacle. After discarding the mask, the wearer must wash and dry the hands thoroughly.

All jewelry should be confined within scrub attire or removed when personnel enter the semirestricted or restricted areas of the surgical suite. Confinement reduces the possibility of jewelry falling into a sterile field or wound. Before handwashing, rings, watches, and bracelets should be removed because organisms can be harbored beneath these pieces of jewelry (Research Highlight 4-3). For safety reasons and to prevent transmission of organisms from the patient to personnel, it may be necessary for personnel to wear PPE. This equipment should provide a barrier that reduces the risk of exposure to potentially infectious materials. Examples of PPE can be found in the Universal Precautions section of this chapter. The two most commonly used PPE items are gloves and protective eyewear or face shields. Gloves should be selected according to the task to be done: sterile gloves for sterile procedures; unsterile gloves for other tasks. Gloves should be changed between patient contacts and after contact with any infectious material. Gloves should be changed as opposed to being washed. Washing may compromise glove integrity and put the wearer at risk for exposure to infectious fluids. Hands should be washed after gloves are removed. To reduce the risk of mouth, nose, and eye mucous membrane exposure, protective eyewear, masks, or face shields should be worn whenever there is opportunity for contamination by splash or aerosols. When the protective devices become contaminated, they should be discarded or decontaminated as soon as possible to prevent contamination to the wearer. Other protective equipment such as liquid-resistant attire, including gowns and shoecovers, should be worn whenever there is a reasonable expectation of exposure to infectious materials.

Surgical Hand Scrub

Skin is a major source of microbial contamination in the surgical environment. Although scrubbed members of the surgical team wear sterile gowns and gloves, the skin of their hands and forearms should be cleaned preoperatively to reduce the number of microorganisms in the event of glove failure. The purposes of the surgical hand scrub are to remove dirt, skin oil, and transient microorganisms from the nails, hands, and forearms; to reduce the resident microbial count to as near zero as possible; and to leave an antimicrobial residue on the skin to prevent growth of microbes for several hours.[16] The skin can never be

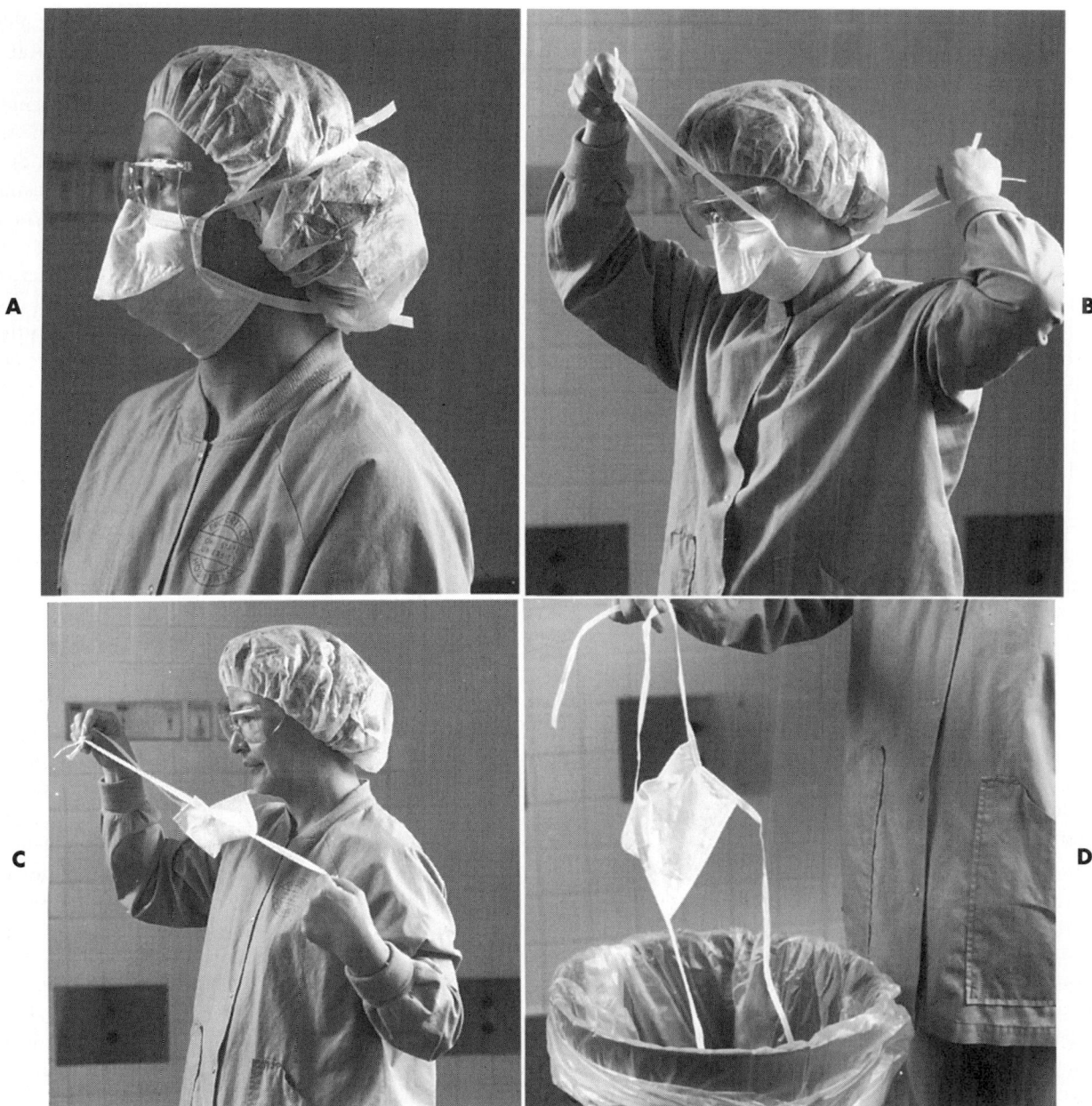

FIGURE 4-12   Proper handling of mask. **A,** Edges of properly worn mask conform to facial contours when mask is applied and tied correctly. **B** and **C,** Personnel should avoid touching filter portion of mask when removing it. **D,** Masks should be discarded on removal.

rendered sterile, but it can be made surgically clean by reducing the number of microorganisms present. A lengthy mechanical scrub, even with strong antiseptics, will fail to remove all microorganisms. Friction and rinsing significantly decrease the number of bacteria on the epidermis, but their numbers are constantly replenished by the continuous secretory activity of the skin glands.

Scrubbed persons should be in good health and possess healthy, intact skin. Cuts, abrasions, and hangnails tend to ooze serum, which is a medium for prolific bacterial growth and can endanger the patient by increasing the hazards of infection. Because microorganisms may be protected from removal and harbored by rings, watches, and bracelets, these items should be removed before scrubbing (see Research Highlight 4-3). Allergic skin reactions from scrub agents or glove powder also may occur if jewelry is not removed. Fingernails of scrubbed persons should be short, clean, and healthy. The subungual region of the nails harbors the majority of microorganisms found on the hands. Vigorous brushing and running water are necessary to clean under the fingernails. Nails that extend beyond the tips of the fingers are more difficult to clean and increase the risk of glove tears. Longer nails may also scratch or gouge patients during the positioning or

4-3 RESEARCH HIGHLIGHT

The hands of healthcare workers provide a route for transmission of nosocomial infection. Historically, handwashing has been emphasized as the most important measure to reduce cross-contamination. Studies have shown persistent colonization of gram-negative bacteria beneath the rings of nurses. This study addressed the following questions:

- Does wearing rings increase the bacterial count on healthcare workers' hands before handwashing?
- Does wearing rings diminish the effectiveness of handwashing in reducing bacterial counts on healthcare workers' hands?

Subjects for this study were selected from healthcare workers providing direct patient care on a medical-surgical patient care unit. Subjects (50) with rings were paired with subjects (50) without rings. Subjects were not matched by any other criteria. Hand cultures were taken both before and after a 10-second hand wash with a nonmedicated soap. Each healthcare worker used his or her normal handwashing technique. Analysis of covariance was used with colony counts after handwashing as the outcome and colony counts before handwashing as the covariate.

Results of this study showed mean colony counts for healthcare workers' hands with rings to be higher than that for workers without rings both before and after handwashing. The study supported previous work indicating that handwashing reduced the presence of skin bacteria. The study also demonstrated a greater reduction in the number of colonies after handwashing for workers without rings.

Authors of this study acknowledge limited generalizability because of the nature of the sample, type of patient care activity, and other variables. Additional studies with larger sample populations, more sophisticated methods of sample collection, and increased control of other variables might increase the generalizability of the study results. Data in this study support the hypothesis that wearing rings affects the bioload of healthcare workers' hands.

From Salisbury, D., Hutfilz, P., Treen, L., Bollin, G., & Gautman, S. (1997, February). The effect of rings on microbial load of healthcare workers' hands. *American Journal of Infection Control*, 24-27.

transfer process. Artificial nails or synthetic nail additives should not be worn. Higher numbers of gram-negative organisms have been cultured from the nails of persons wearing artificial nails or nail additives than from persons with natural nails both before and after handwashing.[32,59] The length of artificial nails may interfere with effective cleaning. Numerous cosmetology boards report that fungal growth occurs frequently under artificial nails as moisture is trapped between the natural and artificial nail.

Institutional procedures govern the selection of materials and the methods used for the surgical hand scrub. The selection of a reusable or disposable brush for scrubbing should be based on realistic considerations of effectiveness and economy. Studies show no significant difference in scrub effectiveness between reusable brushes and disposable brushes or sponges. Individually packaged disposable brushes and sponges provide a cost-effective, labor-saving alternative to reusable brushes. The use of synthetic sponges in place of brushes has gained wide acceptance, especially where long and repeated scrubbing may be traumatic to the skin. Disposable brushes or sponges are available with a variety of antimicrobial soap or detergent solutions infused into the sponge. If a reusable brush is desired, it should be easy to clean and maintain and should be durable enough to withstand repeated heat sterilization without the bristles becoming soft or brittle. A thorough hand wash with an antimicrobial agent may be as effective as the traditional surgical scrub using a brush or sponge (Research Highlight 4-4).

Surgical hand-scrub agent selection should be based on effectiveness of the product, recommended contact time, and user-friendliness of the product. The antimicrobial soap or detergent used for the surgical hand scrub should reduce microorganisms on the skin, be fast acting, have a broad range of activity, not depend on cumulative action, have a minimally harsh effect on skin, and inhibit regrowth of microorganisms. Two popular antimicrobial agents used for surgical hand scrubs are povidone-iodine complex and chlorhexidine gluconate. Both are rapid-acting, broad-spectrum antimicrobials that are effective against gram-positive and gram-negative microorganisms. For individuals who have demonstrated skin sensitivity to these agents, another broad-spectrum antimicrobial agent, parachlorometaxylenol (chloroxylenol, PCMX), may be used as an effective alternative agent for surgical scrubbing. Many persons who previously were unable to use any surgical hand scrub other than hexachlorophene (which is ineffective against gram-negative microorganisms) are now safely using PCMX. It significantly reduces skin flora with an antibacterial effect that persists even after prolonged surgery. Moisturizing agents are now being incorporated into various surgical scrub agents to reduce the potential of skin irritation resulting from multiple scrubs. Persons who are sensitive to all antimicrobial agents may scrub with a nonmedicated soap followed by application of one of the alcohol-based hand-cleansing agents. Many of these agents provide effective skin antisepsis when used according to manufacturers' instructions.

An anatomic scrub, using a prescribed amount of time or number of strokes plus friction, is employed for effective cleansing of the skin. A properly executed surgical hand scrub, using the anatomic, counted, brush-stroke method,

4-4 RESEARCH HIGHLIGHT

In today's economically-driven healthcare environment, methods of cost containment and reduction are continually sought. Quality remains an equally important factor. The purpose of this experimental, crossover design study was to determine the difference between the use of a scrub agent with surgical scrub brush and use of the scrub agent alone on the bacterial hand count of study subjects.

Fifteen subjects were taught a 5-minute surgical scrub procedure. They were then randomized into two groups: those scrubbing with an inert brush and 4% chlorhexidine soap with alcohol and those washing with the 4% chlorhexidine soap and alcohol alone. Specimens were taken immediately after scrubbing and 45 minutes later. A crossover design was used to repeat the experiment after a 1-week washout period. A broad range of baseline hand counts was obtained, and data analysis took into account this occurrence. Three methods of data analysis were used:

- Discord between the presence or absence of hand bacteria within individuals at 45 minutes for each group
- Absolute reduction of hand bacteria from baseline number to 45 minutes for each group
- Proportional change in hand bacteria counts from baseline number to 45 minutes for each group

Results of this study demonstrated a greater reduction in hand bacterial counts for up to twice the number of subjects when they washed with the antimicrobial scrub agent only as opposed to scrubbing with a brush and using the same antimicrobial agent.

The authors conclude that use of the antimicrobial scrub agent alone is as effective as its use with an inert surgical scrub brush. The authors further suggest that the agent can be used alone and the infection rate prospectively monitored. A significant savings can be realized by eliminating the use of scrub brushes.

From Loeb, M., Wilcox, L., Smaill, F., Walter, S., & Duff, Z. (1997, February). A randomized trial of surgical scrubbing with a brush compared to antiseptic soap alone. *American Journal of Infection Control*, 11-15.

usually takes approximately 5 minutes. Individual attention to detail is essential. The prescribed number of strokes with a brush is usually 30 strokes to the nails and 20 strokes to each area of the skin. When scrubbing, the fingers, hands, and arms should be visualized as having four sides; each side must be scrubbed effectively. The number of deeply resident flora is reduced by frequent scrubbing, but the number is increased when the surgical scrub is done only occasionally.

Scrub procedure

Surgical hand scrub procedures should be defined in writing. Before beginning the surgical hand scrub, members of the surgical team should inspect their hands to ensure that their nails are short, their cuticles are in good condition, and no cuts or skin problems exist. All jewelry must be removed from the hands and forearms. The cap or hood is adjusted to cover and contain all hair. A fresh mask is carefully placed over the nose and mouth and tied securely to prevent venting. Goggles or protective eyewear are comfortably adjusted to ensure clear vision and to avoid lens fogging. Personnel confirm that the scrub shirt is fitted, tied, or tucked into the trousers to prevent potential contamination of the scrubbed hands and arms from brushing against loose garments. The basic steps of the scrub procedure follow:

1. Turn on faucet and bring water to a comfortable temperature. Most scrub sinks have automatic or knee controls for the faucets.
2. Dampen hands and forearms.
3. Using a foot control, dispense a few drops of the antimicrobial soap or detergent into the palms. Add small amounts of water to make a lather.
4. Wash hands and forearms using the antimicrobial soap or detergent. Rinse before beginning the surgical hand scrub. The amount of time needed varies with the amount of soil and the effectiveness of the cleansing agent.
5. If a packaged scrub brush or sponge is used, open the package, remove the brush and nail cleaner, and discard the package. Hold the brush in one hand while cleaning the nails on the other hand (Fig. 4-13). Clean all nails and subungual spaces. If a disposable nail cleaner is not available, a metal nail file can be used. Orangewood sticks are prohibited because they cannot be sterilized after use.
6. Rinse the hands and arms thoroughly, exercising care to hold the hands higher than the elbows. Avoid splashing water onto the scrub suit because this moisture may cause subsequent contamination of the sterile gown.
7. If the brush or sponge is impregnated with antimicrobial soap, moisten the brush or sponge and begin scrubbing. If the brush or sponge is not impregnated with soap, apply antimicrobial soap or detergent solution to hands. Starting at the fingertips, scrub the nails vigorously, holding the brush perpendicularly to the nails. Scrub all sides of each digit, including the connecting webbed spaces. Next scrub the palm and back of the hand.
8. Scrub each side of the forearm with a circular motion (see Fig. 4-13) up to the elbows.
9. Hold the hands and arms away from the body, with the hands above the level of the elbows while scrubbing, allowing the water and detritus to flow

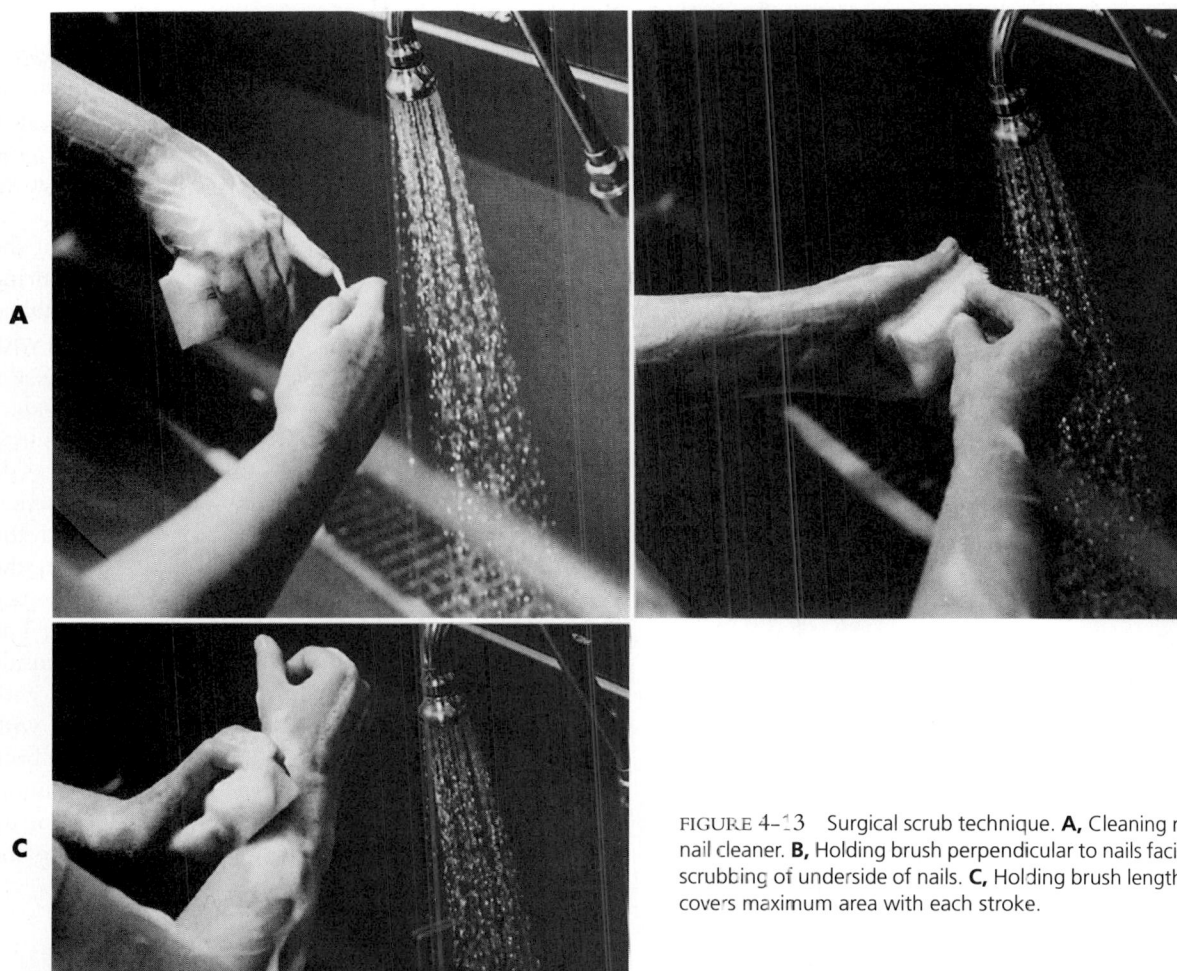

FIGURE 4-13 Surgical scrub technique. **A,** Cleaning nails with plastic nail cleaner. **B,** Holding brush perpendicular to nails facilitates thorough scrubbing of underside of nails. **C,** Holding brush lengthwise along arm covers maximum area with each stroke.

away from the first-scrubbed and cleanest area. Add small amounts of water during the scrub to develop suds and remove detritus.

10. Rinse the hands and arms thoroughly.
11. If the sink is not automatically timed, turn off the faucet by using the knee control or by using the edge of the brush on a hand control. Discard the brush.
12. Hold the hands and arms up in front of the body with elbows slightly flexed and enter the operating room.

Drying the scrubbed area

Moisture remaining on the cleansed skin after the scrub procedure is dried with a sterile towel before a sterile gown and gloves are donned. The gown and gloves should be opened on a flat surface before the surgical scrub is done. A sterile minifield is created by the gown wrapper, which is opened over the flat surface. The gown and gloves should not be opened on the sterile back table because of the increased chance of contamination to the field. The towel must be used with care to avoid contaminating the cleansed skin. The folded towel is grasped firmly near

the open corner and lifted straight up and away from the sterile field without dripping contaminated water from the skin onto the sterile field. The person steps away from the sterile field and bends forward slightly from the waist, holding the hands and elbows above the waist and away from the body. The towel is allowed to unfold downward to its full length and width (Fig. 4-14).

The top half of the towel is held securely with one hand, and the opposite fingers and hand are blotted dry; ensure that they are thoroughly dry before moving to the forearm. To avoid contamination, use a rotating motion while moving up the arm, and do not retrace an area. The lower end of the towel is grasped with the dried hand, and the same procedure is used for drying the second hand and forearm. Care must be taken to prevent contamination of towel and hands. Upon completion, discard the towel without dropping the hands below waist level.

Gowning

Before scrubbed personnel can touch sterile equipment or the sterile field, they must put on sterile gowns

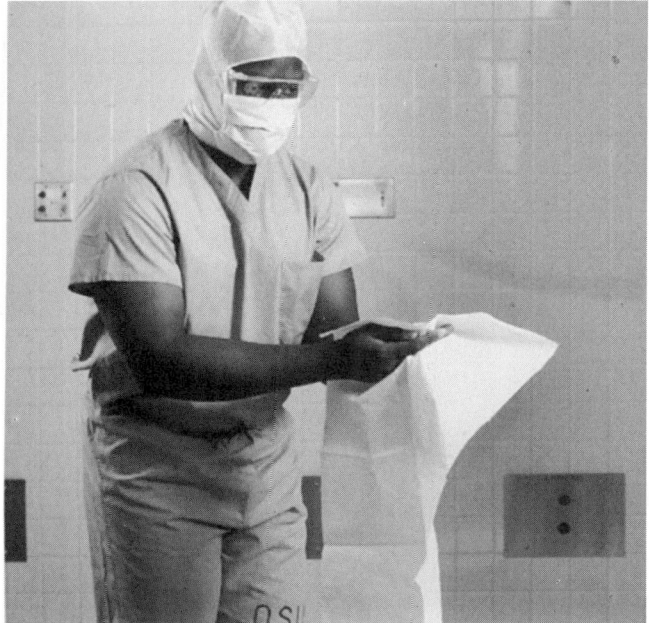

FIGURE 4-14 Drying hands and forearms. Fingers and hand are dried thoroughly before forearm is dried. Extending arms reduces possibility of contaminating towel or hands.

and sterile surgical gloves to prevent microorganisms on their hands and clothing from being transferred to the patient's wound during surgery. The sterile gowns and gloves also protect the hands and clothing of personnel from microorganisms present in the patient or in the atmosphere.

The surgical gown should be made of a combustion-resistant material that establishes an effective barrier to minimize the passage of microorganisms, particulate matter, and fluids between unsterile and sterile areas. Reusable fabrics must allow complete penetration of steam during the sterilization process and should withstand multiple launderings and other processing. Tests indicate that 280-count, water-repellent treated materials lose their barrier quality when subjected to multiple laundering and sterilization, usually at about 75 to 100 cycles. A mechanism should be established to monitor the number of times the fabric is processed. The particular item should be removed from circulation when the maximum number of processings as noted by the manufacturer has been reached. If possible, the item may be used in circumstances where surgical-barrier quality is not needed. With each processing, reusable materials also must be examined for holes or fraying. If these occur, the material should be removed from service. To reduce particle dissemination into the wound and the environment, materials used for surgical gowns should be tear and puncture resistant and as lint free as possible.[19] Regardless of the gown's material, the shape and size should fit the wearer and allow freedom of movement. To provide extra protection, the gown's front from the waist upward and the forearms of the sleeves can be reinforced with additional or different water-repellent material. Each sleeve should be finished with a tight-fitting cuff that prevents the inner side of the sleeve from slipping down onto the outer side of the sterile glove. Cotton tapes, snaps, or Velcro fasteners are attached to the back of the gown to hold it closed. A wraparound gown may be used to achieve better coverage of the back, and you should note that, once donned, the back of the gown is never considered sterile.

Because the outer side of the front and sleeves of the gown come into contact with the sterile field during surgery, the gown must be folded so that the scrubbed person can put it on without touching the outer side with bare hands. For in-house wrapping and sterilization, the gown is folded with the inner side out and the back edges together. The sleeves are not turned inside out; consequently they remain within the folded gown. The side folds of the gown are folded lengthwise toward the center back opening, overlapping slightly at the center. With the open edges of the gown remaining on the inside, the bottom third of the gown is folded upward, and the top third of the gown is folded over the bottom portion. The gown is then folded in half widthwise so that the inside front neckline of the gown is visible on top. Gowns with wraparound backs are prepared in the same manner, with care taken to tie the tape securely on the wraparound back flap to the external side tie of the gown before initial folding. A folded hand towel with its free corners facing up is usually placed on top of the folded gown before the gown is wrapped and sterilized.

Self-gowning procedure

The procedure for donning a wraparound, sterile, surgical gown follows (Figs. 4-15 and 4-16). The scrubbed person should do the following:

1. Grasp the sterile gown at the neckline with both hands and lift from the wrapper. Step into an area where the gown may be opened without risk of contamination.
2. Hold the gown away from the body and allow it to unfold with the inside toward the wearer.
3. Keep hands on the inside of the gown while it completely unfolds.
4. Slip both hands into the open armholes, keeping the hands at shoulder level and away from the body.
5. Push the hands and forearms into the sleeves of the gown, advancing the hands only to the proximal edge of the cuff if the closed gloving technique will be used. If the open gloving technique will be used, advance the hands completely through the cuffs of the gown.

The circulating nurse should do the following:

6. Pull the gown over the scrubbed person's shoulders, touching only the inner shoulder and side seams.
7. Tie or clasp the neckline and tie the inner waist ties of the gown, touching only the inner aspect of the gown. The gown should be completely fastened by the circulator before the scrub person dons gloves to prevent contamination from the gown flapping.

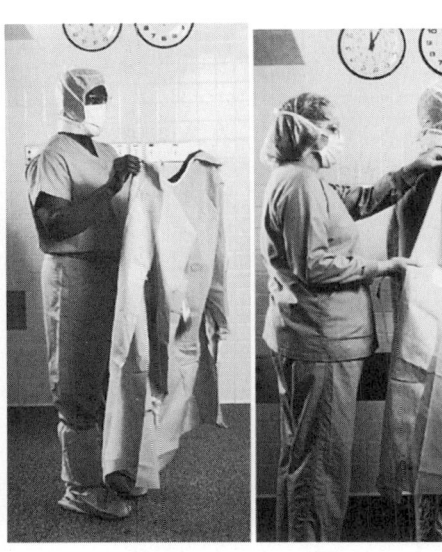
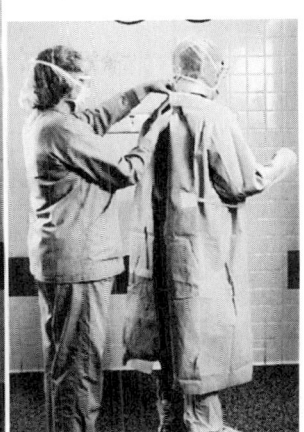

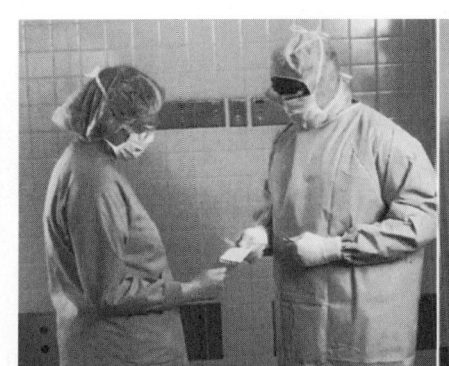
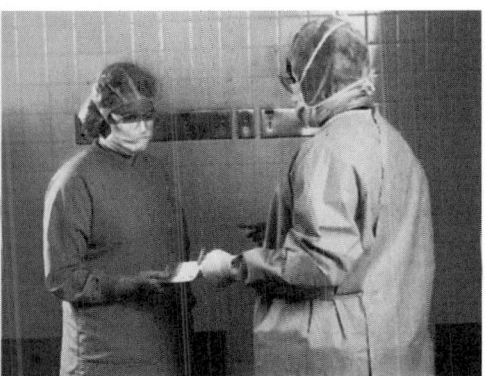

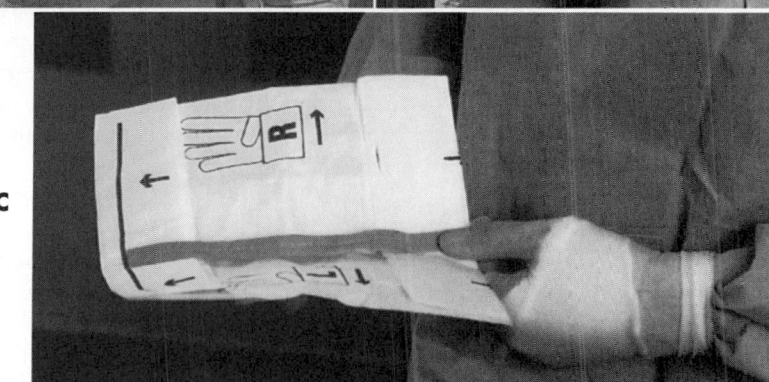

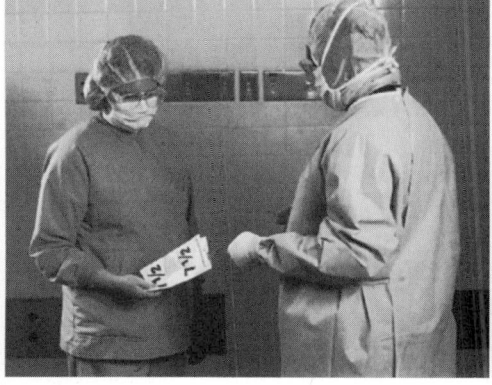
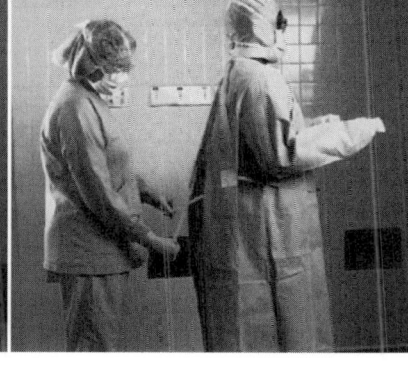

FIGURE 4-15 Gowning procedure. **A,** Scrub person keeps hands on inside of gown while unfolding it at arm's length. **B,** Circulating nurse reaches under flap of gown to pull sleeves on scrub person. **C,** Circulating nurse snaps neckline of gown, touching only snap section of neckline.

FIGURE 4-16 Methods of tying a wrap-around gown. **A,** After handing tab on back tie of gown to circulating nurse, scrub person makes three-fourths turn toward left. **B,** Sterile back panel now covers previously tied unsterile ties; scrub person retrieves back tie by carefully pulling it out of tab held by circulating nurse and ties it securely with other tie. **C,** For gowns having no tab on back tie: using sterile inner glove wrapper, scrub person places end of back tie in crease of wrapper. **D,** After closing wrapper, scrub person hands tie to circulating nurse who grasps it carefully, touching neither tie nor gloved hand of the scrub person. **E,** After making three-fourths turn to left, scrub person carefully pulls back tie from wrapper and ties it with other tie as in step **B** above.

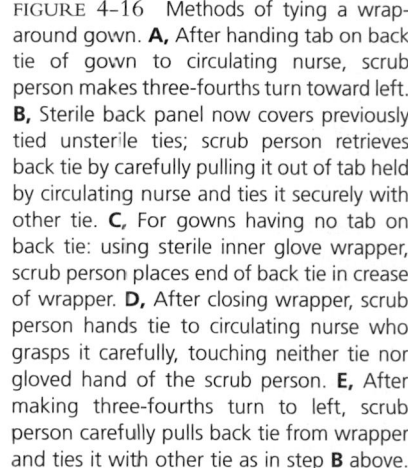

To secure the gown, do the following:

8. After gloving, the scrubbed person hands the tab attached to the back tie of the gown to the circulating nurse. The scrubbed person then makes a three-fourths turn to the left while the circulating nurse extends the back tie to its full length. This action effectively wraps the back panel of the gown around the scrubbed person and covers the previously tied inner waist ties. The scrubbed person retrieves the back tie by carefully pulling it out of the tab held by the circulating nurse and ties it with the other tie, which had been secured to the front top of the gown.

   a. When a reusable gown is used, absence of a tab on the back tie necessitates use of an alternative procedure for securing the gown (see Fig. 4-16, C to E). If the closed gloving technique and commercially prepared, double-wrapped gloves are employed, the inner wrap can be used as a protective extension for the gown tie when the circulating nurse assists with tying a wraparound gown. After gloving, the scrubbed person unties the exterior gown ties (which were tied at the front of the gown before it was folded, wrapped, and sterilized) and holds both in the hands. The end of the back tie is placed in the center crease of the empty glove wrapper, approximately two thirds the way up to the edge of the opened wrapper. The glove wrapper is then closed so that the tie is concealed. The closed wrapper is handed to the circulating nurse, who firmly grasps the folded edge of the wrapper without touching the tie. The scrubbed person then pivots in the opposite direction from the circulating nurse, who extends the back tie to its full length. The scrubbed person grasps the exposed portion of the back tie, pulls it out of the glove wrapper while taking care to avoid touching the glove wrapper or the circulating nurse, and ties both ties. If a sterile glove wrapper is not available, a sterile hemostat or ringed forceps may be clamped to the back tie and used in the same manner as a glove wrapper. After the gowning procedure has been completed, the circulating nurse retains the instrument in the room to avoid problems with the subsequent instrument count.

   b. If another scrubbed person is gowned and gloved, that person, instead of the circulating nurse, may assist with the wraparound procedure. The assisting person must extend the back tie to its fullest length before the scrubbed person turns to avoid any potential contamination.

Assisted-gowning procedure

A gowned and gloved person may assist another person in donning a sterile gown (Fig. 4-17). The gown is opened in the manner previously described. The inner side with

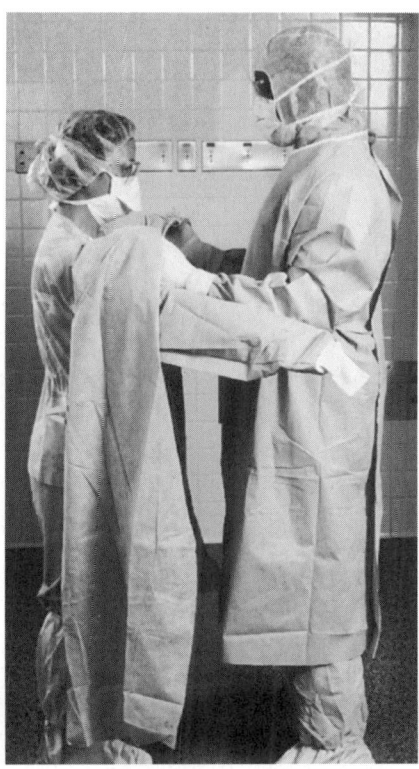

FIGURE 4-17 Gowning another person. Gowned and gloved scrub person cuffs neck and shoulder area of gown over gloved hands to prevent contamination as scrubbed person puts hands and forearms into sleeves.

the open armholes is turned toward the individual who is to be gowned. A cuff is made of the neck and shoulder area of the gown to protect the gloved hands. The gown is held until the person's hand and forearms are in the sleeves of the gown. The circulating nurse assists in pulling the gown onto the shoulders, adjusting the back, and tying the tapes. The wraparound back on the gown is fixed into position by the scrubbed person after gloving is completed.

Gloving

Sterile surgical gloves are worn to provide a bacterial barrier between the patient and the healthcare worker, decreasing the probability of exposing the patient to exogenous organisms with a resulting surgical site infection.

The use of powder as a glove lubricant is not recommended because of two primary hazards: the potential for postoperative complication of powder granulomas and powder fallout from hands and gloves, which provides a convenient vehicle for dissemination of microorganisms throughout the operating room and the facility. For removal of any glove film or powder, the gloves must be wiped thoroughly after they are put on and before the surgical team member approaches the sterile field. To facilitate glove donning, various creams and liquid lubricants have been developed. Oil-based lubricants

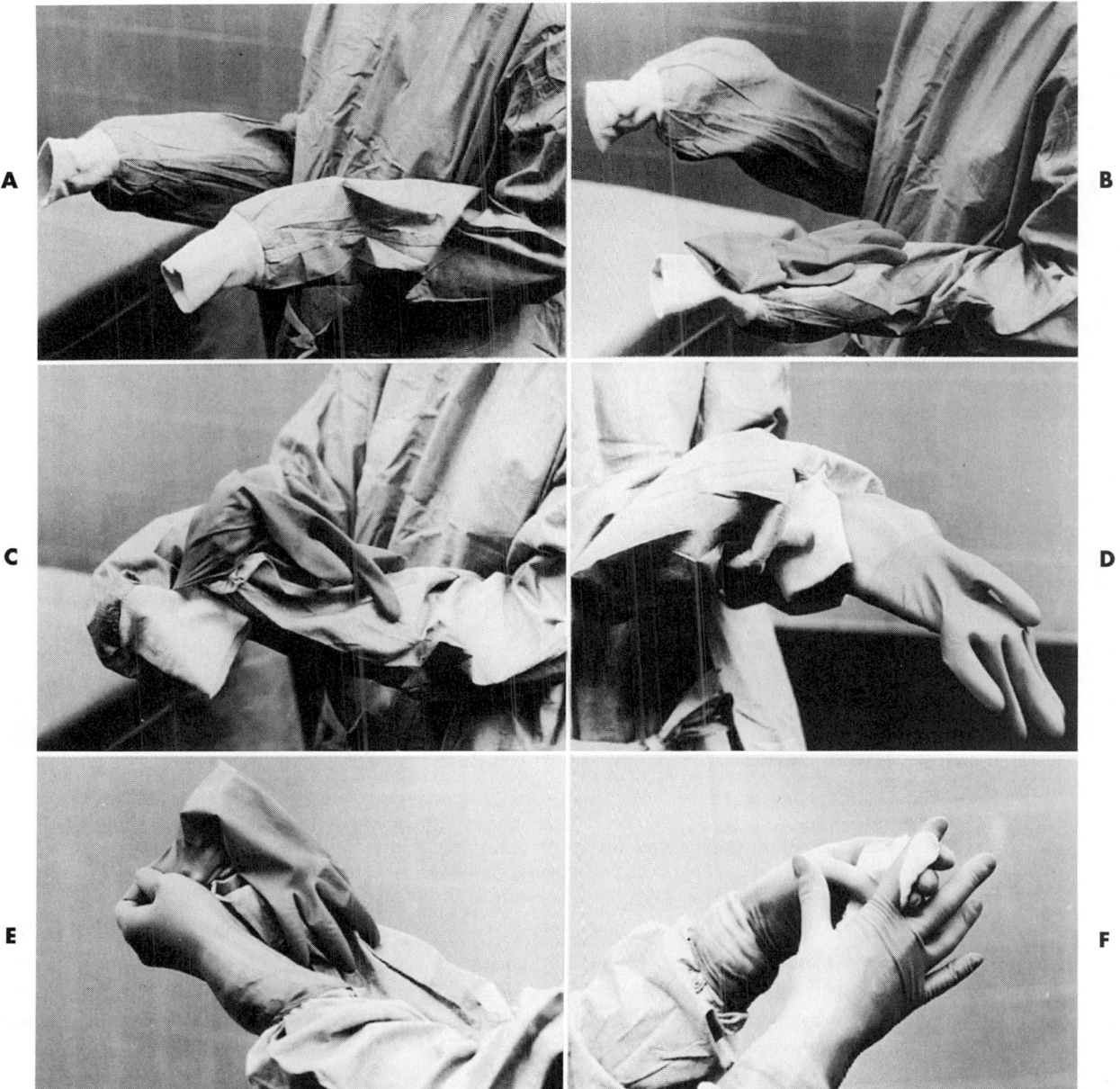

FIGURE 4-18 Closed gloving procedure. **A,** When donning gown, scrub person does not slip hands through wristlets. Hands are not extended from sleeves. **B,** First glove is lifted by grasping it through fabric or sleeve. Cuff on glove facilitates easier handling of glove. Glove is placed palm down along forearm of matching hand, with thumb and fingers pointing toward elbow. Glove cuff lies over gown wristlet. **C,** Glove cuff is held securely by hand on which it is placed, and, with other hand, cuff is stretched over opening of sleeve to cover gown wristlet entirely. **D,** As cuff is drawn back onto wrist, fingers are directed into their cots in glove, and glove is adjusted to hand. **E,** Gloved hand is then used to position remaining glove on opposite sleeve in same fashion. Glove cuff is placed around gown cuff. Second glove is drawn onto hand, and cuff is pulled into place. **F,** Fingers of gloves are adjusted, and gloves are wiped with wet gauze sponge or commercially prepared sterile disposable glove wipe to remove any powder that may be on them.

should not be used because they can cause early glove failure. Some products contain antiseptic or bacteriostatic agents, which assist in keeping the gloved hands relatively free from bacterial growth. Manufacturers of surgical gloves have also used silicone films to eliminate stickiness. Little or no lubrication of the hands is needed to don these gloves easily. Each product should be individually assessed to determine its effectiveness and its affect on patient and personnel tissue.

Closed-gloving technique

The closed method of gloving (Fig. 4-18) is the technique of choice when initially donning sterile gown and gloves. Using this technique, the gloves are handled

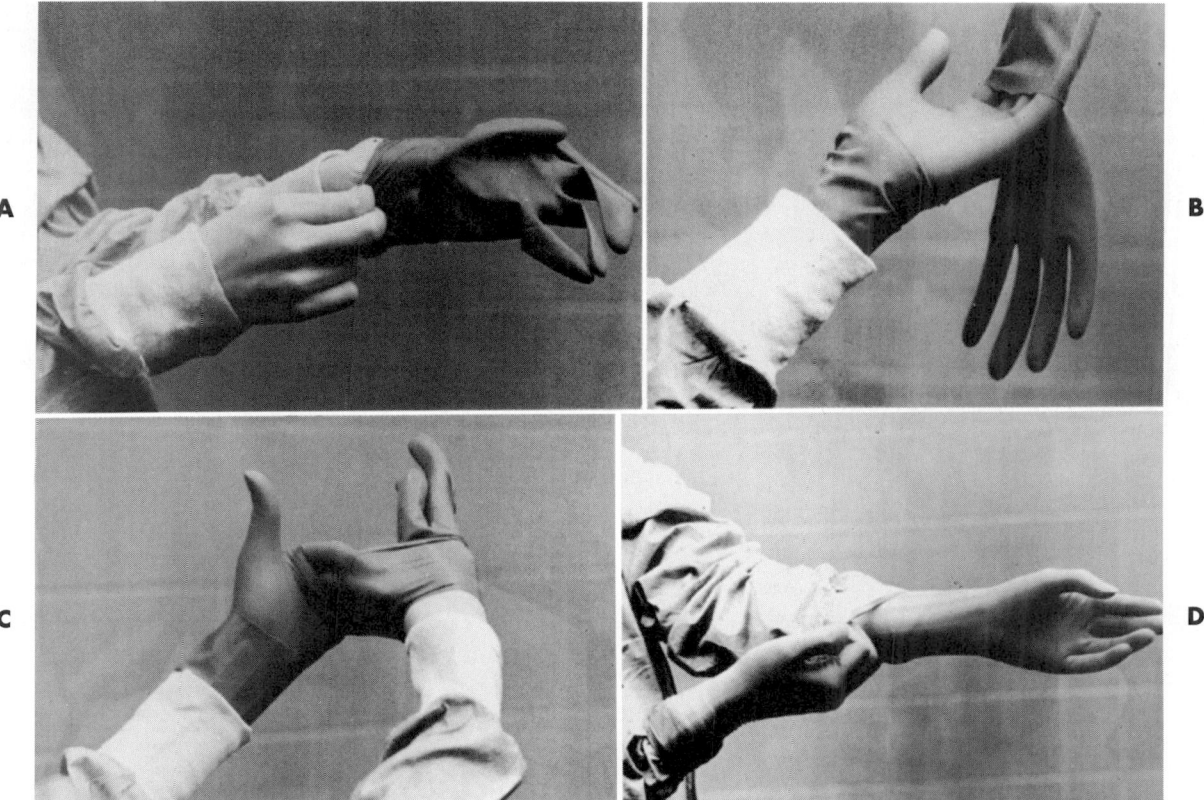

FIGURE 4-19   Open gloving procedure. **A,** Scrub person takes one glove from inner glove wrapper by placing thumb and index finger of opposite hand on fold of everted cuff at a point in line with glove's palm and pulls glove over hand, leaving cuff turned back. **B,** Scrub person takes second glove from inner glove wrapper by placing gloved fingers under everted cuff. **C,** Scrub person, with arms extended and elbows slightly flexed, introduces free hand into glove and draws it over cuff of gown and upper part of wristlet by slightly rotating arm externally and internally. **D,** To bring turned-back cuff on other hand over wristlet of gown, scrub person repeats step **C.**

through the fabric of the gown sleeves. The hands are not extended from the sleeves and cuffs when the gown is put on. Instead, the hands are pushed through the cuff openings as the gloves are pulled into place. Because the cuffs of a sterile gown collect moisture, become damp during wearing, and are considered unsterile, the closed gloving technique can be used only for initial gloving. Cuffs may not be pulled down over the wearer's hand for subsequent gloving. For subsequent gloving an alternative technique must be used. Alternatives include open gloving, assisted gloving, or overgloving, which is the practice of adding an additional sterile glove over the compromised glove.

Open-gloving technique

With the open-gloving technique the everted cuff of each glove permits a gowned person to touch the glove's inner side with ungloved fingers and to touch the glove's outer side with gloved fingers (Fig. 4-19). Keeping the hands in direct view, no lower than waist level, the gowned person flexes the elbows. Exerting a light, even pull on the glove brings it over the hand, and using a rotating movement brings the cuff over the wristlet. Extreme

caution is necessary when using the open method to prevent contamination by the exposed hands. This gloving technique can be used by persons not wearing a gown.

Assisted-gloving technique

A gowned and gloved person may assist another gowned individual with gloving. To assist another, grasp the glove under the everted cuff. Be sure the palm of the glove is turned toward the ungloved individual's hand with the thumb of the glove directly opposed to the thumb of the person's hand. Using thumbs and fingers, stretch the cuff to open the glove. The ungloved individual can then insert his or her hand into the glove. The procedure is repeated for the other hand (Fig. 4-20).

Latex allergies and sensitivities

The increased reporting of latex sensitivity has created concern among operating room personnel. There are three types of reactions to latex people can experience. Irritant contact dermatitis is the most common and is characterized by dry, reddened, itchy, or cracked hands. Irritant contact dermatitis is not a true allergic reaction. Allergic contact dermatitis is considered a class IV allergic

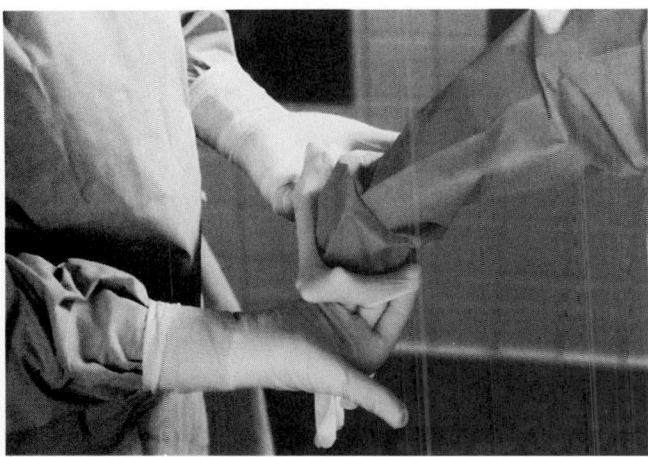

FIGURE 4-20 Gloving another person. Gowned and gloved scrub person places fingers of each hand beneath everted cuff, keeping thumbs turned outward and stretching cuff as gowned person slips hand into sterile glove, using firm downward thrust.

reaction and is a true allergic response. Most often it is caused by chemicals used in the manufacture of latex gloves. Allergic contact dermatitis is a delayed reaction, usually appearing 6 to 48 hours after exposure. Symptoms are similar to those of irritant contact dermatitis except that the reaction may extend beyond the actual point of contact. True latex allergies are classified as type I allergic responses. This is an allergy to water-soluble natural rubber latex (NRL) proteins. True latex allergies are usually seen within minutes of contact with the proteins. Symptoms can range from skin redness and itching to hives to dyspnea to gastrointestinal upset to hypotension, tachycardia, and anaphylaxis. Reactions to latex rarely progress to anaphylaxis because the wearer is treated with appropriate drugs to interrupt the allergic response. Appropriate latex-free gloves should be provided for healthcare workers with known latex sensitivity or for procedures in which patients have known sensitivity or allergy. Some personnel claim allergy to the starch powder in latex gloves. Although this is possible, it is more likely that individuals are allergic to the latex proteins that bind with the starch powder and become aerosolized.[68]

Special nursing protocols should be developed for latex-sensitive patients. To develop a latex-safety protocol, a multidisciplinary team should be assembled. Representative staff from the preoperative holding area, the postanesthesia care unit, and the operating room will be key players. Also required will be representatives from the department of surgery, anesthesia, pharmacy, and any other area involved in the patient's care. To establish a latex-safe patient-care environment, all latex products should be removed from the immediate area. In some instances this may not be possible. In such cases, barriers should be placed between the patient and the latex-containing item. Mobile carts containing latex-free items can be assembled and maintained by the central sterile department. These carts can be accessed for the latex-sensitive patient and can follow the patient throughout the care encounter.[68]

Removing soiled gown, gloves, and mask

To protect the forearms, hands, and clothing from contacting bacteria on the outer side of the used gown and gloves, members of the scrubbed surgical team should use the following steps to remove soiled gowns, gloves, and masks (Fig. 4-21).

1. Wipe gloves clean with a wet, sterile towel.
2. Untie surgical gown. Circulator must unfasten back closures.
3. Grasp gown at one shoulder seam without touching scrub clothing.
4. Bring neck and sleeve of the gown forward, over, and off the gloved hand, turning the gown inside out and everting the cuff of the glove.
5. Repeat steps 3 and 4 for other side.
6. Keep arms and gown away from body while turning the gown inside out and discarding carefully in the designated receptacle.
7. Using the gloved fingers of one hand to secure the everted cuff, remove the glove turning it inside out. Discard appropriately.
8. Using the ungloved hand, grasp the fold of the everted cuff of the other glove and remove the glove, inverting the glove as it is removed. Discard appropriately.
9. After leaving the restricted area, remove the mask by touching the ties or elastic only. Discard in the designated receptacle (see Fig. 4-12).
10. Wash hands and forearms.

Patient Skin Disinfection and Preparation

To prevent bacteria on the skin surfaces from entering the surgical wound, the skin area at and around the proposed incision site must be cleaned and disinfected. Skin preparation methods vary, but all are based on the same principles and share the same objectives: to remove dirt and transient microbes from the skin, to reduce the resident microbial count as much as possible in the shortest time and with the least amount of tissue irritation, and to prevent rapid rebound growth of microbes.

Factors to be considered in skin disinfection are (1) the condition of the involved area, (2) the number and kinds of contaminants, (3) the characteristics of the skin to be disinfected, and (4) the general physical condition of the patient.

Many soaps and detergents are available for skin cleansing. Although most of them produce similar results in the immediate removal of soil and microorganisms, certain factors need further consideration in selecting a product for surgical use. Most soaps and detergents emulsify and peptize waste products and oils that are

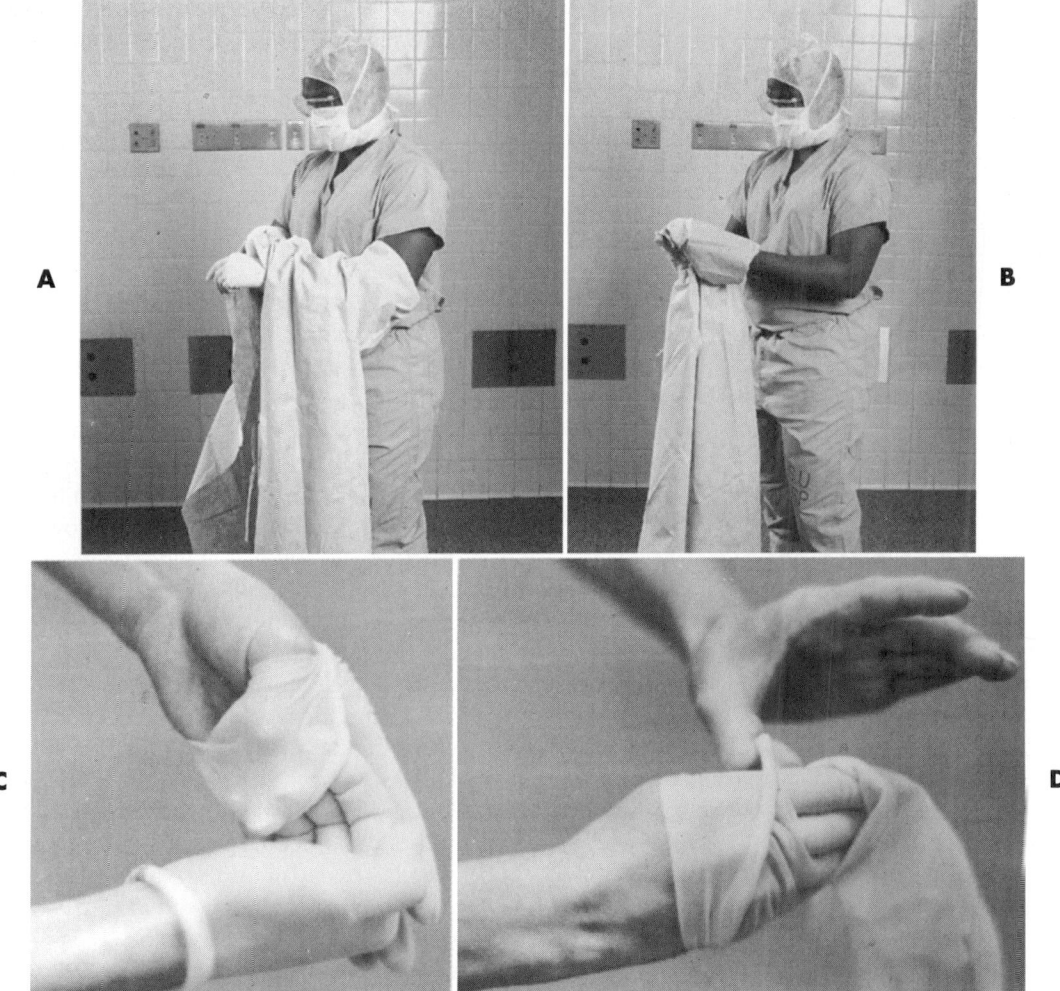

FIGURE 4-21   Removing soiled gown and gloves. **A,** To protect scrub suit and arms from bacteria that are present on outer side of soiled gown, the gown is grasped without touching the scrub clothes. **B,** Scrub person turns outer side of soiled gown away from body, keeping elbows flexed and arms away from body, so that soiled gown will not touch arms or scrub suit **C,** To prevent outer side of soiled gloves from touching skin surfaces of hands, scrub person places gloved fingers of one hand under everted cuff of other glove and pulls it off hand and fingers. **D,** To prevent ungloved hand from touching outer side of soiled glove, scrub person hooks bare thumb on inner side of glove and pulls glove off.

absorbed in surface soil and permit the detritus to be rinsed off the skin with running water. The product selected should become hydrolyzed in the presence of water and yield a pH that corresponds to that of average, normal skin. An odorless agent that produces a good lather for easy, comfortable use is usually preferred. It should not irritate the skin or in any way interfere with normal functioning. Equally important, an effective antimicrobial agent should be used to achieve appropriate disinfection of skin. The antimicrobial agent employed for disinfection of the skin should be selected according to its ability to rapidly decrease the microbial count of the skin, be applied quickly, and remain effective throughout the operation. The agent should not cause irritation or sensitization or be incompatible with or inactivated by alcohol, organic matter, soap, or detergent.

The surgical principle to be followed when preparing the patient's skin for surgery is to prepare the cleanest area first and then move to the less-clean areas. Ordinarily, the skin prep should begin at the point of the incision and proceed to the periphery of the area.

Hair is best left at the surgical site. The necessity for hair removal will depend on the amount of hair, the location of the incision, and the type of surgical procedure to be performed.[13] If hair is to be removed, any of three choices may be used for hair removal: clipping, use of a depilatory, or wet shaving. Studies show that the wound-infection rate is considerably higher for patients who are shaved preoperatively than for patients who have no preoperative shave preparation or a small amount of hair clipped, or for patients on whom a depilatory is used. If a shave is required by the surgeon, the patient should be shaved as close to the time of surgery as is possible. The shave should be performed in an area within the surgical suite that affords privacy and is equipped with good lighting. The amount of time between the preoperative shave and the operation has a direct effect on the surgical site infection rate. Hair removal should be performed by skillful personnel with great care taken to avoid scratching, nicking, or cutting the skin because cutaneous bacteria will proliferate in these areas and increase the chances of infection. The decision of where and by whom hair removal is performed depends on when it is to be done, the facilities and personnel available, the patient's reactions, and the philosophy and policies that have been determined and established by the surgical committee. An electric or battery-operated clipper with a disposable or detachable, reusable head that can be disinfected is the preferred alternative to shaving. Clipping, immediately before surgery, is the simplest and least irritating method of hair removal.

When the patient skin preparation procedure is performed, the antimicrobial agent is applied using sponges or commercially prepared devices or applicators that have handles to distance the operator's hand from the area being prepared. Gloves should be worn. In most instances, the scrub procedure will begin at the operative site and work toward the periphery of the area. The sponges or applicators used in scrubbing are discarded as they become soiled, and fresh ones are used. A soiled sponge or applicator is never brought back over a scrubbed surface. Upon completion of the scrub, the lather is wiped off with dry, sterile sponges or a sterile towel. Depending on the surgeon's preference, a topical, antimicrobial solution or "paint" may be carefully applied to the prepared area, using care to avoid any pooling of solution beneath the patient. All wet drapes should be removed from the patient area after the skin prep is complete.

When a stoma or other contaminated area is involved in the prep procedure, a prep sponge soaked in the antimicrobial agent of choice is placed over the stoma when the prep is initiated. At the completion of the prep the sponge is discarded. Sponges used to cleanse or disinfect an open wound, sinus, ulcer, intestinal stoma, the vagina, or the anus are applied once to that area and discarded. In contrast to the principle of working from the proposed incision to the periphery, open wounds and body orifices are potentially contaminated areas and as such are prepped after the peripheral intact skin is cleansed. The surgical principle is to work from the cleanest to the least clean area.

Creating the Sterile Field with Surgical Draping

To create a sterile field, sterile sheets and towels, known as *surgical drapes*, are strategically placed to provide a sterile surface on which sterile instruments, supplies, equipment, and gloved hands may rest. The patient and operating

room bed are covered with sterile drapes in a manner that exposes the prepared incision site and isolates it from surrounding areas. Objects normally draped and composing the sterile field include instrument tables, trays, basins, the Mayo stand, some surgical equipment, and the patient. It is within this defined sterile area that the actual operative procedure takes place.

Today, both reusable and disposable drapes are used. There are advantages and disadvantages for both reusable (fabric) and disposable (nonwoven, single-use) drapes. Regardless of the type of material used, surgical drapes should have the following characteristics:[19]

- Appropriate barriers to microorganisms, particulate matter, and fluids
- Appropriate to methods of sterilization
- Maintain integrity
- Durable
- Withstand physical conditions
- Resist tears, punctures, fiber strains, and abrasions
- Free of toxic ingredients
- Low linting
- Free of holes or other defects
- Positive cost-to-benefit ratio

In addition to the above characteristics, draping materials should meet or exceed the current requirements of the National Fire Protection Association.

Reusable drapes

Chemically treated cotton or cotton-polyester fabrics provide a barrier to liquids and are abrasion resistant. Quantitative data verifying the impervious quality of any textile drape must be provided by the manufacturer. Care should be taken with reusable drapes to eliminate pinholes caused by towel clamps, needles, or sharp objects. Only nonpenetrating towel clips should be used. Should breaks in the fabric occur, a heat-sealed patch may be used for repair. However, an abundance of heat-sealed patches on any surgical drape may interfere with the sterilization process. The exact percentage of any item that may be successfully patched is unknown. As with reusable gowns, laundering eventually impairs the barrier quality of the drape. Most manufacturers report a loss of barrier quality after 75 to 100 laundry or sterilization cycles. The process of laundering and steam sterilizing swells the fabric fibers, whereas drying and ironing shrink the fibers. Over time, these processes loosen fabric fibers, altering the fabric structure and decreasing the barrier properties and fluid impermeability of the fabric. Just as with surgical gowns, a system to monitor the number of times an item has been processed is essential for control of barrier quality and fluid impermeability.

Disposable drapes

Many synthetic disposable drapes prevent bacterial penetration and fluid breakthrough, also known as *strike through*. These versatile materials can be manufactured to meet different specifications in both absorbent and nonabsorbent forms. Disposable products are packaged and sterilized by commercial sources. Disposable drapes reduce the hazards of contamination in the presence of known infectious microorganisms in body fluids and excretions and in situations in which laundering of grossly contaminated textiles is a problem. The danger inherent in the use of synthetic drapes is that solvents, volatile liquids, and sharp instruments tend to penetrate the barrier. Loss of effectiveness may be caused by cracking at the folds or by pinholes from the use of regular, perforating towel clamps. Manufacturers are continually improving disposable drapes to permit easy handling and adaptability to the body. When considering the purchase of disposable drapes, the buyer must determine whether they will satisfy the needs of surgery, be acceptable to users, and be less expensive than the cost of laundering and processing reusable drapes. Even if the cost of disposables is not lower, other advantages may warrant their use in the healthcare facility. Availability of items, storage facilities, and disposal methods must be analyzed.

Compactors provide a relatively inexpensive method of discarding disposable drapes. They accept any material and reduce its volume substantially. Storage, collection, and transportation of compacted waste materials can be a problem. Hospital engineers must establish methods of controlling odor and maintaining sanitation in the compactor area. Because a portion of the compacted material may be grossly contaminated, city or county codes may prohibit transporting this potentially infectious material through city streets or dumping it at landfills. Incineration is an alternative method for destroying waste disposables. If incinerators are used, they must be properly managed to prevent environmental contamination. Facilities choosing to incinerate must follow specific guidelines established for medical waste incinerators. Many hospital incinerators do not meet federal pollution standards; therefore their use is prohibited.

The environmental effect of disposable items can be only roughly estimated. Each facility must carefully evaluate its capabilities and restrictions for handling both disposable and reusable supplies and equipment to make an informed decision about the products it will use.

Preassembled, sterile, disposable custom packs are used in many operating rooms. Advantages of these packs include reduced setup and room-turnover times, less risk of contaminated waste because fewer individually wrapped items are dispensed, improved inventory control, and fewer lost charges. Although custom packs may be more expensive than multiple separate items, indirect savings related to increased efficiency can offset those costs. Healthcare facilities choosing to use custom packs should determine and document ownership of liability for the function and integrity of individual items within the packs.

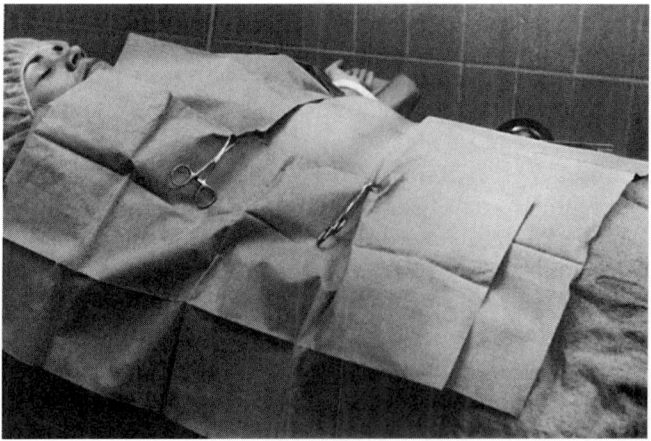

FIGURE 4-22 Abdomen may be draped with four sterile towels, which are secured with nonperforating towel clamps. Standard method of placement of disposable towels is used.

Drape configurations

Careful planning by nursing and surgical departments helps determine the desired types and sizes of surgical drapes required for surgery. The variety of drapes should be kept to a minimum. Standardized draping methods provide management control that ensures patient safety, simplifies staff education, and conserves human and material resources.

A whole, or plain, sheet is used to cover instrument tables, operating tables, and body regions. The sheet should be large enough to provide an adequate margin of safety between the surrounding physical environment and the prepared operative field. Usually two sizes of sheets suffice.

Surgical towels should be available in several sizes to drape the operative site. Four surgical towels of woven or nonwoven material are usually sufficient (Fig. 4-22).

Fenestrated, or slit, sheets are used for draping patients. They leave the operative site exposed. A typical fenestrated (laparotomy) sheet is large enough to cover the patient and operating bed in any position, extend over the anesthesia screen at the head of the bed, and over the foot of the bed (Figs. 4-23 to 4-25). The typical fenestrated laparotomy sheet can be used for most procedures on the abdomen, chest, flank, and back. Other types of fenestrated sheets but with smaller or split fenestrations may be used for the limbs, head, and neck with the patient supine or prone. The size of the fenestration is determined by the use for which the sheet is intended. The fenestrated sheet is fan folded and handled as a typical laparotomy sheet. A perineal drape is needed for operations on the perineum and genitalia with the patient in lithotomy position. A lithotomy drape consists of a fenestrated sheet and two triangular leggings. Although a three-piece drape is less costly and is easier to handle and launder, a single drape with attached leggings may used.

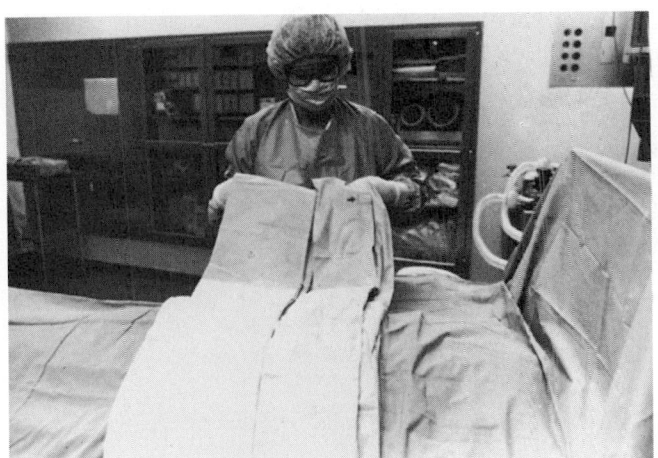

FIGURE 4-23 Placement of laparotomy sheet. Identification of top portion of laparotomy sheet assists scrub person in readily determining correct placement of drape. After placing folded laparotomy sheet on patient, with fenestration of sheet directly over site of incision outlined by sterile towels, scrub person unfolds drape over sides of patient and bed.

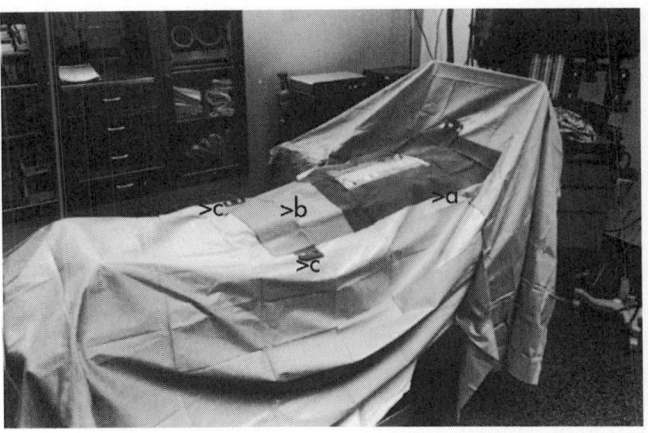

FIGURE 4-25 Laparotomy draping completed. Fenestration provides exposure of prepped operative site. >**a,** Special fabric surrounding fenestration is both absorbent and impermeable. >**b,** Built-in instrument pad prevents instrument slippage. >**c,** Perforated tabs provide means of controlling position of cords and suction tubes.

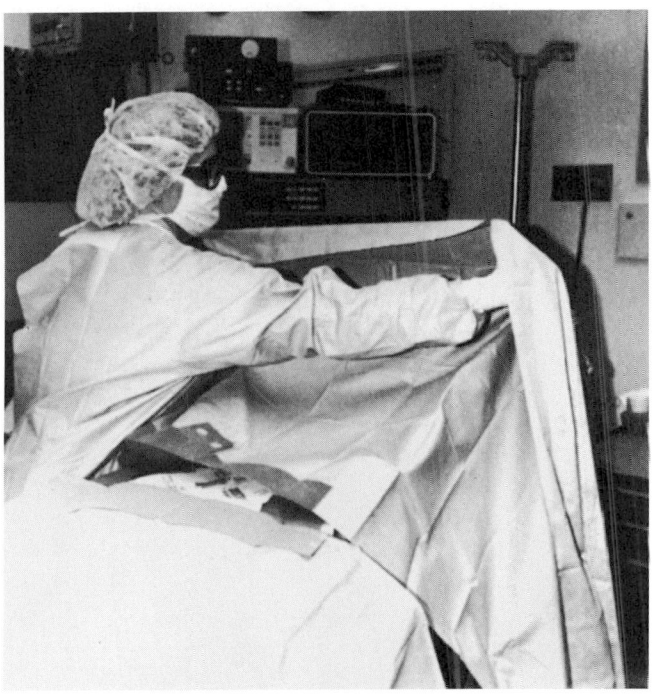

FIGURE 4-24 Laparotomy draping continued. Scrub person protects gloved hands under cuff of fan-folded laparotomy sheet and draws upper section above fenestration toward head of bed, draping it over anesthesia screen. Bottom portion of fan-folded sheet is then extended over foot of bed in similar manner.

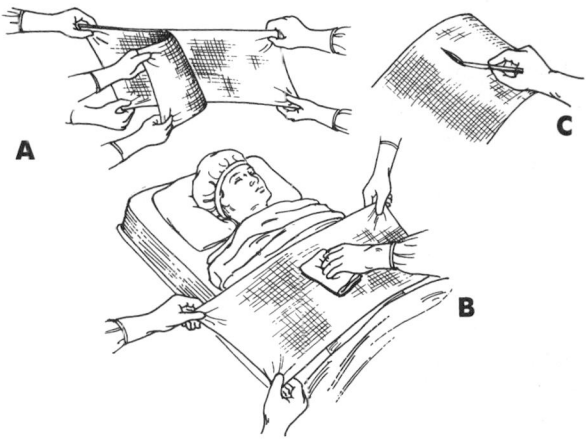

FIGURE 4-26 Sterile impermeable adhesive drape. For maximum sealing to prevent wound contamination, prepped skin must be dry and drape must be applied carefully, preventing wrinkles and air bubbles. **A,** Surgeon and assistant hold plastic drape taut while another assistant peels off back paper. **B,** Surgeon and assistant apply plastic drape to operative site and, using folded towel, apply slight pressure to eliminate air bubbles and wrinkles. **C,** Surgeon makes incision through plastic drape.

Several types of impermeable polyvinyl chloride (PVC) sheeting are available in the form of sterile, prepacked surgical drapes. Plastic incisional drapes are available as a plain impermeable drape or impregnated with iodophor. These plastic drapes are useful adjuncts to the conventional draping procedure. They can be applied after the fabric drape, alleviating the need for towel clamps. They obviate

the need for skin towels and sponges to separate the surgeon's gloves from contact with the patient's skin. Skin color and anatomic landmarks are readily visible, and the incision is made directly through the adherent plastic drape. These materials facilitate draping of irregular body surfaces, such as neck and ear regions, extremities, and joints (Fig. 4-26).

Draping procedure

Drapes should be folded so that the gowned and gloved members of the team can handle them with ease and safety. The larger, regular sheet is usually fanfolded from bottom to top. The bottom folds may be wider than the upper ones. The small sheet is folded in half and then quartered, with the top corners of the sheet turned back or marked for easy identification and handling. To provide for safe, easy handling and a wide margin of safety between the unsterile item and the scrub person's gloved hands, the open end of the Mayo stand cover should be cuffed or folded back on itself (Fig. 4-27). Most fenestrated sheets are fan folded to the opening from the top and the bottom, and then the folds are rolled or fanned toward the center of the opening. The edges of the top and bottom folds of the sheet are fanned to provide a cuff under which the scrub person may place gloved hands. The top and lower sections should be identified by a marking to facilitate easy handling.

When applying drapes to create the sterile field, these principles should be followed:

1. Allow sufficient time and space to permit careful draping and proper aseptic technique.
2. Handle sterile drapes as little as possible.
3. Carry the folded drape to the operative site. Carefully unfold the drape and place it in the proper position. Do not move the drape after it has been placed. Shifting or moving the drape may bring bacteria from an unprepared area of the patient's skin into the surgical field.

4. Hold sterile drapes above waist level until properly placed on the patient or object being draped. If the end of a drape falls below waist level, it should not be retrieved because the area below the waist is considered unsterile.
5. Without contaminating the gloves or other sterile items, immediately discard a drape that becomes contaminated during the draping procedure.
6. Protect the gown by distance and the gloved hands by cuffing drapes over them (Fig. 4-28). Control all parts of the drape at all times during placement, using precise and direct motions.
7. Do not flip, fan, or shake drapes. Rapid movement of drapes creates air currents on which dust, lint, and droplet nuclei may migrate. Shaking a drape causes uncontrolled motion of the drape, which may cause it to come into contact with an unsterile surface or object. A drape should be carefully unfolded and allowed to fall gently into position by gravity.
8. Drape the incisional area first and then the periphery. Always drape from a sterile area to an unsterile area by draping the near side first. Never reach across an unsterile area to drape. When draping the opposite side of the operating room bed, go around the bed to drape.
9. Use nonperforating towel clamps or devices to secure tubing and other items on the sterile field. The low

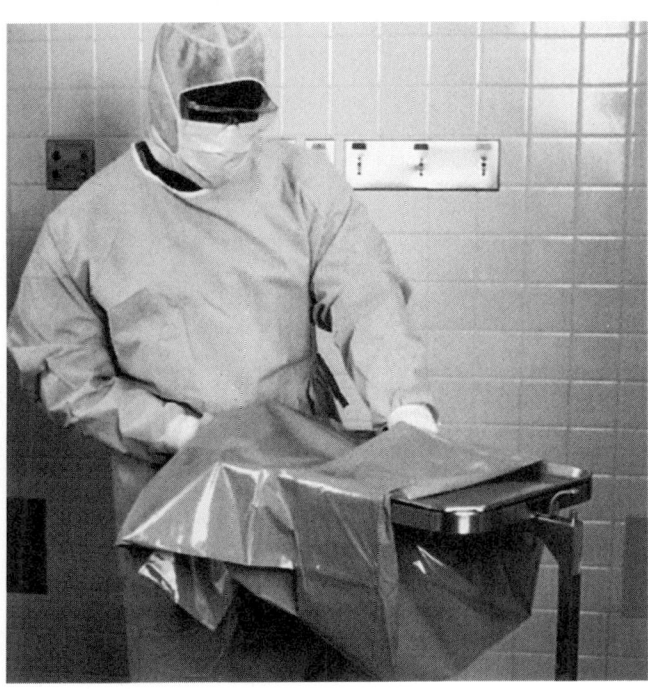

FIGURE 4-27 Draping Mayo stand. Folded cover is slipped over frame. Scrub person's gloved hands are protected by cuff of drape. Cover is unfolded to extend over upright support of stand.

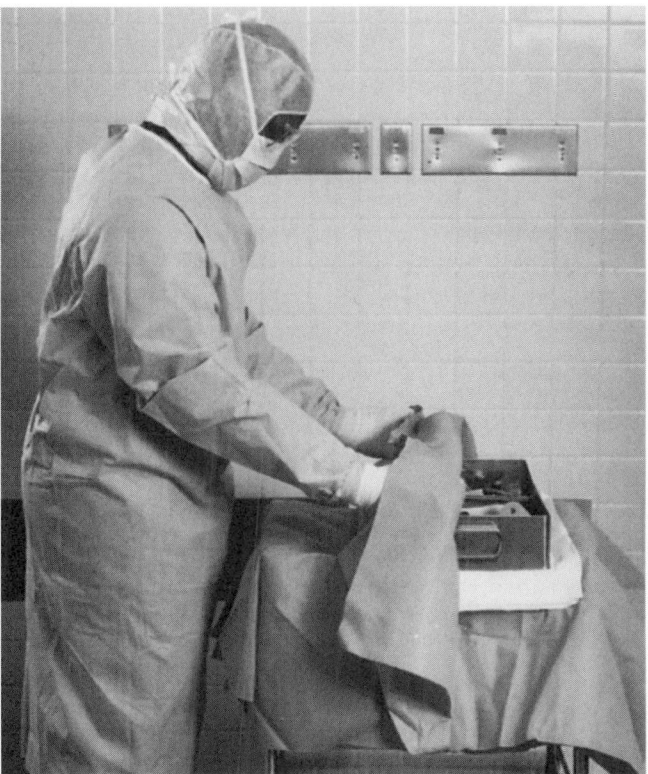

FIGURE 4-28 When placing sterile drape, scrub person rolls corners of drape over hands to avoid contamination.

portion of a sheet that falls below the safe working level should never be raised or lifted back into the sterile area.

10. When sterility of a drape is questionable, consider it contaminated.

The arrangement of instruments, sponges, sutures, and other items on sterile tables should be determined by nursing personnel. Factors to be considered include the surgeon's method of working; ease in handling, preparing, and transporting items; and reduction in human energy. While a standardized setup may be more difficult to define and maintain, its use facilitates personnel assignment and the ability for one scrubbed person to easily substitute for another when procedures continue for an extended period of time.

Operating Room Environmental Cleaning

Contamination in the operating room can occur from various sources. The patient, healthcare workers, and inanimate objects are all capable of introducing potentially infectious material onto the surgical field. Techniques have been established to prevent some of the transmission of microorganisms into the surgical area, such as proper surgical attire and controlled traffic patterns in the surgical suite. During the surgical procedure, traffic within and through the room should be kept to a minimum to reduce air turbulence and to minimize human shedding. All doors in and out of the operating room should be kept closed to decrease air turbulence and the potential for contamination. High-efficiency particulate air filters (HEPA) placed between outside air processing and the operating room vents are used in some institutions. The HEPA filters are capable of screening out particles larger than 0.3 μm.

All surgical patients are potentially infected with bloodborne or other pathogens. For patient and personnel safety, cleaning procedures should be uniform throughout the operating room and for all patients. Using a uniform procedure designed to protect persons from visible or invisible contamination eliminates the need for special cleaning procedures for so-called dirty cases. Cleaning procedures should be carried out in a manner that protects both patients and personnel from exposure to potentially infectious microorganisms. Cleaning measures are needed before, during, and after surgical procedures and at the end of each day. Overall housekeeping procedures such as wall and ceiling washing should be done on a defined, regular basis.[11]

Before beginning the first procedure of the day, horizontal surfaces in the operating rooms should be dusted with a cloth dampened with a facility-approved disinfecting agent. Dust and lint deposited on horizontal surfaces during the night can become airborne vectors for organisms if not removed. During surgery, efforts should be made to confine contamination to as small an area as possible around the patient. Sponges should be discarded in plastic-lined containers. As they are counted, they should be contained in an impervious receptacle. The circulating nurse must use protective eyewear and gloves, instruments, or both when collecting and counting sponges or handling contaminated items. Spills should be cleaned up immediately with a broad-spectrum disinfectant or germicide. Specimens of blood or other potentially infectious tissue should be placed in a container that prevents leakage. The container must be color coded or labeled using the biohazard symbol (see Fig. 4-1). If the outside of the container becomes contaminated, the primary container must be placed within a second container that prevents leakage and is labeled or color coded. Some facilities use biohazard-labeled impervious bags to transport blood or other potentially infectious material.

Upon completion of the surgical procedure, soiled linens should be discarded in fluid-impervious bags, which eliminate potential contamination from wet linen soaking through to the outside of the bag. Contaminated items should be placed in leakproof, color-coded, or labeled containers. Sharps (needles, scalpels, electrosurgical tips, and so forth) are considered infectious and should be placed in special puncture-resistant containers. Bulk blood or suctioned fluid may be carefully poured down a drain connected to a sanitary sewer. Local and state environmental regulations may exist and should be consulted before establishing guidelines for waste disposal. Wall suction units should be disconnected to eliminate contamination of the wall outlet. Suction contents should be disposed of during the flushing of a hopper. Depending on local and state regulations, powder treatments of a chlorine compound are available to solidify liquid material before transport. This chemical may also be tuberculocidal, virucidal, and bactericidal. If used, glass suction containers should be rinsed and terminally sterilized with basins and trays. Suction tubing should be discarded; reusable suction tubing should be avoided because of difficulties in cleaning the lumen properly. Personnel should remove their gowns and gloves and place them in the proper receptacles before leaving the operating room. Instruments and supplies should be contained and taken to the decontamination area, where appropriately educated personnel wearing personal protective attire begin the instrument-decontamination process. Care should be taken to arrange sharp instruments in such a manner that personnel need not reach into basins where sharp instruments are unexposed and could cause injury. Equipment and furniture in the operating room should be cleaned with an EPA-approved disinfecting agent and the floor should be cleaned in a 3 to 4 foot perimeter around the operating bed and where visibly soiled.

Between surgical procedures the scrubbed person should place all instruments directly in wire meshed-bottom trays for processing in a washer-sterilizer. Basins, cups, and trays should also be washed and terminally sterilized. If a washer-sterilizer is not adjacent to the operating room, all these items should be contained for transportation to a central decontamination area, either in the surgical suite or in the central processing department, for terminal sterilization or high-level disinfection. The contaminated instruments should be handled as little as possible. Personnel should avoid reaching into containers to retrieve contaminated instruments.

At the end of each day's operative schedule, operating rooms and support areas should be cleaned by appropriately trained and supervised personnel. Areas to be cleaned include the following:

- Surgical lights and tracks
- Fixed and ceiling-mounted equipment
- Furniture and equipment including wheels
- Halls and floors
- Handles of cabinets and push plates
- Ventilation grills
- Horizontal surfaces
- Substerile areas
- Scrub and utility areas
- Scrub sinks

Refillable liquid soap dispensers should be disassembled and cleaned before being refilled because they can serve as reservoirs for microorganisms. At the conclusion of the housekeeping protocol, cleaning equipment and supplies should be properly cleaned, disinfected, and stored. If a wet vacuum has been used, it should be disassembled and thoroughly washed with a disinfectant before being stored.

SUMMARY

The practice of surgery has evolved over time and with it our knowledge of infection and infection control. This chapter has provided an overview of the causes of infection, including emerging drug-resistant bacteria, and identified a variety of methods to control infection in the perioperative environment. Use of Standard Precautions and Transmission-Based Precautions along with engineering and work-practice controls will assist perioperative practitioners in reducing the transmission of pathogenic organisms. Perioperative nursing practice is based on surgical aseptic principles. Careful adherence to these principles will support infection control in the perioperative arena. Each practitioner must be knowledgeable in aseptic principles and practices and must demonstrate the utmost integrity in application of this knowledge.

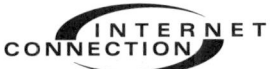

Association for Practitioners in Infection Control (APIC):
http://www.apic.org

National Library of Medicine:
http://www.nlm.nih.gov

Centers for Disease Control and Prevention:
http://www.cdc.gov

Outbreak (Emerging Diseases): http://www.outbreak.org

Microbial Underground:
http://www.lsumc.edu/campus/micr/mirror/public_html/index.html

American Society for Microbiology:
http://www.asmusa.org

Hepatitis B Foundation Home Page: http://www.hepb.org

American Public Health Association: http://www.apha.org

World Health Organization: http://www.who.ch/

HIV Information: http://www.hivpositive.com
http://www.caps.ucsf.edu/capsweb
http://www.thebody.com/
http://www.mlm.nlm.nih.gov/pnr/etc/aidspath.html
http://www.podi.com/aids

News Groups: AIDS treatment/pathology/prevention:
news:sci.med.aids

Association for the Advancement of Medical Instrumentation (AAMI): http://www.aami.org

Occupational Safety and Health Administration (OSHA):
http://www.osha.gov

REFERENCES

1. Agerton, T., Valaway, S., Gore, B., et al. (1997). Transmission of a highly resistant strain (strain WI) of *Mycobacterium tuberculosis*. *JAMA, 278,* 1073-1077.
2. American Health Consultants. (1997). Deadly strep may warrant post-exposure prophylaxis. In *Infection control sourcebook.* Atlanta: American Health Consultants.
3. American Institute of Architects Academy of Architecture for Health with assistance from the U.S. Department of Health and Human Services. (1996). *Guidelines for design and construction of hospital and health care facilities, 1996-97.* Washington, DC: American Institute of Architects.
4. Anderson, R.L., Carr, J.H., Bond, W.W., & Favaro, M.S. (1997). Susceptibility of vancomycin-resistant enterococci to environmental disinfectants. *Infection Control and Hospital Epidemiology, 18*(3), 195-199.
5. Association for the Advancement of Medical Instrumentation (AAMI). (1992). *Good hospital practice: ethylene oxide sterilization and sterility assurance.* Arlington, VA: the Association.
6. Association for the Advancement of Medical Instrumentation (AAMI). (1994). *Good hospital practice: steam sterilization and sterility assurance.* Arlington, VA: the Association.
7. Association for the Advancement of Medical Instrumentation (AAMI). (1995). *Dry heat (heated air) sterilizers.* Arlington, VA: the Association.
8. Association for the Advancement of Medical Instrumentation (AAMI). (1996). *Flash sterilization: steam sterilization of patient-care items for immediate use.* Arlington, VA: the Association.
9. Association for the Advancement of Medical Instrumentation (AAMI). (1997). *Packaging for terminally sterilized medical devices.* Arlington, VA: the Association.
10. Association of Operating Room Nurses (AORN). (1998). Recommended practices for the care and cleaning of instruments and powered

equipment. In *Standards, recommended practices and guidelines*. Denver, CO: the Association, pp. 237-242.

11. Association of Operating Room Nurses (AORN). (1998). Recommended practices for environmental cleaning in the surgical practice setting. In *Standards, recommended practices and guidelines*. Denver, CO: the Association, pp. 209-214.

12. Association of Operating Room Nurses (AORN). (1998). Recommended practices for selection and use of packaging systems. In *Standards, recommended practices and guidelines*. Denver, CO: the Association, pp. 253-258.

13. Association of Operating Room Nurses (AORN). (1998). Recommended practices for skin preparation of patients. In *Standards, recommended practices and guidelines*. Denver, CO: the Association, pp. 283-288.

14. Association of Operating Room Nurses (AORN). (1998). Recommended practices for sterilization in the practice setting. In *Standards, recommended practices and guidelines*. Denver, CO: the Association, pp. 295-306.

15. Association of Operating Room Nurses (AORN). (1998). Recommended practices for surgical attire. In *Standards, recommended practices and guidelines*. Denver, CO: the Association, pp. 159-164.

16. Association of Operating Room Nurses (AORN). (1998). Recommended practices for surgical hand scrubs. In *Standards, recommended practices and guidelines*. Denver, CO: the Association, pp. 225-230.

17. Association of Operating Room Nurses (AORN). (1998). Recommended practices for traffic patterns in the perioperative practice setting. In *Standards, recommended practices and guidelines*. Denver, CO: the Association, pp. 289-292.

18. Association of Operating Room Nurses (AORN). (1998). Recommended practices for use and care of endoscopes. In *Standards, recommended practices and guidelines*. Denver, CO: the Association, pp. 313-316.

19. Association of Operating Room Nurses (AORN). (1998). Recommended practices for use and selection of barrier materials for surgical gowns and drapes. In *Standards, recommended practices and guidelines*. Denver, CO: the Association, pp. 221-224.

20. Bond, W.W., Ott, B.J., Franke, K.A. & McCracken J.E. (1991). Effective use of liquid chemical germicides on medical devices: instrument design problems. In Block, S.S. (Ed.), *Disinfection, sterilization, and preservation* ed 4. Philadelphia: Lea & Febiger.

21. Boyce, J.M. (1998). Are the epidemiology and microbiology of methicillin-resistant *Staphylococcus aureus* changing? *JAMA, 279*, 623-624.

22. Bruning, L.M. (1993). The bloodborne pathogens final rule: understanding the regulation. *AORN Journal, 57*(2), 439-461.

23. Centers for Disease Control and Prevention. (1985). Recommendations for preventing transmission of infection with human T-lymphotropic virus type III/lymphadenopathy–associated virus during invasive procedures. *Morbidity and Mortality Weekly Report, 34*, 681-695.

24. Centers for Disease Control and Prevention. (1994). *Guidelines for preventing the transmission of* Mycobacterium tuberculosis *in health care facilities*. Atlanta.

25. Centers for Disease Control and Prevention. (1995). Recommendations for preventing the spread of vancomycin resistance: recommendations of the Hospital Infection Control Practices Advisory Committee (HICPAC). In *Morbidity and Mortality Weekly Report, 44*(RR-12), 1-13.

26. Centers for Disease Control and Prevention. (1996). Guideline for isolation precautions in hospitals. *Infection Control and Hospital Epidemiology, 17*(1), 53-80.

27. Centers for Disease Control and Prevention.(1997). *Staphylococcus aureus* with reduced susceptibility to vancomycin—United States, 1997. In *Morbidity and Mortality Weekly Report, 46*(33), 765-766.

28. Centers for Disease Control and Prevention, Hospital Infections Program, National Center for Infectious Diseases. (1997). *Creutzfeldt-Jakob disease: epidemiology, risk factors, and decontamination*. Atlanta.

29. Chen C.C. & Willeke, K. (1992). Aerosol penetration through surgical masks. *American Journal of Infection Control, 20*(4), 177-184.

30. Cohen, F.L. & Tartasky, D. (1997). Microbial resistance to drug therapy: a review. *American Journal of Infection Control, 25*(1), 51-64.

31. Cohen, M.L., Dorman, N.J., Kaufmann, C.A. & Thornsberry, C. (1997). Antimicrobial resistance: are the pathogens winning? In *Infection control sourcebook*. Atlanta: American Health Consultants.

32. Edel, E., Houston, S., & LaRocco, M. (1998). Impact of a 5-minute scrub on the microbial flora found on artificial, polished, or natural fingernails of operating room personnel. *Nursing Research, 47*, 54-58.

33. Elpern, E.H., & Girzadas, A.M. (1993). Tuberculosis update: new challenges of an old disease. *MEDSURG Nursing, 2*(3), 176-183.

34. Fogg, D.M. (1997). OR expansions; reuse of single-use devices; universal, standard, and transmission-based precautions. *AORN Journal, 65*(3), 636-639.

35. Grimes, D.E. (1991). *Infectious disease: clinical nursing series*. St. Louis: Mosby.

36. Health Agencies Update. (1998). *JAMA, 279*, 188.

37. Horan, T.C., Gaynes, R.P., Martone, W.J., & Emori, T.G. (1992). CDC definitions of nosocomial surgical site infections, 1992; a modification of CDC definitions of nosocomial surgical site infections. *American Journal of Infection Control, 20*(5), 271-274.

38. Jacobs, P.T. (1989). Plasma sterilization. *Journal of Healthcare Materials Management, 7*(5), 49.

39. Jacobs, P.T. (1993). *Sterrad sterilization system—a new technology for instrument sterilization*. (white paper) Arlington, TX: Johnson & Johnson Medical, Inc.

40. Joslyn, L.J. (1991). Sterilization by heat. In Block, S.S. (Ed.), *Disinfection, sterilization, and preservation* (ed. 4). Philadelphia: Lea & Febiger.

41. LaForce, F.M. (1993). The control of infections in hospitals: 1750-1950. In Wenzel, R.P. (Ed.), *Prevention and control of nosocomial infections* (ed. 2). Baltimore: Williams & Wilkins, pp. 1-12.

42. Lagergren, E. (1995). Gas plasma sterilization. *Surgical Services Management, 1*(2), 18-20.

43. Larson, E. (1989). Innovations in healthcare: antisepsis as a case study. *American Journal of Public Health, 79*(1), 92-99.

44. Laufman, H. (1981). *Hospital special-care facilities: planning for user needs*. New York: Academic Press.

45. Levy, S.B. (1993). Confronting multi-drug resistance: a role for all of us. *JAMA, 269*(14), 1840-1842.

46. Lynch, M.M. (1995). Gas plasma sterilization. *Surgical Services Management, 1*(2), 16-17.

47. Lyons, A.S., & Petrucelli, R.J. II. (1987). Infection. In *Medicine: an illustrated history*. New York: Harry N. Abrams, Inc.

48. Malangoni, M.A., & Hiram, C.P. (1989). Surgical infection, microbiology, and microbial agents. In *Scientific foundations of surgery* (ed. 4). St. Louis: Mosby.

49. Martin, M.A., & Reichelderfer, M. (1994). APIC guideline for infection prevention and control in flexible endoscopy. *American Journal of Infection Control, 22*(1), 19-38.

50. Mayhall, C.G. (1993). Surgical infections including burns. In Wenzel, R.P. (Ed.), *Prevention and control of nosocomial infections* (ed. 2). Baltimore: Williams & Wilkins, pp. 614-664.

51. McCormick, P.J., & Wilder, J.A. 1995). Gas plasma sterilization. *Surgical Services Management, 1*(2), 13-15.

52. Mitchell, N.J., & Hunt, S. (1991). Surgical face masks in modern operating rooms—a costly and unnecessary ritual? *Journal of Hospital Infection, 18*, 239-242.

53. Occupational Safety and Health Administration (OSHA). (1984). Occupational exposure to ethylene oxide, final standard. *Federal Register, 49*(122), 25737-25768.

54. Occupational Safety and Health Administration (OSHA). (1988). Occupational exposure to ethylene oxide, final standard. *Federal Register, 53*(66), 11414-11438.

55. Occupational Safety and Health Administration (OSHA). (1991). Occupational exposure to bloodborne pathogens: final rule. *Federal Register, 56* (235), 64175-64182.

56. O'Toole, M.T., (Ed.), (1997). *Miller-Keane encyclopedia and dictionary of medicine, nursing, and allied health* (ed. 6). Philadelphia: W.B. Saunders Co.

57. Ott, B.J., & Gostout, C.J. (1993). Endoscopic maintenance and repairs. *Gastrointestinal Endoscopy Clinics of North America, 3*, 559-569.

58. Perkins, J.J. (1969). *Principles and methods of sterilization in health sciences* (ed. 2). Springfield, IL: Charles C. Thomas.

59. Pottinger, M., Burns, S., & Manske, C. (1989). Bacterial carriage by artificial versus natural nails. *American Journal of Infection Control, 17,* 340-344.

60. Pugliese, G. & Favaro, M.S. (1997). First isolate of vancomycin-resistant *Staphylococcus aureus*—Japan. *Infection Control and Hospital Epidemiology, 18*(7), 527.

61. Rutala, W.A. (1990). APIC guideline for selection and use of disinfectants. *American Journal of Infection Control, 18*(2) 99-117.

62. Rutala, W.A. (1996). Disinfection and sterilization of patient-care items. *Infection Control and Hospital Epidemiology, 17*(6), 377-384.

63. Rutkow, I.M. (1993). *Surgery: an illustrated history.* St. Louis: Mosby.

64. Saurina, G., Landman, D., & Quale, J.M. (1997). Activity of disinfectants against vancomycin–resistant *Enterococcus faecium. Infection Control and Hospital Epidemiology, 18*(5), 345-347.

65. Schultz, J. K. (1993). Steam sterilization: recommended practices. In Reichert, M., & Young, J.H. (Eds.), *Sterilization technology for the health care facility.* Gaithersburg, MD: Aspen Publications, pp. 115-126.

66. Schultz, J.K. (1997). Steam sterilization: recommended practices. In Reichert, M., & Young, J.H. (Eds.), *Sterilization technology for the health care facility* (ed. 2). Gaithersburg, MD: Aspen Publications, pp. 146-154.

67. Sharbaugh, R.J. (1997). Decontamination: principles of disinfection. In Reichert, M., & Young, J.H. (Eds.), *Sterilization technology for the health care facility* (ed. 2). Gaithersburg, MD: Aspen Publications, pp. 21-28.

68. Shoup, A.J. (1997). Guidelines for the management of latex allergies and safe use of latex in the perioperative practice setting. *AORN Journal, 66*(4), 726-731.

69. Stedman, T.L. (1995). *Stedman's medical dictionary* (ed. 26). Baltimore: Williams & Wilkins.

70. Steelman, V.M. (1994). Creutzfeldt-Jakob disease: recommendations for infection control. *American Journal of Infection Control, 22*(5), 312-318.

71. Steris Corporation. (1995). Peracetic acid sterilization. *Surgical Services Management, 1*(2), 21-23.

72. Tunevall, T.G. (1991). Postoperative wound infections and surgical face masks: a controlled study. *World Journal of Surgery,* 15, 383-387.

73. Weber, D.J., Rutala, W.A. (1997). Role of environmental contamination in the transmission of vancomycin-resistant enterococci. *Infection Control and Hospital Epidemiology, 18*(5), 306-309.

74. Wetle, V.L. (1994). *Bloodborne pathogens: administrative manual for healthcare managers.* Boston: Jones & Bartlett.

75. Young, J.H. (1997). Steam sterilization: scientific principles. In Reichert, M., & Young, J.H. (Eds.), *Sterilization technology for the health care facility* (ed. 2). Gaithersburg, MD: Aspen Publications, pp. 124-133.

76. Young, M.L. (1997). Ethylene oxide sterilization: recommended practices. In Reichert, M., & Young, J.H. (Eds.), *Sterilization technology for the health care facility* (ed. 2). Gaithersburg, MD: Aspen Publications, pp. 209-219.

CHAPTER FIVE

Positioning the Patient for Surgery

Pauline Anne Heizenroth

PROPER PATIENT POSITIONING is essential for safe, successful surgical procedures. Perioperative nurses play a significant role in ensuring uncompromised and physiologically safe patient positioning by understanding the systems affected by positioning and their associated risks. Since surgery may be performed on all anatomic areas, the body may be positioned in multiple and sometimes unnatural configurations to expose a surgical site. Positioning, combined with anesthesia and its physiologic effects, can yield undesirable changes if safety factors are not considered. This chapter discusses some of the risks and prevention strategies associated with standard surgical positions.

The goals of surgical positioning include providing optimum exposure and access to the surgical site, maintaining body alignment, supporting circulatory and respiratory function, protecting neuromuscular and skin integrity, and allowing access to intravenous sites and anesthesia support devices. Meeting these goals while maintaining the patient's comfort and safety is the responsibility of every member of the surgical team.

SURGICAL ANATOMY

The perioperative nurse must thoroughly understand the anatomic and physiologic changes associated with anesthesia, positioning of the patient, and the operative procedure. These changes most frequently involve (1) the integumentary system, (2) the musculoskeletal system, (3) the nervous system, (4) the cardiovascular system, and (5) the respiratory system.

Integumentary System

The integumentary system can be injured by physical forces while establishing and maintaining a surgical position. Those forces include pressure, shear, friction, and maceration.

Pressure can be described as the force placed on underlying tissue by the weight of the body as gravity presses it downward toward the surface of the bed. Pressures above 32 mm Hg (capillary interface pressure) can occlude the flow of the arterioles, which nourish and oxygenate the tissue at the capillary level.[14] If such pressure

is prolonged, it can diminish tissue perfusion and thus result in tissue ischemia. The areas of the body where pressure tends to be greatest are those areas that are dependent and lie beneath a bony prominence. These areas differ depending on the position.

In surgery, the source of pressure is not always limited to the weight of the body by gravity. Pressure can also come from the weight of equipment resting on or against the patient such as drills, Mayo stands, surgical instruments, or operating room (OR) posts for self-retaining retractors. Positioning devices such as stirrup bars, leg or arm holders, and edges of laminectomy frames can rest against the patient under tension. Even surgical team members can lean on the patient and cause various degrees of pressure.

A pressure ulcer can be described as a disruption of normal tissue integrity resulting from the compression of the tissue between a bony prominence and a firm surface for a prolonged period of time. The longer the time of sustained pressure, the greater the risk of pressure ulcer development.

Pressure ulcers are staged according to the degree of observed tissue damage as follows:

- *Stage I.* Nonblanchable erythema of intact skin. In dark-skinned individuals, discoloration, warmth, edema, induration, or hardness may also be indicators.
- *Stage II.* Partial-thickness skin loss involving epidermis, dermis, or both. The ulcer is superficial and clinically presents as an abrasion, blister, or shallow crater.
- *Stage III.* Full-thickness skin loss involving damage or necrosis of subcutaneous tissue that may extend to but not through underlying fascia. These ulcers present as deep craters with or without undermining of adjacent tissue.
- *Stage IV.* Full-thickness skin loss with extensive destruction, tissue necrosis, or damage to muscle, bone, or supporting structures, such as tendon or joint capsule. Undermining and sinus tracts may also be associated with stage IV pressure ulcers.[2]

Stage I or stage II pressure ulcers may be evident immediately after surgery. These areas must be kept free from additional pressure for healing to occur and to keep them from advancing to higher stages. They are sometimes misidentified and thus treated inappropriately. Stage I pressure ulcers can look like normal reactive hyperemia, which generally fades on its own in one half to three fourths the time that the area was under pressure with little or no permanent tissue damage. Reactive hyperemia can be distinguished from a stage I pressure ulcer in that it blanches when compressed and released whereas stage I pressure ulcers are nonblanchable. The blistering that occurs in stage II pressure ulcers are sometimes misidentified as chemical or thermal burns. However, the lack of contact with a chemical or thermal agent in that area and its location under a bony prominence or near where a hard surface had been during surgery can help distinguish it as a pressure ulcer.

It is important to understand that full manifestation of pressure ulcers may be delayed by hours to days after the triggering injurious event. Since tissue damage extends from the bony prominence to the skin, when the deeper necrosis finally erupts to the skin level, what first appeared to be a stage I pressure ulcer, normal reactive hyperemia, or even noninjured skin, may well be a stage III or stage IV pressure ulcer. Lack of postoperative pressure relief can contribute to this advance. Because of the delayed manifestation, the connection may be overlooked that the surgical experience was the triggering event.

As little as 2 to 3 hours of unrelieved pressure on tissues can result in a pressure ulcer. The duration is considered more of a causative factor than the intensity of the pressure. Healthy individuals may tolerate high external pressures such as 100 mm Hg over bony prominences for short periods of time. Higher pressures over nonbony prominences may be tolerated for several hours (such as tourniquets). However, constant, unrelieved pressure is most responsible for microscopic necrosis.[13]

Frequent repositioning of an immobilized patient can protect against the adverse effects of pressure, friction, shear, and maceration. However, surgical procedures that extend beyond two hours may not afford the opportunity for repositioning the patient. The circulator should plan ahead to ensure that preventive measures are taken to reduce pressure ulcer risks. Pressure-relieving OR mattresses or overlays may reduce pressure in dependent areas. Padding applied over or around bony prominences or areas in contact with hard surfaces can reduce localized pressure.

Prolonged local pressure to the scalp during and after surgery can result in a localized postoperative alopecia. Symptoms develop within the first few days to a week postoperatively. Occipital scalp pain, swelling, exudate, crusting, or focal ulceration may precede the actual loss of hair. This is most commonly reported in cases that require prolonged intubation and head immobilization. In cardiac surgery, for instance, the anesthesia induction to extubation time may extend for a long period of time, sometimes even over 24 hours. The longer the time, the greater the risks are that the alopecia will be permanent.[7] Although less common, children undergoing cardiac surgery have also been affected.[6] Recommendations by researchers have been to reposition the patient's head every 30 minutes to reduce the potential for pressure-induced local alopecia (Research Highlight 5-1).

Donut-shaped head rests (ring cushions) are often used for head immobilization during surgery to the head and neck or for protecting the ear when the head is placed in a lateral position. Caution, however, should be taken in using them on a routine basis or for lengthy procedures. Ring cushions, in general, have been known to cause venous congestion and edema.[2] Although few studies have documented their deleterious effects, Crewe[8] determined that with at-risk patients, ring cushions were more likely to

5-1 RESEARCH HIGHLIGHT

Steinmetz and Langemo compared the tissue-interface pressures on the occiput of 25 volunteer patients undergoing coronary artery bypass graft surgery. Pressures were measured by a Gaymar pressure gauge and electropneumatic sensor at various intervals during the intraoperative period. Measurements were taken before and immediately after induction, during onset and conclusion of extracorporeal circulation, every 30 minutes throughout the procedure, and before incision closure. They found that the mean arterial pressures (MAPs) were highest at preinduction; however, all MAP readings were greater than 32 mm Hg, thus high enough to put the patient at risk for impaired occipital circulation and pressure sore development.

From Steinmetz, J.A., & Langemo, D.K. (1996). Changes in occipital capillary perfusion pressures during coronary artery bypass graft surgery, *Advances in Wound Care, 9*(3), 28-32.

cause pressure ulcers than prevent them. When used as a headrest, the weight of the portion of the head that sits inside the hole is supported by the portion of the head that rests on the edge of the inner donut circle causing higher pressures to that area. The weight of the head is more evenly distributed on a soft pillow or a contoured headrest with an induration rather than a hole in the center.

Intrinsic factors can lower a patient's pressure threshold and thus decrease the time and pressure required for tissue breakdown. These factors include respiratory and circulatory disorders, malnutrition (serum albumin levels <3.5 g/dl), advanced age, weight at 20 pounds above or below desirable weight for height and body build, chronic immobility, dehydration, anemia, and chronic emotional stress. Patients on steroids also have diminished tissue tolerance and delayed wound healing. Additionally, pre-existing chronic diseases such as diabetes mellitus also increase the risk of pressure sore development during surgery (Research Highlight 5-2).

Various scales exist for determining pressure sore potential such as the Braden scale,[1] Norton's scale,[16] and Hemphill's Guidelines for Assessment of Pressure Sore Potential.[11] These scales and guidelines score a patient's potential for pressure sore development based on various intrinsic factors. A scale such as the Braden scale (Table 5-1) could be used during the preoperative assessment to guide perioperative nursing interventions.

Shear forces also cause damage to tissue integrity. Shear can be described as the folding of underlying tissue when the skeletal structure moves while the skin remains stationary. This can happen when the head of the bed is raised or lowered and when the patient is placed in Trendelenburg's or reverse Trendelenburg's position.

Shear is created by a parallel force compared to pressure that is created by a perpendicular force. As gravity pulls the skeleton down, the stretching, folding, and tearing of the underlying tissues as they slide with the skeleton occlude vascular perfusion, which leads to tissue ischemia.

When a patient is placed in a shear-producing position before being prepped and draped, measures can be taken to reduce the shear forces. One technique would be to slightly lift the patient momentarily to allow the skin to realign with its surrounding skeletal structures. However, when the patient is placed in these positions during the middle of a surgical procedure, interventions to reduce shearing are limited. Reducing the time that shearing forces are in place is the biggest countermeasure to reduce tissue injury.

Friction is the force of two surfaces rubbing against one another. Friction on the patient's skin can occur when the body is dragged across bed linen instead of being lifted. Friction can denude the epidermis and make the skin more susceptible to higher stages of pressure sore formation as well as pain and infection.

Maceration can exacerbate the effects of pressure, shear, and friction. Maceration occurs when prolonged moisture on the skin saturates the epidermis to the point that it becomes weakened and more vulnerable to the detrimental effects of external forces. In surgery, maceration can occur through the patient perspiring or lying in a pool of prep solution, blood, irrigation, urine, or fecal incontinence. If this moisture is also located in an area of high pressure, the risk of pressure sore expansion into higher stages increases. If friction occurs to macerated skin, it becomes more vulnerable to denuding into the dermal layer. Every effort should be made to avoid pooling of prep solution. Prolonged exposure to the chemicals in the skin prep under the pressure area can also increase the likelihood of chemically induced contact dermatitis.

5-2 RESEARCH HIGHLIGHT

Two research studies focused on pressure sore development in cardiac surgery. Papantonio et al. studied 136 patients undergoing cardiac surgery at The Johns Hopkins Hospital. Significant factors for sacral pressure sore development included diabetes mellitus as well as other preexisting comorbid conditions such as respiratory disease, low hematocrit (in males) and serum albumin levels, transfers from other hospitals (representing poor overall health), longer OR times, and advanced age. They found that patients 60 to 69 years of age had a 2.5-fold greater likelihood of developing pressure sores compared to patients under 60. Patients 70 and older had a 5.3-fold increased likelihood compared to those under 60.

Lewicki et al. studied 337 patients undergoing cardiac surgery at the Cleveland Clinic Foundation to determine significant factors associated with pressure sores of the scapula, sacrum, and heels. Significant factors in their study, which also supported the previous study, included diabetes mellitus and other comorbid conditions as well as low hematocrit and serum albumin levels. Additional significant fators included low preoperative Braden Risk Assessment Scale scores, low hemoglobin, presence of postoperative intraaortic balloon pumps (contributing to immobility), less frequent turning, and more rapid returns to preoperative body temperatures. In both studies, extracorporeal circulation times were not a significant factor.

The findings of these studies support the importance of assessing risk factors such as age, significant lab values, and preexisting comorbid conditions, particularly diabetes mellitus. They also support the need for vigilance in postoperative mobilization and turning.

From Papantonio, C.T., Wallop, J.M., & Kolodner, K.B. (1994). Sacral ulcers following cardiac surgery: incidences and risks, *Advances in Wound Care,* 7(2), 24-36.
From Lewicki, L.J., Mion, L., Splane, K.G., Samstag, D., & Secic, M. (1997). Patient risk factors for pressure ulcers during cardiac surgery, *AORN Journal,* 65, 933-942.

TABLE 5-1 | **Braden Scale for Predicting Pressure Sore Risk**

SCORES	1	2	3	4
Sensory Perception Ability to respond meaningfully to pressure-related discomfort	**Completely Limited:** Unresponsive (does not moan, flinch, or grasp) to painful stimuli, due to diminished level of consciousness or sedation, OR limited ability to feel pain over most of body surface.	**Very Limited:** Responds only to painful stimuli. Cannot communicate discomfort except by moaning or restlessness, OR has a sensory impairment which limits the ability to feel pain or discomfort over ½ of body.	**Slightly Limited:** Responds to verbal commands but cannot always communicate discomfort or need to be turned, OR has some sensory impairment which limits ability to feel pain or discomfort in 1 or 2 extremities.	**No Impairment:** Responds to verbal commands. Has no sensory deficit which would limit ability to feel or voice pain or discomfort.
Moisture Degree to which skin is exposed to moisture	**Constantly Moist:** Skin is kept moist almost constantly by perspiration, urine, etc. Dampness is detected every time patient is moved or turned.	**Moist:** Skin is often but not always moist. Linen must be changed at least once a shift.	**Occasionally Moist:** Skin is occasionally moist, requiring an extra linen change approximately once a day.	**Rarely Moist:** Skin is usually dry; linen requires changing only at routine intervals.
Activity Degree of physical activity	**Bedfast:** Confined to bed.	**Chairfast:** Ability to walk severely limited or nonexistent. Cannot bear own weight and/or must be assisted into chair or wheel chair.	**Walks Occasionally:** Walks occasionally during day but for very short distances, with or without assistance. Spends majority of each shift in bed or chair.	**Walks Frequently:** Walks outside the room at least twice a day and inside room at least once every 2 hours during waking hours.
Mobility Ability to change and control body position	**Completely Immobile:** Does not make even slight changes in body or extremity position without assistance.	**Very Limited:** Makes occasional slight changes in body or extremity position but unable to make frequent or significant changes independently.	**Slightly Limited:** Makes frequent though slight changes in body or extremity position independently.	**No Limitations:** Makes major and frequent changes in position without assistance.

Musculoskeletal System

The musculoskeletal system of the patient may be subjected to unusual stress during operative positioning. Normal range of motion is maintained in the alert patient by pain and pressure receptors that warn against overstretching and twisting of ligaments, tendons, and muscles. The tone of opposing muscle groups also acts to prevent strain and stress to the muscle fibers. When pharmacologic agents such as anesthetics and muscle relaxants depress the pain and pressure receptors and muscle tone, the normal defense mechanisms cannot guard against joint damage and muscle stretch and strain. Obvious resistance to unusual range of motion is often noted only in patients whose arthritic changes prevent even slight exaggeration of the position.

Nervous System

Nervous system depression accompanies the administration of anesthetic agents and many other drugs. The degree of depression depends on the type of regional anesthesia or the level of general anesthesia. Pain and pressure receptors may be affected either regionally or systemically. The most important factor for the perioperative nurse to remember is that when nervous system depression occurs, the body's communication and command system becomes totally or partially ineffective. Compensatory reactions to changes in the physical status no longer respond normally. Lifesaving, physiologic adaptive mechanisms are altered. The stresses of operative positioning are not automatically compensated.

Pressure on superficial nerves can cause temporary or permanent nerve damage resulting in impaired sensory or motor function. Damage is not usually discovered until the patient reaches the postanesthesia care unit (PACU). Sometimes there is a delayed onset of symptoms in which the injury does not manifest itself until days or weeks after the suspected insult. This can lead to some confusion as to whether the injury actually occurred during surgery or convalescence.

The most commonly reported nerve injuries involve

TABLE 5-1 | **Braden Scale for Predicting Pressure Sore Risk—cont'd**

SCORES	1	2	3	4
Nutrition Usual food intake pattern	**Very Poor:** Never eats a complete meal. Rarely eats more than ⅓ of any food offered. Eats 2 servings or less of protein (meat or dairy products) per day. Takes fluids poorly. Does not take a liquid dietary supplement, OR is NPO and/or maintained on clear liquids or IV for more than 5 days.	**Probably Inadequate:** Rarely eats a complete meal and generally eats only about ½ of any food offered. Protein intake includes only 3 servings of meat or dairy products per day. Occasionally will take a dietary supplement, OR receives less than optimum amount of liquid diet or tube feeding.	**Adequate:** Eats over half of most meals. Eats a total of 4 servings of protein (meat, dairy products) each day. Occasionally will refuse a meal, but will usually take a supplement if offered, OR is on a tube feeding or total parenteral nutrition (TPN) regimen, which probably meets most of nutritional needs.	**Excellent:** Eats most of every meal. Never refuses a meal. Usually eats a total of 4 or more servings of meat and dairy products. Occasionally eats between meals. Does not require supplementation.
Friction and Shear	**Problem:** Requires moderate to maximum assistance in moving. Complete lifting without sliding against sheets is impossible. Frequently slides down in bed or chair, requiring frequent repositioning with maximum assistance. Spasticity contractures, or agitation leads to almost constant friction.	**Potential Problem:** Moves feebly or requires minimum assistance. During a move skin probably slides to some extent against sheets, chair, restraints, or other devices. Maintains relatively good position in chair or bed most of the time but occasionally slides down.	**No Apparent Problem:** Moves in bed and in chair independently and has sufficient muscle strength to lift up completely during move. Maintains good position in bed or chair at all times.	

Source: Barbara Braden and Nancy Bergstrom. Copyright 1988. Used with permission.   Total Score _____

If, during preoperative assessment, the patient's score is <20, that patient is at risk for skin breakdown. The perioperative nurse should do the following:

- Prior to positioning, assess skin for evidence of diminished tissue integrity, particularly in areas over bony prominences.
- Pad and protect any fragile skin areas and limit the amount of time these areas are under pressure to the extent possible.
- Pad under and/or around all areas in contact with a firm surface.
- Reassess skin postoperatively. Document findings and communicate any changes to appropriate personnel.

If, during the preoperative assessment, the patient has a score <16, a Stage III or IV pressure ulcer, multiple areas of skin breakdown above knees and over bony prominences, or has had muscle flap surgery, the perioperative nurse should *additionally* do the following:

- Support and protect all existing wound dressings.
- Arrange for the patient to be placed on a specialty bed designed for extreme pressure reduction postoperatively (i.e., alternating air mattress, flotation support bed, etc).

the ulnar nerve, the brachial plexus, the lumbosacral nerve roots, and lower extremity nerves.[3]

The ulnar nerve is a peripheral nerve that passes from the upper arm through the groove of the medial epicondyle of the humerus to the lower arm. Its superficial location as it passes through the condylar groove makes it vulnerable to injury. Ulnar injury can occur from compression close to the elbow region and results in a clawing of the ring and distal fingers.

It is important to remember that certain patients are more vulnerable than others to compression injuries to peripheral nerves. These include patients with diabetes mellitus, cancer, alcoholism, and vitamin deficiencies.

Predisposition specific to ulnar nerve injuries exists in patients whose occupational or personal habits require repeated bending of the elbow. Additionally, there is a 5:1 predominance of ulnar nerve injuries in male versus female patients. This is probably attributable to a more shallow medial epicondylar groove in the male humerus than that in the female.[3]

The brachial plexus is a network of nerves that run beneath the clavicle and down the upper arm. The nerve branches include the ulnar, median, radial, musculocutaneous, and axillary nerves. They innervate the lower part of the shoulder and all of the arm. When the arm is extended on an armboard in excess of a 90-degree angle from the body, the brachial plexus may be stretched and compressed between the clavicle and the first rib. If the head and neck are turned in an opposite direction from the extended arm, even more pressure is exerted so that compression may occur at less than 90 degrees. Distal branches of the nerves can be compressed by tight arm or wrist straps or by resting against the mattress edge or metal frame of the OR bed. Numbness and palsies may affect the entire arm, wrist, and hand.

The most likely cause of brachial plexus injury in cardiac surgery patients, however, is sternal separation and retraction from a medial sternotomy. It may be manifested as an isolated ulnar nerve palsy. In such cases, injury is generally not preventable by padding and positioning techniques.[3]

Potential for nerve injury can also occur in the lumbosacral nerve roots. Long duration of surgery with the patient in lithotomy position can stretch the femoral and lateral cutaneous femoral nerves causing sensory deficit of the anterior thigh and weakness of the quadriceps muscle. Distal lower extremity nerves may also be at risk depending on the type of stirrups used and the associated areas of compression. This is further discussed in the lithotomy section of this chapter.

Vascular System

The vascular system is affected by anesthesia and changes in position. These effects become more dramatic in patients with cardiovascular disease, hypovolemia, or obesity.

General anesthesia causes peripheral vessels to dilate by depressing the sympathetic nervous system. This dilatation causes an overall drop in blood pressure by the pooling of blood in dependent areas of the body. In general anesthesia, these effects are systemic, whereas in regional anesthesia, such as spinals and epidurals, these effects are more limited to the areas anesthetized.

Position changes affect where the pooling of blood occurs. Muscle tone and peripheral vascular resistance are no longer effective in counteracting the forces of gravity on blood pooling. Blood pooling will shift to whatever part of the body is lowest. If the head of the OR table is raised, the lower torso will have increased blood volume and the upper torso will become more compensated. Hypovolemia and cardiovascular disease can further compromise the patient's status.

The anesthesia provider can treat some of the hypotensive effects of positioning through pharmacologic agents and increased intravenous infusion. Vital signs, intravenous intake, and urinary output need to be closely monitored. Position changes may need to be delayed until the blood pressure is stabilized.

Compression to peripheral vessels can occur from the safety strap or wrist restraints being secured too tightly. Such compression can predispose the patient to venous thrombosis. Thrombosis is also a risk of hyperabduction of

the arms beyond 90 degrees. Subclavian and axillary vessels align the brachial plexus so that vessel constriction can occur by compression between the clavicle and the first rib. Radial pulses need to be checked whenever arms are extended to be sure the radial pulse is not obliterated.

Respiratory System

The respiratory system can be compromised during positioning. Movement of the diaphragm may be impeded by abdominal viscera, adversely affecting pulmonary function. Obese patients, pregnant patients, and patients with respiratory insufficiency may have difficulty breathing when lying supine. Any patient who experiences dyspnea should be propped on pillows or have the head of the bed elevated during local, regional, or spinal anesthesia if this does not interfere with surgical access. During general anesthesia, these patients are generally given mechanical ventilation by the anesthesia provider.

The portions of the lung that are perfused with blood are also affected by position. As blood is pumped into the lungs, some of the pulmonary arterial pressure is dissipated in overcoming gravity. This means that the areas of the lung that are most dependent have a greater pulmonary arterial pressure. The greater the pressure, the greater the perfusion. The alveoli in the bases of the lungs are more compliant; thus ventilation is generally highest in those areas. An even distribution of ventilation and perfusion (ventilation-perfusion ratio) is needed for efficient gas exchange.[9]

If the position causes a pathologically compromised area of the lung to be dominant and therefore most perfused, the balance between perfusion and ventilation may be disrupted and respiratory status diminished. The rest of the lung fields may or may not have the capacity to compensate. Oxygen therapy or mechanical ventilation can help compensate, but the amount of time a patient can tolerate a certain position and maintain adequate gas exchange may be limited.

Monitoring of respiratory status should always include pulse oximetry. In some cases, intraoperative arterial blood gas monitoring may be necessary.

PERIOPERATIVE NURSING CONSIDERATIONS

Assessment

The perioperative assessment includes a patient interview, physical examination, and review of medical records. Key points of assessment that are related to surgical positioning include age; weight; height; general health status; activity level; mobility restrictions; skin condition (especially at positional pressure points); respiratory, circulatory, and neurologic status; and presence of implants such as total joints.[4] It should also be determined if there are any particular areas of discomfort that may be affected by a particular position and what interventions might alleviate or reduce that discomfort.[18]

The assessment should also alert the perioperative nurse to patients and situations that could contribute to problems caused by positioning. Vulnerable patients include the following:

- Geriatric patients, whose thin skin layer and increased arteriosclerosis make them more prone to skin breakdown because of pressure.
- Pediatric patients, whose size and weight must be taken into consideration when selecting positioning aids.
- Patients who are malnourished, anemic, obese, hypovolemic, paralyzed, arteriosclerotic, or diabetic, or receiving steroid therapy, because they are more prone to skin breakdown caused by pressure.
- Patients with limitations to mobility through congenital anomalies, preexisting injuries, arthritis, or prosthetic implants who need special considerations during positioning.
- Patients with edema, infection, cancer, or conditions of lowered cardiac or respiratory reserves who have poor general health, making them vulnerable to tissue injury.
- Patients with demineralizing bone conditions, such as malignant metastasis or osteoporosis, which puts the patient at higher risk for skeletal fractures.

Vulnerable situations include the following:

- Lengthy surgical procedures (2 hours or greater).
- Vascular surgery, because optimal blood perfusion may already be compromised as a result of the patient's disease process.
- Excessive sustained pressure to certain body areas because of the surgical procedure or retraction.

Nursing Diagnosis

The general nursing diagnosis for the patient undergoing surgical positioning is the high risk for injury related to positioning. Specific nursing diagnoses might include the following:

- Risk for impaired skin or tissue integrity
- Impaired gas exchange
- Decreased cardiac output
- Impaired physical mobility
- Risk for peripheral sensory alterations

Outcome Identification

The general outcome identified for the nursing diagnosis concerned with patient positioning is that the patient will be free from injury related to positioning. Specific outcomes identified for related nursing diagnoses include the following:

- The patient will maintain normal skin and tissue integrity.
- The patient will maintain adequate gas exchange.

- The patient will not sustain significantly altered cardiovascular status.
- The patient will maintain normal physical mobility.
- The patient will maintain normal peripheral sensory integrity.

Planning

The perioperative nurse needs to plan activities that will protect the patient from injury and provide physiologic support and comfort while allowing for optimal exposure and access to the surgical site. Although carrying out safe surgical positioning involves all members of the surgical team, the circulating nurse plans and coordinates this teamwork.

Knowledge of any preexisting risk factors that may affect positioning strategies (such as obesity, diabetes, paralysis, advanced age) should be taken into account when planning additional staff assistance during positioning as well as support devices or padding.

It is imperative that the exact location of the operative site be identified so that access to that site is not obstructed. If a secondary surgical procedure is involved, such as a graft donor site, that area needs to be exposed and accessible as well. There are times when all the anticipated sites of incision may not be able to be exposed during initial positioning. Plans need to be made for repositioning an anesthetized patient (such as assisting personnel, additional padding devices, and additional sterile drapes) so that repositioning occurs quickly and smoothly without unnecessarily prolonged anesthesia time.

Planning for physiologic support involves collaborating with the anesthesia provider. Sometimes chest rolls are needed for adequate lung expansion while the patient is in prone position. Supports and padding for the head, arms, hands, and axilla should be anticipated and easily accessible.

Planning for the patient's comfort can involve communicating with the patient as to potential areas for discomfort and possible remedies. The awake patient receiving local anesthesia can give feedback on the comfort of the position before, during, and immediately after the procedure. In some cases, all or part of the positioning for an anesthetized patient can be done before the patient is induced if it doesn't interfere with the anesthesia process. For example, a patient could be placed in lithotomy position before induction if he or she has a history of discomfort with leg abduction or lower back pain. If this is done, privacy must be assured by covering the patient with a sheet or blanket and covering or pulling the blinds on room windows.

A Sample Care Plan for the patient undergoing surgical positioning is shown on p. 160.

Implementation

The nursing actions involved in positioning should reflect the individualized care plan, which is designed to

SAMPLE CARE PLAN

Nursing Diagnosis: Risk for injury related to surgical positioning

Outcome: The patient will be free from injury related to surgical positioning

Interventions:

1. Identify surgical sites and determine appropriate position.
2. Identify and document specific risk factors that may predispose patient to position-related injuries.
3. Identify areas of potential discomfort and possible remedies.
4. Check OR bed for proper functioning and availability of all needed attachments.
5. Obtain any needed positioning aids and padding materials.
6. Assure a safe transfer from transport vehicle to OR bed and document mode of transfer.
7. Provide the patient with warmth, privacy, and reassurance.
8. Safely secure the patient to the OR bed.
9. If the patient is repositioned after being anesthetized, support all body parts and maintain body alignment throughout the move.
10. Use slow, smooth movements in making all position changes, utilizing a team approach.
11. Avoid pulling or dragging the patient; utilize lifting techniques instead.
12. Monitor physiologic effects of position changes and be prepared to intervene when necessary.
13. Pad bony prominences and all areas in contact with a solid surface.
14. Protect anatomic areas containing superficial vessels and nerves.
15. Assure access to airway, intravenous catheters, and monitoring devices to the highest degree possible.
16. Prevent pooling of fluids under dependent areas or any area under pressure.
17. Document in detail patient position, including:
    - Position of extremities
    - Type and location of restraints, positioning aids, and padding materials
    - Site of electrosurgical dispersive pad
    - Use and location of warming or cooling blankets or devices
    - Positional changes made during procedure (such as supine to lithotomy to supine)
    - Adverse physiologic responses to position or positions and interventions taken
18. If the patient needs to be repositioned back into supine position at the completion of the procedure, do so slowly and smoothly, supporting body alignment and monitoring physiologic responses.
19. Visually inspect skin for any changes, particularly at areas under pressure; document and communicate any changes.
20. Document method of transfer at time of discharge.

---

assure injury prevention while maintaining optimal surgical access, patient comfort, and physiologic support. Patients who are vulnerable to problems related to positioning (as identified during assessment) need to have their potential for problems documented, which could include data such as mobility limitations or presence of external or internal prostheses.

Patient comfort measures need to include both physical and emotional aspects. Direct communication with the patient regarding his or her positioning concerns can help to reassure the patient as well as provide the nurse with insight into possible comfort strategies. Providing the patient warmth and privacy can help the patient feel more comfortable and relaxed as well as feel respected and cared for.

The OR bed should be positioned in the room in such a way that OR bed relocation after the patient is anesthetized is kept to a minimum. During transfer, the OR bed and transport vehicle should be next to each other and locked. At least one person should stand on either side to assist the patient in the transfer. If the patient is unable to

assist in the transfer, a four-person lift should be done using a draw sheet and securing the head and feet.

Once the patient is on the OR bed the safety strap is placed 2 inches above the knees. The strap should be snug but not so tight as to place pressure on nerves or restrict venous return. One should be able to comfortably slide two fingers beneath the strap. The patient's ankles must not be crossed because vessel and nerve constriction and skin pressure could result. The patient should be reminded of this because many patients automatically cross their ankles while lying down.

Someone should always be directly at the patient's bed. The patient may not appreciate the narrowness of the OR bed and may inadvertently attempt to adjust his or her position and be at risk for a fall or injury.

Assemble all necessary positioning aids such as padding, pillows, bed accessories, and stirrups before the patient's induction because the patient is generally positioned immediately after anesthesia is administered. Make sure extra staff members are available if needed for lifting or turning the patient.

Movement of the patient should be slow and smooth, assuring that the whole body is supported during movements. Quick, jerky movements can cause musculoskeletal injury as well as putting the patient at risk for bruises, pinches, abrasions, fractures, or falls. Any lateral, anterior, or posterior movement of the patient on the OR bed should be done by lifting the patient with the draw sheet rather than by pulling or dragging the patient.

Once the desired position is obtained the patient should be secured so that movement off the OR bed cannot occur from any direction. Safety straps and other support accessories should be checked for pressure against the patient, particularly in areas adjacent to bony prominences. Padding or adjustment needs to be done at this point because it is the last opportunity to do so before prepping and draping are done. Additionally, consider how the position may cause certain body parts to sustain more gravitational weight. For example, if the knees are elevated by a pillow, the heels bear additional weight from the calves. Heel padding may be needed to help dissipate this additional pressure.

After the surgical procedure is completed, all pressure sites, especially those under bony prominences, should be checked before transfer to the PACU. Any changes in the skin integrity should be documented and orally reported immediately so that appropriate interventions can occur right away to reduce further injury.

The mode of transfer, time of discharge, and patient status upon discharge need to be documented.

Evaluation

Actions, observations, and patient responses to treatment should be clearly documented to enable nurses to evaluate and measure the outcomes of the care processes.[18] The evaluation of the nursing care plan should be ongoing during the procedure and conclude with a written and verbal report to the PACU nurse. The outcome of successful implementation of the care plan may be documented as follows:

The patient is free from injury related to positioning, as evidenced by the following:

- No erythema or changes in skin integrity, particularly at bony prominences and pressure areas.
- No patient complaints of strained muscles or ligaments, altered range of motion, or compressed or injured nerves postoperatively
- Circulation in extremities consistent with preoperative status
- No adverse change in hemodynamics related to positioning

Any abnormalities should be documented on the postoperative assessment and reported to the surgeon and the PACU nurse.

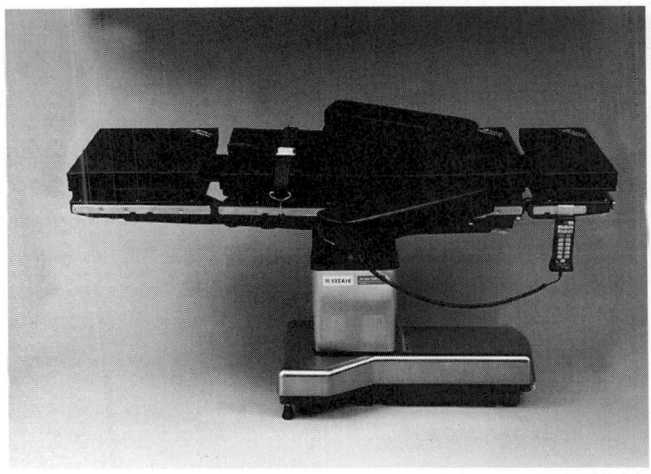

FIGURE 5-1 Surgical OR bed adaptable to a wide range of surgical procedures.

OPERATING ROOM BEDS

Modern operating room beds are designed to support and accommodate the various anatomic configurations required in surgical positioning. Their height can be raised or lowered, they can tilt laterally, and they can be placed in the Trendelenburg's or reverse Trendelenburg's position. They are electrically or battery operated with a manual backup. They have roller wheels, which allow them to be easily moved, and brakes that can lock them in place.

General operating room beds are composed of a flat platform divided into three major sections: the head, body, and foot sections (Fig. 5-1). Each section has a corresponding removable mattress, which usually attaches to the main platform by Velcro or straps. The area between each section is called a *break*. Raising or lowering sections is called *breaking the bed*.

Along the edges of the bed are flat metal side rails that separate at each break and run horizontally along both sides of the entire OR bed. Armboards lock directly onto the side rails at any level of the OR bed. The side rails also accommodate sockets, triclamps, and locks that can secure a multitude of attachments including stirrups, ether screens, elevated armrests, and various retractors.

The OR bed width is narrow to allow ease of access to the operative site. For some patients, this width may not be enough to adequately support their whole body. Armboards can be secured parallel to the OR bed at the waist and hip levels to give additional lateral support to such patients.

Underneath the OR bed platform is a tunnel that runs under the entire body and leg sections to support X-ray cassettes. Additionally, in newer models, the entire OR bed platform is radiopaque to accommodate the use of intraoperative radiologic fluoroscopy.

The body section is attached to the base of the OR bed, since this section supports the heaviest parts of the body: the chest, abdomen, and pelvis. This section also has a break in the center at the hip level that can be flexed or lowered to allow the head and chest areas to be elevated or lowered. At this central break in the body section, there is a crossbar, called a *kidney bridge* (body elevator), that can be raised or lowered for kidney or gallbladder exposure. The kidney bridge is concave and can accommodate lateral braces that slide vertically onto the bridge to maintain the patient in a lateral position. The posterior portion of the body section's platform and mattress have concave cutouts to accommodate access to the perineum when the patient is in lithotomy position.

The head section of the OR bed can be flexed, lowered, or removed. It is connected to the bed by two horizontal posts that fit into corresponding grooves in the front of the body section. Special headrests such as a craniotomy or ophthalmic headrest can slide into these grooves to be used for special procedures.

The leg section of the OR bed can be flexed or lowered to the extent that it folds deeply beneath the lumbar section to allow leg room for a sitting surgeon to gain access to the perineal area when the patient is in lithotomy position. The leg section also has grooves in the distalmost platform to accommodate a footboard for tall patients. The footboard can be flexed to give plantar support if needed. The distal grooves also accommodate the head section in case the patient is to be positioned with the head where the feet usually are. Such positioning allows for movement of C-arm radiologic fluroscopy around the patient's chest and abdomen, since the leg section protrudes farther away from the base than the head section does. Another use for placing the head section at the foot of the OR bed would be to enable the patient to be positioned with the buttocks in the perineal cutout immediately upon transfer to the OR bed. This extends the leg section so that the patient's legs do not hang over the end of the bed and eliminates the need for the patient to be moved down on the bed after induction. This reduces the shearing and friction risks of such a move.

OR mattresses should meet certain basic characteristic requirements. They should be durable, versatile to many intended uses, nonflammable, resistant to bacterial growth, radiolucent with low X-ray attenuation, compatible with warming and cooling devices, be covered with nonallergic antistatic fabric, and have pressure-reduction capabilities.

Durability can lead to increased longevity and thus cost efficiency. The cover should be made of durable but pliable material that is easily washed and resistant to deterioration from various prep solutions and chemical cleaning agents. The covering material should be resistant to the effects of heat from warming blankets and reduce friction and shear. Covers should also be waterproof, and seams and zippers should be water resistant to inhibit entry of solutions into the core of the mattress. The mattress core should also be resistant to both fungal and bacterial growth.

Mattress pad versatility can be evaluated by its ability to easily flex and extend with its accompanying OR bed

platform. The more lightweight it is, the easier it is to remove and shift placement of the pads. Some pads must be stored horizontally because of gel components. This could be a disadvantage if storage space is limited.

Pressure reduction is a prime consideration in OR mattress pads. With more attention being placed on optimal pressure relief, manufacturers are improving OR mattresses to be more protective of tissue integrity. Numerous products are now claiming to reduce the risk of pressure sore development in the OR. Some of the OR mattress materials on the market include solid foam (single or dual layered), segmented foam, combination foam and gel, mattresses with adjustable individual air cells, dry polymer mattress overlays, and static pressure relief surfaces. Since OR mattress compositions vary widely, it is difficult to know which products provide the best results, especially in reducing pressure. It is helpful to refer to studies (preferably by independent researchers) that compare the pressure-reducing features of various products (Research Highlight 5-3). The more recent the study and the more types of products compared, the more helpful the study is as products change and improve continuously.

One pressure-reduction feature is resistance to bottoming out or compacting under the body's weight. This diminishes the cushioning effects between the body and the supporting platform. Generally, the thinner the foam, the easier it is to bottom out.

Another feature is a low measure of interface pressure between the skin and the support platform, particularly under bony prominences. Mattress companies or independent researchers may use interface pressure-monitoring instruments to measure and compare products. The interface pressure can be measured under selected sites by

---

5-3 RESEARCH HIGHLIGHT

Hoshowsky and Schramm studied the relationship between the skin integrity of 505 patients and three OR bed surfaces. These included a standard vinyl-covered 2-inch-thick foam OR bed mattress (SFM), a nylon fabric–covered 2-inch-thick foam and gel OR bed mattress (FGM), and a viscoelastic dry polymer mattress overlay (VEO).

Results of the study showed that skin changes were more likely with an SFM. The VEO was more effective than the SFM or FGM for preventing pressure sore formation. Other factors predictive of pressure sore development included surgery longer than 2.5 hours, age over 40 years, vascular disease, and a high value on a Hemphill scale.

From Hoshowsky, V.M., & Schramm, C.A. (1994). Intraoperative pressure sore prevention: an analysis of bedding materials, *Research in Nursing and Health, 17,* 333-339.

electropneumatic sensors that can convert pressures to mm Hg. Since capillary interface pressure is about 32 mm Hg, the lower the interface pressure sustained by the mattress, the better.

Another type of instrument used to show relative interface pressures is a table in which a computerized image of the table shows as a color-coded scan. The entire surface of the body in contact with the mattress on this table will display various colors ranging from light to dark. The darker the color, the higher the pressure. It can locate areas of highest pressure for selected positions and provide a comparative pressure analysis between different products.

It is important to remember that whatever pressure-reducing properties exist in a mattress these properties can be reduced by a stiff outer covering. Soft nylon coverings may support pressure reduction better than the firmer vinyl coverings of standard OR mattresses.[12] Additionally, the overuse of bedding materials can contribute to increased interface pressures. The more the layers of sheets, absorbent pads, or blankets placed between the patient and the mattress, the more resistance there is to the pliability and thus effectiveness of the padding material. Bedding should be kept to a minimum. With some products, like certain dry polymer overlays, bedding should not be used at all. Check with the manufacturer.

Since the OR bed and accessory devices can accommodate the majority of types of surgical positioning needs, only a few specialty surgical beds are needed. The orthopedic fracture table (Fig. 5-2) has multiple movable and removable parts and suspended frames. However, special orthopedic extensions and accessories that duplicate the functions of the features on traditional orthopedic fracture tables are available for some OR beds. Although urologic procedures can also be done on a general OR bed set up in lithotomy position, specialty urology beds are still a beneficial asset to the OR because they have built-in drainage trays and radiologic equipment.

STANDARD SURGICAL POSITIONS

Supine

The supine (dorsal recumbent) position is the most common. The patient lies with the back flat on the OR bed. The arms may be tucked at the side or placed on armboards. It is the most natural position of the body at rest and is the position in which the patient is usually anesthetized.

The supine position allows access to the major body cavities (peritoneal, thoracic, pericardial). It also allows access to the head, neck, and extremities. Vulnerable pressure areas in the supine position are the occiput, scapula, olecranon, sacrum, coccyx, and calcaneus (Fig. 5-3).

A safety strap should be placed 2 inches above the knees. A sheet or blanket should always be placed between the safety strap and the patient's skin. If the knees are to be flexed, caution should be taken in placing a pillow directly under the patient's knees. The popliteal artery, common peroneal nerve, and tibial nerve all run superficially through the popliteal space. Compression of these structures between a pillow and the safety strap could theoretically cause nerve damage, impaired circulation, and possibly venous thrombosis. Although there is no evidence that such injury has been reported, using a soft pillow under the knees and assuring that the safety strap is not too tight or placing the pillow proximal to the popliteal space will reduce the likelihood of such an occurrence.

The head generally rests on a small pillow or head cushion to support cervical alignment, reduce occipital pressure, and reduce strain on neck muscles. The eyes must be protected from textiles, solutions, and other foreign objects by applying eye patches, eye shields, or taping the eyes closed.

If the arms are placed on armboards, the armboards should be padded with the pad level equal to that of the OR bed. Extension should be less than a 90-degree angle to prevent stretching and compression of the brachial plexus. Wrist restraints should be soft and nonocclusive. The rotational position of the hand on an armboard is controversial. Supination (palms up) theoretically protects

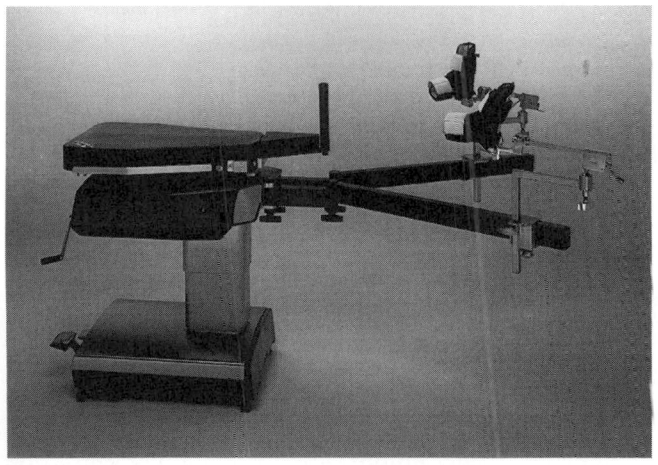

FIGURE 5-2 Orthopedic table with multiple movable and removable parts and suspended frames.

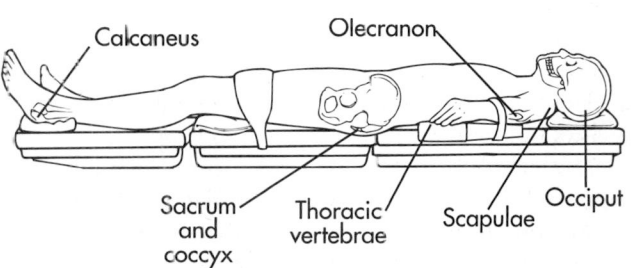

FIGURE 5-3 Supine position. Potential pressure areas shown.

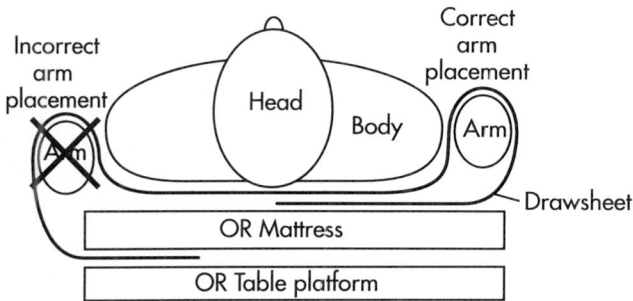

FIGURE 5-4   Correct method for tucking arms in at the patient's side.

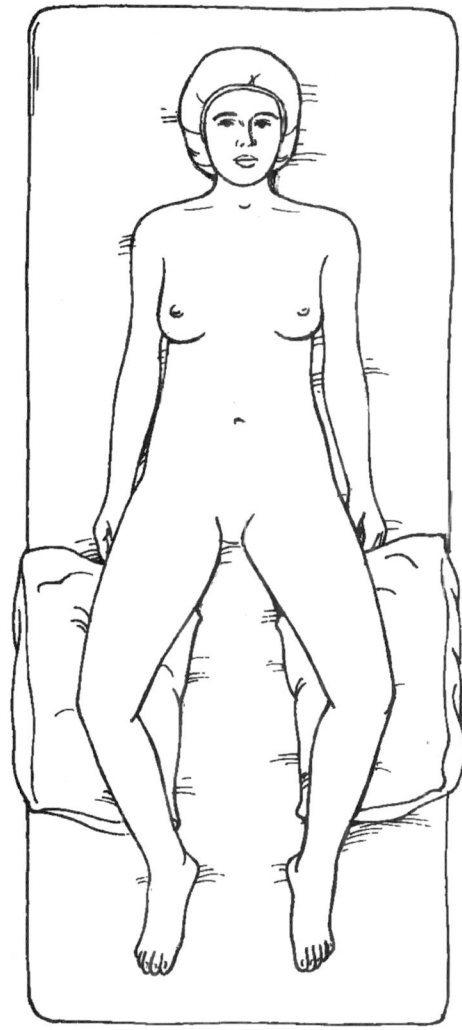

FIGURE 5-5   Supine position with legs flexed.

the ulnar nerve because the bony portion of the condylar groove of the humerus becomes placed against the padded armboard. However, there is no hard evidence that supination actually does protect the ulnar nerve. Supination of the hand may also increase stretch on the brachial plexus of an abducted arm, leading some practitioners to recommend pronation (palms down) rather than supination of the hand. Other factors that may determine the rotational position of the hand include patient comfort, access to intravenous sites, and access for monitoring of neuromuscular blockade with a peripheral nerve stimulator.[3]

If the arms are tucked at the side, the fingers should be straight and the palms should lie neutral against the body. The draw sheet should be brought next to the body, over and around the arm, and then finally tucked under the body. This is best accomplished with an assistant on the other side of the OR bed to roll the patient's body over enough to tuck the draw sheet underneath it (Fig. 5-4). In contrast, using a similar technique of encasing the arm with the draw sheet and then tucking the sheet under the OR mattress instead of the patient's body poses some serious potential risks. The arm can more easily drop over the edge of the bed and become compressed against the mattress or metal sidebars. Such compression could injure the ulnar, radial, or medial nerves.

Sometimes the patient's legs need to be flexed frog-leg fashion to provide access to the groin, perineum, and medial aspects of the lower extremities. The thighs are externally rotated and the knees are flexed and supported with a pillow under each leg (Fig. 5-5). This position is utilized when access to the genitals is required during abdominal gynecologic and urologic procedures. During coronary artery bypass graft procedures, this position allows access for harvesting the saphenous vein. Sometimes a special contoured positioning pad is utilized instead of pillows.

The circulatory system may be compromised in the supine position, not only by a tight safety strap, but also by the overall effect of the horizontal body posture and the changed effects of gravity. Blood volume to the heart and lungs is increased compared to being erect. This increases the cardiac output as well as the cardiac work load. The

weight of the chest in obese patients can cause increased intrathoracic pressure and further increase the cardiac work load. If a patient has cardiovascular deficiencies, this position can further increase their risk for cardiac failure.

Increased pressure on the inferior vena cava from abdominal viscera, abdominal masses, or a fetus in a pregnant woman may decrease blood return to the heart; blood pressure would then be lowered. The vena cava lies slightly to the right of the vertebral column. Tilting the patient slightly to the left by placing a small roll or wedge under the right flank can divert the weight away from the vena cava. An example is tilting the supine cesarean section patient slightly to the left until the baby is delivered.

Respiratory function is compromised in the supine position because functional residual capacity (FRC) is less than that in the erect posture. In general, the supine position does allow a more even distribution of ventilation from the apex to the base of the lungs. Anterior and upward excursion of the chest during inspiration is not

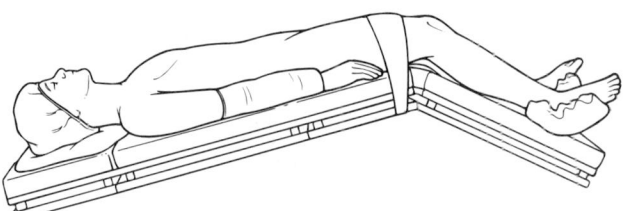

FIGURE 5-6 Trendelenburg's position.

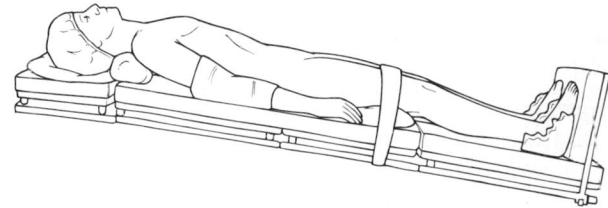

FIGURE 5-7 Reverse Trendelenburg's position, with soft roll under shoulders for thyroid, neck, or shoulder procedures.

greatly impeded except for obese patients whose chest wall weight significantly compresses the rib cage, further diminishing the FRC. Patients who are 100% over normal weight can have as much as a 40% to 50% increase in the mechanical work of breathing.[13] Diaphragmatic excursion may be lessened by the abdominal viscera, particularly when an abdominal retractor is used and packs are placed toward the diaphram.

Trendelenburg's position

Trendelenburg's position is a variation of the supine position in which the upper torso is lowered and the feet are raised (Fig. 5-6). Trendelenburg's position facilitates visualization of the pelvic organs during open or laparoscopic surgeries in the lower abdomen or pelvis. Trendelenburg's position can be utilized to improve circulation to the cerebral cortex and basal ganglia when the blood pressure is suddenly lowered. In this position, the knees are often bent by flexing the leg section of the bed. The patient must have the knees over the break in the bed to maintain safe anatomic positioning. Another modification is that of keeping the trunk level and elevating only the legs by raising the leg section of the bed. As the lower section of the bed is elevated, the Mayo stand should be raised to prevent pressure on the feet.

Shearing is a significant risk in this position. The skeletal structure slides up toward the head of the bed. If the patient is draped, lifting the patient to realign the tissue cannot be done. If necessary, shoulder braces may be used to limit upward sliding. To protect the brachial plexus from compression injury, it is important to make sure that the shoulder braces are well padded and placed above the acromion processes, not the soft tissue of the neck. Additionally they should not be used if the arms are extended on armboards.

Any variation of Trendelenburg's position should be maintained only as long as necessary. In this position blood pools in the upper torso, increasing blood pressure and intracranial pressure. Although the head-down position facilitates drainage of secretions from the bases of the lungs and the oropharyngeal passages, the weight of the abdominal viscera further impedes diaphragmatic movement; as they push the diaphragm up and compress the lung bases, pulmonary compliance and FRC are diminished. Fluid shifts into the alveoli causing edema, congestion, and atelectasis. Slow, smooth postural transitions allow suffi-

cient time for the body to adjust to physiologic changes. If this is not done when the patient is being placed in Trendelenburg's position, blood rapidly shifts from the lower extremities, causing a reflexive decreased cardiac output.[19] Conversely, hypotension may result if the patient is not returned slowly to the supine position.

Reverse Trendelenburg's position

Reverse Trendelenburg's position is described as the head-up, feet-down position (Fig. 5-7). It is frequently used to provide access to the head and neck and to facilitate gravitational pull on the viscera away from the diaphragm and toward the feet. When the foot of the bed is tilted toward the floor, the patient's body is supported by a padded footboard, by nonconstrictive body restraints, or by a liftsheet that supports the arms from above the elbows to the fingers.

For patients having thyroid, neck, or shoulder surgery, a pillow or soft roll is placed horizontally under the shoulders to hyperextend the neck. The hips and knees can be flexed and slightly elevated. The arms are generally tucked at the side to allow for closer access to the surgical site.

When this position is used for shoulder surgery, the arm of the affected shoulder is often prepped and draped to allow for intraoperative shoulder manipulation. The head and cervical spine need to be properly aligned and supported to prevent neuromuscular strain. Rotation of the head in an opposite direction of a shoulder that the surgeon is manipulating can cause injury to the brachial plexus.

For minimally invasive approaches to the esophagus, such as laparoscopic Nissen fundoplication, steep reverse Trendelenburg's position is required. The OR bed is modified by the addition of leg holders and the surgeon stands between the legs. To prevent the patient from sliding as a result of the steep position, a Vac pack (beanbag) is inflated under the patient, and the knees are slightly flexed to a range of 20 to 30 degrees.[17] In this position, the combination of increased abdominal pressure from pneumoperitoneum and steep reverse Trendelenburg's position decrease venous return. Sequential compression stockings are applied as prophylaxis against deep vein thrombosis (DVT).

In the reverse Trendelenburg's position, respiratory function is more like that in the erect position. Venous circulation may be compromised by extended time in the legs-downward position. When this situation is anticipated, the superficial venous return can be aided by the preoperative application of support hose, elastic bandages, or sequentially inflatable stockings. If the legs are wrapped, compression of the common peroneal nerve at the head of the fibula must be avoided.

Return to the supine position from the reverse Trendelenburg's position should be accomplished slowly and smoothly to avoid overload to the cardiovascular system.

Fracture table position

The orthopedic fracture table allows the patient to be positioned for hip fracture surgery or closed femoral nailing. The patient may be brought into the operating room in the hospital bed with traction applied. Before transfer the patient can be anesthetized. During transfer to the fracture table manual traction to the injured leg can be applied.

The patient is positioned supine with the pelvis stabilized against a well-padded vertical perineal post (Fig. 5-8). Pressure on the genitalia from the perineal post

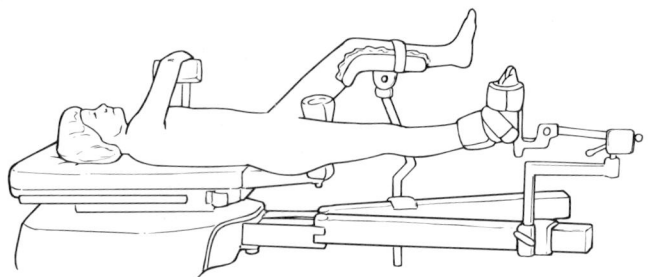

FIGURE 5-8 Fracture table position. The unaffected leg is raised, abducted, and supported in a padded leg rest.

can injure the genital structures. Pressure on the perineal and pudendal nerves can cause fecal incontinence and loss of perineal sensation.[15]

Traction is achieved by restraining the foot of the injured leg in a well-padded bootlike device that is connected to the traction bar so that the leg may be rotated, pulled into traction, or released, as the surgery requires. One method of securing the foot in this device is the use of a boot-shaped cuff that wraps around the entire foot and connects to the traction device. It is inflated with air to secure the foot. Another method is to cushion the foot and then secure it to the device with restraining straps, Ace bandages, or a self-adhering wrap. Whatever method is used, excessive pressure can be placed on the foot and ankle, especially while traction is being applied. It is important to be sure that adequate padding is used. If the boot-shaped cuff is used, care should be taken that it is not inflated beyond the manufacturer's recommendations.

The unaffected leg rests on a well-padded, elevated leg holder or secured in a well-padded bootlike device. C-arm fluoroscopy x-ray examinations can be taken during surgery because the unaffected leg is abducted well out of the field of the x-ray machine.

Lithotomy

The lithotomy position is used for gynecologic, rectal, and urologic procedures and for radical resections of the vulva, groin, and rectal areas (Fig. 5-9).

With the patient supine, the legs are raised and abducted to expose the perineal region. This position is maintained by the legs being placed in stirrups. The stirrups should be checked before use so that they are securely fastened to the sidebars of the OR bed. Slippage of the stirrups once the legs are in place could cause hip dislocation, muscle or nerve injury, or bone fractures. Both

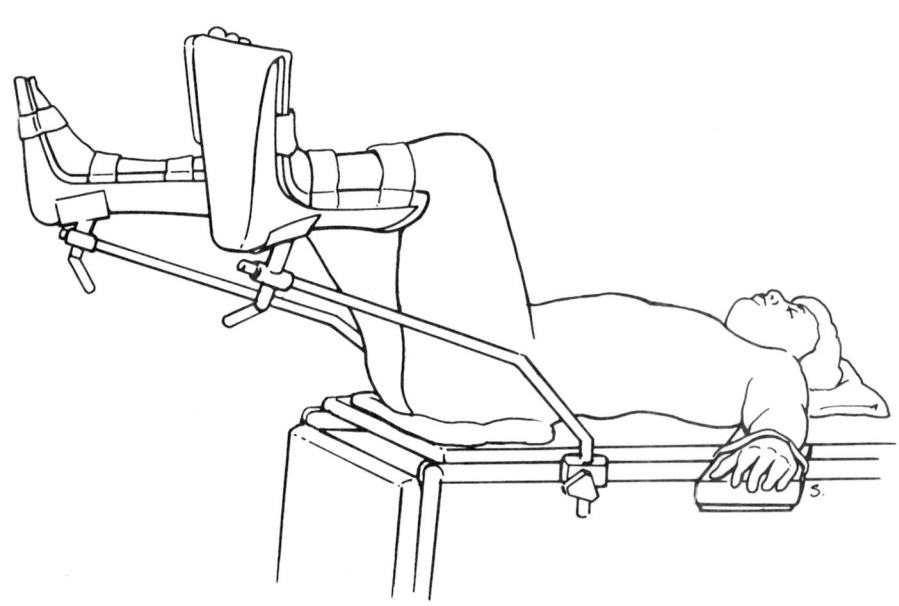

FIGURE 5-9 Lithotomy position utilizing boot type stirrups.

stirrups should be at equal heights and attached to the OR bed at the same level. The legs should be raised simultaneously to prevent strain on the patient's lower back. This requires two people so that both legs are totally supported throughout the move. Each person should grasp the sole of the foot with one hand and support the calf near the knee with the other. The legs should be raised and knees flexed in slow, smooth movements.

Once the legs are secured in the stirrups the mattress of the leg section of the OR bed is removed, and the leg section platform is lowered. The buttocks should be even with the edge of the OR bed to reduce the risk of lumbosacral strain.

The arms are either supported on armboards, placed across the abdomen, or tucked at the patient's side. When the arms are tucked, extreme caution should be taken when the leg section of the bed is elevated back to a horizontal position at the conclusion of the procedure. The hands and fingers can be caught in the break of the bed and pinched or crushed.

Various types of stirrups are used for lithotomy positioning. The most common include candy cane-shaped bars with straps that wrap around the ankles and plantar surface of the foot, posts with knee crutches, and boot type of stirrups that cradle the lower foot and heel and extend to the midcalf area (Fig. 5-10). The type of stirrup used can create unique hazards. The ankle straps of candy cane-shaped stirrups can put pressure on the distal sural and plantar nerves, which could result in neuropathies of the foot. Leaning of the lateral part of the calf against the vertical stirrup bar can put pressure on the common peroneal nerve as it curves laterally over the fibula, resulting in footdrop and a lack of sensation below the knee. If the medial aspect of the knee or calf rests against a stirrup bar, the saphenous branch of the femoral nerve can be compressed against the tibia. Another concern with the candy cane stirrups is the risk of hyperabduction. Hips should not be flexed more than 90 degrees. Exaggerated flexion can stretch the sciatic nerve.

Knee crutch stirrups in which the weight of the leg rests solely on the knee supports can put pressure on the posterior tibial, sural, and common peroneal nerves in the popliteal fossa.

Boot stirrups that support the foot and calf distribute pressure more evenly, reducing the risk of extreme localized pressure on any one area of the foot or leg. They also allow for controlled and limited abduction.

Regardless of the type of stirrup used, hyperabduction of the legs can cause stretching of the femoral, femoral cutaneous, sciatic, and obturator nerves; abductor muscles; and capsule of the hip joint. Abduction should be limited to only the degree needed for adequate surgical access, and the time in this position should be minimized.

Special care is needed for the patient who has a limited range of motion attributable to a hip prosthesis, cast, amputation, or obesity. Severe hip flexion as well as abduction of the joint must be avoided in lithotomy position. The stirrup should be as low as possible and tilted slightly outward. This is a situation in which the patient could be placed in lithotomy position before induction to assess areas of discomfort and implement appropriate therapeutic measures before the procedure begins.

If the patient will be in this position for longer than 2 hours, Ace bandages or antiembolitic stockings should be applied to the patient's legs. The flexing of the knee may impede venous return.

The lithotomy position has significant potential for respiratory and circulatory compromise to the patient. The hazards increase as the position is exaggerated for radical surgery of the groin, vulva, or prostate. Extreme flexion of the thighs impairs respiratory function by increasing intraabdominal pressure against the diaphragm, therefore decreasing the tidal volume. Interference with gravity flow of blood from the elevated legs causes pooling in the splanchnic region during the operative procedure. This effect is greater when the hip and knee flexion are extreme, as in Young's modification (high lithotomy position). Blood loss during surgery may not be immediately manifested because of this increased splanchnic volume. However, when the legs are lowered and 500 ml or more of blood is diverted to more total leg circulation, the circulating volume is depleted, and the blood pressure may decrease. Normal compensatory mechanisms are depressed by the effects of anesthesia on the nervous system, and homeostasis may not be achieved easily.

Arms must not impede chest movement and respiration. The weight of the limbs on the chest, especially in infants and children, may fatigue the muscles used in respiration and induce respiratory problems. Additionally, the elevation of the legs pushes abdominal viscera toward the diaphram. Lowering of the head of the bed

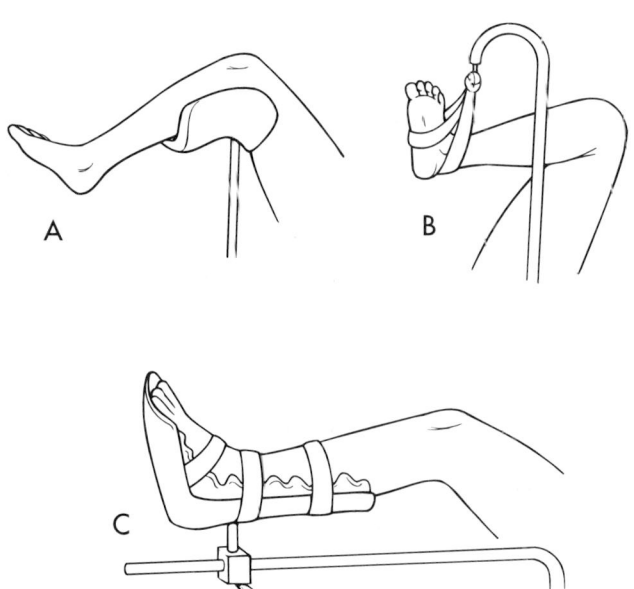

FIGURE 5-10   Types of stirrups used. **A,** Knee crutch. **B,** Candy cane. **C,** Boot type.

can further exaggerate this shift as diaphragmatic excursion is reduced.

Releasing the patient from the position must be done slowly and with adequate assistance. The legs must be taken out of stirrups and lowered simultaneously with support given to the joints to prevent strain on the lumbosacral musculature, which can stretch and tilt, thereby placing the pelvis and limbs in imbalance. The legs should be lowered slowly to allow for gradual hemodynamic adjustment as more blood shifts into the lower extremities.

Semi-Fowler's Position

Semi-Fowler's (lawn-chair) position may be used for some cranial procedures and shoulder or breast reconstruction. This position is accomplished first with the patient supine. The upper body section of the bed is flexed 45 degrees, and the leg section is lowered slightly, flexing the knees. The arms may rest on a pillow in the lap or be secured on armboards parallel to the OR bed. A footboard may be flexed at the bottom of the OR bed to act as a footrest and prevent footdrop. The entire OR bed is tilted so that the head of the bed is not so erect. This can reduce the sliding and shearing effects as well as diminish the hemodynamic effects of anesthesia.

Diaphragmatic excursion is improved in this position compared to the supine position. Although pressure points remain similar to those of supine, additional pressure is placed on the ischial tuberosities, calcaneus, and coccyx.

Fowler's Position

Fowler's (sitting) position is used for some ear and nose procedures and craniotomies involving a posterior or occipital approach (Fig. 5-11). This position is accomplished initially with the patient supine. Slowly, the upper body section of the OR bed is raised 90 degrees while the knees are slightly flexed and the legs lowered. A footrest is used to prevent footdrop. The arms either rest in the lap on a pillow with the elbows flexed 90 degrees or less or are supported on the side with padded armboards. The cervical, thoracic, and lumbar section of the spine should be in alignment once the position is established.

When this position is used for posterior fossa craniotomy or cranial ventricular procedures, a special craniotomy headrest is used to secure and immobilize the head.

The main pressure points include the scapula, ischial tuberosities, calcaneus, and coccyx. There is also increased pressure on the sciatic nerve. There needs to be adequate padding at the lumbar area and under the elbows, knees, buttocks, and heels. The popliteal space needs to be checked to ensure that no pressure is sustained from the edge of the mattress at the bottom of the lumbar section.

This position poses some significant circulatory compromises and risks. Blood pooling occurs in the lower torso and legs, which causes significant orthostatic hypotension as well as diminished perfusion to the brain. Venous return from the lower extremities is impeded, and such hindrance causes an increased threat of venous thrombosis. Antiembolic stockings or Ace bandages along with a sequential venous compression device assist in supporting venous return.

Since the operative site is elevated compared to the heart, gravity causes a negative venous gradient between the operative site and the right atrium. This creates a potential for an air embolism if a venous sinus is opened. During a craniotomy, this potential increases when tissue is dissected free from the cranium, bone is removed, the dura is tacked up, or a highly vascular tumor bed is entered.[10] Prophylactically, a central venous catheter is inserted into the pulmonary artery or right atrium, and a Doppler probe is placed over the chest wall to assist in the diagnosis and treatment of an air embolism. If air embolism is diagnosed, the scrub nurse should quickly irrigate the area with normal saline to prevent further venous aspiration of air. The exposed area should be packed with saline-soaked sponges or cottonoids. If the air embolism occurred during bone entry, bone wax should immediately be placed over the exposed bone to seal it. The anesthesia provider will aspirate air from the right atrium through the central venous line. The circulator should assist and support the endeavors of the anesthesia provider and scrub team.

Respirations are probably least impeded in this position than in any other surgical position. However, it is important to make sure that if the arms are resting on a pillow in the lap and secured with tape, this position does not restrict chest movement. Flexion of the head and neck must be avoided to prevent kinking of the endotracheal tube and subsequent airway obstruction.

When the procedure is concluded, repositioning the patient back to a supine position must be done very slowly

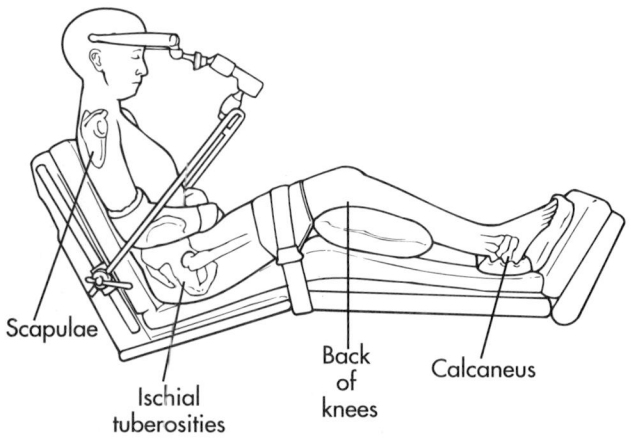

FIGURE 5-11 Fowler's (sitting) position. Potential pressure areas shown.

Scapulae

Ischial tuberosities

Back of knees

Calcaneus

so that the patient can gradually make hemodynamic adjustments.

Prone

In the prone position the patient is lying with the abdomen on the surface of the operating room bed mattress (Fig. 5-12). Modifications of the position allow approaches to the cervical spine, back, rectal area, and dorsal areas of the extremities.

Induction of anesthesia is performed with the patient in the supine position, usually on the transport vehicle. Before the patient is turned, the anesthesia provider secures the endotracheal tube with tape, applies eye ointment in each eye, and then tapes the eyelids closed to prevent corneal abrasions. Turning the supine patient to prone position can be accomplished safely, smoothly, and gently by four persons using the following "log-roll" technique. The transport vehicle is locked adjacent to the locked OR bed. The anesthesia provider supports the head and neck during the turn. A second person stands at the side of the stretcher with hands at the patient's shoulders and buttocks to initiate the roll of the patient. A third person stands at the opposite side of the operating room bed, with arms extended to support the chest and lower abdomen as the patient is rolled forward and over. The fourth person stands at the foot of the stretcher to support and turn the legs. At the completion of the turn, the stretcher is removed.

The arms must not be allowed to hang over the edge of the bed as the radial nerve can be quickly compressed by the weight of the humerus against the OR bed side rails. The arms are either secured at the sides or placed on armboards, in which case the patient's arms are brought down and forward to rest on the armboards with elbows flexed and hands pronated. To prevent shoulder dislocation and brachial plexus injury, there should be minimal abduction of the upper arm and no pressure on the axilla. Elbows should be padded and carefully checked for pressure areas. Other areas that require special attention and padding are the cheek, ear, patella, and toes. The head is turned and positioned on a foam pillow or towels, with the neck kept in alignment with the spinal column. The eyes are carefully protected.

Generally, when the patient is placed in prone position, the patient is placed on a laminectomy frame or chest rolls

that extend lengthwise from the acromioclavicular joint to the iliac crest. These positioning devices raise the chest and permit the diaphragm to move more freely and the lungs to expand. Supports must not press against the female breasts or male genitalia. These areas should be checked after final positioning to ensure that they are free from pressure. A bolster or pillow under the pelvis can decrease abdominal pressure on the inferior vena cava. A cushion or pillow is placed under the ankles to prevent pressure on the toes. The safety strap is placed across the dorsal aspects of the thighs so that the patient is secured but superficial venous return is not impaired. After the patient is positioned, pedal pulses should be checked.

The prone posture is initially hazardous as the anesthetized patient is turned from the supine position to the prone position. Normal compensatory mechanisms are depressed, and the patient cannot readily adjust to imposed hemodynamic changes and the resulting hypotension.

The respiratory system is most vulnerable in the prone position because normal anterior lateral respiratory movement is restricted and normal diaphragmatic movement is inhibited by the compressed abdominal wall. This position requires ventilator assistance.

For spinal operations the prone position may be modified to flex the affected part of the spine. The surgeon specifies the modifications preferred. One method is to increase the arch on the laminectomy frame, which usually can be adjusted by a hand crank. Another method is to place the patient in the knee-chest position without a laminectomy frame or to modify the knee-chest position with the application of chest rolls.

Turning the patient back into supine position onto the PACU stretcher requires a four-person team effort. One person stands at the side of the OR bed, and the other at the side of the stretcher that is adjacent to the OR bed and locked. If a laminectomy frame was used, it can be tilted in the direction of the stretcher to initiate the move. The anesthesia provider supports the head, and a fourth person supports the feet. The patient is "log rolled" onto the stretcher. Skin integrity is checked over all pressure-point areas, particularly the knees and areas that had contact with the laminectomy frame.

Jackknife position

The jackknife (Kraske's) position is a modification of the prone position that is often used for hemorrhoidectomy and pilonidal sinus procedures (Fig. 5-13). The patient's hips are placed on a bolster or pillow over the break in the lumbar section of the OR bed, and the bed is flexed at a 90-degree angle, raising the hips and lowering the head and body. The patient's head, chest, and feet need the usual supports in this position. A small roll placed under each shoulder will relieve pressure on the brachial plexus from the clavicle. A pillow should be placed under the lower legs to prevent pressure on the toes. The restraint strap is placed across the dorsal area of the thighs.

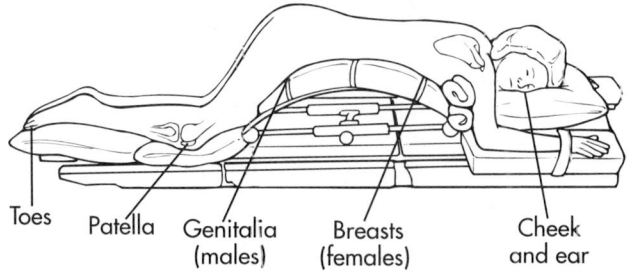

Toes   Patella   Genitalia   Breasts   Cheek
(males)   (females)   and ear

FIGURE 5-12 Prone position using laminectomy frame for spinal procedures. Potential pressure areas shown.

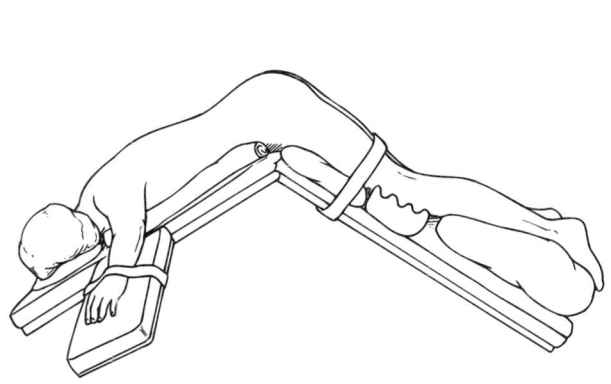

FIGURE 5-13   Jackknife (Kraske's) position.

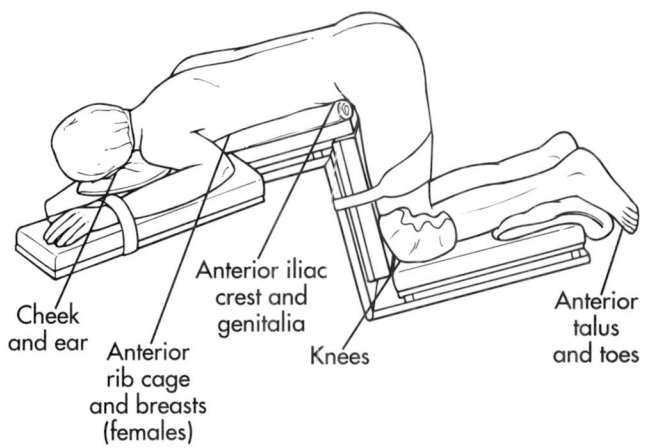

FIGURE 5-14   Knee-chest position. Potential pressure areas shown.

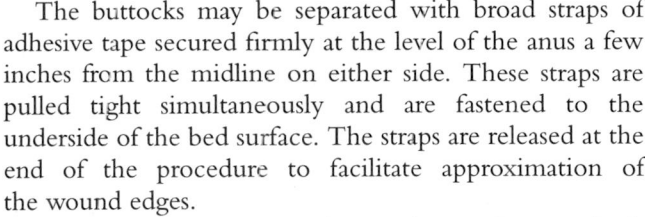

The buttocks may be separated with broad straps of adhesive tape secured firmly at the level of the anus a few inches from the midline on either side. These straps are pulled tight simultaneously and are fastened to the underside of the bed surface. The straps are released at the end of the procedure to facilitate approximation of the wound edges.

This position causes circulatory changes because both the head and the feet are in dependent positions, causing cephalad and caudad venous pooling. Antiembolism stockings assist in venous return and decrease the risk of venous thrombosis.

Respirations are severely compromised because anterior lateral chest movement is restricted. Additionally, pressure is exerted on the diaphragm from the abdominal viscera, and that stress is further exacerbated by the pressure from the flexed OR bed.

If the patient is to be placed on the recovery stretcher in the supine position, the operating room bed is first straightened very slowly so that the body can adjust hemodynamically. The patient is turned by four people using the log-roll technique.

Knee-chest position

The knee chest position, a further exaggeration of the jackknife position, is used primarily for sigmoidoscopies and occasionally for lumbar laminectomy procedures (Fig. 5-14). An extension platform is placed on the end of the foot section. The patient is positioned prone with the hips at the break of the body section. The leg section is lowered, and the extension platform is flexed at a right angle so that the patient kneels on the lower platform. The entire bed is tilted cephalad to expose the posterior pelvis.[5] The safety strap is placed around the posterior area of the thighs.

The arms are placed on armboards and flexed at the elbows to lie adjacent to the head. The chest rests directly on the OR bed. Pressure points are a vital consideration for this position. They include the anterior rib cage, anterior iliac crest, knees, anterior tibial aspects of the calves, anterior talus, and toes. All these areas need to be well padded and supported.

Lateral

In the lateral (lateral recumbent, lateral decubitus, or Sims's) position, the patient is lying on the nonoperative side, providing access to the upper chest, the kidney, or the upper section of the ureter. Reference to right or left lateral position depends on the side on which the patient lies. In the right lateral position, the patient lies on the right side with the left (operative) side facing upward. In left lateral, the patient lies on the left side with the right (operative) side facing upward.

After induction of anesthesia with the patient in the supine position on the operating room bed, the patient is turned to the side. A four-person team uses a lift-sheet from under the patient to facilitate a safe, smooth, gentle turn.

A pillow is placed under the patient's head to maintain good alignment with the cervical spine and the thoracic vertebrae; this alignment also helps to minimize stretching on the dependent brachial plexus. The bottom leg is flexed at the knee and hip to stabilize the patient on the bed. The top leg is straight or slightly flexed. A pillow is placed lengthwise between the patient's legs. The lateral aspect of the bottom knee must be padded to prevent pressure on the peroneal nerve, located superficially at the head of the fibula. One person should remain at the patient's back to steady and support the torso during positioning of the lower extremities.

The torso is supported by pillows, sandbags, rolled blankets, padded kidney braces, or a surgical positioning system, sometimes refered to as a *Vac pack*. A Vac pack is a soft pad filled with tiny beads. When suction is attached to a port on the pad, it conforms to the shape of whatever it is wrapped around. A valve is closed to maintain the vacuum. It acts as an immobilizer until air is reintroduced, and then it softens back into its original shape.

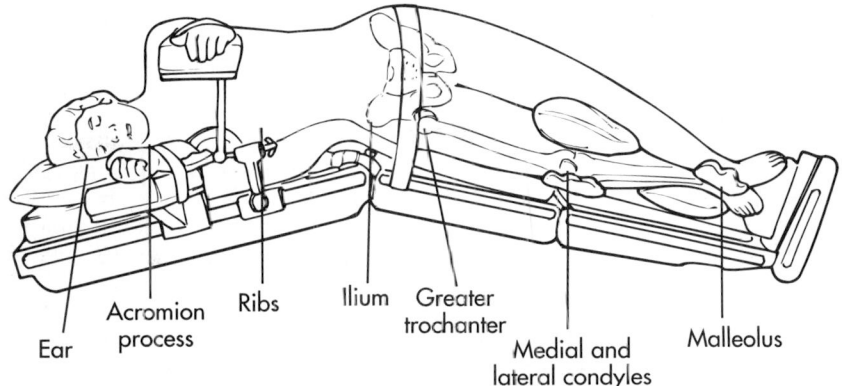

FIGURE 5-15 Lateral kidney position. Potential pressure areas shown.

The shoulders, hips, and legs may be secured with wide tape fastened to the platform of the OR bed. The upper arm is placed on an elevated armboard or rests on a pillow in front of the patient. The lower arm is flexed and rests on an armboard. The lower shoulder should be brought slightly forward, and a small bolster may be placed slightly posterior to the axilla to relieve pressure on the nerves and vessels along the brachial plexus as well as to facilitate chest expansion. Radial pulses should be monitored to confirm adequate circulation in the arms. A pulse oximeter may be used to check perfusion in the dependent hand.[19]

Lateral chest position

The lateral chest position is a modification that allows operative approach to the uppermost part of the thoracic cavity. A variation in the upper arm placement is that it is flexed slightly at the elbow and raised above the head to elevate the scapula, provide access to the underlying ribs, and widen the intercostal spaces. The uppermost arm may still be supported on a raised armboard or pillow.

For torso stabilization, the legs may be positioned in several ways according to the surgeon's preference: (1) both legs may be flexed at a 90-degree angle at the hips and knees, with a pillow placed between them, (2) the lower leg may be extended straight on the bed, with the upper hip and knee flexed at a 90-degree angle with two pillows supporting the thigh and calf, or (3) the lower hip and knee may be flexed at a 90-degree angle, with two or more pillows supporting the extended upper leg.

Slanting the upper section of the bed downward places the trachea and mouth at a lower level than the lungs, a position that enables bronchial secretions and fluids from the lung bases to drain into the mouth and not pass into the unaffected side of the chest.

Lateral kidney position

The lateral kidney position (Fig. 5-15) allows approach to the retroperitoneal area of the flank. While being turned from the supine to the lateral position, the anesthetized patient is positioned so that the lower iliac crest is just below the lumbar break where the kidney bridge is located. To render the kidney region readily accessible, the kidney bridge is raised and the bed is flexed, so that the area between the twelfth rib and the iliac crest is elevated. Raising the kidney bridge depends on the cardiovascular response of the body to the increased pressure transmitted from this area. It should be raised slowly and the blood pressure monitored frequently by the anesthesia provider. The bed is then flexed to lower the patient's head and legs. The patient's affected side presents a straight horizontal line from shoulder to hip. In this position, the gravitational force on the head and torso opposes that on the extended limb to facilitate operative exposure.

For torso stabilization, well-padded kidney braces may be used. A longer one is placed anteriorly, against the iliac crest. A shorter one is placed against the back. Wide adhesive tape is placed across the hips and secured to the undersides of the OR bed. Before wound closure, the adhesive strap is released, the kidney elevator lowered, and the bed straightened to facilitate approximation of the wound edges.

Systolic and diastolic pressures decrease when the lateral position is assumed again because normal compensatory mechanisms are depressed by pharmacologic agents and pathophysiologic processes. The patient may not readily compensate for abrupt postural changes. The acute angulation of the body in the lateral kidney posture and the effect of gravity may also decrease blood return to the right side of the heart.

Respiratory function is compromised by the weight of the body on the lower chest. Chest movements are limited, and the chest size may be decreased. Diaphragmatic movement is limited by the flexion of the lower limbs toward the abdomen. Another respiratory effect of this position is that the dependent lung is more perfused because of the gravitational pooling of blood. The nondependent lung, however, is more easily ventilated because it is less compressed. This results in a ventilation-perfusion mismatch. Applying positive end-expiratory pressure to both lungs helps to compensate for this decrease in functional lung capacity. However, when the nondependent lung is the site of the operation and thus decompressed, functional lung capacity is further aggravated.

SUMMARY

Carefully planned positioning results in maximum patient safety and surgical-site exposure as well as access to the head and neck to administer anesthesia care. All members of the surgical team share the responsibility to protect the patient from injury during positioning. Therefore all members should be familiar with possible risks to maintain patient safety. The following is a summary of important nursing interventions when positioning patients:

- Gather all positioning accessories before the patient is brought into the OR.
- Check with anesthesia provider before moving the patient.
- Determine number of personnel needed to safely and effectively position the patient.
- Pad all bony prominences to prevent disruption to skin integrity.
- Protect all superficial nerves from strain or pressure.
- Ensure that legs are not crossed to prevent pressure on nerves and blood vessels.
- Support and secure extremities to prevent them from falling from the OR bed or resting against any hard surfaces.
- Make certain no equipment, Mayo stand, or personnel are resting on the patient.
- Maintain patient privacy and dignity by avoiding unnecessary exposure.
- Always use slow, smooth movements when changing a patient's position, utilizing a team approach.
- Use good body mechanics.

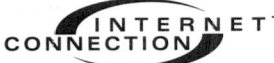

National Library of Medicine: http://www.nlm.nih.gov

Digital Anatomist:
http://www1.biostr.washington.edu/DigitalAnatomist.html

The Visible Human Project:
http://www.nlm.nih.gov/research/visible/visible_human.html

List Serves (to ask questions about patient positioning/ accessories, etc.); e-mail and follow instructions at these sites: listserv@library.umed.edu
listproc@u.washington.edu

REFERENCES

1. Agency for Health Care Policy and Research. (1992, May). *Clinical practice guideline number 3, Pressure ulcers in adults,* Publication no. 92-0047, p. 3. Rockville, MD.
2. Agency for Health Care Policy and Research. (1994, December). *Clinical practice guideline number 15, Treatment of pressure ulcers,* Publication no. 95-0652, pp. 12, 13, 35. Rockville, MD.
3. American Society of Anesthesiologists, Committee on Patient Safety and Risk Management. (1995). *Perioperative peripheral nerve injury,* ASA Patient Safety Videotape Series (Executive Producer: Pierce, E.; Producers: Stoelting, R.K., Warner, M.A., & Blitt, C.D.). Holmdel, NJ: GWF Associates.
4. AORN recommended practices for positioning the patient in the perioperative practice setting. (1998). In *AORN standards, recommended practices, and guidelines.* Denver: Association of Operating Room Nurses, pp. 265-270.
5. Atkinson, L.J., & Fortunato, N.H. (1996). *Berry & Kohn's operating room technique* (ed. 8). St. Louis: Mosby, pp. 442-443.
6. Ben-Amitai, D., & Garty, B. (1993). Alopecia in children after cardiac surgery. *Pediatric Dermatology, 10*(1), 32-33.
7. Boyer, J.D., & Vidmar, D.A. (1994). Postoperative alopecia: a case report and literature review. *Cutis, 54,* 321-322.
8. Crewe, R.A. (1987). Problems of rubber ring nursing cushions and a clinical survey of alternative cushions for ill patients. *Care Science Practice, 5*(2), 9-11.
9. Davey, S.S., & Huether, S.E. (1996). Structure and function of the pulmonary system. In Huether, S.E., & McCance, K.L. (Eds.), *Understanding pathophysiology* (ed. 2). St. Louis: Mosby, pp. 730, 736.
10. Groah, L.K. (1996). *Perioperative nursing* (ed. 3). Stamford, CT: Appleton & Lange, p. 261.
11. Hemphill, B.H. (1986). Time saving assessment and documentation tools that relieve pressure, *Ostomy/Wound Management, Fall,* 50-60.
12. Hoshowsky, V.M., & Schramm, C.A. (1994). Intraoperative pressure sore prevention: ananalysis of bedding materials, *Research in Nursing and Health, 17,* 333-339.
13. Kneedler, J.A., & Dodge, G.H. (1994). *Perioperative patient care: the nursing perspective* (ed. 3). Boston: Jones & Barrtlett, pp. 322, 323.
14. Kosiak, M. (1959). Etiology and pathology of ischemic ulcers, *Physiological Medical Rehabilitation, 40,* 60-69.
15. McEwen, D.R. (1996). Intraoperative positioning of surgical patients, *AORN Journal, 63,* 1059-1061,1067.
16. Norton, D., McLaren, R., & Exton-Smith, A.N. (1962). *An investigation of geriatric nursing problems in the hospital.* London: National Corporation for the Care of Old People (now the Centre for Policy on Aging).
17. Patti, M.G., & Pellegrine, C.A. (1996). Esophageal procedures: minimally invasive approaches. In *Care of the surgical patient* (surgical techniques supplement 8). New York: Scientific American Medicine.
18. Rothrock, J.C. (1996). Generic care planning: AORN patient outcome standards. In Rothrock, J.C. (Ed.). *Perioperative nursing care planning* (ed 2). St. Louis: Mosby, p. 116.
19. Williams, H., & Reeves, F. (1998). Anesthetic techniques and positioning: implications for perioperative nurses. *Seminars in Perioperative Nursing, 7*(1), 14-20.

CHAPTER SIX

Sutures, Needles, and Instruments

Althea Dunscombe

HISTORY AND EVOLUTION OF SURGICAL SUTURES (2000 B.C. TO PRESENT)

The development of surgical sutures has been closely allied with the development of the art of surgery. Medical writing of ancient Egyptian and Assyrian cultures dating back to 2000 B.C. mentions the various materials used, to a limited extent, for suturing and ligating. *Suture* is a generic term for all materials used to sew severed body tissue together and to hold these tissues in their normal position until healing takes place. A *ligature* is a strand of suture material used to tie off (seal) blood vessels to prevent hemorrhage and simple bleeding or to isolate a mass of tissue to be excised (cut out).

The concept of suturing and ligating is also recorded in the writings of the father of medicine, Hippocrates, born in 460 B.C. Gut of sheep intestines was first mentioned as suture material in the writings of Galen, about A.D. 200. The Perisan physician and philosopher Rhazes is credited with employing surgical gut, or catgut, in A.D. 900 for suturing abdominal wounds. The word *catgut* is a misnomer, and its use is inappropriate. According to the *Oxford English Dictionary* it matches the Dutch *kattedarm* 'cat-intestine'. "Catgut" entered English around 1560 to 1600 under obscure conditions, possibly connected humorously with caterwauling.

Despite these promising early beginnings, the science of surgery, including suturing and ligating, progressed and then regressed, with several cultures never advancing much beyond the rudimentary stages. The principal reasons surgery and its allied practices did not progress in early times were the critical problems of hemorrhage, pain, and infection. Even Ambroise Paré, the famous French army surgeon of the middle 1500s who developed the technique for ligating to replace cautery in treatment of war injuries, was confronted with the grim fact that severe pain and subsequent infection greatly curtailed the advancements made possible by surgical repair and correction.

Surgery offered little promise of developing as a truly effective healing science until the nineteenth century, when an American surgeon, Crawford W. Long of Georgia, demonstrated the use of ether as an anesthetic (1842) and Joseph Lister of England first used carbolic acid solution to attempt antiseptic surgery (1865). Lister also experimented with surgical gut as an absorbable suture material and recognized the need for sterile surgical sutures.

Progress in the development of surgical sutures was rapid after the middle 1800s. By 1901 surgical gut and kangaroo gut were available to the surgeon in sterile glass tubes. Since then, numerous materials have been employed as sutures and ligatures. Gold, silver, metallic wire, silkworm gut, silk, cotton, linen, tendon, and intestinal tissue from nearly every creature that walks, swims, or flies have been used at one time or another throughout the evolution of surgery. During the early twentieth century surgical gut, silk, and cotton emerged as the most commonly used suture materials. The last half of this century saw the introduction and increased use of synthetic fibers such as nylon, polyester, polypropylene, and other polymer combinations.

As late as the 1930s the sterility of sutures commercially prepared and sterilized by manufacturers was subject to question. In addition, sutures varied considerably in their physical properties, such as diameter and strength. From the 1940s to the present, great strides have been made in the uniform preparation and sterilization of suture materials. Today the surgical team is assured of sterility, relatively uniform physical properties, and predictable performance in the sutures used in the operating room.

Since the early 1950s the trend has been toward individually packaged and presterilized suture materials, many with preattached (swaged) needles, delivered to the surgical suite in a ready-to-use form. This trend has relieved perioperative nurses of the time consuming and consequently expensive tasks of preparing sutures and needles for sterilization and then sterilizing them.

SUTURE MATERIALS

A variety of suture materials is available for ligating, suturing, and closing the wound. The appropriate suture is selected according to a number of characteristics: whether it is absorbable or nonabsorbable, its breaking (tensile) strength, whether it is monofilament or multifilament, its knot-tying facility, and its tissue reactivity. An understanding of these characteristics of suture materials, as well as knowledge of the risk factors of wound healing and the interaction between the tissues and suture materials, is essential for the perioperative nurse.

Characteristics of Suture Material

The three main features to evaluate the general properties of suture material are (1) physical characteristics, (2) handling characteristics, and (3) tissue-reaction characteristics (Box 6-1).

Physical characteristics

Physical characteristics of sutures are officially defined and described by the *United States Pharmacopoeia* (USP).

They can be measured or visually determined and include the following properties:

- *Physical configuration.* Single-stranded (monofilament) or multistranded (multifilament), containing a number of fibers rendered into a single thread by twisting or braiding (Fig. 6-1).
- *Capillarity.* Ability to soak up fluid along the strand.
- *Diameter.* Determined in millimeters, and expressed in USP sizes with zeroes; the smaller the cross-sectional diameter, the more zeroes; sizes range from #7, the largest, to 11-0, the smallest; sizes 0 to 4-0 are the most commonly used sutures in general surgery. (The surgeon will usually select the finest suture possible for the tissue being closed. The finer diameter provides better handling qualities and small knots. Improved suturing techniques are possible with sutures of finer diameter.)
- *Tensile strength.* The amount of weight (breaking load) necessary to break a suture (breaking strength); varies with type of suture material (Table 6-1).

TABLE 6-1 | **Relative Straight-Pull Tensile Strength of Suture Materials**

		NONABSORBABLE	ABSORBABLE
G	↑	Steel	
R		Polyester	Polyglycolic acid
E		Nylon (monofilamentous)	Polyglactin 910
A		Nylon (braided)	
T		Polypropylene	Polydioxanone
E		Silk	Poliglecaprone
R			Catgut

From Schwartz, S. (1994). *Principles of surgery* (ed. 6). New York: McGraw-Hill Book Co. and *Ethicon wound closure manual.* (1994). Sommerville, NJ: Ethicon, Inc.

BOX 6-1 | **Characteristics of Suture Material**

I. Physical characteristics
   Physical configuration
   Capillarity
   Fluid absorption ability
   Diameter (caliber)
   Tensile strength
   Knot strength
   Elasticity
   Plasticity
   Memory

II. Handling characteristics
   Pliability
   Tissue drag ⎫
   Knot tying ⎬ Related to coefficient of friction
   Knot slippage ⎭

III. Tissue-reaction characteristics
   Inflammatory and fibrous cell reaction
   Absorption
   Potentiation of infection
   Allergic reaction

From Schwartz, S. *Principles of surgery* (ed. 6). New York: (1994). McGraw-Hill Book Co. and *Ethicon wound closure manual.* (1994). Sommerville, NJ: Ethicon, Inc.

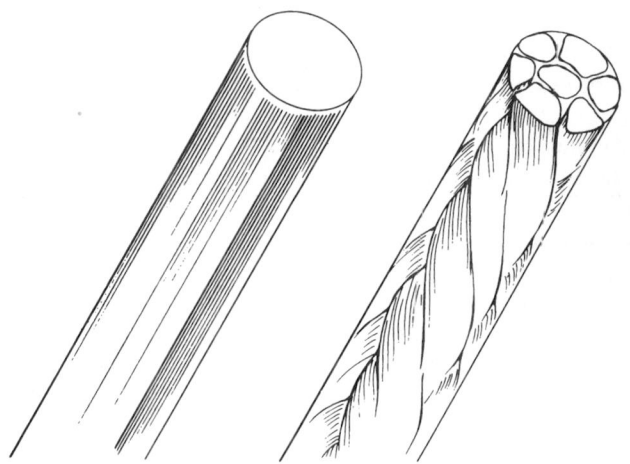

FIGURE 6-1   *Left,* Monofilament suture; *right,* multifilament (braided) suture).

- *Knot strength*. The force necessary to cause a given type of knot to slip, either partially or completely.
- *Elasticity*. Inherent ability to regain original form and length after having been stretched.
- *Memory*. Capacity of a suture to return to its former shape after being re-formed, as when tied; high memory yields less knot security.

Handling characteristics

Handling characteristics of suture material are related both to pliability (how easily the material bends) and coefficient of friction (how easily the suture slips through tissue and can be tied). A suture with a high friction coefficient tends to drag through tissue. It is more difficult to tie because its knots do not set easily. Some suture materials are coated to reduce their coefficient of friction. This coating not only improves the way they pull through tissue on insertion, but also affects the force needed to remove the suture after the wound is healed. The coefficient of friction should not be too low, however, because knots come undone more easily.

Tissue reaction characteristics

Because it is a foreign substance, all suture material causes some tissue reaction. Tissue reaction begins when the suture inflicts injury to the tissue during insertion. In addition, tissue reaction to the suture material itself occurs (Table 6-2). This reaction begins with an infiltration of white blood cells into the area; macrophages and fibroblasts then appear; by about the seventh day fibrous tissue with chronic inflammation is present. The reaction persists until the suture is encapsulated (nonabsorbable material) or absorbed (absorbable material) by the body.

Types of Suture Material

Suture materials are classified into two broad groups: absorbable and nonabsorbable.

Absorbable suture

The *USP* (1996) defines an absorbable surgical suture as a "sterile, flexible strand prepared from collagen derived from healthy mammals, or from a synthetic polymer. . . . It is capable of being absorbed by living mammalian tissue but may be treated to modify its resistance to absorption. . . . It may be modified with respect to body or texture. It may be impregnated with a suitable coating, softening, or antimicrobial agent. It may be colored by a color additive approved by the federal Food and Drug Administration."

Absorbable suture can be digested (by enzyme activity) or hydrolyzed (by reaction with water in tissue fluids to breakdown) and assimilated by the tissues during the healing process. Absorbable sutures vary in treatment, color, size, packaging, and resistance to absorption, according to their purpose. Types of absorbable suture include plain or chromic surgical gut, collagen, and glycolic acid polymers (Table 6-3).

Surgical Gut

Surgical gut is obtained from the collagen of the submucosal layer of the small intestine of sheep or the intestinal serosa of cattle or hogs. The processed strands or ribbons of collagen are either untreated (plain, type A) or treated with chromium salts (chromic, type C).

Chromatization delays absorption of the suture in living mammalian tissue. The strength of the chromium salt content and the duration of the chromatizing process are accurately controlled and tested. Proper chromatizing of gut ensures the integrity of the suture and maintenance of its strength during the early stages of wound healing. It enables a wound with slow healing power to heal sufficiently before the suture is entirely absorbed.

The elaborate processes of mechanical and chemical cleaning of the raw gut are followed by sterilization, usually with ionizing radiation, and storage in hermetically sealed packages. Modern manufacturing processes also ensure tensile strength, more controlled absorption, and more predictable results.

Absorption takes place by digestion of the gut by tissue enzymes. The absorption rate of surgical gut is influenced by the type of body tissue it contacts and, to some extent, by the patient's general physical condition. Studies also show that surgical gut is absorbed faster in serous or mucous membranes than in muscular tissues. When fine chromic gut is properly buried in successive layers of the gastrointestinal tract, for example, it retains its strength long enough for primary union to take place.

Surgical gut suture is wet packaged in an alcohol solution to provide maximum pliability and should be used immediately after removal from the packet. When a gut suture is removed from its packet and is not used at once, the alcohol evaporates, which causes the strand to lose its pliability. If required, the strand's pliability may be restored just before use by immersing it in sterile water or normal saline solution, preferably at body temperature, for only a few seconds. However, this is recommended only for eye sutures, since in other areas tissue fluids will moisten the gut sufficiently as it passes through the tissue when the

TABLE 6-2 | **Relative Tissue Reactivity to Sutures**

	NONABSORBABLE	ABSORBABLE
M		Catgut
O		
S	Silk, cotton	
T	Polyester coated	Polyglactin 910
	Polyester uncoated	Polyglycolic acid
	Nylon	Poliglecaprone
	Polypropylene	

From Schwartz, S. (1994). *Principles of surgery* (ed. 6). New York: McGraw-Hill Book Co. and *Ethicon wound closure manual.* (1994). Sommerville, NJ: Ethicon, Inc.

TABLE 6-3 | Comparison of Absorbable Sutures

TRADE NAME	COMPANY	MATERIAL	CONFIGURATION	TENSILE STRENGTH	TISSUE REACTIVITY
Collagen (plain)	Davis & Geck	Beef flexor tendon	Twisted	Poor (0% at 2-3 weeks)	Moderate
Collagen (chromic)	Davis & Geck	Beef flexor tendon	Twisted	Poor (0% at 2-3 weeks)	Moderate
Surgical gut (plain)	Ethicon; Davis & Geck; U.S. Surgical	Animal collagen	Twisted	Poor (0% at 2-3 weeks)	High
Surgical gut (chromic)	Ethicon; Davis & Geck; U.S. Surgical	Animal collagen	Twisted	Poor (0% at 2-3 weeks)	Moderately high
Monocryl	Ethicon	Poliglecaprone	Monofilament	Fair (20% at 2-3 weeks)	Low
Coated Vicryl	Ethicon	Polyglactin 910 (coated with calcium stearate and polyglactin 370)	Braided	Good (50% at 2-3 weeks)	Low
Dexon S	Davis & Geck	Polyglycolic acid	Braided	Good (50% at 2-3 weeks)	Low
Dexon Plus	Davis & Geck	Polyglycolic acid (coated with poloxamer 188)	Braided	Good (50% at 2-3 weeks)	Low
Polysorb	U.S. Surgical	Glycolide colactide	Braided	Fair (20% at 3 weeks)	Low
PDS	Ethicon	Polydioxanone	Monofilament	Good (50% at 2-3 weeks)	Low
Maxon	Davis & Geck	Polyglyconate	Monofilament	Good (50% at 4 weeks)	Low

From Schwartz, S. (1994). *Principles of surgery* (ed. 6). New York: McGraw-Hill Book Co. and *Ethicon wound closure manual*. (1994). Sommerville, NJ: Ethicon, Inc.

surgeon sews. Excessive moisture will reduce tensile strength.

Collagen Sutures

Collagen sutures are derived from the tendons of cattle. They are chemically treated to remove noncollagenous material, purified, and processed into strands that have physical properties superior to surgical gut. Collagen suture is most often used as a fine suture material for the eye.

Synthetic Absorbable Sutures

To produce synthetic absorbable sutures, specific polymers are extruded into suture strands. The base material for the synthetic absorbables is a combination of lactic and glycolic acid polymers (Vicryl, Dexon, Polysorb). The molecular structure of these products has a tensile strength sufficient for approximation of tissues for 2 to 3 weeks, followed by rapid absorption.

The newer synthetic polymers (PDS, Maxon, Monocryl) provide wound support for longer periods, up to 3 months. They are used when prolonged support for wound healing is desired, as with fascial closure, or for elderly or oncologic patients. Thus they combine the desirable qualities of extended wound support and eventual absorbability.

Synthetic absorbable sutures are absorbed by slow hydrolysis in the presence of tissue fluids. Hydrolysis is the chemical process whereby the polymer reacts with water to cause an alteration of breakdown of the molecular structure. These sutures are degraded in tissue by this process at a more predictable rate than surgical gut (or collagen) and with less tissue reaction. These sutures are dry packaged in sizes 10-0 to #3. They should not be dipped in solutions because moisture reduces their tensile strength. Some polymers have additional coatings to reduce drag in tissue.

Nonabsorbable sutures

Nonabsorbable sutures are strands of material that effectively resist enzymatic digestion in living animal tissue. The *USP* (1996) classifies nonabsorbable surgical suture as follows:

1. Class I suture is composed of silk or synthetic fibers of monofilament, twisted, or braided construction.
2. Class II suture is composed of cotton or linen fibers or coated natural or synthetic fibers where the coating significantly affects thickness but does not contribute significantly to strength.
3. Class III suture is composed of monofilament or multifilament metal wire.

The strand of suture material may be uncoated or coated with a substance to reduce capillarity and friction when passing through the tissue. There are several products used for coating, including silicone, Teflon, and various polymers. Fibers may be uncolored, naturally colored, or impregnated with a suitable dye.

HANDLING	KNOT SECURITY	MEMORY	ABSORPTION	DEGRADATION	COMMENTS
Fair	Poor	Low	Unpredictable (12 weeks)	Proteolytic	Less impure than surgical gut
Fair	Poor	Low	Unpredictable (12 weeks)	Proteolytic	Less impure than surgical gut
Fair	Poor	Low	Unpredictable (12 weeks)	Proteolytic	May be ordered as fast-absorbing gut (Ethicon) for percutaneous sutures
Fair	Fair	Low	Unpredictable (14-80 days)	Proteolytic	Darker, more visible (Davis & Geck); mild or extra chromatization (Davis & Geck)
Good	Fair	Low	Predictable (90 days)	Hydrolytic	Clear
Good	Fair	Low	Predictable (80 days)	Hydrolytic	Clear, violet, coated
Fair	Good	Low	Predictable (90 days)	Hydrolytic	Uncoated
Good	Fair	Low	Predictable (90 days)	Hydrolytic	Clear, green, coated
Good	Fair	Low	Predictable (90 days)	Hydrolytic	Clear, violet
Poor	Poor	High	Predictable (180 days)	Hydrolytic	Violet, clear
Good	Good	Low	Predictable (180 days)	Hydrolytic	Green, clear

Nonabsorbable suture materials are encapsulated or walled off by the tissues around it during the process of wound healing. In suturing skin, for which nonabsorbable materials are often the choice, the sutures are removed before healing is complete.

The most common nonabsorbable suture materials are silk, nylon, polyester fiber, polypropylene, and stainless steel wire (Table 6-4).

Silk

Silk is prepared from thread spun by the silkworm larva in making its cocoon. Top-grade raw silk is processed to remove natural waxes and gum, manufactured into threads, and colored with a vegetable dye. The strands of silk are either twisted or braided to form the suture, which gives it high tensile strength and better handling qualities. Silk handles well, is soft, and forms secure knots.

Untreated silk has a capillary action through which body fluids may transmit infection along the length of the suture strand. For this reason surgical silk is treated to render it noncapillary (able to resist the absorption of body fluids and moisture). It is available in sizes 9-0 to #5, in sterile packets or precut lengths, and with or without attached needles. Silk should be kept dry by the scrub person. Wet silk loses up to 20% in strength.

In the strict sense, silk is not a true nonabsorbable material. When buried in tissue, it loses its tensile strength after about a year and may disappear after several years. Silk sutures, more commonly than less-reactive suture materials, occasionally form tracts as the suture migrates gradually to a wound's exterior surface. This spontaneous migration is called *spitting* and may occur weeks, months, or even years after the suture was placed.[8] Spitting is annoying and sometimes frightening to the patient but has no deleterious effect on wound healing.

Cotton

Surgical cotton sutures are made from individual cotton fibers that are combed, aligned, and twisted to form a finished strand. Because new types of fibers have been introduced, the use of cotton suture is very rare. Some companies no longer manufacture it.

Umbilical tape, although not actually used for suturing, is produced by suture manufacturers and packaged the same as suture is. It consists of long woven ribbons of cotton, $\frac{1}{16}$ to $\frac{1}{8}$ inch wide, and is used for retraction or suspension of small structures and vessels. (Other soft, pliant products such as vessel loops are available and more common for this purpose.)

Nylon

Surgical nylon (Dermalon, Ethilon, Surgilon, Nurolon, Bralon, Monosof) is a synthetic polyamide material. It is available in two forms: multifilament (braided) and monofilament strands. Multifilament nylon is relatively inert in tissues and has a high tensile strength. It is used in conditions similar to those in which silk and cotton are used. Monofilament nylon is a smooth material particularly well suited for closing skin edges and also for tension sutures. Because of its poor knot security, the surgeon usually ties three knots in small sutures and a double square knot in large sutures. It is frequently used in

TABLE 6-4 | Comparison of Nonabsorbable Sutures

GENERIC OR TRADE NAME	COMPANY	MATERIAL	CONFIGURATION	TENSILE STRENGTH
Cotton	—	Cotton	Twisted	Good
Silk	Ethicon; Davis & Geck; US Surgical	Silk	Braided	Good
Ethilon	Ethicon	Polyamide (nylon)	Monofilament	High
Dermalon	Davis & Geck	Polyamide (nylon)	Monofilament	High
Surgamid	Look	Polyamide (nylon)	Monofilament or braided	High
Nurolon	Ethicon	Polyamide (nylon)	Braided	High
Surgilon	Davis & Geck	Polyamide (nylon) (coated with silicone)	Braided	High
Monosof	US Surgical	Polyamide (nylon)	Monofilament	High
Bralon	US Surgical	Polyamide (nylon)	Braided	High
Prolene	Ethicon	Polyolefin (polypropylene)	Monofilament	Fair
Surgilene	Davis & Geck	Polyolefin (polypropylene)	Monofilament	Good
Demalene	Davis & Geck	Polyolefin (polypropylene)	Monofilament	Good
Surgipro	US Surgical	Polyolefin (polypropylene)	Monofilament	Good
Novafil	Davis & Geck	Polybutester	Monofilament	High
Mersilene	Ethicon	Polyester	Braided	High
Dacron	Deknatel; Davis & Geck	Polyester	Braided	High
Polyviolence	Look	Polyester	Braided	High
Ethibond	Ethicon	Polyester (coated with polybutilate)	Braided	High
Ti-Cron	Davis & Geck	Polyester (coated with silicone)	Braided	High
Polydek	Deknatel	Polyester (coated with Teflon-light)	Braided	High
Tevdek	Deknatel	Polyester (coated with Teflon-heavy)	Braided	High
Surgidac	US Surgical	Polyester (coated with silicone)	Braided	High
Stainless steel	Ethicon	Stainless steel	Monofilament, twisted, or braided	High

From Schwartz, S. (1994). *Principles of surgery* (ed. 6). New York: McGraw-Hill Book Co. and *Ethicon wound closure manual.* (1994). Sommerville, NJ: Ethicon, Inc.

ophthalmology and microsurgery because it can be manufactured in fine sizes. Size 11-0 nylon is one of the smallest suture materials available.

Polyester Fiber

Surgical polyester fiber (Ti-Cron, Dacron, Mersilene, Tevdek, Polydek, Ethibond, Surgidac) is available in two forms: a nontreated polyester fiber suture and a polyester fiber suture that has been specifically coated or impregnated with a lubricant to allow smooth passage through the tissue. Polyester fiber is available in fine filaments that can be braided into various suture sizes to provide good handling properties.

Polybutester (Novafil) is a special type of polyester suture that possesses many of the advantages of both polyester and polypropylene. Because it is a monofilament, it induces little tissue reaction.

Polyester material has many advantages over other braided, nonabsorbable sutures. It has greater tensile strength, minimum tissue reaction, and maximum visibility and does not absorb tissue fluids. It is frequently used as a general-closure fascia suture, as well as in cardiovascular surgery for valve replacements, graft-to-tissue anastomoses, and revascularization procedures.

Polypropylene

Polypropylene is a clear or pigmented polymer. This monofilament suture material (Prolene, Surgilene, Surgipro, Demalene) is used for cardiovascular, general, and plastic surgery. Because polypropylene is a monofilament and is extremely inert in tissue, it may be used in the presence of infection. It has high tensile strength and causes minimal tissue reaction. Sizes range from 10-0 to #2.

Stainless Steel

Surgical stainless steel is formulated to be compatible with stainless steel implants and prostheses. This formula, 316L (L for 'low carbon'), ensures absence of toxic elements, optimal strength, flexibility, and uniform size. Monofilament and multifilament surgical stainless steel is known for its strength, inertness, and low tissue reaction. However, stainless steel–suturing technique is very exacting. Steel can pull or tear out of tissue, and necrosis can result from too tight a suture. Barbs on the end of steel can traumatize surrounding tissue or tear gloves. Torn or cut gloves fail to provide an adequate and effective barrier for the patient or the surgeon and assistant and can remain undetected.[7] Kinks in the wire can render it practically

TISSUE REACTIVITY	HANDLING	KNOT SECURITY	MEMORY	COMMENTS
High	Good	Good	Low	Obsolete, use declining
High	Good	Good	Low	Predisposes to infection; does not tear tissue; D & G suture is silicone treated; Ethicon is coated
Low	Poor	Poor	High	Cuts tissue; nylon; black, clear, or green
Low	Poor	Poor	High	Nylon
Low	Poor	Poor	High	Nylon
Moderate	Good	Fair	Medium	May predispose to infection; black or white; waxed; nylon
Moderate	Fair	Fair	Medium	Nylon
Low	Fair	Fair	Medium	Clear, black
Low	Fair	Fair	Medium	Clear, black, coated
Low	Poor	Poor	High	Very low coefficient of friction; cuts tissue; blue or clear
Low	Poor	Poor	High	—
Low	Poor	Poor	High	—
Low	Poor	Poor	High	Clear or blue
Low	Fair	Poor	Medium	Blue or clear
Moderate	Good	Good	Medium	Green or white
Moderate	Good	Good	Medium	—
Moderate	Good	Good	Medium	Green or white
Moderate	Good	Good	Medium	Green or white
Moderate	Poor	Poor	Medium	—
Moderate	Good	Good	Medium	—
Moderate	Poor	Poor	Medium	—
Moderate	Good	Good	Medium	Green or white
Low	Poor	Good	Low	May kink

TABLE 6–5 | **Steel Suture Comparison**

SIZE (USP)	B&S GAUGE	SIZE (USP)	B&S GAUGE
6-0	40	0	26
6-0	38	1	25
5-0	35	2	24
4-0	34	3	23
4-0	32	4	22
000	30	5	20
00	28	7	18

useless. For this reason, packaging has played an important part in the development of surgical stainless steel sutures. Surgical stainless steel is available in packets on spools or in packages of straight, precut, sterile lengths, with or without swaged needles. This packaging affords protection to the strands and delivery in straight, unkinked lengths.

Before surgical stainless steel's availability from suture manufacturers, it was purchased by weight with the Brown and Sharp (B&S) scale for diameter variations. Today the B&S gauge, along with *USP* size classifications, is used to distinguish diameter ranges. Table 6–5 gives comparisons of steel suture sizes.

PACKAGING, STORAGE, AND SELECTION OF SUTURES

Manufacturers now supply suture materials in some form of sterile package ready for immediate use. The *USP* specifies, "Preserve . . . dry or in fluid, in containers so designed that sterility is maintained until the container is opened."

Types of Packaging

For packaging, the suture material is sealed in a primary inner packet, which may or may not contain fluid; then inside a dry, outer, peel-back packet; and then sterilized. This method permits easy dispensing onto the sterile field. Various forms of foil, plastic, and special paper are used for both the inner and outer packets.

Each primary suture packet is self-contained, and its sterility for each patient is ensured as long as the integrity of the packet is maintained. Some suture packets have expiration dates that relate to stability and sterility. Packages should be stored in moistureproof and dustproof containers in units of one size and type.

Suture packets may contain single or multiple strands, with or without a needle attached to the strand. The needle may be permanently attached (swaged) to the suture and may need to be cut off for removal, or it may be designed to separate easily from the suture with a quick tug of the needle holder (Controlled Release, D-Tach, Pop-off). Some sutures may be double armed, with a needle at each end of the strand.

Color codes

Color-coded packaging based on suture fiber is used by most companies to make identification quicker and easier (Table 6-6). Each individual packet is color coded, as the dispenser box is. Although most color codes are universal across companies, there are some exceptions. Ethibond, a coated polyester, is coded orange, whereas most polyesters are coded in shades of green. Dexon, a glycolic acid polymer, is gold colored, whereas Vicryl, a comparable polymer, is coded violet.

Selection of Suture

The choice of suture depends on the procedure, the tissue being sutured, the general condition of the patient, and the surgeon's preferences. An operating room committee or project team may be responsible for establishing standard suture uses for various operations. Current guides published by suture manufacturers should be consulted. These guides list the specific suture materials recommended for various wounds and are based on current clinical practices and research.

To make delivery of sutures to the field more efficient, one can arrange to have custom packets of mixed sutures for specific procedures or surgeons prepared in advance by suture companies.

HEMOSTASIS

Hemostasis is an ongoing process during surgery. In addition to the damaging physiologic effects of blood loss for the patient, bleeding from cut vessels obscures visualization of the operative site for the surgeon and must be controlled.

Hemostasis may be accomplished with suture materials, electrosurgical devices, lasers, and chemical agents. Before wound closure the surgeon carefully checks the operative site to ensure that all active bleeding has been stopped.

TABLE 6-6 | **Suture Packaging Color Codes**

FIBER	COLOR CODE
Plain gut	Yellow
Chromic gut	Tan
Glycolic acid polymers	Violet*
Silk	Medium blue
Cotton	Pink
Polypropylene	Royal blue
Polyester	Medium green*
Nylon	Light green
Stainless steel	Mustard*

*These color codes may change from one manufacturer to another.

Methods of Ligating Vessels

A ligature is a strand of suture material used to encircle and close off the lumen of a vessel to effect hemostasis, close off a structure, or prevent leakage of materials (Research Highlight 6-1). Ties may be on a reel—a spool or disk containing a long length of suture that the surgeon may use to ligate several superficial vessels. Or they may be free ties—precut lengths of suture handed to the surgeon one at a time, usually for bleeders in deeper tissues.

Following are several techniques used to secure a ligature in deep tissues:

1. A hemostat is placed on the end of the structure; the ligature is then placed around the vessel. The knot is tied and tightened with the surgeon's fingers or with the aid of forceps.
2. A slipknot is made, and its loop is placed over the involved structure by means of a forceps or clamp.
3. In deeper cavities, ties are often placed on clamps with the long end extending from the tip. These are sometimes called *ties on a pass*, or *bow ties*. The extending long end is held tightly against the rings by the surgeon (creating the bow), who then passes the tip of the clamp under the vessel or duct to be ligated. The first assistant grasps the extending tie with a forceps, the surgeon releases it, and the tie is pulled under and up to the wound surface and tied.
4. A forceps or a clamp is applied to the structure and then transfixion sutures are applied and tied. A *suture ligature*, *stick tie*, or *transfixion ligature* is a strand of suture material threaded or swaged on a needle. This is usually placed through the vessel and then around it to prevent the ligature from slipping off the end.

When two ligatures are used to ligate a large vessel, usually a free ligature is placed on the vessel and then a suture ligature is placed distally to the first ligature. To ligate a blood vessel situated in deep tissues, the strand must

---

6-1 RESEARCH HIGHLIGHT

Is a square knot tied with one looped end and one free end more secure than one tied with two free ends? Size 4-0 and 6-0 monofilament nylon, polypropylene, and Biosyn sutures were utilized in this evaluation; mechanical performance was judged according to knot-breakage force and number of throws required to attain security. Results indicated that knots with one looped end and one free end require more throws to ensure knot security than knots constructed from two single suture strands of comparable sizes and types do.

From Annunziata, C.C., Drake, D.B., Woods, J.A., et al. (1996). Technical considerations in knot construction. Part I. Continuous percutaneous and dermal suture closure. *Journal of Emergency Medicine, 15*(3), 351-356.

be of sufficient strength and length to allow the surgeon to tighten the first knot.

The preparation of ligatures and suture ligatures is discussed in a later section of this chapter.

Ligating Clips

Ligating clips are small, V-shaped, staplelike devices that are placed around the lumen of a vessel or structure to close it off. They may be made of one of several metals, such as stainless steel, tantalum, or titanium. Stainless steel clips are the most economical to use. Although more expensive, titanium clips are used frequently in specific surgical procedures because the starburst reflection on postoperative radiographic scans is less with titanium than with other metals. Absorbable clips made of synthetic absorbable suture material are also available.

Ligating clips are available in several sizes; each size requires its own applier, which must be loaded by the scrub person (Fig. 6-2). These clips are available in disposable, prepackaged units. Preloaded, disposable clip appliers that can be used in open wounds, or through endoscope trocar cannulas, are available. Ligating clips afford a rapid and secure method of achieving hemostasis when arteries, veins, nerves, and other small structures are ligated.

Metal Cushing or Frazier clips are made of small diameter pieces of stainless steel or silver wire and are heat sterilized. They must be hand loaded onto special rack dispensers. Frazier clips are applied to the ends of severed nerves and blood vessels by means of a forceps designed for the purpose. They are used in neurosurgery and ortho-

pedic procedures. Since the introduction of prepackaged ligating clips, their use is declining.

SKIN STAPLES

Skin staples are one of the most frequently chosen methods of skin closure. They can be used on many types of surgical incisions. The staple appliers are easy to use, and many are disposable. They reduce both operating time and tissue trauma, allowing uniform tension along the suture line and less distortion from the stress of individual suture points. When properly applied (Fig. 6-3), they provide excellent cosmetic results. The length of time the staples stay in place is dependent on the part of the body affected; they are usually removed within 5 to 7 days from chest or abdominal incisions.[6] An extractor is required for their removal.

Most staplers employ a similar anvil type of mechanism for forming the staple, but the applying device varies from company to company. Surgeon's choice is usually determined by the applier's weight, handling characteristics, ease of application, and unobstructed view of the site during application. They are packaged in various assortments of numbers and types of staples, depending on the length of the incision and the type of tissue encountered.

SKIN TAPES

Wounds that are subjected to minimal static and dynamic tension are easily approximated with skin tape. The selection of surgical tape for skin closure is based on the tape's adhesive ability, tensile strength, and porosity. The tape must provide a firm tape-to-skin bond to keep the wound edges closely adherent. The tensile strength must be sufficient to maintain wound approximation. A tape that is too occlusive limits moisture or vapor transmission; fluid may accumulate under the tape and lead to maceration and bacterial growth. Microporous tapes prevent this. The tape must be applied to dry skin; an adhesive adjunct (such as tincture of benzoin or Mastisol) may be applied in a thin film to the skin at the wound edges before tape application. Tapes are applied perpendicularly to the wound edge, first on one side and then the other, so that the edges can be pulled together (Fig. 6-4).

SURGICAL NEEDLES

Surgical needles vary considerably in shape, size, point design, and wire diameter (Fig. 6-5). The appropriate needle is selected depending on the type and location of tissue being sutured. Surgical needles are made from either stainless steel or carbon steel. They must be strong, ductile, and able to withstand the stress imposed by tough tissue. Stainless steel is the most popular, not only because it provides these physical characteristics but also because it is noncorrosive.

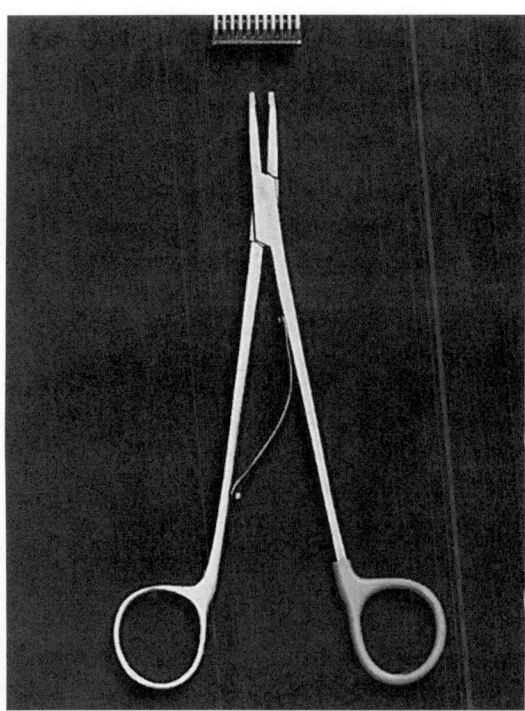

FIGURE 6-2 Ligating clip applier with large, medium, and small clips.

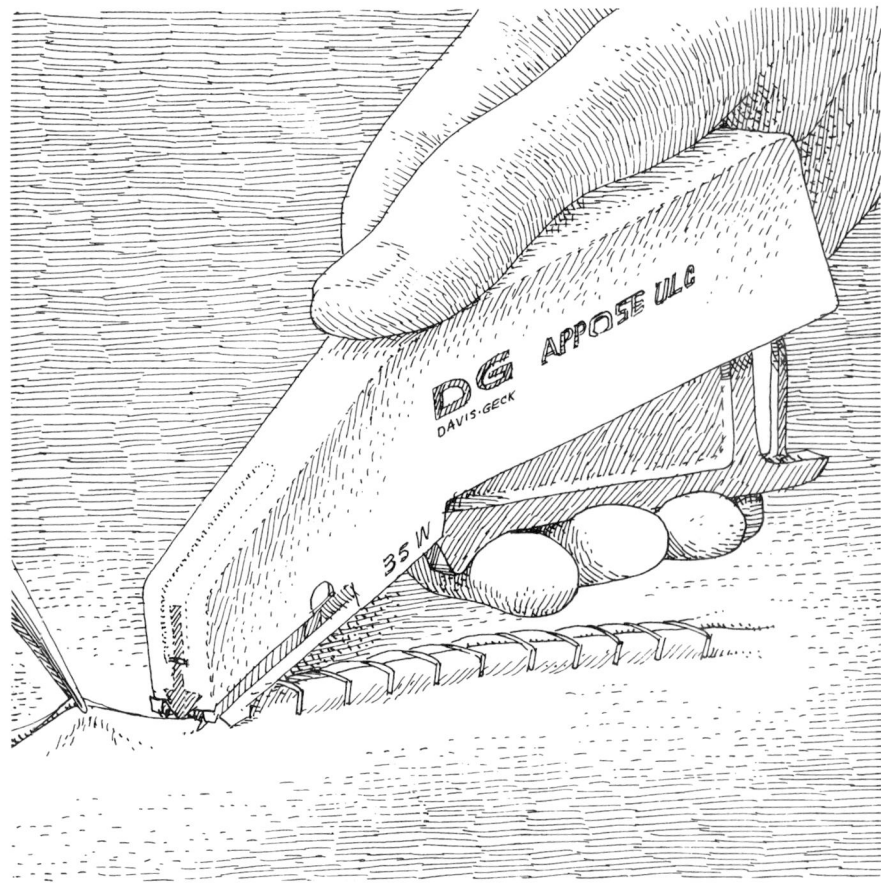

FIGURE 6-3 Application of skin staples. The stapler is lightly positioned over everted skin edges. It is not necessary to press the staple, or stapler anvil, into the skin to get a proper "bite" (just "kiss" the skin). Center the staples over the incision line, using the locating arrow or guideline, and place approximately ¼ inch apart.

There are three basic parts of a surgical needle: the eye, the body, and the point or tip.

Eye

The eye of the surgical needle falls into three general categories: (1) eyed needles, in which the needle, which must be threaded with the suture strand, and two strands of suture must be pulled through the tissue (Fig. 6-6, *A*); (2) spring, or French, eyed needles, in which the suture is placed or snapped through the spring (Fig. 6-6, *B*); and (3) eyeless needles, a needle-suture combination in which a needle is swaged (permanently attached) onto one or both ends of the suture material (Fig. 6-6, *C*).

The swaged needle is the most universally used needle type. Swaged needles eliminate threading eyed needles before and during surgery. The surgeon draws a single strand of suture material through the tissue, and tissue damage is thereby minimized (atraumatic). The swaged needle must be cut off with scissors.

A needle swaged for controlled release of the suture (semiswaged) facilitates interrupted suturing techniques.

The needle remains attached until the surgeon releases it with a straight tug of the needle holder.

Body

The body, or shaft, of the needle may be round, triangular, or flattened (Table 6-7). Surgical needles may also be straight or curved; the curve is described as part of an imaginary circle (see Fig. 6-5). As the radius of the imaginary circle increases, the size of the needle also increases. The body of a round needle gradually tapers to a point.

Point

Choice of needle point relates to density of the tissue to be penetrated. Delicate tissue, such as bowel or kidney, requires a taper or blunted point, whereas skin, which is dense in structure, requires a cutting edge. Taper points tend to tear tissue less than cutting needles do and leave a smaller hole in the tissue. Recently introduced blunt protect-point needles are being recommended as an alternative to taper point needles. Interest in blunt needles

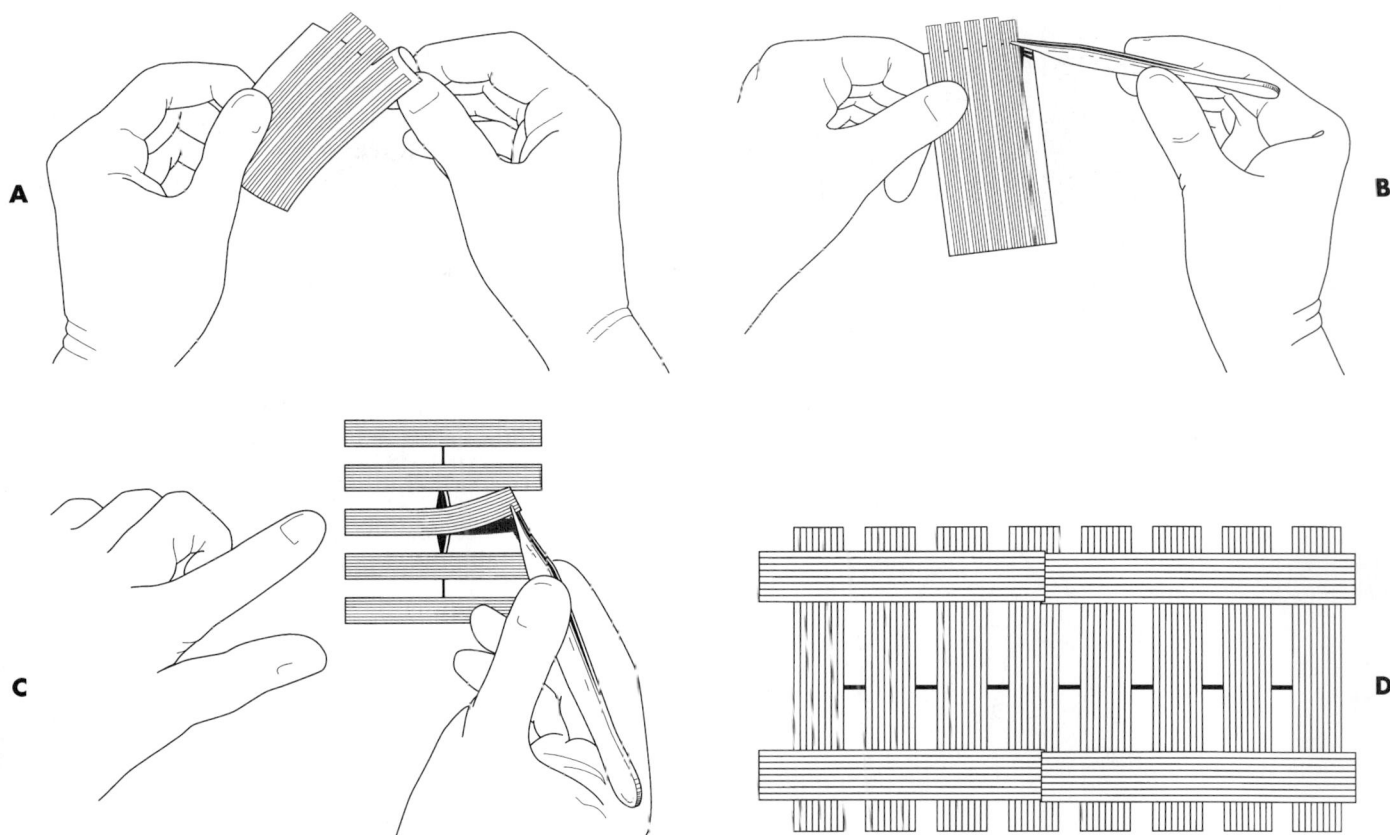

FIGURE 6-4   Application of skin tapes. **A,** Perforated tab is bent and removed. **B,** Tape is peeled from the card. **C,** Tape is applied to wound. **D,** Additional tape is placed parallel to wound to limit shear stress on the skin.

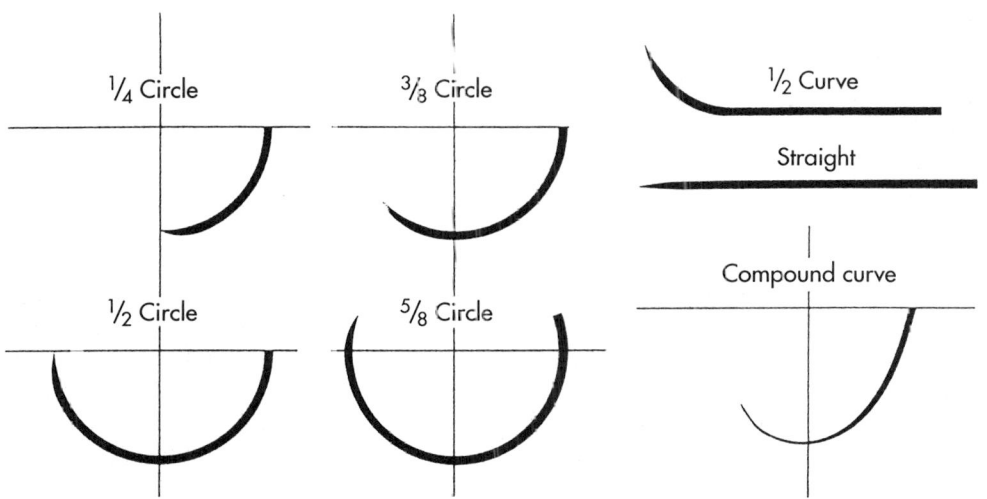

FIGURE 6-5   Surgical needles vary in shape, size, type of point and body, and how the suture is attached.

has evolved because of the risk of bloodborne exposure from percutaneous injuries (PIs). Reports of such injuries have been estimated as occurring in 1% to 15% of surgical procedures, mostly associated with suturing. Some studies have been done to evaluate the effectiveness of blunt needles in preventing PIs and to assess their clinical acceptability by surgeons. Results of these studies indicate that blunt needles are associated with a statistically significant reduction in PIs and can be substituted for conventional curved needles in a variety of surgical procedures.[3] Table 6-7 illustrates the type of points available for various tissues.

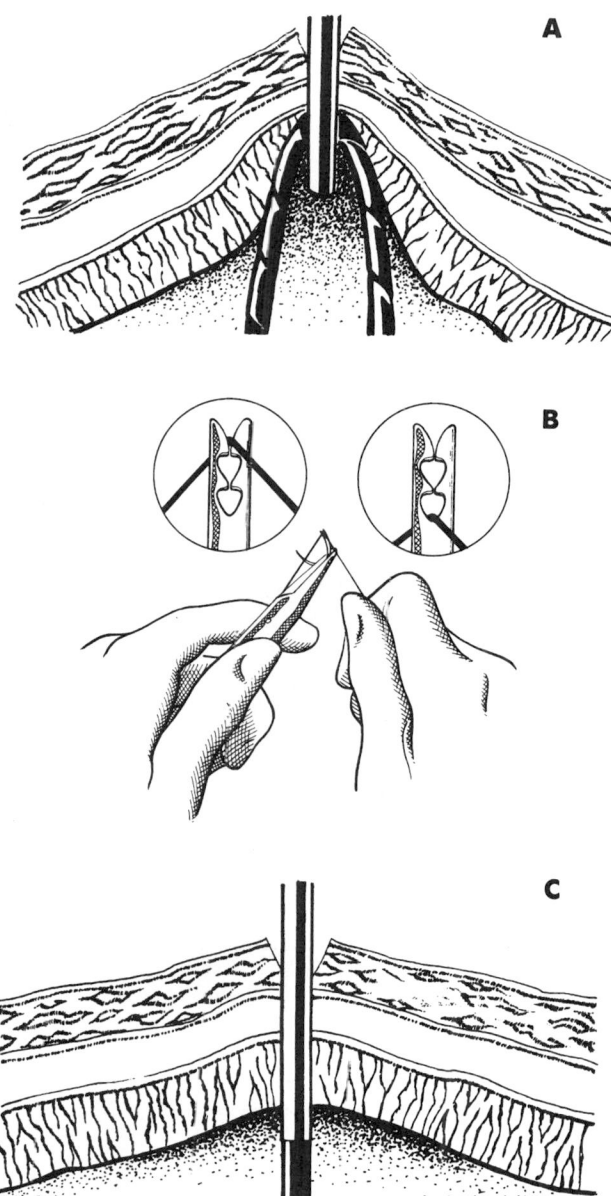

FIGURE 6-6 Types of needles. **A,** Eyed needle. Greater tissue trauma is caused by the double suture strand threaded through eyed needles. **B,** Spring eye. Holding suture strand taut with left hand, bring strand down over top and spring into eye. **C,** Atraumatic needle causes minimum tissue trauma by eliminating the double suture strand.

Triangular needles have cutting edges along three sides. The cutting action may be conventional or reverse. The conventional cutting needle has its cutting edge directed along the inner curve of the needle, facing the wound edge when suturing is performed.

The reverse cutting needle is preferred for cutaneous suturing. When it transsects the skin lateral to the wound, the outside edge is pointed away from the wound edge, and the inside flat edge is parallel to the edge of the wound. This cutting action creates a reduced tendency for the suture to tear through tissue.

For certain types of delicate surgery, needles with exceptionally sharp points and cutting edges are used. Microsurgery, ophthalmology, and plastic surgery require needles of this type; special honing wheels provide needles of precision-point quality for surgeons in these specialties. In some instances the application of a microthin layer of plastic to the needle surface provides for easier penetration and a reduction in drag of the needle through the tissue.

Most surgical services departments have instituted standardization programs to control the variety of needle-suture combinations available for surgical procedures.

SUTURING METHODS
Closure of Wounds

The *primary suture line* refers to the sutures that obliterate dead space, prevent serum from accumulating in the wound, and hold the wound edges in approximation until healing takes place (Fig. 6-7). The *secondary suture line* refers to sutures that supplement the primary suture line. They are placed on each side of the primary suture line, passing through several layers of tissue at once. They help eliminate tension on the primary sutures and reduce the risk of evisceration or dehiscence. Retention sutures are a type of secondary suture line.

An *interrupted suture* is inserted into tissues or vessels in such a way that each stitch is placed and tied individually. This type of suture is widely used and generally considered the strongest and most secure (Fig. 6-8, *A*). The various techniques used for the insertion of interrupted sutures in the tissue are designed to alter the angle of pull and the relationship of the wound's edges to each other. Such maneuvers cause the edges of the wound either to invert or to evert and aid in wound healing because fewer sutures are used. This type of stitch is usually used on skin and may be used on any underlying tissue layer.

A *continuous suture* consists of a series of stitches, of which only the first and last are tied (Fig. 6-8, *B*). With this type of suture a break at any point may mean a disruption of the entire suture line. It is used to close tissue layers where there is little tension but tight closure is required, such as the peritoneum, to prevent the intestinal loops from protruding, or on blood vessels to prevent leakage.

Retention, or *stay*, *sutures* placed at a distance from the primary suture line provide a secondary suture line (Fig. 6-8, *C*), relieve undue strain, and help obliterate dead space. Wound dehiscence is often the result of a combination of factors, including technical problems with closure, local wound factors (infection or hematoma), poor wound healing, and undue stress on the wound (abdominal distention, dilated bowel, vomiting, coughing, chronic obstructive pulmonary disease [COPD]).[4] Predisposing factors such as sepsis, poor nutrition, diabetes, chemotherapy, advanced malignancy, and steroids contribute to poor wound healing. With patients in whom these

TABLE 6-7 | **Atraumatic Needles**

NEEDLE TYPE	DESCRIPTION OF BODY	USE
Taper point	Round shaft, straight or curved, tapered point, no cutting edge	Soft-tissue closure such as gastrointestinal, fascial, vascular, and most soft tissues below the skin surface
Penetrating point	Taper body with finely sharpened point. Optimum penetration with less tissue wound	Ligaments, tendons, calcified, fibrous and cuticular tissue; mostly used for vascular, thoracic, plastic, Ob/Gyn, and orthopedic surgery; excellent penetration through synthetic grafts and scar tissue during repeat surgeries
Blunt point	Taper body with a rounded point, no cutting edge	Friable tissue, fascia, liver, intestine, kidney, muscle, uterine cervix. Note recommendations regarding use of blunt needles, page 183.
Protect-point	Taper body with a blunted point, no cutting edge	Used primarily in fascia and mass closure to minimize the potential of needle sticks
Reverse cutting	Triangular point with cutting edge on the outer curvature	Skin closure, retention sutures, subcutaneous, ligamentous, or fibrous tissues
Cutting taper	Reverse cutting tip with taper shaft	Used in microsurgery for excellent penetration through tough tissue, such as vasovasostomy, tuboplasty
Hand-honed reverse cutting	Same as reverse cutting but hand-honed for added sharpness	Primarily used in plastic surgery for delicate work and where a good cosmetic result is a concern
Spatula side cutting	Two cutting edges in a horizontal plane	Ophthalmic surgery for muscle and retinal repair. Also used for delicate eyelid or plastic surgery; cutting edges "ride" along scleral layers
Regular cutting	Triangular point with cutting edge on the inner curvature	General skin closure, subcutaneous tissue, sometimes for ophthalmic surgery, plastic or reconstructive surgery
Lancet Inverted lancet	Spatula needle with the cutting edge on the inner (lancet) or outer (inverted lancet) curvature	Ophthalmic and microsurgery

Modified from Davis & Geck. (1992). *Surgical atlas and suture selection guide* (ed. 2). Wayne, NJ: American Cyanamid.

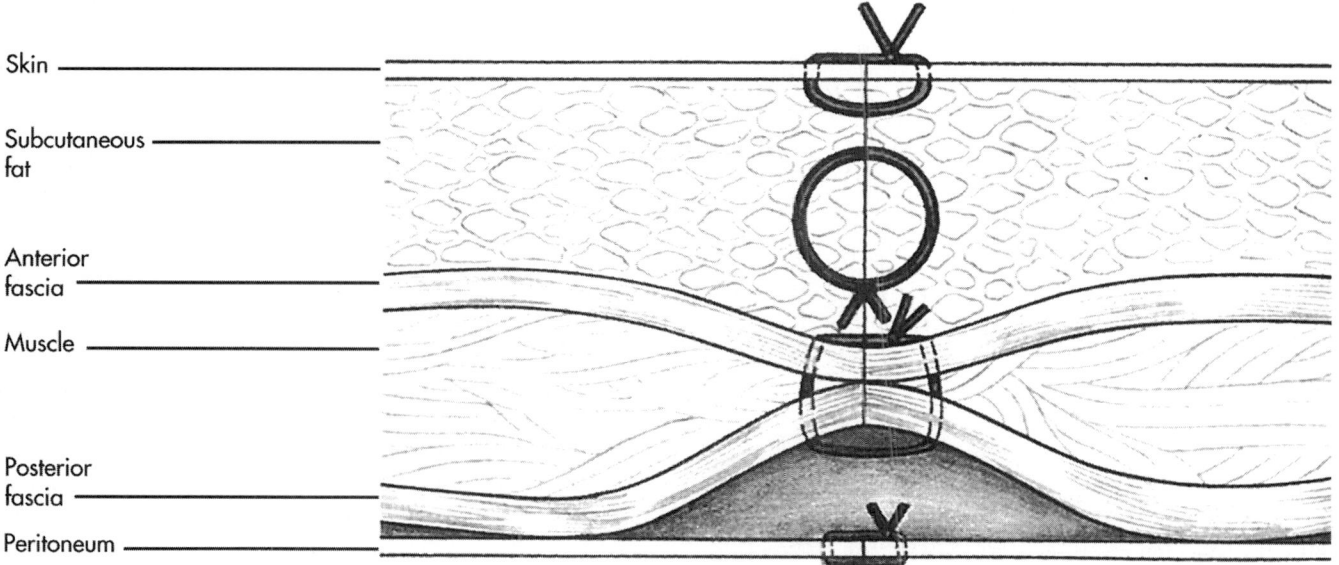

FIGURE 6-7   Primary suture line on the abdominal wall, midline incision.

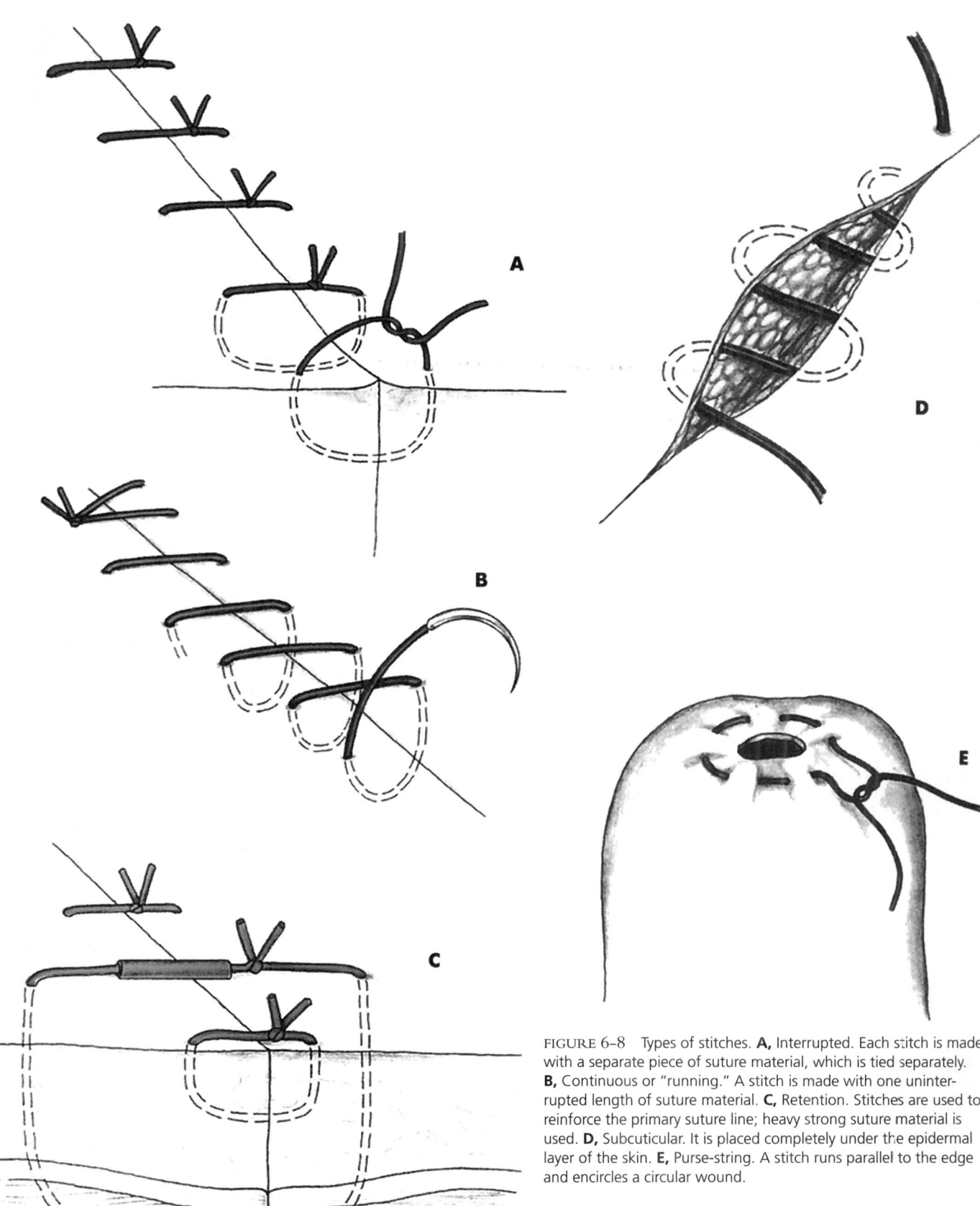

FIGURE 6-8   Types of stitches. **A,** Interrupted. Each stitch is made with a separate piece of suture material, which is tied separately. **B,** Continuous or "running." A stitch is made with one uninterrupted length of suture material. **C,** Retention. Stitches are used to reinforce the primary suture line; heavy strong suture material is used. **D,** Subcuticular. It is placed completely under the epidermal layer of the skin. **E,** Purse-string. A stitch runs parallel to the edge and encircles a circular wound.

factors exist, retention sutures are likely to be used. They are placed in such a way that they include most if not all layers of the wound. A simple interrupted or figure-of-eight stitch is used. Usually heavy, nonabsorbable suture materials such as silk, nylon, polyester fiber, or wire are used to close long, vertical abdominal wounds and lacerated or infected wounds. To prevent the suture from cutting into the skin surface, a small piece of rubber tubing (bumper, bolster, bootie) or other type of device (bridge, button) is passed over or through the exposed portion of the suture. The bridge device allows the surgeon to adjust tension over the wound postoperatively.

Subcuticular sutures, sometimes referred to as buried, are those placed completely under the epidermal layer of the skin (Fig. 6-8, *D*).

A *purse-string suture* is a continuous circular suture placed to surround an opening in a structure and cause it to close (Fig. 6-8, *E*). This type of suture may be placed around the appendix before its removal or in an organ such as the cecum, gallbladder, or urinary bladder before it is opened so that a drainage tube can be inserted, followed by tightening of the purse-string suture around the tube.

Endoscopic Suturing

Suturing through a laparoscope is a learned skill, not an innate talent. The ports must be placed and utilized to maximize the precision and efficiency of the suturing motions. There is an array of needles and suture materials available for laparoscopic suturing so that the surgeon is not disadvantaged by a lack of choice.

Holding a Drain in Place

If a drainage tube is inserted into a wound, the tube may be anchored to the skin with a nonabsorbable suture so that it will not slip in or out. A tube left in a hollow viscus, such as the gallbladder or common duct, may be secured to the wall of that organ with an absorbable suture.

Knot-Tying Technique

The successful use of the many varieties of suture materials depends, in final analysis, on the skill with which the surgeon or first assistant ties the knot. The completed knot should be firm, to prevent slipping, and small, with ends cut short, to minimize the bulk of suture material in the wound.

The suture may be weakened by inappropriate handling. One should avoid excessive tension, sawing, friction between the strands, and inadvertent crushing with clamps or hemostats.

Endoscopic Knot Tying

Knot tying is one of the most challenging aspects of laparoscopic surgery. There are preformed ligature loops used in ligating the appendix or blood vessels. Extracorporeal knots are tied outside the abdomen and slid into the abdomen using a knot pusher. They can be tied rapidly and securely; the square knot is normally used as the locking loop knot. Intracorporeal knotting is done completely within the abdominal cavity whenever fine sutures are being placed in tissues for reconstruction purposes. All suturing and knot-tying techniques performed through the laparoscope require excellent hand-eye coordination, practice and the ability to perform these techniques while the anatomy is being viewed on a television monitor.

PERIOPERATIVE NURSING CONSIDERATIONS

General Considerations

In the preparation and use of sutures in surgery, every precaution must be taken to keep the sutures sterile, to prevent prolonged exposure and unnecessary handling, and to avoid waste. Before perioperative staff prepare the sutures, they should review the sutures listed in the card file or computerized data sheet for a particular procedure and surgeon. The scrub person should prepare only one or two sutures during the preliminary preparation, but the circulator should have an adequate supply of sutures available for immediate dispensing to the sterile instrument table.

Customized suture kits that contain a designated number and variety of sutures for particular procedures, surgeons, or both are available for use when suture preferences are consistently the same. These kits may be more economical than individually packaged sutures because of reduced packaging costs, decreased gathering and dispensing times, and less capital outlay for inventory.

Opening Primary Packets

The scrub person tears the foil packet across the notch near the hermetically sealed edge and removes the suture (Fig. 6-9). Some sutures are now packaged for delivery to the field in their inner folders, ready to load, with no foil wrapper.

Handling Suture Materials

To remove suture strands to be used for ties when they are not on a reel or disk, the loose end is pulled out with one hand while the folder is grasped with the other hand. To straighten a long suture, the free end is grasped (using the thumb and forefinger of the free hand), the kinks, caused by package memory, are removed by gentle pulling with the free end secured, one in each hand, and then the arms are slowly abducted to straighten the strands.

Kinks should never be removed by running gloved fingers over the strand because this action causes fraying. The tensile strength of a gut suture should not be tested

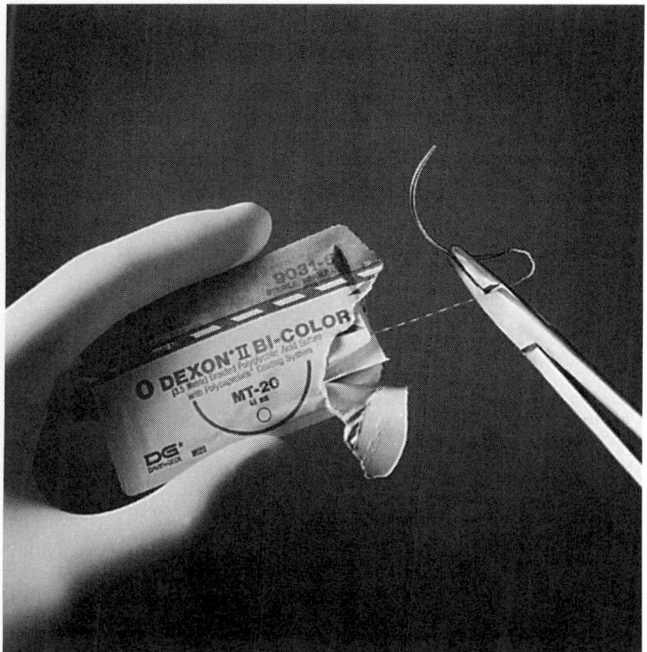

FIGURE 6-9   Loading a suture directly from packet.

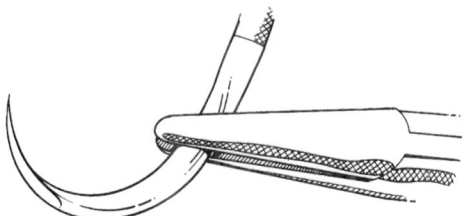

FIGURE 6-10   Loading a needle holder. Clamp needle holder approximately one third the distance from the swage or eye to point of needle.

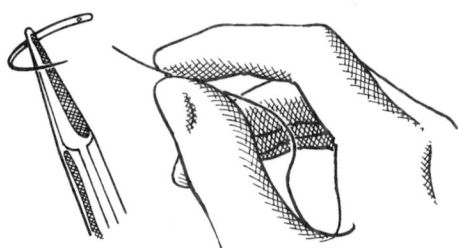

FIGURE 6-11   Eyed needle is threaded from inside curvature. Take care to avoid pricking glove on sharp needle point.

before it is handed to the surgeon. Sudden pulls or jerks used to test the tensile strength may damage the suture so that it will break when in use.

To prepare individual lengths of ligature or suture, the strand is folded in equal parts and held between the fingers and then divided. Standard 54-inch lengths of suture may be cut in quarters, thirds, or halves by the scrub person to meet most procedure needs. For general surgery a continuous suture threaded on a needle is usually about 24 inches long, and its short end is 3 to 4 inches long (half lengths). An interrupted suture is 12 to 14 inches long, with 2 or 3 inches threaded through the needle (quarter lengths). To ligate a vessel in the epidermal and subcutaneous layers, the ligature may be 12 to 14 inches long (quarter lengths). However, vessels or structures deep in the wound are ligated with a suture or ligature that is 24 to 30 inches long (third to half lengths). Sutures are also provided in 12- to 60-inch precut lengths by the manufacturer.

Also supplied are labyrinth packs, where precut strands may be removed one at a time from the package rather than all at once, and the more commonly used 54-inch lengths on reels or disks (discussed earlier).

To remove a suture-needle combination from the package, the scrub person grasps the needle of the suture with a needle holder and gently pulls the strand to remove it. To straighten the suture in a suture-needle combination, the scrub person grasps the suture 1 to 2 inches distal to the needle and pulls gently on the other end of the strand with the other hand to remove kinks. The jaws of the needle holder grasp the flattened surface of the needle to prevent breakage and bending. To facilitate suturing, the needle is

secured about 1/8-inch down from the tip of the needle holder (Fig. 6-10). The holder is placed on the needle about a third of the distance in from the eye or swaged end.

A suture or free ligature should not be too long or too short. A long suture is difficult to handle and increases the possibility of contamination because it may be dragged across the sterile field or fall below it. A short suture makes tying difficult, and if threaded on a needle, it may slip out of the eye.

The depth and distance to the site of tying or suturing guide the scrub person in preparing ties or sutures of the correct length.

Threading Surgical Needles

Free needles, those that come packaged separately from the suture, must be threaded by the scrub person for the surgeon. A curved needle is threaded from within its curvature so that the short end falls away from the outside curvature (Fig. 6-11). This practice helps to prevent accidental pullout. The scrub person pulls the suture about 4 inches through the eye of the needle to prevent the suture from being pulled out of the eye during suturing.

Counting Needles

Institutions vary in their policies regarding needle and sharp counts during operative procedures, but most follow procedure based on AORN Recommended Practices for Sponge, Sharp, and Instrument Counts.[1] Initial counts before the start of the procedure provide the basis for subsequent counts. Items added during the procedure should be counted and documented. The count should be

6-2 RESEARCH HIGHLIGHT

As of June 1996, 51 documented and 108 possible cases of occupationally acquired HIV infection have been reported to the CDC. The estimated risk of acquiring HIV infection after percutaneous exposure to blood from an HIV infection patient is 0.3%. The risk of hepatitis C virus (HCV) transmission to healthcare workers has not been well defined up to now. There is documentation of both HIV and HCV exposure from a single source in which seroconversion to HIV was detected with commercially available assays between 8 and 9½ months after exposure; seroconversion to HCV occurred between 9½ and 13½ months after exposure. These times for seroconversion are unusually long for both viruses; however, the clinical course for the patient was rapid progression to hepatic failure and death. Although the Public Health Service interagency group did not recommend routine HIV serologic follow-up beyond 6 months after exposure, the possible pathogenetic interactions between HIV and HCV warrant further study in the simultaneous occupational exposure to HIV and HCV or in the event of clinical symptoms or signs of infection more than 6 months after exposure to evaluate for late seroconversion.

From Ridzon, R., Gallagher, K., Ciesielski, C., et al. (1997). Simultaneous transmission of human immunodeficiency virus and hepatitis C virus from a needle stick injury. *New England Journal of Medicine, 336*(13), 919-922.

performed audibly and with each sharp visualized by the scrub person and circulator.

During the procedure, needles should be accounted for by the scrub person as they are handed to the surgeon on a one-for-one exchange basis. Subsequent counts should be performed by the scrub person and circulator before closure of a body cavity or deep, large incision, after closure of a body cavity, when either person is relieved by other personnel, and immediately before completion of the surgical intervention. It is imperative that two persons be involved in the count—one counting and the other witnessing that the count is correct.

Many institutions have printed forms to keep track of routinely counted items. Others use erasable count boards visible to all personnel. Recording the count is the responsibility of the circulator. The count sheet may become part of the patient's record. To facilitate counting, used needles should be kept on a needle pad or counter on the scrub person's table. Broken or missing needles must be reported to the surgeon and accounted for in their entirety. Each institution should have established policies for dealing with incorrect counts.

Sharps No-touch Technique

Scalpel blades and suture needles together accounted for 17% of reported injuries from solid (non–hollow bore) devices in a study of 58 hospitals.[5] Most of these injuries occurred in the operating room. Because sharp instruments used in surgery are a frequent cause of injury, recommendations for eliminating hand-to-hand passing have been developed.

Based on OSHA regulations and the Standard Precautions of the Centers for Disease Control and Prevention (CDC),[2] institutions should have written policies regarding the handling of contaminated equipment, including handling contaminated sharp instruments and needles at the surgical field. OSHA recommends passing only clean sharps and needles to the surgeon. After use, the surgeon places the contaminated object in a predesignated basin, tray, collection device, or safe "neutral" zone on the field, from which the scrub person will retrieve it. This technique eliminates hand-to-hand passing of contaminated sharps between the surgeon and the scrub person, such that no two people touch the same sharp at the same time, reducing the chance of accidental needle punctures and cuts (Research Highlight 6-2). All sharps should be accounted for and properly disposed of before the room is prepared for the next patient.

INSTRUMENTS

Historical Perspective

The history of surgical instruments dates back to 2500 B.C. The first instruments were sharpened flints and fine animal teeth. Ancient Greek, Egyptian, and Hindu instruments are amazing in their resemblance to contemporary instruments.

In the late 1700s, to be equipped for the practice of surgery, the surgeon had to employ various skilled artisans such as coppersmiths, steelworkers, needle grinders, turners of wood, bone, and ivory, and silk and hemp spinners. The surgeon had to explain the mechanisms of the instruments and supervise their manufacture. The resulting instruments were crude, expensive, and time consuming to make. Each artisan used hand labor exclusively, devoted time to making only one type of instrument, and thereby gained proficiency. For example, a cutter would keep a small supply of surgical knives. Thus began physician's supply houses and surgical instrument making.

In the mid-1800s, physicians' principal tools were their eyes and ears. Official records show that amputation, the trademark of the Civil War, was the result in three of four operations. Surgeons were scarce and medical instruments almost nonexistent. Kitchen knives and penknives, carpenter saws, and table forks did the job. After the Civil War, the advent of the administration of ether and chloroform brought a demand for new ideas and methods in surgery and instruments. The division of general surgery into specialties took place in the late 1800s and early 1900s. Delicate instruments were seen as more useful than the force of crude and heavy instruments. So that instruments could withstand repeated sterilization, handles of wood, ivory, and rubber were discontinued.

The development of stainless steel in Germany ensured a better material for surgical instruments and other equipment. Today, surgeons and perioperative nurses assist manufacturers in research for new and better instrumentation. Most instrument companies will design an instrument to a physician's specifications.

Composition of Surgical Instruments

Perioperative nurses are responsible for the use, handling, and care of hundreds of surgical instruments a day. A basic knowledge of how these instruments are manufactured can help in their selection and maintenance. Surgical instruments are expensive and represent a major investment for every institution.

Instruments used today are made in the United States and in other countries such as Germany, France, and Pakistan. The United States does not have an agency that reviews or sets standards for surgical instruments. The quality is set by the individual manufacturer. A reputable company stands behind its product. A properly cared for instrument should last 10 years or more.

Most instruments are manufactured from stainless steel. Stainless steel is a compound of iron, carbon, and chromium, which means that stainless steel can have varying qualities. These qualities are designated by grading the steel into series by the American Iron and Steel Institute (AISI). For example, the 400 series stainless steel has some noncorrosive characteristics and good tensile strength. It resists rust, produces a fine point, and retains a keen edge. Hand-held ringed instruments, such as scissors and clamps, should be 400 series stainless steel.

For ringed instruments, the raw steel is converted into instrument blanks by a machinist making an impression of the piece in a stainless steel blank. These blanks are then die forged into specific pieces, male and female halves. The excess metal is trimmed away, and the instrument parts are ready for the final steps.

The two halves are then milled to prepare the box lock fittings, jaw serrations, and ratchets, and the jaws and shanks are properly aligned. After this step is done, the halves are assembled by hand. A hole is drilled through the box lock, and a pin or rivet is inserted through the hole. Final grinding and hardening accomplished by heat-treating bring the object to proper size, weight, spring temper, and balance.

The last part of the process is called *passivation*. The instruments are put into nitric acid to remove any residue of carbon steel. The nitric acid also produces a surface coating of chromium oxide. Chromium oxide is important because it produces a resistance to corrosion in the stainless steel instrument. The instrument is then polished.

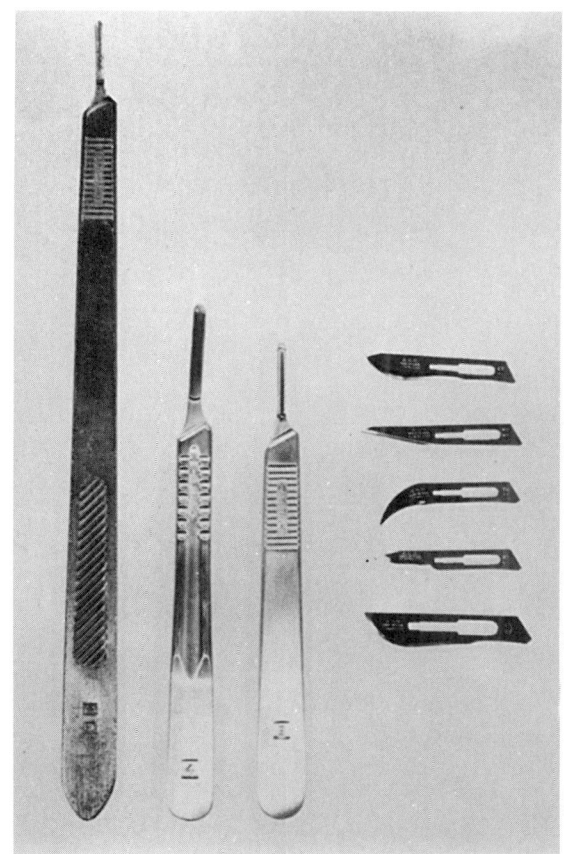

FIGURE 6-12 Long and regular-length knife handles with assortment of blades. Blades, *top to bottom*, numbers 10, 11, 12, 15, and 20.

There are three types of instrument finishes. The first is the bright, highly polished mirror finish, which tends to reflect light and may interfere with the vision of the surgeon. The second is the satin or dull finish, which tends to eliminate glare and lessen eyestrain for the surgeon. The third finish is ebonizing, which produces a black finish. Ebonized instruments are used during laser surgery to prevent deflection of the laser beam. The final inspection and testing are for hardness, proper jaw closure, and smooth lock-and-ratchet action. The instrument is then ready for sale.

Instrument Categories

Although there is no standard nomenclature for specific instruments, there are four main categories: dissectors, clamps, retractors, and accessory or ancillary instruments.

Dissectors

Dissectors, which may be sharp or blunt, are instruments used to cut or separate tissue. The largest categories of sharp dissecting instruments are scalpels and scissors. Scalpels are probably the oldest of all surgical instruments (Fig. 6-12). Most scalpels are handles with one end suited to the attachment of disposable blades. During an

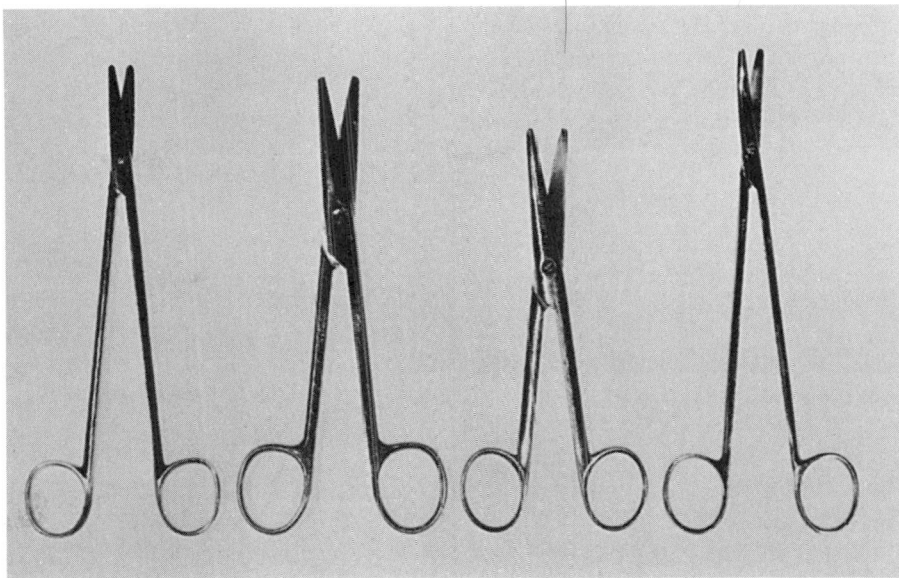

FIGURE 6-13   Commonly used scissors. *Left to right*, Straight, blunt dissecting scissors; heavy or suture scissors; Mayo scissors; Metzenbaum scissors.

operation the blades may be conveniently changed by the scrub person as often as necessary. The blades come prepackaged and sterile and are passed onto the sterile field as needed by the circulator. Careful handling of blades during the procedure and disposal of blades at the end of a procedure are important in the implementation of Standard Precautions.

Scissors are designed in various shapes and sizes for different purposes in cutting body tissues and surgical materials (Fig. 6-13). The basic design consists in two blades, each having a chisel-shaped edge with the bevel consistent with the structure or material it has to cut. Scissor tips may be blunt or sharp, and the blades straight or curved. Conventional scissors require two movements in use: one to open and another to close the jaws. Other scissors may have a spring action in the body design that holds the jaws in an open position. A single movement pressing the spring together closes the jaws to cut. Scissors designed for delicate plastic and eye surgery are often of the latter type. A basic instrument set usually includes a curved Mayo scissors for dissection of heavy tissues, a Metzenbaum scissors for dissection of delicate tissues, and a straight scissors for cutting suture. For surgery in deep areas of the body, scissors with long handles and short blades are used for better control and easier use.

Other sharp dissectors include drills, saws, osteotomes, rongeurs, and other instruments such as adenotomes and dermatomes.

Some instruments in the dissecting category are produced in sharp or blunt form, such as curettes and periosteal elevators.

Instruments or devices used for blunt dissection include peanuts, a sponge on a stick, the back of a knife handle, and the surgeon's finger or hand.

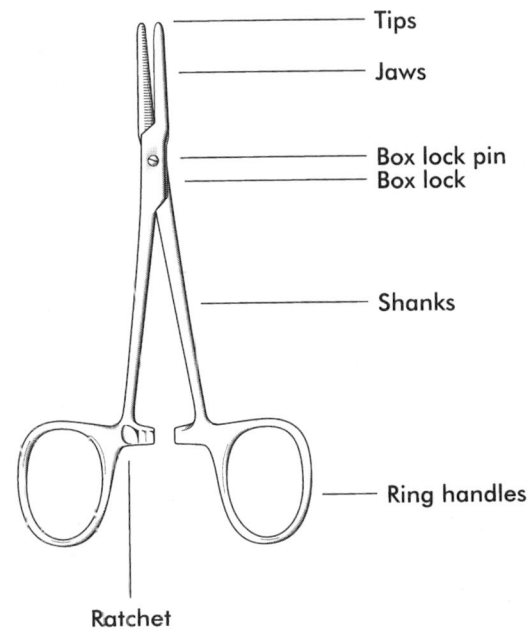

FIGURE 6-14   Anatomy of a clamp.

Clamps

Clamps are instruments specifically designed for holding tissue or other materials, and most have an easily recognizable design. They have finger rings, for ease of holding; shanks whose length is appropriate to the wound depth; ratchets, on the shanks near the rings, which allow for the distal tip to be locked on the tissue or object grasped; a joint, usually a box lock (described later), which joins the two halves of the instrument and allows opening and closing of the instrument; and a jaw, which is the working portion of the instrument and defines its use (Fig. 6-14). Clamps are divided into the following categories.

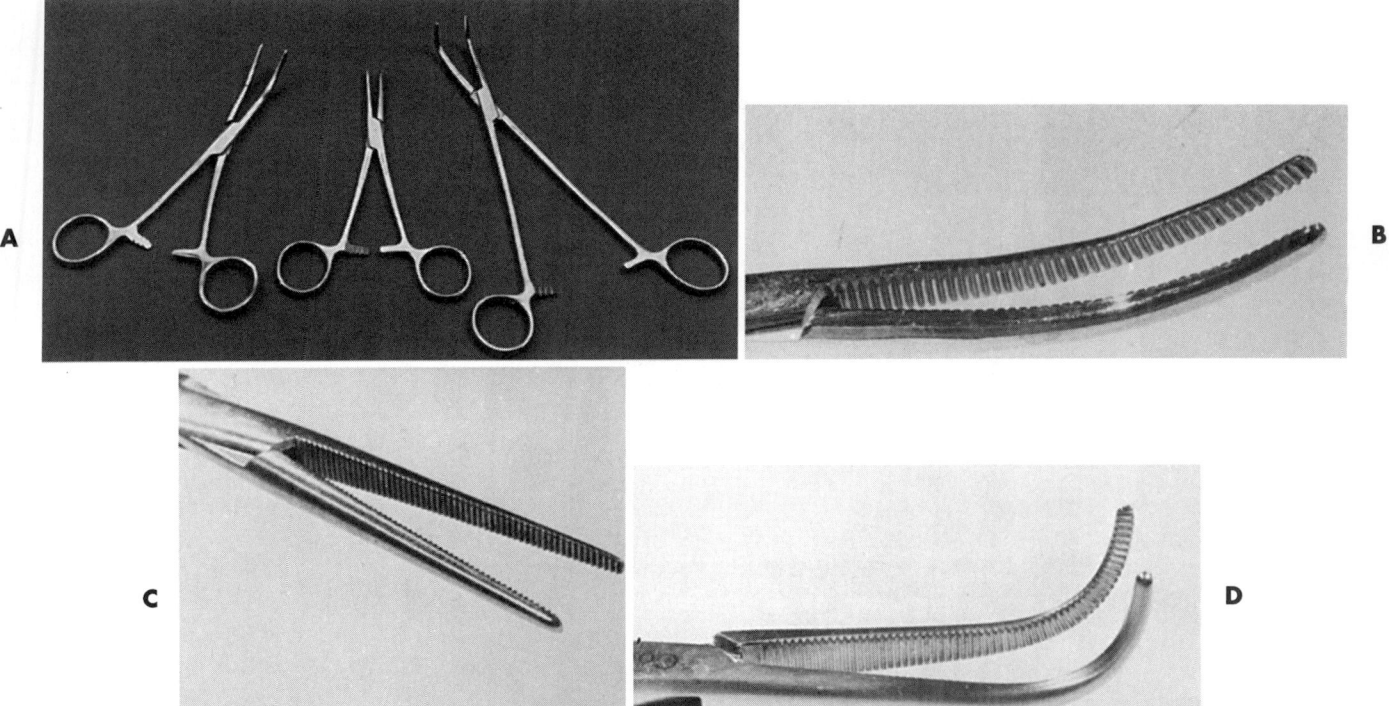

FIGURE 6-15   **A,** Commonly used hemostatic clamps. **B,** Curved Kelly. **C,** Straight Kelly. **D,** Right-angled.

Hemostats are used to close the severed ends of a vessel with a minimum of tissue damage. They prevent the excessive loss of blood in the course of dissection. The jaws must have deep transverse cuts so that the bleeding vessels may be compressed with sufficient force to stop bleeding. The serrations must be cleanly cut and perfectly meshed to prevent the tissue from slipping free from the jaws of the clamp (Fig. 6-15).

Occluding clamps usually have vertical serrations or special jaws that have finely meshed, multiple rows of longitudinally arranged teeth to prevent leakage and to minimize trauma when clamping bowel, vessels, or ducts that are to be reanastomosed. The surgical service usually selects a hemostat or clamp design according to surgeons' preferences.

Graspers and *holders* are used for tissue retraction and generally have jaws of specific design based on their use (Fig. 6-16, *A*). The Allis clamp has multiple, fine teeth on the tip so as not to crush or damage tissue (Fig. 6-16, *B*). The Kocher clamp has transverse serrations as well as large teeth (1 × 2) at its tip to grasp tightly on tough, slippery tissue such as fascia (Fig. 6-16, *C*). The Babcock clamp has curved, fenestrated tips with no teeth, and it grips or encloses delicate structures such as bowel, ureters, or fallopian tubes (Fig. 6-16, *D*). Other holding forceps have handles like clamps with specialized tips or jaws. These jaws may be triangular, straight, angular, or T-shaped.

Nonclamp graspers and holders are known as *forceps*, or *pickups*, because they are used to lift and hold tissue. Often, while the surgeon is cutting with scissors or sewing with a needle, forceps are used in the other hand. The most common kinds are the various two-arm spring forceps (Fig. 6-17). Tweezerlike, they vary in length and thickness and are available with and without teeth. Nontoothed forceps create minimal damage and hold delicate, thin tissues. Toothed forceps hold thick or slippery tissues that need extra grip.

Grasper and holder clamps may hold objects as well. Sponge-holding forceps with ring-shaped jaws are available in 7- and 9-inch lengths. They can be used to grasp or handle tissue but are usually used as sponge holders. A gauze sponge is folded and placed in the jaws and is then used to retract tissue, to absorb blood in the field, and occasionally to perform blunt dissection.

Needle holders (Fig. 6-18), because they must grasp metal rather than soft tissues, are subject to greater damage. As a result, needle holders must be repaired and replaced regularly. For maximum usage, needle holders must retain a firm grip on the needle. Many types of jaws have been designed to meet this need. The so-called diamond jaw needle holder has a tungsten carbide insert designed to prevent rotation of the needle. In needle holders of standard design, a longitudinal groove or pit in the jaw releases tension, prevents flattening of the needle, and holds the needle firmly. Needle holders may have a ratchet similar to that of a hemostat, or they may be of a spring action that may or may not lock.

Towel clamps are also considered holding instruments. Of the two basic types, one is a nonpenetrating towel clamp used for holding barrier draping materials in place.

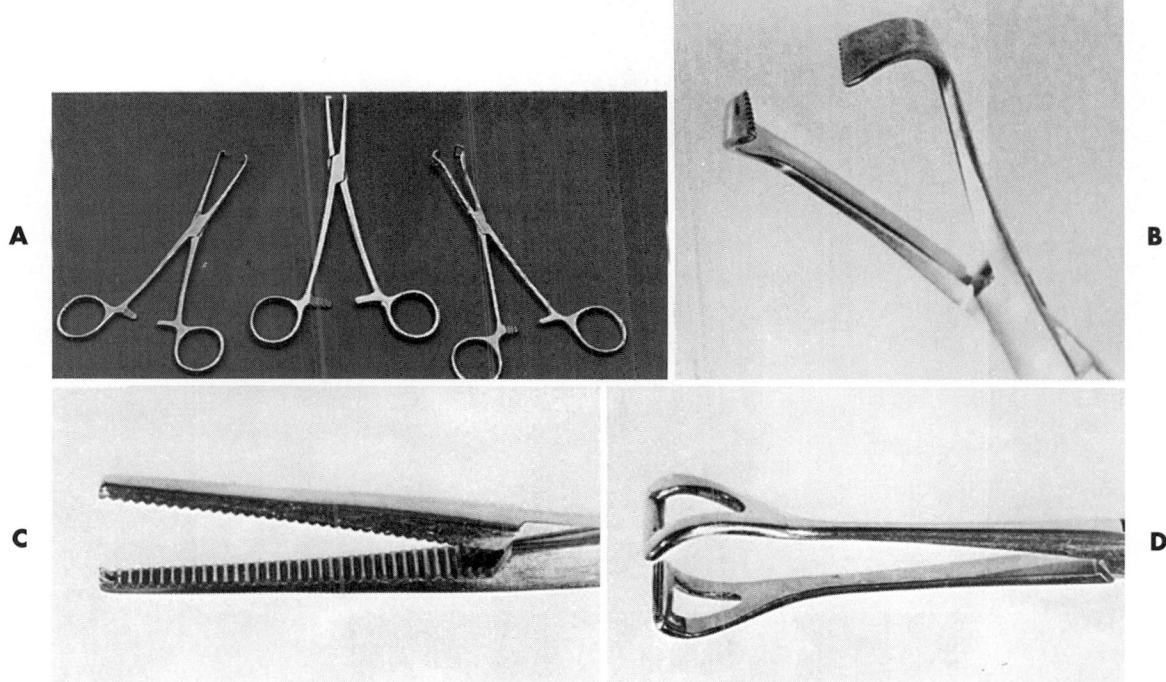

FIGURE 6-16   **A,** Holding forceps with special jaws. **B,** Allis. **C,** Kocher or Ochsner. **D,** Babcock.

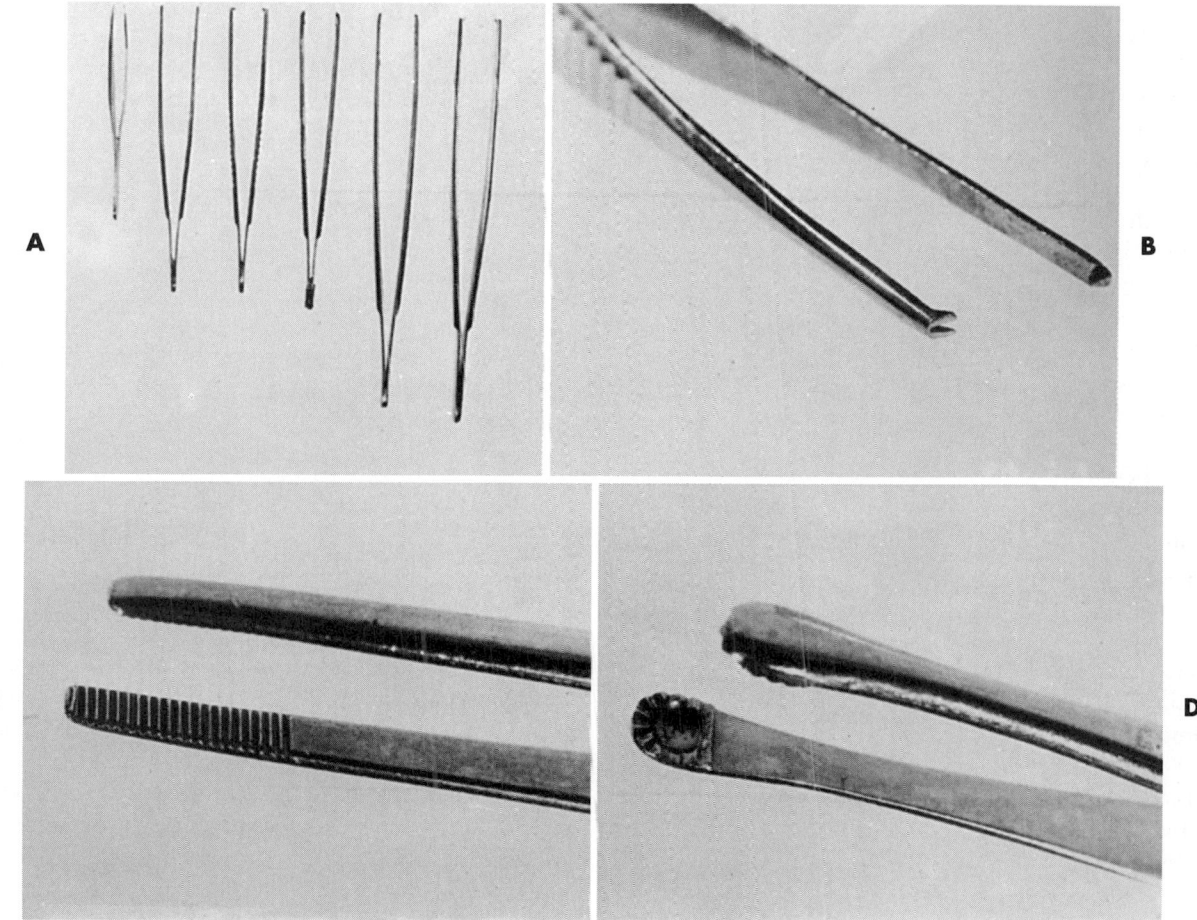

FIGURE 6-17   **A,** Various types of tissue forceps, or "pickups," ranging from those with very fine tips to heavy tips. **B,** Tips with teeth. **C,** Smooth tips. **D,** Tips of Russian forceps.

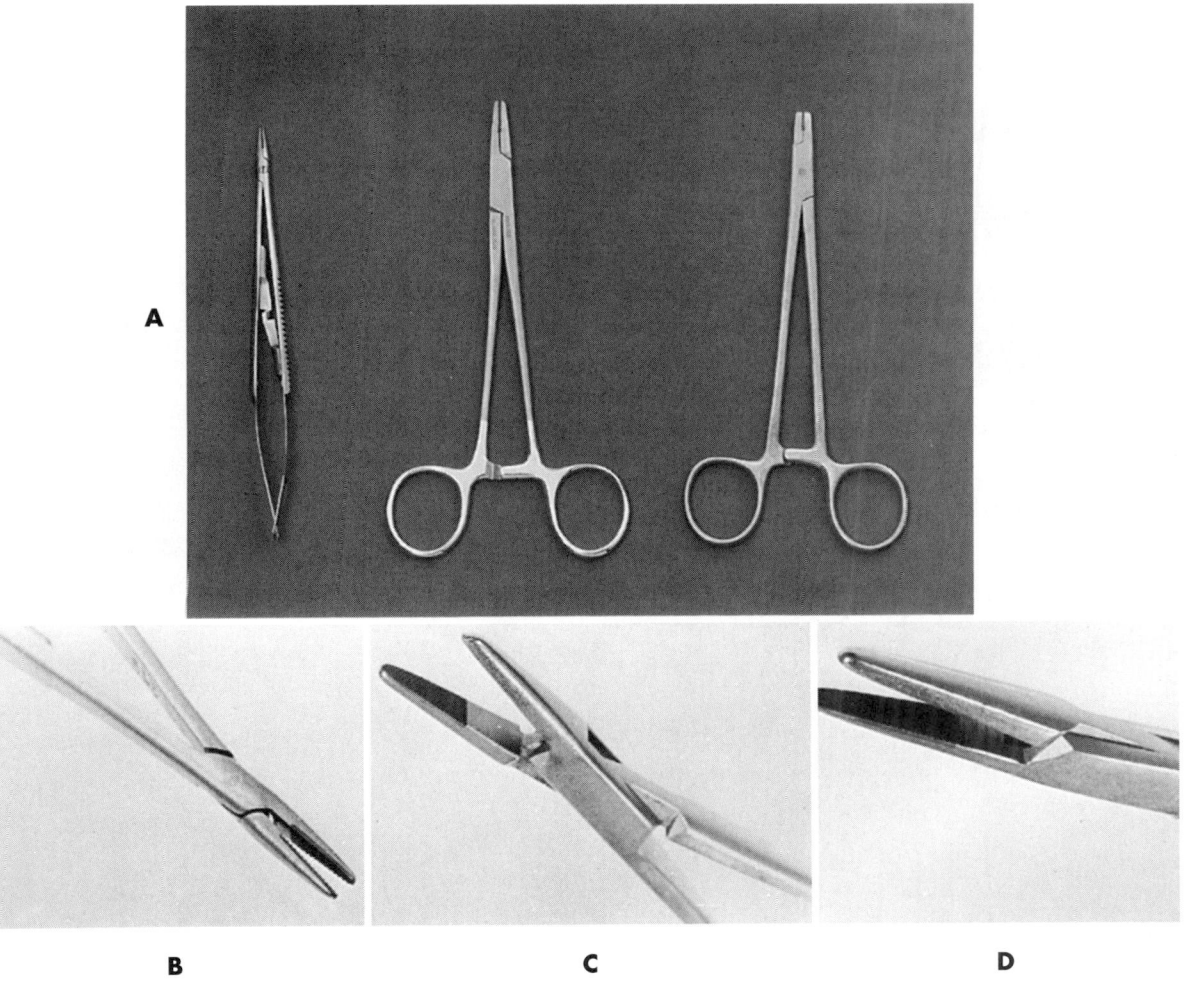

FIGURE 6-18   **A,** Needle holders. **B,** Fine. **C,** Regular. **D,** Heavy.

The other has sharp tips used to penetrate drapes and tissues, but it is damaging to both. The use of sharp towel clamps to penetrate drapes is highly discouraged, since they penetrate the sterile field and can be sources of contamination if removed.

Inspection and Care

The apposition of the clamp tips is necessary for its functioning and must be periodically checked. When a hemostat is held up to the light and the handles are fully closed, no light should be visible between the jaws. These instruments, if used for purposes other than that for which they are intended, can be damaged and need to be repaired. The instrument's joint must also be checked. Instruments made up of two halves may have three types of joints. The most common joint is the box lock, where one arm has been passed through a slot in the other arm and is riveted or pinned. This joint is needed where accurate approximation of the tips is necessary, and it is basic to most ringed instruments.

The second type is the screw joint. The two halves are placed one on top of the other, connected only by a screw. The joint must be checked and tightened periodically because the screw may work itself loose. Screw-joint instruments are easy to make and comparatively inexpensive.

The final and least common type is the semibox, or aseptic, joint. It has the advantage that the two halves can be separated for easy cleaning.

All types of joints must be cleaned regularly, and any protein deposits or rust collecting at the site must be removed to ensure proper functioning.

Retractors

Retractors are used to hold back the wound edges to provide exposure of the operative site. A surgeon needs the best exposure possible that inflicts a minimum of trauma to the surrounding tissue. Retractors are either self-retaining (Fig. 6-19) or manually held in place by a member of the surgical team. The two types of self-retaining retractors are those with frames to which various blades may be attached and those with two blades held apart with a ratchet. An example of the latter is a Weitlaner retractor. With hand-held retractors (Fig. 6-20), the handles may be

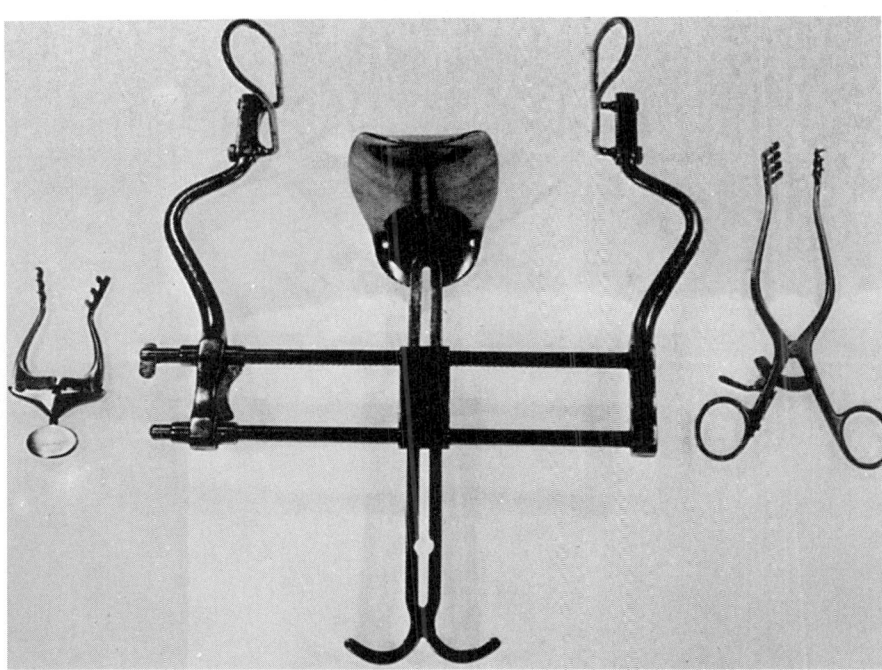

FIGURE 6-19 Self-retaining retractors. *Left to right*, Mastoid, Balfour, and Weitlaner.

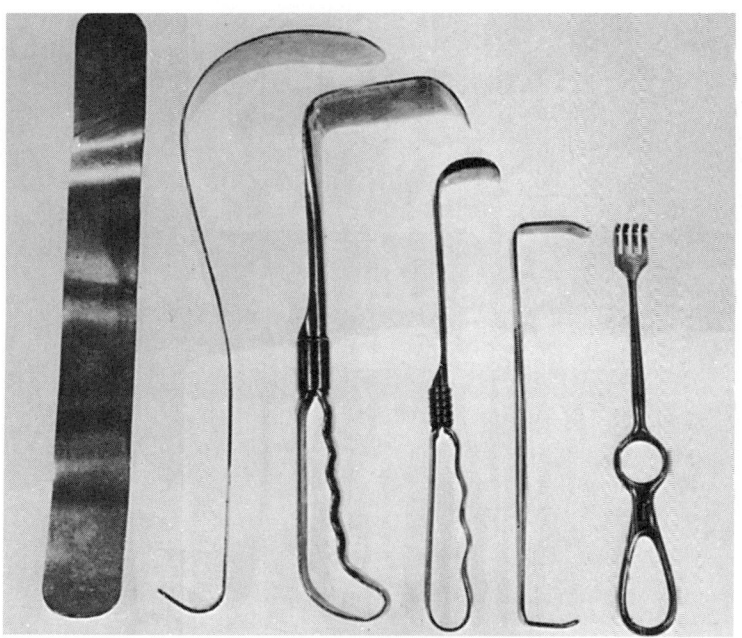

FIGURE 6-20 Handheld retractors. *Left to right*, Ribbon, or malleable; Deaver; Kelly; Richardson; Army-Navy, or USA; and rake.

notched, hook shaped, or ring shaped to give the holder a firm grip without tiring. The blade is usually at a right angle to the shaft and may be a smooth blade, rake, or hook. A malleable (ribbon) retractor is a flat metal ribbon that may be shaped by the surgeon at the field.

Accessory and ancillary instruments

Accessory and ancillary instruments are designed to enhance the use of basic instrumentation or facilitate the procedure. These include suction tips and tubing, irrigators-aspirators, electrosurgical devices, and special-use devices such as probes, dilators, mallets, and screwdrivers.

Many miscellaneous instruments or specialty items are particular to a certain service but generally fall into one of the above categories. Microsurgical instruments are delicate and expensive. They are extremely fine and should be handled separately from other instruments. Instruments used in specialty surgery are discussed in each of the chapters on surgical interventions.

When nursing team members can analyze the planned surgical procedure and approach and identify each instrument and its specific function, they will be able to select instrument sets without omitting necessary items and without including items that will not be used. This intelligent, planned approach ensures economy of time and motion, protects instruments from misuse, and prevents unnecessary handling. During the operation the informed scrub person who anticipates instrument needs becomes a more valuable member of the surgical team.

Endoscopic Instrumentation

Laparoscopy has introduced new equipment and instrumentation to the surgical suite. In addition to insufflation equipment, an optical system, and a documentation system, perioperative personnel must be familiar with the instrumentation utilized by the surgeon to perform surgery through the scope. Basic instrumentation, which may be disposable or reusable, includes trocars, forceps or graspers, clip appliers, stapling devices, scissors, needle holders, and aspiration–irrigation systems.

Verres needles (Fig. 6-21) and trocars (Fig. 6-22)

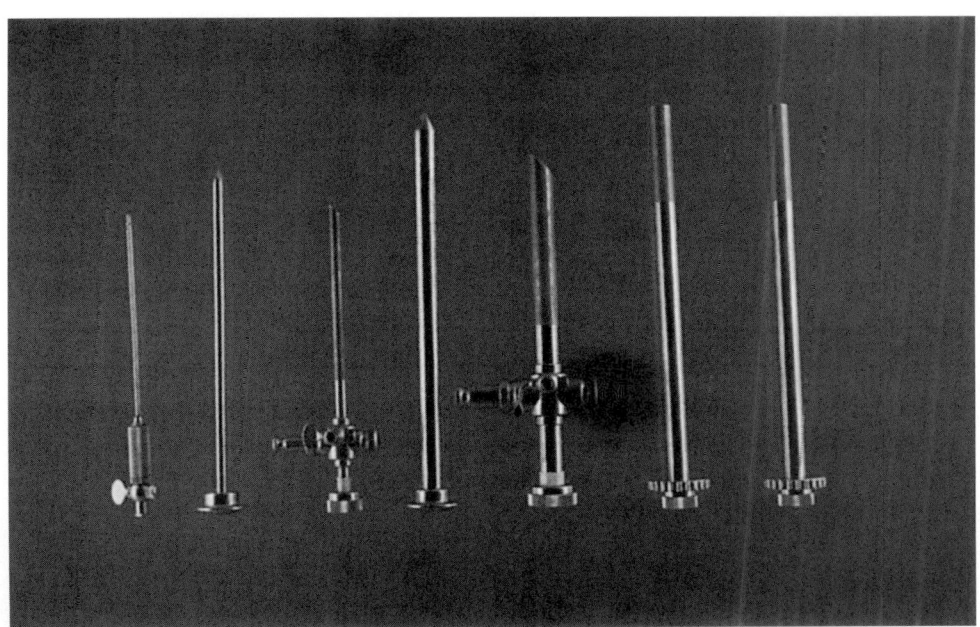

FIGURE 6-21   *Left to right,* Nondisposable: Verres needle; 5.5 mm obturator; 5.5 mm cannula; 10/11 mm obturator; 10/11 mm cannula; reducers, 11 mm to 5.5 mm.

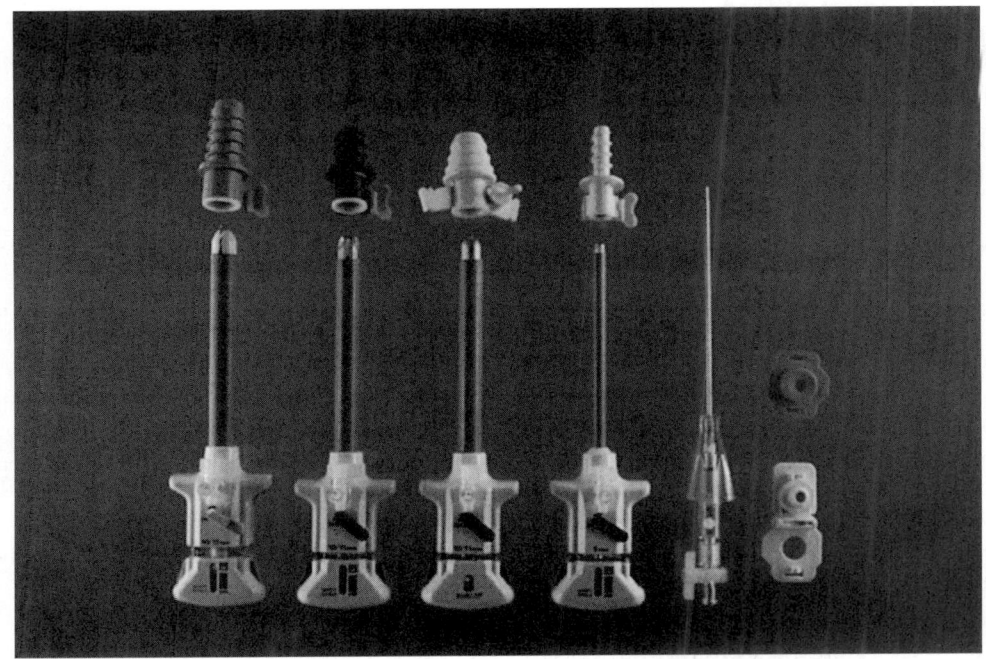

FIGURE 6-22   *Left to right,* Disposable: 10/12 mm cannula with obturator; 10/11 mm cannula with obturator; 10/11 mm Hasson cannula (blunt tip); 5 mm cannula with obturator; Verres needle; 2 reducer caps: *top,* 3-5 mm, and *bottom,* 10/5 mm.

provide access to the peritoneal cavity. A retractable safety shield protects abdominal structures from being inadvertently punctured during insertion. Forceps or graspers are available in 3, 5, and 10 mm sizes. Atraumatic graspers provide appropriate retraction and little risk to tissues. Bipolar coagulation forceps are used to control bleeding. The forceps are available with different tips including ring, paddle, dolphin nose, claw, spoon, DeBakey, Allis, Pollack, Pennington, Glassman, Maryland, Reddic-Saye, Duval, and Babcock. Some dissectors are available with coagulation capability (Fig. 6-23). Scissors also come with

different tips: hook, straight and microtipped, serrated, and curved (Fig. 6-24).

Needle holders come with a hinged-jaw tip to allow easy positioning of the needle before intracorporeal suturing and the sliding sheath. The sliding sheath holds the needle in a distal notch and inner spring loading mechanism. To aid with extracorporeal knot tying, the surgeon may utilize a knot pusher to deliver tied knots into the abdomen (Clarke-Riech). There is also a slide and cinch pusher (Gazayerli) used to deliver and secure the preformed knot. Intraabdominal stapling devices have

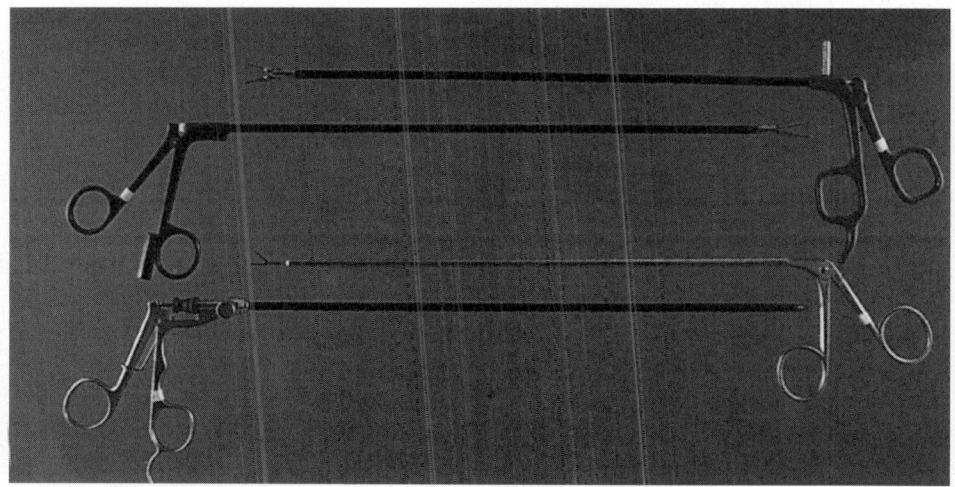

FIGURE 6-23 *Top to bottom,* Nondisposable: curved dissector with cautery capability; straight dissector with cautery capability; microdissector; spring-loaded tapered dissecting forceps.

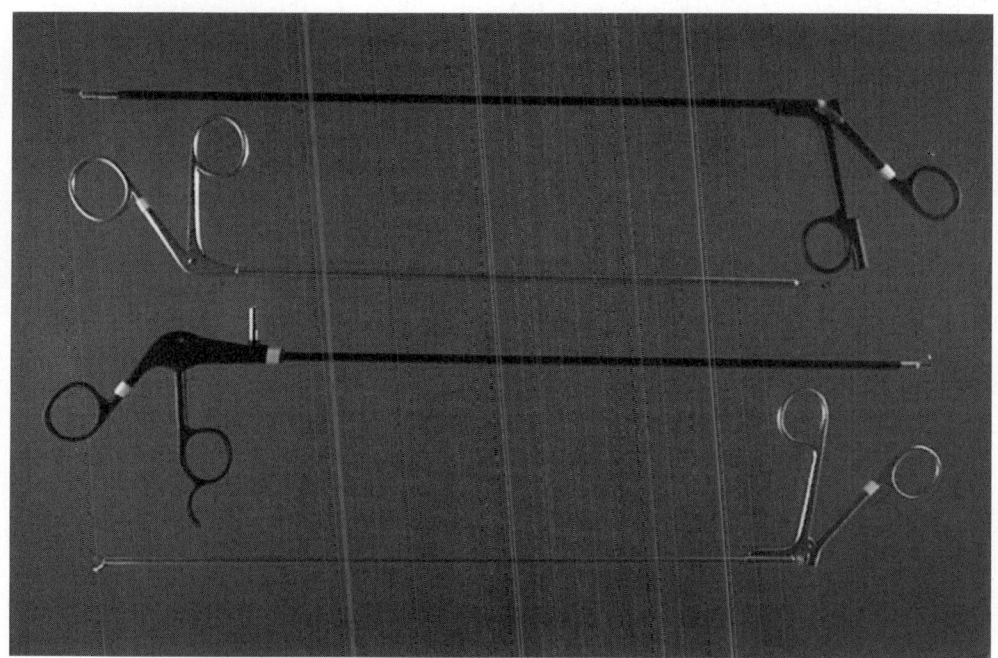

FIGURE 6-24 *Top to bottom,* Nondisposable: straight insulated scissors with cautery capability; Semm microdissecting scissors; serrated hook scissors with cautery capability; small hook scissors.

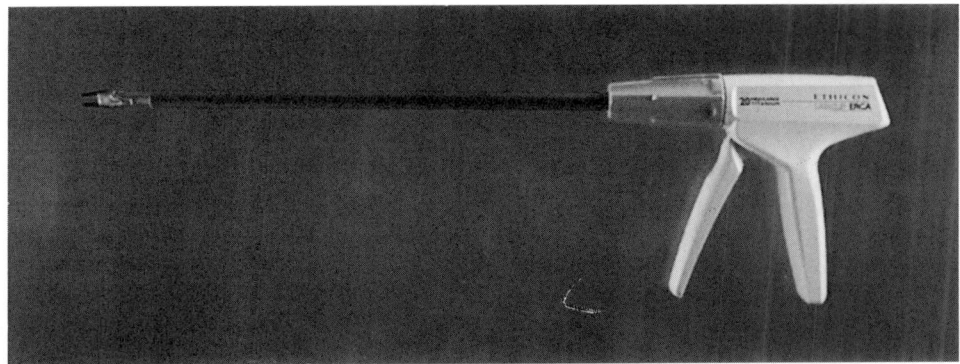

FIGURE 6-25   Disposable: medium/large ligaclip applier with multifire capability.

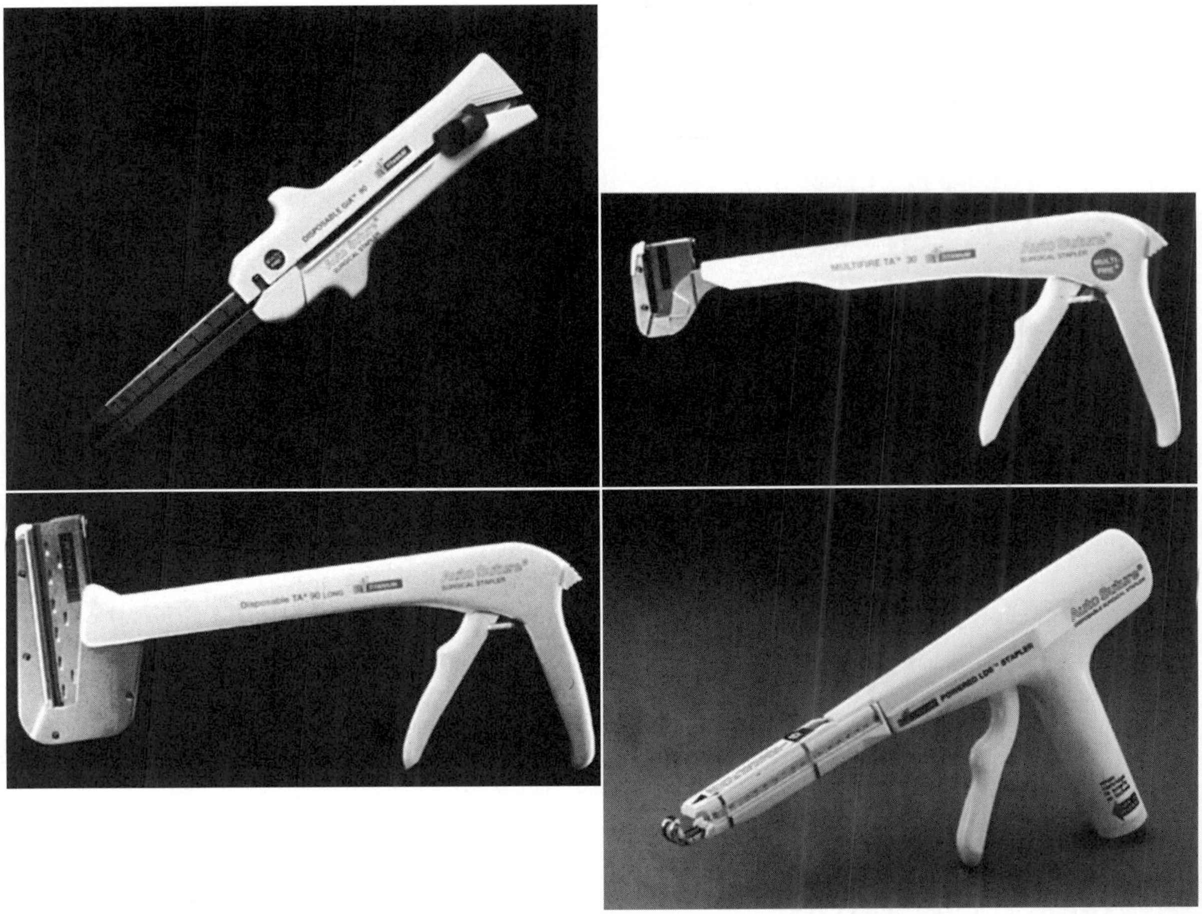

FIGURE 6-26   Set of Auto Suture instruments. **A,** GIA instrument. **B,** TA-30 instrument (TA-55 size instrument is also available). **C,** TA-90 instrument. **D,** LDS instrument.

been modified to fit and perform through the endoscope (Fig. 6-25).

Stapling Instruments

Instrumentation for internal stapling has been refined and is now widely used (Fig. 6-26). Various instruments to suture tissue mechanically are used for ligation and division, resection, anastomoses, and skin and fascia closure (Figs. 6-27 through 6-29). They may be employed in almost every specialty of surgery. Because of the mechanical application of these instruments, tissue manipulation and handling are reduced. The edema and inflammation that usually accompany anastomoses are minimized because the noncrushing B shape of the staples allows nutrients to pass through the staple line to the cut edge of the tissue.

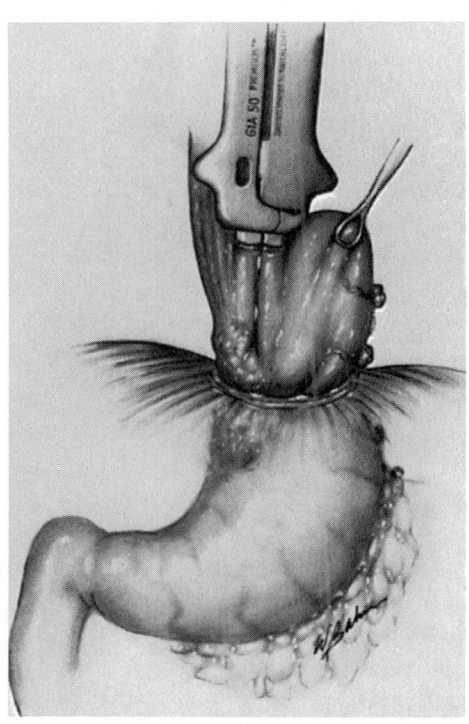

FIGURE 6-27 GIA instrument used to perform esophagogastrostomy. Forks of the instrument are inserted into stab wounds made in the lateral wall of the esophagus and the medial wall of the gastric fundus. The instrument is closed and staples are fired.

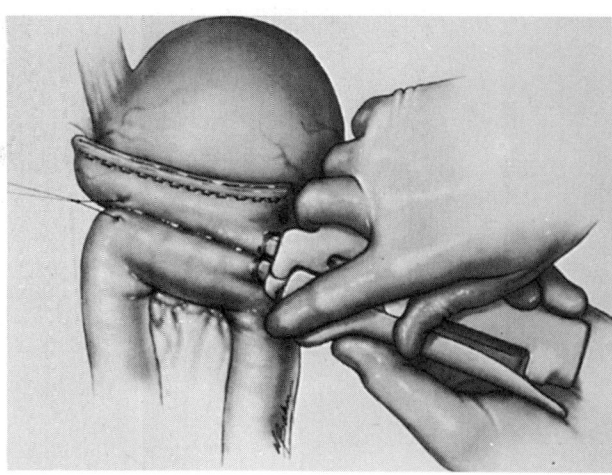

FIGURE 6-28 Using GIA to staple and join stomach and jejunum. At same time, blade in GIA cuts between double staple lines, creating stoma for gastrojejunostomy.

Mechanical staplers (nondisposable and disposable) utilize cartridges of tiny stainless steel, or absorbable, nonmetallic staples that are commercially preloaded, prepackaged, and presterilized. The staples are essentially nonreactive; metal staples will remain permanently in the tissue. They may fire individually or lay down multiple rows in a straight or circular pattern. Devices to cut or anastomose bowel and other structures are available for open-wound use or through endoscopic cannulas. The use of staplers significantly decreases operating time and may shorten postoperative stays.

Selecting and Preparing Instruments for Patient Use

Designated operating room or central supply personnel arrange the various instruments into trays or sets. The trays are named according to their functions. Three basic operating room instrument sets are the basic laparotomy, the minor/plastic, and the D&C. For example, a minor (or plastic surgery) set includes instruments needed for simple superficial incision, excision, and suturing. A basic laparotomy set includes instruments to open and close the abdominal cavity and repair any gross defects in the major body musculature. A D&C set, in addition to its use for dilatation and curettage, is often used as the basic instrumentation for vaginal surgery.

According to each procedure's needs, more individualized instruments or specialty sets such as an intestinal set or

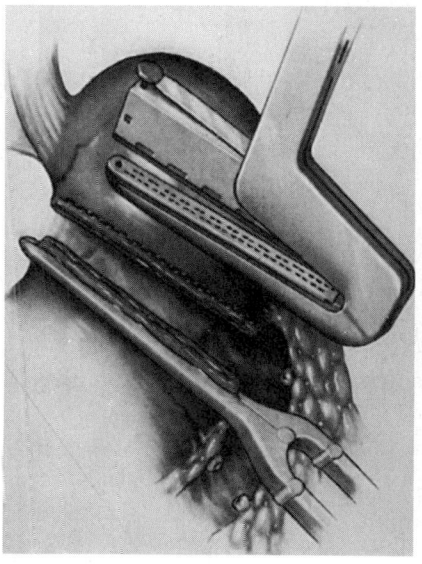

FIGURE 6-29 Using TA-90 to close gastric pouch. Jaws of TA-90 are slipped around stomach at level of transection, the instrument is closed, and staples are fired.

a vascular set may be added. In the same way, basic instrument sets may be selected for opening other body cavities, such as the skull, chest, and pelvis.

Instruments are selected according to the size of the patient's body structures and the nature of the organs involved. Proper selection requires a general understanding of surgical procedures and approaches and knowledge of anatomy, possible pathologic conditions, and the design and purpose of instruments.

This knowledge is reinforced during the orientation of new personnel to the operating room. New personnel learn basic technique first in general surgery and then proceed to the specialty services, where different instru-

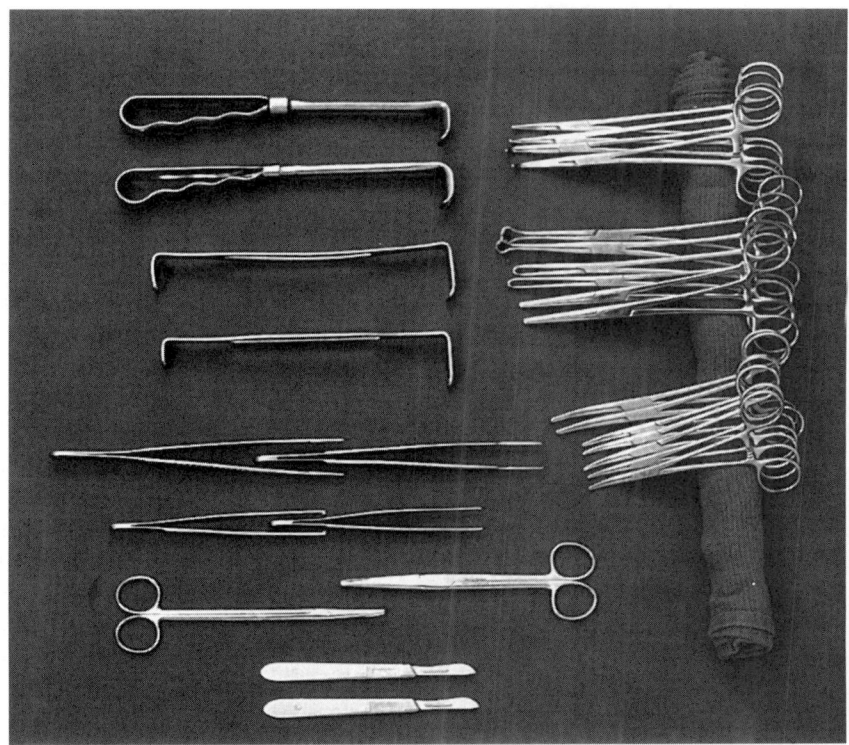

FIGURE 6-30   Mayo stand setup.

ments and devices are added but the same basic principles of perioperative practice are applied.

Basic Table Setups

In most operating rooms the instruments are set up on Mayo stands and back tables in a planned, standardized, organized, functional manner to maintain continuity when the original scrub person is replaced by another. The teaching manual should have illustrations or diagrams to which all personnel may refer. Each item used by the scrub person should have its own placement on the table to prevent the mass clutter that would occur if instruments and supplies were placed randomly.

A proficient scrub person must know the instrument inventory of the department, the routine instruments needed for each type of operation, the individual surgeon's preferences, correct use and handling, method of preparation, and aftercare of the instruments. A file of preference cards or computerized data sheets usually list the procedures each physician performs, the physician's glove size, the preferred skin preparation solution, specific draping instructions, and instruments required for the procedure.

Before an operative procedure, the scrub person may assist the circulator in gathering the needed supplies, equipment, and sutures. The scrub person scrubs, dons gown and gloves (see Chapter 4), and begins to set up the sterile tables with drapes, instruments, supplies, and sutures. Instruments are arranged with those most frequently used on the Mayo stand (Fig. 6-30). Once the patient is on the operating room bed and is draped, the Mayo stand, set up for instrument use at the immediate operative site, is brought across the lower part of the patient's legs.

One or two back tables, according to the number of instruments and supplies, are also set up. The scrub person prepares the sutures and ligatures and places the knife blades on the handles. Other supplies needed are suction tubing and tips, electrosurgical cord and tip, drains, basins, gowns, gloves, drapes, sponges, and needles, all of which are sterile and set up on the back table according to standardized institutional policy (Fig. 6-31).

The scrub person must be attentive to the sterile field to anticipate the surgeon's needs. Instruments should be passed in a positive and decisive manner. Each instrument is placed or slapped firmly into the surgeon's palm in such a manner that it is ready for immediate use with no wasted motion. For example, when a needle holder with a needle is passed to the surgeon, the needle should be pointing in the direction of the surgeon's thumb; there should be no need for readjustment. Knowing if a surgeon or the assistant is left- or right-handed is necessary to load and pass a needle holder correctly.

Often the surgeon or assistant uses hand signals for the type of instrument desired to eliminate unnecessary talking. Scrub persons should become familiar with the basic signals for knife, scissors, suture, forceps, and clamp.

Care and Handling of Instruments

An instrument should be used only for the purpose for which it is designed. Proper use and reasonable care

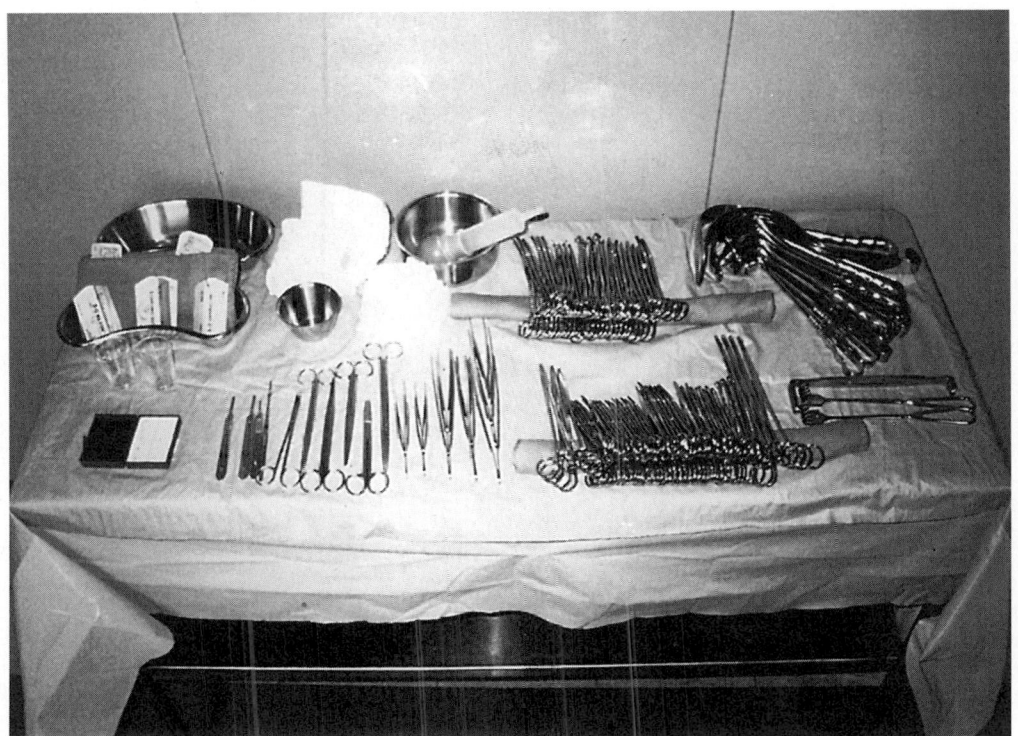

FIGURE 6-31   Back table setup.

prolong its life and protect its quality. Scissors and clamps, which are most frequently misused, can be forced out of alignment, cracked, or broken when used improperly. Tissue scissors should not be used to cut suture or gauze dressings. Hemostatic clamps should not be used as towel clamps or to clamp suction tubing.

Instruments must be handled gently. Bouncing, dropping, and setting heavy equipment on top of them must be avoided. During the procedure, used instruments should be wiped with a damp sponge, or placed in a basin of sterile distilled water to prevent blood from drying on the instruments. Saline solution should never be used on instruments because its salt content is corroding and increases the rusting or deterioration of the metal. As time allows during the procedure, the scrub person should rinse and dry the used instruments and replace them on the back table to facilitate closing counts.

At the end of a procedure, the instruments should not be thrown together in a tangled heap. They should be handled individually or in small groups. Sharp and delicate instruments should be set aside for individual handling and cleaning to avoid damage and accidental injury. Standard Precautions should be applied as dictated by institutional policy. All instruments set up for the procedure should be terminally sterilized or disinfected before reassembly. Instruments must be completely clean to ensure effective sterilization.

Each instrument should be inspected before and after each use to detect imperfections. An instrument should function perfectly to prevent needlessly endangering a patient's safety and increasing operative time because of instrument failure.

Forceps, clamps, and other hinged instruments must be inspected for alignment of jaws and teeth. Instrument jaws and teeth should meet perfectly so that blood flow is occluded without damaging the vein or artery. Ratchets should hold firmly yet release easily. Instrument joints should work smoothly.

The edges of scissors should be tested for sharpness by cutting smoothly through four layers of gauze. All instruments should be checked for worn spots, chips, dents, cracks, or sharp edges.

Damaged instruments should be set aside and sent for repair or replacement. An instrument repair service should be selected carefully and used for regular maintenance, such as sharpening and realignment.

Instrument Counts

Most institutions perform instrument counts as standard practice. Establishing standardized instrument sets with the minimum numbers and types of instruments in them facilitates instrument counts and reduces the amount of time and space required for a setup. Initial counts should be carried out concurrently by the circulator and scrub person before the procedure. Items added during the procedure are counted and documented. Subsequent counts should be taken before closure of a cavity or large, deep incision, when the scrub person or circulator is relieved by other personnel, and at the completion of the procedure. Instruments that are disassembled during surgery, such as certain retractors, must be accounted for in their entirety. All counts are documented by the circulator on the appropriate record.

Storing Instruments

Instruments should be stored safely. Cabinet shelving should be adjustable and properly spaced for storage of various sizes and types of instruments. Most institutions store instruments in presterilized trays or containers. Attached labels and diagrams in cabinets assist personnel. An inventory of all instruments should be taken at periodic intervals.

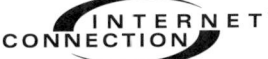

For questions, databases, and links by typing in information you are looking for, try:
Nursing Net: http:/www.communique.net/~nursgnt
Wholenurse: http://www.wholenurse.com/
Medical Matrix: http://www.slackinc.com/matrix
Medscape: http://www.medscpae.com

National Library of Medicine - History of Medicine
Division: http://www.nlm.nih.gov/about_nlm/organization/library_operations/history_of_medicine/history_of_medicine/history_of_medicine.html

REFERENCES

1. AORN recommended practices for sponge, sharp and needle counts. (1998). In *AORN standards, recommended practices, and guidelines*. Denver: Association of Operating Room Nurses, pp. 171-178.
2. Draft Guideline for Infection Control in Health-Care Personnel. (1997). *Morbidity and Mortality Weekly Report, 62*(173), 47276-47314.
3. Evaluation of blunt suture needles in preventing percutaneous injuries among health care workers during gynecologic surgical procedures— New York City, March 1993–June 1994. (1997). *JAMA, 277*(6), 451-452.
4. Gomella, L.G., & Lefor, A.T. (1996). *Surgery on call*. Stamford, CT: Appleton & Lange.
5. Jagger, J. & Balon, M. (1996). Suture needle and scalpel blade injuries. *Infection Control and Sterilization Technology, 2*(9), 13-17.
6. Kidd, P.S., & Stuart, P. (1996). *Mosby's emergency nursing reference*. St. Louis: Mosby.
7. Korniewicz, D.M., & Rabussay, D. (1997). Surgical glove failures in clinical practice settings. *AORN Journal, 66*(4), 660-673.
8. Schrock, T.R. (1994). *Handbook of surgery*. St. Louis: Mosby.

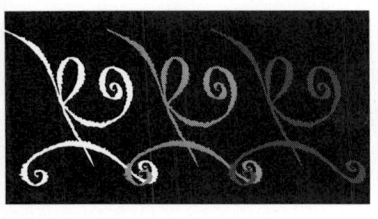

CHAPTER SEVEN | # Anesthesia

J. Lee Hoffer

WITHOUT ANESTHESIA, MOST modern surgical procedures would not be feasible. Therefore the perioperative nurse should be familiar with the principles and practices of anesthesia and the perioperative functions of the anesthesiologist. This chapter presents an overview of the modern practice of anesthesia, the factors involved, and the interrelationship with the perioperative nurse. Included are discussions of the major types of anesthesia, an introduction to the more commonly used drugs, a review of the standards of anesthesia care, and an overview of some of the problems that can occur during the perioperative period. Descriptions of the anesthesia machines and monitoring equipment are also included so that the perioperative nurse can become familiar with their basic functions for potential use during local anesthesia or conscious sedation procedures.

The sections are organized so that they can be referred to independently without reading the entire chapter. Many perioperative nurses are familiar with the commonly used abbreviations employed in this chapter. However, to provide a single reference source, most abbreviations are defined in Box 7-1.

HISTORY OF ANESTHESIA

The early history of modern anesthesia was fraught with controversy. Surgeons in the early nineteenth century frequently used alcohol or opium to intoxicate the patient for procedures involving intense pain or when muscle relaxation was needed. In some cases, hypnotism was also employed. Successful surgery was directly related to the speed of the surgeon.

In March 1842, Crawford W. Long, a physician in Danielsville, Georgia, using ether as an anesthetic, removed a cystic tumor from the neck of James Venable. As confirmed by other physicians in the area, Dr. Long subsequently used ether for other procedures but did not publish reports of his experiences.

In 1844, Horace Wells, a dentist in Hartford, Connecticut, began to use nitrous oxide for anesthesia and communicated his results to his former partner, William T.G. Morton. However, after a death with nitrous oxide, Wells quit the practice of dentistry and later committed suicide. Morton subsequently studied medicine and learned of the anesthetic effects of chloric ether from his preceptor, Charles T. Jackson, a chemist. In 1846, while employing this new drug, Morton was able to fill a tooth without the patient experiencing pain. He later learned

from Jackson that sulfuric ether had similar properties and utilized it while extracting a deeply rooted bicuspid tooth from another patient.

Morton then contacted John C. Warren, a surgeon at the Massachusetts General Hospital, and persuaded him to give the new anesthetic a trial during a surgical procedure. With Morton as the anesthetist, this historic operation took place in the amphitheater (subsequently renamed "The Ether Dome") of Massachusetts General Hospital on October 16, 1846. In 5 minutes, Warren operated on an unconscious, quiet patient and dissected "a congenital but superficial vascular tumor just below the jaw on the left side of the neck." As the patient regained consciousness, Warren exclaimed, "Gentlemen, this is no humbug." The next day, a large fatty tumor on the shoulder of another patient was removed by Haywood with Morton as the anesthetist.

Based on these events, the first medical report of anesthesia was announced to the world on November 18, 1846, by Henry J. Bigelow in the *Boston Medical and Surgical Journal*. An era had ended in which successful surgery was largely predicated on the lightning speed of the surgeon while working on a struggling, distressed patient. Anesthetic techniques gave the surgeon more time

---

BOX 7-1	Abbreviations Used in This Chapter

AA	Anesthesia assistant(s): a physician assistant trained in anesthesia. See section on anesthesia providers.	LPM	liters per minute. This usually relates to the total fresh gas flow from the anesthesia machine.
ABG	Arterial blood gas. Usually includes pH, Pao_2, $Paco_2$, HCO_3^-, O_2 saturation, and base excess. Some units also include Na^+, K^+, and ionized Ca^{++}.	M	Molar.
		MAC	Monitored anesthesia care. See section under types of anesthesia care.
ACLS	Advanced Cardiac Life Support. A protocol for resuscitation from the American Heart Association.	MCAT	Medical College Admission Test.
		μg	microgram; mcg is the nonstandard usage.
ANSI	American National Standards Institute.	mg	milligram; 1×10^{-3} grams
APL	Adjustable pressure limiting valve, a valve on anesthesia machines that limits the maximum pressure in the patient breathing circuit. Frequently referred to as the "pop-off valve."	MH	Malignant hyperthermia. See section on malignant hyperthermia.
		MHAUS	Malignant Hyperthermia Association of the United States
APMS	Acute Pain Management Service.	MMS	Master of Medical Science degree.
ASA	American Society of Anesthesiologists.	MRI	Magnetic resonance imaging.
CD	Computer disk. In this chapter, a 3.5-inch disk on which vital signs are recorded.	MS	Master of Science degree.
		NIOSH	National Institute for Occupational Safety and Health.
cm	Centimeter, 1×10^{-2} meters, 2.54 cm = 1 inch	N_2O	Nitrous oxide.
CRNA	Certified registered nurse anesthetist. See section on anesthesia providers.	nm	nanometer, 1×10^{-9} meters
		NMS	Neuroleptic malignant syndrome. See section on malignant hyperthermia.
CSF	Cerebrospinal fluid. The fluid surrounding the brain and spinal cord. For spinal anesthesia, local anesthetics are injected into the CSF.	NSAID	Nonsteroidal antiinflammatory drug.
		PA	Pulmonary artery
EGTA	Esophageal (gastric tube) airway. A cuffed tube that is blindly inserted into the esophagus and connected to a mask. This permits ventilation through the mask and gastric suctioning through the cuffed tube.	$Paco_2$	Partial pressure of arterial carbon dioxide. The lower case "a" is 'arterial'; a capital "A" is 'alveolar'.
		Pao_2	Partial pressure of arterial oxygen. The lower case "a" is 'arterial'; a capital "A" is 'alveolar'.
		PARS	Postanesthesia recovery score. See section on postanesthesia recovery.
$ETCO_2$	End tidal carbon dioxide reported as a partial pressure. See section on capnography.	PCA	Patient-controlled analgesia. See section on pain management.
ETT	Endotracheal tube.	ppm	parts per million; 1 ppm = 1×10^{-6}.
FDA	U.S. Food and Drug Administration, which must approve all new drugs used in the United States.	psi	pounds per square inch, a measurement of pressure.
		QA	Quality assurance. This function may also be identified as quality improvement (QI), continuous quality improvement (CQI), or similar names.
FiO_2	Fraction of inspired oxygen. This is a fraction (0.00 to 1.00), and it corresponds to the percent (0 to 100%) of inspired oxygen.	SpO_2	Saturation (pulse) of oxygen or in a pulsating vessel, expressed as a percentage. See section on pulse oximetry.
FO	Fiberoptic.		
GRE	Graduate Record Examination.		
kg	kilogram. 1 kg = 2.2 pounds.	$S\bar{v}O_2$	Saturation of mixed venous oxygen in percentage. This measurement is made from a special pulmonary artery catheter.
LED	Light-emitting diode, an electronic device that emits light at a predetermined frequency.		
LMA	Laryngeal mask airway or laryngeal airway. See discussion of typical sequence of general anesthesia, pp. 221-223.	Torr	1 mm Hg

---

to operate and permitted new procedures to be undertaken that would have been impossible before. Thus, many modern surgical techniques have become feasible because of the advances in the art and science of anesthesia.

The word *anesthesia* is derived from the Greek word *anaisthesia*, which literally means 'no sensation.' Anesthesia was listed in *Bailey's English Dictionary* in 1721. When the effects of ether were discovered, Oliver Wendell Holmes suggested *anesthesia* be used as a name for the new phenomenon. Some believed that he coined this term; others believed that he knew of the Greek word that Plato had employed. In any case, anesthesia was, in the memorable phrase of Werr Mitchell, the "death of pain." From these early beginnings, anesthesia has developed into a sophisticated science and "clinical art" that interfaces with many other medical specialties.

ANESTHESIA PROVIDERS

In the United States, anesthesia care is usually provided by (1) an anesthesiologist, (2) a certified registered nurse anesthetist (CRNA) working under the direction of an anesthesiologist or a physician, or (3) an anesthesiologist's assistant (AA; that is, physician's assistant in anesthesia) working under the direction of an anesthesiologist. An anesthesiologist is a physician with 4 or more years of specialty training in anesthesiology after medical school.

Nurse anesthesia programs are now a minimum of 2 years in length. They require a Bachelor of Science (BS) in Nursing or other appropriate field, plus 1 year of acute nursing care experience before acceptance. Many nurse anesthesia programs are at the master's degree level in a school of nursing or allied health, although a number of programs are based in community hospitals.

In recent years, AAs have also been trained. These are physician's assistants to anesthesiologists. Acceptance into an AA program requires a BS degree including a college-level "premed" education and a satisfactory score on the Medical College Admission Test (MCAT) or the Graduate Record Examination (GRE). These AA programs are offered only in medical schools with an approved residency program in anesthesiology. The 2-year training program is based upon the classical premed education. The basic science courses are taught by the regular medical school faculty. The AA are graduate students within the medical school and typically receive a Master of Medical Science (MMS) degree from the medical school. They also take a national certification examination administered by the National Commission on Certification of Anesthesiologist's Assistants under the supervision of the National Board of Medical Examiners.

In this chapter, the term *anesthesia provider* denotes the person *providing* the continuous anesthesia care for the patient. Depending on the practice in a given hospital, this may be an anesthesiologist, a nurse anesthetist, or an AA. In many hospitals, an *anesthesia care team* includes nurse anesthetists with or without AAs supervised by anesthesiologists. In small rural hospitals in some states, there may not be an anesthesiologist, and a CRNA may be the anesthesia provider.

The anesthesia provider is frequently said to be the patient's advocate in the perioperative period; as such, they must be concerned with many divergent factors when the patient's own sensory and cerebral functions are obtunded by anesthesia. The field of anesthesia has become so complex that in many large hospitals an anesthesia provider may further specialize in such areas as obstetric, neurosurgical, pediatric, cardiovascular, regional, or ambulatory anesthesia. Anesthesiologists may also subspecialize in acute and chronic pain management or in critical care medicine.

PATIENT SAFETY

Patient safety is always a concern during surgery and anesthesia. Approximately 26 million anesthetics are administered each year in the United States. Of these, an anesthetic misadventure is the primary cause of death in about 2000 cases. Data from several sources indicate a death rate ranging from 1 per 35,000 to about 1 per

7-1 RESEARCH HIGHLIGHT

ANESTHESIA-RELATED RISKS

One hundred New Yorkers were surveyed, and their greatest fear about anesthesia was not regaining consciousness. Many were also concerned about not getting an adequate amount of anesthesia. Including all types of patients, anesthesiologists often indicate that the risk of major morbidity or death from anesthesia is about 1 in 25,000 to 40,000 anesthetic applications. However, officials at a recent meeting of the New York State Society of Anesthesiologists stated that in 1970 the chance of dying from anesthesia was 1 in 4500, in 1985 it was 1 in 150,000, and today it is probably close to 1 in 400,000. A recent study at Harvard Medical School was stopped after 244,000 surgical patients were tracked and no anesthesia-related deaths occurred. In contrast, the death rate from automobile crashes is 41 per 250,000, from unintentional injuries at home it is 22 per 250,000, and from workplace injuries it is 9 per 250,000.

From Voelker, R. (1995). Anesthesia-related risks have plummeted. *JAMA, 273*, 445-446.

400,000.[7] These rates represent a very significant decline during the past 30 years, despite surgical procedures being performed on increasingly sicker and higher-risk patients than in the past (Research Highlight 7-1).

The general public still considers anesthesia to be a major risk of surgery. This may be attributable to sensationalized reports in the news media and in magazine articles. In addition, people may have a heightened awareness of anesthesia-related deaths, since these often occur acutely in the perioperative period, whereas surgical or medical problems may not result in death until days after the procedure. Also, the American Society of Anesthesiologists (ASA) has been willing to report, analyze, and study anesthetic misadventures in an effort to improve the overall quality of patient care. Awareness of potential problems and constant vigilance are crucial to good patient care.

AWARENESS DURING ANESTHESIA

The possibility of being awake during anesthesia is a concern of both patients and anesthesia providers (Research Highlight 7-2). Some patients are so anxious about being aware of anything during surgery that it affects their reasoning when discussing the options for anesthesia. For example, many procedures such as biopsies, inguinal hernias, or those on the lower extremities, can be done under regional anesthesia or monitored anesthesia care (MAC). However, these patients want only general

WHAT DOES THE PATIENT REMEMBER?

Awareness during anesthesia is a constant concern for anesthesia providers. Although rare, it does occur and recent dramatized accounts in the lay press have caused an increasing number of patients to voice their concern during preoperative interviews. To evaluate this issue, investigators have used a variety of approaches including:

- The effects of intraoperative therapeutic suggestions on the length of postoperative hospitalization or the level of pain.
- Positive suggestions during anesthesia for changes in life style (such as smoking cessation and weight loss).
- Assessment of inadequate amnesia or recall of intraoperative conversation, events, and so on.
- Intraoperative memory analyzed by recall of specific words or phrases spoken during anesthesia.
- Intraoperative physiologic changes or postoperative recall evaluated under hypnosis when a mock crisis was staged during anesthesia.
- Learning of new information during anesthesia.

Bailey and Jones reviewed studies of patients' memories of intraoperative events. Many of these studies employed changes in the latency and amplitude of the middle-latency, auditory-evoked potentials. They found that even under seemingly adequate general anesthesia, implicit memory may be retained along with the ability to subconsciously process auditory stimuli. Based on their review, it would seem prudent to avoid anesthetic techniques that rely solely on receptor-based drugs (that is, benzodiazepines, opioids, N_2O) and to include volatile anesthetics.

Merikle and Daneman conducted a meta-analysis of 2517 patients in 44 studies which involved memory about perceived events during anesthesia. The effect of positive suggestions on postoperative recovery had little influence on the duration of hospitalization or the amount of morphine given with a patient-controlled analgesic system. However, the analysis did show that specific data given during anesthesia may be remembered after surgery if testing occurs within 36 hours.

Studies in these areas are ongoing. Therefore it is important that while the patient is anesthetized all persons in the OR or procedure room should always conduct themselves in a professional manner. There is a possibility that the patient may remember.

From Bailey, A.R., & Jones, J.G. (1997). Patients' memories of events during general anaesthesia (Review article). *Anaesthesia, 52,* 460-476; Merikle, P.M., & Daneman, M. (1996). Memory for unconsciously perceived events: evidence from anesthetized patients. *Consciousness and Cognition, 5,* 525-541.

anesthesia because they do not want to be aware of anything during the procedure. In rare cases during general anesthesia, the patient may be paralyzed but be aware of what is going on and be unable to indicate this to anyone. This situation can be caused by several factors including insufficient level of anesthesia, an empty volatile-anesthetic vaporizer, profound paralysis, or a high drug tolerance.

For many years, the electroencephalogram (EEG) has been the standard for assessing a person's hypnotic and sleep state. However, to routinely employ an EEG for all surgical procedures is unrealistic. For years, investigators have attempted to analyze and mathematically process the EEG to develop a usable monitor. Up to now, their success has been limited. Recently, Aspect Medical Systems has developed the Bispectral Index (BIS). This unit analyzes the relationship and frequency of the signals using a sophisticated algorithm to generate a composite, numerical value that seems to correlate with the cerebral state. Five electrodes are positioned across the forehead, and the monitor gives an index (0 to 100) of the hypnotic state or sedation level. The BIS seems to monitor the effects of anesthetics and sedatives on the hypnotic status of the brain but is less informative about the level of analgesia. This monitor is being used for general anesthesia. Motion artifacts and mental changes cause erratic changes under the lighter level of sedation commonly used with MAC. Use of the BIS monitor will probably become greater in the next few years. Someday, awareness during anesthesia may be a nonissue.

PREOPERATIVE PREPARATION

Patient Evaluation

It is common to perform the preoperative evaluation in advance of the scheduled surgical procedure. One or more days before the procedure a patient will visit a preadmission clinic. (This may also be called preadmission testing, preanesthesia clinic, or anesthesia-assessment unit.) All the admission data and appropriate consent forms are completed, a preoperative history and physical examination may be done, a preanesthesia evaluation and examination are completed, and appropriate diagnostic or laboratory tests are processed. The patient's physical status is assessed, and the most appropriate anesthetic technique is selected. The patient's questions and concerns are resolved and instructions are given to expedite admission on the day of surgery. This preadmission processing has become very popular in the last two decades because third-party payers have agreed to reimbursement for outpatient laboratory testing. In addition, the patient is usually more relaxed and rested after sleeping at home rather than adapting to a strange hospital environment before surgery.

Before elective surgery the patient should be in optimal medical condition. Occasionally, it is believed that a patient's physical status could be improved to reduce the risks involved. In such cases, this is discussed with the patient's primary physician or the surgeon, and if necessary, elective surgery is deferred until the patient's condition is optimized. If, however, the intended surgery is emergent, any benefits gained from a delay must be carefully compared with the hazards of waiting.

The assignment of a physical status classification is based upon the patient's physiologic condition independent of the proposed surgical procedure. The physical-status classification was developed by the American Society of Anesthesiologists (ASA) to provide uniform guidelines. It is an evaluation of the severity of systemic diseases, physiologic dysfunction, and anatomic abnormalities. Intraoperative difficulties occur more frequently with patients who have a poor physical status classification. The ASA classification system is given in Table 7-1.

Preadmission clinics are widely used by many hospitals and ambulatory surgery centers. However, in some metropolitan areas where travel and congestion are problems or for patients in reasonably good health, nurses may conduct preoperative telephone interviews with patients. Then, on the day of surgery, patients arrive 1 or 2 hours before the scheduled surgery time to complete the other preoperative processes. In some facilities, certain ambulatory patients are evaluated just before surgery. These are usually healthy patients having minor procedures or patients with stable, chronic conditions having a procedure (such as cataract removal, skin lesion excision) under monitored anesthesia care (MAC). These preadmission processes have reduced the cost of health care, decreased the risk of nosocomial infections associated with longer hospital admissions, increased the utilization and

efficiency of healthcare resources, improved patient relations, and enhanced the chances of having a well-informed patient in optimal health status.

In larger hospitals and ambulatory surgery centers the person who evaluates the patient in the preanesthesia clinic is often not the anesthesia provider for the surgical procedure. Therefore, immediately before surgery, the anesthesia provider (1) reviews the patient's chart, laboratory data, and diagnostic studies such as the ECG and chest x-ray examination; (2) confirms that the appropriate consent forms (surgery, anesthesia, use of blood products) have been signed; (3) identifies the patient; (4) verifies the surgical procedure; (5) reviews the choice of anesthesia; (6) examines the patient; and (7) gives preoperative medications if appropriate.

Choice of Anesthesia

The choice of anesthesia for a given surgical procedure is made by the patient, the anesthesia provider, and the surgeon. A variety of factors influence this choice including the following:

1. Patient's wishes and understanding of the types of anesthesia that could be used
2. Patient's physiologic status
3. Presence and severity of coexisting diseases
4. Patient's mental and psychologic status
5. Postoperative recovery from various kinds of anesthesia
6. Options for management of postoperative pain
7. Type and duration of the surgical procedure
8. Patient's position during surgery
9. Any particular requirements of the surgeon

TABLE 7-1 | **Physical (P) Status Classification of the American Society of Anesthesiologists**

STATUS*†	DEFINITION	DESCRIPTION AND EXAMPLES
P1	A normal healthy patient.	No physiologic, psychologic, biochemical, or organic disturbance.
P2	A patient with a mild systemic disease.	Cardiovascular disease with minimal restriction of activity. Hypertension, asthma, chronic bronchitis, obesity, diabetes mellitus, or tobacco abuse.
P3	A patient with a severe systemic disease that limits activity but is not incapacitating.	Cardiovascular or pulmonary disease that limits activity. Severe diabetes with systemic complications. History of myocardial infarction, angina pectoris, poorly controlled hypertension, or morbid obesity.
P4	A patient with severe systemic disease that is a constant threat to life.	Severe cardiac, pulmonary, renal, hepatic, or endocrine dysfunction.
P5	A moribund patient who is not expected to survive 24 hours with or without the operation.	Surgery is done as last recourse or resuscitative effort. Major multisystem or cerebral trauma, ruptured aneurysm, or large pulmonary embolus.
P6	A patient declared brain dead whose organs are being removed for donor purposes.	

Adapted from American Society of Anesthesiologists. (1997). *Manual for anesthesia departments.* Park Ridge: ASA.
*In statuses 2, 3, and 4, the systemic disease may or may not be related to the cause for surgery.
†For any patient (P1 through P5) requiring emergency surgery, an E is added to the physical status, such as P1E, P2E. ASA 1 through ASA 6 or I-VI is often used for physical status.

It is often said that there is major and minor surgery but only major anesthesia

Premedications

The primary purpose of premedication before anesthesia is to sedate the patient and reduce anxiety. Medications that may be given preoperatively include sedatives and hypnotics, anxiolytics, amnestics, tranquilizers, analgesics or narcotics, antiemetics, and anticholinergics. A single drug may possess the properties of several classes. Midazolam (Versed) is frequently administered to relieve apprehension and to provide amnesia. An analgesic or narcotic may be ordered if preoperative discomfort is anticipated during invasive procedures or during the administration of a regional anesthetic. An anticholinergic such as atropine or glycopyrrolate may be used to prevent bradycardia in pediatric patients, for controlling secretions in patients undergoing oropharyngeal procedures, or for controlling cardiac reflex that may cause bradycardia as during ophthalmic procedures.

To decrease the risk of aspiration, metoclopramide (Reglan) may be given to empty the stomach and to reduce nausea and vomiting. In addition, an antacid or an H_2 receptor–blocking drug such as cimetidine (Tagamet) or ranitidine (Zantac) may be included to decrease gastric acid production and the acidity of the gastric contents. Should aspiration occur, a gastric pH above 2.5 decreases the resultant pulmonary damage.

Premedications may be administered either intramuscularly, intravenously, or orally with 15 to 30 ml of water. Oral premedication is usually preferred by the patient; the absorption and uptake are more predictable than that with an intramuscular injection; and the small amount of water is readily absorbed directly across the gastric mucosa.

Before a premedication is given, any last-minute questions from the patient concerning surgery and anesthesia should be answered, and proper execution of all consent forms should be verified. Premedications are usually given 30 to 90 minutes before surgery but may be given IV in the peroperative holding area or after the patient arrives in the surgical suite. Except for the small amount of water needed to swallow any medications, adult patients have traditionally been kept NPO (nothing by mouth) for a minimum 4 to 6 hours before elective surgery. However, data indicate that a shorter fasting period for clear liquids may be acceptable.[5,6]

Although premedications are commonly used, studies have shown that visits before surgery by the anesthesia provider and the perioperative nurse are far more important in relieving patient anxiety and concern. Major patient concerns include fear of the unknown, relinquishing control of one's life to someone else, being awake during surgery, and never awakening from anesthesia. Other concerns related to surgery may also be present. Often premedication is not given to older patients because their anxiety levels are lower, their responses to medications are unpredictable, and sedation can be given IV in the operating room if required. Preoperative sedation is usually not given to ambulatory patients because residual effects of most of these drugs may persist for extended periods of time.

Types of Anesthesia Care

A frequently used classification of anesthesia care is the following:

General anesthesia

General anesthesia is a reversible, unconscious state characterized by amnesia (sleep, hypnosis, or basal narcosis), analgesia (freedom from pain), depression of reflexes, muscle relaxation, and homeostasis or specific manipulation of physiologic systems and functions. Most patients think of general anesthesia when they are scheduled to have a surgical procedure; that is, they expect to be "put to sleep."

Regional anesthesia

Regional anesthesia is broadly defined as a reversible loss of sensation in a specific area or region of the body when a local anesthetic is injected to purposefully block or anesthetize nerve fibers in and around the operative site. Common regional anesthesia techniques include spinals (subarachnoid block [SAB]), epidurals, caudals, and major peripheral nerve blocks.

Monitored anesthesia care

Monitored anesthesia care (MAC) is provided when infiltration of the surgical site with a local anesthetic is performed by the surgeon and the anesthesia provider supplements the local anesthesia with IV drugs that provide sedation and systemic analgesia. The anesthesia provider also monitors the patient's vital functions and may use additional medication to optimize the patient's physiologic status. This technique can be used for some procedures for critically ill patients who may poorly tolerate a general anesthetic without extensive invasive monitoring and pharmacologic support. MAC is often used for healthy patients undergoing relatively minor surgical procedures. *Local standby* or *anesthesia standby* are older, less-accurate terms frequently used interchangeably with MAC.

Conscious sedation/analgesia

Conscious sedation/analgesia is increasingly being administered for specific short-term surgical, diagnostic, and therapeutic procedures within a hospital or ambulatory center. The ASA has defined sedation and analgesia as a state that allows patients to tolerate unpleasant procedures while maintaining adequate cardiorespiratory function and the ability to respond purposefully to verbal command and/or tactile stimulation. Patients whose only response is reflex withdrawal from a painful stimulus are sedated to a greater degree than encompassed by sedation/analgesia.[1] The demand for appropriate providers to administer and monitor the patient receiving conscious sedation/analgesia has grown over the past few years, exceeding the supply of anesthesia providers. This has resulted in the increased use of nonanesthesia providers (usually professional registered nurses with additional training in administering conscious sedation/analgesia medications and monitoring these patients) for these function.

Local anesthesia

Local anesthesia refers to the administration of an anesthetic agent to one part of the body by local infiltration or topical application. It is usually administered by the surgeon. Local anesthesia is used for minor procedures, if the patient's cooperation is necessary for the procedure, or the patient's physical condition warrants its use. An anesthesia provider is not involved in the patient's care. A perioperative nurse monitors the patient's vital signs and provides supportive care during the procedure.

PERIOPERATIVE MONITORING

Significant advances in perioperative monitoring have occurred in the last few years. (See also the section on Awareness During Anesthesia.) Among the medical specialties, anesthesiology has been a pioneer in the review and analysis of perioperative mishaps and the implementation of improved monitoring techniques and guidelines. These advances have resulted in significant decreases in mortality and morbidity. In several states malpractice insurance carriers have recognized the significance of these improvements and have decreased their premiums if certain monitors such as pulse oximetry (SpO_2) and end-tidal carbon dioxide ($ETCO_2$) are routinely employed.

The ASA has adopted the Standards for Basic Anesthetic Monitoring (Box 7-2) as guidelines for patient care. The perioperative nurse should be familiar with these standards and understand their significance in patient safety. If routine or frequent deviations from such standards occur, a quality assurance (QA) review should be considered.

Monitors considered appropriate include the following:

- Inspired oxygen analyzer (FiO_2), which is calibrated to room air on a daily basis
- Low-pressure disconnect alarm, which senses pressure in the expiratory limb of the patient circuit
- Inspiratory airway pressure
- Respirometer (these four devices are an integral part of most modern anesthesia machines)
- Electrocardioscope
- Blood pressure (usually measured with a noninvasive automated unit)
- Heart rate
- Precordial or esophageal stethoscope
- Temperature
- Peripheral nerve stimulator if muscle relaxants are used
- SpO_2
- $ETCO_2$

Many facilities also incorporate the analysis of respiratory and anesthetic gases in addition to the other parameters. This is done with an infrared analyzer, a mass spectrometer, or a Raman spectrometer which uses an argon ultraviolet laser.

Recent models of anesthesia machines have most of the basic monitors (excluding ECG) integrated into a computerized system. This system generally includes: FiO_2; inspired and expired CO_2; inspired and expired volatile agents; airway pressure and disconnect alarms; tidal volume, respiratory rate, and minute ventilation; noninvasive blood pressure (systolic, diastolic, and mean); SpO_2 and pulse rate; temperature; and an event marker. A sophisticated, prioritized system displays the caution or alarm condition(s) in one location, making it unnecessary to scan numerous individual monitors with a variety of displays when an alarm sounds. An internal computer system stores the digital data for more than 8 continuous hours. These data can be transferred to a computer disk (CD) for later analysis, or they can be reviewed on the display screen.

Based on the cardiovascular and pulmonary status of the patient, the surgical procedure, and the chance of significant physiologic changes, additional invasive monitors may be used. These include direct arterial and venous pressure measurements, a pulmonary artery (PA) catheter, and continuous mixed-venous O_2 saturation ($S\bar{v}O_2$) measured with a special PA catheter. A recently developed PA catheter can provide a continuous measurement of cardiac output. This new technology employs pulsed thermodilution to provide intermittent heat along a distal segment of the catheter. The small changes in the temperature of the blood are proportional to the blood flow (cardiac output). These changes are sensed by a thermistor on the tip of the catheter.

For certain conditions, other equipment such as transcutaneous O_2 and CO_2, transesophageal echocardiography, evoked potentials, electroencephalogram, and cerebral or neurologic function monitors may be used. For procedures posing a risk of venous air embolism, special monitors (such as a Doppler probe over the right atrium) may be used. An indwelling urinary catheter also provides a useful indication of renal function and hemodynamic status.

Despite some controversy, most anesthesiologists believe that the monitoring employed depends on the physiologic status and stability of the patient, the surgical procedure planned and its potential for sudden changes in cardiopulmonary functions, the anticipated blood loss and major fluid shifts, and the anticipated monitoring needs for postoperative management as opposed to whether a general or regional anesthetic technique will be used. However, monitoring of some parameters may be negated

BOX 7-2 | Standards for Basic Anesthetic Monitoring

These standards apply to all anesthesia care although, in emergency circumstances, appropriate life support measures take precedence. These standards may be exceeded at any time based on the judgment of the responsible anesthesiologist. They are intended to encourage quality patient care, but observing them cannot guarantee any specific patient outcome. They are subject to revision from time to time, as warranted by the evolution of technology and practice. They apply to all general anesthetics, regional anesthetics and monitored anesthesia care. This set of standards addresses only the issue of basic anesthetic monitoring, which is one component of anesthesia care. In certain rare or unusual circumstances, (1) some of these methods of monitoring may be clinically impractical, and (2) appropriate use of the described monitoring methods may fail to detect untoward clinical developments. Brief interruptions of continual† monitoring may be unavoidable. *Under extenuating circumstances, the responsible anesthesiologist may waive the requirements marked with an asterisk (*); it is recommended that when this is done, it should be so stated (including the reasons) in a note in the patient's medical record.* These standards are not intended for application to the care of the obstetrical patient in labor or in the conduct of pain management.

†Note that "continual" is defined as "repeated regularly and frequently in steady rapid succession," whereas "continuous" means "prolonged without any interruption at any time."

Standard I

Qualified anesthesia personnel shall be present in the room throughout the conduct of all general anesthetics, regional anesthetics and monitored anesthesia care.

Objective

Because of the rapid changes in patient status during anesthesia, qualified anesthesia personnel shall be continuously present to monitor the patient and provide anesthesia care. In the event there is a direct known hazard, e.g, radiation, to the anesthesia personnel which might require intermittent remote observation of the patient, some provision for monitoring the patient must be made. In the event that an emergency requires the temporary absence of the person primarily responsible for the anesthetic, the best judgment of the anesthesiologist will be exercised in comparing the emergency with the anesthetized patient's condition and in the selection of the person left responsible for the anesthetic during the temporary absence.

Standard II

During all anesthetics, the patient's oxygenation, ventilation, circulation and temperature shall be continually evaluated.

Oxygenation

Objective

To ensure adequate oxygen concentration in the inspired gas and the blood during all anesthetics.

Methods

1. Inspired gas: During every administration of general anesthesia using an anesthesia machine, the concentration of oxygen in the patient breathing system shall be measured by an oxygen analyzer with a low oxygen concentration limit alarm in use.*
2. Blood oxygenation: During all anesthetics, a quantitative method of assessing oxygenation such as pulse oximetry shall be employed.* Adequate illumination and exposure of the patient are necessary to assess color.*

Ventilation

Objective

To ensure adequate ventilation of the patient during all anesthetics.

Methods

1. Every patient receiving general anesthesia shall have the adequacy of ventilation continually evaluated. While qualitative clinical signs such as chest excursion, observation of the reservoir breathing bag and auscultation of breath sounds may be useful, quantitative monitoring of the carbon dioxide content and/or volume of expired gas is strongly encouraged.
2. When an endotracheal tube or laryngeal mask is inserted, its correct positioning must be verified by clinical assessment and by identification of carbon dioxide in the expired gas. Continual end-tidal carbon dioxide analysis, in use from the time of endotracheal tube/laryngeal mask placement, until extubation/removal or initiating transfer to a postoperative care location shall be performed using a quantitative method such as capnography, capnometry or mass spectroscopy.*
3. When ventilation is controlled by a mechanical ventilator, there shall be in continuous use a device that is capable of detecting disconnection of components of the breathing system. The device must give an audible signal when its alarm threshold is exceeded.
4. During regional anesthesia and monitored anesthesia care, the adequacy of ventilation shall be evaluated, at least, by continual observation of qualitative clinical signs.

Circulation

Objective

To ensure the adequacy of the patient's circulatory function during all anesthetics.

Methods

1. Every patient receiving anesthesia shall have the electrocardiogram continuously displayed from the beginning of anesthesia until preparing to leave the anesthetizing location.*
2. Every patient receiving anesthesia shall have arterial blood pressure and heart rate determined and evaluated at least every five minutes.*
3. Every patient receiving general anesthesia shall have, in addition to the above, circulatory function continually evaluated by at least one of the following: palpation of a pulse, auscultation of heart sounds, monitoring of a tracing of intraarterial pressure, ultrasound peripheral pulse monitoring, or pulse plethysmography or oximetry.

Body Temperature

Objective

To aid in the maintenance of appropriate body temperature during all anesthetics.

Methods

There shall be readily available a means to continuously measure the patient's temperature. When changes in body temperature are intended, anticipated or suspected, the temperature shall be measured.

Reprinted with permission from the American Society of Anesthesiologists (ASA), Park Ridge, Illinois. Approved by ASA House of Delegates on October 21, 1986, and last amended on October 23, 1996.

by the anesthetic technique selected. For example, a low-pressure disconnect alarm is unnecessary with regional anesthesia when a patient is breathing spontaneously. A peripheral nerve stimulator is unnecessary if muscle relaxants are not used.

The perioperative utilization of SpO_2 and $ETCO_2$ has grown exponentially. A brief review will help the reader understand their use.

Pulse Oximetry

Pulse oximetry is based on the principles of spectrometric oximetry, plethysmography, and the Lambert-Beer law, which relates the concentration of solute in suspension to the intensity of light transmitted through the solution. It gives a continuous noninvasive indication of the arterial O_2 saturation of functional hemoglobin and the pulse rate, and thus provides an early warning of hypoxemia.

The O_2-dissociation curve relates the percentage of totally saturated hemoglobin with O_2 on the y axis to the PaO_2 on the x axis. (The curve is sigmoid, and thus the relationship of the O_2 saturation to PaO_2 is nonlinear.) The following values are approximations with the O_2 saturation (and the SpO_2) in percentage (PaO_2 in torr): 98% to 100% (95 torr or greater), 90% (60 torr), 75% (39 torr), 50% (26 torr), and 25% (16 torr). Most pulse oximeters are accurate within ±2% above 70% and ±3% from 50% to 70% but correlate poorly below 50%. On room air, the SpO_2 for a young, healthy person should be 98% to 100%; an elderly patient may be in the low 90s, whereas a heavy smoker or someone with severe lung disease may even be in the 80s. It is wise to note the baseline SpO_2 of a patient before any O_2, medications, or stimulation is introduced. Maintenance of a SpO_2 above 90% corresponds to a PaO_2 of 60 torr or greater.

The sensor combines two low-intensity, light-emitting diodes (LED) as light sources and a photodiode as a receiver or light detector. One LED emits red light (approximately 660 nanometers [nm]), and the other LED emits infrared light (approximately 940 nm). These light sources alternate about 480 times a second. When the two frequencies of light are transmitted through blood and tissue, they are absorbed differently by the tissue components and by the reduced hemoglobin and the oxyhemoglobin. Because absorption by the other tissue components is essentially constant, the major variable is the saturation of the hemoglobin with O_2. The internal microprocessor analyzes the variations in the absorption of light emitted from both LEDs and provides a readout of the percent saturation of hemoglobin with O_2. The pulse rate is also indicated. Many units also display a waveform that correlates with the arterial pulsations.

The pulse oximeter reading can be adversely affected by any event that significantly reduces vascular pulsations such as hypoperfusion, hypotension, hypovolemia, vasoconstriction, or hypothermia. Electrosurgery, motion, or ambient light may also artifactually decrease the readout.

Carboxyhemoglobin (carbon monoxide bound to hemoglobin) falsely elevates the indicated SpO_2 saturation, and methemoglobin (hemoglobin that has an oxidized iron molecule and cannot reversibly combine with O_2) falsely lowers the SpO_2. Intravenous dyes affect the pulse oximeter. Methylene blue may cause a drop to 65% for 1 to 2 minutes, indigo carmine a very slight decrease, and indocyanine green a slightly greater decrease. Nail polish can also decrease the SpO_2. Blue, black, or green polish significantly decreases the SpO_2 reading, whereas red polish has only a slight effect. Opaque, acrylic nail coverings may block the light beam. If nail polish or coverings seem to cause problems, the sensor can be turned sideways so that the fingernail is parallel to the light path.

The sensor is usually placed on the third or fourth finger or on a toe. Some manufacturers have sensors for the ear lobe and the bridge of the nose, as well as smaller ones for soles and palms of infants and children. The pulse oximeter does not require user calibration. Care must be taken to prevent localized neurovascular or ischemic damage. For example, a hard-cased sensor placed on a finger may cause ischemia when the arms are tightly secured at the patient's side during a long procedure.

If trouble with the pulse oximeter is encountered during a local anesthetic, the perioperative nurse should evaluate the patient's ventilatory status, verify proper placement of the sensor, and rule out the items listed above, which adversely affect operation of the unit. Pulsatile blood flow in the extremity may be inadequate because of hypovolemia, decreased cardiac output, malpositioning, constriction by the blood pressure cuff, or hypothermia. As a final step, the pulse oximetry unit, cable, and sensor can be checked by placement of the sensor on the nurse's finger to verify satisfactory function.

Capnography

A capnometer measures CO_2, and a capnograph displays the CO_2 waveform. In patients with normal circulation and pulmonary function, it provides an excellent method to evaluate alveolar ventilation, since there is only a small gradient between the arterial and the alveolar CO_2. With forced expiration, the $ETCO_2$ provides a close approximation of the arterial CO_2 ($PaCO_2$). In an anesthetized patient, expiration is passive, and the point of measurement is near the connection between the patient's circuit and the endotracheal tube. Therefore, the $ETCO_2$ is 5 to 10 torr lower than the $PaCO_2$ measured in arterial blood.

The $ETCO_2$ can be measured by a mass spectrometer, a Raman spectrometer, or an infrared analyzer. Recent advances in the technology of infrared analyzers and microprocessors have resulted in compact units that provide a continuous indication of the $ETCO_2$ and have made these the most widely used units for perioperative monitoring. These units measure the amount of infrared light absorbed by the CO_2 in the sample of gas. Two types of monitors are in use. In the *mainstream* unit, all respired gas passes through the detector, whereas with the *sidestream* unit, a portion of the gas is aspirated at a constant rate (50 to 250 ml/min) through a small-bore tubing into the unit. Each design has advantages. Most units display a waveform of the expiratory CO_2 partial pressure versus time after a short sampling and processing delay. The waveform is important for correctly interpreting the output data. Digital readouts usually give the $ETCO_2$ and respiratory rate. Daily user calibration is rarely required with the newer units. Clinically the units confirm proper endotracheal intubation and are useful to detect anesthesia circuit disconnection, alveolar ventilation, early return of respiratory function after muscle relaxants are used, and acute alterations in metabolic functions such as malignant hyperthermia or thyrotoxicosis.

GENERAL ANESTHESIA

Mechanism of Action

Numerous theories have been proposed to explain the action of general anesthetics. Many of the recent investigations have involved inhalation anesthetics. (The terms *volatile anesthetic, potent agent,* and *inhaled* or *inhalational anesthetic* are synonymous with *inhalation anesthetic.*) Evidence indicates that the synaptic transmission of nerve impulses is reversibly inhibited in several areas of the central nervous system. The extent of inhibition and consequently the progressive depression of function are correlated with the partial pressure of the inhaled anesthetic at various sites. The inhibition is believed to occur at a lipophilic site on the biologic membrane of synapses and possibly on small, unmyelinated nerve fibers. Suppression of spinal reflex activity is believed to produce some relaxation of skeletal muscles. Although no single concept explains all the phenomena, a few theories explain many of the actions that have been observed. The following are some of the more widely accepted theories:

Protein receptor theory

The protein receptor theory proposes that hydrophobic areas of specific proteins in the central nervous system act as receptor sites. The steep dose-response curve of inhaled anesthetics seems to support this theory by indicating that a critical number of receptor sites must be occupied before patient movement in response to noxious stimuli is obtunded.

Meyer-Overton theory

The Meyer-Overton theory is also called the *critical volume hypothesis* to explain the correlation between the lipid solubility (oil-to-gas partition coefficient) and the anesthetic potency. This theory proposes that when enough anesthetic molecules dissolve (that is, a critical volume is reached) at a crucial hydrophobic site, such as

the lipid cellular membrane, anesthesia is achieved. As the cell membrane expands in response to the dissolved anesthetic molecules, changes in the ionic channels occur and alter the sodium flux involved in cellular depolarization. Because some lipid-soluble compounds are not anesthetics, this theory does not give a complete explanation of anesthetic action.

Endogenous endorphins

Endogenous endorphins, or opiate-like substances, suppress various pain pathways. Several classes of endorphins have been identified. The action of beta-endorphins is antagonized by naloxone or nalmefene, specific narcotic antagonists, but the relative potency of inhaled anesthetics is not altered. Although some degree of analgesia may be explained by this mechanism, it does not correlate well with the level of anesthesia achieved by inhaled anesthetics.

Intravenous anesthetics may also function by some of the mechanisms proposed for the inhaled anesthetics. Factors involved in the pharmacokinetics of IV drugs include the volume of distribution, biotransformation, and clearance of the drug by metabolism, excretion, or elimination of the drug and its metabolites.

In summary, no single theory for the mechanism of action can explain all the effects observed with anesthetic agents. The range of anesthetic activity varies with the different anesthetics; the effects on the central nervous system and skeletal muscles are similar but not identical; structural and spatial differences exist among agents; changes at both the membrane and cellular levels occur; and optical isomers produce different responses. Although similar in many respects, anesthetic agents are individually unique and probably work through numerous mechanisms and at multiple sites to produce their effects.

Levels of General Anesthesia

Guedel integrated the signs and stages of ether anesthesia into a system (Fig. 7-1) that was used clinically for more than 60 years. This system applied only to unpremedicated patients breathing spontaneously during ether anesthesia, a technique that is rarely used in modern practice except in developing countries. By evaluating the physiologic changes and reflex responses listed in Fig. 7-1, one can estimate the depth of anesthesia. Stage 1 is from the initial administration of anesthetic agents to loss of consciousness. Stage 2 is from the loss of consciousness to the onset of regular breathing and loss of the eyelid reflex. Stage 2 is also called the *delirium* or *excitement* stage, and thrashing movements may occur. No auditory or physical stimulation should take place during this stage. Stage 3, which begins with the onset of a regular breathing pattern and lasts until cessation of respiration, is divided into four planes and is the stage of surgical anesthesia. Stage 4 is from cessation of respiration to circulatory failure that leads to death.

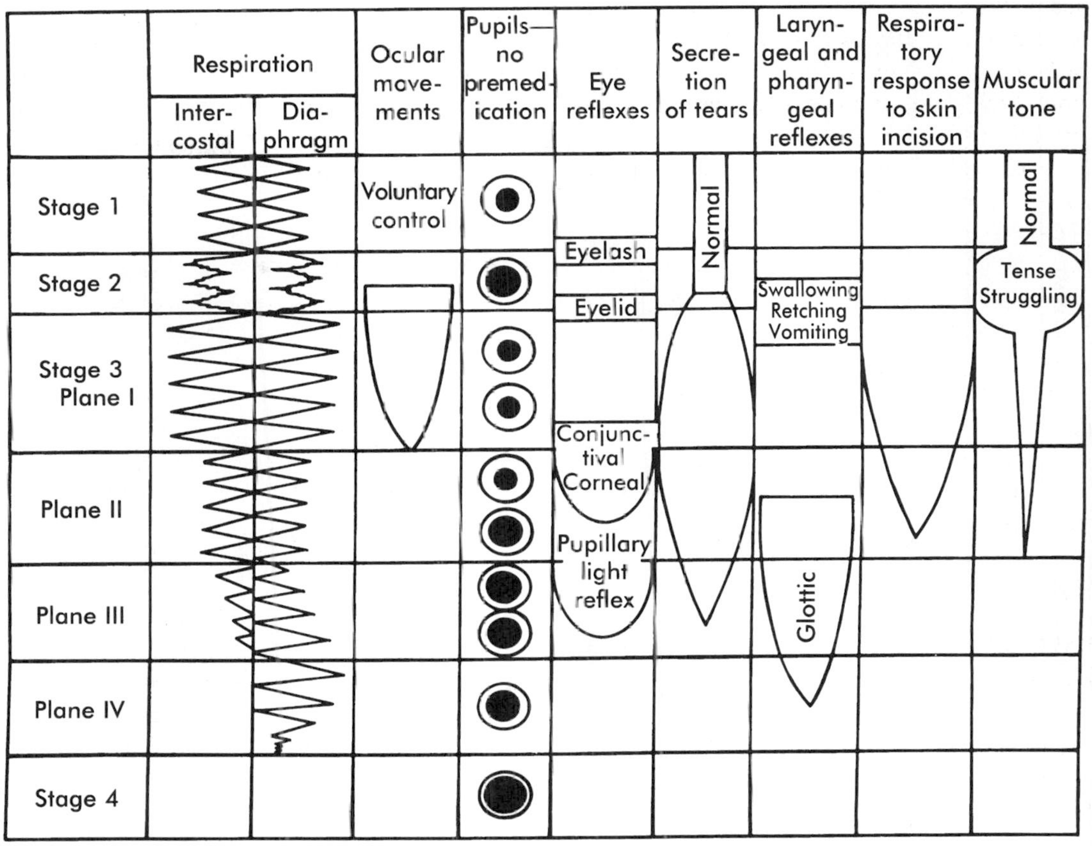

	Respiration		Ocular move-ments	Pupils—no premed-ication	Eye reflexes	Secre-tion of tears	Laryn-geal and pharyn-geal reflexes	Respira-tory response to skin incision	Muscular tone
	Inter-costal	Dia-phragm							
Stage 1			Voluntary control			Normal			Normal
Stage 2					Eyelash / Eyelid			Swallowing Retching Vomiting	Tense Struggling
Stage 3 Plane I									
Plane II					Conjunctival / Corneal / Pupillary light reflex				
Plane III							Glottic		
Plane IV									
Stage 4									

FIGURE 7-1 Changes occurring during ether anesthesia. The actions of different anesthetics vary slightly from this.

Although Guedel's system gives us an appreciation for the interrelationships of numerous signs during anesthesia, the variety of drugs and anesthetic techniques used today do not provide such uniform responses suitable for estimating the exact depth of anesthesia. Narcotics and anticholinergic drugs given as premedicants alter the pupillary responses. Evaluation of respiratory responses and muscle tone is not valid when controlled ventilation and muscle relaxants are used. Today, general anesthesia is usually induced with the IV injection of a rapid-acting drug, such as thiopental or propofol (Diprivan), that takes the patient rapidly to stage 3 and eliminates the untoward responses often seen during stage 2.

For optimal anesthesia and good surgical conditions, several different but interrelated factors are involved. These include hypnosis (sleep), analgesia (freedom from pain), amnesia (lack of recall or awareness), appropriate surgical conditions including muscle relaxation and positioning of the patient, and continued homeostasis of the patient's vital functions. Different drugs and anesthetic agents possess various properties that facilitate the above conditions. Combinations of drugs are therefore used to obtain the desired effects. For example, diazepam and midazolam are hypnotics and amnestics, thiopental and etomidate are hypnotics, morphine and fentanyl are analgesics, and pancuronium and succinylcholine are muscle relaxants.

Muscle relaxants primarily affect only skeletal muscles and not cardiac or smooth muscles; however, some relaxants may have side effects such as tachycardia via the autonomic nervous system or hypotension secondary to the release of histamine. The potent inhalation anesthetics (halothane, enflurane, isoflurane, desflurane, and sevoflurane) provide hypnosis, amnesia, analgesia, and muscle relaxation in varying degrees. Hypotensive or hypertensive drugs and cardioactive agents may also be included to achieve the optimum depth of anesthesia while affecting physiologic homeostasis as little as possible. Some of the drugs commonly used in anesthesia are briefly described in Table 7-2.

Phases of General Anesthesia

General anesthesia may be divided into three phases: *induction, maintenance,* and *emergence. Induction* begins with administration of anesthetic agents and continues until the patient is ready for positioning or prepping, surgical manipulation, or incision. The surgical prep is often started after the induction drugs are given. This end point of induction may vary with the surgical procedure. The *maintenance* phase continues from this point until near completion of the procedure and may be accomplished with inhalation agents or with IV drugs given in titrated doses or by continuous infusions. *Emergence* varies in length

TABLE 7-2 | Commonly Used Anesthetic Gases and Drugs

	COMMON USAGE	ADVANTAGES	DISADVANTAGES	COMMENTS
Inhalation Gases				
Air	Maintenance with O_2; laser surgery near airway	Less support of combustion than N_2O	No anesthetic qualities	Possibly less nausea than N_2O
Oxygen (O_2)	Essential for life	Can slightly ↑ O_2 available to tissues in low-cardiac-output states	Can cause retinopathy in premature infants	High concentrations hazardous with lasers in surgery of head, neck, and pulmonary areas
Nitrous oxide (N_2O)	Maintenance; frequently for induction	Rapid induction and recovery; additive effects to other anesthetics	No relaxation; can depress myocardium	Hypoxia if overdose given; ↑ uptake of other volatile agents
Enflurane (Ethrane)	Maintenance; occasionally for induction	Good relaxation; allows more epinephrine to be used than with halothane; 2.4% metabolized	Can cause ↑ HR and ↓ BP; lowers seizure threshold; slightly irritating odor	Abnormal EEG at high concentrations; used less often today
Desflurane (Suprane)	Maintenance in shorter cases	Very rapid emergence; good relaxation; 0.02% metabolized	May cause transient ↑ HR and ↓ BP; airway irritation; requires heated vaporizer	Rapid recovery phase; can use for emergence after maintenance with another volatile agent; expensive
Halothane (Fluothane)	Maintenance; frequently for induction in pediatrics	Rapid induction and recovery; pleasant, nonirritating odor; fair relaxation	Narrow margin of safety; sensitizes myocardium to epinephrine; rare cause of liver damage; 15% to 20% metabolized	May cause ↓ HR and ↓ BP; PVCs and ventricular fibrillation may occur with epinephrine
Isoflurane (Forane)	Maintenance; occasionally for induction	Good relaxation; allows more epinephrine to be used than with halothane; maintains cardiac output; 0.2% metabolized	↑ HR; slightly irritating odor	Isomer of enflurane; probably most common agent used today
Sevoflurane (Ultane)	Induction and maintenance	Very rapid induction and emergence; good relaxation; ~5% metabolized	A metabolite (compound A) is nephrotoxic in rats; effect in humans unknown	Very rapid and smooth mask induction in children or adults; expensive
Opioid Analgesics				
Morphine sulfate (MS)	Perioperative pain; premedication	Inexpensive; duration of action 4 to 5 hours; euphoria; good cardiovascular stability	Nausea and vomiting; histamine release; postural ↓ BP (↓ SVR); high first-pass effect PO	Used intrathecally and epidurally for postoperative pain; elimination half-life 3 hours
Alfentanil (Alfenta)	Surgical analgesia in ambulatory patients	Duration of action 0.5 hour; used as bolus or infusion		Potency: 750 μg = 10 mg morphine sulfate; elimination half-life 1.6 hours
Fentanyl (Sublimaze)	Surgical analgesia: epidural infusion for postoperative analgesia; add to SAB	Good cardiovascular stability; duration of action 0.5 hour		Most commonly used opioid, potency: 100 μg = 10 mg morphine sulfate; elimination half-life 3.6 hours

Drug	Uses	Advantages	Disadvantages	Comments
Remifentanil (Ultiva)	0.25 to 1.0 µg/kg/min infusion for surgical analgesia; small boluses for brief, intense pain	Easily titratable; metabolized by blood and tissue esterases; very short duration; good cardiovascular stability	New; expensive; requires mixing	Potency: 25µg = 10 mg morphine sulfate; 20 to 30 times potency of alfentanil; elimination half-life 3 to 10 minutes
Sufentanil (Sufenta)	Surgical analgesia	Good cardiovascular stability; duration of action 0.5 hour; prolonged analgesia	Prolonged respiratory depression	Potency: 15 µg = 10 mg morphine sulfate; elimination half-life 2.7 hours
Depolarizing Muscle Relaxants				
Succinylcholine (Anectine, Quelicin)	Intubation; short cases	Rapid onset; short duration	Requires refrigeration; may cause fasciculations, postoperative myalgias, and arrhythmias; ↑ serum K$^+$ with burns, tissue trauma, paralysis, and muscle diseases; slight histamine release	Prolonged muscle relaxation with serum cholinesterase deficiency and certain antibiotics; trigger agent for malignant hyperthermia
Nondepolarizing Muscle Relaxants—Intermediate Onset and Duration				
Atracurium (Tracrium)	Intubation; maintenance of relaxation	No significant cardiovascular or cumulative effects; good with renal failure	Requires refrigeration; slight histamine release	Breakdown by Hofmann elimination and ester hydrolysis
Cisatracurium (Nimbex)	Intubation; maintenance of relaxation	Similar to atracurium	No histamine release	Similar to atracurium
Mivacurium (Mivacron)	Intubation; maintenance of relaxation	Short acting, rapid metabolism by plasma cholinesterase; used as bolus or infusion	Expensive in longer cases	New; rarely need to reverse; prolonged effect with plasma cholinesterase deficiency
Rocuronium (Zemuron)	Intubation; maintenance of relaxation	Rapid onset; elimination via kidney and liver	Vagolytic; may ↑ HR	Duration similar to atracurium and vecuronium
Vecuronium (Norcuron)	Intubation; maintenance of relaxation	No significant cardiovascular or cumulative effects; no histamine release	Requires mixing	Mostly eliminated in bile, some in urine
Nondepolarizing Muscle Relaxants—Longer Onset and Duration				
d-Tubocurarine	Maintenance of relaxation		May cause histamine release and transient ganglionic blockade	Mostly used for pretreatment with succinylcholine
Metocurine (Metubine)	Maintenance of relaxation		Slight histamine release	Large bolus may cause ↓ BP
Pancuronium (Pavulon)	Maintenance of relaxation	Good cardiovascular stability	May cause ↑ HR and ↑ BP	Mostly renal elimination
Intravenous Anesthetics				
Etomidate (Amidate)	Induction	Good cardiovascular stability; fast, smooth induction and recovery	May cause pain with injection and myotonic movements	
Diazepam (Valium, Dizac)	Amnesia; hypnotic; preoperative medication	Good sedation	Prolonged duration	Residual effects for 20 to 90 hours; ↑ effect with alcohol

Continued

TABLE 7-2 | Commonly Used Anesthetic Gases and Drugs—cont'd

	COMMON USAGE	ADVANTAGES	DISADVANTAGES	COMMENTS
Ketamine (Ketalar)	Induction, occasional maintenance (IV or IM)	Short acting; patient maintains airway; good in small children and burn patients	Large doses may cause hallucinations and respiratory depression	Need darkened, quiet room for recovery; often used in trauma cases
Midazolam (Versed)	Hypnotic; anxiolytic; sedation; often used as adjunct to induction	Excellent amnesia; water soluble (no pain with IV injection); short acting	Slower induction than thiopental	Often used for amnesia with insertion of invasive monitors or regional anesthesia
Propofol (Diprivan)	Induction and maintenance; sedation with regional anesthesia or MAC	Rapid onset; awakening in 4 to 8 minutes	May cause pain when injected into small veins	Short elimination half-life (34 to 64 minutes)
Sodium methohexital (Brevital)	Induction	Ultrashort-acting barbiturate	May cause hiccups	Can be given rectally
Thiopental sodium (Pentothal)	Induction	Smooth induction and recovery	Large doses may cause apnea and cardiovascular depression	May cause laryngospasm; can be given rectally
Local Anesthetics				
Bupivacaine (Marcaine, Sensorcaine)	Epidural, spinal, or local infiltration	Good relaxation; long acting	Overdose can cause cardiac collapse	Max. dose: 200 and 150 mg/70 kg with and without epinephrine respectively
Chloroprocaine (Nesacaine)	Epidural anesthesia	Ultrashort acting; good relaxation	May cause neurotoxicity if injected into CSF	Max. dose: 1000 and 800 mg/70 kg with and without epinephrine respectively
Lidocaine (Xylocaine)	Epidural, spinal, peripheral, IV anesthesia, and local infiltration	Short acting; good relaxation; low toxicity	Overdose can cause convulsions; possible transient neurologic changes with spinal anesthesia	Also used for ventricular arrhythmias Max. dose: 7 and 5 mg/kg with and without epinephrine respectively
Tetracaine (Pontocaine)	Spinal anesthesia	Long acting; good relaxation		Max. dose: 1 to 1.5 mg/kg (epinephrine rarely used)
Anticholinergics				
Atropine	Block effects of acetylcholine; ↓ vagal tone; reverse muscle relaxants; treat sinus bradycardia	↑ HR; suppresses salivation, bronchial and gastric secretions	Depresses sweating; may cause dry mouth, flushing, dizziness, CNS symptoms	Quite selective at muscarinic receptor in smooth and cardiac muscle and exocrine glands
Glycopyrrolate (Robinul)	Similar to atropine	Small ↑ HR; does not cross blood-brain barrier; can ↑ gastric pH > atropine	Prolonged duration of effects	Lower incidence of arrhythmias than atropine

and depends on the patient's state and the depth and duration of anesthesia. Emergence starts as the patient begins to "emerge" from anesthesia and usually ends when the patient is ready to leave the operating room (OR). Intubation occurs during the induction phase, and extubation is usually performed during emergence. Recovery from anesthesia can be considered a fourth phase of general anesthesia.

Types of General Anesthesia

The type of general anesthesia employed is often described as IV technique, inhalation technique (with a volatile anesthetic agent), or a combination of both IV and inhalation techniques. For example, an IV technique traditionally includes an induction agent such as thiopental, combined with 30% to 40% O_2 and N_2O, an amnestic drug such as diazepam, an analgesic such as fentanyl or morphine sulfate, and a muscle relaxant.

In contrast, an inhalation technique may utilize thiopental or propofol to facilitate a rapid induction, or patients may "breathe themselves down" with a potent agent such as sevoflurane or halothane plus N_2O and O_2. An inhalation induction is often used with children to avoid inserting an IV catheter when they are awake. Depending on the kind of surgical procedure, maintenance of anesthesia may be accomplished with only inhalation agents and spontaneous, assisted, or controlled ventilation. Effects of the volatile agents are dose related and provide differing levels of anesthesia, amnesia analgesia, muscle relaxation, and hemodynamic responses. If supplemental muscle relaxation is needed, the dose required is significantly less than the dose necessary during IV anesthesia.

In the past, the term *balanced anesthesia* was used when various combinations of IV drugs were "balanced" to provide complete anesthesia. Today, the term is often used to describe a combination of both IV drugs and inhalation agents employed to obtain specific effects for each patient and procedure.

Today, many anesthesia providers may use *total IV anesthesia* (TIVA). This technique may be used in the OR but is commonly employed for pediatric, uncooperative, or trauma patients in remote locations such as the magnetic resonance imaging (MRI), radiology, or surgical laser suite where a waste-gas evacuation system is not available. It is also used in the expanding area of office-based surgical procedures. With TIVA, short-acting drugs such as propofol with remifentanil or alfentanil are used for induction (Research Highlight 7-3). These drugs may be mixed together in one syringe, or separate infusion pumps may be used. Typical infusion pumps are shown in Fig. 7-2. Anesthesia is maintained by an infusion plus O_2 alone or with N_2O. An intermediate-acting muscle relaxant (mivacurium, cisatracurium, atracurium, or vecuronium) may also be given. As surgery nears completion, the maintenance drugs are titrated off, and emergence from anesthesia occurs.

Muscle Relaxants

Muscle relaxants are primarily used by anesthesia providers to facilitate intubation and to provide good operating conditions at lighter planes of general anesthesia. These drugs may be used elsewhere for emergency intubation or less frequently when a patient is being mechanically ventilated. Muscle relaxants primarily affect skeletal muscle and have little effect on cardiac or smooth muscle. Although not always dose dependent, many of these drugs have adverse side effects. The route of metabolism and elimination varies, and this may be important in patients with hepatic or renal disease. Muscle relaxants are classified as *depolarizing* or *nondepolarizing*.

Succinylcholine is the only *depolarizing* muscle relaxant in clinical use. Its action is similar to acetylcholine, and at the neuromuscular junction it causes depolarization of the postjunctional membrane. Generalized skeletal muscle contractions known as fasciculations result from the simultaneous depolarization of all the muscle fibers. These fasciculations and associated postoperative myalgias may be attenuated when a pretreatment dose of a nondepolarizing relaxant (such as *d*-tubocurarine 0.04 mg/kg) is given 3 to 5 minutes before administration of the intubating dose of succinylcholine. Onset of paralysis (30 to 90 seconds) is faster and the duration of action (5 to 10 minutes) is shorter than with other relaxants. The speed of onset makes it the preferred drug for rapid-sequence inductions. Adverse side effects associated with the use of succinylcholine include cardiac arrhythmias, hyperkalemia, myalgias (particularly in young and muscular ambulatory patients), and increases in intraocular, intracranial, and intragastric pressures. It can also trigger malignant hyperthermia in susceptible patients. It can also be infused for longer procedures, but an excessive dose may cause prolonged relaxation (known as phase II blockade). Succinylcholine is hydrolyzed by plasma cholinesterase, and the rare patient with an abnormal or absent enzyme (plasma cholinesterase) will have prolonged muscle paralysis.

Nondepolarizing muscle relaxants competitively block the depolarizing action of acetylcholine at the neuromuscular junction, which results in skeletal muscle paralysis. Fasciculations do not occur. These drugs can be subdivided by the duration of action into *intermediate* (mivacurium, atracurium, cisatracurium, and vecuronium) and *long-acting* (*d*-tubocurarine, metocurine, pancuronium, pipecuronium, and doxacurium). The potency, duration (metabolism and elimination), and side effects of these drugs vary and may be individually altered in patients with hepatic or renal dysfunction, electrolyte imbalance, or hypothermia, or by other drugs administered perioperatively (inhalation and local anesthetics, aminoglycoside antibiotics, calcium-entry blockers, magnesium, and cardiac antiarrhythmics). Generally, nondepolarizing

7-3   RESEARCH HIGHLIGHT

REMIFENTANIL: A NEW NARCOTIC

Adequate analgesia is a vital component of every anesthetic. To provide intraoperative pain relief, fentanyl (a synthetic opioid) is probably the most widely used narcotic. Other synthetic opioids (sufentanil and alfentanil), morphine, and meperidine are also given. Redistribution and metabolism of these narcotics are major factors in the termination of their effects, though several of the metabolites have pharmacologic activity. Dysfunction of the hepatic or renal system can alter the metabolism or excretion of these narcotics.

Remifentanil (Ultiva) is a new, ultrashort-acting synthetic opioid that is chemically related to fentanyl. Its unique characteristic is a propanoic methyl ester that undergoes rapid hydrolysis by nonspecific esterases in blood and peripheral tissues. The short-lived metabolite is less than $\frac{1}{4000}$ the potency of the parent compound.

Remifentanil is a mu-receptor agonist and has the typical side effects of an opioid. It has an elimination half-life of 9.5 minutes compared to 58 minutes for alfentanil. In recent years, alfentanil has been widely used for total intravenous anesthesia (TIVA), but accumulation limits its prolonged use. Since remifentanil has almost no cumulative effect, it is particularly suitable for continuous IV infusion. Combined with a propofol infusion and a muscle relaxant if needed, TIVA can be provided.

With increased emphasis on ambulatory procedures, there is much interest in rapid emergence from anesthesia and discharge to home. A multicenter, randomized, double-blind, parallel group study compared remifentanil with alfentanil for TIVA. In seven medical centers, 200 adults with ASA physical status 1 to status 3 and having laparoscopic surgery scheduled for more than 30 minutes were divided into two groups. All patients received midazolam 1 mg and 5 to 10 ml/kg of lactated Ringer's solution before induction with propofol 2 mg/kg. Anesthesia was maintained with a continuous infusion of propofol 150 μg/kg/min. Group I received a bolus of remifentanil 1 μg/kg followed by an infusion of 0.5 μg/kg/min. Group II received a bolus of alfentanil 20 μg/kg followed by an infusion of 2 μg/kg/min. Vecuronium was used for intubation and muscle relaxation during the procedure. The lungs were ventilated with O_2 or O_2 and air mixtures. Five minutes after trocar insertion, the infusion rates of propofol and the opioid (remifentanil or alfentanil) were decreased by 50%. In a blinded fashion, 10 minutes before the anticipated end of the procedure, the alfentanil infusion was terminated. During the procedure, the level of anesthesia was maintained by prescribed boluses and changes in the infusion rates. After the procedure, the patients were evaluated with psychomotor and cognitive function tests as well as a sedation score.

In summary, fewer remifentanil patients (24%) required intraoperative adjustment of the opioid infusion than the alfentanil patients (41%). Overall, the preinduction awareness, the time to awakening, the alertness score, and the incidences of nausea and vomiting were not significantly different. As expected, postsurgical pain occurred earlier with remifentanil than with alfentanil.

From Cartwright, D.P., Kvalsvik, O., Cassuto, J., et al. (1997). A randomized, blind comparison of remifentanil and alfentanil during anesthesia for outpatient surgery. *Anesthesia and Analgesia, 85,* 1014-1049; Philip, B.K., Scuderi, P.E., Chung, F., et al. and the Remifentanil/Alfentanil Outpatient TIVA Group. (1997). Remifentanil compared with alfentanil for ambulatory surgery using total intravenous anesthesia. *Anesthesia and Analgesia, 84,* 515-521.

relaxants can be used in patients with malignant hyperthermia or plasma cholinesterase deficiencies (except for mivacurium). Side effects vary with the individual drugs. They usually are dose dependent and include alterations in blood pressure and heart rate. The effect of the muscle relaxants (neuromuscular blockade) can be monitored with a peripheral nerve stimulator. Paralysis caused by the nondepolarizing relaxants may be antagonized by IV anticholinesterases such as edrophonium, neostigmine, or pyridostigmine. These antagonists compete for receptor sites at the neuromuscular junction and may be associated with bradycardia, for which atropine or glycopyrrolate is routinely given.

Typical Sequence of General Anesthesia

After arriving in the preoperative area or the OR suite, the patient is identified, the chart is checked for signed consents or an operative permit or both, and the latest results of laboratory tests and diagnostic studies are reviewed. Although the patient may have been evaluated several days earlier in a preanesthesia clinic, certain information must be verified by the perioperative nurse immediately before surgery. The anesthesia provider also reviews the pertinent medical history and data and confirms that there have been no interval changes in the patient's status. Depending on the practice of the anesthesia department and institutional policy, an IV infusion may be started in a preoperative area or after the patient is transferred to the OR. After arrival in the OR the appropriate intraoperative monitors are connected to the patient before induction of anesthesia. In the perioperative period, nearly all anesthesia-related drugs are given IV, except of course the inhalation agents.

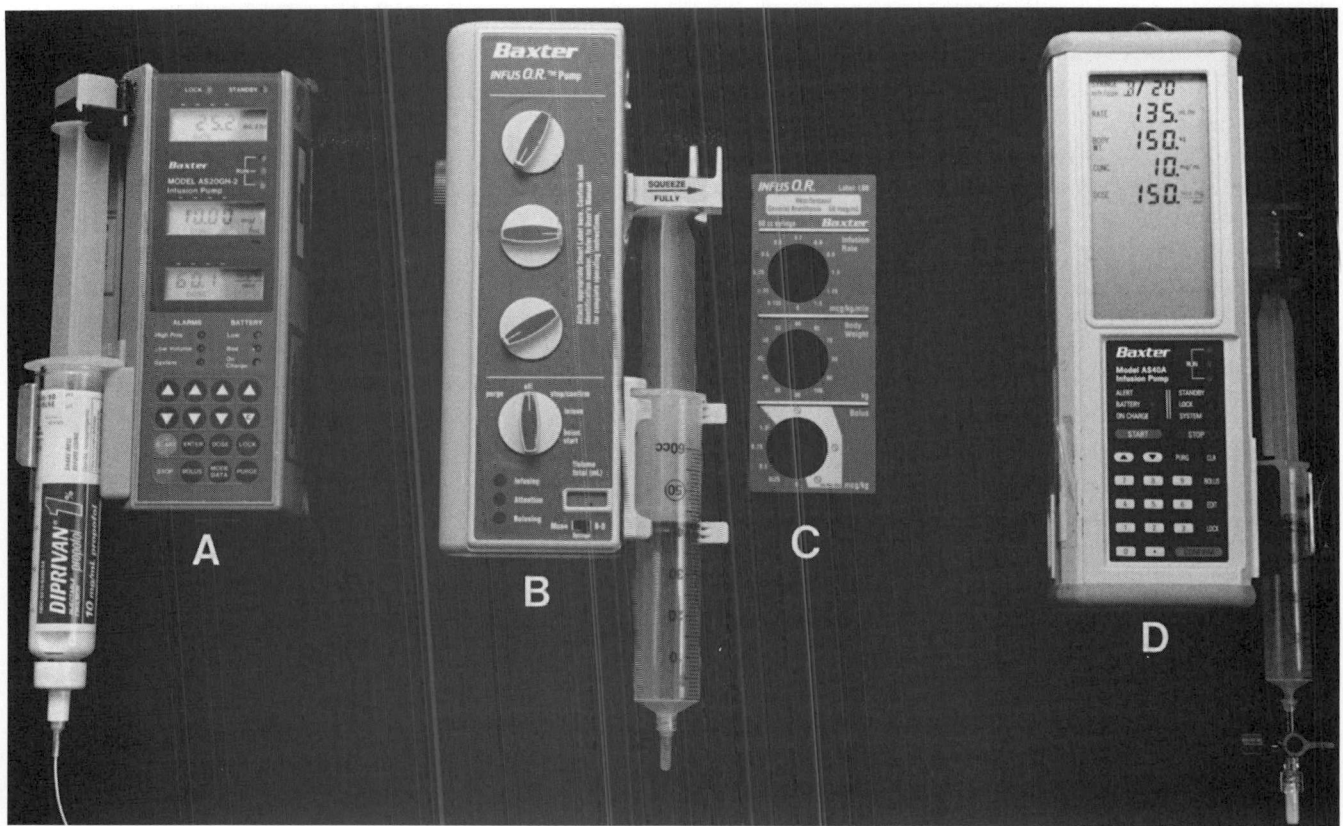

FIGURE 7-2 Typical drug-infusion pumps. These units have rechargeable batteries. After input of body weight and drug concentration, an infusion rate and bolus dose can be programmed. Units **A** and **B** require a 60 ml syringe, whereas **D** can be programed for multiple sizes and brands. A magnetic "smart plate" (**C**) is available for all common drug infusions in specified concentrations. When the plate is placed on **B**, it activates the pump and provides a rapid, simple setup of appropriate infusion rates for that specific drug. As an alternative, many IV pumps can be used, but these usually require special IV tubing sets, the solutions are in a plastic bag, and the total amount infused is less accurate.

Before induction, the patient is usually preoxygenated (actually denitrogenated) using a mask with 100% O_2 for 3 to 5 minutes. This practice permits washout of most of the gaseous nitrogen from the body and provides a large reserve supply of O_2 in the lungs. A test dose of the induction agent (such as 50 mg of thiopental) is often given to check for any unusual or exaggerated response. If succinylcholine is to be used for intubation, a small pretreatment dose of a nondepolarizing muscle relaxant (such as 3 mg of *d*-tubocurarine, or 0.5 to 1 mg of pancuronium or vecuronium) is usually given. If the patient can be safely ventilated with a mask, many anesthesia providers now avoid the adverse effects of succinylcholine and use one of the nondepolarizing muscle relaxants for intubation.

To induce anesthesia, a short-acting barbiturate such as thiopental (2 to 6 mg/kg) or propofol (1.5 to 2.5 mg/kg) is given. When the patient becomes apneic and the eyelash reflex is gone, the airway is checked for patency by ventilating the patient with a mask. Depending on several factors such as the airway and the type and duration of surgery, O_2 and anesthetic gases may be delivered to a spontaneously breathing patient through a mask that is held in place with a head strap. Positioning of the head or insertion of an oral or nasal airway may be used to maintain a patent airway. If spontaneous or assisted ventilation is planned, a laryngeal mask airway (LMA) may be inserted without a muscle relaxant.

If mask anesthesia or an LMA is not suitable or appropriate, an endotracheal tube may be used to facilitate ventilation and to prevent aspiration. (Typical equipment used for intubation as well as airway control and monitoring is shown in Fig. 7-3.) An intubating dose of a muscle relaxant is administered, which results in temporary paralysis.

To facilitate intubation, the patient's head is placed in a "sniffing" position. The laryngoscope is held in the left hand. The laryngoscope blade is inserted into the right side of the mouth and then moved to the midline, "sweeping" the tongue to the left. The endotracheal tube is introduced on the right side of the mouth and gently inserted into the trachea so that the cuff is approximately 1 cm below the vocal cords. The cuff is inflated just enough to occlude any air passage with the peak pressures used for

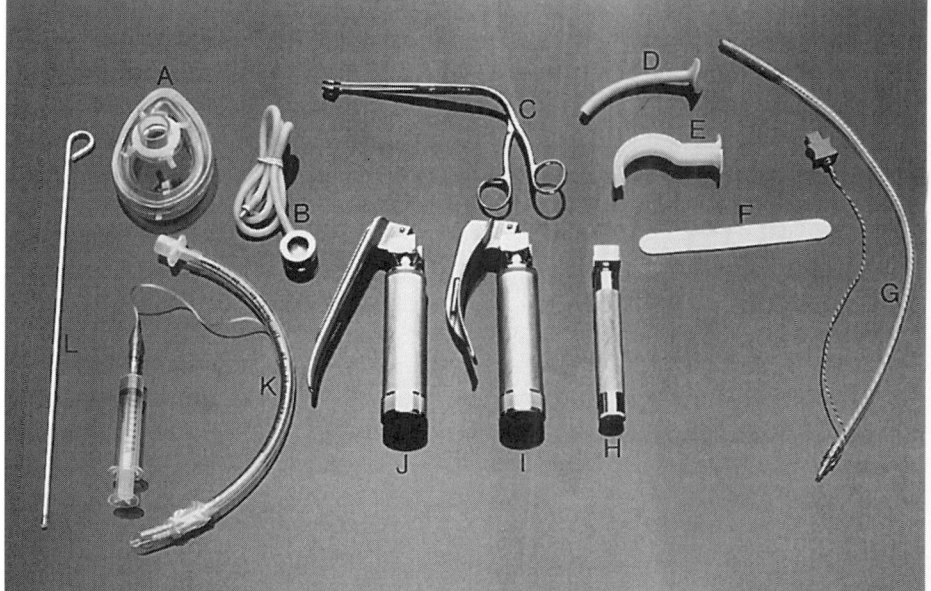

FIGURE 7-3 Commonly used anesthesia equipment. **A,** Mask. **B,** Precordial stethoscope. **C,** McGill forceps. **D,** Nasal airway. **E,** Oral airway. **F,** Tongue blade. **G,** Esophageal stethoscope with esophageal temperature monitor. **H,** Pediatric laryngoscope handle. Fiberoptic laryngoscope blades and handles: **I,** MacIntosh; **J,** Miller. **K,** Endotracheal tube. **L,** Intubating stylet for endotracheal tube.

ventilation. Location of the endotracheal tube in the trachea is verified by an appropriate level and waveform of $ETCO_2$, by listening for bilaterally equal breath sounds with a stethoscope, by absence of sounds over the stomach, by symmetric movement of the thorax with positive-pressure ventilation, and by condensation of moisture from expired air in the endotracheal tube and breathing circuit. Proper placement of the endotracheal tube is shown in Fig. 7-4. The vocal cords are the narrowest portion of an adult trachea; however, the smallest portion of a child's airway is below the vocal cords. Therefore, uncuffed endotracheal tubes are usually selected for children because the internal diameter of cuffed tubes in these small sizes would have too much resistance to ventilation and could easily become obstructed. After the initial paralysis from the muscle relaxant has worn off, the patient may be allowed to breathe spontaneously with intermittent assistance, or additional muscle relaxant may be given and the ventilation controlled mechanically.

If the procedure is an emergency, or the patient is at risk for aspiration (as in cases of a full stomach, intestinal obstruction, hiatal hernia, or significant esophagus reflux), a rapid sequence induction or an awake fiberoptic intubation may be planned. In these instances as well as in routine intubation, the perioperative nurse must be ready to assist by applying cricoid pressure. This is effected when the nurse exerts downward pressure on the cricoid cartilage with the thumb and index finger of one hand (Sellick maneuver) while the other hand is placed under the patient's neck for stability. The cricoid cartilage is the only complete ring in the trachea, and downward pressure occludes the esophagus, which lies immediately posterior (or dorsally) to the trachea. The pressure should not be released until proper placement of the endotracheal tube has been confirmed.

Additional assistance may be provided by the perioper-

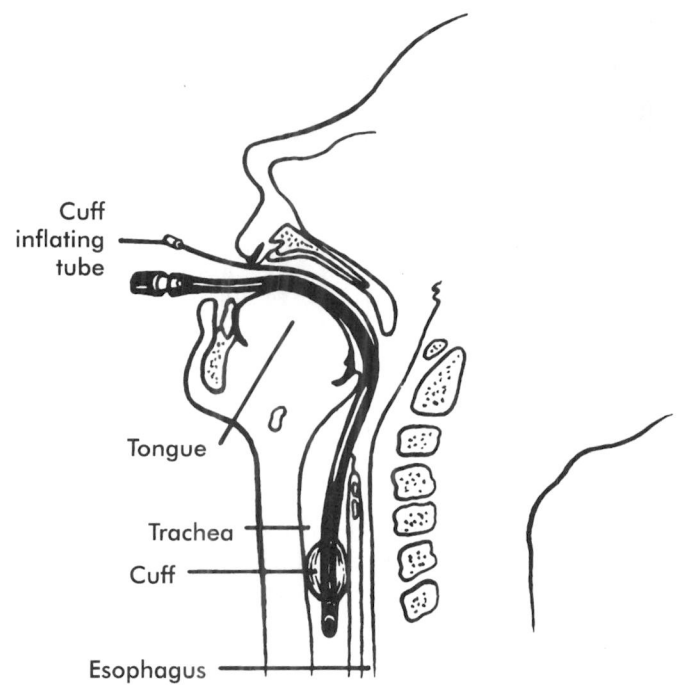

FIGURE 7-4 Endotracheal tube in position.

ative nurse if an unexpected difficult intubation occurs or the patient cannot be adequately ventilated with a mask. Emergency airway equipment should be brought into the room immediately. The nurse should be familiar with the location of the various pieces of equipment and how to assemble them for use and should also assist the anesthesia provider in securing the patient's airway. Contents of a typical difficult-airway cart are listed in Box 7-3. If invasive monitors (such as an arterial line) will be placed after induction, the nurse may assist by properly positioning the patient or extremity and prepping the area or areas;

BOX 7-3 | **Typical Contents of a Difficult-Airway Cart**

Fiberoptic Equipment

- Flexible fiberoptic (FO) bronchoscopes (adult and pediatric)
- Fiberoptic light source
- Bullard scope (FO)
- Siliconized spray

Laryngoscope Equipment

- Assorted pediatric and adult laryngoscope handles and blades
- Extra alkaline batteries

Endotracheal Tubes (ETT)

- Regular ETT: uncuffed, 2.5-6.0 mm
- Regular ETT: cuffed,   5.0-9.0 mm
- Oral RAE ETT: uncuffed, 3.0-7.0 mm
- Oral RAE ETT: cuffed,   6.0-8.0 mm
- Nasal RAE ETT: uncuffed, 3.0-7.0 mm
- Nasal RAE ETT: cuffed,   6.0-8.0 mm
- Reinforced ETT: cuffed,   7.0-8.0 mm
- Controllable-tip ETT (Endotrol)
- Combitube

Airways

- Regular oral: assorted pediatric and adult
- Regular nasal: assorted adult
- Intubating airways: assorted (such as Ovassapian, Williams)
- Nasopharyngeal airway with inflatable introducer
- Laryngeal mask airways (LMA): assorted sizes
- Tongue blades
- Water-soluble lubricant (K-Y)

Intubating Equipment

- Intubating stylettes
- Magill forceps: pediatric and adult
- Esophageal (gastric tube) airway (EGTA)

- Hollow ETT changers with removable Luer-Lok connectors for O_2 insufflation

Suction Equipment

- Assorted flexible suction catheters to fit ETT and LMA
- Stiff suction catheters (Yankauer)

Topical Anesthesia Equipment

- Atomizers and pressurized topical anesthetic spray
- Long Q-Tips
- Lidocaine 4%
- Lidocaine 4% with phenylephrine
- Lidocaine 2%—viscous
- Lidocaine 5%–ointment
- Lidocaine 10%
- Tetracaine 1%

Transtracheal Airway Equipment

- Transtracheal O_2 jet ventilator with pressure regulator, manual control valve, and Luer-Lok male connector
- Assorted large IV catheters
- Assorted long guide wires, epidural needles, and epidural catheters (for retrograde intubation)

Miscellaneous

- Safety glasses
- Heat-moisture exchanger (Humidivent)
- Assorted face masks with port for FO scope
- Right-angled connector (for face masks) with port for FO scope
- $ETCO_2$ chemical indicators (Easy Cap)
- Twill tape (to secure ETT)
- Skin adhesive (Mastisol)
- Adhesive tape

---

and may assist with placement, connection, and calibration of the monitors. If the procedure is emergent, the nurse may also assist by obtaining additional IV access, connecting fluid- or patient-warming units, double-checking blood products, and "pumping" IV fluids as needed. In situations where the anesthesia provider is involved with a critical procedure, the nurse can perform a valuable service by watching the monitors, recording data, and communicating significant changes to the anesthesia provider.

The LMA is a major advancement in airway management. Placement is relatively simple and does not require laryngoscopy or muscle relaxation. When comparing ease of use, invasiveness, and airway protection, the LMA lies between the face mask and an endotracheal tube. It is ideal for a supine patient under general anesthesia with spontaneous ventilation. The LMA may also be useful in a difficult airway situation where tracheal intubation cannot be achieved. It is available in six sizes, is autoclavable, and is reusable. A disposable LMA is also available.

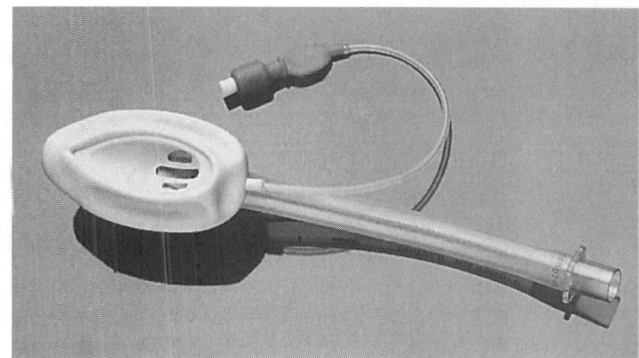

FIGURE 7-5 The laryngeal mask airway deflated and ready for insertion.

Before insertion, the LMA must be carefully deflated so that there are no wrinkles in the cuff (Fig. 7-5). The recommended technique for insertion of the LMA is shown in Fig. 7-6, and correct placement is shown in Fig. 7-7. However, some people insert the LMA rotated

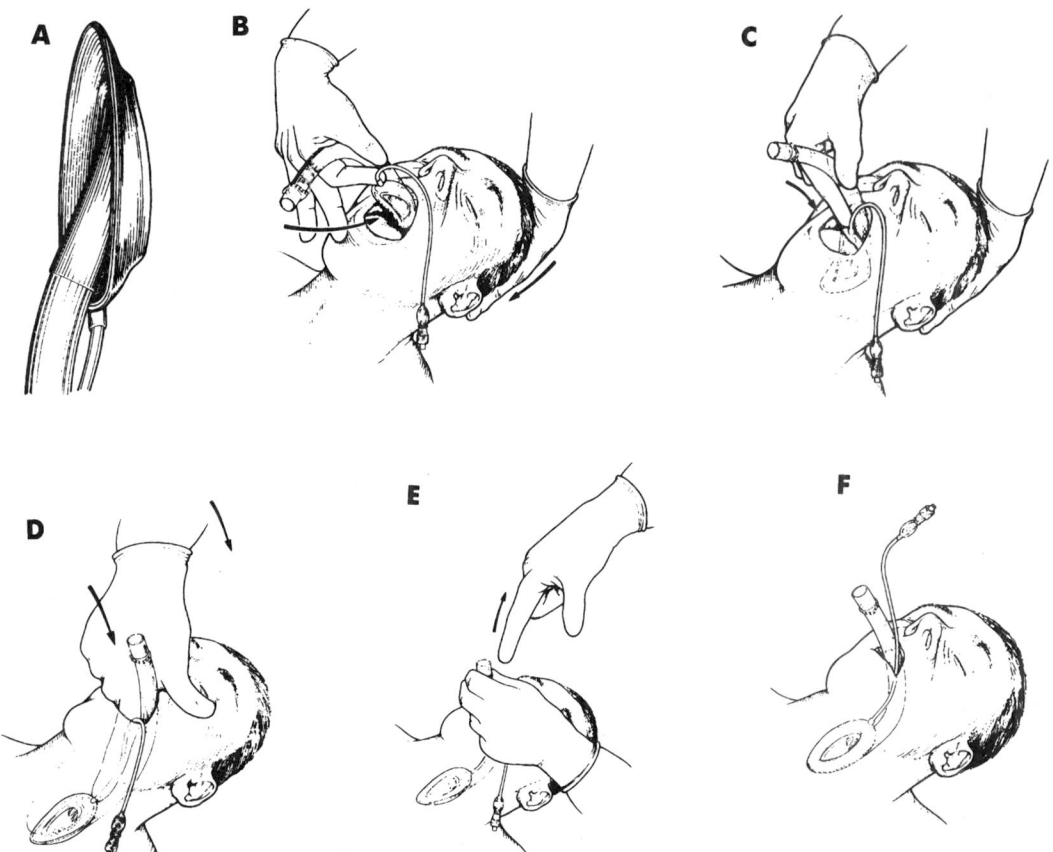

FIGURE 7–6   Insertion of the laryngeal mask airway (LMA). Select the appropriate size of LMA (1: neonate <6.5 kg; 2: infants and children 6.5 to 20 kg; 2½: children 20 to 30 kg; 3: children and small adults >30 kg; 4: normal-sized to large adults; 5: large adults.) **A,** Carefully deflate the LMA as tightly as possible so that the rim faces away from the mask aperture as shown. There should be no folds near the tip. **B,** Under direct vision, press the tip of the LMA cephalad against the hard palate to flatten it out. Using the index finger, continue pressing the LMA against the palate as the LMA is advanced into the pharynx to ensure that the tip remains flattened and avoids the tongue. **C,** Keeping the neck flexed and the head extended, use the index finger to press the LMA into the posterior wall. **D,** Continue pushing with the ball of the index finger guiding the LMA posteriorly into position. By withdrawing the other fingers and slightly pronating the forearm, it is usually possible to push the LMA fully into position in one fluid movement. **E,** Firmly grasp the tube with the other hand and then withdraw the index finger from the pharynx. Gently press the LMA posteriorly to ensure that it is fully inserted. **F,** Carefully inflate the LMA with the recommended volume of air (size 1: 2 to 4 ml; size 2: ≤10 ml; size 2½: ≤14 ml; size 3: ≤20 ml; size 4: ≤30 ml; size 5: ≤40 ml). Do not overinflate. Do not touch the LMA tube while inflating unless it is obviously unstable (as with elderly edentulous patients with loose oropharyngeal tissues). Usually the LMA will move slightly forward out of the hypopharynx as it is inflated. Insert a bite-block (roll of gauze) alongside the LMA tube to minimize occlusion of the tube as the patient is awakening.

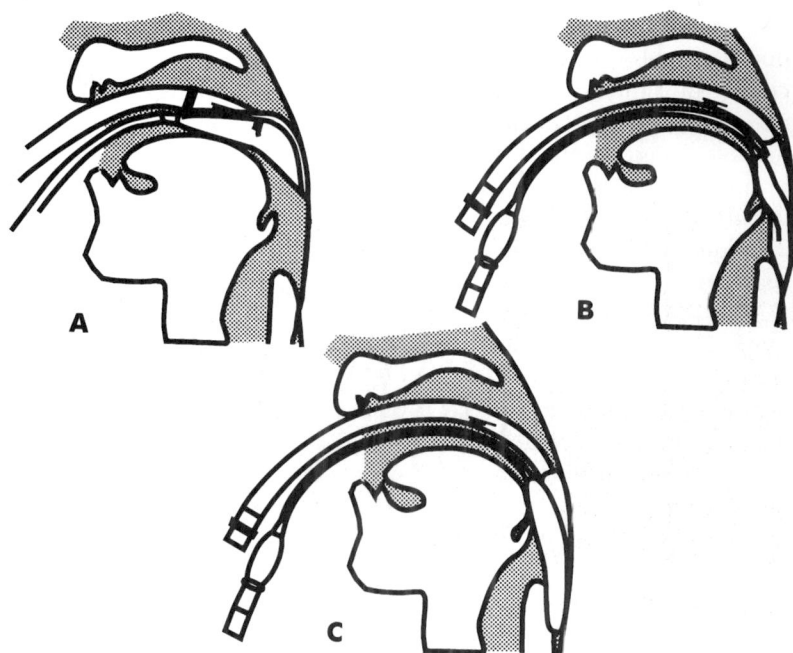

FIGURE 7–7   Sagittal views of insertion and proper placement of the laryngeal mask airway (LMA). **A,** Insertion of LMA. **B,** Proper location of LMA (deflated). **C,** Properly placed and inflated LMA.

180° from that shown in Fig. 7-6. Others find placement is easier if the cuff is inflated to a neutral position (Fig. 7-8). For adults, it is recommended that a 2.5 to 3.0 cm diameter roll of gauze sponges be used as a "bite block" and inserted beside the LMA tube. The LMA and gauze roll can be secured with adhesive tape to the chin.

Maintenance of anesthesia can be accomplished with either IV or inhalational anesthetic techniques or a combination of both, with or without additional muscle relaxation. A variety of factors are considered by the anesthesiologist in selecting the anesthesia technique for each situation.

Many factors influence emergence. The objective is to be able to move the patient from the OR bed to the postanesthesia care unit (PACU) bed as soon as the dressing is applied. During emergence, the anesthesia provider suctions the oropharynx before extubation to decrease the risk of aspiration and laryngospasm after extubation, reverses any residual neuromuscular blockade, and allows the washout of N_2O and volatile agents by giving 100% O_2 for several minutes before extubation. After extubation, the patient is then transported to the PACU to awaken from the anesthetic experience. In some situations the patient may be transferred to the PACU before extubation, and the endotracheal tube is removed when the patient is fully awakened.

Untoward events that can occur with general anesthesia include hypoxia; respiratory, cardiovascular, or renal dysfunction; hypotension; hypertension; fluid or electrolyte imbalance; residual muscle paralysis; dental damage; neurologic problems; hypothermia; and malignant hyperthermia. The anesthesiologist usually directs the treatment and management of such events.

Anesthesia Machines

The first apparatus resembling an anesthesia machine was used in 1905. Since then, innumerable changes and improvements have been incorporated. The anesthesia machines used for general anesthesia look complicated, but the basic functions are similar and simple to understand. Perioperative nurses should be familiar with the basic function of anesthesia machines because they may need to administer O_2 during procedures with local anesthesia or conscious sedation/analgesia. A modern anesthesia machine is shown in Fig. 7-9. A typical generic schema is shown in Fig. 7-10 to help perioperative nurses become familiar with the basic circuit of anesthesia machines.

Oxygen, N_2O, and air are usually supplied from the facility's pipelines to the anesthesia machine at pressures of 50 to 55 psi. The gas hoses going to the machine are color coded: O_2 (green); N_2O (blue); and air (yellow). The

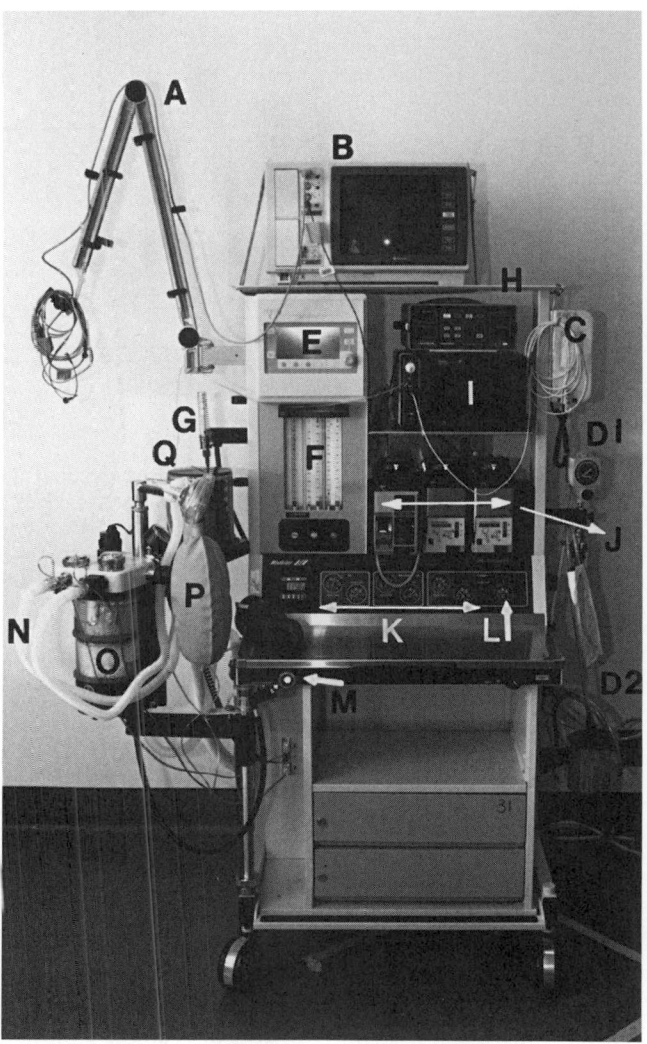

FIGURE 7-9 Modern anesthesia machine (Ohmeda—"Modulus SE," Madison, WI). **A,** Adjustable arm for cables going to patient. **B,** Multichannel physiologic monitor. Channels include ECG, heart rate, temperature, and pressure. Other modules can be inserted for additional pressures, cardiac output, noninvasive BP, and a two-channel recorder. **C,** Custom-mounted telephone. **D1,** Suction regulator. **D2,** Suction cannister. **E,** Integrated ventilator controls, monitor, and displays. **F,** Flowmeters for air, N_2O, and O_2. **G,** O_2 flowmeter for nasal cannula, etc. **H,** Noninvasive blood pressure monitor. **I,** Respiratory gas monitor (RGM) includes patient circuit O_2, FiO_2, percentage of N_2O and inspired and expired anesthetic agents, SpO_2, and alarms. **J,** Flowthrough vaporizers (desflurane, isoflurane, and sevoflurane). **K,** Gauges for pipeline and E-tank pressures (air, N_2O, and O_2). **L,** On/off switch. **M,** O_2 flush valve. **N,** Patient breathing circuit. **O,** CO_2 absorber. **P,** Reservoir ("breathing") bag. **Q,** Ventilator.

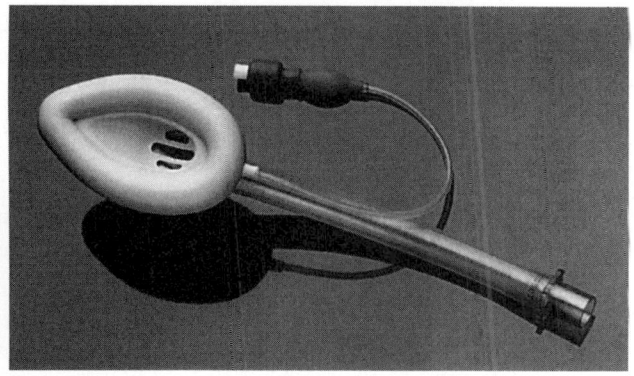

FIGURE 7-8   The laryngeal mask airway inflated to neutral position.

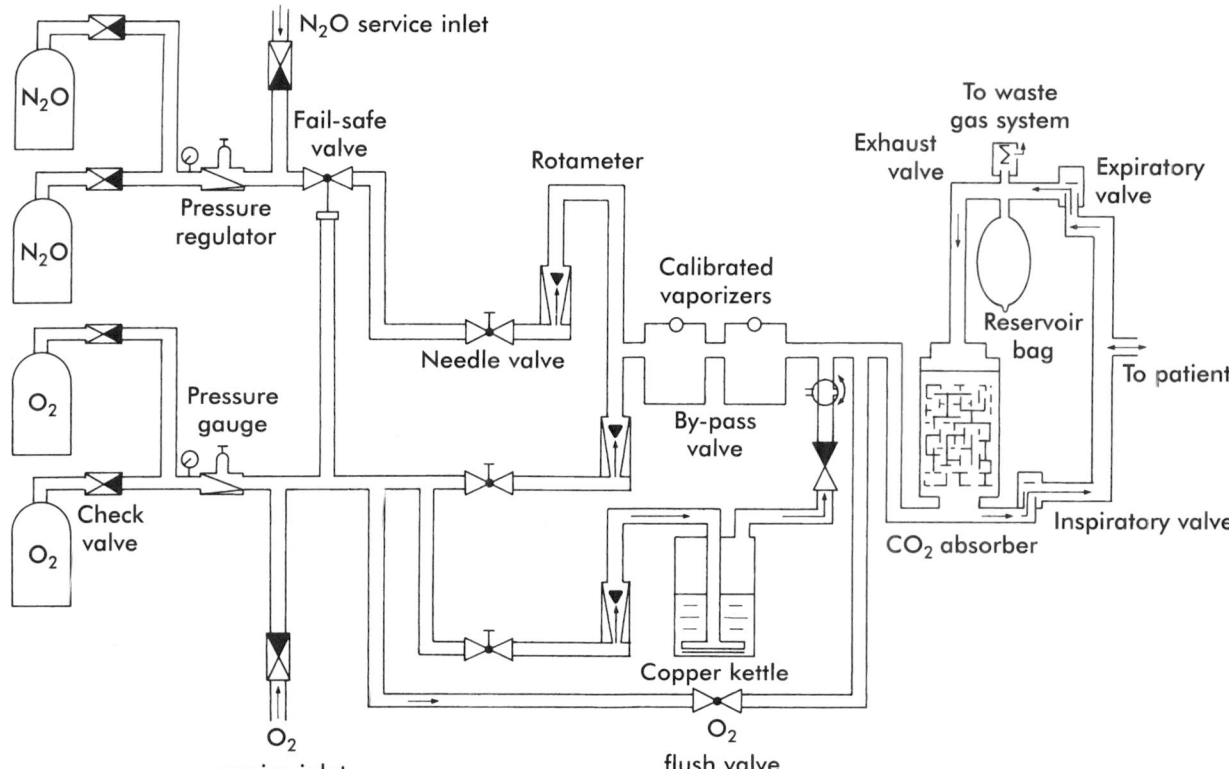

FIGURE 7-10   Generic anesthesia machine circuit. Oxygen and N_2O enter the machine from cylinders or from the hospital service supply. Pressure regulators reduce cylinder pressure to about 45 psi. Check valves prevent transfilling of cylinders or gas flow from cylinders to service line. The fail-safe valve prevents flow of N_2O if the C_2 pressure fails. Needle valves control flows to rotameters. Calibrated vaporizers provide a preselected concentration of volatile anesthetics. An interlock allows only one vaporizer to be on at a time. The Copper Kettle (no longer manufactured) is a "bypass vaporizer" that delivers saturated anesthetic vapor; thus the effluent must be diluted. The bypass valve vents vapor from the Copper Kettle when it is not in service. Gases are delivered to the circle absorber, where unidirectional valves assure flow from patient through carbon dioxide absorber. Excess gas is vented through the exhaust valve into a waste gas–scavenging system. The reservoir bag compensates for variations in respiratory demand.

connectors are specific for each gas so that they cannot be inadvertently cross connected. If a central gas supply is not available or the hospital piping system fails, the machines are equipped with E-size cylinders of O_2 and N_2O. One or two cylinders of each gas are connected to yokes on the machine. These yokes are pin indexed so that only the correct gas can be connected in that position. In the pin-indexing safety system, two steel pins are in a unique location on the yoke assembly. The mating gas cylinder (such as the O_2 tank) has two matching holes in the same locations so that the cylinders cannot be mounted in the wrong place.

In cylinders, O_2 is stored as a compressed gas. A full E-size cylinder contains about 660 L of O_2 at approximately 2000 psi. As the O_2 is used, the pressure falls in direct proportion to the remaining volume. Because the E-size cylinder is used to provide O_2 while patients are being transported, one should know how much O_2 is left in a partially used tank. Thus 1000 psi would indicate 330 L remaining, and 500 psi would indicate 165 L remaining

or sufficient O_2 at 5 L/min flow for more than 25 minutes. When the pressure has dropped to about 250 psi, the cylinder should not be used because it no longer has an adequate reserve.

Nitrous oxide is stored as a liquid in cylinders, and the pressure above the liquid is 745 psi. A full, E-size cylinder contains about 1600 L of N_2O. As the N_2O is used, the pressure above the liquid remains constant. Only when the liquid has been completely vaporized does the pressure begin to fall. Therefore the N_2O can be almost gone but will still show the same pressure. In contrast to O_2, the amount remaining in the tank cannot be readily determined.

The gases in the cylinders flow through regulators that reduce the pressure to about 45 psi. The hoses from the hospital gas sources are connected to the machine at the outlet of these regulators. In machines sold after January 1, 1984, a safety interlock device shuts off the N_2O flow if O_2 pressure is not present or proportionately lowers the O_2 and N_2O flow rates to maintain 30% O_2. The gases then flow through individual flowmeters (or rotameters) on the front of the machine, so that the gas flows and the ratio of O_2 to N_2O or air can be selected by the anesthesia provider. From the top of the flowmeters, the gases are mixed and then flow through a vaporizer in which the inhalational anesthetic of choice is vaporized and added to the gas mixture. The total gas flow is then delivered from the machine to the patient. With a flowthrough vaporizer, by definition, all the fresh gas going from the anesthesia machine to the patient flows through the vaporizer. The control dials are usually located on top of these vaporizers and are calibrated in percentages. The filling ports on the vaporizers are usually key indexed so that only the appropriate volatile agent can be used. Most recently manufactured vaporizers are flow and temperature compensated, meaning that they are reasonably accurate at all flows and temperatures used clinically.

Desflurane (Suprane) is a unque inhalational anesthetic because it is a liquid below 22.8° C and must be heated slightly to ensure vaporization. Therefore the vaporizer for desflurane contains an electric heater. Desflurane also has several other unique characteristics: (1) the solubility in blood (blood-gas partition coefficient) is lower (0.42) than N_2O (0.47), sevoflurane (0.63 to 0.69), isoflurane (1.41), or halothane (2.30), which means that it has a faster "wash-in" (induction) and "wash-out" (emergence) than the other agents; (2) there is far less metabolism (0.02%) as a percentage of the anesthetic taken up than isoflurane (0.2%), sevoflurane (5%), or halothane (15 to 20%); (3) emergence and recovery from general anesthesia and discharge from PACU is significantly faster than with thiopental; (4) the cardiovascular effects are to be similar to those of isoflurane; and (5) the muscle relaxation appears similar to the other inhalational agents. The pungency of desflurane precludes its use as an inhalational induction agent.

Sevoflurane (Ultane) is the newest volatile agent available in the United States. Its pleasant odor and low solubility in blood make it the most popular volatile agent for inhalational induction in pediatric patients. Unlike any of the other volatile agents, it can also provide a rapid, pleasant mask induction in adults (Research Highlight 7-4).

Another important feature of the anesthesia machine is the O_2 *flush valve*. With all new machines and on most earlier models, pushing the O_2 flush valve allows 100% O_2 from the 50 psi line to flow directly to the *fresh gas outlet* on the machine and to the patient. This O_2 flow completely bypasses the flowmeters and vaporizers. Caution must be exercised because the pressure is 35 to 50 psi and the flow rate is 35 to 75 L/min.

In most hospitals and ambulatory surgery centers in the United States, a semiclosed circle system is used to deliver the fresh gas flow (including anesthetic gases) to patients. The circle system is composed of a container filled with a CO_2-absorbing material (such as soda lime or Baralyme),

two *one-way (unidirectional) valves*, an *adjustable pressure-limiting (APL) valve*, a *reservoir bag*, an inlet connection for fresh gas flow, and two connections to the patient through corrugated breathing (or anesthesia circuit) tubing. As the patient inspires, gases are drawn through the CO_2 absorber and from the fresh gas supply through the inspiratory limb of the corrugated tubing. As the patient exhales, the one-way valve on the inspiratory limb prevents backflow, and the exhaled gases flow into the expiratory limb and through the expiratory one-way valve. The expiratory limb and valve are easily identified by the condensation of water vapor along this portion of the circuit. The reservoir bag absorbs the peak flow of expired gases and allows the anesthesia provider to force gas through the CO_2 absorber, along the inspiratory limb of the circuit, and to ventilate the patient. The expired gases flow through the CO_2 absorber where CO_2 is removed. Substances used in the CO_2 absorbent include an indicator that changes color as the soda lime is exhausted. For example, the soda lime may turn from white to blue, indicating that the absorbent material must be changed to prevent a buildup of CO_2 in the patient. Any excess gas is vented through the APL valve into the gas-scavenging system. The APL valve is usually mounted just ahead of the CO_2 absorber. A typical circle system is shown in Fig. 7-11.

The FiO_2 *sensor* is usually mounted in the inspiratory limb just after the one-way valve. It measures the fraction of inspired O_2 (FiO_2) and can be set to alarm if a low concentration is detected. A low-pressure sensor is usually mounted in the expiratory limb near the one-way valve to detect a ventilator malfunction or a circuit disconnection.

On some new machines, flowmeters are mounted in both the inspired and expired limbs where the patient breathing circuit is connected. When the ventilator is used, the electronic circuitry measures the inspiratory and expiratory volumes to ensure that they correspond with the tidal volume and respiratory rate selected. With a cuffed endotracheal tube, the ventilator will compensate for changes in fresh gas flow or small leaks in the breathing circuit and will alarm if a disconnect or inadequate flow occurs.

The advantage of the circle system is that much lower flows of O_2, N_2O, and anesthetic gases can be used. This conserves the patient's body heat and respiratory moisture and reduces the cost of expensive volatile agents. A *semiclosed circuit* (or circle system) is typically used when the fresh gas flows into the system range from 0.5 to 6 L/min. During exhalation, some of the expired gases are recycled through the CO_2 absorber, and the excess gas is scavenged or eliminated (hence *semiclosed*). With a *closed-circle system*, all the CO_2 is absorbed. No gas is vented from the system, and only enough O_2 is added to the system to meet the basal requirements of the patient (approximately 3.5 ml/kg/min). In an *open circuit* (such as the Ayres T-piece, Magill, or Bain circuits), a relatively high flow of fresh gas is used, and most of the exhaled gas is vented from the

7-4 RESEARCH HIGHLIGHT

SEVOFLURANE: A NEW INHALATION ANESTHETIC

Since its introduction in Japan, sevoflurane (Ultane) has been used for more than 1 million anesthetic applications in that country. On June 7, 1995, it was approved by the Food and Drug Administration (FDA) for use in the United States. The blood-gas partition coefficient is 0.63 to 0.69 compared with 0.47 for N_2O. Thus it is not very soluble in blood or other tissues, and it is quickly exhaled from the body during emergence from anesthesia. With sevoflurane, the heart rate and sympathetic nervous system are stable. With these characteristics and its lack of pungency, sevoflurane can provide a smooth inhalation induction, good intubating conditions (or placement of a laryngeal mask airway [LMA]), satisfactory intraoperative anesthesia, and a rapid emergence at the end of the procedure. The postanesthesia recovery time and incidence of side effects are similar to those of propofol.

Compound A is a degradant of sevoflurane formed by interaction with the CO_2 absorbent (soda lime or Baralyme). In high concentrations over time it has been shown to be nephrotoxic in rats; however, this does not seem to be a major problem in normal humans if the total gas-flow rate is greater than 2 L/min and the CO_2 absorbent is not allowed to dry out. Studies are continuing in this area.

Muzi and colleagues (1996) used 20 healthy, nonpremedicated volunteers, 19 to 32 years old, on three separate occasions to determine the time from induction of anesthesia to tracheal intubation or placement of a LMA. Treatment 1 (T_1) was tracheal intubation after induction with 6% to 7% sevoflurane/66% N_2O/O_2. Treatment 2 (T_2) was tracheal intubation after induction with 6% to 7% sevoflurane and O_2. Treatment 3 (T_3) was LMA placement after induction with 6% to 7% sevoflurane/66% N_2O/O_2. The subjects breathed O_2 for 5 minutes before taking three vital-capacity breaths of the treatment gases after a forced expiration to their residual volume. The mean times for acceptable tracheal intubation were 4.7 and 6.4 minutes for T_1 and T_2 respectively. The mean time for acceptable LMA insertion was 1.7 minutes. There were no instances of coughing or laryngospasm during induction, though 25% to 40% of the subjects had some expiratory stridor ("crowing") that did not inhibit mask ventilation. The participants recalled only the first two breaths of gas during induction. There were a few instances of a decrease in mean arterial pressure that quickly resolved after intubation.

In a very similarly designed study, Muzi and his associates (1997) evaluated induction with 8% sevoflurane/66% N_2O/O_2 and intubating conditions in 24 healthy volunteers on three occasions. On the three occasions, 5 minutes before induction, the participants received randomized IV premedications of fentanyl (2.4 μg/kg), midazolam (36 μg/kg), or both fentanyl (0.6 μg/kg) and midazolam (9 μg/kg) respectively. The results showed that pretreatment with midazolam (36 μg/kg) or the combination of midazolam and fentanyl did not shorten the time to achieve loss of consciousness compared to unpremedicated volunteers. However, it nearly halved the time to achieve acceptable intubating conditions.

From Muzi M., Robinson, B.J., Ebert, T.J., & O'Brien, T.J. (1996). Induction of anesthesia and tracheal intubation with sevoflurane in adults. *Anesthesiology, 85,* 536-543; Muzi, M., Colinco, M.D., Robinson, B.J., & Ebert, T.J. (1997). The effects of premedication on inhaled induction of anesthesia with sevoflurane. *Anesthesia and Analgesia, 85,* 1143-1148.

circuit. The fresh-gas flow rate per minute varies from approximately two thirds of the patient's minute volume with the Magill circuit to at least 100 ml/kg for the Bain or T-piece circuits. The open-circuit system is commonly used for neonates, infants, and small children.

With all these circuits, the final connection to the patient is by a mask or endotracheal tube. A mask or LMA may be used for a patient with a good airway who is at minimal risk of aspiration, undergoing a relatively short procedure, and when the surgical site is not located in the head or neck area. Endotracheal intubation ensures a patent airway during surgery. When the patient is paralyzed, the ventilation is controlled during the procedure.

REGIONAL ANESTHESIA

Preoperative preparation for regional anesthesia is essentially the same as that for general anesthesia.

Preoperative medication is ordered frequently before regional anesthesia to blunt any discomfort that may be experienced during placement of the block. The criteria for monitoring during regional anesthesia are similar to general anesthesia. Whenever regional anesthesia is performed, resuscitative equipment and drugs must be immediately available. Regional anesthesia (also called *conduction anesthesia*) can be accomplished by injecting a local anesthetic anywhere along the pathway of a nerve from the spinal cord (spinal anesthesia), epidurally, peripherally, or topically. This provides anesthesia to a region of the body.

During preparation and placement of the regional anesthetic, the perioperative or perianesthesia nurse can provide valuable assistance. This may include placing the appropriate monitors such as pulse oximetry, ECG, and blood pressure; providing supplemental O_2 if indicated; reassuring the patient; administering sedation such

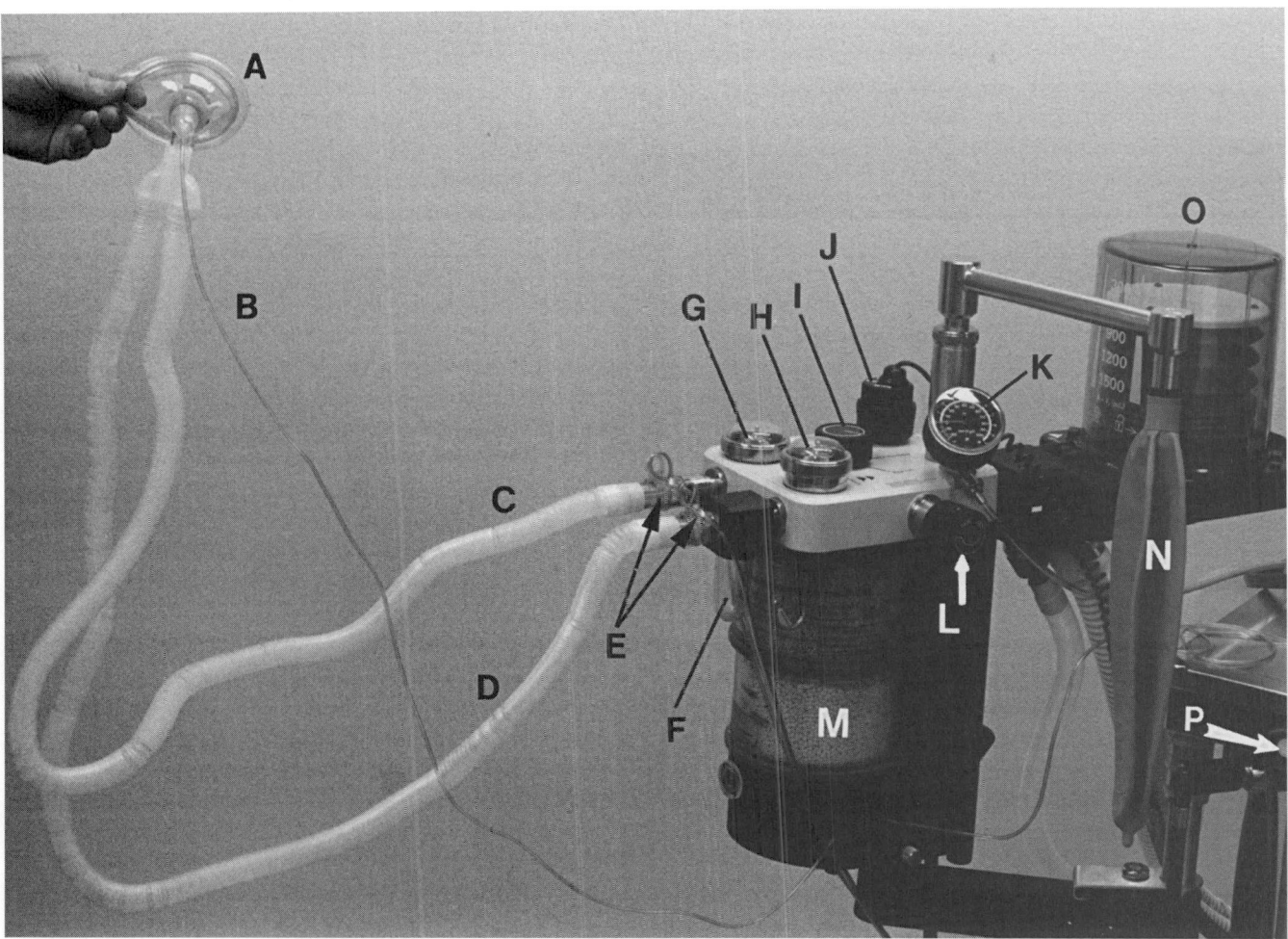

FIGURE 7-11 A typical circle system. **A,** Patient mask. **B,** Sidestream sensing line for respiratory and anesthetic gas monitor. **C,** Inspiratory limb of patient circuit. **D,** Expiratory limb of patient circuit. **E,** Flowmeter sensors for inspired and expired gases. **F,** Moisture trap. **G,** One-way inspiratory valve. **H,** One-way expiratory valve. **I,** Reservoir bag or ventilator selector valve. **J,** FiO$_2$ sensor for circuit. **K,** Airway pressure gauge. A sensing line goes to a pressure transducer in the control module. **L,** Adjustable pressure limiting (APL), or "pop-off," valve. **M,** CO$_2$ absorber. **N,** Reservoir ("breathing") bag. **O,** Ventilator. **P,** O$_2$ flush valve.

as midazolam as directed; and properly positioning the patient, which is crucial for a successful block. Peripheral blocks on the lower or upper extremities or on the head are frequently done in a preoperative holding area to allow adequate time for the local anesthetic to penetrate the peripheral nerve before the patient is transferred to the OR. For peripheral blocks, the perioperative or perianesthesia nurse may aspirate during needle placement (to detect vascular puncture) and inject the local anesthetic while the anesthesiologist is stabilizing the needle in the precise location. After an initial period of evaluation by the anesthesiologist, the nurse monitors the patient for any substantial change in vital signs or untoward reactions until the patient is transferred to the OR. For regional anesthesia as well as general anesthesia, an anesthesia provider continuously monitors the patient during the surgical procedure.

Spinal Anesthesia

A local anesthetic (usually lidocaine, tetracaine, or bupivacaine) injected into the cerebrospinal fluid (CSF) in the subarachnoid space is termed a *spinal anesthetic* or a *subarachnoid block* (SAB). To provide additional analgesia, fentanyl or preservative-free morphine is often added to the local anesthetic. A spinal needle is inserted into a lower lumbar interspace with the patient either lying on one side or in a sitting position. The local anesthetic is generally mixed with a dextrose solution for a total of 1 to 4 ml to make a *hyperbaric* (heavier than the CSF) solution. These hyperbaric mixtures settle in a gravity-dependent manner after injection into the CSF. By changing the patient's position, the block can be directed up, down, or to one side of the spinal cord. For example, with prostate surgery the patient may remain in the sitting position for a minute or so after the local anesthetic is injected. A bilateral block of the S1-S5 dermatomes results.

For surgery in the upper abdomen, the patient may be placed in a slightly (5- to 10-degree) head-down position to allow the anesthetic to move cephalad while the anesthesia provider carefully checks the level of sensory block. When an adequate level is obtained, the bed is leveled to minimize further spread. After 10 to 15 minutes, the block is usually "set" and will not extend farther. The sympathetic nervous system is usually blocked two dermatomes higher and the neuromuscular system two dermatomes lower than the sensory block. The patient may then be positioned as necessary for surgery.

If the local anesthetic is mixed with a larger volume of sterile water, the solution will be *hypobaric*, and the drug will move to the nondependent area. Hypobaric spinal anesthesia is usually done after the surgical site is positioned above the site of injection. An example is perianal surgery in the prone position. By mixing the local anesthetic with some CSF withdrawn from the subarachnoid space, the solution becomes *isobaric*. Distribution of this solution is minimally affected by gravity.

Spinal anesthesia may evoke several physiologic responses that can result in major problems if not properly managed:

Hypotension

Hypotension may occur rapidly after an SAB. It is caused by vasodilatation because the sympathetic nerves that control vasomotor tone are blocked. This causes peripheral pooling of blood resulting in a reduced venous return to the heart and a decrease in cardiac output. The hypotensive response can usually be avoided by infusing 750 to 1500 ml of balanced salt solution immediately before the block and placing the patient in a 5-degree head-down position to improve venous return to the heart. A vasopressor such as ephedrine may also be administered.

Total spinal anesthesia

Total spinal anesthesia (or an inadvertently high block) may cause paralysis of the respiratory muscles and necessitate immediate intubation and ventilation. Any symptom of respiratory distress occurring shortly after instituting spinal anesthesia should alert the anesthesia provider to the possibility of a high spinal block.

Positioning problems

Positioning problems can occur because pain and sensory inputs to a portion of the patient's body are blocked. Care must be taken in positioning the patient intraoperatively to avoid neurologic damage, burns, loss of skin integrity, or other trauma.

Post–dural puncture headache

Post–dural puncture headache (PDPH) (or postspinal cephalgia, spinal headache) is one of the most frequent postoperative complaints after spinal anesthesia. It occurs more commonly in young parturients or other individuals less than 40 years of age. The incidence is about 1% when a 25- or 27-gauge blunt-bevel needle is used. It is unrelated to how soon the patient is ambulated. The headache is believed to result from leakage of CSF through the hole in the dura, and typically occurs when the patient assumes an upright position. The incidence, severity, and duration of the headache appears to correlate with the size of the hole left in the dura. The headache is usually in the occipital area and generally resolves over 1 to 3 days but may last as long as 2 weeks. A variety of treatment modalities have been used to relieve the headache including strict bedrest for 24 to 48 hours; vigorous hydration; abdominal binders; epidural infusion of saline; PO or IV caffeine; and injection of 5 to 20 ml of autologous blood into the epidural space at the puncture site (that is, a "blood patch").

Many anesthesiologists use different spinal needles that have a tip shaped like a sharpened wood pencil with the hole on the side of the needle. These 24- to 26-gauge spinal needles (such as Whitacre, Sprotte, or Gertie Marx) presumably separate or go between the dural fibers as opposed to cutting the fibers, which may occur when a blunt-bevel spinal needle is used. With these "pencil-point" needles, the incidence and severity of PDPHs is extremely low.

Epidural and Caudal Anesthesia

The epidural space is located between the ligamentum flavum and the dura and extends from the foramen magnum to the sacrococcygeal membrane. This potential space is filled with epidural veins, fat, and loose areolar tissue. For epidural anesthesia the local anesthetic is usually injected through the intervertebral spaces in the lumbar region, although it can also be injected into the cervical or thoracic regions. The anesthetic spreads both cephalad and caudad from the site of injection. A comparative location of the needle points and injected anesthetic is shown in Fig. 7-12.

For caudal anesthesia the local anesthetic is also injected into the epidural space, but the approach is through the caudal canal in the sacrum. Compared to a lumbar epidural, this approach requires a greater volume of anesthetic to fill the epidural space. Caudal anesthesia has a 5% to 10% technical failure rate. However, because of the ease of administration, it is often employed for pediatric surgical procedures on the lower extremities or the perineal area.

Several techniques may be used for epidural or caudal anesthesia. A "single-shot epidural" involves administration of the local anesthesia through the needle before its removal. For intermittent injections or continuous infusions, a small catheter is inserted into the epidural space for administration of the local anesthetic.

For a combined spinal and epidural, the epidural needle is inserted into the epidural space and then a

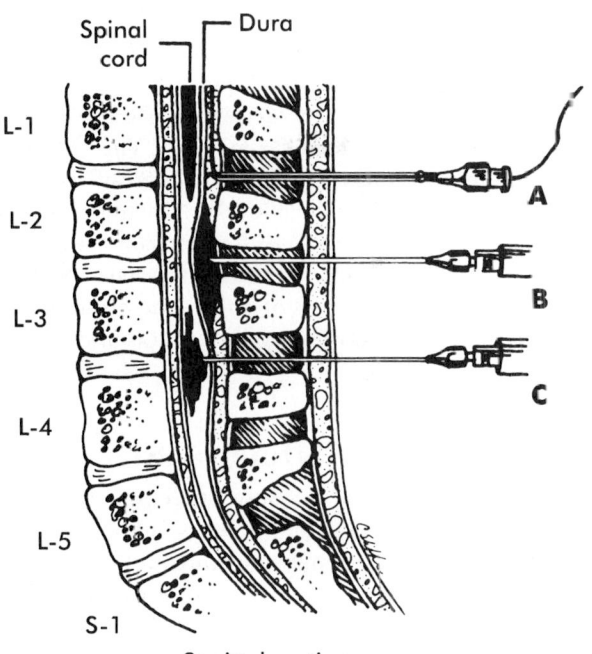

FIGURE 7-12 Location of needle point and injected anesthetic relative to dura. **A,** Epidural catheter. **B,** Single injection epidural. **C,** Spinal anesthesia. (Interspaces most commonly used are L4-5, L3-4, and L2-3.)

special, long, 26-gauge spinal needle is inserted through the epidural needle into the CSF. A small amount of fentanyl or preservative-free morphine is injected and provides very good analgesia for several hours. The spinal needle is removed and an epidural catheter is inserted. This technique is especially useful for obstetrical anesthesia.

Techniques used to identify the epidural space include the "hanging drop" and the "loss of resistance" to injection of either air or liquid (saline or local anesthetic) as the needle is slowly advanced through the ligamentum flavum. With the hanging-drop technique, the needle is filled with liquid to form a meniscus at the needle hub. As the needle is slowly advanced into the epidural space, the negative (less than atmospheric) pressure draws the liquid inward toward the epidural space. Location of the needle tip within the epidural space is verified by injection of an additional 1 to 2 ml of air or saline.

When local anesthetics are injected into the epidural space, the major sites of action are probably the nerve roots as they leave the spinal cord and proceed out the intervertebral foramina beyond the meningeal sheath. However, some of the anesthetic diffuses into the subarachnoid space to the spinal cord. Because local anesthetics diffuse away from the site of injection, segmental anesthesia may be possible in specific areas. In contrast to spinal anesthesia, much larger volumes of local anesthetic are needed with epidural anesthesia; the head-up, head-down, or lateral position of the patient does not have as much effect on the level of the epidural anesthetic; and the onset of anesthesia is much slower with epidural anesthesia. As with spinal anesthesia, hypotension can occur with epidural anesthesia, but the onset is much slower and usually can be managed with the rapid IV infusion of a balanced salt solution or repositioning of the patient.

The local anesthetics most frequently used for epidural anesthesia are lidocaine, bupivacaine, and chloroprocaine. Depending on the concentration of the anesthetic agent, the effect can range from loss of sensory input to complete motor blockade. To help verify that the anesthetic is not being injected into the subarachnoid space or into an epidural vein, a test dose of 3 to 5 ml of lidocaine with a 1:200,000 concentration of epinephrine is frequently used. Injected intravascularly, this test dose causes a transient tachycardia. If injected into the subarachnoid space, it produces a low level of spinal anesthesia. Complications associated with the use of local anesthetics in the epidural and subarachnoid spaces are unique to the agent used. Permanent neurologic sequelae have been reported when chloroprocaine with a preservative was injected into the subarachnoid space. Bupivacaine is associated with pronounced cardiac toxicity if injected intravascularly.

With epidural anesthesia, several complications can occur, including inadvertent dural puncture, subarachnoid injection, and vascular injection.

Inadvertent dural puncture

Inadvertent dural puncture with the epidural needle (that is, a wet tap) can cause a PDPH. This headache is significant in about 50% of patients, and the intensity can be incapacitating. Treatment is essentially the same as that discussed previously under spinal anesthesia.

Subarachnoid injection

Subarachnoid injection occurs if the needle or catheter is unintentionally inserted into the subarachnoid space. If a large volume of local anesthetic is injected as a bolus, it causes "total spinal" anesthesia. This is associated with a rapid onset of hypotension caused by vasodilatation, profound bradycardia as the sympathetic nerves to the heart are blocked, and a totally paralyzed patient. Treatment includes intubation, control of ventilation, support of blood pressure and the cardiovascular system, and administration of amnestic drugs until the block has resolved. If properly managed, this problem is not life threatening, but use of the test dose described previously and injection of only 3 to 5 ml at a time usually averts this problem. With patient movement over time, the epidural catheter may migrate through the dura. Therefore a small test dose should be given each time additional local anesthetic is injected through the catheter. In addition, each subsequent dose should be injected in increments of 3 to 5 ml each.

Vascular injection

Vascular injection of the local anesthetic into an epidural vein may inadvertently occur with the initial dose or with subsequent injections. Intravenously injected bupivacaine is associated with cardiac arrest. Toxicity from other local anesthetics can cause sudden and profound hypotension, convulsions from the effects on the central nervous system, and tachycardia if the solution contains epinephrine. The convulsions usually dissipate rapidly as the local anesthetic is redistributed throughout the body. Intravenous thiopental or a benzodiazepine may be given to reduce these effects. A vasopressor (such as ephedrine or phenylephrine) can be used to restore blood pressure. If the patient becomes paralyzed, this may require intubation and ventilation until the toxic effects are gone. Use of the test dose with each injection usually prevents these problems.

Peripheral Nerve Blocks

A wide variety of peripheral nerves can be effectively blocked by injecting local anesthetic around them to provide adequate surgical anesthesia. Onset and duration of the block are related to the drug used, its concentration and volume, the addition of epinephrine, and the site of injection. Complications are usually caused by an inadvertent intravascular injection or an overdose of the local anesthetic. Rarely, nerve damage may occur from trauma caused by the needle or compression from the volume of local anesthetic injected.

Intravenous Regional Anesthesia

Intravenous regional anesthesia was first described by August Bier in 1908 and is frequently referred to as a *Bier block*. Although it can be used on a lower extremity, it is more often used on the upper extremities. It is highly reliable and easy to accomplish.

A small IV catheter is inserted as distally as feasible, and a single- or double-cuffed pneumatic tourniquet is placed around the limb proximally to the surgical site. The limb is raised upward and is then exsanguinated by wrapping it with an Esmarch bandage. The tourniquet is inflated to approximately 100 mm Hg above the patient's systolic blood pressure, and the Esmarch bandage is removed. Approximately 50 ml of 0.5% lidocaine is injected through the catheter. Onset of anesthesia is rapid and lasts until the tourniquet is deflated.

When a double-cuffed pneumatic tourniquet is used, the proximal cuff is initially inflated. When the patient experiences discomfort from the cuff pressure (usually about 35 to 40 minutes after inflation of the cuff), the distal cuff, which is located over an anesthetized area, is inflated. Then the proximal cuff is deflated. The proximal cuff must remain inflated until the distal cuff has been inflated to prevent loss of the IV anesthetic from the limb. Two single-cuffed tourniquets can be used instead of a double-cuffed tourniquet. If the patient experiences pain from the tourniquet, an IV analgesic or sedative can be used to supplement the block.

Although problems can occur from an overdose or toxic reaction to the lidocaine, these are rare if the tourniquet has been inflated more than 20 minutes. The risk is also minimized by intermittently deflating the cuff for a few seconds at a time for several cycles when the surgical procedure is over. This reduces the transient peak blood level of the local anesthetic in the central nervous system and the heart. Obviously, loss of pneumatic pressure in the tourniquet can cause both a toxic reaction and a loss of anesthesia.

MONITORED ANESTHESIA CARE

A gentle and patient surgeon can safely accomplish minor and even some major procedures with a peripheral nerve block or when the surgical site is infiltrated with a local anesthetic. This technique can be employed for normal, healthy persons as well as sicker, unstable patients who may require extensive invasive monitoring and pharmacologic management if general anesthesia is employed. For these patients, the issue is the relative risks and benefits of monitored anesthesia care (MAC) versus general anesthesia.

During MAC, the anesthesia provider may supplement the local anesthetic with an IV analgesic (such as fentanyl) and with sedative and amnestic drugs (such as midazolam or propofol). In addition, the anesthesia provider carefully monitors the patient's vital signs, respiratory and cardiovascular status, and positioning, and may give supplemental low-flow O_2. Depending on the clinical situation, the anesthesia provider may have to induce general anesthesia or utilize one of the regional techniques described previously if a greater degree of anesthesia is necessary during the procedure.

CONSCIOUS SEDATION/ ANALGESIA

Conscious sedation/analgesia refers to the intravenous administration of certain sedatives and analgesics that produces a condition in which the patient exhibits a depressed level of consciousness but retains the ability to independently maintain a patent airway and respond appropriately to verbal commands or physical stimulation. An anesthesia provider is not involved in the patient's care. Perioperative nurses with additional training and demonstrated competencies in administering conscious sedation/analgesia medications and monitoring these patients perform these functions under the direction of a physician.

Objectives for the patient receiving conscious sedation/ analgesia include: alteration of mood; maintenance of consciousness; enhanced cooperation; elevation of the pain threshold; minimal variation of vital signs; some degree of amnesia; and a rapid, safe return to activities of daily living.[3]

Selection of patients for conscious sedation/analgesia should be based on established criteria developed by an interdisciplinary team of healthcare professionals. It is essential that these patients be thoroughly assessed physiologically and psychologically before the procedure. That assessment should include a review of physical examination findings; current medications taken; existing allergies; current medical problems; history of smoking or substance abuse; current chief complaint; baseline vital signs, height, weight, and age; emotional state; any communication deficits; and the patient's perceptions of the procedure and conscious sedation/analgesia. The monitoring methods used for patients receiving conscious sedation, the medications administered, and the interventions taken must be within the scope of nursing practice as defined by the respective state board of nursing.[8] If the nurse does not feel comfortable managing the care and monitoring of a particular patient, the attending physician and an anesthesia provider should be consulted.

When monitoring a patient who is receiving conscious sedation/analgesia, the nurse should have no other responsibilities that would leave the patient unattended or compromise continuous patient monitoring during the procedure. It is essential that the nurse is clinically competent in the use of monitoring equipment and oxygen-delivery devices, medications used for conscious sedation/analgesia and resuscitation, and airway management. Advanced cardiac life support (ACLS) certification of nurses responsible for monitoring patients receiving conscious sedation/analgesia may be required by some healthcare institutions. If not, healthcare professionals with ACLS skills should be readily available to render support if needed in an emergency situation.

The nurse who administers conscious sedation/analgesia medications should understand their usual dosages, contraindications, interactions with other medications, onset and duration of action and desired effects, and adverse reactions and emergency management techniques. Benzodiazepines (such as diazepam and midazolam) and opioids (such as fentanyl and meperidine hydrochloride) are used for conscious sedation/analgesia.

Equipment that should be present and ready for use in the room where conscious sedation/analgesia will be administered includes noninvasive blood pressure device, electrocardiograph, pulse oximeter, oxygen-delivery devices, and suction.

Before conscious sedation/analgesia is administered, an IV access line should be established to facilitate administration of conscious sedation/analgesia medications and emergency medications and fluids if needed. Parameters that should be monitored during conscious sedation/analgesia are respiratory rate, cardiac rate and rhythm, blood pressure, oxygen saturation, level of consciousness, and condition of skin. An emergency cart with appropriate resuscitative medications and equipment (such as a defibrillator) should be immediately available to every location where conscious sedation/analgesia will be administered.

Nursing documentation of care provided should include the preprocedure assessment; dosage, route, time, and effects of all medications administered; type and amount of fluids administered; physiologic data from continuous monitoring at 5- to 15-minute intervals and upon significant events; level of consciousness; nursing interventions taken and the patient's responses; and any untoward significant patient reactions and their resolution.[3]

Postprocedure monitoring should be provided until the patient has returned to preprocedure baseline parameters as identified by individual institutional policy. Patients and family members or significant others should receive appropriate oral and written discharge instructions and be able to verbalize understanding of those instructions. It is helpful if the instructions can be given both before and after the procedure because conscious sedation/analgesia medications may cause amnesia, which affects recall ability.

Discharge criteria should be established by an interdisciplinary team and should include adequate respiratory function; stable vital signs; return to preprocedure level of consciousness; intact motor reflexes; return of motor and sensory control; absence of protracted nausea; acceptable skin color and condition; absence of significant pain; and satisfactory surgical site and dressing condition when present. A responsible adult must be available at discharge to accompany the patient home.

LOCAL ANESTHESIA

The terms *local anesthesia, local,* and *straight local* are used interchangeably to describe the administration of an anesthetic agent to a specific area of the body by topical application, local infiltration, regional nerve block, or "field" block. Local anesthesia is administered by the surgeon. In addition, other physicians such as cardiologists, pulmonologists, proctologists, or gastroenterologists may perform local procedures in the OR suite. No anesthesia provider is involved in the care of these patients.

Hospitals and ambulatory centers should have established interdisciplinary guidelines for the selection of patients who are appropriate for local anesthesia procedures and monitoring criteria for same. The decision to monitor the patient receiving local anesthesia, the parameters that need to be monitored, and the frequency of observation and monitoring should be tailored to the patient, the surgical procedure, and the medications used.

Patients receiving local anesthesia during a surgical procedure should be assessed preoperatively and continually observed by an RN during the procedure.[4]

Local anesthesia is usually employed for minor, short-term, surgical, diagnostic, or therapeutic procedures. Since the patient does not lose consciousness with local anesthesia, it is frequently preferred when the patient's cooperation is necessary for the procedure. Local anesthesia is economical and eliminates the undesirable effects of general anesthesia. However, adverse reactions may occur from large amounts of local agents. If the agent enters the bloodstream directly, convulsion, circulatory and respiratory distress, cardiovascular collapse, or even death can result.

Local anesthetics are chosen by the surgeon based on the desired duration of action, surgery site, potency potential, and the patient's physical status. Topical agents such as cocaine hydrochloride, tetracaine, or lidocaine may be applied to mucous membranes of the nose, throat, trachea, or urethra. Lidocaine 0.5% to 2%, with or without epinephrine, is the drug most commonly used for local infiltration anesthesia, though bupivacaine (Marcaine) has seen increased use in recent years. Epinephrine may be added to the local anesthesia agent for vasoconstricting properties in the area injected, slower rate of absorption of the local anesthetic agent, and lower incidence of toxicity. This allows for a longer duration of action for the agent and reduces blood flow to the area injected. It should be used with caution in patients with hypertension, diabetes, or heart disease. A general recommendation is that no more than 50 ml of a 1% solution, or 100 ml of a 0.5% solution, of an anesthetic drug such as lidocaine be injected per hour for local anesthesia. For maximum adult dosages see Table 7-2. All local anesthetic containers or syringes should be clearly labeled when on the sterile table.

Preoperatively the perioperative nurse should review the patient's history and physical examination findings and the results of laboratory or other diagnostic tests if indicated. Patients should be carefully assessed to determine their physiologic-baseline and emotional status and if any allergies exist. They may have an IV infusion started before the procedure because adequate venous access can be critical in life-threatening situations when resuscitative drugs must be given immediately.

The perioperative nurse should be clinically competent in the function and use of the monitoring equipment that will be used, the placement of equipment connections to the patient, and the interpretation of data. When indicated, intraoperative monitoring should include heart rate and regularity, respiratory rate, and mental status. Additional monitoring parameters should be based on the patient's condition and may include blood pressure, skin condition, and oxygen saturation.[4] Any changes in the patient's condition should be immediately reported to the surgeon.

The perioperative nurse should be familiar with the drugs to be administered during the procedure. This knowledge should include the usual dosages, limits on both the rate of injection and maximum dosage (usually stated on a per-kilogram basis), the duration of action, the physiologic and psychologic changes to be expected, normal and abnormal reactions to the drugs used, and the appropriate action to take should an untoward reaction occur. The nurse should monitor the dose, route, and time of administration of all local anesthetic medications given to the patient. In addition, the patient should be observed for presence of side effects such as central nervous system disturbances, cardiovascular problems, hypersensitivity to medication, and toxic reaction resulting from high levels of the local anesthetic agent. Emergency drugs, suction apparatus, and resuscitation equipment should be readily available. Symptoms of adverse drug reactions include restlessness, unexplained anxiety or fearfulness, diaphoresis, complaints of nausea, palpitations, disturbed respiration, pallor or flushing, syncope, and convulsive movements. The nurse should also be aware of symptoms of allergic reaction such as urticaria, tachycardia, laryngeal edema resulting in breathing difficulties, nausea, vomiting, and elevated temperature. In some instances, anaphylactoid symptoms, including severe hypotension, can occur. Should any significant change occur in the patient's physiologic or psychologic status, the nurse should immediately notify the physician. Good communication is essential for optimal patient care. Because the patient is awake during the procedure, extraneous or irrelevant conversation and noise pollution should be kept to a minimum.

Documentation of care provided to a patient receiving a local anesthetic should be consistent with the AORN Recommended Practices for Documentation of Perioperative Nursing Care.[2] In addition, the drug dosage, route, and time of administration, and the patient monitoring utilized should also be properly documented.

After completion of the procedure, the patient's postoperative status must be carefully assessed. This evaluation and any special needs of the patient should be properly documented on the chart, and a report should be called to the receiving unit before the patient's transfer. The report should include the type and amount of drugs given as well as any adverse reaction noted, the site and condition of the IV infusion (if applicable), the type and amount of solution infused in the OR, the range of intraoperative vital signs, the surgical procedure performed, and the condition of the dressing. Any special postoperative orders, allergies, and a general statement of the patient's tolerance of the procedure should also be included. The patient may be transferred to the day surgery and discharge area or returned directly to the hospital room. Local anesthesia patients are rarely transferred to PACU for recovery or observation.

PAIN MANAGEMENT

Because of their experience in analgesia and regional anesthesia, many anesthesiologists have applied this expertise to the management of both acute and chronic pain. Chronic pain is often a multifactorial entity that may occur after a discrete injury (or trauma), an amputation, laminectomy, or other surgical procedure. It may also result from prolonged repetitive stress such as "low back pain." Chronic pain frequently has complex psychologic components that are unrecognized by patients or those closely associated with them. Diagnosis and treatment of such chronic pain problems usually involves multiple medical disciplines and prolonged management.

Acute perioperative pain is a different problem. Traditionally, postoperative pain has been treated with IM narcotics every 3 to 6 hours as needed. This treatment is often associated with undesirable side effects including oversedation, respiratory depression, deep venous thrombosis secondary to decreased mobility, and variable degrees of pain relief. Other pain-management modalities are being used successfully. Patient-controlled analgesia (PCA) is a technique that utilizes a programable electronic pump that can continuously infuse a small amount of IV narcotic (at a basal rate) and, in addition, allows the patient to administer a predetermined bolus "on demand." Safety interlocks limit the frequency of the boluses and the total dose per hour.

When spinal or epidural anesthesia is employed for a surgical procedure, a small amount of preservative-free narcotic such as fentanyl, sufentanil, or morphine may be added to the local anesthetic mixture. The narcotic acts via central receptors and provides analgesia for 24 to 36 hours.

More recently, continuous epidural analgesia is used for prolonged postoperative pain management. This technique is employed for extensive procedures including total hip or knee replacements, knee reconstruction, and major abdominal, thoracic, or gynecologic operations. It can also be used for acute trauma such as multiple rib fractures.

Typically, a lumbar or thoracic epidural catheter is inserted before surgery, covered with a transparent occlusive dressing, and injected with local anesthetic. Because of the duration, manipulation, or positioning required for the operative procedure, general anesthesia is often induced for patient comfort. The epidural greatly reduces the analgesic requirements of general anesthesia. For pain control postoperatively, the epidural infusion of local anesthetic is usually one eighth to one sixteenth the concentration used for surgical anesthesia. A small dose of preservative-free narcotic such as fentanyl, sufentanil, or morphine is usually added to enhance analgesia. After the surgical procedure, the infusion rate is adjusted to provide analgesia during the early recovery phase. As the level of pain decreases over time, the infusion rate is reduced. The catheter is removed after 2 to 5 days to minimize the risk of infection. Benefits of epidural analgesia for acute postoperative pain include good analgesia with minimal sedation,

early ambulation and physical therapy, and excellent patient satisfaction. Side effects that may occur include nausea, pruritus, and areas of slight numbness. These are controlled with drugs such as diphenhydramine (Benadryl) or naloxone (Narcan), and by adjusting the infusion rate. A nonsteroidal antiinflammatory drug (NSAID) such as ketorolac (Toradol) is frequently given for any "breakthrough pain" instead of increasing the epidural infusion.

A single caudal injection is often used in pediatric patients having surgery of the lower abdomen, pelvis, or lower extremities. It is usually administered after the induction of general anesthesia, and a long-acting local anesthetic such as bupivacaine with epinephrine is typically used. This provides good analgesia for 8 to 24 hours postoperatively as well as greatly decreasing the intraoperative requirements for general anesthesia. If the procedure will require prolonged recovery, a lumbar epidural can be placed intraoperatively. Postoperatively, it is managed similarly to that of adult patients, except for younger patients the level of analgesia and the presence of side effects must be assessed by someone else.

Epidural infusions have also been used for patients suffering from the intense pain of terminal malignancies. These patients may experience pain that is often so severe that parenteral analgesics provide inadequate pain relief and produce deep respiratory depression. Epidural infusions for prolonged periods of time have been used in these patients. Transdermal fentanyl patches may also be used in these patients as well as for chronic pain.

TEMPERATURE CONTROL

Increased attention has been directed toward maintaining a normal temperature range perioperatively for both pediatric and adult patients. The room temperature can be raised and infrared warming lamps used for pediatric patients. Lower fresh-gas flow rates of cool, dry, anesthetic gases can be used. A heat and moisture exchanger (such as Humidivent) helps to maintain the heat and moisture of inspired gases. A variety of IV fluid warmers are available to warm crystalloid solutions or refrigerated blood products. Some of these units originally designed for major trauma procedures will warm fluids at flow rates up to 500 ml/min. Units that blow heated air onto the upper or lower body surface are also available. These units are usually effective in maintaining body temperature even during a long abdominal procedure and can be used subsequently in the PACU (see Chapter 8).

MALIGNANT HYPERTHERMIA

First identified in the late 1960s, malignant hyperthermia (MH) is a rare, life-threatening complication that may be triggered by drugs commonly used in anesthesia. Inhalational anesthetics and succinylcholine are the most frequently implicated triggering agents. Malignant hyperthermia may also be induced by trauma, strenuous exercise, or emotional stress. It is a multifactorial disease and is genetically transmitted as an autosomal dominant trait with variable expression in affected individuals. There is an increased incidence of MH in patients with central core disease (a congenital myopathy) and some muscular dystrophies.

The syndrome begins with a hypermetabolic condition in skeletal muscle cells that involves altered mechanisms of calcium function at the cellular level. Characteristics of the syndrome include cellular hypermetabolism resulting in hypercarbia, tachypnea, tachycardia, hypoxia, metabolic and respiratory acidosis, cardiac arrhythmias, and elevation of body temperature at a rate of 1 to 2 Celsius degrees every 5 minutes. It must be emphasized that the rise in body temperature is one of the late manifestations of MH. These signs may occur during induction or maintenance of anesthesia, although the syndrome can occur postoperatively or even after repeated exposures to anesthesia. It is most frequently seen in children and adolescents. The signs and symptoms associated with MH are listed in Box 7-4.

It is important to remember that (1) MH is a rare, multifaceted syndrome and can have variable clinical presentations; (2) many of the signs and symptoms associated with MH can have other causes; and (3) other disorders, such as neuroleptic malignant syndrome (NMS), may also have similar presentations. (The NMS occurs after use of neuroleptic drugs, such as haloperidol, and is characterized by muscular rigidity, akinesia, hyperthermia, and autonomic dysfunction.) Because MH is such a life-threatening disorder, many anesthesia providers will initiate a treatment protocol when some of these early signs and symptoms occur that cannot otherwise be readily explained.

Time is crucial when MH is diagnosed. All OR and anesthesia personnel should be familiar with the protocol for its management. In the past, mortality ranged up to 80%, but the immediate infusion of dantrolene (Dantrium) and proper treatment have reduced the incidence of fatalities to about 7%. Dantrolene is a hydantoin skeletal muscle relaxant that also has effects on vascular and heart muscle. In addition to dantrolene, the major modalities of treatment include cooling the patient with ice packs and cold IV solutions, administering diuretics, treating cardiac arrhythmias, correcting the acid-base and electrolyte imbalances, and monitoring fluid intake and output and the body temperature. Many hospitals maintain an emergency MH kit or cart that contains the drugs, laboratory tubes, other supplies, and instructions to treat MH in the OR area. Location of the iced or cold saline and other equipment should also be listed with the emergency kit. Chilled saline is often kept in the refrigeration unit for blood products. An outline for emergency treatment of MH is given in Box 7-5. The Malignant Hyperthermia Association of the United States (MHAUS) has names of on-call physicians available for consultation in MH emergencies at 1-800-MH-HYPER (1-800-644-9737). For patient-referral or nonemergency calls, 1-607-674-7901 should be used.

Patients known or suspected to have this syndrome can be anesthetized with minimal risk if appropriate precautions are taken. If the syndrome is suspected, a muscle biopsy should be done to make a diagnosis before the patient is electively anesthetized. For their own safety, relatives of persons with MH should be evaluated for presence of the syndrome.

SAFETY OF HEALTHCARE WORKERS

The transmission of diseases including hepatitis B and the human immunodeficiency virus (HIV) from body fluids is a major concern for healthcare workers. All healthcare workers should therefore observe the universal precautions for all body fluids. It has been shown that blood, serum, and cerebrospinal fluid have higher concentrations of HIV than saliva, tears, urine, breast milk, amniotic fluid, or vaginal secretions have. Precautions include use of protective eye wear; face mask; gloves; and use of a needleless system, stopcocks, or one-way injection devices for all IV medications given to the patient.

With the implementation of universal precautions among healthcare workers, a new problem has arisen. The increased need to use latex gloves and products has created a rapidly growing segment of healthcare workers who are allergic to latex products. This is most frequently seen in dental or medical (such as anesthesia and perioperative) personnel who repeatedly change inexpensive, disposable latex gloves. Alternatives, such as vinyl gloves, are not very satisfactory. Patients with certain congenital deformities or who require multiple surgical procedures have an increased

---

BOX 7-4	**Signs and Symptoms Often Seen with Malignant Hyperthermia**

1. Hypercarbia
2. Tachycardia
3. Tachypnea (may not be seen in a paralyzed patient)
4. Muscle stiffness or rigidity
5. Hypoxia and dark (desaturated) blood in operative field
6. Unstable or elevated blood pressure
7. Cardiac arrhythmias
8. Changes in CO_2 absorbent (temperature, color)
9. Metabolic and respiratory acidosis
10. Peripheral mottling, cyanosis, or sweating
11. Rising body temperature (1 to 2 Celsius degrees every 5 minutes)
12. Myoglobinuria
13. Hyperkalemia, hypercalcemia, lactic acidemia
14. Pronounced elevation in creatinine phosphokinase (may exceed 20,000 units in initial 12 to 24 hours)

CHAPTER SEVEN | Anesthesia 235

risk of developing a latex allergy. Management of an anaphylactic reaction to latex during anesthesia is described in Research Highlight 7-5. See Chapter 2 for more information on latex allergies.

COST CONTAINMENT IN ANESTHESIA

Decreasing reimbursement for health care and the rise of managed care organizations have stimulated efforts to reduce perioperative expenses. Improving the utilization of expensive OR facilities, equipment, and personnel is a major factor in decreasing costs. It is estimated that the cost of an OR is $15 to $25 a minute. (This includes facility and equipment amortization, utilities, and labor costs but excludes the fees for anesthesia and surgeons.) Anesthesia drug costs and supplies, as well as surgical supplies, are in addition to the OR costs.

Actual savings and improvement are predicated on accurate cost data. Several clinical and management approaches are employed to identify these complex issues. A variety of computer programs have been developed to optimize OR utilization, staff scheduling, patient flow and preoperative preparation, and drug and supply expenses and to correlate these data with patient outcomes. Many organizations and companies are involved in these endeavors. Some examples are described in Research Highlight 7-6.

OPERATING ROOM POLLUTION

Contamination and pollution of the OR environment can come from many sources. Every chemical should be considered harmful until proved otherwise. Reaction to chemicals and irritants may vary with age, sex, race, season of the year, and concurrent exposure to other substances. Disinfectants, antiseptics, soaps, aerosol or pressurized sprays, and other compounds contribute to the pollution potential. Attention is also being paid to noise pollution. Of particular interest in the present context is the pollution of the OR with anesthetic gases such as N_2O and the inhalation anesthetics. Various surveys taken among personnel exposed to these anesthetic gases (anesthesia providers, other anesthesia personnel, perioperative nurses, dentists, and dental assistants who work with anesthetic gases) and their spouses have implicated such pollution as a possible contributing factor to an increased abortion rate and incidence of lymphoma and other conditions. However, the interpretation of these surveys is controversial.

To minimize the hazards of bacteria, other airborne pollutants, and waste anesthetic gases, most OR suites condition and filter their own air and provide more than 15 air exchanges each hour. To minimize contamination, the air pressure inside each OR is usually greater than that in adjacent hallways. To reduce pollution from trace anesthetic gases and to contain costs, many anesthesia providers use "low-flow" anesthetic techniques that

---

| BOX 7-5 | Emergency Management of Malignant Hyperthermia |

1. Immediately discontinue all triggering agents (inhalational anesthetics and succinylcholine).
2. Terminate surgery if possible or continue with safe anesthetic drugs.
3. Hyperventilate with 100% O_2 at highest flow rate. It is not necessary to change any anesthesia equipment.
4. Immediately give dantrolene sodium (Dantrium) 2-3 mg/kg IV. Give additional incremental doses up to 10 mg/kg total or until the signs of MH are controlled.
5. Give sodium bicarbonate IV to correct the metabolic acidosis. Use arterial blood gases (ABG). If ABG are not available, consider 1-2 mEq/kg.
6. If the patient is hyperthermic, begin active cooling.
   a. Inject iced saline (not lactated Ringer's) IV 15 ml/kg every 15 min × 3.
   b. Use iced saline to perform lavage of the stomach, bladder, rectum and open body cavities as feasible.
   c. Cool the body surface with a thermia blanket. Rub with cold, wet towels or ice.
   d. Monitor the temperature to avoid hypothermia.
7. Cardiac arrhythmias usually resolve with correction of acidosis and hyperkalemia. If not, antiarrhythmic agents such as procainamide 3 mg/kg (max. of 15 mg/kg) may be used. Avoid calcium-entry blockers because they may cause hyperkalemia and cardiovascular collapse.
8. Closely monitor temperature, $ETCO_2$, arterial or central venous blood gases, urine output, K^+, Ca^{++}, and coagulation studies. Insert a urinary catheter. Consider arterial line and a central venous or PA catheter.
9. Hyperkalemia is common. Treat with hyperventilation, sodium bicarbonate, or 10 units of regular insulin in 50 ml of D_{50} IV titrated to K^+ level or regular insulin 0.15 units/kg and D_{50} 1 ml/kg. Life-threatening hyperkalemia may also be treated with calcium (such as 2.5 mg/kg of $CaCl_2$).
10. Maintain urine output above 2 mg/kg/hr. Consider volume, mannitol, and furosemide.
11. Children less than 10 to 12 years old who have a sudden cardiac arrest after succinylcholine without hypoxia may have subclinical muscular dystrophy. Treat for acute hyperkalemia first. Give $CaCl_2$ with other treatments in step #9 above.
12. Transfer patient to ICU when stable. Monitor at least 24 hours for recurrence of MH and for late complications.
13. Administer dantrolene 1 mg/kg IV every 6 hours for 24 to 48 hours. Then dantrolene 1 mg/kg every 6 hours for 24 hours may be given orally as necessary.
14. Monitor core body temperature (continuously), ABG, K^+, Ca^{++}, CK, serum and urine myoglobin, and coagulation studies until they return to normal.
15. Counsel the patient and family about MH and further precautions. Refer the patient to MHAUS and complete an Adverse Metabolic Reaction to Anesthesia (AMRA) report to the North American Malignant Hyperthermia Registry at (717) 531-6936.
16. MHAUS 24-hour hotline: 1-800-MH-HYPER (1-800-644-9737).

Modified from Emergency Therapy for Malignant Hyperthermia, revised 1995. Malignant Hyperthermia Association of the United States (MHAUS).

7-5   RESEARCH HIGHLIGHT

LATEX ALLERGY

The incidence of allergic reactions to latex products has rapidly escalated. There are two high-risk groups: (1) healthcare workers (especially those who repeatedly change latex gloves or products to implement universal precautions and (2) compromised patients who are exposed to latex products through multiple surgical or invasive procedures. The risk of latex allergy in healthcare providers is 13.7% for dental personnel, 7.5% for physicians, 5.6% for nurses, and 1.3% for hospital workers compared with 10% for workers in the rubber industry and 0.08% for the general public. Latex allergy occurs in 18% to 40% of patients with spina bifida and in 35% to 83% of patients with a history of atopy (such as allergic response to balloons, rubber gloves, or certain foods or fruits.)

Latex-induced anaphylaxis comprises about 10% of the life-threatening anaphylactic reactions that occur during anesthesia. The intensity of the reactions is variable and may include contact dermatitis, conjunctivitis, asthma, angioedema, anaphylaxis, perioperative hemodynamic collapse, or death. Allergy is an undesirable physiologic response to a foreign substance, which may be nonimmunologic (initial exposure) or immunologic (reexposure). Reactions mediated by IgE antibodies are called "anaphylactic reactions" and can be confirmed by IgE antibody titers or allergy skin tests. Reactions that may be similar but not proved to result from IgE antibodies are called "anaphylactoid reactions."

A careful preoperative evaluation should be done of all "high-risk" patients (such as spina bifida, urogenital abnormalities, multiple surgeries, healthcare workers, and people with atopy, extensive exposure to rubber products, or a history of latex allergy). If indicated by the evaluation, a latex allergy can be confirmed by tests such as radioallergosorbent test (RAST) for latex-specific immunoassays, AlaSTAT test for latex-specific IgE allergens, skin-prick testing (SPT) for IgE-mediated latex hypersensitivity, or a patch test for delayed hypersensitivity reactions.

Preoperative prophylaxis with steroids or histamine (H_1 and H_2) blockers will not prevent IgE-mediated, anaphylactic reactions to latex. Such reactions usually occur 10 to 40 minutes after induction of anesthesia but may happen as long as 290 minutes later. The severity and intensity of the reactions are variable.

Management of an anaphylactic reaction to latex should include stopping all anesthetics, giving 100% O_2 with controlled ventilation, changing to latex-free gloves and products, and infusing IV fluids to sustain blood pressure. Most anesthesia machines that have been recently serviced by factory-authorized personnel should be "latex free," and so changing anesthesia machines should not be required. If necessary, the following IV drugs may be given: epinephrine 3 to 5 $\mu g/kg$, plus an infusion of 1 to 4 $\mu g/kg/min$; diphenhydramine 0.5 to 1 mg/kg; aminophylline 1 to 6 mg/kg over 20 minutes followed by an infusion of 0.5 to 0.9 $\mu g/kg/hr$ if bronchospasm continues; steroids such as methylprednisolone 1 to 2 g, hydrocortisone 1 g, or dexamethasone 4 to 20 mg; and sodium bicarbonate 0.5 to 1 mEq/kg if acidosis or hypotension persists.

Arterial blood gases should be obtained. Blood tests for tryptase and specific IgE antibodies should be made. Urinary methylhistamine should be measured within 3 hours. Since laryngeal edema can occur, the airway should be carefully evaluated. The patient should be monitored in the ICU for 24 to 48 hours after an anaphylactic reaction.

The National Institute for Occupational Safety and Health (NIOSH) released a medical alert titled "Preventing Allergic Reactions to Natural Rubber Latex in the Workplace" on June 23, 1997. One may obtain a copy by calling 1-800-356-4674, or by visiting the NIOSH homepage at http://www.cdc.gov/niosh/homepage.html.

From Hamid, R.K.A. (1996). Latex allergy: diagnosis, management, and safe equipment. *ASA Refresher Courses in Anesthesiology, 24,* 85-96, Philadelphia: Lippincott-Raven.

---

greatly reduce the volume of waste gases. However, air pollution with waste anesthetic gases is still a major concern, and all anesthesia machines should have a waste gas–scavenging system. In modern OR suites, a dedicated vacuum line is used to scavenge such gases. One such scavenging system is shown in Fig. 7-13. It includes (1) a reservoir bag so that less instantaneous vacuum is needed, (2) a positive-pressure relief valve that prevents excessive backpressure in the patient's lungs and that vents excess gas into the room air should the vacuum be occluded or inadequate, (3) a negative-pressure relief valve that prevents excessive vacuum from damaging the patient's lungs, and (4) a needle valve to adjust the vacuum. Evacuation hoses are connected to the ventilator and the adjustable pressure-limiting (APL) valve. When the patient is not intubated, however, air pollution may occur from a loose mask fit on the patient's face. According to the National Institute for Occupational Safety and Health (NIOSH), pollution levels should be less than 25 ppm (time-weighted average) for N_2O and 2 ppm for halogenated agents. These levels are difficult to achieve during induction and emergence.

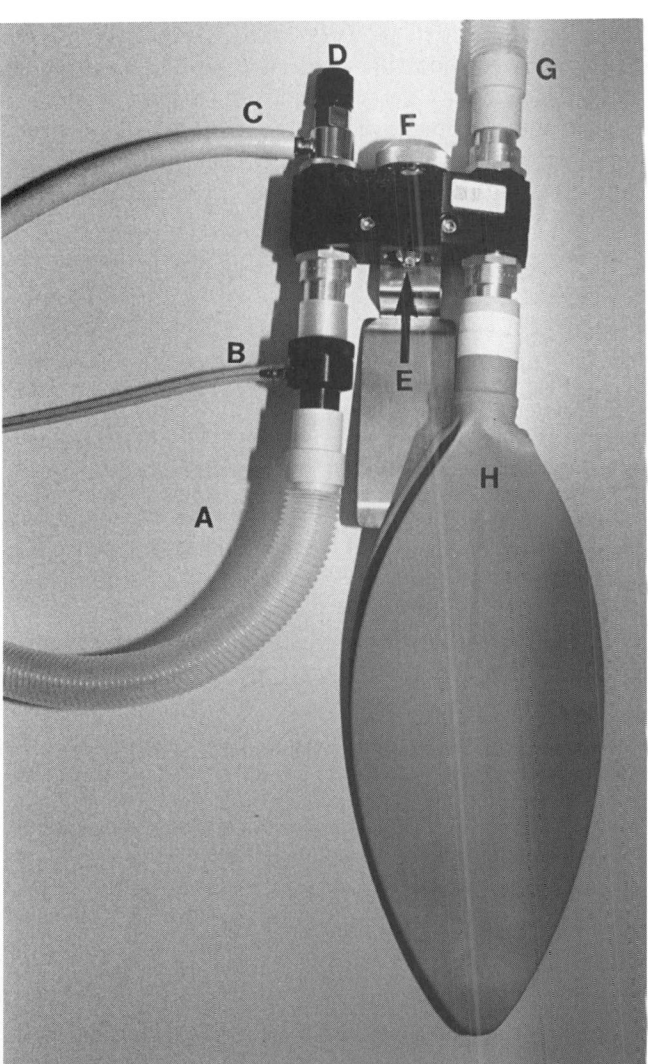

FIGURE 7-13 A typical scavenging system for waste anesthetic gases. **A,** Scavenging hose from ventilator. **B,** Scavenging line from respiratory gas monitor. **C,** Vacuum line to hospital scavenging system. **D,** Vacuum-adjustment valve. **E,** Negative-pressure relief valve. **F,** Positive-pressure relief valve. **G,** Scavenging hose from APL valve. **H,** Reservoir bag.

Chronic occupational exposure to trace concentrations of anesthetic gases is of particular concern to pregnant women. A safe exposure level below which one can be assured that no adverse effects will occur has not been established. Persons with questions about exposure levels should consult a knowledgeable member of the anesthesia department for the latest information.

PERIOPERATIVE NURSING CONSIDERATIONS RELATED TO ANESTHESIA

Care of the surgical patient is a cooperative effort, and personnel involved in the perioperative period should function as a smooth, well-coordinated team. As part of conducting the preoperative patient assessment and

7-6 RESEARCH HIGHLIGHT

COST CONTAINMENT IN THE PERIOPERATIVE ENVIRONMENT

The rising cost of health care and the explosion of managed care organizations have profoundly affected nearly every segment of society. In this new environment, departments and services that utilize the expensive and resource-intensive areas of the hospital (such as the operating rooms and perioperative services) are now considered "cost centers" rather than "profit centers." In health care, common methods of economic analysis evaluate different factors:

1. Cost-benefit analysis compares the pertinent costs with the outcome in monetary terms.
2. Cost-reduction analysis compares the acquisition costs of various drugs or supplies without regard to the outcome or associated side effects. Unless the outcomes are similar, other methods should be used.
3. Cost-effective analysis evaluates the cost of a treatment or intervention in units of outcome or effect. Converting outcomes into monetary values is difficult, and doing so limits the utilization of this method.
4. Cost-utility analysis is similar to factor 3 above but includes patient preferences and the satisfaction with their assessment and treatment. Results are expressed as quality of adjusted life years (QALY).

Freund and colleagues implemented an educational process, practice guidelines, and paperwork barriers to persuade anesthesia care providers to substitute low-cost neuromuscular-blocking (NMB) drugs (pancuronium or a pancuronium-metocurine combination) for more costly vecuronium. This resulted in a 31% reduction ($34,000) in expenditures for NMB drugs during the first year of implementation, and a 47% reduction ($51,000) the second year.

Other studies have taken a more global view. Based on extensive review of the economics of anesthesia practice, Watcha and White showed that better scheduling of procedures, more efficient processing of patients in the PACU, and reduced wastage of anesthetic and surgical supplies lead to greater savings than reducing anesthesia-related drug costs.

Over the next few years in all models of healthcare systems, there will be greater emphasis on cost reduction and increased efficiency in the utilization of a facility's resources. The objective is to provide quality healthcare and patient satisfaction balanced with appropriate therapeutic modalities and QALY.

From Freund, P.R., Bowdle, T.A., Posner, K.L., et al. (1997). Cost-effective reduction of neuromuscular-blocking drug expenditures. *Anesthesiology, 87,* 1044-1049; Watcha, M.F., & White, P.F. (1997). Economics of anesthetic practice. *Anesthesiology, 86,* 1170-1196.

identifying the nursing plan of care, the perioperative nurse checks the chart to verify the patient's identity, the surgeon, and the scheduled procedure; confirm that the operative and anesthesia permits are properly signed; identify any patient allergies; and ensure that current reports of laboratory tests and diagnostic studies are complete and on the chart.

In many OR suites a preoperative preparation or *holding area* is utilized for procedures such as the insertion of arterial, central venous, or pulmonary artery catheters and placement of epidural catheters or peripheral nerve blocks. This area may be staffed by nursing personnel from the OR, PACU, or the department of anesthesiology. The purpose of this area is to improve patient care delivery, optimize the perioperative flow of patients, and provide support services for the above procedures. The minimum requirement for monitoring should be an ECG, noninvasive blood pressure, and pulse oximetry. Equipment for emergency airway management should be readily available. It is important that the nursing staff be familiar with such equipment and be readily available to assist in its utilization.

A patient should never be left alone in the OR suite. When there is an anesthetized patient in the OR, a perioperative nurse should always be immediately available to provide assistance if needed. During the insertion of IV, arterial, central venous, or pulmonary artery catheters, the nurse should assist as appropriate.

During induction of anesthesia, particularly with a traumatized patient or for an emergency procedure, the nurse should be ready to apply cricoid pressure to prevent regurgitation of stomach contents and assist the anesthesia provider in visualizing the vocal cords. When cricoid pressure is used to prevent aspiration, it should not be released until the intubation is accomplished, the cuff on the endotracheal tube is inflated, and proper placement of the endotracheal tube has been verified. However, when two anesthesia providers are present, one of them will usually provide this support.

Operating room personnel should never move an unconscious patient without first coordinating the positioning or move with the anesthesia provider. When the patient is positioned for surgery, the nurse should always check the arms and legs to ensure that no pressure points exist and that the extremities are appropriately positioned and padded (see Chapter 5).

Before transporting the patient from the OR to the PACU, the circulating nurse should call the PACU and give a preliminary status report of the patient's condition. This report includes the surgical procedure performed, type of anesthesia care provided, information specific to the patient's preoperative diagnosis and subsequent outcome related to intraoperative intervention, and any special equipment required (such as a ventilator, T-piece, or arterial pressure monitors).

Postanesthesia recovery care and functions are described in Chapter 8.

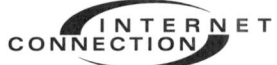

American Society of Anesthesiologists (ASA):
http://www.asahq.org

American Association of Nurse Anesthetists:
http://aana.com

Anesthesia Net: http://www.anesthesia.net/

Gasnet Anesthesiology Home Page:
http://gasnet.med.yale.edu/

Association of Perianesthesia Nurses (ASPAN):
http://www.aspan.org

List Serves (to ask questions about anesthesia); e-mail and follow instructions at these sites:
listserv@ubvm.cc.buffalo.edu

REFERENCES

1. American Society of Anesthesiologists. (1995). *Guidelines for sedation and analgesia by non-anesthesiologists.* Park Ridge, IL: the Society.
2. Association of Operating Room Nurses. (1998). Recommended practices for documentation of perioperative nursing care. In *Standards, recommended practices, and guidelines.* Denver: the Association.
3. Association of Operating Room Nurses. (1998). Recommended practices for managing the patient receiving conscious sedation/analgesia. In *Standards, recommended practices, and guidelines.* Denver: the Association.
4. Association of Operating Room Nurses. (1998). Recommended practices for monitoring the patient receiving local anesthesia. In *Standards, recommended practices, and guidelines.* Denver: the Association.
5. Maltby, J.R., Lewis, P., Martin, A., & Sutherland, L.R. (1991). Gastric fluid volume and pH in elective patients following unrestricted oral fluid until three hours before surgery. *Canadian Journal of Anaesthesia, 38,* 425-529.
6. Shevde, K., & Trivedi, N. (1991). Effects of clear liquids on gastric volume and pH in healthy volunteers. *Anesthesia and Analgesia, 72,* 528-531.
7. Voelker, R. (1995). Anesthesia-related risks have plummeted. *Journal of the American Medical Association, 273,* 445-446.
8. Watson, D.S. (1998). Conscious sedation/analgesia, St. Louis: Mosby.

CHAPTER EIGHT

Postoperative Pain Care and Complications

Jan Odom

THE POSTOPERATIVE PHASE of care begins as soon as the surgical procedure is concluded and the patient is transferred to the postanesthesia care unit (PACU). The PACU has been known in the past as the recovery room, or postanesthesia room.

An assigned area for the care of the postoperative patient is a fairly recent addition to surgical patient care. Even though surgical procedures have been performed for thousands of years and general anesthesia has been available for almost 150 years, PACUs became common only in the last 30 to 40 years. A postanesthesia area was first described by Florence Nightingale[19]: "It is not uncommon, in small country hospitals, to have a recess or small room leading from the operating theater in which the patients remain until they have recovered, or at least recovered from the immediate effects of the operation."

There were a few recovery rooms opened in the 1920s and 1930s. In the 1940s a large number of PACUs opened because of the shortage of nurses during the war years and the need to centralize patients, equipment, and personnel for postoperative care. It was soon discovered that use of the PACU decreased patient morbidity and mortality and shortened the period of hospitalization of some patients.[23] Many hospitals opened PACUs after this discovery was reported.

PACUs have flourished since that time. Technologic innovation has had a profound effect in PACUs, as in other critical care areas. The complexity of anesthesia management demands specially trained nurses who have expertise in the prompt recognition and management of postoperative complications. Most patients who receive general anesthesia, major regional anesthesia, or monitored anesthesia care are transferred to a PACU.

The PACU should be adjacent to the surgical suite with easy access for patient transport. The patient's status should be assessed for needs during transfer (such as oxygen, manual positive-pressure device, a bed instead of a stretcher).

The perioperative nurse in some cases may actually provide care for the patient in the PACU. It is more common, however, for the perioperative nurse to accompany the patient to the PACU with an anesthesia provider and give a report on the status of the patient to a perianesthesia nurse. The nurse in PACU assumes the care of the patient after an initial assessment of the patient and a report from the transferring team.

PERIOPERATIVE NURSING CONSIDERATIONS

Assessment

Admission to PACU

The initial assessment of the postoperative patient begins with an immediate determination of airway and circulatory adequacy. The airway is assessed for patency, humidified oxygen is applied, and respirations are counted. Pulse oximetry is initiated on all patients, and the quality of breath sounds is determined. The patient is then connected to the cardiac monitor, and cardiac rate and rhythm are evaluated. Blood pressure measurement is then obtained by means of a manual cuff or an automatic cuff (such as Dinamap). If the patient has an arterial line, it can be connected to the monitor at this time.

After the PACU nurse has assessed the ABCs (airway, breathing, circulation), the perioperative nurse and anesthesia provider can then provide a comprehensive report on the patient. Even though the report is usually given by the anesthesia provider, the perioperative nurse should collaborate and then add and verify important information about the patient.[20]

The American Society of Perinesthesia Nurses (ASPAN)[3] recommends that the report contain (1) relevant preoperative status, such as vital signs, radiology findings, laboratory values, oxygen saturation, allergies, and disabilities; (2) anesthesia technique; (3) anesthetic agents including muscle relaxants, narcotics, and reversal agents; (4) length of time anesthesia was administered and time reversal agents were given; (5) surgical procedure performed; (6) estimated fluid and blood loss and replacement; and (7) complications occurring during anesthesia course. The patient's American Society of Anesthesiologists (ASA) classification (see Chapter 7) should also be provided during the patient report.

Other useful information that the perioperative nurse can provide includes the status of the airway, presence of tubes, drains and catheters, and intravascular lines. Any postoperative orders to be initiated in PACU can be discussed at this time.

The anesthesia provider should not leave the patient until the PACU nurse accepts responsibility for the patient's care. Standard III-3 of the ASA Standards for Postanesthesia Care[2] states that "the member of the anesthesia care team shall remain in the PACU until the PACU nurse accepts responsibility for the nursing care of the patient."

Initial assessment

After the immediate assessment of ABCs and completion of the report, the PACU nurse begins a more thorough postanesthesia assessment. The assessment is performed quickly and is specific, in part, to the type of operative procedure. ASPAN has recommended elements of an initial assessment in the PACU (Box 8-1).

Some PACUs use a head-to-toe assessment to organize the data obtained (Fig. 8-1). Other PACUs have adopted a major body systems approach to assessment (Fig. 8-2). In any case, the PACU nurse assesses the admitting vital signs and the ABCs beginning with the respiratory system. Respiratory assessment comprises rate, rhythm, ausculta-

---

BOX 8-1 | **Initial Assessment in the PACU**

Initial assessment to include documentation of:
1. Integration of data received at transfer of care
2. Vital signs: (a) airway patent, respiratory rate and competency, breath sounds, type of artificial airway, mechanical ventilator settings and oxygen saturations; (b) blood pressure: cuff or arterial line; (c) pulse: apical, peripheral; (d) temperature: oral, rectal, axillary, digital through dermal sensor, tympanic
3. Level of consciousness
4. Pressure readings: central venous, arterial blood, pulmonary artery wedge, and intracranial pressure if indicated
5. Position of patient
6. Condition and color of skin
7. Patient safety needs
8. Neurovascular: peripheral pulses and sensation of extremity or extremities as applicable
9. Condition of dressings
10. Condition of suture line, if dressing absent
11. Type, patency, and securement of drainage tubes, catheters, and receptacle
12. Amount and type of drainage
13. Muscular response and strength
14. Pupillary response as indicated
15. Fluid therapy, location of lines, condition of intravenous site, and securement and amount of solution infusing (including blood)
16. Level of comfort (physical and emotional)
17. Numerical score if used

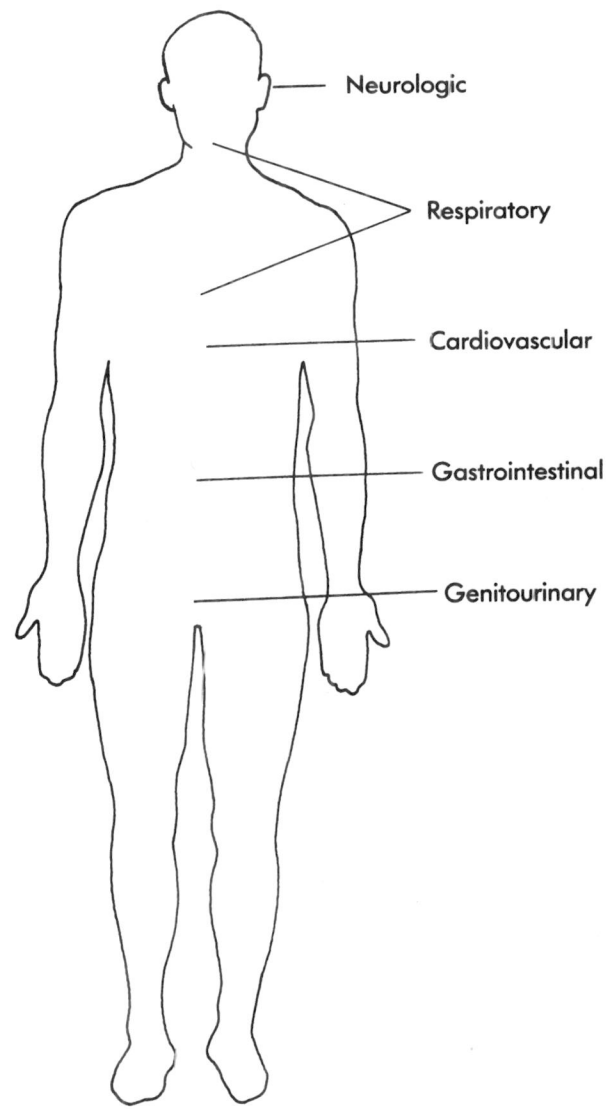

FIGURE 8-1   Head-to-toe assessment.

tion of breath sounds, and an oxygen-saturation level. Presence of an artificial airway and type of oxygen-delivery system are noted.

The cardiovascular system is assessed by monitoring heart rate and rhythm. The patient's initial blood pressure is compared to one or more preoperative readings. Body temperature is obtained, skin condition is examined, and peripheral pulses are checked, if indicated. The patient is then assessed for neurologic functioning. Has the patient reacted (awakened from anesthesia)? Can the patient follow commands? Is the patient oriented, at least to name and hospital? Can the patient move all extremities and lift the head? Are there deviations from preoperative neurologic functioning? Some operative procedures require a more detailed assessment.

To assess renal function, the intake and output are examined. The intraoperative fluid total and estimated blood loss are assessed. The intravenous lines, infusions, and irrigation solutions are recorded. Presence of all lines, drains, and catheters is noted; output is noted for color, amount, and consistency.

All the information obtained from the admission assessment is documented in the PACU record. One example of a PACU record is shown in Fig. 8-3.

Nursing Diagnosis

Common nursing diagnoses related to the care of postanesthesia patients might include the following:

- Ineffective breathing pattern
- Decreased cardiac output
- Risk for altered body temperature
- Altered thought processes
- Pain

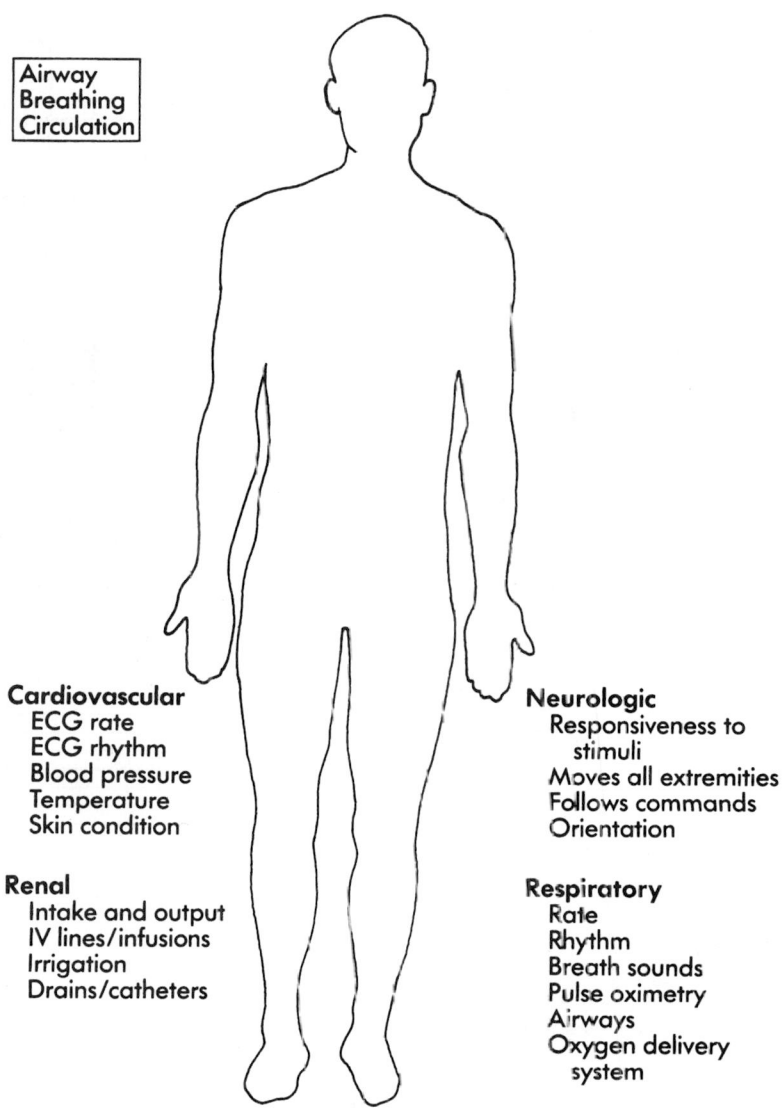

Airway
Breathing
Circulation

Cardiovascular
ECG rate
ECG rhythm
Blood pressure
Temperature
Skin condition

Renal
Intake and output
IV lines/infusions
Irrigation
Drains/catheters

Neurologic
Responsiveness to
  stimuli
Moves all extremities
Follows commands
Orientation

Respiratory
Rate
Rhythm
Breath sounds
Pulse oximetry
Airways
Oxygen delivery
  system

FIGURE 8-2 PACU major body systems assessment.

FORREST GENERAL HOSPITAL
POST ANESTHESIA CARE UNIT RECORD

POST ANESTHESIA RECOVERY SCORE		MINUTES					
		in	30	60	90	out	

Activity
Able to move 4 extremities voluntarily or on command = 2
Able to move 2 extremities voluntarily or on command = 1
Able to move 0 extremities voluntarily or on command = 0

Respiration
Able to deep breathe and cough freely = 2
Dyspnea or limited breathing = 1
Apneic = 0

Circulation
BP ± 20 of Preanesthetic level = 2
BP ± 20-50 of Preanesthetic level = 1
BP ± 50 of Preanesthetic level = 0

Consciousness
Fully Awake = 2
Arousable on calling = 1
Not Responding = 0

O_2 Saturation
Able to maintain O_2 Sat > 92% on room air = 2
Needs O_2 to maintain O_2 Sat > 90% = 1
O_2 Sat < 90% even with O_2 = 0

TOTAL

Pre-op B.P. _____
Allergy

Airway: On Adm.
Jawthrust _____
Chin Hold _____
Endotracheal _____
Oral Airway _____
Mask Oxygen _____
Nasal Oxygen _____
Trach _____
T-Tube _____
Nasal Airway _____
Ventilator Settings _____

Addressograph

Time In _____   Time Out _____
Accompanied by _____
Type of anesthesia _____
Surgical Procedure:

PULSE - RESPIRATION - BLOOD PRESSURE

	15	30	45	15	30	45	15	30	45	15	30	45	
240													
220													
200													
180													
160													
140													
120													
100													
80													
60													
40													
20													

O_2 Sat.
CVP
PAP

CODES   ⊥ A-line   ∨ Manual or   Pulse •   Siderails: Yes   Restraints:: Yes
T B.P.   ∧ NBP   Resp. ○   No   No

IV Type _____

Total IV in OR _____ cc
Blood in OR _____ units
Urinary Output in OR _____ cc
Est. Blood Loss _____ cc

RN Signature _____

RN Signature _____

Foley Cath. _____
Suprapubic _____
Ureteral _____
Levine _____

DRAINS

MEDICATIONS AND TREATMENTS

	AMT.	ROUTE	TIME
Demerol			
Morphine			
Phenergan			
Droperidol			
Zofran			
Toradol			

FIGURE 8–3   PACU record.

FORREST GENERAL HOSPITAL

DATE	TIME	DESCRIPTIVE NOTES (SIGN EACH ENTRY)

FIGURE 8-3, cont'd PACU record.

Continued

FORREST GENERAL HOSPITAL

DATE	TIME	DESCRIPTIVE NOTES (SIGN EACH ENTRY)

Report to Family: Time:	GU IRRIGANT	FOLEY OUTPUT
	TOTAL INFUSED:	TOTAL OUTPUT:

FIGURE 8-3, cont'd   PACU record.

PACU DISCHARGE SUMMARY

VITAL SIGNS ON DISCHARGE	PACU OUTCOME	COMFORT LEVEL
B/P: P: R: T:	UNEVENTFUL ☐	PAIN FREE ☐ PAIN CONTROLLED ☐ SLEEPING BUT C/O PAIN WHEN
OXIMETER: PAR SCORE:	COMPLICATIONS ☐	AWAKEN ☐

REPORT TO: TIME:	SKIN CONDITION WARM COOL DRY MOIST	COLOR PINK PALE JAUNDICED DUSKY

DRESSINGS / SURGICAL SITE / PUNCTURE SITE

X-RAYS TAKEN IN PACU	LABS DRAWN IN PACU	O₂ ORDERED YES NO _____ L/MIN PER _____ O₂ TRANSPORT YES NO

TOTAL IV IN PACU	TOTAL OUTPUT IN PACU		
	URINARY	LEVINE	DRAINS
TOTAL BLOOD IN PACU			
TOTAL PO INTAKE IN PACU	IV SITE: _____ cc LTC		

ORDERS FAXED TO PHARMACY YES NO	EQUIPMENT ORDERED	TRANSPORT BY: AMBASSADOR
		RN LPN TECHNICIAN

DIAGNOSIS (Circle number of any diagnosis made)	GOAL	Goal Achieved	
		YES	NO
1 Alteration in neurological status			
2 Alteration in comfort level			
3 Alteration in emotional status			
4 Alteration in circulation			
5 Alteration in fluid volume			
6 Alteration in mobility			
7 Alteration in respiratory function			
8 Alteration in skin integrity			
9 Alteration in temperature			
10 Alteration in elimination			
11 Alteration in gastrointestinal function			
12 Alteration in injury			
13 Alteration in bleeding			
14 Other			

RHYTHM STRIPS

FIGURE 8-3, cont'd   PACU record.

Outcome Identification

Outcomes identified for the selected nursing diagnoses could be stated as follows:

- Patient will maintain ventilation, perfusion, and adequate expansion of lungs on discharge from PACU.
- Patient will maintain adequate cardiac output on discharge from PACU.
- Patient will maintain normal body temperature (96° to 99.5° F) on discharge from PACU.
- Patient will demonstrate appropriate cognitive functioning on discharge from PACU.
- Patient will exhibit a decreased level of pain or pain will have improved and be at a tolerable level on patient's discharge from PACU.

Planning

Once the nursing diagnoses and desired outcomes are identified for the postoperative patient, the plan of care is designed for the specific patient. Some nursing diagnoses are appropriate for all postanesthesia patients. A Sample Care Plan for the postanesthesia patient is included on p. 247.

Implementation

Dramatic and life-threatening changes can occur rapidly in the perianesthesia setting. Some studies in the PACU have revealed an incidence of complications from 10% to 18%.[9] The following complications are pertinent to the care of all patients during the postoperative period. Prompt recognition and immediate intervention are imperative for the well-being of the patient.

Postoperative complications
Respiratory
Airway obstruction

The first priority in the care of the postanesthesia patient is to establish a patent airway. A common cause of airway obstruction is the tongue, which is relaxed because of the anesthetic agents and muscle relaxants used during surgery (Fig. 8-4). The patient may present with snoring, little or no air movement upon auscultation of the lungs, retraction of intercostal muscles, asynchronous movements of the chest and abdomen, and a decreased oxygen-saturation level. The nursing action taken may be as simple as stimulating the patient to take deep breaths, positioning the patient on the side, or providing supplemental O_2. If the patient is still unresponsive, the nurse may need to open the airway with a chin tilt or jaw thrust. A chin tilt is accomplished by lifting the chin with one hand while tilting the forehead back with the other. A jaw thrust is accomplished by displacing the temporomandibular joint forward bilaterally.

If these actions do not open the airway, an artificial airway may need to be inserted (Fig. 8-5). Either an oral or a nasal airway may be used. An oral airway is indicated for use with an unresponsive patient; a nasal airway is indicated for patients who are arousable, because it is better tolerated by an awake patient.

In certain situations, such as apnea, intubation with ventilation may be required. If intubation is impossible, the patient may require a tracheostomy, although this need is rare.

Laryngospasm

A very serious complication that can occur in the PACU is laryngospasm. The muscles of the larynx contract

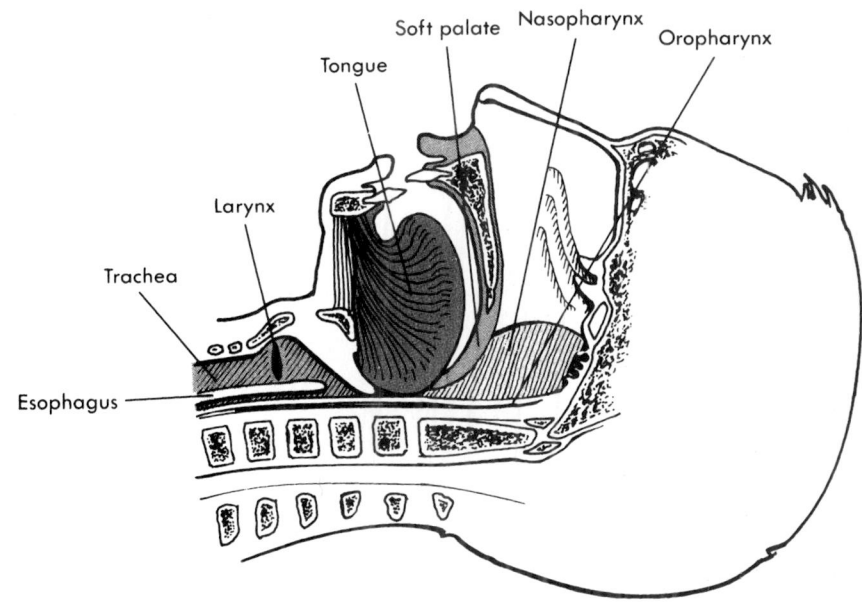

FIGURE 8-4 Obstruction of airway by tongue.

Nursing Diagnosis: Ineffective breathing pattern related to medications associated with anesthesia, type of surgical procedure, pain, tracheobronchial obstruction.

Outcome: Patient will maintain ventilation, perfusion, and adequate expansion of lungs on discharge from PACU: regular respiratory rate and pattern; bilateral breath sounds clear and equal; BP and pulse within preoperative range; oxygen saturation 92% or equal to preoperative status; patent airway; pain controlled.

Interventions:

1. Assess respiratory status on admission to PACU and at intervals until discharge.
2. Determine level of consciousness (to assess for need to reverse narcotic, benzodiazepine, or muscle relaxant).
3. Administer humidified oxygen; assess need for continued oxygen after discharge.
4. Elevate head of bed (if not contraindicated).
5. Encourage patient to take deep breaths or sustained maximal inspiration (SMI).
6. Determine need for chin tilt or jaw thrust if patient nonreactive without patent airway. Insert artificial airway if needed. Call physician for further assistance.
7. Assess patient for level of comfort. Administer pain medication as needed, per order or protocol.

Nursing Diagnosis: Decreased cardiac output related to anesthetic agents and other medications, fluid or blood loss or replacement, peripheral pooling of blood, alteration in preload or afterload, alterations in rate or rhythm.

Outcome: Patient will maintain adequate cardiac output on discharge from PACU: BP within preoperative range, skin warm and dry, oriented to person and place, pulse strong and regular.

Interventions:

1. Monitor vital signs, ECG, central venous pressure, with or without pulmonary artery catheter.
2. Assess level of consciousness to determine effect of medication still in circulation.
3. Monitor and record drainage from surgical site.
4. Monitor and record intake and output.
5. Administer fluid or blood products if indicated.
6. If hypotensive, use Trendelenburg's position unless contraindicated; increase fluid administration.
7. Maintain patency of intravenous lines.
8. Administer medication if needed to improve depressed myocardial contractility, increase cardiac output, and promote diuresis.
9. Administer vasodilators or antidysrhythmics as ordered.
10. Warm patient to temperature 96° F.
11. Administer humidified oxygen.

Nursing Diagnosis: Risk for altered body temperature related to surgical procedure: anesthetic agents, length of surgery, age of patient, environment, irrigation, type of surgery, or genetic predisposition to malignant hyperthermia.

Outcome: The patient will maintain a normal body temperature (oral or tympanic) of 96° to 99.5° F on discharge from PACU.

Interventions:

1. Measure body temperature (oral or tympanic) on admission.
2. Assess peripheral circulation.
3. Monitor vital signs and oxygen saturation.
4. Observe for shivering.
5. Initiate measures to warm the patient if hypothermic: Place warmed blankets on patient's body and head. Utilize forced warm-air device to rewarm patient.
6. Initiate appropriate measures for malignant hyperthermia, if indicated (see Chapter 7).
7. Initiate ongoing temperature monitoring until discharge.

Nursing Diagnosis: Altered thought processes related to the surgical process: anesthetic agents, hypoxia, pain, anxiety, bladder distention.

Outcome: The patient will demonstrate appropriate cognitive functioning on discharge from PACU: oriented to person and place, response to commands, calm appearance.

Interventions:

1. Assess level of consciousness.
2. Determine type of anesthetic agents used.
3. Monitor oxygen saturation level.
4. Evaluate level of anxiety and pain.
5. Offer reassurance; allow anxious patient to ventilate feelings, concerns, or questions.
6. Determine if bladder distention is present; catheterize if appropriate.
7. Reorient patient to person and place.
8. Administer humidified oxygen.
9. Administer sedation for anxiety or appropriate pain medication.

Nursing Diagnosis: Pain related to invasive diagnostic tests or tissue trauma (surgery).

Outcome: The patient will exhibit a decreased level of pain or pain at a tolerable level on discharge from PACU.

Interventions:

1. Assess for subjective signs of pain: The patient reports to the nurse that he or she is in pain; the patient is given a visual analog or numerical scale to determine perception of the level of pain.

Continued

2. Assess for objective signs of pain: Protective guarding behavior, moaning, crying, whimpering, restlessness, irritability, diaphoresis, dilated pupils, facial expression of pain, change in vital signs: BP, respiratory rate, or pulse.
3. Administer pain medication as prescribed: titrate intravenous doses, initiate patient-controlled analgesia (PCA), or continuous epidural analgesia.

4. Initiate alternate methods of pain relief: transcutaneous electrical nerve stimulation (TENS), music, massage, relaxation, guided imagery.
5. Reposition patient if not contraindicated.
6. Assess causes of pain (such as surgical site versus chest pain).
7. Evaluate effectiveness of pain relief.

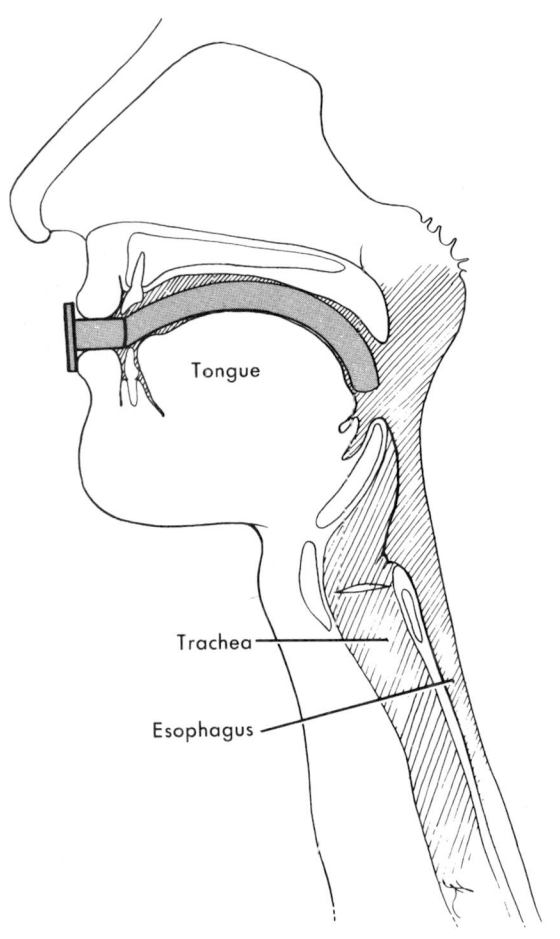

FIGURE 8-5   Oropharyngeal airway in place.

and either partially or completely obstruct the airway; the patient will become hypoxemic quickly. Laryngospasm is usually the result of an irritable airway. Nursing actions include removing the irritating stimulus, suctioning secretions that may be triggering a glottic response, hyperextending the patient's head, oxygenating the patient, and possibly administering an aerosol with racemic (optically inactive) epinephrine. In most cases, positive-pressure ventilation must be delivered per mask and bag. If the symptoms last longer than 1 minute and are unrelieved by positive pressure, administration of a muscle relaxant

such as succinylcholine is required to relax the muscles of the larynx. Reintubation is undesirable and is used only as a last resort.[21] Hemorrhage after neck surgery or carotid endarterectomy can also cause acute obstruction of the airway; the perianesthesia nurse should assess these patients carefully for bleeding.

Bronchospasm

Bronchospasm is a lower airway obstruction caused by spasms of the bronchial tubes. These spasms can cause complete closure because of the lack of cartilaginous support in the bronchioles. Inhaled bronchodilators are the first choice of therapy for these patients, followed by IV aminophylline. Epinephrine and methylprednisolone may also be administered in some cases.

Cardiovascular

Instability of the cardiovascular system is a frequent finding following surgery.[9] Common problems include hypotension, hypertension, and dysrhythmias.

Hypotension

Hypotension has been defined as a blood pressure of less than 20% of baseline or preoperative blood pressure and indicates either relative or absolute hypovolemia.[13] Many times the clinical signs of hypotension are more reliable as an indicator, especially in the patient with only one recorded preoperative pressure.[15] Clinical signs may include a rapid, thready pulse, disorientation, restlessness, oliguria, or cold pale skin.

Cardiac output and vascular resistance determine blood pressure. Hypotension may be caused by a cardiac dysfunction such as myocardial infarction (MI), tamponade, embolism, ischemia, dysrhythmias, congestive heart failure (CHF), valvular dysfunction, or medications, including anesthetic agents. In this case the heart is no longer pumping effectively. Oxygen and cardiac stimulants will be used as needed as well as hemodynamic monitoring.

Hypovolemia

Hypovolemia reduces cardiac output and may be caused by hemorrhage, dehydration (inadequate fluid replacement), or increased positive end-expiratory pressure

(PEEP). Fluid or blood replacement is used to treat hypovolemia. If the patient is hemorrhaging at the surgical site, a return to the operating room is indicated.

Decreased vascular resistance can be related to medications, general and regional anesthesia, or anaphylaxis. Vasodilatation can be treated with fluids, vasopressors, or elevation of the patient's legs. Anaphylactic reactions are treated with epinephrine, antihistamines, and additional fluids.

Hypertension

Systemic arterial hypertension is usually defined as a blood pressure 20% to 30% higher than the patient's baseline or preoperative level.[15] Hypertension is among the most common postoperative complications[13] and often occurs early in the recovery phase. Verification of blood pressure and the rapidity of the change must be noted. Again, clinical signs are the most important indicator of the severity of the hypertension. Headache, mental-status changes, and substernal pain are all indicators of end-organ damage.

Asymptomatic hypertension is a common occurrence in the PACU and is usually considered to be harmless. The solution is usually determined by the cause. Elevated blood pressure does cause increased ventricular wall tension, afterload, and myocardial work. The patient with a history of cardiac disease is more at risk for adverse results.

Hypertension may be caused by volume overload or pulmonary edema, which causes an increase in the cardiac output. In this case the patient is given diuretics, fluids are restricted, and the patient is hemodynamically monitored.

Other causes of hypertension are pain and anxiety, reflex vasoconstriction from hypothermia, hypoxemia, hypercapnia, and viscus distention, all of which cause increased vascular resistance. Patients in pain are medicated, and patients with hypothermia are warmed. Patients are oxygenated well and ventilated if necessary to improve hypoxemia or hypercapnia. Patients are encouraged to void or are catheterized to empty a full bladder.

Antihypertensive drugs are used as necessary to control blood pressure. Patients should resume taking prescribed preoperative antihypertensives as soon as possible after surgery. Ambulatory surgical patients as well as inpatients should be allowed to take their prescribed antihypertensives the day of surgery.

Dysrhythmias

A common dysrhythmia after surgery is sinus tachycardia (a rate greater than 100 in the adult). Frequent causes include pain, hypoxemia, hypovolemia, increased temperature, and anxiety. The underlying cause is treated. Propranolol, metoprolol, or esmolol may be given. Sinus bradycardia (heart rate less than 60 in the adult) is also a common dysrhythmia in the PACU. Causes include hypoxemia, hypothermia, high spinal anesthesia, vagal stimulation, and some medications that are commonly given during or after surgery. The underlying cause is treated. Atropine is the drug of choice to increase the heart rate, and usually no other treatment is required. Temporary or permanent pacemakers may sometimes be required.

Premature ventricular contractions (PVCs) are represented by wide, bizarre-looking QRS complexes. The most common causes in the postoperative period are hypoxemia and hypokalemia. Those underlying conditions should be treated. Many times if cardiac disease or hypotension is not present, the PVCs do not require medication. If intervention is required, lidocaine remains the drug of choice.

Temperature Abnormalities
Hypothermia

Postoperative hypothermia, defined as a temperature less than 36° C (96.8° F), continues to be a widespread problem in the PACU. As many as 60% of patients in the PACU are believed to be hypothermic.[8,22] Often hypothermia is not life threatening; however, it does cause physiologic stress. Hypothermia can prolong recovery time and contributes to postoperative morbidity. Especially vulnerable to the effects of hypothermia are the elderly and children up to 2 years of age.

Prevention of heat loss begins in the operating room. Under general anesthesia the patient does not produce heat and is dependent on ambient temperature. Prevention can include increasing the ambient temperature in the operating room, providing the patient with warm blankets on arrival in the OR, and draping the patient during the procedure to minimize exposure. Heated humidifiers and fluid warmers add heat. A more recent technique of preventing hypothermia in the operating room is the forced warm-air device (Fig. 8-6).

In the PACU tremendous demands are made on the body if the patient begins to shiver. Shivering can increase the need for oxygen by 300% to 400%. Hypothermic patients should have oxygen therapy initiated immediately upon admission. For a patient with a healthy heart, there may be no untoward effects. However, for the patient with coronary artery disease or cardiomyopathy, decompensation can occur. Perioperative normothermia has been associated with a reduced incidence of morbid cardiac incidents and ventricular tachycardia in patients with cardiac risk factors.[24]

There are other problems associated with hypothermia. Intravascular volume loss, attributable to a fluid shift from the extracellular space, is probably related to vasoconstriction. As the patient begins to rewarm, vasodilatation ensues, and the patient can require large amounts of intravenous fluids to avoid hypovolemia.

The central nervous system is depressed by hypothermia. The cold postanesthesia patient will remain more anesthetized than a warm patient while recovering. Nitrogen loss and hypokalemia can cause a predisposi-

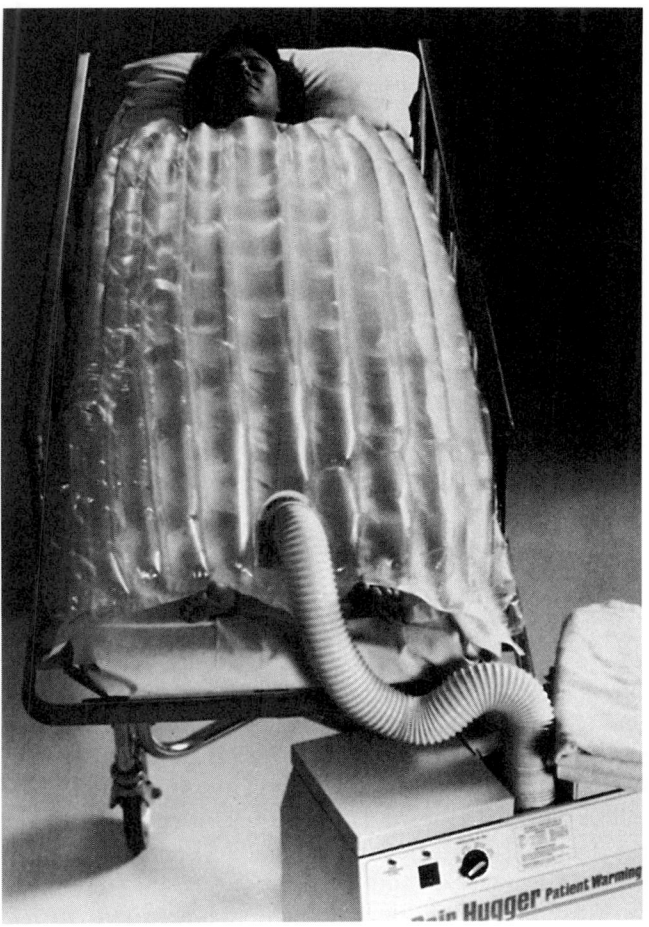

FIGURE 8-6   Bair Hugger; focused thermal environment.

8-1   RESEARCH HIGHLIGHT

Kurz, Sessler, and Lenhardt studied 200 patients undergoing colorectal surgery to test the hypothesis that hypothermia both increases susceptibility to surgical-wound infection and lengthens hospitalization. The patients were randomly assigned to routine intraoperative care (hypothermia group) or additional warming (normothermia group). The anesthetic care was standardized, and all patients received cefamandole and metronidazole. The wounds were evaluated daily until discharge from the hospital and in the clinic after 2 weeks. Wounds containing culture-positive pus were considered infected. Surgical wound infections were found in 18 of 96 patients assigned to hypothermia (19%) but in only 6 of 104 patients assigned to normothermia (6%, $p = 0.009$). The sutures were removed 1 day later in the patients assigned to hypothermia than in those assigned to normothermia ($p = 0.002$), and the duration of hospitalization was prolonged by 2.6 days in the hypothermia group ($p = 0.01$). Based on these data, the researchers concluded that hypothermia itself may delay healing and predispose patients to wound infections.

From Kurz, A., Sessler, D.I., & Lenhardt, R. (1996). Perioperative normothermia to reduce the incidence of surgical-wound infection and shorten hospitalization, *N Engl J Med 334*, 1209-1215.

tion to wound infection[14] (Research Highlight 8-1). Hypothermia delays metabolism and alters effects of some anesthetic drugs. Of special interest is the prolonged elimination of muscle relaxants in hypothermic patients. Clotting abnormalities can occur. Platelet activity declines and fibrinolysis increases with hypothermia. Both of these conditions enhance the tendency to bleed.[24]

Rewarming is a priority in the immediate care of the postoperative patient because normothermia reverses all effects of hypothermia. Wet and cold gowns and blankets should be removed, and warm, dry gowns and blankets applied to head and body. There are several external rewarming techniques available. Application of warm cotton blankets has been the tradition in the PACU. The warm blankets are applied every 5 to 10 minutes until the patient is normothermic. Cotton blankets do gradually increase the patient's temperature. However, they do not actively heat patients and can be a slow process. Continuous fluid-circulating blankets or warm-water mattresses have been shown to have little value in rewarming patients because of the size of surface area in contact with the heat source. Radiant heat lamps depend on exposure of large areas of body surface, which is of limited use to adult patients.

Fluid and blood warmers are useful for large volumes of cool fluids but not to reverse hypothermia. Forced warm-air devices, a new technology, have been very effective in rewarming patients. This device produces a thermal-focused environment that transfers heat to a patient by blowing warm air through a plastic and tissue paper blanket that covers the patient. These forced warm-air devices are now a standard hypothermia treatment in the PACU setting.

Hyperthermia

Hyperthermia may be an indication of an infectious process or sepsis, or it may indicate a hypermetabolic process—malignant hyperthermia. This is a very serious emergency that is genetic in origin and is triggered by volatile anesthetic agents and the depolarizing muscle-relaxant succinylcholine. Death ensues unless malignant hyperthermia is immediately recognized and treated (see Chapter 7).

Altered Thought Processes

The PACU patient may be disoriented, drowsy, confused, or delirious. The cause may range from residual effects of anesthesia to pain and anxiety. Hypoxemia should always be ruled out first; it remains the most common cause of postoperative agitation. Patients who are chemically dependent or substance abusers many times awaken in an agitated state. Viscus distention can also contribute to agitation in a drowsy, confused patient. The PACU nurse should identify and eliminate the cause of the agitation or confusion, if possible. The patient can be engaged in short conversations and reoriented to place and person. Baseline preoperative data are important to determine cause. Persistent changes from preoperative status require thorough assessment and possible intervention from the physician.

Nausea and Vomiting

Nausea and vomiting are postoperative problems that affect a large number of patients in the PACU. The management of nausea and vomiting actually begins preoperatively and continues into the intraoperative period. Preventive therapy has been effective in reducing the incidence. There is no single method of prevention or treatment of nausea and vomiting. Many causative factors are related to anesthesia and surgery.

Antiemetic therapy is planned to reduce GI symptoms without oversedating the patient. A frequently used drug, especially in the ambulatory surgical setting, is droperidol. Other drugs commonly used are metoclopramide (Reglan), prochlorperazine (Compazine), and promethazine (Phenergan). The antiemetic agent odansetron (Zofran) has become popular because of its lack of side effects such as sedation, hypotension, and tremors. Other useful medications include dimenhydrinate (Dramamine), hydroxyzine (Vistaril, Atarax), and scopolamine (Transderm-Scop).

Aspiration

Aspiration, or passage of regurgitated material into the lungs, can occur during the perioperative period, with most aspirations occurring during tracheal intubation or extubation.[25] The PACU nurse must protect the airway of an unconscious or semiconscious patient to prevent the possibility of aspiration of gastric contents. Prevention of aspiration postoperatively includes responding quickly to reports of nausea and vomiting, avoiding conversations that could elicit nausea and vomiting and preventing rapid movement and head elevation of the patient.

The volume and acidity of the aspirate determine the extent of damage to the lungs. The most severe damage seems to be in cases where the pH was less than 2.5 or the volume was greater than 25 ml.[25] Preoperatively patients may receive clear, nonparticulate antacids, such as Bicitra, to raise the gastric fluid pH. Histamine (H_2)–receptor antagonists, such as cimetidine, ranitidine, or famotidine, decrease gastric acid production. Metoclopramide increases gastric-emptying time.[21] Aspiration does not occur in patients with normal protective

TABLE 8-1 | **Risk Factors for Pulmonary Aspiration**

GENERAL RISK FACTORS	SPECIFIC RISK FACTORS
Age (older > younger)	Pregnancy
Sex (female > male)	Recent oral intake
Comorbid diseases	Opioid administration
IDDM	Gastrointestinal obstruction or dysfunction
CNS deficits	Obesity
Peripheral vascular disease	Depressed level of consciousness
Hepatobiliary or gastrointestinal diseases	Previous esophageal dysfunction
Renal dysfunction	Head injury or neurologic dysfunction
	Lack of coordination of swallowing and respiration
	Procedures that increase intraabdominal pressure

CNS, Central nervous system; IDDM, insuline-dependent diabetes mellitus.
From Warner, M. Risks and outcomes of perioperative pulmonary aspiration, *J Perianesth Nurs,* 12(5):355, 1997.

reflexes. Risk factors can be divided into general and specific (Table 8-1).

Signs and symptoms of aspiration include tachypnea and hypoxemia attributable to a decrease in lung compliance. Wheezing, coughing, dyspnea, hypotension, apnea, and bradycardia may occur. Treatment centers around promoting tissue oxygenation. Supplemental oxygen is given. Positive pressure applied by use of a mask or an endotracheal tube may be needed to maintain arterial oxygenation, and a chest x-ray examination may be done. If intubated, the trachea can be suctioned. Bronchoscopy is performed if the particles aspirated are large and causing an airway obstruction. Neither steroids nor antibiotics are warranted.[25] The tracheal secretions can be cultured, and if the results are positive, an appropriate antibiotic started. Recovery of the patient depends on recognition of the problem, quantity of aspirate, pH of the aspirate, physical condition of the patient before the event, and rapidity with which medical care is initiated.[21]

Pain

Pain is a subjective experience and may or may not be verbalized. Many times healthcare providers require objective signs of discomfort in addition to subjective reports of pain from the patient. As a result, it is believed that up to 75% of postsurgical patients are undertreated for pain.[9] McCaffery and Beebe[18] state that pain is whatever the patient says it is. The Agency for Health Care Policy and Research (AHCPR)[1] reports that the single most reliable indicator of the existence and intensity of pain is the patient's self-report. The AHCPR has developed clinical practice guidelines on acute pain management and contends that all patients should be assessed for severity of pain using either a verbal rating scale or a visual analog

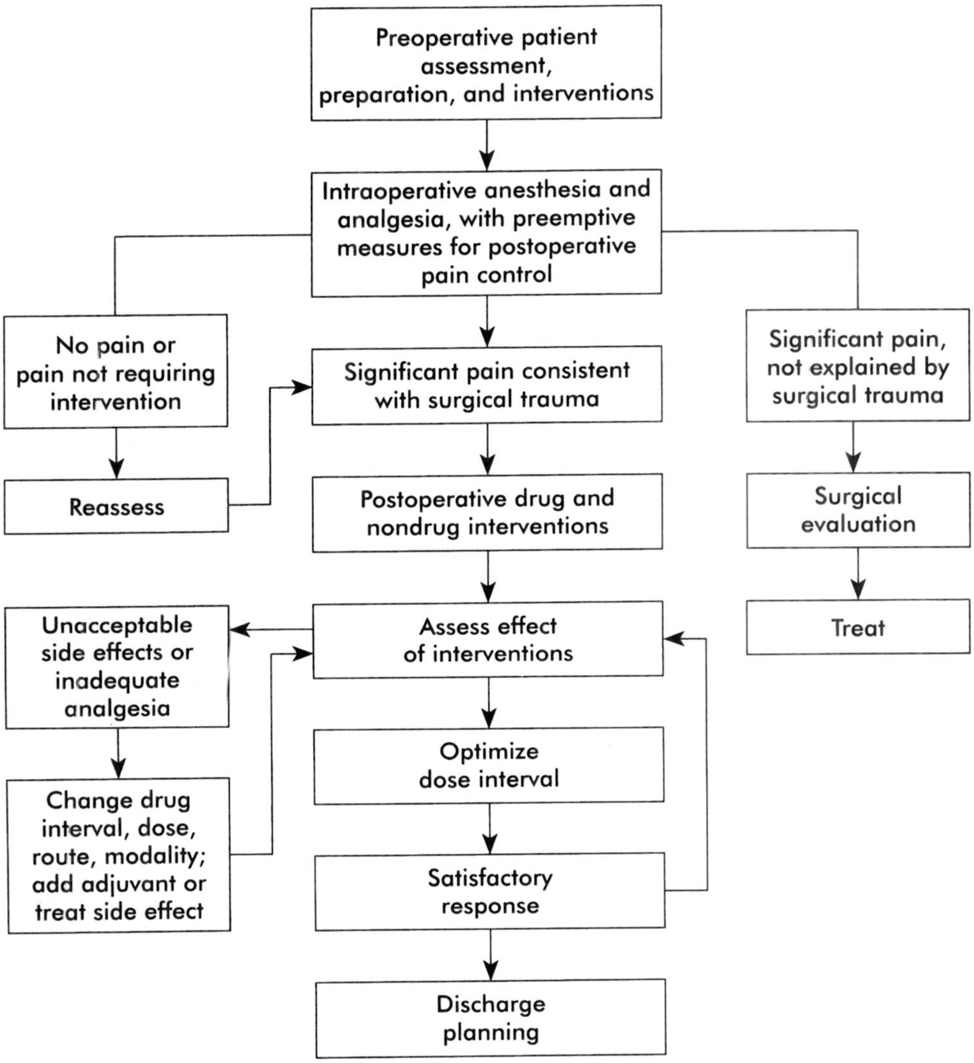

FIGURE 8-7   Acute pain management in adults.

scale (Figs. 8-7 and 8-8). Copies of the guidelines may be obtained by writing to the Center for Research Dissemination and Liaison, AHCPR Publications Clearinghouse, P.O. Box 8547, Silver Spring, MD 20907; or by calling 1-800-358-9295. Patients should be assessed for pain on admission to the PACU and at frequent intervals (Box 8-2). It is also important to remember that not all patients respond to pain in the same manner, despite comparable surgical procedures.

Evidence has indicated that early analgesia reduces postoperative problems. Nonsteroidal antiinflammatory drugs (NSAIDS) and opiates are the analgesics of choice and are usually used in combination in the PACU (Tables 8-2 and 8-3). Traditionally pain has been treated with IM injections of opioids at intervals from 3 to 6 hours as needed. It is now recognized that the inadequate pain relief experienced by postoperative patients using IM injections is attributable to the varying level of opioids in the patients' blood. Other methods of pain relief have fortunately

become more widespread. The most common form of an opioid-delivery system is by way of patient-controlled analgesia (PCA). PCA allows a patient to control the analgesic administration. Dosage, time between doses, and the maximum dosage that can be administered are programed into the machine. This form of analgesia also allows for a basal rate of opioids to infuse continuously, if ordered. When PCA devices are started in the PACU, delays in preventing pain are avoided, its effectiveness can be evaluated, and the patient's understanding and ability to use PCA can be assured.[10]

Other forms of postoperative pain relief may involve use of spinal analgesia, usually in the form of epidural opioid or local anesthetic administration. Patients who have had extensive procedures, including total hip or knee replacements, knee reconstruction, and major abdominal or thoracic operations have been shown to profit from this method of pain control. Benefits of epidural analgesia for acute postoperative pain include good analgesia with

Pain Intensity Scales

Simple descriptive pain intensity scale*

A

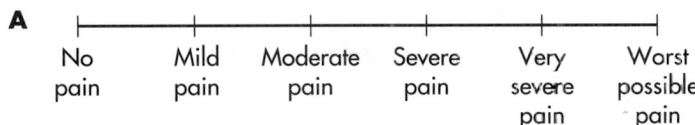

No pain | Mild pain | Moderate pain | Severe pain | Very severe pain | Worst possible pain

0 - 10 Numeric pain intensity scale*

B

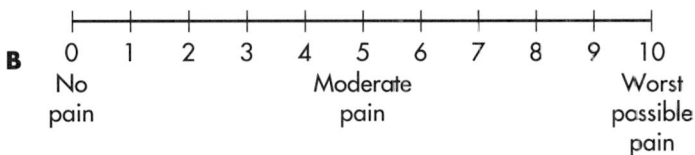

0 1 2 3 4 5 6 7 8 9 10
No pain — Moderate pain — Worst possible pain

Visual analog scale (VAS)†

C

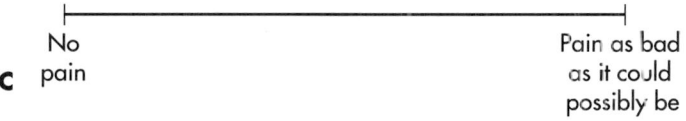

No pain — Pain as bad as it could possibly be

* If used as a graphic rating scale, a 10 cm baseline is recommended.
† A 10 cm baseline is recommended for VAS scales.

FIGURE 8-8　A to C, Examples of pain intensity and pain distress scales. D, FACES Pain Rating Scale.‡
(Wong and Baker, 1988; Wong, 1996)
‡Explain to child that each face is for a person who feels happy because there is no pain (hurt) or sad because there is some or a lot of pain. FACE 0 is very happy because there is no hurt. FACE 1 hurts just a little bit. FACE 2 hurts a little more. FACE 3 hurts even more. FACE 4 hurts a whole lot, but FACE 5 hurts as much as you can imagine, although you do not have to be crying to feel this bad. Ask child to choose face that best describes own pain. Record the number under chosen face on pain assessment record. Recommended for ages 3 and up.

Which Face Shows How Much Hurt You Have Now?

D

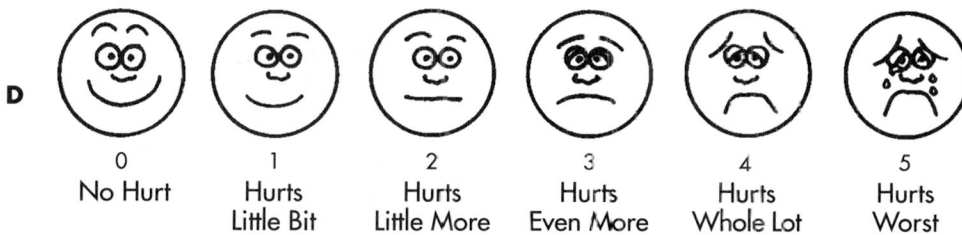

0 No Hurt | 1 Hurts Little Bit | 2 Hurts Little More | 3 Hurts Even More | 4 Hurts Whole Lot | 5 Hurts Worst

minimal sedation, early ambulation and physical therapy, and excellent patient satisfaction. Side effects that may occur include nausea, pruritus, urinary retention, areas of slight numbness, and respiratory depression. These side effects can be controlled with drugs such as diphenhydramine, naloxone, or droperidol, or by adjusting the infusion rate.

Other techniques that have been shown to reduce the level of pain for the surgical patient include infiltration of the site of incision even before the initial incision and use of a long-acting local anesthetic at the site at the conclusion of the surgical procedure.

Nonpharmacologic interventions that may be used to relieve pain include positioning, verbal reassurance, touch, applications of heat or cold, massage, and transcutaneous electrical nerve stimulation (TENS). If the patient was taught preoperatively, other techniques that can be used are relaxation, imagery, music distraction, and biofeedback. The interventions most useful for the postanesthesia patient in the PACU are preoperative education, which reduces the fear of the unknown, relaxation with deep breathing, distraction, and therapeutic massage.[11] Nonpharmacologic interventions are designed to supplement, not substitute, pharmacologic intervention.[1]

Physiologic effects of pain can be very harmful for the postoperative patient and include the following: decreased thoracic movement, increased splinting, reduced lung compliance and volume leading to atelectasis, decreased mobility, increased risk of thromboembolism, exaggerated catecholamine response (which increases cardiac work and myocardial oxygen demand), increased risk for myocardial ischemia, impaired immune system, and delayed return of bowel and gastric function. Physiologic responses with acute pain include increased blood pressure and heart rate, dilated pupils and perspiration, increased respiratory rate

BOX 8-2 | **Pain Assessment and Reassessment**

Principles

- Patients who may have difficulty communicating their pain require particular attention. This includes patients who are cognitively impaired, psychotic or severely emotionally disturbed, children and the elderly, patients who do not speak English, and patients whose level of education or cultural background differs significantly from that of their healthcare team.
- Unexpected intense pain, particularly if sudden or associated with altered vital signs such as hypotension, tachycardia, or fever, should be immediately evaluated, and new diagnoses such as wound dehiscence, infection, or deep venous thrombosis considered.
- Family members should be involved when appropriate.

Pain-Assessment Tools

- The single most reliable indicator of the existence and intensity of pain and any resultant distress is the patient's self-report.
- Self-report measurement scales include numerical or adjective ratings and visual analog scales.
- Tools should be reliable, valid, and easy for the patient and the nurse or physician to use. One may use these tools by showing a diagram to the patient to indicate the appropriate rating. One may also use the tools by simply asking the patient for a verbal response (such as, "On a scale of 0 to 10 with 0 as no pain and 10 as the worst pain possible, how would you rate your pain?").
- Tools must be appropriate for the patient's developmental, physical, emotional, and cognitive status.

Preoperative Preparation

- Discuss the patient's previous experiences with pain and beliefs about and preferences for pain assessment and management.

- Give the patient information about pain management therapies that are available and the rationale underlying their use.
- Develop with the patient a plan for pain assessment and management.
- Select a pain-assessment tool and teach the patient to use it.
- Provide the patient with education and information about pain control, including training in nonpharmacologic options such as relaxation.
- Inform patients that it is easier to prevent pain than to chase and reduce it once it has become established and that communication of unrelieved pain is essential to its relief. Emphasize the importance of a factual report of pain, avoiding stoicism or exaggeration.

Postoperative Assessment

- Assess the patient's perceptions, along with behavioral and psychologic responses. Remember that observations of behavior and vital signs should not be used instead of a self-report unless the patient is unable to communicate.
- Assess and reassess pain frequently during the immediate postoperative period. Determine the frequency of assessment based on the operation performed and the severity of the pain. For example, pain should be assessed every 2 hours during the first postoperative day after major surgery.
- Increase the frequency of assessment and reassessment if the pain is poorly controlled or if interventions are changing.
- Record the pain intensity and response to intervention in an easily visible and accessible place, such as a bedside flow sheet.
- Revise the management plan if the pain is poorly controlled.
- Review with the patient before discharge the interventions used and their efficacy and provide specific discharge instructions regarding pain and its management.

From Acute Pain Management Guideline Panel. Acute Pain Management in Adults: Operative Procedures. Quick Reference Guide for Clinicians. AHCPR Pub. No. 92-0019. Rockville, MD: Agency for Health Care Policy and Research, Public Health Service, U.S. Department of Health and Human Services.

and decreased respiratory excursion.[16,26] Severe pain is one of the most devastating stresses and uses even more body energy than exertion such as weight-lifting.[6] Psychologically the patient still in pain may display fear, helplessness, anxiety, anger, or frustration.[16]

Until healthcare providers become more knowledgeable about pain assessment and management, some patients will continue to unnecessarily suffer from moderate to severe pain (Research Highlight 8-2). Patients of differing cultures express pain differently. Verbal and nonverbal communication differs between cultures. A patient may feel that nonverbal communication is expressing the pain to the nurse, but the nurse may not recognize the clues.[5] Common misconceptions about pain also abound.[4] These misconceptions must be recognized and corrected. A summary of misconceptions is listed in Table 8-4.

In summary, effective management of postoperative

pain will occur if the following requirements outlined by AHCPR are addressed and accomplished:[7]

1. Regular assessment and reassessment of pain intensity and relief
2. Respect for patient preferences for the method of pain management
3. Development of an organized program to evaluate the effectiveness of pain assessment and management

Evaluation

The patient is evaluated based on the outcomes identified as significant after the initial assessment. For the desired outcomes presented previously in this chapter, these might be stated as follows:

- The patient maintained an adequate oxygen saturation while receiving room air.

TABLE 8-2 | Dosing Data for NSAIDs

DRUG	USUAL ADULT DOSE	USUAL PEDIATRIC DOSE*	COMMENTS
Oral NSAIDs			
Acetaminophen	650-975 mg q4hr	10-15 mg/kg q4hr	Acetaminophen lacks the peripheral antiinflammatory activity of other NSAIDs
Aspirin	650-975 mg q4hr	10-15 mg/kg q4hr†	The standard against which other NSAIDs are compared. Inhibits platelet aggregation; may cause postoperative bleeding
Choline magnesium trisalicylate (Trilisate)	1000-1500 mg bid	25 mg/kg q12hr	May have minimal antiplatelet activity; also available as oral liquid
Diflunisal (Dolobid)	1000 mg initial dose followed by 500 mg q12hr		
Etodolac (Lodine)	200-400 mg q6-8hr		
Fenoprofen calcium (Nalfon)	200 mg q4-5hr		
Ibuprofen (Motrin, others)	400 mg q4-6hr	10 mg/kg q6-8hr	Available as several brand names and as generic; also available as oral suspension
Ketoprofen (Orudis)	25-75 mg q6-8hr		
Magnesium salicylate	650 mg q4hr		Many brands and generic forms available
Meclofenamate sodium (Meclomen)	50 mg q4-6hr		
Mefenamic acid (Ponstel)	250 mg q6hr		
Naproxen (Naprosyn)	500 mg initial dose followed by 250 mg q6-8hr	5 mg/kg q12hr	Also available as oral liquid
Naproxen sodium (Anaprox)	550 mg initial dose followed by 275 mg q6-8hr		
Salsalate (Disalcid, others)	500 mg q4hr		May have minimal antiplatelet activity
Sodium salicylate	325-650 mg q3-4hr		Available in generic form from several distributors
Parenteral NSAID			
Ketorolac‡	30 or 60 mg IM initial dose followed by 15 or 30 mg q6hr. Oral dose following IM dosage: 10 mg q6-8hr		Intramuscular dose not to exceed 5 days

From Acute Pain Management Guideline Panel. Acute Pain Management in Adults: Operative Procedures. Quick Reference Guide for Clinicians. AHCPR Pub. No. 92-0019. Rockville, MD: Agency for Health Care Policy and Research, Public Health Service, U.S. Department of Health and Human Services.
Note: Only the above NSAIDs have FDA approval for use as simple analgesics, but clinical experience has been gained with other drugs as well.
*Drug recommendations are limited to NSAIDs where pediatric dosing experience is available.
†Contraindicated in presence of fever or other evidence of viral illness.
‡ODOM'S NOTE: Ketorolac has now been approved by the FDA for intravenous use. Recommended dosing is 30 mg IV for healthy adults and 15 mg IV for adults >65 years. See manufacturer's information for further details.

- The blood pressure and heart rate are within normal range for the patient.
- The patient is normothermic.
- The patient is oriented to time and person.
- The patient's pain decreased to a tolerable level. The patient is relaxed and sleeping at intervals.
- The patient verbalized pain relief.

DISCHARGE FROM THE PACU

The PACU nurse completes a thorough assessment immediately before the patient's discharge and transfer to the surgical unit. The nurse assesses the patient's vital signs, level of consciousness, condition of the operative site, comfort level, intake and output, respiratory function and oxygen saturation, and mobility.

TABLE 8-3 | Dosing Data for Opioid Analgesics

DRUG	APPROXIMATE EQUIANALGESIC ORAL DOSE	APPROXIMATE EQUIANALGESIC PARENTERAL DOSE	RECOMMENDED STARTING DOSE (ADULTS MORE THAN 50 KG OF BODY WEIGHT)		RECOMMENDED STARTING DOSE (CHILDREN AND ADULTS LESS THAN 50 KG OF BODY WEIGHT)[1]	
			ORAL	PARENTERAL	ORAL	PARENTERAL
Opioid Agonist						
Morphine[2]	30 mg q3-4hr (around-the-clock dosing) 60 mg q3-4hr (single dose or intermittent dosing)	10 mg q3-4hr	30 mg q3-4hr	10 mg q3-4hr	0.3 mg/kg q3-4hr	0.1 mg/kg q3-4hr
Codeine[3]	130 mg q3-4hr	75 mg q3-4hr	60 mg q3-4hr	60 mg q2hr (intramuscular/ subcutaneous)	1 mg/kg q3-4hr[4]	Not recommended
Hydromorphone[2] (Dilaudid)	7.5 mg q3-4hr	1.5 mg q3-4hr	6 mg q3-4hr	1.5 mg q3-4hr	0.06 mg/kg q3-4hr	0.015 mg/kg q3-4hr
Hydrocodone (in Lorcet, Lortab, Vicodin, others)	30 mg q3-4hr	Not available	10 mg q3-4hr	Not available	0.2 mg/kg q3-4hr[4]	Not available
Levorphanol (Levo-Dromoran)	4 mg q6-8hr	2 mg q6-8hr	4 mg q6-8hr	2 mg q6-8hr	0.04 mg/kg q6-8hr	0.02 mg/kg q6-8hr
Meperidine (Demerol)	300 mg q2-3hr	100 mg q3hr	Not recommended	100 mg q3hr	Not recommended	0.75 mg/kg q2-3hr
Methadone (Dolophine, others)	20 mg q6-8hr	10 mg q6-8hr	20 mg q6-8hr	10 mg q6-8hr	0.2 mg/kg q6-8hr	0.1 mg/kg q6-8hr
Oxycodone (Roxicodone, also in Percocet, Percodan, Tylox, others)	30 mg q3-4hr	Not available	10 mg q3-4hr	Not available	0.2 mg/kg q3-4hr[4]	Not available
Oxymorphone[2] (Numorphan)	Not available	1 mg q3-4hr	Not available	1 mg q3-4hr	Not recommended	Not recommended
Opioid Agonist-Antagonist and Partial Agonist						
Buprenorphine (Buprenex)	Not available	0.3-0.4 mg q6-8hr	Not available	0.4 mg q6-8hr	Not available	0.004 mg/kg q6-8hr
Butorphanol (Stadol)	Not available	2 mg q3-4hr	Not available	2 mg q3-4hr	Not available	Not recommended
Nalbuphine (Nubain)	Not available	10 mg q3-4hr	Not available	10 mg q3-4hr	Not available	0.1 mg/kg q3-4hr
Pentazocine (Talwin, others)	150 mg q3-4hr	60 mg q3-4hr	50 mg q4-6hr	Not recommended	Not recommended	Not recommended

From Acute Pain Management Guideline Panel. Acute Pain Management in Adults: Operative Procedures. Quick Reference Guide for Clinicians. AHCPR Pub. No. 92-0019. Rockville, MD: Agency for Health Care Policy and Research, Public Health Service, U.S. Department of Health and Human Services.

Note: Published tables vary in the suggested doses that are equianalgesic to morphine. Clinical response is the criterion that must be applied for each patient; titration to clinical response is necessary. Because there is not complete cross tolerance among these drugs, it is usually necessary to use a lower equianalgesic dose when changing drugs and to retitrate to response.

Caution: Recommended doses do not apply to patients with renal or hepatic insufficiency or other conditions affecting drug metabolism and kinetics.

[1] **Caution:** Doses listed for patients with body weight less than 50 kg cannot be used as initial starting doses in babies less than 6 months of age. Consult the *Clinical Practice Guideline for Acute Pain Management: Operative or Medical Procedures and Trauma* section on management of pain in neonates for recommendations.

[2] For morphine, hydromorphone, and oxymorphone, rectal administration is an alternate route for patients unable to take oral medications, but equianalgesic doses may differ from oral and parenteral doses because of pharmacokinetic differences.

[3] **Caution:** Codeine doses above 65 mg often are not appropriate because of diminishing incremental analgesia with increasing doses but continually increasing constipation and other side effects.

[4] **Caution:** Doses of aspirin and acetaminophen in combination opioid/NSAID preparations must also be adjusted to the patient's body weight.

8-2 RESEARCH HIGHLIGHT

Tittle and McMillan studied 44 patients, 20 from an intensive care unit and 24 from a surgical unit, to determine the extent to which nurses manage pain effectively without side effects related to narcotic analgesics. The results determined that patients in both units continued to experience pain even with pain management interventions. The critical care nurses administered an average of 30% of the maximum narcotic dose ordered and the surgical unit nurses 36.8%. Documentation of the effect of the pain medication was minimal on both units. The study indicated that nurses in both intensive care units and surgical units may not appropriately assess, manage, or evaluate pain and pain-related side effects.

From Tittle M, McMillan SC: Pain and pain-related side effects in an ICU and on a surgical unit: Nurses' management, *Am J Crit Care* 3(1):25-30, 1994.

TABLE 8-4 | Common Misconceptions About Pain

MISCONCEPTION	CORRECTION
The nurse is the expert in evaluating a patient's pain.	The patient's self-report of pain is the best indicator of pain.
Patients should expect to have pain.	Pain relief is the goal of pain management. Pain can be reduced significantly by the use of multiple modalities.
Patients always have observable physiologic signs and behavior indicating pain.	Patients can physiologically adapt to pain resulting in lack of observable change in vital signs. Patients are highly variable in behaviorally expressing pain. Lack of pain expression does not indicate lack of pain.
The intensity of pain is directly related to a physical stimulus; that is, the type of surgery determines the amount of pain a patient will experience.	Pain is unique to each individual. Comparable stimuli produce varying pain experiences in different individuals.
Addiction is a likely occurrence in patients receiving opioids.	Addiction occurs in less than 1% of the patients receiving opioids.
Opioids commonly cause respiratory depression.	Respiratory depression is uncommon. Pain can cause respiratory depression in the postoperative patient. Care should be taken in dosing patients older than 75 years because of altered drug metabolism.

From McCaffery M, Beebe A: *Pain Clinical Manual for Nursing Practice,* St. Louis, 1989, Mosby and Watt-Watson JH: Misbeliefs about pain, in Watt-Watson JH, Donovan MI, editors: *Pain Management Nursing Perspective,* St. Louis, 1992, Mosby. In Sullivan L: Factors influencing pain management: a nursing perspective. *J Post Anesth Nurs,* 9(2):83-90, 1994.

The patient is usually discharged from the PACU by an anesthesiologist, who may be present and actually write a discharge order. Alternatively a numeric scoring system approved by the department of anesthesia may be used to determine if the patient is ready for discharge. The most common scoring system in use is the Aldrete Score. Activity, respiration, circulation, consciousness, and oxygen-saturation level are scored from 0 to 2 (see Fig. 8-3). A total score of 8 to 10 is generally acceptable for PACU discharge with exceptions made by the physician's order.

A report on the patient's condition is given to the nurse who will assume care for the patient on the surgical or short procedure unit. This report may be given by telephone before the patient leaves the PACU or person-to-person after the patient reaches the unit. The report should include a preoperative history, pertinent information regarding the patient's surgery and recovery, medications the patient was given, physician's orders, and any other appropriate information.

ADMISSION TO THE SURGICAL OR SHORT PROCEDURE UNIT

The patient's room is prepared for admission, and any necessary equipment is provided. The patient is placed in the bed with adequate help. The bed side rails should remain raised until the patient is fully awake to prevent patient falls. The patient is informed to notify the nurse for assistance to ambulate. The family is also instructed and enlisted to maintain safety for the patient. The equipment and condition of the patient should be explained to the family members who are present. A special concern is the use of PCA. Family members should be instructed that the PCA is for the patient's use only; that pushing the PCA button for the patient can have a detrimental effect on the patient's well-being.

POSTOPERATIVE NURSING CONSIDERATIONS

Assessment

The nurse makes an immediate assessment as soon as the patient is transferred to the bed. The nurse may choose a head-to-toe or systems assessment. Parameters include respiratory, cardiovascular, and neurologic status. The condition of the dressing and surgical site and patient comfort and safety are also assessed (Box 8-3).

| BOX 8-3 | **Patient Assessment on Return from PACU** |

Respiratory Status
  Patency of airway
  Respirations: depth, rate, character
  Breath sounds: presence, character
Circulatory Status
  Pulse, blood pressure
  Skin color, temperature
  Capillary filling
Neurologic Status
  Level of consciousness
  Ability to move extremities
Dressing
  Presence of drainage
  Presence of tubes to be connected to drainage systems
Comfort
  Presence of pain, nausea, vomiting
  Patient positioned for comfort and to facilitate ventilation
Safety
  Necessity for side rails
  Call cord within reach
Equipment
  Monitors connected and functioning
  Intravenous fluids: rate, amount in bag, patency of tubing
  Drainage systems (such as nasogastric, chest, urinary): type, patency of tubing, connection of appropriate container, character and amount of drainage

---

Nursing Diagnosis

Nursing diagnoses related to the care of the postoperative patient might include the following:

- Risk for infection
- Ineffective breathing pattern
- Pain
- Altered nutrition, less than body requirements
- Impaired physical mobility

Outcome Identification

Outcomes identified for the selected nursing diagnoses could be stated as follows:

- The patient will be free from infection as indicated by normal vital signs; temperature within normal range; normal white blood count; clear breath sounds; clear, yellow urine; warm, dry skin.
- The patient's respirations will be easy, unlabored, and adequate.
- The patient will state subjective assertions of comfort ("I am in no pain") and will have no objective signs of discomfort (grimaces, tachycardia).
- The patient eats well from prescribed diet; weight loss is minimal.
- The patient ambulates at appropriate levels and carries out activities of daily living appropriate for condition.

Planning

Planning for the postoperative patient requires not only a knowledge of surgical techniques, but also knowledge regarding underlying medical conditions. Throughout the patient's stay, planning must always involve the family or significant other with measurable goals determined by discharge. A Sample Care Plan for the postoperative patient is included on p. 259.

Implementation
Wound healing

The basis for much of the postoperative nursing care is to promote wound healing. Wound care, nutritional requirements, and need for mobility are all related to the promotion of wound healing.[17] For a detailed discussion of the pathophysiology of wound healing, see Chapter 9.

Adequate respirations

The postoperative patient is at high risk for pulmonary complications because of increased respiratory secretions, decreased lung expansion, depression of the respiratory center, and the possibility of aspiration of gastric contents. The occurrence of these complications can be minimized by appropriate nursing management.

Circulation

Venous stasis in the postoperative patient can lead to thrombophlebitis, which is usually a preventable complication. Platelets adhere to the venous wall and form a thrombus, with a resultant potential for pulmonary embolus.

Prevention may include administration of prophylactic heparin, aspirin, dextran, or warfarin. Application of an intermittent external pneumatic compression device may be ordered, or application of antiembolism (AE) hosiery may be required.

Nursing measures that can prevent formation of a thrombus include using the AE hosiery whether the patient is in or out of bed, teaching the patient not to cross the legs, isometric leg exercises, and encouraging early ambulation.

If thrombophlebitis is suspected (pain or tenderness, presence of Homan's sign, erythema, localized area of warmth), the patient should return to bed, and the physician should be notified. Treatment will be with rest, heat, elastic bandages, and anticoagulant therapy.

Urinary function

One of the priorities during surgery and immediately afterward is to keep the patient well hydrated so that voiding will take place 6 to 8 hours after surgery. Usually intake is greater than output for 48 hours, when the fluid and electrolyte balance returns to normal. Every effort is made to refrain from use of a catheter because of the risk of urinary tract infection. Measures to aid the patient in voiding include a warm bedpan, letting water run, applying warm water to the perineum, and allowing the

SAMPLE CARE PLAN

Nursing Diagnosis: Risk for infection related to altered skin integrity, compromised aseptic technique, or malnutrition.

Outcome: Patient will be free from infection, as indicated by normal vital signs, temperature within normal range, normal white blood count, clear breath sounds, clear yellow urine, and warm, dry skin.

Interventions:

1. Monitor vital signs every 4 hours or as prescribed.
2. Monitor temperature every 4 hours as needed.
3. Monitor laboratory values for evidence of infection.
4. Encourage patient to take deep breaths or sustained maximal inspiration (SMI) or use respiratory aids.
5. Preserve closed urinary system and provide catheter care. Remove catheter as soon as possible.
6. Encourage the patient to eat foods high in protein and vitamin C.
7. Avoid antiinflammatory drugs such as steroids to facilitate healing.
8. Use aseptic technique when changing dressings and change soiled dressings immediately.
9. Monitor suction of wound catheters to provide drainage from wound.

Nursing Diagnosis: Ineffective breathing pattern related to postoperative pain, decreased energy or fatigue, decreased lung expansion, surgery

Outcome: Patient's respirations will be easy, unlabored, and adequate.

Interventions:

1. Monitor respirations and chest expansion frequently for 24 to 48 hours.
2. Place the bed in high Fowler's position if possible.
3. Auscultate lungs and evaluate the productiveness of the cough.
4. Have the patient cough and deep breathe at regular intervals.
5. Encourage use of respiratory aids if appropriate.

6. Treat underlying conditions, such as pain.
7. Splint incisional area with pillow before cough. Encourage the patient to turn and change positions at least every 2 to 3 hours.
8. Ambulate as soon as possible.

Nursing Diagnosis: Altered nutrition, less than body requirements, related to surgery.

Outcome: Patient will eat well from prescribed diet; weight loss will be minimal.

Interventions:

1. Encourage the patient to eat foods high in protein and vitamin C.
2. Offer frequent small amounts of food or high-protein liquids to patients who have little or no appetite.
3. Encourage ambulation (improves appetite).
4. Schedule procedures not to conflict with mealtime.
5. Administer medication for pain and nausea as needed.
6. Refer to nutritional support team if appropriate.

Nursing Diagnosis: Impaired physical mobility related to surgical procedures or pain

Outcome: Patient will ambulate at appropriate levels and carry out activities of daily living (ADL) appropriate for condition.

Interventions:

1. Encourage muscle-strengthening exercises before ambulation. Encourage ambulation or position changes and extremity exercises at least every shift.
2. Have patient dangle legs over side of bed until pulse has stabilized and patient is not dizzy before attempting to ambulate.
3. Use two people to help ambulate if the patient is weak or obese.
4. Encourage patient to walk further with each ambulation.
5. Teach proper use of appropriate devices (such as crutches, slings, Ace bandages) and observe return demonstration.

patient up to the bathroom whenever possible. If discomfort is present and the bladder is palpable, catheterization becomes necessary. In the event several catheterizations are required, an indwelling catheter is inserted. Hydration of the patient becomes a priority. Intake and output are recorded accurately. A urine output of less than 30 ml/hour is reported to the physician.

Bowel elimination

The postoperative patient who has had abdominal or pelvic surgery may have decreased peristalsis for at least 24 hours; this may persist for several days for the patient who has had gastrointestinal surgery. Increased fluid intake and early ambulation can promote the return of peristalsis.

Bowel sounds should be auscultated with a stethoscope to ensure that peristalsis has returned.

Constipation occurs frequently after surgery because of the effects of the anesthetic agents, narcotics, immobility, and decreased gastrointestinal motility. Fluids, roughage, and bulk laxatives can be given to aid in the relief of constipation. Occasionally an enema may be needed to empty the lower bowel.

Early ambulation

Early ambulation can expedite recovery and prevent complications.[17] Benefits are described in Fig. 8-9. Ambulation is usually postponed in the event of severe infection or thromophlebitis.

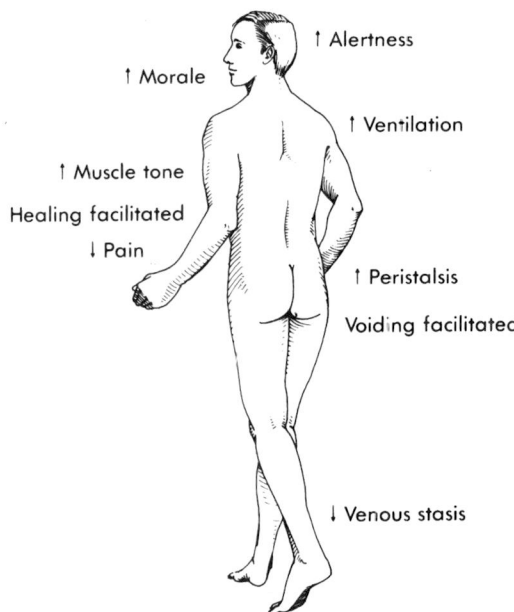

↑ Alertness
↑ Morale
↑ Ventilation
↑ Muscle tone
Healing facilitated
↓ Pain
↑ Peristalsis
Voiding facilitated
↓ Venous stasis

FIGURE 8-9   Benefits from early postoperative ambulation.

Evaluation

Evaluation of the postoperative patient on the surgical unit involves evaluating the outcomes identified as the patient was assessed:

- The patient's vital signs were within normal limits.
- The patient was normothermic.
- The patient's lab values were within normal range.
- The patient's wound is healing properly.
- The patient's breath sounds were clear bilaterally.
- The patient verbalized freedom from pain and was free from facial grimaces, moaning, and other evidence of pain or discomfort.
- The patient was eating well; there were no complaints of nausea or vomiting.
- The patient ambulated as appropriate.
- The patient is capable of performing the appropriate activities of daily living.

Family and Patient Education and Discharge Planning

Ideally, family and patient education and discharge planning should begin before the patient's admission for surgery.[12] The patient and family should be prepared to assume any care that may be needed after discharge. If needed, community resources should be used. Home healthcare is a valuable resource for the patient with treatment needs after discharge. The nurse responsible for the patient's care in the acute care setting collaborates and communicates with the home health team as soon as the need is identified so that the patient's care will be consistent and continue as needed.

The patient and family should be instructed in the proper care of the wound or incision. They should be knowledgeable about every medication that the patient will be using at home. An appointment for the return visit should be scheduled as ordered and the patient taught the importance of the return visit. Normal activities are gradually resumed according to the physician's protocols. Chapter 10 describes patient education and discharge planning in further detail. The chapters on surgical interventions have incorporated important elements for patient and family education and discharge planning. These elements assist the perioperative nurse in identifying and teaching what patients need to know and facilitating safe self-care during recovery from operative and other invasive procedures.

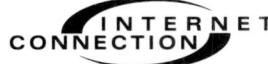

INTERNET CONNECTION

Association of Perianesthesia Nurses (ASPAN):
http://www.aspan.org

American Association of Nurse Anesthetists:
http://www.aana.com

Pain Management:
American Society of Pain Management Nurses:
email aspmn@aol.com
http://www.painnet.com/
http://www.web-shack.com/dee/
http://ww.nauticom.net/www/onsmain (Oncology Nursing Society Netpage)

Diagnostic Test Information Server:
http://dgim-www.ucsf.edu/testsearch.html

Pharmaceutical Information Network Homepage:
http://pharminfo.com

Clinical Discussion Group: http://www.sci.med.nursing

REFERENCES

1. Acute Pain Management Guideline Panel. (1992). *Acute pain management: operative or medical procedures and trauma. Clinical practice guideline.* AHCPR Publ. No. 92-0032. Rockville, MD: Agency for Health Care Policy and Research, Public Health Service, U.S. Department of Health and Human Services.
2. American Society of Anesthesiologists. (1991). *Standards for postanesthesia care* (approved by House of Delegates on October 12, 1988 and last amended on October 23, 1990). Park Ridge, IL: ASA.
3. American Society of Perianesthesia Nurses. (1995). *Standards of perianesthesia nursing practice.* Thorofare, NJ: ASPAN.
4. Coyne, M.L., et al. (1998). Describing pain management documentation, *MedSurg Nursing, 7*(1), 45-51.
5. Davidhizar, R., Shearer, R., & Giger, J.N. (1997). Pain and the culturally diverse patient, *Today's Surgical Nursing, 19*(6), 36-39.
6. Davidson, S.N. (1997). Pain and opiophobia, *Healthcare Forum Journal, 40*(3), 64-67.
7. Dixon, C.L. (1993). Pain management in the recovery room, *Current Review of Post-Anesthesia Care Nursing, 15*(19), 154-160.

8. Frank, S.M., Fleisher, L.A., Breslow, M.J., et al. (1997). Perioperative maintenance of normothermia reduces the incidence of morbid cardiac events: a randomized clinical trial, *JAMA, 277*(14), 1127-1134.

9. Frost, E.A.M. (1992). Complications in the post-anesthesia care unit. Part I, *Current Review of Post-Anesthesia Care Nursing, 14*(14), 113-120.

10. Gates, R.A. (1998). Postoperative patient care, *Seminars in Perioperative Nursing, 7*(1), 67-79.

11. Heffline, M.S. (1990). Exploring nursing interventions for acute pain in the postanesthesia care unit, *Journal of Post-Anesthesia Care Nursing, 5*(5), 321-328.

12. Janikowski, D.L. & Rockefeller, C.A. (1998). Awake and talking: ambulatory surgery and conscious sedation, *Nursing Economics, 16*(1), 37-42.

13. Kahn, R.C. (1996). Approaching common problems in the PACU, *Current Review of Post Anesthesia Care Nursing, 18*(19), 162-168.

14. Kurz, A., Sessler, D., & Lenhardt, R. (1996). Perioperative normothermia to reduce the incidence of surgical-wound infection and shorten hospitalization, *New England Journal of Medicine, 334*, 1209-1215.

15. Litwack, K. (1995). *Post anesthesia care nursing* (ed. 2). St. Louis: Mosby.

16. Litwack, K., & Drain, C. (1995). Pain assessment and management. In Litwack, K. (Ed.), *Core curriculum for post anesthesia nursing practice* (ed. 3). Philadelphia: W.B. Saunders.

17. Long, B.C., Phipps, W.J., & Cassmeyer, V.L. (Eds.). (1993). *Medical-surgical nursing: a nursing process approach* (ed. 4). St. Louis: Mosby.

18. McCaffery, M. & Beebe, A. (1989). *Pain: a clinical manual for nursing practice*. St Louis: Mosby.

19. Nightingale, F. (1863). *Notes on hospitals* (ed. 3). London: Longman, Green, Longman, Roberts, & Green.

20. O'Brien, D. (1996). The perioperative nurse in the postanesthesia care unit. In Rothrock, J.C. (Ed.), *Perioperative nursing care planning* (ed. 2). St. Louis: Mosby.

21. Odom, J.L. (1993). Airway emergencies in the post anesthesia unit, *Nursing Clinics of North America, 28*, 483-491.

22. Patton, C., & Deepika, K. (1991). Selected problems in the recovery room: a commentary, *Current Review of Post-Anesthesia Care Nursing, 13*(7), 49-56.

23. Ruth, H.S., Haugen, F.P., & Grove, A.P. (1947). Anesthesia study commission, *JAMA, 35*, 881-884.

24. Schmied, H., Kurz, A., Sessler, D.I., et al. (1996). Mild hypothermia increases blood loss and transfusion requirements during total hip arthroplasty, *Lancet, 347*(8997), 289-292.

25. Warner, M. (1997). Risks and outcomes of perioperative pulmonary aspiration, *Journal of Perianesthesia Nursing, 12*(5), 352-357.

26. Wenrich, J. (1994). Acute pain management and the nursing process, *Analgesia, 5*(1), 14-18.

CHAPTER NINE

Wound Healing, Dressing, and Drains

Nancye Rue Feistritzer

THE ABILITY TO heal wounds is one of the most powerful defensive properties human beings possess. Wound healing is a complex and highly organized response by an organism to tissue disruption caused by injury. This process is highly reliable in the absence of endogenous and exogenous infections, mechanical interferences, or certain disease processes. Apposition and maintenance of the edges of a cleanly incised wound almost always result in prompt healing. A primary goal of perioperative care is the prevention of surgical wound infections. Surgical wound infections are an important cause of illness, death, and excessive healthcare costs. Recently surgical wound infections have been further complicated by the potential for infection from new strains of antibiotic-resistant bacteria such as methicillin-resistant *Staphylococcus aureus* (MRSA).

Actions taken by perioperative personnel can mean the difference between a postoperative wound infection with associated sequelae and the normal healing process. A clear understanding of wound healing and factors adversely affecting healing is important for the appropriate management of patients undergoing surgery.

ETIOLOGY OF WOUNDS

The causes of wounds can be described as follows:

- *Surgical*: caused by an incision or excision
- *Traumatic*: caused by mechanical, thermal, or chemical destruction
- *Chronic*: caused by underlying pathophysiologic condition (e.g., pressure ulcers or venous leg ulcers) over time

Fig. 9-1 illustrates the layers of the skin corresponding to different wound depths. The amount of tissue loss, the existence of contamination or infection, and damage to tissue are some of the factors determining the type of wound closure. The healing process is inherently related to whether the wound is closed or left open. This process takes place in one of three ways: primary intention, secondary intention (granulation), and delayed primary closure (tertiary intention).

TYPES OF WOUND CLOSURE

Primary Intention

Healing through primary intention occurs when wounds are created aseptically, with a minimum of tissue destruction and postoperative tissue reaction. Wounds closed with sutures, staples, or tape applied as soon after the time of injury as possible fall into this category. Healing by primary intention takes place under the following conditions:

- Edges of an incised wound in a healthy person are promptly and accurately approximated.
- Contamination is held to a minimum by rigid adherence to aseptic technique.
- Trauma is minimal.
- No tissue loss.

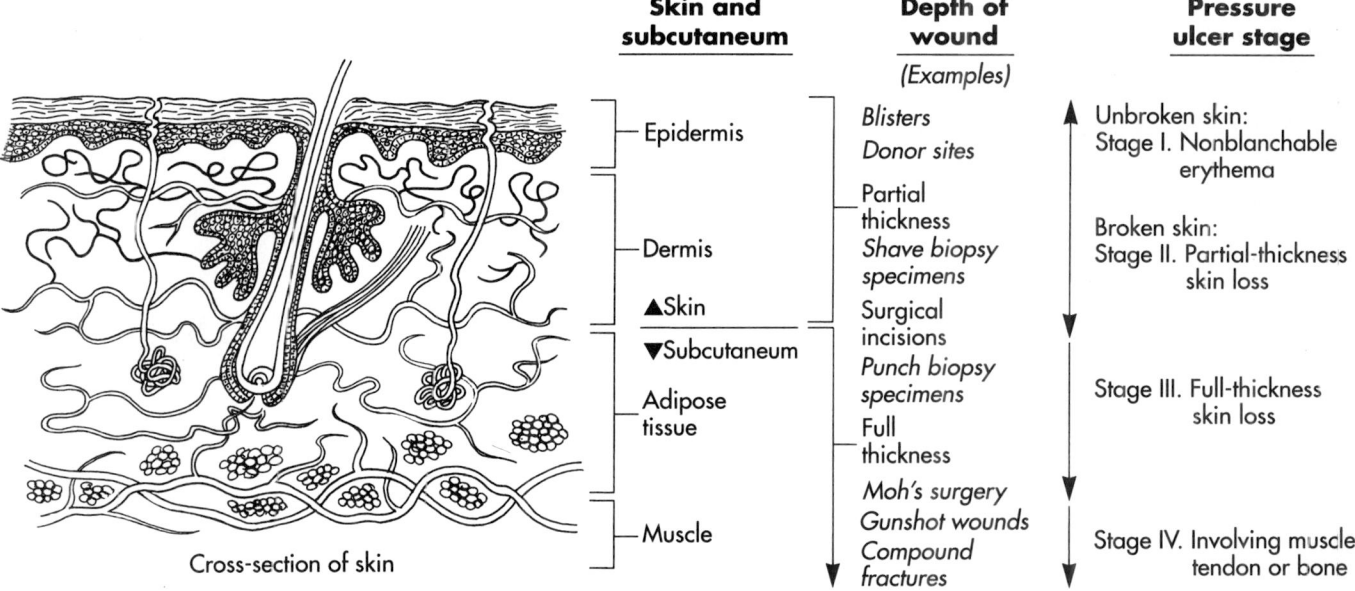

FIGURE 9-1   Layers of the skin corresponding to different wound depths.

- Upon completion of closure, no dead space is left to become a potential site of infection.
- Drainage is minimal.

The healing process in the wound until complete healing occurs is manifested in different ways, one of which is temperature. Research Highlight 9-1 describes this aspect and its implication for clinical practice in greater detail.

Secondary Intention (Granulation)

When surgical wounds are characterized by tissue loss with an inability to approximate wound edges, healing occurs through secondary intention (Fig. 9-2). This type of wound is usually left open and allowed to heal from the inside toward the outer surface. In infected wounds, this process allows the proper cleansing and dressing of the wound as healthy collagen tissue builds up from the inside. The area of tissue loss gradually fills with granulation tissue, comprising fibroblasts and capillaries. Scar tissue is extensive because of the size of the tissue gap that must be closed. The scar is referred to as a *cicatrix*. Contraction of surrounding tissue also takes place. Consequently, this healing process takes longer than primary intention healing does.

Delayed Primary Closure, or Tertiary Intention

As the name implies, this healing process takes place when approximation of wound edges is intentionally delayed by 3 or more days after injury or surgery. These wounds may require debridement and usually require a primary and secondary suture line as when retention

---

9-1 RESEARCH HIGHLIGHT

Cohen and Solomon (1997) conducted a study to establish if there is regularity in temperature changes in wounds healing by primary intention. Thirty patients (27 female, 3 male) admitted for cholecystectomy were studied. Temperature was measured for eight postoperative days at a fixed time and location each day with use of the semiquantitative contact method of liquid-crystal strips. During the first 3 postoperative days, the temperatures rose with few differences between the temperature of the wounds and their wider tissue surroundings. From days 4 to 8 temperatures of the wounds and surroundings gradually fell. When the stitches were removed on day 7, only the narrow zone of the incision site was warmer than the surroundings.

The findings are suggestive that there is a regularity in the course of temperature of the surgical wound in primary healing. The clinical implications are that persistence of a wider zone of infection after day 4 may allow one to predict the possibility of wound infection and disturbed healing.

From Cohen, E.M., & Solomon, R.J. (1997). Surgical wounds, *Primary Care Practitioner, 1*(1), 111-114.

---

sutures are utilized. The conditions leading to a decision for a delayed closure are as follows:

- Removal of an inflamed organ
- Heavy contamination of the wound
- The critical nature of the patient's intraoperative condition such as with hemodynamically unstable trauma patients.

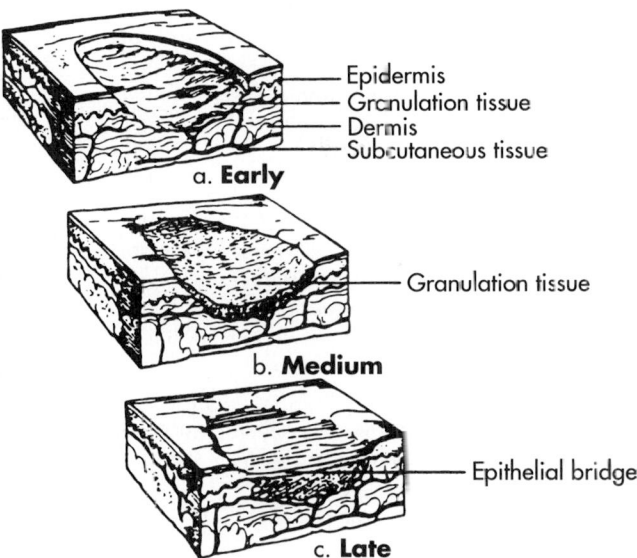

FIGURE 9-2   Three stages in secondary intention healing.

PHASES OF HEALING

Clean, full-thickness wound healing is an intricate biologic process that takes place in three overlapping phases: (1) inflammatory (also known as the catabolic stage), (2) fibroplastic (also known as the proliferative stage), and (3) remodeling (also known as the maturation stage) (Fig. 9-3).

Inflammatory Phase

In the inflammatory phase an exudate containing blood, lymph, and fibrin begins clotting and loosely binds the cut edges together. Blood supply to the area is increased, and the basic process of inflammation is set in motion. Inflammation is a prerequisite to wound healing and is a vascular and cellular response to dispose of bacteria, foreign material, and dead tissue.[5] Leukocytes increase in number to fight bacteria in the wound area and by phagocytosis help to remove damaged tissues. The severed tissue is quickly glued together by strands of fibrin and a thin layer of clotted blood, forming a scab. Plasma seeps to the surface to form a dry, protective crust. This seal helps to prevent fluid loss and bacterial invasion. During the first few days of wound healing, however, the seal has little tensile strength.

Fibroplastic Phase

The fibroplastic phase allows for new epithelium to cover the wound, beginning the process within hours of the occurrence of injury.[3] Epithelial cells migrate and proliferate to the wound area covering the surface of the wound to close the epithelial defect. Epithelialization also provides a protective barrier to prevent fluid and electrolyte loss and to reduce the incidence of infection. While the reepithelialization takes place,

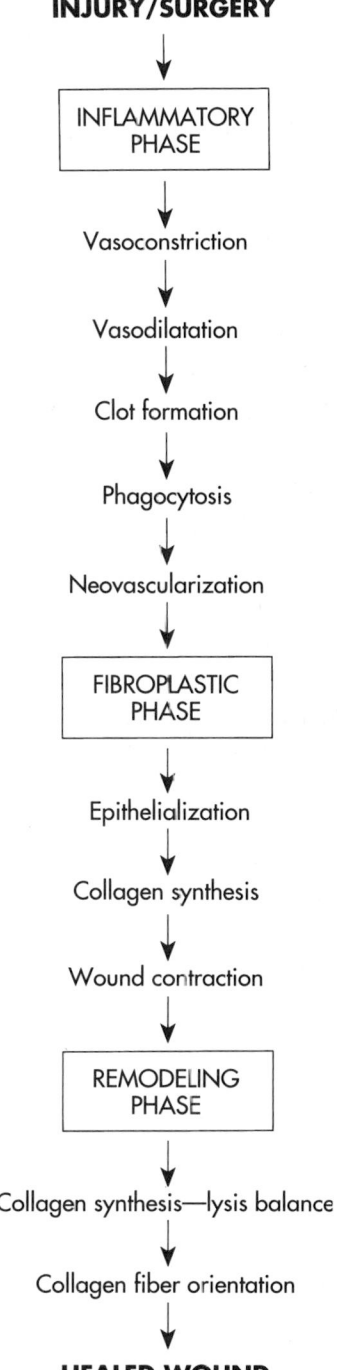

FIGURE 9-3   Flow diagram of normal wound healing.

collagen synthesis and wound contraction are occurring. Contraction begins approximately 5 days after the wound onset and peaks at 2 weeks, gradually pulling the entire wound into a smaller area. Epidermal migration is limited to approximately 3 cm from the point of origin. Larger wounds may require skin grafting because of the limited epidermal migration. Collagen synthesis produces fiber molecules that cross-link to provide strength to the wound.

Remodeling Phase

The remodeling phase begins after approximately 2 to 4 weeks, depending on the size and nature of the wound. It may last up to a year or longer. During the remodeling phase, the scar tissue formed during fibroplasia changes in bulk, form, and strength. Throughout normal wound healing, new collagen is produced while old collagen breaks down in a balanced fashion.[5] This collagen turnover allows randomly deposited connective tissue to be arranged in both linear and lateral orientation. As the scar ages, fibers and fiber bundles become more closely packed and form a crisscross pattern ultimately creating the final shape and function of the wound. At best, the tensile strength of scar tissue is never more than 80% of the tensile strength of nonwounded tissue.

FACTORS AFFECTING WOUND HEALING

Patients who have experienced any sort of wound should be assessed for healing status. The patient's nutritional status, oxygenation, and overall recuperative power are of utmost importance in tissue repair and healing. The nutritional status, inflammatory response, and oxygen tension depend on microcirculation to deliver components to the wound. It is important to maintain body temperature in the operating room to promote healing. If the patient becomes hypothermic, vasoconstriction will occur, leading to compromised wound healing.

Wound healing depends on adequate oxygenation. Decreased oxygen tension to the wound area inhibits fibroblast migration as well as collagen synthesis, resulting in decreased tensile strength of the wound.[5] Nutritional status also has a profound effect on healing because of the need for an adequate supply of protein necessary for the growth of new tissues. Protein is also required for the regulation of the osmotic pressure of blood and other body fluids, and the formation of prothrombin, enzymes, hormones, and antibodies. Other nutritional essentials are water; vitamins A, C, B_6, and B_{12}; iron; calcium; zinc; and adequate calories.

The most common cause of delayed wound healing in the operative patient is wound infection. Box 9-1 summarizes the types and definitions of surgical site infections. There are many possible causes of postoperative wound infections including patient susceptibility and severity of illness, microbial contamination by the patient's microflora, and exogenous wound contamination from the OR environment and personnel. The presence of a foreign body left in place after closure is another factor in wound infections because the body has a diminished capacity to inhibit infection on implanted material. Adherence to strict aseptic principles, careful observation of sterile technique, and thorough antimicrobial preparation of the patient and operative site are essential to minimize the risk of postoperative wound infection.

| BOX 9-1 | Definitions of Surgical Site Infection |

Incisional Surgical Site Infection (SSI)

Superficial incisional SSI
   Within 30 days of surgery
   Skin and subcutaneous tissue
   One of the following: pus, culture, physician's diagnosis, or one symptom (pain, redness, wound separation)
Deep incisional SSI; one of the following:
   Pus from drain into deep tissue not in incision
   Spontaneous dehiscence or being opened by the physician
   Abscess in deep tissues
   Diagnosis of SSI by a physician
Operative field SSI (area contiguous with organ or space of the operating site). Infection within 30 days of surgery and one of the following:
   Pus from drain through stab wound
   Positive culture
   Diagnosis by a physician
Culture obtained by aseptically preparing the site before collection or aspiration of cutaneous tissue or fluid
If an implant is placed, an infection may be linked to the operation for up to 1 year.

From Barrett, T. (1992). Recognition and treatment of surgical wound infections. *Today's OR Nurse, 14* (10), 12.

Wound healing can also be impaired by poor surgical technique. Rough handling of tissue causes trauma that can lead to bleeding and other conditions conducive to infection. Examples of surgical technique promoting wound healing include adequate hemostasis, precise cutting and suturing techniques, efficient use of time to minimize wound exposure to air, elimination of dead spaces, and minimal pressure from retractors and other instruments.

Additional factors affecting wound healing are the patient's age, stress level, immunologic status, and smoking history. Preexisting conditions such as diabetes, anemia, malnutrition, cancer, obesity, and cardiovascular or respiratory impairments also contribute to poor wound healing.

Additional terms used in connection with wound healing are shown in Box 9-2.

WOUND CLASSIFICATION

The Centers for Disease Control and Prevention (CDC) recommends four surgical wound classifications: clean wounds, clean contaminated wounds, contaminated wounds, and dirty or infected wounds.[4] This classification scheme reflects the probability of infection and thus enables appropriate preventive measures to be taken. *AORN Recommended Practices for Documentation of Perioperative Nursing Care* states that the patient record should reflect the surgical wound classification.[1] Following are descriptions of each classification.

BOX 9-2 **Additional Terms Used in Connection with Wound Healing**

The following are additional terms used in connection with wound healing:

keloid Dense, unsightly connective tissue or excessive scar formation that is often removed surgically

"proud flesh" Overgrowth of granulation tissue

gangrene Anaerobic infection process that may occur instead of healing; implies necrosis (death of tissue) and putrefaction (decomposition); usually caused by failure of nutriment or blood to reach a part

adhesions Adherence of serous membranes to one another, causing fibrous tissue to form; sometimes occurring in healing and inflammatory processes; commonly occurring in or about gastrointestinal tract, where adhesions may form bands and cause obstructions and subsequent surgical emergencies

dehiscence Separation of layers of surgical wound (Fig. 9-4)

evisceration Extrusion of internal organs, or viscera, through gaping wound (Fig. 9-4)

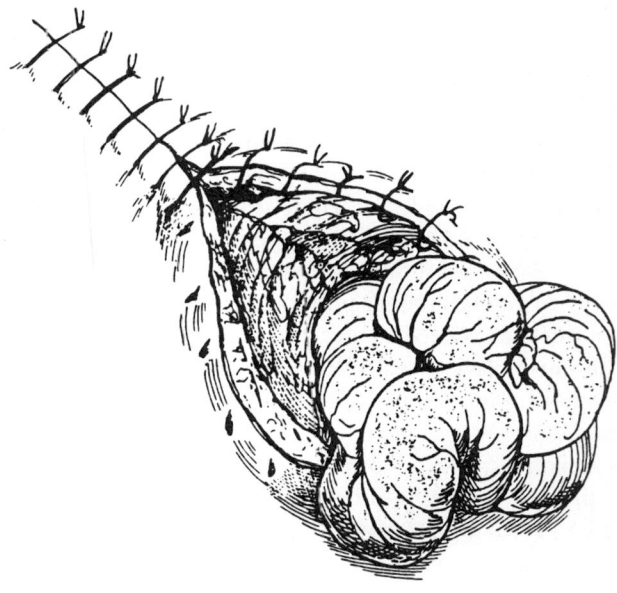

FIGURE 9-4 Wound dehiscence with evisceration of intestines.

Clean Wounds

Clean wounds are uninfected operative wounds in which no inflammation is encountered and the respiratory, alimentary, and genitourinary tracts are not entered. They are primarily closed and can be drained with a closed wound-drainage system. They show no sign of infection. Examples are breast biopsy, total hip replacement, or open-heart surgery.

Clean Contaminated Wounds

Clean contaminated wounds are operative wounds in which the respiratory, alimentary, or genitourinary tract is entered under controlled conditions. There is no sign of infection and no break in surgical aseptic technique. Examples of clean contaminated wounds are nonperforated appendectomy, hysterectomy, or thoracotomy.

Contaminated Wounds

Contaminated wounds are open, fresh, accidental wounds or operations with major breaks in aseptic technique. Incisions with signs of infection or gross spillage from the gastrointestinal tract are also included. Some examples are an appendectomy for ruptured appendix, a penetrating abdominal trauma involving bowel, or a gunshot wound to the abdomen.

Dirty or Infected Wounds

Infected wounds include old physically induced wounds with retained devitalized tissue and wounds that involve an existing clinical infection or perforated viscera. Examples of dirty or infected wounds are excision and drainage of abscess or delayed primary closure of a wound after appendectomy for ruptured appendix.

9-2 RESEARCH HIGHLIGHT

Cardo et al. (1993) prospectively studied the accuracy of circulating nurses in classifying surgical wounds according to the Centers for Disease Control and Prevention (CDC) classification system of clean, clean-contaminated, contaminated, and dirty or infected wounds. One hundred surgical procedures (50 general and 50 trauma) were classified by circulating nurses while a physician simultaneously observed and independently classified each surgical procedure. The overall accuracy of classification by the circulating nurses was 88% compared with the classification of the physician observer. Accuracy increased when surgical wounds were classified into only two categories: clean or clean-contaminated versus contaminated or dirty/infected. The researchers concluded that circulating nurses can classify surgical wounds with a high degree of accuracy utilizing the CDC system and that accuracy increases further when a simplified two-tiered system is utilized.

From Cardo, D.M., Falk, P.S., & Mayhall, C.G. (1993). Validation of surgical wound classification in the operating room. *Infection Control Hospital Epidemiology, 14*(4), 255-259.

An alternative system for classification of surgical wounds exists in the National Nosocomial Infections Surveillance System (NNIS). This risk index utilizes a broader and simpler division of wound class into two categories: clean and clean-contaminated[2] (Research Highlight 9-2).

NURSING DIAGNOSES

The nursing diagnoses—risk for infection (wound), risk for impaired skin integrity, altered nutrition, altered tissue perfusion, and hypothermia—point the nurse toward strategies that can be used to prevent wound infections and promote healing.

Box 9-3 provides a guide to nursing actions for preventing wound infection during the perioperative period. Attention should also be given to maintaining skin integrity through proper positioning, the use of therapeutic mattresses as needed, and the safe use of electrosurgery. The nurse plays a vital role in the prevention of wound infections, pressure ulcers, and burns caused by improper grounding.

A clinical pathway for the assessment and management of pressure ulcers is provided in Fig. 9-5 and is also applicable to surgical wound management. Be aware of the importance of ongoing assessment in the early detection and prevention of further complications. As more patients are discharged from the acute care setting to the home care setting much earlier in their recovery, more surgical wound care will be delivered by patients, their families and home care providers instead of by the hospital nurse. Early planning and teaching regarding wound care, universal precautions, and medical waste disposal have become a vital component of preparing the patient for optimal continuity of care subsequent to discharge. The perioperative nurse must be alert for the presence of predisposing factors contributing to wound infections. The presence of these in a patient should be observed so that early placement on the clinical pathway may be accomplished as appropriate.

DRESSINGS

After surgery a dressing may be applied to the wound. Following are the purposes of a dressing:

1. Cushioning and protection of the wound from trauma and gross contamination
2. Absorption of drainage

| BOX 9-3 | Guide to Nursing Actions for Preventing Wound Infection |

1. Preoperatively assess the patient for preexisting disposition to wound infection. Notice patient's age, weight, nutritional status, history of chronic systemic or metabolic disease, electrolyte values, skin condition at proposed operative site, presence of remote infection (that is, respiratory, urinary), status of immune system, laboratory values.
2. Report deviations in laboratory values, especially white blood cell count.
3. Check the patient's baseline preoperative vital signs.
4. Establish and maintain a sterile field according to principles of basic aseptic technique.
5. Adhere to institutional policy and protocol for OR attire.
6. Follow institutional policy and protocol for surgical hand scrubs.
7. Create effective barriers to transmission of microorganisms through proper gowning, gloving, and draping procedures.
8. Visually inspect room for total cleanliness before opening the case cart/supplies and instrument sets.
9. Inspect sterile items for contamination before opening. Check package integrity and chemical process indicator.
10. Maintain sterility while opening sterile items to preserve the sterility of the item and the integrity of sterile field.
11. Constantly monitor the sterile field.
12. Initiate corrective action when break in technique occurs.
13. Communicate maintenance of a sterile field.
14. Classify surgical wound based on the degree of contamination of the wound and surrounding tissues during the operative procedure (clean, clean-contaminated, contaminated, dirty).
15. Control movement of the patient, personnel, and materials in and out of the OR by adhering to established traffic patterns.
16. Minimize risk of cross infection by cleaning and processing anesthesia equipment and all items that have come into contact with the patient or sterile field properly.
17. Select materials for inhospital packaging that are compatible with the sterilization process, effective barriers, easily presented, and nontoxic.
18. Adhere to OR sanitation policies and protocols.
19. Cleanse skin at the operative site through skin preparation procedures.
20. Utilize methods of sterilization and disinfection to decontaminate needed supplies and equipment.
21. Meticulously wash hands after contact with the patient or any object likely to be contaminated with blood or body fluids.
22. Maintain the OR temperature between 20° and 24° C (68° to 75° F) except where contraindicated for patient care.
23. Maintain relative humidity at 50% ± 10%.
24. Keep OR doors closed to maintain pressure gradients.
25. Requisition, or administer, antibiotics as ordered. Check the patient record for drug allergy and sensitivity. Note drug, dosage, route, and time of administration.
26. Remove soiled linen from around patient before transfer to postanesthesia care unit.
27. Document additional nursing actions related to prevention of wound infection.
28. The following AORN Recommended Practices may be consulted to modify or expand this care plan:
    - Aseptic technique
    - Traffic patterns in the surgical suite
    - Cleaning and processing anesthesia equipment
    - Protective barrier materials for gowns and drapes
    - Selection and use of packaging systems
    - Sanitation in the surgical practice setting
    - Skin preparation of patients
    - Surgical attire
    - Surgical hand scrubs
    - Steam and ethylene oxide sterilization
    - Disinfection

Modified from Rothrock, J.C. (1996). *Perioperative nursing care planning* (ed. 2). St. Louis: Mosby.

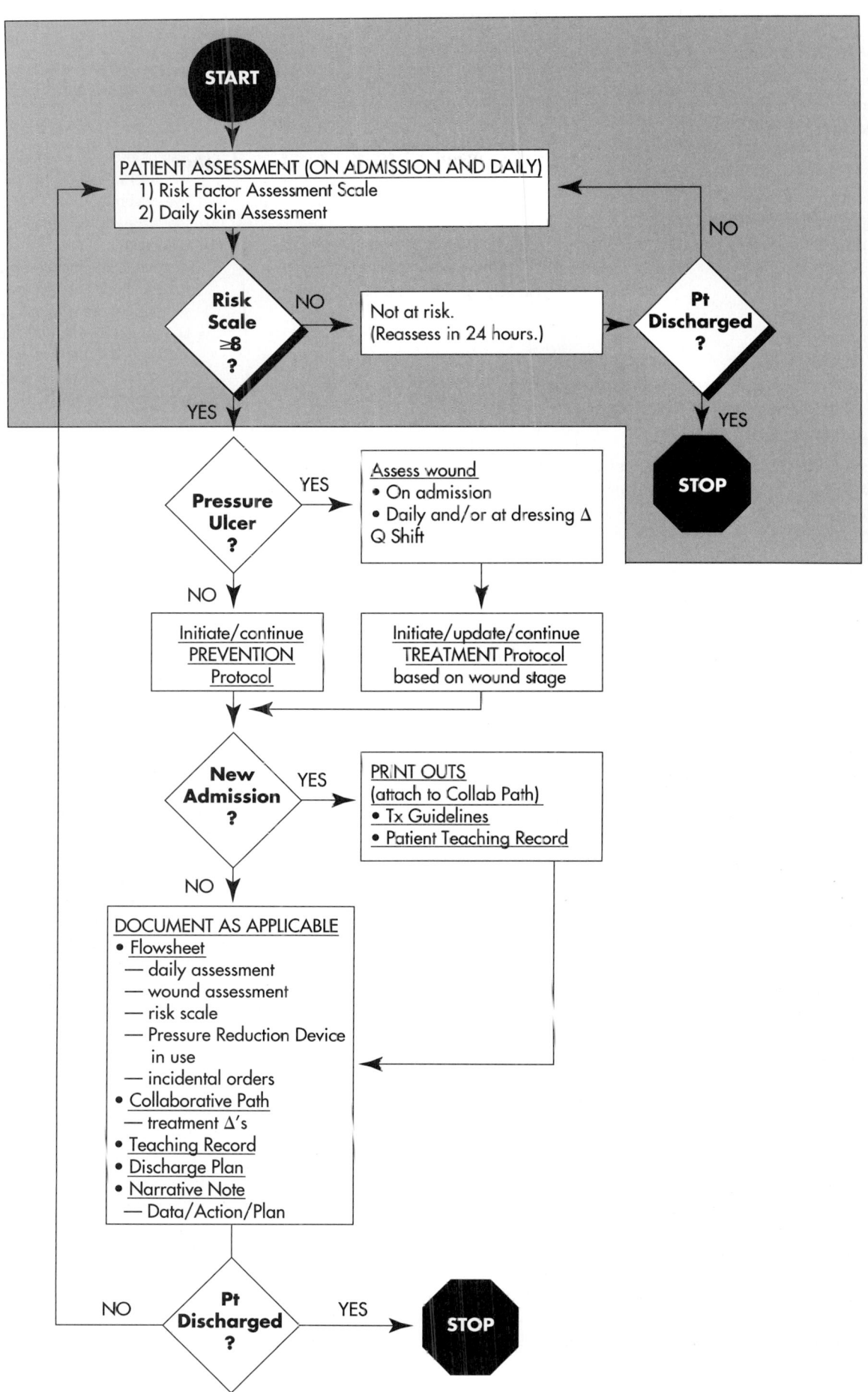

FIGURE 9–5 Clinical pathway for the assessment and management of pressure ulcers.

TABLE 9-1 | **Comparing Wound Dressings**

PRODUCTS	ADVANTAGES	DISADVANTAGES	NURSING CONSIDERATIONS
Cotton Mesh Gauze			
	■ Moderately absorbent	■ Bulky	■ Can be used dry to cover surgical wounds, wet-to-dry to nonselectively debride some wounds, and moist to pack undermining and tunneling ■ Combine with normal saline solution for granulation or antibiotic solutions for infection ■ Use transparent films or occlusive tape to retain moisture, p.r.n. ■ Cover with nonwoven gauzes to increase absorption
Nonadherent Dressing ■ *Nonimpregnated:* ETE Sterile Protective Dressing, EXU-DRY, Metal-line, Release, Telfa ■ *Impregnated:* Adaptic, Scarlet Red, Vaseline Gauze, Xeroflo, Xeroform	■ Occlusive ■ Nontraumatic	■ Minimally absorbent ■ Some impregnated dressings contain antimicrobial agents that harm fibroblasts	■ Nonadhesive ■ Doesn't require secondary dressing ■ Useful for skin tears and other friable wounds, wounds near body hair, donor sites, and skin grafts
Transparent Film ■ ACU-Derm, Bioclusive, BlisterFilm, Ensure-It, Hi/moist, Omiderm, OpraFlex, OpSite, Polyderm Picture Frame Film, Polyskin II, Tegaderm, Tegaderm Pouch, Transite Exudate Transfer Film, UniFlex, Vari/Moist, Visi Derm II	■ Moisture retentive ■ Semipermeable ■ Very comfortable for patient ■ Not bulky ■ Allows for easy wound inspection ■ Water resistant	■ Minimally absorbent ■ Channeling (wrinkling) occurs	■ Adhesive ■ Doesn't require secondary dressing ■ Useful for autolytic debridement, as well as superficial wounds, donor sites, abrasions, and burns

Note: The products included here are representative of what is available; the lists under each category are not meant to be inclusive.
From "Selecting Wound Dressings by Category," *NARD Journal* © 1991, National Association of Retail Druggists, Alexandria, VA, May 1991.
From Krasner, D. (1992). The 12 commandments of wound care. *Nursing '92, 22*(12), 38.

3. Debridement of the wound
4. Support, splinting, or immobilization of the body part and incisional area
5. Aid in hemostasis and minimize edema, as in a pressure dressing
6. Enhancement of the patient's physical comfort and aesthetic appearance
7. Maintenance of a moist environment and prevention of cell dehydration
8. Application of medications

Beyond these clinical needs, dressings should be chosen based on each wound's unique characteristics of site, depth, and area as well as the patient's overall condition.

Several varieties of transparent "biologic" synthetic dressings are available and are quite popular. Most are vapor and oxygen permeable, conform to irregular body surfaces, prevent gross outside contamination, and allow visibility of the wound itself. These transparent semiocclusive films keep the wound moist and thereby enable epidermal cells to move more quickly across the wound and bridge the incision. The "scab" stage of wound healing is avoided. Although these film types of dressings cannot be used on heavily draining wounds, their skinlike qualities seem to aid wound healing and protect delicate healing skin edges. Table 9-1 compares various wound dressings and the nursing considerations for each.

Dressings can be grouped into two main categories: primary and secondary dressings. Primary dressings are placed directly over or in the wound. A variety of dressing materials are available on the market today. The function of these dressings is to absorb drainage and allow it to wick away from the wound edge. Cotton gauze or synthetic dressings may be used for this purpose. Cotton gauze dressings are increasingly less used, as newer, more effective dressing materials have been developed. The layer of dressing directly contacting the wound should be nonadherent unless debridement is desired.

TABLE 9-1 | Comparing Wound Dressings—cont'd

PRODUCTS	ADVANTAGES	DISADVANTAGES	NURSING CONSIDERATIONS
Hydrocolloid			
■ Comfeel, DuoDERM, Hydrapad, Intact, IntraSite, Johnson & Johnson Ulcer Dressing, Restore, Sween-A-Peel, Tegasorb, ULTEC	■ Moisture retentive ■ Occlusive or semipermeable ■ Very comfortable for patient ■ Not bulky ■ Excellent bacterial barriers; high tack ■ Water resistant ■ Moderately absorbent	■ Melt out occurs, resulting in residue in the wound bed and particles on the wound margins	■ Adhesive ■ Doesn't require secondary dressing ■ Useful for autolytic debridement, as well as for covering a variety of acute and chronic wounds ■ Available in powder, wafer, and paste form
Hydrogel			
■ Biolex Wound Gel, Carrington Dermal Wound Gel, ClearSite, Elasto-Gel, Geliperm Wet/Granulate, Hydron Wound Dressing, IntraSite Gel, Nu-Gel, Second Skin, Spand-Gel, Vigilon	■ Moisture retentive ■ Moderately absorbent ■ Cooling, soothing effects ■ Can be used on infected wounds ■ Water resistant (if used with secondary transparent film) ■ Allows for easy wound inspection		■ Adhesive or nonadhesive ■ May or may not require secondary dressing ■ Useful for autolytic debridement, as well as for covering a variety of acute and chronic wounds ■ Available in sheet or gel forms ■ Sheets don't leave a residue; gel easily rinsed off
Exudate Absorber			
■ Algosteril, Allevyn Cavity Wound Dressings, Bard Absorption Dressing, Debrisan, Envisan, Hydragan, Kaltostat, Mesalt, Sorbsan	■ Moisture retentive ■ Highly absorbent		■ Nonadhesive ■ Requires secondary dressing ■ Useful for autolytic debridement and for heavily exudating wounds ■ Available as starches, pastes, beads, hypertonic saline gauzes, and calcium alginate dressings
Foam			
■ Allevyn, EPIGARD, Epi-Lock, LYOfoam, Mitraflex	■ Moisture retentive ■ Very comfortable for patient ■ Moderately absorbent ■ Insulating		■ Nonadherent ■ May or may not require secondary dressing ■ Useful for friable wounds or wounds near body hair

Secondary dressings are placed directly over the primary dressing. These function to absorb excessive drainage, provide hemostasis by compression, and protect the wound from further trauma. These functions are usually accomplished with a bulky dressing such as an abdominal pad. These pads have a cotton filling that provides extra absorbency.

Dressings may be secured with a variety of products including tape, Elastoplast, Ace bandages, or soft roll products. Tape is available with a variety of backing materials (cloth, paper, taffeta, plastic) and with regular or nonallergenic adhesive. The amount of strength and elasticity required, patient allergies, and anticipated frequency of dressing change influence which type is selected. When frequent dressing changes are anticipated, Montgomery straps can be selected to secure the dressing (Fig. 9-6).

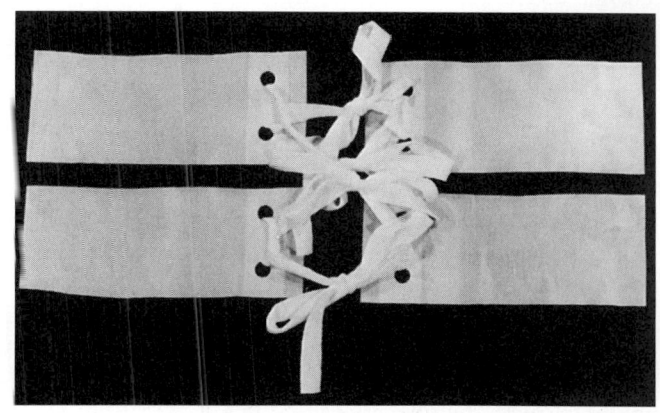

FIGURE 9-6 Montgomery straps.

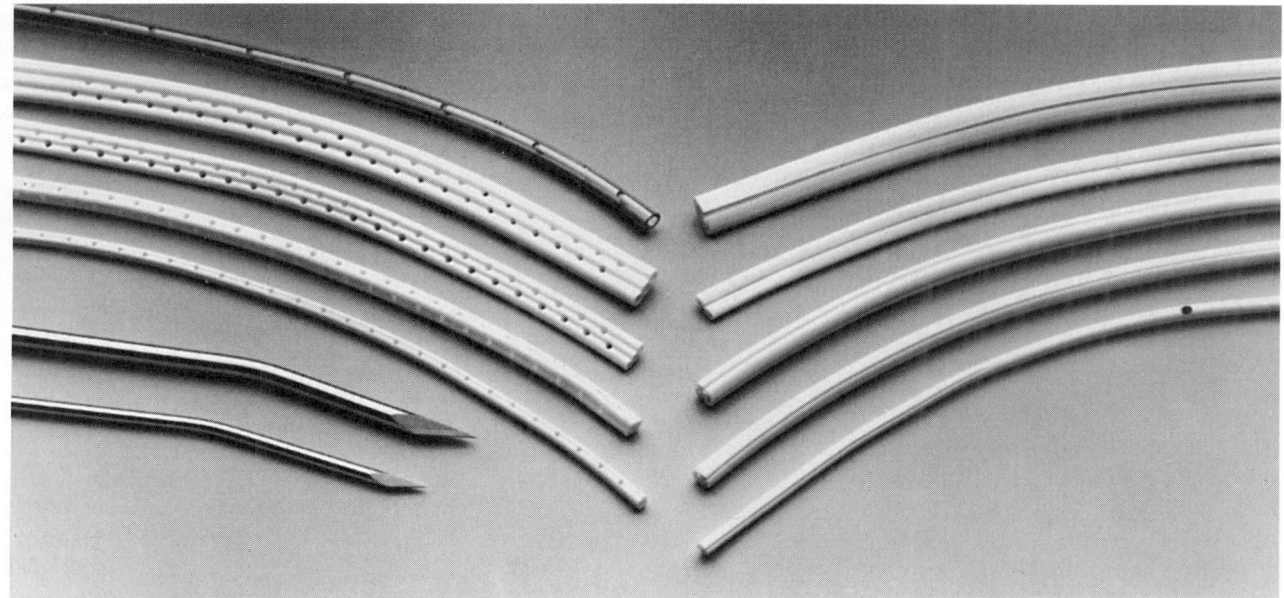

FIGURE 9-7 Drains are available in a variety of styles. Pictured are round polyvinyl chloride, flat and round silicone drains, trocars, and a variety of fluted silicone drains.

When compression of the wound for hemostasis or reduction of edema is desired, a polyurethane dressing, elastic tape, or elastic bandage may be used to secure the secondary dressing. Immobilization is accomplished with the addition of soft padding, splints, elastic bandages, and casting materials. These immobilizing dressings are discussed in greater detail in Chapter 22.

In some situations the wound is not dressed at all. The air-exposed wound will heal, and having no dressing (1) allows for optimum observation of the incisional area, (2) aids bathing, (3) prevents possible adhesive-tape reactions, (4) increases comfort and maneuverability for many patients, and (5) seems to minimize adverse responses by the patient to the operation. Much attention is being paid to the process of wound care management in light of managed care and the need to be as cost effective as possible while maintaining quality outcomes. Research Highlight 9-3 describes a study recently done to compare sterile dressing change with clean dressing change techniques in open surgical wounds. The preliminary results challenge some of the more traditional beliefs and practices about appropriate dressing management techniques.

DRAINS

Drains provide exits through which air and fluids such as serum, blood, lymph, intestinal secretions, bile, and pus can be evacuated from the operative site. Drains may also be used to prevent the development of deep wound infections. They are usually inserted at the time of surgery, primarily through a separate small incision known as a *stab wound*, close to the operative site.

9-3 RESEARCH HIGHLIGHT

Stotts et al. (1997) used a two-group design to conduct a pilot study of 30 patients (15 males and 15 females) undergoing elective gastrointestinal operations with wounds healing by secondary intention. Patients were randomly assigned to receive clean or sterile dressing with the intervention beginning on the first postoperative day and repeated three times a day until discharge from the hospital. The length of stay ranged from 3 to 9 days. The groups were homogeneous at the start of the treatment with respect to age, length of operation, wound volume, nutritional status, and tissue perfusion.

The researchers found no difference in the rate of wound healing between clean versus sterile dressing change technique. The mean cost of care was significantly less for the clean group than for the sterile group. These findings need to be confirmed with a larger sample but provide promising news about how to manage more cost effectively secondary intention wound healing while still maintaining quality outcomes.

From Stotts, N.A., Barbour, S., Griggs, K., et al. (1997). Sterile versus clean technique in postoperative wound care of patients with open surgical wounds: a pilot study. *Journal of Wound Ostomy Continence Nursing, 24*(1), 10-18.

In some instances (chest, common bile duct, bladder), drainage is directly through the lumen of the tube (as with a Foley retention catheter) into a closed drainage system. In other instances (peritoneal cavity or skin wound), drainage of pus or blood is primarily along the outside

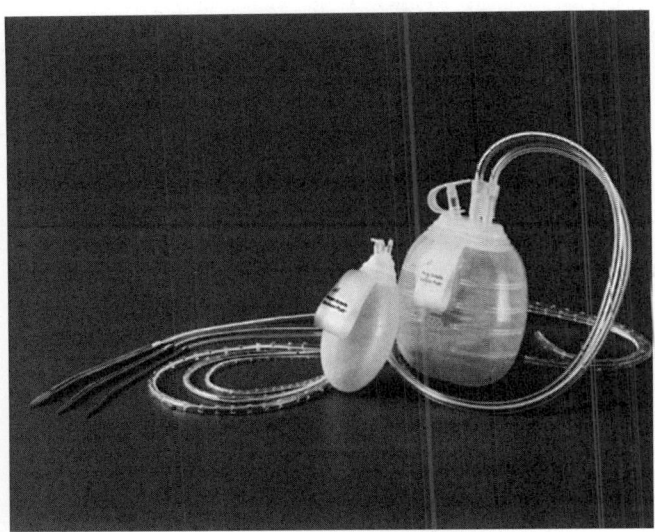

FIGURE 9-8   Portable self-contained wound-drainage system.

surface of the drain by capillary action and gravity (as with the simple Penrose drain). The selection of a simple versus a closed drainage system depends on the needs of the site to be drained, patient activity, and overall healing capability. Many types of drains are available. The most common are made of latex, PVC (polyvinyl chloride), or silicone (Fig. 9-7). Particular care should be taken to ensure that the patient is not allergic to latex when selecting any latex drain. For many wounds, a portable, self-contained, closed wound suction unit is selected. These units create a negative pressure in a reservoir attached to the drain. Fluid is then gently drawn out of the wound and collected in the reservoir (Fig. 9-8).

The perioperative nurse must clearly document the location and type of drains on the operative record. This information is important to nurses caring for the patient in the postanesthesia and postoperative nursing units. Some wounds yield significant amounts of drainage and as such

must be monitored closely during the postoperative course. Closed autologous drains allow for collection of blood from a surgical wound and the return of that blood to the patient. This minimizes the need for transfusion of blood from outside donors thereby reducing the risk of bloodborne pathogen transmission.

SUMMARY

Wound healing is an essential part of the surgical experience. Perioperative nurses should vigilantly guard and enhance their patients' ability to heal with an eye toward prevention of problems before they occur. There is no more important opportunity to prevent surgical wound infections than in the perioperative period.

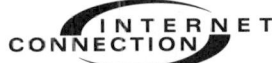
INTERNET CONNECTION

Wound, Ostomy and Continence Nurses Society: http://www.wocn.org

Tissue Engineering: http://www.pittsburgh-tissue.net/

Wound Care Center: http://curative.com

REFERENCES

1. Association of Operating Room Nurses. (1998). Recommended practices for documentation of perioperative nursing care. In *AORN standards, recommended practices and guidelines for perioperative nursing*. Denver: the Association.
2. Cardo, D., Falk, P., & Mayhill, C. (1993). Validation of surgical wound classification in the operating room, *Infection Control Hospital Epidemiology, 14*(4), 255-259.
3. Daly, T. (1990). The repair phase of wound healing: re-epithelialization and contraction. In Kloth, L., McCulloch, J., & Feeder, J. (Eds.). *Wound healing: alternatives in management*. Philadelphia: FA Davis.
4. Garner, J.S. (1985). *Guidelines for prevention of surgical wound infections*. Atlanta: Centers for Disease Control and Prevention.
5. Gogia, P. (1992). The biology of wound healing, *Ostomy/Wound Management, 38*(9), 12-20.

CHAPTER TEN

Patient Education and Discharge Planning

Vicki J. Fox

IMPORTANCE OF PATIENT EDUCATION

Patient education and discharge planning create a vital, emerging role for the perioperative nurse because of the growing emphasis on shortened hospital stays and home care, the increasing number of ambulatory surgery procedures, and managed care and competition. Cross-training between nursing units, such as the operating room, postsurgery units, and perianesthesia care units may become commonplace. The perioperative nurse has the unique opportunity and knowledge base to coordinate efforts to meet the education needs of surgical patients and their families or significant others. This chapter examines four questions about patient education: (1) why teach? (2) when should patient education occur? (3) what is the appropriate content for patient teaching? and (4) how should nurses teach?

Historical Development

One answer to the question "Why teach?" is that patient education is a long-standing nursing tradition. Nursing has used patient education as a tool for providing safe, cost-effective, and quality healthcare since the middle of the nineteenth century. Nurses themselves highly value patient education and consider it an important part of their job.[15,18] Patient education began in an era when the sick were cared for in the home. Operative procedures also were often done at home. Nurses taught families about sanitation and cleanliness when caring for the sick, as well as how to care for those convalescing from home surgery.[38] The National League of Nursing Education, in its 1918 *Standard Curriculum Guide for Schools of Nursing*, considered "preventive and educational factors" an essential element of routine nurse training, especially in new specialties such as public health, school nursing, infant welfare, and industrial welfare. In 1937, the curriculum guide described the nurse as a teacher and an agent for health. In 1950, the guide identified teaching and contributing subject matter, such as psychology, knowledge of principles of teaching and learning, and teaching skills as areas common to all nursing curricula.[30-32]

Legal and ethical mandates

In answering the question "Why teach?" one could argue that, as health care providers, nurses are ethically and legally bound to teach. Illness prevention and patient education have long been nursing priorities. Traditionally, however, the physician's first priority was protecting the patient from harm. Complete disclosure about the disease and treatment was a secondary concern. More recently, the emphasis in medical care has changed from simply treating the disease to health maintenance and wellness. In the 1970s and 1980s, organized medicine recognized patient education as an ethical obligation. The American Hospital Association's *A Patient's Bill of Rights*[4] affirmed the patient's right to information about his or her illness and to give informed consent for treatment. If a healthcare facility adopts that bill of rights as policy, it becomes as legally binding as the hospital's medical bylaws and standards of nursing practice. Several nurse practice acts have made patient education an explicit legal responsibility for the individual nurse.[37,44] Failure to teach or to document that teaching was done is considered below reasonable and prudent nursing practice and has been the basis of malpractice litigation involving nurses.[42] Courts have repeatedly maintained that the right of self-determination in a democratic society is fundamental. To limit it in healthcare decision-making is an injustice. Nowhere is this better demonstrated than in the perioperative setting when obtaining informed consent. In 1993, The Joint Commission for the Accreditation of Healthcare Organizations (JCAHO) *Accreditation Manual for Hospitals* (AMH) consolidated functions of patient and family education from eight chapters in the previous AMH into one new chapter,

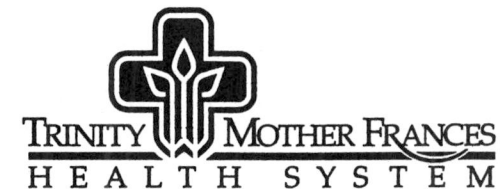

PATIENT/FAMILY CAREMAP

	PRE-OP DAY	DAY OF SURGERY	POST-OP DAY #1	POST-OP DAY #2
Diagnostic Studies	• Lab work • Urine sample • Chest X-ray	• Lab work • Chest X-ray	• Lab work • Chest X-ray when chest drainage tube removed • ECG	• Oxygen level will be checked. If appropriate, oxygen will be removed.
Treatments Nursing Plan	• History taken by nurse • Nurse will ask about special needs	• Skin prep for surgery • Bladder tube placed in surgery • Drainage tubes placed in surgery • Breathing tube placed in surgery • Constant nursing evaluation in intensive care • Family may visit post-op • Elastic stocking on	• Oxygen • Use Incentive Spirometer 10 times per hour while awake • Tubes and IV's removed as your condition improves • Transfer to 4th floor if physician approves • Elastic stocking on	• Blood pressure will be checked every 4 hours • Use Incentive Spirometer 10 times per hour while awake • Dressing will be removed • Daily weight at 6 pm • Elastic stocking on
Physical Therapy/ Rehab Activity	• May continue routine activity	• Bedrest • Bed bath	• Walk 5-50 feet × 4 • Sit in chair for meals • Introduce to cardiac rehab nurse for orientation to post-op activity	• Walk 100 feet, 4 times with assistance from nurse or family member • Sit in chair for meals
Nutrition Diet Fluids	• Cardiac diet — Nothing by mouth after midnight except medications	• Fluids by IV • Ice chips possible after breathing tube removed	• Diet is advanced as tolerated	• Regular cardiac diet
Medications Pain Control	• Take usual medications as ordered by physician • Sleeping pill may be ordered	• IV medications for blood pressure and pain	• As ordered by physician • Pain control by mouth	• It is easier to breathe and walk when free from pain. Ask for pain medication when needed.
Discharge Planning/ Teaching	• Introduction to post-op activity progression • Incentive spirometry instruction — deep breathing exercise • Visit with surgeon and other personnel • Tour Intensive Care Unit • Surgery booklet given to patient	• Nursing staff to provide information to families during surgical procedure and during ICU visit	• Case manager will be available to answer questions • Social Service needs will be evaluated and services offered	• The dietician will talk to you about your diet • Nutrition classes are held twice per week on 4 Center.

FIGURE 10-1   Patient/family coronary artery bypass care map.

"Patient and Family Education" This chapter set a distinct set of standards for patient and family education. It has been revised annually to require an even higher degree of accountability from institutions.[16] In 1997, the Advisory Commission on Consumer Protection and Quality in the Health Care Industry recommended eight measures to promote and ensure healthcare quality and value; among them was the right to receive accurate, easily understood information that would enable participation in treatment decisions.[3]

Definitions and goals

A third answer to the question "Why teach?" comes from the ultimate goal of patient education, which is to enable patients to be responsible for their own healthcare.[44] Patient education is a planned experience designed to change behavior. The goal of patient education is for the patient to improve health behaviors and health status. Patient education may use a combination of methods to accomplish this: behavior modification, counseling, and teaching. Patient teaching is an activity that aims to increase the patient's knowledge. The goals of patient

PROCEDURE:	CORONARY ARTERY BYPASS
DIAGNOSIS:	CORONARY ARTERY DISEASE
SURGEON:	
CLINICAL NURSE SPECIALIST:	

POST-OP DAY #3	POST-OP DAY #4	POST-OP DAY #5	POST-OP DAY #6	DISCHARGE OUTCOMES/ INSTRUCTIONS
	• Lab work		• DISCHARGE Congratulations, you are going home!	• No signs of infection — check temperature at home and call your surgeon if greater than 100 degrees
• Use Incentive Spirometer 10 times per hour while awake • Daily weight at 6 pm • Look at your incisions • Inspect for drainage and redness • Elastic stocking on	• Use Incentive Spirometer 10 times per hour while awake • Daily weight at 6 pm • Look at your incisions • Elastic stocking on	• Use Incentive Spirometer 10 times per hour while awake • Daily weight at 6 pm • Look at your incisions • Elastic stocking on	• Use Incentive Spirometer 4 times a day at home • Continue to look at incisions at home and report any changes to your surgeon. • Daily weight at home • Wear stockings until swelling is gone	• Cardiac rhythm is stable for the last 48 hours. If pulse becomes irregular at home, call your cardiologist or visit your local emergency room • Incisions that have discolored drainage and are reddened or warm to the touch must be reported to your surgeon. • Oxygen level is at least 90% on room air. Weigh yourself daily. If 2 lbs. lost or gained overnight or shortness of breath, call surgeon.
• Walk 250 feet, 4 times with nurse or family • Bathe from basin • Sit in chair for meals	• Walk 450 feet, 4-6 times per day • Sit in chair for meals • Ask nurse when you may shower	• Walk 820 feet, 4-6 times per day • Sit in chair for meals	• Continue walking Increase distance gradually over 4 weeks to one mile per day • Nap after lunch	• You must be able to walk 820 feet before you can go home. Walking is good for you, but don't get too tired. • Allowing yourself a nap only after lunch will help you get back to a regular routine and you will sleep better at night.
• Regular cardiac diet	• Regular cardiac diet	• Regular cardiac diet	• Continue cardiac diet low fat/cholesterol	• You must be eating an adequate diet to help you to heal after surgery.
• It is easier to breathe and walk when free from pain. Ask for pain medication when needed.	• It is easier to breathe and walk when free from pain. Ask for pain medication when needed.	• It is easier to breathe and walk when free from pain. Ask for pain medication when needed.	• Continue pain medications as needed. Extra Strength Tylenol can also be effective	• You must know what medications you will take at home, when they are due and describe warning signs to report to your doctor.
• Your nurse will talk to you about risk factor modification • Social Service needs will be evaluated and services offered.	• A pharmacist will instruct you about the medications you will take at home	• Your nurse will talk to you about activity and incision care and self-care at home	• Your appointment for your return visit with your surgeon will be given to you prior to discharge	• You must be aware of activity restrictions and plan a method to reduce your personal risk factors for heart disease prior to discharge. The Cardiac Rehab nurse can help with this.

FIGURE 10-1, cont'd For legend see opposite page.

teaching are to provide information and to improve knowledge. Changes in knowledge may be needed before the patient is motivated to change behaviors. Teaching is a systematic way of introducing new information, events, skills, or objects into the patient's environment. When viewed as an interpersonal interaction between the patient and nurse, teaching is a distinctive form of communication that is uniquely structured and sequenced to produce learning. Theoretically, teaching should meet the patient's need for new information and skills. Neither the definition of patient education nor patient teaching contains assurance that the patient will actually learn or that behavior will change.[24,37]

Learning, on the patient's part, is demonstrated in changed behavior.[43] Nurses can assess educational needs, provide information, instruction, and resources, and communicate with family and colleagues to enable learning. Nurses cannot, however, force patients to learn. Ultimately patients are responsible for changing their own behaviors.[39]

CARDIAC ACCELERATED RECOVERY FOR HOME CARE
ACTUAL/POTENTIAL PATIENT PROBLEMS

#1	Knowledge deficit related to cardiac disease process.
#2	Knowledge deficit related to medication regimen, diet and activity.
#3	Alteration in functional mobility related to incisional discomfort and deconditioning.
#4	Knowledge deficit re individual behavior modification (Risk factors for CAD).
#5	Potential for wound infection and alteration in skin integrity.

Criteria for Admission to HHC	PROCESS INDICATORS	DATE ____ PRE-ADMISSION	DATE ____ Interaction #1	DATE ____ Interaction #2
☐ Medically cleared for Home Care ☐ Any high risk pt ☐ Care needs can be met by Home Care Services ☐ Pt agrees to participate in Home Care program ☐ Pt/primary caregiver has sufficient mental alertness to learn techniques and activities ☐ Medical condition/fragility precludes treatment on OP basis ☐ Home environment is safe and accessible ☐ Payment source is identified/arranged ☐ Care Management complicated by potential for arrhythmias ☐ Physiological, psychological, social and spiritual support for pt and their families	Dx Studies	⎯ Review dates and times for lab work	⎯ Review lab work schedule with patient. Place dates/times of important events on calendar; place on refrigerator	
	Risk Factors		⎯ Review and discuss individual risk factors ---------------------	--------------
	Assessment/ Monitoring	⎯ Request of service initiated and completed ⎯ Obtain history of dx process	⎯ Complete admission procedure. Assess: VS, wtg, cardiac fx, lung; heart sounds; incisions. Individualize plan of care ⎯ Assess need for SW intervention	⎯ Assess: VS, wtg, cardiac fx, lung; heart sounds; incisions; leg/ankle edema
☐ Care Management complicated by decreased activity tolerance and deconditioned S/P cardiac surgery	Rehab PT/OT	⎯ Obtain range of vital signs from chart	⎯ HR (monitor, other), BP _____. ⎯ Ambulate > 150′ (or 5 mins.) Ft _____. ⎯ Rate of perceived exertion (RPE) _____. ⎯ Assess ROM. ⎯ Strength: 2 lb, hand weights (Reps _____.) ⎯ Terminate activity for intolerance	⎯ BP _____. ⎯ HR _____. ⎯ Ambulate > 175′ (or 6 mins.) Ft _____. ⎯ Rate of perceived exertion (RPE) _____. ⎯ Continue ROM. ⎯ Assess strength (progress from session 1). ⎯ Terminate activity for intolerance
☐ Care Management complicated by nutritional and fluid intake less than body requirements	Nutrition/ Teaching			⎯ Review cardiac diet (add diabetic and/or elderly diet guidelines PRN)
☐ Knowledge deficit of medication regimen	Medications	⎯ List Rx's and sig; # dispensed	⎯ Review med list. ? pharmacy; ? correct and appropriate dosing; reinforce compliance; place schedule of meds. on refrigerator	⎯ Review side effects and precautions
☐ Knowledge deficit of disease process, activity, and self-care	Discharge Planning/ Teaching	⎯ Review discharge instructions MFH. Initiate home care instructions	⎯ Review MD follow-up and "when and why" to call MD	
	Consults			
	Psychosocial/ Emotional Needs		⎯ SW for crisis intervention -------- ⎯ Emotional support for times of depression and feelings of helplessness --------------------	--------------
	Signature of HHC Provider			

FIGURE 10–2 Cardiac accelerated recovery for home care map. *HHC*, Home health care; *wtg*, weight; *fx*, function; *sw*, social work; *ft*, feet; *MFH*, Mother Francis Hospital.

CARDIAC ACCELERATED RECOVERY FOR HOME CARE
ACTUAL/POTENTIAL PATIENT PROBLEMS — cont'd

#6	Potential for arrhythmias.
#7	Limitations in functional capacity (lifting, walking, ADL's).
#8	Alteration in comfort/pain related to surgery.
#9	Depression and sleeplessness.
#10	Alteration in family dynamics, finances, relationships.

DATE _____ Interaction #3	DATE _____ Interaction #4	DATE _____ Interaction #5	DISCHARGE OUTCOMES Discharge may occur when all expected outcomes are met.
			____ Labs are WNL
----------------------------	----------------------------	-------------------------- >	____ Pt knowledgeable re individual risk factors ____ Pt verbalizes plans to modify lifestyle
____ Assess: VS, wtg, cardiac fx, lung; heart sounds; incisions; leg/ankle edema	____ Assess: VS, wtg, cardiac fx, lung; heart sounds; incisions; leg/ankle edema	____ Assess: VS, wtg, cardiac fx, lung; heart sounds; incisions; leg/ankle edema	____ Discharge pt from home care to cardiac rehab ____ Vital signs are WNL ____ HR and rhythm stable ____ Wound healing appropriately ____ No signs of inflammation or infection ____ Breath sounds WNL ____ Weight has returned to pre-op baseline
____ BP_____ . ____ HR_____ . ____ Ambulate > 200' (or 7 mins.) ____ Ft_____ . ____ Rate of perceived exertion (RPE)_____ . ____ Continue ROM. ____ Assess strength (reps only). ____ Terminate activity for intolerance	____ BP_____ . ____ HR_____ . ____ Ambulate > 225' (or 8 mins.) ____ Ft_____ . ____ Rate of perceived exertion (RPE)_____ . ____ Continue ROM. ____ Assess strength (reps only). ____ Terminate activity for intolerance	____ BP_____ . ____ HR_____ . ____ Ambulate > 250' (or 9 mins.) (increase 25' each additional visit or 1 min.) Ft_____ ____ Rate of perceived exertion (RPE)_____ . ____ Continue ROM. ____ Assess strength (reps only). ____ Terminate activity for intolerance	____ Increased activity regimen tolerated ____ Pt ready to participate in Phase II Outpatient cardiac rehab
	____ Discuss increasing kcal/protein necessary for healing		____ Appetite improving ____ Pt understands cardiac dietary restrictions of decreased fat and cholesterol ____ Diabetic and elderly diet regimens are followed appropriately
	____ Review any new meds.		____ Pain managed with medication or resolved ____ Pt knowledgeable re all medications
____ Discuss common problems experienced by CABG pts			____ Coping skills improved or WNL ____ Demonstrates independence in performing ADLs ____ Knowledgeable re accessing community resources/support systems
--------------------------	--------------------------	------------------------ >	____ Resources have been identified and pt/family showing signs of developing adequate coping skills
--------------------------	--------------------------	------------------------ >	

FIGURE 10-2, cont'd For legend see p. 278.

Benefits of preoperative patient education

A fourth answer to the question, "Why teach?" are the benefits for the patient, for the patient's family, support system, and significant others, for nurses, and for institutions. Lindeman and other nurse researchers have confirmed the value of preoperative patient teaching when based on scientific content and structured either for a group or the individual.[8,10,13,21,22,45] The benefits of patient education for the patient undergoing a surgical intervention include the following: (1) it speeds recovery,[28] (2) relieves anxiety,[48] (3) increases self-esteem by increasing self-efficacy,[33] (4) reduces cost of hospitalization, (5) prevents complaints about care, and (6) decreases the amount of perceived immediate and residual pain.

The benefits of education for the patient's family and support system are as follows: (1) it alleviates anxiety and fear, (2) reduces cost, (3) hastens the family's return to normal functioning, (4) increases self-esteem, and (5) develops support for the care giver's efforts.[21,36] A primary benefit of patient education for nurses is increased job satisfaction. Patient education makes the nurse's job easier in the long run by saving time. It reduces the nurse's stress level and increases self-esteem. The institution benefits from patient education by reduced litigation potential, decreased length of hospital stay, and compliance with JCAHO requirements.

Trends in Patient Education

The focus of health care moved from the home to institutions between 1925 and 1975; in the 1990s the focus has returned to the home setting. Ambulatory surgery and shortened hospital stays require creative strategies for preadmission teaching and preparation for convalescence at home.[23] Homes have also become the site of preventive care, such as reducing the risk of highly communicable diseases (such as HIV infection), appropriate nutrition for specific health states (such as diabetes), and early screening for diseases (breast self-examination). The home is the site of follow-up care, such as long-term IV antibiotic therapy and for long-term care of the frail elderly. Home care may involve the use of high-technology equipment. Home care is based on a self-care philosophy aimed at moving the patient from the dependent role limited to compliance with instruction into a more contractual arrangement with the healthcare provider.[37] Self-care philosophy is based on self-reliance, personal responsibility, and individual initiative. Educational support is an integral part of the self-care philosophy. The perioperative nurse has a unique opportunity to manage the educational partnership among healthcare professionals, patients, and their families.[43]

Another trend in patient education is including patient and family education into case management models. Case management is based on the concept of integrating hospital processes among departments to eliminate duplication and draw interdisciplinary care into a coordinated effort. Critical pathways as part of the full case management model are showing promising results in holding down costs while retaining quality. Critical paths can double as an educational tool to facilitate patient and family education (Fig. 10-1). Some facilities are adding an "at-home" path as an adjunct to the inpatient path[48] (Fig. 10-2). Furthermore, critical pathways may be an ideal way to document patient education outcomes and demonstrate compliance with the expanded JCAHO educational standards.[50]

ASSESSMENT

This section examines what content is appropriate for patient teaching and when a patient is ready to learn. This section also introduces the interrelatedness of the nursing process and the process of teaching. The first step in the nursing process and the teaching process is assessment. Table 10-1 illustrates the relationship of these two processes.

Assessment of Individual Patient Education Needs

The most important activity the perioperative nurse can carry out is assessment because it is the foundation for the entire patient education process. Collecting accurate assessment data about what a patient needs to know and the level of readiness to learn assists the perioperative nurse in setting realistic priorities. Not all patient needs are the same, nor do all patients need or desire to know everything. The key question the nurse must ask when assessing the patient's educational needs is, "What does this patient need to know?" The question is not, "What would be nice for this patient to know?" The dramatic increase in ambulatory surgery procedures, drastically shortened hospital stays, and the proliferation of high-tech treatments require that the nurse develop patient and family education prioritized learning needs. The patient needs to know enough to (1) grant informed consent to an invasive procedure, (2) facilitate intraoperative cooperation, (3) provide self-care at home (Research Highlight 10-1), and (4) survive until more teaching can be provided. A patient's admission for a surgical procedure may involve enough discomfort and anxiety to prevent retention of any information on complicated subjects, such as pathophysiology. Highly technical content may actually confuse the patient. Patient compliance has more to do with an understanding of what the patient needs to do and an ability to carry it out than on knowledge. Patients learn information about events directly related to their admission for surgery. The need-to-know assessment should be based on critical activities that the patient will be expected to accomplish in the immediate postoperative period (see Research Highlight 10-1). Naturally the plan is different if the patient actively seeks highly technical information. Assessment should also include determining what the patient already knows.

TABLE 10-1 | **Relationship of the Teaching Process to the Nursing Process**

ASSESSMENT	DIAGNOSIS AND PLANNING	IMPLEMENTATION	EVALUATION
Nursing Process			
General nursing assessment to determine patient's need to learn; if positive, use teaching process	Nursing diagnosis and planning of nursing interventions	Nursing activities may include teaching and learning interactions	Evaluation against outcome criteria
Teaching Process			
Assessment of need to learn Assessment of readiness and motivation	Learning diagnosis; specific content areas to include in other nursing interventions	Teaching and learning interactions	Evaluation of learning

Adapted from Redman, B.K. (1997). *The process of patient education* (ed. 8). St. Louis: Mosby.

10-1 RESEARCH HIGHLIGHT

Kleinbeck and Hoffart conducted a qualitative study designed to examine the personal experiences of 19 adult patients who underwent elective laparoscopic cholecystectomy and were discharged within 23 hours after surgery. The researchers used semistructured postoperative telephone interviews on the second postoperative and fourth or fifth postoperative day. Patients were asked to tell stories that described what they were and were not able to do, how they were managing their problems, what their concerns were, and how close to recovery they estimated themselves to be. In the second interview, they were asked what advice they would give a friend or family member who was scheduled for the same procedure. A single theme emerged from the patient's descriptions of their at-home surgical recoveries: toward the usual self. Two major patterns, progressive activity and self-care, joined to ease the patient to a return to their usual selves. On the trip home, patients feared their "insides" would move around to fill the void left by the removed gallbladder, they may hurt themselves by doing the wrong thing, or "hurt things inside." The first day home, they described being able to move about from place to place slowly and were limited by soreness and tenderness. When describing recovery, responses fit into one of two categories. First was an absence of symptoms such as soreness. Second was resumption of their usual activities with return of strength and energy. Advice for others included recognizing that energy stores will be quickly depleted. They also suggested that nurses give explicit instructions for patients to rest when tired rather than give general instructions like "Take it easy." Since patients define recovery as being able to perform activities they performed before surgery, the researchers recommend detailed teaching on practical matters, such as getting in and out of automobiles, and helping patients recognize alterations to routine daily occurrences, such as picking up an infant or small child. Recovering patients are generally instructed not to lift over 5 pounds of weight. The nurse can suggest that the recovering patient sit and allow the child to sit beside them on a pillow. Postoperative telephone calls to the patient from the perioperative nurse are helpful to those who fear they may do something to interfere with their recovery process.

From Kleinbeck, S.V.M. & Hoffart N. (1994). Outpatient recovery after laparoscopic cholecystectomy. *AORN Journal, 60*(3), 394-402.

Assessment of Individual Readiness to Learn

The timing of preoperative teaching is critical (Research Highlight 10-2). When to teach has more to do with the patient's readiness to learn than the actual number of weeks, days, or hours before a surgical procedure.[20] The literature is replete with articles on the importance of assessing the learner's readiness to learn. Assessment of readiness to learn is similar to other kinds of nursing assessments. A continuous process, it requires expertise in observation, communication skills, especially listening, collaboration with nurse and physician colleagues, and assimilation of chart data.[39] Much of the literature on readiness to learn refers to healthy students in the classroom setting. Although there are some similarities between readiness to learn in an academic setting and readiness to learn in the context of health care, there are notable differences. The differences are time and health.[29] Health affects readiness to learn because the patient and family may be profoundly concerned, rationally or

10-2   RESEARCH HIGHLIGHT

This study is a replication of studies done to identify preoperative teaching content deemed important by patients and nurses in ambulatory surgery settings. The setting was a 200-bed private hospital in a large metropolitan area in the southeastern United States. Thirty patients, ranging from 19 to 68 years of age, participated in the study. Twenty-nine RNs, ranging from 26 to 56 years of age, participated in the study. The instrument used was the Perceptions of Preoperative Teaching Questionnaire, which has items measuring five dimensions of preoperative teaching: (1) psychosocial support, (2) situational information, (3) patient role information, (4) sensation or discomfort information, and (5) skills training. The subjects were asked to rank each item according to its importance of teaching, using a five-point Likert type of scale. Subjects were also asked to rank seven types of preoperative teaching in order of importance on a seven-point Likert type of scale. The seven types were as follows: (1) the preoperative nursing care, (2) the what, when, and why of perioperative events, (3) when the events would occur, (4) what these events would feel like, (5) what patients were expected to do, (6) expressing concern or worries, and (7) new skills to prevent complications. Generally, patients and nurses agreed on the content of what is important to teach in the ambulatory setting. Patients ranked the five dimensions as follows: (1) situational information, (2) psychosocial support, (3) patient role information, (4) sensation or discomfort information, and (5) skills training. On the other hand, RNs ranked the five dimensions as follows: (1) psychosocial support, (2) patient role information, (3) situational information, (4) skills training, and (5) sensation or discomfort information. Both patients and RNs ranked when events will occur as being the most important. Patients ranked what patient is expected to do and the what, when, and why of events as second and third. RNs ranked the what, when, and why of events and what events would feel like as second and third.

After rating the importance of these types of teaching, the subjects were asked to note the time they believed teaching should occur (before admission, after admission but before surgery, or at the time of the event or surgical procedure). Researchers found no significant differences between patients and RNs regarding preferred times for teaching. Most believed that teaching about events, when events would occur, what patients are expected to do, and what events feel like and expressing their concerns or worries should occur before admission to the ambulatory surgery unit. Both believed that learning new skills to prevent complications should occur after admission.

From Brumfield, V.C., Kee, C.C., & Johnson, J.Y. (1996). Preoperative patient teaching in ambulatory surgery settings, *AORN Journal, 64*(6), 941-952.

irrationally, about basic issues such as pain, disability, self-esteem, and dying. Time constraints are very different. In the academic setting the teacher and learner have agreed on a time period: 6 weeks, a semester, or a year. In the healthcare setting the nurse is most often concerned with the patient's readiness to learn at this moment in time. The moment may be the brief span of time the nurse sees the patient preoperatively and postoperatively. The nurse's assessment must be brief, basic, concrete, specific, and useful.

Factors that influence readiness to learn

Nurses do not have time to teach patients who are not physically and emotionally ready. Assessing the patient's readiness to learn should occur before each teaching or learning interaction as a distinct activity, even though it may occur as the nurse is assessing other needs or providing other kinds of nursing care. The assessment may be done quickly. The instruction that follows will be influenced by the patient's readiness to learn. The quality, nature, method, and scope of instruction may well affect the patient's future levels of readiness to learn. Readiness to learn is being both willing and able to make use of instruction.[14] Readiness establishes evidence of motiva-

tion.[29] The degree of readiness to learn depends on the degree of willingness and ability. The difference between teaching and instruction is important to understand. Teaching includes, among other things, both the assessment of readiness and the activities of instruction. Instruction is only a part of teaching.

Several factors influence readiness to learn.[29] The first is comfort, both physical and psychologic. The six most common sources for physical discomfort are pain, nausea or dizziness, itching, fatigue or weakness, hunger or thirst, and the need to urinate or defecate. Since these conditions are not always directly observable, the perioperative nurse may be able to obtain information regarding physcial discomfort from the chart. Asking the patient directly is usually the best way to get the information. One cannot assume that absence of complaints indicates comfort. Psychologic comfort implies that the patient is not currently having uncomfortable emotions to a degree that would impair abilities.

The six most common uncomfortable emotions are fear, anxiety, worry, grief, anger, and guilt. The perioperative nurse may be able to observe behaviors or body language that indicate the present of psychologic discomfort. Any intense emotion, including pleasant ones, will preclude the possibility of effective involvement in learning. One attribute of a skillful perioperative nurse is the ability to modify a planned intervention to accommodate the patient's comfort. If the patient is either physically or psychologically uncomfortable, the appropriate intervention is to relieve the discomfort before proceeding. Patients faced with the prospect of a thoracotomy for a suspected malignant lesion may be so overwhelmed with the fear of cancer that they are unable to listen to procedural information. The wise intervention is to be supportive and wait for patients to advance to a higher level of adaptation to the illness when their level of readiness will be greater than before.

The amount of energy currently available to the learner is a second critical factor. The patient's energy is limited. If large amounts of energy, physical or psychic, are being expended, there may be none available for learning. The amount of energy patients have is closely related to their physical condition, their reaction to the stage of illness, the current number of stressors in their lives, and the degree of the situational or maturational crisis. For example, a patient who is fighting for every breath has no energy for anything else; a person actively denying the illness has little energy to learn about it.

A third factor influencing readiness to learn is motivation. Behaviors that indicate a person is motivated may include leaning forward, asking questions, taking notes, asking for a more complete explanation, seeking out the perioperative nurse for help or information, and requesting books or pamphlets. The perioperative nurse's goal is to help the patient and family learn whatever it is they wish to learn. The goal is to assess the level, not the basis, of motivation. If the behaviors that reflect motivation to learn were placed on a continuum, they would range from an overall posture of eagerness through lack of eagerness and apathy to rejection of any effort to teach. Motivation is discussed in greater depth later in this chapter.

The patient's capability to learn is a fourth critical factor affecting the readiness to learn (Research Highlight 10-3). Obstacles to learning can include vision or hearing problems, limited manual dexterity, vocal or language limitations, or neurologic deficit.[7] The first three factors that influence readiness to learn can be assessed primarily by the use of subjective data. The patient's capabilities can be assessed on more or less objective data. Prerequisite capabilities include physical ability, intellectual ability, knowledge, attitudes, and skill. Capability is influenced or determined by age, maturation, stage of development, past learning, physical and mental health, and environment. Both physical and intellectual capability should be assessed. When assessing physical ability, the perioperative nurse should ask these questions:

1. Are the patient's height and weight adequate to accomplish the task involved? (Can this child reach the light switch?)

2. Is the patient strong enough? (Can this frail elderly woman lift a long leg cast?)

3. Does this patient have the coordination and dexterity to accomplish the task? (Can the patient whose hands are crippled with arthritis manage to change a colostomy bag?)

10-3 RESEARCH HIGHLIGHT

Review of charts at a large southern acute care facility revealed either lack of patient teaching or failure to document teaching activities by various disciplines. These disciplines included physician progress notes, dietary patterns, social services, physical therapy, and nursing. There was no assessment of learning needs, a teaching plan, or follow-up of teaching needs on any patient care forms or nursing flow sheets. Most teaching occurred at the time of discharge with no opportunity to validate that learning occurred. The survey demonstrated a need for a common tool for documenting patient and family education and discharge planning. A multidisciplinary clinical practice committee developed an interdisciplinary *Patient and Family Education and Discharge Plan* teaching system. The system contained three parts. The first was the learner assessment section, which included checklists for obstacles to learning, ability to learn, willingness to learn, how the individual liked to learn, and knowledge of illness or injury. Second was the educational plan, which included teaching and learning objectives, implementation, evaluation, and learner outcomes in six major categories: (1) disease process or conditions, (2) preoperative and postoperative teaching, (3) medications and treatments, (4) nutrition, (5) psychosocial and spiritual needs, and (6) self-care. Third was the discharge plan, which included information about food and drug interaction, postdischarge destination, limitations at discharge, follow-up services, home-care equipment needs, follow-up appointments and special instructions. Extensive in-service and training were conducted over several months preceding hospitalwide implementation. Implementation also occurred in outpatient departments including emergency services, cardiac catheterization labs, same-day surgery units, and endoscopy units. Overall documentation and the evaluation of the effectiveness of patient and family education improved in all disciplines. The process outcomes identified high-priority areas in specific teaching categories that indicated that further improvement could be made. These were in nutrition, psychosocial care, and self-care. Two retrospective chart reviews validated the value of interdisciplinary education and discharge planning.

From Clay, J.C., Wyatt, L.K. & Morris, G.M. (1996). Patient and family education: an interdisciplinary process. *MedSurg Nursing, 5,* 333-338.

4. Can the patient see, hear, smell, taste, and feel well enough to accomplish the task?
5. Can this patient see well enough to adequately compare the color chart on a reagent strip for urinalysis?

Assessment of intellectual ability includes the following:

1. Basic math skills. (Can this patient read a thermometer?)
2. Reading skills. (Can this patient read the directions on a prescription bottle?)
3. Verbal skills. (Can this patient communicate with others who are involved in care and express himself?)
4. Problem-solving skills. (Can this patient recognize situations in which she should seek help and would she know how to seek help? For example, will the patient know what to do if she becomes febrile at home?)
5. Comprehension and ability to follow instructions. (Is there some factor, such as recently administered pain medication, that may impair this patient's ability to receive the instruction the perioperative nurse has to offer?)

Knowledge influences readiness to learn. Does the patient have the basic concepts and facts to understand the new material? For example, does the patient know where the organ to be operated on is located? A related factor influencing the patient's readiness to learn is the patient's acquired skills. Has this patient already acquired skills from past experiences? Will past experiences attract or detract the patient from the goal? Discrepancies between expectations and capabilities should be discovered early as a result of careful assessment rather than later as a result of the patient's failure to reach the goals. The patient's attitude and value system are powerful influences on readiness to learn. These are influenced by factors such as ethnicity, cultural and religious beliefs, values about health care, and socioeconomic status. What is important to the patient? In teaching a new mother about immunizations for her child, does the mother share the belief that immunizations are safe? The discussion on the Health Belief Model in this chapter helps illustrate this.

Motivation

Motivation is the force that "initiates, directs, and maintains behavior."[37] This section looks at general theories of motivation in a teaching-learning context. No single motivation theory, but rather a combination of two or more of these theories, is likely to account for a patient's behavior. The six theories are reinforcement, needs, cognitive dissonance, attribution, personality, and expectancy.[37] Behaviors that have been positively reinforced, rather than punished or ignored, are far more likely to be repeated. The positive social reinforcement a cardiac rehabilitation patient gets from exercising in groups, rather than alone, provides motivation to continue the behavior.

Another reinforcer is the verbal encouragement from other patients and the cardiac rehabilitation nurse.

According to Maslow, people are motivated by a hierarchy of needs, in which higher level needs emerge as lower level needs are met. In other words, unmet needs create motivation. A satisfied need has no power to motivate, but it permits a higher level need to emerge, which in turn motivates the individual. For example, if the patient perceives that a surgical procedure is life threatening, his safety needs motivate him to learn more about it than to interact in meaningful ways with friends, which serves to meet a higher level social need.

Cognitive dissonance theory maintains that people become uncomfortable when a deeply held value or belief is challenged. To resolve the discomfort, a person may rationalize to justify the belief or behavior: "Well, everybody has to die of something. I'll really enjoy smoking while I'm alive and just die a little sooner." The person may also be motivated to change the behavior or belief: "Smoking is less socially acceptable than it used to be. It does contribute to heart disease and lung cancer. I will quit smoking."

Attribution is identifying a cause for what is happening. Patients frequently do this after the diagnosis, an accident, or cure of a disease. Attribution answers the question "Why did this happen to me?" A concept essential to understanding attribution is locus of control. People with an internal locus of control believe that their own efforts contribute to the success or failure of a situation. A postoperative patient with an internal locus of control may be highly motivated to cough, deep breathe, and ambulate. She believes these activities are in her control and will positively affect her health. On the other hand, people with an external locus of control attribute success or failure to causes external to themselves such as luck, the difficulty of the task, or other people's behavior. A postoperative patient with an external locus of control may be poorly motivated to cough, deep breathe, and ambulate. He may see these activities as something the nurse requires of him rather than being in control of them himself. He may not connect participation in those activities to quicker recovery and a shorter hospital stay.

In personality theory, motivation is a relatively stable characteristic that exhibits a tendency toward a desire for one of the following: (1) affiliation, having positive relationships with others, (2) achievement, being productive and reaching goals, or (3) power, influencing and controlling others. Patients with strong affiliation desires may be motivated to learn if they believe it will improve their relationships with their family or health care provider. A patient with strong achievement desires may be motivated to learn because of a sense of accomplishment. This is especially true of learning specific tasks. Coping styles can be a stable personality characteristic. Table 10-2 describes various coping styles people use in the face of illness. Dysfunctional coping occurs when coping styles do

TABLE 10-2 | Coping Styles when Faced with Illness

COPING STYLE	DESCRIPTION	STRATEGY
Confronting	Making an observation about one's behavior	Not useful in dealing with the illness itself; useful in dealing with another's positive or negative response to illness
Distancing	Separating oneself from the problem	Convincing themselves that their problem is unique, therefore they believe that they cannot learn from someone else's experience
Self-control	Taking an active interest in something by taking control	Practicing self-care and participating in decision making; must learn the difference between what can be controlled and what cannot
Seeking social support	Through supportive interaction with friends, family, church groups, etc.	The perception of having support is more important than the actual support received
Accepting responsibility	Buying into the treatment plan	Useful when encouraging life-style changes; harmful when used for blaming
Escape or avoidance	Failure to deal with or address the problem	May be useful as short-term strategy, but harmful in the long run
Problem solving	Critical thinking skills	One of the more useful strategies; most educational programs teach solutions, not the problem-solving process
Positive reappraisal	Reinterpreting or reframing a negative to a positive	Instead of dwelling on what one cannot do, emphasize what one is successful at doing; looking at the illness as a challenge
Activity or distraction	Physical activity such as walking, jogging, swimming, or less activity, such as painting or reading; humor, laughter, and relaxation are other forms	The idea that something is better than doing nothing; especially helping in dealing with pain, depression, and changing habits such as eating or smoking; keeps the mind occupied
Self-talk	A variation of positive thinking	Can be either positive or negative; goal is to change negative self-talk to positive self-talk
Prayer	Private conversations with a higher power; meditation	Useful for segments of the population who find it a source of inner strength

Adapted from Lorig, K. (1992). *Patient education: a practical approach* (ed. 2). Thousand Oaks: Sage Publications.

not change as one matures or adapts in new situations, such as illness.

Expectancy theory maintains that a person's motivation is based on an expectation of success or failure. If the patient expects to go home the morning after a laparoscopic cholecystectomy, she is more likely to do so than a patient who expects to stay in the hospital 2 or 3 days. Learners try to live up to the expectations set both by themselves and by others. Learned helplessness is the idea that one is doomed to failure, no matter what. Depression is a common result. Learned helplessness has three causes.[24] The first separates helplessness caused by the patient himself and helplessness caused by other factors. For example, a smoker may believe he has a personality flaw—lack of will power—that will defeat his efforts to quit smoking. He believes his inability to quit smoking is caused by his own personal failure. He may, however, blame his inability to quit smoking on peer pressure. His inability to quit is caused by factors out of his control or external to himself. Notice how similar these concepts are to locus of control discussed earlier. The second cause of learned helplessness differentiates between global and specific causes. Global helplessness means that the patient

lacks confidence in his ability to do a wide range of things, from losing weight to graduating from school to quitting smoking. Specific helplessness focuses on one activity. The patient may be certain he can quit smoking but does not believe he can graduate from school. The third cause of learned helplessness distinguishes between what occurs occasionally and what occurs consistently, or a trait-state distinction. A trait is a stable personality characteristic. A state is temporary or transitory. Occasional or transient helplessness accounts for the patient's inability to lose weight during the Christmas holidays, even though he may be able to at other times during the year.

Self-efficacy is a concept closely related to learned helplessness and locus of control. Perceived self-efficacy is a person's judgment of her capabilities to organize and follow through a course of action required to achieve a designated level of performance.[24] Perceived self-efficacy has more to do with the person's belief that she is capable of accomplishing the goal than with her actual skill. Judgments about self-efficacy are based on skill mastery, modeling other's behaviors, verbal persuasion from others, and physiologic states. Self-efficacy has been positively related to activities such as coughing, deep breathing, and ambulation to prevent postoperative complications.[33] Self-efficacy theory is the connection between what we believe about ourselves and how we behave. Oetker-Black[33] suggests that self-efficacy is the vehicle by which preoperative teaching affects behavior change.

Stages of psychosocial adaptation to illness

Stages in emotional adjustment occur in all patients; however, the duration of each stage varies depending on the patient, the support system, and coping patterns. Transitions between stages are usually gradual and not clearly defined. The perioperative nurse will be able to assess the correct stage by listening to the patient. Lee[19]

describes these four stages as (1) impact, (2) regression, (3) acknowledgment, and (4) reconstruction. Fig. 10-3 compares Lee's four stages with Maslow's hierarchy of needs.[9,27]

Impact corresponds with the foundation of Maslow's pyramid—physiologic and safety needs. Patients experience fear, anxiety, and loss of control. They may feel threatened. This may be a patient's first encounter with mortality. Patients may be very discouraged and become present oriented, seeing only the here-and-now. They focus all their energy inward because they perceive survival as their primary goal. Those with an external locus of control wonder if they can influence the outcome of the

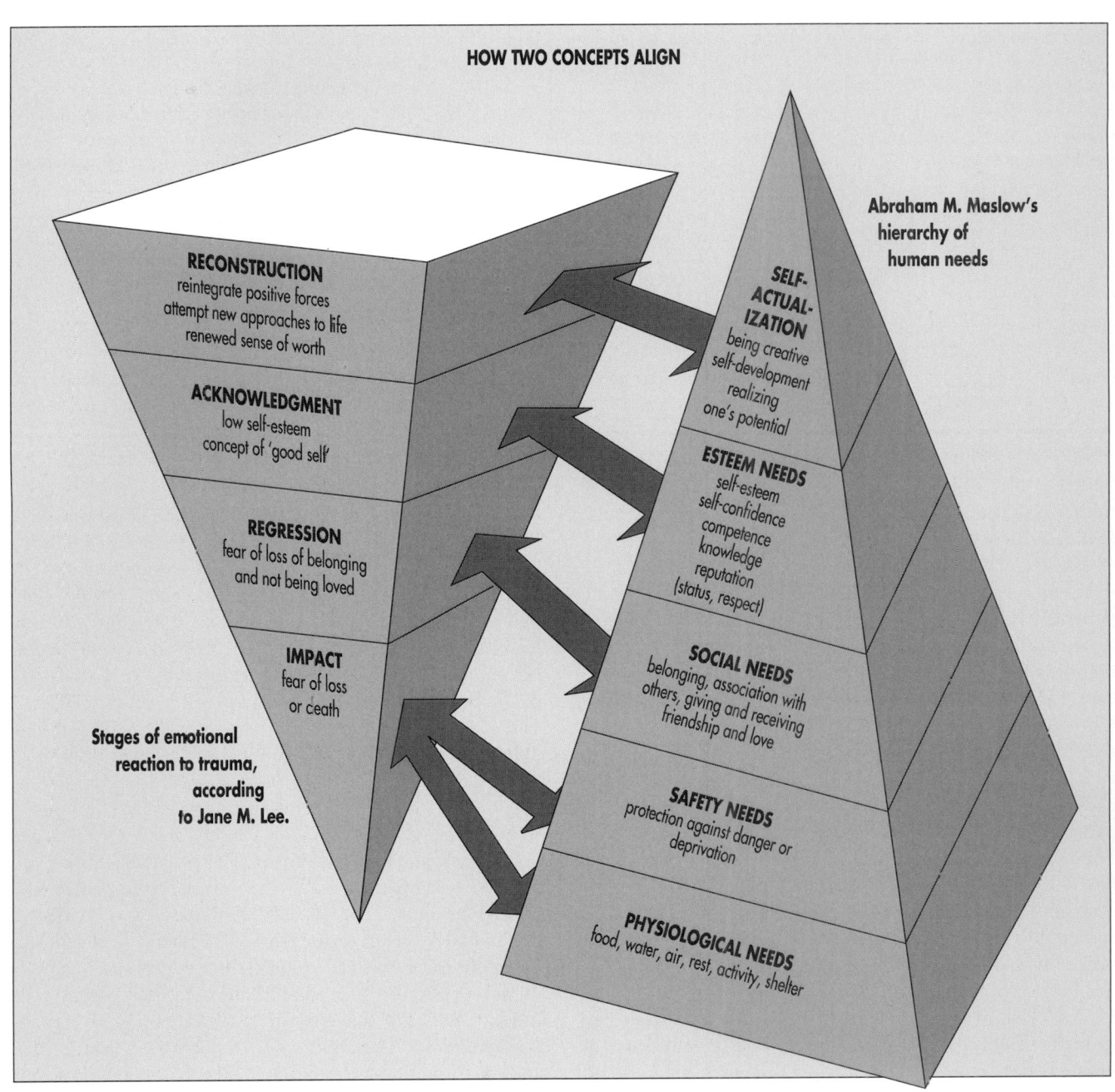

FIGURE 10-3   How two concepts align.

situation. Those with an internal locus of control may begin to operate from a learned helplessness mode.

Regression corresponds to Maslow's third level—social needs. Regression occurs when patients are forced to deal with their present reality and attempt to return to a time when they felt more emotionally comfortable. After regressing for a short time, they will be able to handle this crisis and mourn the loss of body image or self-esteem. In this stage, the sense of belonging is threatened. Patients may lash out in anger at the family or staff. If they succeed in driving people away, their fears of not being able to give or receive love will be reinforced. Accept the patient, but do not support the behavior. To help the patient through this stage, use realistic terms and specific time frames. "It will be 3 or 4 days before your intestines start to work again." They may joke about their illness or reveal unrealistic plans upon discharge. "I plan to play golf with my buddies on Wednesday." Again, respond in realistic terms, but try not to overwhelm them. Having been provided with a measure of psychologic safety, they will move on to the next stage.

Many perioperative nurses do not recognize teaching as such during the impact and regression stages. Although little response is produced, therapeutic instruction helps the patient when moving into subsequent stages. At this point, families may benefit more from teaching than the patient because families may be ahead of patients in terms of adjusting to the crisis. In turn, they will be able to reinforce information when the patient is ready.

Acknowledgment parallels Maslow's fourth level—esteem needs. Patients have little self-confidence and self-respect and may express loss and fear of abandonment: "I'm such a burden to my family like this." As unlikely as it seems, this is the time when effective teaching, in the traditional sense, may begin. Patients realize that they have survived their crisis and are reviewing the events in an attempt to prevent them from recurring. Patients give subtle signs that they have accepted changes in body image: "I thought the colostomy would be bigger." This indicates the patient has actually looked at it. They also begin to make provisions for the future: "Can I get this incision wet? I'd like to take a shower." Soon they will perceive their own need for information, leading them to the last stage.

Reconstruction parallels Maslow's fifth level—self-actualization. This is the most creative and positive stage because patients perceive hope for the future. Even though many patients cannot resume their lives exactly where they left off, they experience a renewed sense of self-worth. Patients start to plan new approaches for old behaviors. They will be very concerned about the future; therefore, instruction should be positive.

Discharge Planning

Even though discharge planning is often considered a postoperative activity, assessment of the patient's needs upon discharge should begin in the preoperative phase, preferably as a preadmission strategy in the ambulatory surgery setting.[6] A preliminary assessment of the patient's and family's understanding of the knowledge and skills required to care for the patient will often make educational needs apparent. Discharge planning must be more than just preparing the patient to leave the healthcare setting. Discharge planning is "preparing for moving the patient from one level of care to another within or outside the current health care agency."[26] Perioperative nurses are becoming more responsible for discharge planning because of the tremendous increase in same-day surgical procedures. The most significant contribution the perioperative nurse can make is to beginning discharge planning early, preferably before or on admission. The perioperative nurse may be the individual who determines if the patient meets the criteria for discharge and then communicates and documents discharge plans. The perioperative nurse is in a unique position to begin the discharge-planning process by asking a single question: "Will this patient go home?" (Fig. 10-4). Taking into account the patient's physical and mental abilities previously discussed, the patient's preferences and rights, and the physician's recommendations, can this patient function well enough after surgery to meet his activities of daily living needs in the environment from which he came? If the answer is yes, a brief appraisal can determine if his existing support systems are adequate (see Fig. 10-4). Does this family have enough resources to assist this patient at whatever level of care he will need on discharge? Required resources may range from providing taxi services to and from the physician's office for follow-up visits to changing dressings, cooking meals, and grocery shopping. Does this family need unskilled assistance such as transportation or housekeeping? What community resources, such as church ministries, are available to this patient and family? Does this patient need skilled care such as complicated wound management provided by a registered nurse? Can this patient get the medications prescribed? Does this patient need home health equipment such as a bedside commode or wheelchair? Discharge activities may include (1) arranging for maintenance or follow-up care with the physician or nurse practitioner, (2) helping the family create a supportive environment at home, (3) encouraging self-care philosophy, (4) coordinating referrals to financial or social services, home care agencies, or outreach programs, (5) evaluating and arranging the need for care giver support, and (6) arranging for discharge.

If the answer to the initial question "Will this patient go home?" is no, the patient needs a more in-depth evaluation of the level of care needed after the surgical intervention (see Fig. 10-4). An in-depth evaluation is more often needed in an inpatient or acute care setting than in a day surgery or ambulatory setting. Once the perioperative nurse suspects that the patient may not be able to return to his presurgical environment, early referral is essential. The perioperative nurse's partners in discharge planning are the case manager and social worker. Early referral to the case manager or social worker shortens the

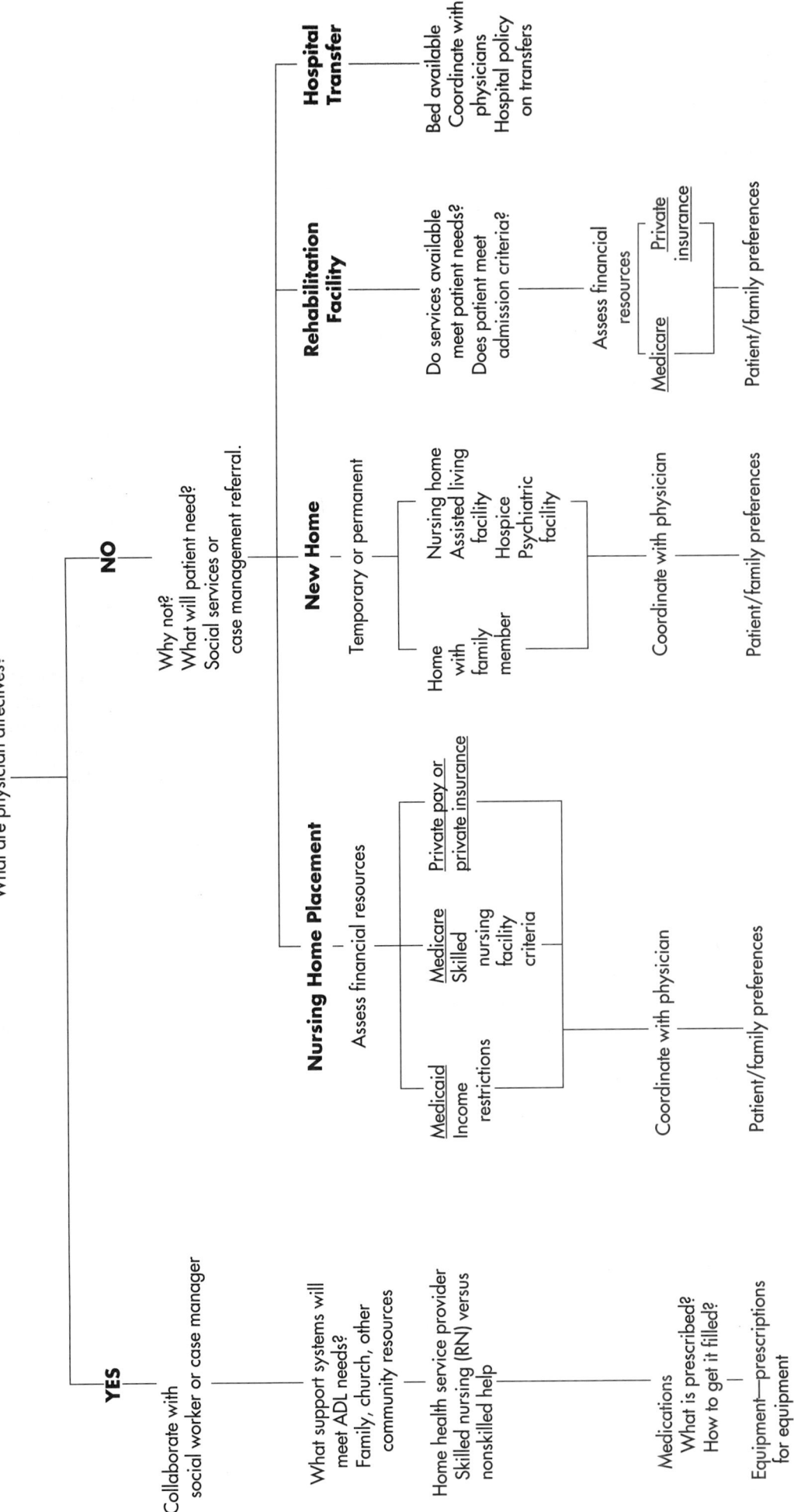

FIGURE 10–4 Discharge screening and planning.

length of stay and prevents readmissions.[11] Perioperative nurses have little information about community resources, Medicare and Medicaid regulations, extended care facilities, and subacute care units. They may find themselves overwhelmed by the maze of rules and regulations faced when discharge planning. Social workers, on the other hand, are familiar with community resources and regulations but know little about the patient's educational needs, physical capabilities, nursing requirements, or home care needs. The case manager coordinates the activities of all hospital services, including social services, and provides clinical expertise about patient physical and psychological needs during an acute care episode. The second most important contribution the perioperative nurse can make is providing clinical information about the surgical procedure and the patient's response. This information helps the social worker and the case manager arrange appropriate placement and follow-up care. Having assessed the patient's discharge needs during the preoperative and postoperative phases, the perioperative nurse helps the patient and family prepare for discharge. This requires collaboration with and coordinating the efforts of the other members of the health care team (see Research Highlight 10-3).

PLANNING

Models for Planning Patient Education

Two models widely used to plan and organize patient education programs are the PRECEDE model and the health belief model.[24] A model is a structure or conceptual framework for organizing things. Models can also help us understand why people behave the way they do and what works when they are changing behaviors. The PRECEDE model is a means of looking at predisposing, enabling, and reinforcing factors when planning an educational program (Fig. 10-5).

Predisposing factors can be either beliefs or benefits. The nurse's goal is to determine what the predisposing factors are and in which category they fall. People generally have rational reasons for doing what they do. We may not agree with the reason, but that doesn't matter. For example, if a patient believes spinal anesthesia always causes headaches, it is not surprising when she chooses general anesthesia instead. To change beliefs, the nurse must first find out what they are. An excellent way to do this is to ask, "What do you think will happen if . . ." (then adding the desired behavior) ". . . you have a spinal anesthetic?" Once you know the belief, the plan can include information to change it: "Headaches after a spinal happen only rarely." Be prepared for those times when you cannot change a belief, particularly if it is a dearly held cultural or religious belief. In these cases, helping a person broaden an interpretation of the belief may accomplish behavior change and improve self-efficacy. The second category of predisposing factors is benefits—the secondary gain from having this illness. Is this illness being used to get out of work or get attention from family and friends? Behavior change is unlikely to occur until the benefits for maintaining cease. For example, the number of smokers

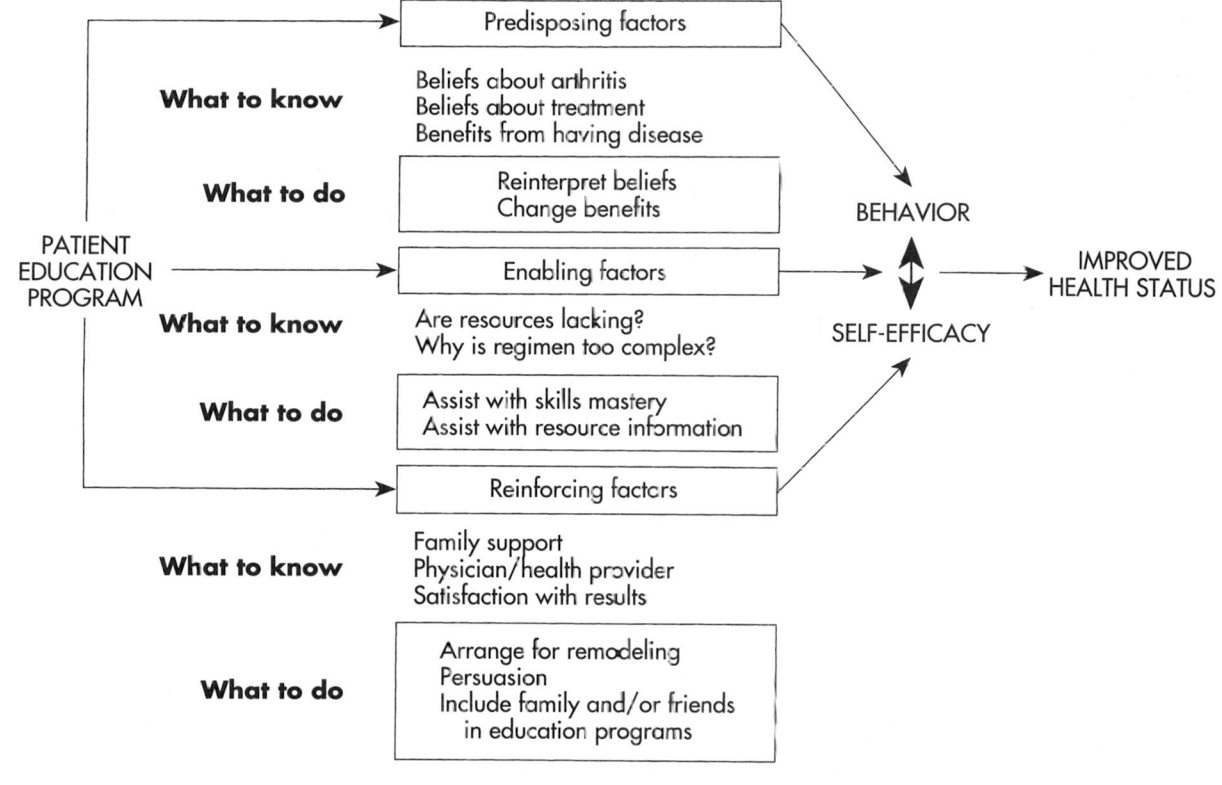

FIGURE 10-5   PRECEDE model.

has decreased with the decline in the social acceptability of smoking.

Enabling factors help people do what they should do and want to do but are unable to do. Two ways to enable people are by finding resources and by skills mastery. Putting resources where the person is can enable learning; skills mastery enables perpetual problem solving rather than simply fixing the situation at hand. Being too helpful too often can encourage dependence.

Reinforcing factors support the person's decision to change. Nurses can provide reinforcement through modeling, persuasion, and including families and friends and other healthcare providers in educational efforts. (More examples of reinforcement are discussed in the facilitating learning section of this chapter, p. 298). One final reinforcing factor is that, if behavior changes, people feel better. If a person consents to a cholecystectomy, the acute attacks of cholecystitis may stop.

The health belief model is one of the oldest and best known educational models (Fig. 10-6). It is based on the concept that people act according to perceived threats or expectations. Perceived threat has two components: perceived susceptibility and perceived severity. For example, although most healthcare providers believe that AIDS is a severe and deadly disease (high perceived severity), many demonstrate low perceived susceptibility by failing to wear gloves when they should. To change behaviors, people must have expectations that the new behavior will reduce their susceptibility or the severity of the condition, that the benefits to changing are

greater than the barriers, and that the behavior change can be accomplished. People engage in a subconscious or conscious cost-to-benefit analysis[34]: "If I have my uterus removed, it will hurt for several days and I will miss several weeks of work. But on the other hand, if I have my uterus out, I will stop bleeding so much. I will feel better and do a better job at work." Difficulty arises when the barriers to behavior change are obvious and the benefits are unpredictable. A good example is exercising and eating properly now to avoid vascular disease later in life.

Nursing Diagnosis

The nursing care plan provides a structured framework through which the nurse delivers nursing care. In the planning phase of the nursing teaching process, the perioperative nurse diagnoses the patient's educational needs, identifies desired outcomes, and plans nursing interventions. Only one of the nursing diagnoses that follow deals directly with an educational need. The other nursing diagnoses indirectly reflect the need for patient teaching. Many nursing diagnoses used by perioperative nurses have an inherent educational component. Killen[17] identified 38 nursing diagnosis used by perioperative nurses that either directly or indirectly required an educational intervention (Research Highlight 10-4). The perioperative nurse cannot isolate planning interventions to meet educational needs from the continuous reassessment and planning that occurs when providing other nursing care.

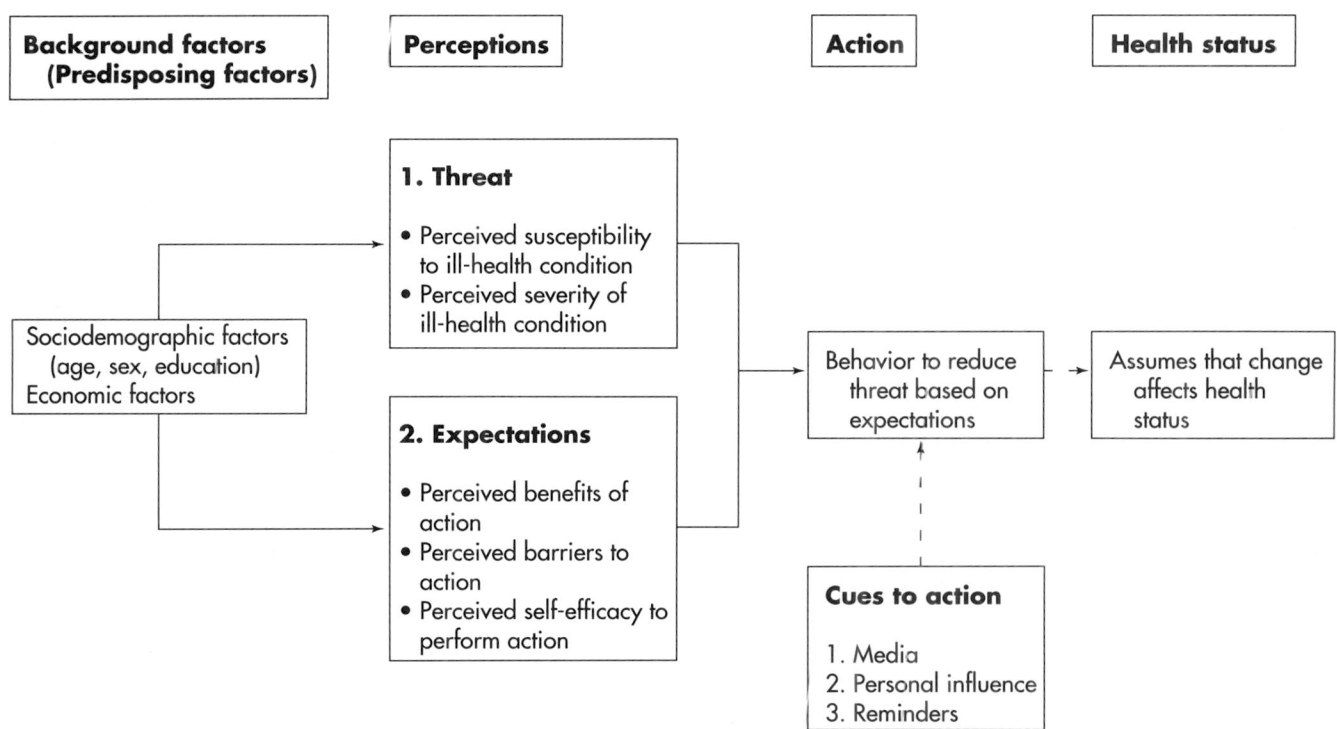

FIGURE 10-6 Health belief model.

Nursing diagnoses related to the educational needs of the preoperative patient may include the following:

- Decisional conflict regarding the treatment options
- Anxiety
- Knowledge deficit regarding planned surgical intervention

A nursing diagnosis related to the educational needs of the postoperative patient may include pain.

10-4 RESEARCH HIGHLIGHT

A clinical judgment about a patient occurs before a perioperative nurse chooses nursing activities and identifies outcomes. The North American Nursing Diagnosis Association (NANDA) nomenclature (nursing diagnosis) is the accepted language for naming the nurse's clinical judgment. Researchers for the Association of Operating Room Nurses, Inc., designed a study that rated the frequency and treatment priority of 60 nursing diagnoses. It also investigated whether, in the percentage of direct care provided, the employment position or the educational background of the perioperative nurse affected the frequency of the nursing diagnosis reported. The sample was drawn from the AORN membership database. Respondents ranked two critical diagnoses (risk for perioperative positioning injury and risk for infection) in the high-frequency and high-priority category more than 50% of the time. Primary diagnoses represent the foundations of perioperative practice. Respondents reported 24 primary nursing diagnoses that occurred less than 50% of the time and that associated conditions required a moderate to high priority of nursing attention. Four primary diagnoses—pain, anxiety, fear, and knowledge deficit—lend themselves readily to patient and family educational interventions. Respondents identified secondary diagnoses that occur infrequently, but associated conditions required a moderate priority of nursing attention. Secondary diagnoses appear to reflect conditions that occur outside the intraoperative phase of the patient's surgical experience but may very well occur in the immediate preoperative or postoperative phases. For example, impaired verbal communication or acute confusion may be diagnoses that require the perioperative nurse to intervene with patient and family education as more ambulatory procedures are performed. Nurses who spent less than 50% of their time in direct patient care, such as educators and clinical nurse specialists, and those with baccalaureates or higher degrees ranked critical diagnoses as occurring significantly more frequently.

From Killen, A.R., Kleinbeck, S.V.R., Golar, G., et al. (1997). The prevalence of perioperative nurse clinical judgments. *AORN Journal, 65*(1), 101-108.

Decisional conflicts arise when the decision maker must consider one or more options. A classic example is the surgical treatment options for breast cancer with a tumor mass less than 2 cm in size and no skin involvement. Different options afford the patient an excellent 10-year survival rate. The options have advantages and disadvantages. The decision maker may take or avoid opportunities to seek further information. Decisional conflict and the accompanying emotional distress occur when one of three conditions is present.[34] First, a conflict can arise when the patient has a treatment preference, such as nutritional or faith healing, but was not offered this option or was discouraged from using it. Second, a conflict can arise when neither treatment option seems to have any advantages from the patient's perspective, and yet the patient must choose one. Third, conflict can occur when the patient prefers one of the offered treatment options, but a significant person prefers the other alternative. For example, when the surgeon strongly recommends mastectomy and the patient prefers lumpectomy and radiation, the situation can be particularly stressful because the patient depends on the physician for medical care. Families can also contribute to the conflict by adding their views regarding what the patient should do. A patient's decision-making ability may be so impaired by anxiety, fear, and interpersonal conflict that she is unable to make the choice and definitive treatment is significantly delayed.

Anxiety is present in most surgical patients to a certain degree. Anxiety is the uneasiness and apprehension the patient feels without being able to identify the precise cause. Anxiety interferes with the patient's ability to concentrate, recall information, and process new information. In the preoperative patient, anxiety may be attributable to threats to the patient's self-concept, socioeconomic status, role functioning, patterns of interacting, or fear of dying. The surgical patient may be anxious about the way the surgical intervention will alter essential values and life goals.[12] Clues that the patient is experiencing high levels of anxiety are increased heart and respiratory rates, elevated blood pressure, voice and hand tremors, insomnia, and poor eye contact. The patient may be able to say that he or she is uptight or nervous or may express concern about changes in his or her life.

Knowledge deficit occurs when the patient lacks specific information. The unknown is often the cause of anxiety in preoperative patients. Signs of knowledge deficit are inappropriate or exaggerated behaviors such as hysteria, overt hostility, agitation, or apathy, inaccurate followthrough of instruction, inadequate return demonstration, a request for more information, or verbalization of the problem. When the knowledge deficit relates directly to the surgical procedure, the surgeon is responsible for informing patients of the nature, risks, and benefits of the procedure. The perioperative nurse's role is to enhance and reinforce this information. The perioperative nurse may be responsible for ensuring that an informed consent has been obtained and documented in the health record according to institutional policy.

Pain for the postoperative patient is most often inadequately controlled incisional pain. Signs of pain include guarding or protecting the incision, facial expression such as grimace or rigid affect, increased respiratory and pulse rates, diaphoresis, and elevated blood pressure. The patient may withdraw from contact with friends and family and focus energy inward in an attempt to deal with the pain. Pain interferes with the patient's perception of time and critical thinking skills. The simplest and most reliable method to diagnose pain is to ask the patient.[2] Behavior or vital signs cannot substitute for a self-report because patients may hide pain from the nurse and family as a coping mechanism. Pain-assessment tools are extremely useful in diagnosing the intensity and affective distress of pain. Samples of commonly used pain-intensity scales appear in Box 10-1.

Outcome Identification

The Association of Operating Room Nurses (AORN) recently revised and expanded their *Patient Outcomes: Standards of Perioperative Care* (Research Highlight 10-5). Standards 3.1 through 3.7 specifically deal with the patient's knowledge of the physiologic responses to the surgical intervention, medication management, pain control, wound healing, and active participation in rehabilitation. Standards 4.1 and 4.4 examine outcomes for informed consent and decision making that require educational interventions. Standards 5.1 and 5.2 address pain control and the uniqueness of every patient. Outcome identification based on these standards should explicitly state the desired behavior; however, as was with diagnoses, outcomes may not explicitly indicate that an educational need was met. For example, the desired outcome for Standard 3.7 "The patient demonstrates knowledge of wound healing,"[5] should be explicitly stated as "The patient communicates anticipated events during wound healing of his or her midline abdominal incision and abdominal drain site." A behavior in the outcome may indicate that the educational need was met. Many outcomes imply that learning occurred and the patient was motivated to change a behavior. Outcomes identified for the selected nursing diagnoses could be stated as:

- The patient will consent to a specific treatment option.
- The patient will verbalize feeling a lower level of anxiety.
- The patient will communicate the sequence of events in the perioperative period.
- The patient will identify a lower level of pain on a pain-intensity scale.

Care Plans Specific to Each Diagnosis

After diagnosing the educational needs and specifying outcomes, the perioperative nurse must plan interventions

---

BOX 10-1 | **Examples of Pain-Intensity Scales**

Simple Descriptive Pain-Intensity Scale*

No pain | Mild pain | Moderate pain | Severe pain | Very severe pain | Worst possible pain

0-10 Numeric Pain-Intensity Scale*

0 1 2 3 4 5 6 7 8 9 10
No pain | Moderate pain | Worst possible pain

Visual Analog Scale (VAS)†

No pain | Pain as bad as it could possibly be

From Acute pain management guideline panel. (1992a). *Acute pain management in adults: operative procedures: quick reference guide for clinicians.* (AHCPR Publication No. 92-0019). Rockville, Md.: Agency for Health Care Policy and Research.
*If used as a graphic rating scale, a 10 cm baseline value is recommended.
†A 10 cm baseline value is recommended for VAS scales.

10-5 RESEARCH HIGHLIGHT

A data element is the smallest unit of information that has meaning and can be electronically measured. The challenge to perioperative nursing is not only to list all data elements that characterize perioperative nursing as a specialty practice, but also to identify data elements that positively affect patient outcomes. In a survey, perioperative nurses were asked to link the Association of Operating Room Nurses, Inc. (AORN) *Patient Outcomes: Standards of Perioperative Care* and nursing action statements in *AORN's Competency Statements for Perioperative Nursing.* The initial survey was revised to contain 91 perioperative nursing actions listed under six patient outcome standards. The second survey asked respondents to indicate whether the nursing actions were relevant to patient outcomes. Respondents in the second survey validated 17 specific nursing actions that directly affected the AORN Outcome Standard 1, *The patient demonstrated knowledge of the physiological and psychological responses to surgical interventions.* They also validated seven specific nursing actions that directly affected the AORN Outcome Standard 6, *The patient participates in the rehabilitation process.* Based on this survey, the researchers recommended that the *Patient Outcomes: Standards of Perioperative Care* be updated and expanded.

From Kleinbeck, S.V.M. (1996). In search of perioperative nursing data elements. *AORN Journal, 63*(5), 926-931.

to help the patient achieve those outcomes. The University of Iowa's Nursing Intervention Classification (NIC) research project defines nursing interventions, nursing activities, nurse-initiated treatments, and physician-initiated treatments as follows:[26]

Nursing interventions

Any direct care treatment that a nurse performs on behalf of the client. Nursing interventions include nurse-initiated treatments and physician-initiated treatments. Nursing intervention labels are at the conceptual level and require a series of actions or activities to carry them out.

Nursing activities

Those behaviors or actions that nurses do to assist clients to move toward a desired outcome. Nursing activities are at the concrete level of action.

Nurse-initiated treatment

Interventions initiated by the nurse in response to a nursing diagnosis: "an autonomous action based on scientific rationale that is executed to benefit the client in a predicted way related to the nursing diagnosis and stated goals."

Physician-initiated treatments

Interventions that are initiated by the physician in response to a medical diagnosis and carried out by the nurse in response to a "doctor's order."

A care plan for the preoperative patient that incorporates the selected diagnoses and outcomes follows. Interventions in these care plans indicate how the nurse may directly or indirectly meet the patient's educational needs for each diagnosis. Again, planning to meet the educational needs of the patient is impossible to separate from planning other

---

SAMPLE CARE PLAN

Nursing Diagnosis: Decisional conflict regarding the treatment options.
Outcome: The patient will consent to a specific treatment option.
Interventions:
Active listening. Attending closely to and attaching significance to a patient's verbal and nonverbal messages.
Cognitive restructuring. Challenging a patient to alter distorted thought patterns and view self and the world more realistically.
Decision-making support. Providing information and support for a patient who is making a decision regarding health care.
Family involvement. Facilitating family participation in the emotional and physical care of the patient.
Referral. Arrangement for services by another care provider or agency.
Self-esteem enhancement. Assisting a patient to increase his or her judgment of self-worth.
Teaching: disease process. Assisting the patient to understand information related to a specific process.
Nursing Diagnosis: Anxiety.
Outcome: The patient will verbalize feeling a lower level of anxiety.
Interventions:
Admission care. Facilitating entry of a patient into a health care facility.
Anxiety reduction. Minimizing apprehension, dread, foreboding, or uneasiness related to the unidentified source of anticipated danger.
Learning-readiness enhancement. Improving the ability and willingness to receive information.
Surgical preparation. Providing care to a patient immediately before surgery and verifying required procedures, tests, and documentation in the clinical record.
Teaching: preoperative. Assisting the patient to understand and mentally prepare for surgery and the postoperative recovery period.
Touch. Providing comfort and communication through purposeful tactile contact.
Nursing Diagnosis: Knowledge deficit with regard to planned surgical intervention.
Outcome: The patient will communicate the sequence of events in the perioperative period.
Interventions:
Learning facilitation. Promoting the ability to process and comprehend information.
Teaching: disease process. Assisting the patient to understand information related to a specific process.
Teaching: preoperative. Assisting a patient to understand and mentally prepare for surgery and postoperative recovery period.
Nursing Diagnosis: Pain.
Outcome: The patient will identify a lower level of pain on a pain-intensity scale.
Interventions:
Pain management. Alleviation of pain or a reduction in pain to a level of comfort that is acceptable to the patient.
Patient-controlled analgesia (PCA). Facilitating patient control of analgesic administration and regulation.
Touch. Providing comfort and communication through purposeful tactile contact.
Simple relaxation therapy. Use of techniques to encourage and elicit relaxation for the purpose of decreasing undesirable signs and symptoms such as pain, muscle tension, or anxiety.

interventions. Each intervention is defined according to the NIC.[26]

IMPLEMENTATION

Nursing Activities: Case Studies

Nursing interventions are conceptual labels that require activities to carry them out. Nursing activities are how nurses help patients reach a specified outcome (see Research Highlights 10-1 and 10-2). They are concrete behaviors. Nursing activities can be either nurse initiated or physician initiated. This section is an analysis of the implementation of nursing activities for selected nursing interventions in the planning section. In the case studies to follow, there may not be a separate nursing intervention that deals with meeting education needs. However, there are nursing activities within every intervention that deal directly or indirectly with meeting educational needs. These nursing activities involve more than merely instructing or informing the patient. Teaching is an interpersonal interaction that includes assessing readiness and current knowledge, facilitating learning, establishing rapport, trust, and mutual respect, reducing anxiety, and evaluating learning and the activities of instruction. The perioperative nurse adjusts nursing activities to meet the educational needs of the individual patient in the following case studies. Many nursing activities specific to one diagnosis will overlap nursing activities specific to another diagnosis.

Decisional conflict regarding treatment options

Mrs. Adams is a 44-year-old bookkeeper who underwent a left breast biopsy 1 week ago. The pathologic diagnosis is invasive intraductal carcinoma. The surgeon discussed treatment options with both Mr. and Mrs. Adams. Mrs. Adams has been scheduled for a quadrantectomy and left axillary lymphadenectomy at a free-standing ambulatory surgery center. The perioperative nurse visits Mr. and Mrs. Adams in the preoperative admitting area. As soon as Mr. Adams leaves the room, Mrs. Adams confides to the nurse that she is not all that sure about having this procedure. She then berates herself for being "wishy-washy" about making a decision. She confesses that she and her mother have had considerable conflict over her original decision to have lumpectomy and radiation rather than mastectomy. Mrs. Adams asks the nurse if she has heard anything about radiation causing cancer rather than curing it.

Nursing Diagnosis

Decisional conflict regarding the treatment options.

Outcome

The patient will consent to a specific treatment option.

Intervention

Active listening. Attending closely to and attaching significance to a patient's verbal and nonverbal messages.

Nursing Activities

Active listening requires undivided attention. Fiddling with IV lines and doing paperwork while listening will send the message that the perioperative nurse is too busy or uninterested. Display interest by maintaining eye contact and leaning toward the patient. Acknowledge understanding by saying "I see" or "I hear you." Encourage the patient to say more by saying "I'm listening" or "Go on." Clarify ambiguous messages from the patient. "You said 'they' don't think lumpectomy is a good choice. Who are 'they'?" Reflecting or repeating the patient's own words back to her can produce more detail.

> Patient: "The idea of radiation really scares me."
> Nurse: "Having radiation scares you?"
> Patient: "Yes, my mother says radiation can cause this problem."

Interpreting what the patient means can also facilitate the active listening process. Notice what words the patient may be avoiding. These are nonverbal clues to underlying fears.

> Patient: "Yes, my mother says radiation caused this problem."
> Nurse: "Are you fearful of getting cancer somewhere else if you choose radiation over mastectomy?"

Reactions that portray disgust, disapproval, embarrassment, impatience, or boredom will block communication. Although the perioperative nurse may be inwardly horrified that the patient may be considering no treatment at all, responses should be unbiased and empathetic. "What you're feeling is understandable. This decision must be very difficult for you." If a series of interactions with the patient is possible, you may identify predominant themes.

Intervention

Cognitive restructuring. Challenging a patient to alter distorted thought patterns and view self and the world more realistically.

Nursing Activities

Help the patient accept that self-statements elicit emotional arousal and that the inability to make this decision may be attributable to irrational self-statements. The self-statement "I'll never be able to make such an awful decision, I'm so wishy-washy" is self-defeating. The self-statement "I'm having difficulty making a decision right now" presents a challenge. Help the patient recognize that some of her beliefs are inaccurate. Overgeneralization, polarized thinking, and magnification of the problem can lead to dysfunctional thinking. "What evidence supports your mother's belief that radiation to the breast will cause you to have cancer somewhere else?" Replace faulty interpretations with accurate information and reality-based interpretations of the situation. Help the patient to label the uncomfortable emotions and identify perceived stressors (such as interactions with family, the diagnosis). "Are you feeling hopeless (angry, fearful, etc.) since you've been diagnosed with breast cancer?"

Intervention

Decision-making support. Providing information and support for a patient who is making a decision regarding health care.

Nursing Activities

These nursing activities build on those used in cognitive restructuring. Establishing a relationship with the patient early in admission may give the perioperative nurse more time. Determine if there is a difference between the patient's view and your view of the patient's condition. The patient may believe the diagnosis of any kind of cancer is an automatic death sentence. The nurse knows that, since the tumor was smaller than 2 cm and there are no palpable axillary nodes, the patient's chances for cure are very high. Determine if the patient understands the difference in the two alternative treatment options for breast cancer. Help the patient identify the advantages and disadvantages of each option. Assist the patient in articulating what she believes the goals of treatment should be. The nurse can serve as a liaison between Mrs. Adams and her husband as well as the surgeon. You should be familiar with the policies of the institution regarding informed consent.

Intervention

Family involvement. Facilitating family participation in the emotional and physical care of the patient.

Nursing Activities

When involving the family in Mrs. Adams's care, you must first determine which family members she prefers, how much information she will allow to be given to the family, and which family members are capable of and desire to be involved in her care. You must also identify what the family expects of Mrs. Adams in this situation and how informed they are about Mrs. Adams's situation and care. In doing so, you will be able to assess the learning needs of the family members to be involved and initiate nursing activities to meet those needs.

Intervention

Referral. Arrangement for services by another care provider or agency.

Nursing Activities

In Mrs. Adams's case, you should refer her to the surgeon. Relate your observations and professional opinion of the causes of the decisional conflict to the surgeon. Decisional conflicts are frequently caused by lack of understanding or misconceptions. The solutions to decisional conflict are often found in patient teaching. Assist the surgeon in knowing what information Mrs. Adams

needs. Furthermore, you can clarify misconceptions and reinforce accurate information after the surgeon leaves. You may be asked to begin physician-initiated interventions, such as teaching about the disease process, after the surgeon and Mr. and Mrs. Adams have talked.

Anxiety

Mr. Caldwell is a 66-year-old retired football coach scheduled for an inguinal herniorrhaphy through the ambulatory surgery department of a small community hospital with two operating rooms. Ambulatory surgery patients are admitted directly to the holding area for admission procedures. Mr. Caldwell is to have local anesthesia and IV sedation monitored by a CRNA. He is accompanied by his wife and adult son. When the perioperative nurse enters the holding area, Mr. Caldwell is pacing beside the stretcher and has refused to change into a hospital gown.

Nursing Diagnosis

Anxiety.

Outcome

The patient will verbalize feeling a lower level of anxiety.

Intervention

Admission care. Facilitating entry of a patient into a health care facility.

Nursing Activities

Begin by introducing yourself and briefly describing the role you will play in Mr. Caldwell's procedure. Pull the drapes around the bed to provide privacy for the patient and family. In the initial interview, document the admission history, nursing assessment (physical exam, psychosocial history, educational needs), and informed consent as required by institutional policy. Ensure that the patient is properly identified. Begin planning for Mr. Caldwell's needs upon discharge. Carry out the admitting physician's orders.

Intervention

Anxiety reduction. Minimizing apprehension, dread, foreboding, or uneasiness related to the unidentified source of anticipated danger.

Nursing Activities

Establish and cement the patient and nurse relationship through active listening while providing admission care. Create an atmosphere of trust by displaying respect. Allow Mr. Caldwell to remain in his street clothes as long as possible. He may feel safer, less vulnerable, and more in control in his own clothes. Begin by making an observation about his behavior and stating what your expectations for his behavior are: "You seem a little jittery. I'd like to help you feel calmer." Explain all procedures, including the sensations likely to be experienced during the procedure. "You will feel a burning sensation while the numbing medicine is being injected. After that, you may feel pressure and pulling. You should not feel anything sharp." Seek to understand Mr. Caldwell's perspective of this stressful situation. Reinforce his behavior when his anxiety level decreases. "You seem calmer. You are sitting down instead of pacing." Judicious use of humor can also lower anxiety levels. "I'm here to take you to the room. That means it's about 5 minutes to kick-off." Stay with the patient as long as possible. Allow time for addressing his concerns.

Intervention

Surgical preparation. Providing care to a patient immediately before surgery and verification of required procedures and tests and documentation in the clinical record.

Nursing Activities

Verify Mr. Caldwell's identity orally and by checking his arm band. Determine his level of anxiety. Reinforce preoperative teaching information. Complete preoperative documentation as required by the institution, such as checklists, consent forms, and nursing assessment. Administer, explain, and document the use of preoperative medications as appropriate. Ensure that required preoperative lab work, ECG, and history and physical are on the chart. Start IV therapy, explaining the procedure, tubing, and equipment as needed. Support the family's needs with reassurance and information. Use supportive touch as appropriate. Solicit family assistance in keeping Mr. Caldwell's personal valuables.

Intervention

Teaching: preoperative. Assisting the patient to understand and mentally prepare for surgery and the postoperative recovery period.

Nursing Activities

Involve both Mr. Caldwell and his family in this intervention. Inform them of the scheduled time of surgery, keeping them updated if delays occur. Ensure that they know the approximate length of the procedure and stay in PACU. Familiarize the family with the locations of the waiting room and cafeteria. Discuss postoperative routines (medication, surgical dressings, ambulation, diet, activity). Discuss how Mr. Caldwell can assist in his own recovery (early ambulation, techniques for incision splinting and getting out of bed, coughing and deep breathing, limits on activity). Determine Mr. Caldwell's expectations of surgery and correct unrealistic expectations. Discuss possible pain control measures. Provide information on what Mr. Caldwell will hear, see, taste, and feel during the procedure and immediately after.

Knowledge deficit regarding treatment options

Mrs. Rhines is a 77-year-old retired English literature professor. She is a widow and has no children. She is accompanied by Mrs. Campbell, a friend who lives across the street. Mrs. Rhines still enjoys an occasional round of golf. She experienced a transient ischemic attack (TIA) that caused her to faint in her kitchen last week. She was admitted through the ambulatory surgery department for carotid arteriograms this morning. She is scheduled for a right carotid endarterectomy this afternoon. During the preoperative assessment Mrs. Rhines says, "I wish I understood more about this block in the vein in my neck. My surgeon explained some of it, but I didn't get it all."

Nursing Diagnosis

Knowledge deficit regarding planned surgical intervention.

Outcome

The patient will demonstrate knowledge of the physiologic and psychologic responses to surgery.

Intervention

Teaching: disease process. Assisting the patient to understand information related to a specific process.

Nursing Activities

Begin by determining what Mrs. Rhines knows about carotid artery disease. Reinforce and elaborate on information provided by other healthcare team members. Show her a drawing of the vessel. Point out on her neck where it is located. Draw in the distribution of plaque around the bifurcation. After the arteriogram, show her the exact location of the lesion. Explain the cause of the TIA. Discuss factors in the cause of vascular disease (genetic, life-style, aging, dietary, and physiologic responses to stress). Provide information about the diagnostic tests, carotid Doppler studies, and digital subtraction arteriography. Determine what she understands about the surgical procedure. Preoperative teaching may be necessary and can be included in this intervention.

Pain

Elliot Chambers is a 54-year-old man who owns his own construction company. He has undergone a sigmoid colon resection for severe diverticular disease. On the first postoperative day the perioperative nurse visits him in the surgical unit. He is pale and tense. When asked, he reports pain relief to be inadequate. He has a PCA pump set to give 3 mg of morphine every 15 minutes. When shown a 0-10 numeric pain intensity scale (see Box 10-1), he chooses the number 8.

Nursing Diagnosis

Pain.

Outcome

The patient will identify a lower level of pain on a pain-intensity scale.

Intervention

Patient-controlled analgesia (PCA). Facilitating patient control of analgesic administration and regulation.

Nursing Activities

Determine if Mr. Chambers received preoperative teaching on the use of the PCA pump. Preoperative teaching in its use enhances the patient's ability to manage postoperative pain.[40,45] Validate that Mr. Chambers and his family understand the use of the PCA pump, how to deliver the medication, the lockout interval, the effect of the medication, and the maximum dose feature. Teach him how to monitor the intensity and duration of pain. Collaborate with the surgical unit nurses in documenting inadequate pain relief at the current dosage. Recommend to the physician a loading dosage of 3 to 5 mg every 5 minutes until current pain is diminished and

then 2 to 3 mg every 10 minutes PRN with a 10 mg hourly maximum dose.[2] Use the pain-intensity scale to evaluate pain after loading dose. Collaborate with unit nurses for ongoing reassessment of pain relief using the pain-intensity scale.

Intervention

Simple relaxation therapy. Use of techniques to encourage and elicit relaxation for the purpose of decreasing undesirable signs and symptoms such as pain, muscle tension, or anxiety.

Nursing Activities

Describe the reason for and benefits of relaxation therapy. Determine if Mr. Chambers has any previous experiences with relaxation therapy. Consider his willingness and ability to participate. Create a quiet, soothing atmosphere by dimming lights and closing the door. Use a slow, rhythmic tone of voice. Use one of the relaxation exercises in Box 10-2, or consider using a guided imagery tape to assist Mr. Chambers in coping and relaxing.[25]

BOX 10-2 | Relaxation Exercises

Example 1: Deep Breathe/Tense, Exhale/Relax, Yawn for Quick Relaxation

1. Clench your fists; breathe in deeply and hold it a moment.
2. Breathe out slowly and go limp as a rag doll.
3. Start yawning.

Additional points: Yawning becomes spontaneous. It is also contagious, and so others may begin yawning and relaxing too.

Example 2: Slow Rhythmic Breathing for Relaxation

1. Breathe in slowly and deeply.
2. As you breathe out slowly, feel yourself beginning to relax; feel the tension leaving your body.
3. Now breathe in and out slowly and regularly, at whatever rate is comfortable for you. You may wish to try abdominal breathing. If you do not know how to do abdominal breathing, ask your nurse for help.
4. To help you focus on your breathing and breathing slowly and rhythmically: Breathe in as you say silently to yourself, "in, two, three." Breathe out as you say silently to yourself, "out, two, three," *or* each time you breathe out, say silently to yourself a word such as peace or relax.
5. You may imagine that you are doing this in a place you have found very calming and relaxing for you, such as lying in the sun at the beach.
6. Do steps 1 through 4 only once or repeat steps 3 and 4 for up to 20 minutes.
7. End with a slow deep breath. As you breathe out, say to yourself, "I feel alert and relaxed."

Additional points: If you intend to do this for more than a few seconds, try to get in a comfortable position in a quiet environment; you may close your eyes or focus on an object. This technique has the advantage of being very adaptable in that it may be used for only a few seconds or for up to 20 minutes.

Example 3: Peaceful Past

Something may have happened to you a while ago that brought you peace and comfort. You may be able to draw on that past experience to bring you peace or comfort now. Think about these questions:

1. Can you remember any situation, even when you were a child, when you felt calm, peaceful, secure, hopeful, comfortable?
2. Have you ever daydreamed about something peaceful? What were you thinking of?
3. Do you get a dreamy feeling when you listen to music? Do you have any favorite music?
4. Do you have any favorite poetry that you find uplifting or reassuring?
5. Have you ever been religiously active? Do you have favorite readings, hymns, or prayers? Even if you haven't heard or thought of them for many years, childhood religious experiences may still be very soothing.

Additional points: Very likely some of the things you think of in answer to these questions can be recorded for you, such as your favorite music or a prayer. Then you can listen to the tape whenever you wish. Or, if your memory is strong, you may simply close your eyes and recall the events or words.

Modified from McCaffery, M., & Beebe, A. (1989). *Pain: Clinical manual for nursing practice,* St. Louis: Mosby.

Selecting Content in Preoperative and Postoperative Teaching

Nursing research has recommended that selection of content for preoperative teaching be based on what the patient wants and needs to know[47] (see Research Highlights 10-1 and 10-2). The perioperative nurse can select content for an individual patient based on input from not only the patient and family and the nurse's own observations, but also from other healthcare team members. Selecting educational content specifically for families and significant others is also important. In addition to the procedural, sensory, temporal, coping, and reassurance content that the patient receives, families and significant others need information about what they can do as helping care givers.[41] Preoperative information falls into four broad categories:[47] (1) procedural, (2) sensory and temporal, (3) coping, and (4) reassurance. Not every patient needs or wants to know everything. Content should be selected on a need-to-know basis. The perioperative nurse selects the content appropriate for each patient, the institution, the amount of time allotted, and resources available.

Procedural information is a concrete description of which procedures are to be carried out and why. Box 10-3 lists possible procedural information that could be included in preoperative and postoperative content. Sensory and temporal information includes how the procedures will feel and how long they will take (Box 10-4). Table 10-3 has procedural, sensory, and temporal content for specific surgical procedures. Coping suggestions inform the patient of ways to control the emotional responses. These can include any of those listed in Table 10-2. Perioperative nurses frequently give global reassurances rather than specific information they believe the patient will find alarming or when time is extremely limited, as in emergency situations like trauma. "Your surgical team is highly skilled at this procedure. This hospital has the latest equipment." A combination of the salient points of all categories is the appropriate content. Booklets that provide simple procedural information, sensory and temporal experiences, suggestions on how to cope, as well as practical information about hospital admission procedures are welcomed by patients.[47]

Facilitating Learning

Facilitating learning can take a variety of forms. Since readiness to learn is an essential factor, nurses can enhance readiness to learn by addressing the patient's specific concerns first, minimizing sensory overload in the environment, providing time for the patient to ask questions, assisting the patient to realize what ability he has

Text continued on p. 304

BOX 10-3	Procedural Information in Preoperative Teaching

Location of surgery suite
Location of holding area
Location of surgery waiting area
Location of PACU
Location and tour of postsurgical unit and waiting area
Incision site
Planned alterations to anatomy and physiology by surgical intervention
Use of PCA pump
Splinting of the incision
Technique for getting out of bed postoperatively
Coughing and deep breathing
Use of incentive spirometer
Leg exercises
Description of preoperative routines
    Bowel preparation
    Diet and NPO
    Preoperative lab tests and diagnostic procedures
    Voiding
    Skin preparation
    ECG
    Preoperative sedation
Anesthesia
Description of postoperative routines
    Support hose
    Surgical dressings
    Diet
    Medications
    Respiratory treatments
    Machines
    Drains
    Nature of postoperative nursing assessments

BOX 10-4	Sensory and Temporal Information in Preoperative Teaching

Date and time of surgery
Time patient will leave room or ambulatory surgical unit (ASU)
Amount of time spent in the preoperative holding area
Length of surgical procedure
Length of stay in PACU
Length of hospital or ASU stay
Estimated time to full recovery
When diet can resume
When drains, cast, dressings, etc. will be removed
Hours of family visitation
Sights, sounds, and smells of preoperative holding area, OR, and PACU
Sensations during administration of local anesthesia
Sensations produced by preoperative medications
Taste of certain drugs used in anesthesia induction
Postoperative pain sensations
Sensations of the stretcher transport to and from surgery
Postoperative sensations specific to certain procedures (sore throat from endotracheal intubation)

TABLE 10-3 | Selecting Content for Teaching

	INGUINAL HERNIORRHAPHY	SIGMOID COLECTOMY	THORACOTOMY	CHOLECYSTECTOMY (OPEN OR LAPAROSCOPIC)	CAROTID ENDARTERECTOMY
Preoperative Pointers					
Medical diagnosis	Inguinal hernia	CA of sigmoid colon; diverticulitis	CA, primary or metastatic; for diagnosis; drain abscesses	Cholecystitis; cholelithiasis	Carotid stenosis
Diagnostic tests	History and physical exam	Barium enema, colonoscopy	CT of chest; bronchoscopy; needle biopsy; CME; thoracoscopy	Sonogram; HIDA scan; oral cholecystogram; blood amylase and bilirubin	Dopscan; arteriogram; CT of head
Routine preop tests	CBC, ECG if > 50	SMA 6/20, T&C if H&H low, bowel prep, ECG	Pulmonary functions, SMA 20, T&C, ECG	SMA 20, ECG	SMA 6/20, ECG
Incision site	Right or left lower quadrant	Lower midline or transverse	Lateral chest, fourth or fifth interspace	Open: right subcostal; lap: umbilicus, rt subcostal, RLQ, upper midline	Neck
Resume eating	ASAP	4-5 days when ileus resolves	2-3 days	Open: 2-3 days; lap: 2-6 hr	ASAP
Pain control	PO or IM	IM or PCA	PCA or epidural	IM, PCA, or PO	IM or PO
Estimated length of procedure	1-1½ hr	2½-3 hr	3-4 hr	1-1½ hr	1-1½ hr
Estimated length of hospital stay	Day surgery or 23 hr	6-8 days	7-8 days	Open: 3-5 days; lap: 12-23 hr	2-4 days
Long-term effects of surgery	Return to normal activities	Potential for temporary colostomy	Potential for reduced pulmonary functions	Rare bile salt imbalance	Potential for permanent or temporary neurologic deficit
Drains or tubes	None	Potential for colostomy bag; Foley catheter	2 chest tubes and suction; needed 2-4 days	Open: potential for T-tube/surgical drain; lap: drainage tube rare	Potential for drain; needed 1-2 days
Postoperative Pointers—Home Instructions					
Food	ASAP	Regular or low-residue diet	Regular diet	Regular diet	Regular or cardiac diet
Wound care	Change dressing PRN × 1-2 days, then none required except for comfort; ice pack is OK	Shower daily	Shower daily	Bathe or shower daily	Bathe or shower daily
Bathing	24-48 hr	Shower	Shower	Daily	Daily
Driving	2 to 4 weeks; and by limits of pain	In 10-14 days when soreness less	2-3 weeks when soreness less	Open: 1-2 wks when soreness less; lap: 2-4 days	In 5-7 days when soreness less

Modified from Fox, V.J. (1993, June). Preop and postop pointers. In *Getting ready for RNFA certification*. Association of Operating Room Nurses, Inc. Symposium, Lake Tahoe, NV. *ASAP*, As soon as possible; *CA*, cancer; *CBC*, complete blood cell count; *CEA*, carcinoembryonic antigen; *CME*, cervical mediastinal exploration; *CT*, computerized tomography; *ECG*, electrocardiogram; *ERCP*, endoscopic retrograde cholangiopancreatography; *H&H*, hematocrit and hemoglobin; *HIDA* is the acronym for the radioisotope hepato-iminodiacetic acid used in a hepatobiliary scan); *IOL*, intraocular lens; *IVP*, intravenous pyelogram; *lap*, laparoscopic; *MRI*, magnetic resonance imaging; *PCA*, patient-controlled analgesia; *PSA*, prostate-specific antigen; *PT*, prothrombin time; *PTCA*, percutaneous transluminal coronary angioplasty; *PTT*, partial thromboplastin time; *RLQ*, right lower quadrant; *T&C*, type and crossmatch.

Continued

TABLE 10-3 | Selecting Content for Teaching—cont'd

Postoperative Pointers—Home Instructions—cont'd

	INGUINAL HERNIORRHAPHY	SIGMOID COLECTOMY	THORACOTOMY	CHOLECYSTECTOMY (OPEN OR LAPAROSCOPIC)	CAROTID ENDARTERECTOMY
Sex	Restricted 2-3 wks and by limits of pain	Restricted 3-4 wks and by limits of pain	Restricted 3-4 weeks and by limits of pain	Restricted 2-3 weeks and by limits of pain for open; Lap: Restricted within limits of pain	Restricted within limits of pain
Return to work	2-6 weeks, depending on nature of work	6 weeks	6 weeks		2 weeks
Medications	Oral analgesics	Oral analgesics	Oral analgesics	Oral analgesics	Oral analgesics: aspirin
Follow-up	7-10 days	7-10 days	10-14 days	7-10 days	7-10 days
Special restrictions	Heavy lifting 4-6 weeks	Within limits of pain and energy; heavy lifting 4-6 weeks	Walking within limits of pain and energy; heavy lifting 4-6 weeks	Walking within limits of pain and energy	Within limits of pain and energy
Worrisome but normal	Swelling and bruising of penis and scrotum	Temporary colostomy closure 6-8 weeks	Noticeable incision pain 3-6 months		Temporary or permanent numbness of earlobe

	MASTECTOMY	VENTRAL HERNIORRHAPHY	SMALL BOWEL RESECTION	ABDOMINAL PERINEAL RESECTION	OPEN COMMON DUCT EXPLORATION
Preoperative Pointers					
Medical diagnosis	CA of breast	Incisional hernia	Small bowel obstruction; small bowel strangulation	CA of rectum	Common duct stone; common duct stricture
Diagnostic tests	History and physical exam; mammogram; breast biopsy	History and physical exam	History and physical exam; abdominal radiograph	Digital rectal exam; colonoscopy; rigid sigmoidoscopy	History and physical exam; ERCP
Routine preop tests	CBC, ECG if >50	CBC, ECG if >50	CBC, ECG if >50	CEA, SMA 6/20, CBC, ECG, T&C, bowel prep	SMA 6/20, ECG, CBC, amylase, bilirubin
Incision site	Right or left upper chest	Previous abdominal incision site	Midline or transverse	Midline or transverse	Right subcostal
Resume eating	ASAP	ASAP	4-5 days or when ileus resolves	4-5 days or when ileus resolves	1-3 days
Pain control	PO or IM	PO, IM, or PCA	IM or PCA	IM, PCA, or epidural	IM or PCA
Estimated length of procedure	1-1½ hr	1½-2 hr	1-2 hr	3-4 hr	1-1½ hr
Estimated length of hospital stay	24-48 hr	24-48 hr	5-7 days	6-8 days	1-3 days
Long-term effects of surgery	Potential for restricted movement in arm, lymphedema	Possibility of recurrence	Possibility of recurrence	Permanent colostomy	Potential for common duct stricture
Drains or tubes	1-2 Jackson-Pratt drains to stay 2-5 days	Jackson-Pratt drain to stay 2-5 days		Colostomy bag: Jackson-Pratt to stay 2-4 days; Possible posterior wound drain	T-tube to stay 10 days; potential for other surgical drain to stay 2-3 days
Postoperative Pointers—Home Instructions					
Food	Regular diet	Regular diet	Regular diet	Regular diet	Regular diet
Wound care	Empty drain and redress daily for comfort; ice pack is OK	Shower daily and redress	Bathe or shower daily	Shower daily; change perineal pad to posterior wound PRN	Shower daily; redress T-tube daily

Bathing	Daily—lower body	Shower	Shower	Shower	Shower
Driving	7-10 days when soreness less	7-10 days when soreness less	10-14 days when soreness less	2-3 weeks when soreness less	7-10 days when soreness less
Sex	Restricted within limits of pain	Restricted 4-6 weeks and by limits of pain	Restricted 2-3 weeks and by limits of pain	Restricted 2-3 weeks and by limits of pain	Restricted 2-3 weeks and by limits of pain
Return to work	4-6 weeks	6-10 weeks	4-6 weeks	6-10 weeks	2-4 weeks
Medications	Oral analgesics	Oral analgesics	Oral analgesics	Oral analgesics	Oral analgesics
Follow-up	7-10 days; 2-4 days if discharged with drain	7-10 days; 2-4 days if discharged with drain	10-14 days	10-14 days	10-14 days
Special restrictions	Begin arm and shoulder exercises within prescribed limits	Heavy lifting 6-10 weeks; walking within limits of pain and energy	Walking within limits of pain and energy; heavy lifting 2-3 wks	Walking within limits of pain and energy; heavy lifting 2-3 weeks	Walking within limits of pain and energy
Worrisome but normal	Numbness and tingling from elbow to axilla		Drainage from posterior wound particularly if left open	Drainage from posterior wound particularly if left open	Leaking of bile around T-tube

	CESAREAN DELIVERY	VAGINAL HYSTERECTOMY	TOTAL HIP REPLACEMENT	CATARACT EXTRACTION	CRANIOTOMY
Preoperative Pointers					
Medical diagnosis	Cephalopelvic disproportion; cord prolapse; fetal distress; abruptio placentae; placenta previa; breech presentation; previous cesarean section	Uterine prolapse; dysfunctional uterine bleeding; benign or malignant lesions	Degenerative joint disease	Cataracts	Subdural hematoma; malignant or benign lesions
Diagnostic tests	History and vaginal exam; fetal monitor	History and pelvic exam; biopsy of lesions; transvaginal sonogram	History; physical exam; x-ray film	History and slitlamp eye exam; keratometer, A scan	CT of head; neurologic assessment
Routine preop tests	CBC, T&C blood	SMA 6/20, T&C if H&H low	SMA 20, T&C, ECG	SMA 6, ECG if warranted	SMA 20, ECG
Incision site	Vertical or transverse	Through the vaginal opening; abdominal punctures if lap-assisted	In line with vertical axis of joint	Conjunctival flap	Head, depending on location of lesion
Resume eating	ASAP	1 day postop	ASAP	ASAP	ASAP
Pain control	PO or IM	IM or PO	PCA; epidural; IM; PO	PO, nonnarcotic	IM, PO, PCA
Estimated length of procedure	1 hr	1-1½ hr	2-3 hr	½-1 hr	1-1½ hr
Estimated length of hospital stay	3 to 4 days	2-4 days	7-8 days	4-6 hr	Variable depending on diagnosis and neurologic status
Long-term effects of surgery	May require subsequent cesarean delivery	Permanent sterilization	Reduced pain; potential for dislocation of prosthesis	Improved or restored vision; rarely change IOL	Potential for permanent or temporary neurologic deficit
Drains or tubes	Foley catheter	Foley catheter	Hemovac for 2 days	None	None
Postoperative Pointers—Home Instructions					
Food	Regular diet	Regular diet	Regular diet	Regular diet	Regular diet
Wound care	Change dressing PRN × 1-2 days; then none required	Bathe or shower daily	Shower may be easier than bathing	Eye patch and shield for 24 hr; then shield at night	Bathe or shower daily

Continued

TABLE 10-3 | Selecting Content for Teaching—cont'd

	CESAREAN DELIVERY	VAGINAL HYSTERECTOMY	TOTAL HIP REPLACEMENT	CATARACT EXTRACTION	CRANIOTOMY
Postoperative Pointers—Home Instructions—cont'd					
Bathing	12-24 hr	Daily	Shower	Bathe or shower after 24 hr	Daily
Driving	1 to 4 weeks	7-14 days when soreness less	Varies with MD preference; may be 2-6 weeks	2-7 days because of impaired depth perception	Depends on existence and extent of neurologic deficit
Sex	Restricted within limits of pain	3-6 weeks and by limits of pain	MD preference; limited by restrictions on internal and external rotation of joint	Restrictions by limitations on rigorous activity	Restricted within limits of pain
Return to work	6 weeks, depending on nature of work	2-4 weeks	6-12 weeks	3-7 days if work does not require rigorous activity	6-12 weeks
Medications	Oral analgesic	Oral analgesic	Oral analgesics; anticoagulant	Antibiotic and antiinflammatory drops; artificial tears	Oral analgesics
Follow-up	7-10 days	7-10 days	7-10 days	First day postop; then 7 days; then in 3-4 weeks	7-10 days
Special restrictions	Within limits of pain and energy; heavy lifting 4-6 weeks	Within limits of pain and energy; heavy lifting 2-4 weeks	Must keep knees lower than hips; may recline but may not sit in low chair or commode seat if lower than knees	Heavy lifting, bending, or rigorous activities for 7 days	Within limits of pain and energy
Worrisome but normal	Vaginal drainage	Vaginal drainage	Prolonged discomfort	Foreign-body sensation; dry eye; may see floaters	Lingering neurologic deficit

	RETROPUBIC PROSTATECTOMY	NEPHRECTOMY	RADICAL NECK DISSECTION	ARTHROSCOPY OF KNEE	CORONARY ARTERY BYPASS GRAFT
Preoperative Pointers					
Medical diagnosis	Malignant lesions	Malignant lesions; infectious or inflammatory processes that destroy kidney function	Malignant lesions of the mouth and neck	Torn meniscus; diagnostic purposes	Coronary artery occlusive disease
Diagnostic tests	Rectal sonogram control for needle biopsy	Arteriogram; sonogram; CT; IVP with retrograde pyelogram; radio-nucleotide renogram	Physical exam; CT; nasopharyngoscopy	Physical exam; MRI	ECG; stress test; chest radiograph; thallium scan; cardiac catheterization; interventions: PTCA, atherectomy, laser
Routine preop tests	CBC, ECG, T&C blood, PSA, and acid phosphatase	Renal functions (creatinine and electrolytes)	SMA 20, ECG	SMA 6, ECG if indicated	SMA 20, ECG, T&C, pulmonary function, PT, PTT

Incision site	Pfannenstiel or midline	Lateral for inflammatory disease; anterior for malignant lesions	T shape; horizontal extends along underside of mandible; vertical from jaw to sternal notch	3-4 stab incisions around patella	Midsternal, multiple leg incisions for vein harvest
Resume eating	ASAP	Lateral: ASAP; anterior: 2-3 days	ASAP	ASAP	2-3 days after removal of endotracheal and nasogastric tubes
Pain control	PO or IM	IM or PCA	IM or PO	PO	IM; PO, PCA
Estimated length of procedure	2-2½ hr	2 hr	2-2½ hr	1-2 hr	4-6 hr
Estimated length of hospital stay	4-6 days	5-7 days	3-5 days	4-6 hr	6-8 days
Long-term effects of surgery	Probably impotence; possibly incontinence	Remaining kidney hypertrophies up to ⅓ in size	Poor cosmetic effect; possible loss of trapezius muscle	Possibility of arthritic changes	Loss of saphenous vein, possible intermittent lower leg edema
Drains or tubes	Jackson-Pratt for 2-4 days; Foley catheter	Jackson-Pratt or other surgical drain for 2-4 days	Jackson-Pratt for 2-4 days	None	2 days: mediastinal chest tube; 2-3 days: pleural chest tube; 2-3 days: Hemovac in leg wounds

Postoperative Pointers—Home Instructions

Food	Regular diet	Regular diet	Regular diet	Regular diet	Cardiac diet
Wound care	Shower daily	Bathe or shower daily	Bathe or shower daily	Bathe or shower daily	Wounds covered it draining; redress after shower or bathe
Bathing	Shower	Shower	Shower	Daily	Daily
Driving	2-3 weeks when soreness less	2-3 weeks when soreness less	5-10 days when soreness less	2-4 days when soreness less	4-6 weeks (automatic shift only)
Sex	Restricted 2-3 weeks and by limits of pain and ability	Restricted 2-3 weeks and by limits of pain	Restricted within limits of pain	Restricted within limits of pain	Restricted by limits of ability to bear weight on upper arms and chest
Return to work	6-8 weeks	4-6 weeks	3-4 weeks	2-4 days, depending on nature of work	8-12 weeks
Medications	Oral analgesics	Oral analgesics	Oral analgesics	Oral analgesics	Aspirin anticoagulant; cardiac drugs
Follow-up	7-10 days	7-10 days	7-10 days	7-10 days	7-14 days
Special restrictions	Within limits of pain and energy	Within limits of pain and energy; should always avoid dangerous contact sports	Within limits of pain and energy	Limited weight bearing as tolerated	Upper body movement restricted for 6 weeks for sternal healing
Worrisome but normal	Impotence; incontinence		Inability to raise shoulder		Fatigue, swelling in leg, leg discomfort 4-6 weeks

to control the illness, and helping him to have confidence in his judgment.[35]

The perioperative nurse can use basic principles of motivation to enhance teaching and learning interactions.[37] Use the environment to focus the patient's attention on what he needs to know. A warm yet businesslike atmosphere is a successful strategy. Visual and tactile aids, such as a drawing of the biliary system or a sample of a vascular prosthesis, capture and hold the learner's interest. Incentives stimulate the motivation to learn. For some persons the payoff for learning is approval and praise from their family or healthcare providers. For others the enjoyment of reaching a goal is motivation enough. Others need more concrete incentives such as having special food as a treat. Internal, self-directed motivation to learn will last longer than external motivation. External motivation requires frequent positive reinforcement. Assessment data can give the nurse a place to start, but unless the patient buys into the plan, behavior change will be short lived or not occur at all.

A person will learn most effectively when he or she is ready to learn. Factors affecting readiness to learn and ways to enhance readiness have been discussed. If the need for change is urgent, the perioperative nurse is in a good position to encourage the development of readiness and supervise the patient's progress. Motivation is enhanced by structured educational materials. Better organized material is more meaningful and more effective. Success motivates better than failure. Design a learning experience that allows the learner to succeed. Learning takes place in small increments. The patient can easily be overwhelmed by too much, too soon. Practice and return demonstrations done in sequence allow the patient to succeed one step at a time. Learning is likely to create anxiety because it may require changes in beliefs and behavior. During high anxiety or stress periods, keep teaching and learning interactions to a minimum.

The perioperative nurse must help the learner set personal goals and provide feedback information about progress toward those goals. Goals are more likely to be met if the patient's behavior is reinforced and praised, if the content is tailored to the individual, if the perioperative nurse helps the patient take action, if the content is relevant, and if the teaching methods are meaningful and appealing to the patient.

As discussed earlier, there are three ways to enhance self-efficacy that, when used properly, can enhance learning.[24] First, skills mastery is based on the principle that success motivates better than failure. Skills mastery is accomplished by breaking the task into small manageable subtasks and ensuring that each subtask is completed successfully. Modeling is another way to enhance self-efficacy. Ideally the model should be an ordinary person who has the same problem as the patient and has to cope with it daily. An excellent example of learning enhancement through modeling is the American Cancer Society's Reach for Recovery program. Women who have had mastectomies teach new mastectomy patients how to do arm and shoulder exercises. A third way of facilitating learning by enhancing self-efficacy is through persuasion. This is probably the most used and least effective. It can be used to urge patients to do more than they are currently doing.

Teaching materials are divided into two major categories: printed and nonprinted materials. Printed materials include booklets, brochures, and pamphlets. Although printed material can limit feedback, it is useful for relaxing the time requirements. Printed material is always available to the learner and can be referred to as often as needed. The following are considerations in selecting printed material:[39]

Is the content written at the appropriate skill level of the target audience? The mean literacy level in the United States is the eighth-grade level or below; 20% of adult learners are functionally illiterate; 34% have marginal reading skills. Materials should be written for a sixth-grade level. Simplify printed material by eliminating medical jargon and pathophysiology. In addition, illness or stress can lower one's ability to comprehend even more. For patients with higher levels of literacy and the desire to know, additional information can be provided. Are sentences clear, short, and concise? Material presented should be the very least needed to convey the message. The content should be essential material. Focusing on required behaviors, such as "Do not eat or drink anything after midnight the day of your surgery," increases the chances the patient will follow through. Is the material logically organized? The most important points should be presented first and highlighted. Headings and graphics can draw attention to important content. The purpose and summary should be clearly stated. Are the visual and graphic elements pleasing, and do they help convey the message? Visuals should relate to the topic and not detract from the message. Is the content accurate? Is the type large and easy to read? Does the material foster interaction between the nurse and patient? This helps develop the nurse-patient relationship and assists the patient to individualize and personalize the instructions.

Nonprinted materials include audio and visual programs, such as videotapes, television, flip charts, pictures and slides, cassette tapes, and models. Videotapes and television are very effective tools for instructing hospitalized patients.[37] These may be rented or purchased. Some hospitals are part of a nationwide satellite network that televises patient-education programs, and some produce their own videotapes and live broadcasts. Audiotapes and phone teaching are available in some hospitals by means of a toll-free dial-access system. Another technique is to tape an educational session and give it to the patient when the session is completed. Cassette tapes or videotapes of the teaching session can be replayed at the patient's convenience. Select audio or video programs that are appropriate to the subject matter, accurate in content, simple, and appealing to the target audience.

Documentation

Unfortunately, patient education is often not thoroughly documented. Perioperative nurses may not recognize the value of teaching and learning interactions or not consider the interaction with patient education because it was not a formal process with written objectives.[39] As the JCAHO focuses on quality of care and outcomes, standardized documentation of all kinds of patient education is becoming very important. A simple narrative in the nursing notes is adequate for informal teaching and learning interactions. Be sure to include the outcomes of the interaction as well as assessment data and content. Effective forms for documentation combine teaching protocols, objectives, and outcomes on a single page. Equally as important to document are those times when the patient was not ready to learn. It should include the assessment data that indicated lack of readiness and what the nurse did to enhance readiness. Be sure to document when portions of the content are referred to another provider. Referral is an important nursing intervention for perioperative nurses, given the limited amount of time available to spend with patients. Fig. 10-7 provides an

EXAMPLE OF CHECKLIST DOCUMENTATION

GENERIC CARE PLAN   The patient demonstrates knowledge of the physiologic and psychologic responses to surgery

KEY ASSESSMENT POINTS

Physiologic condition
Presence of anxiety/fear/concern
Level of formal education
Cultural/ethnic/language barriers
Current knowledge and understanding
Psychologic response to current condition
Interest in learning
Motivation/readiness to learn
Experience with surgery

NURSING DIAGNOSIS

Risk for knowledge deficit regarding planned surgical intervention

PATIENT OUTCOMES

The patient will demonstrate knowledge of the physiologic and psychologic responses to the planned surgical intervention as evidenced by:
1. Remaining oriented to person, place, and time
2. Confirming, in writing or orally, consent for the operative procedure
3. Describing the sequence of events during the perioperative period
4. Stating outcomes in realistic terms
5. Expressing feelings about the surgical experience

NURSING ACTIONS

	Yes	No	N/A
1. Patient identified?	☐	☐	☐
2. Sensory aids/prosthetic devices removed?	☐	☐	☐
3. Sensory impairments?	☐	☐	☐
4. LOC: Alert?	☐	☐	☐
5. Verbal verification of operative site?	☐	☐	☐
6. Consent signed? Advance directive?	☐	☐	☐
7. Language barrier?	☐	☐	☐
8. Special religious/spiritual needs?	☐	☐	☐
9. Special cultural/ethnic needs?	☐	☐	☐
10. Perioperative routine explained?	☐	☐	☐
11. Patient expressed understanding?	☐	☐	☐
12. Patient has additional questions?	☐	☐	☐

Document additional nursing actions/care plan revisions here:

_____

_____

_____

EVALUATION OF PATIENT OUTCOMES

	Outcome met	Outcome met with additional outcome criteria	Outcome met with revised nursing care plan	Outcome not met	Outcome not applicable to this patient
1. The patient remained oriented to person, place, and time.	☐	☐	☐	☐	☐
2. Physical and emotional factors which affected the patient's response to the planned surgical intervention were alleviated.	☐	☐	☐	☐	☐
3. The patient was physically and emotionally prepared for the planned surgical intervention.	☐	☐	☐	☐	☐
4. The patient correctly reviewed anticipated perioperative events.	☐	☐	☐	☐	☐
5. The patient signed the operative permit.	☐	☐	☐	☐	☐

Signature: _____ Date: _____

FIGURE 10-7 Example of checklist documentation.

TABLE 10-4 | **Methods of Evaluating Learning**

TECHNIQUE	ADVANTAGES	DISADVANTAGES
Direct observation	Performance under real or simulated conditions can be assessed.	Awareness of the observer may affect performance.
	Task is credible to patient.	Training, supervising, using observers is costly.
	Measure has good content validity.	Number of patients who may be studied and their locale may be restricted because of the high per-patient cost of observing.
Observational checklist	Simple, objective task to record observations.	Checklist may be long if a multifaceted behavior is measured.
	Observer error low.	
Anchored rating scale	Simple, objective task to record observations.	Difficult to write behavioral descriptions that differ by equal amounts over an ordered scale.
	Observer error low.	
	More gradations of judgment allowed than typical of an observational checklist.	Descriptions may introduce several dimensions into a single rating.
Observational record	Permits routine recording of simple, repetitive behaviors.	Inferences depend on sample of time and fineness of recording unit.
Anecdotal notes	May provide unique insights, illustrations.	May be irrelevant to outcomes of interest.
Critical incidents	Characterize adaptive and maladaptive behavior.	Time consuming to collect and analyze.
	May serve as the basis for more structured measurement.	Focus on behavioral extremes; ignore typical behavior that is not outstandingly adaptive or maladaptive.
Physiologic measures	Measure is accurate.	Measure may be multiply determined; not affected by teaching outcomes alone.
	Measure is a good indicator of health status.	
	Measure is responsive to compliance with healthcare regimen.	Measure may depend on patient's willingness and ability to perform routine self-testing and recording.
		Measurement may be costly to obtain and analyze.
		Measurement may be invasive.
Self-report	Provides data and insights not available for other sources.	Subject to faking, socially desirable response set.
	Measures cognitive, affective, and performance outcomes directly.	Requires skill in construction of instrument.
Oral self-report	Little reading and no writing required of patient.	Recording burden for interviewer.
	Contingent questions, probing, and question clarification possible.	Responses may be biased by interviewer.
		Data collection individualized and costly.

From McSweeney, M. (1981). *Diabetes Educ* 7, 3, 9-15.

example of how to document the nursing diagnosis, activities, and outcomes in an easily used checklist format. To meet JCAHO requirements, some institutions are creating interdisciplinary documentation forms (Research Highlight 10-3).

EVALUATION

Evaluation of patient education activities should be considered early in the teaching process. Evaluation measures if and how well a patient learned the desired behavior. Does the patient willingly change behavior? Desired patient outcomes are identified during the planning phase. Evaluation can serve many purposes. It can motivate continued learning or behavior change because it provides concrete evidence that the patient accomplished or failed to accomplish the goal. It reinforces desired behavior on the part of the patient and helps the perioperative nurse determine the adequacy of the instruction and teaching materials. Evaluation may also

serve to identify an especially beneficial or particularly worthless educational process. In evaluation, the evidence of learning is compared to the outcome criteria. Although there is a variety of methods to measure learning (Table 10-4), the most frequent method used by the perioperative nurse is some form of observation. Direct observation is more effective in evaluating learning in health care than in other areas. Whereas it may be difficult to evaluate cognitive skills and thinking processes by direct observation, we know that motor skills rely on and reflect cognitive processes. For example, for the outcome criterion "The patient will consent to a specific treatment option" the nurse can directly observe whether the patient signed the operative permit.

Recording observations or documenting outcomes is essential when using observation as the evaluation method. Narrative form is the best method to document critical incidents or anecdotal events that do not lend themselves to a simpler, quicker method of documentation. Checklists and rating scales save time and produce uniform documen-

TABLE 10-4 | **Methods of Evaluating Learning—cont'd**

TECHNIQUE	ADVANTAGES	DISADVANTAGES
Written self-report	Cost-effective group administration of instruments is possible.	Reading and recording burdens are placed on patient. Questions are fixed; probes and clarifications cannot be introduced. Possible reduction in response rate of quality resulting from respondent burden.
Open-ended questions	Respondent free to shape reply.	Extent of reply depends on verbal fluency of respondent. Heavy recording burden for respondent or interviewer. Inconsistent dimensions of response across patients. Responses difficult to code and analyze.
Closed, fixed-alternative questions	Easy recording, coding, processing of data. Limited dimensions for replies. Relative insensitivity to verbal fluency.	Construction of instrument is time consuming. Dimensions on which choices will vary must be anticipated. Choices may be forced among nonsalient options.
Single questions per topic	Speed, ease of response.	Instability of response.
Scales of questions per topic	Stability of response.	Increased length of instrument.
Self-monitoring	Recording occurs concurrently with behavior. Access to all behaviors, covert and overt, is possible.	Recording process may be reactive. Quality of record is dependent on patient's cooperation. Self-monitored data may differ from externally observed data.
Records	*Noninvasive*—supply data without added demands on patients. *Nonreactive*—relatively insensitive to external manipulation to claim desired outcomes. Relatively low cost of collection.	May not be organized to permit easy access retrieval. Incomplete or inconsistent records. Indirect measures; may not be directly relevant to teaching outcomes.
Patient charts, physician records		May require healthcare professional to record and interpret relevant data. Privacy considerations may restrict access to records or require hierarchy of obtained consents.
Agency service records, public records and reports	Data may be collected by relatively unskilled workers.	Data come from a variety of sources with varying degrees of accessibility, reporting standards, and variable conceptualization.

tation. Fig. 10-7 provides an example of a checklist format. Rating scales are another useful way to document outcomes. Box 10-1 illustrates three types of pain rating scales. Rarely will the perioperative nurse be able to evaluate using more extensive self-reports and self-monitoring methods. Although these are excellent methods of evaluation, they are time consuming. Time is a resource in critically short supply. These methods are best used for group educational programs. Although evaluation is the final step in the teaching and nursing process, it rarely means the end of the process. Evaluation frequently points the perioperative nurse back to other steps in the process.

SUMMARY

This chapter is an examination of four basic questions about patient education for the perioperative nurse. Why teach? Teach because it is the right thing to do for the patient, family, nurse, and institution. When should patient education occur? Teach when the patient is ready learn. What is the appropriate content for patient teaching? Teach what patients and families want and need to know to accomplish the tasks of daily living and return to their "usual self." How should nurses teach? Teach so that patients and families can actively participate in what they are learning.

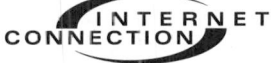

Sources for Consumers/Patients:
http://www.aorn.org/patient

http://www.mediconsult.com/

http://wellweb.com/

http://www.achoo.com/

http://www.healthyideas.com

http://wwwicic.nci.nih.gov/patient.htm

http://www.ama-assn.org

http://healthfinder.gov

http://www.healthtouch.com

http://www.virtualhospital.org

http://www.wilmington.net/dees ("Ask the pharmacist")

http://www.infolane.com/pamp/

http://www.cc.emory.edu/WHSCL/medweb.consumer.html

http://www.nova.edu/Inter-Links/health/consumer.html

http://www.social.com/health/index.html

http://medhlp.netusa.net/index.htm

http://infonet.welch.jhu.edu/advocacy.html

http://www.vh.org/Patients/THB/DiagnosticRad.html

http://cancernet.nci.nih.gov

http://www.housecall.com/

http://www.falk.med.pitt.edu/subjects/consumer.html

REFERENCES

1. Acute Pain Management Guideline Panel. (1992a). *Acute pain management in adults: operative procedures: quick reference guide for clinicians* (AHCPR Publ. No. 92-0019). Rockville, MD: Agency for Health Care Policy and Research.

2. Acute Pain Management Guideline Panel. (1992b). *Acute pain management: operative or medical procedures and trauma: clinical practice guidelines* (AHCPR Publ. No. 92-0032). Rockville, MD: Agency for Health Care Policy and Research.

3. Advisory on Consumer Protection and Quality in the Health Care Industry. (1997). *Consumer bill of rights and responsibilities.* Washington, DC: the Commission.

4. American Hospital Association. (1992). *A patient's bill of rights.* Chicago: the Association.

5. Association of Operating Room Nurses. (1998). Patient outcomes: standards of perioperative care. In *Standards, Recommended Practices and Guidelines.* Denver: the Association

6. Brumfield, V.C., Kee, C.C., & Johnson, J.Y. (1996). Preoperative patient teaching in ambulatory surgery settings, *AORN Journal, 64*(6), 941-952.

7. Clay, J.C., Wyatt, L.K., & Morris, G.M. (1996, October). Patient and family education: an interdisciplinary process. *MedSurg Nursing, 5,* 333-338.

8. Devine, E.C., & Cook, T.D. (1983). A meta-analytic analysis of effects of psychoeducational interventions on length of hospital stay. *Nursing Research, 32,* 267-274.

9. Fox, V.J. (1986). Patient teaching: understanding the needs of the adult learner. *AORN Journal, 44,* 234-242.

10. Good-Reis D.V., & Pieper, B.A. (1990). Structured vs unstructured teaching: a research study. *AORN Journal, 51*(5), 1334-1339.

11. Haddock, K.S (1994). Collaborative discharge planning: nursing and social services. *Clinical Nurse Specialist 8*(5), 248-252.

12. Hankela, S., & Kiikkala, I. (1996). Intraoperative nursing care as experienced by surgical patients. *AORN Journal, 63,* 435-442.

13. Hathaway, D. (1986). Effect of preoperative instruction on postoperative outcomes: a meta-analysis. *Nursing Research, 35,* 269-275.

14. Johnson, E.A., & Jackson, J. (1989). Teaching the home care client. *Nursing Clinics of North America, 24,* 267.

15. Johnson, S. (1989). Preoperative teaching: a need for change. *Nursing Management, 20,* 80B-80H.

16. Joint Commission for the Accreditation of Healthcare Organizations. (1996). *1997 Accreditation Manual for Hospitals.* Chicago: the Commission.

17. Killen, A.R., Kleinbeck, S.V.R., Golar, G. et al. (1997). The prevalence of perioperative nurse clinical judgements. *AORN Journal, 65*(1), 101-108.

18. Kruger, S. (1991). The patient educator role in nursing. *Applied Nursing Research, 4,* 19-24.

19. Lee, J.M. (1970). Emotional reactions to trauma. *Nursing Clinics of North America, 5,* 577-587.

20. Lepczyk, M., Raleigh, E.H., & Rowley, C. (1990). Timing of preoperative patient teaching. *Journal of Advanced Nursing, 15,* 300-306.

21. Lindeman, C.A. (1972). Nursing intervention with the presurgical patient. *Nursing Research, 21*(3), 196-209.

22. Lindeman, C.A. (1973). Influencing recovery through preoperative teaching. *Heart and Lung, 2*(4), 515-521.

23. Lookinland, S., & Pool, M. (1998). Study on effect of methods of preoperative education in women. *AORN Journal, 67,* 203-213.

24. Lorig, K. (1992). *Patient education: a practical approach.* St. Louis: Mosby.

25. Mathias, J.M. (1998). Guided imagery tapes help surgical patients. *OR Manager, 14*(2), 18-19.

26. McCloskey, J.C., & Bulechek, G.M. (Eds.). (1996). *Nursing classification interventions (NIC)* (ed. 2). St. Louis: Mosby.

27. McHatton, M. (1985). A theory for timely teaching. *American Journal of Nursing, 85,* 798-800.

28. Midgley J.W., & Osterhage, R.A. (1973). Effect of nursing instruction and length of hospitalization on postoperative complications in cholecystectomy patients. *Nursing Research, 22,* 69-72.

29. Narrow, B.W. (1979). *Patient teaching in nursing practice: a patient and family centered approach.* New York: John Wiley & Sons.

30. National League for Nursing Education. (1918). *Standard curriculum for schools of nursing.* Baltimore: The Waverly Press.

31. National League for Nursing Education. (1937). *A curriculum guide for schools of nursing.* New York: the League.

32. National League for Nursing Education. (1950). *Nursing organization curriculum conference.* Glen Gardener, NJ: Libertarian Press.

33. Oetker-Black, S.L. (1996). Generalizability of the preoperative self-efficacy scale. *Applied Nursing Research, 9,* 40-43.

34. Pierce, P.F. (1993). Deciding on breast cancer treatment: a description of decisional behaviors. *Nursing Research, 42,* 22-28.

35. Rakel, B.A. (1992). Interventions related to patient teaching. *Nursing Clinics of North America, 24,* 397-423.

36. Raleigh, E.H., Lepczyk, M., & Rowley, C. (1990). Significant others benefit from preoperative information. *Journal of Advanced Nursing, 15,* 941-945.

37. Redman, B.K. (1997). *The process of patient education* (ed. 8). St. Louis: Mosby.

38. Rothrock, J.C. (1996). Generic care planning: AORN patient outcome standards. In Rothrock, J.C. (Ed.), *Perioperative nursing care planning.* St. Louis: Mosby.

39. Ruzicki, D.A. (1989). Realistically meeting the educational needs of hospitalized acute and short-stay patients. *Nursing Clinics of North America, 24,* 629-637.

40. Shade, P. (1992). Patient-controlled analgesia: can client education improve outcomes? *Journal of Advanced Nursing, 17,* 408-413.

41. Silva, M.C. (1987). Needs of spouses of surgical patients: a conceptualization within the Roy adaptation model. *Scholarly Inquiry for Nursing Practice: An International Journal, 1,* 29-44.

42. Smith, C.E. (1987, July). Patient teaching: it's the law. *Nursing, 87,* 67-68.

43. Smith, C.E. (1989). Overview of patient education: opportunities and challenges for the twenty-first century. *Nursing Clinics of North America, 24,* 583-587.

44. Sundeen, S.J., Stuart, G.W., Rankin, E.A.D., & Cohen, S.A. (1994). *Nurse-client interaction: implementing the nursing process* (ed. 5). St. Louis: Mosby.

45. Timmons, M.E., & Bower, F.L. (1993). The effect of structured preoperative teaching on patients' use of patient-controlled analgesia (PCA) and their management of pain. *Orthopaedic Nursing, 12,* 23-31.

46. Van Aernam, B., & Lindeman, C.A. (1971). Nursing intervention with the presurgical patient: the effects of structured and unstructured preoperative teaching. *Nursing Research, 20*(4), 319-332.

47. Wallace, L.M. (1985). Surgical patients' preferences for preoperative information. *Patient Education and Counseling, 7,* 377-387.

48. Wells, S. (1996). Adding an "at home" path to your discharge plan. *American Journal of Nursing, 96,* 73-74.

49. Wolfer, J.A., & Davis, C.E. (1970). Assessment of surgical patient's preoperative emotional condition and postoperative welfare. *Nursing Research, 19,* 402-414.

50. Worried about complying with patient education standards? Critical paths can help. (1994, Sept.). *Hospital Case Management, 2,* 145-146.

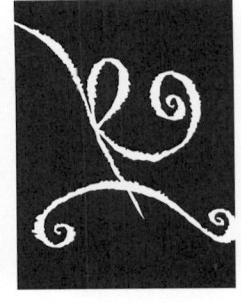

UNIT II | SURGICAL INTERVENTIONS

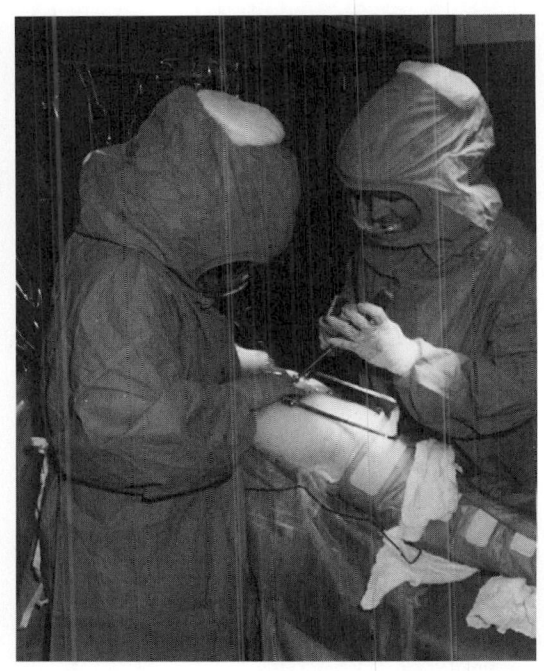

CHAPTER ELEVEN | # Gastrointestinal Surgery

Lynda R. Petty

MANY GASTROINTESTINAL (GI) diseases are treated by surgery, and many surgical procedures of the abdomen begin with an exploratory laparotomy as a means of diagnosis, assessment of extent of disease, and treatment. In several diseases, such as cancer, the planned procedure may be changed because of the laparotomy findings. In other instances a first plan of care is made only after laparotomy findings are ascertained. Many different procedures involving the abdominal viscera are performed by means of a laparotomy approach; examples include resection of a portion of the bowel because of disease or obstruction, procedures performed on the stomach such as gastrectomy, and procedures performed to diagnose a problem that has resulted in physiologic symptoms.

Surgical procedures involving the GI tract are usually performed through an abdominal incision; however, endoscopic possibilities and laparoscopic procedures are rapidly changing the approach to surgical interventions. Diagnostic laparoscopy with intraoperative laparoscopic ultrasonography is a less invasive means of assessing the abdominal viscera for bleeding, tumor, and extent of disease. Many new advances in technology and minimally invasive instrumentation permit the surgeon to explore the abdominal cavity and manipulate and biopsy suspicious sites, thus reducing the morbidity associated with laparotomy. When laparotomy is indicated, the surgeon chooses an incision that affords maximum exposure of the involved structures, ensures minimal trauma and postoperative discomfort, and provides for primary wound healing with maximal wound strength. Although surgical interventions have changed drastically over the years, the types of laparotomy incisions used to expose the affected organs of the GI tract have remained relatively constant. In few other types of surgery can attention to detail and technique so profoundly affect the ultimate result as in the opening and closing of abdominal incisions.

The abdominal wall consists of various tissue layers through which dissection is necessary to enter the abdominal cavity (Figs. 11-1 and 11-2). Beneath the skin and subcutaneous fat, the layers include fascia, muscles (external and internal oblique, rectus abdominis, and transversus abdominis), preperitoneal fat, and peritoneum. Fascia, which consists of bands of tough, fibrous connective tissue, surrounds the muscles anteriorly and posteriorly (Fig. 11-3). The peritoneum is a serous membrane lining the abdominal cavity. Incision of this tissue layer exposes abdominal cavity contents.

ABDOMINAL INCISIONS

Vertical Midline Incision

The vertical midline is the simplest abdominal incision to perform. It is an excellent primary incision and generally preferred because it offers good exposure to any part of the abdominal cavity. With this incision hemostasis is easily achieved, and fewer layers are traversed. The incision can be extended from just below the sternal notch, distally around the umbilicus (which is avascular, tough connective tissue), back to the midline, and down to the symphysis pubis (Fig. 11-4). The peritoneum is incised, and the round ligament of the liver may be divided.

To close the wound, the peritoneum and posterior fascia are usually sutured as a single layer. Sometimes the suture line is supported by using retention sutures, which extend through most or all layers of the wound. Anterior fascia, subcutaneous tissue, and skin are closed as layers. An alternative closure uses figure-of-eight, monofilament, nonabsorbable sutures, for one-layer closure of peritoneum and fascia.

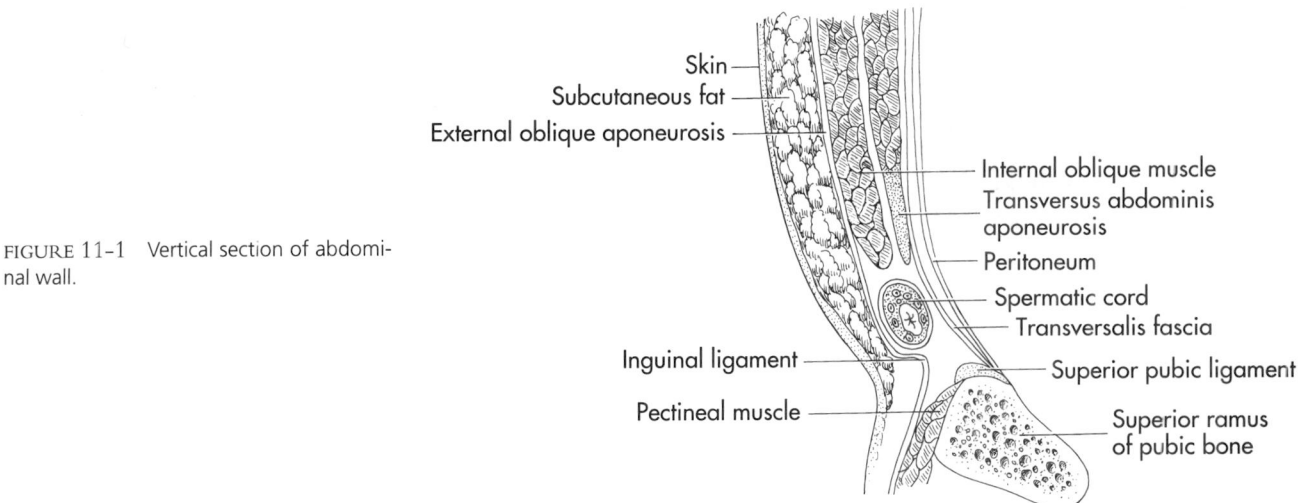

FIGURE 11-1   Vertical section of abdominal wall.

Skin
Subcutaneous fat
External oblique aponeurosis

Internal oblique muscle
Transversus abdominis aponeurosis
Peritoneum
Spermatic cord
Transversalis fascia
Superior pubic ligament
Superior ramus of pubic bone

Inguinal ligament
Pectineal muscle

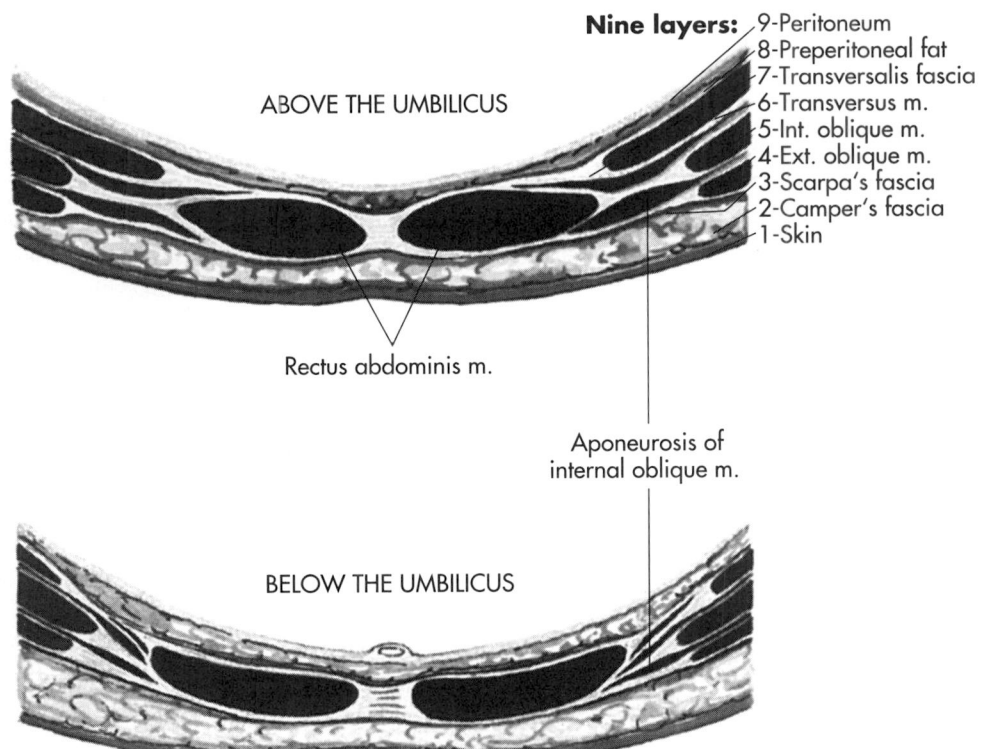

Nine layers:
9-Peritoneum
8-Preperitoneal fat
7-Transversalis fascia
6-Transversus m.
5-Int. oblique m.
4-Ext. oblique m.
3-Scarpa's fascia
2-Camper's fascia
1-Skin

ABOVE THE UMBILICUS

Rectus abdominis m.

Aponeurosis of internal oblique m.

BELOW THE UMBILICUS

FIGURE 11-2   Horizontal section of abdominal wall. Aponeurosis of internal oblique muscle splits into two sections, one lying anterior and the other posterior to rectus abdominis muscle, thereby forming an encasing sheath around muscle above umbilicus. Below umbilicus, aponeuroses of all muscles pass anterior to rectus.

Oblique Incisions
McBurney muscle-splitting incision

The McBurney muscle-splitting incision is used for removal of the appendix. It is an 8 cm oblique incision that begins well below the umbilicus, goes through McBurney's point, and extends upward toward the right flank (see Fig. 11-4). The external oblique muscle and fascia are split in the direction of their fibers and are retracted. The internal oblique muscle, transversalis muscle, and fascia are split and retracted. The peritoneum is incised transversely. This incision is quick and easy to close and allows a firm wound closure. However, it does not permit good exposure and is difficult to extend. To extend the incision medially, the inferior epigastric

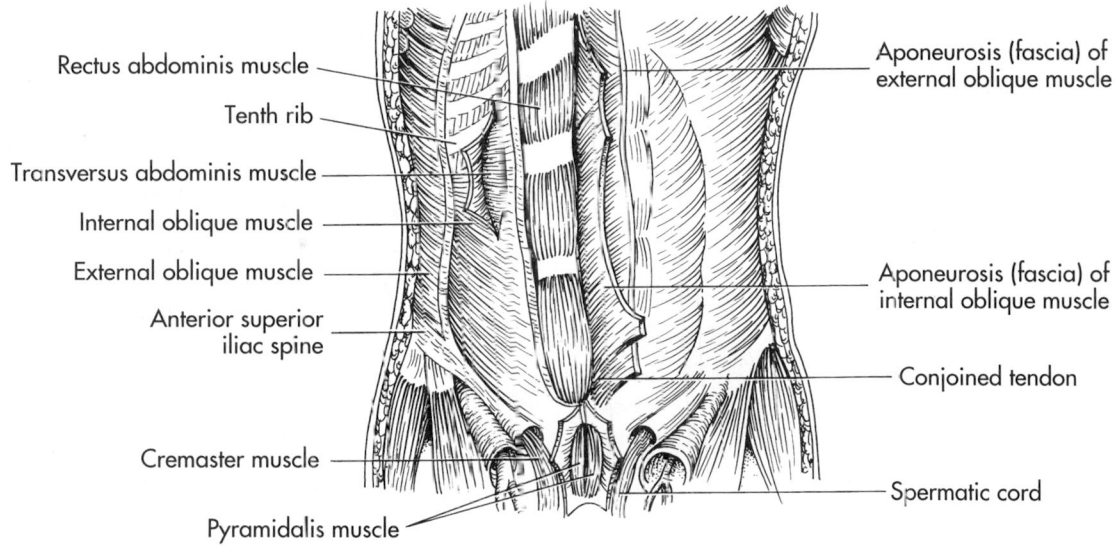

Rectus abdominis muscle

Tenth rib

Transversus abdominis muscle

Internal oblique muscle

External oblique muscle

Anterior superior iliac spine

Cremaster muscle

Pyramidalis muscle

Aponeurosis (fascia) of external oblique muscle

Aponeurosis (fascia) of internal oblique muscle

Conjoined tendon

Spermatic cord

FIGURE 11–3 Superior muscles of abdominal wall.

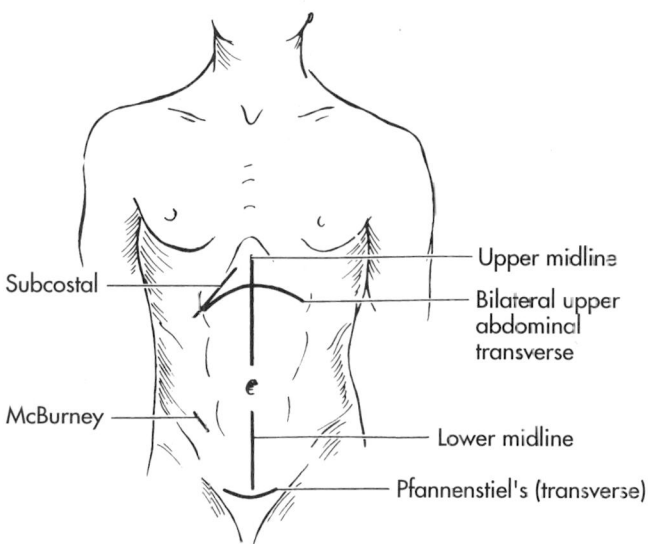

Subcostal

McBurney

Upper midline

Bilateral upper abdominal transverse

Lower midline

Pfannenstiel's (transverse)

FIGURE 11–4 Incisions made through the abdominal wall.

vessels are ligated, and the rectus sheath is incised transversely.

Subcostal incision

The subcostal incision is usually made on the right side and may be used for operations on the gallbladder, common duct, or pancreas. When made on the left side, it is used for splenectomy. This incision usually gives only limited exposure unless the patient is short with a wide abdomen and wide costal margins. The advantages of this type of incision are that it provides good cosmetic results because it follows the skin lines and the nerve damage is limited because only one or two nerves are cut, most commonly the eighth intercostal nerve. Also, tension on the incisional edges is less than in a vertical incision, it can

readily be extended for wide exposure, and it causes less respiratory impairment.

This oblique incision begins in the epigastrium, extending laterally and obliquely downward to just below the lower costal margin (Fig. 11–5). Each muscle contains veins and arteries requiring ligation. If more exposure is needed, the incision is extended across the rectus muscle of the other side. The rectus muscle is either retracted or transversely divided. Vessels in the muscle must be ligated.

The closure of this incision includes approximation and closure of the falciform ligament, peritoneum, posterior rectus sheath, and anterior rectus sheath with interrupted, nonabsorbable sutures. The subcutaneous tissue and skin are closed as described for a vertical midline incision. Absorbable sutures may be used with staples.

Transverse Incisions
Pfannenstiel's incision

Pfannenstiel's incision is used frequently for pelvic surgery. It is a curved transverse incision across the lower abdomen through the skin, subcutaneous tissue, and rectus sheaths (Fig. 11–6). This incision is made approximately ½ inch above the symphysis pubis. The rectus muscles are separated in the midline, and the peritoneum is entered through a midline vertical incision. This incision provides for a strong closure; when the rectus muscles contract, there is minimal strain on the fascial sutures.

Midabdominal transverse incision

The midabdominal transverse incision is used on the left or right side or for a retroperitoneal approach. The incision begins slightly above or below the umbilicus on either side and is carried laterally to the lumbar region at an angle between the ribs and crest of the ilium. The skin

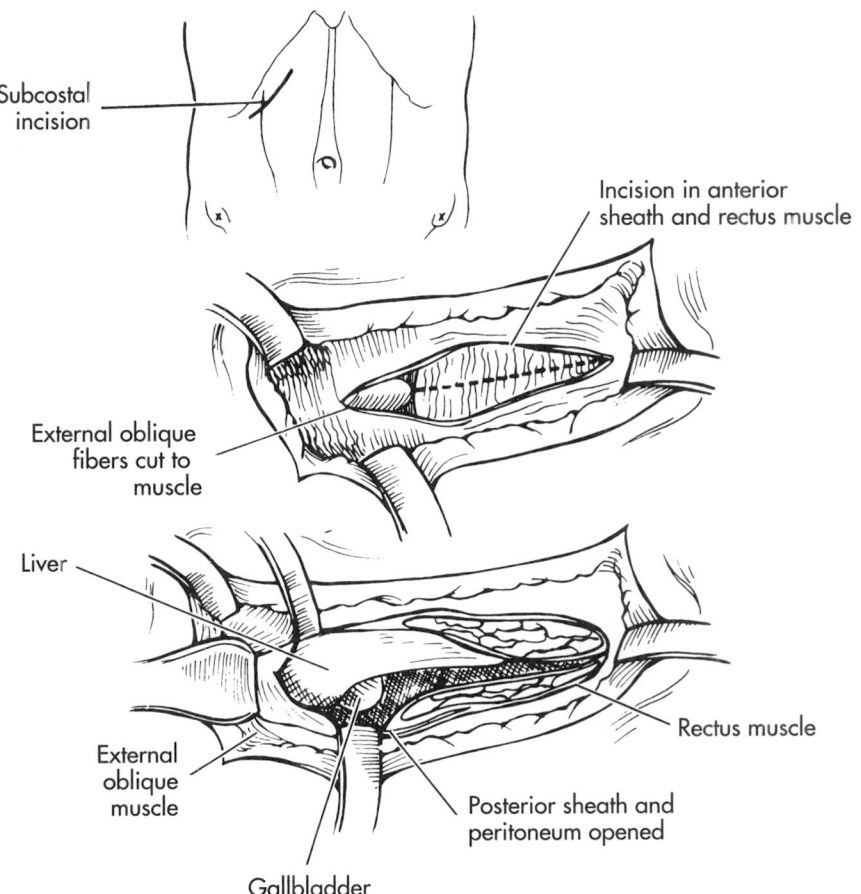

Subcostal incision

Incision in anterior sheath and rectus muscle

External oblique fibers cut to muscle

Liver

External oblique muscle

Gallbladder

Rectus muscle

Posterior sheath and peritoneum opened

FIGURE 11-5   Subcostal incision in upper right quadrant. Anterior sheath has been divided transversely, and muscle is exposed. Posterior sheath and peritoneum have been opened transversely.

and subcutaneous tissue are incised, the anterior rectus sheath is split, the rectus muscle is divided, and the vessels within the rectus are clamped and ligated. The posterior rectus sheath and peritoneum are cut in the direction of the fibers, preserving the intercostal nerves. The peritoneum is incised near the midline, and the incision is extended laterally to the oblique muscle. The lateral muscles are incised to provide wide exposure. The closure is in layers with interrupted sutures; the subcutaneous tissue and skin are closed as for laparotomy (see pp. 334-335). The rectus muscle usually cannot be closed because its fibers run vertically. Approximation of the rectus sheath brings the edges of the rectus muscle into excellent apposition, thus eliminating the need to suture the muscle itself.

Thoracoabdominal incision

The thoracoabdominal incision is used for operations on the proximal portion of the stomach and the distal section of the esophagus. Often the abdominal part of the incision is made first for exploration and then if necessary is extended across the costal margin into the chest. The incision begins at a point midway between the xiphoid process and the umbilicus and extends across to the seventh

or eighth interspace and to the midscapular line. The rectus and oblique abdominal muscles are divided in the line of the incision down to the peritoneum and pleura. The costal cartilage and the diaphragm are then divided (Fig. 11-7).

The wound is closed in layers with interrupted sutures. Absorbable sutures may be used for the peritoneum and intercostal muscles. Nonabsorbable suture may be used for the muscle and fascial layers. Skin edges are approximated with staples or a nonabsorbable suture.

Upper inverted-U abdominal incision

An upper inverted-U abdominal incision is seldom used today; however, it can be used for gastrectomy, transverse colon resection, transverse colostomy, and biliary and pancreatic procedures. The incision extends from a point below the costal margin on one side in the anterior axillary line to the same point on the opposite side. It is curved, with the midpoint lying midway between the xiphoid process and the umbilicus. The intercostal nerves are preserved.

An upper abdominal transverse incision is closed by placement of interrupted sutures in the peritoneum and anterior and posterior rectus sheaths. The muscle and fat

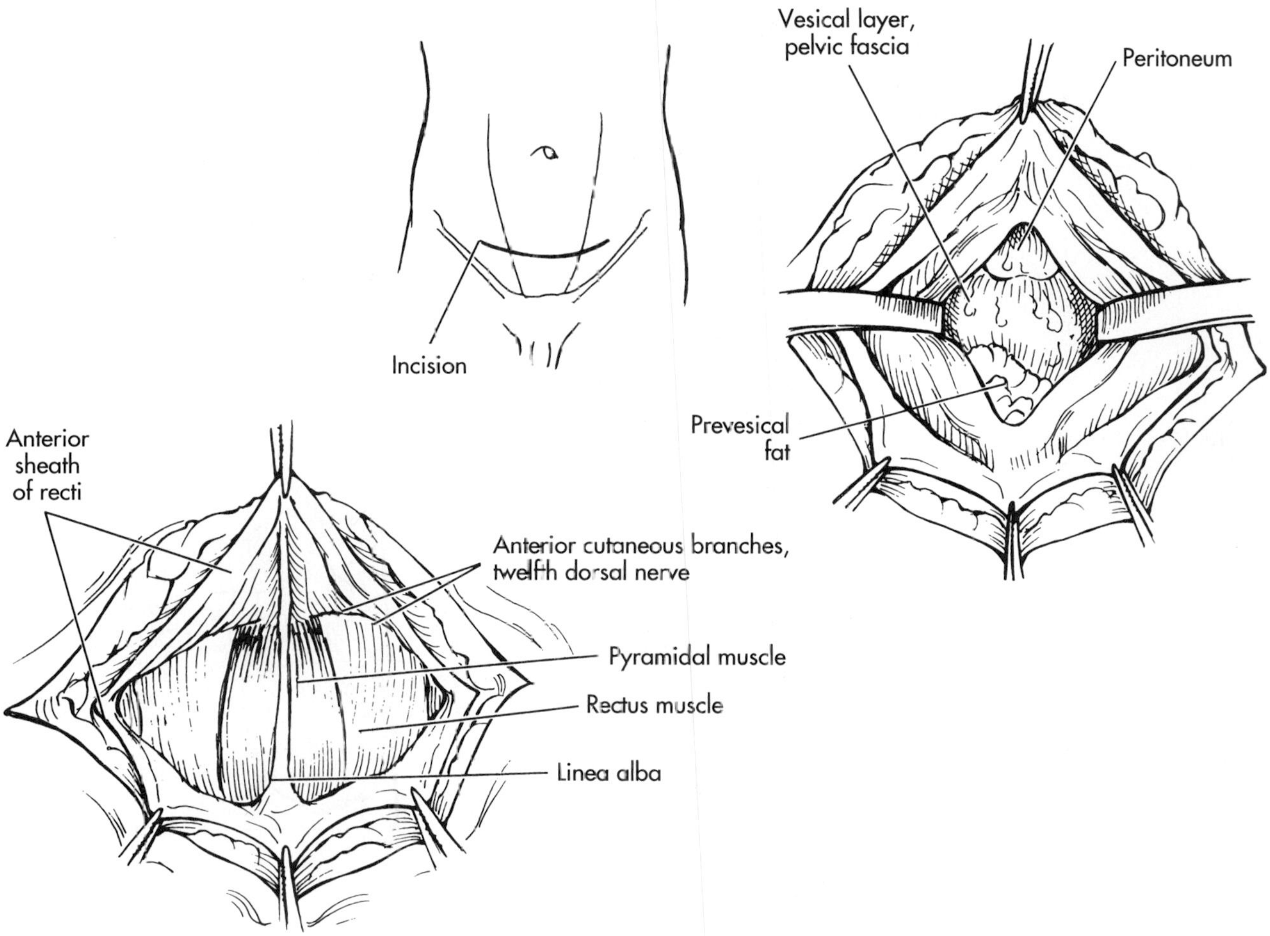

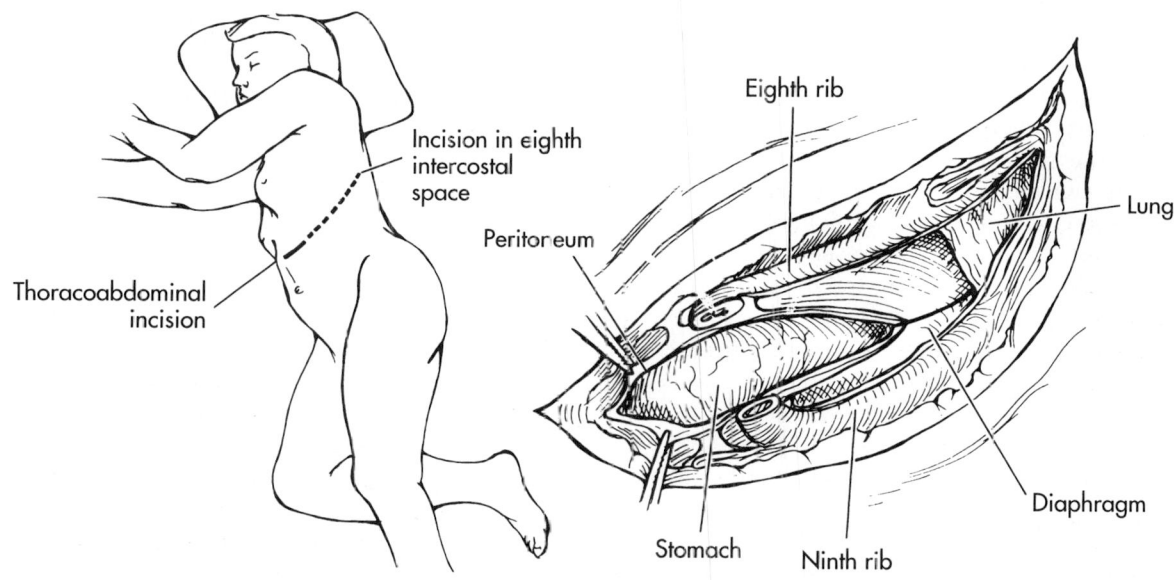

Incision

Vesical layer,
pelvic fascia

Peritoneum

Prevesical
fat

Anterior
sheath
of recti

Anterior cutaneous branches,
twelfth dorsal nerve

Pyramidal muscle

Rectus muscle

Linea alba

FIGURE 11-6   Pfannenstiel's incision (transverse).

Incision in eighth
intercostal
space

Eighth rib

Lung

Peritoneum

Thoracoabdominal
incision

Stomach

Ninth rib

Diaphragm

FIGURE 11-7   Thoracoabdominal incision. Patient is placed on unaffected side. Incision is usually made from point midway between xiphoid process and umbilicus to costal margin at site of eighth costal cartilage. Dissection is carried down to peritoneum and pleura. Costal cartilage and diaphragm are divided, and stomach is exposed.

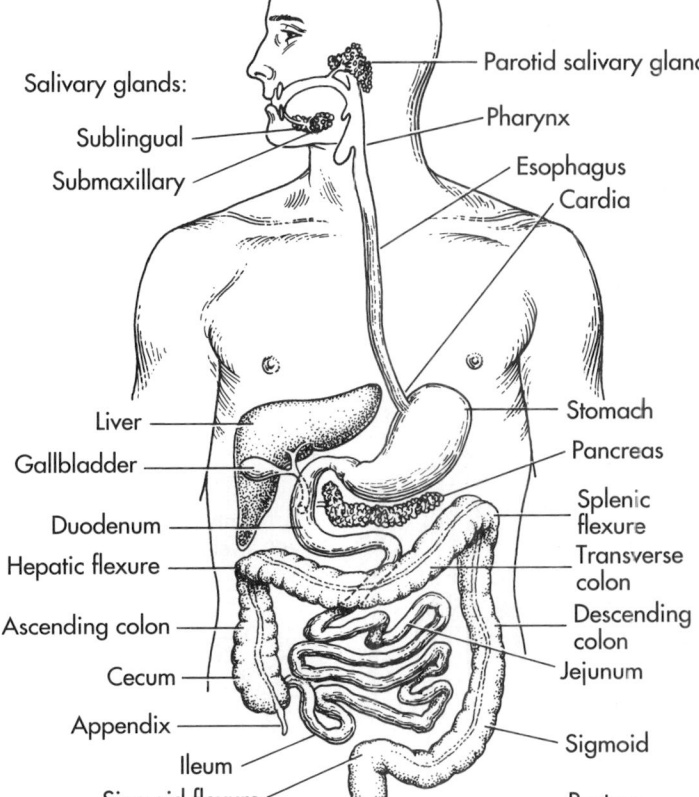

FIGURE 11-8   Alimentary canal and its appendages.

need not be sutured. The skin edges are approximated and closed using suture or a mechanical staple applier according to the surgeon's preference.

SURGICAL ANATOMY

The alimentary canal comprises a series of organs joined to form a tubelike structure that extends the entire length of the trunk (Fig. 11-8). The alimentary tract includes the mouth; pharynx; esophagus; stomach; small intestine, consisting of the duodenum, jejunum, and ileum; and large intestine, which comprises the cecum, ascending colon, transverse colon, descending colon, sigmoid colon, rectum, and anus. These organs are responsible for the supply of nourishment to the body and the elimination of solid wastes.

The esophagus extends from the pharynx, at the level of the sixth cervical vertebra, and passes through the neck, posterior to the trachea and heart and anterior to the vertebral column. The lower portion of the esophagus passes in front of the aorta and through the diaphragm, slightly to the left of the midline, to join the cardia of the stomach.

Blood is supplied to the esophagus from branches of the inferior thyroid, thoracic aorta, and celiac arteries. The nerve supply comes from branches of the vagi and sympathetic chain. The esophagus of an adult is about

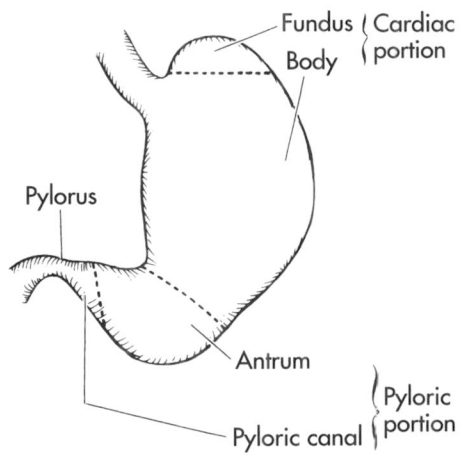

FIGURE 11-9   Regional anatomy of stomach.

10 inches in length and is a collapsible musculomembranous tube.

The stomach is situated between the esophagus and the duodenum and lies in the upper left abdominal cavity, slightly to the left of the midline and beneath the diaphragm. The stomach is divided into three parts: the fundus, the body, and the antrum (Fig. 11-9). The fundus lies beneath the left dome of the diaphragm, behind the apex of the heart, and the body and antrum lie in an oblique direction within the abdominal cavity. The stomach is stabilized indirectly by the lower portion of the esophagus and directly by its attachment to the duodenum, which is anchored to the posterior parietal peritoneum. The omentum, the peritoneal ligaments, and branches of the celiac vessel provide additional support to the stomach.

The convex, or lower, margin of the stomach is known as the greater curvature; the concave, or upper, margin is the lesser curvature. Attached to the greater curvature is the greater omentum, which is a double fold of peritoneum containing fat. It covers the intestines loosely and is not to be confused with the mesentery, which connects the intestines with the posterior abdominal wall. The left gastroepiploic branch of the splenic artery and the right gastroepiploic branch of the hepatic artery run through the greater omentum. The lesser omentum, which is attached to the lesser curvature of the stomach, contains the left gastric artery, a branch of the celiac axis, and the right gastric branch of the hepatic artery (Fig. 11-10). During a gastrectomy, these vessels are clamped and ligated.

The small intestine begins at the pylorus and ends at the ileocecal valve (Fig. 11-11). It is also divided into three parts: the duodenum, which is about 10 inches long; the jejunum, which is about 7½ feet long; and the ileum, which is about 10½ feet long in an adult. The small intestine varies in size with the degree of contraction but is usually about 20 feet in length and 1 inch in diameter (Fig. 11-11). The duodenum, the proximal portion of the small intestine, begins at the pylorus, is continuous with the jejunum, and is stabilized by a fusion between the pancreas and the posterior parietal peritoneum. The duodenum is divided into four portions: superior (I), descending (II), transverse (III), and ascending (IV) (Fig. 11-12). Nearly all of the first portion mucosa is characterized by the lack of folds; it appears slightly dilated, and is referred to as the *duodenal bulb*. The characteristic circular folds of the small intestine mucosa begin just proximal to the end of the first portion of the duodenum and extend through the jejunum. They become less prominent in the ileum. The purpose of the circular mucosal folds, called *plicae circulares of Kerckring,* or *valvulae conniventes*, is to provide greater mucosal surface area.[2]

The common duct enters the pancreas posterior to the duodenal bulb. The common bile duct and the main pancreatic duct enter the medial wall of the middle of the second portion of the duodenum at the ampulla of Vater. The first, second, and third portions of the duodenum curve in a C-loop concavity in which the head of the pancreas lies. The fourth portion of the duodenum ascends to the duodenojejunal flexure. The duodenojejunal flexure is stabilized by the ligament of Treitz, which suspends the duodenum from the posterior body wall. The ligament of Treitz serves as an important landmark during any abdominal exploration because it provides the surgeon with a reliable orientation of the patient's anatomy.

The blood supply of the duodenum comes from the arterial branches of the celiac axis. The gastroduodenal artery branches off the hepatic artery and is located behind the duodenal bulb. At the inferior margin of the bulb the gastroduodenal artery divides into the right gastroepiploic artery and a superior pancreaticoduodenal branch. The superior pancreaticoduodenal artery supplies blood to the proximal duodenum and head of the pancreas. The inferior pancreaticoduodenal artery branch of the superior mesenteric artery supplies blood to the third and fourth portions of the duodenum as well as to the head and body of the pancreas (Fig. 11-13).

The jejunum, which is situated in the upper portion of the abdomen, joins the ileum, which is situated in the lower portion of the cavity. The ileum empties into the large intestine through the ileocecal valve. The jejunum and ileum are suspended by the mesentery, which is attached to the posterior abdominal wall (Fig. 11-14). The free border of the mesentery, which is about 18 feet long, contains branches of the superior mesenteric artery, many veins, lymph nodes, and nerve fibers. The blood supply to the jejunum and ileum comes entirely from the superior mesenteric artery. The small bowel contains major deposits of lymphatic tissue, known as *Peyer's patches*, in the ileum. The rich lymphatic drainage of the small bowel plays a major role in fat absorption. Lymphatic drainage from the mucosa proceeds through the wall of the small intestine to lymph nodes adjacent to the mesentery. Lymphatic drainage then proceeds to larger lymphatics that communicate to the retroperitoneal cisterna chyli and from there to the thoracic duct. The lymphatics of the intestine play a major role in the body's immune defense as well as in the spread of cells arising from intestinal neoplasms.[2]

The jejunum has a larger circumference and is thicker than the ileum. The mesenteric vessels usually form only one or two arcades, a series of anastomosing arterial arches, in comparison to the multiple vascular arcades of the ileum. The jejunal mucosa is thick and has prominent plicae circulares. The ileum mucosa is thinner with few plicae[2] (Fig. 11-15).

The large intestine begins at the ileocecal valve and terminates at the anus. It is divided into the cecum, colon, and rectum. The cecum is attached to the ileum and extends about 2½ inches below it (Fig. 11-16). The cecum in an adult is usually adherent to the posterior wall of the peritoneal cavity and has a serosal covering on its anterior wall only. The cecum forms a blind pouch from which the appendix projects.

The colon is divided into four parts: the ascending colon, the transverse colon, the descending colon, and the sigmoid colon (see Fig. 11-16).

The ascending colon is about 6 inches long and extends upward from the ileocecal valve to the hepatic flexure. The upper portion of the ascending colon lies behind the right lobe of the liver and in front of the anterior surface of the right kidney.

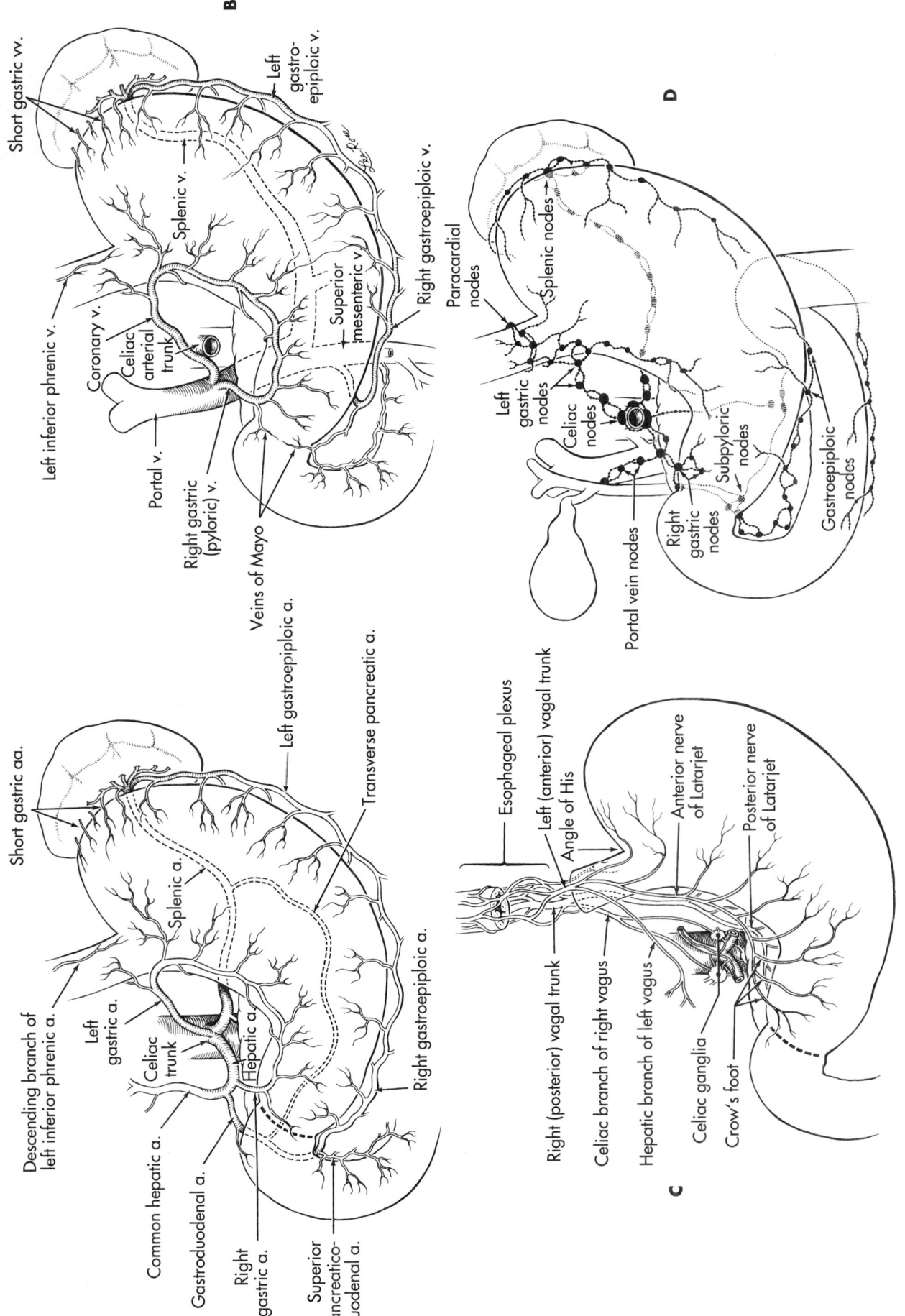

FIGURE 11–10 **A**, Arterial supply of stomach. **B**, Venous supply of the stomach. **C**, Innervation of the stomach and distal esophagus. **D**, Lymphatic drainage of the stomach, duodenum, and periportal region.

The transverse colon, which is about 20 inches long, begins at the hepatic flexure and ends at the splenic flexure. It lies below the stomach and is attached to the transverse mesocolon.

The descending colon extends downward from the splenic flexure to the area just below the iliac crest and is about 7 inches long. The iliac portion of the sigmoid colon, which is about 6 inches long, lies on the inner surface of the left iliac muscle. The remaining portion of the colon passes over the pelvic rim into the pelvic cavity and lies partly in the abdomen and partly in the pelvis. It then forms an S curve in the pelvis and terminates in the rectum at the level of the third segment of the sacral vertebrae.

The blood supply to the ascending colon, hepatic flexure, and transverse colon comes from the superior mesenteric artery, whereas the blood supply to the descending colon and rectum comes from the inferior mesenteric artery (Fig. 11-17).

The wall of the colon is made up of taeniae coli, epiploic appendices, and haustra. The taeniae coli are three longitudinal, or axial, strips of muscles distributed around the circumference of the colon. They represent the longitudinal muscle layer, which is not complete in the colon. The small intestine and rectum have both circular and complete longitudinal muscle layers. The epiploic appendices are fatty appendages along the bowel that have no particular function; the haustra are sacculations that are the outpouchings of bowel wall between the taeniae coli. The diameter of the colon varies in size from about 3½ inches in the cecum to an average of about ½ inch in the sigmoid colon.

The rectum originates at the sigmoid colon and terminates in the anus. A slightly curved passage about 6 inches long, it is surrounded by the pelvic fascia as it lies on the anterior surface of the sacrum and coccyx. In the male the rectum lies behind the prostate gland, seminal vesicles, and the bladder. In the female the rectum lies behind the uterus and the vagina. A septum rectovesicale, also called *Denonvilliers' fascia*, separates the rectum from the urogenital structures. The rectum is suspended in the pelvis by fascia extending from the right and left pelvic sidewalls. Rectosacral fascia extending from the sacrum to the anorectal junction suspends the rectum posteriorly. The

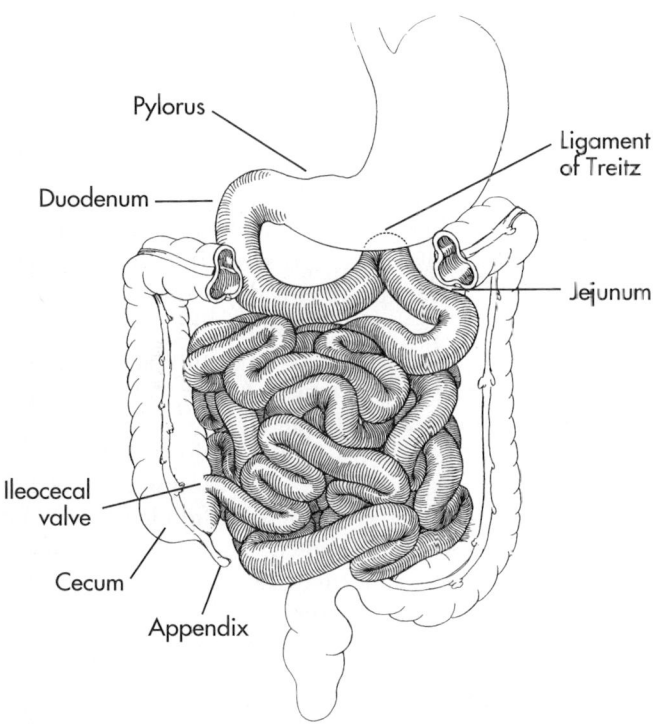

FIGURE 11-11 Illustration of the small bowel; the duodenum originates at the pylorus and flexes at the ligament of Treitz where the jejunum begins. The jejunum extends into the ileum, which terminates at the ileocecal valve at the cecum.

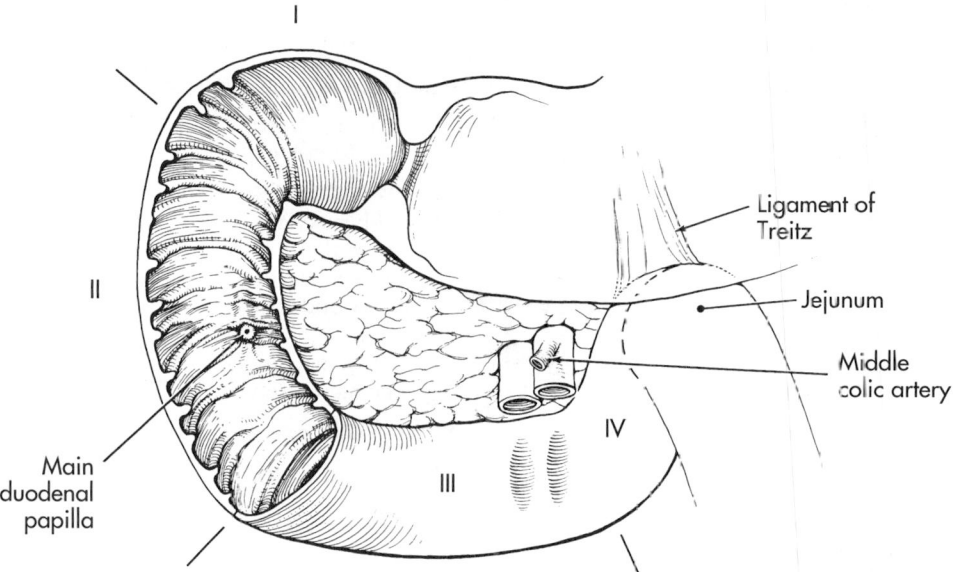

FIGURE 11-12 The duodenum consists of four portions, as illustrated.

rectum dilates just before it becomes the anal canal, and this dilatation, or ampulla, presents folds called *Houston's valves*. The wall of the rectum consists of four layers, similar to those of the small intestine.

The anal canal is a narrow passage about 1 inch long, which passes downward and slightly posteriorly. It is surrounded and controlled by two circular muscle groups, which form the external and internal anal sphincters. The internal sphincter is a continuation of the longitudinal muscle layer.

The esophagus serves as the route from which food enters the stomach from the mouth. When food enters the stomach, it undergoes chemical and mechanical changes and then enters the duodenum, where it is mixed with bile and pancreatic juices. The stomach is never entirely empty because it always contains some gastric juice, which is acid in nature and produced by numerous tubular glands in the wall of the stomach.

Food enters the stomach by passing through the lower esophageal sphincter and leaves by passing through the pyloric sphincter. When food is in the stomach, the stomach becomes distended and the rugae, or folds, flatten out. Little absorption takes place in the stomach, and liquid enters the duodenum within 30 minutes after ingestion. Food is moved through the stomach and intestines by peristalsis, which consists in waves of motion caused by successive contractions of the muscles in the walls of the stomach and intestines.

Absorption of nutrients is a function of the small intestine. The large intestine absorbs water from the contents and expels the indigestible residue from the body. The residue is composed primarily of cellulose from carbohydrates, connective tissue, and undigested fats. The act of defecation is accomplished by contraction of the rectal and abdominal muscles, the descent of the diaphragm, and the relaxation of the anal sphincter muscles.

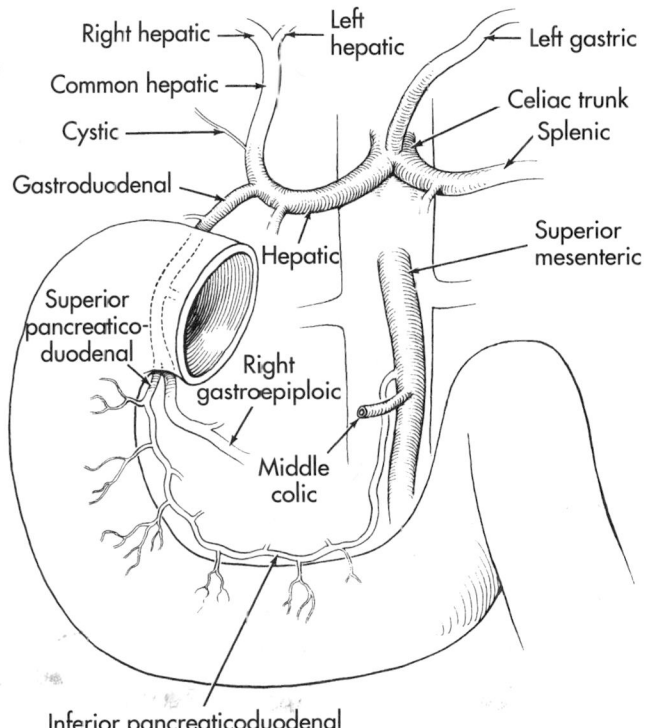

FIGURE 11–13   Blood supply of the duodenum.

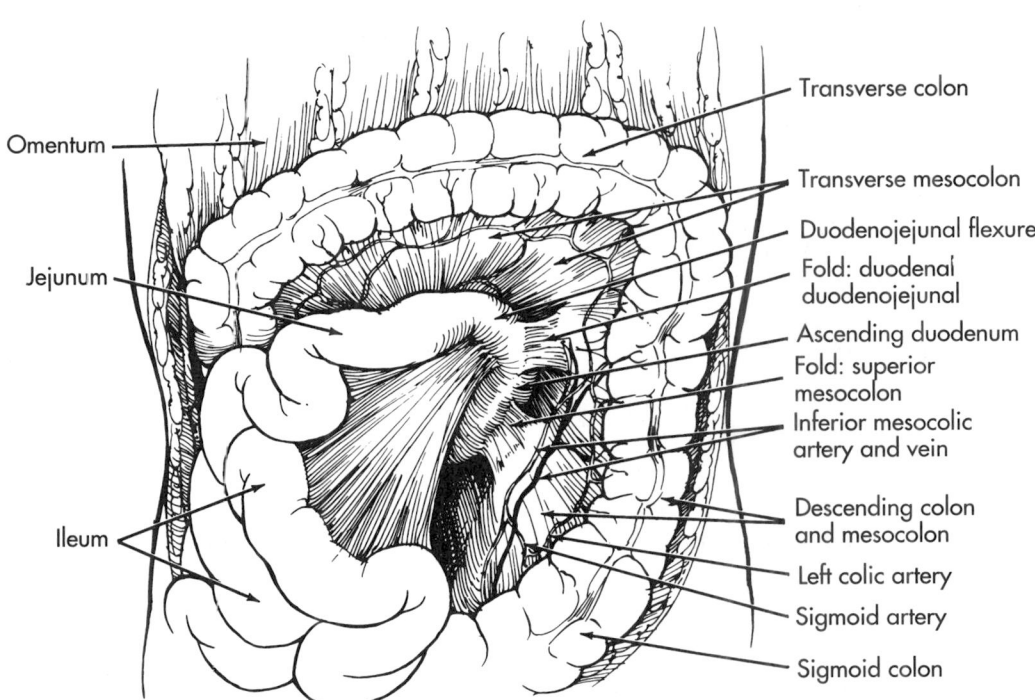

FIGURE 11–14   Mesentery, as seen when intestine is pulled aside.

The GI tract is probably affected by psychologic factors at least as much as other body systems are. In our high-pressured society, people tend to overeat or undereat, and the pressures of everyday living frequently show their effects on the GI tract. Although there is no conclusive evidence, some disease entities—such as pylorospasm, peptic and duodenal ulcers, colitis, and obesity—seem to be exacerbated by psychologic factors. Some of these diseases can be treated medically; others require adjunctive psychotherapy. All of them necessitate diagnostic studies, and many require surgery.

PERIOPERATIVE NURSING CONSIDERATIONS

Assessment

Nursing care for patients undergoing GI surgery begins with assessment. Individualized care, integrating physiologic with psychologic preparation, is given to each patient. Patients undergoing GI surgery should understand why they need preoperative preparation, what the intended surgical intervention will be, and how it will affect them postoperatively. A preoperative nursing assessment of the patient is essential for appropriate planning and implementation of intraoperative nursing care and evaluation of patient outcomes. The nurse should ensure that the patient understands the nature of the surgery and the site of the incision. Turning, coughing, and deep breathing are taught preoperatively and reinforced after surgery. If an ostomy is anticipated, an enterostomal nurse specialist should be consulted to prepare the patient for the realization of an abdominal stoma. The enterostomal specialist can also assist in allaying fears and anxieties for the patient and the family. The patient's abdomen can be marked preoperatively, indicating the most optimal placement for the abdominal stoma.

The nursing assessment of the patient having GI disease should include the following information:

- Demographic data
- Present problems, chief complaint, or symptoms that lead the patient to seek medical attention (Box 11-1)
- Medical history
- Family history
- Personal and social history

Examination of the patient's abdomen should include inspection, palpation, and auscultation of bowel sounds.

Pertinent serum studies related to the patient with GI disease might include a complete blood count (CBC) with differential, serum electrolytes, platelet count, serum osmolality, cholesterol level, vitamin and mineral levels,

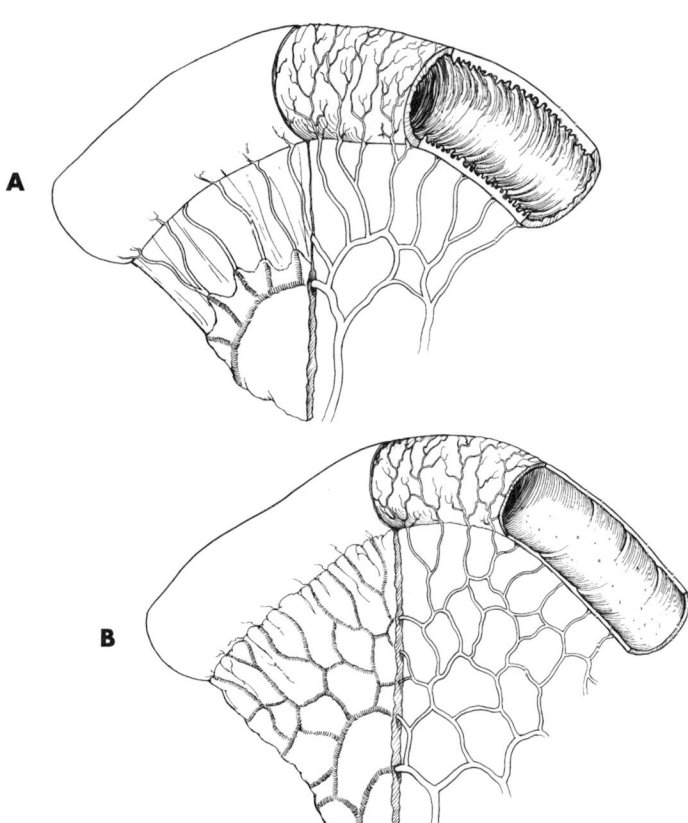

FIGURE 11-15 Comparison of jejunum to ileum. **A**, Jejunum has larger circumference, thick mucosa, and one or two vascular arcades. **B**, Ileum has smaller circumference, thin mucosa, and multiple vascular arcades.

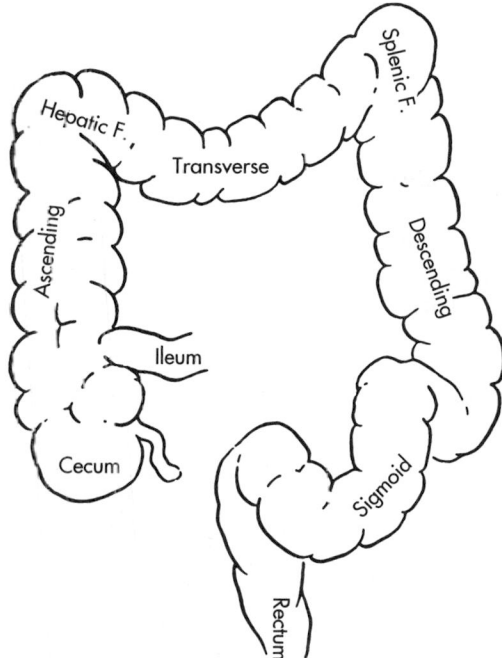

FIGURE 11-16 Anatomic division of large intestine, showing placement of ileocecal valve, hepatic flexure, and splenic flexure.

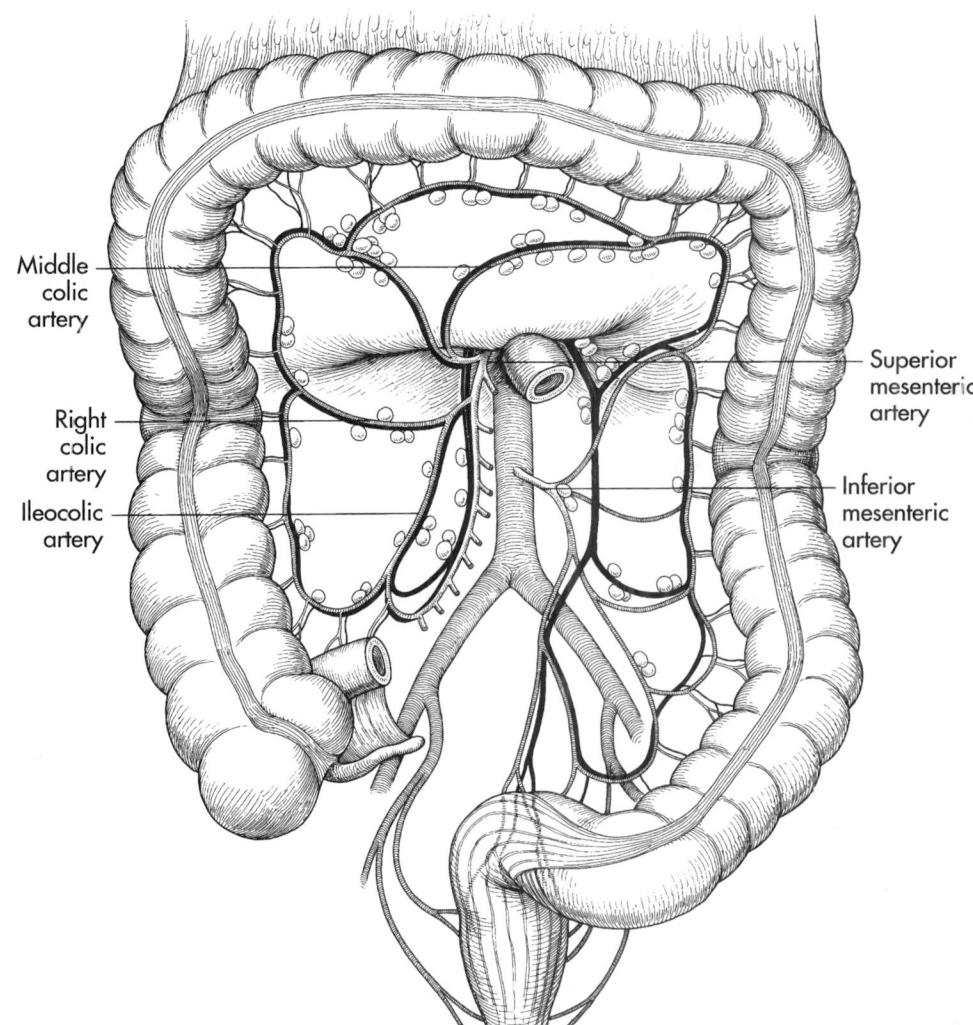

Middle
colic
artery

Right
colic
artery

Ileocolic
artery

Superior
mesenteric
artery

Inferior
mesenteric
artery

FIGURE 11-17   Blood supply of the colon.

serum enzymes, bilirubin metabolism, serum proteins, and pancreatic function studies (Table 11-1). Laboratory indices of nutritional status may also be relevant for patients with GI disease (Table 11-2).

Carcinoembryonic antigen (CEA) is a serum tumor marker that has been found to be a valuable monitoring tool for patients having a history of colon or rectal cancer. CEA is a glycoprotein found in the cell membranes of many tissues, including tumors of the GI tract. It is not used as a screening tool because patients with primary colon or rectal cancer may have normal CEA levels. The normal range is 0 to 5 ng/ml. A baseline CEA is usually obtained on patients diagnosed with cancer of the colon or rectum so that their levels can be closely followed after surgery. Any rise in the patient's CEA level after resection of the primary tumor is cause for concern and will be closely monitored. When a definite pattern of elevation is established, the patient will be advised to undergo an aggressive regimen of diagnostics to detect possible metastasis. A laparoscopic assessment of the patient's

peritoneal cavity with or without a CEA-directed second-look laparotomy may be indicated even if scans are negative. This procedure is reviewed later in this chapter (see pp. 364, 365, and 368).

Nursing Diagnosis

The value of nursing care plans has been well documented in the literature. Perioperative nurses are challenged to diagnose, plan, implement, and evaluate care in a very short time. They must have the ability to prioritize patient needs and act accordingly. The first step in this process, patient assessment, leads to the formulation of nursing diagnoses and identification of desired outcomes and is essential to all other steps.

Nursing diagnoses related to the care of patients undergoing GI surgery might include the following:

- Anxiety related to fear of the unknown
- Body image disturbance related to potential postoperative ostomy

---

BOX 11-1 | **Assessment Data**

General Data

Usual height and weight

Nutrient intake:

    Types of food usually eaten at each meal or snack

    Food likes and dislikes

    Religious or medical food restrictions

    Food intolerances

    Patient's perception and concerns pertaining to diet and weight

    Effects of life-style on diet, weight gain or loss

    Vitamins and nutritional supplements used

Oral hygiene

Bowel elimination patterns

Use of medications or laxatives

    Stool softeners

    Antiemetics

    Antidiarrheals

    Antacids

    Frequent or high doses of aspirin, acetaminophen, or ibuprofen

Specific Data

Oral lesions

Appetite

Digestion or indigestion

Dysphagia

Nausea

Vomiting

Hematemesis

Change in stool

    Color (clay color, black)

    Contents (undigested food, blood, mucus)

Constipation

Diarrhea

Flatulence

Hemorrhoids

Abdominal pain

Hepatitis

Jaundice

Ulcers

Gallstones

Polyps

Tumors

Anal discomfort

Fecal incontinence

Exposure to infectious disease

TABLE 11-1 | **Common Nonspecific Serum Studies**

TEST NAME	NORMAL VALUES
Complete Blood Count with Differential Count (CBC and Diff)	
Red blood cell count (RBC)	Men: 4.7-6.1 million/mm^3
	Women: 4.2-5.4 million/mm^3

- Low values indicate anemia resulting from blood loss, hemolysis, dietary deficiency, drug ingestion, bone marrow failure, or chronic illness.
- High values may indicate compensation for high altitudes, chronic anoxia, or polycythemia vera

Hemoglobin (Hb) concentration	Men: 14-18 g/dl
	Women: 12-16 g/dl

- Low and high values tend to be caused by the same processes that cause low or high values for RBC
- Dehydration causes an artificially high value

Hematocrit (Hct)	Men: 42%-52%
	Women: 37%-47%

- Low and high values tend to be caused by the same processes that cause low or high RBC and Hb values

Mean corpuscular volume (MCV)	Adults: 80-95/mm^3

- High values may be seen in megaloblastic anemias (such as vitamin-B_{12} deficiency)
- Low values may be seen with iron-deficiency anemia or thalassemia

Mean corpuscular hemoglobin (MCH)	Adults: 27-31 pg

- Low and high values tend to be caused by the same processes that cause low or high values for MCV.

Mean corpuscular hemoglobin concentration (MCHC)	Adults: 32-36 g/dl

- Low values indicate hemoglobin deficiency and are seen in iron-deficiency anemia and thalassemia

White blood cell count (WBC) differential	Adults: 5000-10,000/mm^3
	Neutrophils: 55%-70%
	Lymphocytes: 20%-40%
	Monocytes: 2%-8%
	Eosinophils: 1%-4%
	Basophils: 0.5%-1%

From Doughty, D.B., & Jackson, D.B. (1993). *Gastrointestinal disorders.* St. Louis: Mosby.

Continued

TABLE 11-1 | **Common Nonspecific Serum Studies—cont'd**

TEST NAME	NORMAL VALUES

- Elevated WBC commonly indicates infection or leukemia.
- Decreased WBC may indicate bone marrow failure, overwhelming infection, dietary deficiency, or autoimmune disease.
- Elevated neutrophil count may be seen in acute suppurative infection.
- Decreased neutrophil count may be seen with overwhelming bacterial infection (especially in the elderly) or dietary deficiency.
- Elevated lymphocyte count may be seen with chronic bacterial infection or viral infection.
- Decreased lymphocyte count may be seen with sepsis.
- Elevated eosinophil count may be seen with parasitic infestation, allergic reactions, or autoimmune diseases.
- A "shift to the left" means there is an increased percentage of neutrophils and immature leukocytes, which occurs with infection.

Platelet count   150,000-400,000/mm³

- Reduced levels of platelets may result from decreased platelet production, increased sequestration (as is seen in hypersplenism), increased platelet destruction or consumption (such as disseminated intravascular coagulation), or loss of platelets through hemorrhage.
- Elevated levels may be seen with severe hemorrhage, polycythemia vera, postsplenectomy syndromes, and some malignant disorders.

Serum Electrolytes

Sodium (Na)   136-145 mEq/L

- Elevated levels may be seen with excessive sweating, extensive burns, osmotic diuresis, and excessive sodium intake or reduced sodium excretion.
- Reduced levels may be seen with inadequate sodium intake, increased sodium losses (such as vomiting, nasogastric suction, diarrhea, renal disease, or third-space losses of sodium).

Potassium (K)   3.5-5 mEq/L

- Elevated levels may be seen with excessive intake or reduced excretion of potassium (such as renal failure), crushing injuries causing release of intracellular potassium, or with metabolic acidosis.
- Reduced levels may be seen with inadequate intake or excessive losses (such as diarrhea, vomiting, use of diuretics, hyperaldosteronism) or as a result of metabolic alkalosis or administration of glucose, insulin, or calcium (which causes a shift of potassium from the bloodstream into cells).

Chloride (Cl)   90-110 mEq/L

- Changes in chloride concentration usually parallel changes in sodium concentration.

Carbon dioxide (CO_2)   23-30 mEq/L

- Elevated levels are seen with acidosis.
- Reduced levels are seen with alkalosis.

Blood Gas Studies

(ARTERIAL)

pH   7.35-7.45

- High levels indicate alkalosis.
- Low levels reflect acidosis.

Partial pressure of carbon dioxide (P_{CO_2})

- High levels indicate carbon dioxide retention caused by respiratory depression or pulmonary disease (respiratory acidosis).
- Low levels reflect excessive loss of carbon dioxide through hyperventilation (such as respiratory alkalosis from overventilation or emotional trauma; may also be seen as compensatory response in metabolic acidosis).

Bicarbonate (HCO_3)   22-26 mEq/L

- Low levels indicate metabolic acidosis caused by excessive acid production, resulting in depletion of HCO_3 (such as diabetic acidosis); failure to eliminate H⁺ ions, resulting in depletion of HCO_3 (such as renal failure); or excessive loss of HCO_3 (such as intestinal losses through diarrhea or fistula drainage). Low levels may also be seen with insulin overdose, insulinoma, hypothyroidism, hypopituitarism, Addison's disease, and extensive liver disease.
- High levels indicate metabolic alkalosis resulting from bicarbonate overdose or excessive gastric losses; may also be seen as a compensatory response in a patient with prolonged respiratory acidosis; pancreatic disorders (such as adenoma, pancreatitis), corticosteroid therapy, diuretics, Cushing's disease, and hyperthyroidism.

- Risk for fluid volume deficit related to loss of blood and electrolyte-rich gastric and intestinal juices
- Risk for infection related to invasive GI procedures
- Hypothermia related to room temperature, skin exposure, and an open wound

Outcome Identification

Outcomes identified for the selected nursing diagnoses could be stated as follows:

- The patient will verbalize knowledge of the perioperative experience.

TABLE 11-2	Laboratory Indices of Nutritional Status

TEST NAME	NORMAL VALUES
Albumin (serum)	3.5-5.5 mg/dl

- Decreased levels are seen in protein malnutrition and with hepatocellular injury.

Transferrin (serum) 250-300 mg/dl

- Decreased levels are seen in protein malnutrition; transferrin levels may be used to monitor a patient's response to nutritional support therapy because the half-life of transferrin is 8 to 10 days, whereas the half-life of albumin is 19 to 20 days (this means that transferrin levels reflect changes in the patient's visceral protein status much faster than albumin levels do).

Prealbumin (serum) 15-32 mg/dl

- Decreased levels are seen in protein malnutrition. Because the half-life of prealbumin is 2 to 3 days, these values reflect changes in the patient's visceral protein status even faster than transferrin levels do.

Total lymphocyte count (serum) >150,000/mm³

- Decreased levels may be seen in protein malnutrition; however, many other conditions affect the total lymphocyte count (such as infection or conditions affecting WBC production).

24-hour urine for urea nitrogen (UUN)

- Reflects renal excretion of nitrogen; used to determine nitrogen balance, which should be present.

Formula:

$$\frac{\text{24-hour nitrogen intake (g of protein)}}{6.25} - (\text{24 hours UUN} + 4) = \text{Balance}$$

From Doughty, D.B., & Jackson, D.B. (1993). *Gastrointestinal disorders.* St. Louis: Mosby.

- The patient demonstrates knowledge of the ostomy and a desire to perform self-care.
- The patient's fluid and electrolyte balance is maintained.
- The patient will demonstrate no clinical signs of wound infection.
- The patient will be free from injury related to heat loss.

Planning

Preoperative assessment enables the perioperative nurse to plan for the specific needs of the individual patient. For example, the size of the patient influences positioning during surgery and may necessitate additional instruments, such as deeper retractors and longer forceps and scissors. The perioperative nurse has to provide the patient with reassurance and emotional support for effective management of anxiety. The perioperative nurse must also understand the potential for altered body image with some GI procedures.

Once the nursing diagnosis is made, desired outcomes are identified and the care plan is developed to assist the patient to meet the outcomes. The care plan is an essential component in ensuring high-quality perioperative nursing

care. A typical care plan for a patient undergoing GI surgery follows.

Implementation

Preoperative mechanical preparation of the GI tract is often employed for elective surgery, and often bactericidal and bacteriostatic agents are used in an attempt to eliminate pathogenic microorganisms, especially in the lower GI tract. Many patients require nasogastric tubes. Fluid and electrolyte balance must be maintained before, during, and after surgery. Often an indwelling urinary catheter is inserted preoperatively or immediately after induction to monitor output and renal function during surgery and to keep the bladder empty, thereby allowing more space in the lower abdomen for the surgeon to perform the operation.

If required, hair removal from the proposed incisional site should be accomplished as close to the time of incision as possible, especially if removal is by shaving so that there is no time for bacteria to grow in the disturbed hair follicle. A wet shave is performed to reduce the abrasion to the skin surface and prevent hair from becoming airborne and possibly contaminating the sterile fields. Hair should be removed according to the protocol for the type of surgery the patient is to have, as well as the surgeon's preference.

If the surgeon anticipates the need to replace blood, the patient's blood is typed and crossmatched before the operation. Preadmission arrangements may have been made for the availability of autotransfused blood or donor-directed units.

The circulating nurse should be well informed of what the procedure will entail and should ensure that all necessary supplies and equipment are on hand and that the integrity of the equipment is uncompromised. An electrosurgical unit and accessories are usually used for the cutting and coagulation of tissue.

As in all surgery, careful consideration should be given to positioning the patient so that the surgeon can gain optimum exposure without compromising the respiratory, circulatory, and nervous systems and without producing undue pressure on any body part (see Chapter 5). Instruments for GI surgery should include a basic laparotomy set combined with instruments specifically designed for use with GI tissue. The basic laparotomy set contains basic knife handles, scissors (Fig. 11-18), holding instruments and grasping forceps (Fig. 11-19), hemostatic clamps and clamping instruments (Fig 11-20), and various types of retractors (Fig. 11-21). A mechanical retractor system such as a Balfour retractor, Omni retractor, or Bookwalter retractor set may be used according to the type and size of incision and the surgeon's preference. For procedures that will include resection and anastomosis of the GI structures, long forceps, long scissors, and noncrushing clamps designed to gently cross-clamp the lumen of the esophagus, stomach, or bowel should be available (Fig. 11-22). Surgeon preference and the

S A M P L E   C A R E   P L A N

Nursing Diagnosis: Anxiety related to fear of the unknown

Outcome: Patient will verbalize knowledge of the perioperative experience.

Interventions:

Explain preoperative procedures that will facilitate the surgery, such as intravenous lines, skin preparation, bowel preparation.

Explain all procedures done in the OR before induction.

Explain postoperative drains, catheters, dressings.

Minimize stimuli in the OR.

Remain with the patient during induction.

Allow time for the patient to verbalize feelings and fears.

Nursing Diagnosis: Body image disturbance related to potential postoperative ostomy

Outcome: Patient demonstrates knowledge of the ostomy and a desire to perform self-care.

Interventions:

Participate in therapeutic communication during the preoperative visit; include family members if appropriate.

Be aware of nonverbal cues.

Refer patient to ostomy nurse.

Encourage patient participation in all aspects of care.

Nursing Diagnosis: Risk for fluid volume deficit related to loss of blood and electrolyte-rich gastric and intestinal juices

Outcome: The patient's fluid and electrolyte balance is maintained.

Interventions:

Obtain baseline data from the chart relating to fluid and electrolyte balance.

Assess nutritional status, skin turgor, or medications affecting fluid and electrolyte balance.

Periodically inform the surgical team of estimated blood loss.

Record all solutions being administered from the surgical field.

Nursing Diagnosis: Risk for infection related to invasive gastrointestinal procedure

Outcome: Patient will demonstrate no clinical signs of wound infection.

Interventions:

Check the integrity and expiration date of all sterile packages and containers.

Ensure aseptic technique is maintained; communicate and correct breaks in asepsis.

Contain contaminants appropriately.

Nursing Diagnosis: Hypothermia related to room temperature, skin exposure, and an open wound

Outcome: Patient will be free from injury related to heat loss.

Interventions:

Provide the patient with a warm blanket before induction. Place forced warm-air blanket over patient's upper body and head.

Ensure that irrigating solutions are warm.

Keep room temperature at a level that provides for maintenance of body temperature.

Cover patient with a warm blanket before transport to postanesthesia care unit (PACU).

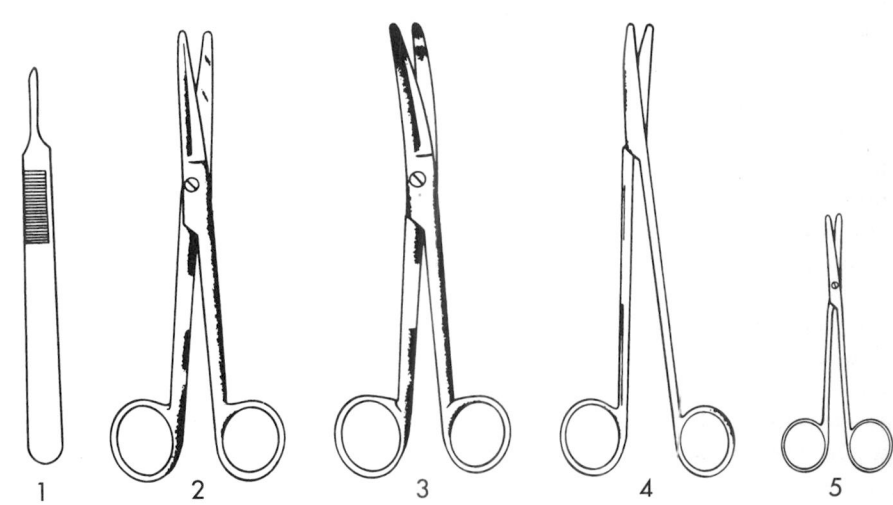

FIGURE 11-18 Basic cutting instruments for laparotomy. *1,* Knife handle; *2,* Mayo scissors, straight; *3,* Mayo scissors, curved; *4,* Metzenbaum scissors, curved; *5,* suture scissors, straight.

1   2   3   4   5

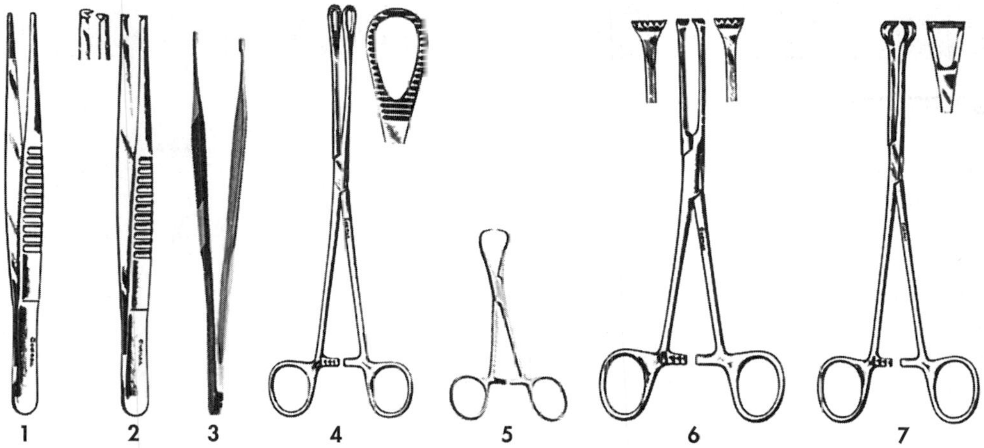

FIGURE 11-19   Basic holding instruments for laparotomy. *1*, Tissue forceps, smooth; *2*, tissue forceps with teeth; *3*, Adson tissue forceps; *4*, sponge-holding forceps; *5*, towel clamps; *6*, Allis forceps; *7*, Babcock intestinal forceps.

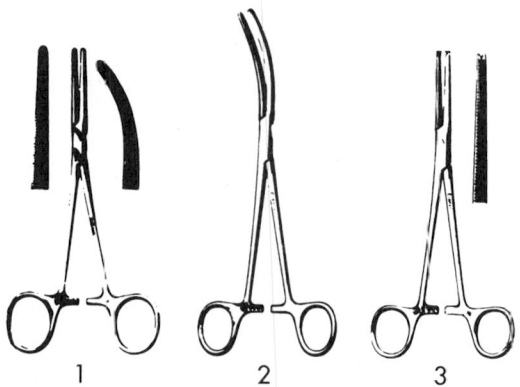

FIGURE 11-20   Basic clamping instruments for laparotomy. *1*, Crile hemostatic forceps; *2*, Rochester-Pean hemostatic forceps; *3*, Ochsner or Kocher hemostatic forceps.

resection site dictate the type and design of the clamp. To reduce tissue trauma, the jaws of heavy intestinal forceps may be protected by pieces of soft rubber tubing or other smooth material. These guards (shods) should fit the jaws firmly but not tightly and should extend slightly beyond the tips of forceps. Before sterilization the rubber shods must be separated from the forceps to facilitate and ensure steam penetration.

A Poole suction tip with tubing or Yankauer suction tip with tubing (Fig.11-23) is commonly used during GI procedures. Whenever a portion of the GI tract is entered, bowel technique should be performed. Bowel technique means that any instrument coming into contact with the GI mucosa is used only on that mucosa, not on any other tissue. These instruments may be discarded into a separate basin so that they do not come into contact with other instruments. For closure, some surgeons may desire a new set of instruments, additional draping materials, and a change of gown and gloves.

For hemostasis an electrosurgical unit with accessories is commonly available for GI procedures. Argon beam, Cavitron Ultrasonic Surgical Aspirator (CUSA), Harmonic scalpel, and laser may also be used for GI surgical interventions.

Suture materials used on GI tissue have traditionally been chromic and silk. With the increased number of synthetic absorbable and nonabsorbable suture materials available, surgeons have a variety of materials from which to choose. Polyester fiber sutures and polyglycolic acid sutures are frequently employed on GI tissue. Generally, 3-0 and 4-0 sutures on a semicircular taper needle are used on intestinal tissues. Ligatures for small vessels usually require a 3-0 or 4-0 braided material, whereas 0 or 2-0 braided ligatures are used for larger vessel occlusion. For closure or anastomosis of GI layers, 3-0 or 4-0 synthetic absorbable suture with a curved atraumatic intestinal needle is commonly used on the mucosa. A 3-0 or 2-0 continuous synthetic absorbable suture and 4-0 or 3-0 nonabsorbable suture with curved or straight atraumatic intestinal needles may be used for the seromuscular layer. Some surgeons may prefer interrupted silk sutures on intestinal (semicircular taper) needles for anastomosis procedures. For abdominal closure #1 or 0 braided or monofilament suture is commonly used. Retention sutures may be indicated when there is potential for compromised tissue or wound healing. Checking the surgeon's preference card for appropriate suture materials not only ensures the availability of necessary supplies but also is a cost-effective measure.

Surgical stapling instruments have had a great influence on the technical aspects of GI surgery. For some surgeons the use of these devices has to an extent replaced conventional suturing techniques. The stapling instruments can be employed to divide and ligate, resect and anastomose. The B design of the implanted staple does not compromise the vascularity of the resected tissue edges.

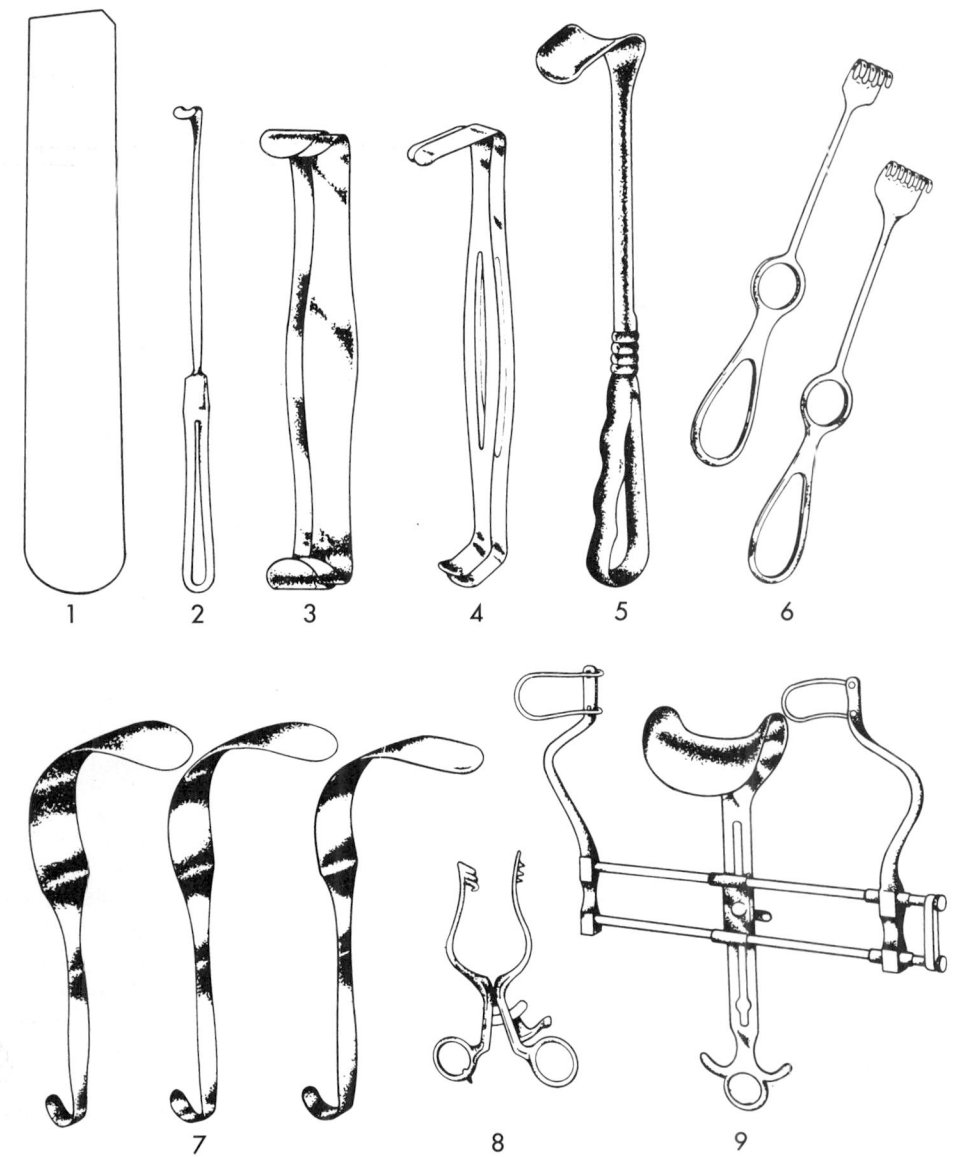

FIGURE 11-21 Basic exposing instruments for laparotomy. *1*, Malleable retractor; *2*, vein retractor; *3*, Parker retractors; *4*, Army-Navy retractors; *5*, Richardson retractor; *6*, Volkmann rake retractors; *7*, Deaver retractors; *8*, Weitlaner retractor; *9*, Balfour self-retaining retractor with blades.

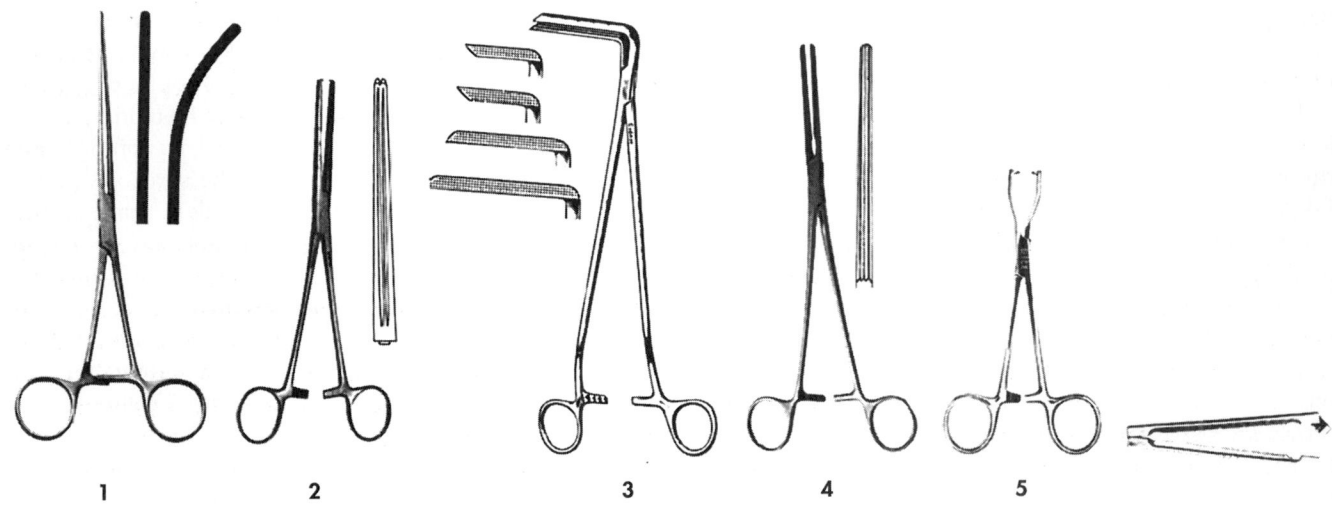

FIGURE 11-22 Instruments for stomach and intestinal operations. *1*, Doyen intestinal forceps, straight and curved; *2*, Allen intestinal anastomosis clamp; *3*, Best colon clamps; *4*, Dennis intestinal clamp, *5*, Pace-Potts clamp.

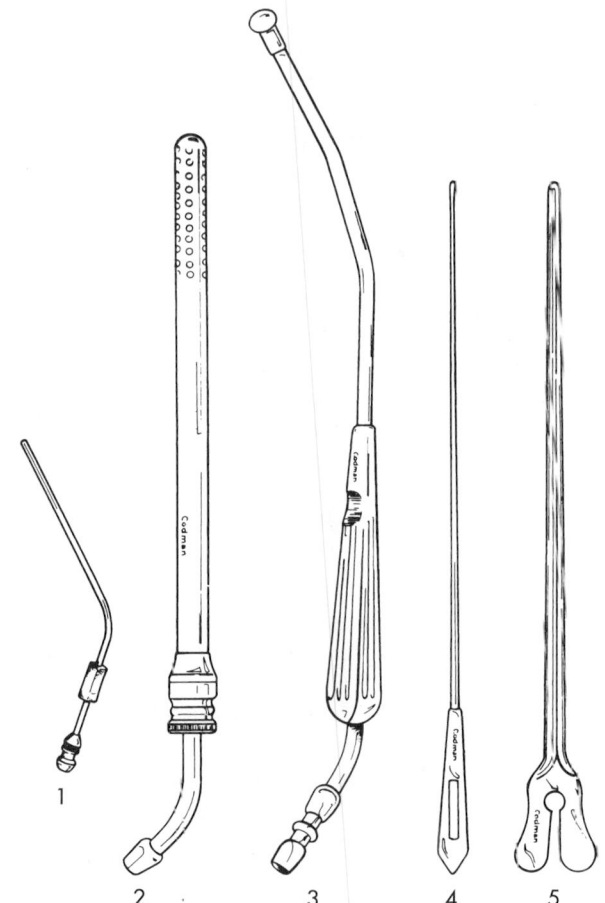

FIGURE 11-23 Accessory items. *1*, Frazier suction tip; *2*, Poole suction tube; *3*, Yankauer suction tube; *4*, silver probe; *5*, grooved director.

TABLE 11-3 | **Mechanical Linear Stapling Devices★**

U.S. SURGICAL	ETHICON	INSTRUMENT APPLICATION AND PURPOSE
LDS		Ligating and dissecting vascular tissue such as that in the omentum and mesentery. This instrument applies two ligating clips and cuts the tissue between them.
GIA	ILS	Applies two parallel linear rows of staples against an anvil and severs the tissue between the two staple lines. Available in sizes 60 and 80. Used to transect bowel, stomach, or lung and bronchi while providing hemostasis and, in the case of the gastrointestinal tract, confinement of luminal contents.
TA		Applies two parallel linear rows of staples against an anvil for anastomosing tissues and tissue closure. Available in sizes 30, 50, and 90. Length of staple is 3.5 or 4.8 mm. The roticulating head provides flexibility in angling the instrument to better access deep pelvic tissues.
CEEA	ILA	Applies a circular ring of staples for intraluminal end-to-end or end-to-side anastomosis of two segments of gastrointestinal tract. A small amount of tissue is resected at the firing of the instrument. Available in 21, 25, 28, 31 straight or curved.

★The mechanical linear stapling devices serve the surgeon with timely efficiency over manually suturing anastomoses.

These devices are available in reusable and disposable models. Personnel must be familiar with the types of available stapling equipment, applications, assembly if indicated, and proper loading (Table 11-3). Ligating clips are also used in GI procedures. Irrigating solution is frequently used during GI procedures. The surgeon specifies the solution of choice, which frequently contains a broad-spectrum antibiotic. Normal saline, an isotonic solution, may be used to moisten laparotomy sponges and for irrigation. Moist packs are used to isolate open and diseased portions of the stomach and bowel from the abdominal cavity and to protect other viscera. Solutions should be warm when used for these purposes.

As in all operations, the excised specimen is handled carefully and prepared for examination by the pathologist. The surgeon usually determines how the specimen will be handled before examination. It may be sent to the pathology department fresh, in saline, or in a preservative solution. Tissue also may be sent for frozen-section examination to verify the pathologic condition and determine whether tissue margins are free from malignant cells.

Drains may be indicated for evacuation of the gastric juices. A Malecot, Pezzer, or Foley catheter in desired size may be inserted for gastrostomy tube drainage until normal bowel peristalsis returns. A 12 or 14 French Robinson catheter or Baker jejunostomy tube may be placed in the jejunum after gastric resection for purposes of nutrition. Closed wound drainage systems may be indicated if infection is present.

Evaluation

As with any surgical procedure, evaluation of nursing care must be done throughout the surgery and before the patient is transported to the postanesthesia care unit (PACU) or a surgical intensive care unit (SICU) if indicated. The dressing and drains are securely placed to avoid damage during transfer to the PACU stretcher or SICU bed. Skin is assessed for reddened or bruised areas; if such areas are present, treatment is initiated immediately. The electrosurgical dispersive pad is removed, the site is inspected, and the condition of the skin is documented. The circulating nurse ensures that the patient is covered with a clean, warm blanket before being transported to PACU or SICU. Any variances postoperatively are reported to the surgeon, documented in the nursing notes, and included in the report given to the nurse in PACU or SICU. Patient outcomes, based on the perioperative nursing diagnoses, should be reviewed. Based on the nursing diagnoses selected for the patient undergoing GI surgery, documenting and reporting perioperative patient care might include the following statements:

- The patient verbalized knowledge and expressed feelings about the perioperative experience.
- The patient verbalized feelings about body image disturbance.
- The patient's fluid volume status was maintained.
- The patient will demonstrate no clinical signs of wound infection postoperatively. Contamination related to the invasion of the GI tract was confined.
- Normothermia was maintained.

Patient and Family Education and Discharge Planning

Patients undergoing surgical intervention for GI disorders will vary greatly in the length of time and complexity of recovery depending on the type of procedure and site of surgery.

GI structures may have varying degrees of edema, decreased peristalsis, alterations in tissue oxygenation and lymphatic drainage depending on the amount of manipulation, resection and trauma to the normal anatomic structures of the GI tract. General anesthesia is commonly administered to the patient undergoing surgical interventions of the GI tract. Smooth muscle relaxation is imperative for most major GI procedures. The patient will usually experience decreased GI peristalsis for 2 to 5 days after laparotomy and intestinal resection. A nasogastric tube or gastrostomy tube is inserted to evacuate the large volumes of gastric juices. Diet is introduced only after bowel sounds return. The patient may experience nausea and vomiting if food or drink is introduced too early for the GI system to function with normal absorption and motility.

Coughing and deep breathing is important for the patient recovering from general anesthesia. Splinting of the abdominal muscles and the use of an incentive spirometer will assist the patient in postoperative coughing and deep breathing initiatives. Early ambulating will assist the patient in regaining overall muscle tone and preventing deep venous thrombosis in the lower extremities.

Pain management is a very important factor in the patient's recovery. An epidural catheter may be placed immediately prior to surgery for postoperative pain control. For most major GI procedures patient controlled analgesia (PCA) is utilized for consistent control of pain and discomfort in the first 1 to 3 postoperative days of hospital recovery. Narcotics may add to the length of time after which normal bowel peristalsis returns and so are monitored closely after the third postoperative day.

The patient having a newly created ostomy will require consultation with an enterostomal therapist to assist both the patient and his or her family or significant others in the care and management of the ostomy and surrounding skin. Many life-style changes are associated with an ostomy. The enterostomal therapist consultation is an essential factor in the successful recovery and rehabilitation of the patient with a new ostomy. The enterostomal therapist first teaches the patient and his or her family acceptance of the ostomy. Skin care, appliance application, ostomy irrigation, diet, and bowel training are but a few of the topics that must be taught for care and management of an ostomy. Clothing, self-esteem, body image, sex and intimacy, travel, public toileting, and controlling odor are some of the social issues for which the enterostomal therapist will provide the patient and his or her family or significant others with strategies to ensure quality and fulfillment in their lives.

Patients with resected small bowel may require total parental nutrition (TPN) because their ability to absorb nutrients from ingested food is compromised. Referral to homecare agencies that are expert in administering TPN is essential for this patient population.

General discharge instructions for the patient undergoing GI surgery may include the following:

- Swelling inside the GI tract may produce a feeling of tightness; this should dissipate in 6 to 8 weeks.
- Solid foods should be added to the diet gradually. Chew solid foods well and avoid gulping or eating fast or swallowing large bulk portions.
- Avoid carbonated beverages for 3 to 4 weeks to help prevent gas bloating.
- Plan small frequent meals because the feeling of fullness will come quickly.
- Keep the incisional area clean and dry.
- Increase exercise gradually to return to activities of daily living. Exercise regularly.
- Make an appointment for follow-up care with the surgeon.
- Have written instructions with phone numbers as to who to call and when. The patient should call the doctor if any of the following develop:
  - Persistent fever (101° F) or higher
  - Bleeding
  - Increased abdominal swelling or pain
  - Persistent nausea or vomiting
  - Chills
  - Persistent cough or shortness of breath

Procedure-specific instructions may be necessary to fully assist the patient and his or her care givers with recovery and rehabilitation outside of the hospital setting.

SURGICAL INTERVENTIONS
ENDOSCOPIC PROCEDURES

Endoscopic procedures that permit direct visual inspection of the contents and walls of the esophagus, stomach, and colon may be pertinent to establishing a diagnosis or determining preferred treatment of a disease process. A neodymium:yttrium–aluminum–garnet (Nd:YAG) laser may also be used with endoscopic procedures as a treatment modality for ulcers, esophageal varices, malignancies, and GI bleeding (see Chapter 3).

Care must be taken in handling fiberoptic equipment. Flexible scopes can be easily damaged if handled improperly. The OR personnel should be educated as to the proper care and handling of each specific endoscope. Flexible endoscopes should not be bent at a severe angle. Leak-testing must be performed before perfusion of disinfectant or sterilant is begun. Flexible scopes placed in endoscope washers or Steris sterilization units may be crushed if not contained within the appropriate troughs or groove patterns. Diagrams are useful in guiding personnel as to the proper arrangement of the flexible scopes in washers or Steris units. The endoscopic equipment is terminally cleaned according to the manufacturer's instructions and stored so that drainage of liquid from the lumens can occur. See Chapter 3 for more information on endoscope processing.

Endoscopic procedures may be performed with local anesthesia, with IV conscious sedation/analgesia, or during the course of a procedure being performed with general anesthesia. Although medications may be used for sedation, the nurse must be immediately available to provide emotional support and appropriately monitor the patient's physiologic and psychologic status.

Gastroscopy

Gastroscopy is visual inspection of the stomach, with aspiration of contents and biopsy, if necessary, by an instrument known as a *gastroscope* (Fig. 11-24). When gastroscopy is performed with local anesthesia or sedation, the patient is usually not allowed to eat solid food 4 to 6 hours before the procedure but may take liquids up to 2 hours before it.

Procedural considerations

The patient's position for gastroscopy depends on the areas of the stomach to be visualized. For inspection of lesions in the gastric fundus and cardia, an upright sitting position may be used. A protective bite block should always be placed in the patient's mouth to protect the scope from injury. Instrumentation will include a gastroscope and video camera (optional) and biopsy forceps.

Local anesthesia may be used. This could be in the form

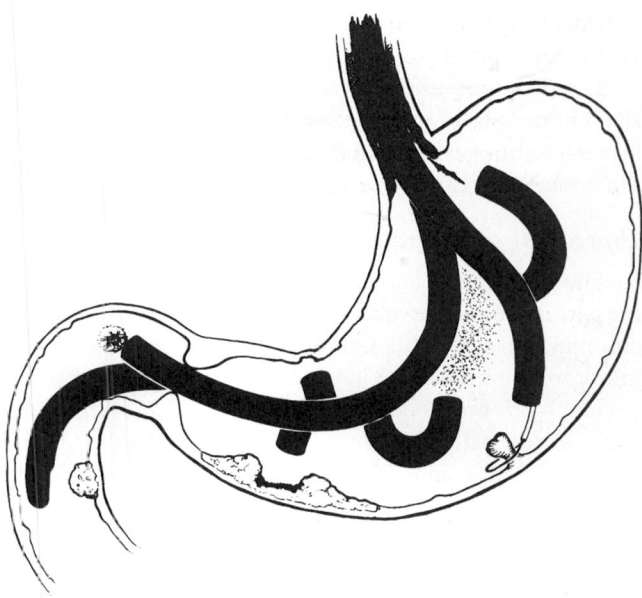

FIGURE 11-24 Gastroscope in lumen of stomach illustrating the visualization capabilities and potential uses that gastroscopy affords.

of viscous lidocaine gel that is swallowed, or in the form of a spray. A light source with air-infusion capability and a water bottle for irrigation is required. Suction, aspiration tubes, and a cup of saline for the biopsy should be available. Lubricating jelly is placed over the sheath of the gastroscope for ease in placement. An electrosurgical unit and cord should be available if fulguration of a lesion is necessary.

Operative procedure

1. The gastroscope is thinly but completely covered with water-soluble lubricating jelly.
2. During introduction of the gastroscope, the patient's head and neck must remain in the sagittal plane of the spine so that the axis of the mouth is in line with the esophagus.
3. The gastroscope is slowly passed into the stomach.
4. The stomach is inspected, and stomach contents may be aspirated for cytologic analysis. A biopsy can be performed. Laser treatment may be carried out as indicated.

Colonoscopy and Sigmoidoscopy

Colonoscopy is the visual inspection of the entire large intestine by means of a colonoscope. Sigmoidoscopy is the direct visualization of the sigmoid colon and rectum. The colonoscope is an important diagnostic tool and may be used for biopsy, removal of polyps, or laser treatment of tumors or bleeders. Colonoscopy and sigmoidoscopy may be performed in the OR just before the abdominal colon/sigmoid resection to mark the tumor site with India ink. This is helpful for the surgeon to define the tumor site, viewing from the serosal side of the colon by laparotomy or laparoscopy access.

The patient must receive a liquid diet for 2 days before the colonoscopy and sigmoidoscopy and may receive bowel-cleansing agents such as citrate of magnesium or GoLytely. Enemas may be necessary before the procedure.

Procedural considerations

The instruments and equipment that must be available for performing colonoscopy and sigmoidoscopy include a colonoscope or flexible sigmoidoscope, video camera and monitors (optional), a light source, an air-insufflation device with water bottle for irrigation, a biopsy forceps, snares, cytology brush, electrosurgical-fulguration-desiccation unit and appropriate accessories, lubricating jelly, and suction. For efficiency and rapid accessibility, these items are commonly mounted on a designated procedure cart.

Analgesia is induced intramuscularly or intravenously.

Operative procedure

1. The well-lubricated colonoscope is passed slowly into the anal canal and advanced continuously until it reaches the cecum for colonoscopy. With sigmoidoscopy, only the left colon is examined.
2. After the endoscopic examination, the patient should be observed carefully to ensure that neither postprocedural bleeding nor signs of perforation occur.

Laparoscopy

A small incision is made in the fold of the umbilicus through which a percutaneous needle or trocar and sheath are placed. The peritoneal cavity is insufflated with CO_2, and a rigid wide-angled laparoscope is placed into the operative sheath for direct visualization of the abdominal viscera. This can be for diagnostic purposes or to assist or accomplish surgical interventions when additional operative ports are established. Specific laparoscopic procedures are described later in this chapter.

Laparotomy

An opening made through the abdominal wall into the peritoneal cavity is called a *laparotomy*. Surgical intervention may be necessary to repair or remove traumatized tissue, to cure disease processes by organ removal, or to examine by biopsy or otherwise visualize internal organs for diagnosis. Surgery may be indicated for diagnostic, therapeutic, palliative, or prophylactic reasons. Most procedures requiring a laparotomy involve the organs of the alimentary canal.

Procedural considerations

A basic laparotomy instrument set is used. An electrosurgical unit and suction are basic to performing laparotomy. The patient is positioned supine with arms extended at less than a 90-degree angle. General anesthesia with endotracheal intubation is the usual choice of anesthesia although spinal or epidural anesthesia may administered for laparotomy. An indwelling urinary catheter may be inserted before the abdominal prep. For laparotomy, the patient is commonly prepped from above the nipple line to above the symphysis pubis. A forced warm-air blanket may be applied over the patient's upper body, arms, and head for thermoregulation. Synchronous compression leggings may be ordered and applied before induction as a means to prevent deep venous blood pooling in the lower extremities.

Operative procedure

Laparotomy Opening

1. The skin incision is made and carried to the fascia (Fig. 11-25, *A*).
2. Hemostats or ligating clips are used to control bleeding vessels. Clamped vessels are ligated with fine absorbable ligatures or nonabsorbable suture, or they are electrocoagulated.
3. The wound edges are retracted with small retractors.
4. With tissue forceps and scalpel, the external fascia is incised (Fig. 11-25, *B*).
5. With Metzenbaum or curved Mayo scissors, electrocautery, or a knife, the external oblique muscle is split the length of the incision. Bleeding vessels are controlled with hemostats, ligating clips, or medium or fine ligatures.
6. The external oblique muscle is retracted.
7. The internal oblique and transverse muscles are split, parallel to the fibers, up to the rectus sheath with a scalpel or scissors. These muscles are then retracted.
8. The peritoneum is exposed, grasped with smooth tissue forceps, and nicked with a no. 10 blade (Fig. 11-25, *C*).
9. Sponges, laparotomy pads, and suction are used as needed. Culture samples may be taken at this time.
10. The peritoneal incision is extended the length of the wound with Metzenbaum or Mayo scissors.
11. The peritoneum is retracted with large Richardson retractors for initial exploration.
12. Once the affected organs are identified, a self-retaining retractor, such as the Bookwalter retractor system, may be used to ensure adequate exposure.

Laparotomy Closure

1. Two tissue forceps or clamps are used to approximate the peritoneal edges, and the peritoneum is closed with a continuous synthetic absorbable suture or interrupted nonabsorbable sutures. The internal oblique fascia is usually closed with the peritoneum. Muscle tissue is approximated and may or may not be sutured.
2. The external oblique fascia is closed with interrupted sutures, staples, or both. Retraction is necessary as the

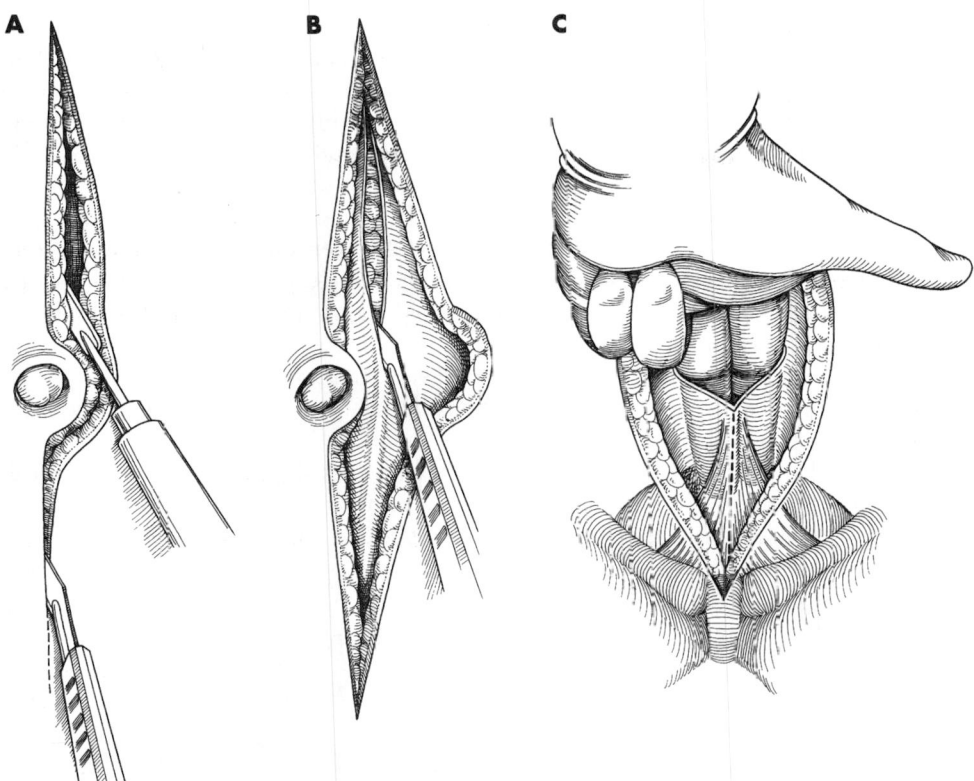

FIGURE 11-25   **A**, Midline laparotomy incision around the umbilicus. **B**, External fascia is excised. **C**, Entry into the peritoneal cavity.

various layers are closed. Richardson retractors are commonly utilized.

3. Fine (3-0 or 4-0), absorbable sutures are usually employed to close the subcutaneous or subcuticular tissue. Retraction is provided with laparotomy pads or small retractors.

4. Skin edges are held with Adson forceps and approximated with interrupted fine silk, nylon, or other nonabsorbable sutures on a cutting needle. Skin staples or clips are often used to approximate skin edges. Retention sutures of heavy nonabsorbable material may be used. Usually prepackaged retention bridges or rubber tubing bolsters are used to protect the incision site.

SURGERY OF THE ESOPHAGUS

Esophagectomy and Intrathoracic Esophagogastrostomy

Esophagectomy and intrathoracic esophagogastrostomy involve the removal of diseased portions of the stomach and esophagus through a thoracoabdominal incision in the left side of the chest—including a resection of the seventh, eighth, or ninth rib or separation of the two appropriate ribs—and establishment of an anastomosis between the esophagus and the stomach. These procedures are performed to remove strictures in the distal esophagus that may develop after trauma, infection, or corrosion or to remove tumors in the cardia of the stomach or in the distal esophagus.

Procedural considerations

Instrumentation would include a basic thoracotomy set (Chapter 25), basic laparotomy set, and GI set. Linear stapling devices (see Table 11-3) and vascular ligating clips should also be available. The patient is placed in lateral position after induction of general anesthesia. An indwelling urinary catheter is inserted. Measures are taken to ensure that the patient's body temperature is maintained.

Operative procedure

1. The skin incision is carried downward midway between the vertebral border of the scapula and the spinous processes to the eighth rib and then forward along this rib to the costochondral junction. The extent of the vertical portion of the incision depends on the location of the tumor.

2. The wound is retracted, and bleeding vessels are ligated or coagulated.

3. The chest cavity is opened, and the rib spreader is placed. Moist packs are placed, and the lung is retracted with a Deaver or Harrington retractor.

4. The mediastinal pleura is incised with long Metzenbaum scissors and long plain forceps in line with the esophagus and the lesion.

5. The esophagus is dissected free from the aorta with dry dissectors.
6. Suture ligatures of 2-0 and 3-0 nonabsorbable material are used for controlling bleeding vessels.
7. The diaphragm is opened, and a series of traction sutures is attached.
8. The stomach is mobilized by dissection of its ligamental attachment with long scissors and curved thoracic clamps.
9. The left gastric artery is clamped, cut, and doubly ligated with 2-0 nonabsorbable suture and a suture ligature of 3-0 nonabsorbable material. The sterile field is prepared for the open method of anastomosis.
10. The stomach is transsected well below the lesion with the selected resection instruments.
11. Closure of the stomach is completed with two rows of intestinal sutures of 2-0 synthetic absorbable suture and sometimes with an additional row of 3-0 nonabsorbable sutures for reinforcement.
12. A separate circular opening is usually made in the upper portion of the stomach for anastomosis to the esophagus.
13. Two Allen clamps or a stapler type of clamp is applied above the stricture, and the freed esophagus is divided.
14. The circular opening in the stomach and the transsected end of the esophagus are anastomosed. The mucosal layers are approximated. The muscular layers of the esophagus and stomach are closed by two rows of interrupted sutures. A mechanical end-to-end anastomosing surgical stapling device may also be used to accomplish the gastroesophageal anastomosis.
15. The stomach is anchored to the pleura, and the edges of the diaphragm are sutured to the wall of the stomach with interrupted sutures of 3-0 or 2-0 nonabsorbable material.
16. The pleura is cleansed with warm, normal, saline irrigation that is suctioned off.
17. A thoracic catheter is inserted for closed drainage. The chest wall is closed as described for thoracotomy (see Chapter 25).

Excision of Esophageal Diverticulum

Excision of an esophageal diverticulum, sometimes referred to as *Zenker's diverticulum*, is removal of a weakening in the wall of the esophagus that collects small amounts of food and causes a sensation of fullness in the neck. Because diverticula usually occur in the cervical portion of the esophagus, excision gives complete relief of symptoms.

Procedural considerations

Instrumentation would include a thyroid set (see Chapter 16) with the addition of two Pennington clamps, six Halsted curved mosquito hemostats, two 5-inch Adson forceps, and two lateral retractors. The patient is commonly positioned supine with a shoulder roll placed to assist with hyperextension of the patient's neck. The patient's head may be turned to the side and held in place with a padded headrest or donut.

Operative procedure

1. An incision is made over the inner border of the sternocleidomastoid muscle and is extended from the level of the hyoid bone to a point 2 cm above the clavicle.
2. The sac of the diverticulum is freed and ligated.
3. The pharyngeal muscle and surrounding tissues are closed.
4. In conjunction with this procedure, an esophageal myotomy is often performed distally to the diverticulum. A myotomy seems to lessen the likelihood of recurrence.

Esophageal Hiatal Hernia Repair and Antireflux Procedure

Hiatal herniorrhaphy is performed to restore the cardioesophageal junction in its correct anatomic position in the abdomen, to secure it firmly in place, and to correct gastroesophageal reflux. A hiatal hernia is a special type of hernia in which a defect, either congenital or accidental, in the diaphragm permits a portion of the stomach to enter the thoracic cavity.

Hiatal hernias are usually of two distinct types—paraesophageal and sliding. Symptoms vary from none to severe heartburn, reflux (backward flow), regurgitation, and dysphagia. When symptoms are severe, a repair of the hernia is done, usually through a transabdominal approach. A transthoracic approach is used in patients who previously had left upper quadrant surgery or are extremely obese, or if a Belsey Mark IV procedure is selected. Nissen fundoplication is being performed laparoscopically by some surgeons.

An antireflux procedure, which prevents reflux of gastric juices into the esophagus, is also done when the hernia is repaired. The three most frequently performed antireflux procedures are the Nissen (Fig. 11-26), Hill, and Belsey Mark IV procedures.

Procedural considerations

The patient is commonly positioned supine but may need to be repositioned to lateral if the gastroesophageal sphincter cannot be accessed through a high midline position. An indwelling urinary catheter is inserted after induction of general anesthesia.

Instrumentation would include a basic laparotomy set, Maloney or Hurst dilators in 32 to 42 Fr, a self-retaining retractor system, and a 1-inch Penrose drain. If a transthoracic approach is contemplated, a basic thoracic set would be required.

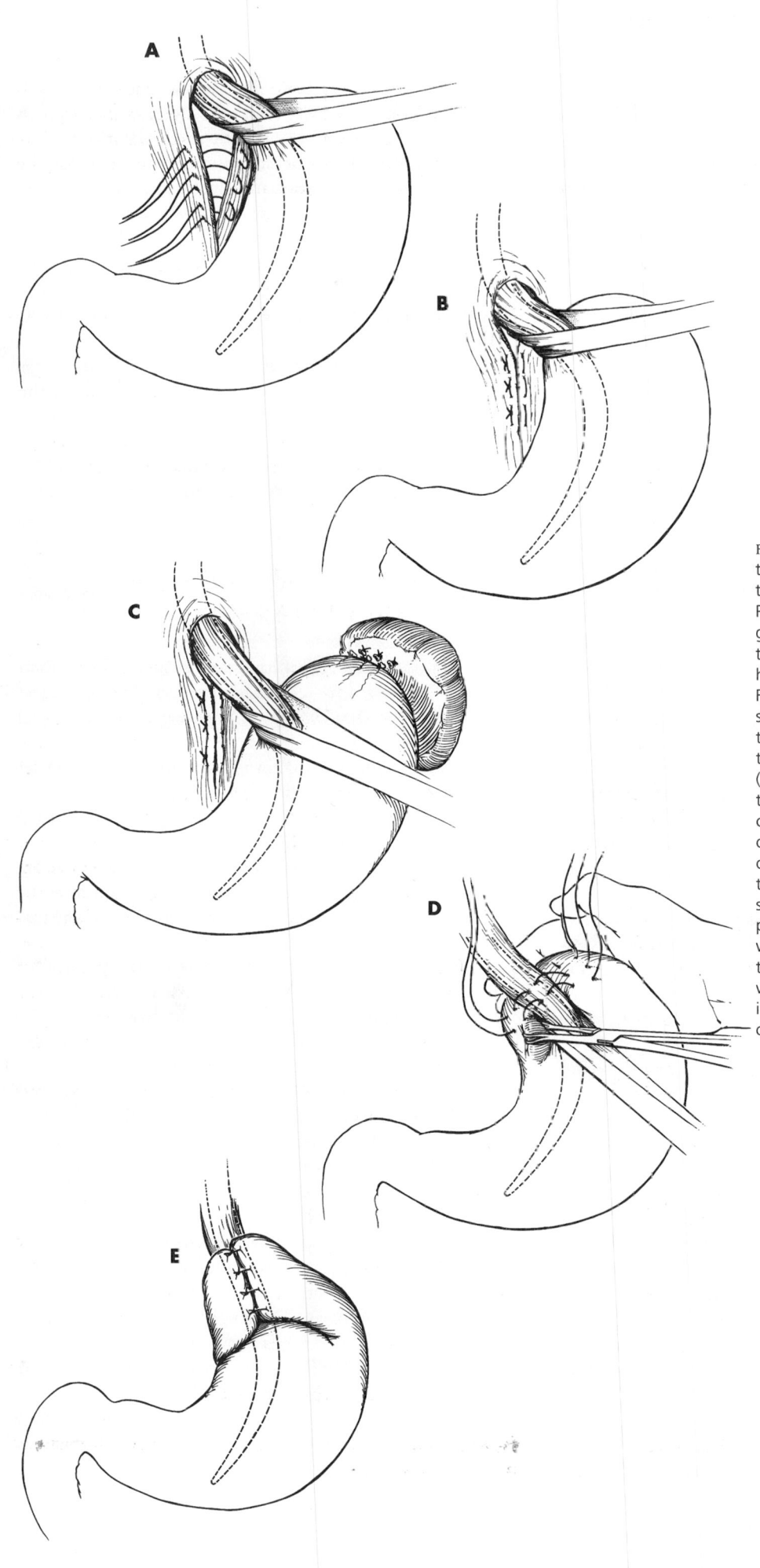

FIGURE 11-26 The Nissen fundoplication procedure begins with, **A**, Mobilization of the esophagus and placement of a Penrose drain around the gastroesophageal junction to allow for traction to pull the esophagus downward and out of the hernia after a Maloney dilator (40 to 48 Fr) has been passed into the lumen of the stomach from the patient's oral cavity in the same manner as passing a nasogastric tube. **B**, Shown are three heavy sutures (#0 braided absorbable) placed to narrow the hiatal aperture but not so tight as to constrict the esophagus, thus the purpose of stenting the esophagus with the Maloney dilator. **C**, Further traction is applied to the distal esophagus while the proximal stomach and fundus are freed from all peritoneal attachments. **D**, The posterior wall of the stomach is brought up around the distal esophagus. **E**, The stomach walls are wrapped and sutured around the intraabdominal esophagus, with the Maloney stent in place.

Operative procedure

1. Through a transabdominal incision, the hernia is located, and a crural repair is done.
2. The fundus of the stomach is wrapped around the lower 4 to 6 cm of the esophagus and is sutured in place (Nissen fundoplication); the upper part of the lesser curvature of the stomach and the cardioesophageal junction are sutured to the median arcuate ligament (Hill procedure), or the stomach is plicated around approximately 270 degrees of esophageal circumference (Belsey Mark IV procedure). The Nissen fundoplication procedure is illustrated in Fig. 11-26.
3. Vagotomy, pyloroplasty, or both may be performed at the same time.
4. The wound is closed.

Laparoscopic Nissen Fundoplication

Recent advances in minimal-access surgery, using laparoscopic visualization, have prompted adaptations of laparotomy procedures to be developed. The Nissen fundoplication previously described was developed in the early 1990s.[1] The Nissen-Rosetti fundoplication, the Toupet operation, the Lind technique, the Thal fundoplication, the Belsey Mark IV procedure, and the Watson technique are other laparoscopic procedures developed for the management of gastroesophageal reflux disease (GERD).

The patient having laparoscopic Nissen fundoplication is commonly admitted the day of surgery. The patient's surgery is performed through 5 stab wounds in the abdomen, which greatly reduces the postoperative recovery period. The healthy patient is expected to be discharged on the second postoperative day, barring no complications. A postoperative upper GI series is performed to verify the functioning of the newly constructed antireflux valve. The patient is discharged after the x-ray interpretations indicate that all is well.

Procedural considerations

The patient's surgery is performed under general anesthesia. A nasogastric tube and urinary drainage catheter is placed after induction and intubation. The patient is positioned supine or in the modified lithotomy position.

Instrumentation and supplies required for a laparoscopic Nissen fundoplication would include a basic laparotomy set, laparoscope, laparoscopic camera, two 5 mm trocars, one 10 mm trocar, two 11 mm trocars, a light cord, filtered insufflation tubing, and an electrosurgery cord. Laparoscopic instruments commonly used for the procedure include grasping forceps, endoscissors, endo-Babcock forceps, endodissecting forceps, endoclip appliers, and an endosuturing device. Endoretractors should be available. Suction and a suction-irrigator is commonly used. A Penrose drain or a 12 Fr red Robinson catheter is used to assist in isolating and retracting the distal esophagus.

Bougie dilators size 40 to 60 Fr may be used to act as an esophageal stent in which to secure the fundoplication. A water-based lubricating jelly is used to assist the anesthesiologist in placing the bougie. Equipment needed for the procedure would include an electrosurgical unit, an insufflation unit with CO_2 gas, and two video monitors placed on both sides of the patient.

Operative procedure

1. A stab wound is made in the infraumbilical fold with a #11 blade.
2. The 11 mm trocar is placed, and insufflation is achieved. This may be performed before placing the trocar by inserting a Verres needle for purpose of insufflation.
3. The laparoscope is placed through the infraumbilical sheath. The camera is attached to the laparoscope.
4. The 5 mm trocars are placed below the xiphoid process, lateral to the midline in the right upper quadrant of the abdomen. The 10 mm trocar is placed on the lateral plane to the midline in the left abdomen. The second 11 mm trocar is placed in the lateral abdominal wall for use by the assistant.
5. An endoretractor, fan shaped, is inserted through the 11 mm trocar and used to retract the left lobe of the liver for exposure of the gastroesophageal junction.
6. An endo-Babcock forceps is inserted through the 10 mm port and is used to grasp the upper aspect of the fundus of the stomach. The stomach is retracted laterally and downward.
7. The surgeon mobilizes the distal esophagus by opening the hiatus and employs a endodissector forceps to bluntly dissect the tissue along the right and left crura.
8. Endoclips are used to ligate the most distal portion of the pericardiophrenic vessel before it is divided.
9. The posterior vagus is identified but left intact.
10. The dissection is continued to expose the posterior esophagus.
11. The upper aspect of the greater curvature of the stomach is mobilized, and dissection is continued to the posterior esophagus.
12. The Penrose or Robinson catheter is inserted through a sheath and is passed behind the gastroesophageal junction. The catheter and Penrose drain ends are brought together and secured with an endoclamp that is then locked. This catheter and Penrose drain will be used as a traction retractor during the procedure.
13. Another grasping forceps is used to grasp the apex of the gastric fundus and retract it downward to expose the short gastric vessels. The vessels are ligated with endoclips and divided with endoscissors.
14. The upper portion of the mobilized greater curvature is grasped and passed through the opening that has been created at the hiatus.

15. Tension and adequate mobilization of the greater curvature of the stomach are assessed. The portion of the greater curvature of the stomach that has been brought around the posterior esophagus at the proximal part of the gastroesophageal junction is then manipulated over the anterior distal esophagus.

16. A nonabsorbable endosuture is passed through a 5 mm port and used to place a row of interrupted sutures to join the aspects of the greater curvature of the stomach in a 2 to 3 cm "wrap" around the esophagus.

17. A large bougie is passed down the lumen of the esophagus by the anesthesiologist. The sutures are secured with the bougie in place.

18. The catheter and Penrose drain is removed. The bougie is removed. The abdomen is deflated.

19. Closure of the trocar sites is performed. Dressings are applied.

Esophagomyotomy

Esophagomyotomy (Heller cardiomyotomy) is myotomy of the esophagogastric junction and is done to correct esophageal obstruction resulting from cardiospasm.

Procedural considerations

Selection of a transthoracic or transabdominal incision depends on the patient's general condition and other existing pathologic factors. The surgeon may elect to perform a pyloroplasty to prevent reflux. Instrumentation would include a basic laparotomy set and instruments to enter and retract the thorax, if necessary.

Operative procedure

1. A midline abdominal incision is made from the xiphoid process to the umbilicus.
2. After exposure of the esophagogastric junction, a Maloney dilator is inserted through the patient's oral cavity to distend the esophagus.
3. A scalpel with a #15 blade is used to make a longitudinal incision through the muscular wall of the distal esophagus and proximal stomach, leaving the mucosa intact.
4. A small portion of the fundus of the stomach may be plicated to the lateral wall of the esophagus.
5. The wound is closed.

ESOPHAGEAL DILATATION

Esophageal dilatation may be indicated in patients having esophageal stricture related to past surgery, chemical or thermal injury, or anatomic anomalies. An upper GI series is required before the procedure to determine the location of the stricture.

Procedural considerations

Esophageal dilatation is a clean procedure performed in the operating room because general anesthesia is required.

An esophageal perforation is a complication that could require an open repair if indicated.

The patient is positioned supine after induction and intubation.

A flexible gastroscope and light source with video camera and monitor, bougie dilators (Hurst or Maloney dilators are commonly used) in graduated sizes, water-soluble lubricant, gauze sponges, and gloves are required to perform the procedure. An esophageal stent that can be inserted through a large-channel gastroscope or along a guidewire may be requested. The surgeon may utilize fluoroscopy to demonstrate that the dilatation site is accurate by combining esophagoscopy with fluoroscopy and marking the site of stricture distally and proximally with radiopaque markers taped to the patient's skin.

Operative procedure

1. The perioperative nurse has the bougies arranged in graduated order beginning with the smallest (24 Fr) and progressing to the largest size (60 Fr).
2. The surgeon may first perform gastroscopy and pass a guidewire through the esophageal stricture.
3. The bougies are then passed one at a time gently but firmly through the strictures in an attempt to dilate the esophageal lumen.
4. Continuation of the dilatation to the largest bougie depends on ease of passage and patient tolerance.
5. Laser therapy may be indicated for palliation if a tumor mass is causing the stricture. The Nd:YAG laser energy may be delivered to the mass or stricture via a flexible quartz fiber passed through the operative channel of the gastroscope.
6. An esophageal stent may be placed at the stricture site to decrease the chance of recurrence.

SURGERY OF THE STOMACH

Vagotomy

Truncal vagotomy

Truncal vagotomy is the identification of the two vagal trunks on the distal esophagus and resection of a segment of each, including any additional nerve fibers running separately from the trunks. By interrupting the parasympathetic innervation, this procedure reduces the gastric acid secretion in patients with duodenal ulcers. When truncal vagotomy was initially performed alone, a high incidence of gastric stasis resulted from the loss of cholinergic innervation to the smooth muscle of the stomach; thus pyloroplasty or another gastric drainage procedure almost always accompanies truncal vagotomy. Truncal vagotomy deprives not only the stomach but also the liver, gallbladder, bile duct, pancreas, small intestine, and half of the large intestine of the parasympathetic nerve supply (Fig. 11-27). Truncal vagotomy with antrectomy or

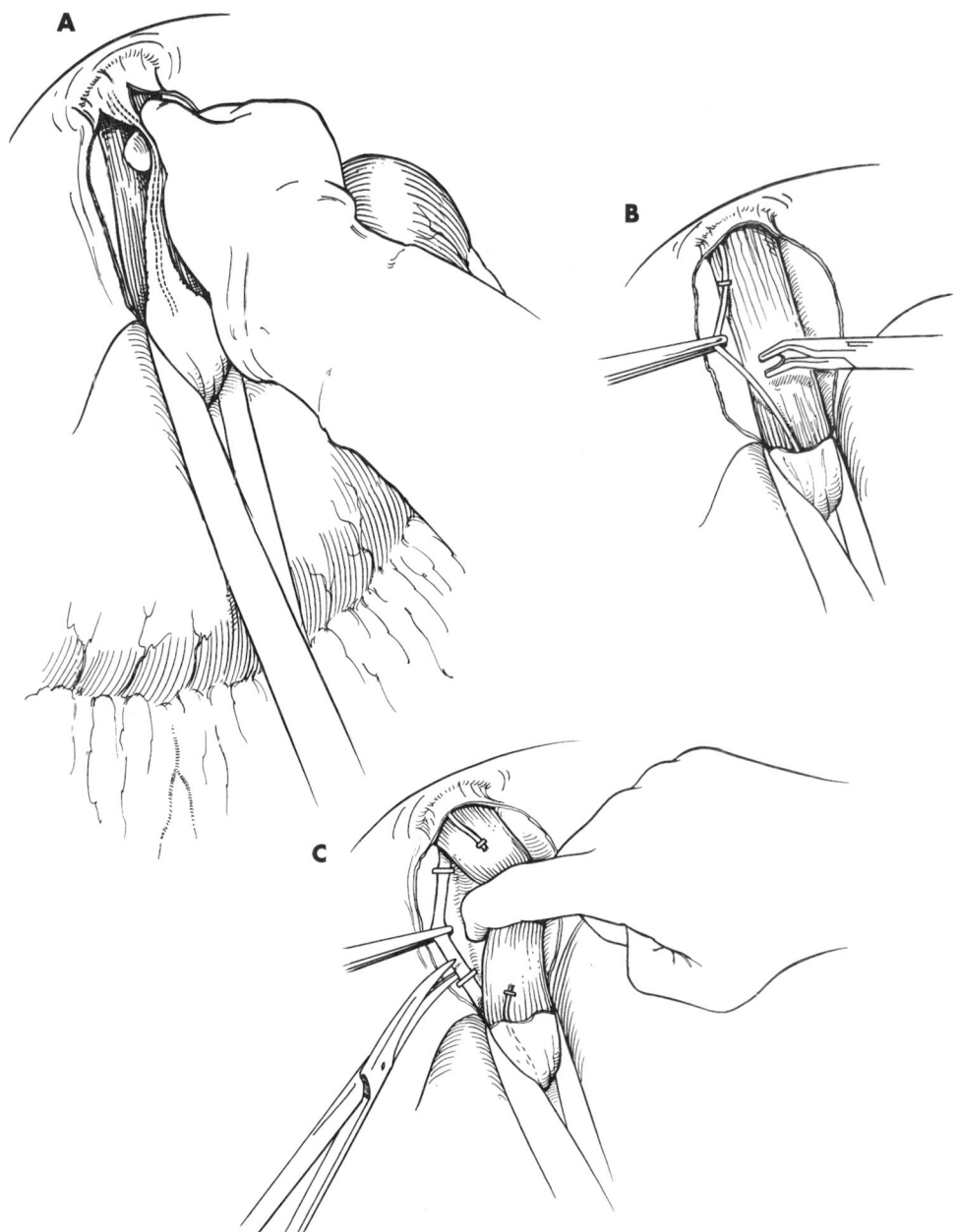

FIGURE 11-27 Truncal vagotomy. **A,** The phrenoesophageal ligament is lifted from the surface of the esophagus, and the vagal trunks are identified. **B,** Ligating clips are applied to the vagus nerve. **C,** Ligating clips have been applied to the larger posterior nerve in preparation for resecting a 2 cm segment between the clips.

drainage procedure is the most common operation for duodenal ulcers.

Selective vagotomy

Selective vagotomy is the transection of each abdominal vagus at a point just beyond its bifurcation into the gastric and extragastric divisions. Thus the hepatic branch of the anterior vagus and the celiac branch of the posterior vagus are preserved. Selective vagotomy possesses theoretical advantages over truncal vagotomy because vagal innervation of the viscera other than the stomach is preserved. However, selective vagotomy also denervates the entire stomach, so the addition of a drainage procedure is still necessary. Selective vagotomy may cause less postvagotomy diarrhea than truncal vagotomy does, but the incidence of dumping syndrome is probably the same or even higher. Both procedures are about equally effective in controlling duodenal ulcers.

Parietal cell vagotomy

Parietal cell vagotomy is the vagal denervation of only the parietal cell area of the stomach. The technique spares the main nerves of Latarjet but divides all vagal branches that terminate on the proximal two thirds of the stomach.

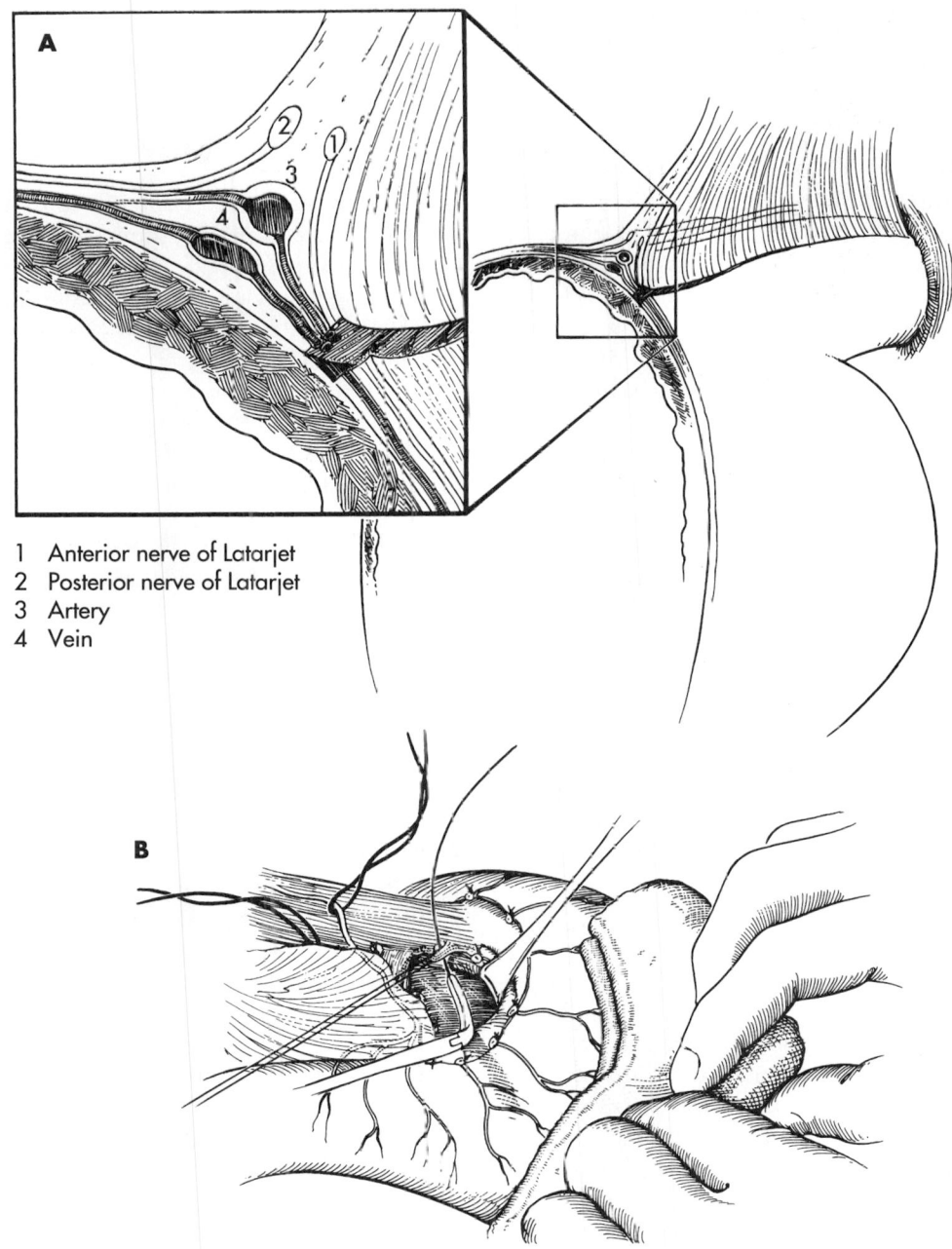

1 Anterior nerve of Latarjet
2 Posterior nerve of Latarjet
3 Artery
4 Vein

FIGURE 11-28   Selective proximal vagotomy. **A**, Illustrates the junction of the gastrohepatic ligament with the lesser curve of the stomach and demonstrates the anterior (*1*) and posterior (*2*) nerves of Laterjet, along with the artery (*3*) and vein (*4*). **B**, The lesser curve is lifted with a vein retractor to facilitate serial ligation of the intermediate and posterior neurovascular attachments.

The operation has also been called *proximal gastric vagotomy* (Fig. 11-28) and *highly selective vagotomy*. Because antral innervation is preserved, gastric emptying is unimpaired, and a drainage procedure is unnecessary. The incidence of dumping and diarrhea after parietal cell vagotomy is much lower than after truncal or selective vagotomy.

Procedural Considerations

Instrumentation for vagotomy would include a basic thoracotomy set (if a thoracoabdominal incision is to be used), a laparotomy set, GI set, 2 blunt nerve hooks (Smith-Wick), 2 10-inch vessel clip appliers with clips, and 10-inch Metzenbaum dissecting scissors. A 1-inch Penrose drain will be used to retract the esophagus. The patient is positioned supine under general anesthesia.

Operative Procedure

1. A midline incision is made, and the esophagus is identified and retracted with a 1-inch wide Penrose drain.
2. The vagus nerves or their branches, depending on which type of vagotomy is being done, are identified,

clamped with either a ligature or a hemostatic clip, and resected.

3. The wound is closed in layers.

Pyloroplasty

Pyloroplasty is the formation of a larger passageway between the prepyloric region of the stomach and the first or second portion of the duodenum with excision of peptic ulcer, if present. A pyloroplasty may be performed for the treatment of a peptic ulcer under selected conditions but is more frequently employed to remove cicatricial bands in the pyloric ring, thus relieving spasm and permitting rapid emptying of the stomach. In adults a vagotomy is usually performed with a pyloroplasty.

Procedural considerations

A laparotomy set and a GI instrument set are required. The patient is positioned supine after general anesthesia. A nasogastric tube is placed by the anesthesiologist. An indwelling urinary catheter is inserted.

Operative procedure

1. The abdominal cavity is opened through a midline incision.
2. The pylorus of the stomach is isolated.
3. An incision is made through the stomach and the duodenum.
4. The pyloroplasty is closed with nonabsorbable or synthetic, absorbable intestinal sutures.
5. The abdominal wound is closed in layers, and a dressing is applied.

Gastrostomy

Through a high left rectus abdominal or midline incision, a temporary or permanent channel is established from the gastric lumen to the skin. This lumen permits liquid feeding or retrograde dilatation of an esophageal stricture. Gastrostomy is a palliative procedure performed to prevent malnutrition and starvation, which may be caused by a lesion or stricture situated in the esophagus or in the cardia of the stomach. A temporary procedure is done when the obstruction is capable of being corrected.

For an extensive lesion of the esophagus, some surgeons advise a permanent gastrostomy in which a stomach flap is formed around the catheter. The catheter is brought out of the abdomen through a separate stab wound. When the incisional area is avoided, tissue healing is improved, and the incidence of postoperative wound-healing problems decreases.

Procedural considerations

The patient is positioned supine under general anesthesia or IV conscious sedation/analgesia with local anesthesia. A basic laparotomy set of instruments and a catheter and drainage reservoir are required.

Operative procedure

1. The abdominal cavity is opened through an upper midline or transverse incision.
2. The stomach is held with an Allis or Babcock forceps, and a purse-string suture is placed at the proposed site for the catheter.
3. A scalpel with a #15 blade is used to make an incision within the purse-string suture, and the contents of the stomach are suctioned.
4. Bleeding points are controlled using electrocautery.
5. The catheter is inserted, and the purse-string suture is tied around it.
6. The catheter is brought through a stab wound in the area of the left rectus muscle.
7. The stomach may be sutured to the peritoneal layer, and the abdominal wound is closed in layers

Percutaneous Endoscopic Gastrostomy

Percutaneous endoscopic gastrostomy (PEG) utilizes a flexible gastroscope and a uniquely designed gastrostomy tube for placement through the abdominal wall. The patient may remain awake with sedation while the procedure is performed in the operating room or endoscopy suite. There are push-and-pull techniques to insert a PEG tube. The pull technique is reviewed here.

Procedural considerations

A PEG tube kit containing the following is required: a percutaneous needle, a long silk suture with end strengthened for feeding it down the lumen of the needle, a percutaneous gastrostomy tube, and a bolster. A flexible gastroscopy system is required as well as snare forceps.

The patient is positioned supine under IV conscious sedation. A bite block should be inserted into the patient's oral cavity to avoid damage to the gastroscope.

Operative procedure

1. The gastroscope is passed into the stomach through the patient's oral cavity and down the esophagus.
2. The end of the scope is angled anteriorly to the left anterolateral wall of the stomach's fundus so that the light from the gastroscope can be seen through the abdominal wall.
3. The stomach is insufflated with air through the gastroscope.
4. Local anesthesia is injected at the site of the intended gastrostomy if the patient is awake.
5. A small stab wound is made with a #11 blade.
6. The percutaneous needle is inserted into the abdominal wall and into the stomach lumen under direct visualization of the gastroscope.
7. The long silk suture is threaded into the lumen of the needle and passed into the stomach where it is snared with the forceps.

8. A clamp is applied to the exterior distal end of the suture after the needle is removed.
9. The gastroscope is removed and the suture extends out of the patient's oral cavity.
10. The suture is then attached to the tapered end of the gastrostomy tube.
11. The gastrostomy tube is gently guided into the patient's oral cavity, down the esophagus, and into the lumen of the stomach and pulled through the abdominal wall.
12. The tube is secured with an internal bolster by reinserting the gastroscope and snugging it up to the gastric wall under direct visualization.
13. An external bolster is applied over the tube and snugged to the abdominal wall. Care is taken to ensure the bolsters are not compressing the tissues because such compression could compromise tissue integrity and perfusion.
14. The distal end of the tube is cut, and a connector is applied.
15. The patient's stomach is deflated, and the procedure is complete.

Gastrotomy

Gastrotomy is the opening of the anterior stomach wall through a left paramedian abdominal incision and exploration of the interior. This procedure is usually done to explore for upper GI tract bleeding, perform a tissue biopsy, or remove a gastric lesion or foreign body.

Procedural considerations

A laparotomy set and GI instrument set are required.

Operative procedure

1. A longitudinal incision is made through the anterior wall of the stomach, halfway between the curvatures.
2. The stomach wall is grasped and elevated by an Allis or Babcock forceps.
3. An incision is made, and a suction tube is inserted into the stomach to remove gastric contents.
4. The lesion or foreign body is removed.
5. The stomach wall and abdominal wall are closed.

Closure of Perforated Gastric or Duodenal Ulcer

Closure of a perforation in the stomach or duodenum is performed through a high right rectus or midline abdominal incision.

Procedural considerations

A perforated gastric or duodenal ulcer is treated as a surgical emergency, and the operation is performed as soon as the diagnosis is made. The patient's blood should be typed and crossmatched so that an adequate supply will be available for emergency replacement. A gastric lavage is not performed, but continuous suction is used. A laparotomy set and GI set are required. Linear stapling instruments are available.

Operative procedure

1. Through a right rectus or midline abdominal incision the perforation is located.
2. Suction is used to remove exudate in the peritoneal cavity.
3. The perforation is closed with a purse-string suture by inverting the raw edges and suturing a piece of omentum over the closure.
4. The ulcerated area may be resected using linear stapling devices.
5. The abdomen is copiously irrigated with warm saline, which may contain a broad-spectrum antibiotic.
6. The abdominal wound is closed in layers, and a dressing is applied.

Gastrojejunostomy

Gastrojejunostomy is the establishment of a permanent communication, either between the proximal jejunum and the anterior wall of the stomach or between the proximal jejunum and the posterior wall of the stomach, without removing a segment of the GI tract (Fig. 11-29). It is accomplished through a midline or a paramedian abdominal incision.

Gastrojejunostomy may be performed to treat a benign obstruction at the pyloric end of the stomach or an inoperable lesion of the pylorus when a partial gastrectomy would not be feasible. It also provides a large opening without sphincter obstruction.

Procedural considerations

A laparotomy and GI instrument set are required. Linear stapling instruments should be available. The patient is positioned supine under general anesthesia. A nasogastric tube is inserted by the anesthesiologist after intubation. An indwelling catheter is placed into the urinary bladder before abdominal skin prep.

Operative procedure

1. Through an upper midline or paramedian abdominal incision exploration of the peritoneal cavity is completed, as described for routine laparotomy.
2. The pathologic condition is confirmed.
3. Warm, moist packs are placed, and the self-retaining retractor is positioned.
4. A loop of proximal jejunum is grasped with a Babcock forceps and freed from the mesentery.
5. The loop of jejunum is approximated to either the anterior or posterior stomach wall several centimeters from the greater curvature of the stomach.
6. 2-0 nonabsorbable traction sutures are placed through the serosal layers at each end of the selected portion of the jejunum and stomach.

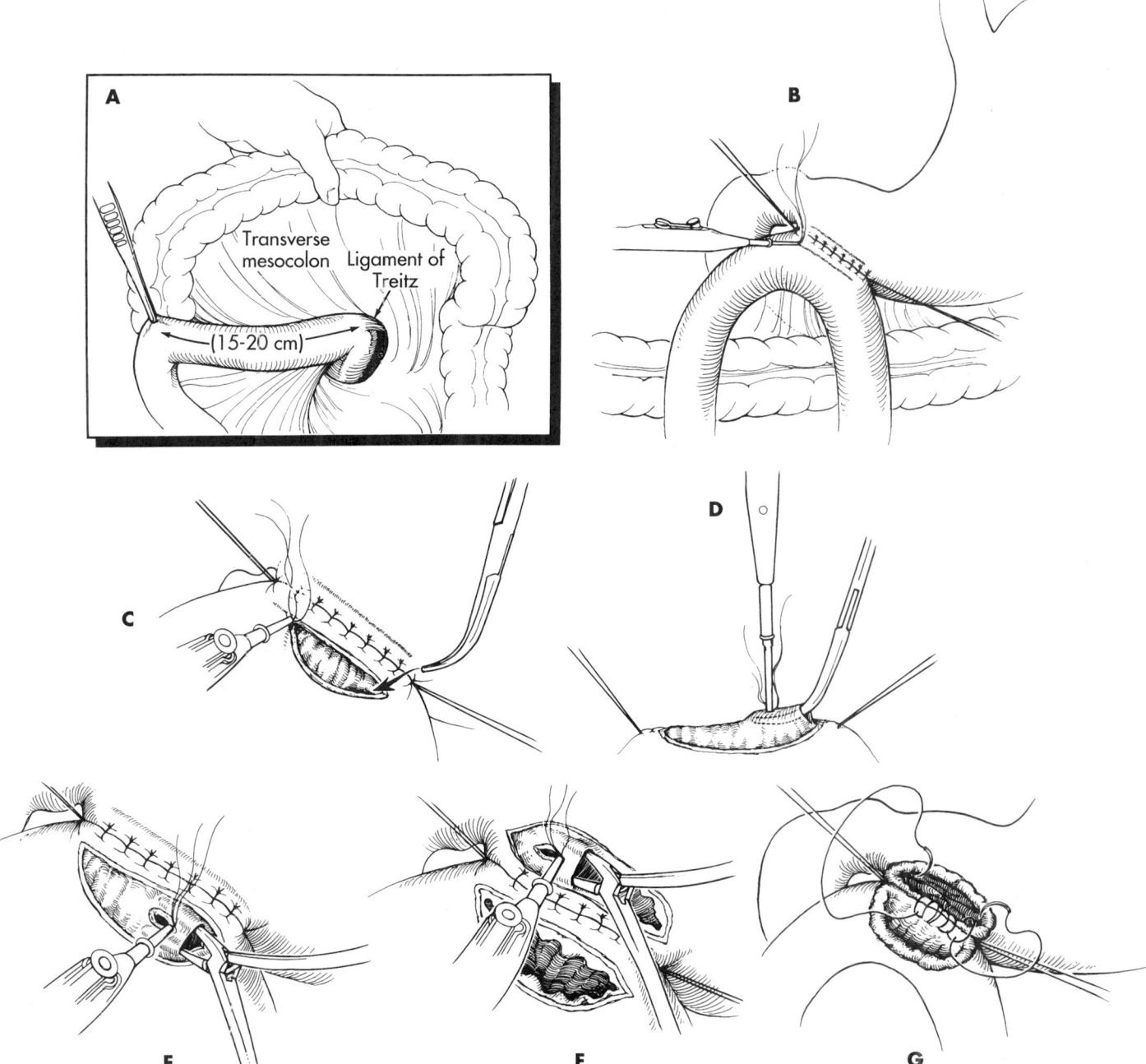

FIGURE 11-29 Gastrojejunostomy. **A,** Illustrates the selection of a segment of jejunum that will be anastomosed to the stomach; the distance between the ligament of Treitz and the anastomosis should not be excessively long or under any tension. **B,** A posterior row of interrupted sutures is placed between the gastric and jejunal serosae and the sites of the gastric and jejunal stomas are scored with the electrosurgical pencil. **C,** The jejunal stoma is created by dissecting through the serosa, and muscularis with the electrosurgical pencil. An opening is made in the mucosa and a right-angled clamp is inserted into the lumen. **D,** The clamp is opened and elevated. **E,** Electrosurgery is applied between the two jaws of the clamp. **F,** The procedure is repeated for creating the gastric stoma. **G,** Full-thickness anastomosis is begun posteriorly.

7. Gastroenterostomy clamps may be placed before insertion of the posterior interrupted 3-0 or 2-0 nonabsorbable serosal sutures.

8. The field is draped for open anastomosis.

9. The jejunum and stomach are opened.

10. Bleeding points are clamped with mosquito or Crile hemostats and ligated with 3-0 synthetic absorbable sutures.

11. The inner posterior row of sutures is placed, using continuous 2-0 or 3-0 synthetic absorbable suture

with atraumatic intestinal needles, and continued for the first anterior row.

12. The anastomosis is completed with anterior serosal sutures of 3-0 or 2-0 nonabsorbable material.

13. Traction sutures are removed.

14. Interrupted 4-0 nonabsorbable sutures may be used for reinforcement.

15. The contaminated instruments are discarded into a basin.

16. The abdominal wound is closed in layers and a dressing applied.

Partial Gastrectomy

Billroth I

A Billroth I gastrectomy is the resection of the diseased portion of the stomach through a right paramedian or midline abdominal incision and the establishment of an anastomosis between the stomach and duodenum. It is performed to remove a benign or malignant lesion located in the pylorus, or upper half of the stomach. One of several techniques may be followed to establish GI continuity, including the Schoemaker, the von Haberer-Finney, and other modifications of the Billroth I procedure (Fig. 11-30).

Procedural Considerations

A laparotomy set and GI instrument set are required. Linear stapling instruments should be available. The patient is positioned supine under general anesthesia. A nasogastric tube is inserted by the anesthesiologist after intubation. An indwelling urinary catheter is inserted before the abdominal skin prep.

Operative Procedure

1. The abdominal wall is incised, and the peritoneal cavity is opened and explored.

2. Bleeding vessels are clamped and ligated or coagulated.

3. The abdominal wound is retracted, and the surrounding organs are protected with warm, moist packs.

4. The gastrocolic omentum is freed from the colon mesentery to prevent injury to the middle colic artery.

5. With hemostats and Metzenbaum scissors, the right and left gastroepiploic arteries and veins are clamped, divided, and ligated with 2-0 nonabsorbable sutures and 2-0 and 3-0 suture ligatures, thereby freeing the greater curvature of the stomach.

6. The gastric vessels are also clamped, divided, and ligated to free completely the diseased portion of the stomach.

7. The operative field is prepared for open anastomosis.

8. After sectioning of the stomach from the greater to lesser curvature, two Allen intestinal anastomosis clamps or other suitable clamps are placed on the upper portion of the duodenum just distal to the pylorus.

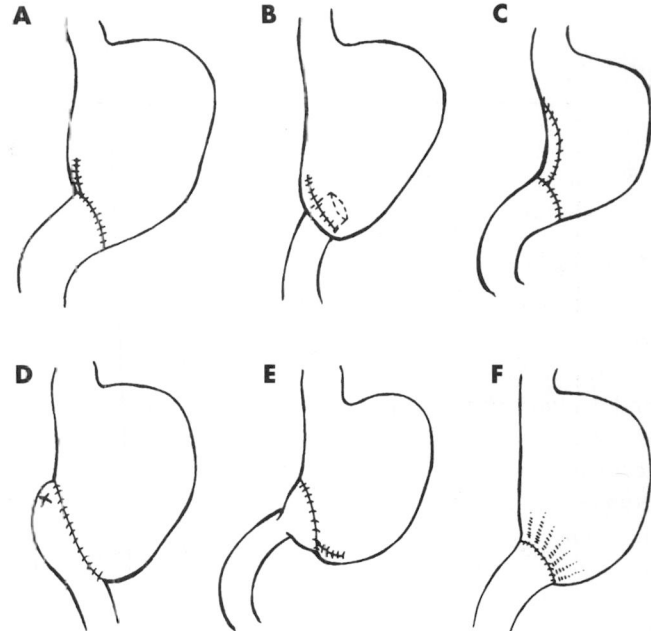

FIGURE 11-30 Diagrams illustrating resections of stomach with anastomosis of stomach and duodenum (gastroduodenal anastomosis). All are modifications of Billroth I technique, in which stomach is brought to duodenum. **A,** Billroth I: after pylorus is removed, lesser curvature is partially closed, and duodenum is sutured to open end of stomach at its lower margin. **B,** Kocher: distal end of stomach is closed, and duodenum is brought up to posterior margin of closed stomach. **C,** Schoemaker: lesser curvature of stomach is sutured and brought down to same size as duodenum, and end-to-end anastomosis is done. **D,** Von Haberer-Finney: side of duodenum is brought up to end of stomach so that entire end of stomach is open for direct anastomosis. **E,** Horsley: lesser curvature end of stomach is used to suture to duodenum and closes greater curvature end. **F,** Von Haberer: modification of operation shown in **D.** Stomach is, so to speak, narrowed or puckered so that it fits end of duodenum. Modification of this is done by some as follows: duodenum is split longitudinally, and its ends are flared open so that opening is large enough to fit open end of stomach.

9. Division of the duodenum is accomplished by scalpel or electrosurgery, as preferred. A linear cutting and stapling device (such as GIA) may be used to divide the tissues.

10. Additional moist packs are placed for protection, and two sets of anastomosis clamps are placed across the stomach.

11. Division of the stomach is completed by the surgeon's preferred method.

12. At the lower margin the opened stomach is approximated to the duodenum by a series of interrupted sutures placed in the serosa layers. 3-0 nonabsorbable suture on an atraumatic intestinal needle is used. Suture ends are held with hemostats, and the intestinal clamps are removed.

13. Stumps of the stomach and duodenum are cleansed with moist sponges, and bleeding vessels are ligated with fine suture or coagulated.

14. During the anastomosis of the stomach and remaining duodenum, the involved segments may be held with rubber-shod clamps. The excess of the lesser curvature of the stomach is closed on completion of the anastomosis.
15. Soiled instruments are discarded into a separate basin.
16. Routine laparotomy closure is completed.

Billroth II

A Billroth II gastrectomy is a resection of the distal portion of the stomach through an abdominal incision and the establishment of an anastomosis between the stomach and jejunum. It is performed to remove a benign or malignant lesion in the stomach or duodenum. This technique and modifications may be selected because the volume of acidic gastric juice will be reduced, and the anastomosis can be made along the greater curvature or at any point along the stump of the stomach. Modifications of the Billroth II procedure include the Polya and Hofmeister operations, which also establish GI continuity through bypassing the duodenum.

After surgery, duodenal and jejunal secretions empty into the remaining gastric pouch. The stomach empties more rapidly because of the larger opening, and a limited amount of gastric juice remains.

Procedural Considerations

A laparotomy set and GI instrument set are required. Linear stapling instruments should be available. The patient is positioned supine under general anesthesia. A nasogastric tube is inserted by the anesthesiologist after intubation. An indwelling urinary catheter is inserted before the abdominal skin prep.

Operative Procedure

1. The abdominal wall is incised, and the peritoneal cavity opened and explored.
2. Bleeding vessels are clamped and ligated or coagulated.
3. The abdominal wound is retracted, and the surrounding organs are protected with warm, moist packs.
4. The gastrocolic omentum is freed from the colon mesentery to prevent injury to the middle colic artery.
5. With hemostats and Metzenbaum scissors, the right and left gastroepiploic arteries and veins are clamped, divided, and ligated with 2-0 nonabsorbable suture and 2-0 and 3-0 suture ligatures, thereby freeing the greater curvature of the stomach.
6. The distal portion of the stomach is isolated.
7. Moist packs are placed for protection of the viscera, and two sets of anastomosis clamps are placed across the distal stomach.
8. The stomach is resected just distal to the pylorus using a scalpel, electrocautery, or a linear stapling and cutting device (GIA)(Fig. 11-31, *A*).
9. A proximal loop of jejunum is positioned for anastomosis to the posterior wall of the remaining stomach.
10. An anastomosis is established between the stomach and jejunum using mechanical linear stapling devices (GIA and TA instruments)(Fig. 11-31, *C*).
11. The abdomen is closed.

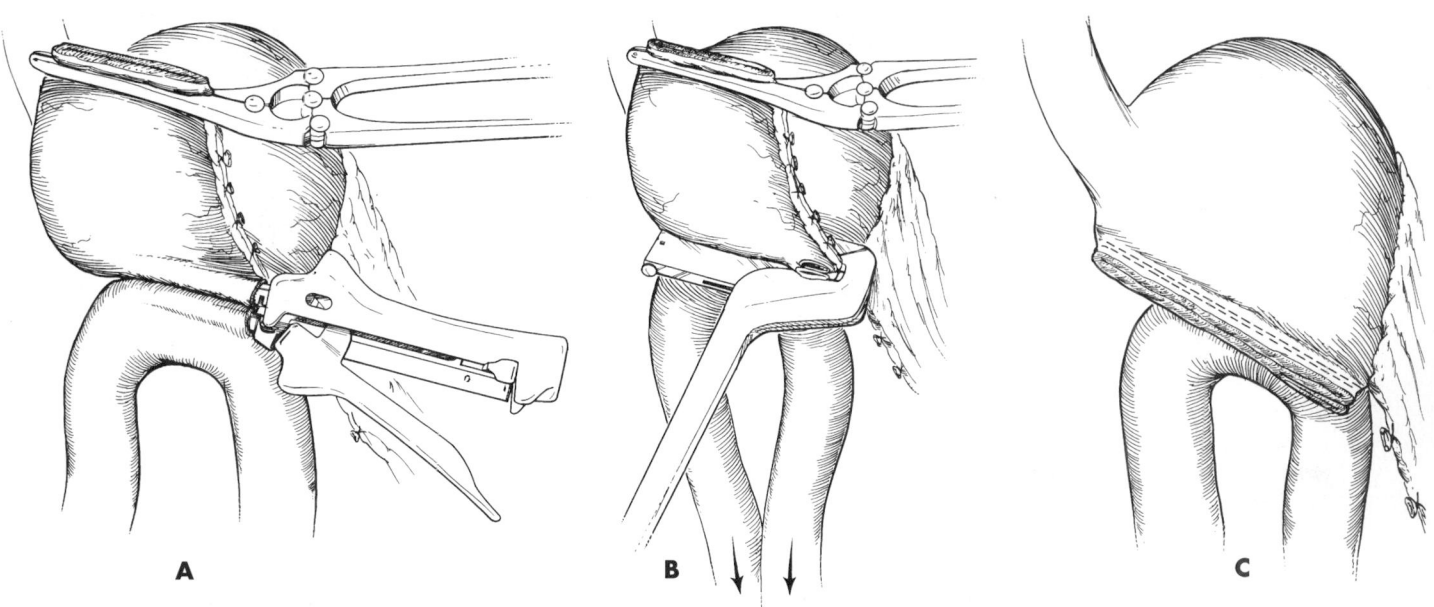

A   **B**   **C**

FIGURE 11-31 Subtotal gastrectomy with stapled Billroth II anastomosis. **A,** The distal stomach has been dissected free and resected just distal to the pylorus. A proximal limb of jejunum is brought up to anastomose to the posterior wall of the stomach with a linear stapling instrument that transsects between two parallel staple lines. **B,** The stomach is elevated and a 90 staple mechanical stapling device is placed across the distal stomach. **C,** Illustration of the completed subtotal gastrectomy with stapled antecolic gastrojejunostomy.

Total Gastrectomy

Total gastrectomy is the complete removal of the stomach and establishment of an anastomosis between the jejunum and the esophagus (Fig. 11-32). It may include an enteroenterostomy, if indicated. Total gastrectomy is done as a potentially curative or palliative procedure to remove a malignant lesion of the stomach and metastases in the adjacent lymph nodes.

Procedural considerations

The incision may be bilateral subcostal, long transrectus, long midline, or thoracoabdominal. A basic thoracotomy set, a GI set, and a laparotomy set are necessary. Mechanical linear stapling devices should be available. In addition, two long, blunt, nerve hooks and two 10-inch needle holders are used. The patient is positioned supine under general anesthesia. A nasogastric tube is inserted by

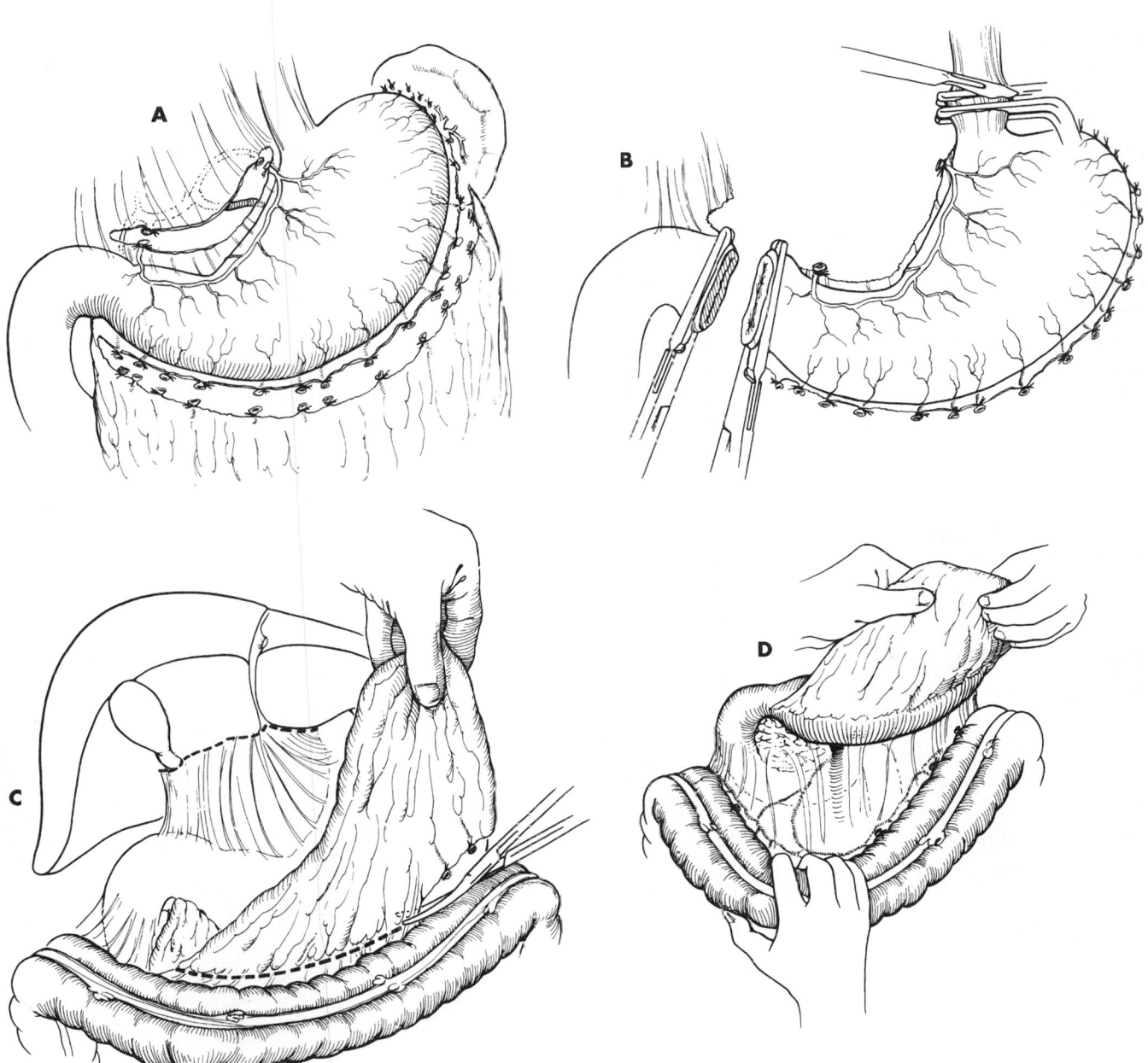

FIGURE 11-32 Total gastrectomy may be performed for benign or malignant disease. **A** demonstrates the mobilization of the stomach for benign disease. Serial division of the vessels in the gastrocolic ligament and gastrohepatic ligament are performed to free the greater and lesser omentum. The short gastric vessels connecting the stomach to the spleen are divided, and the spleen is preserved. **B,** The duodenum is divided distally to the pylorus, and the proximal line of division is at the distal intraabdominal esophagus. **C,** For malignancies, the line of resection includes both the lesser and greater omentum. **D,** The retrogastric area is inspected for tumor involvement. The spleen and tail of the pancreas may be included in the resection.

Continued

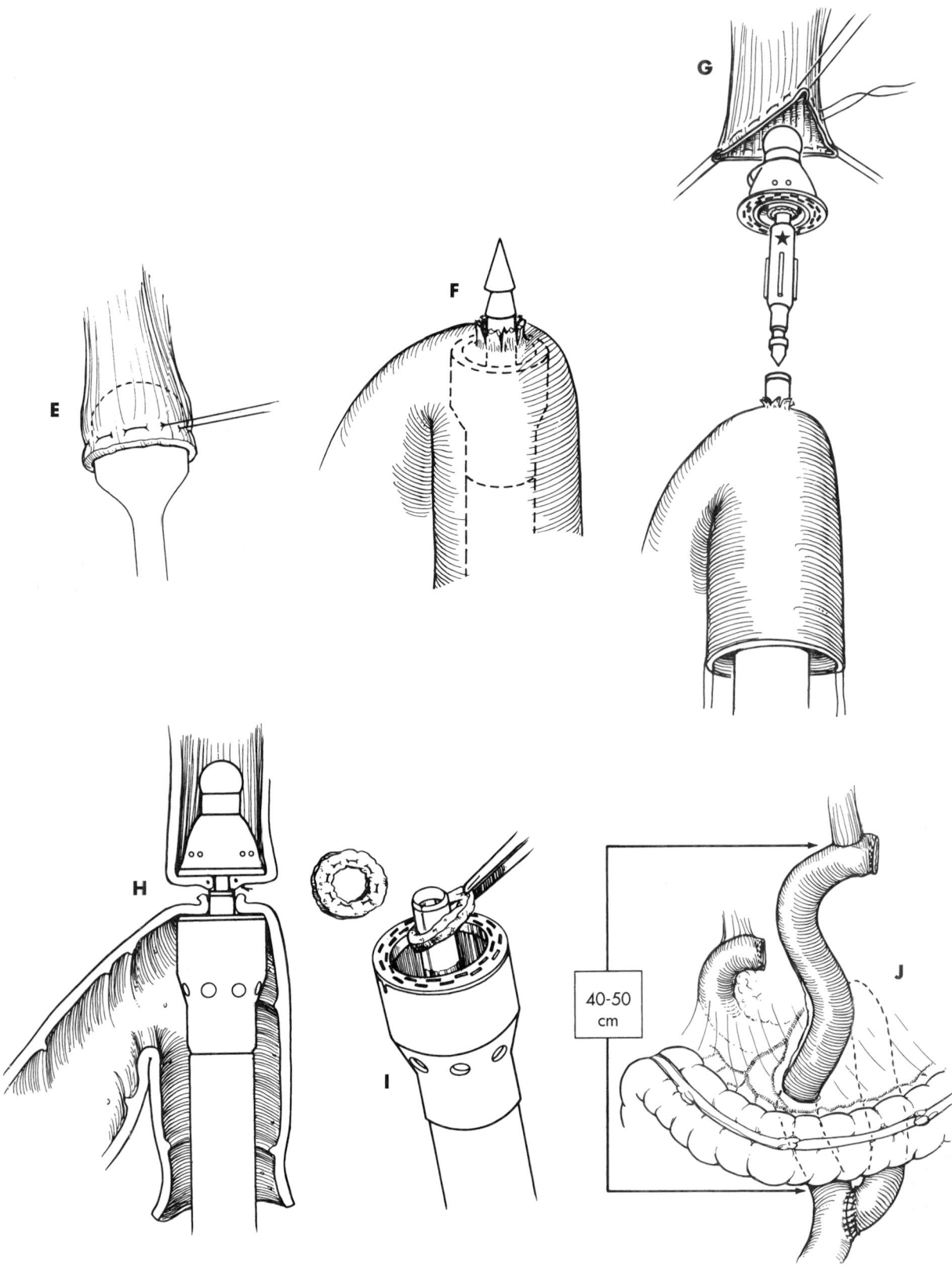

FIGURE 11-32, cont'd   **E**, A sizer is inserted into the lumen of the distal esophagus. **F**, The EEA or ILA is inserted into the lumen of the jejunum to facilitate esophagojejunostomy. **G**, The anvil is inserted into the distal esophagus where purse-string sutures will be snugged around the protruding arm of the anvil. **H**, The distal esophagus and the jejunum are brought together by the mechanism of the stapling device, and the interluminal anastomosis will be performed. **I**, The "donuts," distal esophagus and jejunal tissues, are examined for integrity and completeness. **J**, Illustration of the esophagojejunostomy completed.

the anesthesiologist after intubation. An indwelling urinary catheter is inserted before the abdominal skin prep.

Operative procedure

1. Through an incision of choice, the abdomen is opened.
2. The wound edges are protected and retracted.
3. Careful and complete exploration for the extent of metastasis is performed.
4. The omentum is freed from the colon, using sharp dissection; vessels are ligated with 2-0 nonabsorbable suture.
5. The splenic vessels are ligated and transfixed with 2-0 and 3-0 nonabsorbable suture at the tail of the pancreas; the spleen is left attached to the omentum.
6. The duodenum is mobilized, intestinal clamps are applied, and the operative field is protected for transection and closure of the distal duodenum.
7. The right gastric artery is ligated and transfixed with 2-0 and 3-0 nonabsorbable suture, and the gastrohepatic omentum is separated from the liver.
8. After ligation of the left gastric artery, the mobilized stomach, spleen, omentum, and lesser and greater curvature ligamentous attachments are delivered into the wound.
9. Division of the coronary ligament of the left lobe of the liver permits exposure of the diaphragmatic peritoneum over the esophagogastric junction.
10. The liver is protected by moist packs, and gentle retraction is maintained with a Harrington, Deaver, or malleable retractor.
11. A flap of peritoneum is freed from the diaphragm, and branches of the vagus nerves are divided.
12. A loop of jejunum is selected and delivered antecolic to the esophagogastric junction for anastomosis.
13. With the specimen for traction, the posterior layer of interrupted 3-0 nonabsorbable sutures is inserted or stapling devices are utilized.
14. As the jejunum and the esophagus are incised, bleeding is controlled by mosquito or Crile hemostats and ligatures of 3-0 synthetic absorbable suture.
15. The posterior layer is reinforced with 3-0 intestinal, synthetic absorbable sutures or a linear staple line.
16. Division of the esophagus is completed, and the entire specimen is removed.
17. 4-0 interrupted, synthetic absorbable sutures also are used to approximate the mucosal anterior wall of the anastomosis. An end-to-end anastomosis circular stapling device may be used to complete the anastomosis between the esophagus and jejunum.
18. A second layer of sutures, 3-0 nonabsorbable or synthetic absorbable, is placed anteriorly in the seromuscular and muscular coat of the intestine.

19. A flap of the peritoneum is attached to the jejunum with interrupted 3-0 nonabsorbable sutures to relieve traction on the anastomosis.
20. A lateral jejunojejunal anastomosis is completed to permit irritating bile and pancreatic fluids to bypass the anastomosis line, thereby preventing esophageal regurgitation.
21. The alternative to using suture materials is the use of mechanical stapling devices. Another method of establishing continuity is a combination of a Roux-en-Y jejunojejunostomy and a jejunoesophagostomy.
22. The abdominal wound is closed in layers. If retention sutures are used, they must be placed extraperitoneally because of the absence of omentum to protect the small bowel.

SURGERY OF THE SMALL BOWEL

Operation for Meckel's Diverticulum

Meckel's diverticulum is removed to prevent inflammation and obstruction from intussusception of the diverticulum. Meckel's diverticulum consists of an unobliterated congenital duct at the umbilicus that is attached to the distal ileum (Fig. 11-33). The diverticulum may contain gastric mucosa, which may ulcerate, perforate, or bleed.

Procedural considerations

A laparotomy set and GI instrument set are required. Linear stapling devices should be available. The patient is positioned supine under general anesthesia. A nasogastric tube is inserted by the anesthesiologist after intubation. An indwelling urinary catheter is inserted before the abdominal skin preparation.

Operative procedure

1. The abdomen is opened through a midline incision, and the diverticulum is identified.
2. If the diverticulum is long and narrow with a narrow base, the procedure is similar to that of an appendectomy. If the base is broad, the loop of bowel containing the diverticulum is isolated from the mesentery, and a limited small bowel resection is performed.
3. An anastomosis of the divided ends is completed with an inner continuous layer of 3-0 synthetic absorbable suture and an interrupted outer layer of 4-0 nonabsorbable sutures.
4. The abdominal wound is closed.

Appendectomy

Appendectomy is the severance and removal of the appendix from its attachment to the cecum through a right lower quadrant muscle-splitting (McBurney) incision. This procedure is performed to remove an acutely inflamed appendix, thereby controlling the spread of infection and reducing the danger of peritonitis. A normal

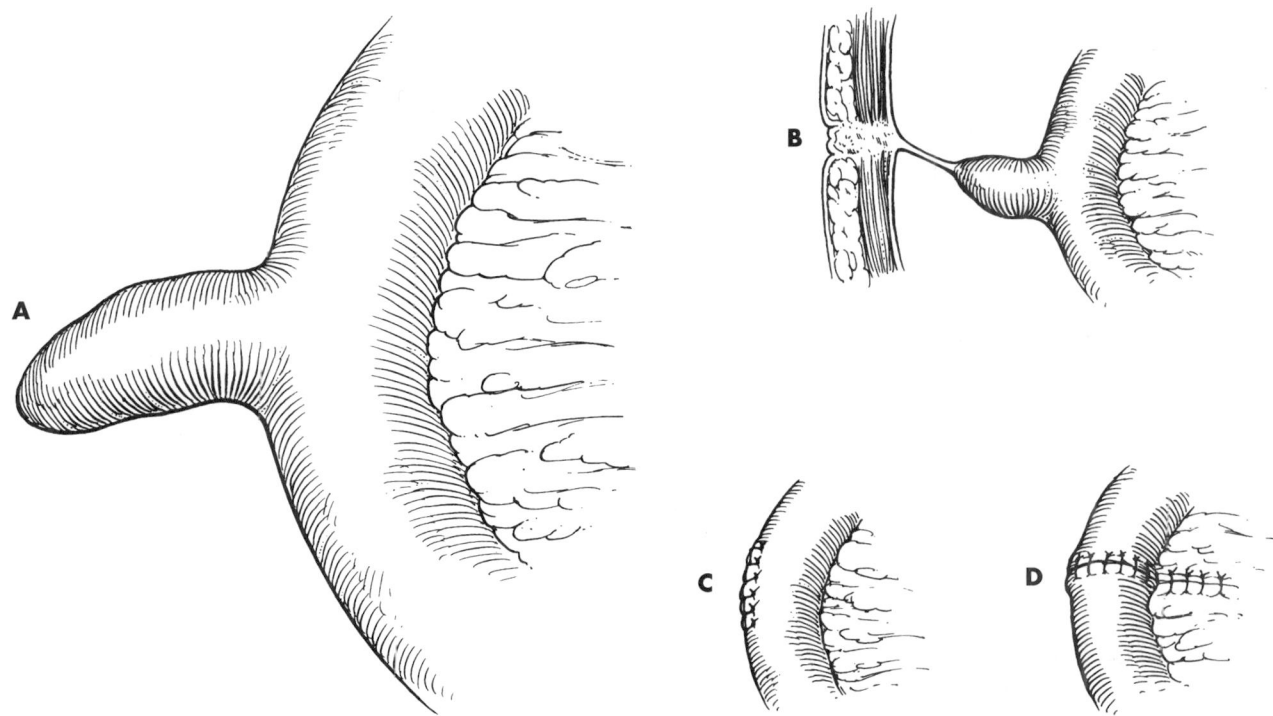

FIGURE 11-33 **A**, The most common nonpathologic appearance of Meckel's diverticulum arises from the antimesenteric border of the distal ileum. **B**, A persistent fibrous band of tissue connects the apex of the diverticulum to the anterior abdominal wall at the umbilicus. **C**, Demonstrates the suture line of a local Meckel's diverticulectomy. **D**, Illustration of completed ileoileal anastomosis after excision of 1 to 2 cm of ileum on each side of a Meckel's diverticulum.

appendix is sometimes removed when the abdomen is opened for another procedure.

Procedural considerations

A basic laparotomy instrument set is utilized. The patient is positioned supine under general anesthesia.

Operative procedure

1. A right lower quadrant muscle-splitting incision (McBurney) usually is made.
2. Muscles are retracted with Richardson or Parker retractors to expose the peritoneum.
3. The peritoneum is grasped with tissue forceps or an Allis forceps, and a small incision is made with a scalpel using a #15 blade.
4. A culture sample may be taken.
5. The incision is completed with a Metzenbaum scissors.
6. The mesoappendix is grasped near the tip with a Babcock forceps or a hemostat for gentle traction.
7. The mesoappendix is dissected from the appendiceal wall by hemostats and ligated with 3-0 nonabsorbable suture. If a suture ligature is required, 2-0 synthetic absorbable suture on an atraumatic GI needle is preferred.
8. The appendix is elevated as a purse-string suture of 2-0 synthetic absorbable suture is placed in the cecal wall at the appendiceal base.

9. The base of the appendix is crushed with a straight hemostat, a 3-0 synthetic absorbable suture tie is placed over the crushed area, and a hemostat is placed above the ligature.
10. A basin is provided for the specimen and discarded instruments that have come into contact with GI mucosa.
11. Protective gauze sponges are placed over the cecum around the base of the appendix.
12. The appendix is amputated between the clamp and synthetic absorbable suture with a scalpel. Sometimes the stump is swabbed with alcohol or Betadine solution to reduce bacterial flora.
13. The appendiceal stump may be inverted into the lumen of the cecum as the purse-string suture is tightened and tied by means of a fine straight hemostat and a small sponge on a holder. Soiled instruments are discarded into the basin.
14a. The abdomen is closed in the usual manner.
14b. If the appendix has ruptured, copious amounts of warm fluids are used to irrigate the peritoneal cavity. A drain may be inserted down to the appendiceal bed to allow continuous drainage. Deeper layers are closed, leaving the subcutaneous tissue and skin open. The wound may then be packed open with moist, fine-meshed gauze, and healing by secondary intention is permitted. This packing method may be used in any case in which bowel contamination or abscess

formation is present. It allows clean healing and prevents pocketing of pus.

Laparoscopic Appendectomy

A laparoscopic approach to appendectomy has gained popularity and may be the surgeon's preferred technique at many institutions.

Procedural considerations

The procedure involves the placement of three trocars with the standard laparoscopic instrumentation, equipment, and supplies available. The patient is positioned supine under general anesthesia. An indwelling urinary catheter may be placed before the abdominal skin prep.

Operative procedure

1. Pneumoperitoneum is obtained by a Verres needle or through the periumbilical trocar.
2. An 11 or 12 mm trocar is placed in the umbilicus for insertion of the laparoscope.
3. An 11 or 12 mm trocar is placed in the right upper quadrant (RUQ) to serve as the working port.
4. The 5 mm trocar placed in the midline suprapubic site serves as the traction trocar.
5. A laparoscopic Babcock instrument is inserted into the RUQ trocar to grasp the cecum and retract it toward the liver.
6. The appendix is grasped at its tip by a grasping forceps that has been inserted through the suprapubic trocar and is held in an upward position.
7. The Babcock forceps is removed, and a dissecting instrument is inserted through the RUQ trocar to create a mesenteric window in the mesoappendix.
8. Dissection is performed in proximity to the appendix, beginning directly under the base and progressing to a 1 to 2 cm length.
9. Depending on the surgeon's preferred technique, the appendix may be transsected in several different ways: (a) by an endoscopic linear stapling instrument, (b) a ligating loop instrument, or (c) a suturing instrument.
10. If an endoscopic linear stapling instrument is used, the lower jaw of the stapling device is passed through the mesenteric window previously created via the RUQ trocar.
11. The grasping forceps are used to rotate the tip of the appendix so that the stapling device can be snugged to the base of the appendix and closed.
12. The stapling instrument is fired and withdrawn, and the staple line is inspected.
13. The remainder of the mesoappendix is dissected, hemostasis is achieved, and the appendix is removed through the RUQ port.
14. If the appendix is too thick, a specimen pouch may be necessary to facilitate its extraction.
15. The abdomen is irrigated, the irrigation fluid is aspirated with a suction and irrigation device, and then the abdomen is deflated.
16. Trocar sites are closed and dressed in the usual fashion.

Resection of the Small Intestine

Resection of the small intestine involves excision of the diseased intestine through an abdominal incision and frequently includes some type of bowel reanastomosis. It is performed to remove certain tumors, a gangrenous portion of the intestine caused by strangulation from bands of adhesions, a herniation of the intestine, or a volvulus.

Procedural considerations

A laparotomy set and GI instrument set are required. Linear stapling instruments should be available. The patient is positioned supine under general anesthesia. A nasogastric tube is inserted by the anesthesiologist after intubation. An indwelling urinary catheter is inserted before the abdominal skin prep.

Operative procedure

1. The abdominal wall is incised through a midline incision and retracted.
2. The peritoneal cavity is explored and protected with moist, warm saline packs.
3. Intestinal clamps are placed above and below the diseased segment of the small bowel and mesentery.
4. The involved area is removed with a linear stapling instrument such as a GIA, electrosurgical blade, or a scalpel.
5. The continuity of the GI tract is established by an end-to-end, end-to-side, or side-to-side anastomosis.
6. The wound is closed and dressed.

An alternative approach to a traditional suture anastomosis is the use of a mechanical stapling device. The device allows the surgeon to perform an end-to-end, end-to-side, or side-to-side anastomosis. An enterotomy is made close to the anastomosis site. The stapler is inserted, and the distal bowel is secured between the anvil and the head of the stapler. The anvil is then inserted into the proximal loop of bowel and secured to the center rod. The gap is closed, and the stapler is fired. The stapler is extracted through the enterotomy. The integrity of the anastomosis is verified, and the enterotomy is closed with sutures.

Ileostomy

Ileostomy is the formation of a temporary or permanent opening into the ileum. This procedure is generally done when an extensive lesion is present either to reduce activity in the colon by means of diversions or when all the large bowel has been resected.

Procedural considerations

A laparotomy set and GI instrument set are required. Linear stapling instruments will be used. The patient is positioned supine under general anesthesia. A nasogastric tube is inserted by the anesthesia care provider after intubation. An indwelling urinary catheter is inserted before the abdominal skin prep. An ostomy appliance for the stoma should be available.

Operative procedure

1. Through a midline incision the peritoneal cavity is explored, and the pathologic condition is determined.
2. The ileum is mobilized with a Metzenbaum scissors and hemostatic clamps.
3. The mesentery is clamped, divided, and ligated with 3-0 nonabsorbable sutures at the proposed site, usually about 15 cm from the ileocecal junction.
4. Two intestinal clamps are placed on the bowel, and the ileum is divided with a scalpel or linear stapling instrument (GIA) between the two clamps.
5. The distal end of the ileum is closed with 2-0 synthetic absorbable suture on a taper needle if a stapling device has not been used.
6. The proximal end is brought out to the skin through an opening on the right side and is held in place by clamps, making sure that the ileum is not over-stretched or its blood supply compromised.
7. The mesentery of the ileum is sutured to the parietal wall to eliminate a potential internal hernia.
8. The abdomen is then closed.
9. The stoma is sutured to the skin after the ileum is everted to form a protective cover over the exposed ileal serosa.
10. A disposable ostomy appliance is placed over the stoma to collect small bowel contents.

An alternative to a conventional ileostomy for selected patients is the Kock pouch, or continent ileostomy. The internal pouch is constructed of small intestine with an outlet to the skin. When it is functioning properly, no stool spontaneously leaves the stoma. A catheter is inserted into the stoma three or four times daily to evacuate the contents. This procedure eliminates the need for an external appliance.

SURGERY OF THE COLON

Laparoscopic Colectomy

Resection of a segment of bowel and an anastomosis can be accomplished using laparoscopic techniques.[3] The advantages of laparoscopic colectomy are the reduction of postoperative ileus and a potential shortening of the recovery period.

Procedural considerations

Depending on the intended segment of bowel to be resected, the patient may be positioned supine or in a modified lithotomy for access to the rectum for end-to-end anastomosis. A nasogastric tube is inserted by the anesthesiologist after intubation. An indwelling urinary

catheter is inserted before the abdominal skin preparation. Laparotomy instrumentation should be available. Mechanical stapling devices and endostapling devices should be readily available. To assist the surgeon in accurately identifying the segment of bowel to be resected, a colonoscope may be used preoperatively or during the laparoscopic procedure to tattoo the lesion with methylene blue.

Operative procedure

1. Pneumoperitoneum is created, and the 10 mm umbilical trocar is placed for insertion of the laparoscope.
2. Usually two 12 mm trocars are placed in locations dependent on the anatomic segment of colon that will be resected.
3. A dissecting forceps is used to establish a mesenteric window as the bowel segment is held with a Babcock forceps.
4. A multifire endoscopic linear stapling device (GIA) is positioned appropriately over the segment of bowel and fired to both transsect and staple the segment.
5. Unless an end-to-end anastomosis can be performed, as in a low sigmoid or rectal resection, a small incision is made over the area of the abdomen so that it will provide the best access to the segments for anastomosis.
6. The segment of bowel to be resected is brought through the small laparotomy incision and transsected, and anastomosis is performed by the surgeon's preferred manner.
7. The anastomosed bowel is then dropped back into the peritoneal cavity, the cavity is well irrigated and suctioned, and closure commences after hemostasis is ensured.

Colostomy

Colostomy is the mobilization of a loop of colon through a right rectus incision to expose the transverse colon. A left rectus incision can also be made to expose the descending sigmoid colon. The layers of the wound beneath or around the colostomy are subsequently closed. A colostomy is performed to treat an obstruction in the sigmoid colon resulting from a malignant lesion. Another possible indication for this procedure is advanced inflammation or trauma that has caused distention or obstruction of the proximal portion of the colon. A temporary colostomy is often done to decompress the bowel or to give the bowel a rest (Fig. 11-34).

Procedural considerations

A laparotomy set and GI instrument set are required. Linear stapling instruments may be used. Stoma appliances as determined by the surgeon are required. These items may include a colostomy rod, rubber tubing, or a loop ostomy bridge.

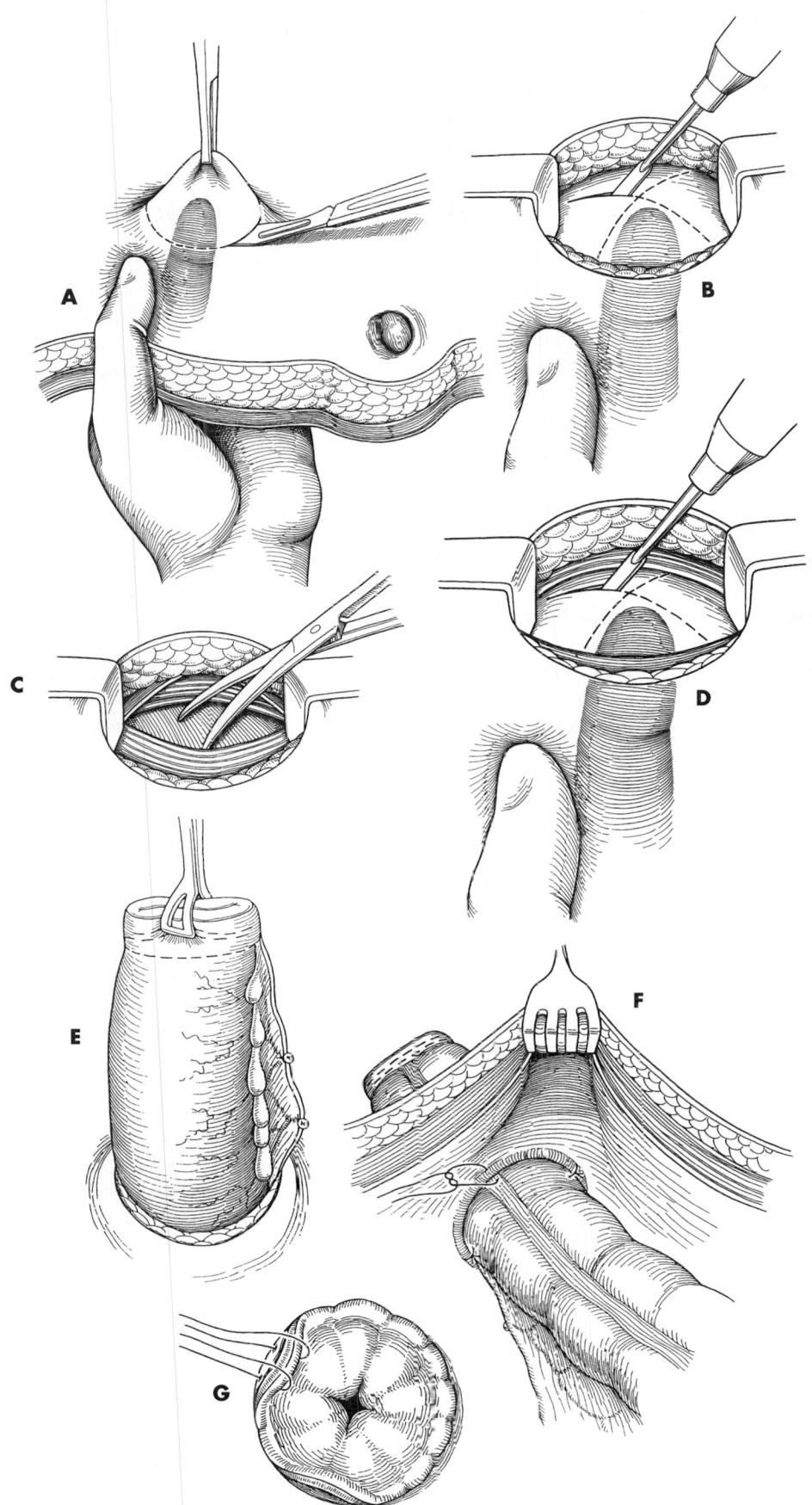

FIGURE 11–34   Construction of a colostomy through the anterior abdominal wall. **A**, A core of subcutaneous tissue is removed after making a circular skin incision with a #10 blade and using an electrosurgical pencil to dissect down to the anterior fascia. **B**, Muscle fibers are split. **C**, Tissues are dissected to the posterior layers, and, **D**, the peritoneum is opened. **E**, The colon is delivered through the abdominal wall so that it extends 2 to 3 cm beyond the skin surface. **F**, The bowel is tacked internally to the peritoneal defect. **G**, Four sutures are placed in each quadrant, incorporating the full-thickness cut end of the colon, the serosa surface approximately 1 to 2 cm below the open end of the colon, and up to the dermis. Additional sutures are used to mature the stoma, which refers to the procedure of everting the mucosa to create a stable opening through which feces can be evacuated.

The patient is positioned supine under general anesthesia. A nasogastric tube is inserted by the anesthesiologist after intubation. An indwelling urinary catheter is inserted before the abdominal skin preparation.

Operative procedure

First-Stage Loop Colostomy

1. The abdomen is opened, and the wound edges are protected and retracted.
2. The peritoneal cavity is opened and walled off with moist laparotomy packs, and appropriate retractors are inserted.
3. A small opening is made in the mesentery near the bowel with curved hemostats and a Metzenbaum scissors.
4. A piece of tubing or Penrose drain is passed around the colon, and the two ends are held with a hemostat to maintain gentle traction.
5. The loop of colon is brought out through an incision made on the left side of the midline. The abdominal incision is closed.
6. A loop ostomy bridge is used to keep the loop of colon in proper position.
7. The loop of intestine is dressed with petrolatum gauze.

Second-Stage Loop Colostomy

After 48 hours the loop of colon is completely severed by an electrosurgical blade. By this time, if there is no tension, healing has advanced sufficiently to allow protection from feces contamination onto the wound. This procedure is simple and painless and is usually performed in the patient's room or in a treatment room.

Transverse Colostomy

1. A short incision, vertical or preferably transverse, is made to reach the transverse colon.
2. A loop of transverse colon, freed of omentum, is withdrawn (Fig. 11-35).
3. A loop ostomy bridge is passed through an avascular area of the mesocolon, preventing the loop from returning to the peritoneal cavity.
4. A mushroom catheter, which is held in place with a purse-string suture, brings about immediate decompression.
5. The bowel is opened 24 to 36 hours later.
6. The bridge may be removed in about 7 to 10 days.

Closure of a Colostomy

Closure of a colostomy involves the reestablishment of internal intestinal continuity and repair of the abdominal wall.

Procedural considerations

When the loop has been completely divided, a closed or open anastomosis may be performed. A laparotomy set and GI instrument set are required. Linear stapling instruments may be used.

The patient is positioned supine under general anesthesia. A nasogastric tube is inserted by the anesthesiologist after intubation. An indwelling urinary catheter is inserted before the abdominal skin prep.

Depending on the location of the bowel to be reanastomosed, the patient may be placed in low lithotomy position to facilitate transanal access for a circular stapling device. An end-to-end anastomosis of the left colon or ileal pouch to the rectal stump can then be achieved.

Operative procedure

1. A circumferential incision is made around the colostomy to free the skin margin.
2. Moist packs, a scalpel with a #10 blade, a Metzenbaum scissors, and Crile hemostats are used as the layers of the abdominal wall are identified and dissected free.
3. An end-to-end anastomosis is completed in two layers, the inner with 3-0 synthetic absorbable suture and the outer with 3-0 nonabsorbable suture on an intestinal needle, using interrupted sutures. This anastomosis may be completed with a surgical stapling device.
4. The abdominal wound is closed in layers. A dressing is applied.

The surgeon may elect to leave the subcutaneous tissue and skin open. In this instance the wound is packed and permitted to heal by secondary intention.

Right Hemicolectomy and Ileocolostomy

Right hemicolectomy and ileocolostomy involve the resection of the right half of the colon—including a portion of the transverse colon, the ascending colon, and the cecum—and a segment of the terminal ileum and mesentery (Fig. 11-36, *A*). An end-to-end, side-to-side, or end-to-side anastomosis is done between the transverse colon and the ileum. A right hemicolectomy and ileocolostomy are performed to remove a malignant lesion of the right colon and in some cases to remove inflammatory lesions involving the ileum, cecum, or ascending colon. A clinical pathway for primary colon resection is shown in Fig. 11-37.

Procedural considerations

When a side-to-side anastomosis is carried out, the transsected stumps of the ileum and the transverse colon are closed before the anastomosis is done. It is completed between the side portions of the ileum and the transverse colon. A side-to-side anastomosis can also be performed by inserting the GIA stapler into both colon segments and firing the device. The stumps are then closed using a TA linear stapling device.

When an end-to-end anastomosis is performed, the

Text continued on p. 359

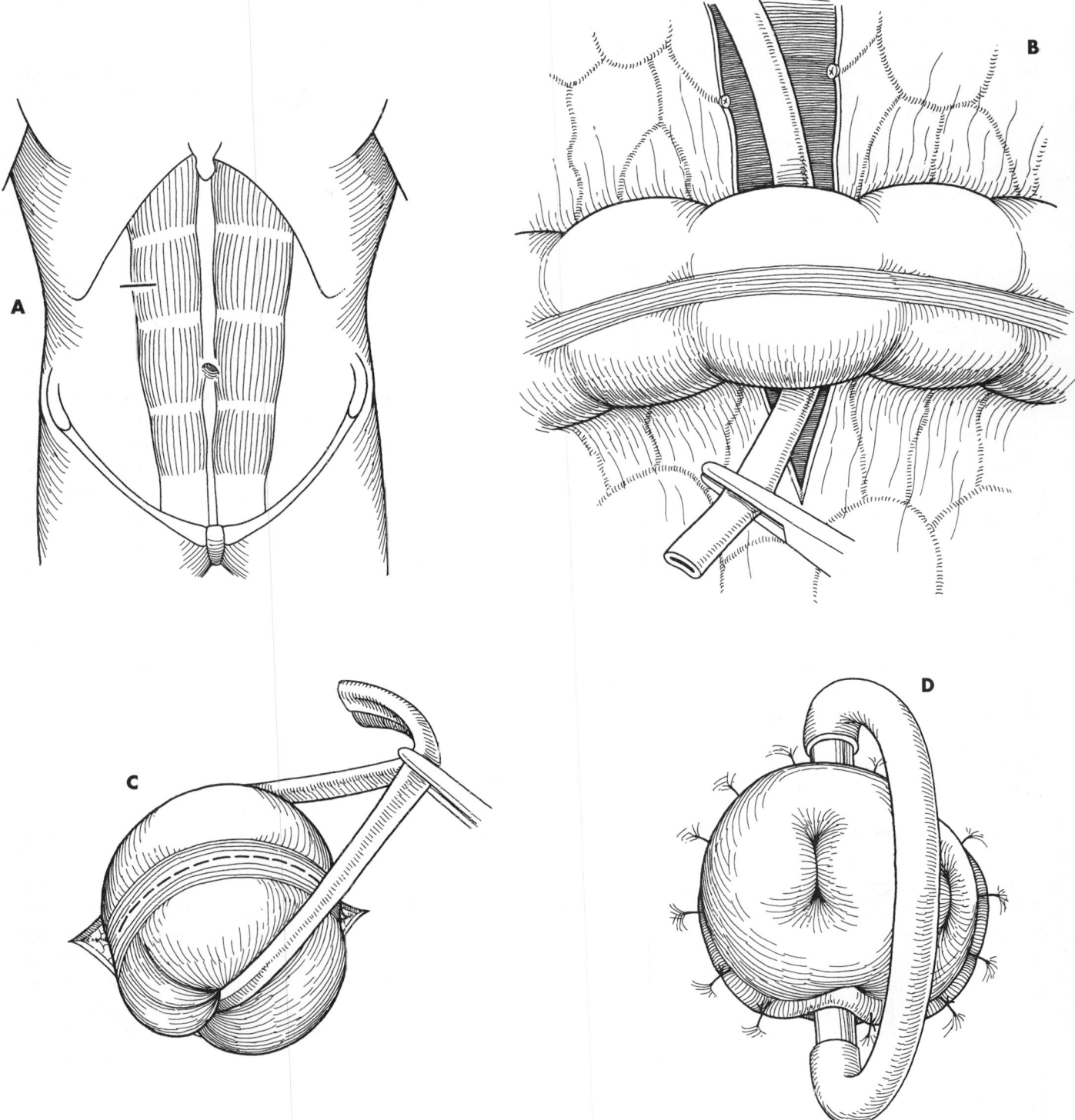

FIGURE 11-35 Transverse loop colostomy. **A**, Small transverse incision into the abdomen. **B**, The mesentery adjacent to the colon is taken down so that a Penrose drain may be passed beneath the colon. **C**, The colon is pulled through the transverse incision and opened longitudinally along the taeniae. **D**, An apparatus or rod is placed underneath the stoma; sutures are used to mature the colostomy. The rod can be removed after the seventh postoperative day.

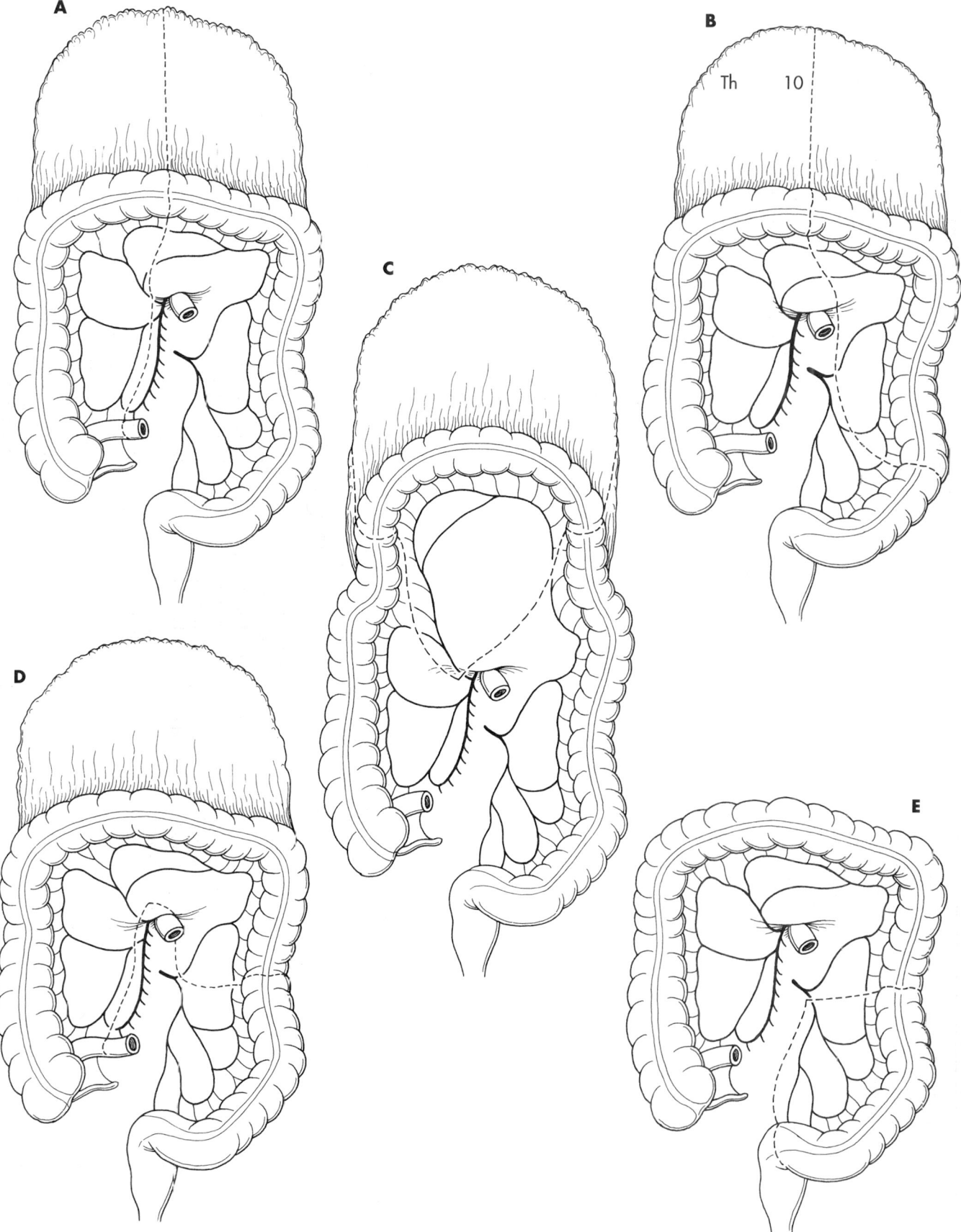

FIGURE 11-36 The resection lines for various types of colon resection. **A**, Right hemicolectomy and ileocolostomy; **B**, Left hemicolectomy. **C** and **D**, Transverse colectomy. **E**, Anterior resection of sigmoid colon and rectosigmoidostomy.

CLINICAL PATHWAY FOR THE PATIENT WITH COLON CANCER UNDERGOING PRIMARY COLON RESECTION

	PREOPERATIVE	INTRAOPERATIVE	CLOSURE	POSTOPERATIVE	DISCHARGE
ASSESSMENTS Evaluations Consults	• History and physical • Nursing assessment • Anesthesia assessment • Preop medications • Vital signs, O_2 saturation • Allergies listed • Consent	• Continuous reassessment by RN and anesthesia provider • Physiological monitoring by anesthesia provider during entire procedure • Monitor peripheral pulses after positioning patient • Urinary output and fluid administration monitored • Blood loss monitored	• Reassessment and evaluation	• Vital signs, O_2 saturation • Lungs assessed • Breathing patterns assessed • Dressings checked • IV site assessed • NG tube drainage monitored • Urinary output and fluid administration monitored • Pain management assessment/evaluation • Consult pain management team if indicated	• Consultation with dietician • Nutritional support assessment • Enterostomal therapist consultation if indicated • Bowel function assessment • Assessment/evaluation of skin integrity/ostomy site • Bowel sounds • Ability to eat and defecate
TESTS	• Laboratory results reviewed, especially Hgb and electrolytes • Barium studies, X-rays, scans reviewed • Preadmission testing per standards • Baseline carcinoembryonic antigen (CEA) serum level	• Intraoperative ultrasound of liver • Intraoperative colonoscopy or sigmoidoscopy if indicated to mark tumor	None	• Hemoglobin and hematocrit • Electrolytes	
SAFETY/ TREATMENTS	• Transport gurney appropriate • Sensory aides with patient if necessary for cure — Hearing aide — Eyeglasses • Jewelry/prosthetics removed • Patient gown donned • Pulsatile antiembolism system/leggings applied as ordered	• Bowel prep if necessary • Initiate pulsatile antiembolism system as ordered • Insert indwelling urinary catheter-attach to urimeter/drainage bag • Electrosurgical set up per standard • Shave/skin prep per standard • Draping per standard • Incision made • Care, handling and labeling of specimens	• Correct sponge/sharp/instrument counts • Application of ostomy appliance if indicated • Application of dressing to incisional wound • Extubation • Transfer of patient to PACU or SICU bed • Transport to PACU/SICU — Siderails up — O_2 — Monitor if necessary	• Postprocedure status documented — Postop phase I — Postop phase II • Support for patient breathing/oxygenation • Medications administered as ordered • Pain control/management • NG tube to suction if necessary • Hemodynamic/thermodynamic stabilization • Vital signs, O_2 saturation monitored • Chest sounds assessed • Bowel sounds assessed • Nausea/vomiting assessed — medications administered as indicated • Pulsatile antiembolism system administered if ordered	• Coughing and deep breathing exercises • Ambulation and return to activities of daily living • Pain management • Nutritional support • Care and irrigation of ostomy (if applicable) • Follow-up appointment with surgeon • Removal of skin staples and assessment of incision

FIGURE 11–37   Clinical pathway for primary colon resection.

Continued

CLINICAL PATHWAY FOR THE PATIENT WITH COLON CANCER UNDERGOING PRIMARY COLON RESECTION

	PREOPERATIVE	INTRAOPERATIVE	CLOSURE	POSTOPERATIVE	DISCHARGE
MEDICATIONS	• Comprehensive list of all medications taken at home • Bowel prep is adequate • Oral antibiotic prophylaxis regimen • IV broad spectrum antibiotic administered 20-30 minutes prior to start of surgery • IV sedation as appropriate • Epidural catheter may be placed for postoperative pain • Management/control	• Anesthesia agents per standards • Induction of general anesthesia • Irrigation solutions — May include antibiotic or antiseptic agent per surgeon's preference	• Wound irrigation prior to closure • Anesthesia agents per standards	• IV/IM medications for pain control and management • Antiemetics if needed • Patient's daily medications resumed and administered	• Diet supplements • Daily medications • Pain management
DISCHARGE PLANNING/ TEACHING	• Patient and family member teaching/orientation — Explanation of perioperative events — Orientation to environment — Family members directed to waiting area, time frame expectations discussed, expectations of communication from the OR — Patient belongings — Anticipated patient Discharge from PACU to nursing unit	• Communicate with family members: — Delays — Surgery begins — Updates — Surgeon to meet with family • Transport cart readily available with necessary support equipment: — IV pole — O$_2$ — Ambu bag — Monitor (if indicated) • Skin closure supplies and dressings are readily available • Wound classification is documented	• Call report to receiving unit: — PACU — SICU • Communicate with family • Inform surgeon of family's location • Arrange for special equipment: — Respirator — Warming unit — Pulsatile Antiembolism system as ordered — O$_2$	• Patient will demonstrate effective coughing and deep breathing exercises • Pain control/management if patient controlled analgesia (PCA) pump • Purpose and importance of NG tube and drainage • Purpose of indwelling urinary catheter • Ambulation • Ostomy care	• Ostomy care and management • Ambulation and self care plan • Home health care support if indicated • Follow-up visit • Who to contact with concerns • Signs and symptoms that may require immediate attention • Medications/ prescriptions • Diet
EXPECTED OUTCOMES	• Maintain patient safety and comfort • Patient and family members understand preoperative teaching and perioperative events	• Maintain patient's hemodynamic and thermodynamic stability • Maintain skin integrity • Patient will not experience neurovascular compromise related to positioning • Patient is free of infection	• Maintain patient's hemodynamic and thermodynamic stability • Establish functional ostomy for fecal excretion if indicated	• Maintain patient's hemodynamic and thermodynamic stability • Patient's pain is controlled • Skin integrity is intact • Patient is free of infection	• Patient will return to activities of daily living • Quality of life will be preserved

FIGURE 11-37, cont'd Clinical pathway for primary colon resection.

layers of the transsected stumps of the ileum and the transverse colon are sutured together. Circular linear stapling devices such as an EEA may be used for anastomosis.

A laparotomy set and GI instrument set are required. The patient is positioned supine under general anesthesia. A nasogastric tube is inserted by the anesthesiologist after intubation. An indwelling urinary catheter is inserted before the abdominal skin prep.

Operative procedure

1. The abdomen is opened, and the peritoneal cavity is retracted and packed with warm, moist sponges.
2. The mesentery of the transverse colon and the terminal ileum is incised at the points where the resection is to be done.
3. Moist packs are placed to isolate the viscera to be resected. A Metzenbaum scissors, hemostats, and 3-0 nonabsorbable ligatures are used to clamp, cut and ligate mesentery vessels.
4. The lateral peritoneal fold along the lateral side of the right colon is incised, and the right colon is mobilized medially. Metzenbaum scissors, hemostats, and sponges on holders are used.
5. The ureter and duodenum are carefully identified.
6. The same procedure is carried out on the terminal ileum. The mesenteric vessels are clamped and ligated with 2-0 nonabsorbable ligatures.
7. The operative field is prepared for anastomosis.
8. Intestinal clamps are placed on the transverse colon and ileum.
9. Division is completed with a scalpel, and the specimen is removed.
10. An end-to-end anastomosis is completed between the severed ends of the terminal ileum and the transverse colon.
11. Instruments and supplies that have come into contact with bowel mucosa are discarded.
12. The mesentery and posterior peritoneum are closed with interrupted 3-0 nonabsorbable sutures.
13. The abdominal wound is closed. A dressing is applied.

Transverse Colectomy

Transverse colectomy is excision of the transverse colon through an upper midline or transverse incision (Fig. 11-36, *C* and *D*). Bowel integrity is reestablished by an end-to-end anastomosis. A transverse colectomy is performed for malignant lesions of the transverse colon. A more radical procedure may be required when the lesion has perforated the greater curvature of the stomach. If the entire lesion is resectable, a partial gastrectomy may also have to be performed.

Procedural considerations

A laparotomy set and GI instrument set are required. Linear stapling instruments should be available. A self-retaining retractor system is an asset. The patient is positioned supine under general anesthesia. A nasogastric tube is inserted by the anesthesiologist after intubation. An indwelling urinary catheter is inserted before the abdominal skin prep.

Operative procedure

1. The abdomen is opened, and the peritoneal cavity is explored to determine the extent of the pathologic area.
2. Moist packs are used to wall off surrounding structures to expose the hepatic and splenic flexures of the colon.
3. The colon is mobilized by incising the lateral peritoneum on either side and transsecting the transverse mesocolon. Hemostats, a Metzenbaum scissors, and 3-0 nonabsorbable ligatures are used.
4. The operative field is prepared for resection by placing towels or laparotomy sponges around the colon to isolate any contamination from the lumen of the bowel.
5. Two intestinal resection clamps are applied.
6. Transection is completed with a scalpel or mechanical linear stapling device.
7. An end-to-end or side-to-side stapled anastomosis is completed.
8. Contaminated articles are discarded.
9. Approximation of mesentery and lateral peritoneum is completed with 3-0 nonabsorbable sutures.
10. The abdominal wound is closed. Retention sutures may be used.
11. The wound is dressed.

Anterior Resection of the Sigmoid Colon and Rectosigmoidostomy

Anterior resection of the sigmoid colon and rectosigmoidostomy involve the removal of the lower sigmoid and rectosigmoid portions of the rectum (Fig. 11-36, *E*). This is usually done through a laparotomy incision, and an end-to-end anastomosis is completed. This operation is selected to treat lesions in the lower portion of the sigmoid and rectum that permit excision with a wide margin of safety and still retain sufficient tissues with adequate blood supply for a viable rectosigmoid end-to-end anastomosis.

Procedural considerations

A laparotomy set and GI instrument set are required. Linear stapling instruments as well as the end-to-end curved mechanical stapling instruments (EEA) are used. Long instruments for dissecting into the pelvis may be necessary. A rigid sigmoidoscope is utilized before patient preparation and after the anastomosis. A self-retaining retractor set is required. The patient is placed in a modified lithotomy position with legs extended into Allen universal stirrups.

An indwelling urinary catheter is inserted before the abdominal and perineal preps.

If there is an assisting surgeon, a table with a basic minor set and rectal instruments should be available to facilitate the end-to-end stapling of the anastomosis. Cross-contamination from the table of instruments utilized on the patient's rectum to the table of laparotomy instruments is prevented. A table with closure instruments may be the surgeon's preference. This should require only a laparotomy set of instruments.

Identification of the ureters during extensive deep abdominal procedures may best be achieved by the preoperative placement of ureteral catheters by a transurethral approach. If the tumor is believed to involve the ureters, the surgeon may have consulted a urologist to perform the ureteral catheter placement at the start of the patient's scheduled procedure. Provision of transurethral endoscopes, supplies, and equipment is necessary.

Operative procedure

1. The abdomen is entered through a laparotomy incision.
2. The peritoneal cavity is explored for metastasis and resectability of the lesion.
3. Before the colon is mobilized, the tumor-bearing segment is isolated by ligatures to the lymphovenous drainage (that is, provided that these structures are accessible).
4. A loop of sigmoid colon is elevated as the small intestines are walled off with moist packs; retractors are placed.
5. The peritoneum on the left side of the colon is incised with a long scalpel, scissors, hemostats, and sponge forceps.
6. Traction sutures of 2-0 nonabsorbable may be used as the peritoneum is reflected.
7. Bleeding vessels are ligated with 2-0 or 3-0 nonabsorbable ligatures.
8. The pelvic peritoneum is exposed and dissected free to form the left side of the reconstructed pelvic floor. Long dissecting instruments are used.
9. Vessels are ligated with 30-inch nonabsorbable ligatures.
10. Extreme care must be exercised throughout to protect the ureters from injury.
11. The sigmoid colon is turned toward the left, and incision and dissection of the peritoneum is performed on the right side of the pelvis.
12. The two incisions are then curved and joined in front of the rectum.
13. The rectum is freed anteriorly and posteriorly from the adjacent structures.
14. The sigmoid colon is clamped with intestinal clamps after mobilization of the proximal portion. A right-angled intestinal clamp or a roticulating linear stapling device may be commonly used to clamp the distal portion of the rectosigmoid.
15. As the sigmoid colon is divided distally to the clamp, the transsected rectal edges are grasped with Allis or Ochsner forceps, and the rectal opening is exposed.
16. The diseased portion is removed, and the soiled instruments are discarded into a separate basin.
17. Continuity is established by an end-to-end anastomosis of the proximal colon and the rectum using a curved mechanical stapling instrument (EEA) (Fig. 11-38).
18. "Donuts" of tissue removed from the EEA stapling device are examined closely for thickness and continuity and then sent as separate specimens to the pathology laboratory.
19. The assisting surgeon passes a rigid sigmoidoscope into the lumen of the bowel transanally.
20. Warm irrigating solution is poured into the peritoneal cavity, and the lumen of the bowel is insufflated.
21. The surgeon observes for air leak from the anastomosis and oversews the site if indicated.
22. The pelvic floor is reperitonealized, and drains may be placed.
23. The abdominal wound is closed in the routine manner, and a dressing is applied.

Abdominoperineal Resection

Abdominoperineal resection is the mobilization and division of a diseased segment of the lower bowel through a midline incision. The proximal end of bowel is exteriorized through a separate stab wound as a colostomy. The distal end is pushed into the hollow of the sacrum and removed through the perineal route (Fig. 11-39).

An abdominoperineal resection is performed for malignant lesions and inflammatory diseases of the lower sigmoid colon, rectum, and anus that are too low for the use of EEA stapling devices.

Procedural considerations

The choice of patient position depends on the surgeon. Some surgeons prefer to start with the patient in the supine position and move the patient to the lithotomy position for the perineal portion of the operation. Others initially place the patient in a modified lithotomy position; thus surgery may be performed simultaneously by two teams, which may require two scrub nurses with two different setups. An indwelling urinary catheter is inserted after induction. A nasogastric tube will be inserted by the anesthesiologist following intubation.

A GI set and an ostomy appliance are required for the abdominal portion of the procedure. A perineal set is used for the perineal portion of the procedure;

Identification of the ureters during extensive deep abdominal procedures may best be achieved by the preoperative placement of ureteral catheters via transurethral approach. If the tumor is believed to involve the ureters, the surgeon will have consulted a urologist to perform the ureteral catheter placement at the start of the

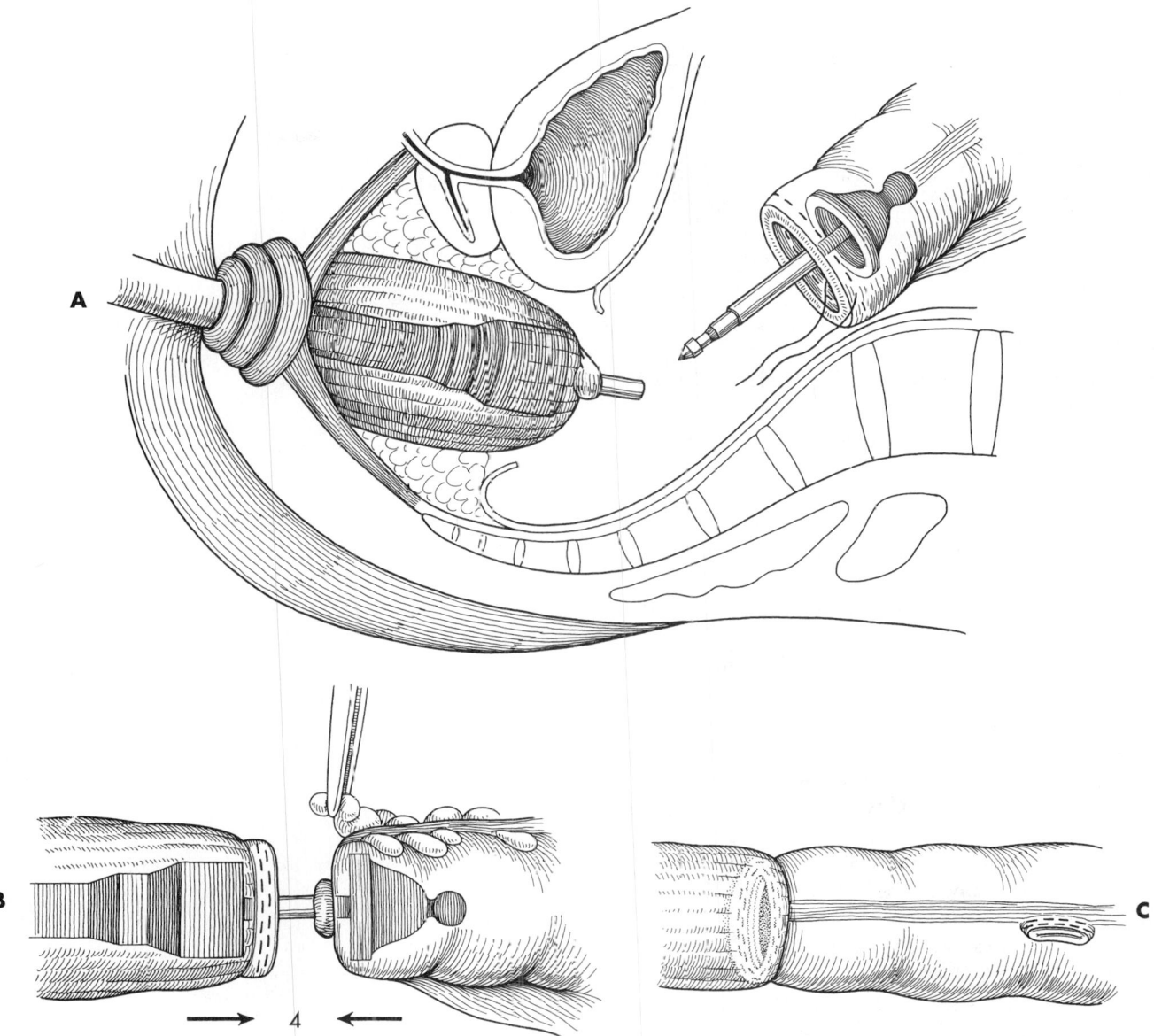

FIGURE 11-38   EEA stapling device, used to perform low anterior anastomosis. **A,** Stapler is introduced into anus, and the anvil is placed into the proximal colon loop. **B,** EEA is advanced to level of the anvil, and the EEA is closed and fired. **C,** Circular double-staggered row of staples joins bowel; simultaneously, circular blade in instrument cuts stoma. Instrument is gently removed. The resulting anastomosis is illustrated with bowel wall transparent to depict reconstruction.

patient's scheduled procedure. Preparation and assembly of transurethral endoscopes, supplies, and equipment are necessary.

Operative procedure

1. A midline incision is made.
2. After thorough exploration of the abdominal cavity, the surgeon determines the extent and operability of the lesion.
3. If a resection is to be done, the surgeon retracts the sigmoid colon to the right side.
4. The peritoneum on the left of the mesocolon is divided. The incision into the peritoneum is made

opposite the main branches of the inferior mesenteric vessels and extended into the pelvis and around anterior to the rectum.

5. The pelvic peritoneum is mobilized by blunt dissection to form the left side of the new pelvic floor and permit early visualization of the left ureter.
6. The peritoneum is incised on the right side until the incision connects with that made on the left.
7. The right ureter is identified and protected.
8. The blood supply of the portion of intestine to be removed is isolated and ligated.
9. Care must be taken not to damage the left colic artery, which will supply the blood to the colostomy.

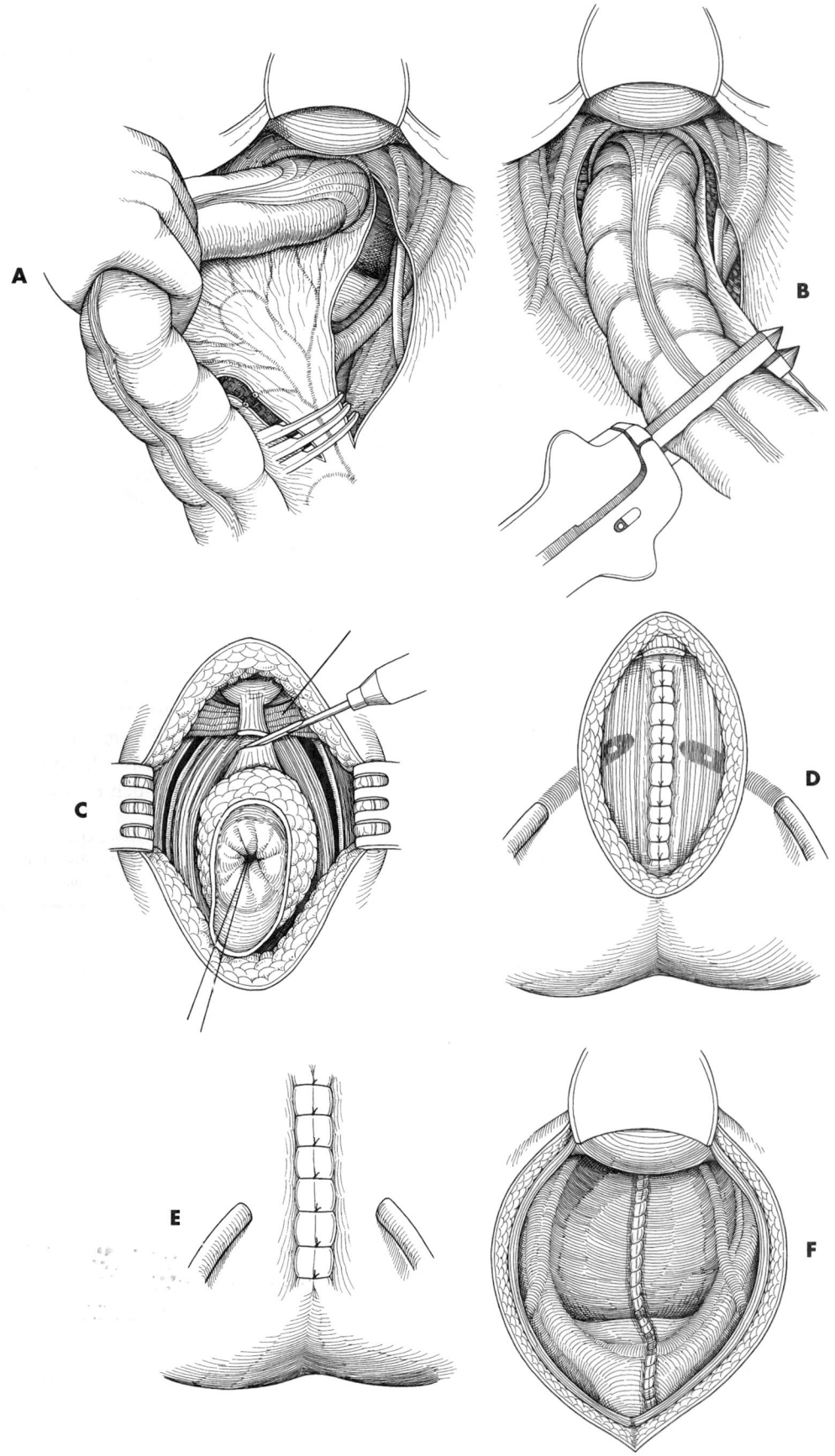

FIGURE 11-39 Abdominoperineal resection for cancer of the rectum. **A,** The sigmoid colon is deflected to the right to complete the rectosigmoid peritoneal detachment. **B,** The distal sigmoid is transected to allow for better access to mobilize the rectum from the sacrum. **C,** The rectal stump is excised from the perineal approach. **D,** Drains are placed and brought through stab wounds; the levator tissues are reapproximated with 2-0 synthetic absorbable sutures. **E,** The perineal skin is closed. **F,** The pelvic peritoneal floor is closed from the abdominal approach.

10. The mesentery is tied to permit greater exposure in the operative field.
11. The surgeon frees the rectum, usually as low as the sacrococcygeal junction. Care is taken to avoid injury to the presacral nerves, which could result in sexual and bladder dysfunction.
12. After the bowel is freed, the distal segment is transsected with a linear stapling instrument (Fig. 11-39, B).
13. The proximal margin of resection is examined and transsected. The bowel and mesentery are removed from the abdominal cavity.
14. The surgeon prepares the permanent colostomy by extending the stump through the abdominal wall.
15. The colostomy will be "matured" (sutured externally to the abdominal wall tissues so that the mucosa is everted into a raised and secured ostomy) after abdominal closure.
16. The combined excision and perineal dissection is initiated when the lesion is determined to be resectable.
17. To prevent contamination, the anus is often closed with a purse-string suture.
18. An incision is made around the anus in an elliptical manner outside of the sphincter muscles with a generous margin of perianal skin.
19. The anus is grasped with an Allis or Ochsner forceps and tipped upward to enable its attachment to the coccyx to be severed more readily.
20. Electrodissection is used. The levator ani muscle is exposed; while the finger of the surgeon is held beneath it, it is divided as far from the rectum as possible.
21. All bleeding points are clamped and tied.
22. The Foley catheter allows the surgeon to get as close to the bladder as possible without damaging it.
23. After the anococcygeal raphe is divided, the surgeon's hand is thrust up into the hollow sacrum to free the rectum by blunt dissection, grasp the upper end of the distal fragment, and deliver the stump through the perineum.
24. Drains may be placed into the pelvic cavity and exteriorized through stab wounds in the buttocks (Fig. 11-39, D).
25. The surgeon is regowned and gloved before returning to the abdominal wound.
26. When all bleeding is controlled, the incision is closed.

If two teams are not available for synchronous excision of the perineum, the perineal portion of the operation is performed after the abdominal resection is complete. In this case the abdomen is closed and the remaining rectosigmoid stump is excised perineally.

Ileoanal Endorectal Pullthrough

Ileoanal endorectal pullthrough is the removal of the entire colon and the proximal two thirds of the rectum. It

---

11-1 RESEARCH HIGHLIGHT

The effect of systemic steroids on ileal pouch–anal anastomosis in patients with ulcerative colitis was the topic of study from researchers at The Cleveland Clinic Foundation, Department of Colorectal Surgery. The purpose of the study was to determine the incidence of early septic complications in patients having ileal pouch–anal anastomosis and who were undergoing long-term steroid therapy. A chart review of 692 patients undergoing ileal pouch–anal anastomosis for ulcerative colitis was the methodology. The incidence of septic complications within 30 days after surgery and sepsis-related reoperations in patients receiving a high dose (>20 mg of prednisone per day) and in patients receiving a low dose (<20 mg of prednisone per day) for more than 1 month before surgery, was compared with patients who were not receiving steroid therapy. The three groups were similar in sex composition, age at surgery, types of anastomosis (handsewn or stapled), and incidence of diabetes mellitus, peripheral vascular disease, and obesity.

The study demonstrated that prolonged steroid therapy before surgery for patients undergoing ileal pouch–anal anastomosis for ulcerative colitis did not have clinically or statistically significant effect on early septic complication rate, sepsis-related reoperation rate, or need for sepsis-related pouch excision.

From Ziv, Y., Church, J.M., Fazio, V.W., et al. (1996). Effect of systemic steroids on ileal pouch–anal anastomosis in patients with ulcerative colitis, *Diseases of Colon and Rectum, 39*(5), 504-508.

---

includes a mucosectomy of the remaining distal rectum, creation of a pouch from the distal small bowel, and anastomosis of the pouch to the anus. The operation is performed to relieve the symptoms of ulcerative colitis and familial polyposis (diarrhea, pain, cramping, bleeding, and others) and to prevent colon malignancies (Research Highlight 11-1). This procedure is an anal sphincter–saving operation that is done to avoid the need for a traditional ileostomy.

Procedural considerations

The patient is usually placed in a modified lithotomy position. Some surgeons prefer to perform the mucosectomy with the patient in a jackknife position and then place the patient in a modified lithotomy position for the remainder of the procedure. A nasogastric tube is inserted by the anesthesiologist after intubation. An indwelling urinary catheter is inserted before the abdominal skin prep.

A GI set, a perineal set, and rectal instrumentation are required. A self-retaining retractor system is an asset. Separate instrument tables are used for the rectal and abdominal approaches. Additional draping and gowning supplies should be available because redraping and regowning occur after the mucosectomy and after the ileoanal anastomosis. An epinephrine solution should be available for injection into the submucosal tissue, proximal to the anus, to separate the mucosa from the muscularis layer. An ileostomy appliance is applied immediately postoperatively.

Operative procedure

1. The anal canal is dilated and inspected through an anoscope.
2. Starting at the dentate line, the anorectal junction, the epinephrine solution is injected circumferentially, separating the mucosa from the muscularis layer.
3. The mucosectomy is then performed by making a circular incision at the dentate line, cutting only through mucosa.
4. The mucosa is peeled off the muscularis tissue for a distance of 2 to 8 cm and resected.
5. When all bleeding is controlled, the patient is repositioned, if necessary, for the abdominal approach.
6. A midline incision is made, and the abdomen is explored.
7. The entire large intestine from the ileocecal junction through the upper two thirds of the rectum is freed and immobilized.
8. All vessels are ligated.
9. The terminal ileum is separated from the cecum using a mechanical cutting and stapling device (GIA).
10. The mesocolon is ligated using suture ligatures or a ligating, dividing, and stapling instrument.
11. The rectum is resected down to the level of the mucosectomy.
12. The colon and resected portion of the rectum are removed en bloc.
13. The pouch is created. Most surgeons use either the J pouch or the S pouch.
14. The J pouch is created at the terminal ileum by folding two adjacent loops of small bowel, approximately 10 to 15 cm each, parallel with each other and anastomosing them using a GIA. An opening is made at the bottom of the pouch, and the pouch is pulled through the rectal stump. The bottom of the pouch is anastomosed to the anus with interrupted absorbable sutures (Fig. 11-40).
15. An S pouch is created by aligning the distal ileum in an S configuration with each of the three limbs approximately 10 cm in length. The most distal 2 cm of the ileum is not incorporated into the pouch but is preserved for the anastomosis to the anus. The three limbs are manually incised and anastomosed to create a pouch. Mucosal tissue is approximated with absorbable suture, and nonabsorbable suture is used for the serosal layer. The preserved distal end of the ileum and the pouch are pulled through the rectal stump and anastomosed to the anus (Fig. 11-41).

16. This completes the anal portion of the procedure.
17. The scrubbed team changes gowns and gloves, redrapes, and completes the abdominal procedure by creating a loop ileostomy on a previously designated site through the abdominal wall.
18. The abdominal incision is closed in the usual manner.

Approximately 2 to 6 months are required after the initial operation for adequate healing of the ileoanal anastomosis to occur and to ensure the absence of postsurgical complications. When the patient's status is determined to be satisfactory, a second procedure is performed to restore bowel continuity and close the loop ileostomy.

Carcinoembryonic Antigen-Directed Second-Look Laparotomy

Carcinoembryonic antigen (CEA) serum levels are followed closely in patients with a history of adeno-carcinoma of the colon or rectum. When a persistent rise in the patient's CEA level is demonstrated, noninvasive diagnostics such as CT scan or MRI scans are obtained. Colonoscopy may be performed to directly visualize the anastomotic site for recurrence or a secondary primary tumor. CT scans and MRI scans may not detect tumor metastasis less than 0.5 cm in size. Lymph nodes in the periportal area may, however, be identified as enlarged or suspicious. Negative diagnostic workup does not negate the justification for exploratory laparotomy when the patient's CEA level rises persistently 2 standard deviations above the individual's baseline level. Normal CEA levels vary according to the type of assay conducted to measure CEA serum levels. Generally, CEA levels are normal in the 0 to 5 ng/ml range. A patient's baseline value may be 0.2 ng/ml, but a rise to 4.2 ng/ml is cause for alarm. Thus obtaining baseline CEA levels in all patients undergoing surgical intervention for the primary resection of adenocarcinoma of the colon or rectum is extremely important. These patients can be educated as to the importance of periodic monitoring of CEA serum levels and readily accept this as justification to undergo laparotomy.

Potential findings upon exploratory laparotomy vary (Research Highlight 11-2). If carcinomatosis is found, a simple biopsy specimen may be taken to confirm diagnosis. The patient signing an informed consent for CEA-directed second-look laparotomy understands the potential for extensive radical resection, which may include hysterectomy with bilateral salpingo-oophorectomy, partial or total cystectomy, retroperitoneal lymph node dissection, hepatic resection, gastrohepatic lymph node dissection, colon resection, small bowel resection, omentectomy, and abdominal wall resection. For patients with a history of rectal adenocarcinoma, pelvic exenteration may be performed. The informed surgical consent should

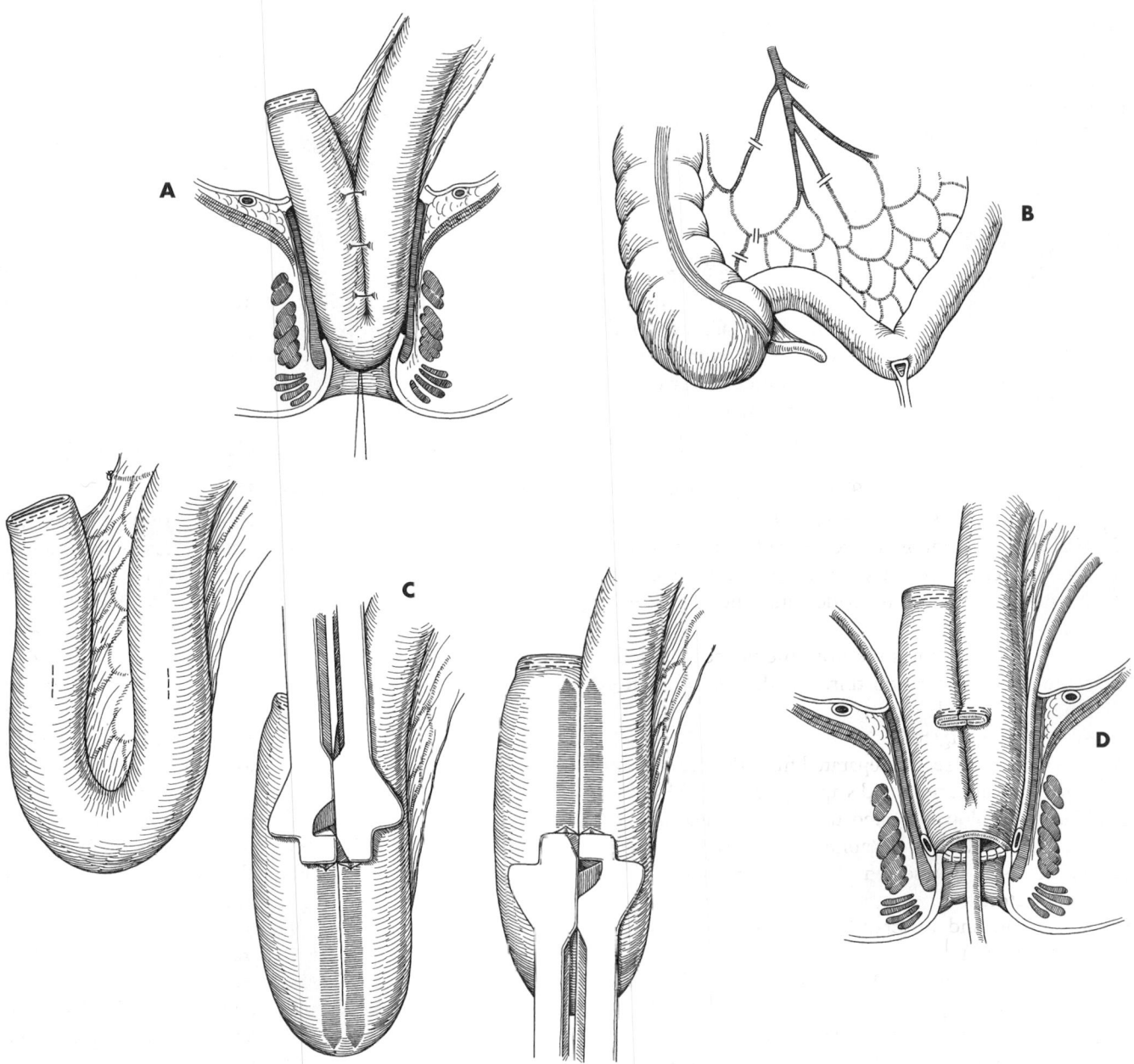

FIGURE 11–40   J pouch for ileoanal endorectal pullthrough. **A**, The J pouch is created at terminal ileum by folding two adjacent loops of small bowel, approximately 10 to 15 cm each, parallel with each other. **B**, Mesenteric vascular arcades may need to be divided to provide adequate length for anal anastomosis. **C**, The two loops are anastomosed using mechanical cutting and stapling device (GIA). **D**, Opening is made at bottom of pouch, and pouch is pulled through rectal stump. Bottom of pouch is anastomosed to anus.

reflect the possible interventions, as well as the potential for blood loss and complications.

Procedural considerations

A basic laparotomy instrument set is required as well as Richardson retractors and a Bookwalter retractor system. GI instruments, vascular instruments and linear stapling instruments should be readily available. Intraoperative ultrasonography and the Cavitron Ultrasonic Surgical Aspirator (CUSA) should also be available.

The patient is positioned supine under general anesthesia. A Foley catheter is inserted into the urinary bladder, and the patient's abdomen is prepped from the nipple line to the midthigh. A nasogastric tube is inserted for stomach decompression.

Operative procedure

1. A midline incision is made from the xiphoid, around the umbilicus, to the pubis.
2. The peritoneum is entered after removal of any sutures from earlier surgical procedures.

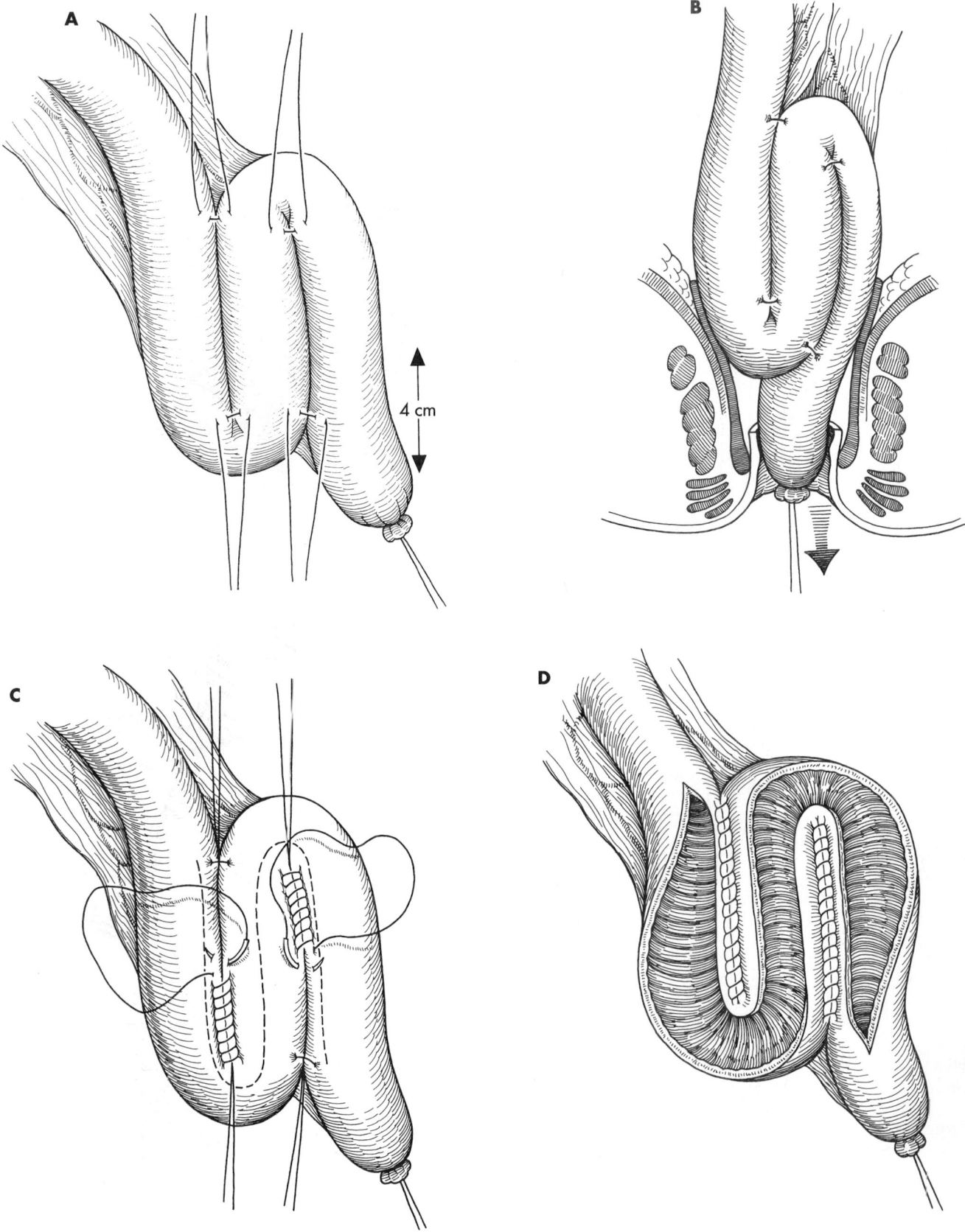

FIGURE 11–41   S pouch for ileoanal endorectal pullthrough. **A**, Pouch is created by aligning distal ileum in S configuration with each limb (three in total) approximately 12 cm in length. **B**, The length is measured before anastomosis begins. **C**, Three limbs are incised and anastomosed to create pouch. **D**, Incision is made as illustrated.

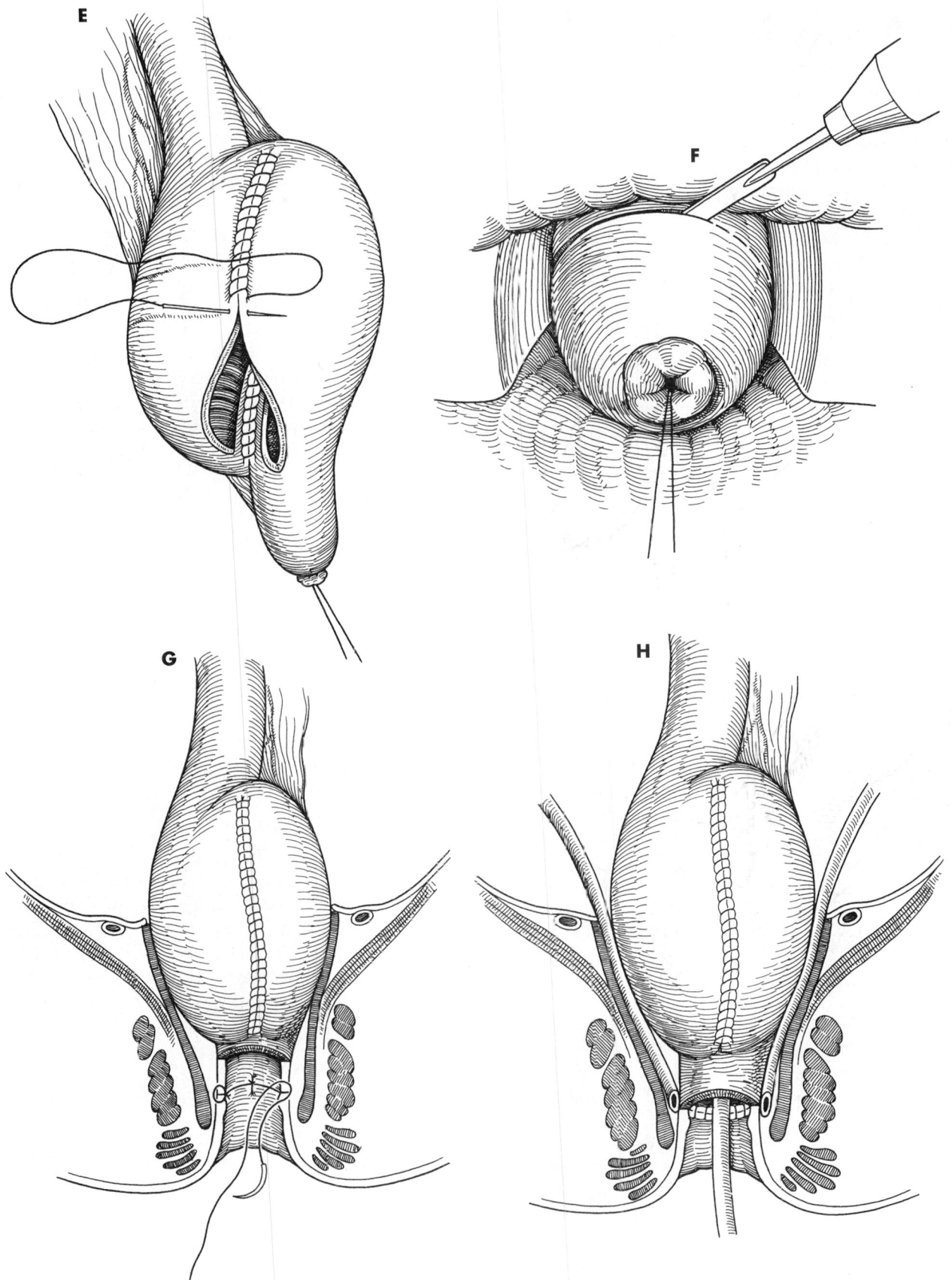

FIGURE 11–41, cont'd   **E,** The pouch is closed using suture for the formation of the reservoir. **F,** Distal ends of ileum and pouch are pulled through the rectal stump, and the lower outflow tract is trimmed. **G,** With 3-0 absorbable sutures, the outflow tract is anastomosed to the anus at the dentate line. **H,** Drain in place in the lumen of the newly created ileoanal-rectal canal.

11-2 RESEARCH HIGHLIGHT

The detection of the extent of tumor metastasis and the patterns of tumor dissemination for patients with colon and rectal cancer continues to be problematic. Micrometastatic disease is undetectable by direct visual examination and palpation of tissues. Most studies have examined tumor metastasis retroactively and have depended largely on computerized tomographic (CT) scans that have been ordered because of a demonstrated increase in serial carcinoembryonic antigen (CEA) levels in patients after surgical intervention for their colon or rectal cancer. These scans are compared with available preoperative scans.

A study at the Ohio State University Medical Center, Department of Surgery, evaluated two selected populations of colorectal cancer patients (86 evaluable patients in total) who had been screened and injected with a radiolabeled monoclonal antibody (MAb) for radioimmunoguided surgery (RIGS). The method of study was to perform exploratory laparotomy with traditional examination of selected anatomic sites and then perform exploration and examination of those same sites using a hand-held gamma ray–detecting probe that would detect the radiolabeled MAb that is known to target colorectal cancer cells.

Results. In 41 patients with primary colorectal cancer, traditional examination detected 45 sites of disease. In these same patients, the use of the hand-held gamma ray–detecting probe for RIGS demonstrated 153 RIGS-positive sites. In 45 patients with recurrent colorectal cancer, traditional examination found 116 sites. In these same patients, the use of RIGS demonstrated 184 RIGS-positive sites. Moreover, areas not usually included in traditional exploration for colorectal cancer were proportionately highest for RIGS-positive tissue. This included lymphatics in the gastrohepatic ligament area, celiac lymph nodes, and retroperitoneal lymph nodes.

monoclonal antibody (MAb) before surgery, abdominal exploration using the Neoprobe is performed. The Neoprobe is a hand-held gamma ray–detecting probe used to detect the minute amount of radioactive ^{105}I bonded to an MAb that is injected intravenously 2 to 3 weeks before the patient's scheduled surgery. The MAb is a glycoprotein that will bind to the antigen on cancer cell membranes. Remaining circulating MAb is excreted from the body through the kidneys during the weeks before surgery. During exploration with the Neoprobe, an audible tone sounds when the instrument is in proximity with tissues in which the MAb-antigen bonding has occurred. The surgeon can then detect an occult tumor that might otherwise remain concealed. The radioimmunoguided surgery concept is currently being tried with several carrier substances such as the MAb. Future applications may apply to malignancies other than adenocarcinoma.

8. Necessary resection of organs and tissues is performed.
9. The abdomen is closed according to surgeon preference.
10. Retention sutures may be used.

SURGERY OF THE RECTUM

Hemorrhoidectomy

Hemorrhoidectomy is the excision and ligation of dilated veins in the anal region to relieve discomfort and control bleeding. The frequency of hemorrhoidectomies performed in the operating room has decreased because of banding procedures now being done on an ambulatory surgery basis.

Procedural considerations

Preoperative anal dilatation aids in exposing the vessels and contributes to the patient's comfort in the immediate postoperative period. Many surgeons prefer to precede the operation with a sigmoidoscopy. Spinal, caudal, epidural, or local anesthesia may be used. The CO_2 laser may also be used for vaporization and coagulation of hemorrhoidal tissue. The patient is usually placed in the lithotomy or jackknife position.

Operative procedure

1. The anal canal is dilated and inspected through an anoscope.
2. Four Allis forceps are applied several centimeters from the anal margin to expose the anus.
3. The base of the hemorrhoid and tissue are grasped with Allis forceps and held.
4. An intestinal suture of 2-0 synthetic absorbable suture is placed and tied at the proximal end of the hemorrhoid, and a Buie pile forceps is applied across the base and above the proposed incision line.
5. Excision is completed with a scalpel.

3. Abdominal adhesions may be extensive and require hours of tedious dissection using Metzenbaum scissors, Debakey forceps, gauze dissectors, and electrodissection.
4. An extensive inspection and palpation of all the abdominal viscera is required in a systematic approach.
5. Samples of suspicious tissues are collected for biopsy. Frequent specimens may be sent for frozen section to confirm diagnosis.
6. The liver is examined by palpation, inspection, and intraoperative ultrasonography.
7. If the patient has been prepared for radioimmunoguided surgery (RIGS) by receiving a radiolabeled

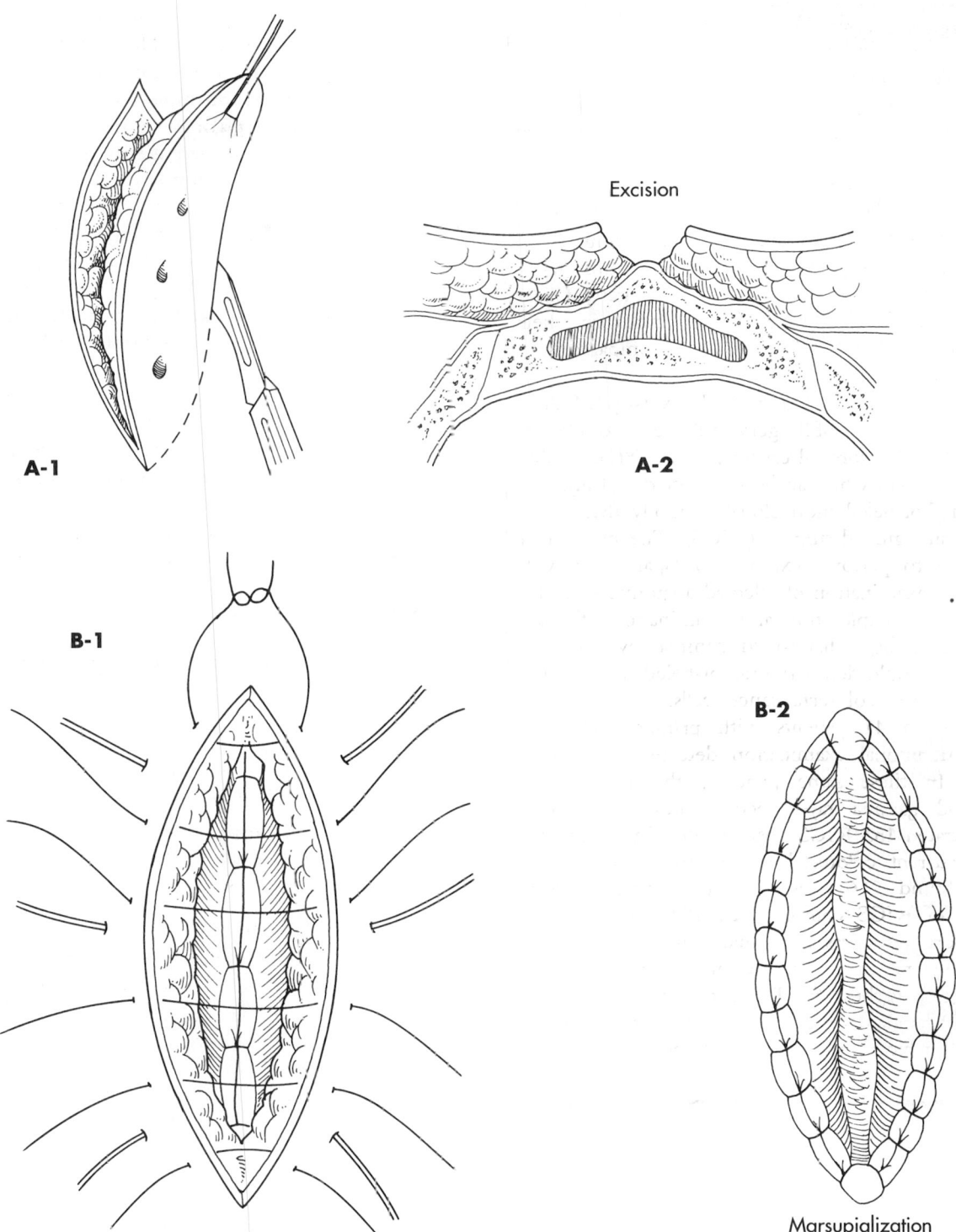

Excision

A-1

A-2

B-1

B-2

Marsupialization

FIGURE 11–42   Pilonidal cyst. The pilonidal sinus tract is identified with injection of methylene blue into the tract. **A**, Wide elliptical incision (*A-1*) is made to include all the subcutaneous tracts and tissue to the fascia overlying the sacrum and coccyx (*A-2*). **B**, Closure of the wound can be primary (*B-1*) or secondary (*B-2*).

6. Suturing is completed by loosely placed continuous sutures over the Buie forceps.

7. The suture is tightened as the forceps are removed, and the suture ends are tied.

8. Traction may be maintained as hemostatic forceps are applied and dissection is completed segmentally.

9. Suture ligatures of 2-0 synthetic absorbable suture are used as each hemostat is removed.

10. Remaining hemorrhoids are excised in a similar manner.

11. Petrolatum gauze packing may be placed in the anal canal. A dressing is applied.

Excision of Anal Fissure and Lateral Sphincterotomy

Excision of an anal fissure involves the dilatation of the anal sphincter and removal of the lesion. Anal fissures are benign lesions of the anal wall.

Procedural considerations

A minor set and rectal instruments are required. The patient is placed in the lithotomy or jackknife position.

Operative procedure

1. Dilatation of the anal sphincter is completed.
2. The fissure is excised, and bleeders are ligated or electrocoagulated.
3. A lateral incision is made, and the internal sphincter is incised.
4. The mucosa is approximated over the incision.
5. A drain or packing is inserted. A dressing is applied.

Excision of Pilonidal Cyst and Sinus

Excision of a pilonidal cyst and sinus is removal of the cyst with sinus tracts from the intergluteal fold on the posterior surface of the lower sacrum (Fig. 11-42). A pilonidal cyst and sinus, which may have a congenital origin, rarely become symptomatic until the individual reaches adulthood. Inflammatory reaction varies from a mild, irritating, draining sinus tract to an acute abscess with secondary recurrences. Treatment consists of drainage in the acute stage and total surgical excision during remission.

The excision of the cyst and sinus tracts must be complete to prevent recurrence. The defect resulting from recurrences may become too large for primary closure. In this case the wound is left open to heal by granulation.

Procedural considerations

A minor set and rectal instruments are required, as well as methylene blue, a 10 or 20 ml syringe, and a blunt-tipped needle. The patient is placed in the jackknife position.

Operative procedure

1. The sinus tracts are identified with probes.
2. The tract is marked by injecting methylene blue with a blunted needle into the tract.
3. An elliptical incision is made down to the fascia.
4. A curette is used to remove gelatinous tissue.
5. Excision of cyst and sinus tracts is completed.
6. Bleeding is controlled.
7. If the wound is to be left open, it is packed, and a pressure dressing is applied.
8. If the wound is closed, 2-0 nonabsorbable sutures are used for stay sutures on the deeper tissue, and fine nonabsorbable suture is used on the skin.

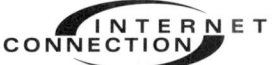

American Cancer Society: http://www.cancer.org

Oncolink: http://oncolink.upenn.edu

Crohns and Colitis Foundation: http://www.ccfa.org

National Digestive Disease Clearinghouse:
e-mail nddic@aerie.com

Patient Info Documents on Digestive Diseases:
http://www.niddk.nih.gov/health/digest/digest.htm

Society for Gatroenterology Nurses and Associates:
http://www.sgna.org

Laparoscopy: http://www.laparoscopy.com

McGill General Surgery Home Page:
http://www.mcgill.ca/surgery

REFERENCES

1. Brooks, D.C. (1994). *Current techniques in laparoscopy.* Philadelphia: Current Medicine.
2. Thompson, J.C. (1992). *Atlas on surgery of the stomach, duodenum, and small bowel,* St. Louis: Mosby.
3. Quilici, J.P. (1992). *New developments in laparoscopy,* Norwalk, Conn: The U.S. Surgical Corp.

CHAPTER TWELVE

Surgery of the Liver, Biliary Tract, Pancreas, and Spleen

Lynda R. Petty

DISEASES OF THE liver, biliary tract, pancreas, and spleen have a great influence on the wellness of the patient. Because these organs are highly vascular and control many of the metabolic and immune functions of the body, a pathologic condition in one or more of them requires urgent intervention. Surgical interventions relating to the liver, biliary tract, pancreas, or spleen may be indicated for tumor, infection, cystic anomalies, congenital anomalies, metabolic diseases, or trauma.

In the past decade, surgeries of the liver and biliary tract have become more advanced as research and new technology have permitted more complete diagnosis of pathologic conditions involving this complex organ and portal system. A resection of the liver for carcinoma has achieved a recognized role for cure or substantial palliation with safety and low morbidity.

Cholecystectomy is the most common nonemergency abdominal operation performed. In the United States approximately 500,000 cholecystectomies are carried out each year and it is expected that this number will increase because of the aging population.[5]

Laparoscopic cholecystectomy has become the most common mode of surgical intervention for the treatment of cholecystitis. It offers the advantages of reduced trauma to tissues as well as a significant reduction in the length of postoperative recovery. The introduction and success of laparoscopic cholecystectomy have evolved into numerous abdominal procedures now being performed or assisted through the laparoscope.

New diagnostic technology and the intraoperative use of ultrasonography, biliary endoscopy, and radiography have enabled surgeons to better treat diseases of the biliary tract. Solid organ transplantation, as with the liver, pancreas, and kidneys, has achieved commonality as a means of treatment for primary hepatic tumors, end-stage liver disease, and insulin-deficient diabetes. Liver transplant now offers the patient the option of living-related organ donation. The pioneers in transplantation are now attempting animal-to-human organ transplants as a possible means of providing more organs for the ever-growing list of waiting recipients.

This chapter contains information pertaining to the most common and innovative procedures and technology related to surgery of the liver, biliary tract, pancreas, and spleen.

SURGICAL ANATOMY

The liver is in the right upper quadrant of the abdominal cavity, beneath the dome of the diaphragm and directly above the stomach, duodenum, and hepatic flexure of the colon. The external covering, known as *Glisson's capsule*, is composed of dense connective tissue.

The visceral peritoneum extends over the entire surface of the liver, except at the point of posterior attachment to the diaphragm. This connective tissue branches at the porta hepatis into a network of septa that extends into an intrahepatic network of support for the more than one million hepatic lobules. The porta hepatis is located on the

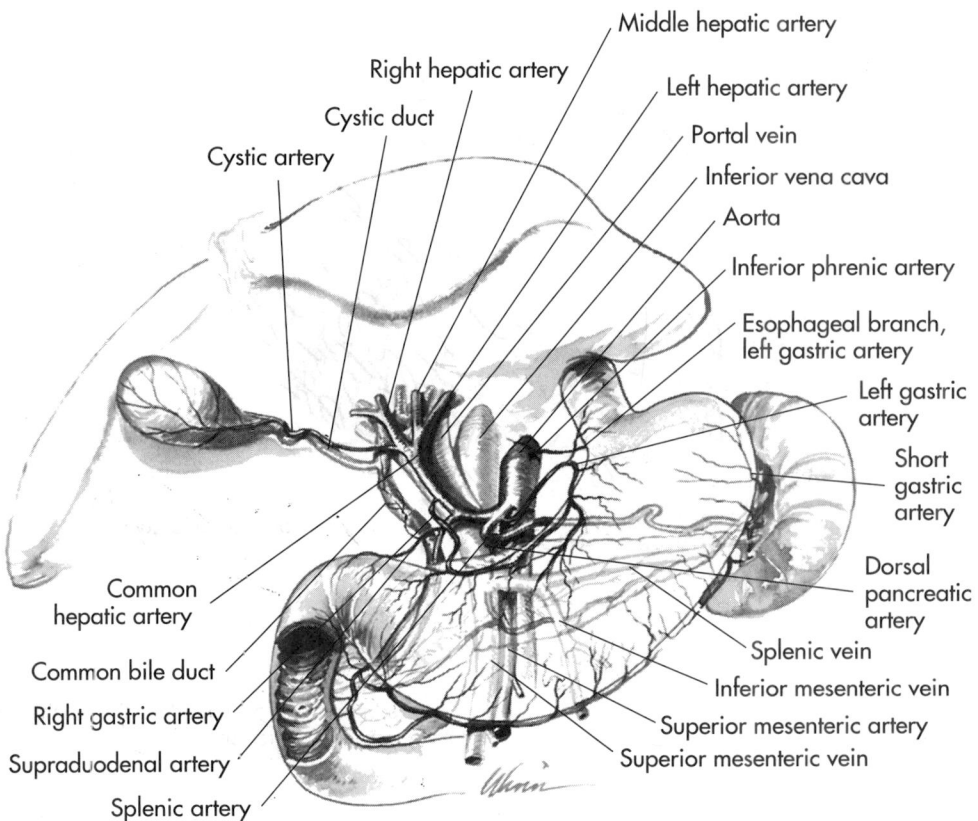

FIGURE 12-1   Intricate relationships of the arterial and venous blood supply of the liver, gallbladder, pancreas, spleen, and the biliary ductal system.

inferior surface of the liver and is the location of entry and exit for the major vessels, ducts, and nerves. The arterial blood supply is maintained by the hepatic artery, and venous blood from the stomach, intestines, spleen, and pancreas is carried to the liver by the portal vein and its branches (Fig. 12-1). The hepatic venous system returns blood to the heart by way of the inferior vena cava.

The lobules are the functional units of the liver. Each lobule contains a portal triad that consists of a hepatic duct, hepatic portal vein branch, a branch of the hepatic artery, nerves, and lymphatics. A central vein is located in the center of each lobule and provides for venous drainage into the hepatic veins.

The lobules also contain hepatic cords, hepatic sinusoids, and bile canaliculi. The hepatic cords comprise numerous columns of hepatocytes, the functional cells of the liver. The hepatic sinusoids are the blood channels that communicate between the columns of hepatocytes. The sinusoids have a thin epithelial lining composed primarily of Kupffer's cells, phagocytic cells that engulf bacteria and toxins. The sinusoids drain into the central vein.

Bile is manufactured by the hepatocytes. The bile canaliculi are tiny bile capillary vessels that communicate between the columns of hepatocytes. The bile canaliculi collect bile and transport it to the bile ducts in the portal triad of each lobule, and subsequently it flows into the hepatic ducts at the porta hepatis. These ducts join

immediately to form one common hepatic duct that merges with the cystic duct from the gallbladder to form the common bile duct (Fig. 12-2). The common bile duct opens into the duodenum in an area called the *ampulla*, or *papilla, of Vater,* located about 7.5 cm below the pyloric opening from the stomach.

Bile contains bile salts, which facilitate digestion and absorption, and various waste products. The liver is essential in the metabolism of carbohydrates, proteins, and fats. It metabolizes nutrients into glycogen stores for regulation of blood glucose levels and energy sources for the brain and body functions.

The liver plays several important roles in the blood-clotting mechanism: It is the organ that synthesizes plasma proteins, excluding gamma globulins but including pro-thrombin and fibrinogen. Vitamin K, a cofactor to the synthesis of prothrombin, is absorbed by the metabolism of fats in the intestinal tract as a result of bile formation by the liver. Patients with liver disease may have alterations in their blood-coagulation abilities.

The liver also synthesizes lipoproteins and cholesterol. Cholesterol is an essential component of the blood plasma. It serves as a precursor for bile salts, steroid hormones, plasma membranes, and other specialized molecules. A diet high in cholesterol reduces the amount that must be synthesized by the liver. When the diet is deficient in cholesterol, the liver increases synthesis to maintain the

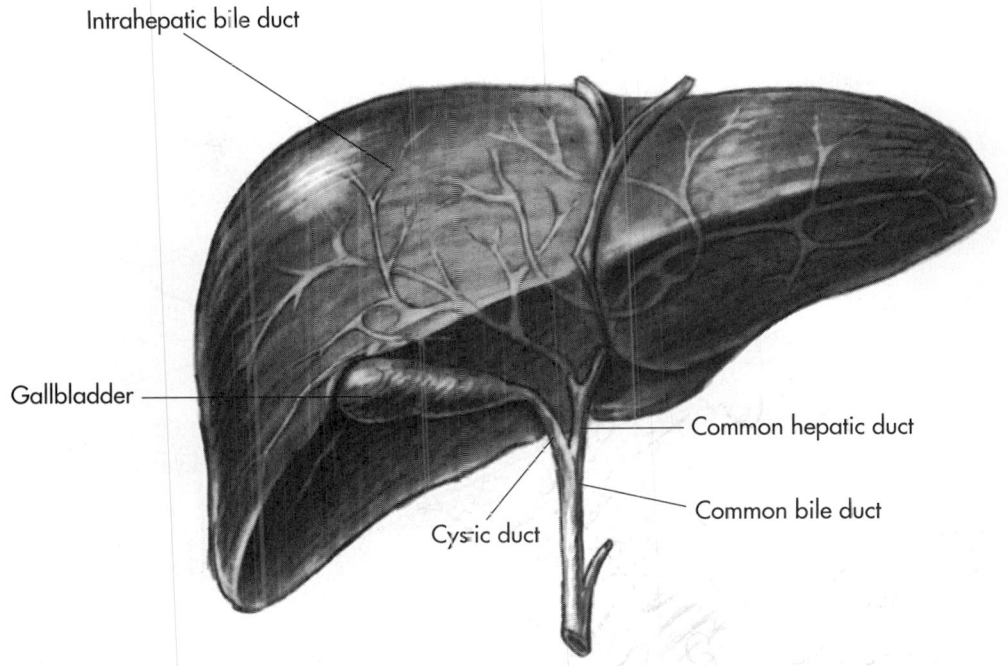

FIGURE 12-2   Biliary system can be divided into three anatomic areas: the intrahepatic bile duct, the extrahepatic bile duct (common hepatic and common bile ducts), and the gallbladder and cystic duct.

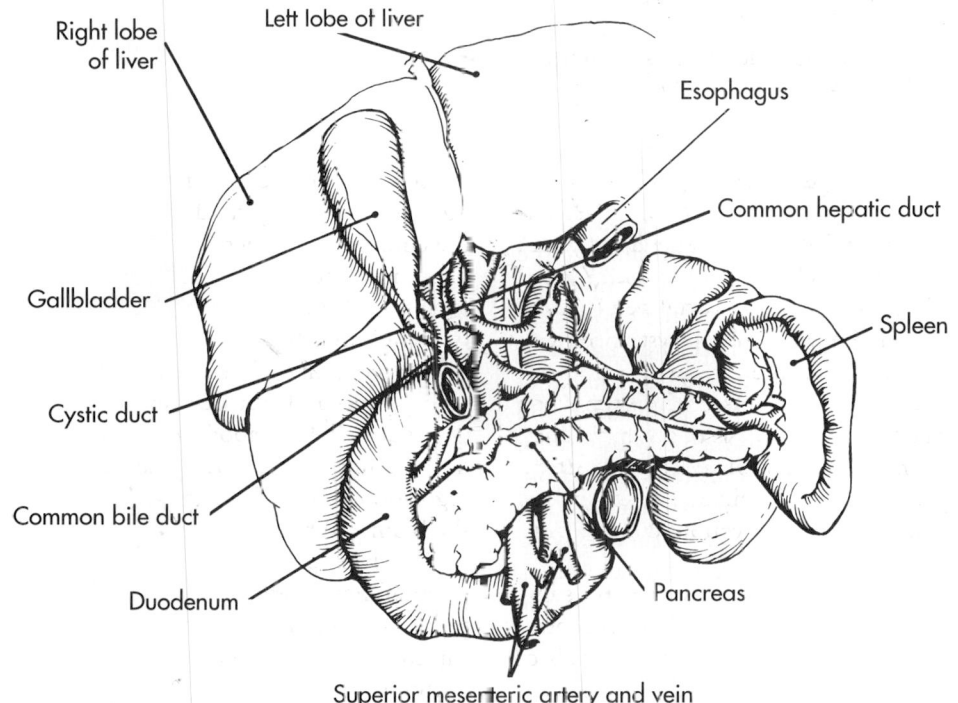

FIGURE 12-3   Gallbladder and surrounding anatomy.

levels necessary for the production of the vital chemical molecules.

The liver also serves in the metabolic alteration of foreign molecules or biotransformation of chemicals. The microsomal enzyme system (MES) plays a major role in the body's response to foreign chemicals such as pollutants, drugs, and alcohol. Patients with liver disease may have alterations in their response to chemical substances. This consideration is most important in the induction and management of general anesthesia for patients with liver disorders.

The gallbladder, which lies in a sulcus on the undersurface of the right lobe of the liver, terminates in the cystic duct (Fig. 12-3). This ductal system provides a

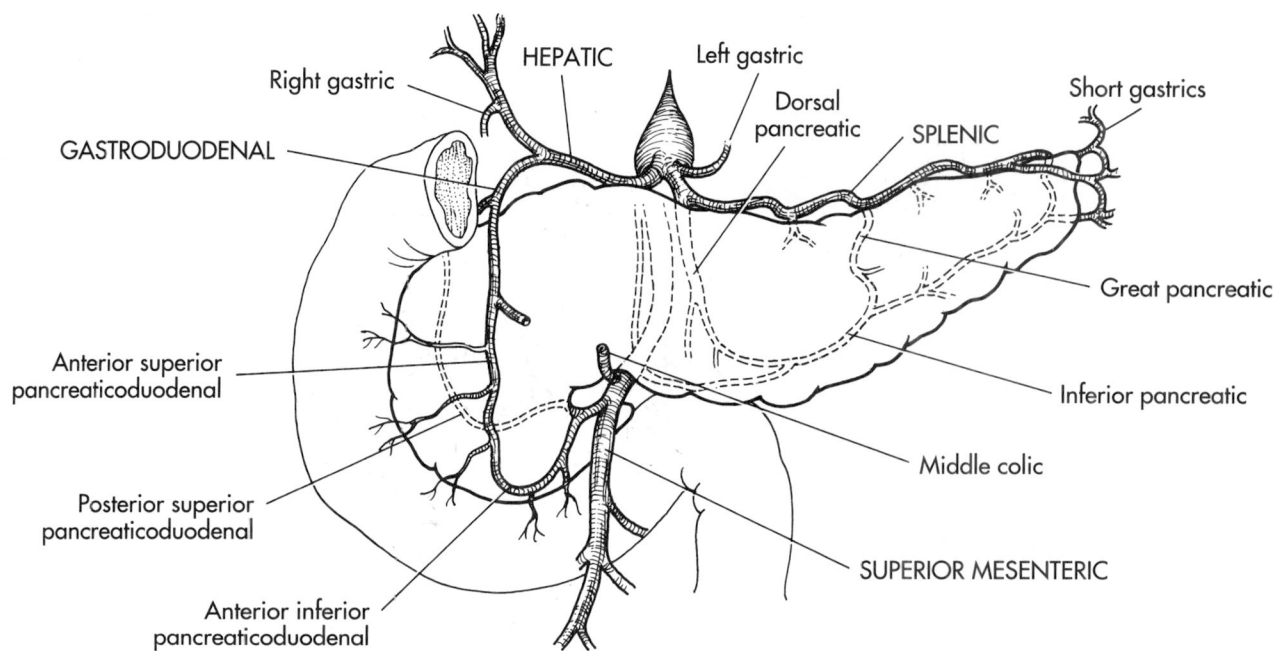

FIGURE 12-4   Arterial supply to the pancreas arises from the celiac axis (hepatic and splenic arteries) and the superior mesenteric artery. The blood supply to the head of the gland is via the pancreaticoduodenal (anterior and posterior) arcades, which arise from the gastroduodenal artery (superior) and superior mesenteric arteries (inferior).

channel for the flow of bile to the gallbladder, where it becomes highly concentrated during the storage period. Approximately 600 to 1000 ml of bile are produced by the liver daily. The gallbladder's average storage capacity is 40 to 70 ml. As food, especially fats, is ingested, cholecystokinin is released by the duodenal cells when food enters the small intestine. The musculature of the gallbladder contracts, forcing bile into the cystic duct and through the common duct. As the sphincter of Oddi in the ampulla of Vater relaxes, bile pours forth, flowing into the duodenum to aid in digestion by emulsification of fats. The gallbladder receives its blood supply from the cystic artery, a branch of the hepatic artery. Innervation for the gallbladder and biliary tree is controlled by the autonomic nervous system. The parasympathetic innervation stimulates contraction, whereas sympathetic innervation inhibits contraction.

The pancreas (see Fig. 12-3) is a fixed structure lying transversely behind the stomach in the upper abdomen. The head of the pancreas is fixed to the curve of the duodenum. Blood is supplied to the pancreas and the duodenum via the celiac axis and the superior mesenteric artery (Figs. 12-4 and 12-5). The body of the pancreas lies across the vertebrae and over the superior mesenteric artery and vein. The tail of the pancreas extends to the hilum of the spleen. In total, the pancreas extends approximately 25 cm. The pancreatic secretions, containing digestive enzymes, are collected in the pancreatic duct, or duct of Wirsung, which unites with the common bile duct to enter the duodenum about 7.5 cm below the pylorus. The ampulla of Vater is formed by the dilated junction of the two ducts at the point of entry.

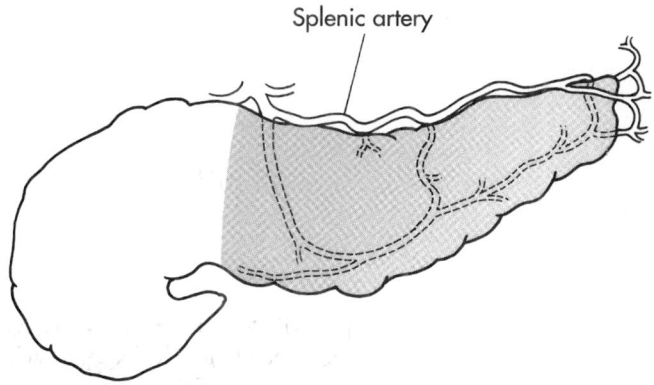

FIGURE 12-5   Major arterial supply to the body and tail of the pancreas is derived from branches of the splenic artery.

The pancreas also contains groups of cells, called *islets*, or *islands*, *of Langerhans*, that secrete hormones into the blood capillaries instead of into the duct. These hormones are insulin and glucagon, and both are involved in carbohydrate metabolism.

The spleen (Fig. 12-6) is in the upper left abdominal cavity, with full protection provided by the tenth, eleventh, and twelfth ribs; the lateral surface is directly beneath the dome of the diaphragm. The anterior medial surface is in proximity to the cardiac end of the stomach and the splenic flexure of the colon. The spleen is covered with peritoneum that forms supporting ligaments. The arterial blood supply is furnished by the splenic artery, a branch of the celiac axis. The splenic vein drains into the portal system.

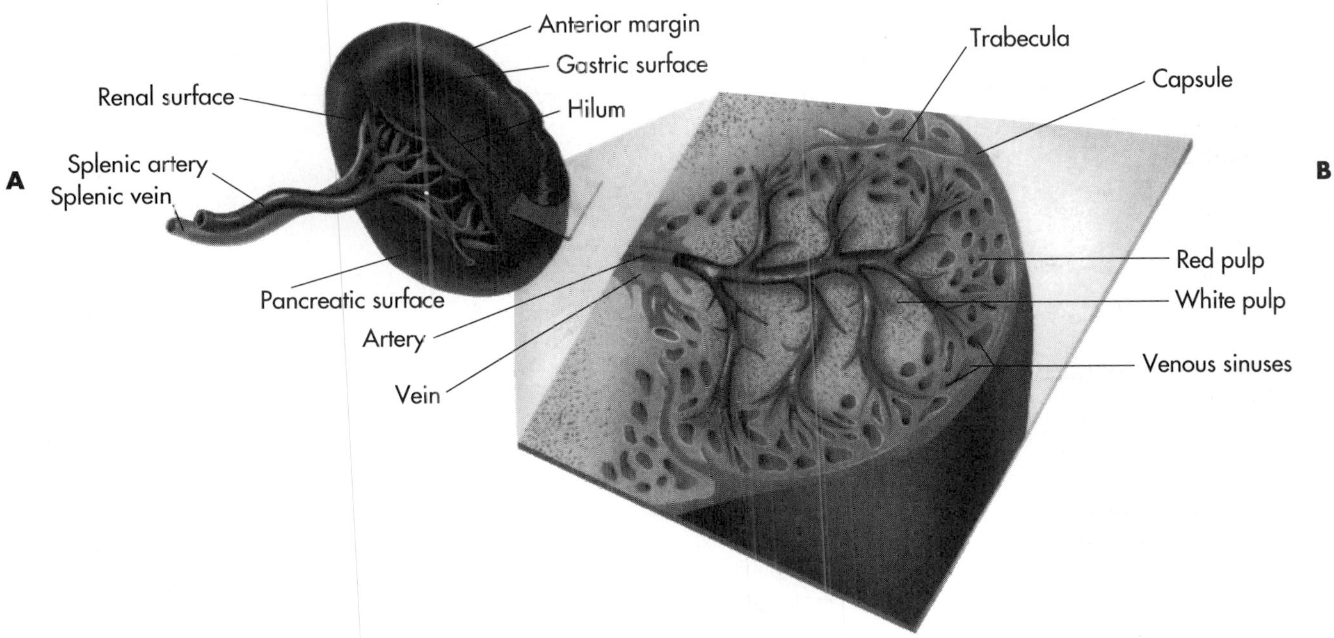

FIGURE 12-6   Spleen. **A**, Medial aspect. Arrangement of vessels at hilum is highly variable. **B**, Section showing the internal organization of the spleen.

The spleen has many functions. Among them are the defense of the body by phagocytosis of microorganisms, formation of nongranular leukocytes and plasma cells, and phagocytosis of damaged red blood cells. It also acts as a blood reservoir.

PERIOPERATIVE NURSING CONSIDERATIONS

Assessment

The patient with hepatobiliary disease may have extreme jaundice, urticaria, petechiae, lethargy, and irritability. Depending on the extent of the disease, the patient may have increased bleeding and coagulation times and a decreased platelet count, thus predisposing to bruising easily. A thorough nursing history is necessary for proper assessment of the health status of patients with dysfunctions of the hepatobiliary system, the pancreas, or the spleen. Assessment should include data pertaining to the patient's perception of his or her disease, comfort status, nutritional status, fluid and electrolyte balance, bowel and elimination patterns, energy level and independence, and exposure to toxins.

Establishing the objective database for a person with hepatobiliary or pancreatic dysfunction requires comprehensive assessment. Particular attention should be directed toward observing for characteristic signs of dysfunction. Increased abdominal girth and distention, palmar erythema, distended periumbilical veins, hemorrhagic areas, spider nevi, muscle wasting, and dry mucous membranes are a few of the characteristic signs and symptoms of dysfunction. Vascular volume can be assessed by monitoring of vital signs, including orthostatic changes, assessment of skin turgor, temperature, appearance, and weight gain or loss.

Physical examination of the patient's abdomen should include palpation and percussion to evaluate tenderness, ascites, and organ enlargement.

The common laboratory tests to assess liver function are those that provide an evaluation of fat metabolism, protein metabolism, blood coagulation properties, bilirubin metabolism, and antigens and antibodies of hepatitis (Table 12-1). Radiographic studies commonly used to evaluate function of the liver, pancreas (Table 12-2), and spleen include ultrasound studies, computerized tomography (CT) scan, radioisotope scanning, nuclear magnetic resonance imaging (MRI), angiography, cholecystography, and cholangiography. An abdominal flatplate x-ray examination and upper gastrointestinal (GI) series may also aid in diagnosing gross anomalies of the liver, pancreas, and spleen.

Endoscopy and biopsy are more invasive diagnostic procedures that may be used in evaluation of the liver, pancreas, and spleen. Endoscopic retrograde cholangiopancreatography (ERCP) is a procedure that allows for direct visualization of the biliary tract, the injection of radiographic dye into the ductal system, and biopsy when indicated. Percutaneous transhepatic cholangiography (PTC) involves percutaneous insertion of a long flexible needle into a bile duct of the liver. Contrast medium is injected and serial x-ray examination is performed. Arteriography of the liver, biliary tree, pancreas, and spleen is accomplished by femoral arteriotomy and the placement

TABLE 12-1 | **Liver Function Studies**

TEST NAME	NORMAL VALUES
Serum Enzymes	
Alkaline phosphatase	13-39 U/ml
	Elevated levels are seen with biliary obstruction and cholestatic hepatitis.
Aspartate aminotransferase (AST; previously SGOT)	5-40 U/ml
	Elevated levels are seen with hepatocellular injury.
Alanine aminotransferase (ALT; previously SGPT)	5-35 U/ml
	Elevated levels are seen with liver dysfunction; the ratio of AST/ALT usually is more than 1 in alcoholic cirrhosis and liver congestion and less than 1 in acute hepatitis, viral hepatitis, and infectious mononucleosis.
Lactate dehydrogenase (LDH)	200-500 U/ml
	Elevated levels are seen with hepatitis and untreated pernicious anemia, as well as in several other conditions (such as acute myocardial infarction, renal disease, muscle disease, or malignant tumors).
5-Nucleotidase	2-11 U/ml
	Elevated levels may be an early indication of metastasis to the liver.
Leucine aminopeptidase (LAP)	*Men:* 80-200 U/ml; *women:* 75-185 U/ml
	Elevated levels may be seen with liver metastasis and choledocholithiasis.
Gamma-glutamyltranspeptidase (GGTP)	*Men:* 8-38 U/L; *women 45 yr:* 5-27 U/L
	Elevated levels are seen in 75% of chronic alcoholics.
Bilirubin Metabolism	
Serum bilirubin	
Indirect (unconjugated)	0.8 mg/dl
	Elevated levels are seen with hemolysis (lysis of RBCs).
Direct (conjugated)	0.2-0.4 mg/dl
	Elevated levels are seen with hepatocellular injury or obstruction.
Total	1 mg/dl
	Elevated levels may be seen with biliary obstruction.
Urine bilirubin	0
	Bilirubin in the urine may be seen with hepatic disease or biliary obstruction; only conjugated bilirubin spills into the urine because unconjugated bilirubin is bound to albumin in the serum and thus cannot pass the glomerular membrane.
Urine urobilinogen	0-4 mg/24 h
	Increased levels are seen with hemolytic processes, shunting of portal blood flow, or increased intestinal bacteria.
Fecal urobilinogen	40-280 mg/24 h
	Reduced levels cause clay-colored stools and are seen in biliary obstruction.
Ammonia	*Adult:* 15-110 mg/dl
	Elevated levels may be seen with liver dysfunction, hepatic failure, or congestive heart failure.
Serum Proteins	
Albumin	3.5-5.5 g/dl
	Reduced levels are seen with hepatocellular injury.
Globulin	2.5-3.5 g/dl
	Increased levels are seen with hepatitis.
Total	6-7 g/dl
	Decreased levels may be seen with hepatocellular injury.
Albumin/globulin (A/G) ratio	1.5/1 to 2.5/1
	Ratio may be reversed with chronic hepatitis or other chronic liver disease.
Transferrin	250-300 mg/dl
	Reduced levels may be seen with liver damage; increased levels may be seen with iron deficiency.
Blood-Clotting Functions	
Prothrombin time (PT)	11.5-14 sec or 90%-100% of control
	Increased levels may be seen with chronic liver disease (such as cirrhosis) or vitamin K deficiency.
Partial thromboplastin time (PTT)	25-40 sec
	Increased levels may be seen with severe liver disease or heparin therapy.

From Doughty, D.G., & Jackson, D.B. (1993). *Gastrointestinal disorders.* St. Louis: Mosby.

TABLE 12-2 | Tests of Pancreatic Function

TEST NAME	NORMAL VALUES
Serum amylase	60-180 Somogyi units/ml Elevated levels are seen with pancreatic inflammation.
Serum lipase	1.5 Somogyi units/ml Elevated levels may indicate pancreatic inflammation.
Urine amylase	35-260 Somogyi units/h Elevated levels are seen with pancreatic inflammation.
Secretin test	Volume 1.8 ml/kg/h HCO_3^- concentration >80 mEq/L HCO_3^- output >10 mEq/L/30 sec Reduced volumes are seen with pancreatic disease.

of a catheter into the celiac branch of the abdominal aorta under fluoroscopic visualization. Contrast medium is then injected and serial x-ray examination is performed as the vessels are visualized during the perfusion and drainage phases.

Nursing Diagnosis

After a thorough nursing assessment of all subjective and objective data related to the patient with dysfunction of the liver, biliary tract, pancreas, or spleen, nursing diagnoses are formulated. Nursing diagnoses related to the care of patients undergoing surgery of the liver, biliary tract, pancreas, or spleen might include the following:

- Anxiety related to impending surgical procedure and knowledge deficit
- Risk for fluid volume deficit related to hemorrhage or large-volume blood loss
- Risk for altered body temperature
- Risk for infection related to invasive GI procedure
- Risk for injury related to positioning and length of surgical procedure

Outcome Identification

Outcomes identified for the selected nursing diagnoses could be stated as follows:

- The patient will maintain a manageable level of anxiety as evidenced by the ability to communicate appropriately and to verbalize knowledge and understanding of the perioperative events.
- The patient will maintain fluid volume equilibrium throughout the operative procedure.
- The patient will demonstrate a consistent core body temperature of 96° to 99° F.
- The patient will demonstrate no clinical symptoms of wound infection.
- The patient will maintain neuromuscular function and tissue integrity normal for him or her.

Planning

Planning for the care of the patient having surgery of the liver, biliary tract, pancreas, or spleen requires assimilation of knowledge of the anatomy and subsequent physiologic complications that may occur with surgical interruption of tissues. Principles of proper positioning of the patient, maintenance of asepsis, prevention of biologic and electrical hazards, and providing proper instrumentation and equipment are a few constituents of the plan of care.

Assessment and patient interview will give insight as to the specific needs of the individual patient. The patient's past medical and surgical history as well as age, size, and nutritional status will assist the perioperative nurse in developing an effective plan of care. A Sample Care Plan for a patient undergoing surgery of the liver, biliary tract, pancreas, or spleen follows.

Implementation

Patients having surgery of the liver, biliary tract, pancreas, or spleen are usually given general anesthesia. The following pertinent factors are to be considered in caring for the patient undergoing biliary surgery.

Positioning the patient

The patient is placed in a supine position. A small positioning aid placed under the lower right side of the thorax may be requested by the surgeon. This elevates the lower rib cage to provide better exposure and access to the viscera in the right upper quadrant of the abdomen.

Positioning the patient for laparoscopic procedures requires the nurse to exercise caution when applying the safety strap or straps. Because of the potential for the patient to be placed in a severe side tilt or reverse Trendelenburg's position, the nurse must ensure the security of the safety strap placement. Attention is given to proper alignment of the patient's body and extremities. Areas of pressure and bony prominences are padded well to prevent interruption of circulation and pressure injury to tissues. This precaution is especially important with diabetic, circulatory impaired, and elderly patients. Close monitoring of the patient is essential during positional changes because of the decreased lighting in the room.

When an operative cholangiogram is anticipated, the operating room bed is prepared with an x-ray cassette holder before the patient is positioned. A preliminary x-ray film may be taken to ensure correct placement of the cassette. The holder must be directly beneath the patient's right upper quadrant because correct positioning is imperative to ensure accurate visualization of the biliary tract. The use of fluoroscopy for an operative cholangiogram is becoming more prevalent. If it is the technology of choice for the operative cholangiogram, the nurse must ensure that the OR bed has been equipped and positioned so that C-arm image intensification can be efficiently accomplished.

S A M P L E   C A R E   P L A N

Nursing Diagnosis: Anxiety related to impending surgical procedure and knowledge deficit

Outcome: Patient will maintain a manageable level of anxiety as evidenced by the ability to communicate appropriately and to verbalize knowledge and understanding of the perioperative events.

Interventions:

Complete as much of the setup as possible before the patient's arrival to the OR suite, especially those activities that create noise.

Greet the patient positively and professionally.

Introduce the patient to the OR team.

Avoid hasty movements or gestures of indecision.

Speak slowly and clearly when addressing the patient, and use terminology the patient can understand.

Offer emotional reassurance through touch, facial expression, and allowing the patient to talk about feelings.

Nursing Diagnosis: Risk for fluid volume deficit related to hemorrhage or large volume of blood loss

Outcome: Patient will maintain fluid volume equilibrium throughout surgical procedure.

Interventions:

Have available blood products in close-by, refrigerated storage for timely access.

Measure and record accurate fluid volume loss throughout surgical procedure.

Anticipate and communicate potential for fluid volume deficit to blood bank personnel.

Check lab values intraoperatively.

Nursing Diagnosis: Risk for altered body temperature

Outcome: Patient will demonstrate a consistent core body temperature of 96° to 99° F.

Interventions:

Adjust room temperature and humidity to accommodate preservation of body temperature.

Cover all possible body surfaces to maintain body heat.

Use only warm irrigation solutions.

Warm IV fluids and blood products before infusion.

Use forced warm-air system for supporting body temperature maintenance.

Nursing Diagnosis: Risk for infection related to invasive gastrointestinal procedure

Outcome: Patient will demonstrate no clinical symptoms of wound infection

Interventions:

Ensure that aseptic technique is maintained; communicate and correct breaks in asepsis.

Ensure that preoperative antibiotics are administered as ordered.

Contain contaminants appropriately.

Ensure that all sterilization procedures have been properly observed.

Ensure that the integrity of sterile supply packaging is intact before dispensing items to the sterile field.

Nursing Diagnosis: Risk for injury related to positioning and length of surgical procedure

Outcome: Patient will maintain neuromuscular function and tissue integrity normal to the individual.

Interventions:

Ensure patient is in optimal anatomic alignment after induction of anesthesia.

Adequately pad all bony prominences.

Secure limbs with nonflexible safety strap to ensure position is maintained and to prevent limb from falling from positioning device.

Ensure safe and proper placement of electrosurgical dispersive pad.

Ensure that no weight or stress is placed on body parts and structures.

Ensure padding is in place beneath all self-retaining retractors.

Thermoregulation of the patient

When laparotomy is performed, a patient is at risk for hypothermia. The perioperative nurse ensures that measures are taken to maintain body temperature in the operating room. The environmental temperature and humidity are set to prevent body heat loss caused by evaporation and convection. A forced-air warming blanket placed over the patient's upper body, head, and neck will assist in maintenance of body temperature. Minimizing body exposure to ambient air and the use of warm prep and irrigating solutions also supports thermoregulation for the patient. A blood and fluid warming device may be utilized by the anesthesia care provider to deliver intravenous fluids at a temperature greater than room air.

The patient entering the operating room will usually welcome a warm blanket before and after surgery.

The patient's core temperature is commonly monitored by the anesthesia care provider by use of an esophageal temperature probe or indwelling urinary catheter with probe when the duration and complexity of the surgical procedure places the patient at risk for hypothermia. Temperature dots are a means utilized in some operating rooms for monitoring peripheral body temperature in a noninvasive manner.

Application of sequential compression leggings

Patients undergoing laparotomy under general anesthesia may be at risk for venous dilation and blood pooling in

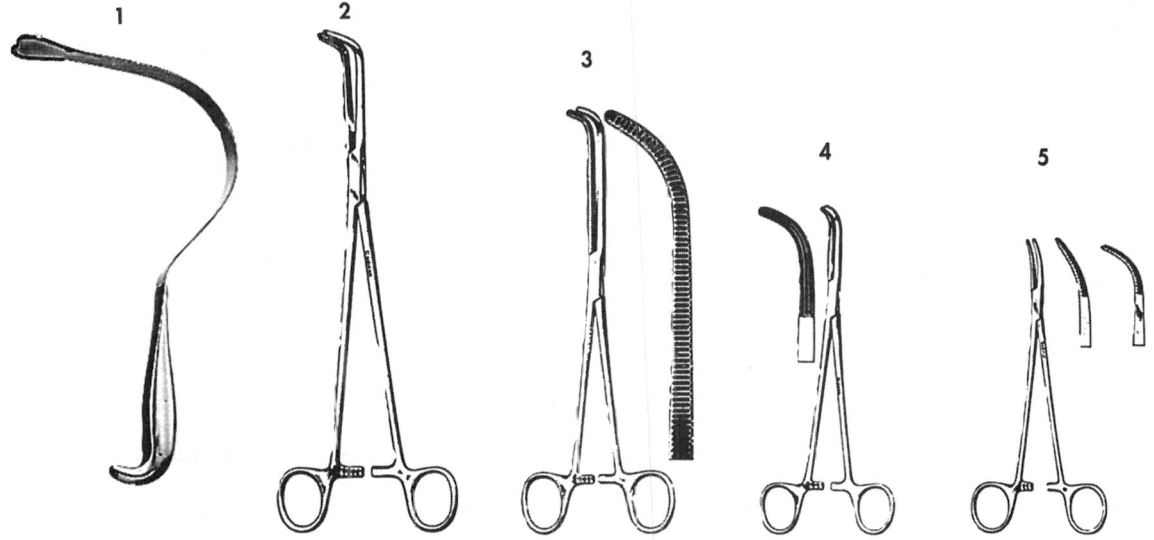

FIGURE 12-7 Clamping and exposing instruments for gallbladder surgery. *1*, Harrington retractor; *2*, Mixter (right-angled) gallbladder forceps; *3*, Johns Hopkins gallbladder forceps; *4*, Lahey gall duct forceps; *5*, Schnidt gall duct forceps.

the lower extremities. This may predispose the surgical patient for deep venous thrombosis in the postoperative period. The surgeon may order the patient to have sequential compression leggings applied in the operating room before induction of general anesthesia and commencing of the surgical procedure. It remains controversial as to which type is best. Both thigh-high and knee-high leggings are available on the market. Use of sequential compression leggings on the lower extremities will usually be discontinued in the postoperative recovery period when the patient resumes active ambulation.

Draping the patient

After the abdominal prep, sterile towels are arranged to accommodate the intended incision. A sterile drape sheet may be applied over the patient's lower torso, and a laparotomy sheet is then placed to provide a wide sterile field and cover all exposed body surfaces except the incisional site.

Instrumentation

Instrumentation for surgeries of the liver, biliary tract, spleen, and pancreas, if performed through a laparotomy incision, would include a basic laparotomy set, biliary probes and forceps for dilating and exploring the ducts of the pancreas and biliary tract (Figs. 12-7 to 12-9), vascular clamps, GI clamps, ligating clips of all sizes with appliers, and linear stapling instruments should be available. A self-retaining system such as the Bookwalter Retractor set (Fig. 12-10) could enhance exposure for the surgeon and allows optimal safe retraction of tissues and excellent exposure of the abdominal viscera. In addition, a flexible choledochoscope, Cavitron Ultrasound Suction Aspirator (CUSA), intraoperative ultrasound, laser, argon beam coagulator, harmonic scalpel, and an electrosurgical unit

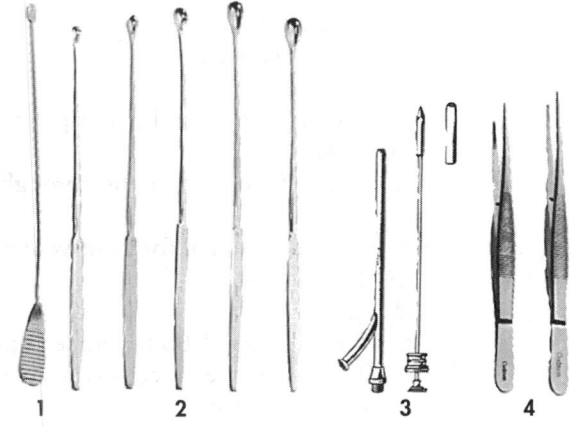

FIGURE 12-8 Duct instruments. *1*, Mayor common duct scoop; *2*, gall duct spoons; *3*, Ochsner gallbladder trocar; *4*, Potts-Smith tissue forceps.

may be required to perform certain procedures on the hepatobiliary system.

Thrombin, Gelfoam, Surgicel, Avitene, and other hemostatic agents should be available in the operating room suite. Radiographic dye and supplies for intraoperative radiography or angiography may also be required.

Drainage materials

Tubes and catheters must be in optimal condition and suitable for the areas to be drained. If a defective drain is used, a free fragment may remain in the wound on removal of the tube.

The scrub nurse should note the condition of all drainage materials and should test them for patency before they are placed into the patient.

Soft rubber or latex tissue drains may be used after a cholecystectomy or a choledochostomy. A latex rubber

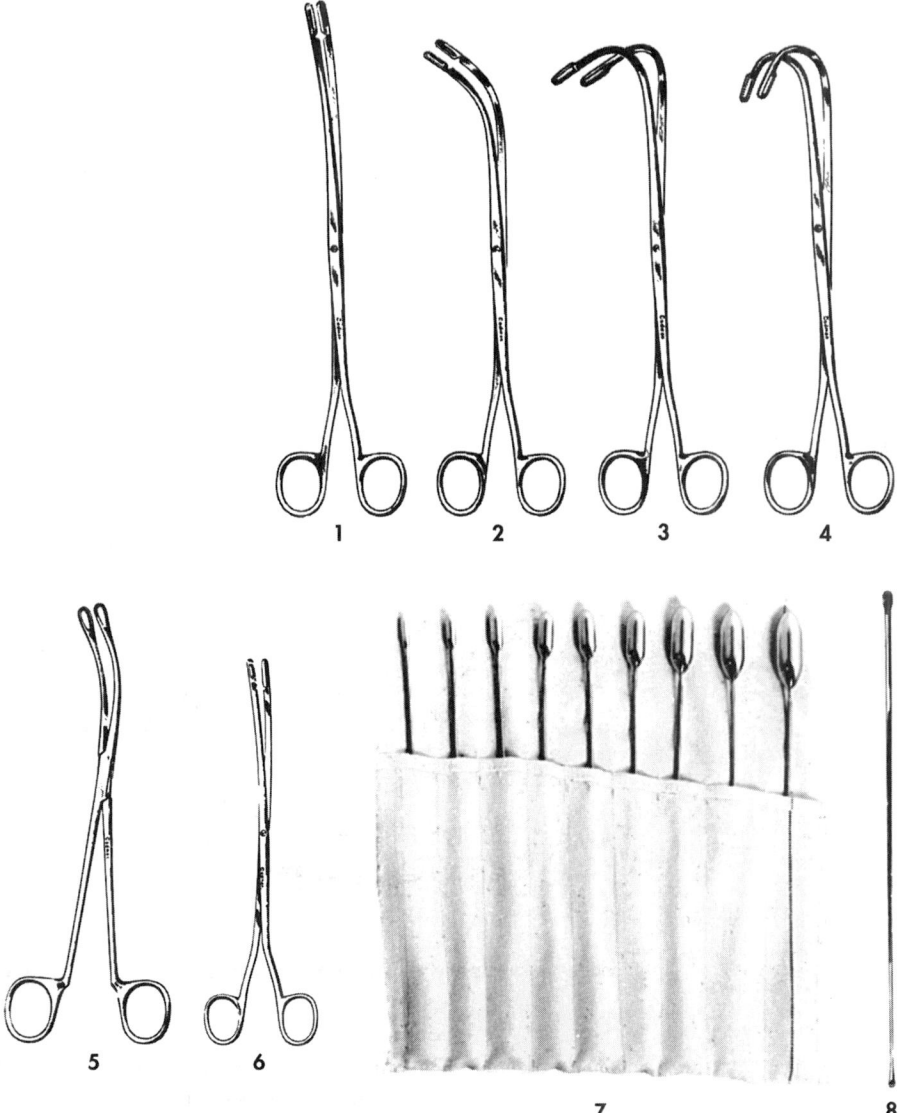

FIGURE 12-9   Stone instruments. *1* to *4*, Randall kidney stone forceps (four shapes); *5*, Blake gallstone forceps; *6*, Desjardin gallstone forceps; *7*, Bakes common duct dilators; *8*, Moynihan gall duct probe and scoop.

T-tube drain of suitable size is prepared by the surgeon after the duct has been explored. The center of the crossbar is notched opposite the junction of the vertical limb so that its ends will bend more readily during removal. The ends are beveled and tailored to fit the duct.

Drains are usually exteriorized through separate stab wounds and anchored to skin edges to prevent their retraction. The perioperative nurse should document the types of drains and reservoirs inserted during the operative procedure and identify them with an applied label. All drains and their locations should be included in the perioperative nurse's report to the nursing unit to which the patient is transferred postoperatively.

Aseptic considerations

When the common duct is opened or an anastomosis is established between a duct and other parts of the tract, it may be the institution's policy or the surgeon's preference to isolate contaminated instruments and materials from the remainder of the operative field, as described for GI surgery. Instruments and materials used for the exteriorization of a drain should be treated as contaminated.

Blood products

The perioperative nurse should be aware of the type and amount of blood products available for the patient having surgery of the liver, biliary tract, pancreas, or spleen. Constant evaluation of blood loss is communicated to the anesthesia and surgical team as well as to the blood bank personnel so that blood products are readily available.

Autologous blood or donor-directed blood products may be used in elective procedures involving the liver, pancreas, spleen, and biliary tract. Cell-saver devices may

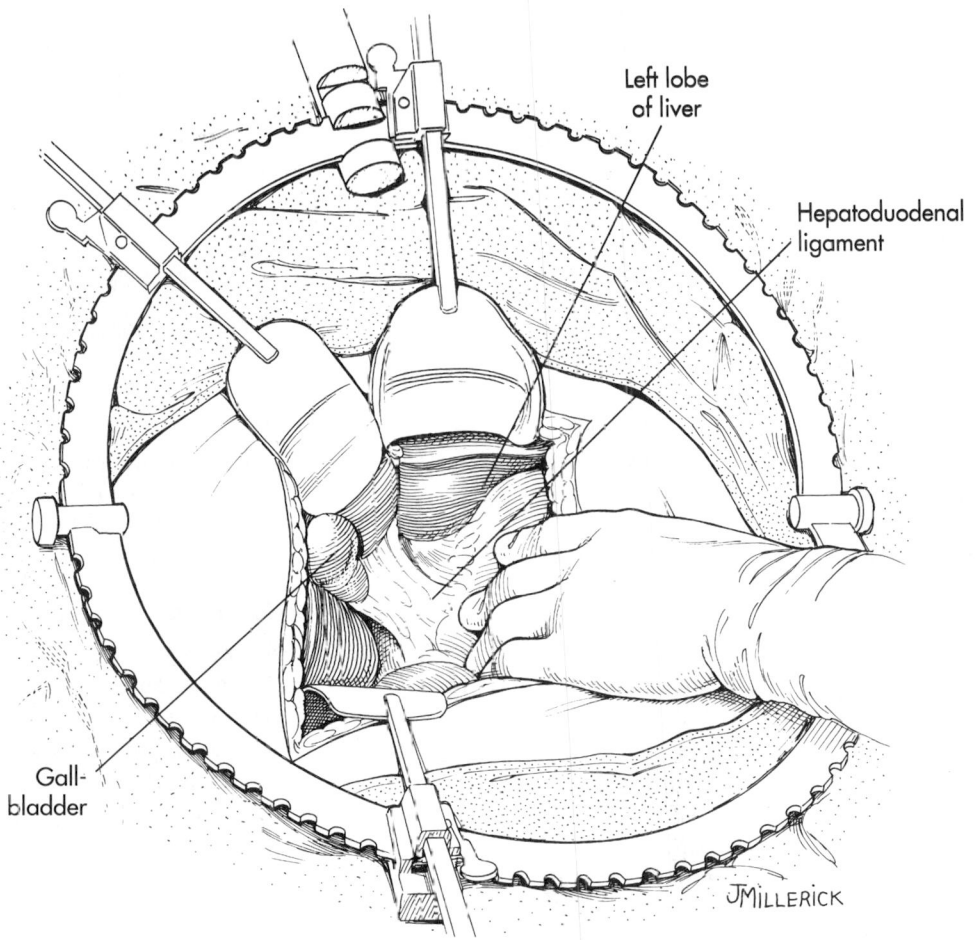

FIGURE 12-10   Bookwalter self-retaining retractor in place to provide optimal exposure to the abdominal viscera.

be used when the potential for contamination of the blood from bile or bowel does not exist.

Evaluation

Evaluation of the patient after surgery includes examination of all skin surfaces and comparison to the preoperative assessment data. Abdominal drains, chest drainage systems, urinary drainage systems, and peripheral infusion lines are assessed for patency and labeled appropriately. Fluid volume use and loss are documented and communicated appropriately. A thorough report of the patient's history, preoperative assessment, intraoperative events, and postoperative evaluation is communicated to the PACU or SICU nurse.

The evaluation of patient status can be phrased as outcome statements such as the following:

- The patient expressed a positive recollection of perioperative events upon postoperative visit.
- The patient's hematocrit is in the 30% to 35% range; vital signs are stable.
- The patient's core body temperature remained consistently in the 96° to 99° F range.

- The patient's surgical incision is dry and intact. There are no clinical signs of infection.
- All skin surfaces are clear, intact, and free from stress markings; capillary filling is noted after blanching of tissues. The patient demonstrates normal range of motion in extremities. Pulses are palpable in all distal extremities.

Patient and Family Education and Discharge Planning

Patients undergoing surgical intervention for disorders of the liver, pancreas, spleen, or biliary tract will vary greatly in the length of time and complexity of recovery. Laparoscopic cholecystectomy may be performed on an outpatient basis with extended recovery and observation of 6 to 8 hours. In contrast, patients undergoing liver transplantation or resection may require extensive recovery that includes a stay in the surgical intensive care unit.

Patients undergoing laparotomy for surgical intervention of the liver, pancreas, spleen, or biliary tract may have varying degrees of postoperative edema, decreased GI peristalsis, and alterations in tissue oxygenation and lymphatic drainage depending on the amount of manipulation, resection, and trauma to the normal anatomic structures of these viscera. General anesthesia is commonly administered to the patient undergoing surgical intervention for disorders of the liver, pancreas, spleen, or biliary tract. Smooth muscle relaxation is imperative for most major abdominal viscera interventions. The patient will usually experience decreased peristalsis for 2 to 5 days after laparotomy. A nasogastric tube or gastrostomy tube is inserted during the surgical event to evacuate the large volumes of gastric juices. Diet is introduced only after bowel sounds return. The patient may experience nausea and vomiting if food or drink is introduced too early for the GI system to function with normal absorption and motility.

Coughing and deep breathing is important for the patient recovering from general anesthesia and abdominal surgery. Splinting of the abdominal muscles and the use of an incentive spirometer will assist the patient in postoperative coughing and deep breathing initiatives. Early ambulation will assist the patient in regaining overall muscle tone and preventing deep venous thrombosis in the lower extremities.

Pain management is a very important factor in the patient's recovery and discharge planning. For most patients undergoing abdominal surgery, Patient-controlled analgesia (PCA) or epidural analgesia may be utilized for better and more consistent control of pain and discomfort in the first 1 to 3 postoperative days of hospital recovery. Narcotics may, however, add to the length of time at which normal bowel peristalsis returns and so are monitored closely after the third postoperative day.

General discharge instructions for the patient undergoing surgery for disorders of the liver, pancreas, spleen, or biliary tract may include the following:

- Keep incisional area clean and dry.
- Swelling inside the GI tract may produce a feeling of tightness; this should dissipate in 6 to 8 weeks.
- Solid foods should be added to the diet gradually. Chew solid foods well and avoid gulping or eating fast or swallowing large bulky portions.
- Avoid carbonated beverages for 3 to 4 weeks to help prevent gas bloating.
- Plan small frequent meals because the feeling of fullness will come quickly.
- Increase exercise gradually to return to activities of daily living. Exercise regularly.
- Make an appointment for follow-up care with the surgeon.
- Have written instructions with phone numbers as to whom to call and when. The patient should call the doctor if any of the following develop:
  - Persistent fever (101° F or higher)
  - Bleeding

- Increased abdominal swelling or pain
- Chills
- Persistent cough or shortness of breath

Procedure-specific instructions may be necessary to fully assist the patient and his or her caregivers with recovery and rehabilitation outside of the hospital setting.

SURGICAL INTERVENTIONS SURGERY OF THE BILIARY TRACT
Cholecystectomy

Cholecystectomy is removal of the gallbladder. It is performed for the treatment of diseases such as acute or chronic inflammation (cholecystitis), stones (cholelithiasis), or the presence of polyps or carcinoma.

Procedural considerations

A basic laparotomy set and biliary instruments are utilized when cholecystectomy is performed through an open abdominal incision. The patient is positioned supine and usually receives general anesthesia. After intubation, a nasogastric tube is inserted by the anesthesiologist. Antibiotic prophylaxis may be ordered to be administered in the immediate preoperative period (Research Highlight 12-1).

Operative procedure (Fig. 12–11)

1. Through a right subcostal, right paramedian, or midline incision the abdominal cavity is opened.
2. Hemostasis of capillary vessels is achieved with electrocoagulation. Larger vessels are clamped with hemostats and tied with suture material.
3. Retractors and laparotomy packs are employed as the abdominal cavity is carefully examined.
4. The common duct is palpated for evidence of stones, and the pathologic conditions are determined.
5. Harrington, Deaver, or automatic retractors such as an upper-hand or Gomez retractor are placed to provide exposure. Long tissue forceps, and suction are used to manipulate tissues. The surrounding organs are walled off from the gallbladder region by laparotomy packs and deep retractors.
6. To facilitate gentle traction, Pean forceps are usually placed on the body of the gallbladder (Fig. 12-11, *A*).
7. The peritoneal fold overlying the junction of the cystic and common duct is incised with a #7 knife handle and a #15 blade, long Metzenbaum scissors, and forceps. Suction is available, and bleeding points are clamped and ligated or electrocoagulated.
8. Adhesions are separated by blunt dissection with small, round, dry dissector sponges, sponges on holders, and blunt right-angled clamps.

12-1 RESEARCH HIGHLIGHT

Cholecystectomy for chronic calculus cholecystitis by either laparoscopic or open technique is the only clinical implication for antibiotic prophylaxis in surgery of the biliary tract. Operations for acute cholecystitis, empyema of the gallbladder, ascending cholangitis, or liver abscess require treatment with antibiotics rather than prophylaxis. The healthy biliary tract rarely harbors significant concentrations of bacteria. Aerobic gram-negative bacilli such as *Escherichia coli* are the most common bacterial inhabitant cultured from the biliary tract. Positive cultures collected at the time of cholecystectomy are an indicator of potential for high risk for infection postoperatively.

Controlled studies have demonstrated decreased post-operative infection rates when antibiotic prophylaxis is administered to patients with one or more clinical risk factors. Cephalosporin is the most commonly used broad-spectrum antibiotic for prophylaxis.

The primary controversy is whether to administer prophylaxis to all patients undergoing cholecystectomy or only to those who have clinical risk factors. Studies have been inconclusive. A concentrated effort to study antibiotic prophylaxis including the timing of initial administration, appropriate choice of agents, and clinical risk factors is suggested. At this time it appears that a single-dose systemic regimen of an appropriately chosen cephalosporin given during the immediate preoperative period is the safe and indicated practice.

From Nichols, R.L. (1996). Update: antibiotic prophylaxis in surgery, *Infectious Diseases in Clinical Practice, 5*(2), S77-S84.

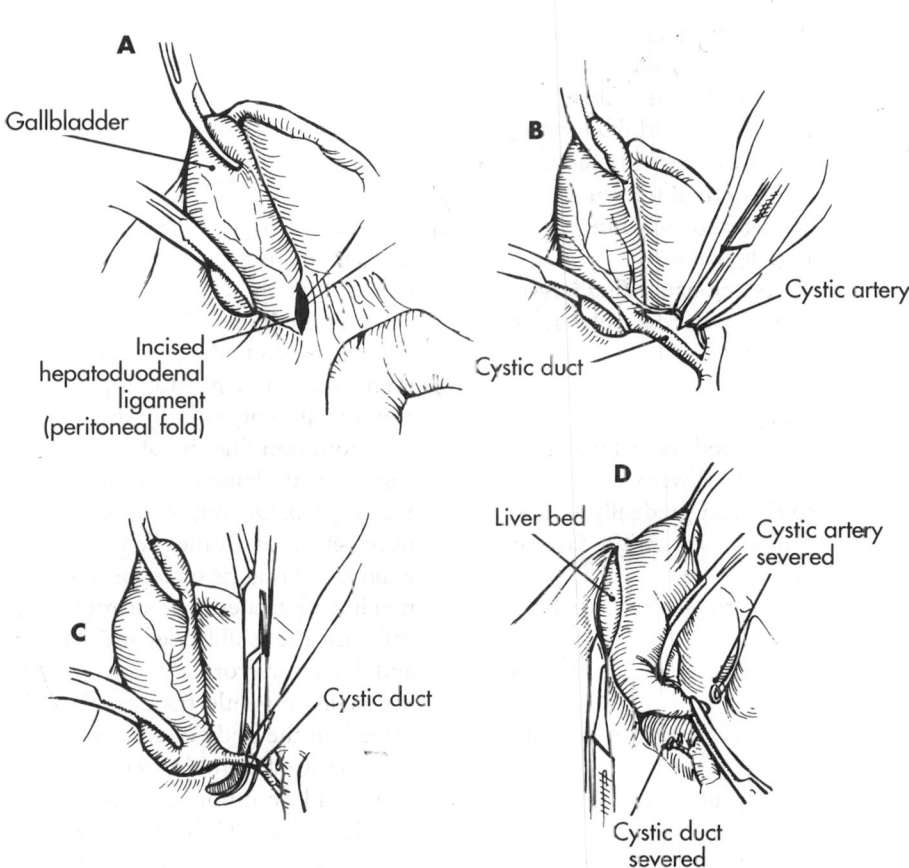

FIGURE 12-11   Cholecystectomy. **A,** With Pean forceps in place, gentle traction is maintained as peritoneum over Calot's triangle is incised. **B,** Cystic artery is clearly visualized, doubly ligated, and divided. **C,** Cystic duct is carefully dissected and identified before forceps and ligatures are applied **D,** Dissection of gallbladder from liver bed is completed.

9. Dissection is continued to expose the neck of the gallbladder, the cystic artery, and the cystic duct (Fig. 12-11, *B* and *C*).

10. Dissection is continued to expose the cystic artery as it enters the wall of the gallbladder.

11. On complete exposure and visualization of the branches, the cystic artery is doubly ligated with silk or clamped with ligating clips and divided (Fig. 12-11, *B*).

12. Occasionally a third ligature or clip may be used. If the cystic artery has more than one branch, each is ligated and divided separately.

13. Abnormalities of the arterial and ductal anatomy are common (Fig. 12-12), and the surgeon works with meticulous care to identify these structures.

14. The true junction of the cystic duct with the common bile duct is visualized.

15. The cystic duct is identified and carefully dissected down to its junction with the hepatic duct.

16. Any stones in the cystic duct are milked back into the gallbladder, and a tie is placed around the proximal part of the cystic duct.

17. If necessary, a cholangiogram is performed at this time (see procedure for intraoperative cholangiogram). If a cholangiogram is not done, the cystic duct is doubly ligated and divided (Fig. 12-11, *C*). A transfixion suture of fine absorbable suture may be used on the stump of the cystic duct near the common bile duct.

18. Free gallbladder from the liver, working upward to the fundus, and remove it (Fig. 12-11, *D*).

19. In some cases working from the fundus downward to the neck of the gallbladder may be necessary.

20. All bleeding is controlled; reperitonealization of the liver bed, if indicated, is accomplished with interrupted or continuous fine, absorbable intestinal sutures.

21. A drain may be inserted near the cystic duct stump. The free end of the drain is exteriorized through a stab wound in the lateral abdominal wall.

22. The wound is closed in layers and a dressing applied.

Intraoperative Cholangiogram

An intraoperative cholangiogram is usually performed with cholecystectomy to visualize the common bile duct and the hepatic ductal branches and to assess patency of the common bile duct.

Procedural considerations

An intraoperative cholangiogram requires the use of an x-ray machine. The OR bed should be prepared with radiographic attachments that permit easy insertion of the x-ray film cassette beneath the patient. If the surgeon prefers fluoroscopy to visualize the filling of the ducts, the OR bed is prepared before the patient's arrival in the OR suite with an image-intensification attachment.

The perioperative nurse should ensure that the patient has not had previous allergic reactions to the x-ray medium before dispensing the pharmaceutical agent to the sterile field.

Protection such as x-ray aprons or leaded shields should be readily available for all members of the surgical team. Because the patient's abdomen remains open while the x-ray equipment is positioned directly over the operative site, appropriate draping to maintain asepsis is necessary.

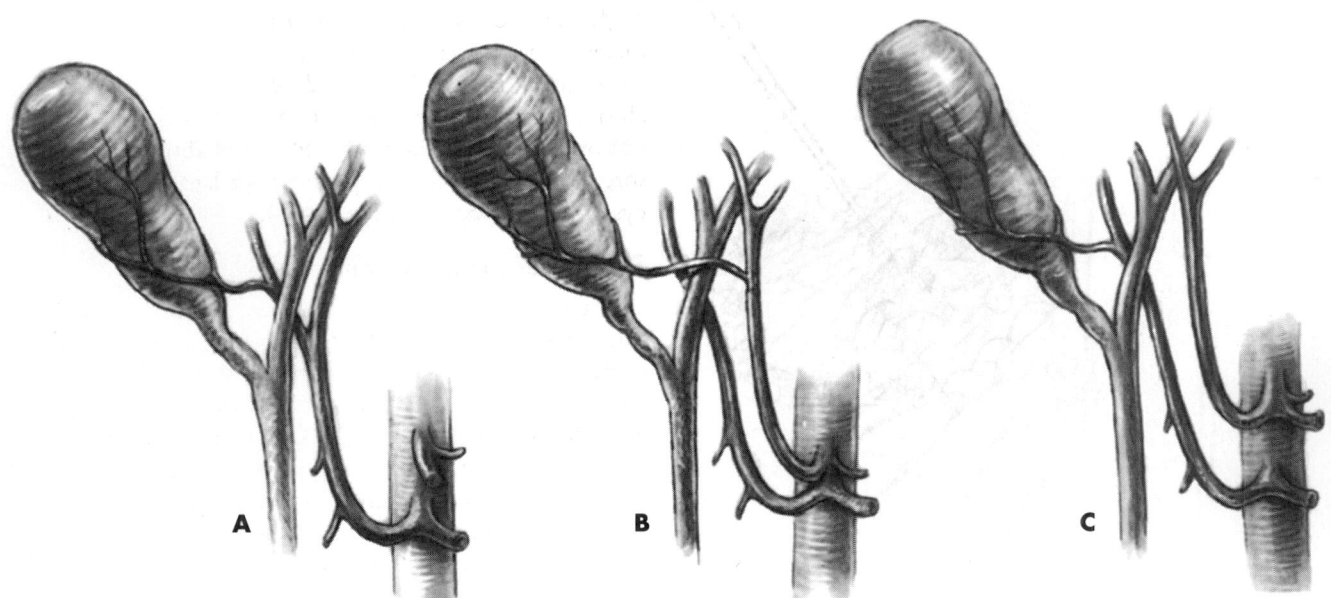

FIGURE 12-12   Arterial blood supply of the liver and biliary system is quite variable. **A**, The most common anatomic arrangement is a cystic artery arising from the right hepatic artery. **B**, A dual hepatic blood supply is found in 15% to 20% of patients, with the right hepatic artery arising from the superior mesenteric artery in a significant number, as in **C**.

Radiopaque sponges and any unnecessary instrumentation are removed from the abdominal site to avoid obscuring the view of the contrast medium filling the ducts.

The scrub nurse prepares a cholangiocath by attaching a stopcock with a 20 ml syringe of saline and a 20 ml syringe of contrast medium to the Luer-Lok ports. All air bubbles are removed because they might be misinterpreted as gall duct stones on the x-ray film.

Operative procedure

1. The cholangiocath is irrigated with saline before and during the insertion of the catheter into the cystic and common bile ducts (Fig. 12-13).
2. The cholangiocath is inserted into the duct using a traumatic grasping forceps. Irrigation during insertion facilitates dilatation and reduces trauma to the ductal lumen.
3. The cholangiocath is anchored in the lumen of the common bile duct by the surgeon's preferred method. The more common methods are applying a ligaclip proximal to the insertion site, tying or suturing the catheter in place, or using a ring-jawed holding clamp, such as a Swenson clamp, that has been designed specifically for this purpose.
4. With placement of the cholangiocath confirmed and anchored, the surgeon informs the surgical team that x-ray examination is now required.
5. All radiopaque sponges, instruments, and obstructing equipment are removed from the field.

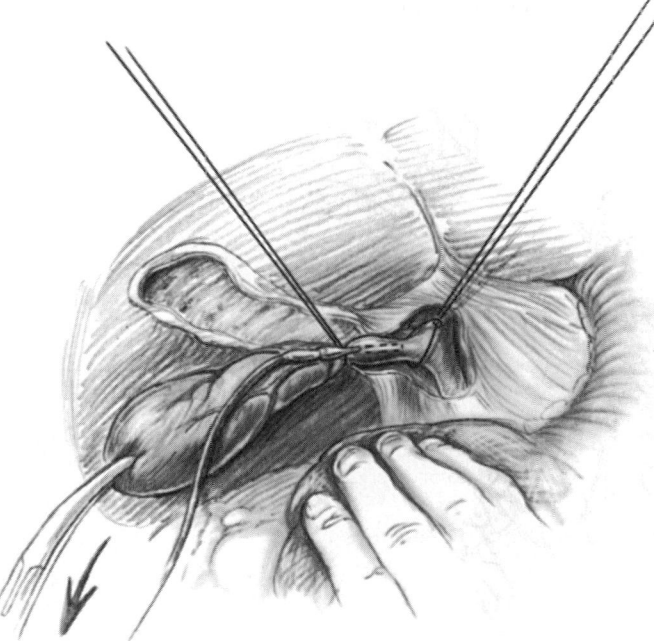

FIGURE 12-13 Cholangiocath inserted into the cystic duct through a small opening proximal to a silk tie placed at the cystic duct–gallbladder junction. The gallbladder has been dissected from the liver bed, and the cystic duct is dissected down to its junction with the hepatic duct.

6. The surgical field is draped with a sterile drape sheet to maintain asepsis of the wound and field. The x-ray equipment is positioned, as the surgeon redirects the stopcock to allow for injection of the contrast medium.
7. The surgeon directs the radiology technician as to the precise time to perform the x-ray examination.
8. The x-ray equipment is removed from the operative site, and the drapes covering the incisional site are carefully removed and discarded. The x-ray film is developed immediately to ensure that appropriate visualization of the ductal structures has been achieved. Once the surgeon studies the x-ray film hung on the x-ray view box in the OR, the decision is made to repeat the intraoperative cholangiogram, to explore the common bile duct, or to proceed with the conclusion of the patient's surgery.

Laparoscopic Cholecystectomy

Laparoscope-guided cholecystectomy using electrodissection for detachment of the gallbladder from the liver bed has gained popularity as the surgical treatment of choice in patients with gallbladder disease who meet the appropriate criteria for safe laparoscopic intervention. The preoperative evaluation of patients having laparoscopic cholecystectomy differs little from that for patients scheduled for laparotomy. An abdominal ultrasonogram may be performed to document the presence or absence of gallstones as well as intrahepatic or extrahepatic bile duct dilatation, which may suggest intraductal stones. If stones are not present and the patient does not have a history of pancreatitis or jaundice, the patient becomes a candidate for the laparoscope-guided procedure. For patients with a history of peptic ulcer disease, a flexible esophagogastroduodenoscopy may be performed to rule out existing disease. In patients with suspected ductal stones, a preliminary ERCP is advised. A laparoscopic procedure always has the potential to be converted to a laparotomy, an option the patient should be informed about before their surgical event. A clinical pathway for laparoscopic cholecystectomy is shown in Fig. 12-14.

Procedural considerations

Patients are generally admitted to the ambulatory surgery unit of a hospital facility or outpatient surgery center on the morning of surgery and will commonly require less than a 24-hour stay or admission to an extended recovery unit (ERU). General anesthesia is commonly utilized; however, a combination of regional and local anesthetics with IV sedation may be requested. Antibiotic prophylaxis may be ordered to be administered in the immediate preoperative period (Research Highlight 12-1).

The following instrumentation, supplies, and equipment are required for laparoscopic cholecystectomy: laparoscope, three 5 mm trocars and sheaths or two 5 mm trocars and sheaths and one 7 mm trocar and sheath, two

1. Focus of clinical path: Laparoscopic cholecystectomy
2. Timeline: Preoperative: 120 minutes   Intraoperative: 60-90 minutes   Postoperative: 2-23 hours

3. Patient Care Problems	4. INTERVENTIONS	Preoperative:	Intraoperative:	Postoperative:
A. Knowledge deficit		• Reinforce patient/family teaching; use materials/booklet PRN • Review clinical pathway • Discuss informed consent • Reinforce Patient Bill of Rights	• Reinforce knowledge; explain new events in OR • Answer questions • Provide emotional support	• Reinforce and provide details of postop care • Answer questions • Provide emotional support • Reinforce discharge teaching: diet, activity, medications, wound care, and follow-up
B. Risk for injury		• Confirm patient ID • Confirm NPO status • Nursing assessment for risk factors • Allergies documented • Check equipment and supplies in OR	• Assist with induction • Supine position • Prepare incision site • Monitor CO_2 insufflation/expulsion • Antibiotic irrigation • Heparin irrigation • Insert NG • Urinary catheter PRN • Place electrodispersive pad	• Safe transfer of patient to PACU • Postop assessment • DC, NG, and urinary catheter • PACU discharge criteria met
C. Risk for altered physiologic function		• H&P, preop lab, ECG, x-rays complete (as needed) and documented • Nursing assessment documented	• Physiologic monitoring • Warm IV/irrigation fluids • DVT prophylaxis	• Physiologic monitoring • OOB to chair with assistance • Progress ambulation • Ice chips/liquids; advance as tolerated • VS q 15 min × 2 hrs, then q 4 hrs • Turn, cough, deep breathing
D. Pain		• Pain assessment and intervention as needed (biliary colic) • Patient/family teaching regarding postop pain (shoulder and incisions) and control options	• Provide comfort/privacy measures • Local anesthetic agent at incision sites	• Provide comfort/privacy measures • Pain assessment and intervention • Reinforce preop teaching regarding types of pain and home pain management options

5. EXPECTED OUTCOMES

Immediate:
A. The patient verbalizes understanding of procedures and sequence of events.
B. The patient is free of electrical, chemical, or mechanical injury.
C. The patient is free of significant alterations in physiologic functioning.
D. The patient has adequate pain control.

Discharge:
A. Patient/family understands postop care of incisions, activity level, and time and location of clinic follow-up.
B. The patient remains free of injury.
C. Vital signs within normal limits; free of nausea; able to perform ADL with little assistance.
D. Adequate pain control; understands use of home pain medicines; understands activity limits.

6. VARIANCES

For concurrent intervention:
A. Knowledge deficit: Consent signed/correct; patient/family perception of adequacy of preop/postop teaching.
B. Injury: Skin integrity; neuromotor integrity; oral/pharyngeal/dental integrity; visceral integrity.
C. Presence of assessment data on chart at time of surgery (e.g., H&P, preop lab, ECG, x-rays, nursing assessment); significant changes in physiologic function; DVT; significant VS changes associated with pneumoperitoneum; significant VS changes associated with reverse Trendelenburg's position.
D. Adequacy of pain control; adequacy of teaching regarding use of home pain meds.

For retrospective analysis:
A. Knowledge deficit: Patient/family perception of adequacy of preop/postop teaching within 3-6 weeks after surgery.
B. Injury: Neuromotor integrity within first postop week.
C. DVT within 24-48 hours postoperative.
D. Adequacy of pain control 24-72 hours postop; adequacy of teaching regarding use of home pain meds within 3-6 weeks of surgery.

FIGURE 12–14 Clinical pathway for laparoscopic cholecystectomy.

10 or 11 mm trocars and sheaths to adapt sheath size to instrument size, a #7 knife handle with a #11 blade, multiple clip appliers, blunt grasping forceps (an assortment of alligator, Babcock, and spatula), and laparoscopic scissors. A laparoscopic video unit and secondary "slave" monitor, laparoscopic camera and control unit, light source, CO_2 tank and insufflation unit, electrosurgical unit, filtered insufflation tubing (disposable), electrocautery or electrocautery suction-irrigator (disposable), and a pressure bag for IV saline 0.9% are items commonly used by the surgeon. Laparotomy instrumentation and supplies should be readily available in the operating room if needed.

The patient is positioned supine with the usual comfort and safety measures observed. The surgeon may prefer to have a Foley catheter or red Robinson catheter inserted into the urinary bladder through the urethra for bladder decompression. A nasogastric tube is inserted for decompression of the stomach. The patient is then placed in a reverse Trendelenburg's position of 10 to 20 degrees.

Open laparoscopy, sometimes termed the *Hasson technique*, which is the surgical opening into the peritoneum and placement of the operative sleeve to which the insufflation tubing is then attached and pneumoperitoneum is achieved. This technique is suggested in patients who have had a prior abdominal incision near the umbilicus or those having potential for intraperitoneal adhesions. The Hasson technique may also involve the use of sutures placed on either side of the sleeve to anchor and hold the sleeve in place. CO_2 is commonly the gas of choice for pneumoperitoneum. Gas flow is initiated at 1 to 2 L/min. Because CO_2 diffuses into the patient's bloodstream during laparoscopy, elevated CO_2 levels and respiratory acidosis may occur. The intraabdominal pressure is normally in the 8 to 10 mm Hg range and is commonly used as an indicator for proper Verres needle placement by the surgeon. If the pressure gauge indicates a higher pressure, the needle may be in a closed space such as fat, buried in the omentum, or be in the lumen of the intestine. The perioperative nurse should set the insufflation unit to a maximum pressure of 15 mm Hg. When intraabdominal pressure reaches 15 mm Hg, the flow will stop. Pressure higher than 15 mm Hg may result in bradycardia or a change in blood pressure or may force a gas embolus into an exposed blood vessel during the operative procedure. Most insufflation units are equipped with an alarm mechanism to alert the operative team if the intraabdominal pressure is exceeded. The surgeon may frequently ask what the pressure reading is, as the anesthesiologist might.

Operative procedure

1. A small skin incision is made in the folds of the umbilicus with a #11 blade on a #7 knife handle.
2. Pneumoperitoneum is accomplished by two options: A Verres needle is placed percutaneously through the umbilicus into the peritoneal cavity, and insufflation is performed with CO_2 gas before the introduction of the trocar. When 3 to 4 liters of gas have been infused and the abdomen is rounded, the insufflation needle is removed, and the trocar is inserted. The second technique requires the surgeon to grasp the abdominal flesh and pull upward as the trocar and sheath are placed through the umbilicus at an angle so as to avoid visceral puncture. The insufflation tubing is then attached to the port on the sleeve and insufflation commences as in the Hasson technique.
3. The skin incision is extended using the #11 blade so that a 10 or 11 mm trocar and sheath can be inserted.
4. The surgeon grasps the abdominal skin cephalad to the trocar and sheath and in a firm motion inserts the sharp trocar point slightly angled toward the pelvis. The trocar is removed, leaving the sheath in place.
5. The laparoscope is then placed through the sheath, and the camera is attached to view and explore the peritoneal cavity on the video screen.
6. The surgeon usually stands on the left side of the patient while the first assistant stands on the right. Video monitors are positioned at eye level at both the right and left sides of the operative field.
7. The patient is then placed in a 30-degree, reverse Trendelenburg's position and tilted slightly to the left.
8. Three additional skin incisions are made for the insertion and placement of the operative sheaths (Fig. 12-15).
9. The trocar and sheaths are inserted into the peritoneal cavity under the direct visualization of the laparoscopic view.
10. Two sheaths are usually 5 mm and one is 10 mm to accommodate the accessory instrumentation. A fifth trocar and sheath may be needed to accomplish grasping or retracting during the procedure.
11. Blunt grasping forceps are inserted through the 5 mm sheaths.
12. The gallbladder is manipulated with one pair of forceps while the porta hepatis is exposed with the other.
13. Using the midline sheath, the surgeon dissects the cystic duct and artery with blunt forceps beginning at the gallbladder and proceeding toward the cystic and common bile duct junction. (Fig. 12-16, *A*).
14. The cystic artery and the cystic duct are dissected free from the surrounding tissues (Fig. 12-16, *B*).
15. Two clips are applied proximally and distally to the intended line of division on both the duct and artery (Fig. 12-16, *C*). The use of a disposable, preloaded multiple clip applier assists in the placement of ligating clips in a more efficient manner than a singly loaded reusable applier. A pretied suture loop may be used if the surgeon desires.
16. The cystic duct and artery are divided. Attention is then given to dissection of the gallbladder from the

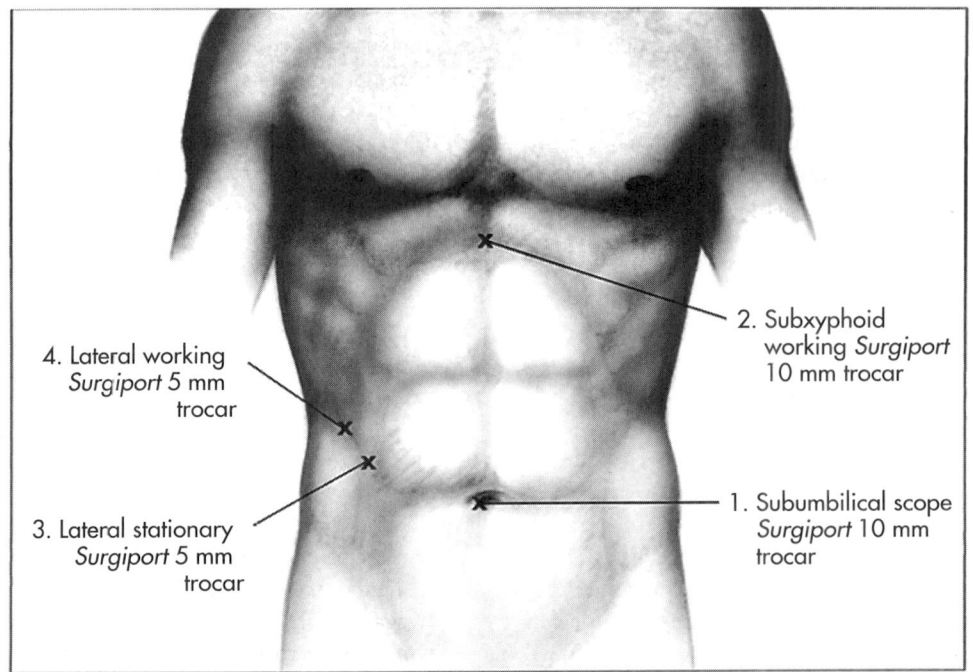

FIGURE 12-15   Trocar placement for laparoscopic cholecystectomy demonstrating anatomic placement and the usual size of trocar used at each site.

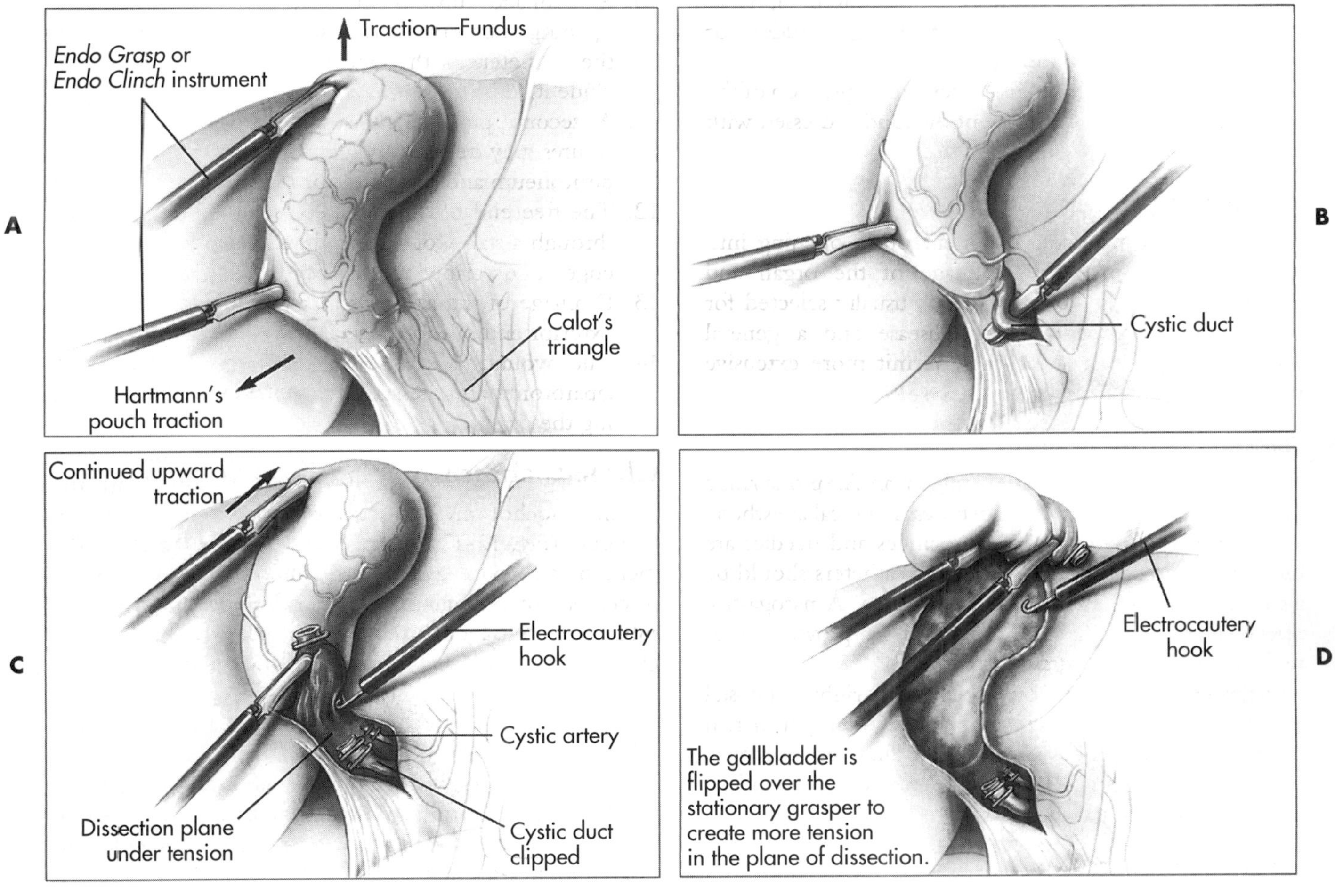

2. Subxyphoid working *Surgiport* 10 mm trocar

4. Lateral working *Surgiport* 5 mm trocar

3. Lateral stationary *Surgiport* 5 mm trocar

1. Subumbilical scope *Surgiport* 10 mm trocar

A

Endo Grasp or *Endo Clinch* instrument

↑ Traction—Fundus

Calot's triangle

Hartmann's pouch traction

B

Cystic duct

C

Continued upward traction

Electrocautery hook

Cystic artery

Dissection plane under tension

Cystic duct clipped

D

Electrocautery hook

The gallbladder is flipped over the stationary grasper to create more tension in the plane of dissection.

FIGURE 12-16   Laparoscopic cholecystectomy. **A,** The gallbladder is grasped with blunt grasping forceps, and the cystic duct and artery are identified by gentle retraction anteriorly. **B,** The cystic duct and artery are isolated from the surrounding tissue. **C,** Ligating clips are applied by means of an endoscopic multiple-clip applier. **D,** The gallbladder is dissected from the liver bed.

liver. This is accomplished by use of an electrosurgical unit set at 25 to 35 W. The electrosurgical instrument may have a channel through which suction can be applied. This is particularly useful in evacuating the smoke plume during the procedure. Some disposable instruments employ suction, electrocoagulation, and irrigation through the same instrument.

17. The gallbladder is retracted using the forceps inserted through the 5 mm sheaths. It is manipulated to allow the medial and lateral attachments to be dissected with the electrosurgical instrument (Fig. 12-16, *D*).
18. Irrigation of the liver bed is performed before the detachment of the gallbladder.
19. Once it is determined to have no visible bile leak or bleeding in the liver bed, the laparoscope and camera are moved to the upper midline sheath.
20. Large grasping forceps are inserted through the umbilical sheath and are placed on the neck of the gallbladder.
21. An endobag or similar specimen-containing accessory may be used to secure the gallbladder for extraction, or the gallbladder may be brought out through the umbilical incision. If the gallbladder is too large to be extracted, the neck is brought above the surface of the incision, Kelly clamps are applied, and bile is suctioned out of the gallbladder for decompression.
22. The stab wounds are closed after decompression of the peritoneal cavity. The patient's wound is dressed with Steri-Strips.

Cholecystostomy

Cholecystostomy is establishment of an opening into the gallbladder to permit drainage of the organ and removal of stones. This procedure is usually selected for patients with acute gallbladder disease and a general physical condition that does not permit more extensive surgery.

Procedural considerations

A large Toomey syringe (50 ml) or an Asepto syringe may be needed for irrigation purposes. If a local anesthetic is used, the anesthetic drug and syringes and needles are necessary. Specified drainage tubes or catheters should be available. The patient is positioned supine. A nasogastric tube may be inserted by the anesthesia provider after general anesthesia and intubation.

Although many surgeons prefer the right subcostal incision, cholecystostomy procedures are often performed as emergencies, and so a quicker midline or transverse incision may be used. Instrumentation would include a basic laparotomy set and gallbladder specials.

Operative procedure

1. After incision into the abdominal cavity the gallbladder is isolated by retraction of the surrounding viscera.

2. The fundus of the gallbladder is grasped with an Allis or Babcock forceps, and the proposed opening is encircled by means of an absorbable purse-string suture, leaving the ends long.
3. To protect the abdominal cavity from contamination, the gallbladder is isolated with laparotomy packs, and suction is available.
4. An incision may be made into the gallbladder for insertion of a trochar with sheath.
5. Within the purse-string suture the gallbladder contents are aspirated by means of a suction tubing attached to a trocar sheath.
6. As the contents are aspirated, culture specimens should be taken. The contaminated trocar and sheath are removed and discarded.
7. The opening into the gallbladder can be enlarged with Metzenbaum scissors; gallstones are removed with malleable scoops and stone forceps.
8. Irrigating the gallbladder with isotonic saline solution is necessary to remove small stones, grit, or pastelike material. A syringe with a catheter or an Asepto syringe may be used for irrigation.
9. Contaminated instruments are placed into a basin on the operative field.
10. A drainage tube is inserted into the gallbladder opening. The purse-string suture is tightened around the catheter, with care being taken not to occlude it.
11. A second purse-string suture or separate mattress sutures may be used to secure the gallbladder to the peritoneum and the posterior rectus fascia.
12. The free end of the catheter or tube is exteriorized through a stab wound and then anchored to the skin edges, as described for cholecystectomy.
13. Drainage of the abdominal cavity is established. The exterior end of each drain is secured.
14. The wound is closed in layers, as described for laparotomy, and dressings are applied without disturbing the drains.

Choledochotomy and Choledochostomy

Choledochotomy is an incision made into the common bile duct (Fig. 12-17). Choledochostomy is the establishment of an opening into the common bile duct with placement of a drainage T-tube. Choledochotomy with subsequent choledochostomy are performed to treat choledocholithiasis or to relieve an obstruction in the common bile duct.

Procedural considerations

The patient is positioned supine under general anesthesia. A nasogastric tube is inserted by the anesthesiologist after intubation. An indwelling urinary catheter may be inserted before the abdominal prep.

Instrumentation would include a basic laparotomy set with gallbladder specials. T-tubes of assorted sizes should be available. A flexible choledochoscope may be requested.

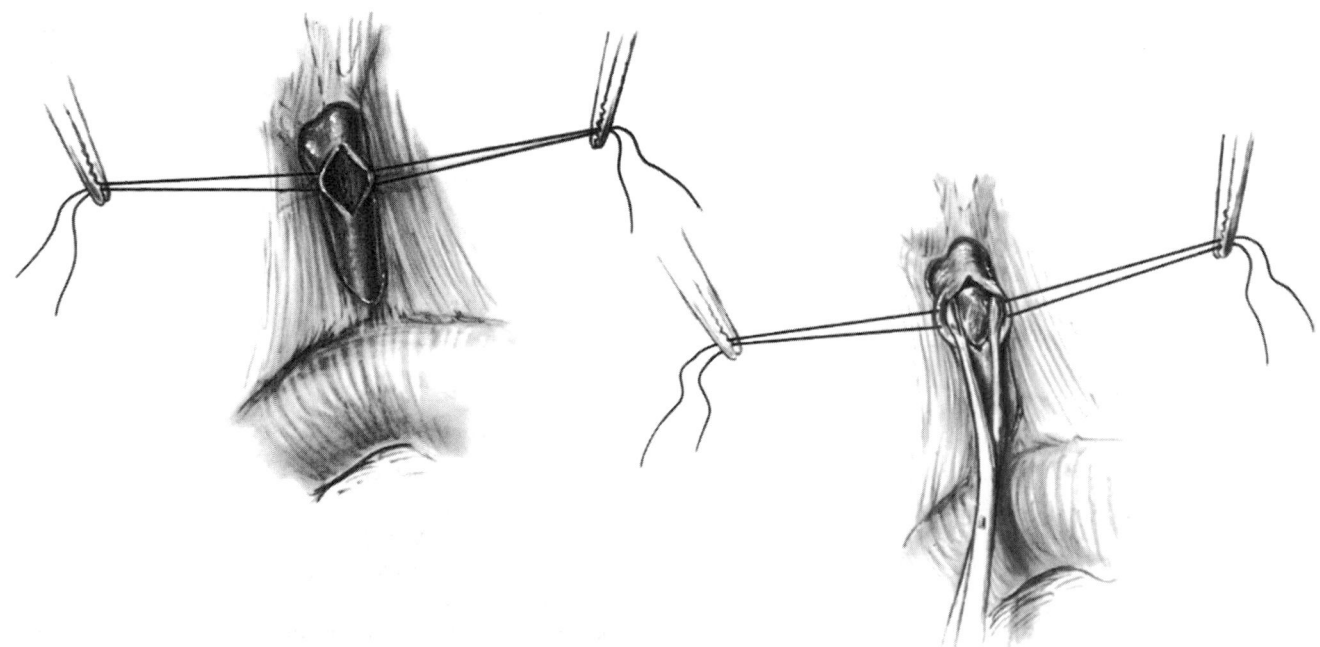

FIGURE 12-17 During choledochotomy, the common bile duct is opened longitudinally between two traction sutures. Any stones in the duct can then be extracted with stone forceps or removed by irrigation of the duct with saline solution.

Intraoperative cholangiography will most likely be used to confirm that all stones have been removed. A biliary Fogarty catheter and the surgeon's preference for cholangiocatheter should be available.

Before exploration is begun, operative cholangiography may be performed to locate all stones within the ductal system. X-ray films are repeated after the T-tube drain is in place to confirm the successful evacuation and patency of the ducts. A subcostal or upper right rectus incision is made.

Operative procedure

1. The abdomen is opened through a subcostal incision or midline incision.
2. If the gallbladder has not been previously removed, it is exposed and removed or retracted by means of laparotomy packs and retractors.
3. The common duct may be identified by means of an aspirating syringe and fine-gauge needle to make certain that the suspected duct is not a blood vessel.
4. Culture specimens may be obtained.
5. Two fine traction sutures are placed in the wall of the duct, below the entrance of the cystic duct.
6. The common duct region is walled off with laparotomy packs and narrow-blade retractors. A discard basin for contaminated instruments is placed at the lower end of the operative field; a suction apparatus is made ready for immediate use.
7. A longitudinal incision is made in the common duct (Fig. 12-18, A), between the traction sutures, with a long no. 3 knife handle and a no. 15 or no. 11 blade.

8. Constant suction is maintained with a Yankauer suction tube to keep the field free from oozing bile as the incision is enlarged with Potts angled or Metzenbaum scissors.
9. Additional stay sutures may be applied to the ductal opening.
10. Visible stones are removed with gallstone forceps, after which exploration of the duct is begun with small malleable scoops proximal and then distal to the opening.
11. Probing is continued as stones are removed from both the common and hepatic ducts.
12. Isotonic saline solution in an Asepto syringe and a small-lumen catheter or a Fogarty-type, balloon-tipped catheter are used to facilitate the removal of small stones and debris as well as to demonstrate patency of the common bile duct through to the duodenum (Fig. 12-18, B to D). A duodenotomy may be performed if patency of the sphincter of Oddi and ampulla of Vater cannot be demonstrated.
13. An area of the duodenum is walled off with laparotomy packs.
14. The incision is made longitudinally, using a scalpel with a #15 blade and Metzenbaum scissors.
15. Bleeding vessels are clamped with mosquito hemostats and ligated with fine silk or absorbable sutures or electrocoagulated.
16. Fine silk traction sutures (4-0) are inserted, and exploration is continued.
17. The duodenal opening is usually closed transversely in two layers with fine absorbable and silk intestinal sutures.

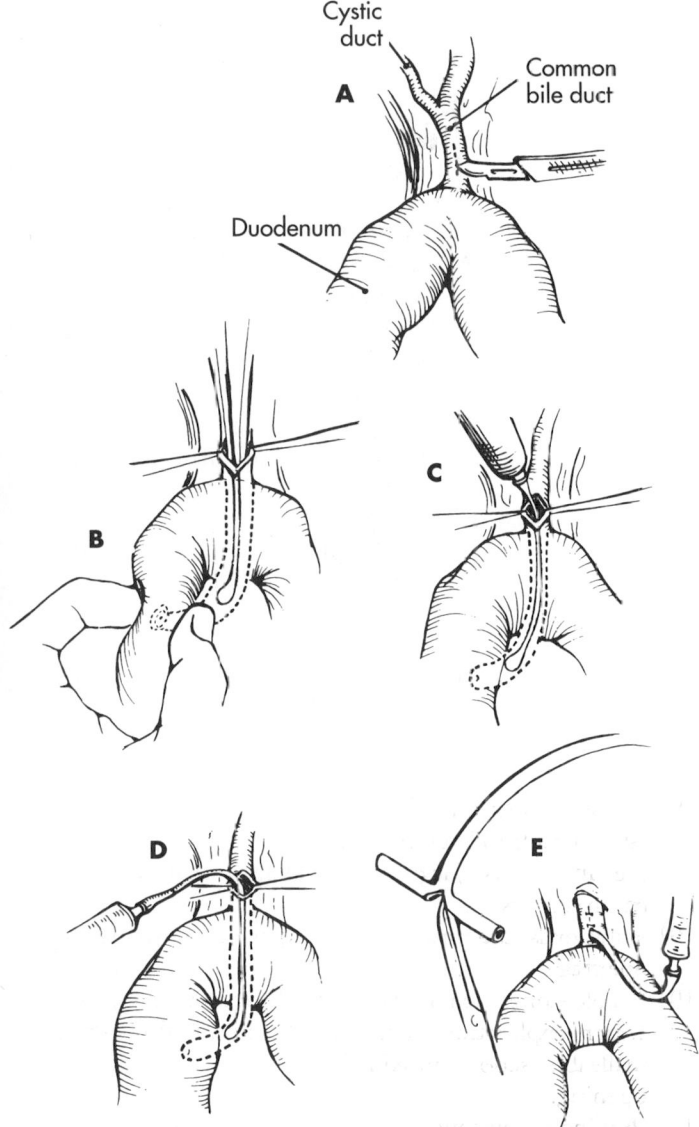

FIGURE 12-18 Choledochotomy with choledochostomy. **A,** Opening common duct. **B,** Introducing stone forceps. **C,** Probing common duct. **D,** Irrigating duct. **E,** Preparing and irrigating T-tube.

18. The T-tube is prepared by the surgeon (Fig. 12-18, *E*), irrigated for patency, and introduced into the common duct with fine vascular forceps.
19. The common duct incision is closed with fine (4-0) absorbable intestinal sutures.
20. Contaminated instruments are placed into the discard basin.
21. The T-tube is irrigated to demonstrate patency (Fig. 12-18, *E*), and a cholangiogram is done.
22. The gallbladder may be removed as described for cholecystectomy.
23. A drain is introduced into the foramen of Winslow.
24. Both drain and T-tube are exteriorized through a stab wound.
25. The wound is closed in layers; the T-tube and drain are carefully anchored to the skin, and each wound is

dressed individually to prevent undue tension, which could result in displacement of the tube and drain. Sterile tubing is used to connect the T-tube to a small drainage container or bag.

Choledochoscopy

Choledochoscopy is direct visualization of the common bile duct by introduction of a choledochoscope. Surgeon's preference may require a rigid or flexible scope. Choledochoscopy may take the place of operative cholangiography. It provides a means for extraction of stones that are difficult to remove.

Procedural considerations

The patient is positioned supine under general anesthesia. A nasogastric tube is inserted by the anesthesiologist after intubation. An indwelling urinary catheter may be inserted before the abdominal prep.

Distending the common duct is necessary for better visualization and is accomplished by irrigating the duct with copious amounts of sterile saline. A pressure bag is placed around an IV bag of 0.9% saline, and pressure to 300 mm Hg is applied. Sterile tubing is then passed from the sterile field and attached to the saline bag. The scrub nurse attaches the distal end of the sterile IV tubing directly to the irrigating stopcock on the scope.

Instrumentation is as described for biliary surgery, with the addition of the following instruments:

- Choledochoscope with accessories: biopsy forceps, stone-grasping forceps, and a sheath that can be used to direct other instruments into various portions of the biliary tract
- Video camera and viewing screen
- Light cord
- 0.9% normal saline (1000 ml bag)
- Sterile IV tubing
- Pressure bag
- Light source for the choledochoscope.

Operative procedure

1 to 5. As described for choledochotomy.
6. The choledochoscope is inserted into the common duct, which is then flushed with saline.
7. Stones are grasped with the stone forceps and removed. The choledochoscope allows visualization of the entire duct to ensure that no stones remain. After all stones are removed, the common duct is again thoroughly flushed with saline.
8. Closure of the duct and wound is completed.

Cholecystoduodenostomy and Cholecystojejunostomy

Cholecystoduodenostomy and cholecystojejunostomy are the establishment of continuity by creating an anastomosis between the gallbladder and duodenum or the gallbladder and jejunum to relieve an obstruction in the distal end of the common duct.

An obstruction in the biliary system may be caused by a tumor of the ducts involving the head of the pancreas or the ampulla of Vater, the presence of an inflammatory lesion, a stricture of the common duct, or the presence of stones.

Procedural considerations

Instrumentation includes a basic laparotomy set, gallbladder specials with two Doyen intestinal forceps, curved with guards, or similar nontraumatic holding forceps, and a self-retaining retractor system.

The patient is positioned supine under general anesthesia. A nasogastric tube is inserted by the anesthesiologist after intubation. An indwelling urinary catheter may be inserted before the abdominal prep.

Operative procedure

1. The abdomen is opened, the gallbladder is exposed, the contents are aspirated, and the pathologic condition is confirmed, as described for cholecystostomy.
2. The anastomosis site is prepared, posterior serosal silk sutures are placed, and open anastomosis is performed.
3. The surgical technique for anastomosis of the gallbladder to the duodenum or loop of jejunum is usually performed as a two-layer anastomosis.
4. The serosa of the duodenum or loop of jejunum is sutured to the full thickness of the fundus of the gallbladder.
5. A 1 to 1.5 cm opening is made into the small bowel and gallbladder in corresponding positions.
6. Interrupted 4-0 sutures of surgeon's preference are then placed around the entire circumference.
7. Contaminated instruments are placed into the discard basin, and the operative field is prepared for closure.
8. A drain may be introduced; the wound is closed in layers, and dressings are applied.

Choledochoduodenostomy and Choledochojejunostomy

Choledochoduodenostomy is anastomosis between the common duct and the duodenum, and choledochojejunostomy is anastomosis between the duct and the jejunum. These procedures may be necessary in postcholecystectomy patients to circumvent an obstructive lesion and reestablish the flow of bile into the intestinal tract.

Procedural considerations

Surgical approaches are similar to those for choledochostomy and cholecystojejunostomy.

The patient is positioned supine under geneneral anesthesia. A nasogastric tube is inserted by the anesthesiologist after intubation. An indwelling urinary catheter may be inserted before the abdominal prep.

Instrumentation and supplies necessary for this procedure would include a basic laparotomy set, gallbladder specials, a self-retaining retractor system, linear stapling devices, T-tubes in varying sizes, with or without a Silastic biliary stent.

Operative procedure

Choledochoduodenostomy

1. The abdomen is opened through a midline incision.
2. The common duct and duodenum are exposed.
3. The common duct is identified and dissected free using forceps and Metzenbaum scissors.
4. The common duct and duodenum are approximated, either side-to-side or the end of the common duct to the side of the duodenum, and an anastomosis is established.
5. An intraluminal catheter is inserted.
6. The wound is closed in layers, and dressings are applied.

Choledochojejunostomy

1. The abdomen is opened through a midline incision.
2. The jejunum is mobilized, and the common duct is identified and opened (Fig. 12-19, *A*).
3. Anastomosis is established between the common duct and the transected jejunum.
4. A catheter is introduced, as described for cholecystoduodenostomy.
5. Jejunal continuity is reestablished by jejunojejunostomy (Fig. 12-19, *B*).
6. As an alternative, anastomosis may be fashioned from the end of the severed duct to the side of a loop of jejunum, with a side-to-side jejunal anastomosis.
7. Contaminated instruments are removed from the operative field.
8. A drain is exteriorized, the wound is closed in layers, and dressing are applied.

Transduodenal Sphincteroplasty

Transduodenal sphincteroplasty is a method of producing a choledochoduodenostomy between the distal end of the common duct and the side of the duodenum. The sphincters normally affecting the distal common and pancreatic ducts are rendered functionless because the stoma is noncontractile and remains permanently open. Indications for transduodenal sphincteroplasty include a history of recurrent bile stones, impacted distal common duct stones, papillary stenosis, distal common bile duct strictures, recurrent idiopathic pancreatitis, and postcholecystectomy pain.

Procedural considerations

Instrumentation is as described for choledochotomy, with the addition of a GI set, since the duodenum is entered through a longitudinal incision. The patient is positioned supine under geneneral anesthesia. A nasogastric tube is inserted by the anesthesiologist after intubation.

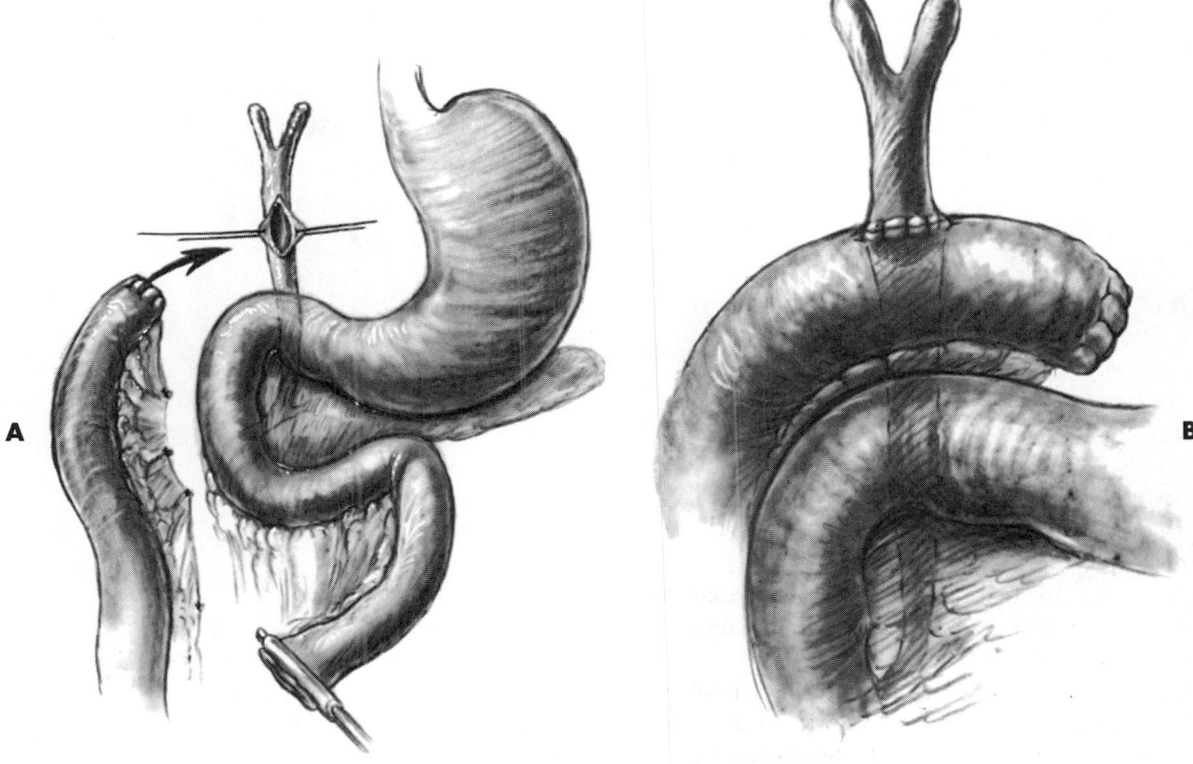

FIGURE 12-19   Choledochojejunostomy. **A**, The divided end of the jejunum is closed, and an end-to-side choledochojejunostomy is made in two layers to the jejunum. **B**, A jejunojejunostomy completes the operative procedure.

An indwelling urinary catheter may be inserted before abdominal preparation. The abdomen is prepped from nipple line to pubis.

Operative procedure

1. A right subcostal or midline incision is made, and exposure of the biliary tract is achieved.
2. All structures are inspected, and the normal configuration is established before any structure is tied, clamped, or divided during biliary tract dissection.[7]
3. Operative cholangiography is then performed by placing a cholangiocath through a small incision made with a #11 blade into the cystic duct.
4. The surgeon examines the films and makes the final decision to proceed with the sphincteroplasty.
5. If the gallbladder is present, cholecystectomy is performed.
6. The duodenum is mobilized by dividing the peritoneal reflection that covers the lateral portion of the second part of the duodenum and holds it in place.[7]
7. The common duct is incised longitudinally between two stay sutures and explored.
8. Any residual stones are removed. Duodenotomy is performed with a longitudinal incision, and the location of the papilla of Vater is identified (Fig. 12-20, *A*).

9. The sphincter of Oddi is divided at the 11 o'clock position with angled Potts scissors, and the ductal mucosa is sutured to the duodenal mucosa with a fine absorbable suture on a small urologic needle (Fig. 12-20, *B*).
10. The duodenum is then closed in two layers.
11. The common bile duct is joined to the apex of the mobilized duodenum in a two-layer anastomosis.
12. A T-tube is inserted to splint the anastomosis (Fig. 12-20, *C*).
13. The abdominal cavity is drained, and the wound is closed.

SURGERY OF THE PANCREAS

Drainage or Excision of Pancreatic Cysts

Pancreatic cysts may be drained internally into the small intestine or stomach or may require excision or external drainage (marsupialization).

Cysts of the pancreas have been classified according to the following etiologic factors: developmental or congenital, inflammatory, traumatic, neoplastic, and parasitic. Their causes, size, location, and anatomic relationships are important factors in the selection of the surgical procedure. Pancreatic pseudocysts are an encapsulated collection of pancreatic fluid exudate that has escaped from the

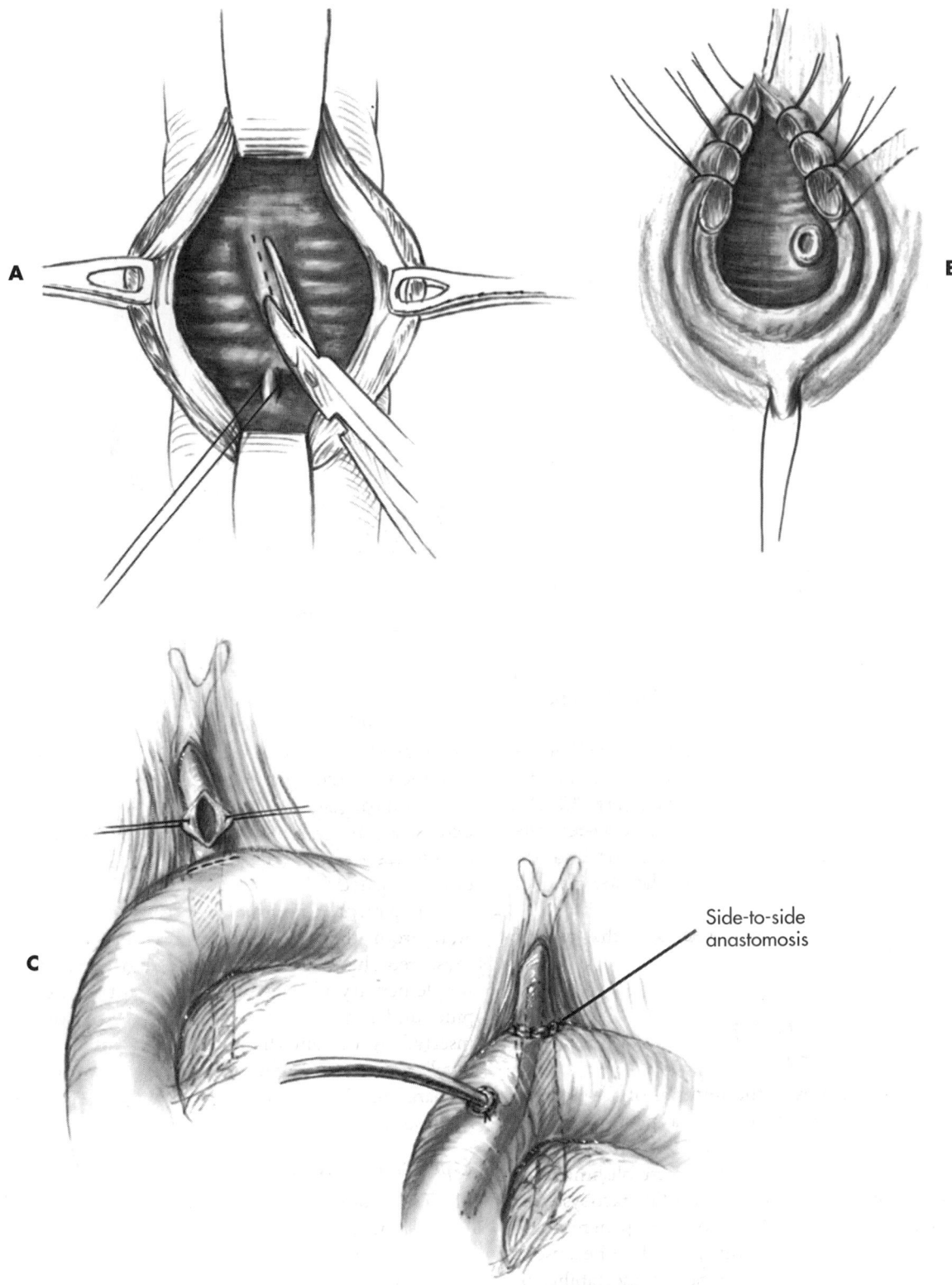

FIGURE 12–20   Tranduodenal sphincteroplasty. **A,** The duodenum is opened longitudinally. **B,** The sphincter of Oddi is divided at 11 o'clock with angled Potts scissors, and the ductal mucosa is then sutured to the duodenal mucosa with 4-0 absorbable suture. The duodenum is then closed longitudinally in two layers. **C,** Choledo-choduodenostomy. The common bile duct is joined to the apex of the mobilized duodenum in a two-layer anastomosis. A T-tube is placed to stent the anastomosis with the external stem of the tube brought out through the bile duct or through the wall of the duodenum.

pancreas. Inflammation of the serosal surfaces of the surrounding viscera causes fibrosis to occur, creating the walls of the pseudocysts. Pancreatic pseudocysts most commonly occur in the lesser sac of the peritoneum.

Procedural considerations

The patient is positioned supine under geneneral anesthesia. A nasogastric tube is inserted by the anesthesiologist after intubation. An indwelling urinary catheter may be inserted before the abdominal prep.

Instrumentation and supplies necessary for this procedure would include a basic laparotomy set, gallbladder specials, GI set, and a self-retaining retractor system.

Internal or external drainage of the cyst is the preferred procedure. Appropriate drains must be available.

Operative procedure

1. A midline incision is made into the abdomen.
2. A self-retaining retractor system is utilized to provide exposure of the pancreatic area.
3. The pancreatic cysts are examined, and the area is isolated with moist packs.
4. Simple external drainage is established by direct introduction of a retention catheter into the cyst, after decompression and inspection.
5. Internal drainage may be accomplished by an incision into the anterior wall of the stomach, directly opposite the cyst as it adheres to the posterior wall.
6. A fistula is established between the anterior wall of the cyst and the posterior wall of the stomach, thereby providing drainage through the GI tract (Fig. 12-21).
7. Many surgeons prefer an anastomosis between the cyst and a Roux-en-Y loop of jejunum or into the duodenum directly, depending on the location of the cyst.
8. The anterior gastrotomy is closed, and the wound closure is completed.

Pancreatoduodenectomy (Whipple Procedure)

Pancreatoduodenectomy is the removal of the head of the pancreas, the entire duodenum, a portion of the jejunum, the distal third of the stomach, and the lower half of the common bile duct, with the reestablishment of continuity of the biliary, pancreatic, and GI tract systems.

Radical excision of the head of the pancreas for carcinoma is a technically hazardous procedure because it involves many vital structures and organs. Resectability of the tumor in the presence or absence of metastasis and the general overall condition of the patient are evaluated carefully before resection.

Procedural considerations

A basic laparotomy set, GI instruments, a self-retaining retractor system (such as Bookwalter), linear stapling

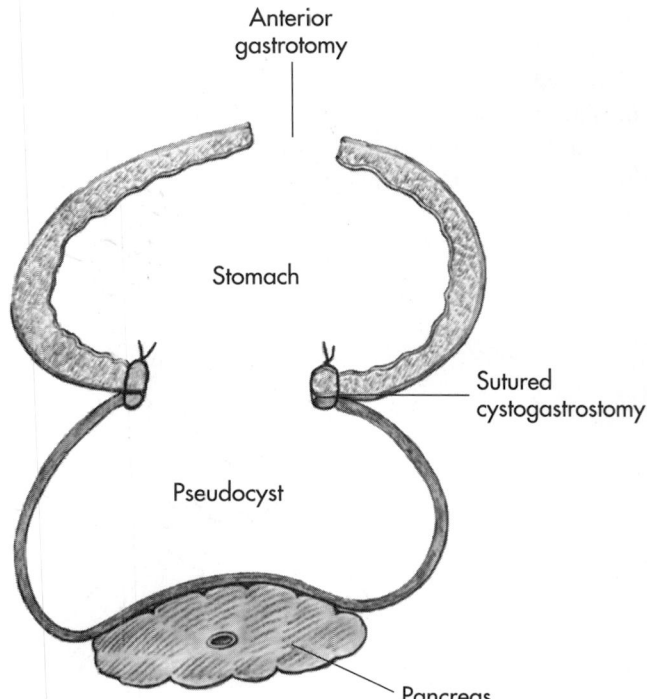

FIGURE 12-21 Cross-section diagram of cystogastrostomy for drainage of pseudocyst of the lesser sac.

devices, and appropriate drains and catheters are used for this procedure. After the surgeon opens and explores the abdomen, including the liver, pancreas, and biliary tree, the blood bank should be advised if the patient will require extensive surgery. Pancreatoduodenectomy may require 5 to 6 hours and the transfusion of many units of blood or blood products.

The patient is commonly sent to the SICU immediately from the OR suite. After surgery the surgeon must reevaluate the patient's insulin requirements and supplementary pancreatin. The patient is positioned supine under geneneral anesthesia. A nasogastric tube is inserted by the anesthesiologist after intubation. An indwelling urinary catheter is inserted before abdominal preparation. The abdomen is prepped from nipple line to midthigh.

Operative procedure

1. The abdomen is entered through an upper transverse, bilateral subcostal, or long paramedian incision.
2. Laparotomy packs and retractors are used to expose the operative site and protect vital structures.
3. Mobilization of the duodenum is achieved with an adequate Kocher maneuver, which comprises incision of peritoneal reflection, lateral to the second portion of the duodenum, with Metzenbaum scissors and subsequent blunt dissection of loose areolar tissue.
4. Mobilization of the duodenum continues, and bleeding vessels are ligated with silk.

5. The gastrocolic ligament and the gastrohepatic omentum are divided between curved forceps and are ligated or transfixed.
6. The gastroduodenal and right gastric arteries are clamped, divided, and ligated.
7. The prepyloric area of the stomach is mobilized.
8. The operative field is prepared for open anastomosis by isolating the area with laparotomy sponges.

9. By placing two long Allen or Payr clamps near the midportion of the stomach, the transection is completed.
10. The duodenum is reflected, the common duct is divided, and the hepatic end is marked or tagged for later anastomosis.
11. The jejunum is clamped with two Allen forceps, and the duodenojejunal flexure is divided.

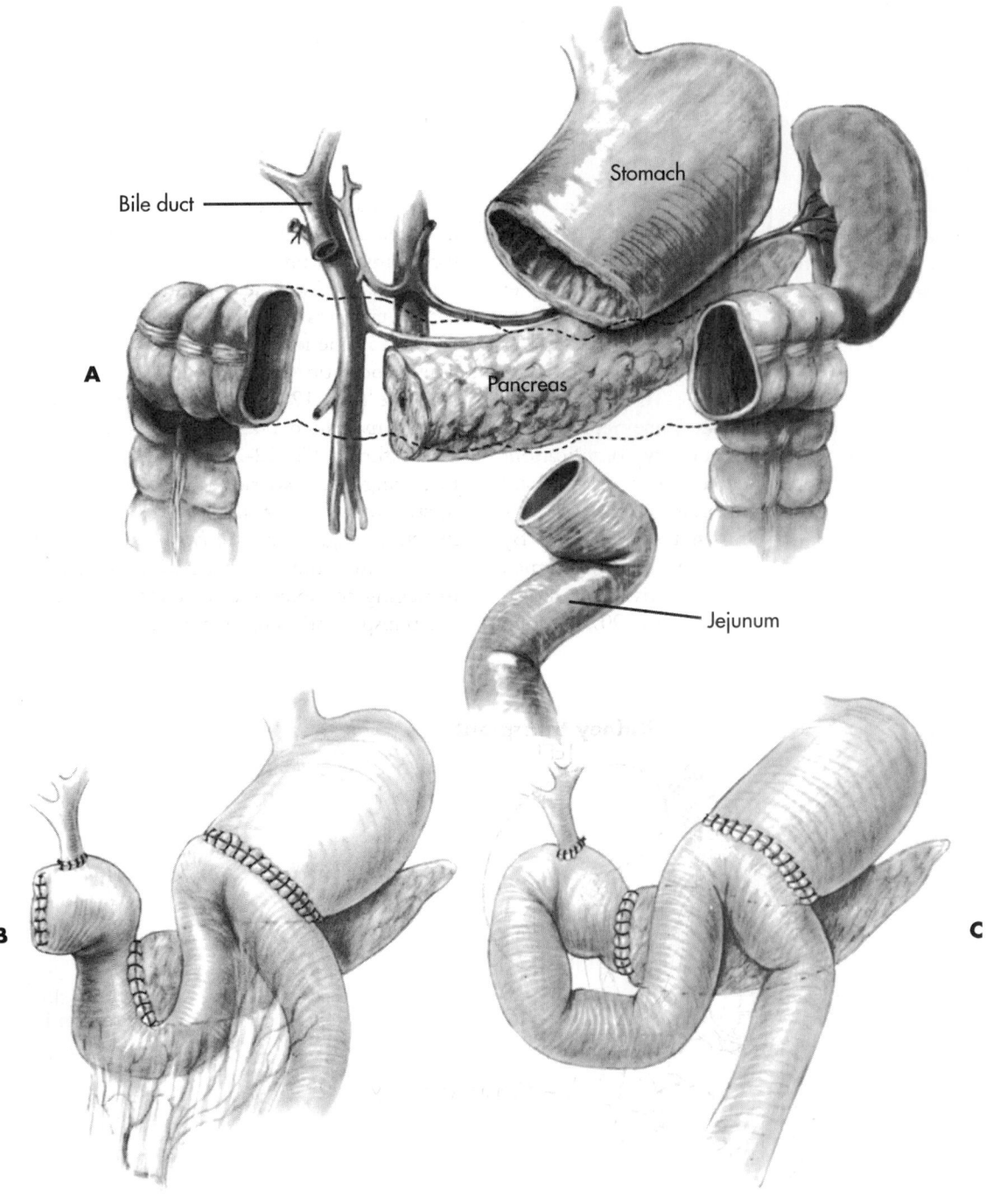

FIGURE 12-22 **A**, Resection margins of bile duct, pancreas, stomach, and jejunum following a Whipple procedure. **B**, Reconstruction after a Whipple procedure showing biliary anastomosis preceding pancreas and stomach. **C**, Reconstruction showing pancreatic anastomosis preceding bile duct and stomach.

12. The pancreas is divided, and the duct is carefully identified.

13. Further mobilization of the duodenum and division of the inferior pancreatoduodenal artery are done to permit complete removal of the specimen.

14. Reconstruction of the GI tract is completed by the following anastomoses: retrocolic end-to-end pancreatojejunostomy, retrocolic end-to-side choledochojejunostomy, and an antecolic long-loop isoperistaltic gastrojejunostomy (Fig. 12-22).

15. Drains are introduced, as for cholecystostomy. Some surgeons prefer to place a sump drain near the pancreatic anastomosis.

16. The wound is closed in layers. An abdominal dressing is applied.

Pancreatic Transplantation

Pancreatic transplantation is the implantation of a pancreas from a donor into a recipient. This procedure is considered a possible means of treatment for type I diabetes. Pancreatic transplantation differs from other organ transplants in that it does not have immediate life-saving results. Insulin therapy is a more common alternative medical treatment. Pancreatic transplantation is indicated for long-established, totally insulin-deficient diabetics with end-stage renal disease. Since nephropathy, retinopathy, and neuropathy are secondary complications to long-established, insulin-deficient diabetes, pancreatic transplantation may interrupt their progression.

Pancreatic transplantation was first tried in 1967. By 1989, more than 500 transplants were being performed annually in the United States. The operative mortality is low, and the 1-year survival is greater than 90%. Insulin independence is achieved in up to 70% of the patients receiving pancreas transplants at 1 year.[2]

Procedural considerations

The majority of pancreatic transplantations performed in the United States are part of a simultaneous pancreas and renal transplant procedure with both organs procured from the same cadaveric donor. Combined kidney-pancreas transplants (Fig. 12-23) seem to prevent recurrence of diabetic nephropathy in the transplanted kidney as well as some other microvascular complications.[2] Serial transplantation is an alternative for patients who have already received a transplanted kidney.

The surgical technique for pancreatic transplantation varies between segmental pancreatic grafting and whole-organ transplantation. With either procedure, vascular anastomosis and management of the pancreatic duct are performed. Managing pancreatic ductal exocrine secretions remains one of the major technical problems with the transplantation procedure. The segmental pancreatic graft can be placed into a paratopic position just superior to the native pancreas of the recipient or into a heterotopic position in the retroperitoneum or in an intraperitoneum. The pancreatic duct is then routed into the stomach, intestine (Fig. 12-24, *A*), or urinary bladder (Fig. 12-24, *B*). A pancreaticocutaneous fistula, with external drainage via a catheter (Fig. 12-24, *C*), may also be an alternative for managing the exocrine secretions from the pancreatic duct. Occlusion of the pancreatic duct with polymer injection (Fig. 12-24, *D*) before transplantation or 3 to 6 weeks after the transplantation is another means of managing the exocrine secretions. Whole-organ pancreatic transplantation has achieved popularity over segmental

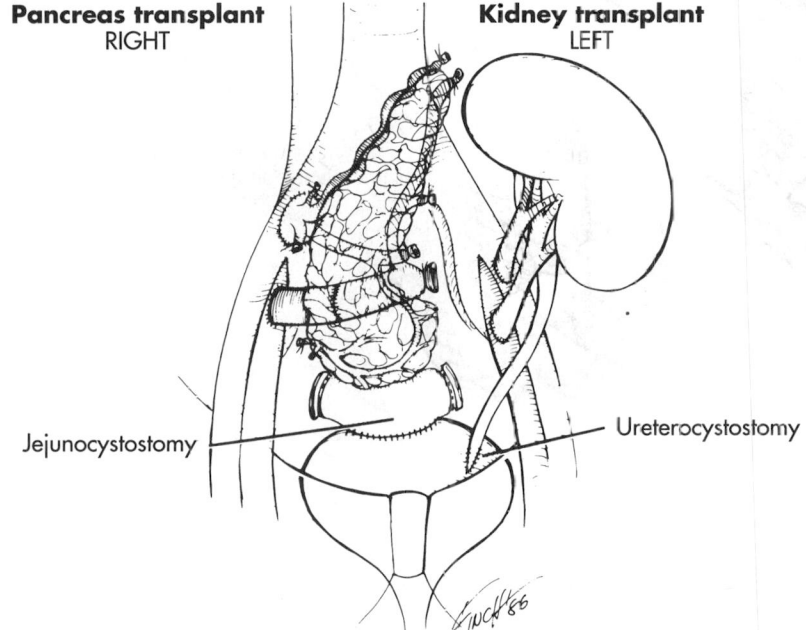

Pancreas transplant
RIGHT

Kidney transplant
LEFT

Jejunocystostomy

Ureterocystostomy

FIGURE 12-23   Whole pancreas transplantation with simultaneous or serial kidney transplantation illustrating the position of the two donor grafts in the recipient.

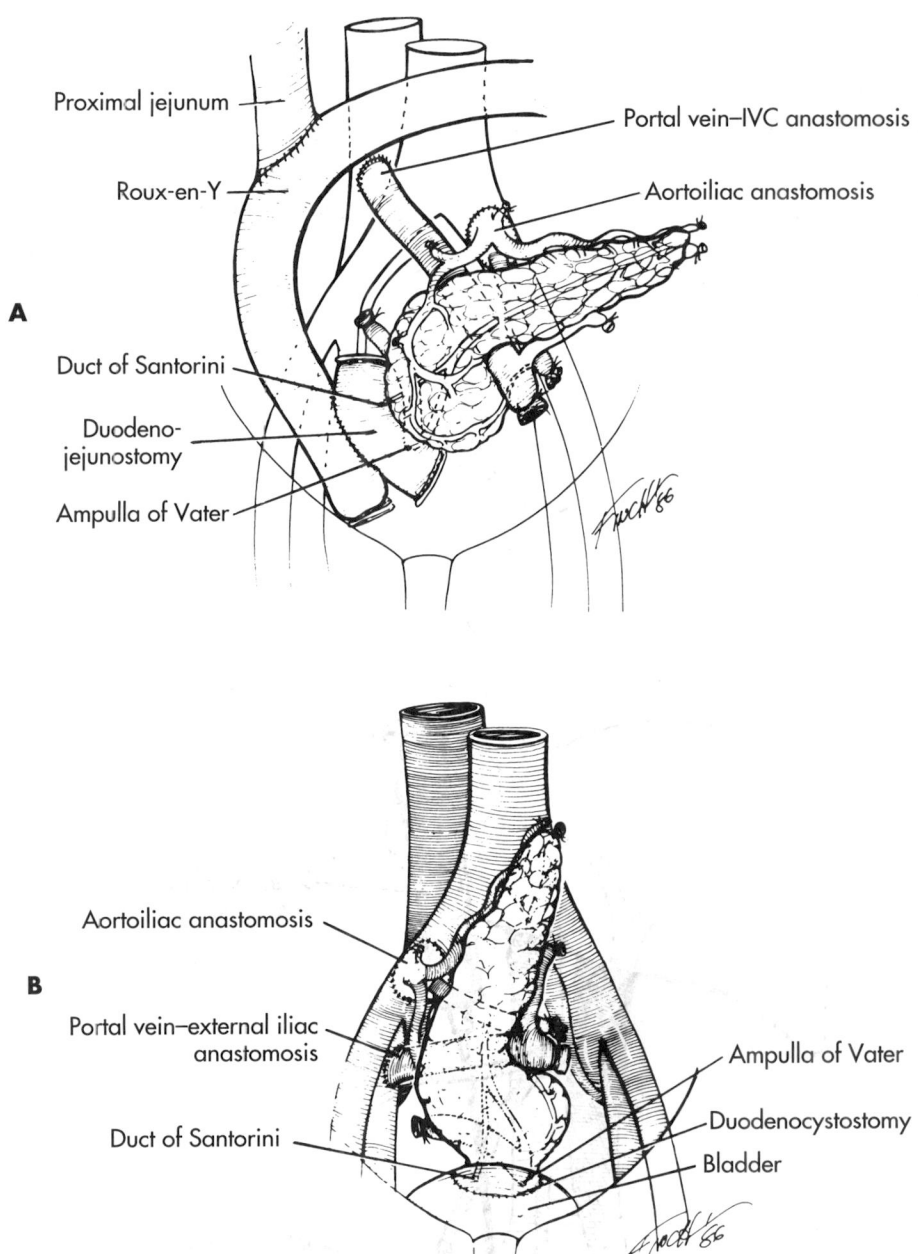

Proximal jejunum

Roux-en-Y

Portal vein–IVC anastomosis

Aortoiliac anastomosis

Duct of Santorini

Duodeno-
jejunostomy

Ampulla of Vater

A

Aortoiliac anastomosis

Portal vein–external iliac
anastomosis

Duct of Santorini

Ampulla of Vater

Duodenocystostomy

Bladder

B

FIGURE 12-24   **A,** Enteric drainage of a whole-pancreas graft showing a side-to-side anastomosis of the donor duodenal patch and the recipient's jejunal segment of a Roux-en-Y. **B,** Whole-pancreas transplantation showing donor duodenal patch anastomosed to dome of urinary bladder.

pancreatic transplantation. Better blood supply of the whole-organ graft and an increased number of islet cells for insulin production are the advantages that have changed the trend to whole-organ pancreatic transplantation in recent years.

Instrumentation for pancreatic transplantation includes a transplant set as described for kidney transplantation in Chapter 15. In addition to the transplant set, consideration must be given to the resection of the duodenal segment and the management of the pancreatic duct. A GI instrument set and linear stapling devices with two loads are required for grafting the duodenal segment that contains the pancreatic duct into an enteric route of drainage.

The patient is positioned supine under geneneral anesthesia. A nasogastric tube is inserted by the anesthesiologist after intubation. An indwelling urinary catheter is inserted before the abdominal prep.

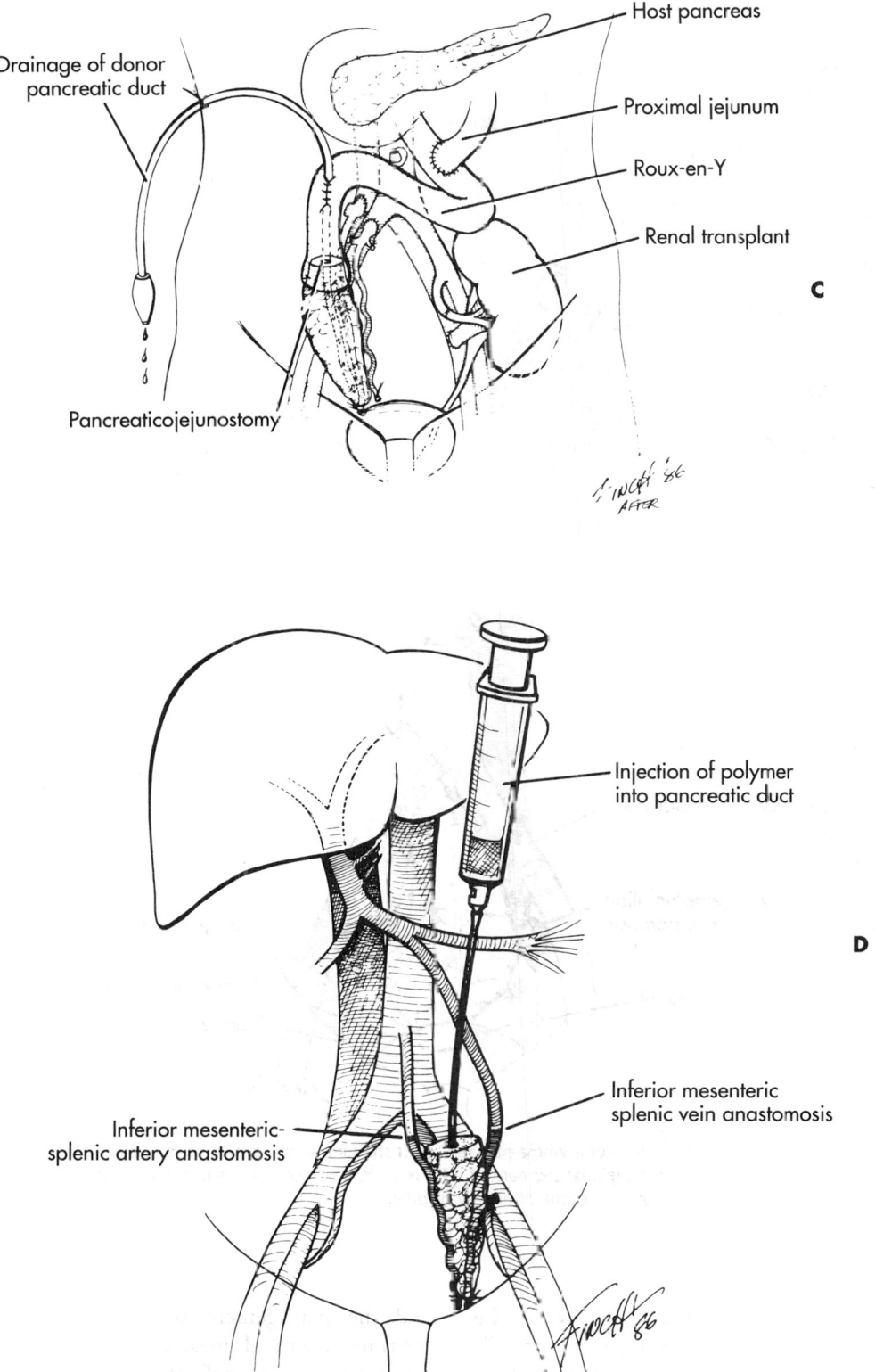

FIGURE 12-24, cont'd   **C**, Enteric drainage of a segmental pancreas graft to a Roux-en-Y limb of the recipient jejunum, showing an external drain exteriorized through the abdominal wall. **D**, Segmental pancreas transplantation showing polymer injection into pancreatic duct of graft.

Operative procedure

1. The whole-organ pancreatic transplantation procedure is performed through an oblique incision opposite the side of the renal transplant in the lower abdominal quadrant. A midline incision may also be used for pancreatic transplant.
2. The external iliac artery and vein are skeletalized, and lymphatics are tied off with 4-0 silk strands.
3. The external iliac vein is clamped with noncrushing vascular clamps, and venotomy is achieved with a #11 blade.
4. The venotomy incision is extended with Potts scissors.
5. An end-to-side anastomosis of the donor portal vein to the recipient's external iliac vein is achieved with four double-armed 5-0 polypropylene sutures.
6. The external iliac artery is then clamped, and arteriotomy is achieved with an aortic punch.
7. An end-to-side anastomosis of the recipient's external iliac artery with the donor aortic patch containing the origin of the superior mesenteric artery and the celiac axis is performed with four double-armed 6-0 polypropylene sutures.
8. Management of the pancreatic duct is then performed.
9. The whole-organ pancreatic transplantation may also be performed as a pancreaticoduodenal transplantation or a pancreaticoduodenal-splenic transplantation.
10. Management of the pancreatic duct depends on the type of en bloc procedure performed.
11. Various enteric procedures for drainage of pancreatic duct secretions have been performed with whole-organ transplants en bloc with a segment of duodenum and the spleen. They include cutaneous jejunostomy, drainage into an ileal loop, and duodenojejunostomy with an end-to-end or side-to-side anastomosis.
12. Direct grafting of the pancreatic duct into the enteric or urinary system is also performed for management of exocrine secretions. Surgical procedures would include pancreaticojejunostomy with an established Roux-en-Y loop of jejunum, pancreaticoductoureterostomy, and pancreaticocystostomy.

SURGERY OF THE LIVER
Drainage of Intrahepatic, Subhepatic, or Subphrenic Abscess

Abscesses of the liver may require incision and drainage. Hepatic abscesses may be pyogenic or parasitic and single or multiple.

Extreme care is used in removal of an *Echinococcus* (hydatid) cyst because the fluid is under high tension, and any spillage into the peritoneal cavity may result in an anaphylactic reaction. Even more important is the possible escape of daughter cysts, which can spread through the abdomen and produce multiple cysts, an extremely difficult condition to treat. Hydatid cysts of the liver are rare in the United States.

Procedural considerations

A basic laparotomy set is used. Biliary instrumentation, drainage materials, and aerobic and anaerobic culture tubes should be available.

The patient is positioned supine under genneral anesthesia. A nasogastric tube is inserted by the anesthesiologist after intubation. An indwelling urinary catheter may be inserted before the abdominal prep.

Operative procedure

1. The incision and type of procedure selected depend on the cause and location of the abscess.
2. For the anterior approach, a right transperitoneal incision is made.
3. For the posterior approach, the patient is prepped and the incision selected as described for a posterior thoracotomy.
4. Drainage of an abscess may be treated in one or two stages. In the one-stage procedure, the approach is through the outer third of the right twelfth rib to reach the liver abscess retroperitoneally and extrapleurally. A two-stage operation, which is rarely done, obliterates the right pleural cavity. The objective of the first stage is to seal off the pleural cavity by stimulating adhesions with the insertion of iodoform packing. When the second stage is performed at a higher level, the chest cavity does not become contaminated.

Hepatic Resection

The liver is divided into the left lobe and the right lobe, with the caudate lobe lying in the dorsal segment. Resection of the liver is according to the lobe and segment involved (Figs. 12-25 to 12-27); a small wedge biopsy, excision of simple tumors, or a major lobectomy may be performed. Increased knowledge of liver function and circulatory physiology as well as improved methods of hemostasis now permit the surgeon to offer safe, definitive treatment to the patient with liver disease or trauma.

Procedural considerations

Supplies and equipment should be available for thermoregulation, electrosurgery, measurement of portal pressure, thoracotomy drainage, and replacement of blood loss. Special blunt needles for suturing liver tissue are also necessary.

The patient is placed in the supine position. A nasogastric tube will be inserted by the anesthesiologist after induction of general anesthesia and intubation. An indwelling urinary catheter is inserted before the abdominal prep. The abdomen is prepped from nipple line to midthigh. A midline abdominal incision, occasionally with division of the lower sternum, provides access to the liver. Vertical abdominal incisions are advantageous because

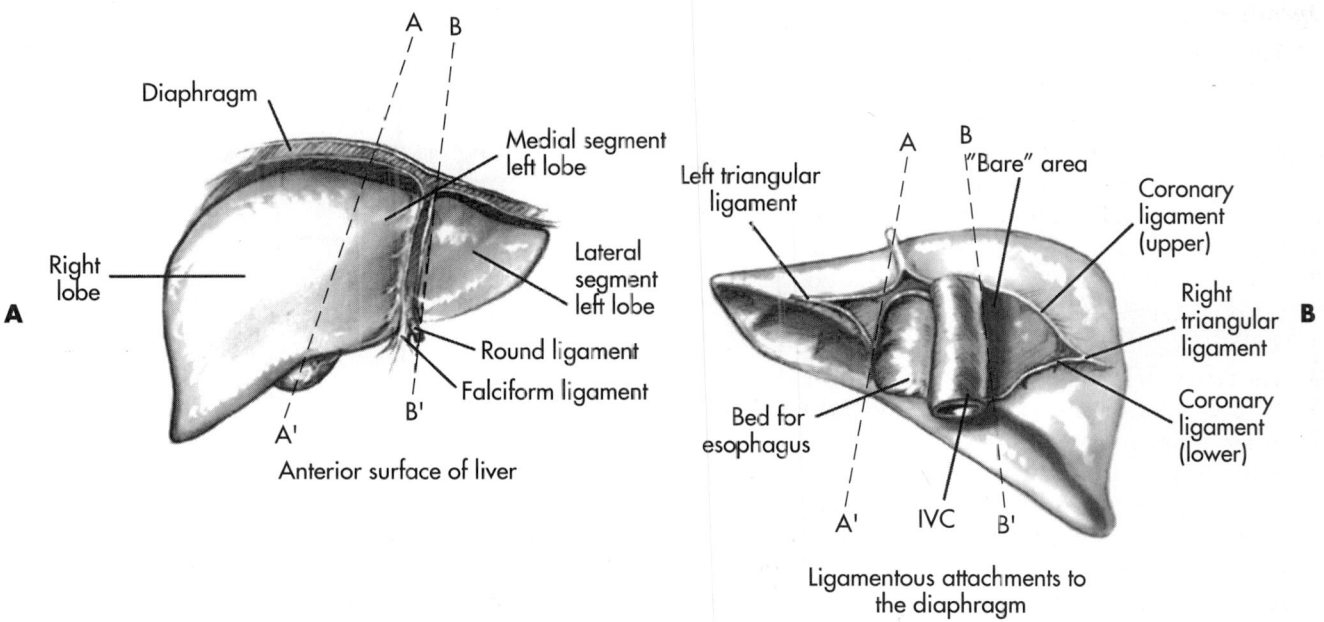

FIGURE 12-25 **A**, Anterior surface of the liver. Plane A-A' divides the liver into the right and left lobes. Plane B-B' divides the left lobe into the medial and lateral segments. **B**, The ligamentous attachments to the diaphragm.

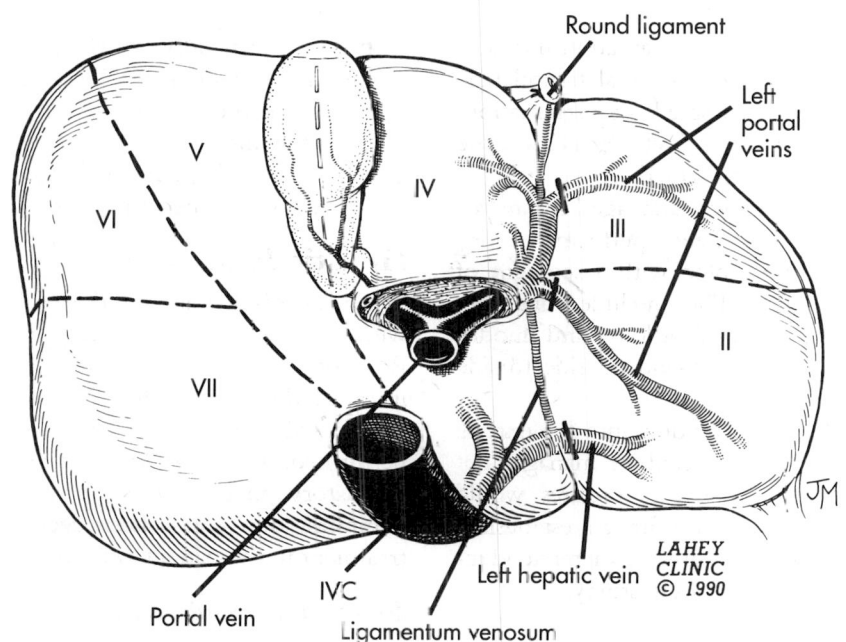

FIGURE 12-26 Seven segments of the liver.

they can be made and closed more rapidly and permit better exposure of all abdominal organs than nonvertical incisions can.

Instrumentation includes a basic laparotomy set, biliary instruments, vascular instruments, and additional items such as long clamps and a self-retaining retractor system (such as the Bookwalter retractor system).

Liver sutures, absorbable or nonabsorbable, according to surgeon's preference, vessel loops, and umbilical tapes should be available on the sterile field.

Hemostatic material, such as Gelfoam, Surgicel, or Avitene, and absorbable collagen sheets should be readily available when the resection is begun.

Equipment needed for hepatic resection includes an intraoperative ultrasound 7 mHz probe and unit, CUSA unit and handpiece, electrosurgical unit (set on blend 3 and coagulation at 100 to 110 during resection), two suction tubes and tips, smoke-evacuation system, surgeon's headlight, and an argon-beam coagulator unit and handpiece if this is the surgeon's preference.

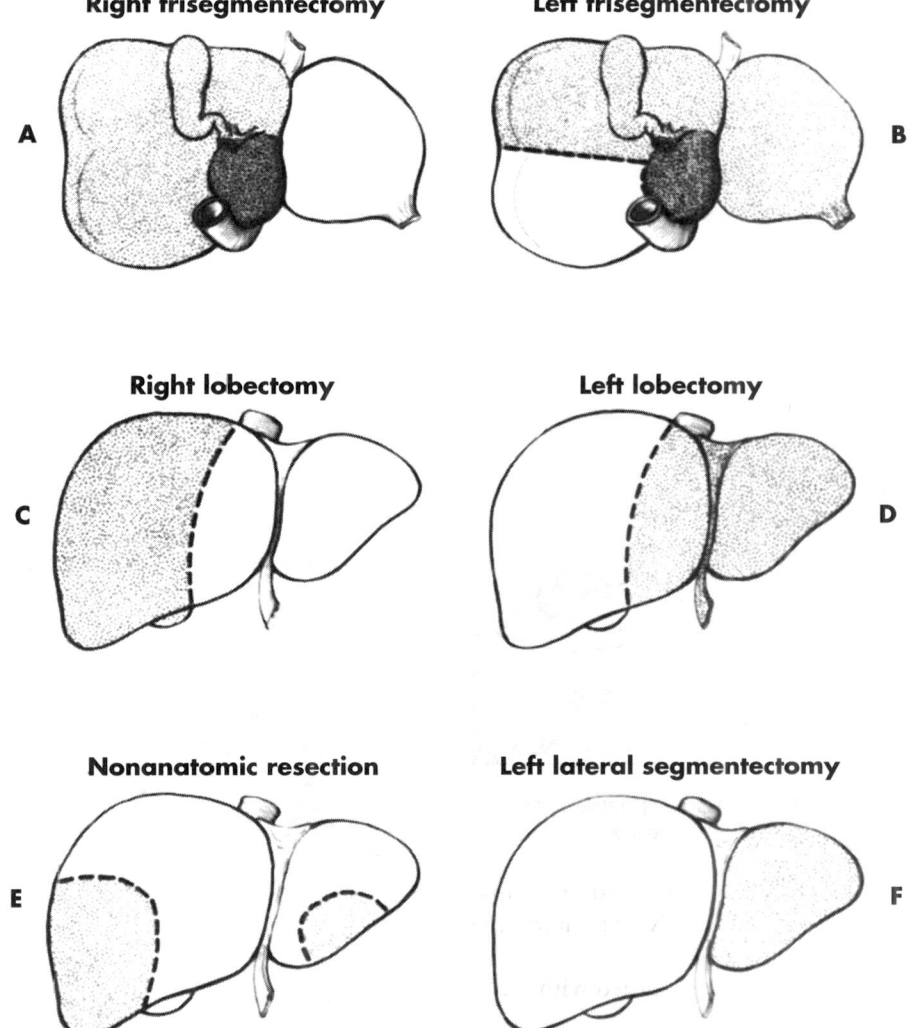

Right trisegmentectomy

A

Left trisegmentectomy

B

Right lobectomy

C

Left lobectomy

D

Nonanatomic resection

E

Left lateral segmentectomy

F

FIGURE 12-27 Techniques for hepatic resection. **A**, Right trisegmentectomy. **B**, Left trisegmentectomy. **C**, Right lobectomy. **D**, Left lobectomy. **E**, Nonanatomic resection such as a wedge resection. **F**, Left lateral segmentectomy.

The surgeon may use various methods to remove liver tissue. The CUSA allows the surgeon to dissect tissue using ultrasonic waves incorporated with fluid and suction. The ultrasonic waves cut through liver tissue, emulsifying it and diluting the tissue with fluid so that it can be suctioned away. The electrosurgical pencil uses electrical current to cut through and desiccate liver tissue. Finger-fracture of the liver tissue is performed by applying digital pressure against the parenchyma to fracture the tissue. This method is performed only after the larger vessels have been addressed. Hemostasis of the fractured parenchyma will be necessary.

Operative procedure

1. Through an upper midline or chevron type of incision, the abdominal cavity is opened and examined.

2. Pathologic condition is determined, and resectability evaluated.
3. Moist laparotomy packs are inserted, and a self-retaining retractor is placed.
4. Intraoperative ultrasonography is performed to assess all segments of the liver (Fig. 12-28).
5. If the tumor appears to be confined to one lobe, the procedure will proceed. If the tumor is diffuse or unresectable, a simple biopsy is performed for diagnostic confirmation.
6. Lymph nodes in the porta hepatis and along the gastrohepatic ligament are then assessed by palpation to determine extrahepatic metastasis.
7. Exposure of the hilar structures is obtained by upward displacement of the right lobe toward the right chest cavity.

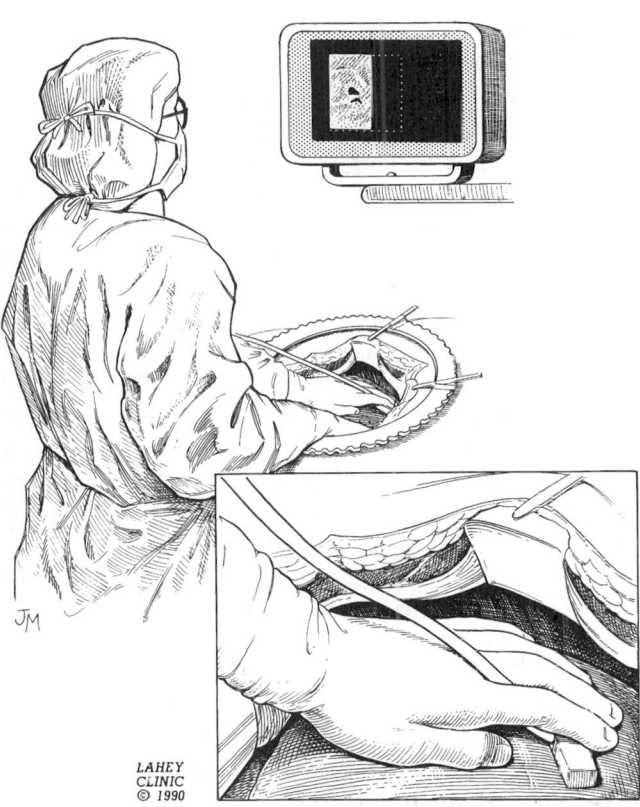

FIGURE 12-28 Demonstrating the use of intraoperative ultrasound using a 7 mHz T-probe to permit assessment of the liver.

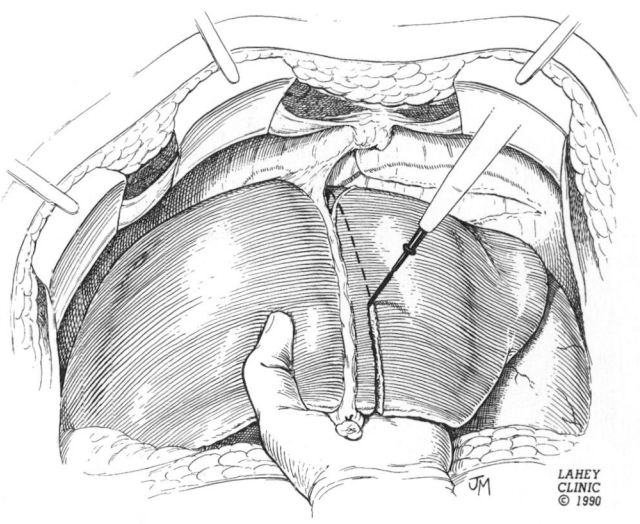

FIGURE 12-29 Use of electrosurgical pencil with blade tip to score the line of resection on the surface of the liver.

8. The falciform ligament is disconnected using electro-dissection until it approaches division into the triangular ligament.

9. Displacement of intestines is accomplished with moist packs and retractors.

10. The cystic duct is carefully exposed using Metzen-baum scissors, vascular forceps, small dry dissectors on curved clamps, and fine right-angled forceps. It is clamped, transsected, and double ligated with chromic or silk ligatures and transfixion sutures.

11. The involved hepatic duct, branch of hepatic artery, and branch of the portal vein are also transsected and doubly ligated with silk ligatures and transfixion sutures.

12. The liver is rotated forward, and the multiple hepatic veins are assessed and isolated.

13. The intended resection line is scored with an electrosurgical pencil with blade tip and coagulation set at the surgeon's preferred setting. (Fig. 12-29).

14. The liver parenchyma is then delicately resected using the CUSA handpiece set at 5 (Fig. 12-30).

15. Large vascular structures are identified and clamped, ligaclips are applied, and the structures are ligated (Fig. 12-31). The surgeon may choose suture material for vessel occlusion.

16. Use of the CUSA handpiece continues for dissection through the parenchyma.

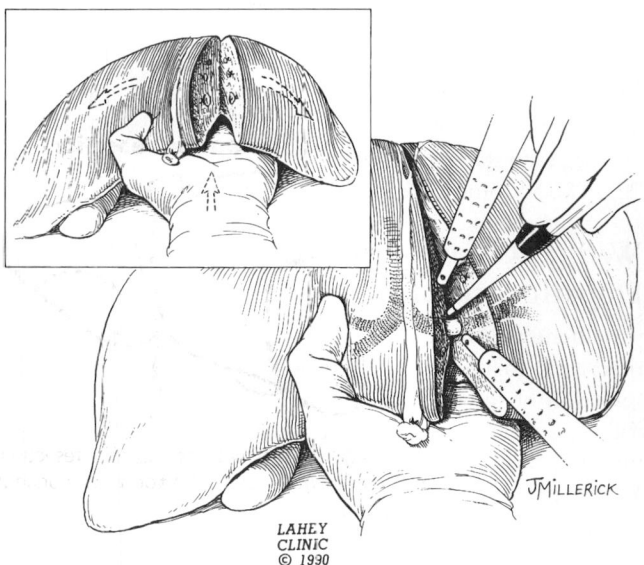

FIGURE 12-30 Use of the Cavitron Ultrasonic Surgical Aspirator (CUSA) handpiece to dissect through the hepatic parenchyma.

17. Electrosurgical charring of surfaces or use of the argon beam coagulator is intermittent.

18. Once the portion of the liver is resected, the remaining liver resection margins are assessed for bleeding and bile leakage.

19. A laparotomy sponge is placed against the transsected surface for several minutes. The laparotomy sponge is gently rolled from the surface and examined for bile leakage.

20. Areas may then be oversewn with 2-0 or 3-0 absorbable suture or an intended layer of eschar applied using electrocoagulation or the argon beam coagulator.

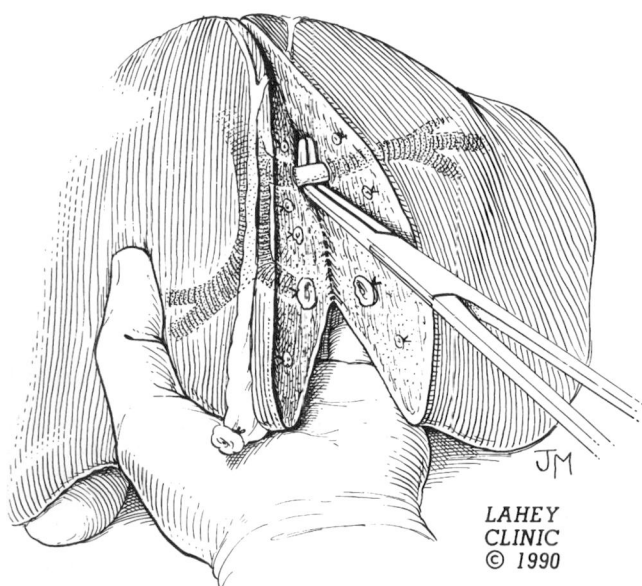

LAHEY
CLINIC
© 1990

FIGURE 12-31 Large intrahepatic vascular structures are isolated with blunt dissection, clamped, and ligated before division. Ligating clips or suture may be used to ensure hemostasis.

21. Abdominal drains may be placed along the liver bed and brought out through the abdominal wall through separate stab wounds.
22. The abdominal wound is then closed.

Wedge Resection of Metastatic Hepatic Tumors

Patients with primary colon or rectal cancer can have metastasis to the liver occur within 5 years of primary resection of the colon or rectal lesion. These patients are followed closely by monitoring of CEA levels in their blood at scheduled intervals that depend on the findings. When a rise in CEA levels is noted, x-ray examination, MRI, and CT scans are often used for diagnosis.

Wedge resection of metastatic hepatic lesions is an abbreviated procedure for isolated lesions in which lobectomy or segmentectomy is not indicated. The criteria for candidacy exclude those patients who have metastases outside the abdominal cavity, in lungs, or in bones.

Procedural considerations

Intraoperatively the surgeon can confirm suspicion of liver metastasis by bimanual examination of each lobe, intraoperative ultrasonography, biopsy, or Neoprobe scanning of the liver (see p. 407). This is sometimes scheduled as a CEA-directed second-look procedure, and equipment and supplies for bowel or liver resection should always be available. This procedure and considerations are discussed in depth in Chapter 11.

An elongated electrosurgical blade with the unit set on a high blend 2 setting is used to begin the resection of the metastatic tumor. The CO_2 laser with smoke evacuator or the CUSA aspirator and the argon beam coagulator

provide valuable technologic assistance for resection of metastatic lesions of the liver.

The surgeon's intent is to achieve a 1 cm margin of normal liver tissue dissection around each lesion.

Metastatic lesions may range from 0.5 to 20 cm in diameter. After resection or excision of the metastatic lesions from the liver, localized chemotherapy lines may be indicated for postoperative, self-administered chemotherapy. A Broviac catheter is inserted into the hepatic artery, and a Hickman catheter is inserted into the portal vein via a gastroepiploic artery and vein. The catheters exit the skin in the right upper quadrant of the abdomen and are labeled accordingly. A continuous-flow hepatic artery pump may also be inserted after wedge resection if continuous-flow chemotherapy is planned for postoperative adjuvant treatment. The patient is placed in the supine position. A nasogastric tube will be inserted by the anesthesiologist after induction of general anesthesia and intubation. An indwelling urinary catheter is inserted before the abdominal prep. The abdomen is prepped from nipple line to midthigh. A midline abdominal incision, occasionally with division of the lower sternum, provides access to the liver. Vertical abdominal incisions are advantageous because they can be made and closed more rapidly and permit better exposure of all abdominal organs.

Instrumentation includes a basic laparotomy set, biliary instruments, vascular instruments, and additional items such as long clamps and a self-retaining retractor system (such as the Bookwalter retractor system).

Liver sutures, absorbable or nonabsorbable, according to the surgeon's preference, vessel loops, and umbilical tapes should be available on the sterile field.

Hemostatic material, such as Gelfoam, Surgicel, or Avitene, absorbable collagen sheets should be readily available when the resection is begun.

Procedure for wedge resection of metastatic carcinoma lesions follows the hepatic resection technique.

Operative procedure

1. The liver is examined by palpation and visualization.
2. Intraoperative ultrasonography is used to assess all eight segments of the liver.
3. Procedures are taken to mobilize the intended lobes of the liver from which the wedge resection will be performed.
4. Electrocautery is used to score the surface of the resection line (Fig. 12-32).
5. The CUSA is then used for dissection of the parenchyma (Fig. 12-33).
6. Hemostasis is achieved by electrocoagulation, application of ligaclips, and the use of Surgicel or Avitene sheets.
7. Once the wedge resection is accomplished, the margins are assessed for remaining tumor, hemostasis, and bile leakage.

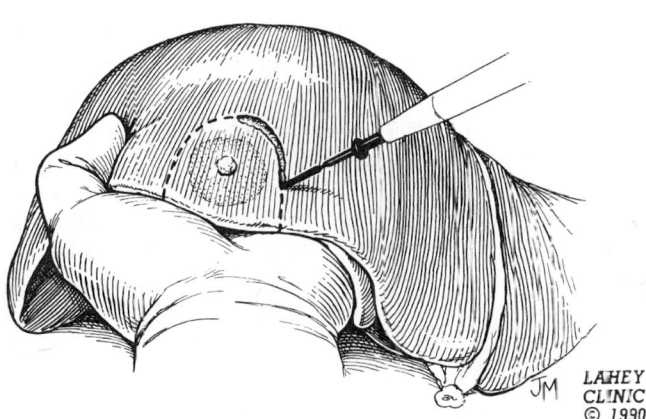

FIGURE 12-32 Hepatic wedge resection demonstrating the use of electrocautery to score a reasonable clear margin around the liver lesion.

8. If no further resection is indicated, a layer of eschar may be applied to the parenchymal margin.
9. The abdominal wound is then closed.

Right Hepatic Trisegmentectomy

As the field of extensive surgical procedures for treatment of liver diseases evolves, an aggressive approach to the resection of hepatic metastases has also become more common. Trisegmentectomy refers to an extensive resection of the liver. With right trisegmentectomy, the right lobe of the liver and the medial segment of the left lobe are removed. The caudate lobe may be included in the right trisegmentectomy if indicated by tumor involvement. In left trisegmentectomy the left lobe of liver and the anterior segment of the right lobe are resected. Again, the caudate lobe may or may not be included in the resection.

Procedural considerations

Supplies and equipment should be available for hypothermia, electrosurgery, measurement of portal pressure, thoracotomy drainage, and replacement of blood loss. Special blunt needles for suturing liver tissue are also necessary.

The patient is placed in the supine position. A nasogastric tube will be inserted by the anesthesiologist after induction of general anesthesia and intubation. An indwelling urinary catheter is inserted before the abdominal prep. The abdomen is prepped from nipple line to midthigh. A midline abdominal incision, occasionally with division of the lower sternum, provides access to the liver. Vertical abdominal incisions are advantageous because they can be made and closed more rapidly and permit better exposure of all abdominal organs than nonvertical incisions can.

Instrumentation includes a basic laparotomy set, biliary instruments, vascular instruments, and additional items such as long clamps and a self-retaining retractor system (the Bookwalter retractor is the system of choice).

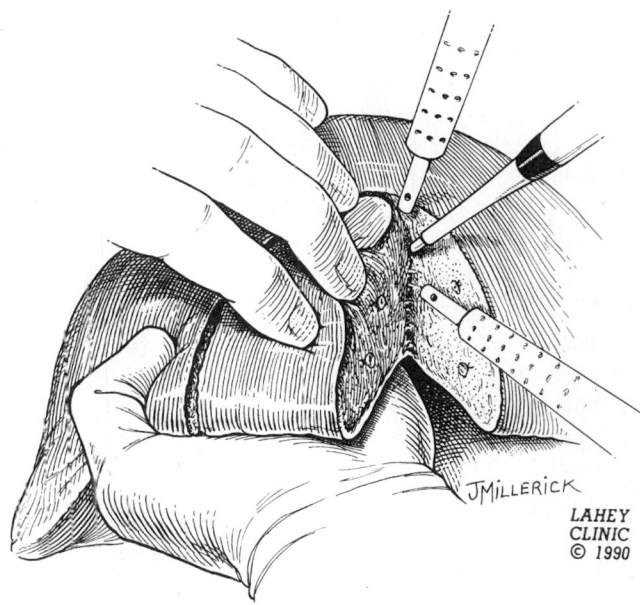

FIGURE 12-33 The surgeon places a hand beneath the liver lobe while using the CUSA handpiece to dissect through the parenchyma. The assistant affords gentle manual retraction and suction to the site.

Liver sutures, absorbable or nonabsorbable, according to surgeon's preference, vessel loops, and umbilical tapes should be available on the sterile field.

Hemostatic material, such as Gelfoam, Surgicel, or Avitene, absorbable collagen sheets should be readily available when the resection is begun.

Equipment needed for hepatic resection includes an intraoperative ultrasonic 7 mHz probe and unit, CUSA unit and handpiece, electrosurgical unit (set on blend 3 and coagulation at 100 to 110 during resection), two suction tubings and tips, smoke-evacuation system, surgeon's headlight, and an argon-beam coagulator unit and handpiece if this is the surgeon's preference.

Operative procedure

1. Various types of incisions may be performed according to the surgeon's preference: a basic bilateral subcostal with an upper midline extension; the right subcostal incision is longer; a J-shaped incision, beginning at the xiphoid process and extending down and across the rectus abdominis muscle and then anteriorly and laterally; a midline incision extending from the xiphoid to the pubis. Variations in these incisions may be applied.
2. Once the patient's abdomen is opened, the liver is assessed for resectability.
3. Intraoperative ultrasonography must confirm an absence of tumor in the segment of liver that is to remain.
4. The vascular structures supporting the remaining segment must also have margins free from tumor involvement.

5. The surgeon then assesses the porta hepatis and foramen of Winslow by palpation for extrahepatic disease. Should enlarged or suspicious lymph nodes be found along the gastrohepatic ligament or in the area of the celiac axis, a decision to abandon resection of the liver may be made. It is critical for the surgeon to carefully weigh this decision. Suspicious tissue may be sampled and sent for frozen-section analysis to assist in deciding the best plan of treatment for the patient.

6. Lymph node dissection may be performed in an attempt to remove all extrahepatic disease or for pathologic confirmation of lymph node metastasis. Surgeons' philosophies differ in regard to extrahepatic disease–defining resectability. Radioimmunoguided surgery (RIGS) is an innovative intraoperative technology that has been developed to better assist the surgeon in assessing lymph node metastasis. This technique is discussed later in this chapter.

7. When a decision to resect is made, the surgeon begins with mobilization of the liver (Fig. 12-34).

8. The falciform ligament is disconnected, and the attachment of the hepatocolic ligament and the renohepatic ligament is separated from the inferior surface of the right lobe of the liver.

9. The right lobe of the liver is then manipulated so that the triangular ligament can be dissected using long Metzenbaum scissors.

10. For right trisegmentectomy, the hilar dissection is the same as that for right lobectomy.

11. The cystic duct and artery are dissected, ligated, and divided.

12. The peritoneum and lymphatics are then dissected clear for access to the right branch of the portal vein. If applicable, clamps are applied for ligation and division of the vessel. Suture may be required to close the proximal end of the vessel, depending on the length.

13. Care is taken to identify the biliary ducts that are to be included in resection and especially to identify the duct that passes into the segment that will be retained.

14. The exact location of the umbilical fissure is then identified. It is the landmark to identify vascular structures and hepatic ducts that will be ligated and divided and those that must remain intact for viability of the remaining segment.

15. The right lobe of the liver is retracted anteriorly and to the left to expose the vena cava.

16. A vessel loop is placed to encircle the right hepatic vein. Small branches are ligated and divided, and the right hepatic vein is then clamped, ligated, and divided with care.

17. The resection line is scored with the electrosurgical pencil.

18. For right trisegmentectomy the falciform ligament on the anterior surface and the umbilical fissure or

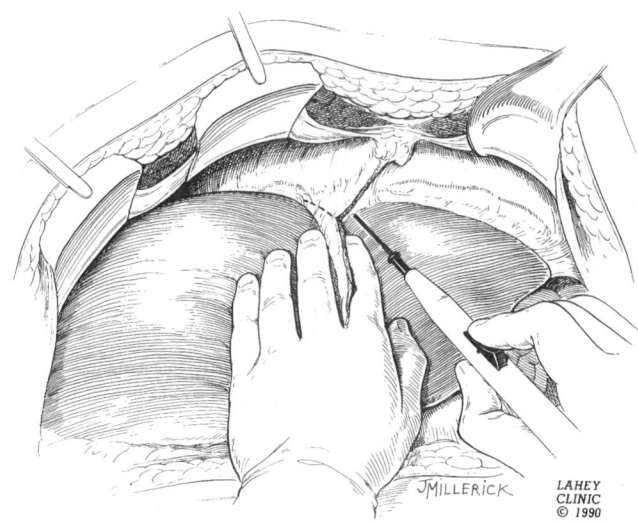

FIGURE 12-34 With the Bookwalter self-retaining retractor in place the liver is mobilized by separating the falciform ligament using electrocautery. Curved Metzenbaum scissors may also be used.

round ligament on the inferior surface mark the transsection line.

19. The CUSA is used to dissect through the parenchyma.

20. Devascularization of the three segments is achieved, and those become cyanotic. Upon removal of the liver segments, the remaining segment is assessed for vascularization and hemostasis.

21. Appearance of the remaining left segment is almost alarming, considering that 75% to 80% of the patient's liver has been removed.

22. The abdominal wound is closed.

Left Hepatic Trisegmentectomy

Left hepatic trisegmentectomy refers to the resection of the left lobe and right anterior lobe of the liver. As with right trisegmentectomy, decision is contemplated only after inspection, palpation, and ultrasonic examination of the liver indicate that the remaining right inferior segment is free from tumor. Extrahepatic disease is also assessed.

Procedural considerations

Procedural considerations are the same as that for right trisegmentectomy.

Operative procedure

1. A midline incision is made extending from xiphoid to pubis.

2. The liver is isolated and the Bookwalter retractor is placed.

3. The liver is closely examined for extent of disease by visualization, palpation, intraoperative ultrasonography, and possibly RIGS.

4. The ligament teres hepatis is divided, and the falciform ligament is disconnected.

5. The left triangular and coronary ligaments are divided.

6. The left lobe of the liver can be lifted anteriorly and retracted to the right to expose the vena cava and left hepatic vein (Fig. 12-35).

7. The left branch of the portal vein, left hepatic artery, and the left hepatic duct are identified, ligated, and divided.

8. Parenchymal transsection begins in front of the vena cava at the ductus venosus.

9. Using the CUSA, an intersegmental plane is transsected from the hilum of the liver toward the diaphragm (Fig. 12-36, *A* to *D*).

10. Complete hemostasis and attention to bile leaks is achieved. Abdominal drains may be placed.

11. The abdomen is closed.

Radioimmunoguided Surgery (RIGS)

RIGS is an innovative technique used intraoperatively to detect cancer that may not be readily detected by inspection or palpation. This technique has been found to be very useful in determining safe margins of resection for metastatic colon cancer lesions in the liver. Current studies have also identified RIGS to be efficacious in assessing extrahepatic disease and occult tumor in patients with rising serum CEA levels.

About 2 to 3 weeks before surgery, patients receive an intravenous injection of radiolabeled monoclonal antibody, which binds reactive antigen on or near the surface of tumors cells. The antigen-antibody bond keeps minute amounts of radioactivity, or gamma emissions, localized in tumor tissue. An intraoperatively used, hand-held, gamma ray–detecting probe connected to a microcomputer emits an audible signal when the radioactive waves hit the crystal in the distal end of the probe.[3] The Neoprobe instrument (Fig. 12-37) gives a digital reading as well as an audible pitch that rises or falls when placed on the gamma ray–emitting tissue. This advance in the intraoperative detection of adenocarcinoma and metastases can greatly assist in decision making and resection of diseased tissue.

Procedural considerations

Instrumentation includes a basic laparotomy set, biliary instruments, vascular instruments, and additional items such as long clamps and a self-retaining retractor system (the Bookwalter retractor is the system of choice). Minimal suture (2-0 and 3-0 silk ties, 2-0 suture ligature) is added to the sterile field until the abdomen is explored, and the extent of disease is assessed. The patient is placed in the supine position. A nasogastric tube will be inserted by the anesthesiologist after induction of general anesthesia and intubation. An indwelling urinary catheter is inserted before the abdominal prep. The abdomen is prepped from nipple line to midthigh. A midline abdominal incision provides access to the liver. Vertical abdominal incisions are advantageous because they can be made and closed more rapidly and permit better exposure of all abdominal organs.

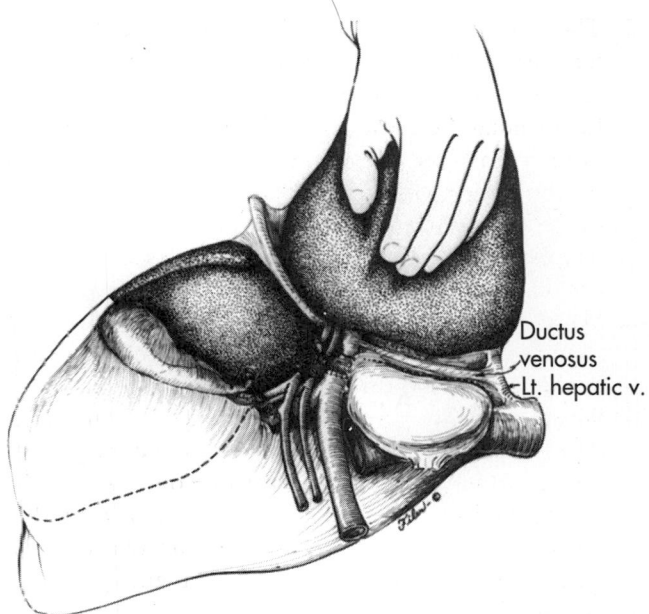

Ductus venosus

Lt. hepatic v.

FIGURE 12-35 Left trisegmentectomy. The lobe of the liver is retracted anteriorly to demonstrate the ductus venosus and the intended resection line through the right lobe.

Operative procedure

The operative procedure is identical to the second-look laparotomy procedure as described previously.

1. A midline abdominal incision is made from the xiphoid process to the pubis.

2. Intraoperative scanning of the liver and abdominal viscera is performed using the probe.

3. The digital readings as well as the anatomic structures being scanned are recorded.

4. Great care is taken to scan mesenteric, pelvic, and periaortic lymph nodes individually.

5. The liver is scanned, and areas emitting strong-pitched tones are marked with a sterile marking pen. A very distinct change in pitch may be noted on liver tissue within a 2 to 3 cm radius of the tumor site.

6. Intraoperative ultrasonography and a review of the CT and MRI scans of the patient's liver are used to further confirm the liver lesions.

7. Margins for resection are drawn using an electrosurgical knife on a blend 2 setting at 40.

8. Resection of the lesion may be segmental, circumferential, or lobar.

9. After each resection the margins of healthy liver tissue adjacent to the resection site are scanned, and readings are recorded. This procedure continues until all tissue emitting high gamma-ray waves has been resected.

10. Specimens are sent to the pathology lab for further pathologic and histologic analysis. The perioperative nurse greatly enhances the correlation of pathologic diagnosis with the intraoperative RIGS findings by specifically and accurately identifying the tissue specimens.

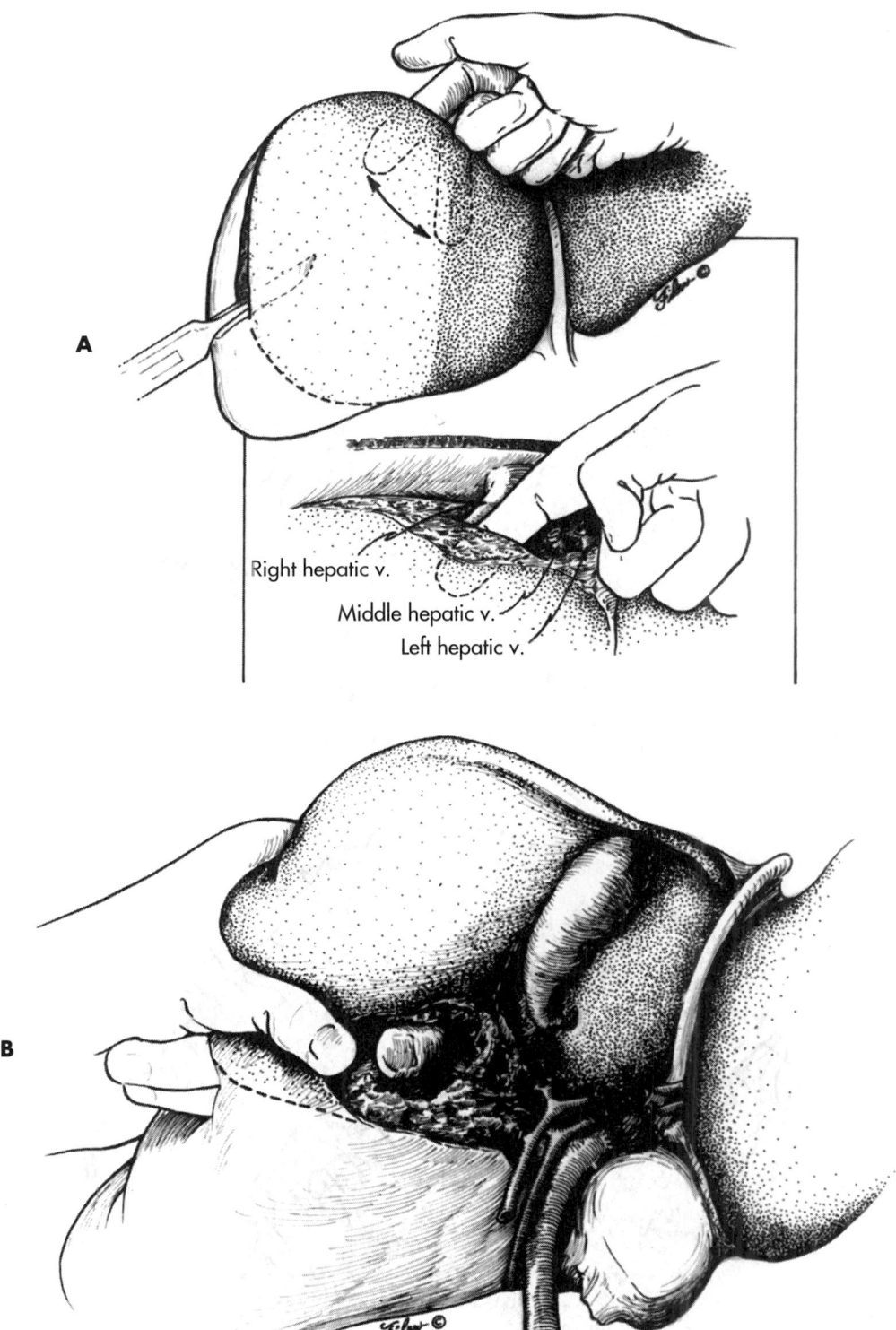

Right hepatic v.

Middle hepatic v.

Left hepatic v.

FIGURE 12–36   Left hepatic trisegmentectomy. **A,** Demonstrates the intended resection from the anterior viewpoint. **B,** Manual retraction of the segments included in left trisegmentectomy and finger-fracture through the parenchyma.

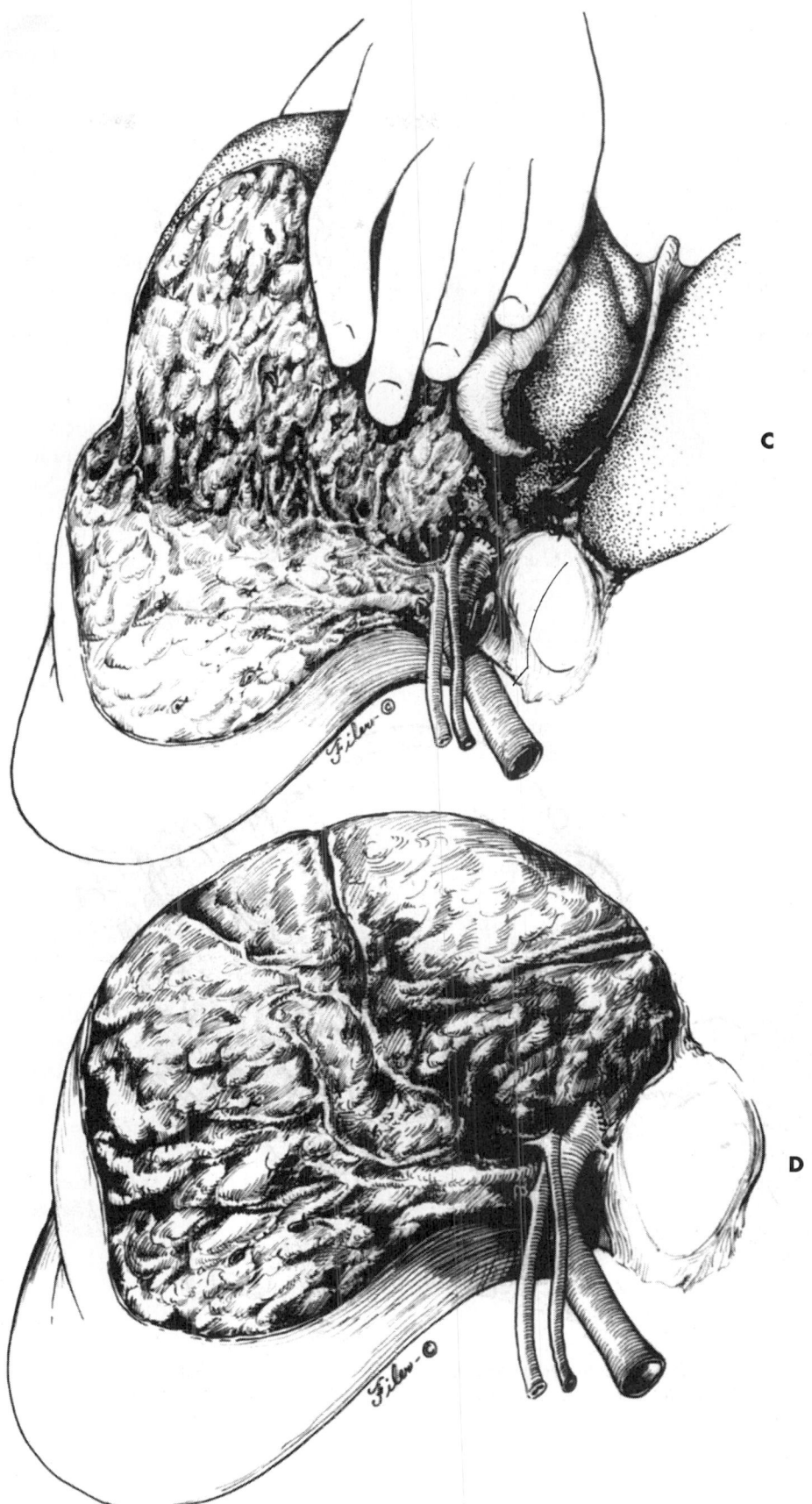

FIGURE 12–36, cont'd   **C,** The liver parenchyma s transsected in the right lobe. **D,** Illustration of the remaining liver after left trisegmentectomy.

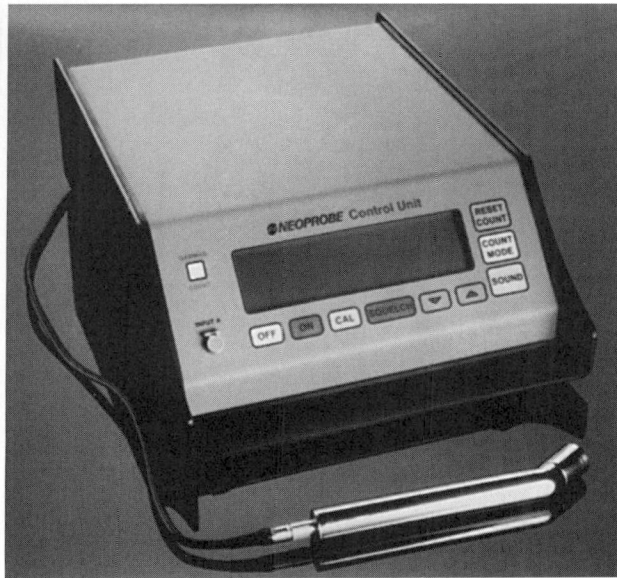

FIGURE 12-37   Neoprobe instrument.

11. The surgeon determines the best plan of treatment for the patient based upon the information obtained from intraoperative assessment of the extent of the patient's disease. Resection of RIGS-positive tissue may result in an extensive retroperitoneal lymphadenectomy, liver resection, gastrohepatic ligament lymphadenectomy, or the resection of colon, uterus, or bladder. Information gained by use of the probe and subsequent pathologic confirmation of sampled tumor sites may indicate that the best plan of care for the patient is to close the abdomen and encourage a speedy return to home.

Hepatic Artery Pump Insertion

Insertion of a continuous-flow hepatic artery pump is performed when the patient with a carcinoma in the liver may benefit from direct intrahepatic infusion of chemotherapy. The patient may have a primary hepatoma that is malignant or may have metastatic disease from a primary site such as a colon cancer.

The use of hepatic artery chemotherapy is based on the pharmacologic principle that regional administration of certain drugs can lead to higher concentrations at the site of the tumor.[6] In the 1970s and 1980s intrahepatic chemotherapeutic agents were administered into the hepatic artery through a catheter placed into the gastroduodenal branch or the gastroepiploic branch and then exteriorized through the right lateral abdominal wall for port access. Implantable continuous-flow pumps have made this a more efficient procedure for patients to endure. The pumps are accessed with noncoring needles through which the pump is loaded with the prescribed dosage of chemotherapeutic drug. The pump then delivers a prescribed dosage continuously over a 14-day period (Research Highlight 12-2).

12-2 RESEARCH HIGHLIGHT

Approximately 140,000 people in the United States were diagnosed with colon or rectal cancer in 1996, and 40% of those patients will ultimately die of metastasis from that disease. The liver is the dominant metastatic site in the majority of colorectal cancer patients. More than 80% of patients with liver metastasis succumb to liver failure. In some patients metastasis is confined to the liver. The use of regional chemotherapy of certain drugs administered via the hepatic artery has been in practice since the 1980s. Higher drug concentrations at the site of the tumor has been the premise for administering intrahepatic artery chemotherapy.

Dr. Alan P. Venook (Associate Professor of Clinical Medicine, Division of Hematology and Oncology at The University of California, San Francisco) summarized an update on the use of intrahepatic artery chemotherapy and studies that support future applications of adjuvant therapy by the intrahepatic artery route.

Venook cited four large randomized studies that failed to demonstrate a survival advantage of regional versus systemic treatment, though two meta-analyses confirmed an improvement in response rate and suggest a trend upward in survival. Two randomized trials have shown improved survival in patients treated with intrahepatic artery chemotherapy as compared with those given supportive care. Quality of life also appeared to be superior in those patients treated with intrahepatic artery chemotherapy. Complications in the studies included hepatobiliary toxicity and varied surgery-related occurrences including catheter dislodgment and gastrointestinal misperfusion. Improved and standardized surgical techniques for pump and catheter placement and newer chemotherapy combinations have demonstrated improved phase II study results. A randomized trial is currently being conducted by the Cancer and Leukemia Group B (CALGB) to better ascertain the utility of intrahepatic artery therapy.

Venook concluded that the regional advantage gained by the intrahepatic artery route may prove to be most advantageous for the delivery of newer biologic agents.

From Venook, A.P. (1997). Update on hepatic intra-arterial chemotherapy, *Oncology, 11*(7), 947-954.

Procedural considerations

Patients scheduled for hepatic artery pump insertion will have had angiographic studies to define the anatomy of that particular patient's arterial flow and to confirm the patency of the portal vein. Portal vein occlusion is an absolute contraindication to any manipulation of the hepatic artery. Confirmation that extrahepatic disease is absent may be performed radiographically and by exploration of the abdomen at the time of insertion.

A basic laparotomy set of instruments is used. Instrumentation may also include biliary instruments and a self-retaining retractor system (the Bookwalter retractor is the system of choice). Minimal suture (2-0 and 3-0 silk ties, 2-0 suture ligature) is added to the sterile field until the abdomen is explored and the extent of disease is assessed. The patient is placed in the supine position. A nasogastric tube will be inserted by the anesthesiologist after induction of general anesthesia and intubation. An indwelling urinary catheter is inserted before the abdominal prep. The abdomen is prepped from nipple line to midthigh. A midline abdominal incision provides access to the liver. An additional horizontal incision is made lateral to the midline incision for the implantable pump.

The perioperative nurse will need to have the pump available in the OR. Heparin and saline warmed to 40° C is also needed. The pump is treated as an implantable device for reasons of manufacturer's tracking and institutional policies. Before insertion, the pump is tested at the sterile field to ensure that it works properly.

Operative procedure

1. A midline incision is made.
2. An exploratory laparotomy is performed to exclude unresectable extrahepatic tumor.
3. The porta hepatis, celiac axis, and common hepatic artery areas are examined for lymph node involvement.
4. When extrahepatic disease is ruled out, a cholecystectomy is performed. Cholecystectomy is performed to prevent drug-induced cholecystitis.
5. Vascular dissection is then performed. The hepatic artery is identified, and the gastroduodenal branch is isolated using vessel loops distally and proximally. The common hepatic artery may be isolated with a vessel loop to ensure that the potential for vascular accident is controlled.
6. Small collateral branches off the gastroduodenal artery are dissected and either clipped or tied off to prevent GI ulceration and hemorrhage.
7. An incision is made in the right side of the abdomen to place the pump into a subcutaneous pocket. The pocket should be deep enough to ensure that the drum of the pump is well below the incisional line. Accessing the pump through normal subcutaneous tissues is much more comfortable and efficient for the patient than attempting to penetrate granulation tissue.
8. The pump is secured in the pocket using 2-0 polypropylene sutures placed through the anchoring loops.
9. The hepatic artery catheter is inserted through the muscular and fascial layers into the right upper abdominal cavity.

10. The hepatic artery catheter is then measured, cut to the appropriate length, and prepared with heparinized saline for insertion into the gastroduodenal artery.
11. Silk 2-0 ties are placed proximally and distally to the site of the intended arteriotomy and are secured with a hemostat.
12. The vessel loops are tightened to prevent hemorrhage during catheter insertion.
13. Arteriotomy is made with a #11 blade. The catheter is inserted using vascular forceps as the proximal vessel loop and silk tie are opened to facilitate insertion.
14. The catheter is inserted through the gastroduodenal artery so that its tip lies just at the juncture of the gastroduodenal artery. The 2-0 silk ties are secured snuggly on either side of the intraluminal lead.[6]
15. To check liver perfusion, 5 ml of fluorescein is administered through the pump as a bolus injection. A Wood's lamp is used to observe perfusion into the lobes of the liver. The stomach and duodenum are also examined to ensure that these viscera are not perfused.
16. Hemostasis is completed, and the abdominal cavity is irrigated with warm saline.
17. The abdomen is closed.
18. The subcutaneous pocket incision is closed.
19. Dressings are applied.

Liver Transplantation

Liver transplantation is the implantation of a liver from a donor into a recipient. The total procedure involves retrieving, or procuring, the liver from a donor, transporting the donor liver to the recipient's hospital, performing a hepatectomy on the recipient, and implanting the donor liver, including reanastomosis of suprahepatic vena cava, infrahepatic vena cava, portal vein and hepatic artery, biliary reconstruction with end-to-end anastomosis of donor and recipient common bile ducts, or Roux-en-Y anastomosis if the recipient bile duct is absent as a result of biliary atresia.

Liver transplantation is indicated for patients with end-stage liver disease resulting from postnecrotic cirrhosis, primary biliary cirrhosis, sclerosing cholangitis, Budd-Chiari syndrome, biliary atresia, metabolic disorders, and sometimes alcoholic cirrhosis. Patients with primary hepatic malignancies and metastatic malignancies confined to the liver are also candidates for liver transplantation. When malignancies are the cause of the end-stage liver disease, intraoperative radiation of the right upper quadrant after hepatectomy and before the transplantation may be performed in institutions employing this advanced technology.

Procedural considerations

Successful transplantation requires the cooperative efforts of the organ-procurement agency and the staffs of the donor and recipient hospitals. Usually two members of the surgical team from the recipient's hospital travel to the donor's hospital to procure the donated liver. Multiple transplant teams may arrive at the donor hospital to procure the various organs available and viable for transplantation.

The donor operating room is set up for a major laparotomy procedure. Basic instrumentation and equipment include a basic laparotomy set, cardiovascular instruments, power sternal saw, and nephrectomy instruments.

The procurement team provides special Collins solution for flushing the organs, sterile plastic containers and ice chests for organs, and in situ flush tubing. The liver is generally placed in two Lahey bags immediately after procurement. The common practice is to procure the heart and kidneys as well as the liver; other organs, tissues, and bone may also be procured.

Each transplantation surgeon has preferred instruments, supplies, and sutures. In general, the following are needed in the recipient operating room: a basic laparotomy set, cardiovascular instrument set, an assortment of T-tubes, slush unit or means of providing iced lactated Ringer's solution, 2 electrosurgical units, Bair Hugger unit and blanket, temperature probe, intravenous volumetric pumps on stands, 2 blood warmers or water baths, a urinary Foley catheter, insertion tray, and urinometer.

A medium sterile draped instrument table is needed for preparation of the liver away from the main sterile operative field and instrument tables.

Large-bore cannulas for intravenous monitoring and fluid or blood replacement lines are placed in addition to an arterial line and central venous line.

Two surgeon headlights and light sources will be necessary to augment visualization of the abdominal site. A venovenous bypass system may be used to support peripheral blood flow. Extra drape sheets, table covers, gowns, towels, gloves, sponges, and laparotomy pads, cold intravenous Ringer's solution, sterile intravenous administration set for flushing the new liver, umbilical tape, booties, and vessel loops should be available to support the many steps of the transplantation procedure.

A cart containing sutures and the numerous other small items should be set up and placed into the room for each procedure. This practice eliminates the circulating nurse running for extra supplies.

The procedure requires a bilateral subcostal incision with possible midline extension and removal of the xiphoid. The right side of the chest may be entered to provide more exposure when needed.

In addition to previously noted nursing diagnoses, patient goals, and nursing interventions, the following aspects of implementing the perioperative care plan deserve special attention.

Patient Positioning

The patient is placed in the supine position with knees slightly flexed and padded. Accurate body alignment is essential. Foam padding should be used under all poten-tial pressure areas. Heel protectors are applied. The safety strap is placed over the lower part of the thighs and secured. A forced warm-air blanket is applied over the upper body, neck, and head to assist in maintaining the patient's temperature. Fluid warmers will be used to warm the blood products and IV solutions that will be infused during the procedure.

Blood Loss and Replacement

Blood loss may be extensive, and replacement must be timely. Blood products normally available at the beginning of the procedure include 10 units each of packed cells, fresh-frozen plasma, and platelets. Sufficient clot should be available in the blood bank to process additional blood products if needed. As in all surgical procedures, care must be exercised by all members of the surgical team in handling bloody sponges and instruments. Universal precautions should be strictly enforced. Nursing and medical team members should have previously been tested for immunity to hepatitis B and should have received Heptavax or another appropriate vaccine if indicated. Needle sticks must be reported and treated according to hospital policy.

Intraoperative Laboratory Testing

Thirty to 50 blood specimens can be drawn for analysis during the procedure. This blood must be recorded on the blood-loss record and calculated into replacement needs. The specimens are delivered to the laboratory immediately. A telephone in the operating room is most useful for receiving reports directly from the laboratory.

Length of Procedure

Procedures may last from 6 to 20 hours but normally last 8 to 10 hours. Special attention must be directed toward maintaining the integrity of the sterile environment from the standpoint of time and the numbers of people moving in and out of the room.

Communication with Family

Frequent reports to the family are important. Family members usually are knowledgeable about liver function tests and laboratory values and want this information, in addition to reports on the condition of their loved one. One person should be assigned in advance to make regular contacts with family and support persons.

Communication between Teams

The perioperative nurse will ensure that communication occurs between teams. The procurement team, the anesthesiology team, and the surgical team must all be "in sync" for a successful transplantation procedure. The perioperative nurse assists with tracking issues and communicating necessary information between the teams. The perioperative nurse will communicate blood-loss volume in suction canisters and on sponges, will communicate the availability of blood and blood products, lab results, and time of organ arrival, will track ischemic time, and so on.

Operative procedure

1. Bilateral subcostal incisions are made with a midline incision extended toward the umbilicus.
2. Initial dissection of the underlying tissues is achieved with electrosurgery and suture ligatures.
3. Isolation of all hilar structures and dissection to mobilize the lobes of the native liver are performed.
4. The retrohepatic vena cava is skeletalized, as are the hepatic artery, portal vein, common bile duct, and inferior vena cava.
5. Nothing irreparable is done to the native liver before the arrival and examination of the donor liver.
6. After the arrival of the donor organ, the patient is prepared for venovenous bypass, if indicated, by incision into the left external iliac vein and the left axillary vein.
7. Cannulation into both the femoral and axillary sites allows for bypass of the portal system and inferior vena cava.
8. The infrahepatic vena cava and the suprahepatic vena cava are clamped, as are the portal vein, the hepatic artery, and the common bile duct.
9. Native hepatectomy is then performed.
10. Revascularization of the donor organ begins with an end-to-end anastomosis of the suprahepatic vena cava with double-armed 3-0 vascular suture.
11. The infrahepatic vena cava anastomosis is performed, followed by the end-to-end anastomosis of the portal vein.
12. At this point, all venous clamps are removed, and blood flow through the vena cava and portal vein is restored.
13. Hemostasis of the anastomosis sites is then achieved.
14. Venovenous bypass is discontinued, and the cannulation sites are closed.
15. In situations in which the portal vein anastomosis may obstruct the ability to anastomose the hepatic artery, the hepatic artery anastomosis may be performed before that of the portal vein.
16. Clamps are removed from the vena cava sites, the portal vein, and the hepatic artery simultaneously.
17. Modifications in the method of arterial reconstruction may be necessary, depending on the anatomic structure of the donor organ and the recipient's remaining hepatic arterial stump.
18. The postrevascularization phase focuses on achieving hemostasis. Complete hemostasis may require extensive time at this point. Bleeding may be exacerbated by a fibrinolytic episode associated with the reperfusion of the donor organ.
19. Biliary reconstruction varies with the status of the recipient's biliary tract. If biliary atresia is the cause of the patient's end-stage liver disease, choledochoenterostomy into a Roux-en-Y loop of jejunum is performed (Fig. 12-38, *A*). Sclerosing cholangitis also necessitates this biliary reconstruction procedure. An end-to-end reconstruction of the common bile duct may be possible if the recipient's biliary tract is free from disease and a T-tube can be placed into the native duct (Fig. 12-38, *B*).
20. Drains are inserted and leave through the right abdominal wall. The abdomen is then closed.

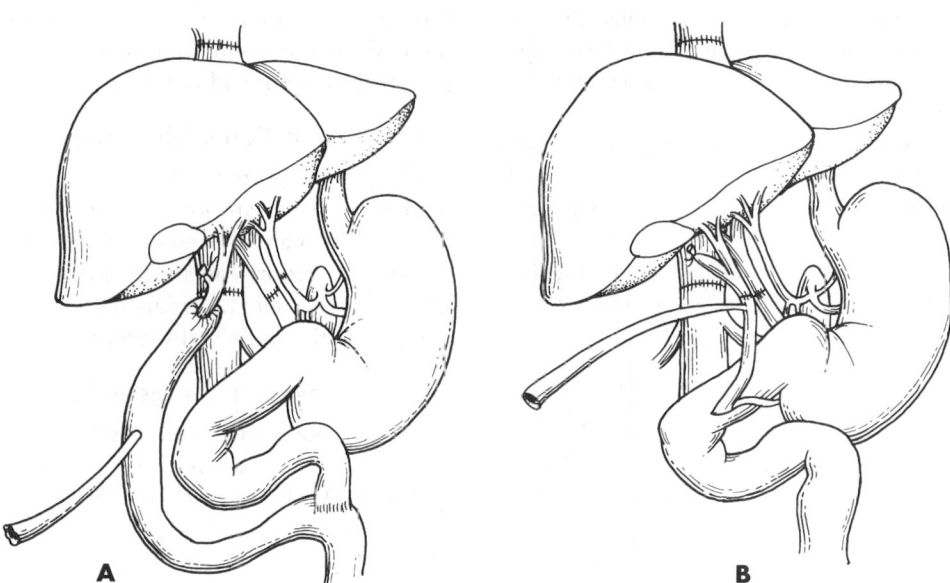

FIGURE 12-38   Completed orthotopic liver transplant with Roux-en-Y biliary reconstruction (**A**), and end-to-end anastomosis of the donor-to-recipient common bile ducts (**B**).

Donor Hepatectomy

Donor hepatectomy is performed for procurement of a healthy liver for transplant into a patient suffering from end-stage liver failure. This procedure occurs only after the donor patient has been determined to be brain dead and family consent for organ donation has been obtained. Donor hepatectomy can be performed at any hospital. Organ procurement agencies arrange contact with transplant centers when a viable organ donor has been identified. Candidates for liver transplantations are placed on a national-network waiting list and are matched according to urgency of need, blood type, and body size.

Procedural considerations

Once the liver transplant candidate has been identified, the procurement team from that transplant center travels to the institution where the organ donor is hospitalized. If multiple organs are being donated, surgeons from several transplant centers may arrive to procure the organs they will be transplanting at their respective centers.

The procedure for procurement of multiple organs may differ according to the transplant centers represented. Most commonly the systemic cooling of the donor's body temperature is started before the procurement of the heart. Cannulation sites may also vary according to which organs are procured.

The perioperative nurses at the donor hospital are responsible for supplying a basic laparotomy setup with instrumentation to open the sternum. Basic vascular clamps are also required for clamping the major vascular structures. Cold lactated Ringer's solution for parenteral infusion and cold Ringer's solution for irrigation are usually used in large amounts.

Perioperative nurses involved in organ procurement procedures must first consider their ethical and moral beliefs. Often the organ donor is a young and otherwise healthy individual who does not exhibit outward signs of death. The donor is brought to the surgical suite on life-support systems. The donor may appear as any patient would under general anesthesia. Strong feelings of uncertainty, denial, and internalization of fear for one's own loved ones must be dealt with appropriately. Perioperative nurses involved with organ procurement procedures must support and respect each person's feelings, since that individual may be grieving for the donor and his or her family during and long after the procedure is completed.

Operative procedure

1. The donor is positioned supine on the OR bed. The skin area from neck to midthigh is prepped and draped.
2. A midline incision is made from the suprasternal notch to the pubis.
3. A subcostal incision is performed bilaterally on the abdomen for better exposure of the abdominal viscera.
4. Retractors are placed to provide optimal exposure of the organs that will be procured.
5. The aorta and vena cava, superior and inferior to the liver and kidneys, are skeletalized by dissection and ligation of the lymphatics and smaller vasculatures.
6. The porta hepatis is dissected; the superior mesenteric artery and celiac trunk are dissected and delicately exposed as close to the aorta as is convenient.
7. The superior mesenteric vein is dissected and prepared for cannulation. The donor is heparinized and systemically cooled.
8. If the heart is to be procured, at this point the procurement of the heart is achieved.
9. Further cooling and flushing of the pancreas, liver, and kidneys are achieved by cannulation and infusion of cold lactated Ringer's solution through the inferior vena cava just superior to the bifurcation.
10. One to 2 liters of lactated Ringer's solution are infused before the organs have been properly cooled.
11. The liver, pancreas, spleen, and a segment of the duodenum harboring the pancreatic duct are procured en bloc by placing clamps on the suprahepatic and infrahepatic venae cavae.
12. The superhepatic vena cava is transsected with a surrounding cuff of diaphragm intact.
13. The infrahepatic vena cava is transsected above the level of the renal veins.
14. The celiac axis is detached from the aorta with an aortic patch or taken with a full aortic circumference.
15. The duodenal segment is procured, using a linear stapling device at opposite ends of the segment.
16. The en bloc organs are taken to a back table for further dissection and ligation to separate the liver from the en bloc pancreas, spleen, and duodenal segment graft. Meanwhile, other members of the procurement team continue working to free the kidneys and ureters if they are to be taken.
17. The liver is placed in a basin of very cold Ringer's solution, double-bagged in sterile Lahey bags, and placed in an ice chest for transport to the recipient's hospital.
18. The kidneys are placed in sterile cassettes and mechanically perfused.
19. The pancreatic en bloc graft is also placed in a basin of cold Ringer's solution, bagged, and transported in a thermal chest of ice.
20. The abdomen is closed with a single layer of 1 or 0 nonabsorbable suture.
21. Drapes are removed, and the body is cleaned and washed. Tubes and infusion lines are tied off or clamped. Sometimes the family of the donor re-

quests to view the body after organ donation. This factor may be important in helping them face the loss of their loved one. The perioperative nurse can assist them in their grieving process by providing them with a quiet and private environment in which to say good-bye to their family member. Removing the donor's body from the OR where the surgical procedure took place is best. The nurse should make sure that the donor is clothed and covered with a warm blanket and then stay with the family to support them through this most painful realization.

22. Morgue care is performed, and the donor is transported by stretcher to the morgue.

Living-Related Liver Transplantation

Just as kidney transplantation has evolved into cadaveric donor and living-related donor possibilities, so too has liver transplantation. On November 27, 1989, a 21-month-old girl received the left lobe of her mothers liver at the University of Chicago Medical Center. The capacity of the liver to regenerate provided the scientific basis for development of the living related donor transplantation procedure. Surgeons in Australia, Brazil and Japan had attempted such operations before in an attempt to save desperately ill children in end-stage liver failure.[1] In Japan, a study of 56 living-related liver transplant patients demonstrated an 88% survival after 5 years.[4]

Reduced-size and split-liver transplants have been performed successfully. Reduced-size liver transplantation has been performed for infants, children, or very small adults. Initial results of reduced-size and split-liver transplantations from the pioneering centers were disappointing. This was attributable, at least in part, to the critical clinical condition of the patients undergoing transplantation. The improvements in technique and growing experience have led to satisfactory results comparable to those obtained with whole-organ transplantation.[4]

Where the field of transplantation will go is an ethical question. As cloning, biogenetic engineering, techniques, and technology increase the possibilities, the only limiting factor in transplantation may be our ever-changing social paradigms.

SURGERY OF THE SPLEEN

Splenectomy

Splenectomy is removal of the spleen. It is usually performed for trauma to the spleen, for specific conditions of the blood such as hemolytic jaundice or splenic anemia, or for tumors, cysts, or splenomegaly. Another common indication for splenectomy is accidental injury to the spleen during vagotomy or other gastric procedures or operations involving mobilization of the splenic flexure of the colon. If accessory spleens are present, they are also removed, because they are capable of perpetuating hypersplenic function.

Procedural considerations

Massive splenomegaly may occasionally require a thoracoabdominal approach. Abdominal suction apparatus should be available throughout all splenectomies. A cell saver may be requested.

Instrumentation is as described for a basic laparotomy, plus two large, right-angled pedicle clamps, long instruments, and hemostatic materials or devices. The patient is placed in the supine position. A nasogastric tube will be inserted by the anesthesiologist after induction of general anesthesia and intubation. An indwelling urinary catheter is inserted before the abdominal prep. The abdomen is prepped from nipple line to midthigh. A midline abdominal incision provides access to the spleen. Vertical abdominal incisions are advantageous because they can be made and closed more rapidly and permit better exposure of all abdominal organs.

Operative procedure

1. The abdomen is opened through an upper midline or left subcostal incision.
2. Retractors are placed over laparotomy packs, and gentle retraction is employed as exploration is carried out.
3. The costal margin is retracted upward.
4. The splenorenal, splenocolic, and gastrosplenic ligaments are clamped and divided with long dressing forceps, long hemostats, sponges on holders, and long Metzenbaum or Nelson scissors.
5. Adhesions posterior to the spleen are freed.
6. The spleen is delivered into the wound after these attachments are freed.
7. The short gastric vessels are now easily identified, clamped, divided, and ligated.
8. The cavity formerly occupied by the spleen is packed with moist laparotomy pads, if necessary.
9. The splenic artery and vein are dissected free with fine dissecting scissors and forceps.
10. The artery is clamped and double ligated with silk. The artery is ligated first and then the vein; such ligation permits disengorgement of blood from the spleen and facilitation of the return of venous blood to the circulatory system.
11. The splenic vein is clamped, divided, and ligated.
12. The specimen is removed; all bleeding vessels are controlled. The wound is closed in layers, as described for laparotomy, and dressings are applied.
13. Drainage is usually required only if many adhesions to the diaphragm were divided or if significant clotting abnormalities exist.

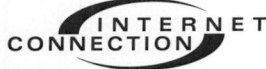

American Liver Foundation Homepage:
http://sadieo.ucsf.edu/alf/alffinal/homepagealf.html

Atlas of Liver Pathology:
http://indy.radiology.uiowa.edu/Providers/Textbooks/Liver
Pathology/Text/AtlasLiverPathology.html

Disease of the Liver:
http://cpmcnet.columbia.edu/dept/gi/disliv.html

Hans Popper Hepatopathology Library:
http://zapruder.path.med.umich.edu/users/hepatopath/

Laparoscopy: http://www.laparoscopy.com/index.html

REFERENCES

1. Fox, R.C., & Swazey, J.P. (1992). *Spare parts.* New York: Oxford University Press.
2. Flye, M.W. (1995). *Atlas of organ transplantation.* Philadelphia: W.B. Saunders.
3. Martin, E.W. Jr., Mojzisik, C.M., Hinkle, G.H. Jr., et al. (1988). Radioimmunoguided surgery using monoclonal antibody. *American Journal of Surgery, 156,* 386–392.
4. Mazziotti, A., Cavallari, A. (1997). *Techniques in liver surgery.* London: Greenwich Medical Media.
5. McNulty, J.G. (1994). *Minimally invasive therapy of the liver and biliary system.* New York: Thieme Medical Publishers, Inc.
6. Venook, A.P. (1997). Update on hepatic intra-arterial chemotherapy, *Oncology, 11*(7), 947–954.
7. Way, L.W., & Pellegrini, C.A. (1987). *Surgery of the gallbladder and bile ducts.* Philadelphia: W.B. Saunders.

CHAPTER THIRTEEN

Repair of Hernias

Dale A. Smith

> *NO DISEASE OF the body, belonging to the province of the surgeon, requires in its treatment, a better combination of accurate, anatomical knowledge with surgical skill than hernia in all its varieties.* Sir Astley Paston Cooper, 1804

According to Eubanks,[6] a hernia is an abnormal protrusion of a peritoneum-lined sac through the musculoaponeurotic covering of the abdomen. The word *hernia* is a Latin term that means 'rupture' of a portion of a structure. Weakness of the abdominal wall, congenital or acquired, results in the inability to contain the visceral contents of the abdominal cavity within their normal confines.

Groin hernias were originally documented 3500 years ago, with surgical intervention starting approximately 1500 years after that.[7] Before the intervention of surgical repair of the hernia, external supports called *trusses* were used to contain hernias that protruded from the body. In the late nineteenth century, Edoardo Bassini introduced a surgical technique that is still the foundation for modern hernia repair.[3] Approximately 75% of all hernias occur in the inguinal region. Approximately 50% of hernias are indirect inguinal hernias, and 24% are direct inguinal hernias. Incisional and ventral hernias account for approximately 10% of all hernias; as the frequency and magnitude of abdominal surgeries have increased in recent years, so has the incidence of incisional hernia. Femoral hernias account for 3%, and unusual hernias account for the remaining 5% to 10%.

Most hernias occur in males. The most common hernia in males and females is the indirect inguinal hernia. Femoral hernias occur much more frequently in females, and only 2% of females will develop inguinal hernias in their lifetime. Also, hernias occur more commonly on the right side than on the left. Herniorrhaphy is one of the most common operative procedures performed and is the preferred treatment when a defect is detected.

Hernias have a tremendous economic significance in the United States. The amount of work days lost is substantial. The trend toward ambulatory surgery with local anesthesia for hernia repair is one of many attempts to provide cost-effective healthcare than also leads to patient satisfaction.[5]

A hernia can occur in several places in the abdominal wall, with protrusion of a portion of the parietal peritoneum and often a part of the intestine. The weak places or intervals in the abdominal aponeurosis are (1) the inguinal canals, (2) the femoral rings, and (3) the umbilicus. Any number of conditions causing increased pressure within the abdomen can contribute to the formation of a hernia. Contributing factors to hernia formation include age, sex, previous surgery, obesity, nutritional state, and pulmonary and cardiac disease. Loss of tissue turgor occurs with aging and in chronic debilitating diseases.

SURGICAL ANATOMY

A hernia is a sac lined by peritoneum that protrudes through a defect in the layers of the abdominal wall. Generally a hernial mass is composed of covering tissues, a peritoneal sac, and any contained viscera. Hernias may be acquired or congenital.

Depending on their location, hernias are classified as direct inguinal, indirect inguinal, femoral, umbilical, or epigastric. Hernias in any of these groups are either reducible or irreducible; that is, the contents of the hernia sac either can be returned to the normal intraabdominal position or are trapped in the extraabdominal sac

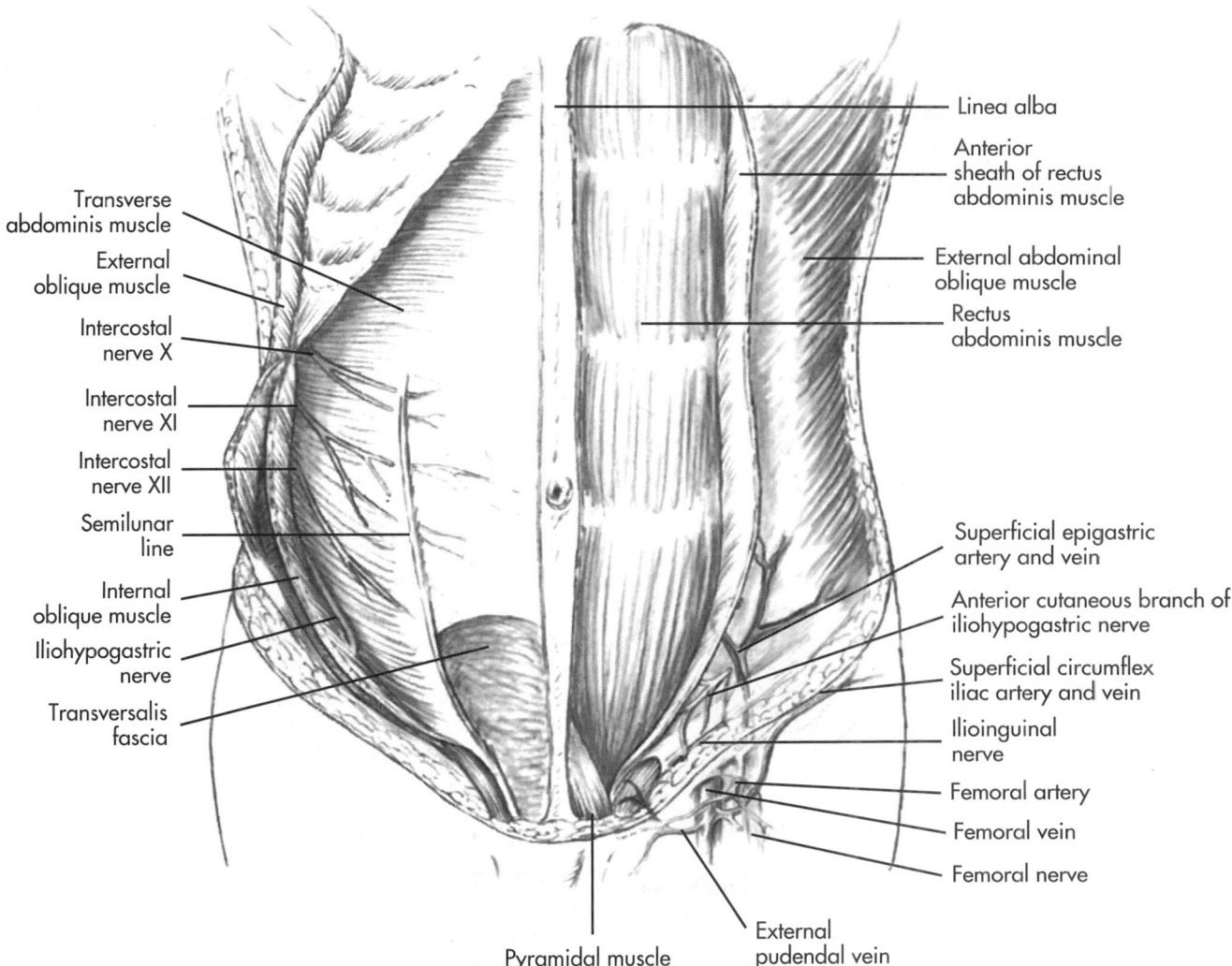

FIGURE 13-1 Perspective of the anterior abdominal wall illustrating the layers of musculature, aponeurotic extensions, vasculature, and innervation.

Labels in figure:
- Linea alba
- Anterior sheath of rectus abdominis muscle
- External abdominal oblique muscle
- Rectus abdominis muscle
- Superficial epigastric artery and vein
- Anterior cutaneous branch of iliohypogastric nerve
- Superficial circumflex iliac artery and vein
- Ilioinguinal nerve
- Femoral artery
- Femoral vein
- Femoral nerve
- External pudendal vein
- Pyramidal muscle
- Transversalis fascia
- Iliohypogastric nerve
- Internal oblique muscle
- Semilunar line
- Intercostal nerve XII
- Intercostal nerve XI
- Intercostal nerve X
- External oblique muscle
- Transverse abdominis muscle

(incarcerated). The conditions preventing the return of the hernial contents to the abdomen can result from (1) adhesions between the contents of the sac and the inner lining of the sac, (2) adhesions among the contents of the sac, or (3) narrowing of the neck of the sac. Patients with incarcerated hernias may have signs of intestinal obstruction, such as vomiting and distention. The great danger of an incarcerated hernia is that it may become strangulated. In a strangulated hernia the blood supply of the trapped sac contents becomes compromised, and eventually the sac contents necrose. When bowel is trapped in such a hernia, resection of necrosed bowel, in addition to the repair of the hernia defect, becomes mandatory.

Inguinal Hernias

The anterolateral abdominal wall consists of an arrangement of muscles, fascial layers, and muscular aponeuroses lined interiorly by peritoneum and exteriorly by skin (Figs. 13-1 and 13-2). The abdominal wall in

the groin area is composed of two groups of these structures: a superficial group (Scarpa's fascia, external and internal oblique muscles, and their aponeuroses) and a deep group (internal oblique muscle, transversalis fascia, and peritoneum).

Essential to an understanding of inguinal hernia repair is an appreciation of the central role of the transversalis fascia as the major supporting structure of the posterior inguinal floor. The inguinal canal, which contains the spermatic cord and associated structures in males and the round ligament in females, is approximately 4 cm long and takes an oblique course parallel to the groin crease. The inguinal canal is covered by the aponeurosis of the external abdominal oblique muscle, which forms a roof (Fig. 13-3). A thickened lower border of the external oblique aponeurosis forms the inguinal (Poupart's) ligament. This ligament stretches from the anterior superior iliac spine to the pubic tubercle. Structures that traverse the inguinal canal enter it from the abdomen by the internal ring, a

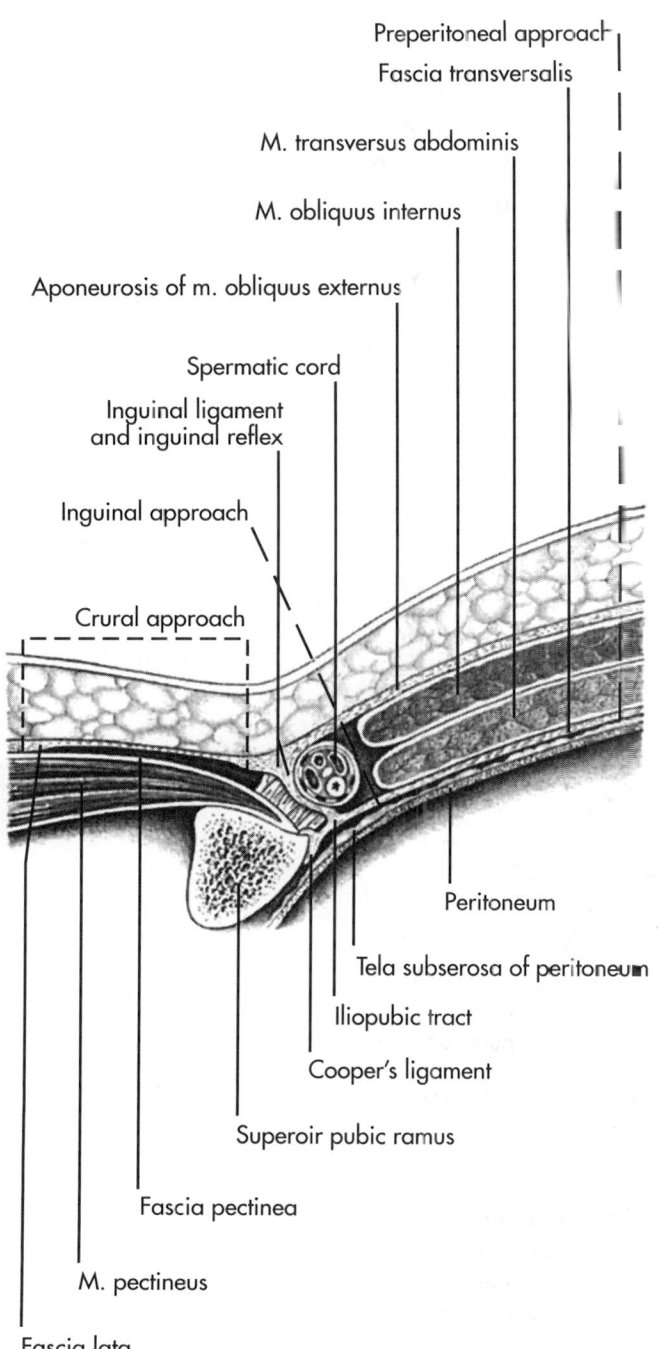

Preperitoneal approach

Fascia transversalis

M. transversus abdominis

M. obliquus internus

Aponeurosis of m. obliquus externus

Spermatic cord

Inguinal ligament
and inguinal reflex

Inguinal approach

Crural approach

Peritoneum

Tela subserosa of peritoneum

Iliopubic tract

Cooper's ligament

Superoir pubic ramus

Fascia pectinea

M. pectineus

Fascia lata

FIGURE 13-2 Anatomy and approach routes (*broken lines*) to the inguinal and femoral region in cross section.

associated aponeurosis and fascia. The posterior inguinal floor can be divided into two areas. The superior lateral area represents the internal ring, whereas the inferior medial area represents the attachment of the transversalis aponeurosis and fascia to Cooper's ligament (iliopectineal line). Cooper's ligament is the site of the insertion of the transversalis aponeurosis along the superior ramus from the symphysis pubis laterally to the femoral sheath. Notice that the inguinal portion of the transversalis fascia arises from the iliopsoas fascia and not from the inguinal ligament.

Medially and superiorly the transversalis muscle becomes aponeurotic and fuses with the aponeurosis of the internal oblique muscle to form anterior and posterior rectus sheaths. As the symphysis pubis is approached, the contributions from the internal oblique muscle become fewer and fewer. At the pubic tubercle and behind the spermatic cord or round ligament, the internal oblique muscle makes no contribution, and the posterior inguinal wall (floor of the inguinal canal) is composed solely of aponeurosis and fascia of the transversalis muscle.

None of the three groin hernias develops in the presence of a strong transversus abdominis layer and in the absence of persistent stress on the connective tissue layers. When a weakening or a tear in the aponeurosis of the transversus abdominis and the transversalis fascia occurs, the potential for development of a direct inguinal hernia is established.

Femoral Hernias

When the transversus abdominis aponeurosis and its fascia are only narrowly attached to the Cooper's ligament, a femoral hernia may develop. Dilatation of the femoral ring and canal, which allows for the prominence of the iliofemoral vessels, can also result in femoral herniation.

The walls of the femoral sheath are formed anteriorly and medially from the transversalis fascia, posteriorly from the pectineus and psoas fascia, and laterally from the iliaca fascia. The pelvis ostium consists of a relatively fixed rim of bone and connective tissue: anteriorly and medially the iliopubic tract, posteriorly the superior ramus, and laterally the iliopectineal arch.

The femoral sheath is subdivided into three compartments. The lateral compartment contains the femoral artery, and the intermediate compartment the femoral vein. The medial compartment is the smallest and constitutes the femoral canal, which is formed anteriorly and medially by the iliopubic tract. Laterally this opening is bound by the iliofemoral vessels and posteriorly by the superior pubic ramus and pectineus fascia. Superiorly, laterally, and inferiorly the fossa is formed by the falciform margin of the fascia lata.

Abdominal Hernias

The anterior abdominal wall is composed of external abdominal oblique muscles attached to a thick sheath of connective tissue called the *rectus sheath*. The linea alba

natural opening in the transversalis fascia, and exit by the external ring, an opening in the external oblique aponeurosis, to go to either the testis or the labium. If the external oblique aponeurosis is opened and the cord or round ligament is mobilized, the floor of the inguinal canal is exposed. The posterior inguinal floor is the structure that becomes defective and is susceptible to indirect, direct, or femoral hernias (Figs. 13-4 and 13-5).

The key component of the important posterior inguinal floor is the transversalis muscle of the abdomen and its

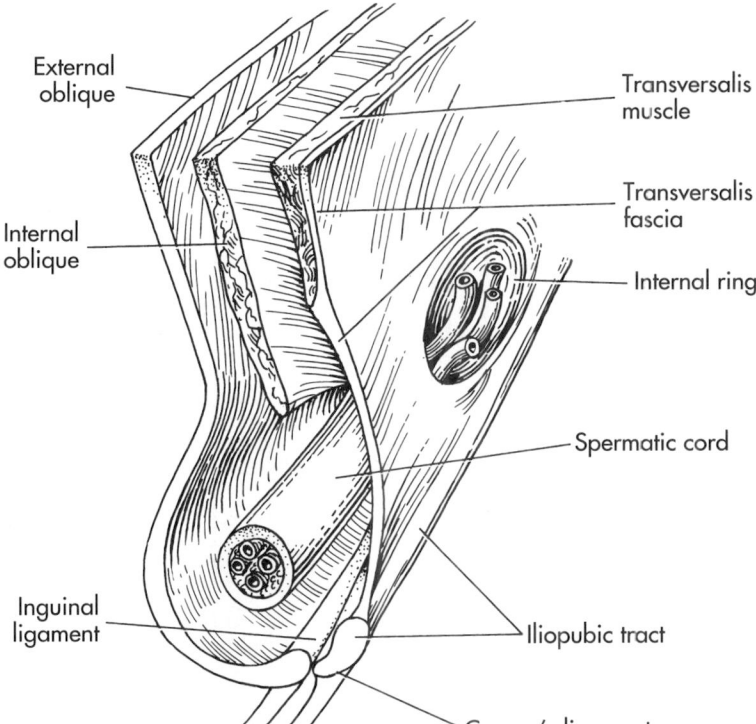

FIGURE 13-3 Right inguinal region, parasagittal section. Roof of inguinal canal is formed by external oblique aponeurosis, and floor is formed by transversalis aponeurosis and fascia.

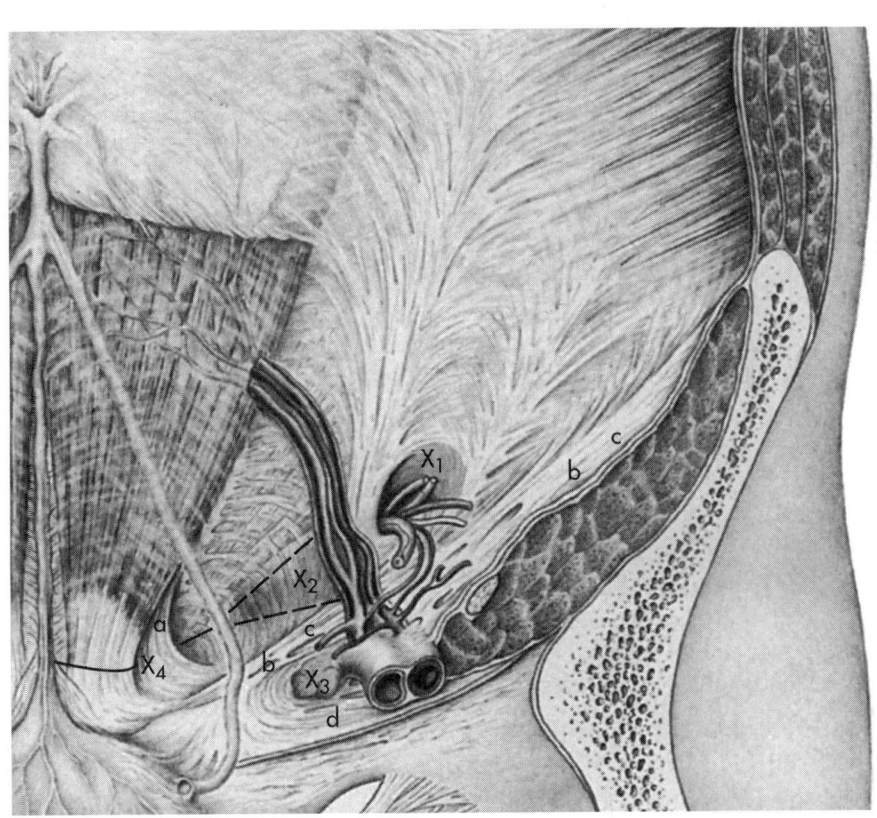

FIGURE 13-4 Anatomic representation of the abdominal wall. Internal view in the area of the hernia orifices, showing the hernial orifice of the indirect and direct inguinal hernia, the femoral hernia, and the supravesical hernia (X_1 to X_4). a, Falx inguinalis; b, inguinal ligament; c, iliopubic tract; d, pectineal ligament; X_1, indirect hernia; X_2, direct hernia; X_3, femoral hernia; X_4, supravesical hernia.

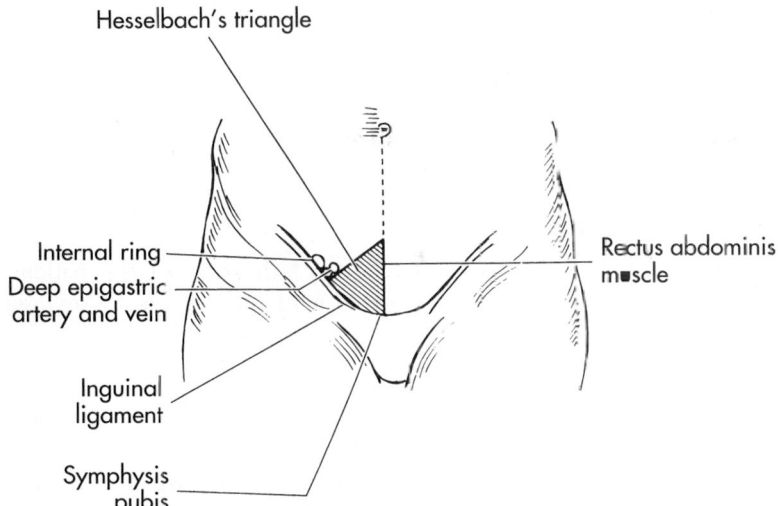

FIGURE 13-5   Schema of Hesselbach's triangle. Boundaries of Hesselbach's triangle are deep epigastric vessels laterally, inguinal ligament inferiorly, and rectus abdominis muscle medially.

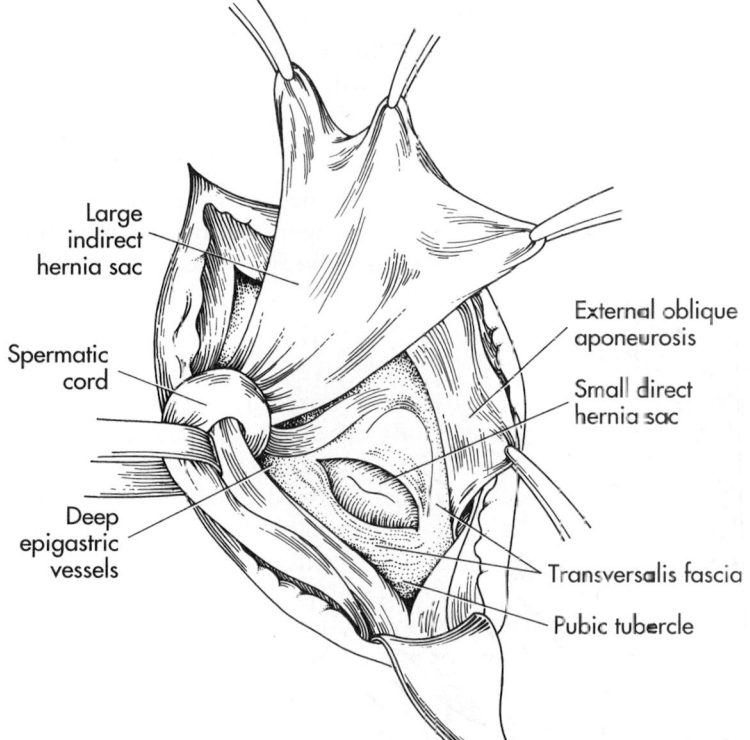

FIGURE 13-6   Defect in transversalis fascia, medial to deep epigastric vessels, gives rise to direct hernia. Defect lateral to deep epigastric vessels results in indirect hernia.

extends superiorly and inferiorly from above the xiphoid process to the pubis. Beneath the rectus sheath lies the rectus abdominis muscles, laterally to the right and left of the linea alba. Lateral to the rectus abdominis is the linea semilunaris. The transversus abdominis muscles originate from the seventh to the twelfth costal cartilages, lumbar fascia, iliac crest, and the inguinal ligament and insert on the xiphoid process, the linea alba, and the pubic tubercle. The third layer of abdominal wall includes the internal abdominal oblique muscles originating from the iliac crest, inguinal ligament, and lumbar fascia and inserting on the tenth to twelfth ribs and rectus sheath.

Direct And Indirect Inguinal Hernias

The deep epigastric vessels (inferior epigastric) arise from the external iliac vessels and enter the inguinal canal just proximal to the internal ring. The triangle formed by the deep epigastric vessels laterally, the inguinal ligament inferiorly, and the rectus abdominis muscles medially is referred to as *Hesselbach's triangle* (see Fig. 13-5).

Hernias that occur within Hesselbach's triangle are called *direct inguinal hernias*. Indirect inguinal hernias occur laterally to the deep epigastric vessels. Therefore both direct and indirect hernias represent attenuations or tears in the transversalis fascia (Fig. 13-6).

Direct hernias protrude into the inguinal canal but not into the cord and therefore rarely into the scrotum. Direct inguinal hernias usually result from heavy lifting or other strenuous activities. Indirect hernias leave the abdominal cavity at the internal inguinal ring and pass with the cord structures down the inguinal canal. Consequently the indirect hernia sac may be found in the scrotum. Indirect hernias may be either congenital, representing a persistence of the processus vaginalis, or acquired. In a congenital hernia, the hernia sac has a small neck, is thin walled, and is closely bound to the cord structures. In an acquired indirect hernia the neck is wide, and the sac is both short and thick walled. When both direct and indirect hernias are present, the defect is called a *pantaloon hernia* after the French word for 'pants', which this situation suggests.

PERIOPERATIVE NURSING CONSIDERATIONS

Assessment

Assessment of the patient with a hernia begins with a nursing history of past surgeries related to the herniated area. The patient's occupation and physical activities may be contributing factors to the development of the hernia. A thorough nursing history includes information relating to a familial history of hernias, the patient's nutritional status, when the symptoms occurred, a history of obesity, increased intraabdominal pressure, chronic cough, constipation, a history of benign prostatic hypertrophy, intestinal obstruction, colon malignancy, and, for women, pregnancy.[12]

Pain is often a notable symptom for the patient. An accurate description of the type and degree of pain is included in the assessment. Patients often describe the feeling of a foreign body at the hernia site.

Physical examination is the most common means for diagnosis. Palpation of the herniated area reveals the contents of the hernia sac. Fingertip palpation allows the nurse to feel the edges of the ring or abdominal wall. Having the patient stand and cough during the examination also assists in the evaluation of the herniated area.

The diagnosis of hernias is almost always accomplished by a clinical physical examination and a thorough health history. If a definitive diagnosis is not confirmed, ultrasonic scanning and imaging techniques (such as computerized tomography [CT], herniography, and standard radiography) may be employed.

A hernia may cause no symptoms; its only sign may be a swelling or protrusion in a restricted area of the abdominal wall. If the hernia is unilateral, the patient notes the lack of a protrusion on the other side in comparison. The area may be visible when the patient stands or coughs and may disappear on reclining. Femoral hernias can be difficult to diagnose and may resemble an enlarged lymph node.

Preoperative testing for a hernia repair facilitates safe and efficient perioperative care. Baseline data are obtained by a complete blood count. Before surgery, patients over 40 years of age may need an ECG and chest radiograph. Patients with a history of more complex medical problems must be fully evaluated with appropriate laboratory tests.

Nursing Diagnosis

Nursing diagnoses related to the care of the patient undergoing hernia surgery might include the following:

- Activity intolerance related to pain
- Risk for urinary retention
- Altered tissue perfusion of the scrotal area causing scrotal edema and ecchymosis
- Knowledge deficit related to disease process (hernia) and convalescence.

Outcome Identification

Outcomes identified for the selected nursing diagnoses could be stated as the following:

- The patient will return to previous level of activity.
- The patient will not experience urinary retention.
- The patient will not experience scrotal edema.
- The patient and family or significant other will verbalize knowledge regarding disease process (hernia) and convalescence.

Planning

The perioperative nurse formulates a plan of care for the patient undergoing herniorrhaphy by assimilating knowledge pertaining to the anatomy involved and principles of asepsis. Instrumentation, draping, and positioning for the patient's surgery depend on the type of hernia and repair to be performed, open versus laparoscopic, for example.

A typical care plan for a patient having surgery for repair of a hernia is shown in the Sample Care Plan.

Implementation

The patient may undergo general anesthesia, spinal or epidural block, regional anesthesia with sedation, or local anesthesia with sedation. Routine monitoring equipment such as a three-lead ECG, oxygen-saturation monitor, and blood pressure cuff are utilized for a hernia repair. An IV line is inserted for fluid replacement and medication administration. During inguinal herniorrhaphy the surgeon may want the patient to cough or bear down.

The patient is usually positioned supine (see Chapter 5) with basic prepping and draping procedures followed (see Chapter 4). Instruments used for herniorrhaphies are those found in standard laparotomy sets, laparoscopy sets, or minor sets.

A self-retaining retractor, such as a Weitlaner, facilitates the separation of tissue layers. A moistened Penrose drain is

SAMPLE CARE PLAN

Nursing Diagnosis: Activity intolerance related to pain

Outcome: The patient will return to previous level of activity.

Interventions:

Determine the patient's baseline activity level.

Encourage early postoperative ambulation.

Instruct the patient to use prescribed pain medications before physical activity and as needed.

Advise the patient to gradually increase activity as tolerated.

Explain the anticipated postoperative activity recommendations and limitations (see Box 13-1).

Nursing Diagnosis: Risk for urinary retention.

Outcome: The patient will not experience urinary retention.

Interventions:

Encourage patient to void before surgery.

Monitor and record intake and output status.

Postoperatively assess bladder for signs of urinary retention (palpable bladder or patient discomfort).

Encourage and assist patient with early ambulation as soon as choice of anesthesia permits.

Maintain adequate oral fluid intake without nausea or vomiting before discontinuing IV fluids.

Catheterize the patient if urinary retentions occurs.

Nursing Diagnosis: Altered tissue perfusion of the scrotal area causing scrotal edema and ecchymosis.

Outcome:

The patient will not experience any scrotal edema or ecchymosis.

Interventions:

Preoperatively discuss the possibility of swelling and ecchymosis.

Apply scrotal support intraoperatively.

Assess scrotum for evidence of swelling, ecchymosis, and redness.

Apply ice packs as prescribed.

Reassure the patient and instruct him on the importance of wearing the scrotal support.

Reassure the patient that the swelling and ecchymosis will subside.

Nursing Diagnosis: Knowledge deficit related to disease process (hernia) and convalescence.

Outcome: The patient and family or significant other will verbalize an understanding of the disease process (hernia) and convalescence.

Interventions:

Review possible contributing factors (as individualized for type of hernia and specific patient) to hernia formation.

Discuss postoperative pain-management strategies during recovery at home.

Describe and verify patient understanding of surgical site or incision care and reportable signs and symptoms (temperature, wound redness, tenderness at incision site, swelling, drainage).

Determine patient's dietary habits; discuss importance of roughage (fruits, vegetables, grains) to prevent constipation.

Provide written discharge instructions. Review these with patient and family or significant other to validate understanding.

Provide opportunity for questions and expression of concern.

Verify that patient has or knows how to schedule follow-up appointment.

---

used to retract the spermatic cord structures for better exposure. Because the peritoneal cavity may be entered in this procedure, accurate sponge, sharp, and instrument counts must be performed.

With a sliding hernia or an incarcerated hernia, the possibility of having to enter the peritoneal cavity must be considered. If the hernia is strangulated, necrotic bowel must be resected, and instruments for doing a bowel anastomosis must be ready. Antibiotics may be added to the irrigation to prevent an infection.

Repair of an inguinal hernia includes approximation of the transversalis fascia with a heavy, nonabsorbable type of suture. With some indirect hernias, only two or three sutures may be necessary. In other cases, however, up to 10 sutures in succession may be needed. Numerous types of needles are used for hernia repair. Scarpa's fascia is approximated with absorbable sutures, and the skin is closed by one of several methods.

Implementation of a laparoscopic hernia repair is technically similar to the open laparotomy, but the instrumentation includes laparoscopic equipment. There is always a possibility that a laparoscopy may become a laparotomy, and instrumentation for this change in procedure must always be available.

Evaluation

Evaluation of the patient having repair of a hernia should include examination of all skin surfaces to assess variances with the preoperative assessment data. The patient should awaken from general anesthesia in a reasonable amount of time without exhibiting signs of anxiety or extreme disorientation. Extubation should be timely to avoid stress on the repaired hernia site. The evaluation of the patient's status can be phrased in outcome statements such as the following:

- The patient will return to previous level of activity.
- The patient will not experience urinary retention or scrotal edema.
- The patient and family or significant other will verbalize understanding of hernia and recommendations for convalescence.

The perioperative nurse gives a detailed report to the PACU nurse pertaining to the relative events and patient status during the operative procedure.

Urinary retention may occur after a herniorrhaphy, and measures must be taken to prevent overdistention of the bladder. Early ambulation is encouraged to facilitate resumption of bladder and bowel functions. If the bowel has been resected because of strangulation, a nasogastric tube and suction may be required to reduce the incidence of postoperative vomiting and distention with subsequent strain on the suture line.

Patient and Family Education and Discharge Planning

In their report to the President of the United States, the Advisory Commission on Consumer Protection and Quality in the Health Care Industry noted that greater involvement of consumers in their care increases the likelihood of achieving the best outcomes and simultaneously supports a quality-improved, cost-conscious environment.[1] In order for the hernia patient to assume such responsibilities, plans for patient and family education along with plans for discharge and home recovery need to be designed. With options such as open or laparoscopic repair techniques, surgical and recovery times, analgesic requirements, complication rates, and times for return to full activity become part of informed consent.[13] Once the patient and surgeon have decided on the surgical approach, the perioperative nursing responsibilities for teaching the patient initial postoperative management strategies become crucial. Discharge planning is desirably begun before admission. This becomes increasingly important because hernia repair is commonly performed as an ambulatory procedure. Anticipated postoperative care, including incision care, incisional splinting as appropriate to the repair approach, and the importance of early ambulation and deep breathing are reviewed. Pain management is important as a part of discharge planning; it has been estimated that 50% or more of surgical patients report inadequate pain management during their postoperative recovery and convalescence.[4] Specific home care requirements are presented in Box 13-1. Perioperative nurses may also participate in the development of critical paths for specific diagnoses or surgical procedures such as hernia repair;

these have the goals of reducing patient complication rates, controlling resource utilization, decreasing errors, and enhancing patient education and satisfaction.[8] A sample critical path for the patient undergoing hernia repair is shown in Fig. 13-7.

SURGICAL INTERVENTIONS
SURGERY FOR REPAIR OF GROIN HERNIAS

Repair of inguinal hernias

Several operative procedures for repair of inguinal hernias are currently used. Approaches that reestablish the integrity of the transversalis fascia and simultaneously reestablish and strengthen the posterior inguinal floor are favored. A surgical repair in which transversalis fascia is sewn to transversalis fascia accomplishes this goal.

Procedural considerations

The patient is in the supine position for abdominal wall and inguinal or femoral hernia repairs. The patient's skin surface area from above the umbilicus to midthigh is exposed, prepped with antimicrobial solutions, and draped with sterile drapes. A sterile drape should be placed under the scrotum if it becomes necessary to enter the scrotum.

Operative procedures
McVay, or Cooper's, Ligament Repair

A McVay, or Cooper's, ligament repair approximates transversalis fascia superior to the inferior insertion of the transversalis fascia along Cooper's ligament.

1. An oblique incision is made parallel to the inguinal ligament, ending two fingerbreadths lateral to the pubic tubercle (Fig. 13-8).
2. The incision is carried through the superficial and deep (Scarpa's) fascia to the external oblique aponeurosis. Hemostasis is maintained with fine ties or electrocoagulation.
3. The external oblique aponeurosis is opened in the direction of its fibers to the external ring, and the aponeurotic flaps are reflected back along the iliohypogastric and ilioinguinal nerves, which are identified and preserved from injury (see Fig. 13-8). The ilioingunial nerve is a sensory nerve that innervates the medial thigh and the scrotum.
4. The cremaster muscles that form an envelope around the spermatic cord and represent the continuation of the internal oblique muscles are opened and the cord is exposed. The medial fibrous portion of the internal oblique is called the *conjoined tendon*.
5. By gentle dissection the spermatic vessels and the vas deferens are separated. A moistened Penrose drain is then used to gently retract the vessels and vas deferens.

BOX 13-1 | **Home Care for the Hernia Patient**

Home Care

- Give both the patient and the caregiver *oral* and *written* instructions. Provide them with the name and telephone number of a physician or nurse to call if questions arise:
- *General information*
  — Review any explanation about the procedure and specific follow-up care.
  — Explain and discuss the development of hernias, causes or contributing factors, care and treatment, and prevention.
- *Wound/incision care*
  — Discuss and demonstrate proper wound management and dressing changes: procedures, frequency, and signs to report.
- *Warning signs*
  — Review the signs and symptoms that should be reported to a physician or nurse.
    Infection: fever, pain, edema, erythema, warmth, purulent drainage, foul odor from the incision
    Abdominal distention, nausea, vomiting
    Hernia recurrence: firm, tender, globular, irreducible swelling in the groin
- *Special instructions*
  — Apply and demonstrate to the male patient scrotal support or ice packs to decrease scrotal edema and discomfort.
  — Assist the patient in obtaining appropriate supplies, such as sterile dressings.
- *Medications*
  — Explain the purpose, dosage, schedule, and route of administration of any prescribed drugs, as well as side effects to report to a physician or nurse.
    Analgesics
    Stool softeners
    Laxatives
- *Activity*
  — Encourage the patient to discuss allowances and limitations with respect to occupation, recreation, or activities.

—Instruct the patient to avoid coughing, straining, stretching, constipation, heavy lifting (>10 pounds), strenuous exercise, and sports for 6 weeks.
— Demonstrate splinting incision manually or with a pillow during coughing, sneezing, or hiccups.
— Stress the importance of activity restrictions and splinting the incision for up to 6 weeks after surgery.
— Demonstrate proper body mechanics for moving and lifting.
— Advise returning to work in 2 weeks for desk workers and 6 weeks for heavy laborers.
— Advise that sexual activity should be avoided for several weeks to avoid strain on the incision and discomfort to the scrotum, if edematous.
- *Diet*
  — Advise the patient to plan a high-fiber diet to help prevent constipation; provide the patient with a list of high-fiber foods.
  — Advise the patient to drink plenty of fluids, up to 2-3 liters per day, unless contraindicated.
  — Stress the importance of weight loss if the patient is obese.

Follow-Up Care

- Stress the importance of regular follow-up visits. Make sure the patient has the necessary names and telephone numbers.
- Stress the importance of smoking cessation to eliminate the smoker's cough as a contributing factor to hernia development.

Psychosocial Care

- Encourage the verbalization of fears and concerns about altered sexual function secondary to impaired blood supply to the vas deferens.

Referrals

- Provide information and refer the patient to community resources for weight loss and smoking cessation, if indicated.

From Canobbio, MM. (1996). *Mosby's handbook of patient teaching.* St. Louis: Mosby.

The cord is then examined for an indirect hernia, which arises from the internal ring lateral to the inferior epigastric vessels, and is initially adherent to the cord.

6. If an indirect sac is identified, it is carefully dissected away from the cord until the neck of the hernia is clearly delineated (Fig. 13-9).

7. The sac is opened, and any abdominal contents are returned to the peritoneal cavity.

8. A suture ligature or purse-string suture is placed high in the neck of the sac, and the excess peritoneum of the hernia is excised. The ligated stump quickly retracts into the peritoneal cavity. The inguinal floor is then inspected for evidence of a direct hernia. If only a

direct sac is present, usually no resection of the hernia is done because the sac easily returns to the abdominal cavity.

9. If transversalis fascia is present on both sides of the hernia defect, it is sutured together (Fig. 13-10). Suturing begins at the symphysis pubis and continues laterally to the internal ring. If the inferior transversalis fascia is weak or not present, the superior portion is sutured to Cooper's ligament, the site of insertion of the transversalis fascia. In this case, suturing again begins at the pubic tubercle and is continued laterally along Cooper's ligament to the medial border of the femoral sheath, where a transition stitch is placed. The repair is then carried

	PREOPERATIVE	INTRAOPERATIVE	CLOSURE	DISCHARGE
Assessments Evaluations	Nursing assessment Anesthesia assessment/preoperative medications	Continuous reassessment	Reassessment and evaluation of desired outcomes	Pain management per standard
Tests	Per institutional standards	Awake patient may be asked to cough to check adequacy of repair		
Safety and treatments	Consent/advance directive Hernia procedure card Endotracheal intubation Regional and local with IV conscious sedation Monitoring devices per institutional standard	Position and prep patient per standard Electrosurgical setup per standard Drape per standard Incision made _____ Implant material or suture (as applicable)	Closure of wound	Dressing applied Document implant material (implant log) Finalize perioperative documentation Warm blankets on
Medications	Surgical field per standard: Local (such as lidocaine) Long acting (such as bupivacaine for preemptive analgesia)	Anesthesia agents per standard Local	Anesthetic agents per standard	Pain management per standard
Discharge plans and teaching	Patient and family member teaching and orientation: Anticipated perioperative events Patient to OR environment Location of surgical waiting area Anticipated postoperative care Pain management Incision care Scrotal support and icepacks Splinting for coughing or sneezing Early ambulation Signs and symptoms to report Activity limitations Proper body mechanics for moving or lifting Return to work Follow-up appointment		Call to report to PACU Family called at waiting area	Anesthesia nurse transports patient to PACU
Expected outcomes	Maintain patient safety/comfort Patient and family members understand preoperative teaching/discharge plans	Maintain patient safety and comfort	Maintain patient safety and comfort	Skin integrity intact Pain controlled Patient voided and ambulated Discharge instructions provided (written) Questions and concerns addressed

FIGURE 13-7 Clinical pathway for hernia repair.

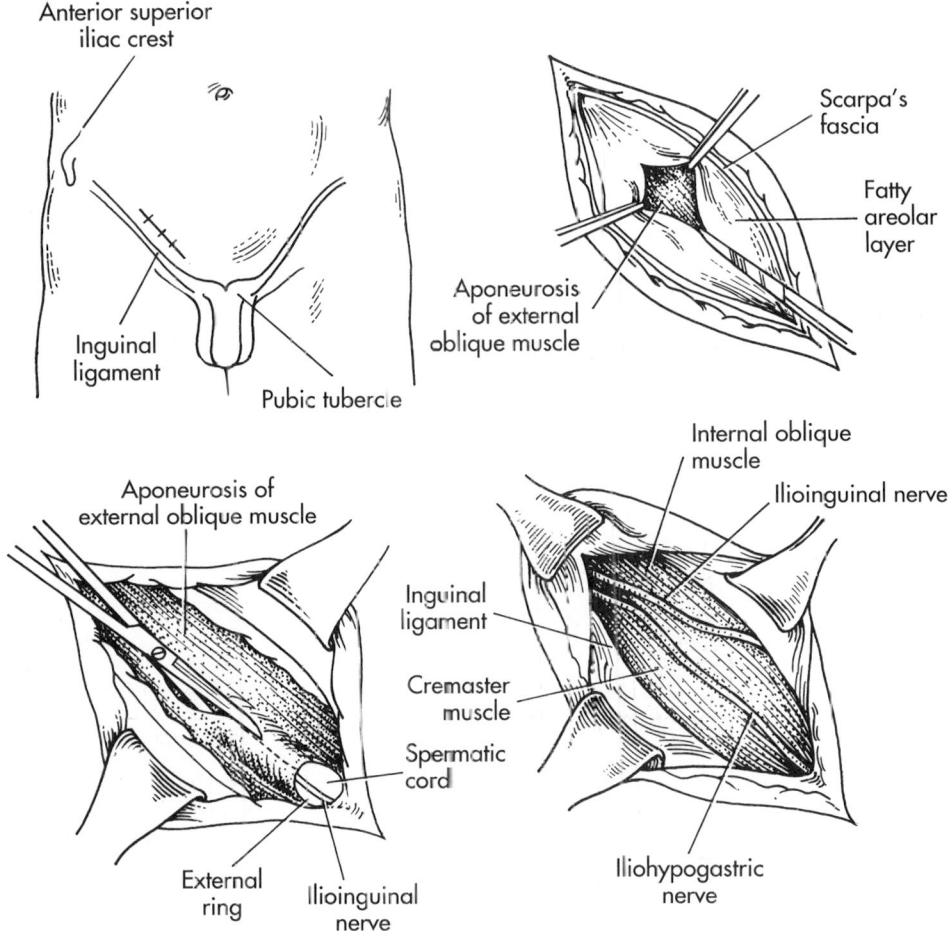

Anterior superior
iliac crest

Inguinal
ligament

Pubic tubercle

Scarpa's
fascia

Fatty
areolar
layer

Aponeurosis
of external
oblique muscle

Aponeurosis of
external oblique muscle

Internal oblique
muscle

Ilioinguinal nerve

Inguinal
ligament

Cremaster
muscle

Spermatic
cord

External
ring

Ilioinguinal
nerve

Iliohypogastric
nerve

FIGURE 13-8   Skin incision with division of superficial muscle and fascial layers.

laterally, approximating transversalis fascia to inguinal ligament (Fig. 13-11).

10. When the transveralis fascia is pulled down to Cooper's ligament, a relaxing incision in the rectus sheath is sometimes necessary to relieve excess tension. Essentially this incision is 5 to 7 cm long in the anterior rectus sheath. The incision begins immediately above the pubic crest, approximately 1 cm from the midline, and extends cephalad, following the line of fusion of the external oblique aponeurosis with the rectus sheath. The posterior rectus sheath and the rectus muscle itself guard against later herniation at the point where the relaxing incision is made. If too much tension makes direct approximation undesirable, a synthetic surgical mesh may be sutured in place as the new inguinal floor ("tension-free" mesh repair).[11]

11. After the integrity of the posterior inguinal floor has been reestablished, the cremaster muscles are reapproximated around the cord. Repair is completed with the approximation of the external oblique aponeurosis, Scarpa's fascia, and the skin.

Bassini Repair

The Bassini repair approach to the hernia and the treatment of the sac is identical to that previously described. The major difference with this repair is that the superior transversalis fascia is sutured to the inguinal ligament with no attempt made to approximate it to the inferior portion of the transversalis fascia or Cooper's ligament (pectineal ligament). Critics of this procedure claim that it is not anatomic because layers that originally are not one (transversalis fascia and inguinal ligament) now are approximated. Nonetheless, this repair is extremely popular and is used successfully by many surgeons.

Shouldice Repair

Again, the approach to the hernia is the same as previously described, but in the Shouldice repair a double layer of transversalis fascia is sutured to the inguinal ligament. It is reinforced by a layer of internal oblique muscle and conjoined tendon approximated to the undersurface of the fascia of the external oblique. Proponents of this repair have reported very low recurrence rates in a large series of patients. Although the

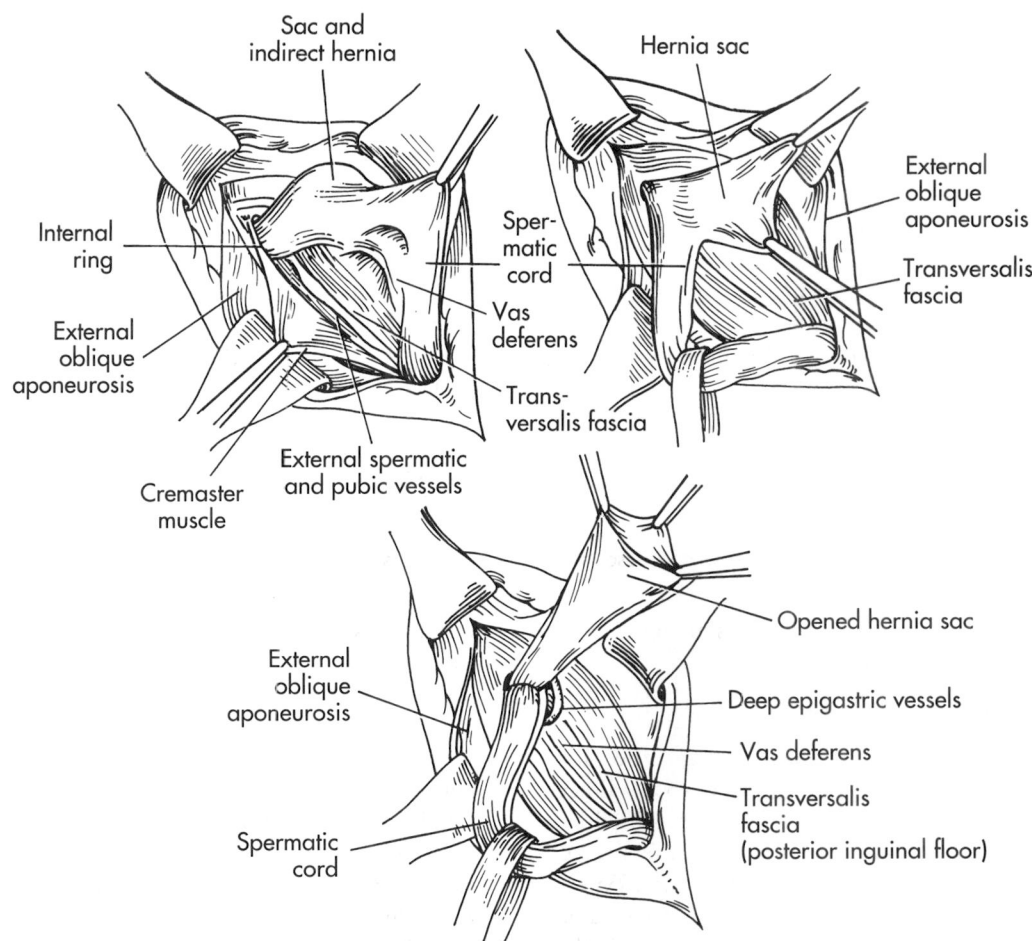

FIGURE 13-9   Indirect hernia sac is identified along with cord structures and dissected away from cord. Neck of hernia sac is clearly delineated, and sac is opened to check for abdominal contents.

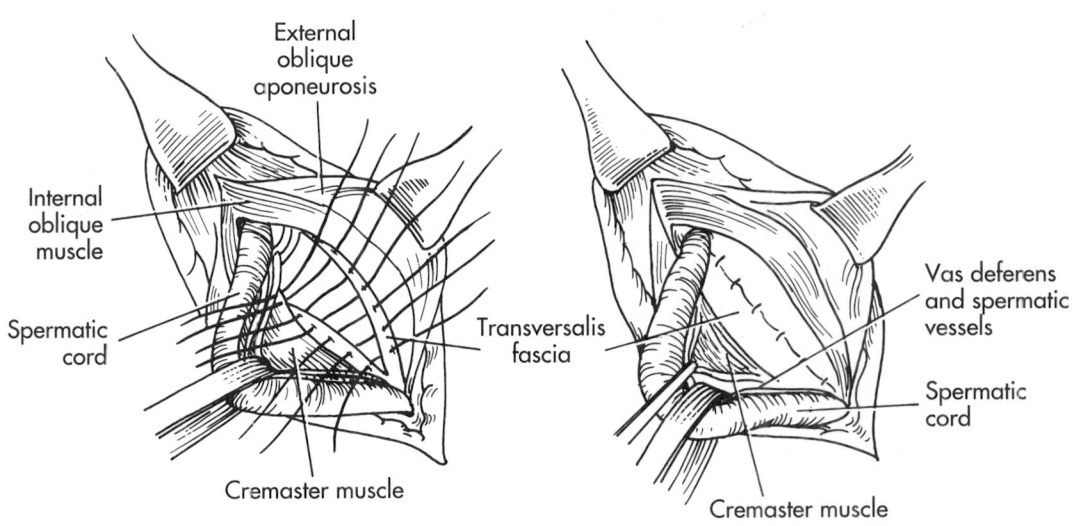

FIGURE 13-10   Transversalis fascia on either side of large hernia defect is approximated.

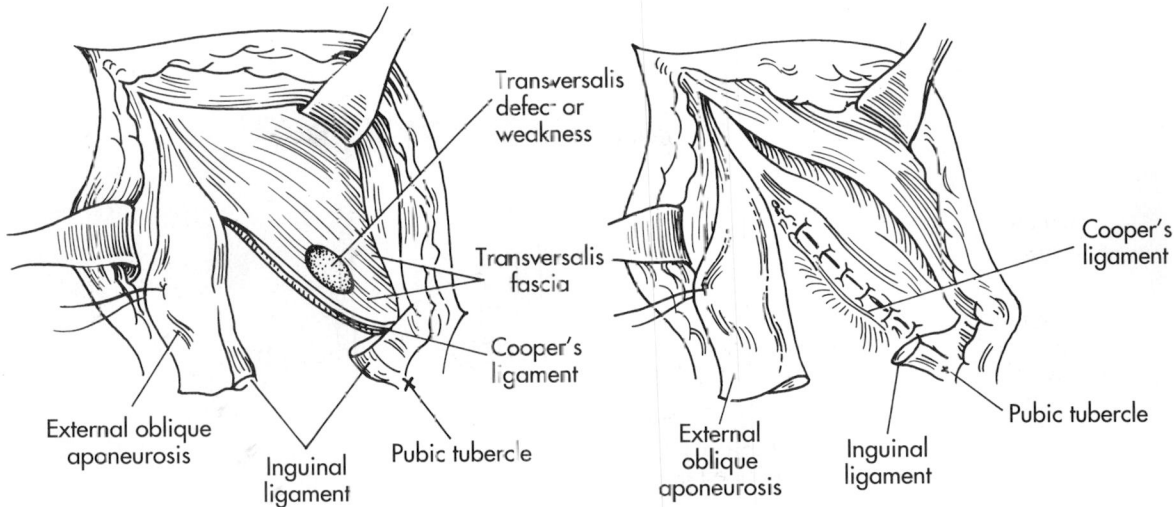

FIGURE 13-11   Defect in transversalis fascia repaired by approximation of fascia to Cooper's ligament.

Shouldice repair is controversial, it remains an alternative for surgeons who have studied the technique.

Mesh-Plug Repair

The mesh-plug technique has been recommended for the treatment of primary and recurrent direct and indirect inguinal hernias. The various hernia types as classified by Gilbert have a corresponding relationship to the use of mesh plugs.[9] Types I, II, and III are indirect hernias. Type I is characterized by a tight internal ring through which any size peritoneal sac can pass. The sac, when surgically reduced, is held within the abdominal cavity by the intact internal ring. Type II hernias have a moderately enlarged internal ring, 4 cm or smaller. Type III hernias have a patulous internal ring greater than 4 cm. In this type, the sac can have a sliding component that impinges upon the direct space. Type IV and Type V hernias are direct hernias. In type IV hernias, the defect involves virtually the entire flow of the inguinal canal. Type V is a diverticular defect of the floor and is generally in a suprapubic position, resembling a punched-out recurrent hernia. Type VI includes components of both indirect and direct hernias. Femoral hernias are classified as type VII.

Regardless of the hernia type, the mesh-plug technique is performed on an ambulatory basis. Repair of the inguinal hernias with mesh-plug technique has provided significant advantages when compared with conventional suture technique. A plug repair requires less overall dissection and ensures tension-free hernioplasty. These factors increase patient comfort, speed rehabilitation, and contribute to a very low recurrence rate, that is, 1% for primary and 2% for recurrent hernias.[14]

Surgical technique using the PerFix Plug

1. An oblique incision, 6 cm in length, is made and the external oblique fascia is opened through the external ring. Exposure is obtained by use of a self-retaining retractor (such as a Beckmann); a hand-held retractor such as Gouley may also be required. Hemostasis is usually achieved with the use of electrocoagulation.

2. The spermatic cord is mobilized, as previously described in the McVay repair. The ilioinguinal and genital femoral nerves are identified and preserved. The medial external oblique fascia is separated from the underlying transversus abdominis aponeurosis with a sweeping motion of the index finger.

3. An indirect sac and any lipoma of the cord are dissected free (Fig. 13-12, *A*). The sac and lipoma are allowed to drop back through the internal ring and into the abdominal cavity. Rarely is the sac opened except for incarcerated hernias.

4. Using the Gilbert classification, the internal ring is sized and the tapered end of the mesh plug is inserted through the internal ring and positioned just beneath the crura. The plug is designed such that its fluted outer layer, combined with its inside configuration of eight mesh petals, maintains its overall contour while allowing it to conform tension-free to the configuration of the internal ring (Fig. 13-12, *B*).

5. *Repair of indirect hernias.* Type I indirect hernias require 1-2 synthetic, absorbable sutures; in type II and III hernias, more sutures are required due to the increased size of the internal ring. *Repair of direct hernias.* In direct hernias, the fusiform or saccular defect is circumscribed near its base with an electrosurgical device and the hernia is reduced, providing a surrounding margin of intact tissue for securing the plug. The plug is then inserted through the floor of the defect (Fig. 13-12, *C*). With Type IV and V (direct) hernias, the mesh plug is routinely secured with up to 8-10 interrupted sutures of synthetic, absorbable. Where there are both indirect and direct hernias (Type VI) two mesh plugs may be needed. Type VII defects are treated similarly with mesh plugs.

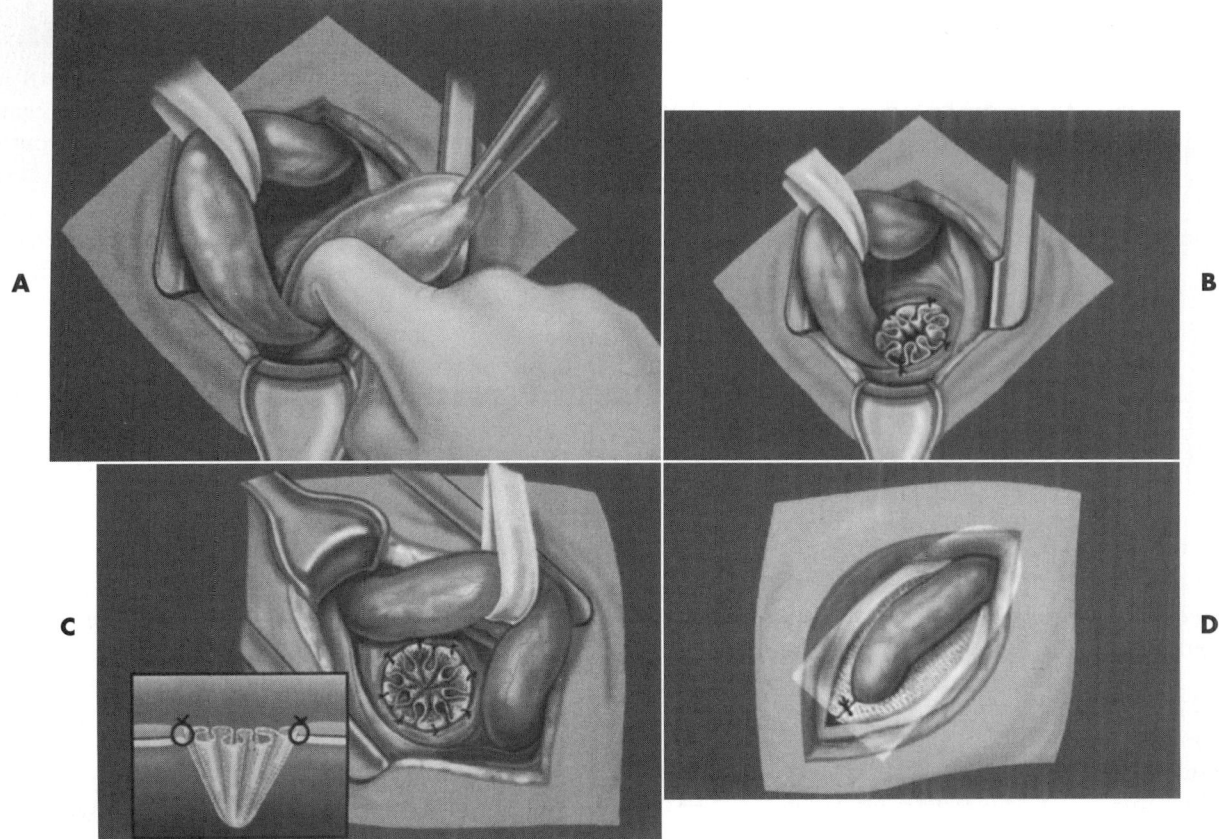

FIGURE 13-12   Mesh plug repair using the PerFix Plug. **A**, The hernia sac is dissected free of the cord structure to the level of the internal ring. **B**, A large plug is typically used. Some of the internal petals may be removed if the plug is too bulky. **C**, Large or extra large PerFix Plug is inserted. The plug should not be stretched to fill the defect. Eight to ten sutures are typically used. **D**, Sutureless onlay patch. The tails of the onlay patch are taken around the cord and sutured together. The onlay patch is not sutured to the floor of the inguinal canal.

6. Repair of femoral hernias. In femoral hernias, a small or medium-sized plug is secured in position after the sac has been reduced.

7. In most types of mesh-plug hernia repairs, a second piece of flat mesh is used for reinforcement. The piece is cut to match the shape of the inguinal canal and then placed without sutures on the anterior surface of the posterior wall of inguinal canal. The proximal portion is split to provide an opening for the spermatic cord, and the mesh tails are brought together with sutures to form a new internal ring (Fig. 13-12, *D*).

8. With the spermatic cord structures placed on top of this flat mesh, the external oblique fascia is reapproximated over the structures with a running, synthetic, nonabsorbable suture.

9. An interrupted suture of a similar size is used to bring the subcutaneous tissue together, and the skin is closed with a subcuticular stitch. A transparent dressing is used to cover the wound site.[15]

Laparoscopic Hernia Repairs

Ger was the first surgeon to perform a laparoscopic herniorrhaphy. In 1982 he described a laparoscopic transabdominal hernia approach. Variations in techniques for laparoscopic hernia repair continue to develop as surgeons gain experience with these procedures.

Two similar techniques are being used today for laparoscopic herniorrhaphy. These are the transabdominal preperitoneal (TAPP) approach and the totally extraperitoneal approach (TEPA). The difference between the two approaches is the manner in which access is gained to the preperitoneal space. The TAPP uses intraperitoneal trocars and the creation of a peritoneal flap over the posterior inguinal region. TEPA provides access to the preperitoneal space without entering the peritoneal cavity.[6]

Studies indicating long-term postoperative hernia recurrence and complication rates are not yet available (Research Highlight 13-1). A laparoscopic hernia repair has the advantages of a quicker return to normal activity and some reduction of postoperative adhesions. The disadvantages of a laparoscopic repair include longer operating times, the potential for nerve injury, and the need for a general anesthetic (Research Highlight 13-2). Evaluation of long-term outcomes of laparoscopic hernia repair continue. It may be anticipated that as the surgeon's laparoscopic skill level improves and the patient receives

13-1 RESEARCH HIGHLIGHT

To compared the short-term effects of open herniorrhaphy (OH) and laparoscopic repair (LH), this study randomized 130 patients after stratifying for age and type of hernia (direct or indirect). The technique for OH was individualized and based on operative findings, type of hernia, and the strength of the inguinal floor. Laparoscopic repair was performed under general anesthesia, usually with the transabdominal preperitoneal (TAPP) approach. An endoscopic staple tacker and reinforcement with mesh were employed in the LH repair. Outcomes analysis revealed that total operative times were similar, but anesthesia time was longer for LH. Length of stay and time needed to convalesce were similar for both groups. The LH patients used less narcotics, but about half of each group reported discomfort 7 days after repair. Complications developed in 22.5% of the LH group compared to 12% of those having OH. Total direct costs were $1,224 for OH and $1,718 for LH. Although the study supports the feasibility of LH repair, it also suggests that comparable results might be achieved by use of a tension-free open repair.

From Barkin, J.S., Wexler, M.J., Hinchey, E.J., et al. (1995). Laparoscopic versus open inguinal herniorrhaphy: preliminary results of a randomized controlled trial. *Surgery, 118,* 703-710.

13-2 RESEARCH HIGHLIGHT

Recurrence rates for open repair of inguinal and femoral hernias may be below 1% in specialized centers or as high as 10% to 17% when performed outside specialized centers. Laparoscopic techniques for hernia repair have been introduced. However, the initial promise of these procedures has been tempered by complication reports, including nerve injury and postoperative bowel obstruction. The experience with a series of laparoscopic herniorrhaphies was studied prospectively.

Two hundred laparoscopic hernia repairs were performed in 175 patients under general anesthesia. The median follow-up was 12 months (range, 5 to 24 months). Intraoperative and postoperative complications, recovery, and results of the procedures were studied.

Operative times for the procedures were a median of 67 minutes for unilateral hernias and 130 minutes for bilateral hernias. Two patients had anesthesia-related rising carbon dioxide tension in the expired gas. There were 19 postoperative complications, which included bowel obstruction in 2 women, inguinal seromas in 9 patients, portsite hematomas in 3, transient neuralgia in 1, hydrocele in 1, incisional hernia in 1, periostitis in 1, and orchitis in 1 patient. There were 7 recurrences; 6 occurred in patients treated early in the series. Of the 175 patients. 70 were discharged within 12 hours, and an additional 76 were discharged within 24 hours. The patients had a median length of stay of 1 day (range, 0 to 27 days). Sixty patients (52%) could return to work within 1 week, 87 (75%) within 2 weeks, and 109 (94%) within 1 month. The median recovery period before return to work was 7 days (range, 0 to 91 days).

Because of the use of general anesthesia for laparoscopic procedures, risk, and cost are greater than those associated with open techniques, which are usually performed with local, spinal, or epidural anesthesia. Cost is also increased by the use of disposable instruments in laparoscopic hernia repairs. Operative time was longer with the laparoscopic than with open repair. However, discomfort and morbidity were not increased, and both sides could be repaired in 1 operation. The convalescent period was significantly shorter with laparoscopic repair than is usually true after open repair. Further study is needed to determine whether the patient benefits and reduced postoperative costs associated with laparoscopic hernia repair justify its significantly higher intraoperative cost.

From Kald, A., Smedh, K., & Anderberg, B. (1995). Laparoscopic groin hernia repair: results of 200 consecutive herniorrhaphies. *British Journal of Surgery, 82,* 618-620; as reviewed in *Capsules and Comments in Perioperative Nursing, 1*(3), 249-250.

less pharmacologically involved anesthesia, outcomes, efficiency, and cost will similarly improve.

Repair of Inguinal Hernias in Females

Regardless of the specific technique used, the initial approach to the repair of a hernia in the female is the same as that used in the male. After the cremaster muscles are opened to expose the round ligament, variations that may be encountered include the following: (1) with the sac exposed and cleared from the round ligament, the round ligament and accompanying vessels are dissected free from the inguinal floor to the labium; (2) at the labium the round ligament is clamped, ligated, and divided; (3) the sac at the internal ring is opened, checked to be sure that no abdominal contents are present, and ligated at its neck, together with the round ligament and associated vessels; or (4) the sac distal to the ligature is removed with the distal round ligament, while the ligated stump retracts promptly into the abdomen. The remainder of the repair is the same as that previously described.

Repair of Femoral Hernias

A femoral hernia protrudes from the groin below the inguinal ligament into the thigh (Fig. 13-13). In its most obvious form, a femoral hernia is an inflamed, tender mass

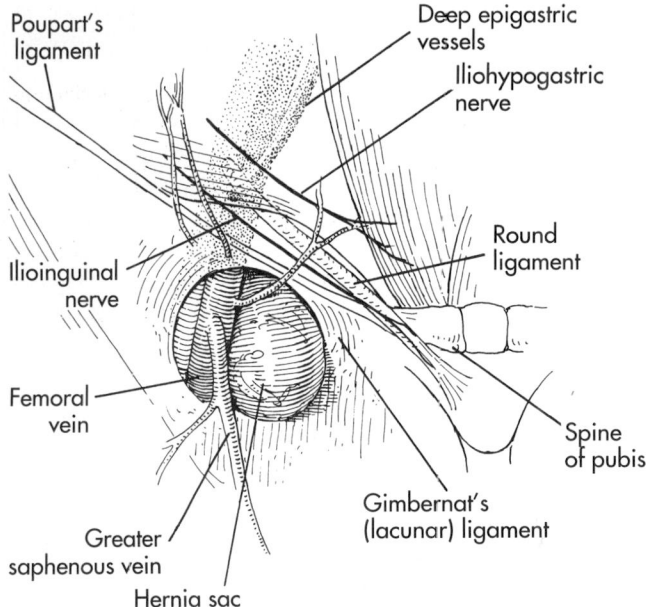

FIGURE 13-13   Bulge from femoral hernia occurring below inguinal ligament.

with bowel sounds below the inguinal ligament. Unfortunately, the presentation is frequently more subtle, and the diagnosis is completely missed or confused with enlarged inguinal lymph nodes, a psoas muscle abscess, a saphenous varix, or a lipoma. The defect is usually small and frequently irreducible. Femoral hernias are highly likely to become incarcerated and strangulated; elective repair is clearly indicated unless serious contraindications to surgery exist.

Operative procedure

The general approach is surgical treatment to free the tightly bound hernia, closely examine the contents of the hernia for ischemic change, and repair the hernia defect. The principles for repair of this type of hernia are the same as those described for inguinal herniorrhaphies. Ultimately, repair of the transversalis fascia must be accomplished. Repair of femoral hernia requires approximating the aponeurotic margins of the femoral canal. The sutures are placed through the iliopubic tract superiorly and through the Cooper's ligament and pectineus fascia inferiorly. Care is taken to not compromise the femoral artery and vein.

Preperitoneal (Properitoneal) Repair

Preperitoneal (properitoneal) repair also is based on the essential role of the transversalis fascia in the cause and subsequent correction of a hernia. This repair is suitable for direct, indirect, and femoral hernias. It is particularly applicable in dealing with recurrent hernias because exposure is obtained by operating through virgin surgical fields rather than through previous scars.

Operative procedure

1. A transverse incision is made 2 cm above the symphysis pubis, through the rectus abdominis muscle on the affected side (Fig. 13-14, A).
2. The wound is deepened by cutting the external oblique, internal oblique, and transversalis muscles.
3. The transversalis fascia is then cut, and the preperitoneal space is entered. This is the proper plane of dissection for the remainder of the operation.
4. Retraction on the lower side of the incision reveals the posterior inguinal wall and the hernia defect.

Variations in the procedure are performed for different types of hernias.

1. If the hernia is direct, it can be reduced easily, and the superior edge of the hernia defect (the transversalis fascia) is sutured to the iliopubic tract (origin of the transversalis fascia) (Fig. 13-14, B).
2. In an indirect hernia, the sac is gently retracted from the inguinal canal. A purse-string suture is placed around the peritoneal defect as the sac is excised (Fig. 13-14, C). The lateral aspect of the internal abdominal ring is closed, and the posterior wall is reinforced as with the direct hernia.
3. In repair of a femoral hernia, the sac is again reduced by traction. After the sac is inspected for contents, a high ligation is performed. As it approaches Cooper's ligament, the defect in the posterior inguinal floor is clearly identified and is repaired by direct approximation (Fig. 13-14, D). After repair of any of the aforementioned hernias the preperitoneal space is irrigated with saline solution, and the appropriate layers are approximated.

Repair of Sliding Hernias

Direct or indirect hernias may occur as sliding hernias. A sliding inguinal hernia occurs when the wall of a viscus forms a portion of the wall of the hernia. The most common sliding hernias involve the bladder in direct hernias, the sigmoid colon in left indirect hernias, and the cecum in right indirect inguinal hernias (Fig. 13-15). This hernia must be recognized early in the repair because attempts at surgical removal of the entire sac will injure the sliding viscus.

Operative procedure

All operations designed to repair sliding hernias adhere to the basic principle of repairing the defect in the transversalis fascia. To free the bowel from the sac, the following steps must be taken:

1. The sac is opened in an area where no bowel is present and is excised medially and laterally to a point at which the bowel can be mobilized (Fig. 13-16).

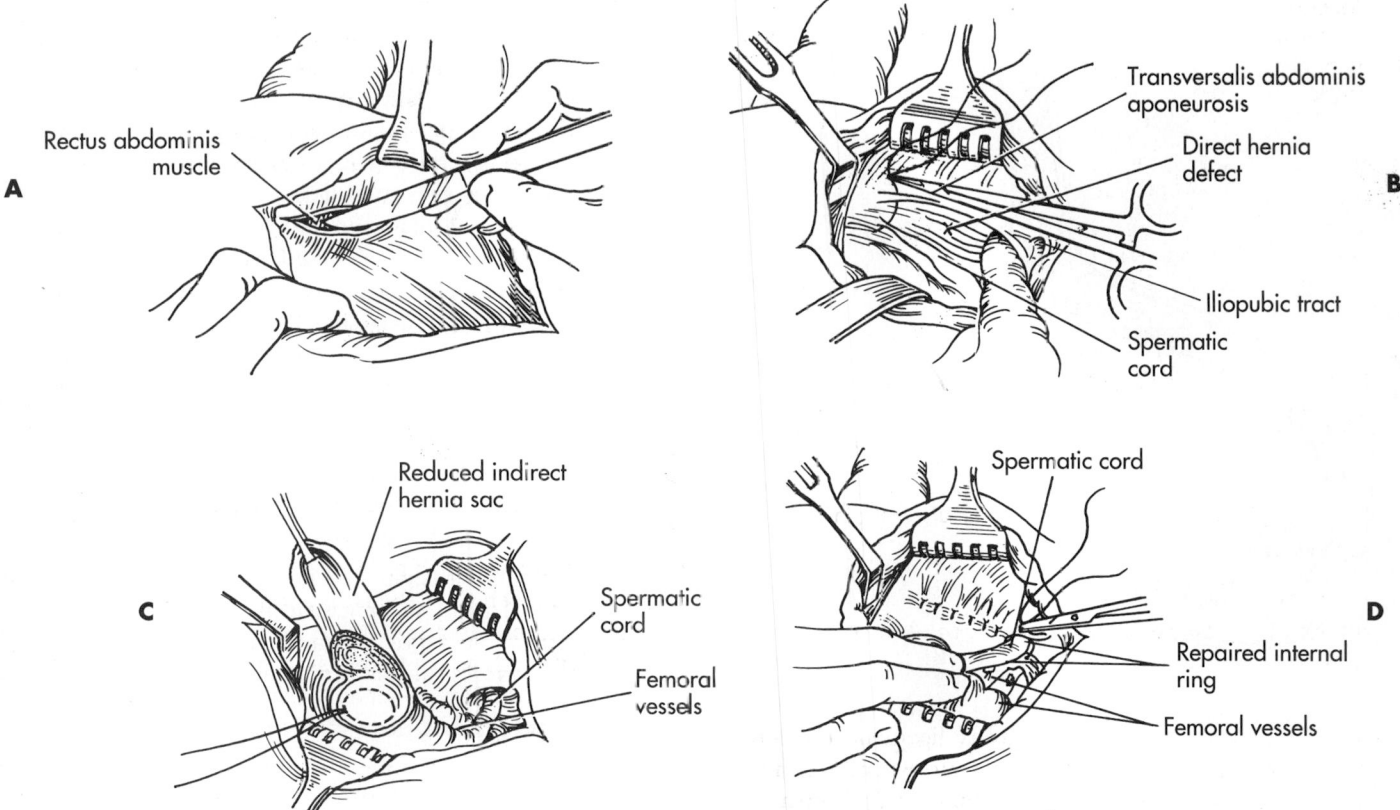

FIGURE 13–14   Preperitoneal repair. **A**, Skin incision starts 2 cm above symphysis pubis and is extended through external oblique, internal oblique, and transversalis muscles. **B**, With finger in direct hernia defect, surgeon sutures transversalis abdominis aponeurosis to iliopubic tract. **C**, In case of indirect defect, sac is reduced and then excised, with high ligation being achieved by use of a purse-string suture. **D**, Internal ring is tightened after transversus abdominis aponeurosis has been approximated to iliopubic tract.

2. The lateral and medial peritoneal margins are approximated.
3. The bowel is reduced to the peritoneal cavity, and high ligation of the sac is performed.
4. Repair of the transversalis fascia is done by one of the methods previously described.

Littre's Hernia, Maydl's Hernia, and Richter's Hernia

An inguinal hernia containing a Meckel's diverticulum is called *Littre's hernia*, and one containing two loops of bowel is called *Maydl's hernia*. A special type of strangulated hernia is Richter's hernia (Fig. 13-17). In this hernia only a part of the circumference of the bowel is incarcerated or strangulated in the hernia. Frequently it is described as a knuckle of bowel that becomes trapped and ischemic. Because initially a very small area is necrotic, diagnosis may be delayed; the probability of death then becomes significant. Richter's hernia most frequently occurs in femoral hernias because of the small size and sharp, relatively inflexible nature of the fascial ring in this area. A strangulated Richter's hernia may be reduced spontane-

ously, and the gangrenous piece of intestine may be overlooked at the time of operation. Most commonly, the distal ileum is involved in Richter's hernia; however, omentum is frequently encountered in the sac. The favored approach for repair is through the preperitoneal space.

SURGERY FOR REPAIR OF HERNIAS OF THE ANTERIOR ABDOMINAL WALL

Ventral or Incisional Hernias

Ventral hernias can appear either spontaneously or after previous operations. Spontaneously occurring ventral hernias include epigastric and umbilical hernias. Postoperative ventral hernias, called *incisional hernias*, appear more frequently when the original incision was T shaped or a vertical midline. Operations that involve a potential for contamination, such as that for acute perforated ulcer or other perforated abdominal viscera, are more prone to developing subsequent ventral hernias. A poor nutritional

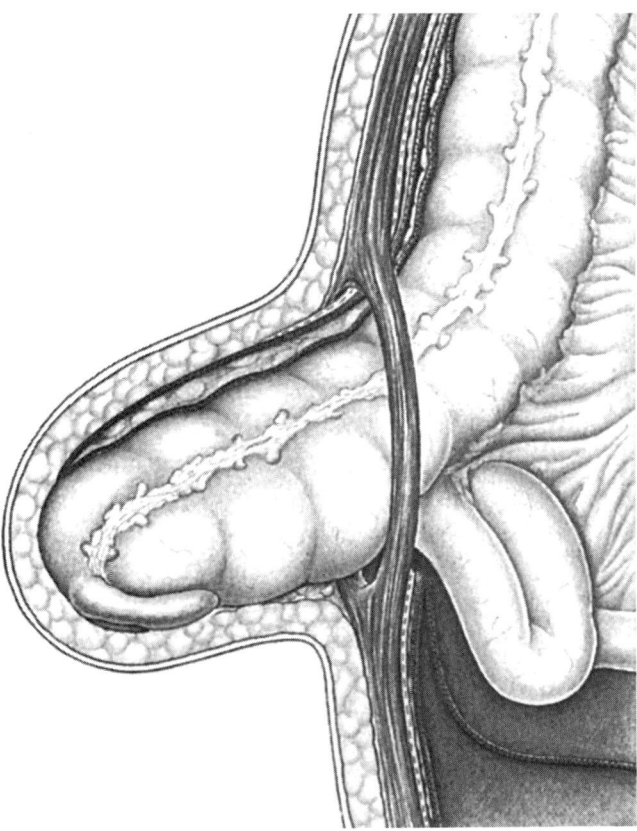

FIGURE 13-15 Sliding hernia.

state with resulting hypoproteinemia predisposes some individuals to ventral hernia formation.[10] Finally, faulty surgical technique, such as the choice of inappropriate suture materials, may result in the ultimate appearance of a ventral hernia.

Several methods have been developed for repairing ventral hernias. If all layers of the abdominal wall are easily identified, anatomic layer-by-layer repair may be done. Frequently a type of overlap method for repair is employed. Vertical and transverse overlap procedures are referred to as *vest-over-pants repairs*. For large defects, in which approximation of tissue would result in closure with excessive tension or would cause either circulatory or respiratory compromise, synthetic materials such as surgical mesh or patches are employed.

When a very large fascial defect is present, a technique that extrapolates on the principles of tissue expansion may be used. A Tenckhoff catheter is placed percutaneously into the peritoneal cavity. Gradual expansion of the abdominal fascia is accomplished by insufflation of the abdomen with 1 to 2 liters of nitrous oxide gas, similar to the procedure for laparoscopy. The patient's vital signs are monitored during and after the insufflation procedure, which may be performed on a nursing unit or possibly in an outpatient clinical setting. The graduated expansion of the tissues sometimes allows for primary closure of the defect without the use of synthetic mesh or a patch.

Umbilical Hernias

Umbilical hernias are extraperitoneal and occur as small fascial defects under the umbilicus. They are common in children and frequently disappear spontaneously by 2 years of age. If the defect is persistent, a simple approximation of the overlying fascia is all that is necessary for repair. (See Chapter 29 for a description of hernia repair in children.) In adults, umbilical hernias represent a defect in the linea alba just above the umbilicus. These hernias tend to occur more frequently in obese people, making diagnosis more difficult. Umbilical hernias are potentially dangerous because they have small necks and frequently become incarcerated. Surgical repair is indicated for all adults with asymptomatic umbilical hernias.

Epigastric Hernias

Epigastric hernias are protrusions of fat through defects in the abdominal wall between the xiphoid process and the umbilicus. Patients with epigastric hernias can have nausea, vague abdominal pain, or epigastric pain similar to that observed with cholecystitis or duodenal ulcers. Surgical repair of epigastric hernias is simple and very successful.

Spigelian Hernias

The linea semilunaris, often referred to as *Spigelius's line*, marks the transition from muscle to aponeurosis in the transversus abdominis muscle. The area of aponeurosis that lies between the linea semilunaris and the lateral edge of the rectus muscle is referred to as the *spigelian zone*. Protrusion of a peritoneal sac, preperitoneal fat, or other abdominal viscera through a congenital or acquired defect in this area is called a *spigelian hernia*. It is usually located between the different muscle layers of the abdominal wall. For this reason the spigelian hernia may be referred to as an *interparietal*, *interstitial*, or *intramuscular hernia*.

Spigelian hernias are uncommon and are generally difficult to diagnose. Ultrasonic scanning has improved the diagnosis of such intramural hernias. When ultrasonic scanning is not conclusive, CT can better visualize the hernia orifice.

Interparietal Hernias

An interparietal hernia lies between the layers of the abdominal wall. These hernias may be classified by dividing them into those that present with ventral swelling and those without ventral swelling. Diagnosis is often made during an exploratory laparotomy for symptoms of intestinal obstruction.

Repair follows the same procedure as that done for a strangulated hernia. The sac contents are closely examined for ischemia, the sac is resected, and the defect is repaired.

Synthetic Mesh and Patch Repairs

Synthetic meshes, such as Mersilene, Marlex, Prolene, and Dacron, have been particularly helpful in repairing recurrent or large ventral hernias. Closure of the defect is

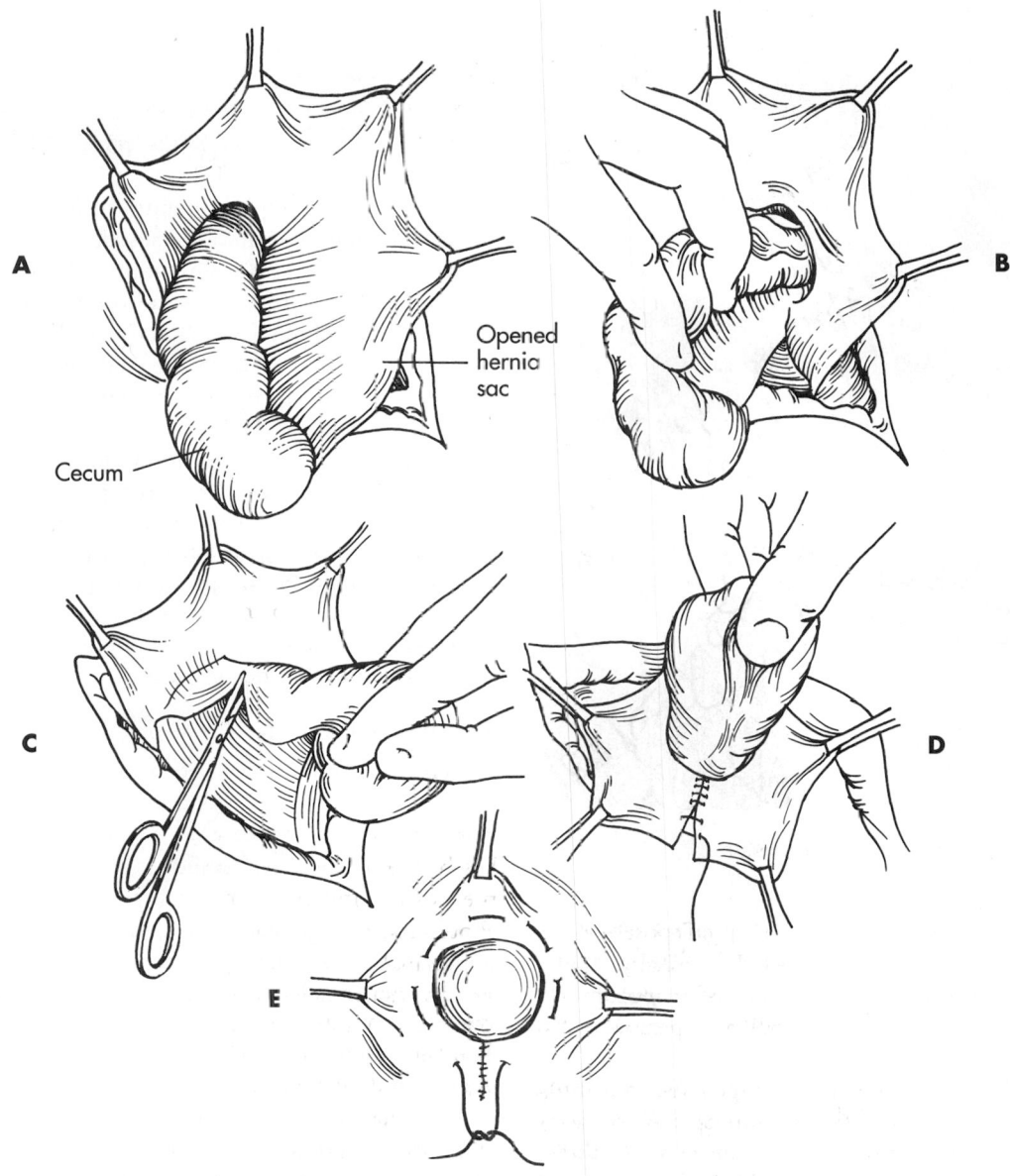

FIGURE 13-16   Right sliding hernia. **A**, Cecum forms posterior wall of hernia sac. **B**, Peritoneum is excised medially (**C**), and laterally (**D**), to allow mobilization of cecum for subsequent reduction to peritoneal cavity. Lateral and medial margins are approximated. **E**, After reduction, high ligation is accomplished by using purse-string suture.

obtained with minimal or no tension on the suture line. These synthetic materials are strong and durable, promoting fibrovascular growth within their pores, which lends extra strength to the repair.

A major criticism of synthetic meshes is that, as with any foreign-body implant, the risk of infection is increased.

Another synthetic material, the Gore-Tex patch, has become popular for the reconstruction of abdominal wall defects and repair of soft tissue. Gore-Tex soft-tissue patches come in both 1 cm and 2 cm thicknesses. Impregnation of Gore-Tex patches with an antimicrobial agent has been associated with reduced incidence of infection. Gore-Tex is, however, very expensive, and surgical services departments should evaluate products such as surgical mesh with consideration to its performance, cost, effect on quality patient care, and value analysis.[2]

Essential to the use of mesh or patch in a hernia repair are the identification and cleaning of tissue planes to which the mesh or patch will be attached (Fig. 13-18, *A*). In a ventral hernia the peritoneum is dissected from the undersurface of the rectus abdominis muscle, and the mesh or patch is placed between the peritoneum and the rectus

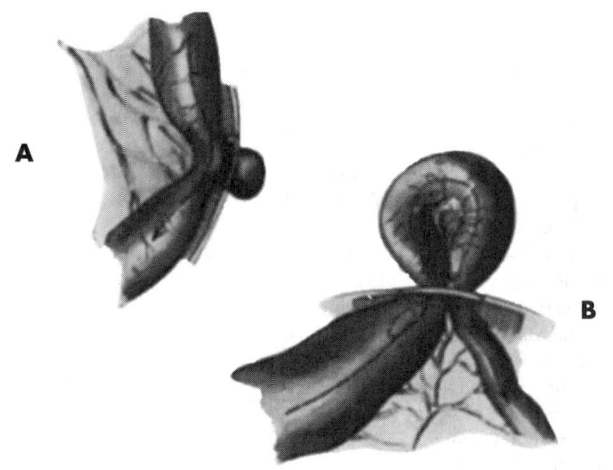

FIGURE 13-17   **A**, Richter's hernia. Only a portion of bowel passes through hernial ring; *arrow* indicates that bowel need not be obstructed mechanically even with strangulation. **B**, Incarcerated hernia. Distended bowel in hernia cannot return to abdomen through narrow fascial defect.

(Fig. 13-18, *B*). After the mesh or patch is positioned, it is sutured in place on one side, using the synthetic suture material compatible with the type of mesh or patch employed (Fig. 13-18, *C*). After the mesh is in place, the surgeon often sprinkles an antibiotic powder over the mesh.

At this point the peritoneum can be closed, if possible. If the peritoneum cannot be closed, mesh or patch can be placed directly over the omentum. The mesh or patch is then placed and sutured to the other side of the defect, with moderate tension maintained (Fig. 13-18, *D*). If possible, the mesh or patch is then covered with a fascial or muscular layer before the subcutaneous fat and skin are closed. Closed-wound drainage catheters may be placed in the wound, and antibiotics are frequently used prophylactically. Using mesh or patch to repair inguinal hernias is based on the same principles used for closing ventral hernias. With inguinal hernias, the mesh or patch is sutured to transversalis fascia on both sides of the defect.

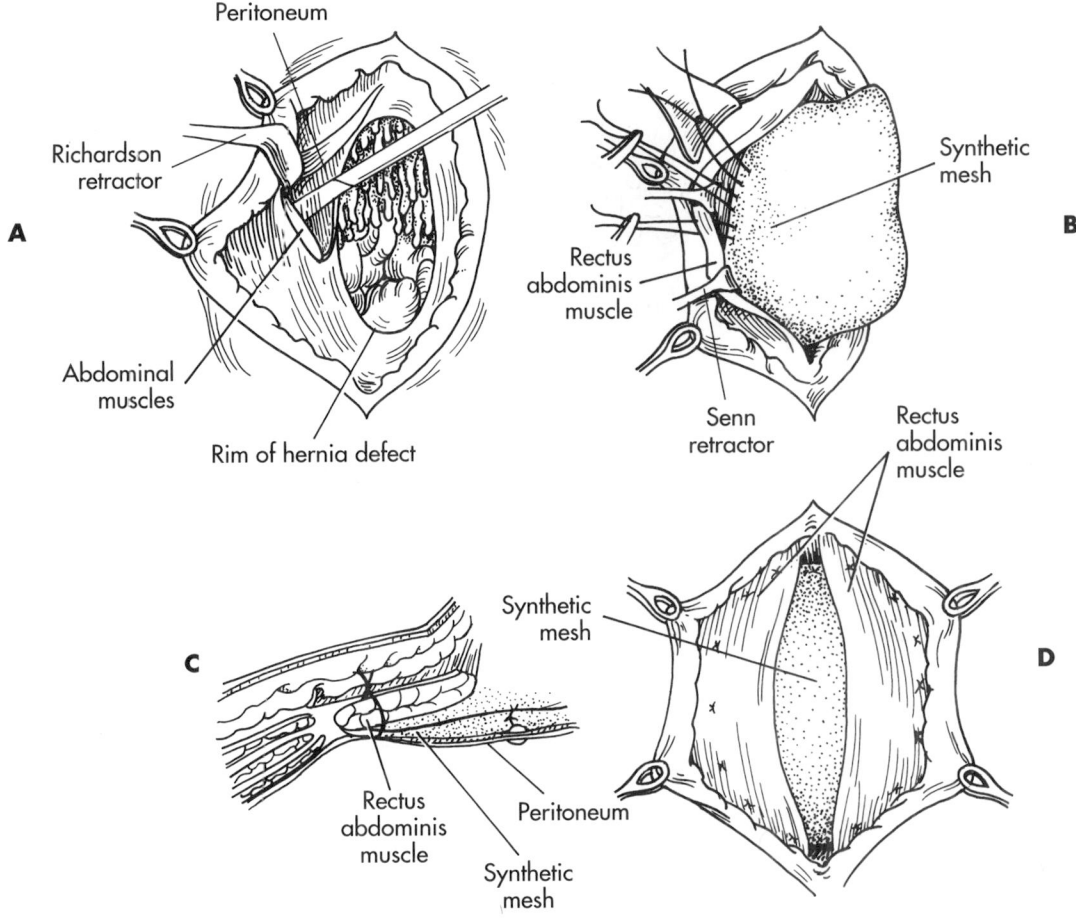

FIGURE 13-18   Use of mesh in hernia repair. After layers of abdominal wall surrounding ventral hernia are identified (**A**), mesh is inserted between rectus and peritoneum (**B**). **C**, Mesh is sutured into place on one side. **D**, With moderate tension, mesh is inserted between appropriate layers on opposite side and is sutured into place.

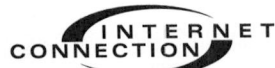

http://www.davol.com/groin.htm (mesh plug technique)

http://www.laparoscopy.com

http://www.theherniacenter.com

For links and clinical information, use this database and type in the information you are looking for:
Medical Matrix: http://www.medicalmatrix.com

REFERENCES

1. Advisory Commission on Consumer Protection and Quality in the Health Care Industry. (1997). *Consumer bill of rights and responsibilities* (Report to the president of the United States). Washington, D.C.: the Commission.

2. Association of Operating Room Nurses Recommended Practices for the evaluation and selection of products and medical devices in perioperative practice settings. (1998). In *AORN standards, recommended practices & guidelines.* Denver: the Association, pp. 271-274.

3. Bascom, J. (1996). Inguinal hernia. In Harken, A.H., & Moore, E.E., (Eds.), *Abernathy's surgical secrets.* Philadelphia: Hanley & Belfus.

4. Coyne, M.L., Smith, J.F., Stein, D., et al. (1998). Describing pain management documentation, *MEDSURG Nursing,* 7(1), 45-51.

5. Embrey, J.P. (1996). [Commentary]. *Capsules & Comments in Nurse Anesthesia,* 1(1), 33.

6. Eubanks, S. (1997). Hernias. In Sabiston, D.C., (Ed.), *Textbook of surgery: the biological basis of modern surgery practice.* Philadelphia: W.B. Saunders.

7. Fogel, S. (1992). Groin hernia. In Cameron, J.S. (Ed.), *Current surgical therapy.* St. Louis: Mosby.

8. Forkner, D.J. (1996). Clinical pathways—benefits and liabilities, *Nursing Management,* 27(11), 35-38.

9. Gilbert, A. (1989). An anatomical and functional classification for the diagnosis and treatment of inguinal hernia, *American Journal of Surgery,* 157, 331-335.

10. Mäkelä, J.T., Kiviniemi, H., Juvonen, T., & Laitinen, S. (1995). Factors influencing wound dehiscence after midline laparotomy, *American Journal of Surgery,* 170, 387-390.

11. Mann, B.D., Seidman, A., Haley, T., & Sachdeva, A.K. (1997). Teaching three-dimensional concepts of inguinal hernia in a time-effective manner using a two-dimensional paper-cut, *American Journal of Surgery,* 173, 542-545.

12. Penman, E.L., Baker, R.J. (1995). Operations for groin hernia. In Ritchie, W.P., Steele, G., & Dean, R.H. (Eds.), *General surgery.* Philadelphia: J.B. Lippincott.

13. Rudkin, G.E., Maddern, G.J. (1995). Peri-operative outcome for day-case laparoscopic and open inguinal hernia repair, *Anaesthesia, 50,* 586-589.

14. Rutkow, I.M., Robbins, A.W. (1995). Groin hernia. In Cameron, J.S. (Ed.), *Current surgical therapy,* St. Louis: Mosby.

15. Sabiston, D.C. (1997). *Textbook of surgery: the biological basis of modern surgical practice,* Philadelphia: W.B. Saunders.

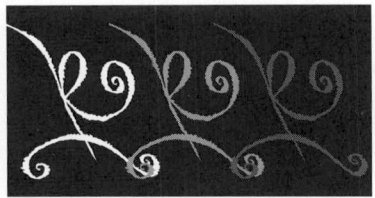

CHAPTER FOURTEEN

Gynecologic Surgery and Cesarean Birth

Gwen Lynn Nelson

HISTORICAL ADVANCEMENTS IN gynecology have been based on increasing the quality of health care provided for women. Descriptions of gynecologic examinations have been traced back to the time of Hippocrates. For years the midwife performed the roles of gynecologist and obstetrician in society. As knowledge increased regarding female anatomy and its abnormalities, surgeons began to develop techniques in abdominal and pelvic surgery. In 1794 Jesse Bennett is recorded as having performed one of the earliest pelvic surgeries. Effective surgical corrections of gynecologic disorders continued into the nineteenth century. Through the years, the efficiency of laparoscopy, along with improvements in diagnostic techniques and surgical interventions, has evolved to promote the health care of women.

Today's gynecologic surgery has been built on this foundation. Some of the gynecologic specialties that have evolved are oncology, endocrinology, and infertility. The numerous developments and techniques within each of these specialty areas represent challenges for today's perioperative nurse.

Operations on the structures of the female reproductive system are performed for diagnostic or therapeutic purposes, for conditions such as abnormal bleeding from the reproductive organs, for suspected malignant or benign neoplasms, and for infertility. Procedures are also done to remove or repair weakened anatomic structures.

SURGICAL ANATOMY

The female reproductive organs and their relationships are shown in Fig. 14-1. The adult female structures associated with the process of reproduction are the bony pelvis, the associated ligaments and muscles, the soft tissues and contents of the pelvic cavity, the external organs (vulva) (Fig. 14-2), and the breasts (mammary glands).

Bony Pelvis

The Latin word *pelvis* means 'basin'. The pelvis is that portion of the trunk below and behind the abdomen. The bony pelvis is composed of the ilium, symphysis pubis, ischium, sacrum, and coccyx. The so-called pelvic brim divides the abdominal false portion, located above the arcuate line, from the true portion of the pelvis, located below this line. It forms the passageway through which the fetus passes during parturition.

The true pelvis may be considered as having three parts: inlet, cavity, and outlet. The muscles lining the pelvis facilitate movement of the thighs, give form to the pelvic cavity, and provide firm elastic lining to the bony pelvic framework (Fig. 14-3). All organs located in the pelvis are covered by pelvic fascia, which is extremely important in the maintenance of normal strength in the pelvic floor.

The fascia covering the muscles is usually dense and firm, whereas that covering organs is often thin and elastic. The nerves, blood vessels, and ureters coursing through the anatomic structures are closely associated with muscular and fascial structures.

The pelvic fascia may be divided into three general groups: parietal, diaphragmatic, and visceral. The parietal pelvic fascia covers the muscles of the true pelvic wall and perineum. The diaphragmatic fascia covers both sides of the pelvic diaphragm, which is made up of the levator ani and coccygeal muscles. The visceral fascia is thin and

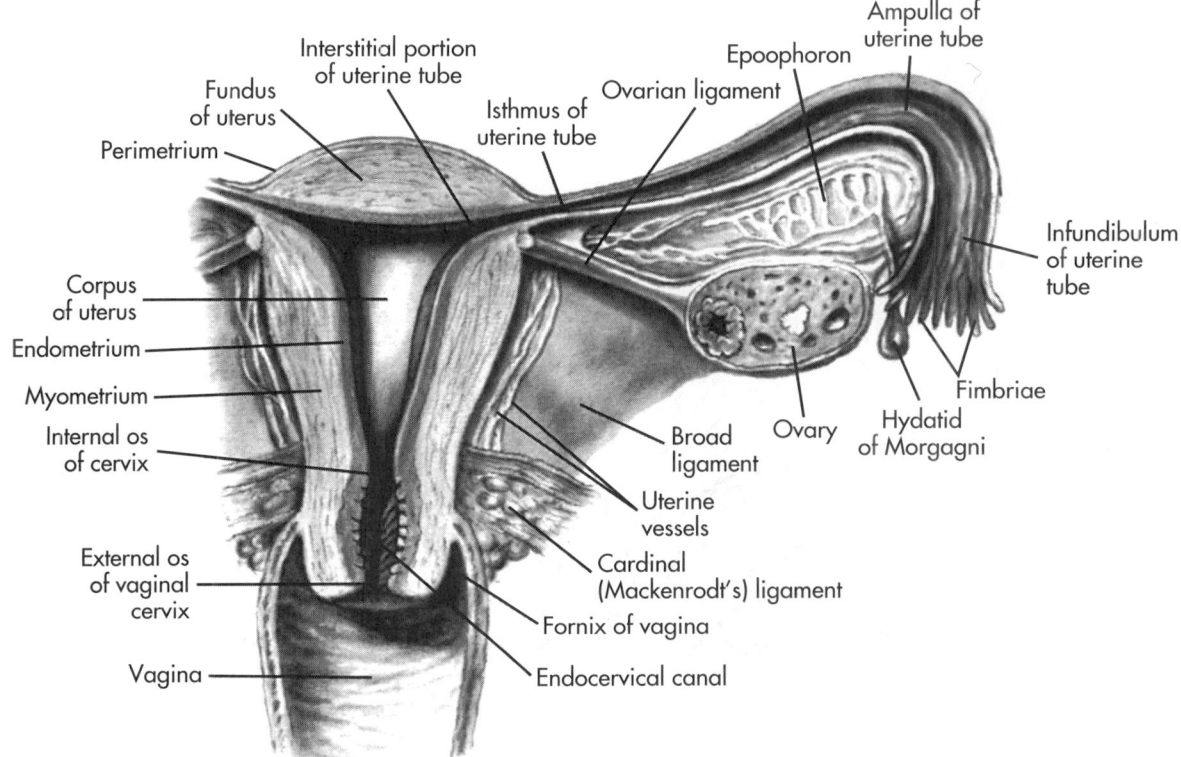

FIGURE 14–1 Female reproductive organs.

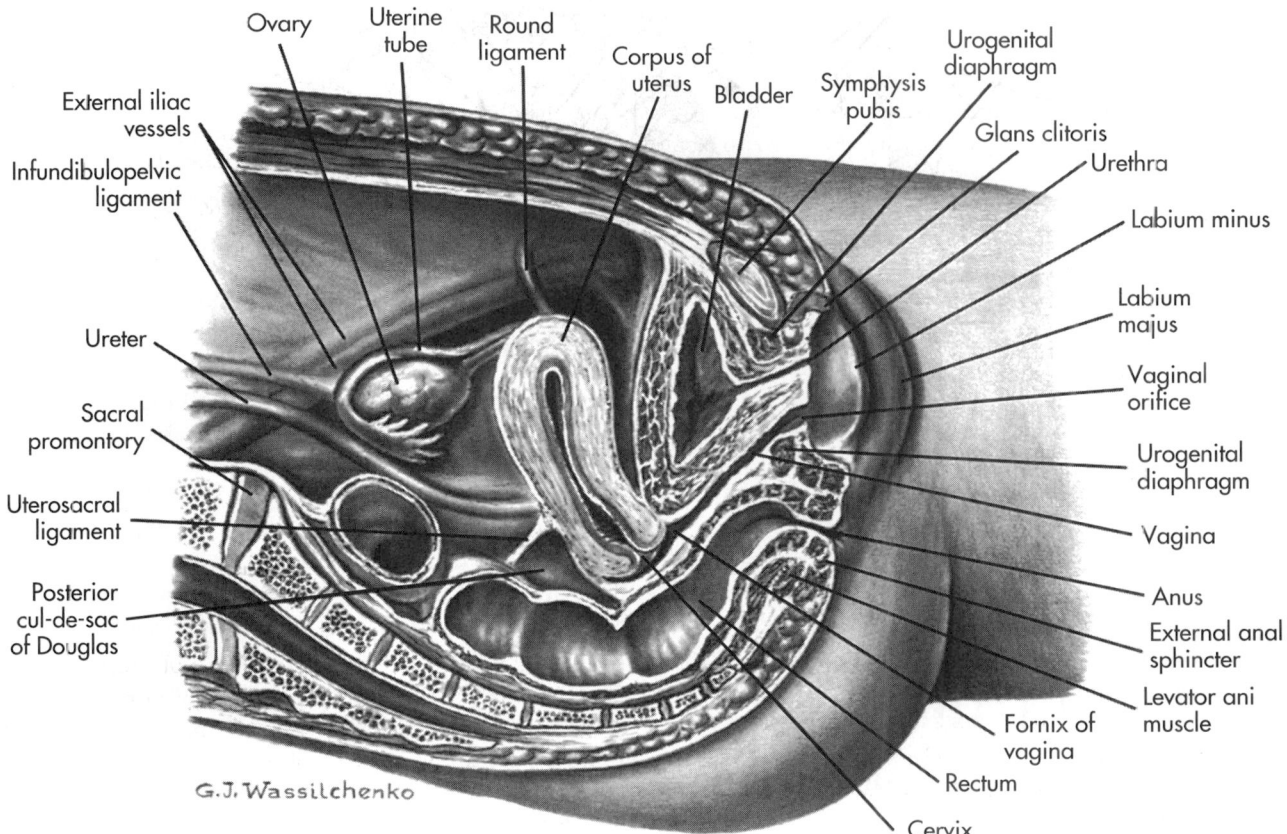

FIGURE 14–2 Female pelvic organs as viewed in midsagittal section.

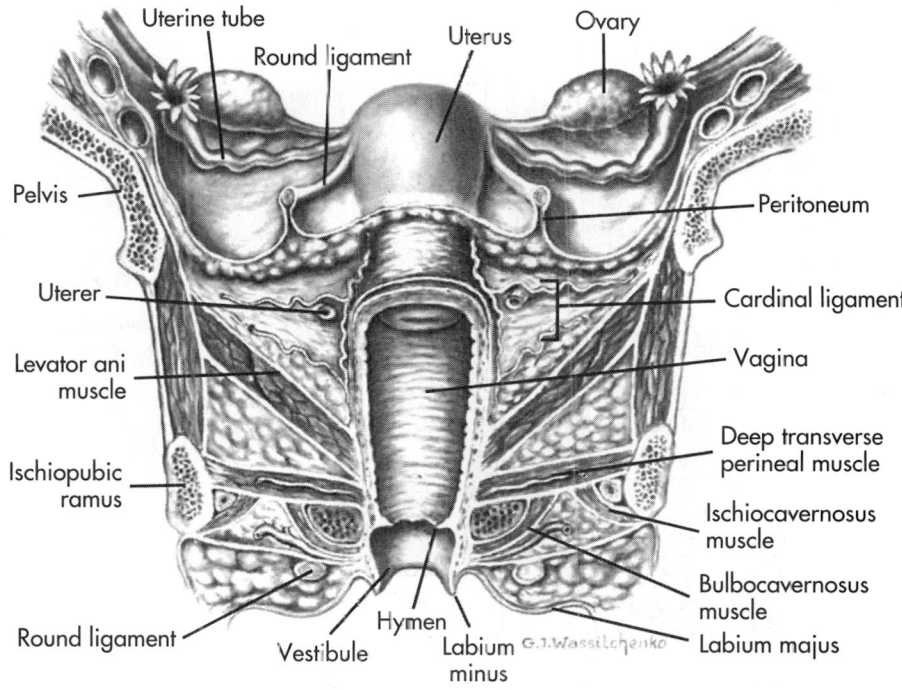

FIGURE 14-3   Relationship of female sexual organs to anterior abdominal wall.

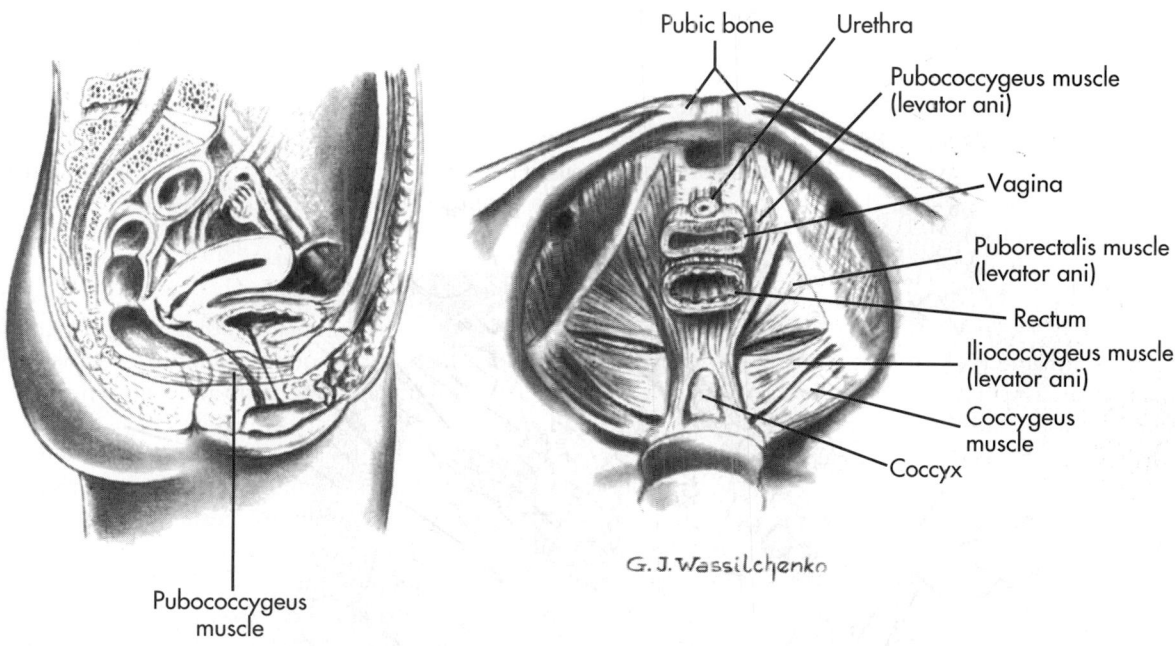

FIGURE 14-4   Perineal musculature.

flexible and covers the pelvic organs. The floor of the pelvis, known as the *pelvic diaphragm*, gives support to the abdominal pelvic viscera in this region. It consists of the levator ani and coccygeal muscles with their respective fascial coverings and separates the pelvic cavity from the perineum (Fig. 14-4, *A*).

The levator ani muscles, varying in thickness and strength, may be divided into three parts: the iliococ-

cygeal, the pubococcygeal, and the puborectal muscles (Fig. 14-4, *B*). The fibers of the levator ani muscles blend with the muscle fibers of the rectum and vagina. The pubovaginal fibers of the pubococcygeal portion of the levator ani muscles, lying directly below the urinary bladder, are involved in the control of micturition. The pubococcygeal fibers of the levator ani muscles control and pull the coccyx forward and assist in the closure of the

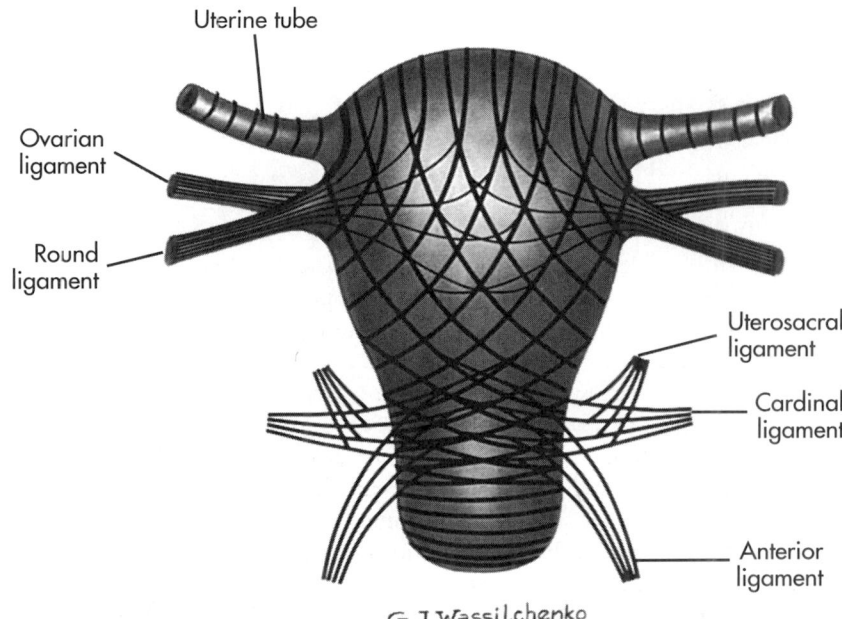

FIGURE 14-5   Schema to show relative positions of eight uterine ligaments formed by folds of peritoneum: two broad ligaments, double folds extending from uterus to side walls of pelvic cavity; two uterosacral ligaments, foldlike extensions of peritoneum from uterus to sacrum; posterior ligament, fold between uterus and rectum; and two round ligaments, folds from uterus to deep inguinal ring.

pelvic outlet. The fibers pull the rectum, vagina, and bladder neck upward toward the symphysis pubis in an effort to close the pelvic outlet and are responsible for the flexure at the anorectal junction. Relaxation of the fibers during defecation permits a straightening at this junction. During parturition the action of the levator ani muscles directs the fetal head into the lower part of the passageway.

Pelvic Cavity

Uterus

The uterus (from the Greek word *hystera*) is a pear-shaped organ situated in the pelvic cavity between the bladder anteriorly and the rectum posteriorly. It gains much of its support by its direct attachment to the vagina and by indirect attachments to nearby structures such as the rectum and pelvic diaphragm. The uterus is supported on each side by the broad, round, cardinal, and uterosacral ligaments and levator ani muscles (Fig. 14-5). The upper lateral points, the uterine cornua, receive the fallopian tubes. The fundus of the uterus is the upper rounded portion situated above the level of the tubal openings and just below the pelvic brim. Below, the body of the uterus joins the cervix, from which it is separated by a slight constriction canal called the *isthmus*. The cervix lies at the level of the ischial spines. The body of the uterus communicates with the cervical canal at the internal orifice, called the *internal os*. The constriction (canal) ends at the vaginal portion of the cervix at the external orifice, called the *external os*. This is a small oval aperture situated between two lips.

The uterine body has three layers: (1) the outer peritoneal, or serous, layer, which is a reflection of the pelvic peritoneum; (2) the myometrium, or muscular layer, which houses involuntary muscles, nerves, blood vessels, and lymphatics; and (3) the endometrium, or mucosal layer, which lines the cavity of the uterus.

Fallopian tubes (oviducts)

The Greek word *salpinx*, meaning 'trumpet' or 'tube', is used to refer to the fallopian tubes (see Fig. 14-1). Bilateral tubes, each consisting of a musculomembranous channel about 4 to 5 inches long, form the canals through which the ova from either ovary are conveyed to the uterus. The outer surfaces of the tubes are covered by peritoneum. Each tube receives its blood supply from the branches of the uterine and ovarian arteries. Each fallopian tube leaves the upper portion of the uterus, passes outward toward the sides of the pelvis, and ends in fringelike projections called *fimbriae*. These fimbriae are situated just below the ovaries.

It has been theorized that the transfer of the ova from the ruptured follicles into the uterus is accomplished through vascular changes, which occur with contraction of the smooth muscle fibers of the tube. The peristaltic movements of the tube then push the ova toward the uterus.

The right tube and ovary are in close relationship to the cecum and appendix; the left tube and ovary are situated near the sigmoid flexure. The proximity of the fallopian tubes to the ureters should be noted.

Ovaries

The ovaries are situated on each side of the uterus. Each ovary lies within a depression (ovarian fossa) on the lateral wall of the pelvic cavity and above the broad ligament (see Fig. 14-1). The anterior border of each ovary is attached to the posterior layer of the broad ligament by a peritoneal fold (mesovarium) and is suspended by the ovarian ligament.

The ovaries, small, almond-shaped organs, are composed of an outer layer, known as the *cortex*, and an inner vascular layer, known as the *medulla*. The medulla consists of connective tissue containing nerves, blood, and lymph vessels. The ovary is covered by epithelium, not peritoneum. The cortex contains ovarian (graafian) follicles in different stages of maturity. After ovulation the corpus luteum arises from the graafian follicle that expelled the ovum.

The ovaries are homologous with the testes of the male. They produce ova after puberty and also function as endocrine glands, producing hormones, such as estrogen, secreted by the ovarian follicles. Estrogen controls the development of the secondary sexual characteristics and initiates growth of the lining of the uterus during the menstrual cycle. Progesterone, which is secreted by the corpus luteum, is essential for the implantation of the fertilized ovum and for the development of the embryo.

Ligaments of the uterus

The uterine ligaments are the broad, round, cardinal, and uterosacral ligaments (see Figs. 14-3 and 14-5).

From each side of the uterus the pelvic peritoneum extends laterally, downward, and posteriorly. A double fold of pelvic peritoneum forms the layers of the broad ligament, enclosing the uterus (see Fig. 14-3). These layers separate to cover the floor and sides of the pelvis. The fallopian tube is situated within the free border of the broad ligament. The free margin of the upper division of the broad ligament, lying immediately below the fallopian tube, is termed the *mesosalpinx*. The ovary lies behind the broad ligament.

Round ligaments are fibromuscular bands attached to the uterus (see Figs. 14-2 and 14-3). Each round ligament passes forward and laterally between the layers of the broad ligament to enter the deep inguinal ring.

Cardinal ligaments are composed of connective tissue with smooth muscle fibers and provide strong support for the uterus.

Uterosacral ligaments are a posterior continuation of the peritoneal tissue. The ligaments pass posteriorly to the sacrum on either side of the rectum (see Fig. 14-5).

Vagina

The vagina is like a collapsed tube and is lined with mucous membrane. It functions as the organ for copulation, the excretory duct for products of menstruation, and the birth canal. The anterior wall measures 6 to 8 cm in length and the posterior wall 7 to 10 cm (see Figs. 14-1 and 14-2). The anterior wall of the vagina is in proximity to the bladder and urethra. The lower posterior wall is anteriorly adjacent to the rectum. The upper portion of the vagina lies above the pelvic floor and is surrounded by visceral pelvic fascia. The lower half is surrounded by the levator ani muscles.

The cervix consists of a supravaginal portion, which is closely associated with the bladder and the ureters, and a vaginal portion, which projects downward and backward into the vaginal vault. The projection of the cervix into the vaginal vault divides the vault into four regions, called *fornices*: anterior and posterior and right and left lateral.

The posterior fornix is in contact with the peritoneum of the pouch of Douglas, or cul-de-sac. The rectovaginal septum lies between the vagina and rectum. The dense connective tissue separating the anterior wall of the vagina from the distal urethra is termed the *urethrovaginal septum*.

Female External Genital Organs (Vulva)

The external organs, referred to collectively as the *vulva*, include the mons pubis, the labia majora and minora, the clitoris, the vestibule, the urethral orifice, the hymen, and various glandular structures (Fig. 14-6).

The mons pubis is a rounded elevation of tissue covered by skin and, after puberty, by hair. It is situated over the anterior surface of the symphysis pubis.

The labia majora are two folds of skin that extend downward and backward from the mons pubis. They unite below and behind to form the posterior commissure and in front to form the anterior commissure. The labia minora are the two delicate folds of skin that lie within the labia majora. Each labium splits into lateral and medial parts. The lateral part forms the prepuce of the clitoris, and the medial part forms the frenulum. The posterior folds of the labia are united by a delicate fold extending between them. This forms the fossa navicularis.

The clitoris is the homolog of the penis in the male. It hangs free and terminates in a rounded glans (small, sensitive vascular body). Unlike the penis, the clitoris does not contain the urethra.

The vestibule is a smooth area surrounded by the labia minora, with the clitoris at its apex and the fossa navicularis at its base. It contains openings for the urethra and the vagina.

The urethra, which is about 4 cm long, is close to the anterior vaginal wall and connects the bladder with the urethral meatus. On either side of the urethral meatus lie two small paraurethral ducts, which are commonly known as *Skene's ducts*.

The vaginal orifice lies below the urethral meatus. This opening extends through the hymen, which was originally a septum. The configuration and size of the opening vary and cannot be used as a determinant of a virginal state.

Bartholin's glands and ducts lie one on each side of the lower end of the vagina. They are homologs of the

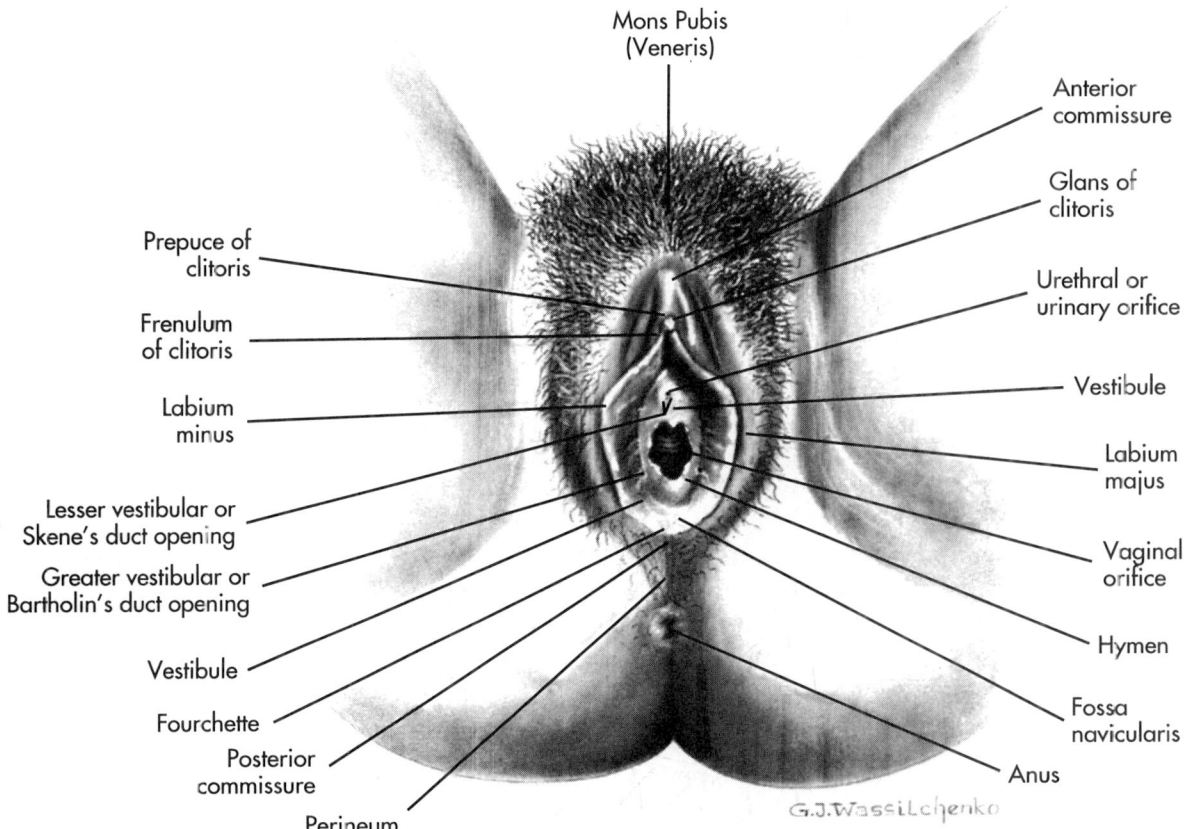

Mons Pubis
(Veneris)

Anterior
commissure

Glans of
clitoris

Prepuce of
clitoris

Urethral or
urinary orifice

Frenulum
of clitoris

Vestibule

Labium
minus

Labium
majus

Lesser vestibular or
Skene's duct opening

Vaginal
orifice

Greater vestibular or
Bartholin's duct opening

Hymen

Vestibule

Fourchette

Fossa
navicularis

Posterior
commissure

Anus

Perineum

G.J.Wassilchenko

FIGURE 14-6   External female reproductive organs.

bulbourethral glands in the male. These narrow ducts open into the vaginal orifice on the inner aspects of the labia minora.

Vascular, Nerve, and Lymphatic Supply of the Reproductive System

The blood supply of the female pelvis is derived from the internal iliac branches of the common iliac artery and is supplemented by the ovarian, superior rectal, and median sacral arteries—branches of the aorta.

The nerve supply of the female pelvis comes from the autonomic nerves, which enter the pelvis in the superior hypogastric plexus (presacral nerve). The lymphatics of the female pelvis either follow the course of the vessels to the iliac and preaortic nodes or empty into the inguinal glands (Fig. 14-7).

PERIOPERATIVE NURSING CONSIDERATIONS

Assessment

The provision of quality perioperative nursing care depends on thorough perioperative assessment and care planning. Data are gathered on the gynecologic patient through the review of systems, physical examination, nursing and medical histories, and diagnostic test results located in the patient record.

Initial review of the patient record permits the perioperative nurse to prioritize and validate information on which the care plan is formulated. Through review of the history and physical exam the perioperative nurse interprets and applies information to the plan of care for the individual patient and the surgical interventions to be performed.

Application of interpersonal communication techniques is vital during nursing assessment. The interview may be conducted on the patient care unit or in the holding area of the surgical suite. Open-ended questions, progressing from general to specific, are incorporated throughout this process. For example, the perioperative nurse may initially inquire about the patient's understanding of the surgical intervention to be performed and then proceed to questions pertaining to intraoperative positioning, which would include the presence of back pain and limitations in joint mobility.

The assessment includes identification of the gynecologic patient's chief complaint, present problem, social history, sexual history, and relevant medical and surgical histories. A family history includes such information as maternal use of diethylstilbestrol and deaths related to gynecologic disorders, cancer, hypertension, diabetes, and heart disease. Cultural, psychologic, and religious beliefs

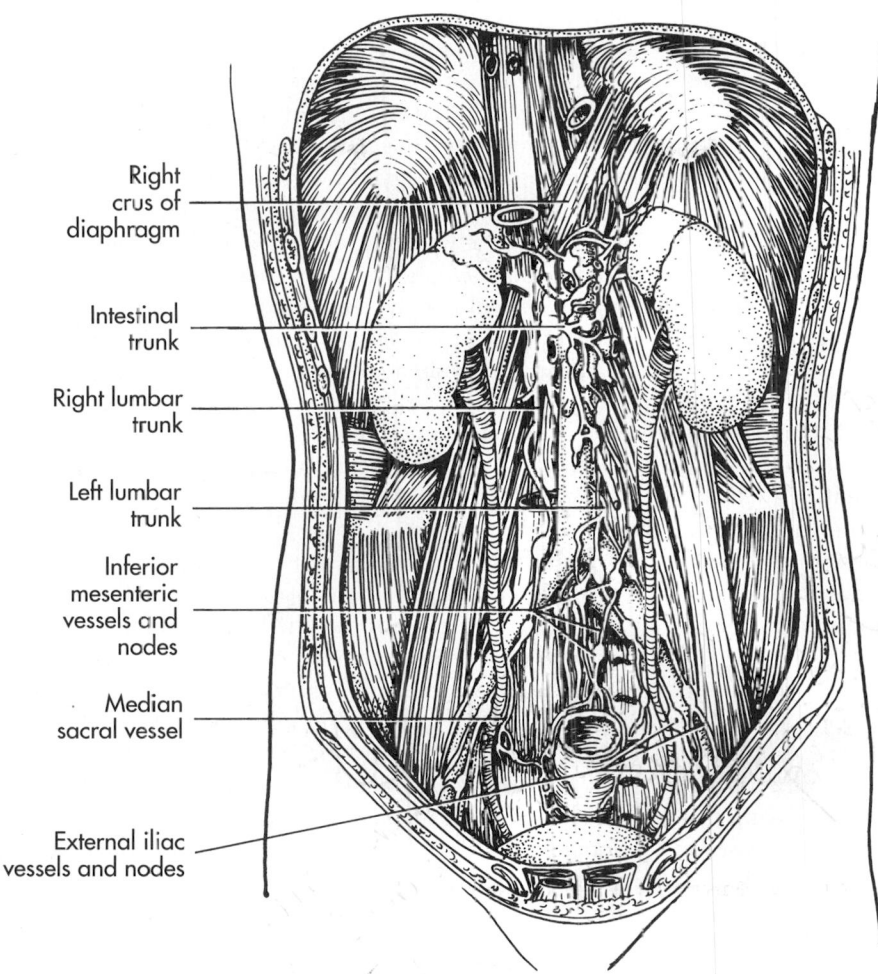

Right
crus of
diaphragm

Intestinal
trunk

Right lumbar
trunk

Left lumbar
trunk

Inferior
mesenteric
vessels and
nodes

Median
sacral vessel

External iliac
vessels and nodes

FIGURE 14-7   Lymphatic system of abdomen and pelvis.

are identified and incorporated into the care plan. Throughout this process the perioperative nurse must remain open and supportive to assist in establishing a trusting therapeutic relationship. These factors can greatly affect the patient's perception of her intended surgery and play a major role in patient outcomes.

The gynecologic patient's history includes a chronologic listing of each pregnancy with length of gestation, type of delivery, complications during pregnancy, duration of labor, and fetal weight. The menstrual cycle is discussed to include age at onset, length of each cycle, amount of flow, duration of bleeding, and pain or discomfort associated with menses. The amount of flow is described in relation to the number of sanitary napkins and tampons used. The perioperative nurse should inquire about a history of vaginal infections or discharge and sexually transmitted diseases. If bleeding is present, the duration, color, and consistency of blood are noted. Questions about use of vaginal douches, creams, and contraceptives are included in the assessment.

A medication history is taken, including use of analgesics, oral contraceptives, estrogen therapy, diuretics, antihypertensives, and cardiac medications. Medication frequency, dosage, and duration of use are noted.

Gynecologic disorders may be associated with urinary problems. Stress incontinence or loss of urine while coughing, sneezing, or laughing should be identified. Pain or burning sensations upon urination are noted. The gynecologic patient may have urologic studies ordered preoperatively, especially in the presence of uterine prolapse.

Results of the physical examination are reviewed by the perioperative nurse. Baseline vital signs, height, weight, and findings from assessment of the thyroid, chest, heart, lungs, breasts, abdomen, pelvis, and rectum are analyzed for their relationship to intraoperative care planning.

The gynecologic patient may undergo numerous diagnostic studies. The studies performed depend on the gynecologic problem or disorder. A laparoscopy may be performed for diagnostic or therapeutic reasons, such as infertility, pelvic pain, pelvic inflammatory disease, ova retrieval for in vitro fertilization (IVF), lysis of adhesions, evaluation of pelvic mass, removal of ectopic pregnancy, or tubal sterilization.

Gynecologic surgery is performed in proximity to the kidneys, ureters, and bladder and may warrant preoperative studies such as an intravenous pyelogram (IVP) and barium enema (BE) to establish an anatomic baseline.

Pelvic ultrasonography helps diagnose ectopic pregnancy and adnexal and uterine disease. Uterine fibroids and blood or fluid in the pelvis may be identified by means of ultrasonography. Computerized tomography (CT) scanning and magnetic resonance imaging (MRI) may be utilized in evaluation of the patient with suspected malignancy in the retroperitoneal lymph nodes or bone.

Preoperatively the gynecologic patient may have a hysterosalpingogram to identify abnormalities in the uterine cavity and occlusions in the tubal folds. This diagnostic tool is useful in detecting potential reasons for infertility.

A colposcopy, with colpomicroscopy, is often performed in the physician's office. This examination is indicated for the patient with an abnormal Papanicolaou (Pap) smear suggestive of dysplasia. It identifies cellular abnormalities that may involve the vulva, vagina, or cervix and helps identify areas of dysplasia and carcinoma in situ. Endocervical curettage may be obtained during the colposcopic procedure to rule out invasive carcinoma or to detect early adenocarcinoma.

Nursing Diagnosis

Comprehensive perioperative nursing care is a planned process that is implemented to ensure safe, quality patient care. Nursing diagnoses are formulated after reviewing the patient record and conducting a complete patient assessment. All significant data collected are reviewed and prioritized and then incorporated into the perioperative care plan. The gynecologic patient may have multiple nursing diagnoses that warrant perioperative nursing intervention. Nursing diagnoses for the gynecologic patient may include the following:

- Anxiety related to surgery and surgical outcome
- Risk for urinary retention
- Risk for impaired skin integrity
- Body image disturbance
- Risk for injury related to surgical position

Outcome Identification

Outcomes identified for the selected nursing diagnoses could be stated as the following:

- The patient will experience reduced anxiety.
- The patient will maintain or regain normal patterns of urinary elimination.
- The patient's skin will remain intact.
- The patient will effectively cope with disturbance in body image.
- The patient will be free from injury related to the surgical position.

Planning

Planning determines the ability of the perioperative nurse to provide patient care in an organized and individualized manner. Planning involves preparation for both the psychosocial and physiologic needs of the gynecologic patient. Part of the nursing care plan is therefore the gathering of the required equipment and supplies and the positioning of accessories, devices, and adjuncts requisite to gynecologic surgical interventions. For example, if the gynecologic patient is undergoing a lengthy surgical intervention, the perioperative nurse will plan to have a warming device, gel-filled mattress, and antiembolic stockings available. These will aid in maintaining the patient's body temperature,[7] in promoting skin integrity, and in preventing venous stasis. Once nursing diagnoses and desired outcomes are established, nursing interventions that will assist the gynecologic patient to reach the desired outcomes are identified. Some examples of interventions for the gynecologic patient are shown in the Sample Care Plan.

Implementation

During implementation of the plan of care, the perioperative nurse performs the identified nursing interventions. Part of perioperative care plan implementation includes selecting the appropriate instruments and patient care supplies, patient positioning on the OR bed, antimicrobial skin preparation, insertion of urinary catheters, draping, creation and maintenance of a sterile field, initiation of safety measures, and patient monitoring. Data continue to be collected, the care plan is documented, and reports are given to relief personnel, ensuring continuity of the patient's plan of care.

Principles and methods of patient positioning for different types of surgical procedures are described in Chapter 5. Stirrups with padding promote maintenance of skin integrity and assist in preventing nerve injury. Patient positions may be modified based on the surgical procedure and surgeon preference. The patient is placed in the lithotomy position for most vaginal and vulvar surgery. For abdominal gynecologic surgery, Trendelenburg's position may be used. Some surgeons use the low lithotomy position with Trendelenburg's position for abdominal oncology procedures to facilitate access to pelvic and paraaortic nodes. Patients placed in Trendelenburg's position for prolonged gynecologic procedures are at increased cardiovascular risk because of decreased pulmonary compliance and functional residual capacity (FRC).[21] Care should be taken to protect all patients from integumentary, musculoskeletal, and nerve injury and ensure adequate circulatory, renal, and respiratory functions.

Because pelvic and vaginal procedures involve manipulation of the ureters, bladder, and urethra, indwelling urinary drainage systems are frequently established before or during surgery. Either an indwelling urethral catheter or a suprapubic cystostomy catheter may be used, depending on the surgeon's preference and the type of procedure. The size of sutures, needles, and drains also varies, depending on surgeon preference and patient needs.

Skin preparation and routine draping procedures are

SAMPLE CARE PLAN

Nursing Diagnosis: Anxiety related to surgery and surgical outcome

Outcome: The patient will experience reduced anxiety.

Interventions:

Introduce self and establish rapport.

Determine signs and symptoms indicating presence of anxiety:

Diaphoresis

Restlessness

Hyperventilation

Tachycardia

Urinary frequency

Nausea

Identify maladaptive and adaptive responses to anxiety.

Encourage use of adaptive coping mechanisms.

Evaluate strengths and resources available to assist patient in coping with anxiety.

Encourage use of relaxation techniques, guided imagery, or music when appropriate for patient.

Identify patient's readiness to learn and provide individualized teaching based on these findings.

Describe sequence of perioperative events to patient in a brief, clear manner.

Use short, simple sentences.

Use calm, firm tone of voice.

Minimize environmental stimuli.

Encourage patient to ventilate feelings and concerns.

Develop therapeutic relationship with patient.

Use active listening skills.

Offer, clarify, and further validate information as needed.

Nursing Diagnosis: Risk for urinary retention

Outcome: The patient will maintain or regain normal patterns of urinary elimination.

Interventions:

Instruct patient on importance of adequate postoperative fluid intake and early ambulation.

Before surgery, explain that indwelling urinary catheter will be inserted (as applicable). Review important elements of catheter care, management of drainage system, catheter removal, and signs and symptoms of urinary tract infection.

Encourage patient to verbalize feelings and concerns regarding ability to void postoperatively, presence of indwelling catheter, and catheter removal.

Clarify any misperceptions the patient may have.

Insert indwelling urinary catheter using aseptic technique.

Obtain urine specimen as required. Connect catheter to closed drainage system.

Document size of catheter inserted and specimens obtained.

Secure tubing to patient to prevent inadvertent stretching or stress on catheter.

Place urinary drainage bag where it is readily observable.

Keep drainage bag below level of bladder.

Check patency of catheter and drainage system whenever patient is repositioned.

Observe color and amount of urine; report abnormalities.

Record urinary output; report amount of urine to anesthesia provider.

Nursing Diagnosis: Risk for impaired skin integrity

Outcome: The patient's skin will remain intact.

Interventions:

Notice the presence of any skin rashes, bruises, lacerations, ecchymoses, petechiae, or other alterations, and record them.

Select an appropriate site of placement for electrosurgical dispersive pad (close to the operative site, on area with good muscle mass, free of excessive hair or skin oil).

Verify that the patint has no known allergies to antimicrobial skin-preparation agents.

Prepare operative site according to institutional procedure.

Keep dependent skin areas around preparation site and electrosurgical pad dry; do not allow solutions to pool.

Keep OR bed surface free from wrinkles.

Pad bony prominences, which may include the heels, ankles, and buttocks, depending on patient position.

Place safety and restraining straps so that they are snug but not tight.

Apply dressings to surgical incision line and drain exit sites before surgical drapes are removed to prevent contamination of the incision; use aseptic technique.

After dressing has been applied, cleanse area surrounding incision and drain sites of blood and exudate.

Apply tape gently but firmly to secure dressing in place; allow room for postoperative swelling to prevent tape burns.

Document location of electrosurgical dispersive pad site and ECG leads, antimicrobial skin preparation solution, placement of safety and restraining straps, and presence of drains.

Continued

SAMPLE CARE PLAN—CONT'D

Nursing Diagnosis: Body–image disturbance

Outcome: The patient will effectively cope with disturbance in body image.

Interventions:

Encourage patient to express feelings about her diagnosis and surgery and how she believes it will affect her body image.

Clarify any misconceptions.

Maintain the patient's privacy.

Express understanding and assurance to the patient that her feelings and concerns are normal.

Determine patient's readiness to learn, and teach patient information relevant to her body-image alteration.

Be nonjudgmental.

Demonstrate empathy and positive regard.

Identify effective coping skills previously used by patient and encourage use of these if appropriate in current situation.

Assist patient to value her present self realistically.

Encourage patient to identify her strengths.

Encourage attendance at self-help groups when appropriate.

Nursing Diagnosis: Risk for injury related to surgical position.

Outcome: The patient will be free from injury related to the surgical position.

Interventions:

Notice the presence of any preexisting patient conditions (nutritional status, weight, preoperative chemotherapy, limitations in mobility or range of motion, neurovascular impairments) that place the patient at risk for positional injury. Document them.

Preoperatively assess and document condition of dependent skin areas.

If possible, have the patient assume the planned surgical position before induction of anesthesia. Modify plan for patient positioning in presence of pain or discomfort.

Gather positioning accessories appropriate to the planned position.

Pad OR bed (foam, water, or gel-filled mattress) as appropriate to identified patient risk factors.

Pad dependent pressure sites.

Protect vulnerable neurovascular bundles from injury.

Reassess padding and protection on any positional changes.

Maintain body alignment.

Secure patient in position with safety and body straps.

Accomplish all positioning and positional changes slowly, gently, and gradually.

Document position (and positional changes), safety measures, and accessories used.

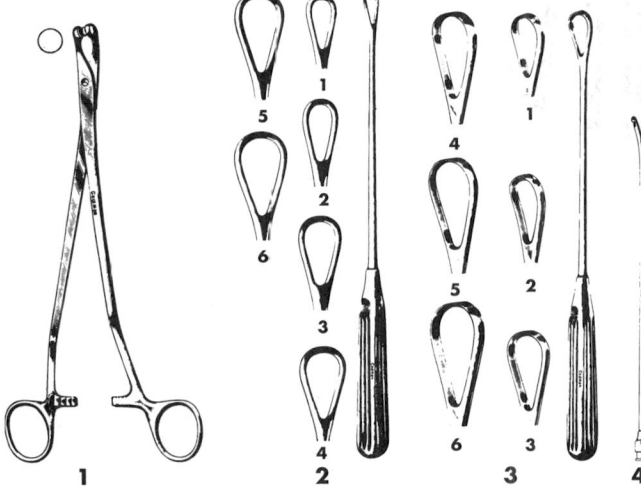

FIGURE 14–8 Vaginal instruments, cutting: *1*, Gaylor biopsy forceps; *2*, Thomas uterine curettes (blunt); *3*, Sims uterine curettes (sharp); *4*, endometrial biopsy suction curette.

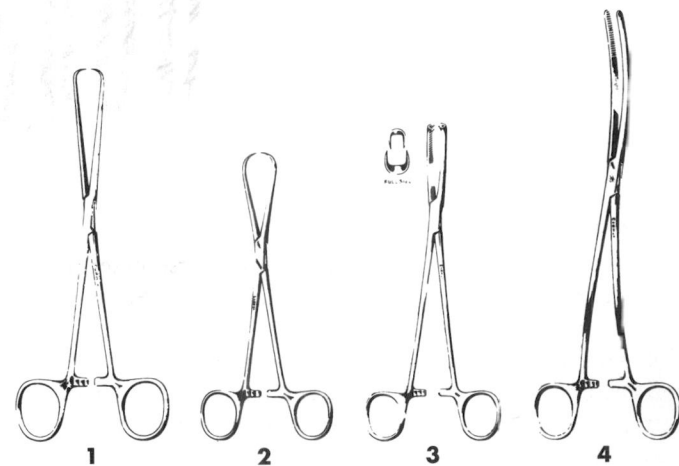

FIGURE 14–9 Vaginal instruments, holding: *1*, uterine tenaculum; *2*, Staude uterine tenaculum; *3*, Jacobs vulsellum forceps; *4*, Bozeman dressing forceps.

described in Chapter 4. The vaginal prep setup should be separate from an abdominal prep setup. A basic vaginal instrument set is required for vaginal and vulvar surgery (Figs. 14-8 to 14-11). A basic abdominal gynecologic instrument set is required for abdominal gynecologic

surgery (Figs. 14-12 to 4-14). Surgeons' instrument preferences may vary, and instrument lists described in this chapter are not meant to be all inclusive.

For most abdominal gynecologic procedures, a dilatation and curettage set should be available.

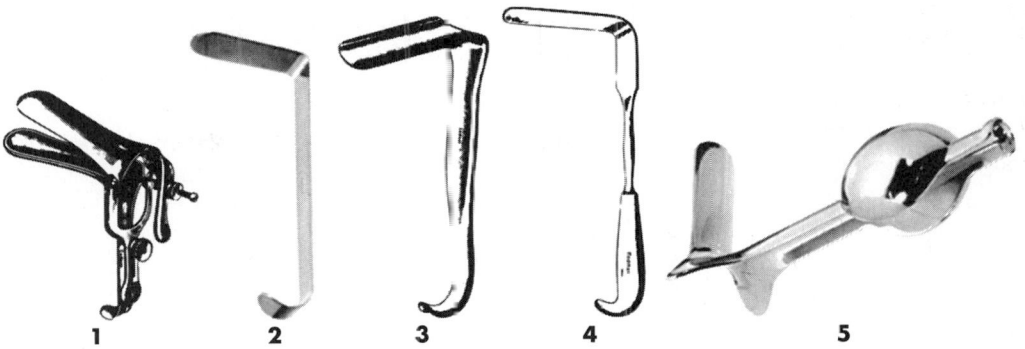

FIGURE 14-10 Vaginal instruments, exposing: *1*, Graves self-retaining vaginal speculum; *2*, Heaney hysterectomy retractor; *3*, Doyen vaginal retractor; *4*, Glenner vaginal retractor; *5*, Auvard vaginal speculum (weighted).

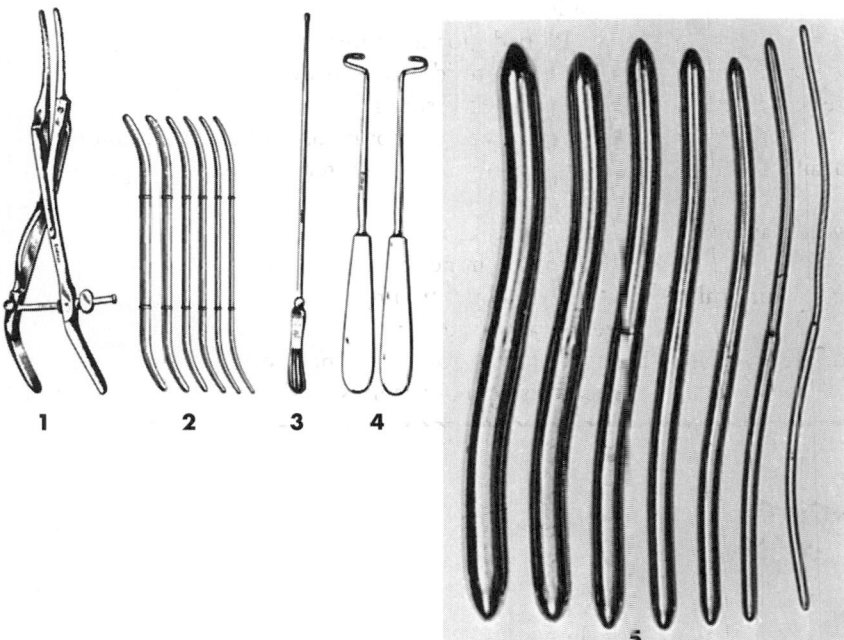

FIGURE 14-11 Vaginal instruments, exposing: *1*, Goodell uterine dilator; *2*, Hank uterine dilators; *3*, uterine sound (graduated); *4*, Deschamp ligature carriers (right and left); *5*, Hegar dilators.

Evaluation

During evaluation the perioperative nurse determines whether the patient met the established goals. Some goals can be reached during the preoperative and intraoperative phases of care; they are evaluated before the patient's discharge from the operating room. Others require ongoing monitoring and measurement in the postoperative phase; these are denoted by the word "will" to indicate their ongoing nature. Part of the perioperative nursing report to the recovery area (PACU, ambulatory recovery) should include the goals of the nursing care plan. They can be phrased as outcome statements, as follows:

- The patient's anxiety was reduced; she verbalized concerns and used personally effective coping strategies.
- Urinary elimination patterns were maintained; urinary output was adequate, and catheter patency was maintained.

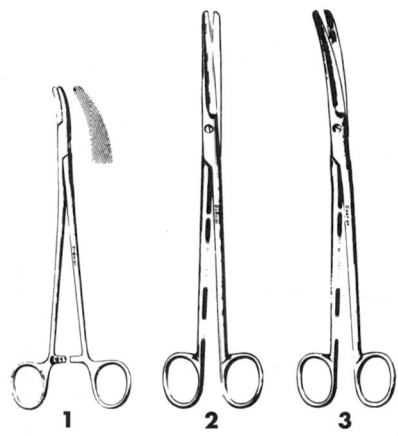

FIGURE 14-12 Abdominal gynecologic instruments, cutting and suturing: *1*, Heaney needle holder; *2*, Mayo dissecting scissors (straight, 6¾ inches); *3*, Mayo dissecting scissors (curved, 6¾ inches).

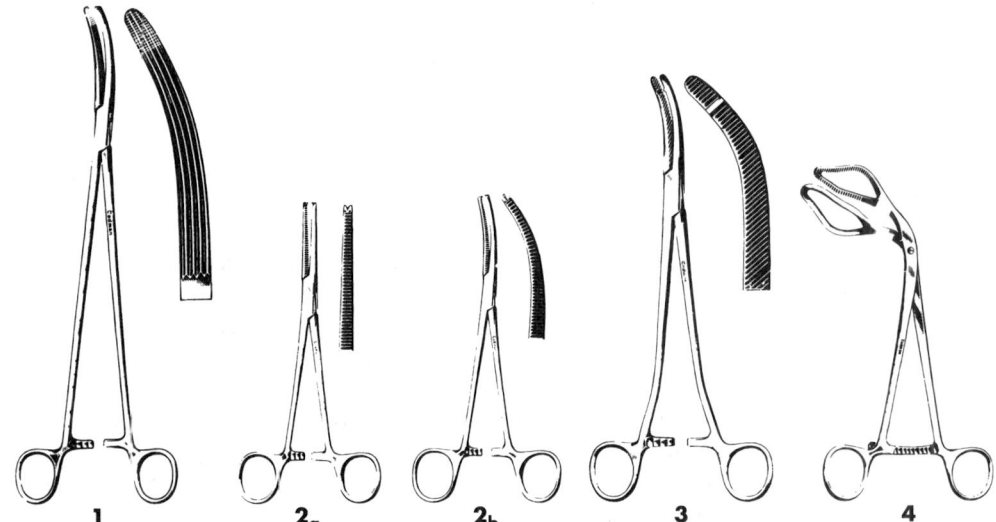

FIGURE 14-13   Abdominal gynecologic instruments, clamping: *1*, Rochester-Pean forceps; *2a*, Rochester-Ochsner (straight) forceps; *2b*, Rochester-Ochsner (curved) forceps; *3*, Heaney hysterectomy forceps; *4*, Somer uterus-elevating forceps.

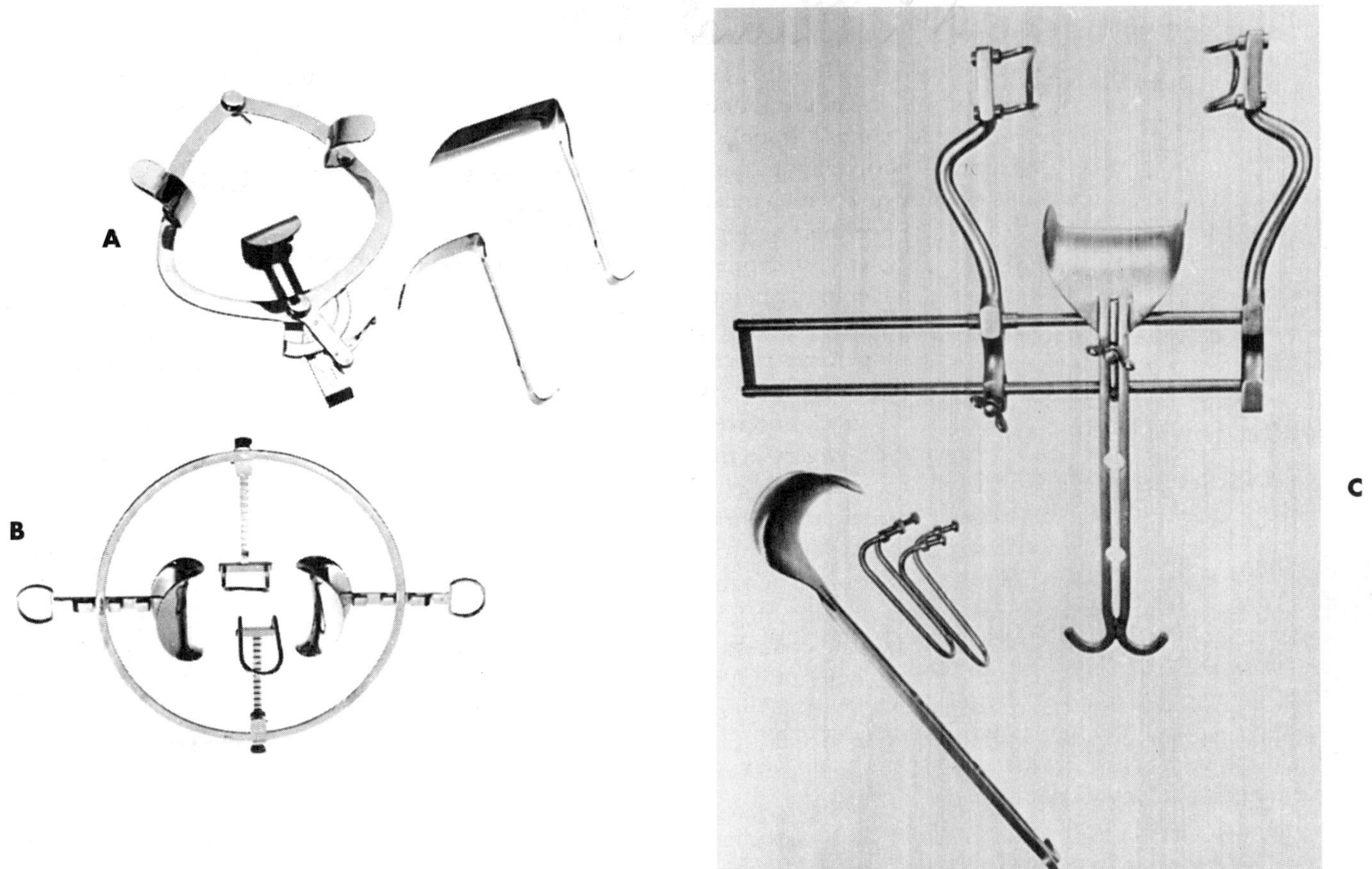

FIGURE 14-14   Abdominal gynecologic instruments, exposing: **A**, O'Sullivan-O'Connor self-retaining abdominal retractor. **B**, Martin self-retaining abdominal ring retractor. **C**, Balfour self-retaining retractor with blades.

- Skin integrity was maintained; there were no reddened areas at dependent pressure sites or at the placement site of the dispersive pad; the incision was aseptically dressed.
- The patient will effectively cope with her disturbance in body image; questions will continue to be answered and misconceptions clarified.
- There was no evidence of injury related to surgical positioning; range of motion and neurovascular status were consistent with preoperative levels.

Patient and Family Education and Discharge Planning

Patient and family education, along with discharge planning, has become a priority perioperative nursing activity in the late 1990s. No longer is this a nursing intervention that is begun after the patient is admitted to an acute care setting. Many gynecologic surgical procedures are performed on an ambulatory basis, and for those that require an inpatient admission, length of stay continues to decrease. Thus, patient education and discharge planning often begin before any admission, be it

---

14-1 RESEARCH HIGHLIGHT

In this study, 30 women scheduled for laparoscopic tubal ligation were randomly assigned to either routine, unstructured preoperative education (control group) or a structured educational session (experimental group). Both groups had a preadmission interview with a nurse and anesthesiologist 1 to 2 weeks before their surgery. The experimental group also received structured teaching during the preadmission screening appointment, which consisted of a slide-sound tape describing preoperative, intraoperative, and postoperative procedural and sensory information. A 6-page brochure was also given to the patients. The control group received unstructured teaching on the day of their surgery in the preoperative holding area. A comparison of vital signs, patient satisfaction, analgesic and antiemetic administration, and length of stay in phase I and phase II recovery showed that the only significant difference between the two groups was related to analgesics. Patients in the experimental group reported less pain and requested and received less pain medication. Although the study was limited by a small sample size, the measurement of clinical outcomes mediated by nursing interventions is important in quantifying the contributions of nurse care to improvements in patient care.

From Franzen-Coslow, B.I., & Eddy, M.E. (1998). Effects of preoperative ambulatory gynecological education: clinical outcomes and patient satisfaction. *Journal of Perianesthesia Nursing,* 13(1), 4-11.

---

ambulatory or inpatient (Research Highlight 14-1). Regardless of the gynecologic procedure performed, the perioperative nurse should begin patient and family education with routine postoperative care information. The goal of this information is to restore normal body function and may include such areas as early ambulation, prevention of respiratory complications, incision care and anticipated postoperative discomfort, managing postoperative pain, any restrictions in activity, diet, and any other concerns the patient has. Following "need-to-know" information (see Chapter 10 for a full discussion of patient education), home-care management and an assessment of the patient's resources for it guide discharge planning and requirements for referral or follow-up. Such areas as progression of activities, emotional and physical issues, sexual activity, general nutritional needs, and health maintenance guide this planning. For gynecologic patients, other specific information should include signs and symptoms to report, especially in relation to vaginal bleeding and the surgical site, and restrictions related to douching and vaginal penetration (tampons or sexual intercourse). With the growth in same-day surgery, many types of hysterectomies, some myomectomies and even laparotomies are now same-day, 23-hour stay procedures. In these cases, it is likely that a visit or visits by a nurse in the home will be part of discharge planning.[19] Simple, clearly written information and instructions such as those presented in Box 14-1 are helpful, and perioperative nurses should consider participating in their development.

LASERS IN GYNECOLOGIC SURGERY

The carbon dioxide (CO_2) laser, neodymium:yttrium-aluminum-garnet (Nd:YAG) laser, and argon laser have been used in gynecology to treat extrauterine disease such as pelvic endometriosis, cervical dysplasia, condylomata acuminata, pelvic adhesive disease, and premalignant diseases of the vulva and vagina. Lasers are usually used in conjunction with the colposcope and operating microscope, or the laparoscope. A laser plume evacuator or suction system is necessary to remove smoke and fumes from the operative field.[12] All accessories and instrumentation used should be laser safe, secure, and tested or examined for working order before use. Safety precautions must be implemented by the OR team when the laser is used (see Chapter 3).

SURGICAL INTERVENTIONS
VULVAR SURGERY

The treatment of early malignant disease of the vulva is accomplished by a skinning technique, local wide excision, or, for more multicentric or extensive lesions, simple vulvectomy. These procedures may also be accomplished by use of a laser.

| BOX 14-1 | Before and After a Hysterectomy |

I have been advised to have a hysterectomy to remove my uterus. Will my ovaries be removed, too?

Your first impression was right. A *hysterectomy* is an operation to remove the uterus. Sometimes the ovaries are taken out at the same time. Removal of the ovaries is called oophorectomy. It's important to know the difference between these two operations because each has a different effect on your body. If you have only a hysterectomy, your periods will stop. But if you have your ovaries removed as well, the effects on your body will be greater. If your ovaries are removed, your body will no longer produce sufficient estrogen. This is called surgical menopause. It's just like natural menopause, except it happens more suddenly. And sometimes the effects are more severe because of the sudden loss of estrogen.

Will I notice any physical differences, such as change in abdominal shape, after surgery?

There is no change in body appearance, especially if surgery is performed through the vagina or navel. Once the incision has healed, your abdomen should return to normal. A hysterectomy usually involves the removal of the cervix, and the innermost part of the vagina is sutured. Even though the cervix is gone, the vaginal space remains unchanged. Sexual intercourse should feel the same.

What kind of reactions will my body have after an oophorectomy?

Most women (about 85%) feel some of the effects of the sudden, complete loss of estrogen immediately. At first you can probably expect hot flashes and night sweats. The hot flashes spread over the chest and neck area; the night sweats may wake you up from a sound sleep. This sleep disturbance may result in tiredness, depression, and nervousness. These may continue for several years. Some problems caused by estrogen loss may crop up later, but these can often be prevented by taking estrogen.

What's so important about estrogen?

Estrogen, a hormone made by your ovaries, prepares the uterus for either pregnancy or a menstrual period. It's needed, along with calcium, to keep bones strong; it also helps protect your vaginal and urinary tract tissues against thinning and drying.

What are the other health problems of surgical menopause besides hot flashes and night sweats?

One problem—changes in cholesterol levels—can slowly build up for years. After menopause it is very likely that cholesterol levels will

increase more rapidly. Surgical menopause may also cause the lining of your vagina to become thin and dry, causing pain sometimes during or after intercourse. Over time, changes in the urinary system may cause bladder control problems, such as the need to urinate more frequently or some leakage of urine when coughing or sneezing.

Can anything be done to cure or prevent these problems?

Taking estrogen can help relieve or prevent many of these problems. It certainly relieves hot flashes and night sweats, helps prevent vaginal and urinary tract tissue from thinning and drying, and is the single best way to prevent osteoporosis. Replacing lost estrogen greatly lowers a woman's chances of breaking a bone or developing a humped back. Estrogen has no effect on rising cholesterol levels, but it does not affect them adversely.

I've heard that estrogen can cause cancer. Is this true?

Some studies have suggested a possible increased incidence of breast cancer in women taking *higher* doses of estrogen for prolonged periods of time, but most of these studies do not link breast cancer with taking the *usual* doses of estrogen *after* menopause. However, if anyone in your family has had breast cancer, let your doctor know before you start taking estrogen. Your doctor may very well recommend that you continue taking estrogen, even after any obvious symptoms have vanished. Taking estrogen continually lessens your chances of breaking a bone by as much as 50% to 60%. Taking estrogen along with calcium helps your bones stay strong. Almost half of the bone loss a woman suffers occurs in the first 7 years after surgical menopause. And if you have a hysterectomy at age 35 or 40, you can expect to live another 40 years or more without producing natural estrogen.

On the other hand, since taking any drug has some chance of side effects, estrogen may not be right for you. It's important to consult your physician about the best treatment for you to counter the effects of surgical menopause.

This guide may be copied for free distribution to patients and families. All rights reserved.

From Mosby. (1997). *Mosby's Patient Teaching Guides.* St. Louis: Mosby, p. 208.

Simple Vulvectomy

Simple vulvectomy is removal of the labia majora and labia minora, possibly but not preferably the glans clitoris, and occasionally tissue from the perianal area, with a plastic closure. A simple vulvectomy is usually done to treat carcinoma in situ of the vulva when it is multicentric. Occasionally a vulvectomy is necessary for the treatment of either leukoplakia or intractable pruritus, especially when a skinning procedure is impractical or has failed.

Procedural considerations

The basic vaginal instrument set is required, plus an electrosurgical unit, if desired. The patient is positioned in lithotomy.

Operative procedure

1. The affected skin is incised, usually starting anteriorly above the clitoris. The incision is continued laterally to the labia majora, to the midline of the perineum, and around the anus, if it is involved. A knife, hemostats, gauze sponges on sponge-holding forceps, tissue forceps, and Allis forceps are needed. Bleeding vessels are clamped. Bleeding is also controlled by electrocoagulation or sutures.

2. Periurethral and perivaginal incisions are made. Bleeding of this vascular area can be controlled by means of Kelly or Crile hemostats and electrocoagulation. Ligation of blood vessels should be minimal. Allis-Adair forceps are used for holding diseased tissues.

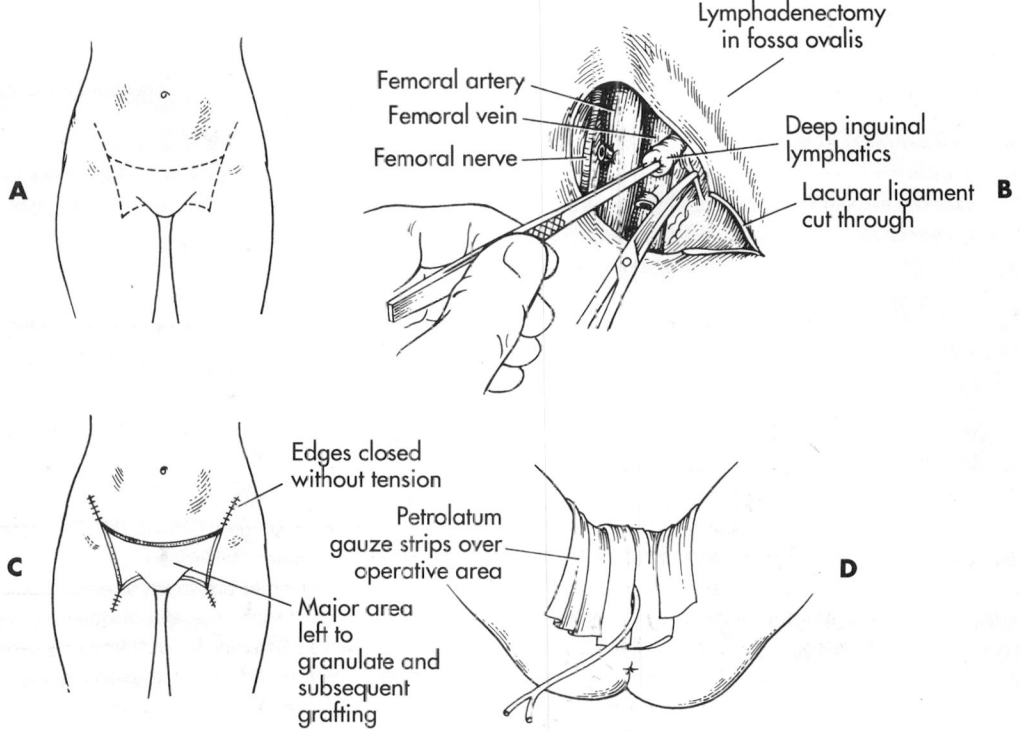

FIGURE 14-15 **A**, Outline of incisional lines for simple or radical operations for vulvar cover. **B**, Dissection is completed, involving nerves, saphenous veins, and muscles, when dissection of distal half of femoral canal has been completed. **C**, Upper edges of abdominal incisions may be partially closed. **D**, With indwelling catheter in bladder, wound is dressed with layers of gauze and held in place with light pressure dressing.

3. All skin and subcutaneous tissues are undermined and mobilized with curved dissecting scissors, tissue forceps, Allis forceps, and sponges on holding forceps.
4. The wound is closed, usually by simple bilateral Z-plasty or other plastic closure. In some cases skin is excised around the anus to accomplish a sliding skin flap.
5. Closed wound drainage catheters may be placed in the dependent areas, an indwelling urinary catheter is inserted, and vaginal gauze packing may be placed in the vagina. Dressings are applied.

Skinning Vulvectomy

Skinning vulvectomy is the simple removal of the external skin from the affected area, which has been previously identified with a stain such as toluidine blue. The purpose of this procedure is to preserve the underlying structures of the external genitalia. A skinning procedure may be done to treat leukoplakia, intractable pruritus, or other types of skin lesions, such as kraurosis, vitiligo, and chronic venereal granulomas.

Procedural considerations

The instrumentation required and patient position are as described for simple vulvectomy.

Operative procedure

The external skin is simply excised from the affected area.

Groin Lymphadenectomy and Radical Vulvectomy

Groin lymphadenectomy and radical vulvectomy are the en bloc dissection of the following structures: a large segment of skin from the abdomen and groin, labia majora, labia minora, clitoris, mons veneris, and terminal portions of the urethra, vagina, and other vulvar organs, as well as the superficial and deep inguinal nodes, portions of the round ligaments, portions of the saphenous veins, and the lesion itself. It also involves reconstruction of the vaginal walls and pelvic floor and closure of the abdominal wounds (Fig. 14-15). Placement of full-thickness pinch or split-thickness grafts may be done if the denuded area of the vulva appears too large for normal granulation. A plastic surgeon may immediately complete skin grafts or rotation flaps to cover defects (see Chapter 24).

Groin lymphadenectomy and radical vulvectomy involve abdominoperineal dissection and groin dissection, which may be performed as a one- or two-stage operation. When performed as a one-stage operation, it is optimally done by a four-person team. The skin prep is extensive, including the abdomen and thighs; if a skin graft will be done, the donor site will also need to be prepped.

Procedural considerations

The patient lies supine and may be placed in Trendelenburg's and low lithotomy positions, as required for the various stages. The skin prep includes the abdomen, vulva, and thighs. An indwelling urinary catheter is often inserted to act as a urethral marker and to prevent postoperative urethral trauma. As in other radical surgery, the nursing team should be prepared to measure blood loss and anticipate procedures to combat shock.

For groin lymphadenectomy the basic abdominal gynecologic instrument set is required, with the addition of Schnidt tonsil forceps, Kantrowitz thoracic clamps, ligating clips and appliers and closed-wound drainage systems.

For radical vulvectomy the basic vaginal instrument set is required, with the addition of assorted sizes of Richardson retractors, Richardson appendectomy retractors, Volkmann rake retractors, skin hooks, and closed-wound drainage systems.

Operative procedures

Groin Lymphadenectomy

1. The first skin incision is made on the side opposite the primary lesion. The end of the incised skin is grasped with Allis forceps. The incision is carried down to the aponeuroses of the external oblique muscle.
2. The fascia over the inguinal ligament and the fascia lata of the upper thigh are exposed, separated, and freed with retractors, knife, scissors, hemostats, and sponges.
3. Bleeding vessels, including the superficial iliac artery and vein, the epigastric artery and vein, and the superficial external pudendal artery and vein, are clamped and ligated. Smaller bleeding vessels are controlled by electrocoagulation.
4. The fibers of the inguinal, hypogastric, and femoral nerves are resected using Metzenbaum scissors, tissue forceps without teeth, and long-bladed retractors.
5. The lymphatic node beds may be identified with silk sutures or metal clips. Fine, long, sharp dissection scissors are needed.
6. The large tissue surfaces are exposed for complete dissection by means of retractors and are protected by warm, moist laparotomy packs. High saphenous vein ligation is performed with scissors, forceps, and hemostats and should be doubly tied with nonreactive suture.
7. The femoral canal is cleaned of its lymphatics; the round ligament is clamped, cut, and ligated.
8. The peritoneum is freed from the muscles; the fascia is dissected free; deep lymphatic nodes and areolar tissue are removed; and vessels and their attachments are clamped, cut, and ligated, using long curved scissors,

long tissue forceps, hemostats, and ligatures (Fig. 14-15, *B*).
9. The lesion is removed. In deep pelvic lymphadenectomy, the ureter may be exposed and the area drained.
10. The inguinal canal is reconstructed, and the wound is partially closed with a nonabsorbable suture (Fig. 14-15, *C*). An indwelling urethral catheter is inserted, and the wound is dressed (Fig. 14-15, *D*).

Radical Vulvectomy

1. The skin incisions of the abdomen and thigh join with those for vulvectomy. The incisions in the vulva encircle the urethra.
2. In the vulvar dissection, terminal portions of the urethra and vagina, the mons veneris, the clitoris, the frenulum, the prepuce of the clitoris, Bartholin's and Skene's glands, and fascial coverings of the vulva are removed with the specimen.
3. Reconstruction of the vaginal walls and the pelvic floor is completed. An indwelling urinary catheter is inserted, closed wound drainage catheters are placed in the denuded area, and the wound is dressed with a pressure dressing.

VAGINAL SURGERY

Plastic Reconstructive Repair of the Vagina (Anterior and Posterior Repair; Colporrhaphy)

A vaginal repair is done to correct a cystocele or a rectocele and to reestablish the support of the anterior and posterior vaginal walls, restoring the bladder and rectum to their normal positions. A cystocele is a herniation of the bladder that causes the anterior vaginal wall to bulge downward (Fig. 14-16). A defect in the anterior vaginal wall is usually caused by obstetric or surgical trauma, age, or an inherent weakness. A large protrusion may cause a sensation of pressure in the vagina or present a mass at or through the introitus; it may also cause voiding difficulties.

A rectocele is formed by a protrusion of the anterior

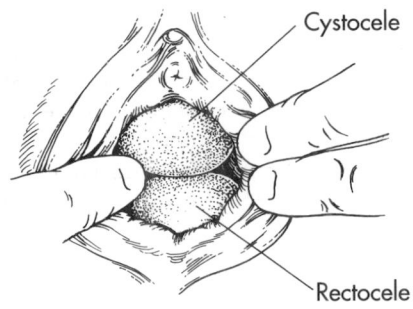

FIGURE 14-16 Cystocele and rectocele resulting from unrepaired tears of muscles of pelvic floor and those under bladder, usually resulting from childbirth, surgical trauma, age, or inherent weakness.

rectal wall (posterior vaginal wall) into the vagina. In general, the anterior rectal wall forms a bulging mass beneath the posterior vaginal mucosa (see Fig. 14-16) As the mass pushes downward into the lower vaginal canal, the rectum may be torn from the fascial and muscular attachments of the urogenital diaphragm and the pelvic wall. The levator ani muscles (see Fig. 14-4) become stretched or torn. The symptomatic signs are a mass protruding into the vagina, difficulty in evacuating the lower bowel, hemorrhoids, and a feeling of pressure.

An enterocele is a herniation of Douglas's cul-de-sac and almost always contains loops of the small intestine. An enterocele herniates into a weakened area between the anterior and posterior vaginal walls.

Procedural considerations

The basic vaginal instrument set is required.

Operative procedures

1. Dilatation and curettage may be done in conjunction with the repair.
2. Vaginal retractors are used for exposure. The labia may be sewn back if the exposure is inadequate.

Anterior wall repair

1. The bladder may be drained, or an indwelling urinary catheter or suprapubic cystostomy catheter may be inserted (surgeon's preference). Areolar tissue between the bladder and vagina at the bladder reflection is exposed. The full thickness of the vaginal wall is separated up to the bladder neck by a knife, curved scissors, tissue forceps, Allis–Adair or Allis forceps, and gauze sponges. Bleeding vessels are clamped and tied with ligatures or electrocoagulated.
2. The urethra and bladder neck are mobilized with a knife, gauze sponges, and curved scissors.
3. Sutures are placed adjacent to the urethra and bladder neck in such a manner that, after they have been tied, a narrowing of the bladder neck and a delineating of the posterior urethrovesical angle occur (Fig. 14-17, A).
4. The connective tissue on the lateral aspects of the cervix is sutured into the cervix to shorten the cardinal ligaments.
5. Allis–Adair forceps are applied to the edges of the incision, and the left flap of the vaginal wall is drawn across the midline. Edges are trimmed according to the size of the cystocele. This process is repeated on the right flap of the vaginal incision.
6. The anterior vaginal wall is closed in a manner resulting in reconstruction of an anterior vaginal fornix (Fig. 14-17, B).

Rectocele repair

1. Allis forceps are placed posterior at the mucocutaneous junction on each side, at the hymenal ring, and just above the anus (Fig. 14-18, A).

2. Skin and mucosa are incised and dissected from the muscles beneath with a knife, tissue forceps, curved scissors, and gauze sponges.
3. Allis–Adair forceps are placed on the posterior vaginal wall, scar tissue (from obstetric trauma) is removed, and dissection is continued to the posterior vaginal fornix and laterally, depending on the size of the rectocele (Fig. 14-18, A and B).
4. The perineum is denuded by sharp dissection, and the trimming of the posterior vaginal wall is carried out

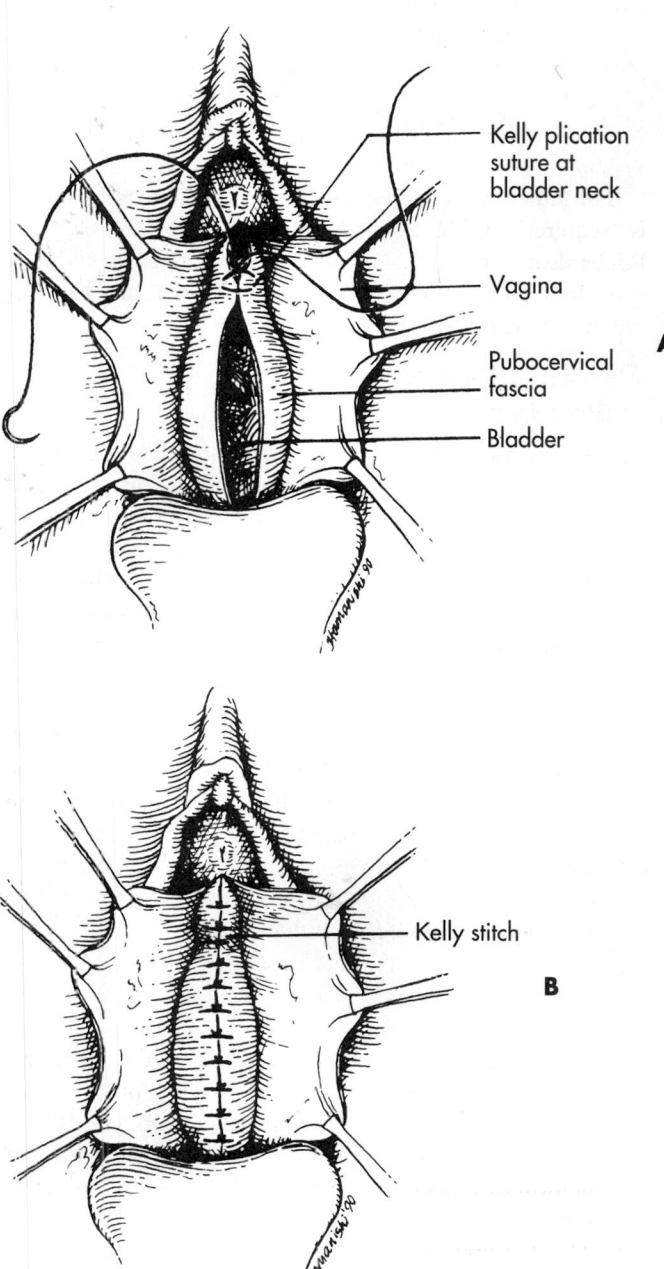

FIGURE 14-17   Cystourethrocele repair. **A**, The placement of Kelly stitch in the pubocervical fascia at the junction of the urethra with the bladder neck. **B**, The repair of the cystocele as the pubocervical fascia is sutured. Thus the cystocele is plicated.

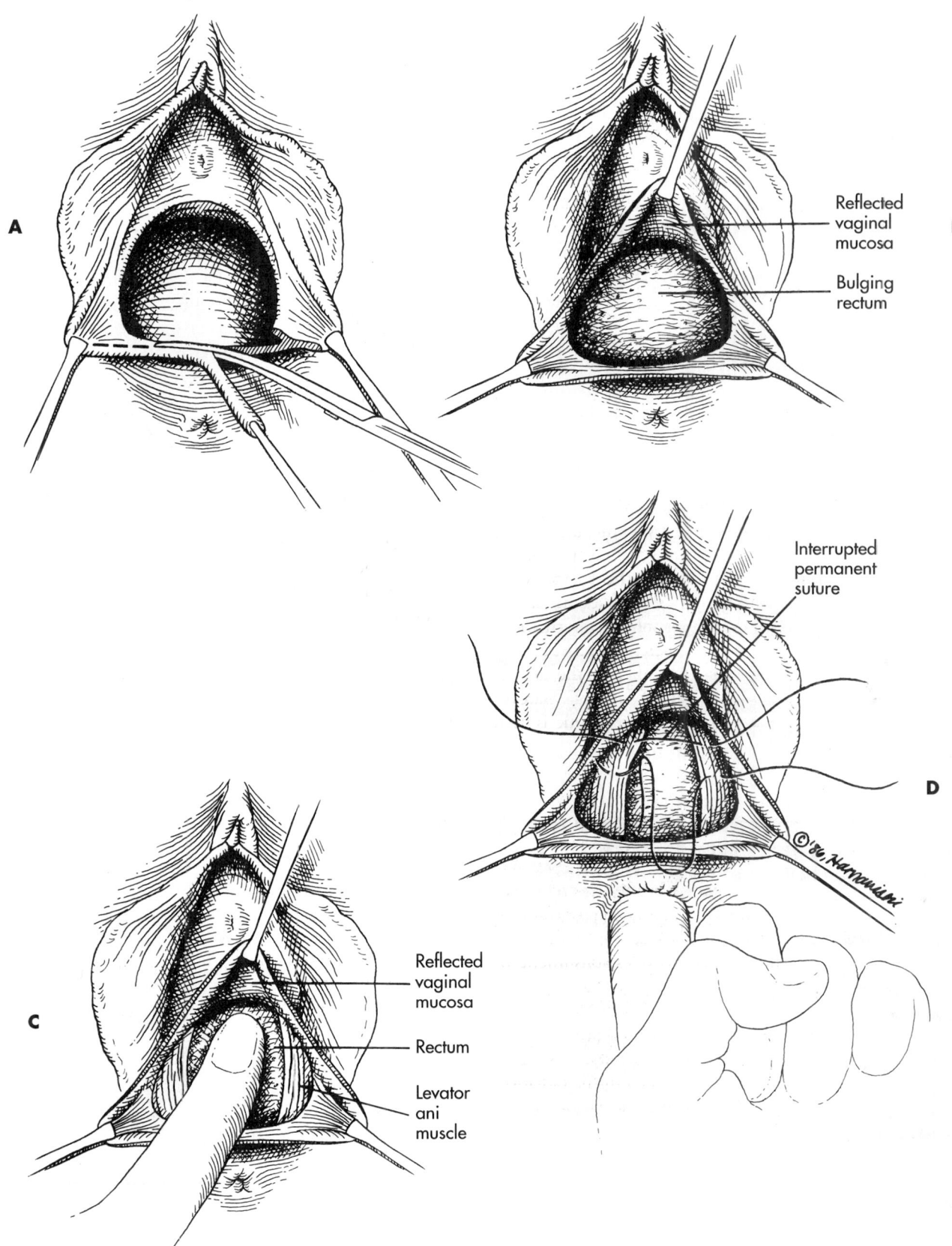

FIGURE 14–18   Rectocele repair. **A**, Placement of Allis clamps at margins of perineal incision; perineal incision is being made. **B**, Reflected vaginal mucosa with rectum bulging. **C**, Depression of rectum identifying margins of levator ani muscle. **D**, Placement of sutures in perirectal tissue and levator ani bundles.

with Allis forceps, curved scissors, and gauze sponges (Fig. 14-18, C).

5. The rectal wall proximal to the puborectal muscle is strengthened by placement of sutures.
6. Bleeding is controlled, and the vaginal wall is closed from above, downward to the anterior edge of the puborectal muscle. The rectocele is repaired from the posterior fornix to the perineal body. Remains of the transverse perineal and bulbocavernosus muscles are used to build up the perineum. The anterior edge of the levator ani muscle may be approximated (Fig. 14-18, D).
7. The mucosa and skin are trimmed, and the remaining closure is effected by interrupted sutures.
8. The vagina may be packed with 2-inch vaginal gauze packing to which sulfonamide cream may be added. An indwelling urinary catheter or suprapubic cystostomy catheter is inserted, according to the surgeon's preference.

Enterocele repair

The procedure is illustrated in Fig. 14-19. The peritoneal sac must be carefully dissected from the underlying rectum, the overlying bladder, or both, so that the peritoneal tissues are completely freed from the surrounding structures. The sac is opened to establish true identification and is then closed as high as possible by permanent purse-string sutures. The portion of peritoneal tissue distal to the purse-string ties is then excised, and the area is reinforced locally by transverse suture closures of whatever supportive tissues may be available. This technique is used to prevent recurrence.

Perineal repair

The procedure is illustrated in Fig. 14-20.

Vesicovaginal fistula repair

A vesicovaginal fistula is repaired by free dissection of the mucosal tissue of the anterior vaginal wall, closing of the fistula tract, and repair of the fascial attachments between the bladder and vagina, with establishment of urinary drainage. Fistulas vary in size from a small opening that permits only slight leakage of urine into the vagina to a large opening that permits all urine to pass into the vagina (Fig. 14-21). They may result from radical surgery in the management of pelvic cancer, from radiation therapy without surgery, from chronic ulceration of the vaginal structures, from penetrating wounds, or from obstetric trauma.

A urethrovaginal fistula usually causes constant incontinence or difficulty in retaining urine. This condition occurs after damage to the anterior wall and bladder or after radiation therapy or parturition. A ureterovaginal fistula develops as a result of injury to the ureter. In some cases reimplantation of the ureter in the bladder or ureterostomy may be done.

Urethrovaginal fistula repair (vaginal approach)
Procedural Considerations

The basic vaginal instrument set is required, with the addition of Kelly fistula scissors, dressing forceps, probes, skin hooks, Frazier suction tips, ureteral catheters, and sterile water for irrigation.

Operative Procedure

1. Traction sutures are placed about the fistulous tract; tissues are grasped with Allis-Adair forceps and plain tissue forceps.
2. The scar tissue around the fistula is excised, cleavage between the bladder and vagina is located, and flaps are mobilized with scissors, forceps, and gauze sponges.
3. The bladder mucosa is inverted toward the interior of the bladder with interrupted sutures. The sutures are passed through the muscularis of the bladder down to the mucosa.
4. A second layer of inverting sutures is placed in the bladder and tied, thereby completely inverting the bladder mucosa toward the interior.
5. The vaginal wall is closed with interrupted sutures in a direction opposite the closure of the bladder wall.
6. The bladder is distended with sterile water to determine any leaks. An indwelling urinary catheter is left in place.

Vesicovaginal fistula repair (transperitoneal approach)

In the presence of a high vesicovaginal fistula, a suprapubic incision is used. The opening from the bladder into the vagina is closed, and the fascial attachments are repaired.

Procedural Considerations

The patient is placed in slight Trendelenburg's position. Ureteral catheters may be inserted just before surgery (see Chapter 15). The vagina is cleansed and packed with moist gauze saturated with an antibiotic or antimicrobial solution. The abdominal operative site is prepped, and the patient is draped.

An abdominal gynecologic instrument set is required.

Operative Procedure

1. A midline abdominal incision is usually made, as described for laparotomy.
2. The fistulous tract is identified; the vaginal vault and the adjacent adherent bladder are separated with scissors, forceps, and sponges.
3. The vesicovaginal septum is dissected down to the healthy tissue beyond the site of the fistula.
4. The fistulous tract is mobilized. The bladder site of the fistula is inverted into the interior of the bladder with two rows of inverting sutures. The muscularis and

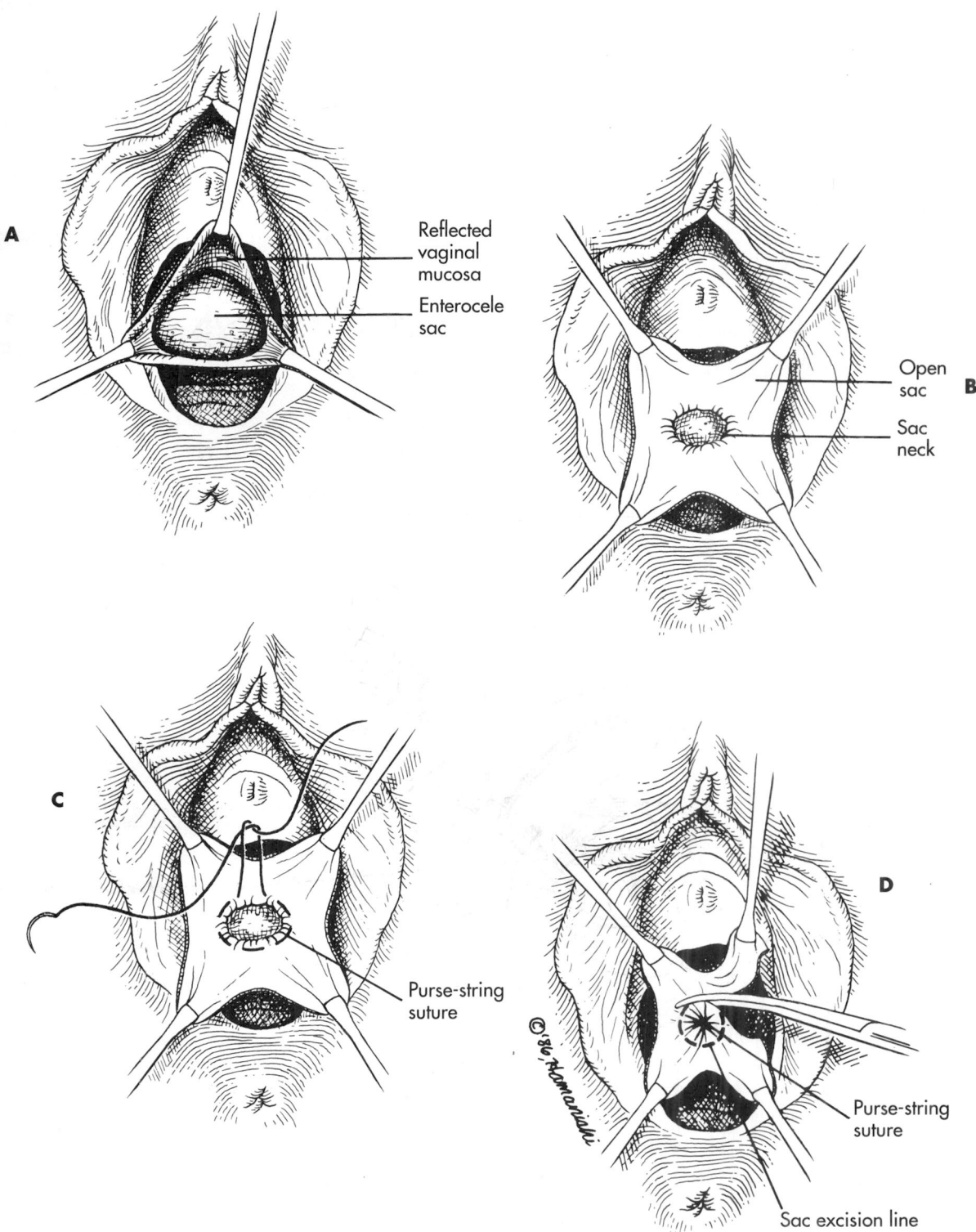

FIGURE 14–19   Enterocele repair. **A,** Appearance of enterocele sac with vaginal wall reflected. **B,** Appearance of open enterocele sac with sac neck identified. **C,** Placement of purse-string suture at neck of enterocele sac. **D,** Excision of enterocele sac.

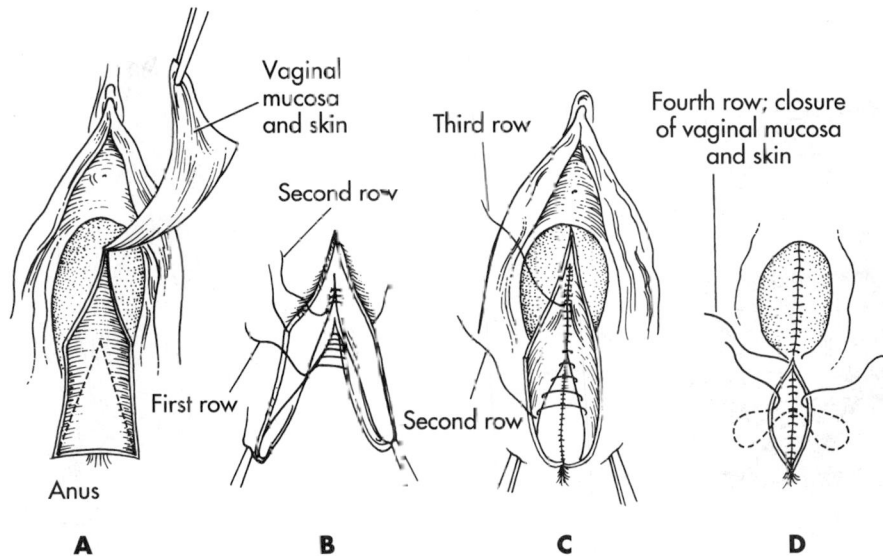

FIGURE 14-20   Repair of complete lacerations of the perineum. **A**, Lower margins of incision. **B**, Placement of first and second rows of sutures. **C**, Second and third rows of sutures. **D**, Fourth row of sutures.

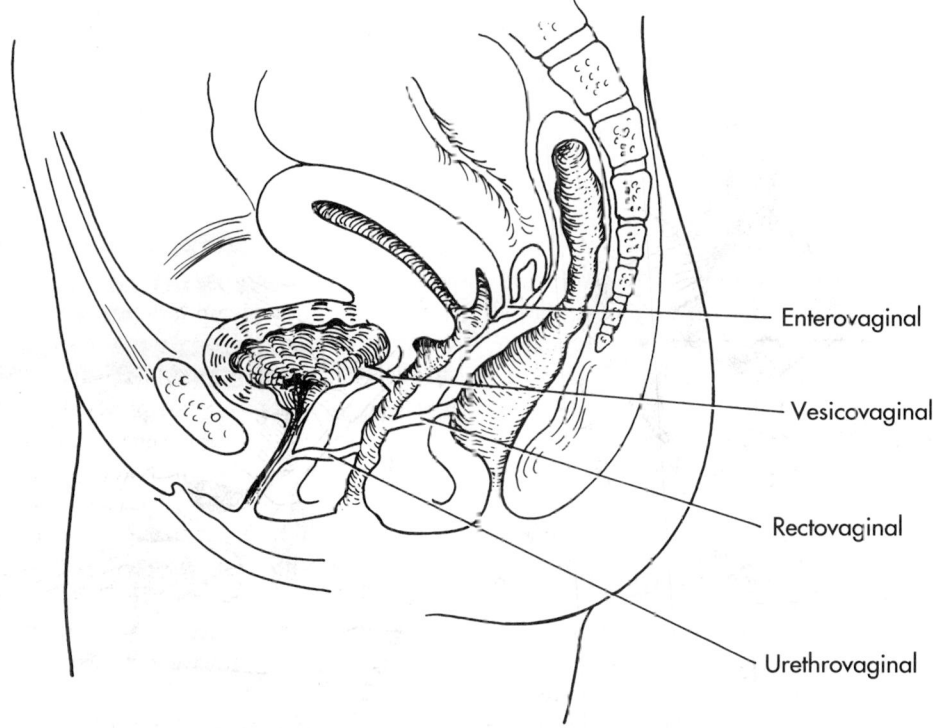

FIGURE 14-21   Genital fistulas may present as communications between the urethra, bladder, one of the ureters, or the bowel and some part of the genital tract. Two of the most common types are urethrovaginal and vesicovaginal, both of which empty into vaginal canal.

mucosa layers of the vagina are inverted into the vaginal vault by means of two rows of sutures.

5. The flaps of peritoneum are mobilized, both from the bladder and from the adjacent vaginal vault, and are closed to form a new vesicovaginal reflection of peritoneum below the site of the old fistulous tract.

6. The wound is closed in layers, as for laparotomy.

Abdominal dressings are applied. An indwelling urinary catheter is left in the bladder.

Rectovaginal fistula repair (vaginal approach)

Rectovaginal fistula repair by the vaginal approach includes repair of the perineum, fascia, and muscle-supporting structures between the rectum and vagina,

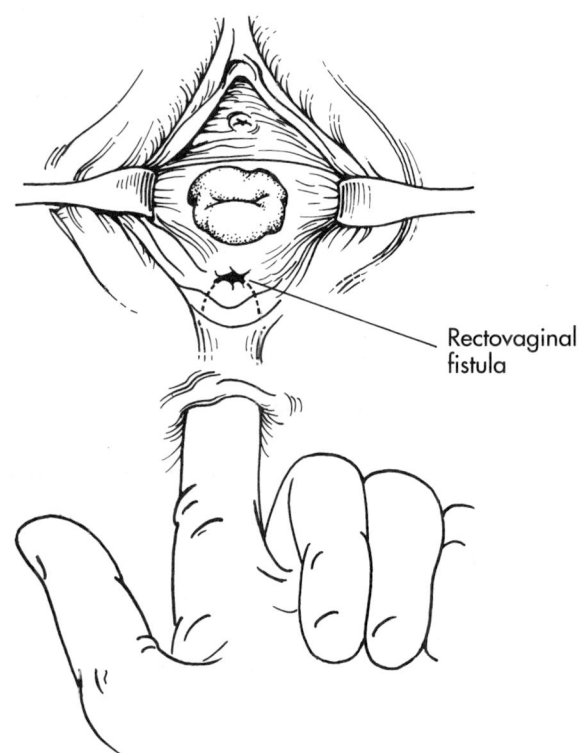

FIGURE 14-22　Rectovaginal fistula. Examiner's finger puts tension on rectovaginal septum.

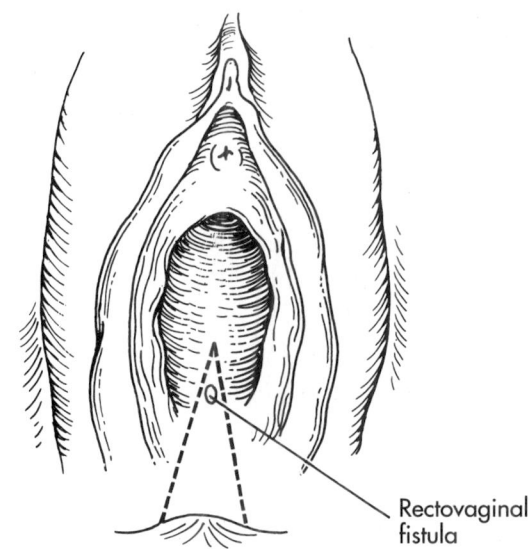

FIGURE 14-23　Repair of rectovaginal fistulas of all types essentially same as shown here. Portion of scar tissue to be excised is included within *dotted lines*; repair is as described for complete lacerations of perineum (see Fig. 14-20).

thereby closing the fistula formed between the rectum and the vagina (Fig. 14-22). In the presence of a large rectovaginal fistula, as in patients who have incurable cancer, a colostomy may be done (see Chapter 11).

Procedural Considerations

The basic vaginal instrument set is required for a rectovaginal fistula repair.

Operative Procedure

1. The scar tissue and tract between the rectum and vagina are excised (Fig. 14-23); edges of fresh tissue are approximated with absorbable sutures.
2. The rectum and vaginal walls are mobilized; the rectum is closed with inversion of the mucosa into the rectal canal.
3. The vagina is closed transversely or in a sagittal plane different from that of the rectal canal. The vaginal mucosal layer is inverted into the vaginal wall; an indwelling urinary catheter is inserted.

Operations for Urinary Stress Incontinence

Surgery for urinary stress incontinence entails repair of the fascial supports and the pubococcygeal muscle (see Fig. 14-4) surrounding the urethra and the bladder neck through a vaginal or abdominal approach.

The proper operative approach for the treatment of stress incontinence must be selected specifically for each patient. Normal micturition depends on a finely coordinated group of voluntary and involuntary movements. As a result of volitional impulses, voiding may be inhibited or stopped by the intrinsic muscles of the bladder neck and proximal urethra and the puborectalis division of the levator ani muscle (see Chapter 15).

The type of operation selected depends on the severity of stress incontinence, the extent of the condition causing it, the patient's ability to use the anatomic mechanism for voluntary inhibition of urination, and the operations that have previously been performed. States of stress incontinence are classified in relation to frequency and degree of incontinence, the presence of other diseases, and the function of the pubococcygeus muscle (levator ani) (see Fig. 14-4).

Previous pelvic operations may have resulted in scarring and distortion, with displacement of the bladder neck to an unfavorable position for proper functioning. Conditions such as uterine prolapse, cystocele, urethrocele, cystourethrocele, or urogenital fistulas after radiation therapy may be associated with stress incontinence.

The outcome of any operation for urinary stress incontinence is to improve the performance of a dislodged or dysfunctional vesical neck, to restore normal urethral length, and to tighten and restore the anterior urethral vesical angle. The Agency for Health Care Policy and Research developed clinical practice guidelines for the treatment of female stress incontinence in 1992. These are presented in Box 14-2.

Operative procedures
Vaginal Approach

1. An indwelling urinary catheter or suprapubic cystostomy catheter is inserted, according to the surgeon's preference. The posterior vaginal wall is retracted, and an incision is made through the anterior vaginal wall down to the urethra and bladder.
2. The vaginal wall is dissected from the bladder and urethra; the neck of the bladder is sutured together. The wound is closed, as described for anterior vaginal wall repair.

Vesicourethral Suspension

See the Marshall-Marchetti procedure (Chapter 15). Basic steps of the procedure follow.

1. Through a suprapubic abdominal incision the space of Retzius is entered, and the bladder and urethra are freed from the underlying structures.
2. Mattress sutures are inserted through the perivaginal fascia on either side of the vesicourethral angle area and preferably at a right angle to the long axis of the urethra and bladder. These are then passed through the central portion of the undersurface of the symphysis pubis under direct vision. The application of the sutures to the perivaginal connective tissue is done with the surgeon's hand in the vagina to ensure that the suture material is not passed through the vaginal mucosa (see Figs. 14-2 and 14-4).
3. The wound is closed and may be drained if the vascularity of the area warrants. An abdominal dressing is applied.

Excision of Fibroma of the Vagina

Excision of fibroma of the vagina involves the removal of the lesion through a transverse or longitudinal incision of the vaginal wall. Small cysts or small benign tumors that distort the vagina or those that are ulcerated and infected are treated surgically.

Procedural considerations

A dilatation and curettage set is required, plus six Halsted mosquito hemostats.

Operative procedure

1. The vaginal vault is retracted with lateral retractors. Sutures may be placed on each side of the tumor. The posterior lip of the cervix is grasped with a tenaculum and is drawn anteriorly to expose the operative site.
2. The vaginal wall is incised, and the edges are grasped with traction sutures on curved, taper-point needles or with Allis forceps.
3. The base and its capsule are then excised with a knife and curved scissors; bleeding vessels are clamped with Halsted mosquito hemostats and ligated with fine sutures.
4. The vaginal incision is closed with interrupted sutures.

Construction of a Vagina

Two basic approaches are used for repairing or overcoming a congenital or surgical defect of the vagina: obtaining a skin graft, which is applied to a mold and placed in the area of vaginal reconstruction, and a simple opening of the area of vaginal reconstruction and the placing of a mold to permit the spontaneous epithelialization of the area.

Procedural considerations

For a skin graft the plastic instrument set (Chapter 24) is required, with the addition of a dermatome, marking pen, and nonadherent gauze dressing.

For vaginal construction the basic vaginal instrument set is required, with the addition of iris scissors, skin hooks, a vaginal mold, Halsted mosquito hemostats, and a ruler.

Operative procedure

1. The skin graft is taken from the abdomen or anterior thigh. The donor site is dressed in the routine manner with nonadherent gauze and a pressure dressing.
2. The skin graft is kept in a moist gauze sponge until it is ready to be used.
3. A vaginal orifice is created by sharp dissection. Great care must be taken to prevent damage to the rectum and bladder. A mold is used to apply the donor skin or simply to hold the dissected area open to permit spontaneous epithelialization.

Trachelorrhaphy

Trachelorrhaphy is removal of torn surfaces of the anterior and posterior cervical lips and reconstruction of the cervical canal. It is performed to treat deep lacerations of a cervix that is relatively free from infection.

Procedural considerations

The basic vaginal instrument set is required, plus a conization loop electrode, if desired. An indwelling urinary catheter may be inserted into the bladder, depending on the surgeon's preference.

Operative procedure

1. The labia may be retracted with Allis-Adair tissue forceps or sutures. The cervix is grasped with a tenaculum.
2. The infected tissue of the exocervix is denuded with a knife. The flaps are undermined by means of a knife and curved scissors. Bleeding vessels are clamped and ligated. The mucosa is dissected from the cervix.
3. A small distal portion of the cervical canal is coned with a knife or a loop electrode to remove infected tissue. Bleeding vessels are clamped and ligated.
4. The denuded and coned areas are covered by transversely suturing the mucosal flaps of the exocervix, using interrupted sutures. Tissue forceps, hemostats, and gauze sponges are needed. The sutures are placed in such a manner that the fibromuscular tissue of the

BOX 14-2 | **Algorithm Recommendations for Treatment of Female Stress Incontinence**

In a broad-based review of the literature, the Agency for Health Care Policy and Research (AHCPR) concluded that the following steps be implemented in making decisions regarding treatment of female stress incontinence:

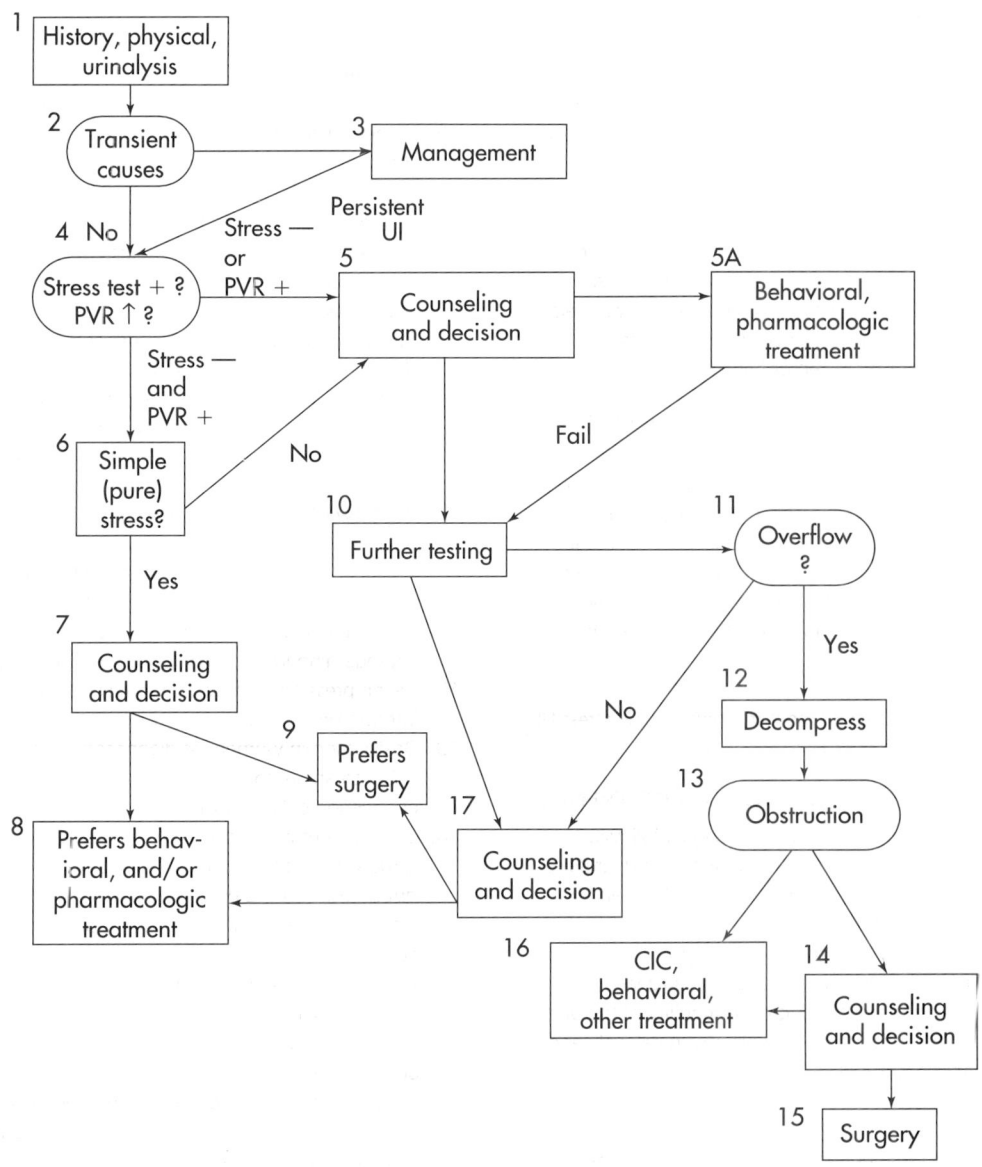

1. History, physical, and urinalysis.
2 and 3. Transient causes are identified and managed. If urinary incontinence (UI) persists, go to node 4.
4. Provocative stress testing and measurement or estimation of postvoid residual (PVR) volume should be performed at this point.

Possibilities include:
- Stress test positive for leakage and PVR normal—simple stress (pure), go to node 6.
- Abnormal PVR regardless of stress test result—not simple stress, mixed stress, and urge symptoms, go to node 5.
- Stress test negative and PVR normal, go to node 5.

From Urinary Incontinence Guideline Panel. (1992). *Urinary incontinence in adults: clinical practice guideline.* AHCPR Pub. No. 92-0038. Rockville, Md.: Agency for Health Care Policy and Research, Public Health Service, U.S. Department of Health and Human Services.

BOX 14-2	Algorithm Recommendations for Treatment of Female Stress Incontinence—cont'd

STRESS URINARY INCONTINENCE OTHER THAN SIMPLE

5. After stress testing and PVR estimation/measurement, all patients except those with simple stress UI will need further counseling and evaluation of disposition. The types of patients that will be encountered include:
   - Stress test negative and PVR normal
   - Stress test positive and PVR normal and symptoms are mixed/other/not simple stress UI
   - PVR elevated regardless of stress test result or symptom
   - Anatomically reversible condition including prolapsing cystocele, rectocele, enterocele, or uterus

5A. Stress test negative and PVR normal

If the symptom of stress UI is simple and the PVR volume is low but incontinence cannot be documented with the stress test, the patient can be counseled either for a trial of behavioral therapy and/or pharmacologic treatment. Perform further testing, if the initial therapy is not preferred or has failed.

Stress test positive and PVR normal and symptoms are mixed/other/not simple stress

If the patient has mixed symptoms (stress/urge) or other symptoms and the stress test is positive and the PVR is low, the patient can be counseled for either trial of behavioral or pharmacologic therapy or surgical therapy. Further testing is recommended for patients who already failed initial therapeutic trial or have other comorbid conditions complicating the UI symptom.

PVR abnormal

If the PVR is elevated regardless of the symptoms (simple stress UI, complex or mixed), further testing is recommended.

SIMPLE (PURE) STRESS URINARY INCONTINENCE

6. Simple stress urinary incontinence is defined as follows:
   - Urine loss only with physical exertion (history and stress test)
   - Normal voiding habits (less than or equal to 8×/d and no more than 2× at night)
   - No neurologic history or neurologic findings
   - No prior antiincontinence or radical pelvic surgery
   - Pelvic examination documenting hypermobility of the urethra and bladder neck, pliable and compliant vaginal wall, and adequate vaginal capacity
   - PVR normal
   - Not pregnant

Any patient with stress incontinence who fails any of these criteria will be considered not to have simple or pure stress UI; go to node 5.

7. Patients with simple stress UI may be counseled regarding behavioral, pharmacologic, and surgical treatment options.
8. Treatment. If the patient prefers behavioral therapy, the recommended techniques are pelvic muscle exercises or bladder training with or without biofeedback and/or vaginal cones.
   If the patient prefers pharmacologic therapy, the recommended agent is an alpha-adrenergic agent. For women with vaginal atrophy, a trial of estrogen therapy may be initiated alone or in combination with an alpha agonist.
9. In patients with simple stress incontinence who prefer surgery, preoperative evaluation should include a comprehensive history, physical examination, urinalysis, urine culture, and PVR volume

measurement. Document incontinence directly (positive stress test). For further corroboration, cystoscopy, cystogram with straining, Valsalva leak point pressure, and/or dynamic urethral profilometry may be used. The goal of surgical intervention in this case is to correct urethral hypermobility.

Anatomically reversible conditions such as prolapsing cystocele, uterine prolapse

If an anatomically reversible condition is present, see the algorithm for urge UI (node 8).

10. Numerous specialized diagnostic tests are available, and the choice of tests must be tailored to the question to be answered. Tests for bladder and urethral function include filling cystometry, stress cystourethrogram, dynamic profilometry or Valsalva leak-point pressure, pressure flow, and/or cystoscopy. Tests should be performed according to the need of the patient as described below.

Suspected condition	Recommended test
Unstable bladder	Filling cystometry
Stress UI	Dynamic profilometry or Valsalva leak-point pressure and/or stress cystourethrogram or videourodynamics
Overflow UI	Voiding cystometrogram (pressure flow study), cystoscopy, and/or stress cystourethrogram, videourodynamics is another option

11. If overflow incontinence is found, the patient will need counseling regarding initial decompression of the bladder.
12. Decompression of the bladder may be accomplished with either intermittent self-catheterization or indwelling Foley catheter.
13. Obstruction in women, as diagnosed in node 10, is usually due either to an anatomically reversible condition or to postsurgical obstruction of the urethra.
14. If the patient is a good surgical risk and is willing to undergo surgery, relief of obstruction is an option with the risk of recurrent stress UI. If the patient is a poor risk or prefers nonsurgical therapy, clean intermittent catheterization (CIC) and other nonsurgical treatments should be instituted.
15. The patient should be counseled regarding the procedure for repair of the prolapse or relief of postsurgical urethral obstruction and told whether suspension of the bladder neck will be performed.
16. If there is no obstruction, as determined in node 10, and the patient has an acontractile or underactive detrusor, or if obstructed and the patient is either not a surgical candidate or prefers nonsurgical treatment, counseling regarding the use of CIC, behavioral voiding techniques, use of pessary, etc., is necessary. If bladder neck suspension is a consideration in the face of persistent abnormal residual volume, the patient must be counseled that persistent retention may result after the suspension procedure.
17. If the patient is found to have no overflow incontinence in node 10, the specific condition identified after testing and the patient preference will determine treatment option. Options include behavioral, pharmacologic, and surgical treatment. For surgical treatment of intrinsic sphincter deficiency (ISD), recommend bulking technique, sling, or artificial urinary sphincter. If hypermobility is found, see node 7.

cervix is included, thereby eliminating dead space where a hematoma may form and providing a complete reconstructed cervical canal.

5. A vaginal pack may be inserted.

Dilatation of the Cervix and Curettage

In this procedure, instruments are introduced through the vagina for the purpose of dilating the cervix. Dilatation of the cervix can also take place by inserting laminaria tents into the cervical os before surgery; these tents are removed immediately before the procedure. Dilatation and curettage are done either for diagnostic purposes or as a form of therapy for a variety of pelvic conditions such as incomplete abortion, therapeutic abortion, abnormal uterine bleeding, or primary dysmenorrhea. Dilatation and curettage may also be performed when carcinoma of the endometrium is suspected, in the study of infertility, or before amputation of the cervix or an operation for prolapse of the uterus.

Procedural considerations

The dilatation and curettage set includes the following:

EXPOSING INSTRUMENTS

2 Jackson vaginal retractors	1 Uterine sound, graduated (see Fig. 14-11)
1 Sims vaginal retractor	1 Set Hegar or Hank uterine dilators (see Fig. 14-11)
1 Auvard vaginal speculum, weighted (see Fig. 14-10)	1 Goodell uterine dilator (see Fig. 14-11)
2 Deaver retractors	

HOLDING INSTRUMENTS

2 Barrett tenaculum forceps (see Fig. 14-9)	2 Backhaus towel clamps, 5¼ inches
1 Jacobs vulsellum forceps (see Fig. 14-9)	1 Tissue forceps with 1 × 2 teeth, 5½ inches
2 Foerster sponge-holding forceps	1 Russian tissue forceps, 8 inches
1 Bozeman dressing forceps (see Fig. 14-9)	1 Dressing forceps, 7¼ inches
1 Fletcher–Van Doren polyp forceps	2 Allis forceps, 6 inches

CUTTING INSTRUMENTS

1 Bard-Parker knife handle #3 with blade #10	1 Set Thomas uterine curettes, blunt (see Fig. 14-8)
2 Mayo dissecting scissors, 1 curved and 1 straight, 6¾ inches	1 Heaney uterine curette
1 Set Sims uterine curettes, sharp (see Fig. 14-8)	1 Gaylor biopsy forceps (see Fig. 14-8)

CLAMPING INSTRUMENTS

2 Crile hemostats, 5½ inches	2 Pean forceps, 6¼ inches

SUTURING INSTRUMENTS

1 Mayo-Hegar needle holder, 8 inches	Suture of surgeon's preference, if desired

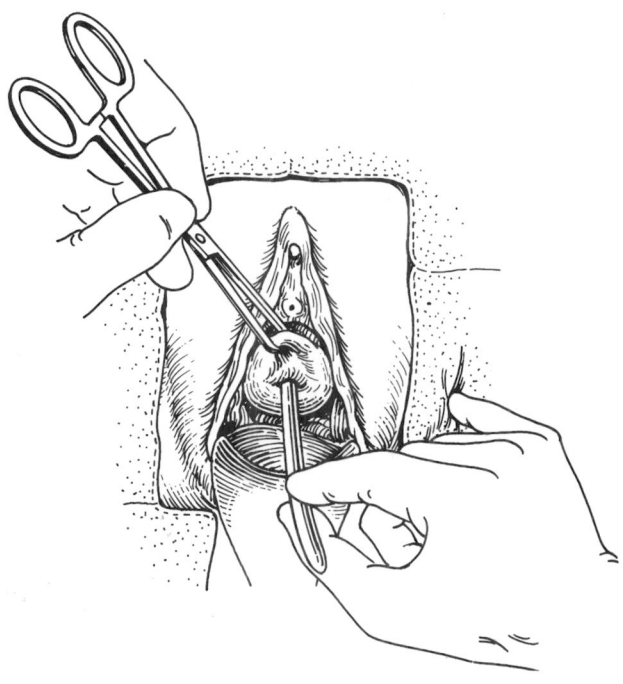

FIGURE 14-24 Dilatation of cervix and curettage. Vaginal wall retracted; cervix held by tenaculum; cervix dilated with dilator. Uterine cavity curetted with sharp curettes.

ACCESSORY ITEMS

1 Urethral catheter, 16 or 18 Fr	Iodoform or plain gauze packing, as desired
1 Telfa dressing	Vaginal gauze packing, as desired
1 Ampule oxytocic drug, if desired	

Operative procedure

1. A Jackson or Auvard retractor is placed posteriorly in the vagina. A Sims or Deaver retractor is placed anteriorly to expose the cervix. The anterior lip of the cervix is grasped with a tenaculum (Fig. 14-24).
2. The direction of the cervical canal and the depth of the uterine cavity are determined by means of a blunt probe or graduated uterine sound.
3. The cervix is gradually dilated by means of graduated Hegar or Hank dilators and possibly a Goodell uterine dilator.
4. Exploration for pedunculated polyps or myomas may be done with a polyp forceps.
5. The interior of the cervical canal and the cavity of the uterus are curetted to obtain either a fractional or a routine specimen. For specific identification of the site of specimens, the endocervix is scraped with the curette first, and the specimen is separated from the curettings of the uterine endometrium. In a routine curettage, all curettings are sent together for identification of tissue cells.
6. Fragments of endometrium or other dislodged tissues may be removed with warm, moist gauze sponges on

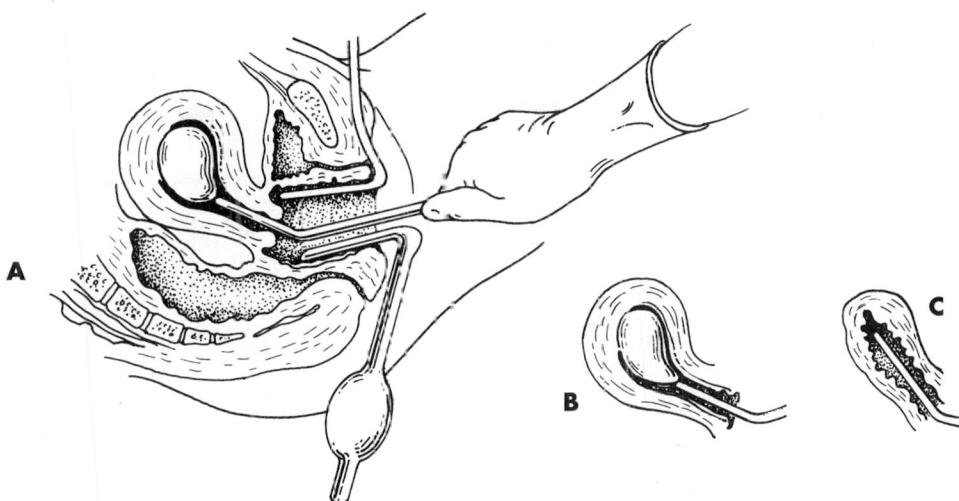

FIGURE 14-25   Suction curettage. **A,** Insertion of cannula. **B,** Gentle suction motion to aspirate contents. **C,** Uterine contents evacuated.

sponge-holding forceps or with a teaspoon and are then collected on Telfa.
7. Multiple-punch biopsies of the cervical circumference (at the 3, 6, 9, and 12 o'clock positions) may be taken with the Gaylor biopsy forceps to supplement the diagnostic studies.
8. Retractors are withdrawn; iodoform or plain gauze packing may be inserted into the uterus, using dressing forceps. The tenaculum is removed from the cervix. A vaginal pack may be inserted.

Suction Curettage

Suction curettage is vacuum aspiration of the uterine contents. Aspiration has proved to be a safe and effective method for early termination of pregnancy and for use in missed and incomplete spontaneous abortions. Advantages are smaller dilatation of the cervix, less damage to the uterus, less blood loss, less chance of uterine perforation, and reduced danger of infection. Laminaria tents may be inserted approximately 4 to 24 hours before suction curettage to dilate the cervix.

Procedural considerations

The instrumentation required includes the dilatation and curettage set, with the addition of one set of Pratt, Hawkin, or Hank uterine dilators, placenta forceps, urethral catheter, sterile cannulas, aspirator tubing, a vacuum aspirator unit, and oxytocic drugs.

Operative procedure

1. The cervix is exposed with an Auvard weighted speculum and an anterior retractor; then the cervix is grasped with a sharp tenaculum and is drawn toward the introitus.
2. The laminaria tents are removed, and the cervix can be further dilated in the routine manner, allowing 1 mm of cannula diameter for each week of pregnancy.

3. The appropriate-sized cannula is inserted into the uterus until the sac is encountered. The suction is turned on with immediate disruption and aspiration of the contents. Continued gentle motion of the cannula removes the uterine contents (Fig. 14-25). Use of uterine curettes may supplement suction in removing the entire uterine contents.
4. Retractors and tenaculum are removed.
5. The specimen, contained in the suction bottle, is removed for pathologic examination.

Removal of Pedunculated Cervical Myoma (Cervical Polyps)

Cervical polyps (small pedunculated lesions) stem from the endocervical canal and consist almost entirely of columnar epithelium with or without squamous metaplasia. They may vary in size and are soft, red, and friable. Bleeding may result from the slightest trauma. Pedunculated lesions may be removed by the snare method or by dissection from the cervical canal with a knife, cold-knife conization, or resectoscope. Usually the surgeon performs an endometrial and endocervical curettage, and a cytologic smear is taken.

Procedural considerations

A dilatation and curettage set, a tonsil snare with medium-sized snare wire, glass slides, an electrosurgical unit, and a blade electrode or resectoscope are required.

Operative procedure

1. The anterior lip of the cervix is grasped with a Jacobs vulsellum or a tenaculum. The canal is sounded and dilated either to visualize or palpate the base of the pedicle.
2. If the pedicle of the tumor is thin, a tonsil snare may be placed over the body of the tumor, permitting the snare

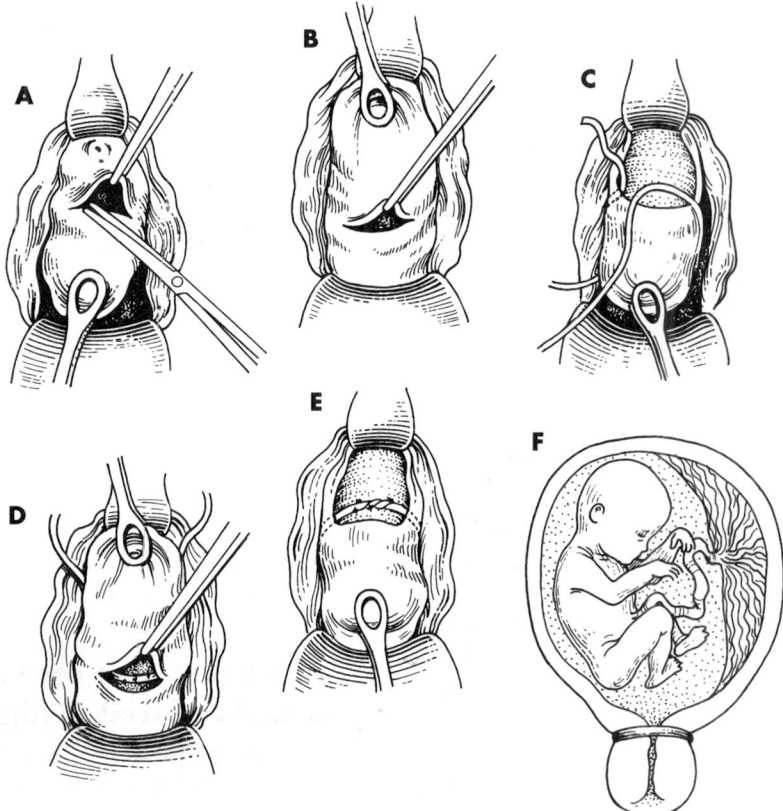

FIGURE 14-26 Principles of Shirodkar operation for treatment of incompetent internal cervical os during pregnancy.

to crush the base of the tumor and to control bleeding. If the tumor is large, its base is dissected out with a knife. Bleeding may be controlled by the use of warm, moist gauze sponges with or without electrocoagulation. A resectoscope with the use of electrosurgery may be used to dissect the tumor.

3. Iodoform or plain gauze packing may be introduced into the cervical os. The tenaculum is removed from the cervix, and the retractors are withdrawn. A vaginal pack may be inserted for hemostasis.

Shirodkar Operation (Postconceptional)

Incompetence of the cervix is a condition characterized by habitual midtrimester spontaneous abortions. Surgical intervention is designed to prevent cervical dilatation that results in the release of uterine contents. The postconceptional Shirodkar operation is placement of a collar type of ligature of Mersilene, Dacron tape, heavy nylon suture, or plastic-covered braided-steel suture at the level of the internal os to close it.

Procedural considerations

Gentle vaginal preparation is carried out. The instrumentation includes the basic vaginal instrument set, with the addition of Deschamps ligature carriers, right and left, trocar needles, sutures for the internal os, and the surgeon's preference for closure of the mucosal incisions.

Operative procedure

1. Anterior and posterior vaginal retractors are placed, and the cervix is pulled down with smooth ovum or sponge-holding forceps. With smooth tissue forceps and dissecting scissors, the mucosa over the anterior cervix is opened to permit the bladder to be pushed back (Fig. 14-26).

2. The cervix is lifted, and the posterior vaginal mucosa is similarly incised at the level of the peritoneal reflection. The corners of the anterior and posterior incisions are bilaterally approximated in the area of the lateral mucosa with curved tonsil or Allis forceps.

3. The prepared ligature is placed at the desired level by passage of the material through the approximated tissue and is drawn tight posteriorly to close the cervix. The suture material for the ligature is then tied. It is not necessary to suture the ligature to the underlying tissues. The suture material used for this ligation is 5 mm Dacron or Mersilene tape. The anterior and posterior mucosal incisions are usually closed with 2-0 absorbable suture to complete the procedure.

Conization and Biopsy of the Cervix

Cervical cancer is the second most common malignancy of the female reproductive tract, reaching a peak between 45 and 55 years of age. Eighty percent of cervical cancers are squamous cell; the remainder are adenocarci-

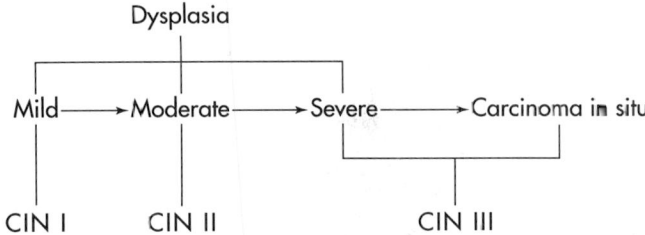

Dysplasia

Mild ──→ Moderate ──→ Severe ──→ Carcinoma in situ

CIN I   CIN II   CIN III

FIGURE 14-27 The spectrum of intraepithelial neoplasia of the cervix. *CIN,* Cervical intraepithelial neoplasia.

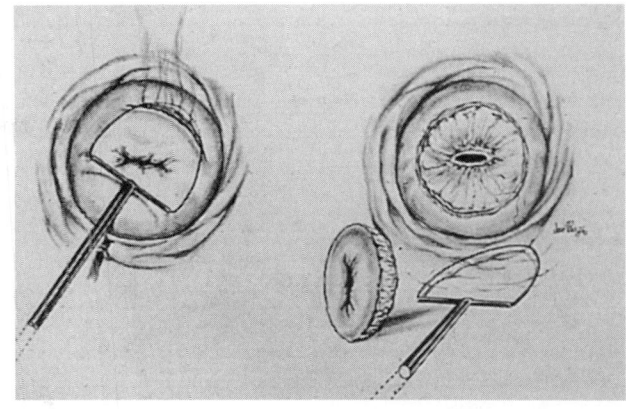

FIGURE 14-28 The electrical loop (0.2 mm) vaporizes across at 1.5- to 2-cm front; therefore it cuts more rapidly than a laser.

nomas, mixed type of sarcomas, or metastatic lesions. Abnormal vaginal bleeding or discharge may be the only presenting symptoms. Dysplasia, a disorder of the maturation of the squamous endothelium of the cervix, is graded cytologically and histologically as mild, moderate, or severe cervical intraepithelial neoplasia (CIN) (Fig. 14-27). There are usually no signs or symptoms of dysplasia or carcinoma in situ. When Pap smear results indicate dysplasia, mild dysplasia is usually managed by careful observation and repeated clinical and cytologic examination. Persistent mild, moderate, and severe dysplasia, as well as carcinoma in situ, are treated by the eradication of the abnormal tissue. This may be initiated with colposcopy and punch biopsy, followed by electrocoagulation, cryosurgery, cold-knife cone biopsy, loop electrosurgical excision cone (LEEC) (Fig. 14-28), or laser excisional cone (Fig. 14-29), the latter two of which appear to provide adequate histologic specimens while promoting hemostasis and eradication of abnormal tissue.[17]

Procedural considerations

The instruments required include a dilatation and curettage set. An electrosurgical unit or laser, conization electrical loop, and ball-tipped electrodes will be required, depending on the procedure.

Operative procedure

1. The posterior vaginal wall is retracted by a speculum and the anterior vaginal wall by lateral retractors. The outer portions of the cervix are grasped with a tenaculum, and the cervix is drawn toward the introitus. Cystic areas of the cervix may be treated with a needle electrode or laser. Endometrial biopsy may be done (Fig. 14-30, *A*). Bleeding points are coagulated or lasered.
2. For cauterization the electrode is passed into the cervical canal, and the diseased tissue is treated. Ferrous subsulfate (Monsel's solution) may be used for hemostasis.
3. The electrical loop (Fig. 14-30, *B* and *C*) or the laser may be used to remove the diseased tissue and provide a histologic specimen, which is sent to the pathology lab for examination.
4. If a wide conization is performed, the cervix may be

sutured and vaginal packing may be used. An indwelling urinary catheter may be inserted.

Cesium Insertion for Cervical and Endometrial Malignancy

Cesium has generally replaced radium insertions for treatment of malignancy of the cervix and endometrium.

Procedural considerations

The patient is brought to the operating room for insertion of the applicators. The cesium is loaded into the applicators later in the radiation department or in the patient's room under controlled conditions, in which all personnel are monitored by use of a dosimeter.

The bladder is drained with an indwelling urinary catheter. The catheter balloon is inflated with a radiopaque medium for radiographic visualization after insertion of the cesium. An indwelling rectal marker is also placed by the surgeon for radiographic visualization. Various cesium applicators may be used according to the surgeon's preference and the area of malignancy.

Interstitial therapy

Cesium needles are available in various lengths with small diameters for insertion into the tissue surrounding the cervix. They are inserted vaginally with a needle applicator and are used as a supplement to intravaginal or intrauterine sources. To facilitate removal, the needles have wires or threads attached to their distal ends.

Culdocentesis and Posterior Colpotomy (Culdotomy)

Needle culdocentesis is insertion of an aspirating needle through the posterior fornix of the vagina. Posterior colpotomy (culdotomy) is incision through the vagina and peritoneum into the cul-de-sac.

Diagnostic needle culdocentesis is done to diagnose ectopic pregnancy and to detect intraperitoneal bleeding

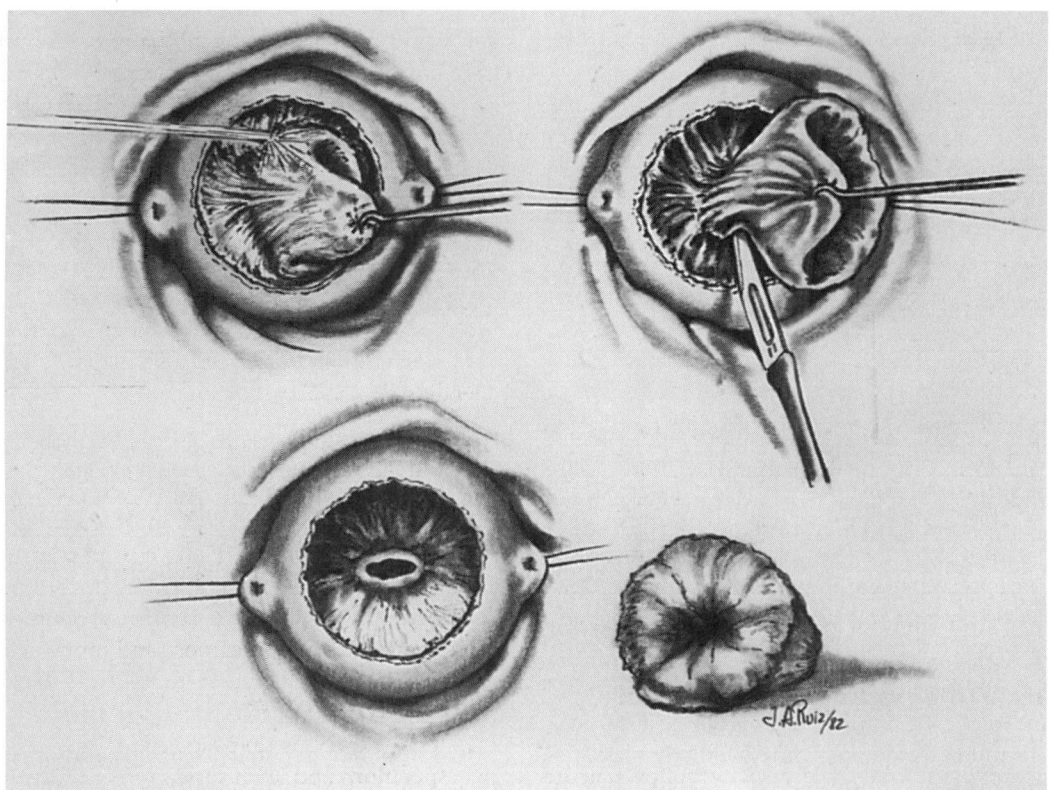

FIGURE 14–29   The laser creates a 0.3- to 0.5-mm spot, which cuts as it is swept across the tissue plane. A hook provides traction as the laser cuts and permits shaping of the cone.

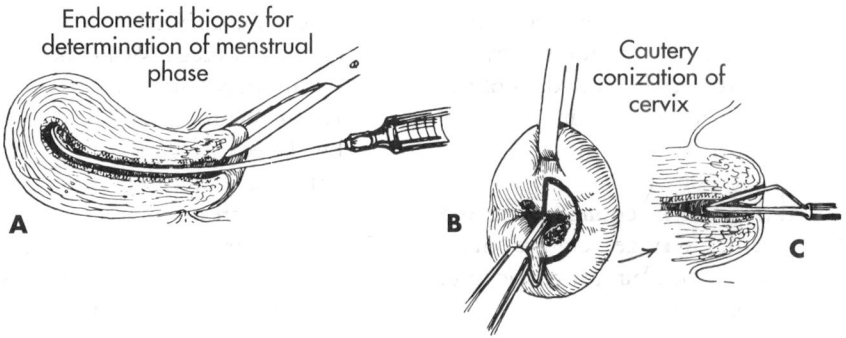

FIGURE 14–30   **A**, Endometrial biopsy technique. **B** and **C**, Methods of treating cervical conditions or obtaining specimens for diagnostic tests.

or cul-de-sac hematoma. This procedure is rarely done today as a result of advancements in diagnostic laparoscopy. Posterior colpotomy can be done to carry out definitive operative procedures: various kinds of tubal ligations, aspiration or the removal of ovarian cysts, the occasional management of an ectopic pregnancy, and exploratory diagnostic operative procedures.

Procedural considerations

The basic vaginal instrument set is required, with the addition of a 15-gauge needle, syringe, culture tubes, drains.

An abdominal gynecologic instrument set should be available in case laparotomy is indicated.

Operative procedures
Needle Culdocentesis

1. A 15-gauge needle attached to a syringe is inserted through the posterior fornix of the vagina. Suspected intraperitoneal bleeding is confirmed if dark or red blood flows freely into the syringe. Failure to obtain blood does not rule out the possibility of intraperitoneal bleeding.
2. Any bleeding of the vaginal wall is controlled by

sutures. Vaginal packing and an indwelling urinary catheter may be inserted.

Posterior Colpotomy

1. A transverse incision is made through the posterior vaginal wall with curved scissors. This incision is carried into the peritoneum, behind the cervix at the superior point of the posterior fornix.
2. Allis forceps are used to facilitate exposure, and hemostasis is obtained by placing a number of sutures into the corners or angles of the wound.
3. The posterior vaginal wall is held open with a weighted retractor.
4. In case of infection in the cul-de-sac, the opening is enlarged enough to permit drainage from the cul-de-sac. The cavity is explored; drains may be inserted.
5. Bleeding of the vaginal wall is controlled by sutures. The peritoneum and the vaginal mucosa are closed with a continuous suture. Vaginal packing and an indwelling urinary catheter may be inserted.

Marsupialization of Bartholin's Duct Cyst or Abscess

A cyst in a Bartholin's gland usually follows acute infection and is treated by marsupialization when it is quiescent. Such cysts are not neoplastic but result from retention of glandular secretions caused by blockage somewhere in the duct system. Marsupialization of Bartholin's duct cyst or abscess entails removal or incision of the cyst through the vaginal outlet and drainage of the area. In true marsupialization the cyst is surgically exteriorized by resecting the anterior wall and suturing the cut edges of the remaining cyst to the adjacent edges of the skin.

Procedural considerations

The basic vaginal instrument set is required, with the addition of a 15-gauge needle, syringe, culture tubes (aerobic and anaerobic), iodoform or plain gauze packing, and a drain, if desired by the surgeon.

Operative procedure

1. The labia minora may be sutured to the perineal skin on each side to expose the vaginal introitus.
2. An elliptic incision is then made into the mucosa, which is distended over the cyst.
3. The cyst wall is dissected, and, if indicated, removal of the gland is completed with blunt-pointed scissors. The tissue may be everted with sutures and left open. A drain or packing may be inserted, and a dressing is applied.

Hysteroscopy

Hysteroscopy is endoscopic visualization of the uterine cavity and tubal orifices. A fiberoptic hysteroscope is introduced vaginally and aids in the diagnosis and treatment of intrauterine disease. The common indications for hysteroscopy include evaluation of abnormal uterine bleeding, with possible endometrial ablation, location and removal of "lost" intrauterine devices (IUDs), evaluation of infertility, diagnosis and surgical treatment of intrauterine adhesions, verification of submucous leiomyomas or endometrial polyps, resection of uterine septa or submucous leiomyomas, and tubal sterilization. Laparoscopy may be done in association with hysteroscopy to assess the external contour of the uterus. Contraindications to either diagnostic or operative hysteroscopy include pelvic infection, cervical malignancy, and in some instances heavy bleeding.

Procedural considerations

The instrumentation required includes a dilatation and curettage set, with the addition of a hysteroscopy set (Fig. 14-31), 50 ml syringes, polyethylene tubing, fiberoptic light source, electrosurgical unit if desired, laser if desired, hysteroscopic insufflator if desired, pressure-infusion pump if desired, and a video camera and monitor if desired.

Operative procedure

1. The cervix is exposed with an Auvard weighted speculum and an anterior retractor; the anterior lip of the cervix is grasped with a tenaculum and is drawn toward the introitus.
2. The direction of the cervical canal and the depth of the uterine cavity are determined by means of a graduated uterine sound.
3. The endocervical canal is dilated by means of graduated Hegar or Hank uterine dilators to 6, 7, or 8 mm, depending on the size of the hysteroscope.
4. A self-retaining vacuum cannula with obturator may be placed into contact with the cervix. The cannula is firmly applied to the cervix by vacuum created with a negative pressure.
5. The obturator is withdrawn and the hysteroscope is introduced to the level of the internal cervical os.
6. To achieve satisfactory visualization and sustained intrauterine pressure, the uterine cavity must be distended with one of the following media: 32% dextran 70 in dextrose (Hyskon), dextrose 5% in water (D_5W), sorbitol, mannitol, saline (NSS), or sterile water, or by CO_2 gas insufflation. Air or gas used for uterine insufflation may result in gas or air embolism. Therefore CO_2 pressures must be monitored closely. Injection of liquid media may be under continuous pressure from a 50 ml syringe or delivered by means of a pressure-controlled fluid-infusion (hysteroscopic) pump into the irrigating channel of the hysteroscope. When the syringe is used, care must be taken to prevent air bubbles, which distort the view or could lead to air embolism. Uterine distention with D_5W may be achieved by inserting a 500 ml plastic bag containing the medium into an intravenous pressure

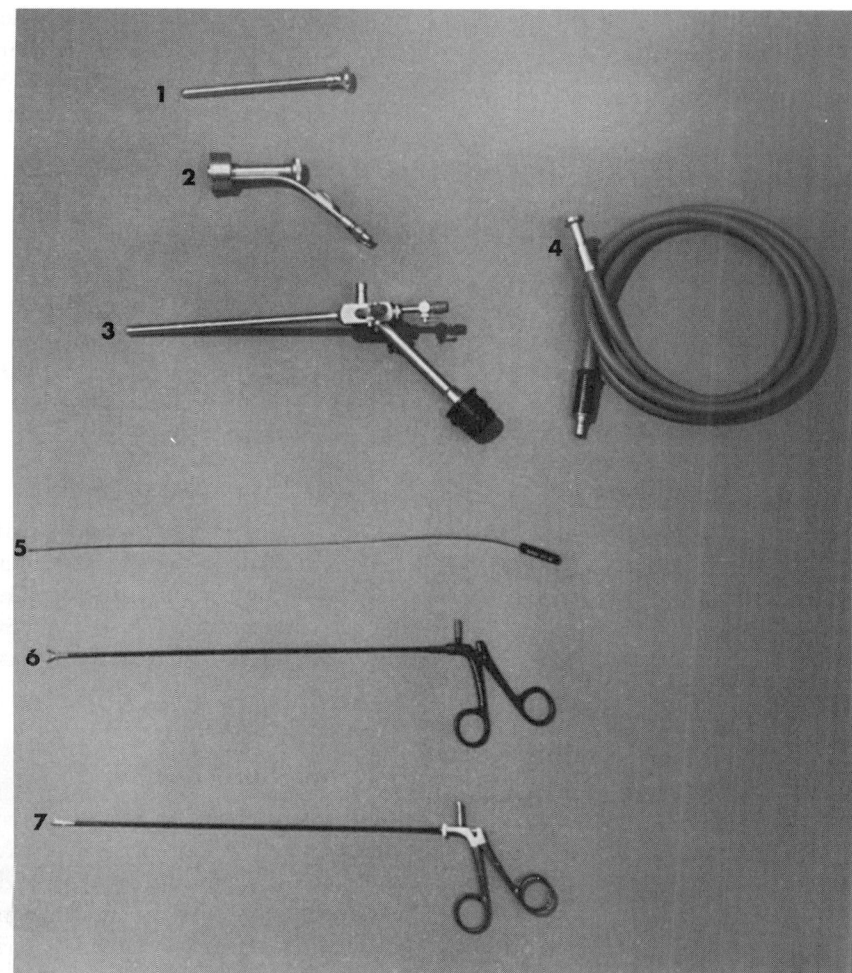

FIGURE 14-31   Instruments for hysteroscopy. *1*, Obturator for cannula; *2*, self-retaining vacuum cannula, small; *3*, hysteroscope; *4*, fiberoptic light cord; *5*, coagulation electrode; *6*, grasping forceps; *7*, scissors.

infusor or the infusion pump. The fluid runs freely through polyethylene tubing through the channel of the hysteroscope. Nursing research has indicated that the mean arterial pressure (MAP) should be monitored during this procedure and fluid-infusion pump pressures maintained at or below the MAP to decrease the risk of fluid overload in the patient.[1]

7. Exploration of the uterine cavity is begun. A video camera monitor may be used to enhance visibility for the OR team, and the procedure may be videotaped for record keeping and reevaluation.

8. Ancillary instruments such as rigid and flexible biopsy forceps, scissors, grasping forceps, insulated coagulation electrodes, resectoscope with "rollerball" electrode, laser fiber tips, and tubal occlusive devices may be introduced for intrauterine manipulation or surgical intervention through the operating channel of the hysteroscope.

9. Upon completion of the procedure, the hysteroscope is withdrawn, and the self-retaining vacuum cannula is removed.

10. If 32% dextran 70 in dextrose (Hyskon) is used for uterine distention, the instruments must be rinsed immediately and cleaned in hot water because dextran has a tendency to harden and is difficult to remove if permitted to dry.

Endometrial Ablation

Endometrial ablation is performed to treat abnormal uterine bleeding. The overall goal of endometrial ablation is to create amenorrhea or to reduce menstrual bleeding to a normal, tolerable flow for the patient (Research Highlight 14-2). It may be an alternative to hysterectomy in some patients with chronic menorrhagia. Endometrial ablation may be performed after unsuccessful dilatation and curettage, or during it. This procedure is performed through the hysteroscope with the use of energy from either the laser or the electrosurgical unit.

The Nd:YAG laser destroys the endometrium and results in scarring of the uterine lining. It is often the laser of choice for this procedure because of its ability to penetrate deep into the tissue, which results in greater

14-2 RESEARCH HIGHLIGHT

In this study operative hysteroscopy was employed in over 1000 women (15% postmenopausal). Ninety percent of the premenopausal patients received some type of preoperative endometrial suppression. All patients had a laminaria tent placed before surgery. All surgery was performed under general anesthesia. Follow-up examination occurred from 6 months to 4 years. Success was based on the patients' satisfaction with the overall results. In women with normal to slightly enlarged uteri (that is, in under 10 weeks), over 95% reported being satisfied. Complications in less than 0.05% were reported in this study. Success rates, however, cannot be determined until 2 years after the surgical intervention because patients experience bleeding sometimes as late as 3 years after the procedure. As a result, operative hysteroscopy, when properly performed, is a safe, effective option for managing women with abnormal uterine bleeding.

From Townsend, D.E., Fields, G.A., & McCausland, A.M. (1992). Operative hysteroscopy: results in 1,000 patients. *American Association of Gynecologic Laparoscopists Annual Meeting Proceedings.* Santa Fe Springs, Ca.: the Association.

tissue destruction. The Nd:YAG, argon, and KTP 532 lasers may be used hysteroscopically.

There are two endometrial ablation techniques when the Nd:YAG laser is used: blanching and dragging. In the blanching technique the tip of the laser fiber is held away from tissue. In the dragging technique the laser fiber tip is in direct contact with the endometrium. The endometrial lining is treated from the fundus to approximately 4 cm above the external cervical os. Air or gas is not used in cooling the laser fiber because of the risk of air or gas embolism. Because of the systemic effects of fluid absorption through open capillaries, 32% dextran 70 in dextrose (Hyskon) is not generally used as an irrigant for endometrial laser ablation.

Electrical energy delivered through an adapted urologic resectoscope, using continuous-flow irrigation, either coagulates or resects the endometrium. Endometrial ablation with the use of a resectoscope, with a rollerball electrode attached, is not an option for a patient who desires to remain fertile. When using the resectoscope, often 32% dextran 70 in dextrose is chosen as the distending medium because it is electrolyte free and compatible with electrosurgery.

Reported complications associated with endometrial ablation using the Nd:YAG laser and electrosurgery have included hemorrhage, fluid overload, uterine perforation, recurrent bleeding, injury to bowel and bladder, cervical lacerations, and rupture of a fallopian tube.

The patient usually has general anesthesia, yet endome-trial ablation can be performed using a local anesthetic. The patient is placed in the lithotomy position, and all potential pressure points are padded. If the Nd:YAG laser is to be used, all laser safety precautions for the patient and the OR team are followed (see Chapter 3). If electrosurgery is being used for the procedure, an electrosurgical dispersive pad is applied. The perioperative nurse must keep an accurate intake and output of irrigating fluid to avoid fluid overload. Discrepancies of greater than a 1500 ml intake versus output should be communicated to the OR team. The length of the procedure is typically less than that for a hysterectomy. Therefore the patient requires less anesthesia and may be discharged the same day, provided that her condition remains stable.

Vaginal Hysterectomy

Vaginal hysterectomy is removal of the uterus through an incision made in the vaginal wall and the pelvic cavity. Contraindications to a vaginal approach are (1) when a large uterine tumor is present, (2) in pelvic malignancy because of an associated inflammatory process involving the fallopian tubes and ovaries, and (3) the possibility of missing metastatic disease that might be present.

Procedural considerations

The instrumentation includes the basic vaginal instrument set with the addition of 2 22-gauge needles, 1½ or 3 inches, and 2 10 ml syringes. An abdominal gynecologic instrument set should be available in case laparotomy is indicated. To facilitate dissection and decrease bleeding, the vaginal walls may be infiltrated with normal saline or a local anesthetic (vasoconstrictors are optional).

Operative procedure

1. The labia may be retracted with sutures. A vaginal retractor is inserted to retract the vaginal wall.
2. Dilatation and curettage may be performed, as previously described (see Fig. 14-24).
3. A Jacobs vulsellum, tenaculum, or suture ligature is placed through the cervical lips to permit traction on the cervix (Fig. 14-32).
4. The vaginal wall is incised with a knife anteriorly through the full thickness of the wall. The bladder is freed from the anterior surface of the cervix by sharp and blunt dissection. The bladder is then elevated to expose the peritoneum of the anterior cul-de-sac, which is entered by sharp dissection (Fig. 14-32, *B*).
5. The peritoneum of the posterior cul-de-sac is identified and incised.
6. The uterosacral ligaments containing blood vessels are clamped, cut, and ligated (Fig. 14-32, *C* and *D*). The ends of the ligatures are left long and are tagged with a clamp.
7. The uterus is drawn downward, and the bladder is held aside with retractors and moist, small laparotomy packs.

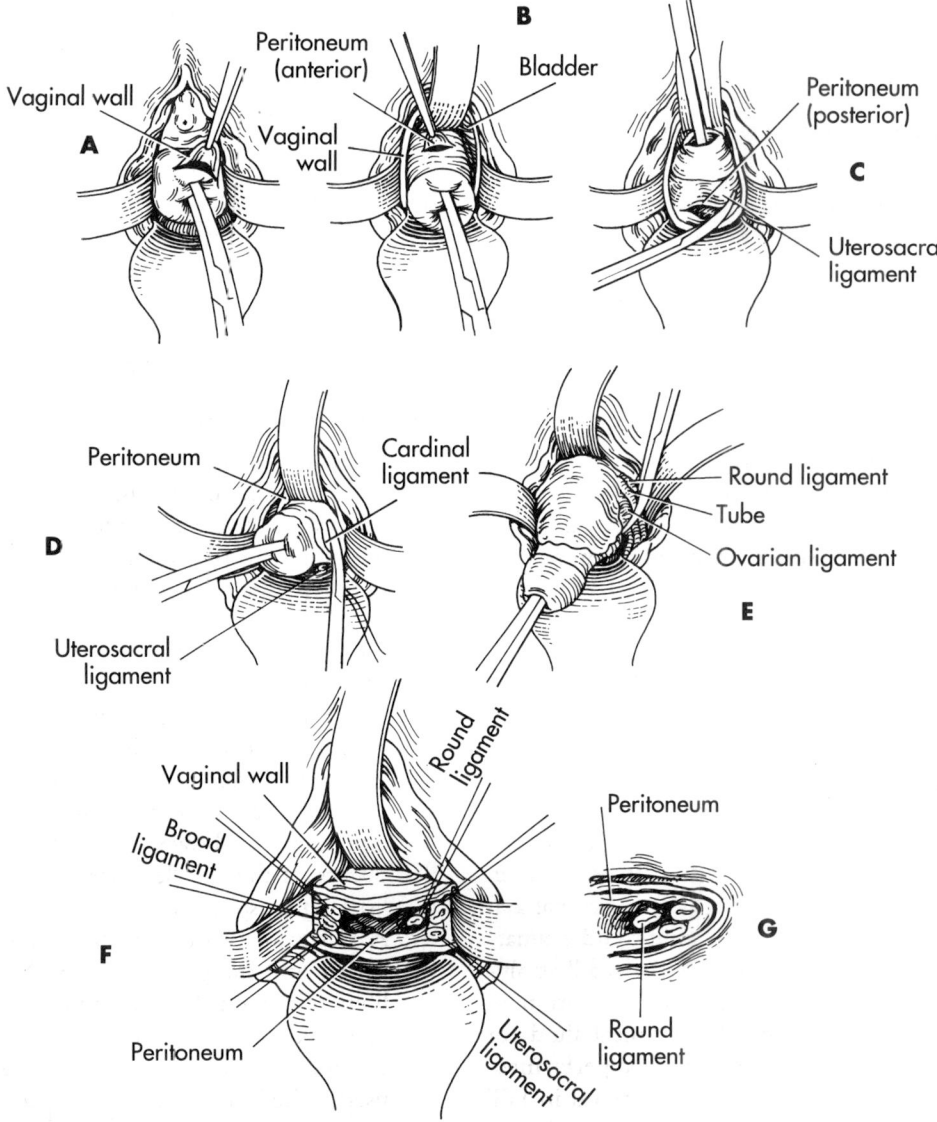

FIGURE 14-32 Vaginal hysterectomy. **A,** Incision of vaginal wall around cervix. Anterior vaginal wall slightly elevated. **B,** Deaver retractor on each side; one Deaver retractor under bladder. Peritoneum opened. **C,** Posterior cul-de-sac opened. Heaney clamp applied to left uterosacral ligament. **D,** Left uterosacral ligament cut and tied. Clamp applied to left cardinal ligament. **E,** Clamp applied to ovarian ligament, round ligament, and fallopian tube. **F,** Uterosacral ligament, broad ligament, and round ligament shown in their respective normal positions. **G,** Peritoneum closed and cardinal broad ligament and uterosacral ligaments reattached to angle of vagina. Left uterosacral and broad ligaments anchored.

8. The cardinal ligament on each side is clamped, cut, and ligated. The uterine arteries are doubly clamped, cut, and ligated.
9. The fundus is delivered with the aid of a uterine tenaculum.
10. When the ovaries are to be left, the round ligament, the uterovarian ligament, and the fallopian tube on each side are clamped together (Fig. 14-32, *E*) and cut, and the uterus is removed. These pedicles are then ligated.
11. The peritoneum between the rectum and vagina is approximated with a continuous suture. The retro-peritoneal obliteration of the cul-de-sac is done by sutures that pass from the vaginal wall through the infundibulopelvic ligament and round ligament, through the cardinal ligament, and out the vaginal wall. The sutures are tied on the vaginal aspect of the new vault (Fig. 14-32, *F* and G). The round, cardinal, and ureterosacral ligaments may be individually approximated for additional support.
12. Any existing cystocele and rectocele and the perineum are repaired, as described for vaginal plastic repair. In the presence of prolapse, reconstruction of the pelvic floor may be required.

13. An indwelling urethral or suprapubic catheter is usually inserted. The vagina may be packed, and a drain may be inserted.

Uterine Balloon Heat Therapy

Excessive menstrual bleeding, responsible for close to 25% of the hysterectomies performed in the United States, can now be treated with a uterine balloon heat therapy device.[6] The balloon is inserted through the vagina and cervix into the uterus, connected to a console with a microprocessor, and inflated and heated. The microprocessor controls the temperature, pressure, and time as the heat ablates the endometrium. Performed on an ambulatory basis, often under local anesthesia, the procedure takes approximately 10 minutes. Other technology for hysterectomy alternatives continues to be developed, and perioperative nurses can anticipate the need to constantly learn new techniques and their implications for gynecologic patient care.

ABDOMINAL GYNECOLOGIC SURGERY

Laparoscopy

Laparoscopy is endoscopic visualization of the peritoneal cavity through the anterior abdominal wall after the establishment of a pneumoperitoneum. It is used in investigating and diagnosing the causes of abdominal and pelvic pain, determining causes of infertility, and evaluating pelvic masses. Ancillary procedures such as adhesiolysis, fulguration of endometriotic implants, aspiration of cysts, biopsy of tissue, aspiration of peritoneal fluid for cytologic study, and tubal sterilization may be performed. Laparoscopy also can be used for oocyte retrieval in IVF procedures. Lasers and electrosurgery may be used with the laparoscope.

Procedural considerations

A general or local anesthetic is administered. The patient is placed in lithotomy position. The abdomen, perineum, and vagina are prepped. The abdomen and perineum are then draped for a combined procedure. Specially designed drapes with openings for the umbilical and perineal areas may be used. The bladder should be emptied.

Dilatation and curettage may be done with laparoscopic procedures when indicated. After the cervix is exposed and the position and depth of the uterus are confirmed, Hulka forceps or a uterine dilator may be introduced into the cervix to manipulate the uterus during the laparoscopy so that the surgeon has better visibility. If chromotubation to evaluate the patency of the fallopian tubes will be performed during the laparoscopy, an intrauterine cannula is placed in the cervical canal at the time of dilatation and curettage.

The usual instrumentation for the vaginal portion of the procedure includes a dilatation and curettage set, with the addition of Hulka forceps, intrauterine cannula, diluted methylene blue or indigo carmine solution, and a syringe. Laparoscopy instruments are shown in Fig. 14-33.

An abdominal gynecologic instrument set should be readily available in the event that a laparotomy is indicated. Common complications that may lead to laparotomy are (1) perforation of a hollow viscus, such as the intestine, (2) hemorrhage from a punctured vessel or biopsy site, (3) gas embolism from intravascular injection, and (4) burns of the bowel and abdominal wall.

Operative procedure

1. A small incision (0.7 to 1.2 cm) is made at the inferior margin of the umbilicus.
2. Elevating the skin with a towel clamp on either side of the umbilicus or grasping below the umbilicus with a gauze sponge for traction, the surgeon inserts a Verres needle through the layers of the abdominal wall into the peritoneal cavity.
3. Once the Verres needle is inserted into the peritoneal cavity, a 10 ml syringe partially filled with sterile saline is attached to the needle for aspiration. If the needle has entered a blood vessel, blood is aspirated. If a loop of intestine or the stomach has been entered, aspiration of bowel contents or malodorous gas occurs. If the needle is free in the peritoneal cavity, nothing is aspirated.
4. A plastic or Silastic tubing is attached to the Verres needle and the gas insufflator. Approximately 2 to 3 liters of carbon dioxide or nitrous oxide gas are then delivered into the peritoneal cavity to achieve pneumoperitoneum. Carbon dioxide is commonly used as the insufflation medium because it is nontoxic, highly soluble in blood, and rapidly absorbed from the peritoneal cavity. The intraabdominal pressure must be closely monitored to prevent overdistention of the abdomen and to ensure free passage of gas into the peritoneal cavity.
5. After insufflation is completed, the Verres needle is withdrawn.
6. The trocar covered by the trocar sleeve is inserted boldly through the abdominal wall into the peritoneal cavity. The angle taken by the trocar is approximately 45 degrees toward the concavity of the pelvis. The plastic or Silastic tubing is attached to the trocar sleeve and insufflation is resumed. Some surgeons prefer a direct trocar-insertion technique or open laparoscopy technique of Hassan to establish the pneumoperitoneum through the valve of the trocar sleeve rather than through a Verres needle.
7. With the trocar sleeve in place, the trocar is withdrawn and the laparoscope is introduced (Fig. 14-34). Visualization of the pelvis and lower abdomen and the visceral contents is begun. If the lens of the

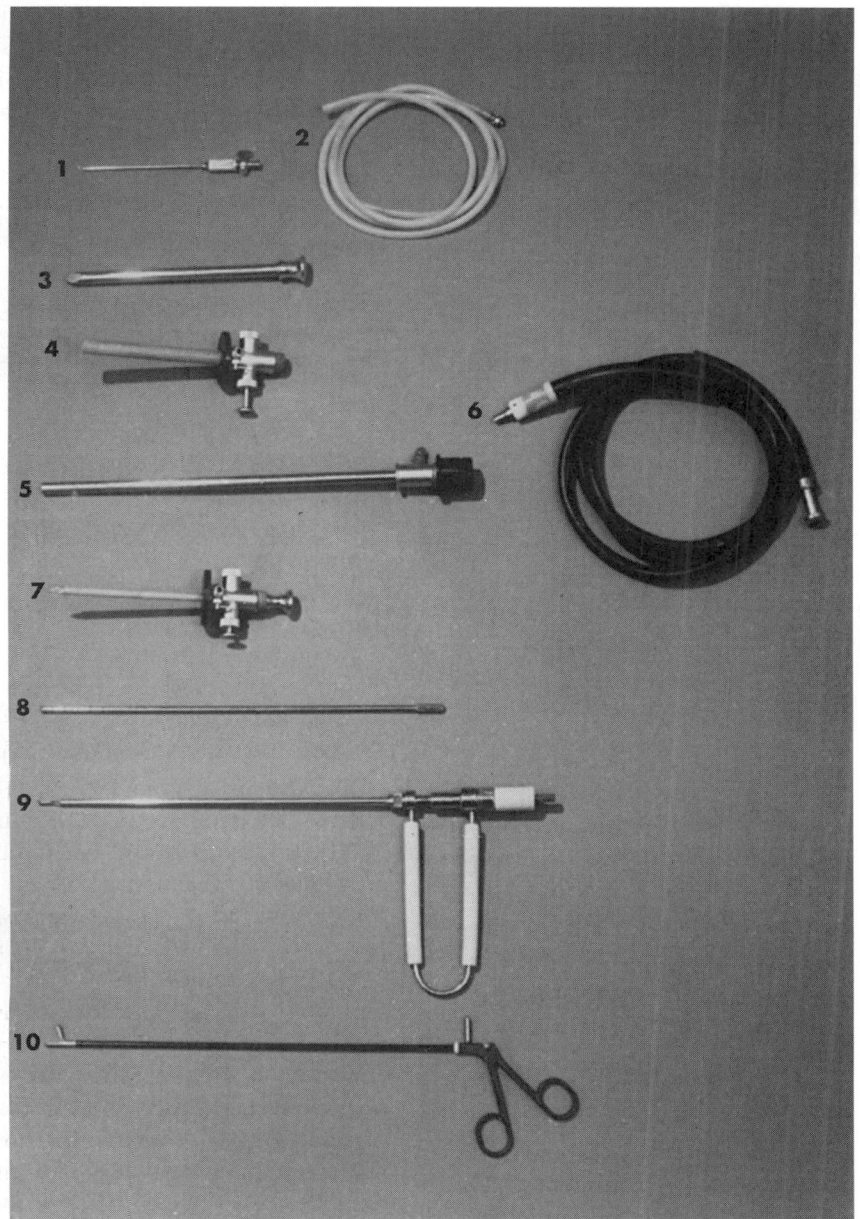

FIGURE 14-33 Instruments for laparoscopy. *1*, Verres needle; *2*, Silastic tubing with connector; *3*, trocar with pyramidal tip; *4*, trocar sleeve with trumpet valve; *5*, laparoscope; *6*, fiberoptic light cord; *7*, secondary trocar sleeve and trocar; *8*, calibrated probe; *9*, bipolar forceps; *10*, biopsy forceps.

laparoscope becomes foggy, touching the lens to a loop of intestine is one method of clearing it. Before use, warming the tip of the scope in warm saline or towels may prevent fogging of the distal lens.

8. The patient is placed in Trendelenburg's position.

9. The video camera may be attached to the scope to aid in the OR team's visualization, and the procedure may be recorded for future reference. If an ancillary instrument such as biopsy forceps or bipolar forceps is needed, a second trocar with sleeve is inserted under direct laparoscopic visualization through an incision made suprapubically.

10. To test for tubal patency, diluted methylene blue or indigo carmine solution is injected through the intrauterine cannula into the cervical canal. If the fallopian tubes are patent, dye can be seen at the fimbriated ends.

11. On completion of the intraabdominal procedure the laparoscope is withdrawn and the insufflated gas is allowed to escape from the trocar sleeve. The trocar sleeve is removed.

12. Application of skin clips or subcuticular closure of the primary skin incision is followed by placement of a Band-Aid or Steri-Strip.

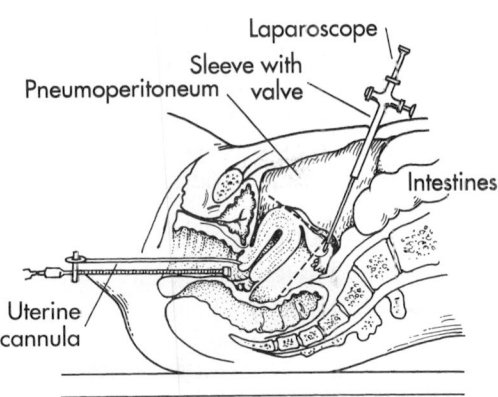

FIGURE 14-34   Technique of laparoscopy.

Pelviscopy

Pelviscopy has become a fast-growing alternative to abdominal surgery for many procedures.[14] Pelviscopic surgery historically was utilized in treating infertility in younger women but is now being used with older women as well. Some benefits associated with pelviscopic surgery have been shown to be shorter hospital stay, decreased total cost, lower morbidity, and quicker return to full activity (Research Highlight 14-3). Pelviscopy is an endoscopic approach to pelvic and intraabdominal examination or surgery. It differs from operative laparoscopy in two ways: (1) a 10 mm pelviscope with a 30-degree angle replaces the standard 7 mm laparoscope with a 0-degree angle; (2) the instrumentation utilized is capable of intraabdominal hemostasis and suturing. A 30-degree angle telescope is used to visualize the intrapelvic and intraabdominal structures. There is a wide field of vision, and the size, depth, and mobility of the organs can be assessed throughout the procedure.

Procedural considerations

Many of the procedural considerations for pelviscopy are similar to those associated with laparoscopy. The patient may be typed and crossmatched for blood preoperatively, as in the instance of ectopic pregnancy. If the pelviscopic surgery is elective, autologous blood donation may be an alternative. The patient may be placed in the supine position, with a warming blanket in place. An indwelling urinary catheter is inserted, and antiembolic stockings are applied. Bony prominences are padded, and a dispersive electrosurgical pad is applied. In the instance of possible ectopic pregnancy, dilatation and curettage may be performed to rule out an intrauterine pregnancy. There are usually two or three puncture sites established for the necessary accessory instrumentation.

The surgeon and assistants manipulate instruments through trocar sheaths, as described with laparoscopy. The OR team utilizes the video screens placed on opposite sides of the operating room bed for visualization. Accessory instruments used with the pelviscope include dissecting forceps, grasping forceps, scissors, sponge

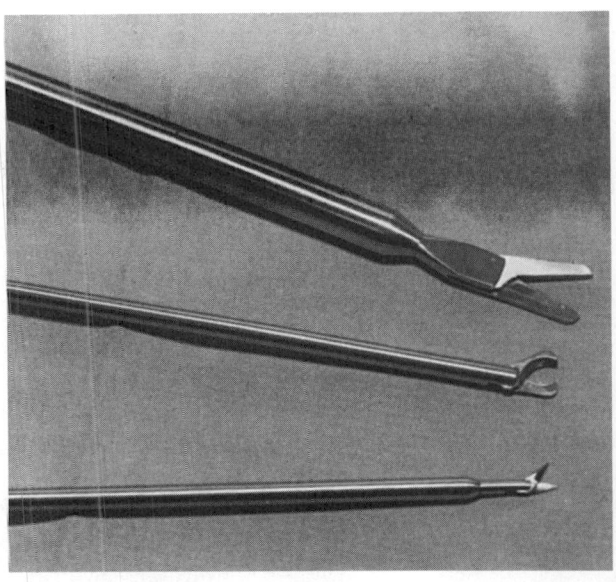

FIGURE 14-35   Scissors range from microscissors with delicate tips to heavy scissors designed to go through an 11-mm trocar.

14-3 RESEARCH HIGHLIGHT

One hundred seventy women who underwent operative pelviscopy over a 67-month period were evaluated in this study. Each participant followed a preoperative screening, involving CA-125 and ultrasonography, to decrease the risk of affecting the prognosis of potentially malignant ovarian tumors. CA-125 is a tumor marker that has a high degree of sensitivity and specificity for ovarian cancer. Forty-four women were over 40 years of age. Participants' ages ranged up to 68 years. The mean age was 45 years. The operations performed ranged from pelviscopic lysis of adhesions to bilateral oophorectomy. Eighty-six percent of the patients were hospitalized for 2 days or less; 45% were outpatients, and 36.4% were 23-hour admission patients. Many postmenopausal women undergo laparotomy with its high financial cost and increased morbidity. Women of this age group may now have a choice, provided that they have adequate preoperative screening, and may be spared the long recovery time and increased cost with little, if any, increased risk.

From Levine, R.L. (1990, June). Pelviscopic surgery in women over 40. *Journal of Reproductive Medicine, 35,* 597.

holders, needle holders, suture forceps, knot tiers, appendix extractors, suction manipulators, fulgurating electrodes, laser probes, and applicators for loop ligature (Figs. 14-35 to 14-37). A tissue morcellator may be used to slowly fragment the tissue using jaws; the tissue is then loaded into the barrel of the morcellator for removal.

Endocoagulation and endoligation may be accomplished (Fig. 14-38). Intraabdominal ligation is accomplished using loops of synthetic and natural suture materials.

Procedures performed through the pelviscope include adhesiolysis, ovarian biopsy, ovarian cystectomy, oophorectomy, adnexectomy, enucleation of intramural myomas, appendectomy, fimbrioplasty, removal of ectopic tubal pregnancy, tuboplasty, uterosacral neurectomy, and lymphadenectomy. The complications associated with pelviscopy are similar to those described with laparoscopy. An abdominal gynecologic instrument set should be readily available in case laparotomy is indicated.

Ectopic Tubal Pregnancy

A majority of tubal pregnancies occur in the ampullary region of the fallopian tube, and nearly 67% are within the lumen of the fallopian tube.[13] The selection of an operation is determined by (1) location of the pregnancy within the fallopian tube, (2) the capabilities of the surgeon, and (3) the availability of special instrumentation.[13] The overall goal is tubal preservation. Adhesion formation and tubal damage may be minimized by ensuring hemostasis, atraumatic tissue handling, prevention of serosal drying, and the use of fine nonreactive sutures throughout the pelviscopic surgery.

Pelviscopic Salpingostomy

Pelviscopic salpingostomy may be used in the treatment of unruptured ampullary gestations.

Operative procedure

1. After successful pelviscopic entry, the distal end of the fallopian tube is mobilized, and the adhesiolysis is completed. Grasping forceps are placed on either side of the fallopian tube, and gentle traction is applied.

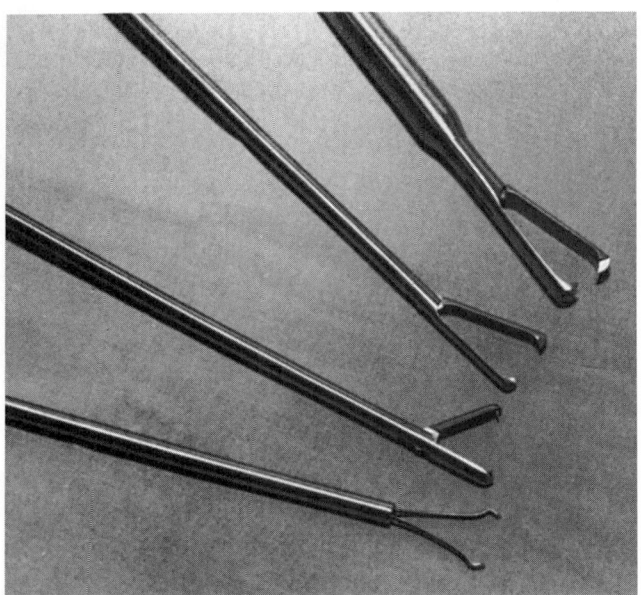

FIGURE 14-36   Graspers have been designed for work on various pelvic organs.

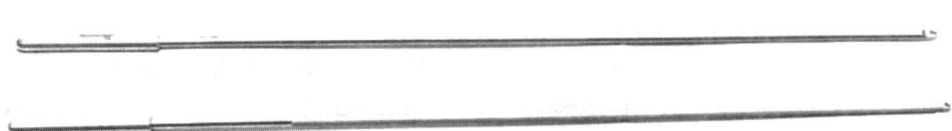

FIGURE 14-37   Suturing technique can be aided by extracorporeal ties with the knot pushed by ligating devices such as the Clarke-Reich ligators.

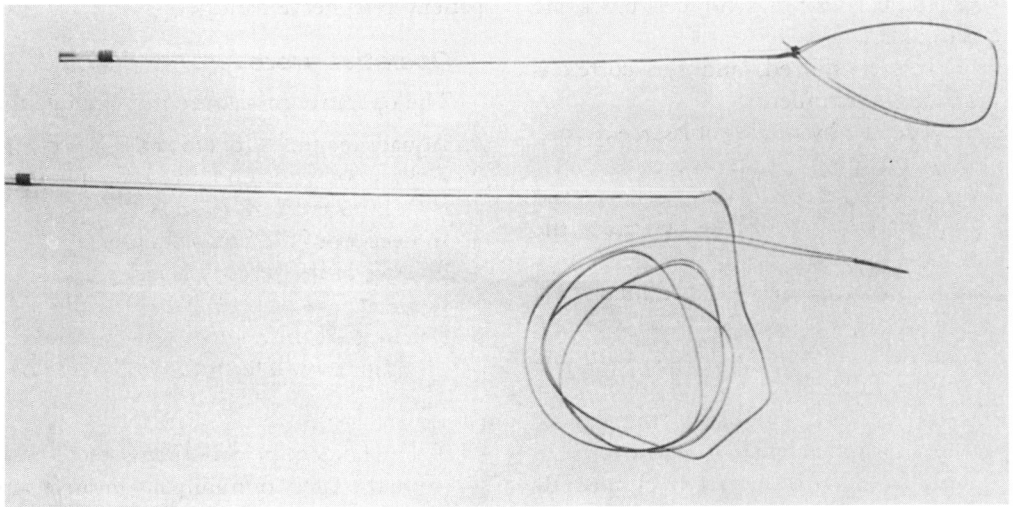

FIGURE 14-38   Endoloops and Endoknots (Ethicon, Inc.) have been easy to place and use at laparoscopy.

2. Before making an incision, cauterization of the serosal vessels on both sides of the anticipated incision may be performed. A dilute solution of vasopressin may also be injected into the mesenteric margin to avoid excessive bleeding.

3. A single incision is made with scissors from the mesenteric to the antimesenteric side of the fallopian tube, where the products of conception are exposed.

4. The tissue is removed gently with forceps while constant irrigation is maintained with an isotonic solution. Care needs to be taken to avoid vigorous evacuation, so that the highly vascular underlying interstitium is not disturbed.

5. Small bleeding vessels can be ligated with a fine, nonreactive suture, or simple atraumatic compression of bleeding margins will promote hemostasis. Mesosalpingeal vessel ligation may be performed.

6. The tubal incision may be closed by second intention or, as in the instance of salpingotomy, the incision may be closed in one or two layers, with 6-0, interrupted, nonreactive sutures. Upon completion, the pelviscope and instrumentation are removed. The insufflated gas is permitted to escape from the trocar sleeves. Trocar sleeves are then removed. Application of skin clips, or subcuticular closure of the primary skin incisions, is followed by placement of Band-Aids, Steri-Strips, or dressings.

Other methods to pelviscopically treat ectopic pregnancy include salpingotomy, segmental resection, fimbrial expression, and salpingectomy.

Ovarian Cystectomy

Ovarian cystectomy is frequently performed via pelviscopic surgery.

Operative procedure

1. After successful pelviscopic entry, adhesiolysis is achieved.

2. Upon entry, peritoneal washings for cell block are obtained, if indicated.

3. The ovarian cyst is mobilized, and the cortex is grasped with a biopsy instrument.

4. The cortex is then incised by scissors or laser, exposing the cyst wall.

5. The incision is then enlarged with scissors, and aquadissection is used to separate the cyst from the ovarian stroma.

6. The cyst is dissected and may be removed intact by a culdotomy incision, or the cyst may be opened, evacuated, thoroughly cleaned by lavage with the aquadissector, and removed.

7. If the cyst is opened intraperitoneally, the patient should be taken out of Trendelenburg's position while the fluid is removed, and the pelvis is cleaned by lavage.

8. Arterial bleeders are identified and desiccated.

9. The ovary usually does not require suturing; however, if the edges gape widely, they may be loosely approximated with interrupted, 4-0, synthetic absorbable suture.

10. Upon completion, the pelviscope and accessory instrumentation are removed. The insufflated gas is permitted to escape from the trocar sleeves. Trocar sleeves are then removed.

11. Application of skin clips or a subcuticular closure of the primary skin incisions is followed by placement of Band-Aids, Steri-Strips, or dressings.

Laparoscope-Assisted Vaginal Hysterectomy

Laparoscope-assisted vaginal hysterectomy (LAVH) or pelviscope-assisted vaginal hysterectomy (PAVH) offers an alternative to total abdominal hysterectomy (TAH) and vaginal hysterectomy (VH). The patient does not have the large abdominal incision, long hospital stay, and long recovery period that would be necessary with a total abdominal hysterectomy. Patients who are not candidates for traditional vaginal hysterectomy may be candidates for laparoscope-assisted vaginal hysterectomy.

The surgeon uses laparoscopy to visualize the pelvis and thereby determine whether disease is present. This is not possible with traditional vaginal hysterectomy. Conditions leading to LAVH include postmenopausal bleeding, pelvic pain, uterine leiomyomas, and adnexal masses. Indications for LAVH may be absence of genital prolapse, required adnexectomy, history of abdominopelvic surgery, salpingitis or endometriosis, lymphadenectomy, and endometrial cancer.

Procedural considerations

Procedural considerations and accessory instrumentation and approach are similar to that used in other pelviscopic surgical procedures. The patient may be placed in lithotomy position or with legs spread; padding is applied to bony prominences and all potential pressure areas to prevent pressure at vulnerable sites and protect the patient from nerve damage.

Operative procedure

The operative procedure may include the following:

1. Aquadissection of the broad ligament

2. Dessication of round and infundibulopelvic ligaments with bipolar coagulation

3. Dissection of the broad ligaments

4. Freeing of the urinary bladder from the lower uterine segment

5. Opening of the vaginal vault with endoscopic scissors or monopolar electrode, and removal of the uterus vaginally.

Advancements in endoscopic technology continue to promote the safety of minimally invasive surgical interventions just as an ongoing emphasis on research related to women's health does.[4]

Total Abdominal Hysterectomy

Total abdominal hysterectomy (TAH) is removal of the entire uterus, including the corpus and the cervix. When TAH is combined with bilateral salpingo-oophorectomy, the procedure is commonly termed *panhysterectomy*, or *complete hysterectomy*. TAH may be performed for symptomatic pelvic relaxation or prolapse, pain associated with pelvic congestion, pelvic inflammatory disease, endometriosis, recurrent ovarian cysts, fibroids (myomas), bleeding with no apparent cause in postmenopausal women, adenomyosis, or dysfunctional uterine bleeding. TAH, usually with bilateral salpingo-oophorectomy, is also indicated in anatomic disease, malignancy, premalignant states, and conditions of high risk for development or recurrence of malignancy. The procedure can also be used to accomplish sterilization. It has been estimated that one out of every three women undergo hysterectomy by 60 years of age and a large percentage of these are performed by the abdominal approach.[10] A clinical pathway for TAH is shown in Fig. 14-39.

Procedural considerations

Diagnostic dilatation and curettage usually have already been performed. However, an instrument set should be readily available. Before the abdominal skin prep, an internal vaginal prep is done. An indwelling urinary drainage catheter is inserted to provide constant bladder drainage during the operation. The supine position, modified during the procedure with Trendelenburg's position, is used. Instrumentation includes the abdominal gynecologic set. Provisions are made to remove from the abdomen and field those instruments used in separating the cervix from the vagina, thereby avoiding vaginal contamination of the pelvis.

Operative procedure

1. In an obese patient or for exploration of the upper abdominal cavity, a left rectus or midline incision may be made. For simple hysterectomy a Pfannenstiel incision may be used. The abdominal layers and the peritoneum are opened as described for laparotomy.
2. As the peritoneal cavity is opened, the patient is usually placed in Trendelenburg's position to provide better visualization of the pelvic organs.
3. The round ligament is grasped with forceps, clamped, and ligated with sutures on long needle holders. Pedicles are cut with a knife or Metzenbaum scissors; sutures are tagged with a hemostat to be used as traction later. This procedure is done on both sides (Fig. 14-40, *A*).
4. By use of the surgeon's fingers, the layer of the broad ligament close to the uterus is separated on each side, bleeding vessels are clamped and ligated, and a moist laparotomy pack is inserted behind the flap. The fallopian tube and the uteroovarian ligaments are double-clamped together, incised, and double-tied with suture ligatures (Fig. 14-40, *B*).

5. The uterus is pulled forward to expose the posterior sheath of the broad ligament, which is incised with a knife or Metzenbaum scissors. Ureters are identified. The uterine vessels and uterosacral ligaments are double-clamped, divided by sharp dissection at the level of the internal os, and ligated with suture ligatures (Fig. 14-40, *C*).
6. The severed uterine vessels are bluntly dissected away from the cervix on each side with the aid of sponges on sponge-holding forceps, scissors, and tissue forceps.
7. The bladder is separated from the cervix and upper vagina with sharp and blunt dissection assisted by sponges on sponge-holding forceps. The bladder may be retracted with a moist laparotomy pack and a retractor with an angular blade. The vaginal vault is incised close to the cervix with a knife or scissors (Fig. 14-40, *D*).
8. The anterior lip of the cervix is grasped with an Allis, Kocher, or tenaculum forceps. With scissors, the cervix is dissected and amputated from the vagina. The uterus is removed. Potentially contaminated instruments used on the cervix and vagina are placed into a discard basin and removed from the field (including sponge-holding forceps and suction). Bleeding is controlled with hemostats and sutures.
9. The vaginal vault is reconstructed with interrupted sutures. Angle sutures anchor all three connective tissue ligaments to the vaginal vault. The pedicles, fallopian tubes, and ovarian ligaments are left free of the vault.
10. Vaginal mucosa is approximated with a continuous suture on a long needle holder. The muscular coat of the vagina may be closed with figure-of-eight sutures to make the vault of the vagina firm and provide resistance against prolapse. A drain may be placed in the vagina.
11. The peritoneum is closed over the bladder, vaginal vault, and rectum (Fig. 14-40, *E*). The laparotomy packs are removed, and the omentum is drawn over the bowel.
12. The abdominal wound is closed as described for laparotomy closure (see Chapter 11).

Abdominal Myomectomy

Uterine fibroids are benign tumors that arise from the muscular wall of the uterus. Abdominal myomectomy is removal of fibromyomas, or fibroid tumors, by carefully separating each fibroid from the uterine wall and its blood supply. Myomectomy is usually done in young women who have symptoms that indicate the presence of tumors and who wish to preserve their potential fertility. Also, tumors may be removed because of infertility, habitual abortion, excessive bleeding during menses, pain, or pressure on the bladder or bowel. Myomectomy may be performed as a prophylactic measure with other abdominopelvic surgery.

Text continued on p. 485

CLINICAL PATHWAY: TAH/TAH BSO
COOPER HOSPITAL/UNIVERSITY MEDICAL CENTER
DRG: 358/359

Goal LOS 3-4 days

DATES:					
TIME FRAME:	Day 1				
UNIT:	Preadmission	Post OP (Day of Surgery)	Post OP DAY 1	Post OP DAY 2	Day of Discharge
GOALS	Admission criteria met. M☐ NM☐ NA☐	Early Ambulation M☐ NM☐ NA☐	------>		Discharge when clinically stable and no longer requiring acute level of care. M☐ NM☐ NA☐
Met (M)	Advance Directive/Code Status obtained within 24 hours of admission. M☐ NM☐ NA☐	Maintain Afebrile M☐ NM☐ NA☐	------>	------>	Patient/Parent/Care Giver verbalizes understanding of discharge plan and the need for follow-up. M☐ NM☐ NA☐
Not Met (NM)	Pt/Family has understanding of plan of care and treatment. M☐ NM☐ NA☐	Pain Management M☐ NM☐ NA☐	------>	------>	
Not Applicable (NA)	PAT completed M☐ NM☐ NA☐	Absence of infection M☐ NM☐ NA☐	------>	------>	
	Cleared for OR M☐ NM☐ NA☐	Wound Condition M☐ NM☐ NA☐	------>	------>	
	Consent signed M☐ NM☐ NA☐ Surgical consent Anesthesia consent Blood consent				
ADDRESSOGRAPH:					

*Goals are evaluated at the end of the day as Met, Not Met, or N/A

*Circle indicates not done

*Cross-out indicates not applicable to this patient

FIGURE 14-39 Clinical pathway for total abdominal hysterectomy.

Continued

DATES:					
TIME FRAME:		Day 1			
UNIT:	Preadmission	Post OP	Post OP DAY 1	Post OP DAY 2	Discharge DAY
CLINICAL ASSESSMENTS	H&P completed Nursing Assessment Admission criteria met	**PACU** Systems Assessment Pain Assessment Vital Signs q 15 min until stable Evaluate wound Status (Check Abdominal Dressing for drainage) Assess vaginal discharge with VS checks **Post OP-Med/Surg Unit** VS q 15 minutes × 4, then q 30 minutes × 2, then q 4 hours Check Vaginal Discharge with VS checks I&O Pain Assessment Systems Assessment Evaluate Bowel Sounds Evaluate IV site Evaluate Incision Assess drain status if indicated	Vital Signs q8hours; assess vaginal bleeding with VS & pad count Evaluate Breath Sounds and Bowel Sounds q8hours Pain Assessment Systems Assessment Monitor Abdominal incision Check for spontaneous voiding after Foley removal	Vital Signs q shift Assess incision for S/S of infection Assess for BM ----------> ---------->	----------> ----------> ----------> ----------> ---------->
CONSULTS	Gyn Oncology if indicated General Surgery if indicated Urology/UroGyn if indicated Anesthesia Medicine if indicated	PM&R if necessary Social Service if indicated Home Care if indicated	----------> ----------> ---------->	----------> ----------> ---------->	----------> ----------> ---------->
TESTS (Incl. Labs & Diag. Tests)	CBC with differential Type & Screen UA EKG if indicated CXR if indicated Preg test if indicated		CBC with Diff		
ADDRESSOGRAPH:					

FIGURE 14-39, cont'd   Clinical pathway for total abdominal hysterectomy.

Continued

		Preadmission	Day 1 Post OP	Post OP DAY 1	Post OP DAY 2	Discharge DAY
DATES:						
TIME FRAME:						
UNIT:						
MEDICATIONS/IV, ALLERGIES:		Prophylactic Antibiotics Other medications: ___ ___ ___	Analgesics Antibiotics if indicated Antiemetic	--------> Stool Softeners -------->	--------> --------> Bowel Stimulants as indicated	--------> --------> -------->
INTERVENTIONS (Procedures/Supportive Tx)		DVT Prophylaxis if indicated	Foley or Suprapubic Urinary Catheter TEDS/Kendalls Cough & Deep Breath Incentive Spirometry q1hour while awake Perineal care q4hours W/A Continuous IV fluids Reinforce Abdominal dressing as needed Emotional Support	Remove Foley --------> --------> Perineal care q8hours (pt may do on own) --------> Emotional Support; encourage ventilation of feelings about surgery and body image effects	Start Clamping S/P tube (per MD's Order) D/C Kendalls if ambulating TEDS --------> --------> D/C IV fluids when tolerating po fluids and no nausea Determine timing of staple removal -------->	--------> D/C Staples if indicated
NUTRITION		NPO	NPO	Clear Liquids advance as tolerated	Regular diet	-------->
ACTIVITY (Incl. PT/OT)		Bedrest	Bedrest	Out of Bed to chair Advance as tolerated	Ambulate May Shower	Ambulate
ADDRESSOGRAPH:						

FIGURE 14-39, cont'd   Clinical pathway for total abdominal hysterectomy.

Continued

DATES:					
TIME FRAME:		Day 1			
UNIT:	Preadmission	Post OP	Post OP DAY 1	Post OP DAY 2	Discharge DAY
PATIENT/FAMILY EDUCATION & COMMUNICATION	Advance Directive Discussion Y/N RN/MD Y/N Copy on chart Y/N Family spokesperson Benefits Reviewed Financial counseling as indicated Spirometry PCA	Inform family of progress Review with pt and family as to limitations and expectations of progress to normal ADL Orient to hospital and unit Teach and demonstrate procedure for Cough & Deep Breath and incentive spirometry Remind pt to expect vaginal bleeding and to report passing large clots or having severe pain Reinforce basic understanding of surgical procedure	Review S/S infection Wound Care Medications Teach perineal care procedure Initiate S/P tube education if indicated	-------> -------> -------> -------> -------> Review follow up and restrictions	Review discharge instructions regarding Wound care Pain management Physical activity Sexual activity Complications Physical changes Meds Restrictions S/S of infection Appropriate medication teaching sheets discussed with and given to patient.
ADDITIONAL PATIENT INFORMATION	Consideration of Estrogen Replacement Therapy Effect on Sexuality	Inform as to expected course of recovery			
DC PLANNING & REFERRALS	Home Assessment	Assess home situation for support systems & financial status consider VNA	Reassess home needs & support	Home health referral if patient is unable to provide self care F/U visits with Gyn or other consultant's	-------> Instruct to arrange for follow-up appointment as MD specific
ADDRESSOGRAPH:					

FIGURE 14–39, cont'd   Clinical pathway for total abdominal hysterectomy.

Continued

DATES:				
TIME FRAME:	Day 1			
UNIT:	Preadmission	Post OP	Post OP DAY 1	Post OP DAY 2	Discharge DAY
EQUIPMENT		IMED	IMED	TEDS	
		O2 flow meter	Kendalls/TEDS		
		Kendalls/TEDS			
		Incentive Spirometry			

ADDRESSOGRAPH:

Initials/Signature/Title: _____ Committee Approval: _3/7/96_ Committee Review: _____

Discharge RN: _____

Physician: _____

_____

_____

_____

_____

DISCLAIMER:

The parameters contained in this carepath should not be considered inclusive of all proper methods of care or exclusive of other methods of care reasonably directed to obtaining the same results. The majority of the patients will progress according to the goals and activities on this outline. However, each patient may have individual variations and or needs in his/her progress. This pathway represents guides for clinical decision making and should not be viewed as rigid standards which dictate defined courses of treatment. Rather, the pathway should be recognized as a tool which describes key events in the process of patient care and has been agreed upon by a consensus of physicians and other healthcare disciplines.

FIGURE 14-39, cont'd   Clinical pathway for total abdominal hysterectomy.

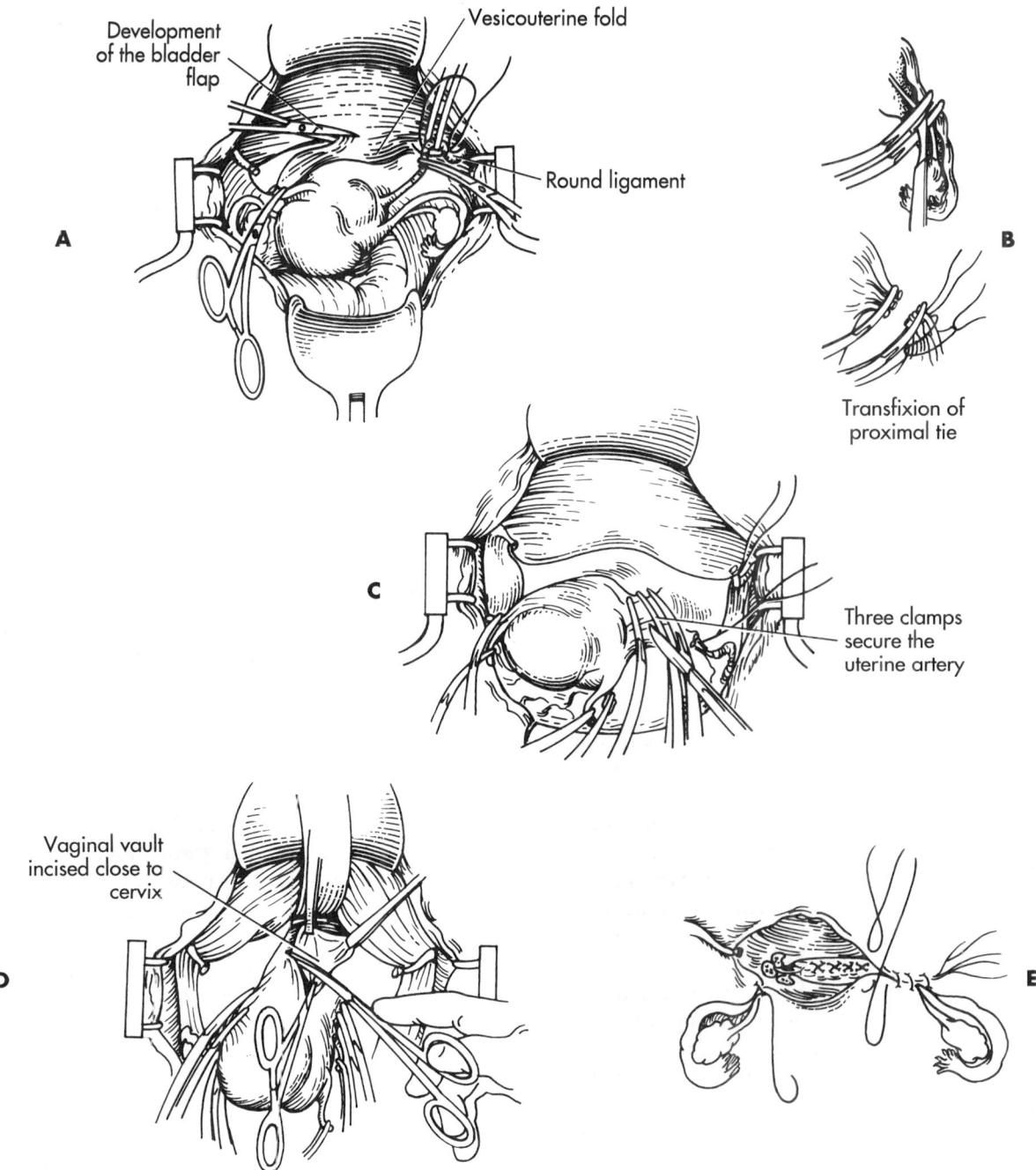

Development of the bladder flap

Vesicouterine fold

Round ligament

A

B

Transfixion of proximal tie

C

Three clamps secure the uterine artery

Vaginal vault incised close to cervix

D

E

FIGURE 14-40   Abdominal hysterectomy for single fibroid uterus. **A**, Peritoneum retracted with self-retaining retractors, and organs protected with laparotomy packs saturated in warm normal saline solution. Transverse incision made through uterine peritoneum and carried to each side of uterine attachments of round ligaments. Bleeding vessels clamped and ligated. Round ligament grasped, ligated, and cut. **B**, Tube and ovarian ligaments clamped, cut, and sutured. **C**, Uterus pulled forward, posterior sheath of broad ligaments divided, and uterine artery and veins secured by three heavy curved clamps. Pedicle divided, leaving two hemostats on proximal pedicle. **D**, Bladder separated from cervix and upper vagina. Vaginal vault opened and grasped with Allis forceps. Allis forceps placed on anterior lip of cervix, and dissection of cervix carried out to complete its amputation from vagina. **E**, Three connective tissue thickenings anchored to vaginal vault, vaginal mucosa approximated, and vault closed. As shown, peritoneum closed with continuous suture.

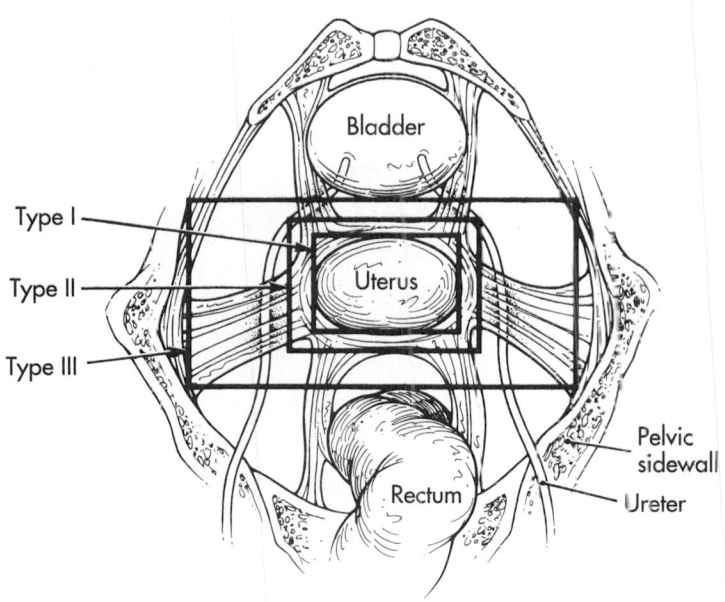

FIGURE 14-41   Different types of hysterectomy: type I simple hysterectomy, type II modified radical hysterectomy, type III radical hysterectomy.

Procedural considerations

The basic abdominal gynecologic instrument set is required.

Operative procedure

1. The patient is prepared as described for abdominal hysterectomy. A midline or Pfannenstiel incision is used, and the uterus is exposed.
2. To contract the musculature of the uterine wall, a suitable drug may be injected into the fundus.
3. The fibroid tumor is grasped with a tenaculum. The broad ligament may be opened with curved hemostats and Metzenbaum scissors to determine the course of the ureter or to free the bladder.
4. Each tumor is shelled out of its bed, using blunt and sharp instruments, or lasered. Bleeding vessels are clamped and ligated or electrocoagulated.
5. The uterus is reconstructed with interrupted or continuous sutures.
6. The perimetrium is closed over the operative site. The abdominal wound is closed.

Radical Hysterectomy (Wertheim)

Radical hysterectomy is en bloc dissection with careful removal of all recognizable lymph nodes in the pelvis, together with wide removal of the uterus, tubes, ovaries, supporting ligaments, and upper vagina (Fig. 14-41). Extensive dissection of the ureters and of the bladder is also involved.

Radical abdominal hysterectomy is performed in the presence of cervical carcinoma, with or without attendant radiation therapy. Abdominal exploration determines lymph node involvement. With no lymph node involvement, a wide-cuff hysterectomy is performed. The uterus, tubes, and ovaries, together with most of the parametrial tissues and the upper portion of the vagina, are dissected en bloc. Dissection of the ureters from the paracervical structures takes place so that the ligaments supporting the uterus and vagina can be removed. Radical abdominal hysterectomy can also be used in certain cases of endometrial carcinoma.

Procedural considerations

Careful estimation of blood loss and calculation of urinary output are needed throughout the operative procedure. The patient is prepped as described for total abdominal hysterectomy. An indwelling urinary catheter is inserted. The basic abdominal gynecologic instrument set is required, plus long and deep instrumentation and a self-retaining retractor may be used.

Operative procedure

1. The skin is incised, and the abdominal layers are opened, as described for laparotomy.
2. The peritoneum is cut at its reflection on the anterior surface of the uterus between the round ligaments (Fig. 14-42, A). By blunt dissection, the bladder surface is freed from the cervix and vagina.
3. The right round and infundibulopelvic ligaments are clamped, cut with a knife or Metzenbaum scissors, and ligated with sutures to expose the external iliac artery. The ureter is identified and retracted with a vein retractor (Fig. 14-42, B).
4. The lymph and areolar tissues are dissected from the iliac artery, obturator fossa, and ureter with Lahey forceps, Kitner sponges, and Metzenbaum scissors. A complete lymph gland dissection removes the tissue from Cloquet's node to the bifurcation of the iliac arteries bilaterally. The uterine artery and vein are clamped, cut, and doubly ligated.

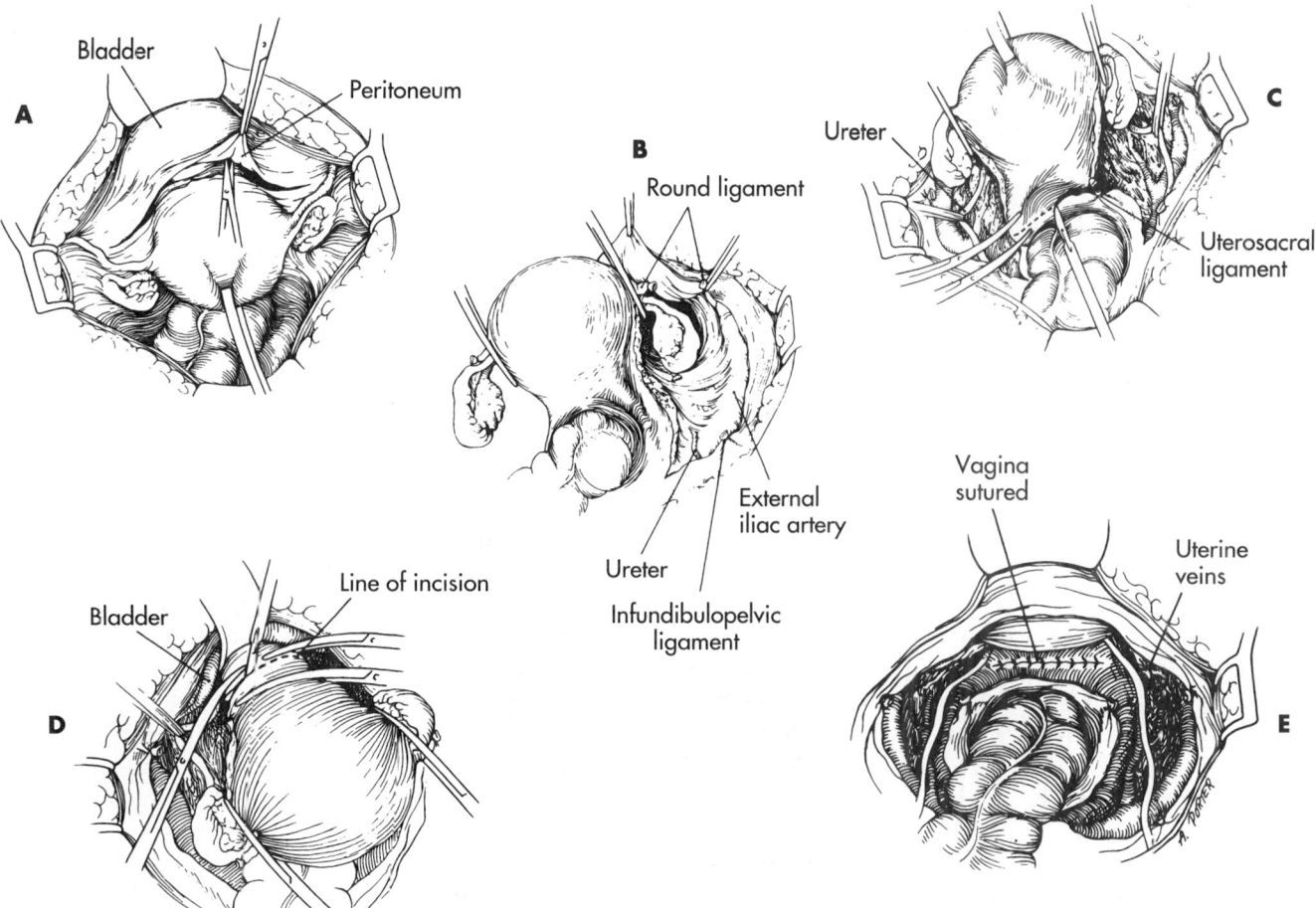

FIGURE 14-42 Wertheim radical hysterectomy. **A**, With upward traction applied on uterus, peritoneum is incised from round ligament to round ligament. **B**, Right round and infundibulopelvic ligaments are ligated and cut, thus exposing right external iliac artery. **C**, Uterus is held upward and forward, exposing cul-de-sac, which is incised as shown by *dotted line*. **D**, After dissection is completed, vagina is doubly clamped preparatory to transsection, after which entire specimen is lifted out en masse. **E**, Vagina is closed. Peritoneum remains to be reperitonealized.

5. The uterus is elevated, the cul-de-sac is opened (Fig. 14-42, *C*), and the uterosacral and cardinal ligaments are clamped, cut with scissors, and doubly ligated with suture ligatures. The pararectal and paravesical areolar tissues are dissected free to skeletonize the upper vagina, and the paraurethral tissues are removed as near to the pelvic walls as possible.
6. The upper third of the vagina is cross-clamped with Heaney forceps (Fig. 14-42, *D*) and divided with a long #4 knife handle and #20 blade. The uterus and surrounding tissues are removed. Electrocoagulation is useful in minimizing venous oozing from small venules and capillaries. Lowering the head of the operating bed 15 degrees is also helpful in reducing the oozing of blood and serum. Careful apposition of the skin edges with interrupted mattress sutures must take place to prevent overlapping of the skin edges and a resulting delay in healing.
7. The vagina is sutured open with a running locked stitch, and closed wound drainage is provided from above (Fig. 14-42, *E*). The pelvis is peritonealized with a continuous suture.
8. The abdominal wound is closed (retention sutures may be used) and dressed in the usual manner. Vaginal packing and drains may be used. A suprapubic indwelling catheter may be placed. The catheter helps prevent postoperative bladder spasm and allows for bladder drainage if the patient is unable to void after removal of the urinary catheter.

Pelvic Exenteration

Pelvic exenteration is en bloc removal of the rectum, distal sigmoid colon, the urinary bladder and the distal ureters, the internal iliac vessels and their lateral branches, all pelvic reproductive organs and lymph nodes, and the entire pelvic floor with the accompanying pelvic peritoneum, levator muscles, and perineum. A partial exenteration, either anterior or posterior, may be performed, depending on the origin of the carcinoma and the extent of local tissue invasion.

The success of modern deep pelvic surgery for malignant abdominoperineal lesions is attributable to increased knowledge regarding aseptic and surgical techniques, anesthesia, transfusions, intravenous antibiotic therapy, and the pathophysiology of involved organs. Current therapeutic techniques evolved after determination of the modes of metastasis, resective possibilities, and means of reestablishing modified physiologic function.

Pelvic exenteration is the preferred treatment for recurrent or persistent carcinoma of the cervix after radiation therapy; it is also applicable to carcinomas of the endometrium or rectum. Exenteration is considered only after a thorough investigation of the patient and disease status to determine if there is a reasonable chance of cure and of return to a productive life. The surgeon can determine with finality the chance of resectability with cure at the time of abdominal exploration.

The need for creation of urinary and bowel diversions must also be considered, together with the patient's ability to cope with these diversions postoperatively. Plastic surgery may be required for creation of a neovagina. Total pelvic exenteration has been advocated as the definitive procedure of choice in a critical clinical situation.

Psychologic preparation of the patient and family by the perioperative nurse and physician is a prime requisite. Perioperative nursing care should be directed toward supporting the patient during therapy and helping the patient maintain personal dignity.

Procedural considerations

The bowel is cleansed preoperatively with antibiotics and enemas. A nasogastric tube, indwelling urinary catheter, and rectal tube are inserted before or during surgery. Antiembolic stockings are placed on both legs. A warming device and radiant hat, leg, and arm covers are applied to maintain body temperature. Cardiac and central venous pressure monitoring is maintained throughout the procedure.

Utmost care must be taken in positioning the patient, because of the duration of surgery. Strict attention should be paid to the knees, hips, and lower back to prevent vascular and nerve damage. The patient is placed in the supine position with legs abducted in the ski position or elevated in a modified lithotomy position to allow access to the perineum without disruptive position changes; antiembolic devices are applied. Skin prepping includes the abdomen, thighs, perineum, and the internal vaginal vault.

The circulating nurse and scrub person must be alert to fluid and blood loss, irrigation solutions must be accurately measured, laparotomy packs must be weighed to assess blood volume loss, and the anesthesia provider and surgical team must be apprised of the measurements.

When the colon is transsected or ureteral drainage is diverted into an ileosegment, the gastrointestinal technique as described in Chapter 11 should be followed.

Separate instrument setups are required for the abdominal and perineal approaches. Extra drapes, gowns, and gloves should be available. For the abdominal approach, the basic abdominal gynecologic instrument set and instrumentation described previously for abdominoperineal resection (see Chapter 11) are required.

For the perineal approach, the basic vaginal instrument set is required. To prevent contamination, the anus may be closed with a purse-string suture.

Operative procedure

1. A long midline incision from the symphysis pubis to the umbilicus is made, and the abdomen is opened in the usual manner. A second incision within the perineum encircling the vestibule and anus is also made.
2. The peritoneal cavity is explored for metastasis to the liver, the nodes of the celiac axis, the superior mesenteric artery, and the paraaortic tissues.
3. The pelvis is explored, and the peritoneum along the brim of the pelvis examined for lymph node involvement. Frozen sections may be indicated. The obturator fossa and the region of the uterosacral ligaments are explored. When findings at exploration are negative, retractors are placed and the small bowel is packed off with moist laparotomy packs (Fig. 14-43).
4. The sigmoid mesocolon is freed and sectioned by means of intestinal clamps and a scalpel or a stapling device. The proximal end is exteriorized through an opening in the left side of the abdomen; an intestinal clamp is left across the lumen until later, when the permanent colostomy will be secured to the skin.
5. The remaining sigmoid mesentery is clamped with Rochester-Pean forceps, cut, and ligated down to and including the superior hemorrhoidal vessels. Long instruments and sutures are used to facilitate reaching the deep pelvic structures.
6. The distal sigmoid colon is closed with an inverting suture. The sigmoid colon and rectum are freed from the sacrococcygeal area by blunt and sharp dissection.
7. The lateral pelvic peritoneum is cut along the iliac vessels; the ovarian vessels and round ligaments on each side are clamped with Rochester-Pean forceps, cut, and doubly ligated.
8. The peritoneum is incised over the dome of the bladder with a long knife and Metzenbaum scissors, and the bladder is separated from the symphysis pubis down to the urethra.
9. The ureters are identified and divided 2 to 3 cm below the brim of the pelvis. The proximal end is left open to allow urinary drainage, whereas the distal end is ligated.
10. The hypogastric artery, the internal iliac vein, and the superior and inferior gluteal vessels are exposed, clamped with hemostats, doubly ligated, and cut. The external iliac vein is retracted to allow evacuation of

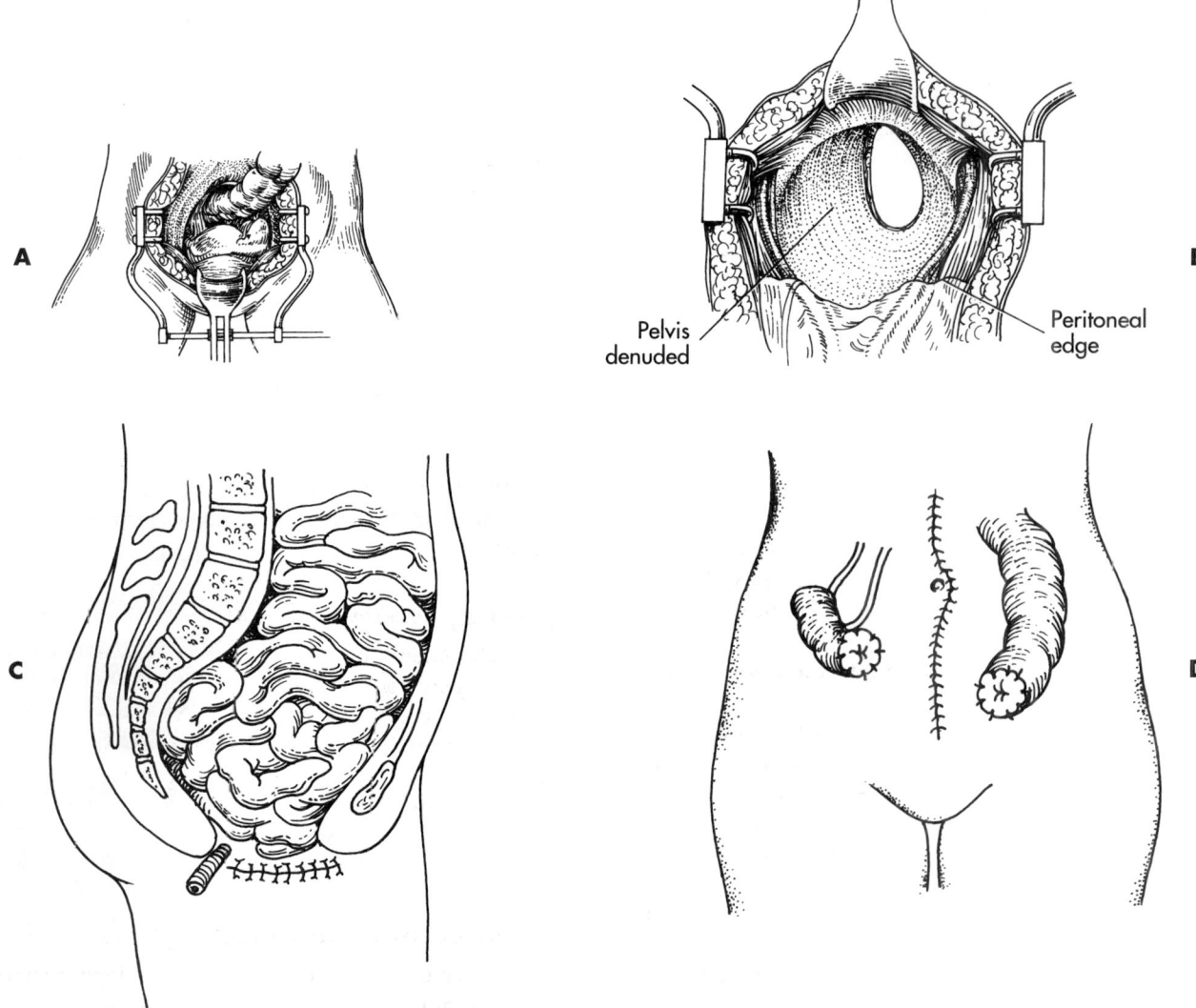

FIGURE 14-43   Pelvic exenteration. **A**, Pelvic viscera in situ as viewed from operating surgeon's vantage point after retractors are placed and small bowel is packed off. **B**, Empty pelvis after dissection of paravesical and paravaginal tissues and removal of specimen en bloc. **C**, Sagittal view of small bowel above pelvic defect. Perineal packing or drain may be used. **D**, After closure of abdominal wall, colostomy and ileostomy stomas are sutured to skin edges.

the contents of the obturator fossa, leaving the obturator nerve intact. Care must be taken in dissection not to damage the sacral plexus and sciatic nerve.

11. The internal pudendal vessels are isolated, ligated with transfixion sutures, and cut. The remaining soft-tissue attachments of the pelvis are clamped and cut. Steps 10 and 11 are then performed on the opposite side.

12. The perineum is incised by an elliptic incision that includes the clitoris and anus. The ischiorectal fat is incised up to the area of the levator muscle.

13. The coccygeal attachment of the rectum is severed. The levator muscles are severed at their lateral attachments by means of a long #4 knife handle with #20 blade; hemostasis is maintained by pressure and traction.

14. The paravesical and paravaginal tissues are resected from the periosteum of the symphysis pubis and superior pubic rami by means of a knife. The specimen is completely freed and removed from the pelvis (Fig. 14-43, *B*).

15. After residual bleeding vessels are identified and controlled by transfixing ligatures, the subcutaneous tissue is closed by interrupted sutures. A drain is placed in the wound, and the skin is closed.

16. In the abdomen, further residual bleeding vessels are controlled. Packs may be left in the pelvis to be removed through the perineum after 48 hours.

17. The ileosegment is then fashioned, and the ureters are anastomosed to it. The external stoma of the ileosegment is placed on the right side of the abdomen.

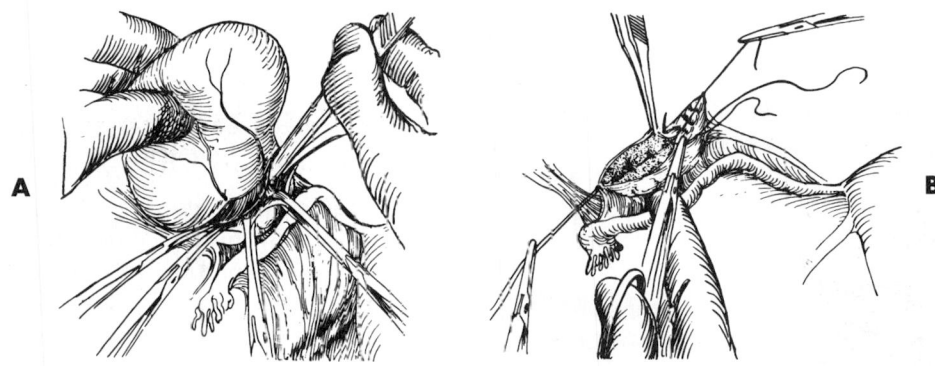

FIGURE 14-44   Resection of small cyst from ovary. **A**, Incision made around ovary near junction of cyst wall and normal ovarian tissue. Knife handle is convenient instrument for shelling out cyst. **B**, Wound in ovary closed.

18. A red, rubber, multieyed tube, size 16 Fr, is inserted into the proximal jejunum for the length of the jejunum and the ileum to aid in postoperative bowel decompression. It is connected to the bowel with a purse-string suture and brought out to the skin, where it is sutured in place.
19. A gastrostomy tube is placed into the stomach in the same manner.
20. Hemostasis is checked. The small intestines are carefully repositioned into the pelvis. Packs and retractors are removed (Fig. 14-43, *C*).
21. The peritoneum, rectus muscles, and fascial sheaths are closed with interrupted figure-of-eight sutures. The skin is closed with interrupted sutures.
22. The colostomy stoma is prepared by removing the intestinal clamp from the sigmoid colon, opening the colon, and suturing the stoma to the skin edges (Fig. 14-43, *D*).
23. The abdominal wound and tube sites are dressed in the usual manner. Drainage bags are applied to the colostomy and ileostomy stomas. A perineal dressing may be secured by means of a T binder.

SURGERY FOR CONDITIONS THAT AFFECT FERTILITY

Uterine Suspension

Uterine suspension is shortening of the ligaments of the uterus and positioning them retroperitoneally. The ligaments are then sutured bilaterally to the undersurface of the abdominal fascia in the corners of the transverse incision to ensure the maintenance of an anterior position of the uterus. This prevents the fallopian tubes and ovaries from entrapment in the cul-de-sac. Uterine suspension is done as part of a conservative surgical treatment of pelvic inflammatory disease or endometriosis. It is also indicated in patients who require lysis of extensive pelvic adhesions, for the correction of the symptoms of uterine retroversion, and for uterine prolapse in young women.

Procedural considerations

The basic abdominal gynecologic instrument set is required.

Operative procedure

1. The abdomen is opened as described for myomectomy.
2. The suspension is accomplished. If it is being done to correct uterine prolapse, a strip of Mersilene material is placed retroperitoneally to elevate the uterus at the level of the internal os posteriorly and to correct the prolapse into the vagina.
3. The wound is closed in layers, as described for laparotomy.

Oophorectomy and Oophorocystectomy

Oophorectomy is removal of an ovary. Oophorocystectomy is removal of an ovarian cyst (Fig. 14-44). Functional cysts constitute the majority of ovarian enlargements, with follicular cysts being the most common. Functional cysts develop in the corpus luteum; these cysts are usually larger than other functional cysts. The true ovarian epithelial tumors, serous cystadenomas and pseudomucinous cystadenomas, are prone to malignant change.

The choice of operation depends on the patient's age and symptoms, findings during physical examination, and direct examination of the adnexa during exploration. If the ovarian tumor is recognized as benign, only the visibly diseased portions of the adnexa are removed. In the presence of dermoid, follicular, and corpus luteum cysts, the cyst is usually enucleated, and most of the ovarian parenchyma is preserved. In tubal pregnancy the ectopic pregnancy may be removed from the tube, or the pregnant fallopian tube may be removed and, in some instances, the ovary.

Procedural considerations

The basic abdominal gynecologic instrument set is required, with the addition of a trocar and cannula, suction tubing, 10 ml syringe, and 21-gauge needle.

Operative procedure

1. The abdominal cavity is opened, as described for laparotomy.

2a. For *removal of a large ovarian cyst,* a purse-string suture may be placed into the cyst wall, and a trocar is introduced in its center; the suture is tightened around the trocar as the fluid is aspirated. The trocar is removed, and the purse-string suture is tied. All normal ovarian tissue is preserved.

2b. For *removal of a dermoid cyst,* the field is protected with laparotomy packs because the contents of such cysts produce irritation if they are spilled into the peritoneal cavity. An incision is made along the base of the cyst between the wall and normal ovarian tissue. The cystic wall is dissected away. The ovary is closed with interrupted or continuous sutures.

2c. For *decortication of the enlarged ovary and wedge resection,* a large segment of the ovarian cortex opposite the hilum is removed. The cysts are punctured with a needlepoint and collapsed. A wedge of ovarian stroma, extending deep into the hilum, is resected with a small knife; the cortex of the ovary is closed with interrupted or continuous sutures.

3. To prevent prolapse of the tube into the cul-de-sac, it may be sutured to the posterior sheath of the broad ligament.

4. The abdominal wound is closed as described for laparotomy.

Salpingo-Oophorectomy

Salpingo-oophorectomy is removal of a fallopian tube and all or part of the associated ovary. Unilateral salpingo-oophorectomy may be done to cure chronic salpingo-oophoritis, in patients with ectopic tubal gestation, or in those with certain disease conditions of the adnexa or large adnexal cysts. If both tubes and ovaries are diseased, they are removed with total hysterectomy.

Procedural considerations

The basic abdominal gynecologic instrument set is required.

Operative procedure

1. The abdominal cavity is opened, as described for laparotomy.

2. The affected tube is grasped with Allis or Babcock forceps. The infundibulopelvic ligament is clamped with hemostats, cut, and ligated.

3. The mesosalpinx is grasped with hemostats and divided with the suspensory ligament of the ovary.

4. The cornual attachment of the tube is excised with a knife or curved scissors. Bleeding vessels are clamped and ligated.

5. The edges of the broad ligament are peritonealized from the uterine horn to the infundibulopelvic ligament, as described for total hysterectomy.

6. The wound is closed, as described for laparotomy; dressings are applied.

Microscopic Reconstructive Surgery of the Fallopian Tube

The obstructed portion of a fallopian tube may be removed and the tube reconstructed to create patency of the remaining portion of the tube to promote the possibility of fertilization. Reconstructive surgery of the tube, categorically called *tuboplasty,* includes reanastomosis, salpingoneostomy, fimbrioplasty, and lysis of adhesions.

The development of microsurgical techniques has advanced surgical reconstruction of fallopian tubes. Microsurgical tubal anastomosis permits atraumatic, accurate alignment of fallopian tube segments. After surgery the fallopian tubes are shorter in length yet remain normal in other aspects. A common approach using microsurgical techniques with minilaparotomy or laparoscopy, or both, has been successful in restoring tubal patency in many women.[11] The laser may be adapted to the operating microscope, or the free-hand approach may be utilized, in tubal reconstructive surgery.

Procedural considerations

The patient is placed in the supine position. The vagina is prepped as described previously. An indwelling urinary catheter is inserted into the bladder. A Kahn, Calvin, Rubin, Hui, or Humi cannula or a pediatric Foley catheter may be placed into the uterine cavity for intraoperative chromotubation with diluted methylene blue or indigo carmine solution. Intraoperative chromotubation can also be achieved by applying a Buxton uterine clamp around the lower segment of the uterus and inserting an Angiocath catheter through the fundus into the cavity. A vaginal pack may be inserted to help elevate the uterus.

The basic abdominal gynecologic instrument set is required, with the addition of Iris scissors (1 curved and 1 straight), Adson forceps without teeth, Halsted mosquito hemostats, a set of Bowman lacrimal probes, Webster needle holders, Frazier suction tip, Kirschner retractor (if desired), and Buxton uterine clamp (if desired).

Basic microsurgical instruments include microscissors (1 curved and 1 straight), bayonet microscissors, Jeweler's forceps, microforceps, fallopian tube forceps, petit-point mosquito hemostats, microneedle holders (1 curved and 1 straight), ball-tipped nerve hook, and glass or Teflon rods.

Accessory items include microneedle electrodes, electrosurgical pencil, bipolar forceps with cord, irrigator, syringes and blunted needles for irrigation of the tissues, plastic or Silastic tubing and connectors, diluted methylene blue or indigo carmine solution, diluted heparinized lactated Ringer's solution, microscope drape, microscope or operative loupes, electrosurgical unit with monopolar and bipolar capabilities, and a video monitoring system (if desired).

Operative procedure

Operative procedures for correction of postsurgical tubal occlusion are usually performed under the operating microscope. Other reconstructive procedures vary according to the nature of the pathologic condition of the tube and may be done under the operating microscope or by use of operative loupes.

In microsurgery the surgeon must make sure that virtually no instruments are used in contact with the fallopian tube except those necessary to carry out the surgical technique. Microsurgery for infertility requires the use of specialized and delicate instruments. Each of these instruments is designed to permit gentle, atraumatic handling of tissues and prevent abrasions, lacerations, and vascular damage.

The tissues must be continually irrigated to prevent drying of the serosal surfaces. Lactated Ringer's solution alone or with heparin added may be used as the irrigating solution. Meticulous hemostasis is required in microsurgery. Irrigation is used to identify the bleeders. Hemostasis can be achieved by electrocoagulation with a microneedle electrode or very fine bipolar forceps. When a CO_2 laser beam is used, the smoke from laser vaporization should be evacuated through suction to prevent carbon deposits on the tissue.

Tubal Ligation

Tubal ligation is interruption of fallopian tube continuity, resulting in sterilization of the patient. In general, the indication for sterilization depends entirely on the desire of the patient. Certain medical indications and concern for the psychosocial needs of the patient are factors, and occasionally an obstetric indication exists, such as inherited fetal deformity. However, at least in the United States, sterilization is entirely a voluntary procedure. Depending on state law, a sterilization permit may or may not have to be signed by the husband. Good presurgical counseling is needed for the patient and her husband or significant other because this procedure is not predictably reversible. Approximately 1% of sterilized women seek reversals as a result of sterilization performed at an early age, death of a child, or remarriage. Patients may elect to have the procedure performed on an ambulatory surgery basis at a time that is convenient for them.

The optimal time for sterilization is approximately 24 hours after vaginal delivery. This method may not delay the normal discharge time for the patient. An objection to this practice is that the danger of hemorrhage still exists soon after delivery. With a normal delivery, tubal ligation is done on the first or second postpartum day. If a cesarean section is done, the tubes may be ligated at that time.

Operative procedures

Many surgical methods and techniques are available for tubal ligation. The objective of each method is to achieve complete closure of the fallopian tube so that conception is prevented. When a segment of each fallopian tube is excised, it is preserved for pathologic examination. General surgical considerations are directed to excising a section of each fallopian tube, ligating the severed ends, achieving hemostasis, and incorporating the proximal stump within layers of the mesosalpinx.

Laparoscopic Tubal Occlusion

1. Operative procedure is the same as that for laparoscopy.
2. An accessory suprapubic incision may be made for the occluding instrument.
3. Sterilization may take place by electrocoagulation or thermal coagulation, or by the placement of a spring clip or Silastic band after the tube has been identified and isolated in the grasping forceps.
   a. *Bipolar coagulation* occurs when electrical current passes only through the tube from prong to prong (Fig. 14-45). At least 3 cm of the tube is destroyed, which therefore prevents spontaneous recanalization. It has been recommended that the tube be grasped at least 2 to 3 cm away from the uterocornual junction at the time of this procedure so that a stump of isthmus remains to absorb the intrauterine fluid under pressure and minimize fistula formation, which could result in an ectopic pregnancy for the patient in the future. A spring clip offers a mechanical alternative to electrocoagulation.
   b. The *spring clip* occludes the isthmus of the tube by two plastic jaws (Fig. 14-46, *A* and *B*). The tube is compressed by a stainless steel spring that presses the jaws together. Spring clip application requires careful surgical technique to assure that the clip is completely across the isthmus of the tube (Fig. 14-46, *C*). Some surgeons may prefer to apply two spring clips positioned close together on each tube when utilizing this approach.
   c. The *Silastic band* offers another mechanical alternative to electrocoagulation. The tube is drawn 1.5 cm into a 0.5 cm diameter metal cylinder, which destroys approximately 3 cm of the tube (Fig. 14-47, *A*). A Silastic ring stretched on the outside of the cylinder is released to form an occlusion (Fig. 14-47, *B*). In time about 3 cm of the constricted tube undergoes necrosis and the tubes separate (Fig. 14-47, *C*).

Vaginal Approach (Posterior Colpotomy)

1. Operative procedure is the same as that for posterior colpotomy.
2. Sterilization can take place by the placement of a spring clip or Silastic band, by fimbriectomy, or by ligation of the proximal portion of the fallopian tubes with a permanent suture.

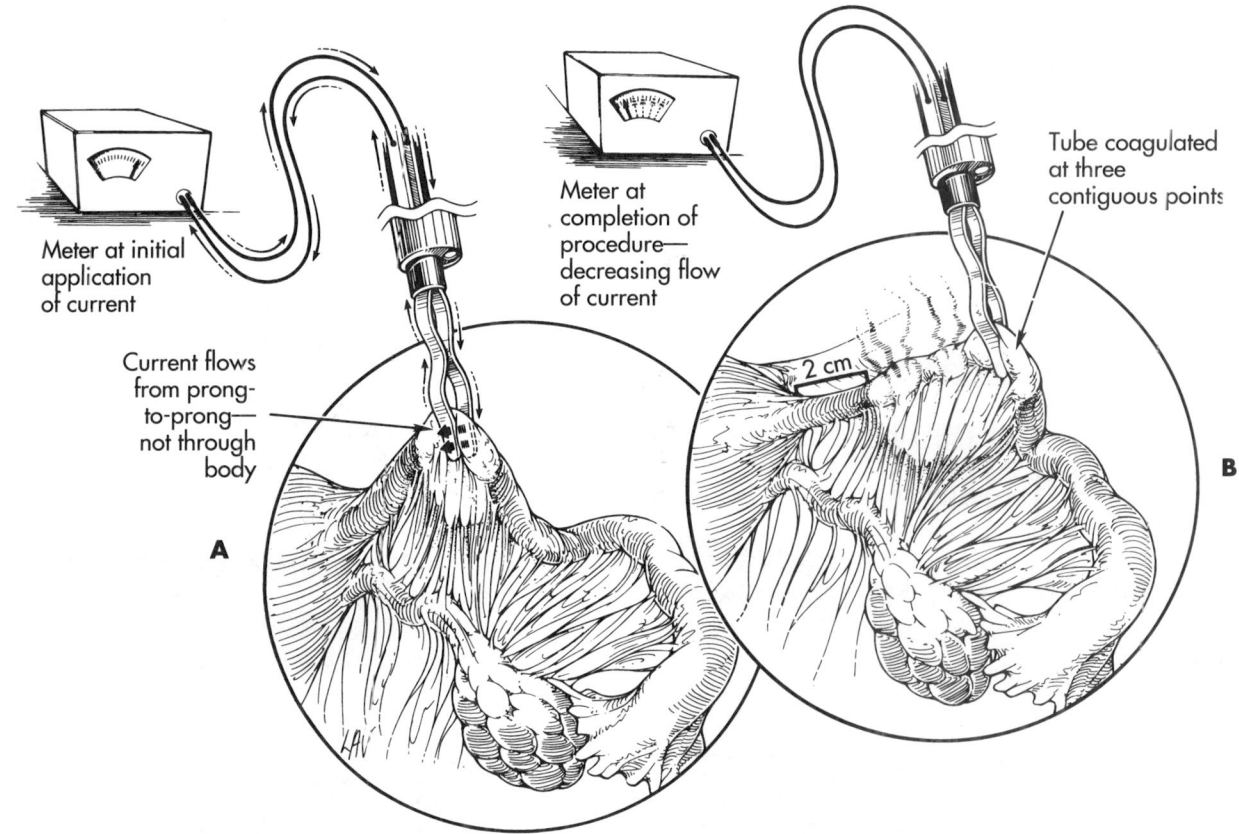

FIGURE 14-45 Bipolar coagulation. **A**, Current passes only through the tube from prong to prong of the forceps. **B**, Three contiguous burns are needed to prevent spontaneous recanalization. The end point for coagulation is tissue desiccation, at which point current ceases to flow through the dry, nonconducting tube. A meter on the generator to monitor current flow is therefore necessary.

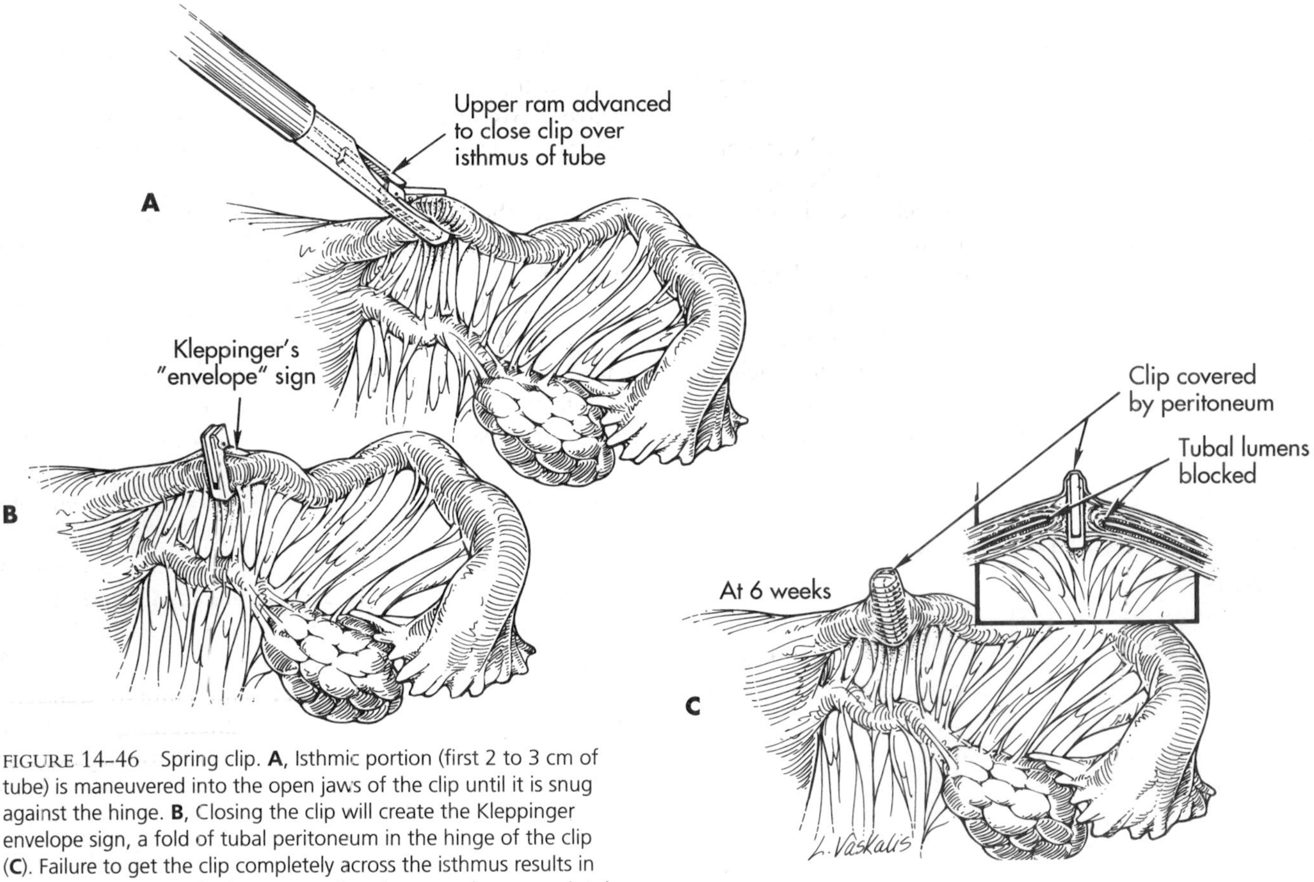

FIGURE 14-46 Spring clip. **A**, Isthmic portion (first 2 to 3 cm of tube) is maneuvered into the open jaws of the clip until it is snug against the hinge. **B**, Closing the clip will create the Kleppinger envelope sign, a fold of tubal peritoneum in the hinge of the clip (**C**). Failure to get the clip completely across the isthmus results in pregnancy. Some routinely use two clips close together on each tube.

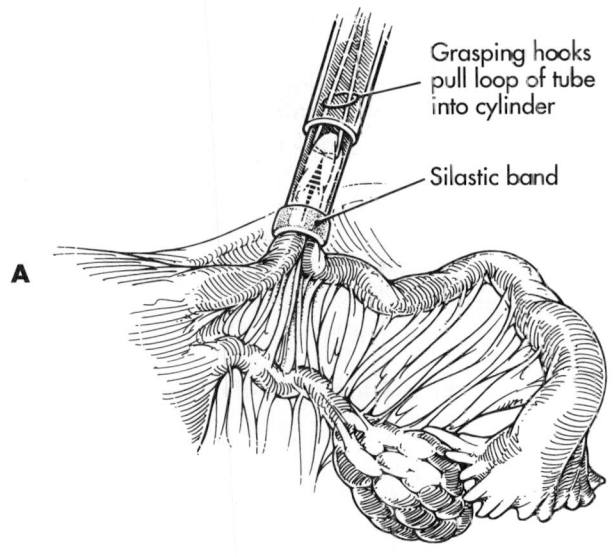

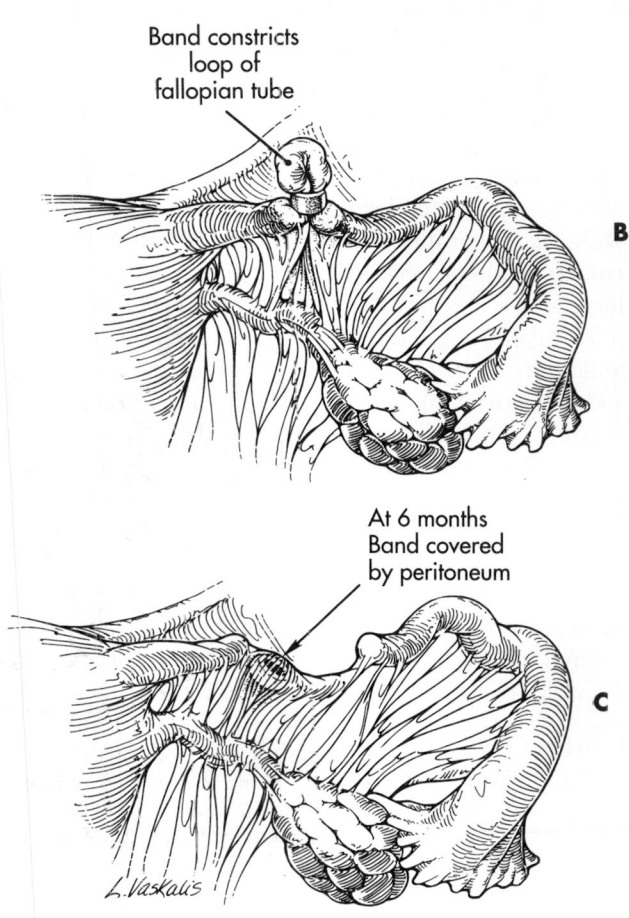

Grasping hooks
pull loop of tube
into cylinder

Silastic band

Band constricts
loop of
fallopian tube

At 6 months
Band covered
by peritoneum

L. Vaskalis

FIGURE 14-47   Silastic band. **A**, About 3 cm of tube are drawn into a 5 mm cylinder over which a Silastic band has been stretched. **B**, Releasing the band constricts the knuckle of tube with eventual necrosis. **C**, As with the Pomeroy, 6 months later the stumps are about 3 cm apart.

Minilaparotomy Approach

1. A 2 cm transverse incision is made above the pubic hairline.
2. A large bivalved speculum may be placed through the incision and into the peritoneal cavity. The large Graves bivalve speculum serves as a small abdominal retractor and permits easy access to the tubes.
3. Spring clips or Silastic bands can be applied, or the original Pomeroy method of ligation can be carried out. The Pomeroy technique provides a tissue specimen of each tube. Suture material is tied around each tube, and a section of tube is removed. Over time the tubes pull apart, destroying the passage between the ovary and the uterus.

In Vitro Fertilization and Embryo Transfer

Infertility may be described as the inability of a couple to conceive a biologic child after a year or more of repeated attempts. This is an emotionally stressful process for both partners. There are various coping strategies utilized by individuals with infertility, and the perioperative nurse needs to be aware of these in providing effective care (Research Highlight 14-4).

Both partners undergo extensive testing to identify possible organic or functional causes for their infertility. For example, there may be a structural defect in either partner, past or present infections, genetic or immunologic abnormalities, or endocrine imbalance or deficit.

Today there are options couples may select to assist them in the reproduction process. Fertilization may be achieved by retrieval of oocytes from the ovary, followed by IVF with sperm and implantation of the fertilized oocytes (embryos) into the uterine cavity.

IVF and embryo transfer are indicated for women who have had bilateral absence or irreparable obstruction of the fallopian tubes, for women who have undergone tubal reconstructive surgery and have not conceived within 1 year after surgery, for women who have cervical or immunologic factors and have not conceived after treatment or for whom no treatment is available, for women who have failed to conceive after conservative surgery and hormone-suppressive therapy for endometriosis, for couples who have unexplained infertility, and for oligospermia as a cause of infertility.

To be a candidate for IVF and embryo transfer, a woman must have at least one functioning ovary. The ovaries must be physically accessible for laparoscopic follicular aspiration unless aspiration is done under ultrasound-guided transabdominal or transvaginal puncture. The uterus must be normal and have functioning

---

14-4 RESEARCH HIGHLIGHT

A study was conducted to examine the coping patterns of women who were infertile. The sample consisted of 30 infertile women who were clients of a physician specializing in infertility. Each participant had a private interview in which she was asked what she had done to cope with feelings and experiences associated with her infertility. The researchers identified six common coping strategies used by the women: (1) increasing space between themselves and reminders of infertility, (2) regaining control, (3) being the best, (4) looking for hidden meaning, (5) giving in to feelings, and (6) sharing the burden. These findings may be utilized in providing nursing care in a sensitive yet informed manner. Nurses can promote an atmosphere in which the woman can give in to her feelings and share her burden. The nurse can assure the woman that her feelings are normal and might direct the couple to an organized support group for couples experiencing common concerns. Further research to examine the coping strategies of males and couples experiencing infertility will aid the nurse in caring for these persons.

From Davis, D.C., & Dearman, C.N. (1991). Coping strategies of infertile women. *Journal of Obstetric, Gynecologic, and Neonatal Nursing, 20*(3), 221.

---

endometrium. The partner's semen must have sufficient motile sperm for insemination.

The treatment cycle for IVF and embryo transfer can be divided into five stages: follicular development, aspiration of the mature preovulatory follicles, sperm preparation, IVF, and embryo transfer. Laparoscopic aspiration of the follicles is the only stage that may occur in the operating room. Embryo transfer may or may not take place in the operating room. The treatment cycle is extremely stressful, and both partners need emotional support from all members of the IVF team.

Follicular development

Although a spontaneous ovulatory cycle was used for recovery of the oocyte in the early development of IVF, all programs at present use a stimulated cycle to obtain multiple oocytes. With a stimulated cycle, induction of ovulation is achieved by one of three regimens. The first is clomiphene citrate (Clomid) and human chorionic gonadotropin (HCG). The patient receives 50 to 150 mg/day of Clomid for 5 days starting at a specified point in her menstrual cycle. On the day after the last dose of Clomid, the patient begins daily ultrasonic scanning and determination of serum level of estrogen to monitor follicular growth. The timing for HCG administration is based on the size and rate of growth of the follicles and the level of serum estradiol. To ensure follicular maturation, 4000 to 10,000 units of HCG are then administered to the patient.

The second regimen is human menopausal gonadotropin (HMG) and HCG. The patient receives 1 to 3 ampules of HMG daily starting on day 3 or day 5 of her menstrual cycle, depending on the protocol. Monitoring methods and timing of the HCG are similar to the Clomid regimen.

The third regimen is a combination of Clomid, HMG, and HCG. The patient receives Clomid for 5 days, followed by daily administration of HMG. In all three regimens, oocyte retrieval is performed 34 to 36 hours after the administration of HCG.

Aspiration of the mature preovulatory follicles

Follicular aspiration may be performed through an ultrasound-guided transabdominal or transvaginal puncture or by laparoscopic technique. When the laparoscopic follicular aspiration technique is used, a regular laparoscopic instrument setup is utilized. In addition, grasping forceps, an aspirating needle with needle sleeve, a trap to collect the follicular fluid and ovum, a suctioning device, and a warming unit for the traps may be needed. A closed-circuit television monitoring system may be used, and the procedure videotaped or portions photographed.

In preparation for the procedure the operating room temperature may be increased. Perioperative considerations when opening sterile supplies and setting up the sterile field include the elimination of talc powder and antimicrobial solutions from the instrument setup. These substances may be toxic if they are permitted to contact the follicular fluid or ovum.

The laparoscopy is performed with the patient in the supine or modified lithotomy position. Routinely, instruments are not placed in the cervix or vagina. The pneumoperitoneum may be achieved with 100% carbon dioxide or a gas mixture of 90% nitrogen, 5% oxygen, and 5% carbon dioxide.

1. Follicular aspiration may be performed using a double-puncture or a triple-puncture technique.
2. The ovary is stabilized against the pelvic side wall by grasping the uteroovarian ligament with grasping forceps.
3. The aspirating needle is placed into contact with the surface of the follicle.
4. Suction is applied as the follicle is punctured. The needle tip is moved within the follicle in an attempt to dislodge the cumulus mass from the follicle wall.
5. After the follicle has collapsed, suction is disconnected before the needle is removed from the follicle; this disconnection prevents aspiration of carbon dioxide.
6. After the needle is outside the peritoneal cavity, suction is reapplied to empty the fluid contained within the tubing into the ovum trap.
7. The ovum trap is changed, and the culture medium is aspirated into another ovum trap to rinse the needle and ensure that the oocyte is not retained within the tubing.

8. The follicular aspirate is transferred immediately to the embryo laboratory where it is inspected microscopically for the presence of an oocyte. If an oocyte is not identified, the aspirating needle is reintroduced into the follicle. The follicle is redistended with culture medium and is reaspirated.

9. The laparoscopic procedure is completed after all available follicles are aspirated.

Sperm preparation

A semen sample is obtained from the partner. After liquefaction, the semen is washed of seminal plasma by centrifugation twice in culture medium and incubated at 37° C until the time of insemination.

In vitro fertilization

The oocytes and surrounding cumulus are transferred to culture medium to complete maturation. The oocytes are incubated for different periods of time, depending on the degree of maturation of the oocytes before insemination. Oocytes may be inseminated with 50,000 to 200,000 motile sperm to each oocyte.

Evaluation of fertilization in the tissue culture dish requires visualization of the oocyte approximately 18 hours after insemination. The presence of two pronuclei is taken as presumptive evidence of fertilization, and the oocyte is transferred to a growth medium. The embryo should be at the four-cell stage by 32 to 40 hours after insemination.

Embryo transfer

No anesthesia is required. The patient may be placed in the knee-chest or lithotomy position. A Graves vaginal speculum is inserted into the vagina. A single-tooth tenaculum may be used to grasp the cervix.

As soon as the patient is ready, the embryos are loaded into the transfer catheter with a minute amount of transfer medium and two small air bubbles. The catheter is carefully introduced into the uterine cavity, and the embryos are expelled. The catheter is withdrawn and returned to the laboratory, where it is examined for retained embryos. If the embryos have not been retained in the catheter, the speculum is removed.

After embryo transfer, the patient is placed in the supine or modified jackknife position, depending on the position of the uterus, for 4 to 24 hours.

Gamete intrafallopian transfer

Another approach to IVF is the gamete intrafallopian transfer (GIFT). It has been proved successful for partners with long-standing infertility. The female requires at least one patent fallopian tube. This procedure involves placement of a prepared semen specimen with retrieved oocytes into the fallopian tubes by laparoscopic approach. Fertilization occurs inside the patient.

The GIFT procedure consists of two stages: the oocyte retrieval and the gamete transfer. General anesthesia is initiated after the oocyte retrieval to minimize oocyte exposure to anesthesia. The abdomen and vagina are prepped and draped. Often the prep solution is rinsed off with lactated Ringer's solution. A laparoscope is used to view the fallopian tubes, and a 6 mm trocar is placed to manipulate the fallopian tubes. The catheter system is then used to insert the egg-and-sperm mixture into the fallopian tubes. The patient is awakened and transferred to the PACU where she will have her vital signs monitored until stable. The patient will remain supine and still for a few hours after this procedure.

Zygote intrafallopian transfer

Zygote intrafallopian transfer (ZIFT) procedure involves placement of fertilized eggs into the right and left fallopian tubes of the patient. The patient is placed in the lithotomy position before general anesthesia. The abdomen is prepped and draped followed by rapid induction of general anesthesia to minimize oocyte exposure to anesthesia. A laparoscope is used to visualize the fallopian tubes, a 5 mm trocar is used to manipulate the fallopian tubes. When the transfer is complete, the IVF technician examines the syringes to verify successful transfer. The patient is awakened and transferred to the PACU. Complications from GIFT and ZIFT include ectopic pregnancy and spontaneous abortion.[20]

Abdominal Surgery During Pregnancy

The incidence of the immediate need for abdominal surgery occurs as frequently among pregnant women as among nonpregnant women of childbearing ages. Diagnosis of the abdominal problems in the pregnant woman is challenging because of the enlarged uterus and displaced organs. Mild leukocytosis and increased levels of alkaline phosphatase and amylase are normal during pregnancy and may also be indicative of surgical intraperitoneal processes. Abnormally high or rising laboratory values should be noted. X-ray evaluation is contraindicated in most instances during pregnancy.[15]

The surgical team is faced with the challenge of caring for a patient with both a surgical problem and obstetric concerns. Laparotomy or laparoscopy may be required for conditions such as appendicitis and intestinal obstruction. Acute suppurative appendicitis complicates about 1 in 1500 pregnancies.[16] The second most common nonobstetric abdominal emergency in the pregnant woman is intestinal obstruction.[9]

Hazards of performing abdominal surgery on the pregnant patient include abortion and premature labor. In addition to monitoring of the pregnant patient, the fetal vital signs, activity and uterine contractility should be monitored throughout the perioperative period.[8] The patient will be placed under regional or general anesthesia. The pregnant woman is considered to have a full stomach, and a rapid induction is therefore indicated with general anesthesia. The surgical team should be prepared for an obstetric emergency. Support for the pregnant woman and her family is essential throughout the perioperative period because they may have concerns regarding the fetal well-being as a result of the surgery and anesthesia.

Fetal Surgery

Developments in prenatal diagnosis have progressed to the point where clinicians may consider the fetus to be the patient. Serious congenital anomaly is diagnosable by ultrasonography, alpha-fetoprotein specimen, amniocentesis, chorionic vili sampling, or percutaneous umbilical blood sampling. When an anomaly is identified, the mother's complete medical history and prenatal ultrasonograms are reviewed by a multidisciplinary team.

Depending on the anomaly and the immediate danger posed to the fetus, the family will be counseled on their options. If no treatment is available and the condition is fatal, the family may elect to terminate the pregnancy if it is earlier than 24 weeks of gestation or may choose to carry the fetus to term. If postnatal correction is possible, the family may consider terminating the pregnancy or may continue the pregnancy with monitoring for management after delivery. A lethal anomaly may be treated with prenatal surgery. If a family elects this option, both the mother and fetus will be evaluated to determine if they will be acceptable surgical candidates. Currently, prenatal surgery is used to treat anomalies that would result in fetal death before term or during the immediate postnatal period, such as urinary obstruction, congenital cystic adenomatoid malformation of the lung, and sacrococcygeal teratoma of the lower spine.[3]

Postoperatively the mother is monitored in the fetal intensive care unit. Preterm labor is of great concern, and uterine contractions, fetal heart rate, and fetal ECG are closely assessed. Tocolytic medications are titrated to control uterine contractions. The mother is educated in self-monitoring of uterine contractions, and tocolytic therapy is continued on an outpatient basis. Frequent fetal ultrasonic scans are performed postoperatively to monitor fetal growth, amniotic fluid volume, and the adequacy of the surgical repair.

As fetal surgery continues to evolve, investigators are focusing on minimally invasive procedures to correct cleft lip before birth and twin-twin transfusions. In utero stem cell therapy and gene therapy are also being investigated.

Cesarean Birth

Cesarean birth, also referred to as *cesarean section*, or *C-section*, is delivery of the fetus or fetuses through abdominal (laparotomy) and uterine (hysterotomy) incisions. In general, cesarean birth is employed whenever further delay in delivery may seriously compromise the fetus, the mother, or both, and vaginal delivery cannot be safely accomplished. In recent years the use of cesarean birth has increased as a result of fetal monitoring, fetal scalp blood sampling for pH determination, and the widespread emphasis on recognition of actual or suspected impairment of fetal well-being if delivery were delayed or vaginal delivery attempted. Reasons for cesarean birth include malposition and malpresentation, cephalopelvic disproportion, abruptio placentae, toxemia, fetal distress, uterine dysfunction, placenta previa, prolapsed cord, previous pelvic surgery, cervical dystocia, active herpes progenitalis, and diabetes. Multiple pregnancy may also be an indication for cesarean delivery.

Cesarean delivery is one of the most frequently performed major surgical operations in the United States. Approximately 25% of all births are cesarean deliveries. From the mid-1960s to the late 1980s, the cesarean delivery rate has increased from less than 5% to approximately 25%. Reasons include increased use of electronic fetal monitoring, an increase in the number of first-time pregnancies, pregnancy at an older age, and a high incidence of repeat cesarean deliveries.[2] There are institutional differences in primary cesarean delivery rates, and these, along with national trends towards shorter lengths of stay (LOS) for maternal and newborn care, have prompted interest in mechanisms to streamline and improve coordination of care without sacrificing the quality of that care.[18] Critical paths and variance tracking are two strategies used to plan and manage a patient's care. The critical path presents a "blueprint" of care designed to decrease variation in practice patterns,[5] combining patient outcomes in specified time frames with the patient interventions required to reach them.

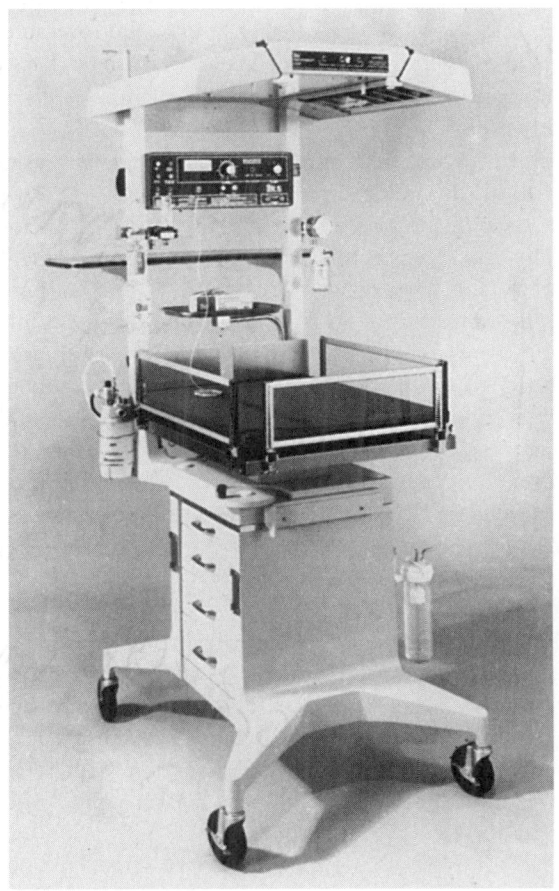

FIGURE 14-48   Radiant warmer for neonate.

Cesarean delivery may take place in the obstetric labor delivery suite or in the OR suite. Patients about to undergo cesarean birth need careful assessment and emotional support. Because cesarean birth frequently involves emergency situations, the patient may express grave concern for the infant's well-being. If the patient has participated in childbirth classes, she may believe that she has failed in some way. The nurse must be aware of the psychologic as well as physiologic needs of this patient population. Mothers may choose to remain awake under regional anesthesia; her significant other may be permitted to accompany and support her in the OR and witness the birth (based upon hospital policy). The significant other may need the perioperative nurse's assistance in preparing for the delivery by washing hands and donning scrub attire or a protective gown. The perioperative nurse may need to reassure and encourage the significant other to coach and lend support to the mother during this intensely stressful time. The significant other can be included in the bonding process that is initiated at birth. The mother, if awake and stable, is shown and encouraged to hold the infant. The perioperative nurse promotes a positive family-oriented experience.

If the cesarean delivery is performed as an emergency, the family-oriented approach may not be feasible. In this emergency situation the mother's support people need to be directed to the surgical waiting area. The nurse and physician need to communicate the condition of the mother and infant. Support people may then be able to accompany the infant as he or she is transferred to the nursery.

Procedural considerations

The patient should be in a supine position with elevation of the right side to displace the uterus and prevent aortocaval compression.[21] Bony prominences are padded, and the patient is positioned in good body alignment with a safety strap above the knees. It may be necessary to assist the anesthesia team with the administration of regional anesthesia before placing the patient in the supine position. Throughout this process the maternal vital signs are monitored and recorded according to the institutional protocol. Fetal heart tones are also monitored and recorded per institutional protocol. The perioperative nurse is caring for two patients.

If a general anesthetic is to be employed, all preparations, including skin prep, bladder drainage, draping, suction connection, counts, and gowning and gloving of all scrubbed personnel, must be done before induction. In many hospitals, healthcare providers qualified to deliver newborn care and resuscitation are in attendance for the delivery. A radiant warmer (Fig. 14-48) and resuscitative equipment for immediate postdelivery care of the infant are available in the operating room because these infants are considered to be at risk until there is evidence of physiologic stability.

In preparation for delivery, if indicated, the mother's hair is clipped or shaved from the abdomen above the umbilicus to the level of the mons pubis and laterally to above the level of the iliac crests. The skin is prepped for abdominal surgery. The vagina is not prepared. An indwelling urinary catheter is inserted. Instrumentation includes the basic abdominal gynecologic set (Fig. 14-49),

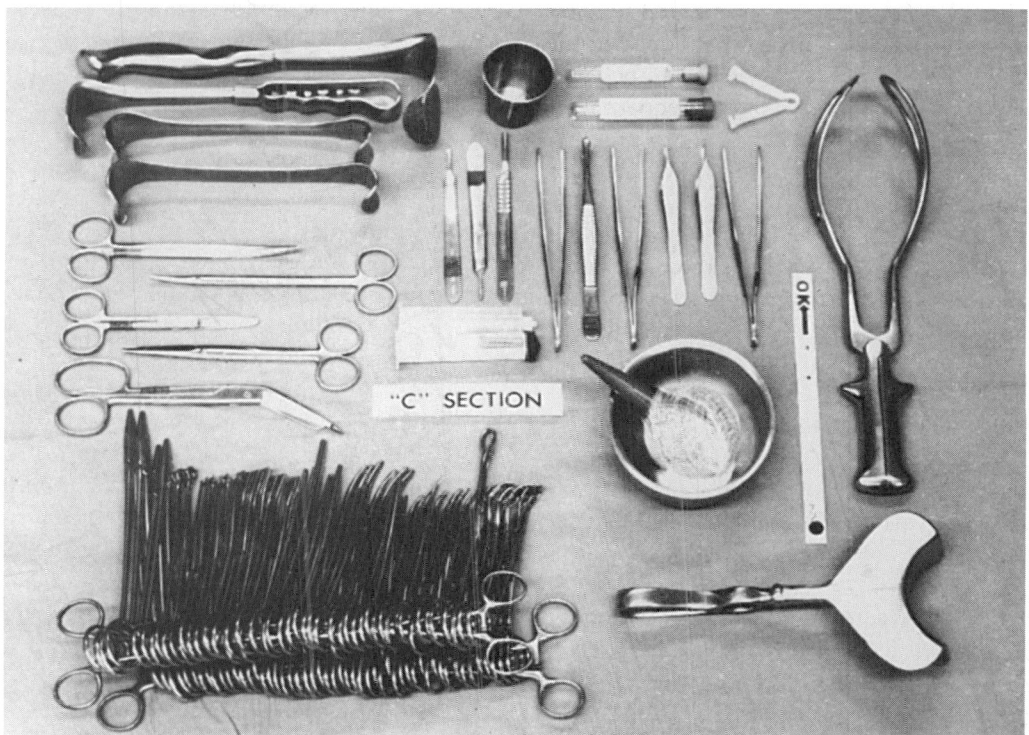

FIGURE 14-49   Instrument setup for cesarean birth.

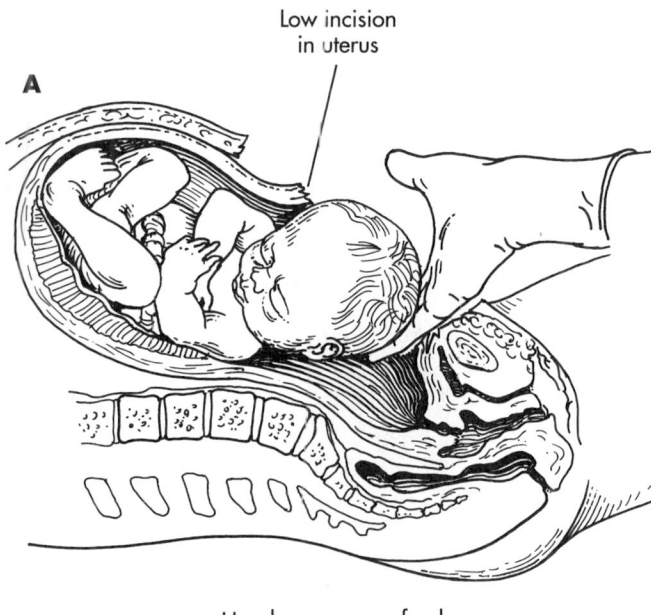

Low incision
in uterus

A

Hand pressure on fundus

B

FIGURE 14-50   Manual delivery of fetal head at low uterine segment cesarean section. **A**, Lateral view. **B**, Anterior view.

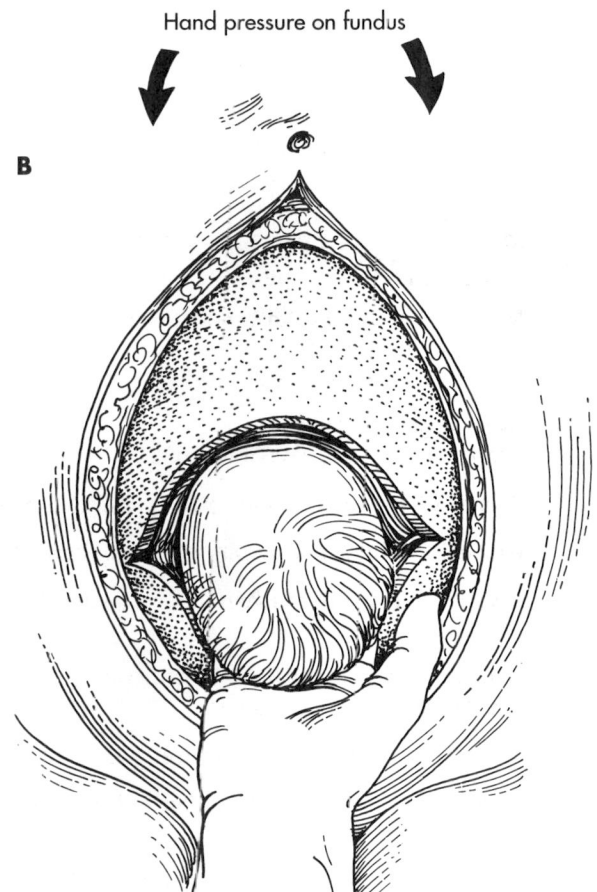

with the addition of Lister bandage scissors, Foerster sponge-holding (ring) forceps, Pennington forceps, cord clamps, DeLee retractor, delivery forceps, a head extractor (if desired), laboratory tubes for cord blood, a drain (optional), and a bulb syringe.

Operative procedure

1. An infraumbilical vertical incision or lower transverse Pfannenstiel incision is made. The incision should be long enough to allow the infant to be delivered without difficulty but no longer. Therefore the length of the incision varies with the estimated size of the fetus.

2. The abdominal wall is opened in layers. The rectus and pyramidalis muscles are separated in the midline by sharp and blunt dissection to expose the underlying transversalis fascia and peritoneum.

3. The peritoneum is elevated with two Crile hemostats about 2 cm apart. The peritoneum between the two clamps is palpated to rule out the inclusion of bowel, omentum, or bladder. The peritoneum is opened and the abdominal cavity entered.

4. Bleeding sites anywhere in the abdominal incision may be clamped but not ligated until later, unless the clamps obstruct exposure. When the patient is under general anesthesia, speed is important to prevent an anesthetized infant. Electrosurgery may be used at this point to stop bleeding, especially if the patient is awake and under regional anesthesia.

5. The uterus is quickly but carefully palpated to determine the size and presenting part of the fetus as well as the direction and degree of rotation of the uterus.

6. The reflection of the peritoneum (serosa) above the upper margin of the bladder and overlying the anterior lower uterine segment is gently separated by sharp and blunt dissection.

7. The developed bladder flap is held downward beneath the symphysis with a bladder retractor such as the DeLee.

8. The uterus is opened with a knife through the lower uterine segment about 2 cm above the detached bladder. Once the uterus is opened, the incision can be extended by cutting laterally with a large bandage scissors or by simply spreading the incision by means of lateral pressure applied with each index finger when the lower uterine segment is thin.

9. The presenting membranes are incised. Suction is imperative here, and many surgeons prefer no suction tip (only the large open end of the suction tubing) during the expulsion and suctioning of amniotic fluid.

10. All retractors are removed. The fetal head is gently elevated, either manually or by use of obstetric forceps, through the incision, aided by transabdominal fundal pressure (Fig. 14-50). The pressure helps expel the fetus.

11. As soon as the head is delivered, a bulb syringe or aspirator tip is used to aspirate the exposed nares and mouth to minimize aspiration of amniotic fluid and its contents (Fig. 14-51).

12. About 20 units of oxytocin per liter of fluid may be

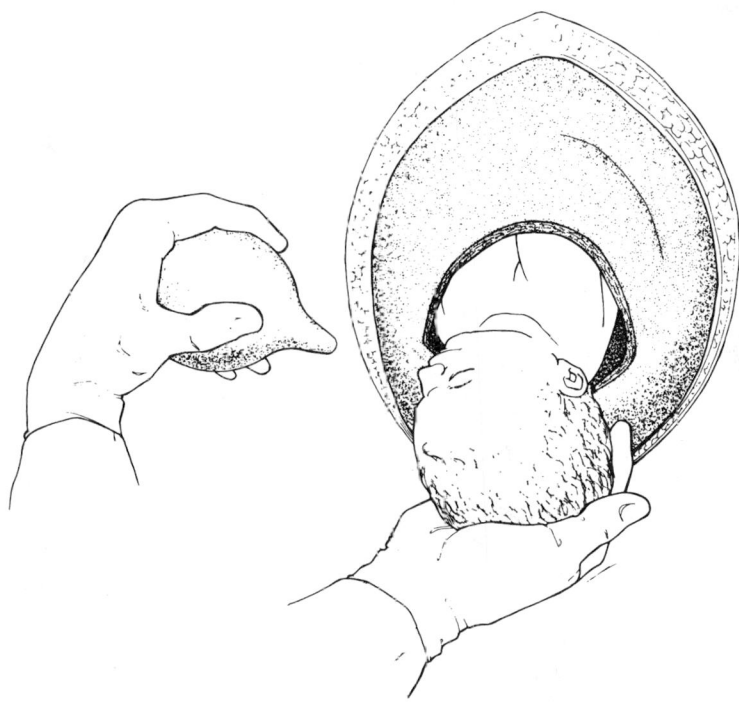

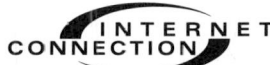

FIGURE 14-51　Cesarean birth. Delivery of head. Bulb syringe used to clear nares and mouth of amniotic fluid.

administered intravenously as soon as the shoulders are delivered (or after delivery of the infant), so that the uterus contracts. This use of oxytocin minimizes blood loss.

13. On delivery of the entire infant, the cord is clamped and cut, and the infant given to the member of the team who is responsible for resuscitation efforts as needed. A sterile gown or sheet should be provided to the individual receiving the infant to avoid any break in aseptic technique and to maintain universal precautions during transfer of the infant.

14. The edges of the uterine incision are promptly clamped with Pean forceps, ring forceps, or Pennington clamps.

15. The placenta is delivered and placed in a large receptacle provided from the back table. Fundal massage or manual removal may be employed to hasten delivery of the placenta and reduce bleeding.

16. One or two separate layers of suture may be used to close the uterine incision.

17. After determination that there is no further bleeding after closure of the uterine incision, the cut edges of the serosa overlying the uterus and bladder are approximated with a continuous suture.

18. Any blood, blood clots, vernix, and amniotic fluid in the pelvis and peritoneal cavity are removed. The fallopian tubes and ovaries are also inspected. Tubal ligation may be carried out at this point.

19. The peritoneum and each abdominal layer are closed.

INTERNET CONNECTION

National Women's Health Information Center:
http://www.4woman.org/
http://www.obgyn.net

Gynecologic Oncology:
http://gynoncology.obgyn.washington.edu/

Women's Health Hotline Homepage: www.libov.com

Women's Health Resources: http://timon.sir.arizona.edu/

Association of Reproductive Health Professionals:
http://www.arhp.org

National Association of Nurse Practitioners in Reproductive Health: email nanprh@aol.com

American College of Nurse-Midwives: http://www.acnm.org

Association of Women's Health, Obstetric and Neonatal Nurses: http://www.awhonn.org

Laparoscopy: http://www.laparoscopy.com/index.html

Obstetrics & Gynecology News Group: news:sci.med.obgyn

REFERENCES

1. Bennett, K.L., Ohrmundt, C., & Maloni, J.A. (1996). Preventing intravasation in women undergoing hysteroscopic procedures. *AORN Journal, 64*, 792-799.

2. Bobak, I.M., & Jensen, M.D. (1993). *Maternity and gynecologic care: the nurse and the family* (ed. 5). St. Louis: Mosby.

3. Brazzino, J. (1997). New developments in neonatology. *Nursing Spectrum, 6*(12), 4-6.

4. Cannon, C.M. (1998, March). The business of women's health. *Working Woman,* 39-42.

5. Comried, L.A. (1996). Cost analysis: initiation of HBMC and first CareMap,™ *Nursing Economics, 14*(1), 34-39.

6. FDA clears uterine balloon to treat excessive bleeding (1998). *OR Manager, 14*(2),10.

7. Frank, S.M. (1998). *Body temperature and clinical outcome in the perioperative period.* Paper presentation, Consensus Conference on Perioperative Thermoregulation, Bethesda, MD, February 7, 1998.

8. Gabrielse, L., & Boosamra, S. (1997). Obstetrical patient postanesthesia management. *Journal of Perianesthesia Nursing, 12*(4), 245-251.

9. Gleicher, N. (1992). *Principles and practice of medical therapy in pregnancy.* Norwalk, CT: Appleton & Lange.

10. Graff, B.M. (1997). Caring for women experiencing hysterectomy. *Nursing Spectrum, 6*(15), 12-14.

11. Haspel-Siegel, A. (1997). Fallopian tube anastomosis procedures to restore fertility. *AORN Journal, 65*(1), 75-86.

12. Lanfranchi, J.A. (1997). Smoke plume evacuation in the OR. *AORN Journal, 65,* 627-633.

13. Leach, R.E., & Ory, S.J. (1989). Modern management of ectopic pregnancy. *Journal of Reproductive Medicine, 34,* 324-335.

14. Levine, R.L. (1990). Pelviscopic surgery in women over 40. *Journal of Reproductive Medicine, 35,* 597.

15. Lowdermilk, D.L., Perry, S.E., & Bobak, I.M. (1997). *Maternity and women's health care.* St. Louis: Mosby.

16. Mishell, D.R. & Brenner, P. (1994). *Management of common problems in obstetrics and gynecology.* Boston: Blackwell Scientific.

17. Mishell, D.R., Herbst, A.L., & Kirschbaum, T.H. (1997). *Yearbook of obstetrics, gynecology, and women's health.* St. Louis: Mosby.

18. Oberer, D., & Auckerman, L. (1996). Best practice: clinical pathways for uncomplicated births. *Best Practices and Benchmarking in Healthcare, 1*(1), 43-50.

19. Patterson, P. (Ed.). (1995). Same-day hysterectomy beneficial for some patients. *OR Manager, 11*(7/8), 39-41.

20. Robinson, B.J. (1997). The perioperative nurse's role in assisted-fertility procedures. *AORN Journal, 65*(1), 87-93.

21. Williams, H., & Reeves, F. (1998). Anesthetic techniques and positioning implications for perioperative nurses. *Seminars in Perioperative Nursing, 7,* 14-20.

CHAPTER FIFTEEN | # Genitourinary Surgery

Gratia M. Nagle

OVER THE PAST decade major advances in genitourinary surgery have occurred. The influences of the neodymium:yttrium-aluminum-garnet (Nd:YAG), potassium titanyl phosphate (KTP, frequency-doubled YAG), carbon dioxide (CO_2), holmium:YAG, and pulse–dyed lasers, ultrasonography, the Swiss lithoclast, electrohydraulic (EHL), ultrasonic, and electrocorporeal shock-wave lithotriptors (ESWL), as well as other innovative diagnostic measures and minimally invasive surgical approaches have expanded treatment options. Urologic surgery continues to become more complex and far more precise.

The perioperative urology nurse has new challenges to face with these advancements. For the perioperative urology nurse to function optimally, up-to-date knowledge, documented competence, and superb technical skills are priorities.[2] Pressures to contain the rising costs of healthcare are resulting in more procedures being done on an ambulatory or short-stay basis, and with limited time being available for patient and family education and discharge planning. Frequently this critical intervention falls to the perioperative nursing team. The success of surgical intervention and patient outcomes depends greatly on the perioperative nurse's ability and knowledge in developing a perioperative plan of care.

SURGICAL ANATOMY

A comprehensive understanding of the anatomic structures involved in genitourinary surgery is required to facilitate safe patient positioning and proper selection of instrumentation and equipment. Collaboration with the urologist's plan of care is necessary in preparing the patient for surgery. As technology expands and new procedures are developed, genitourinary surgery finds itself crossing paths with other specialties.

The normal genitourinary system includes one pair of kidneys, two ureters, the urinary bladder, the urethra, and the prostate gland in the male. Also considered essential to the genitourinary system are the adrenal glands, male reproductive organs, and the female urogynecologic system.

Urine is excreted by the kidneys and conveyed to the bladder through the ureters. Urine is stored in the bladder, which serves as a reservoir until its full capacity (350 to 700 ml) is reached, and is eliminated from the body by way of the urethra. Normal urinary output ranges from 0.5 to 1 ml/kg of body weight per hour for the average adult.

Kidneys

The kidneys are located in the retroperitoneal space along the lateral borders of the psoas muscle, one on each side of the vertebral column at the level of the twelfth thoracic to the third lumbar vertebrae. Usually the right kidney is several centimeters lower than the left because the liver rests above and anterior to the right kidney (Fig. 15-1).

Each kidney is surrounded by a mass of fatty and loose areolar tissue known as *perirenal fat*. A capsule enclosing the renal space is known as the *fascia renalis*, or *Gerota's fascia*. These structures help keep the kidneys in their normal anatomic position. The anterior and posterior relationships of the kidneys are shown in Fig. 15-2.

On the medial side of each kidney is a concave area known as the *hilum* through which the renal artery and vein enter and leave. The renal pelvis, a funnel-shaped structure that lies within the kidney and posterior to the renal vascular pedicle, divides into several branches called *calyces* (Fig. 15-3). When surgery is indicated in these

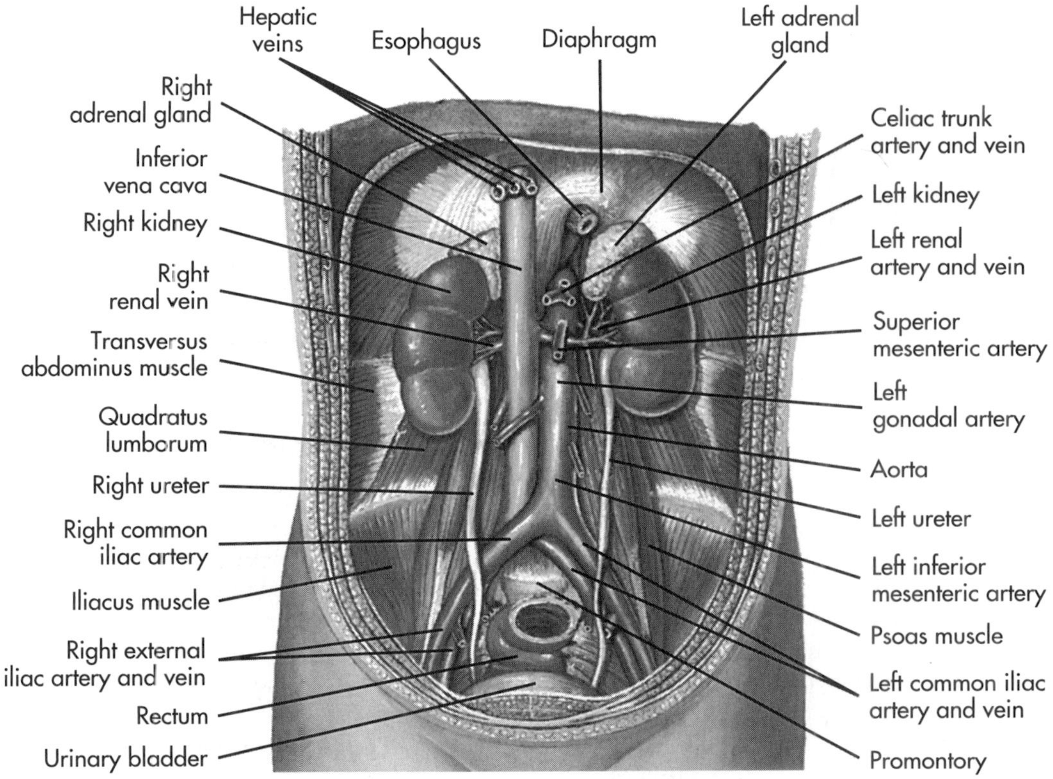

FIGURE 15-1   Location of urinary system organs.

structures, a posterior flank approach is preferred. When surgery for removal of a mass is anticipated, a transabdominal or thoracoabdominal incision is often chosen.

The kidneys are highly vascular organs that process approximately one fifth of the entire volume of blood at any one time. The blood supply to the kidney is conveyed through the renal artery, a large branch of the aorta, and leaves through the renal vein. On entering the kidney, the renal artery divides into anterior and posterior sections. These undergo further division into interlobular arteries from which smaller afferent branches pass to the glomeruli. Efferent arterioles in the glomeruli then pass to the tubules of the nephron. Renal arteriography is commonly performed preoperatively to help identify the patient's renal vascular anatomy when renal hypertension and horseshoe kidney are suspected and as part of the routine workup before renal transplantation.

The renal lymphatic supply originates beneath the capsule of the kidney and empties into the lumbar lymph nodes at the junction of the renal vascular pedicle and aorta. The nerves of the autonomic (involuntary) nervous system come from the lumbar sympathetic trunk and from the vagus. Removal of the nerve pathways does not impair renal function. The renal artery and vein with their accompanying nerves and lymphatics are referred to as the *pedicle* of the kidney.

Adrenal Glands

The adrenal glands lie retroperitoneally beneath the diaphragm capping the medial aspects of the superior pole of each kidney. On the right side the triangular gland is adjacent to the inferior vena cava; on the left side it is a rounded, crescent-shaped gland posterior to the stomach and pancreas. Each adrenal gland has a medulla, which secretes epinephrine (adrenaline), and a cortex, which secretes steroids and hormones. Secretions from the adrenal cortex are influenced by the activity of the pituitary gland. The adrenal glands are liberally supplied with arterial branches from the inferior phrenic and renal arteries and from the aorta. Venous drainage is accomplished on the right side by the inferior vena cava and on the left by the left renal vein. The lymphatic system accompanies the suprarenal vein and drains into the lumbar lymph nodes.

Ureters

Each ureter is a continuation of the renal pelvis. The ureter extends in a smooth S curve from the renal pelvis to the base of the bladder. It is approximately 25 to 30 cm long and 4 to 5 mm in diameter in the adult. This fibromuscular cylindrical tube is lined by transitional epithelium (urothelium) and lies on the psoas muscle, passing medially to the sacroiliac joints and laterally to the

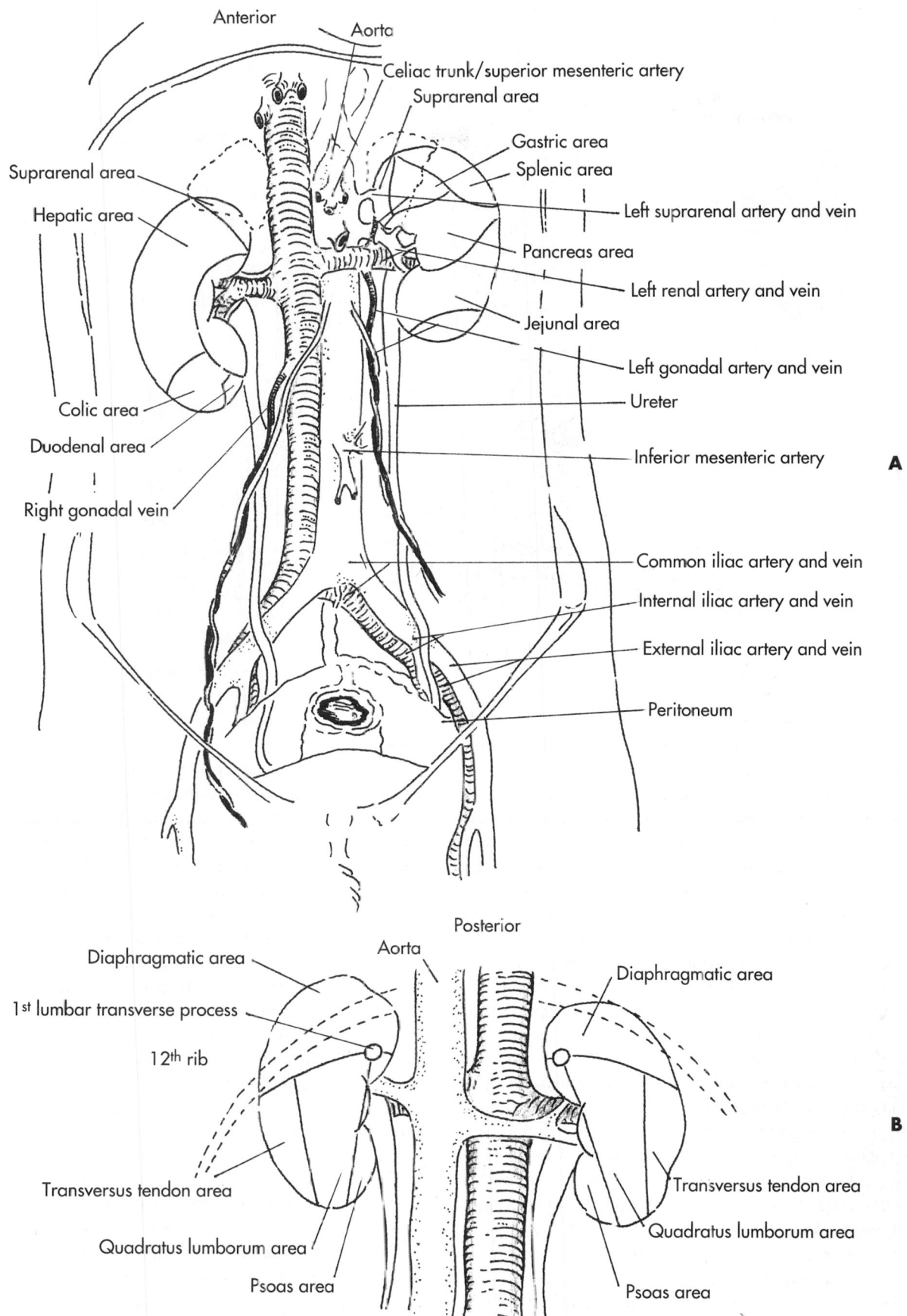

Anterior

Aorta

Celiac trunk/superior mesenteric artery

Suprarenal area

Suprarenal area

Hepatic area

Gastric area

Splenic area

Left suprarenal artery and vein

Pancreas area

Left renal artery and vein

Jejunal area

Left gonadal artery and vein

Colic area

Ureter

Duodenal area

Inferior mesenteric artery

A

Right gonadal vein

Common iliac artery and vein

Internal iliac artery and vein

External iliac artery and vein

Peritoneum

Posterior

Aorta

Diaphragmatic area

Diaphragmatic area

1st lumbar transverse process

12th rib

B

Transversus tendon area

Transversus tendon area

Quadratus lumborum area

Quadratus lumborum area

Psoas area

Psoas area

FIGURE 15-2   **A,** Blood supply of kidneys and relationship of kidneys and ureters to the main arteries and veins and the intraperitoneal organs. **B,** Relationship of the kidneys and ureters to the spinal column.

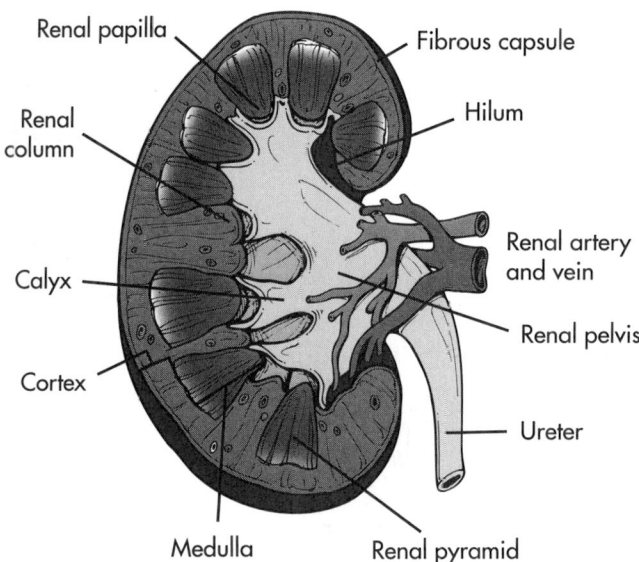

FIGURE 15-3   Normal kidney.

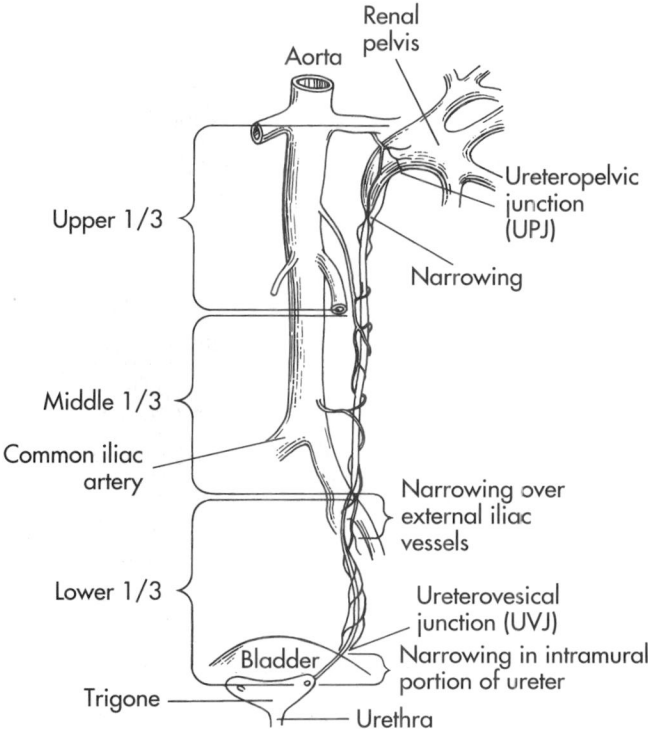

FIGURE 15-4   Anatomy of ureter.

ischial spines. As urine accumulates in the renal pelvis, slight distention initiates a wave of muscular contractions. This peristaltic activity continues down the ureter, propelling urine into the bladder.

The ureter has three areas of narrowing where calculi may become lodged and pose a potential problem with pain and obstruction: (1) the ureteropelvic junction, (2) the crossing of the ureter over the external iliac vessels, and (3) the ureterovesical junction (Fig. 15-4). Urine may sometimes cause calculi to be washed down the ureter to produce severe ureteral colic. Of all renal calculi, 90% are spontaneously passed into the bladder. However, if they become lodged in the ureter, an ESWL, ureteroscopy, stone manipulation, lithotripsy, or ureterolithotomy may be indicated. During pelvic or intestinal surgery, ureteral catheters or stents are often inserted to facilitate positive identification of the ureters and reduce the potential for severing or ligating them. These stents are frequently removed postoperatively, although some surgeons prefer to leave them in place through the early recovery period.

Urinary Bladder

The adult urinary bladder is a hollow muscular viscus that acts as a reservoir for urine until micturition (voiding) occurs. It has an outer adventitial and inner urothelial layer. The trigone, a triangular area, forms the base of the bladder. The three corners of the trigone correspond to the orifices of the ureters and the bladder neck (opening of the urethra) (Fig. 15-5). The ureteral orifices, on the proximal trigone at the interureteric ridge, are 2.5 cm apart. The bladder neck (internal sphincter) is formed from converging detrusor muscle fibers of the bladder wall that pass distally to form the smooth musculature of the urethra. Physiologically the bladder fills with urine and expands into the abdominal cavity. The extraperitoneal

location is advantageous because a suprapubic (above the pubic arch) incision may be performed without violating the peritoneum and potentially causing intraperitoneal complications.

The main arterial supply of the bladder comprises the superior, middle, and inferior vesical arteries. These vessels are derived from the internal iliac (hypogastric) artery, the obturator and inferior gluteal arteries, and in females the uterine and vaginal arteries. The bladder has a rich venous supply that drains into the internal iliac (hypogastric) vein. The lymphatic system is served by the vesical, external and internal iliac, and common iliac lymph nodes.

The bladder's size, position, and relation to the bowel, rectum, and reproductive organs vary according to the bladder's distention. In a female the vagina lies dorsally to the base of the bladder and parallel to the urethra (Fig. 15-6). In a male the prostate gland is interposed between the bladder neck and the urethra (Fig. 15-7). These anatomic relationships influence the symptoms that a patient experiences preoperatively and are important landmarks during pelvic surgery.

The process of bladder evacuation appears to be initiated by nerve cells from the sacral division of the autonomic nervous system. These sacral reflex centers are controlled by higher voluntary centers in the brain. Stimulation of the sacral centers results in contraction of the bladder muscles and relaxation of the bladder outlet sphincters. Muscles inside and adjacent to the urethral wall and from the pelvic floor maintain closure of the sphincters of the bladder, thus enabling continence.

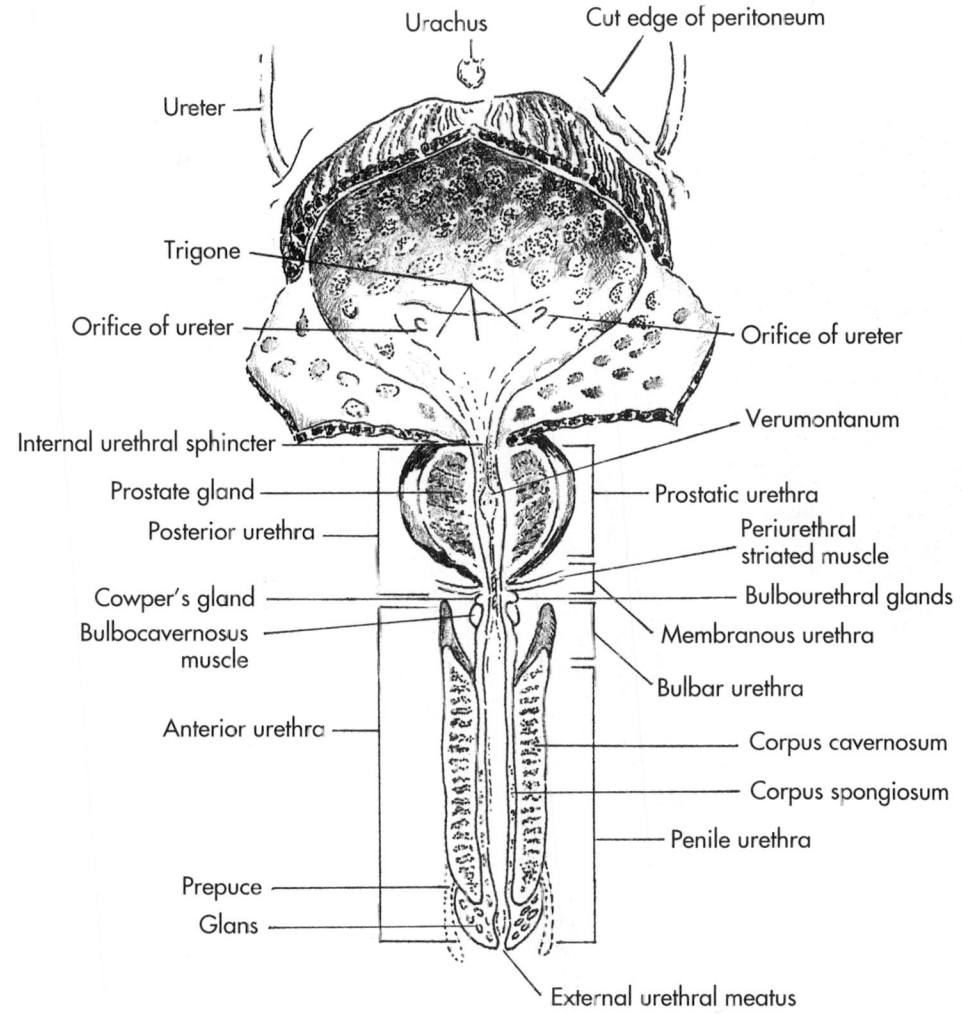

FIGURE 15-5 Anatomy of male urinary bladder, prostate gland, and urethra.

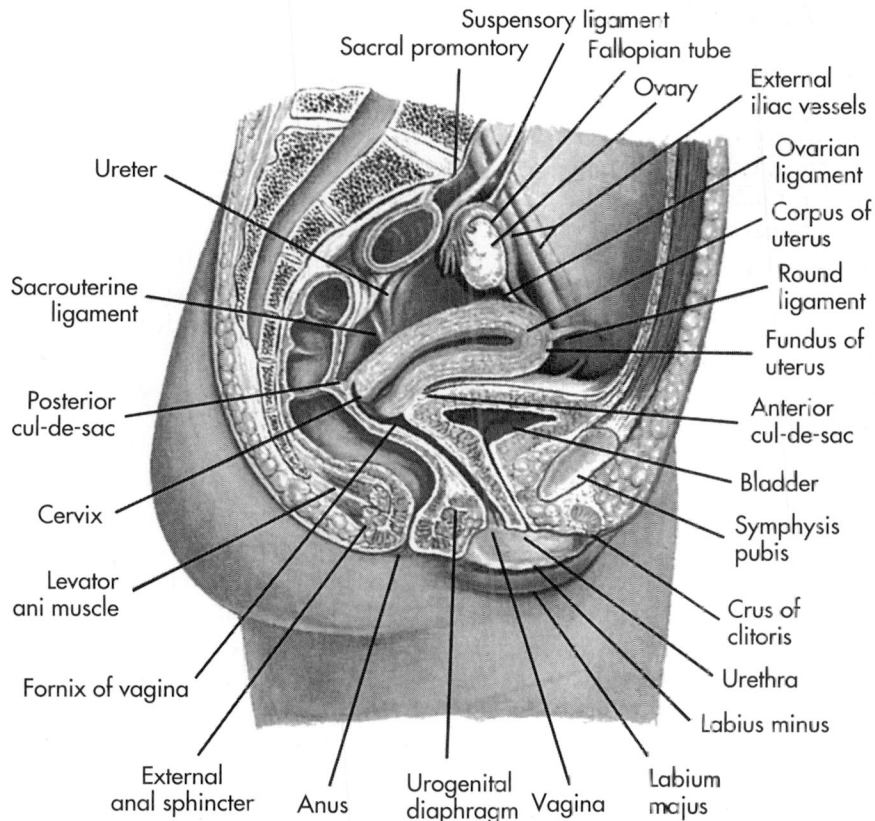

FIGURE 15-6 Female genitourinary and reproductive anatomy.

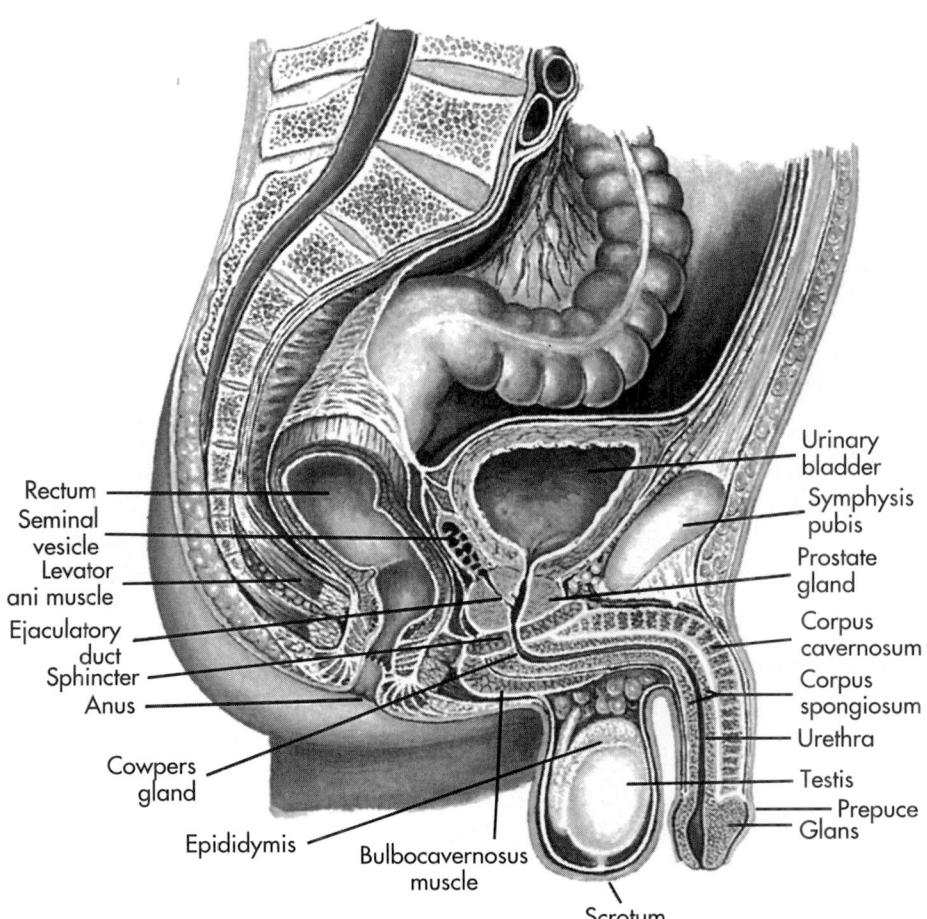

Rectum
Seminal vesicle
Levator ani muscle
Ejaculatory duct
Sphincter
Anus
Cowpers gland
Epididymis
Bulbocavernosus muscle
Scrotum
Urinary bladder
Symphysis pubis
Prostate gland
Corpus cavernosum
Corpus spongiosum
Urethra
Testis
Prepuce
Glans

FIGURE 15-7   Male genitourinary and reproductive anatomy.

Urethra

The male urethra, normally 20 to 25 cm long, extends from the bladder neck to the tip of the penis and varies in diameter from 7 to 10 mm. It is divided into two portions: the proximal (sphincteric) and the distal (conduit or anterior) urethra, both of which undergo further subdivision. The proximal urethra is commonly referred to as the *posterior urethra*, where it is elevated by the verumontanum, extending from the bladder neck through the prostate and the membranous portion. Within the posterior urethra lie the prostatic and membranous portions (see Fig. 15-5). As the urethra exits the prostate and crosses the pelvic (urogenital) diaphragm, it is called the *membranous urethra*. The distal urethra, commonly called the *anterior urethra*, is subdivided into the bulbar, pendulous (penile), and glandular urethras. The bulbar urethra is the area most prone to urethral strictures in the male. The prostatic urethra is approximately 3 cm long and is the widest portion of the urethra. On the floor of the prostatic urethra is the verumontanum, which contains the openings of the ejaculatory ducts. The membranous urethra is the shortest portion, measuring approximately 2.5 cm and extending from the external sphincter to the apex of the prostate. The penile, or pendulous, urethra lies within the corpus spongiosum. The urothelium of the urethra is continuous with that of the bladder.

The female urethra is a narrow, membranous tube about 3 to 5 cm in length and 6 to 8 mm in diameter. Slightly curved, it lies behind and beneath the symphysis pubis, anterior to the vagina. It passes through the internal and external sphincter and the urogenital diaphragm. The periurethral glands of Skene open on the floor of the urethra just inside the meatus. Because the female urethra is so short and in proximity to the anal and vaginal areas, microorganisms find easy access to the bladder and can cause urinary tract infections (UTIs).[11]

Prostate Gland

The prostate gland is a donut-shaped organ composed of fibromuscular and glandular components. It is located at the base of the bladder neck and completely surrounds the urethra. The gland is about 4 cm at its base and about 2 cm in depth and weighs approximately 20 g (see Figs. 15-5 and 15-7).

There are four glandular regions within the prostate: two major regions, the peripheral zone and central zone, and two minor regions, the transitional and periurethral zone. Many clinicians still prefer to divide the prostate into the intraurethral lobe (right and left lateral) and the extraurethral lobe (posterior and median). The posterior lobe is readily palpable during rectal examination and prone to cancerous degeneration. Benign prostatic hypertrophy generally occurs in the transitional zone (intraurethral lobe).

Behind the prostatic capsule is a fibrous sheath known as the *true prostatic capsule*, which separates the prostate gland and the seminal vesicles from the rectum. This fascia is an important landmark during perineal prostatectomy.

The lobes of the prostate gland secrete highly alkaline fluid that dilutes the testicular secretion as it is excreted from the ejaculatory ducts. These secretions are believed to be essential to the passage of spermatozoa and helpful in keeping them alive. The arterial supply to the prostate is derived from the pudendal, inferior vesical, and hemorrhoidal arteries.

Male Reproductive Organs

The male reproductive organs include several paired structures: the testes, epididymides, seminal duct (vas deferens), seminal vesicles, ejaculatory ducts, and bulbourethral glands. Other organs of the reproductive tract are the penis, prostate gland, and urethra.

The *scrotum* is located behind and below the base of the penis and in front of the anus. Each loose sac contains and supports a testis, an epididymis, and some of the spermatic cord. The two sides of the scrotum are separated from each other by a median raphe (septum). Within the scrotum are two cavities or sacs that are lined with smooth, glistening tissue, the tunica vaginalis. Normally, a small amount of clear fluid is contained in the tunica vaginalis. The condition known as *hydrocele* is an abnormal accumulation of this fluid.

The *testes* manufacture the spermatozoa and also contain specialized Leydig's cells that produce the male hormone testosterone. Each testis consists of many tubules in which the sperm are formed, surrounded by dense capsules of connective tissue. The tubules coalesce and continue into the adjacent epididymis, where the sperm mature and are stored. At the upper pole of the testis is the appendix testis, a small body that may be pedunculated (stalked) or sessile (flat).

The *epididymis* is a long, convoluted duct located along the posterolateral surface of the testis. It is closely attached to the testicle by fibrous tissue and secretes seminal fluid, which gives the sperm a liquid medium in which to migrate. The vas deferens (ductus deferens, or seminal duct) is a distal continuation of the epididymis as it enters the prostate gland and conveys the sperm to the seminal vesicle.

The *vas deferens* extends from the epididymis into the abdomen and lies within the spermatic cord in the inguinal region. The spermatic cord also contains veins, arteries, lymphatics, nerves, and surrounding connective tissue (cremaster muscle), which give support to the testes. The terminal portion of each vas deferens is called the *ejaculatory duct*; it passes between the lobes of the prostate gland and opens into the posterior urethra.

The *accessory reproductive glands* include the seminal vesicles, prostate gland, and bulbourethral gland. The seminal vesicles unite with the vas deferens on either side, are situated behind the bladder, and produce protein and fructose for the nutrition of the sperm cell. Sperm and prostatic fluid are discharged at the time of ejaculation.

Cowper's glands (bulbourethral glands) are located on each side at the juncture of the membranous and bulbar urethras. Each gland, by way of its duct, empties mucous secretions into the urethra.

The *penis* is suspended from the pubic symphysis by the suspensory ligaments. The penis contains three distinct vascular spongelike bodies surrounding the urethra: two outer bodies called the *right corpus cavernosum* and *left corpus cavernosum*, and an inner body, the *corpus spongiosum urethrae*. These tissues contain a network of vascular channels that fill with blood during erection (see Fig. 15-5). At the distal end of the penis the skin is doubly folded to form the prepuce, or foreskin, which serves as a covering for the glans penis. The glans penis contains the urethral orifice.

PERIOPERATIVE NURSING CONSIDERATIONS

Assessment

Patients entering a hospital or ambulatory surgery unit for genitourinary surgery exhibit many emotions and reactions. These feelings encompass fear, embarrassment, helplessness, hostility, anger, and grief. To most, a successful surgical outcome is of prime importance. The urology patient population varies from infants with congenital anomalies to the elderly with physiologic impairments. Because of the dramatic increase in ambulatory surgery, the nursing staff must prepare to meet patients' specific needs, from preoperative teaching to postoperative home care. The families of patients need to be involved in this preparation process. Patient education begins in the urologist's office. Communication between the office and perioperative nursing staff allows continuity of care and increases the efficiency and effectiveness of surgical procedures.

In addition to routine admission information, urologic and cardiac histories are usually obtained. This information includes but is not limited to vital signs, allergies (including latex), the patient's primary problem, history of the present illness, nature of symptoms, and limitations imposed by the disease condition. All data pertinent to the proposed operative procedure should be reviewed. Nursing observation should include the patient's general

TABLE 15-1 | **Common Preoperative Laboratory Analyses for Patients with Genitourinary Disorders**

LABORATORY STUDIES	NORMAL RANGE (ADULT VALUES)	LABORATORY STUDIES	NORMAL RANGE (ADULT VALUES)
Coagulation Profiles		**Serum Profiles (Low: Female; High: Male)—cont'd**	
Bleeding time	1-9 min	Creatinine	0.5-1.2 mg/dl
Partial thromboplastin time (PTT)	60-70 sec	Glucose (blood sugar)	70-105 mg/dl
Platelet count	150,000-400,000/mm^3	Osmolality	285-295 mOsm/kg H$_2$O
Prothrombin time (PT)	11-12.5 sec	Potassium (K)	3.5-5 mEq/L
		Phosphorus (P)	3-4.5 mg/dl
Fertility Profiles (Male)		Prostate specific antigen (PSA)	<4 ng/ml
Follicle-stimulating hormone (FSH)	1-15 mIU/ml	Prostatic acid phosphatase (PAP)	0.11-0.6 U/L
Luteinizing hormone (LH)	7-24 mIU/ml	Protein	6-8 g/dl
Testosterone (total)	300-1000 ng/dl	Sodium (Na)	136-145 mEq/L
Sperm count	50-200 million/ml, 60%-80% motile	Uric acid	2-8.5 mg/dl
		Urine Profiles (Values Not Listed Should Be Negative)	
Hematologies (Low: Female; High: Male)		Calcium (Ca)	100-300 mg/day
Hematocrit (Hct)	37%-52%	Chloride (Cl)	110-250 mEq/L/day
Hemoglobin (Hgb)	12-18 g/dl	Creatinine clearance	88-137 ml/min
Red blood cells (RBCs)	4.2-6.1 million/mm^3	Glucose (24 hr)	0.5 g/day
White blood cells (WBCs)	5000-10,000 million/mm^3	Hyaline casts	Occasional
		Osmolality (random)	50-1400 mOsm/kg H$_2$O
Serum Profiles (Low: Female; High: Male)		Phosphorus	0.4-1.3 g/24 hr
Bicarbonate	21-28 mEq/L	Potassium (K)	25-120 mEq/L/day
Blood urea nitrogen (BUN)	10-20 mg/dl	Protein	30-150 mg/day
Calcium (Ca)	9-10.5 mg/dl	Red blood cells (RBCs)	0-2
Chloride (Cl)	90-110 mEq/L	Sodium (Na)	40-220 mEq/L/day
Cholesterol	150-200 mg/dl	Uric acid	250-750 ml/day
HDL (High-density lipids)	>45-55 mg/dl	White blood cells (WBCs)	0-4
LDL (Low-density lipids)	60-180 mg/dl	pH	4.6-8 (ave.: 6)
VLDL (triglycerides)	25%-50%	Specific gravity	1.005-1.030

Data from Pagana, K. (1997). *Diagnostic and laboratory test reference* (ed. 3). St. Louis: Mosby; Tanagho, E. (1992). *Smith's general urology.* Norwalk, Conn.: Appleton & Lange; and Gray, M. (1992). *Genitourinary disorders.* St. Louis: Mosby.

physical appearance as well as nonverbal behaviors such as restlessness, which may indicate discomfort or anxiety. Any limitations in mobility or sensory deficits should be noted. Urologic procedures frequently require positions that create unusual stress for the patient, both anatomic and physiologic. Assessment must provide the perioperative nurse with data adequate to support preoperative planning and postoperative evaluation.

Many urologic surgical interventions require the patient to be in a flank position, causing compression of the vena cava. Additionally, large amounts of irrigating fluids are frequently used intraoperatively. For these reasons a current cardiac and electrolyte status should be available for review. Studies that have been done preoperatively may include serum and urine electrolytes, blood glucose, blood urea nitrogen (BUN), urinalysis and urine cultures, cardiac enzymes, complete blood count (CBC), prothrombin time (PT) and partial thromboplastin time (PTT), blood chemistry profiles (Table 15-1), electrocardiogram (ECG), and chest x-ray examination. The medical history, including a list of medications and any infectious processes or chronic diseases, should be reviewed. Specific geni-

tourinary studies can also be found in the patient's medical record. They may encompass all or some of the following: computerized tomography (CT) scans, magnetic resonance imaging (MRI), intravenous pyelograms or urograms (IVPs, IVUs), KUBs (genitourinary flat plate), urinary flow studies, fluoroscopic examinations (angiography, cavernosography), prostatic specific antigen (PSA), and ultrasonography. After the medical record is reviewed, assessment information is compiled, perioperative nursing diagnoses are identified, and the perioperative plan of care is formulated.

Nursing Diagnosis

Nursing diagnoses related to the care of patients undergoing genitourinary surgery might include the following:

- Anxiety
- Risk for injury
- Altered patterns of urinary elimination
- Fluid volume excess or deficit
- Impaired gas exchange

Outcome Identification

Outcomes identified for the selected nursing diagnoses could be stated as follows:

- The patient will verbalize a reduced anxiety level to the perioperative nurse.
- The patient will be free from injury related to the surgical position.
- The patient will maintain or regain a normal pattern of urinary elimination.
- The patient will maintain adequate fluid volume and electrolyte balance.
- The patient will maintain adequate oxygen supply and alveolar ventilation.

Planning

Care plans are the organizing framework for perioperative nursing activities, wherein nursing interventions are clinical processes in a quality health outcome model.[12] Frequently the urology patient presents a complex medical picture. Any alterations in the patient's physical or emotional status may greatly influence both the surgical and the postoperative course. A review of the patient record, communication with the patient or family, recognition of specific psychosocial, cultural, ethnic, and spiritual needs of the patient and family, and knowledge gained from other members of the patient care team are all used to formulate the nursing data base. A sample care plan for a patient undergoing genitourinary surgery follows.

Implementation

Care plan implementation begins during the patient interview. Patient education that is concise and simply explained enhances the final surgical outcome. Meeting the patient's emotional needs is a nursing priority. A calm patient retains more information and is cognitively and emotionally more receptive to perioperative teaching. Explanations of what to expect throughout the operative period allay fears and nurture confidence in the nursing care provided, assisting patients to minimize the effect of the surgical experience on their coping ability and to be emotionally comfortable.[9] Perioperative nursing care requires not only the collection of pertinent patient data, but also the coordination of numerous supplies and equipment to support the smooth implementation of the care plan.

Clinical pathways (paths) are structured outlines or plans for patient care based on research and desired outcomes of care. Although these tools require extensive interdisciplinary cooperation and data collection they facilitate standardized and consistent approaches to patient problems and diagnoses. As such, they have the potential for improving quality, and increasing both the efficiency and cost-effectiveness of patient care.[3] In 1997, AORN developed a template for a perioperative clinical path, and it can be found in Chapter 1. A clinical pathway for a patient undergoing radical perineal prostatectomy is shown in Fig. 15-8.

Positioning

Thorough understanding of the urologic OR bed and its functions is essential for optimum patient positioning. The position in which the patient is placed for surgery is determined by the particular operation to be performed. For urologic operative procedures the patient may be placed in the lateral, supine, prone, or lithotomy position, which may be exaggerated to give optimum access to the organ involved, particularly in radical surgery of the prostate and bladder. Considerable care must be taken to ensure that the patient's position does not interfere with respiration or circulation. It is essential to avoid displacement of the joints and undue tension on neurovascular bundles or ligaments.

A patient positioned laterally (flank position) for renal surgery has the spine extended for greater access to the retroperitoneal space. Padding and stabilized support with gel pads, pillows, sandbags, and straps should be available for precise anatomic positioning and safety. When an electrosurgical unit is to be used, care must be taken that the patient does not contact metal parts of the OR bed.

In some procedures involving stones of the kidneys or ureters, intraoperative x-ray examinations or fluoroscopy may be required. If x-ray examination is to be done, the patient must be on an operating room bed with an x-ray cassette holder. If the OR bed design does not accommodate x-ray cassettes, an x-ray cassette holder must be placed under the patient who is in the supine, prone, or lithotomy position before the procedure begins. If the patient is in the lateral position with the bed flexed and kidney rest elevated, the x-ray cassette, encased in a sterile bag, is held laterally to the patient's flank at the time of x-ray exposure. When fluoroscopy (C-arm) is to be employed, the patient must be placed on an OR bed compatible with its use. Whenever possible, the patient should be protected from undue radiation exposure to the thyroid and chest areas by the use of small leaded shields. In urologic procedures it is not generally feasible to shield the reproductive organs.

Aseptic techniques and safety measures

Prevention of infection is an important nursing goal in the care of the genitourinary patient. It is, however, seldom possible to confirm freedom from infection intraoperatively or immediately postoperatively. Aseptic techniques must be carefully maintained and monitored. Skin preparation and draping procedures (see Chapter 4) vary, depending on the surgery to be performed and institutional protocols. Special care must be taken when cleansing the perineal area to avoid contamination from the rectum to the urethra. Prepping solutions should be applied with downward strokes and the sponge discarded once it has contacted the inner vaginal or anal areas. Transurethral passage of instruments and catheters requires

SAMPLE CARE PLAN

Nursing Diagnosis: Anxiety

Outcome: The patient will verbalize reduced anxiety level to the perioperative nurse.

Interventions:

Provide an accepting and supportive environment.

Use touch (as appropriate) to convey caring and support.

Encourage expression of feelings.

Promote feelings of self-worth.

Offer suggestions to cope with anxieties.

Facilitate or assist patient in using coping strategies (relaxation, deep breathing, music, imagery).

Maintain patient privacy.

Encourage participation of patient and family in plan of care.

Nursing Diagnosis: Risk for injury

Outcome: The patient will be free from injury related to surgical position.

Interventions:

Maintain proper body alignment.

Assess range of motion and musculoskeletal, peripheral vascular and cardiovascular status preoperatively.

Pad all bony prominences.

Avoid compression of vulnerable nerves and neurovascular bundles.

Secure patient to operating room bed without friction or pressure.

Provide support stockings or antiembolism device as indicated.

Initiate measures to warm patient and maintain normothermia.

Nursing Diagnosis: Altered pattern of urinary elimination

Outcome: The patient will maintain or regain a normal pattern of urinary elimination.

Interventions:

Include catheter care and measures to facilitate voiding (intermittent catheterization) after catheter removal as part of preoperative teaching to patient and family.

Instruct patient in importance of any postoperative antibiotic or anticholinergic therapy.

Follow aseptic technique during catheter insertion and connection to drainage device.

Maintain closed urinary drainage system.

Note color and character of urine; report abnormalities.

Keep drainage tubing and collection device below the level of the patient's bladder.

Keep urine draining freely; avoid kinks in tubing.

Check patency of catheter after all positional changes.

Anchor drainage tubing to patient to prevent pulling or retraction of tubing.

Assess bladder for distention.

Record intake and output daily.

Provide patient with information on preventing recurrent UTI.

Nursing Diagnosis: Fluid volume excess or deficit

Outcome: The patient will maintain adequate fluid volume and electrolyte balance.

Interventions:

Provide appropriate intravenous solutions, volumetric pumps, warmers.

Monitor patency of all intravenous lines.

Record volume of intravenous or irrigating fluids instilled.

Monitor ECG, vital signs, cardiopulmonary status as appropriate.

Monitor blood loss and volume replacement.

Monitor urinary output, note color, report output less than 30 ml/hour and changes in color or clarity.

Maintain accurate intake and output records.

Monitor serum electrolyte status.

Monitor pH and specific gravity of urine.

Nursing Diagnosis: Impaired pulmonary gas exchange

Outcome: Patient will maintain adequate oxygen supply and alveolar ventilation.

Interventions:

Review breathing exercises with patient preoperatively.

Position patient to provide maximum lung perfusion.

Apply cardiac monitor, blood pressure cuff, and pulse oximeter.

Monitor and report alterations from preoperative status in ventilation or perfusion.

Administer oxygen as required; assist with intubation and maintenance of airway during positioning.

Assist with collection of arterial blood gases; report results promptly.

---

meticulous technique to prevent retrograde infections of the urinary tract, which account for close to 40% of all nosocomial infections.[11]

Visualization of the bladder during transurethral procedures is enhanced by darkening the room. Provision should be made for proper adjustments to lighting. Electrosurgical units and fiberoptic light systems are frequent adjuncts in urologic surgery. The staff must be familiar with the

manufacturer's safety precautions and recommendations during their use.

Use of irrigating fluids

When the bladder is entered, sterile distilled irrigating fluid is administered to distend the bladder for effective visualization. Commercially prepared sterile irrigation solutions with appropriate closed administration sets are

CLINICAL PATHWAY FOR RADICAL PERINEAL PROSTATECTOMY

DRG#: 334/335
LOS: 3 DAYS

	Preoperative (outpatient 3-14 days)	Day of surgery	Postoperative day 1	Postoperative day 2	Postoperative day 3	Follow-up 7-14 days
Outcome	Verbalizes fears Understands ambulation and ROM exercises Return demonstrate pulmonary therapy	Free of anxiety, positional injury, and infection Foley patent Pain <3 on 1-10 scale Participates in ROM and pulmonary therapy	Foley output pink at >30 ml/hr Minimal pain Performs pulmonary therapy and ROM with PCA	Foley output clear at >30 ml/hr No spasms or nausea Pain <3 Performs pulmonary therapy and ROM with PO pain medication VS stable Lungs clear	Drain removed Foley output clear at >30 ml/hr Pain <2 on 1-10 scale ROM without pain medication	BMs normal Foley output clear at >30 ml/hr No pain or fever Wound clean
Labs	CBC/diff, chemistry 18 Bleeding time, PT/PTT, Ua/C&S, PSA/PAP, Electrolytes, T&S	Repeat abnormals preoperatively Repeat CBC, electrolytes, chemistry 18 postoperatively		Urinalysis, CBC/diff, chemistry 18, electrolytes if appropriate		
Tests	Biopsy prostate CT/bone scans/MRI H&P CXR/ECG	Radial and pedal pulses				
Treatments	Assess pulmonary, peripheral, and cardiovascular status Assess ROM musculoskeletal status	O₂, VS q4h, I&O Drain Foley/dressing care PRN Foley irrigation sequential stockings Pulmonary therapy	Pulmonary therapy: I&O, VS q4 to 8 per 24 hr Drain/Foley/dressing care, PRN Foley irrigation Remove sequential stockings	VS q8h, I&O Drain/Foley/dressing care PRN Foley irrigation Pulmonary therapy D/C PCA and IV	VS q8h PRN Foley irrigation Drain/Foley/dressing care	D/C narcotic Voiding trial at 2 weeks
Activity	Ad lib	Bedrest to chair in morning	Ambulate tid Chair ad lib. Shower	Ambulate/chair ad lib. Shower	Ambulate ad lib. Shower	No lifting or driving Shower Sitz bath after drain site healed
Diet	Day before: increase oral fluid, light lunch, clear liquid supper, NPO after 12 midnight	NPO to ice chips in morning	Clear liquid to full liquid Force fluids	Full liquid to soft to regular as tolerated Force fluids	Regular Force fluids	Regular Force fluids

FIGURE 15-8   Clinical pathway for radical perineal prostatectomy.

Continued

	Preoperative (outpatient 3-14 days)	Day of surgery	Postoperative day 1	Postoperative day 2	Postoperative day 3	Follow-up 7-14 days
Consultations	Anesthesia, oncology, medical	Clergy if appropriate	Home health care, social services		Home health care, social services	
Equipment and supplies	Preoperative testing supplies Preop medications	OR/anesthetic supplies IV and tubing Sequential stockings Foley with bag Wound drain, dressings	Nursing care supplies	Nursing care supplies	Nursing care supplies	Dressings
Medications by IV	Hormone deprivation for 12 weeks preoperatively PO antibiotic/ metronidazole if LPLND	$D_5\frac{1}{2}NS$ at 100 ml/hr IV IV sedative/ antibiotic/ anesthetic/ crystalloids IV narcotic/ antiemetic/ antispasmodic Toradol IM Tylenol q4h for temp. >101° F Start PCA	$D_5\frac{1}{2}NS$ at 75 ml/hr IV PCA to IM narcotic IM to PO Toradol IV to IM antibiotic/ antiemetic/ antispasmodic Tylenol q4h for temp. >101° F Stool softener	Antibiotic/ antiemetic/ antispasmodic IM to PO IM to PO narcotic Toradol PO Stool softener Tylenol q4h for temp. >101° F	Antibiotic/ Toradol/ narcotic PO Tylenol q4h for temp. >101° F Stool softener	Continue antibiotic/ Toradol/stool softener Begin multivitamins Antibiotic/vitamin E or aloe vera ointment to wound after incision closed
Teaching and discharge plan	Procedure/Foley/ drain/dressing care Medication regimen Postoperative recovery	Pulmonary therapy, Foley/drain/ dressing care Instruct 0-10 pain scale	Reinforce preoperative teaching Begin home care plan	Catheter and drain care Foley irrigation Dressing care Pain control Antibiotic therapy Bowel regime	Prescriptions for narcotic/ Toradol/ antibiotic/ stool softener Leg bag Review all teaching	Review Foley irrigation, restrictions, and diet
Patient flow	Complete tests/labs Comply with preoperative order	Admit 1½ hr preoperatively EBL <500 ml General anesthesia, lithotomy	Pain <3 on 1-10 scale Bowel sounds, no flatus	Pain <3 on 1-10 scale No spasms or nausea Bowel sounds ± flatus Lungs clear	Bowel sounds with flatus Discharge to home	Returns to office 2, 7, and 14 days after discharge

BMs, Bowel movements; *C&S,* culture and sensitivity; *CBC/diff,* complete blood cell count with differential; *chemistry 18,* full chemistry panel; *CXR,* chest radiograph; *D-NS,* dextrose titer in normal saline; *D/C,* discontinue; *DRG,* diagnosis related groups; *EBL,* estimated blood loss; *ECG,* electrocardiogram; *H&P,* history and physical examination; *I&O,* intake and output; *IM,* intramuscular; *IV,* intravenous; *LPLND,* laparoscopic pelvic lymph node dissection; *LOS,* length of stay; *MRI,* magnetic resonance imaging; *NS,* normal saline; *OR,* operating room; *PCA,* patient-controlled anesthesia; *PO,* per os, by mouth; *PSA/PAP,* prostate specific antigen/prostatic acid phosphatase; *PT/PTT,* prothrombin time/partial thromboplastin time; *ROM,* range-of-motion exercises; *T&S,* type and screen; *tid,* thrice a day; *Ua,* urinalysis; *VS,* vital signs.

FIGURE 15-8, cont'd   Clinical pathway for radical perineal prostatectomy.

highly recommended. Such closed systems prevent the inherent risks of cross-contamination. Large volumes of irrigating solutions are frequently used, particularly during more extensive endoscopic procedures. When these solutions are at the room temperature of the OR, they are a shock to the patient's internal body temperature and can cause hypothermia. Solution-warming units are available commercially and are a useful tool to help decrease this risk.[5] The drawback to these units may be that the warmth delays clotting, thus increasing the risk of blood loss.

For simple observation cystoscopy, retrograde pyelography, and simple bladder tumor fulgurations, sterile distilled water may be used without complication. However, during transurethral resection of the prostate (TURP), venous sinuses may be opened, and varying amounts of irrigant are invariably absorbed into the bloodstream. Studies indicate that the use of distilled water during TURP may result in hemolysis of erythrocytes and possible renal failure. Other important complications include dilutional hyponatremia and cardiac decompensation.

Ideally a clear, nonelectrolytic, and isosmotic solution should be used. The most widely used urologic irrigating fluids are 3% sorbitol, an isomer of mannitol, and 1.5% glycine, an aminoacetic solution. Other acceptable solutions include 5% mannitol, 1.8% urea, and 4% glucose. In dilute solutions sorbitol and glycine have many properties that make them particularly useful for irrigation during transurethral prostatectomy. At slightly hypotonic concentrations they do not produce hemolysis. Because the solutions are nonelectrolytic, they do not cause dispersion of high-frequency current with consequent loss of electrosurgical cutting capacity, as occurs with normal saline.

Commercially prepared sterile irrigation solutions are available in collapsible bags and rigid plastic containers, both of which have the same advantage; neither depends on air, and each may be hung in series, thus providing continuous irrigation without interruption. Air bubbles, a problem that distorts visibility during the procedure, are eliminated with these systems.

Thorough knowledge of the potential hazards encountered intraoperatively during transurethral surgery is extremely important. Although complications are more prevalent in the postoperative stage, close observation during the intraoperative period is essential. Symptoms such as sudden restlessness, apprehension, irritability, confusion, nausea, slow pulse, seizures, dysrhythmias, and rising blood pressure may be suggestive of TURP, a severe hyponatremia caused by systemic absorption of irrigating fluid used during surgery.[14] Minimum amounts of fluids should be given and urine output carefully monitored. Irrigation fluid should be under as little pressure as possible, and the bladder emptied before it reaches full capacity to prevent intravesical pressure. Serum electrolyte values should be obtained without delay. If a low serum sodium value is reported, hypertonic sodium chloride is administered by means of a slow intravenous drip, often on a volumetric pump. Intravenous diuretics such as furosemide (Lasix) may be required to prevent possible pulmonary edema associated with the administration of hypertonic saline. If the patient's reaction is severe, surgery may have to be terminated.

Endoscopic and ancillary equipment

Cystoscopic and ancillary equipment often varies from one institution to another. Therefore it is valuable to have a reference manual or Kardex system that illustrates and describes in detail the required instrumentation for each specific procedure.

The basic cystoscopy tray should include instruments and accessory items that are routinely used for all cystoscopy procedures. If ureteral catheterization is planned, catheterizing telescopes or an Albarran bridge, which can be packaged and sterilized separately, may be easily added to the basic cystoscopy setup. Instruments for transurethral surgery and other special procedures may be wrapped, sterilized, and placed on separate trays so that they are available on request. This concept minimizes handling of the delicate lensed instruments and ultimately reduces costly repairs.

Cystoscopic procedures frequently require additional instrumentation. Instruments of various types and sizes, such as a visual obturator, biopsy forceps, urethral sounds, Phillips filiforms and followers, and Ellik evacuators, are available as prepackaged, sterile, disposable items. The reusable products may also be packaged separately and sterilized.

Urethral and ureteral catheters

A variety of urethral and ureteral catheters is necessary in the management of urologic disease. Catheters are designed for specific procedures to meet the individualized needs of particular patients. Ureteral catheters are manufactured of polyurethane material and are graduated so that the urologist may determine the exact distance the catheter has been inserted into the ureter. Most manufacturers provide disposable catheters double-wrapped in peel-open packages to allow aseptic handling during ureteral insertion. Some indications for the use of ureteral catheters are to (1) perform retrograde pyelography, (2) identify the ureters during pelvic or intestinal surgery, and (3) bypass partial or complete obstruction that may be present as a result of ureteral tumors, calculi, or strictures.

Frequently used ureteral catheters include the whistle tip, round, Braasch bulb, spiral, cone, open ended, and olive tip (Fig. 15-9). The spiral Blasucci is useful when difficulty occurs in introducing a ureteral catheter past the ureterovesical junction. When a retrograde ureterogram is indicated, a Braasch bulb or cone-tipped ureteral catheter may be helpful in occluding the ureteral orifice to accomplish the x-ray study effectively. When a ureteral catheter is left indwelling, a special adapter (Fig. 15-10) can be connected to the end of the ureteral catheter to facilitate connection to a closed urinary drainage system. A small slit may also be created in the Foley catheter and the distal end of the ureteral catheter can be slipped into it and taped in place.

Indwelling double-pigtail or double-J stents are available and are passed cystoscopically to reside within the ureter (Fig. 15-11). When the guidewire is removed from the core of the stent, a proximal and distal J, or pigtail, forms in the tubing to retain the stents. Many of these stents have nonabsorbable suture attached to the distal end, which extends through the urethral meatus. A suture may be easily tied to the distal end of those that do not. The surgeon can then remove the stent in the office setting postoperatively without needing to perform a cystoscopy.

Urethral catheters have a multitude of functions as stents, as drainage tubes, and in diagnostic studies in the operating room. They are generally divided into two categories, plain and indwelling (retention), and range in different French sizes, most commonly 10 through 30. The Foley catheter is the most frequently used retention catheter and is manufactured with a variety of balloon sizes, tip styles, lengths, and eye arrangements.

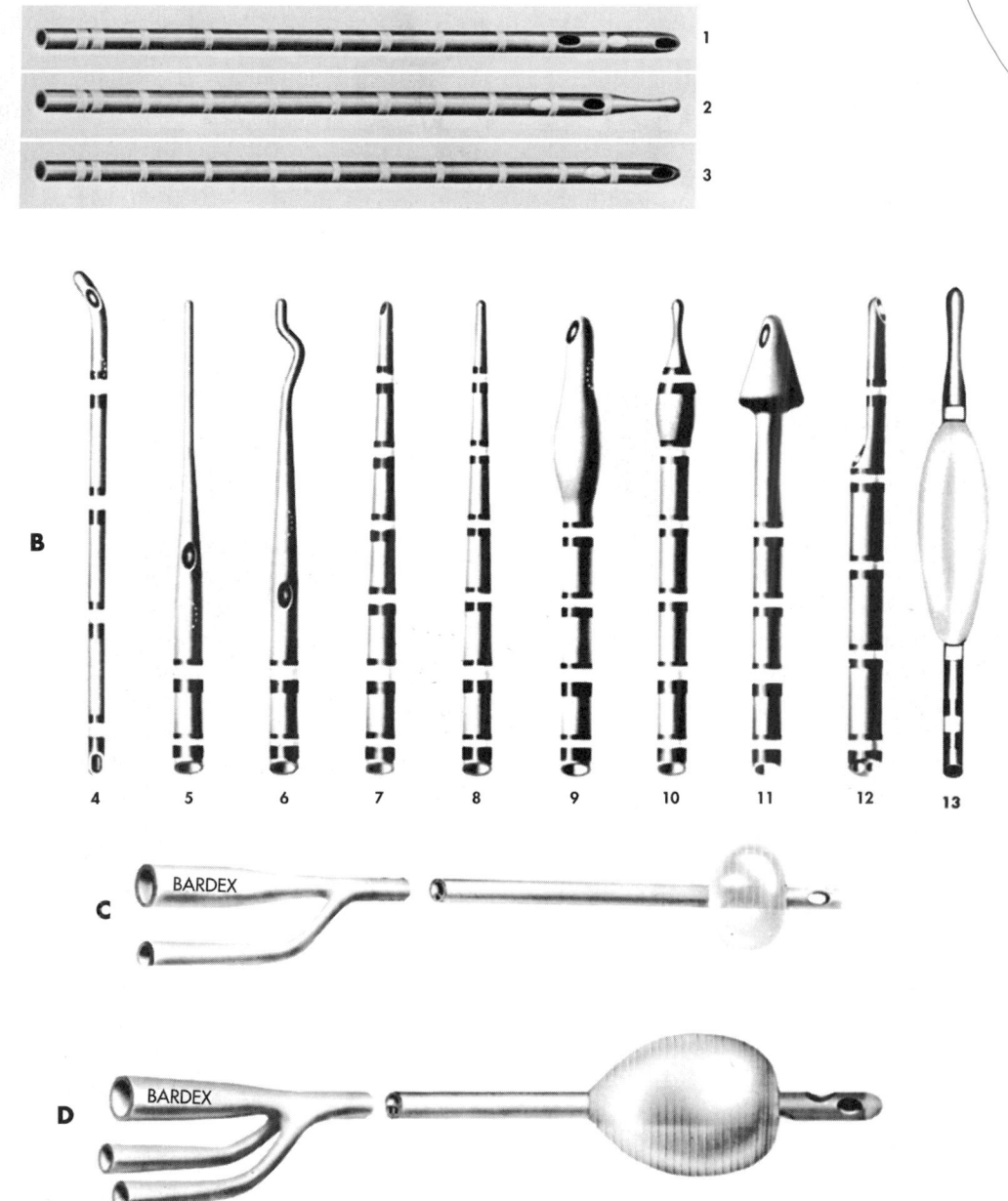

FIGURE 15-9 **A**, X-ray image of graduated woven ureteral catheters of nylon or polyurethane material with outer surfacing to provide flexibility for easy entry without kinking. Eyes provide adequate high-flow rate. Catheter tips constructed for specific procedures as shown. *1*, Whistle tip, *2*, olive tip, *3*, round tip. **B**, X-ray image of graduated woven ureteral catheters and bougies. *4*, Wishard catheter with flat, coude tip; *5*, Blasucci catheter with flexible filiform tip; *6*, Blasucci catheter with flexible spiral filiform tip; *7*, Garceau catheter, tapered for dilatation, with whistle tip; *8*, Garceau bougie, tapered for dilatation, with conical tip; *9*, Braasch bulb catheter with whistle tip; *10*, Braasch bougie with bulb tip; *11*, cone-tipped catheter (for ureteropyelography); *12*, Hyams double-lumen catheter; *13*, Dourmashkin dilator with inflation balloon and olive tip. **C**, Foley retention catheter. **D**, Bard three-way hemostatic catheter.

After transurethral prostatic surgery a three-way Foley catheter with a 30 ml balloon capacity may be left indwelling. This type of catheter is preferred because it facilitates continuous bladder irrigation (CBI), and the large balloon aids in achieving hemostasis in the prostatic bed. The urologist may apply light traction on the Foley catheter, with tape or a leg strap. This causes pressure against the bladder neck and aids in hemostasis (Fig.

15-12). A hematuria catheter, a three-way Foley specifically for patients with excessive clot formation, is also available. This catheter is reinforced with a stretch spiral wire within the catheter lining that permits vigorous aspiration without fear of lumen collapse.

Diagnostic studies are also performed in the cystoscopy suite and require special catheters for specific studies. For example, the Davis double-balloon urethrographic cath-

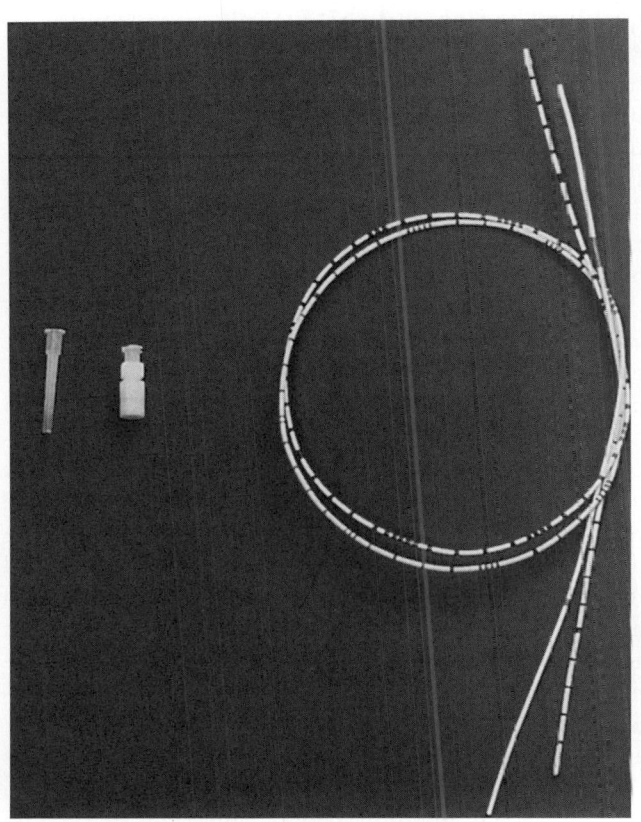
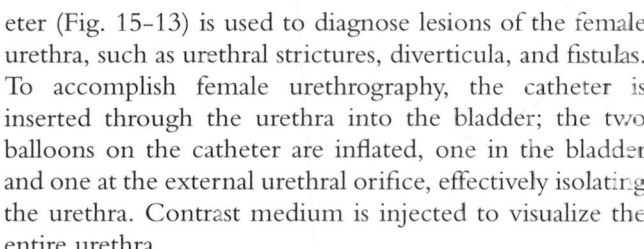

FIGURE 15-10   Ureteral catheters and adapters.

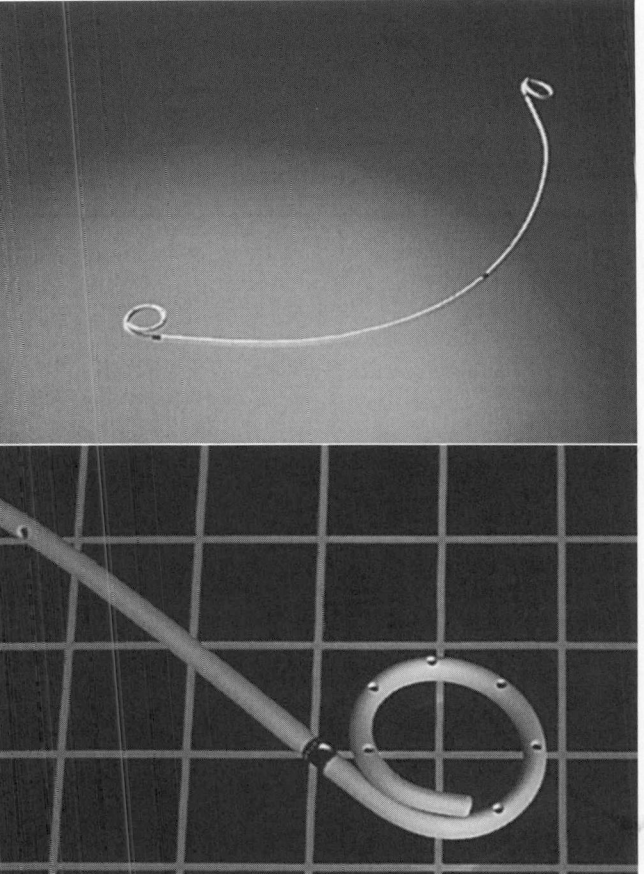
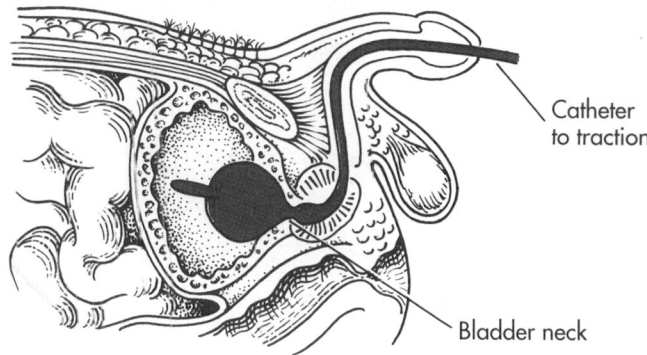

FIGURE 15-11   Double-pigtail stent set.

eter (Fig. 15-13) is used to diagnose lesions of the female urethra, such as urethral strictures, diverticula, and fistulas. To accomplish female urethrography, the catheter is inserted through the urethra into the bladder; the two balloons on the catheter are inflated, one in the bladder and one at the external urethral orifice, effectively isolating the urethra. Contrast medium is injected to visualize the entire urethra.

Another type of self-retaining catheter frequently used in the operating room is a Pezzar, also known as a mushroom catheter (Fig. 15-14). It may be straight or angulated with a large single channel and a preformed tip in the shape of a mushroom. The flexible mushroom tip helps keep the catheter in place. This catheter is used primarily for suprapubic bladder drainage, often for poor-risk patients who have uremia, neurogenic bladder syndrome, or possibly long-standing urinary retention. The catheter is inserted in the bladder through a midline or small transverse abdominal wall incision and secured to the abdomen with suture or tape. The Malecot four-winged catheter, often used as a nephrostomy tube to provide temporary or permanent diversion of urine after kidney surgery and when renal tissue needs to be restored, may also be used for suprapubic drainage (see Fig. 15-14). A Foley catheter of preferred size is frequently chosen for either purpose. Nephrostomy tube replacement is accom-

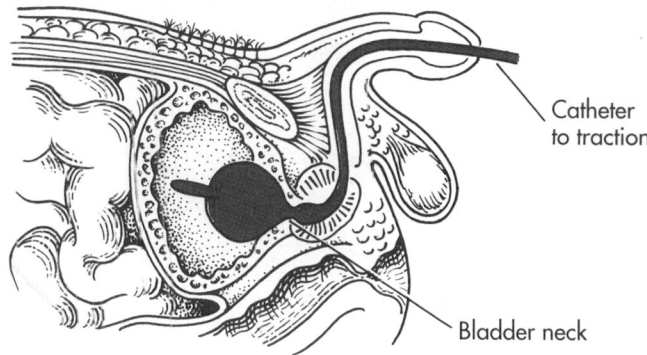

Catheter
to traction

Bladder neck

FIGURE 15-12   Balloon of Foley catheter inflated to size that prevents catheter from being pulled into prostatic fossa.

plished by introducing the catheter into the surgical tract with a straight catheter guide and securing it in place with a suture or a nephrostomy retention disk that is one size smaller than the nephrostomy tube being used. The flanges of the disk are taped or sutured to the skin. The use of other variations of urethral catheters is described later in the text.

Photography in urology

The use of photographic and video imaging equipment in urologic surgery serves to document the patient's disease, the progress of a disease process, and long-term follow-up study. It is also an important teaching resource. Video equipment adapts to endoscopic instrumentation and has the capability of projecting an enhanced image on a television monitor, permitting members of the surgical team to observe and learn during the actual surgical procedure. Other visual aids, such as slides and photographs, are used in teaching, as visual references in publication, and as documentation in patient records.

When any form of photography or video imaging is used, the patient's privacy must be ensured and an informed consent should be obtained. Special release forms should also be signed preoperatively by the patient for any videotapes or photographs to be used in teaching or publications.

Evaluation

Before the patient is taken to the postanesthesia care unit (PACU) or observation unit, his or her general

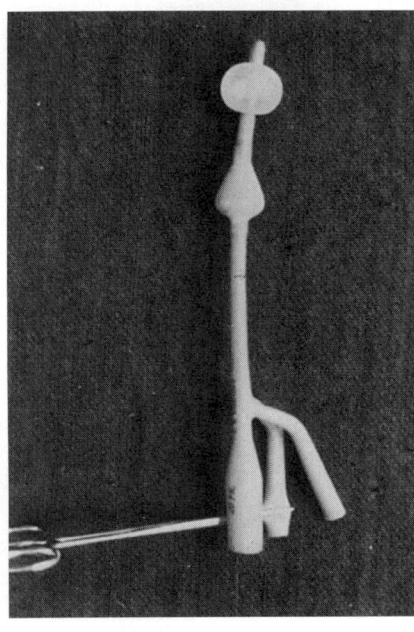

FIGURE 15-13 Double-balloon Davis urethrographic catheter.

condition is evaluated. The skin is assessed, and bony prominences, prepped and draped areas, and areas contacted by the attachment of ancillary equipment are observed for signs of pressure, irritation, or other changes from the preoperative status. Ancillary attachments include but are not limited to the electrosurgical dispersive pads or indifferent electrode (ESU) pad and ECG lead pads. Because many urology patients are nutritionally deficient and consequently have friable tissues, the trend has been to minimize the use of tape and to coat the skin with a protective sealant before the use of tapes.

Many urology patients are discharged to the PACU with drains inserted, including urethral, ureteral, suprapubic, and wound drains. Local anesthesia may have been used for either primary analgesia or postoperative pain management (preemptive analgesia); preoperative or intraoperative infiltration of the surgical site blocks sensory input, resulting in postoperative analgesia.[8] A complete report to the PACU nurse should include intraoperative position, problems encountered specific to the patient, and the patient's preoperative physical status as well as comprehension and anxiety levels. Documentation of medications administered from the sterile field or by the perioperative nurse intraoperatively should include time of administration, medication, dosage, site and route of administration, and who performed the application or injection. Drains should be documented as to size and type, insertion site, time and date of insertion, type of collection device, who performed the insertion, and character of drainage. When several drains are in place, additional labeling on the collection devices is beneficial. Any postoperative observations before or during transport should be recorded. Evaluation should also address whether the patient met the identified outcomes related to specific nursing diagnoses in the perioperative nursing care plan. Attainment of identified desired outcomes, included in the documentation and report to the PACU, may be phrased:

- The patient verbalized a reduced anxiety level to the perioperative nurse.
- The patient had no evidence of positional injury;

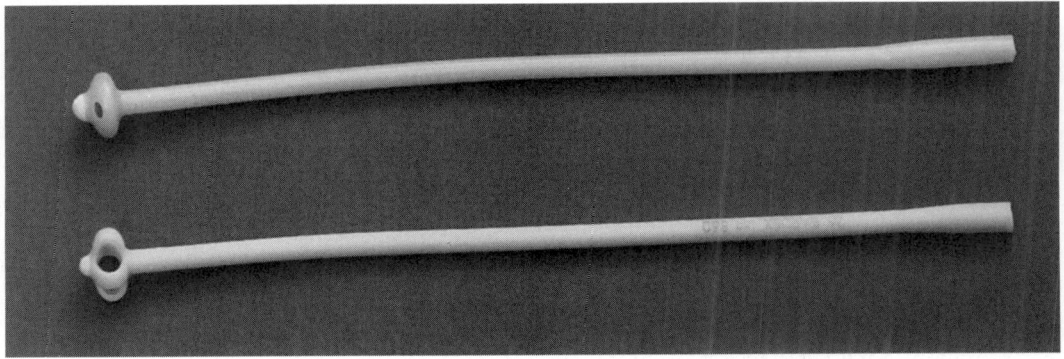

FIGURE 15-14 Pezzar (mushroom) catheter and Malecot (bat-winged) four-winged catheter.

neurovascular status was consistent with preoperative level, and skin integrity was intact.

- The patient maintained patency of the urinary catheter with no signs of infection, blockage, or retention. Urinary output remained within normal limits. The patient should void without difficulty after catheter removal.
- The patient evidenced no signs of fluid volume or electrolyte imbalance; vital signs were stable, arterial blood gases were within normal limits, and urinary output was maintained at acceptable levels.
- The patient maintained adequate gas exchange; lung expansion and O_2 saturation were satisfactory.

Patient and Family Education and Discharge Planning

Patient and family education and preparation for discharge allow perioperative nurses to plan for the urologic surgery patient's care across a continuum. General guidelines for preoperative education are presented in Box 15-1. Information provided should be presented in language the patient can understand ("lay terms") and clarified with the patient. When possible and with the patient's approval, family members or others who will serve as care givers should be included in the educational process at the outset. Because of the wide variety of urologic surgery, institutions may find it helpful to inventory the patient education materials available for select surgical procedures. An example of patient education content after nephrectomy is presented in Box 15-2.

Discharge instructions should be printed and include community resources and support groups as appropriate for the surgical intervention and the patient's diagnosis. These too should be presented in easily understood terms and reviewed. Any requisite skills that the patient or family will be responsible for should be demonstrated, with return demonstrations as time permits. Perioperative nurses may find it helpful to involve institutional resource persons or departments such as the social services

---

BOX 15-1	Teaching: Preoperative

Definition

Assisting a patient to understand and mentally prepare for surgery and the postoperative recovery period

Activities

Inform the patient and significant other(s) of the scheduled date, time, and location of surgery

Inform the patient/significant other(s) how long the surgery is expected to last

Determine the patient's previous surgical experiences and level of knowledge related to surgery

Appraise the patient's/significant other(s) anxiety relating to surgery

Provide time for the patient to ask questions and discuss concerns

Describe the preoperative routines (anesthesia, diet, bowel preparation, tests/labs, voiding, skin preparation, IV therapy, clothing, family waiting area, transportation to operating room) as appropriate

Describe any preoperative medications, the effects these will have on the patient, and the rationale for using them

Inform the significant other(s) of the location to wait for the results of the surgery as appropriate

Conduct a tour of the postsurgical unit(s) and waiting area(s) as appropriate

Introduce the patient to the staff who will be involved in the surgery/postoperative care as appropriate

Reinforce the patient's confidence in the staff involved as appropriate

Provide information on what will be heard, smelled, seen, tasted, or felt during the event

Discuss possible pain control measures

Explain the purpose of frequent postoperative assessments

Describe the postoperative routine and equipment (medications, respiratory treatments, tubes, machines, support hose, surgical dressings, ambulation, diet, family visitation) and explain their purpose

Instruct the patient on the technique of getting out of bed as appropriate

Evaluate the patient's ability to return-demonstrate getting out of bed as appropriate

Instruct the patient on the technique of splinting his or her incision, coughing, and deep breathing

Evaluate the patient's ability to return-demonstrate splinting incision, coughing, and deep breathing

Instruct the patient on how to use the incentive spirometer

Evaluate the patient's ability to return-demonstrate proper use of the incentive spirometer

Instruct the patient on the technique of leg exercises

Evaluate the patient's ability to return-demonstrate leg exercises

Stress the importance of early ambulation and pulmonary care

Inform the patient how he or she can aid in recuperation

Reinforce information provided by other healthcare members as appropriate

Determine the patient's expectations of the surgery

Correct unrealistic expectations of the surgery as appropriate

Provide time for the patient to rehearse events that will happen as appropriate

Instruct the patient to use coping techniques directed at controlling specific aspects of the experience (e.g., relaxation, imagery) as appropriate

Include the family or significant others as appropriate

From McCloskey, J.C., & Bulechek, G.M. (1992). *Iowa intervention project: nursing interventions classification (NIC)* St. Louis: Mosby.

BOX 15-2 | **Postprocedure and home care education for the nephrectomy patient**

Review of Postprocedural Care

- Tell the patient that the hospital stay after surgery will be 3-5 days.
- Stress the importance of turning, coughing, and deep breathing.
- Discuss the purpose of the incentive spirometer and demonstrate its use.
- Explain the purpose of wearing thigh-high elastic compression stockings and alternating pressure stockings while in bed.
- Emphasize the importance of getting out of bed (usually the second day) and moving about.
- Explain that drainage tubes may be needed after surgery and describe the various possibilities: chest tube, nasogastric tube, urinary drainage tube from bladder, nephrostomy tube from kidney through flank, Penrose drain, or Jackson-Pratt drain from incisional area.
- Explain the need for frequent dressing changes soon after the procedure.
- Inform the patient that the urine will be blood colored (pink to red) but will become normal appearing in a few days.
- Discuss the need for pain relief medication, antibiotics, and stool softeners.

Home Care

- Give both the patient and the caregiver *oral* and *written* instructions. Provide them with the name and telephone number of a physician or nurse to call if questions arise.
- *General information*
  — Review the purpose and explain the type of procedure performed: partial or total nephrectomy.
- *Wound or incision care*
  — Instruct the patient on caring for the incision and changing the dressing.
    Wash hands.
    Inspect the incision for signs of infection.
    Cleanse the area with antiseptic agent.
    If there is no evidence of drainage, leave the site open to the air. Otherwise, cover the incision with sterile gauze squares held in place with tape.

If Steri-Strips were used, do not remove them; allow them to drop off.
  — Teach the patient how to care for the nephrostomy tube, if present.
- *Special instructions*
  — Inform the patient that showering and bathing may be resumed as recommended by the physician.
  — Explain how to measure urine output as indicated.
- *Warning signs*
  — Review the signs and symptoms that should be reported to a physician or nurse.
    INFECTION: incision red, warm to touch, painful, with increased or purulent drainage (define)
    URINARY TRACT INFECTION: fever, chills, hematuria ("blood in urine"), flank pain, sudden increase in urinary output
- *Activity*
  — Discuss the need to exercise to tolerance and to plan frequent rest periods. Explain that fatigue is common.
  — Encourage the patient to discuss allowances and limitations with respect to occupation, recreation, and activities.
  — Tell the patient to avoid heavy lifting (>10 pounds) for at least 6 weeks.
  — Advise the patient to avoid contact sports (e.g., wrestling, football) that could endanger the remaining kidney.
- *Diet*
  — Inform the patient that a regular diet can be followed unless there are restrictions related to the underlying reason for nephrectomy.
    Encourage the patient to drink 8-10 glasses of fluids per day unless restrictions of the underlying disease apply. Half of these should be fruit juices (to maintain electrolyte balance).

Follow-up Care

- Stress the importance of regular follow-up visits. Make sure the patient has the necessary names and telephone numbers.

Modified from Canobbio, M.M. (1996). *Mosby's handbook of patient teaching*, St. Louis: Mosby.

---

department in developing information related to home care services, durable medical equipment, and transfers to postdischarge facilities other than home (skilled nursing center, rehabilitation facility, other long-term care facility). Patients and their families need preparation for mastering information and tasks that need to be performed. The goal of such interdisciplinary discharge planning is to provide information for the patient that is comprehensive and easy to use. This is part of perioperative nursing's ethical and professional responsibility to patients; it also meets the Joint Commission's requirements of providing consistent, interdisciplinary patient and family education (see Chapter 10).

SURGICAL INTERVENTIONS
DIAGNOSTIC AND ENDOSCOPIC PROCEDURES
Cystoscopy

Cystoscopy is an endoscopic examination of the lower urinary tract, including visual inspection of the interior of the urethra, the bladder, and the ureteral orifices. In a male patient special attention is given to the examination of the verumontanum (which contains the ejaculatory duct), the bladder neck, and the median and lateral lobes of the prostate. In a female patient the urethra, bladder neck, and bladder are examined.

15-1 RESEARCH HIGHLIGHT

The genital and lower urinary tracts in women have a common origin and similar hormonal sensitivities. Research has demonstrated the existence of estrogen receptors in the bladder and urethra; estrogen-mediated effects such as increased sensitivity to α-adrenergic stimulation have also been described in the human urethra. Estrogen has been used clinically for the treatment of stress urinary incontinence and other urogenital symptoms in women. The reported beneficial effects of estrogen in postmenopausal women suffering from stress incontinence can partly be explained by recent findings showing that estrogen can cause an increase in urethral blood flow, an increase in adrenergic receptor density, and an increase in urethral cell mass. Administration of estrogen to postmenopausal women produces an increase in urethral pressure and mucosal thickness, and blood vessel engorgement. On the other hand, the extent to which estrogen is able to influence smooth muscle function in the urinary bladder is not clearly known. Moreover, estrogen could alter the response of the bladder to α-adrenergic agonists.

The low estrogen production during and after menopause produces symptoms from the autonomic nervous system such as flushing, perspiration, atrophy of the mucous membrane of the genitourinary tract, and irritative voiding symptoms. Such women usually show stable detrusor function, with a tendency toward an early first sensation of filling and a low functional capacity as assessed urodynamically. Sensory urgency is attributable to hypersensitivity of the bladder or urethra, causing either a constant desire to void, which is unrelieved by voiding, or a desire to void at a low bladder volume because of pain or discomfort. Hypersensitivity of the urethra or bladder may be caused by atrophy of the mucous membranes of the lower urinary tract in this low estrogen state.

In this study, estrogen replacement therapy produced subjective and objective improvements. Chronic irritative voiding symptoms were relieved during the treatment period. After hormonal replacement therapy (HRT), the volume at first sensation and maximum cystometric capacity had significantly increased. These findings, combined with previous reports, indicate that estrogen treatment would improve atrophic changes of the lower urinary tract, and that such improvements would relieve hypersensitivity of the bladder and urethra. Urodynamically, these improvements may be reflected in a finding that the volume at first desire to void was increased. The muscarinic receptor density of the bladder may be reduced by estrogens, which could result in a reduction in detrusor contractility and an increase in bladder capacity. Although the incidence of side effects was relatively high (most such reactions were not long lasting) and the long-term continuous use of estrogen may induce a fear of occurrence of uterine body cancer, estrogen replacement therapy in the short term seemed to be useful in the treatment of postmenopausal women with chronic irritative voiding symptoms and could be repeated when symptoms recurred.

From Ishigooka, M., Hashimoto, T., Tomara, M., et al. (1994). Effect of hormonal replacement therapy in postmenopausal women with chronic irritative voiding symptoms, *International Urogynecology Journal, 5* 208-211.

Cystoscopy is an important diagnostic tool that provides the urologist with valuable information concerning the patient's urologic condition. Indications for cystoscopy include hematuria, urinary retention, urinary tract infection, cystitis, tumors, fistulas, vesical calculus disease, and urinary incontinence. Urinary incontinence in postmenopausal women may be related to estrogen deprivation (Research Highlight 15-1).

Procedural considerations

Once in the OR, before entering the cystoscopy suite, all patients should be greeted by name and identified by their identification bracelet and number. The perioperative nurse should check the chart for operative consent and pertinent laboratory reports; IVPs and any diagnostic x-ray studies ordered preoperatively should also be available for review. Customarily the patient voids immediately before transport to the OR. The time of urination and the output volume should be documented for ruling out residual urine in the bladder.

After the patient is placed on the cystoscopy bed, correct positioning requires optimum relaxation of muscles of the legs and perineum. Proper positioning of the knee crutches on the cystoscopy bed is a vital consideration for patient safety and comfort. When knee crutches are properly positioned, the curve of the yoke suspension should flow outward from the perineum, as the patient's legs do. Padding the knee crutches is beneficial in reducing pressure on the popliteal areas. If sling stirrups that support only the feet are employed, the post should be padded and positioned to prevent pressure on the peroneal nerve. There are special pads designed for use with both of these stirrups. Allen stirrups are a boot style that supports the foot and calf. These have thick gel padding within the stirrup and provide optimum patient comfort and protection, relieving pressure on the popliteal

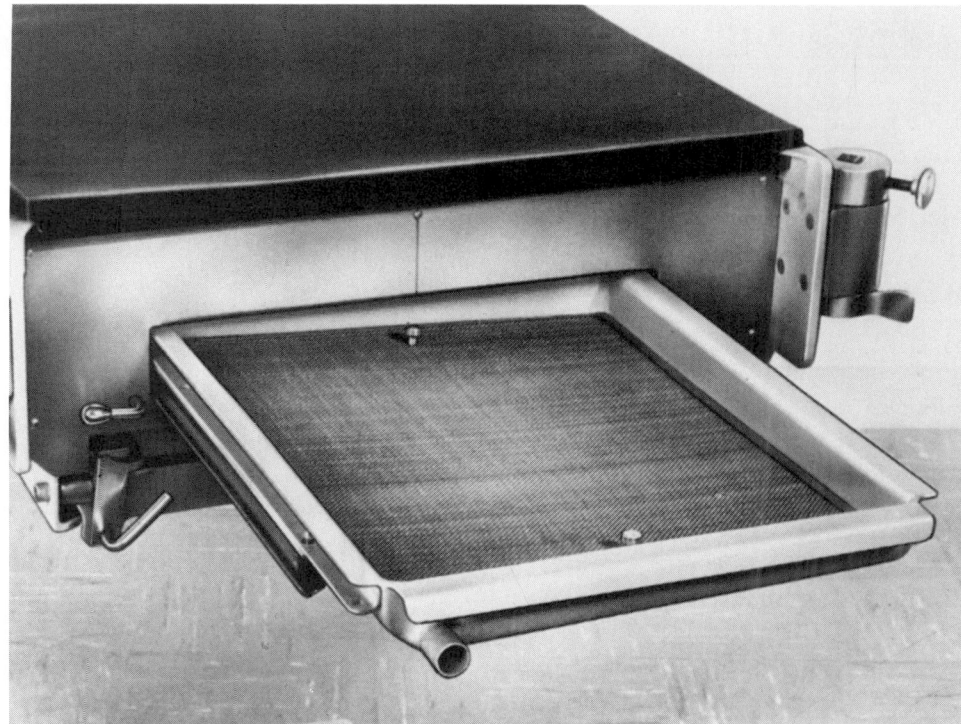

FIGURE 15-15   Screen over drainage drawer on cystoscopy bed.

space. They are especially beneficial for the patient who has limited hip mobility and altered peripheral circulatory status. Bilateral pedal pulses should be assessed preoperatively and postoperatively when using any stirrups. Care must be taken to adjust the stirrups so that there is no undue pressure on the calf.

After the patient is properly positioned, the bed may be tilted so that the patient's head is slightly higher than the buttocks to allow the prep solution to drain into the collecting pan. Pooling of solutions beneath the patient may cause skin reaction and severe irritation, as well as the potential for burns if an electrosurgical unit is used. If the cystoscopic procedure requires the use of an ESU, the dispersive pad is placed on the patient in direct contact with the skin as close to the operative site as practical and accessible to the circulating nurse, usually on the upper thigh. When placing the ESU pad, it is important to avoid hairy areas, bony prominences, scar tissue, and proximity to prosthetic metal implants or pacemakers.[1]

After properly positioning the patient, the nurse or urologist dons gloves and preps the entire pubic area, including the scrotum and perineum, with an antimicrobial solution. A screen is placed over the drainage pan on the cystoscopy bed (Fig. 15-15). Disposable draping systems with a sterile screen material incorporated into them are available. The patient is then draped to ensure that aseptic technique is maintained during the urologic procedure. If a general or spinal anesthetic is required, it is administered before prepping and draping. If a local anesthetic is preferred, it is instilled into the urethra of the male patient after prepping and draping but before instrumenta-

tion. For a female patient, a cotton applicator that has been dipped into the anesthetic solution is placed in the urethral meatus. Viscous lidocaine (Xylocaine), 1% or 2%, is usually used. If the patient is allergic to lidocaine, instillation of 50 to 60 ml of lubricant accompanied by anesthesia-monitored sedation is often adequate to afford painless access to the urethra and bladder. The patient should be informed that a sensation of pressure is to be expected.

The basic cystoscopy setup requires a cystoscopy pack, a sterile gown or apron, sterile gloves, a fiberoptic light source, a prep cup and solution, gauze sponges, the cystourethroscope (Fig. 15-16), a short bridge and fiberoptic light cord, lateral and Foroblique telescopes, a Luer-Lok stopcock, irrigation tubing and sterile water irrigant, and water-soluble lubricant. Additional items that should be sterile and available include a calibrated container to measure residual urine, test tubes with screwtops for urine specimens, an Albarran bridge and rubber catheter nipples or adapters, a medicine glass for dye, anesthetic solution, disposable 10 and 20 ml syringes, a penile clamp (to occlude male urethra after local anesthetic is instilled), contrast material, an ESU, a patient dispersive pad, and a Bugbee electrode.

The flexible cystoscope (Fig. 15-17) is used for patients with obstructive symptoms resulting from prostatic hyperplasia and rigid prostatic urethra. In addition, the flexible cystoscope can be used for patients who cannot assume a lithotomy position, such as those with spinal cord injuries or severe arthritis. Flexible cystoscopy may be accomplished with the use of a local anesthetic, although it is not usually necessary. It affords the patient a higher degree of

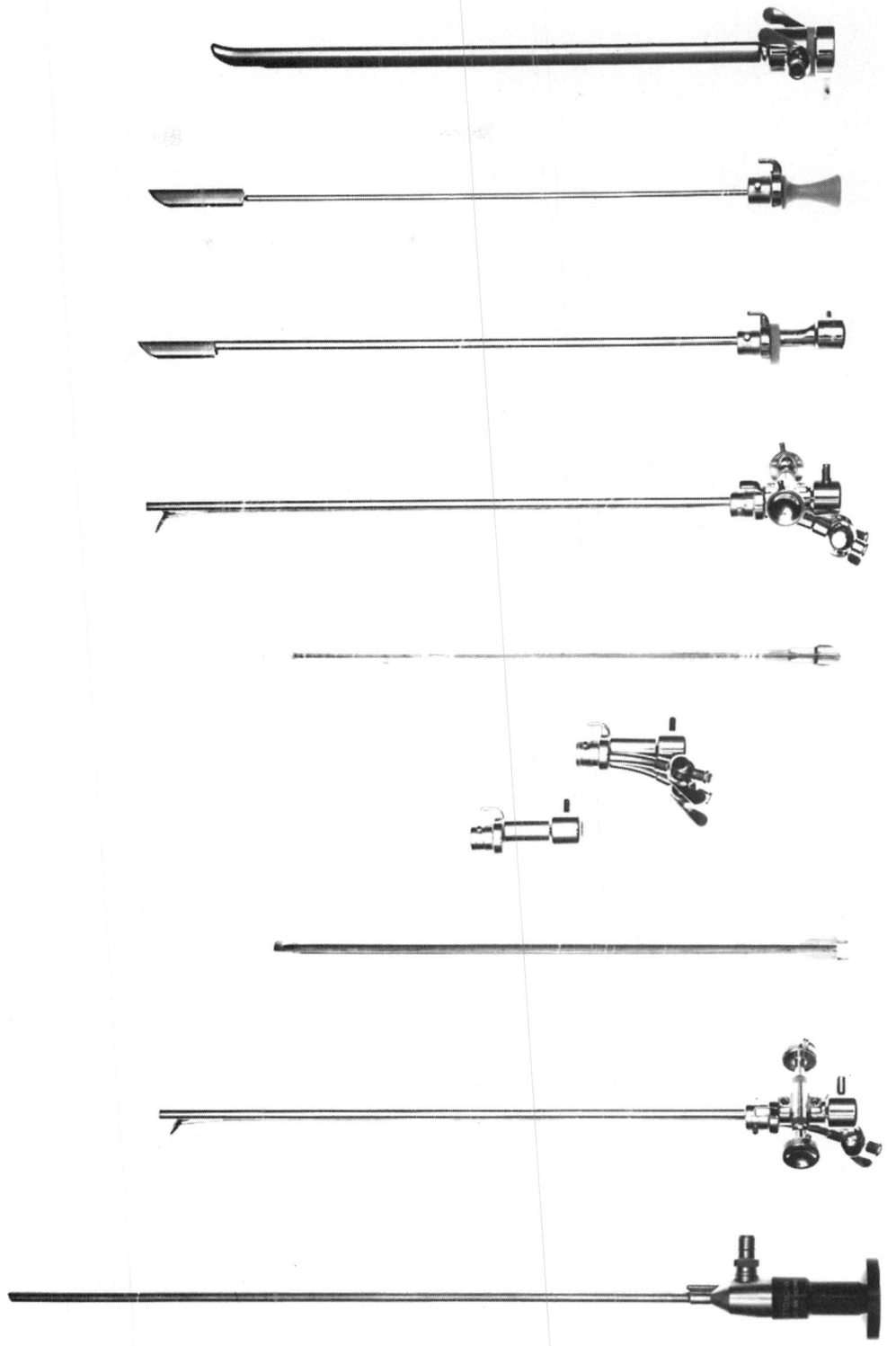

FIGURE 15–16 Instruments for cystoscopy, catheterization, and retrograde ureteral pyelography. *Top to bottom,* Cystoscope sheath, obturator, visual obturator, double-catheterizing Albarran bridge, double-catheterizing fin, double-catheterizing bridge, examining bridge, stationary deflector, operating Albarran bridge, telescope.

comfort, is less traumatic to the urethra, and can be performed in the patient's bed on the nursing unit.

Cleaning, sterilization, disinfection, and maintenance of endoscopic equipment are important procedures in the care of fiberoptic lensed instruments. Ultimately this process reduces costly repairs and ensures the availability of properly functioning instruments.

Protective padding should be placed on the countertop and on the bottom of the sink in the instrument decontamination area to prevent possible damage to lensed

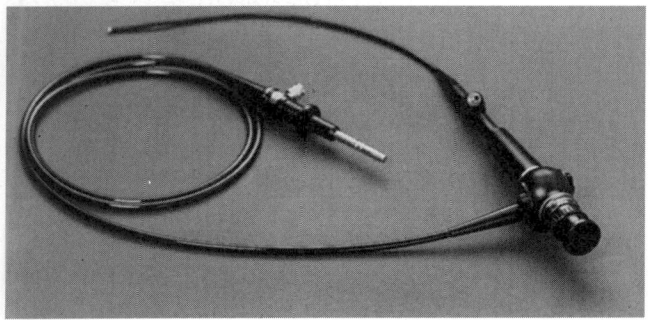

FIGURE 15-17 Flexible cystoscope.

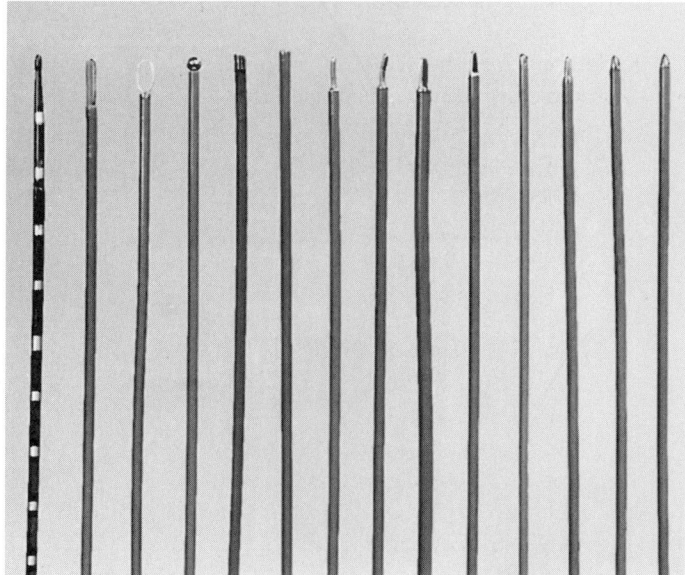

FIGURE 15-18 Flexible fulgurating electrode tips.

telescopes. After each surgical procedure, components of each cystoscopic set should be disassembled and washed in a solution of warm water and germicidal detergent with enzymatic action (breaks down proteins). All stopcocks and sheaths should be cleaned thoroughly with a soft brush to remove blood, dried lubricant jelly, or other debris. Instruments should then be thoroughly rinsed in warm water, placed on protective padding, and allowed to dry. Although warm water is appropriate for washing the instrumentation, lensed instruments should not be allowed to soak in warm water for too long. Lengthy soaking can cause the seals to loosen, allowing water to leak into the scope, resulting in cloudiness and bubbles. All moving parts must be individually evaluated for mobility. A lubricating-instrument milk solution may be applied as required. The patency of all outlets must be maintained to ensure proper sterilization or disinfection. Fiberoptic light cords must not be tangled, twisted, or sharply angulated because the fibers inside the cord are easily broken.

Endoscopy of the genitourinary tract is considered a class II (clean-contaminated) procedure and, according to CDC and APIC guidelines, presently requires disinfection rather than sterilization. High-level disinfection with an agent such as activated glutaraldehyde or dialdehyde that can destroy vegetative microorganisms, most fungal spores, tubercle bacilli, and small nonlipid viruses is recommended. In most situations, the routine of meticulous cleaning of endoscopic instruments and making sure that all channels are accessed, followed by appropriate high-level disinfection, provides reasonable assurance that the items are safe to use.[13] The level of disinfection is based on the contact time, temperature, and concentration of the active ingredients of the disinfectant, as well as the nature of microbial contamination. Many institutions are, however, treating endoscopic interventions as sterile procedures because the sterilization of instruments provides the greatest assurance that the risk of infections transmitted by contaminated instruments has been eliminated (see Chapter 4). Options available include glutaraldehyde (Cidex) solution, hydrogen peroxide solution (Sporox), a combination of peracetic acid and hydrogen peroxide (Peract 20), an ETO (ethylene oxide, "gas") sterilizer, a hydrogen peroxide or plasma sterilizing unit, and high-vacuum or gravity steam autoclaving for those components that may be sterilized in this manner. The manufacturer's recommendations should always be followed. If soaking is chosen, it is imperative that the instrumentation be thoroughly rinsed in sterile distilled water after immersion and before use.[4] Residue of Cidex remaining in the channels or on the lens can result in chemical burns for the patient and the surgeon. For sterilization or disinfection, instruments should be assembled on a covered tray and protected with padding. Because the lens system is delicate and costly, a plastic covering available from some manufacturers may be used to protect the lens. Various instrument manufacturers provide sterilization containers for endoscopy equipment and have written recommendations for the cleaning, sterilization, and disinfection of their equipment.

Stone removal, bladder biopsy, and bladder fulguration may be performed by using special cystoscopic accessories such as the Hendrickson-Bigelow lithotrite, which crushes large bladder calculi. This procedure is called a *litholapaxy*. Lowsley forceps, Wappler rigid cup forceps, and flexible foreign body forceps may also be employed. Bladder fulguration requires the use of flexible-stem electrodes available in various French sizes and tip configurations such as the ball, cone, dome, and bayonet (Fig. 15-18).

Operative procedure

1. After the urologist has scrubbed, gowned, and gloved, the fiberoptic light cord is connected to the light source and tested for proper intensity.
2. The irrigating system is set up, and, if required, the high-frequency cord is connected to an electrosurgical unit.
3. The cystourethroscope is lubricated and introduced into the urethra, the obturator withdrawn, and residual urine obtained, provided that the patient has voided

before the examination. The specimen may be saved for cultures or cytologic studies.

4. The cystourethroscope is connected to the irrigating system, and the telescope is inserted and locked in place. If the patient is awake, telling him or her to try to urinate also helps facilitate passage of the scope. The urologist controls the flow and volume of fluid by adjusting the stopcock on the scope. If difficulty is encountered during insertion, the visual obturator may be used to introduce the scope under direct vision. This accessory is constructed to smooth the fenestrated edges of the cystourethroscope. It requires the use of the telescope for direct vision and permits irrigation during introduction.

5. For retrograde ureteral catheterization and pyelography, ureteral catheters are passed through the cystoscope sheath and directed by the Albarran bridge deflector through the ureteral orifice and into the ureter. A radiopaque substance, such as 30% Renografin or 50% Hypaque, is then injected, and an x-ray film is taken to outline the entire upper urinary collecting system.

Periurethral–Transurethral Injection of Collagen

Collagen injection was developed as an outpatient procedure achievable under local anesthesia with or without sedation. Collagen (Contigen) consists of live bovine extract and is prepackaged in a sterile syringe of the collagen material. Female patients with intrinsic sphincter deficiency (ISD) demonstrated by urodynamic evaluation, and male patients (usually after prostatectomy) with incontinence lasting more than 1 year often benefit from this procedure. Other indications for collagen injection include stress urinary incontinence secondary to previous stricture treatment, trauma, or myelodysplasia.

Procedural considerations

Collagen must be kept under refrigeration and the FDA guidelines for its use and documentation followed. Patients selected for collagen injection must be skin tested with collagen 1 month before periurethral injection. A urine culture and sensitivity will be done approximately 10 days preoperatively. An alternative, somewhat less effective, but less costly approach is the injection of subcutaneous fat. Both procedures generally need to be repeated at periodic intervals over time. It is optimal to utilize a video system for the procedure. A basic cystoscopy set is required. The patient will generally be in lithotomy position.

Operative procedure

1. Urethral anesthetic is instilled and a perineal block of 1% or 2% lidocaine is injected. Cystoscopic examination is performed before collagen injection to rule out any associated findings. It is recommended that the irrigation be instilled by use of a pressure bag to minimize extravasation of the material by increasing the intraurethral pressure.

2. The injection needle provided by the manufacturer is introduced through the cystoscope and the tip placed, transurethrally, below the urethral mucosa, just distal to the bladder neck. In the female the needle provided is shorter and is introduced periurethrally. Positioning of the needle tip is accomplished when the surgeon sees the indentation of the urethra by the tip while he or she manipulates the needle.

3. Contigen is injected until the urothelium coapts in the midline, approximating the appearance of lateral lobe enlargement of the prostate. It may not be possible to achieve coaptation of the urothelium during the first injections; however it may be possible to do so on subsequent injections, once the pockets of collagen established originally have congealed and become compact.

4. The alternative technique is the injection of subcutaneous fat, aspirated under sterile technique much as in suction lipectomy. A large-bore needle or a suction lipectomy probe on a 50 to 60 ml syringe or Lukens trap is inserted into the lower abdomen subcutaneously after the application of an antiseptic prepping solution. The aspirated material is transferred to a 3 to 5 ml syringe and attached to a Williams injection needle. The same procedure is then carried out.

Transurethral Ureteropyeloscopy

Transurethral ureteropyeloscopy is an endoscopic examination of the ureters and renal pelvis. The use of rigid or flexible ureteroscopes or ureteropyeloscopes provides the opportunity to diagnose filling defects in the ureter and renal pelvis, congenital anomalies, hematuria, ureteral obstruction, and damage from trauma. Manipulation, fragmentation, basketing of ureteral and renal calculi, and retrieval of foreign bodies are possible with transurethral ureteropyeloscopy. Often ESWL, EHL, or sonic or laser lithotripsy accompanies the procedure. It may also be used to manage residual sludge and *Steinstrasse* (German for 'street of stones') after these treatments. ESWL and EHL are addressed in more detail later in the chapter.

Ureteral strictures may be treated transurethrally, and biopsies of tumors of the ureter and renal pelvis are performed under direct visualization. Internal ureteral stents may also be inserted for ureteral patency. These range in size from 3 to 8.5 Fr and are available in single J, double-J, and pigtail configurations.

Procedural considerations

The setup is similar to that for a cystoscopy with the addition of a rigid or flexible ureteroscope system (Fig. 15-19). A critical factor in this procedure is allowing enough time for careful dilatation of the ureter under C-arm fluoroscopy. The flexible ureteroscope has gained popularity because of its inherent tip mobility, which

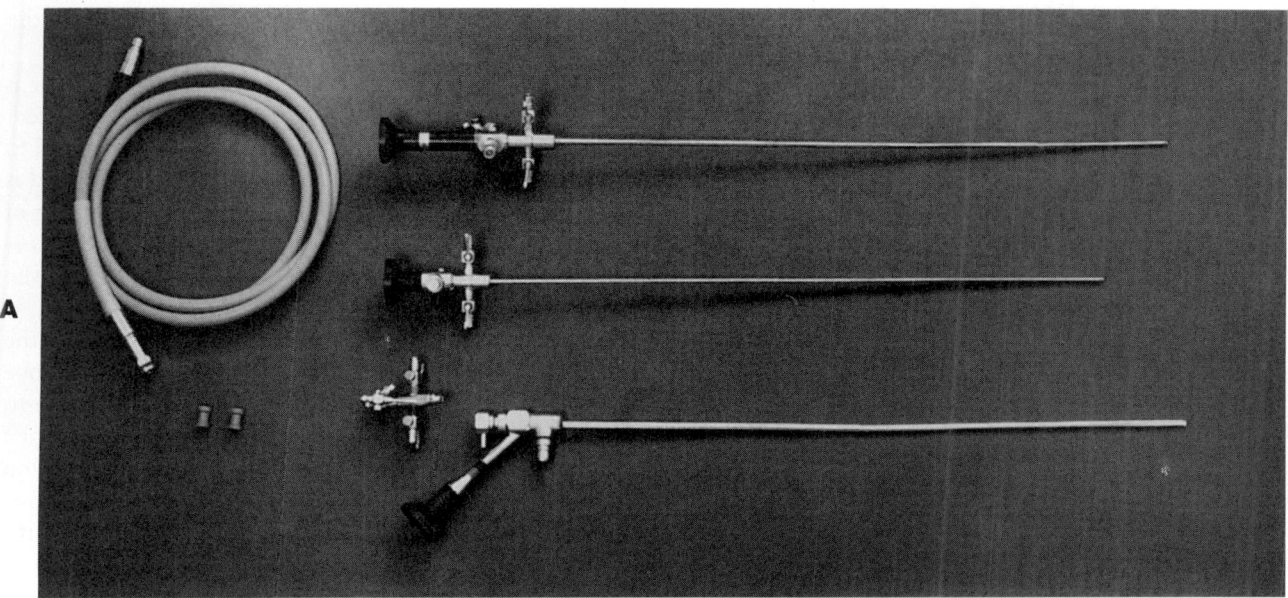

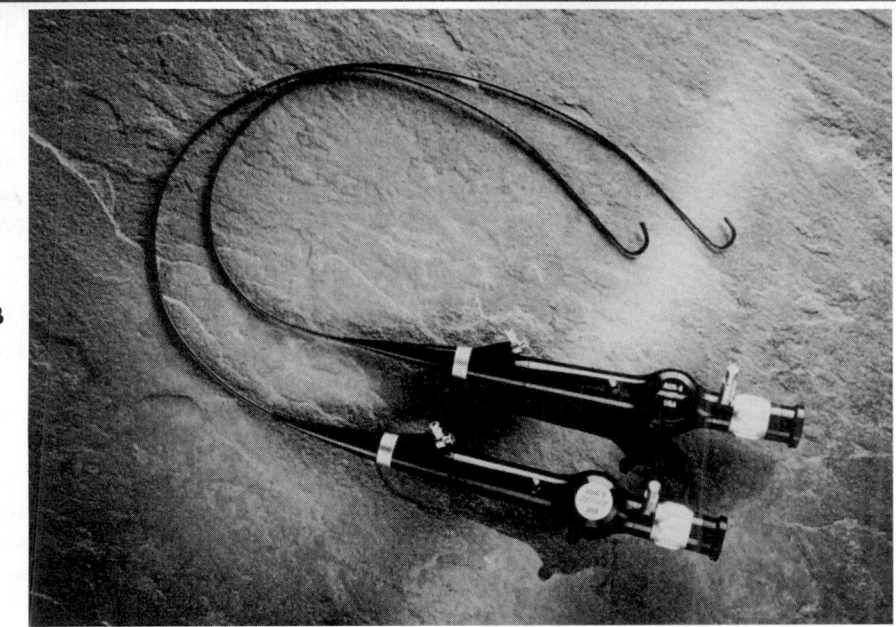

FIGURE 15-19 **A**, Rigid ureteroscope system. **B**, AUR8 and AUR9 flexible ureteropyeloscopes.

provides a more panoramic view of the entire circumference of the ureter. The perioperative nurse must be able to tilt the radiolucent operative bed at head and foot and laterally, as well as raise the bed.

In addition to the standard cystoscopy setup, the following items should be available: a rigid or flexible ureteroscope, ureteral dilators of graduated sizes and styles, size 3 to 5 Fr ureteral stone baskets of various styles, a ureteral grasping forceps, a ureteral biopsy forceps, a ureteral snare, ureteral scissors, ureteral catheters of various styles and sizes, ureteral stents, ureteral guidewires, ureteral balloon dilators, and radiographic contrast material.

Operative procedure

1. Once the ureteropyeloscope has been inserted, access to the ureter is gained when a guidewire is passed under fluoroscopic control. The ureter should be irrigated as the guidewire is advanced. The assistance of a scrub person to hold the wire on slight tension will allow for a smoother course of operation.

2. The ureter is dilated to 10 to 12 Fr with a balloon dilator or coaxial dilators. If a balloon dilator is chosen, the balloon should be inflated with contrast material and a pressure syringe to ensure that it not exceed the maximum allowable ATM (burst pressure).

3. A working guidewire to be used as a safety wire is placed in addition to the initial guidewire.

4. The ureteroscope is passed over the working guidewire to the location of interest. Biopsy of suspicious lesions, diagnostic pyeloscopy, and ureteroscopy is performed. The characteristics of calculi are observed to determine the best treatment approach. Urine may be obtained for

cytologic and microbiologic examination. If a calculus is small enough to be delivered through the ureter, it is engaged in a retrieval basket and removed under visual as well as fluoroscopic control. If, after ureteral dilatation, the calculus does not appear to be small enough for delivery, lithotripsy (fragmentation) must be performed through the ureteroscope, or ESWL may be performed later. Lithotripsy may be performed with the ultrasonic (through a rigid ureteroscope) or electrohydraulic lithotriptors, or with the pulse-dyed or holmium:YAG lasers. Appropriate laser precautions must be enforced. Chapter 3 discusses laser safety issues in more depth.

5. After the completion of the procedure, the ureter is assessed for integrity (perforation or laceration) with retrograde pyelography. A ureteral stent is placed over the remaining safety guidewire, and the guidewire is removed.

SURGERY OF THE PENIS AND THE URETHRA

Laser Ablation of Condylomas and Penile Carcinoma

Laser ablation of condylomas or penile cancer is the eradication of diseased tissue by means of a laser beam. Laser therapy has been determined, through clinical trials, to be effective therapy for condylomas and penile cancers that are refractory to other treatments. One of the major advantages of the laser is that heat is distributed evenly to the tissue underlying the lesion. When any laser is being used, precautions appropriate to that system must be initiated (see Chapter 3).

Procedural considerations

Laser treatment may be performed successfully with a local infiltration of anesthetic. A U-shaped craterlike lesion of predetermined depth with a 2 mm radius can be created. A power setting ranging from 2 to 20 W on continuous or superpulse mode is commonly used. With laser ablation less edema and necrosis occur, fibrosis is minimized, and rapid healing is facilitated. The argon, CO_2, KTP, and Nd:YAG lasers are all suitable for this therapeutic application.

Operative procedure

1. The operator moves the beam transversely across the tissue and then in a crosshatch matrix, thereby treating all perimeters of the lesion. Periodically the area should be wiped with a sponge moistened in acetic acid (3% to 5% vinegar). This treatment causes diseased tissue to stand out and allows therapy to deeper layers.
2. Postoperatively the affected areas may be coated with an antibiotic ointment. Wounds are generally left uncovered. A mild oral pain medication is usually adequate for postoperative discomfort.

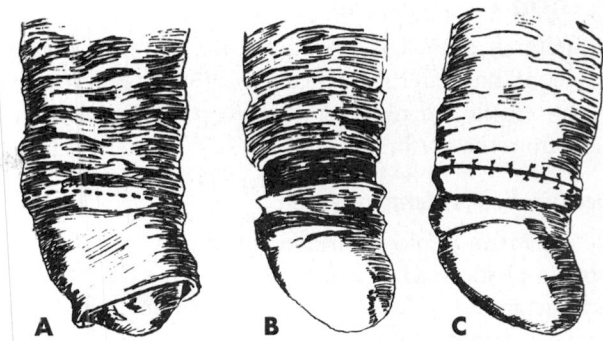

FIGURE 15-20 Circumcision.

Circumcision

Circumcision is the excision of the foreskin (prepuce) of the glans penis. Circumcision in adult males is performed for the relief of phimosis, a condition in which the orifice of the prepuce is stenosed or too narrow to permit easy retraction behind the glans. Another condition, balanoposthitis, results in an inflamed glans and mucous membrane with purulent discharge and may require circumcision. In addition, circumcision may be done to prevent recurrent paraphimosis, a condition in which the prepuce cannot be reduced easily from a retracted position. (See Chapter 29 for pediatric considerations during circumcision.)

Procedural considerations

The patient is placed in the supine position. A plastic or minor instrument set and a local anesthetic with IV sedation is sufficient. The ESU should be available.

Operative procedure

1. If the prepuce is adherent, a probe or hemostat may be used to break up adhesions. The prepuce is clamped in the dorsal midline and incised toward the coronal margin (Fig. 15-20, A), leaving about 5 cm of coronal mucosa intact.
2. A similar procedure is performed ventrally. The two incisions are then joined circumferentially. Alternatively, a superficial, circumferential incision is made in the skin with a scalpel at the level of the coronal sulcus and the mucosa at the base of the glans.
3. The redundant skin is undermined between the circumferential incisions and removed as a complete cuff (Fig. 15-20, B).
4. Bleeding vessels are coagulated or clamped with mosquito hemostats and tied with fine absorbable ligatures.
5. Before closure, the area may be cleansed with an appropriate antiseptic solution.
6. The raw edges of the skin incision are approximated to a coronal cuff of mucosal prepuce, generally with 4-0 or 5-0 absorbable sutures on atraumatic, plastic cutting, or fine gastrointestinal needles (Fig. 15-20, C).
7. The wound is usually dressed with petrolatum gauze.

Excision of Urethral Caruncle

A urethral caruncle is a benign lesion or inflammatory prolapse of the external urinary meatus in the female. Excision entails the removal of these papillary or sessile tumors from the urethra.

Procedural considerations

The patient is placed in the lithotomy position. A minor or plastic set, an electrosurgical unit, and a local anesthetic are used. A urethral catheter of an appropriate size may be required if the distal urethral prolapse is severe.

Operative procedure

1. With a small, fine-tipped Metzenbaum or plastic scissors the tumor is exposed and excised within a wedge of ventral urethral tissue.
2. Figure-of-eight 4-0 absorbable sutures at the edge of the incision are usually sufficient to achieve good hemostasis.

Urethral Meatotomy

Urethral meatotomy is an incisional enlargement of the external urethral meatus to relieve congenital or acquired stenosis or stricture at the external meatus.

Procedural considerations

A male patient is placed in the supine position. Prepping and draping are as described for urethral catheterization. For a female patient the lithotomy position is used. Local anesthesia is generally employed. A plastic instrument set is required.

Operative procedure

1. A straight hemostat is placed on the ventral surface of the meatus.
2. An incision is made along the frenulum to enlarge the opening and overcome the stricture. Bleeding vessels are clamped and ligated with fine absorbable sutures.
3. The mucosal layer is sutured to the skin with fine absorbable sutures. A dressing of petrolatum gauze may be applied.

Urethral Dilatation and Internal Urethrotomy

Urethral dilatation and internal urethrotomy entail the gradual dilatation and lysis of a urethral stricture to provide relief of distal lower urinary tract obstruction. Urethral strictures or narrowing of the urethra may be caused by a congenital malformation that is usually found at the external urinary meatus. Infection or trauma may also contribute to stricture of the membranous and pendulous urethra. Urethral stricture disease may be treated by periodic dilatation with Phillips filiforms and followers, Van Buren sounds, and balloon dilatation catheters.

Procedural considerations

The male patient may be placed in a supine position for routine urethral dilatation and in lithotomy position for other procedures. Prepping and draping are as required for male catheterization. A local anesthetic such as viscous lidocaine (Xylocaine) should be used. The female patient is placed in the lithotomy position. A cotton-tipped applicator dipped into the local anesthetic or a urethral syringe filled with anesthetic is placed in the urethral opening. Female urethral dilatation is performed with short, straight metal dilators or with hollow McCarthy dilators. The latter allows a urine specimen to be obtained.

In addition to a cystoscopy setup required instrumentation includes urethrotomes (Fig. 15-21), the resectoscope working element with sheath, obturator, and cold knives, urethral dilators, Phillips filiforms and followers, Van Buren sounds, and a silicone Foley catheter.

Operative procedures
Gradual Dilatation

1. In a male patient the urethra is lubricated and anesthetized with a viscous anesthetic that is instilled into the urethra with a urethral or Uro-Jet syringe. A penile clamp occludes the penile urethra at the coronal sulcus and keeps the anesthetic within the urethra.
2. Phillips filiforms of various tips and sizes are introduced first in an attempt to pass an instrument beyond the urethral stricture. Followers of increasing size are connected to the filiforms and passed through the strictured portion of the urethra, stretching the scarred area (Fig. 15-22).
3. Slow dilatation is also achieved with a small catheter or follower left in the urethra. It leads to softening of the stricture over the course of several days. Before use or sterilization, the filiforms and followers should be carefully inspected for damaged or weak points, particularly around the scored-threaded end.

Internal Urethrotomy

1. The assembled visualizing urethrotome is inserted under direct vision into the urethra.
2. When necessary, a filiform or ureteral catheter is fed into the catheterizing channel to help identify the patent portion of the urethra.
3. The urethrotome is advanced to the desired position, and the blade is used to incise the urethral scar. The normal urethra must be incised 1 cm proximally and distally beyond the stricture to achieve optimum results.
4. A silicone Foley catheter is usually left in place for 3 to 5 days after surgery.

Urethroplasty

Urethroplasty is reconstructive surgery of the urethra for strictures, urethral fractures, or narrowing of the urethral lumen that are congenital, inflammatory, or traumatic in origin. Urethral grafts are generally required

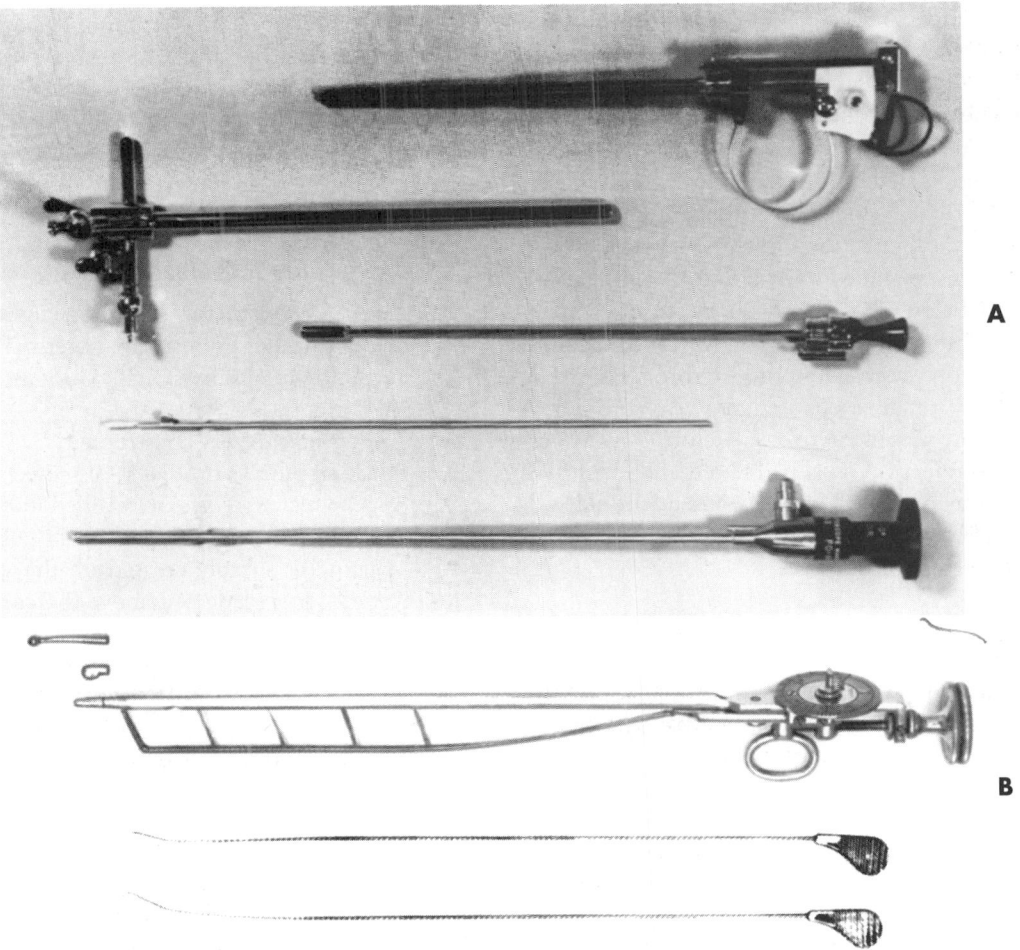

FIGURE 15-21 **A**, Circon Corporation internal urethrotome components. **B**, Otis urethrotome components.

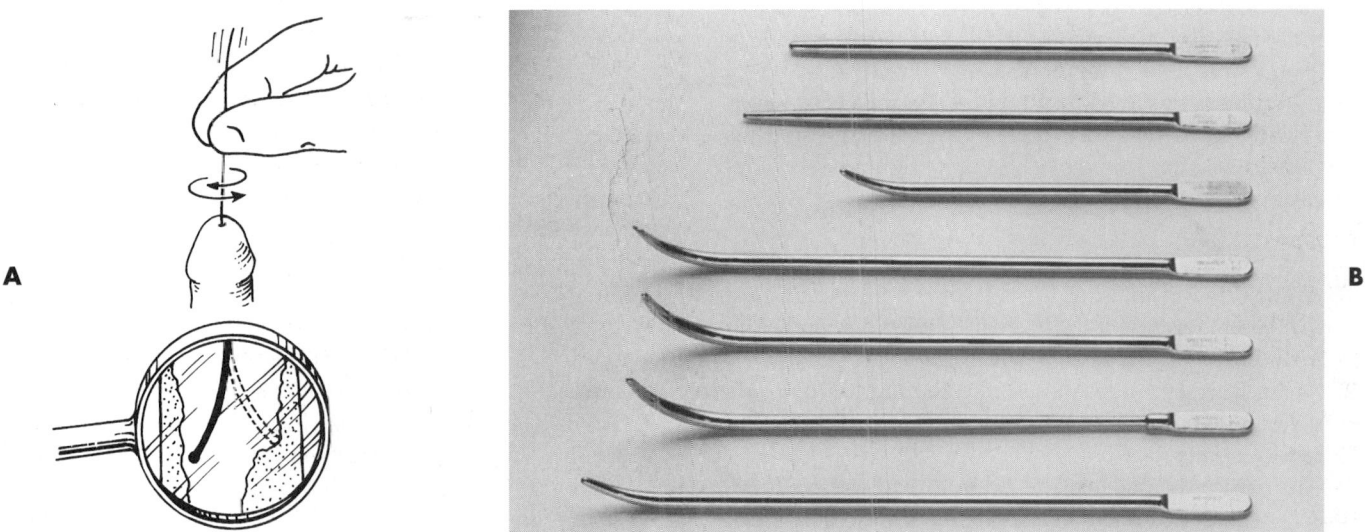

FIGURE 15-22 **A**, Method of using couce-tipped bougie for passing stricture. **B**, Variety of urethral sounds (dilators).

and may include free skin grafts and mobilized vascular flaps. There are many combinations of these procedures, and in all of them some type of temporary urinary diversion may be used, depending on the location and severity of the condition.

Evaluation preoperatively is initiated from the patient's complaint of obstructive symptoms, frequently associated with a urinary tract infection. Techniques utilized to determine diagnosis include urodynamics (voiding pressures above and below the site of obstruction), urinary flow cytometry, intravenous urography (IVU) to rule out an upper tract lesion, cystoscopy, and urethrography. The length and density of diseased urethra is determined to plan the appropriate reconstructive procedure. Any associated urinary tract infection must be treated and eradicated before surgical intervention. Definitive repair should wait for 10 to 12 weeks after diagnostic instrumentation until the inflammatory reaction subsides.

Procedural considerations

The patient is placed in the exaggerated lithotomy position. Routine prepping and draping procedures are employed with precautions for protecting the anus (that is, the use of an impervious plastic adherent drape). The setup includes a minor instrument set with fine plastic instruments for dissection and plastic repair. Strictures may be located deep, requiring fiberoptic lighting. An ESU may be required.

Operative procedures
Johanson Urethroplasty

The Johanson urethroplasty is a two-stage procedure, for severe urethral stricture disease, to repair and reconstruct the urethra. Approximately 3 months after the first stage, if the operative site is healing and the patient is voiding adequately, a second-stage procedure is performed. Vascularized flaps of preputial or penile skin may be mobilized to the ventrum by leaving them attached to the outer surface of the prepuce or as an island flap. One modification is the transverse preputial island flap neourethra with glans channel positioning for the meatus. Preputial skin is preferred because of its rich reliable blood supply and non–hair bearing characteristics.

First-stage

1. An inverted U incision is made in the perineum from the inner borders of the ischial tuberosities up to and including the base of the scrotum.
2. A Van Buren sound is passed into the urethra up to the stricture. The bulbocavernosus muscle is dissected and retracted laterally.
3. An incision is made in the urethra over the strictured area and is extended in each direction at least 1 cm beyond the diseased area. The abnormal scar tissue is excised or simply incised, because scrotal skin ultimately increases the lumen.

4. A #28 sound is passed through both the proximal and the distal urethral lumens to rule out further stricture.
5. The remaining urethral mucosa is sutured with 4-0 absorbable suture to the scrotal skin.
6. A cystotomy tube to divert the urinary stream may be left indwelling and removed in 5 to 7 days.

Second-stage (mobilized vascular flap)

1. A red rubber catheter is temporarily inserted into the bladder through the proximal urethral stoma.
2. The penoscrotal skin is incised longitudinally, adjacent to the urethra.
3. A new urethra is constructed by developing the ventral preputial skin that is dissected free and fanned out. The rectangle of skin is rolled into the neourethra and measured.
4. A channel is sharply created on the ventral aspect of the glans, in a plane just above the corpora.
5. The glans tissue is removed forming a groove approximately 14 Fr in diameter.
6. Layers of subcutaneous tissue are dissected free from the dorsal penile skin to create an island flap that is spiraled to the ventrum. The flaps are brought together in the midline and closed with a continuous or interrupted 4-0 absorbable suture.
7. The neourethra is anastomosed proximally to the urethra and carried to the tip of the glans.
8. The dorsal penile flaps are transposed laterally to the midline, and excess skin is excised.
9. Closure is with 4-0 absorbable interrupted mattress sutures around the glans and down the penile shaft. A bulky pressure dressing is applied.
10. Suprapubic cystostomy drainage is an option, but a urethral catheter usually suffices.

Horton-Devine Urethroplasty (Urethral Patch Graft)

Urethral patch graft is a one-stage operative procedure that incorporates a free skin graft to correct a urethral stricture. Free skin grafts should be at full thickness. Since the free graft must be revascularized, it is important that it have a perfect skin cover of dorsal, preputial, penile skin that is well vascularized. This type of graft is generally used with a one-stage repair.

1. A 17 Fr panendoscope is passed into the posterior urethra, and a #20 urethral dilator is passed into the posterior urethra.
2. A perineal vertical midline incision is made into the urethral lumen. The panendoscope is reinserted, and the incision is examined to determine if it crossed the stricture.
3. The defect is measured, and a circumferential incision is made on the posterior penile shaft to harvest an oval piece of skin the size of the defect.

4. The epidermal side of the graft is defatted, and absorbable sutures of 4-0 are placed at the apex and base.

5. The apex is sutured into position at the proximal and distal ends of the stricture with the epidermal side toward the urethral lumen.

6. The graft is anastomosed proximally to the urethra with the suture line of the graft next to the corpus. The middle glans dart is fixed to the corpus. The graft is formed into a neourethra over a Silastic stenting catheter.

7. The panendoscope is again inserted, and the urethra is irrigated to check for suture-line leaks.

8. A Foley or fenestrated catheter is inserted to serve as a stent.

9. The corpora spongiosum is approximated and closed over the patched area as a separate layer with interrupted 3-0 absorbable sutures. Subcutaneous 4-0 absorbable sutures are placed.

10. The skin and the graft site are closed with interrupted 4-0 sutures.

11. A suprapubic catheter is inserted to divert urine for healing. Petrolatum gauze is wrapped around the penis and covered with gauze sponges and fluffed dressings. A scrotal supporter is applied to provide support and pressure.

Insertion of a Urolume Endoprosthesis

The Urolume endoprosthesis is a braided wire-meshed implant intended to relieve urinary obstruction distal to the external sphincter and proximal to the bulbar scrotal junction (Fig. 15-23, A). It is an alternative for men with stricture disease secondary to bulbar urethral strictures less than 3 cm in length where other treatments have failed. The prosthesis should not be used in patients at significant risk for bleeding. The device has also been beneficial in the treatment of men suffering from prostatic obstruction as a result of BPH.

Procedural considerations

The patient is placed in the lithotomy position. Routine prepping and draping procedures are employed with precautions for protecting the anus (that is, the use of an impervious plastic adherent drape). The setup includes urethral sounds or filiforms and followers, urethrotomy instrumentation, a 12 Fr 0- to 12-degree telescope, an irrigation setup, a 17 or 21 Fr cystoscope, the urethra measuring catheter, and the Urolume endoprosthesis kit. An ESU may be required.

Postvoid dribbling, pain, and hematuria are common during the first few weeks after the procedure. Transurethral instrumentation and sexual activities must be avoided for approximately 6 to 8 weeks postoperatively.

Operative procedure

1. A diagnostic cystoscopy is performed to visualize the site of the stricture.

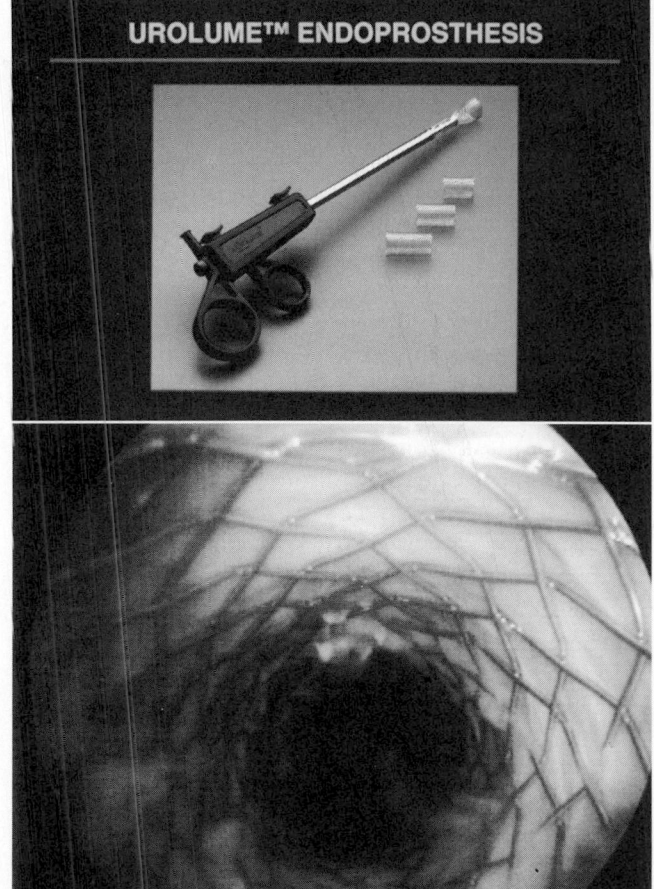

FIGURE 15-23 **A**, Urolume endoprosthesis and inserter. **B**, Urolume in urethra.

2. The stricture length is measured, and a prosthesis that is 1 cm longer than the measured length is selected.

3. The Urolume deployment system is prepared according to the manufacturer's guidelines.

4. The stricture is then opened by means of dilatation or a 3-incision internal urethrotomy to a minimum diameter of 26 Fr.

5. The delivery instrument is positioned approximately 5 mm proximal to the stricture.

6. The prosthesis is exposed and, after confirmation of its position, is released to cover the entire length of the stricture without covering the external sphincter (Fig. 15-23, B). More than one stent may be placed.

7. A suprapubic catheter may be placed to facilitate voiding during the initial recovery period.

8. Prophylactic antibiotics are provided postoperatively.

Penectomy

Penectomy is the partial or total removal of a cancerous penis. The procedure selected depends on the extent of involvement and disease stage. Invasive penile cancer not suited for irradiation because of its size, depth, or location is best dealt with by penectomy. Excision of a 2 cm gross tumor margin is adequate for local management. Partial penectomy may afford a sufficient length for directable and upright urination. At least 3 cm of viable proximal shaft is necessary for consideration of a partial penectomy. If the residual stump is inadequate in length, detachment and mobilization of the suspensory ligaments may be an option in selected patients. A total penectomy is generally required when tumor margins are beyond a 2 cm retrievable length from the penoscrotal junction.

Options are available to limit the extent of the disfiguring surgery previously indicated for penile cancer. Chemotherapy agents, often combined with irradiation, are proving effective in shrinking penile carcinomas that would have previously mandated radical penectomy. Bleomycin, usually combined with irradiation, is showing great success in patients with known metastasis. Methotrexate is another relatively new and effective agent. A third therapy involves the use of cisplatin.

Reconstruction is possible after penectomy. Evaluation must take into account sexual, urinary, and cosmetic factors. Extensive or proximally invasive lesions that include the scrotum, perineum, abdominal wall, and pubis necessitate emasculation as well as expanded resection of involved tissues.

Procedural considerations

The setup necessary is similar to that for any inguinal surgery, with the addition of a medium Penrose drain for use as a tourniquet.

Operative procedures
Partial Penectomy

1. The lesion is excluded by a towel attached to the planned amputation line. A penile tourniquet is applied at the base (Fig. 15-24, A).
2. After circumferential skin incision, the cavernous bodies are divided to the urethra with a 2 cm gross margin (Fig. 15-24, B).
3. Dorsal vessels are ligated, margins of the tunica albuginea are approximated, and the urethra is dissected proximally and distally (spatulated) to obtain a 1 cm redundant flap (Fig. 15-24, C).
4. Without sacrificing the tumor margin, the urethra is then divided. Interrupted sutures are placed on the opposite margins of the tunica albuginea to secure the corpora. The tourniquet is removed, and hemostasis is achieved.
5. After the dorsal urethrotomy, a skin-to-urethra anastomosis is performed. The redundant skin flap is then dorsally approximated (Fig. 15-24, D).
6. A small urinary catheter is inserted, and a nonadherent dressing is applied. They are generally removed in 3 or 4 days.

Total Penectomy

1. A vertical elliptic incision is made around the penile base (Fig. 15-25, A).

2. The distal urethra and its ventral traction are divided through an incision in Buck's fascia, mobilizing the urethra and aiding its dissection, which extends from the corpora to the bulbar region.
3. The corpora are then separated and ligated (Fig. 15-25, B). The suspensory ligaments and dorsal vessels are divided as corporal dissection is carried out.
4. The urethra is transsected from the corpora (Fig. 15-25, C).
5. An ellipse of skin approximately 1 cm in size is taken from the perineal area. A tunnel is fashioned in the perineal subcutaneous layer of tissue. A traction suture through the tunnel, at the penile base, aids dissection for transposition of the urethra to the perineum (Fig. 15-25, D).
6. The urethra is grasped with forceps and transferred to the perineum. The urethra is spatulated, and a skin-to-urethra anastomosis is performed through a buttonhole incision in the perineum (Fig. 15-25, E).
7. The primary incision is closed horizontally, elevating the scrotum away from the urethral opening (Fig. 15-25, F).
8. A urinary catheter is inserted, and the wound is covered with a nonadherent dressing.

Penile Implant

A penile prosthesis is implanted for treatment of organic sexual impotence. Sexual impotence may be caused by (1) diabetes mellitus, (2) priapism, (3) Peyronie's disease, (4) penile trauma, (5) pelvic surgery, (6) neurologic disease (in selected cases), (7) vascular disease, (8) hypertension, and (9) idiopathic impotence (in carefully screened patients). The penile implant serves as a stent to enable vaginal penetration for sexual intercourse.

Procedural considerations

Spinal or general anesthesia is required. The patient is placed in either the supine or lithotomy position. Routine skin prepping and draping are carried out. To prevent urethral injury and potential urinary retention, a 14 or 16 Fr Foley catheter may be inserted to identify the urethra intraoperatively. The ESU may be required. Often, a penile block is instilled intraoperatively, before the incision, into the corpus cavernosum and the incisional sites. This enables the surgeon to evaluate erectile size and provides some postoperative pain management.

A separate sterile Mayo stand or small table covered with a plastic drape is generally set up for the implants. It is recommended that the implants not be in contact with paper or cloth, which may shed fiber particles.

The instrument setup includes a minor set with fine instruments, plus Hegar dilators, the penile prosthesis of choice (Fig. 15-26), the Furlow inserter (Fig. 15-27, A and B), the closing tool (Fig. 15-27, C), the assembly tool for clamping connectors (Fig. 15-28, A), and the connectors of choice (Fig. 15-28, B). Medications needed in the operative field include 50 ml of 1% lidocaine, 150 ml of

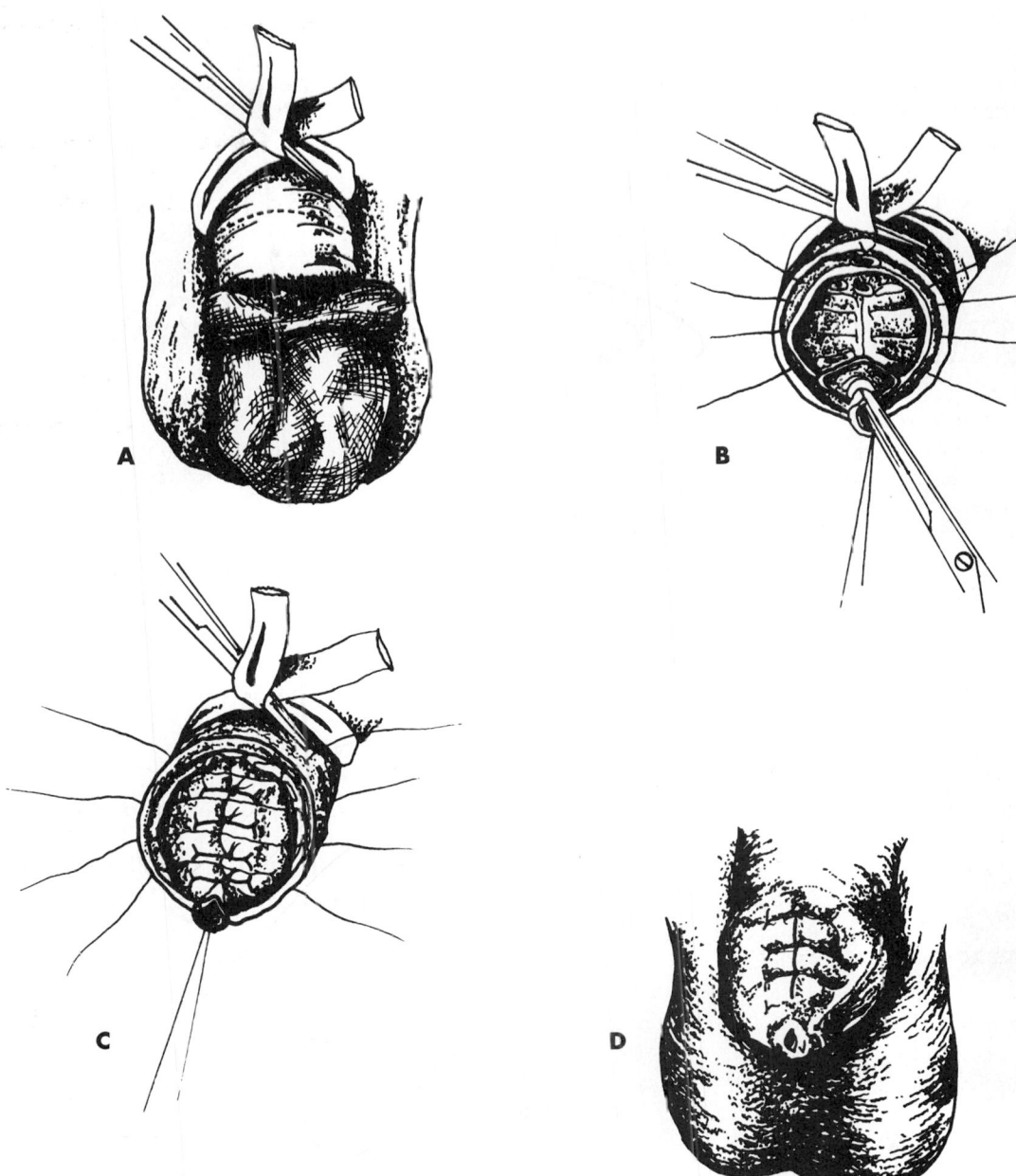

FIGURE 15-24 Partial penectomy.

injectable 0.9% normal saline, 1 ml of methylene blue, 2 ml of papaverine, 50 ml of 0.5% bupivacaine (Marcaine) or 1% etidocaine (Duranest), 50,000 U of bacitracin, and 80 mg of kanamycin.

A serious complication to a penile implant is infection. Meticulous aseptic technique and careful draping are essential. The sterile team should be double gloved throughout the procedure. Some surgeons coat their hands with Betadine (povidone-iodine complex) just before donning sterile gloves. A 5-minute Betadine scrub of the operative area is critical in reducing skin flora. The anus should be isolated in the perineal approach. Intraoperatively and before insertion of the implant components, a prophylactic antibiotic irrigant of bacitracin and kanamy-cin in normal saline is used on the implants and in the insertion sites. Systemic antibiotics may also be required. As with any implant procedure, it is vital to maintain an environment conducive to infection prevention. Traffic in and out of the room should be minimized.

Operative procedures

Implantation of Noninflatable (Semirigid) Prosthesis

1. A midline incision is made from the base of the penis into the scrotum for approximately 3 cm. Some surgeons may choose a suprapubic or dorsal penile approach.

2. The tunica albuginea is incised over the most proximal

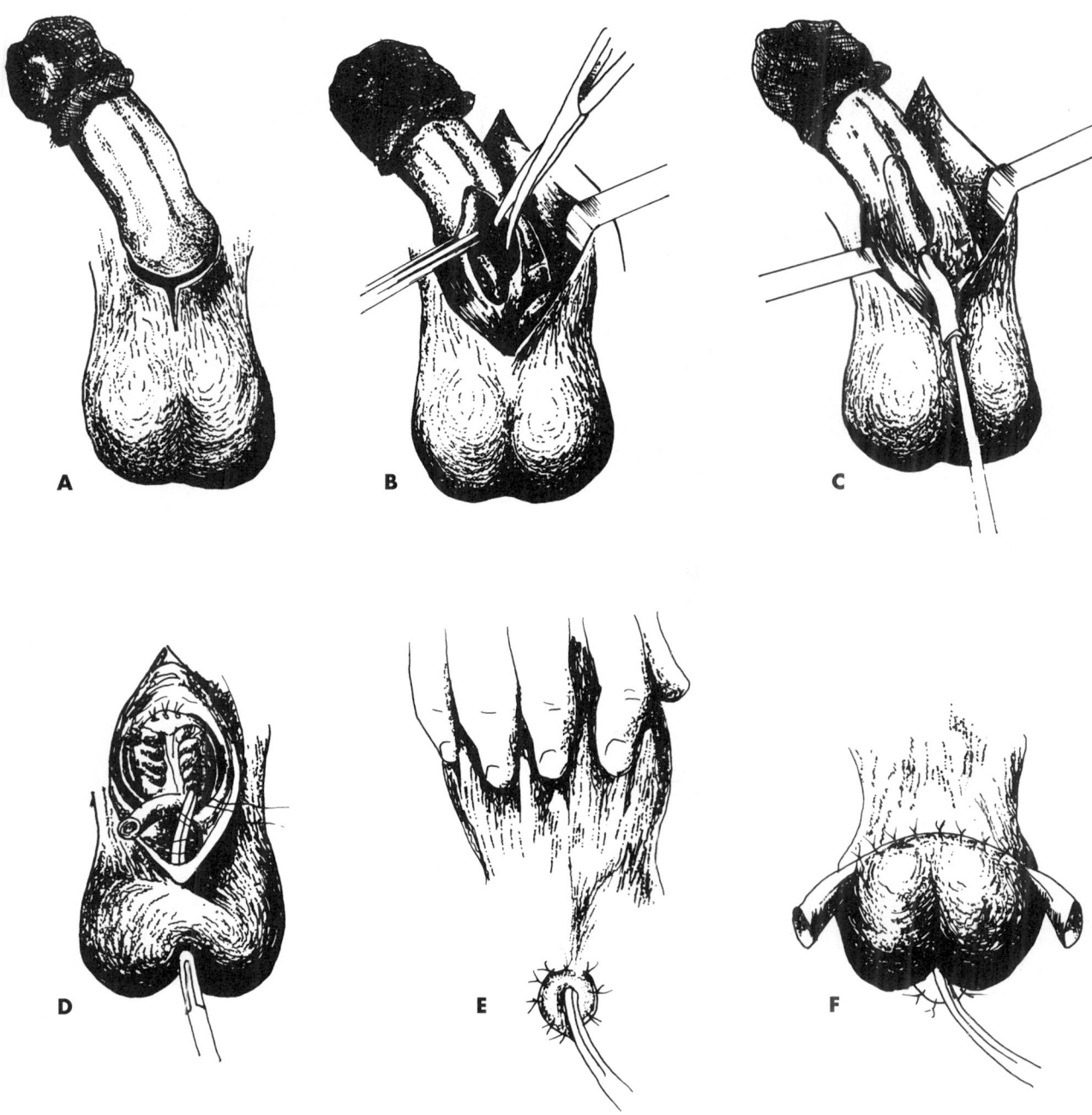

FIGURE 15-25 Total penectomy.

portion of the corpora in a longitudinal manner, and stay sutures are placed.

3. The corpora are dilated proximally and distally with 7 to 11 mm Hegar dilators. Care must be taken to not perforate the urethra.

4. Measurements of the entire corporal length are taken with the Furlow inserter or sizing instrument.

5. After placement of the closure sutures, the prostheses are inserted into the corpora. Proper placement is evident immediately by a change in the configuration of the penis with no buckling of the glans.

6. The tunica albuginea is then closed with the previously

placed 2-0 absorbable continuous suture; 3-0 or 4-0 absorbable interrupted sutures are used for skin closure.

7. Petrolatum gauze or 2-inch Kling tube gauze may be used for the dressing.

8. A Foley catheter is inserted, and the amount and color of urine are noted. Some surgeons divert the urine intraoperatively.

Implantation of Inflatable Prosthesis

1. A midline incision is made from the base of the penis into the scrotum for approximately 3 cm (Fig. 15-29, *A*).

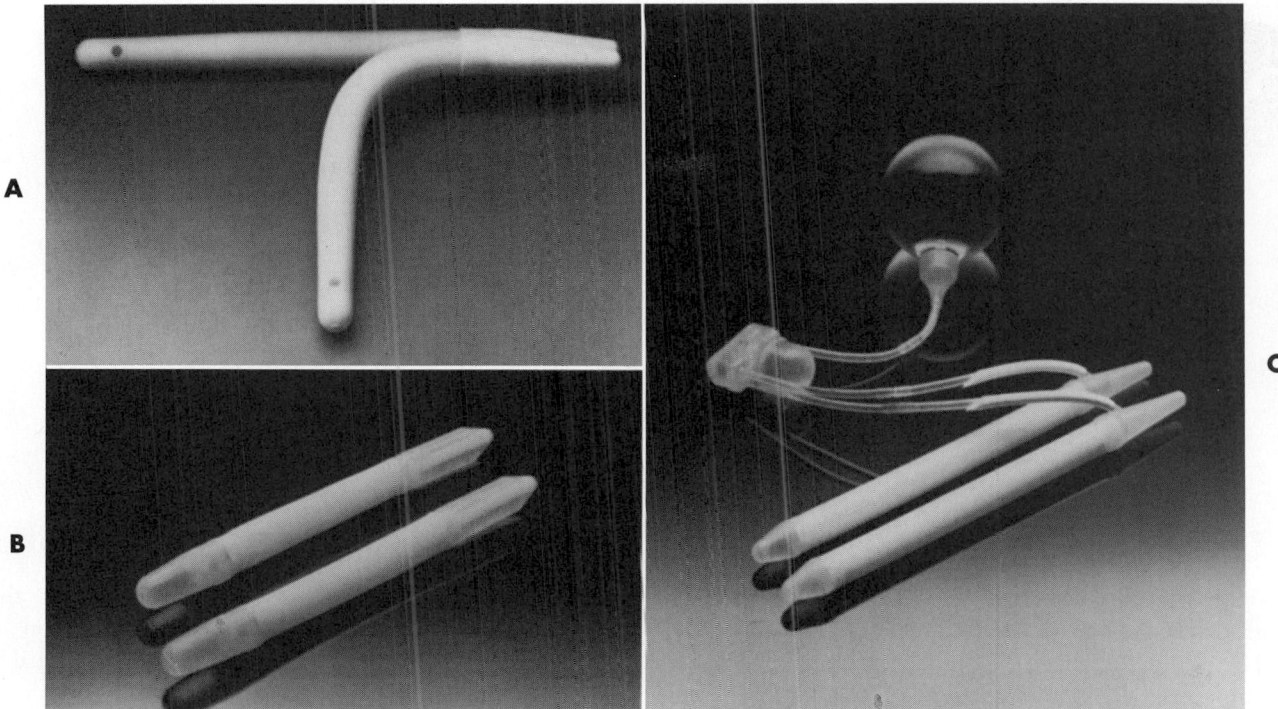

FIGURE 15-26   **A**, AMS malleable 600 penile prosthesis. **B**, AMS Hydroflex penile prosthesis. **C**, AMS 700CX inflatable penile prosthesis.

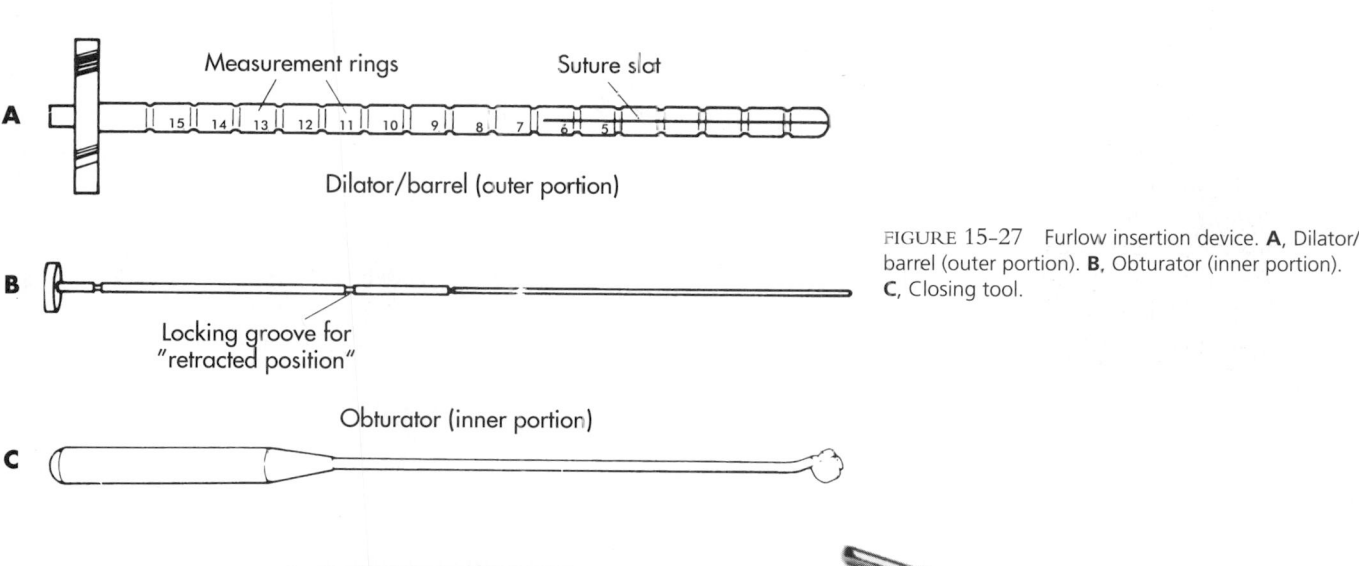

FIGURE 15-27   Furlow insertion device. **A**, Dilator/barrel (outer portion). **B**, Obturator (inner portion). **C**, Closing tool.

2. A Foley catheter is inserted to identify and retract the urethra out of the operative field.
3. The tunica albuginea of each corpus is incised in the most proximal portion, and stay sutures are placed.
4. The corpora are dilated distally and proximally with 7 to 11 mm Hegar dilators.
5. The Furlow inserter is used for measuring the entire corporal length.
6. Corporal sutures of 2-0 absorbable material are placed along the tunica incision, left uncut with needle attached, and tagged.
7. The cylinders are packaged with attached traction sutures at the distal end. These are placed through the

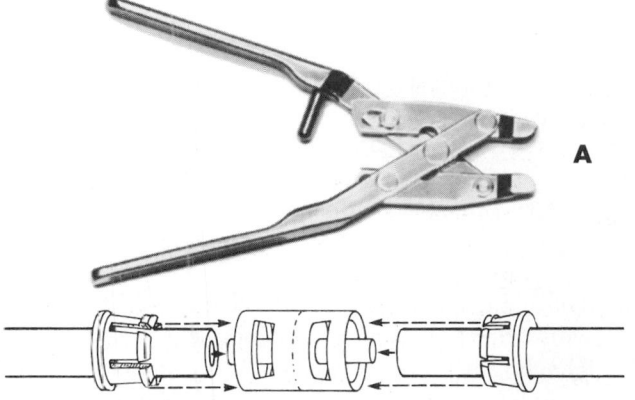

FIGURE 15-28   **A**, Assembly tool. **B**, Quik-connectors.

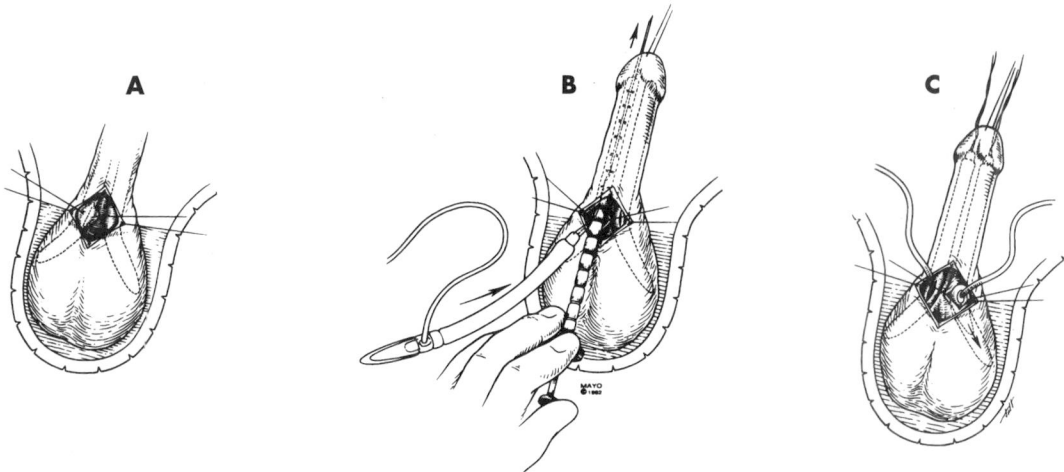

FIGURE 15-29   Penoscrotal approach for inflatable penile implant.

eye of a Keith needle, and the needle is slid into the groove of the Furlow inserter.

8. The Furlow inserter is guided along the corporal tunnel, and the plunger is pushed to release the Keith needle, which punctures the glans (Fig. 15-29, *B*).

9. The needle is grasped with a heavy hemostat and pulled through the glans, allowing the cylinders to slide to the channel opening. The Furlow inserter is removed, and the cylinder is inserted and guided to its proper position beneath the glans penis (Fig. 15-29, *C*).

10. If necessary, rear tip extenders are added to the proximal end of the cylinder. The proximal end is positioned in the crus.

11. The procedure is repeated on the other side.

12. The external inguinal ring is palpated and a path bluntly created. Dissecting scissors are used to separate the transversalis fascia on the inguinal floor.

13. The perivesical space is enlarged to allow palpation of Cooper's ligament. The reservoir is then positioned into the perivesical space.

14. The reservoir is filled with the appropriate amount of solution for its capacity (with different sizes being available) and pulled against the floor of Hesselbach's triangle.

15. The pump is then placed into the most dependent portion of the scrotum. It is generally positioned on the patient's dominant side. The space is created by blunt dissection lateral to the testicle.

16. The rods and reservoir tubings are connected to the pump with the connectors of choice, using the assembly tool to clamp them in place, and tested for inflation and deflation.

17. The tunica of the scrotum is closed over the pump with a running stitch of 3-0 absorbable suture.

18. The prosthetic device is left in a partially inflated position to reduce bleeding and promote healing (Fig. 15-30).

19. The Foley catheter is left in place during the immediate postoperative period. The incision is closed in a subcuticular fashion with 4-0 absorbable suture and a dressing is applied.

20. The penis is positioned flush with the lower abdomen for patient comfort. Mesh pants are useful as a nonadherent support dressing.

Deep Dorsal and Emissary Vein Ligation

This procedure entails the ligation or elimination of the penile deep dorsal vein and its tributaries. It is a treatment undertaken for vascular compromise–related impotence. Care is taken to avoid damage to the arteries and nerves lying alongside the deep dorsal vein. A common cause of erectile dysfunction in patients with organic impotence is vascular compromise. Before surgical intervention is undertaken, a definitive diagnosis of a corporal leak is made through dynamic infusion cavernosometry and cavernosography. Diagnostic results may indicate failure-to-store or failure-to-fill impotence. Patients with vascular compromise in a given anatomic region tend be compromised elsewhere as well. Many are diabetic or hypertensive. Because of this, the perioperative nurse must exercise great care in positioning the patient to prevent further damage to the patient's altered tissue perfusion. The cavernous and crural veins are suture ligated. All circumflex and emissary branches are ligated or coagulated. The suspensory ligament is detached, and the entire deep and accessory dorsal vein is removed.

Revascularization of the Penile Arteries

The relationship of focal arterial occlusive disease to sexual dysfunction has prompted efforts to rectify the resulting impotence. Investigational reconstructive surgery is taking place in patients who demonstrate correctable vascular disease in the large arteries. The most widely attempted repairs are end-to-end and end-to-side microscopic anastomosis of the distal inferior epigastric artery to

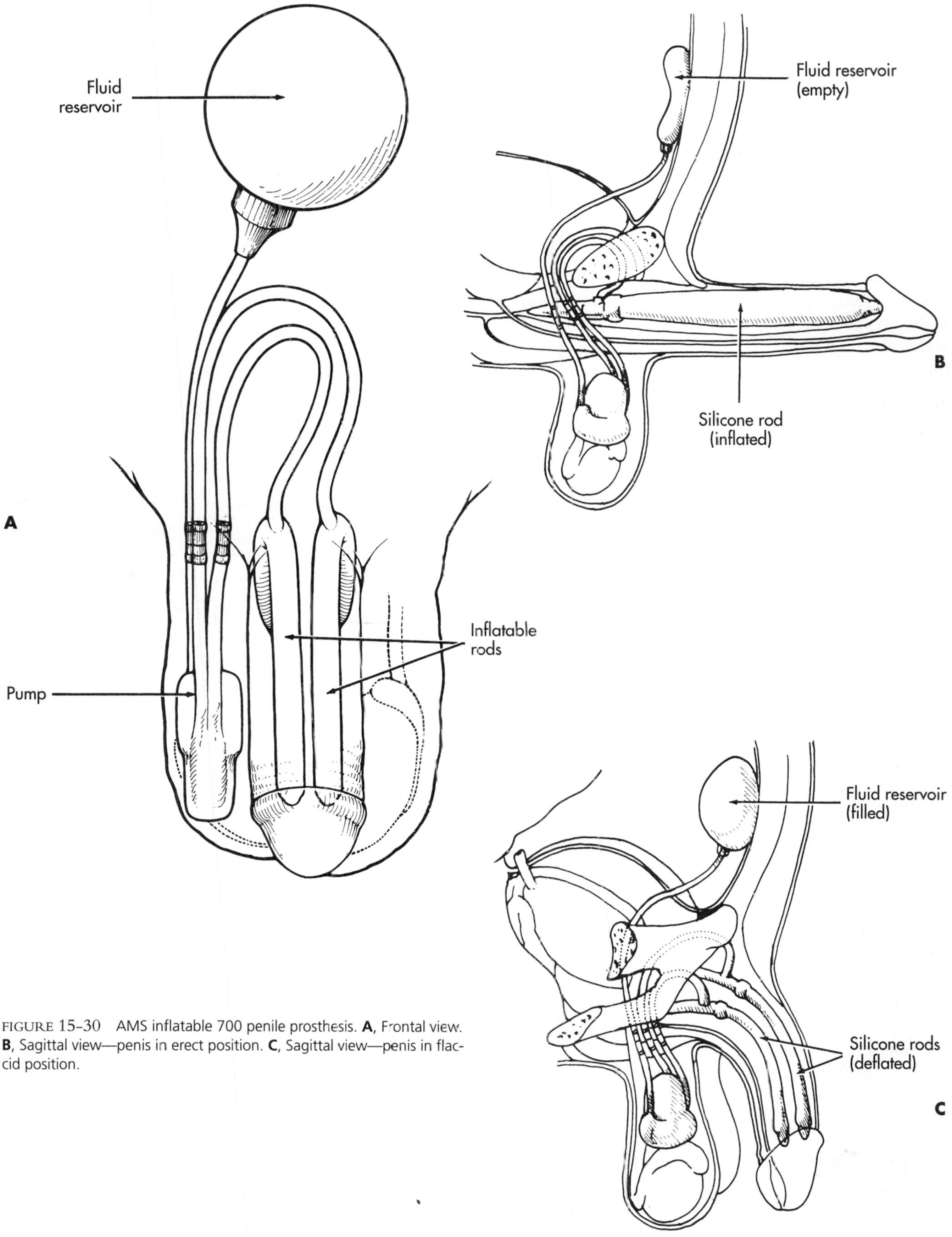

Fluid
reservoir

Fluid reservoir
(empty)

Silicone rod
(inflated)

B

A

Inflatable
rods

Pump

FIGURE 15-30   AMS inflatable 700 penile prosthesis. **A**, Frontal view.
B, Sagittal view—penis in erect position. **C**, Sagittal view—penis in flac-
cid position.

Fluid reservoir
(filled)

Silicone rods
(deflated)

C

the proximal deep dorsal artery near the pubic level, below the rectus muscle and Buck's fascia. Paramedian and infrapubic incisions are made, and the arteries are freed and tunneled. This procedure requires both a urologist and a vascular surgeon.

SURGERY OF THE SCROTUM AND TESTICLES

Hydrocelectomy

A hydrocele is an abnormal accumulation of fluid within the scrotum. The fluid is contained within the tunica vaginalis. Excessive secretion or accumulation of hydrocele fluid may be the result of infection or trauma. A hydrocelectomy is the excision of the tunica vaginalis of the testis to remove the enlarged, fluid-filled sac.

Procedural considerations

The patient is placed in the supine position. Preparation and draping of the patient include routine cleansing of the external genitals and draping with a fenestrated sheet. A minor instrument set is required, plus a small drain, a 30 ml syringe with a 20-gauge, 2-inch aspirating needle, and a suspensory dressing.

Operative procedure

1. Local anesthetic is instilled by grasping the cord in one hand and placing the thumb and index finger of the other hand over the scrotum. The cord is infiltrated at the base of the scrotum with 10 to 15 ml of plain lidocaine 1%.
2. An anterolateral incision is made in the stretched skin of the scrotum over the hydrocele mass with a #10 or #15 blade.
3. Bleeding is controlled with Crile hemostats, electro-coagulation, or vessel ligation with 3-0 absorbable ligatures. Stretching the skin of the scrotum com-presses the scrotal vessels.
4. An incision is then made between the blood vessels. The fascial layers are incised to expose the tunica vaginalis.
5. The hydrocele is dissected free with fine scissors, forceps, and blunt dissection.
6. The sac is opened, and Martius clamps are placed on each side incorporating the tissue adjacent to the tunica vaginalis and the skin.
7. The incised edges are everted under tension with the Martius clamps. The tension placed by the Martius clamp compresses the incised edge, controls bleeding, and prevents dissection between the tissue layers.
8. A pouch is created by dissecting between the tunica vaginalis and the dartos layer. Scrotal pressure is re-leased. This pouch will hold the testis after the repair.
9. The tunica vaginalis is opened, and the fluid contents are aspirated or drained.

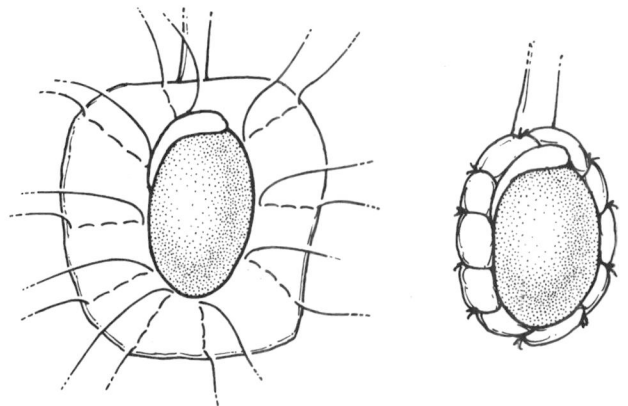

FIGURE 15-31   Hydrocelectomy.

10. The testis is lifted, and the sac is inverted so that it surrounds the testicular attachments and epididymis.
11. Excess tunica vaginalis may be excised. The tunica edges are sutured along the peritoneal surface with 3-0 absorbable suture in an interrupted fashion to the juncture of the testis. Six to eight sutures are placed around the circumference of the testis (Fig. 15-31). Some surgeons elect to sew the sac behind the spermatic cord in an interrupted fashion, and others may choose a continuous radial stitch around the posterior testis and epididymis.
12. The testis is replaced into the scrotum.
13. A drain may be placed into the scrotum and brought out through a stab wound in its most dependent portion. The drain is loosely sutured to the external scrotal wall to prevent migration.
14. The scrotal incision may be closed with 3-0 absorbable sutures in a full-thickness, continuous manner, or in layers with 3-0 and 4-0 continuous absorbable sutures.
15. A fluff compression dressing contained in a scrotal support or mesh underwear aids in reducing postoperative scrotal edema.

Vasectomy

A vasectomy is the excision of a section of the vas deferens. The operation may be performed selectively as a permanent method of sterilization and also before prostatectomy to prevent possible postoperative epididymitis. Because of the serious implications of permanent sterilization, particular attention must be paid to acquiring informed consent. Although studies have raised the question of a correlation between prostate cancer and vasectomy, a definitive causal relationship has not been established.

The patient having elective sterilization for birth control is encouraged to return to the office setting for sperm-count analysis. Generally two successive negative counts are sufficient to indicate that sterility has been achieved. Elective vasectomies are seen less frequently in operating room settings because more surgeons perform the procedure in the office setting.

Procedural considerations

The patient usually lies in the supine position, although the patient can be in the lithotomy position if vasectomy is performed before transurethral prostatectomy. The patient is given regional anesthesia for this procedure. A minor instrument set and scrotal suspensory are needed.

Operative procedure
No-Scalpel Approach

The no-scalpel technique was devised in China and has five fundamental principles:

- Fixation of the vas deferens without entering the scrotal skin
- Performance under direct vision to prevent damage from blind sharp scrotal penetration
- Simplified instrumentation
- Decreased operative time by simplification of the procedure
- Elimination of an incision or use of a scalpel

1. The right vas deferens is fixed under the scrotal skin with three fingers.
2. Using the local syringe and needle, a small wheal is raised in the median raphe of the scrotum. The needle is advanced along the vas toward the external inguinal ring. Plain lidocaine 1% or 2%, 3 to 5 ml is injected into the perivasal region.
3. The procedure is repeated on the left side. Pressure is applied to the wheal site to minimize edema.
4. Once adequate anesthesia is accomplished, the right vas is again fixed with three fingers.
5. A vas ring clamp is applied over the scrotal skin, encircling the vas. Lifting the clamp upward, the skin over the vas is stretched as thin as possible leaving minimal tissue between the vas and the clamp.
6. The ring clamp is locked in place, and the scrotal skin cephalad to the clamp is stretched with an index finger.
7. The skin is punctured, with the inner prong of the pointed dissecting hemostat, directly into the vas deferens. Both prongs of the dissecting hemostat are placed into the puncture site and spread directly on top of the vas.
8. When the surface of the vas is visualized, one prong is used to penetrate the vas itself. The vas is brought out of the wound by twisting the hemostat 180 degrees.
9. The ring clamp is moved to directly encircle the vasal tissue. The vas may then be divided and occluded by intraluminal electrocoagulation, clips, or suture ligation. Fascia should be placed between the severed ends of the vas.
10. The procedure is repeated on the left side. It is usually possible to place the ring clamp around the left

vas through the initial entry site. Sutures are not necessary.
11. After ensuring that there is no bleeding, antibiotic ointment, pressure dressings, and a scrotal support are applied.

Vasovasostomy

Vasovasostomy is the surgical reanastomosis of the vas deferens, using the operative microscope. The number of vasal reanastomosis procedures has increased dramatically. Reanastomosis may often alleviate chronic testicular pain, a not infrequent complication after vasectomy. Additionally, a significant number of men who have had a vasectomy want to regain their fertility. A precise reconnection can be performed with the use of a microscope and a modified two-layer anastomosis. Success rates vary from 40% to 70%. When there are no longer two viable segments of vas deferens, a similar procedure, the epididymovasostomy, may be performed. This involves anastomosis of a vas deferens to a segment of the epididymis.

Procedural considerations

A minor instrument set is required, with the addition of selected microsurgical instruments and sutures.

Operative procedure

1. After the vas deferens has been located by external manipulation, a vertical scrotal incision is made.
2. The testicle, epididymis, and vas are displaced from the scrotum. The vasectomy site is identified, and the scarred area is excised.
3. The proximal end of the vas deferens is cut back until fluid is expressed. Fluid is collected on a glass slide and examined for the presence of live sperm. Surgery continues even if results for sperm are negative unless an epididymal obstruction exists.
4. The distal end of the vas is resected until a normal lumen is visible.
5. The distal and proximal lumens are then dilated.
6. The two portions of the vas are placed in an approximator clip with background material placed underneath. Six stitches of 10-0 nonabsorbable microsuture are placed in the inner layer. The proximal end is sutured through the serosa to the mucosa, and the distal end through the mucosa to the serosa (Fig. 15-32).
7. A second layer of 8 to 10 stitches of 9-0 nonabsorbable suture is placed without penetrating the lumen of the vas.
8. The incision is closed in two layers with interrupted 3-0 and 4-0 absorbable sutures.
9. Gauze sponges and a suspensory support are placed on the patient to provide a pressure dressing. Postoperative precautions include no lifting or ejaculation for a minimum of 2 weeks. The sperm count and viability of sperm are rechecked at 3- and 6-month intervals.

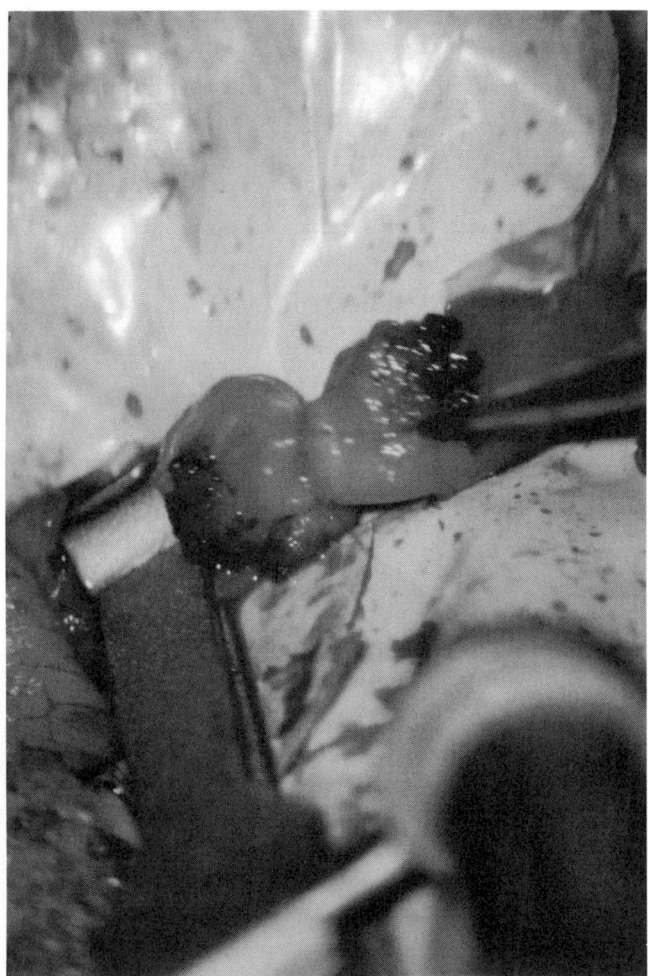

FIGURE 15-32 The two portions of the vas in approximator clip with background material as the proximal end is sutured through the serosa to the mucosa with 10-0 nylon.

Microscopic Epididymal Sperm Aspiration

Microscopic epididymal sperm aspiration (MESA), requires the availability of an in vitro fertilization team, so the aspirated sperm may be immediately processed and used for the selected in vitro technique, or frozen for later use. The procedure must be timed according to the partner's cycle of ovulation. Ova are aspirated as an office procedure just before MESA is performed.

Microscopic epididymal sperm aspiration should be done using the micropipette technique. The tip of a 250- to 350-micrometer pipette is inserted into an epididymal tubule to retrieve sperm cells without contamination by red blood cells. After aspiration, the fluid is given to the in vitro fertilization team to process the sperm cells. Processing involves washing debris from the cells, retrieving the most active cells from the sample, and removing any red blood cells, if possible. This is critical because red blood cells significantly interfere with sperm cell function.

After aspirating the sperm cells, the epididymal tubule is closed using microscopic technique. If adequate numbers of sperm cells can be obtained from one testis, the other side may be aspirated to add to the sperm bank if this is desirable. It may be necessary to aspirate sperm cells from the rete testis, tubules between the testicles and the epididymal head that carry cells to the head of the epididymis, if sperm cells are not found in tubules closer to the vas deferens.

The sperm cells retrieved may be used for intracytoplasmic injection into the partner's egg (ICSI), the most successful of the in vitro techniques available. This technique is not as dependent on the quality of the sperm as earlier techniques of in vitro fertilization.

Using sperm cells from the epididymis and intracytoplasmic injection techniques, pregnancy rates may approach 50%. It may be possible to retrieve sperm cells by percutaneous aspiration of the testis, but the numbers of sperm cells retrieved by this technique are not as high as with MESA.

Epididymectomy

An epididymectomy is the excision of the epididymis from the testis. Epididymectomy lacks the general support of the urologic community and is rarely performed. It may, however, still be indicated as a last choice treatment for degenerative cystic disease, chronic infection, and intractable pain of the epididymis.

Procedural considerations

The patient is placed in the supine position with the legs slightly abducted. A general, spinal, or regional anesthetic is required. Setup is as described for hydrocelectomy, plus an electrosurgical unit, if desired.

Operative procedure

1. An anterolateral incision is made over the testis in the scrotum to expose the tunica vaginalis. The tunica is incised to expose the testis and overlying epididymis.
2. An incision is made along the superior head of the epididymis, which is then sharply dissected from the testis. A portion of the vas deferens may also be excised.
3. Bleeding is controlled by electrocoagulation and absorbable ties.
4. The skin wound is closed with 4-0 absorbable sutures.
5. A small drain may be left intrascrotally for 24 to 48 hours.

Spermatocelectomy

Spermatocelectomy is removal of a spermatocele, a lobulated intrascrotal cystic mass attached to the superior head of the epididymis. It is usually caused by an obstruction of the tubular system that conveys the sperm. This complication after vasectomy is not infrequent and does not exhibit itself immediately.

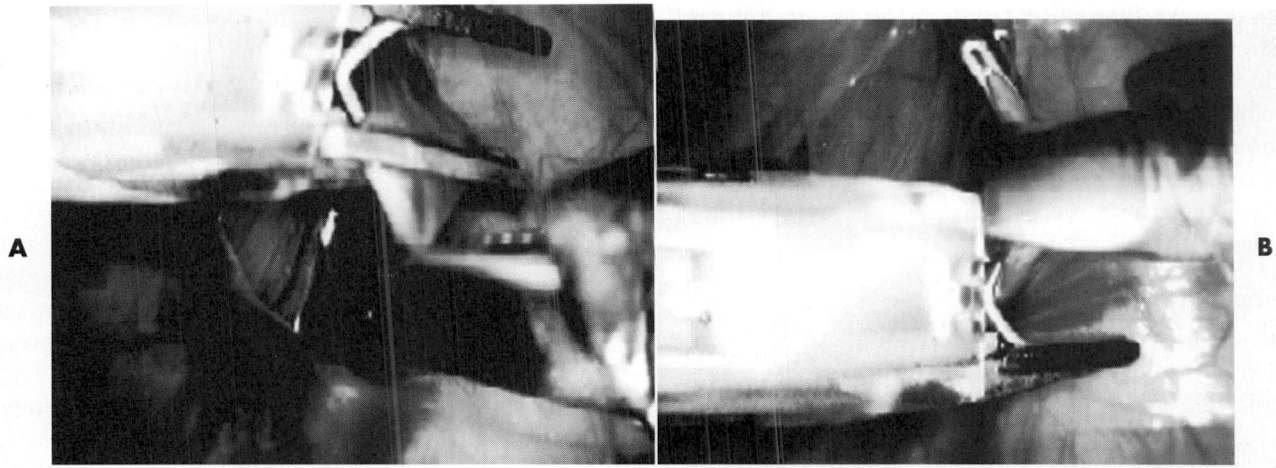

FIGURE 15-33 **A**, Applying second proximal clip to first vein. **B**, Applying distal clip to vein.

Procedural considerations

The setup for a spermatocelectomy is as described for a hydrocelectomy, plus a microscope and slides, if desired.

Operative procedure

1. The mass is approached through a scrotal incision as described for hydrocelectomy.
2. The structures of the testis and spermatic cord are identified, and the cystic structure is dissected free.
3. Bleeding is controlled with electrocoagulation.
4. The wound is closed and dressed as described for hydrocelectomy.

Varicocelectomy

A varicocelectomy is the high ligation of the gonadal veins of the testes. Varicocelectomy is done to reduce venous backflow of blood into the venous plexus around the testes and to improve spermatogenesis. When surgery for this condition was originally devised, the veins of the pampiniform plexus were ligated and divided individually.

Varicoceles occur more frequently on the left side because the gonadal vein of the left testis unites retroperitoneally with the renal vein at a 90-degree angle and is consequently under greater backpressure. As a result of this unusual backpressure, the pampiniform plexus of the spermatic cord becomes tortuous and engorged, resembling a bag of worms.

A variation of the standard inguinal or scrotal approaches is the laparoscopic varicocelectomy. Often this procedure may be combined with a laparoscopic herniorrhaphy.

Procedural considerations

The setup for inguinal varicocelectomy is as described for an inguinal hernia repair (see Chapter 13). The setup for laparoscopic varicocelectomy is as for a laparoscopic hernia repair with the exclusion of the mesh implant.

Operative procedures

Inguinal Approach

1. The incision may be through a suprainguinal approach or an oblique inguinal approach over the external inguinal ring.
2. The structures of the spermatic cord are identified, and the vessels are dissected free from the vas deferens.
3. The abnormal dilated veins in the inguinal canal are clamped and ligated. The redundant portions are excised. A drain may be placed.
4. The incision is closed in layers.

Laparoscopic Approach

1. Intraabdominal instillation of CO_2 through an umbilical incision and the insufflation needle is accomplished. The procedure is performed through primary 10 to 11 mm umbilical and suprapubic ports and a 5 mm ipsilateral port.
2. The peritoneum is entered laterally to the spermatic cord and incised in a T configuration across the cord.
3. The spermatic cord is elevated and its major components separated with blunt dissection after identification of the spermatic artery. Irrigation of the area with papaverine mixed with 0.9% injectable saline will cause the artery to pulsate and make identification easier.
4. The involved veins are ligated with small and medium vascular endoclips (Fig. 15-33).
5. The incisions are closed and dressed as for other laparoscopic procedures with Steri-Strips, Telfa, and Tegaderm.

Testicular Biopsy

A biopsy of the testicle involves a wedge excision of suspicious tissue for diagnostic confirmation. Men suffering from infertility, who are azoospermatic or oligospermatic, with normal or minimally elevated follicle-stimulating hormone, may be evaluated through this means. Although controversial, if a surgeon is prepared to proceed with an orchiectomy, he or she may choose to first take a biopsy specimen and evaluate a testicular lesion with a frozen-section microscopic examination. This occurs in a circumstance where a suspicion of carcinoma is questionable and the patient refuses an orchiectomy without diagnostic confirmation.

Procedural considerations

If required, hair may be removed from the scrotum, which is then aseptically cleansed. General, regional, or spinal anesthesia may be selected. A minor instrument set is used. Special fixatives, such as Bouin's or Zenker's solution, must be available. Formalin destroys the germinal epithelium and should not be used.

Operative procedure

1. The scrotum is held firmly on its posterior aspect. This causes the skin on the anterior aspect to stretch tightly over the incisional site, forcing the epididymis to remain posterior and allowing the scrotal skin to part without retraction.
2. A 1 to 2 cm vertical incision is made, with care taken to avoid injury to the epididymis.
3. The incision is continued to the tunica vaginalis. As the tunica is incised, there should be a normal efflux of clear fluid.
4. Absorbable 4-0 stay sutures are placed in the tunica vaginalis. Two more are placed in the tunica albuginea.
5. A small ellipse of tunica is resected, with its tubules, with a scalpel in a shaving action, with no-touch technique. The tissue is placed in the fixative or sent to the histology department as a fresh specimen.
6. The wound is closed in three layers with 3-0 and 4-0 absorbable suture.
7. Gauze sponges and fluffed dressings are placed over and around the scrotum. A suspensory support is applied to provide pressure and support.

Orchiectomy

An orchiectomy is the removal of the testis or testes. Removal of both testes is castration and renders the patient sterile and deficient in the hormone testosterone, which is responsible for development of secondary sexual characteristics and potency. This operation, like vasectomy, has legal implications that require attention to acquiring informed consent for surgery. Bilateral orchiectomy is usually performed to control symptomatic metastatic carcinoma of the prostate gland. A unilateral orchiectomy is indicated because of testicular cancer, trauma, or infection. Presently, silicone gel testicular implants have been removed from the market. Saline-filled implants are in development.

Procedural considerations

The patient is placed in the supine position and draped according to established procedure. A minor instrument setup is required.

Operative procedures

Scrotal Approach

1. For benign conditions the incision is made over the anterolateral surface of the midportion of the scrotum.
2. The skin incision is carried through the subcutaneous and fascial layers through the tunica vaginalis, exposing the testicle.
3. Retractors are placed, and bleeding vessels are clamped and tied.
4. The spermatic cord is divided into two or three vascular bundles. Each vascular bundle is doubly clamped, cut, and ligated, first with 0 absorbable suture ligature and then with a proximal free 0 absorbable tie.
5. The vas is separately ligated with a 0 absorbable tie. The testis is removed.

This procedure has recently been approached through laparoscopic techniques, usually in conjunction with laparoscopic herniorrhaphy.

Inguinal Approach

1. For malignant conditions the incision is begun just above the internal ring, extending downward and inward over the inguinal canal to the external inguinal ring.
2. The inguinal canal is exposed, and the spermatic cord is dissected free, cross-clamped, and divided into vascular bundles at the internal ring.
3. Gentle forward traction is applied to the cord, which is dissected from its bed.
4. The testis is everted into the wound from the scrotum and excised.
5. Bleeding is controlled with electrocoagulation. A small drain may be placed in the empty hemiscrotum if desired.
6. The external oblique fascia is reapproximated with 2-0 absorbable interrupted sutures.
7. Subcutaneous tissue, including Scarpa's fascia, is closed with 4-0 absorbable sutures.
8. The skin is reapproximated with surgical staples or 4-0 subcuticular suture.

Radical Lymphadenectomy (Retroperitoneal Lymph Node Dissection)

Radical lymphadenectomy is a bilateral resection of retroperitoneal lymph nodes. Dissection usually includes lymph nodes, channels, and fat around both renal pedicles, the vena cava, and the aorta, including the bifurcation of the aorta. Lymph node dissection is performed for treatment of nonseminomatous testicular tumors. The procedure is performed after radical inguinal orchiectomy.

Procedural considerations

The patient is placed in the supine position. If the dissection is unilateral, the patient is supine with the operative side tilted upward. Routine skin preparation from nipples to midthigh and draping procedures are carried out. Long fine dissection instruments along with basic laparotomy instruments are required.

Operative procedure

1. A midline abdominal incision is made from the xiphoid process to the symphysis pubis.
2. The abdominal contents are explored to determine the degree of gross nodal involvement. The colon is either packed within the abdominal cavity or mobilized and kept moist outside the abdomen.
3. The posterior peritoneum is opened between the aorta and the vena cava.
4. The lymphatic structures and fat are removed en bloc from around both renal pedicles, the vena cava, and the aorta from above the renal hilum to beyond the bifurcation of the iliac vessels on the side of the original testicular neoplasm, by blunt and sharp dissection.
5. The spermatic vessels of the affected side are removed down to and including the stump of the previous orchiectomy.
6. The inferior mesenteric artery may be sacrificed if technically necessary, but the superior mesenteric artery is not disturbed.
7. The ureter on the affected side is skeletonized to remove any perilymphatic tissue.
8. If reperitonealization is desired, the posterior peritoneum is closed with a 2-0 absorbable continuous suture.
9. The viscera are repositioned into the abdominal cavity, and the wound is closed, usually without placement of a drain.

SURGERY OF THE PROSTATE GLAND

Glandular hyperplasia of the prostatic urethra usually manifests itself after 50 years of age. Prostatic enlargement may occur in one or more lobes of the prostate but most frequently occurs in the lateral or median lobes. Progressive growth of the hyperplastic gland compresses the remaining normal prostatic tissue, forming what is called a *surgical capsule*. The growth of adenomatous tissue slowly encroaches on the prostatic urethral lumen, causing obstruction of urinary outflow.

Prostatic enlargement may be benign or malignant. In BPH only the periurethral adenomatous portion of the gland is removed. Operable prostatic malignancy requires radical prostatectomy, which includes removal of the entire prostate gland and the seminal vesicles.

A blood sample is drawn to determine the prostatic specific antigen (PSA) level, followed by a digital rectal examination. The blood is often drawn first, since manipulation of the gland has been known to alter the efficacy of the PSA test. The PSA test is considered the most valuable tool available for early detection of carcinoma of the prostate. If this test is elevated, the patient is at risk for carcinoma of the prostate; a PSA value above 10 ng/ml is highly suggestive of prostatic carcinoma.[6] Clinical evaluation and an elevated PSA usually indicate the need for a transrectal ultrasound needle biopsy to confirm the diagnosis. When the results of the biopsy are positive for malignancy, a bone scan and skeletal survey are necessary to rule out metastasis. A more precise blood study. the free total PSA (PSA II) has proved to be quite accurate in delineating those patients at increased risk for prostate cancer (Research Highlight 15-2). An older blood study, which is still being used, is the prostatic acid phosphatase level (PAP). When elevated, it usually indicates that tumor extension beyond the prostatic capsule has occurred. The possibility of hemolytic anemia, Gaucher's disease, or Paget's disease of the bone should be evaluated if diagnostic measures are negative for carcinoma.

In an attempt to provide cost-effective, curative treatment with a low morbidity, treatment protocols that provide alternatives to the open surgery approach have been developed. A thorough workup procedure includes a digital rectal examination, freetotal serum PSA II, bone scans, CT and MRI scans of the pelvis, and transrectal, ultrasonically guided biopsies with histologic grading of the malignancy. After these evaluations, select patients with well or moderately differentiated lesions may be candidates for transperineal, ultrasonically guided implantation of radium seeds (brachitherapy) or cryoablation of the prostate (cryotherapy).

Three open surgical approaches are possible in removing the benign hyperplastic obstructive prostate gland: retropubic prostatectomy, suprapubic prostatectomy, and perineal prostatectomy. Of these, the one most commonly employed is the suprapubic prostatectomy. All open prostatectomies hold the risk for loss of sexual potency.

Transurethral prostatectomy (TURP) is the endoscopic (closed) surgical approach that may be performed on most patients. Alternative modalities that have had some success in the treatment of benign prostatic hypertrophy (BPH) are the transurethral incision of the prostate (TUIP), transurethral laser incision of the prostate (TULIP), visual laser ablation of the prostate (VLAP), and transurethral microwave therapy (TUMT) with the Prostatron. The TULIP and VLAP require the use of the Nd:YAG laser, and specially designed fibers. Results seem to indicate a

15-2 RESEARCH HIGHLIGHT

In serum and prostatic fluid, PSA exists in six molecular forms. The predominant forms of PSA in the serum are free PSA (f-PSA), PSA bound to α-antichymotrypsin (PSA-ACT), and PSA bound to α_2-macroglobulin (PSA-MG). Since the PSA-MG form cannot be measured by currently available methodology, for practical purposes total serum PSA represents f-PSA and PSA-ACT. Of these, PSA-ACT is the most abundant form of PSA. The development of monoclonal antibodies that accurately measure f-PSA has permitted an exploration of variabilities in the levels of free and total PSA in men with BPH and cancer. Most studies have consistently demonstrated that the amount of PSA-ACT in serum is higher in men with prostate cancer than in men with BPH or normal glands and, in addition, that cancer is associated with a reduced amount of f-PSA. Prestigiacomo et al. report on the performance of free-to-total PSA ratio as a predictor for prostate cancer. They compared preoperative serum PSA levels in 51 men with clinically significant prostate cancer (based on pathologic cancer volume) and 48 men with BPH. Mean serum PSA levels in both groups were similar at the time of the study. In the clinically relevant PSA range of 4 to 10 ng/mL an f/t ratio of ≤0.15 was the most reliable diagnostic cutoff and correctly identified 95% of the men with prostate cancer. However, in the total serum PSA range of 2 to 4 ng/mL, no ratio of free-to-total PSA discriminated BPH from prostate cancer. Along with previously published data, this study indicates that using the f/t ratio can reduce the incidence of unnecessary prostate biopsies in men with PSA levels ranging from 4 to 10 ng/mL.

From Klein, E.A. (1997). Can free PSA or other PSA derivatives reduce the frequency of unnecessary prostate biopsies? In Lynch, J.H. (Ed.). *Prostatic disease: insights and innovations.* Deerfield, Ill.: Discovery International.

decrease in postoperative blood loss and a low recurrence rate of BPH.

If the prostate gland is cancerous, a radical retropubic or radical perineal prostatectomy, in conjunction with open or laparoscopic pelvic lymph node dissection, is performed.[7] Many patients desire to retain sexual function. The surgeon may attempt to save the neurovascular bundles in what is termed a nerve-sparing approach. The site and size of the prostatic lesion, however, often determines if this can be achieved successfully and without undue risk to the patient.

Several factors must be taken into account to determine the best route for removal of the prostatic obstruction:

the age and medical condition of the patient, the size of the gland and location of the pathologic condition, and the presence of associated medical disease.

Prostatic Core Needle Biopsy

Needle biopsy of the prostate is indicated for patients in whom prostatic cancer is clinically suspected. It may be accomplished transperineally or transrectally with a needle designed for this purpose.

Procedural considerations

Needle biopsy of the prostate has the risk of both intraoperative and postoperative bleeding. Although seldom needed, an ESU should be available. A cystoscopic examination may accompany a needle biopsy. More and more frequently, needle biopsies are being performed in the office or ultrasound department of the hospital.

The most significant potential complication of a biopsy is systemic infection. This risk can be decreased with antibiotic coverage before and after the procedure and the use of an enema before the examination. The patient is placed on antibiotic therapy twenty-four hours before the procedure and is advised to use a Fleet enema 2 to 3 hours before the test is performed. Before the examination, an antiseptic solution mixed with a viscous local anesthetic is often instilled into the rectum and allowed to coat the tissues for 5 to 15 minutes.

Operative procedures
Transrectal, Ultrasonically Guided Biopsy

This procedure is commonly performed in the urologist's office using a high-frequency transrectal ultrasound transducer to assess the prostate gland. The size, volume, and shape of the prostate may be assessed in addition to the likelihood of the presence of a malignancy. Suspicious areas or lesions may be biopsied with a needle passed under ultrasound guidance across the rectal wall. The needle penetrates the rectal mucosa with spring-loaded biopsy guns or a core biopsy system. Color-flow imaging may also be used to help in the identification of areas that are likely invaded with prostatic carcinoma or have acute and chronic inflammation. A full bladder helps delineate the base of the prostate.

The prostate is visualized in three dimensions, allowing more accurate localization of abnormalities and extent of disease. For the axial view, the transrectal transducer is placed deeply into the rectum, just proximal to the seminal vesicles, to about 10 cm above the anal verge. Here the vas deferens may be distinguished. The transducer is slowly withdrawn to the level of the base of the gland, enabling visualization of the inner gland. Seminal vesicles are seen in cross section. To evaluate the prostate in the sagittal planes the probe may be rotated clockwise or counterclockwise. A series of "sextant" (six) biopsy specimens are generally taken with the disposable "core biopsy" needle. These are taken from the right and left apex, the right and left

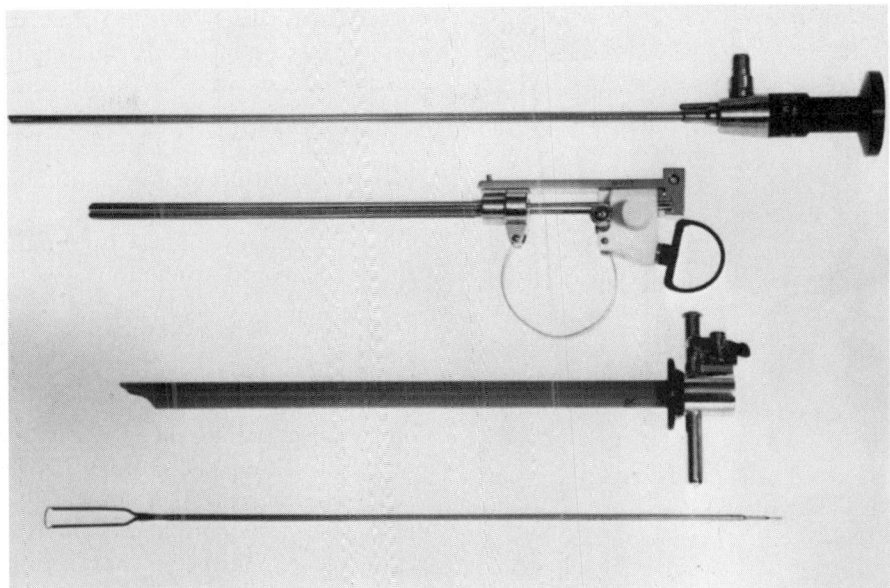

FIGURE 15-34   Resectoscope components: Foroblique telescope, Iglesias operating element, postresectoscope sheath, and cutting loop.

midline, and the right and left base. Lesions as small as 2 to 3 mm are visible with this procedure.

Transrectal Approach without Ultrasound Guidance

The patient is placed in the lateral or dorsal-lithotomy position. The biopsy needle is inserted into the rectum along the volar aspect of the surgeon's index finger. The needle is advanced to the border of the nodule. The obturator is removed, and the cutting blades are inserted or advanced. When the blades are in position, the outer sheath is advanced over them and twisted to receive a slender thread of prostate tissue. This technique is believed to be easier to accomplish than a transperineal approach is.

Transperineal Approach

The patient is placed in the lithotomy position. The examining finger is inserted into the rectum and the induration identified. The needle is inserted through the perineal skin and guided ahead until the tip is against the lesion. The biopsy specimen is taken in the same fashion as described for the transrectal approach. Transperineal biopsy is believed to hold less risk of infection and postoperative bleeding. Some surgeons may incise the site with a #11 or #15 scalpel blade and place a 4-0 absorbable closing suture.

Transurethral Resection of the Prostate Gland

In this procedure, a resectoscope is passed into the bladder through the urethra, and successive pieces of tissue are resected from around the bladder neck and the lobes of the prostate gland, leaving the capsule intact. The resectoscope uses a stabilized cutting loop to resect tissue and coagulate blood vessels by means of electric current. The electric current that powers the electrode is supplied by a high-frequency ESU. The current settings are specified by the urologist, who activates the cutting or coagulating current with a foot pedal during the course of the procedure.

TURP is one surgical method of treating benign obstructive enlargement of the prostate gland. Several factors influence the surgical approach: size of the gland and location of the pathologic condition, age and condition of the patient, and presence of associated diseases.

Controversy continues in regard to the efficacy of prophylactic vasectomy to prevent the postoperative complication of epididymoorchitis. If vasectomy is to be done, it should be performed immediately before the transurethral procedure. The patient must be well informed and have full understanding of the implications of the procedure. Operative consent is mandatory.

Procedural considerations

The instrument setup for transurethral resection of the prostate is as described for cystoscopy with additional necessary instruments. The four principal types of resectoscopes are McCarthy, Nesbit, Iglesias, and Baumrucker. Adult resectoscopes range in size from 24 to 28 Fr and have the following components: Foroblique telescope, operating element, cutting loops, and postresectoscope sheaths and obturators (Fig. 15-34). A transurethral resection of the prostate requires a resectoscope (multiple working elements), a Foroblique telescope as well as a backup

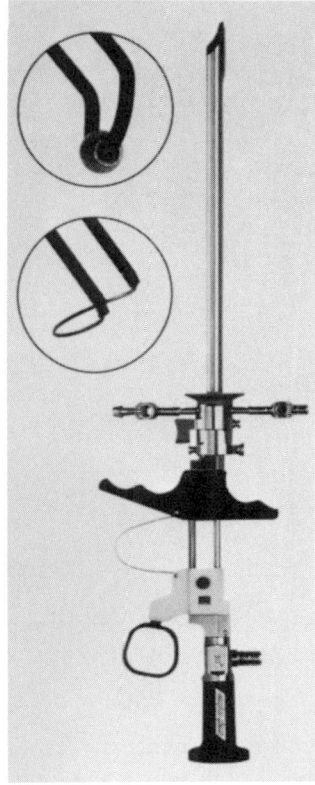

FIGURE 15-35   CFR resectoscope.

telescope, stabilized or unstabilized cutting loops, a postre-sectoscope sheath with its corresponding articulated obturator, a high-frequency cord, a short bridge, a Toomey syringe or the Ellik or Urovac evacuator, Van Buren sounds, a #22 or #24 30 ml three-way Foley catheter, a disposable urologic drape with rectal sheath, and a system for continuous bladder irrigation and urinary drainage. Supplementary instruments include a resectoscope adapter and a lateral telescope.

The continuous-flow resectoscope (CFR) (Fig. 15-35) has unique components that include an outlet stopcock to which a suction tube is attached, an inflow tube on the inner sheath, and outflow holes on the outer sheath. These features enable the urologist to resect tissue without interruption to empty the bladder, as must be done with the standard resectoscope. In addition to the CFR, which replaces the standard resectoscope, the setup includes a thick-walled Silastic suction tubing and a continuous-flow pump. The continuous-flow technique decreases intravesical pressure on the bladder during the procedure, provides a clearer field of vision because of the constant inflow and outflow of irrigant, reduces the operating time because the resection process need not be interrupted to evacuate the bladder, and provides a "still" bladder for the resection of bladder tumors.

A continuous flow of isotonic and nonelectrolytic irrigating fluid is necessary to ensure transmission of electrical current and clear visualization throughout surgery. Irrigating solution such as 1.5% glycine or 3% sorbitol, 3 to 6 liters, may be connected in tandem to provide a constant flow. Warming units, available for these solutions, help to eliminate the hypothermia often experienced when large amounts of cold irrigants are employed. On the other hand, when solutions are warm, the patient may show a tendency to bleed more intraoperatively. At all times perioperative nursing personnel must be alert to replace the irrigation solution as required.

During transurethral prostatic surgery, return of irrigation fluid must be monitored because extravasation and absorption of fluid into open prostatic venous sinuses or bladder perforation may occur. The perioperative nurse should be aware of the early symptoms and measures employed to remedy these complications. The patient usually experiences significant respiratory changes and abdominal discomfort. Other important observations are rigidity and swelling of the lower abdomen, coupled with changes in sensorium. If extravasation of irrigating fluid is evident, the surgical procedure is discontinued, and a cystogram is obtained immediately to determine if bladder perforation has occurred. Insertion of a Foley catheter is generally all that is necessary to control the situation. In the rare instance of a major perforation, surgical closure may be accomplished through a cystotomy incision.

Operative procedure

1. In transurethral prostatic surgery the urethra is usually first dilated with sounds from 20 to 30 Fr.
2. Cystourethroscopy is performed to assess the degree of prostatic obstruction and to inspect the bladder. Some urologists perform this diagnostic procedure several days before surgery, whereas others perform the examination in the operating room immediately before surgery.
3. A well-lubricated postresectoscope sheath with its fitted Timberlake obturator is passed into the urethra.
4. The Timberlake obturator is removed, and the working element (resectoscope), assembled with the Foroblique telescope and cutting loop, is inserted through the sheath.
5. The irrigation tubing, light cord, and high-frequency cord are appropriately connected, and irrigation fluid is allowed to fill the bladder.
6. Initial inspection of the prostatic urethra and bladder trigone is carried out.
7. After determining the location of the ureteral orifice, the urologist initiates electrodissection, alternating cutting and coagulating currents as required (Fig. 15-36).
8. The bladder is drained, washing out prostatic tissue and small blood clots. At times it is necessary to employ the Ellik evacuator to remove resected prostatic tissue. To do this the urologist must remove the working element of the resectoscope. The nozzle of the evacuator is fitted onto the resectoscope sheath,

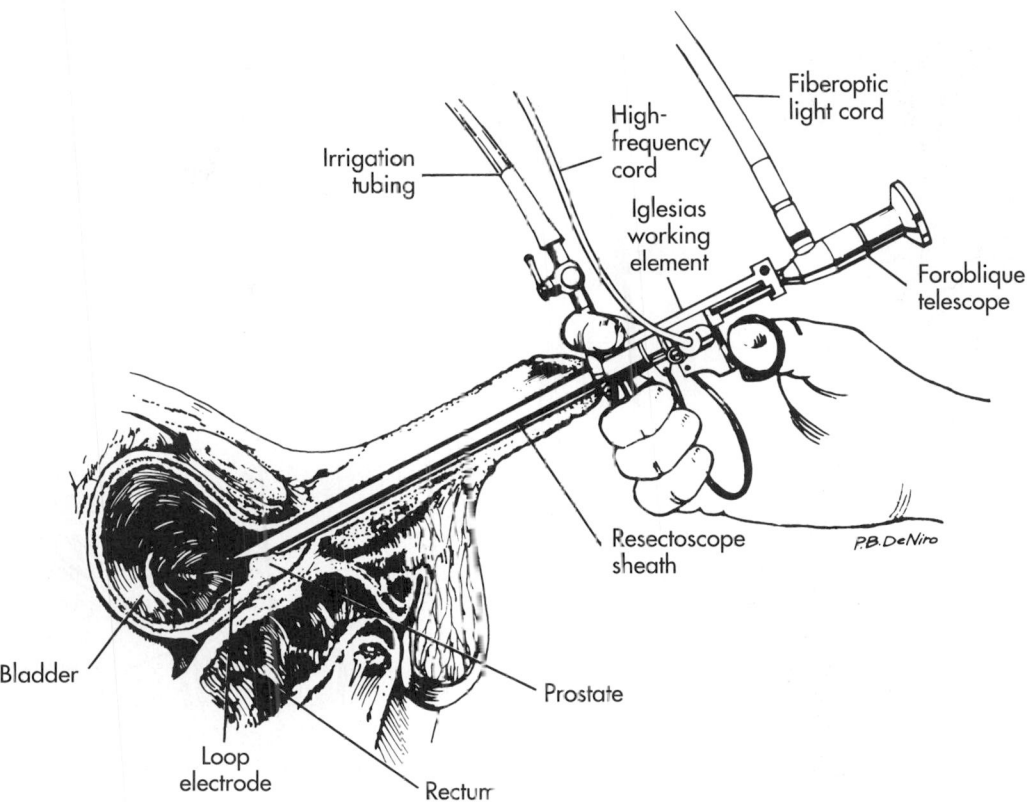

FIGURE 15–36   Sectional view illustrating removal of portion of hypertrophied middle lobe of prostate gland with Iglesias resectoscope.

and by manual pulsatile pressure the bladder contents are removed. An Ellik or Urovac evacuator or Toomey syringe should be readily available for manual irrigation. Fluid may be drawn from the irrigant directly into the resectoscope sheath through the already attached tubing.

9. When the prostatic resection is completed, the prostatic fossa is inspected to ensure that all bleeding points have been coagulated.

10. The resectoscope is then removed, and a Foley catheter (22 or 24 Fr, two- or three-way, 30 ml balloon) is inserted into the bladder for urinary drainage. The balloon is inflated (Fig. 15-37, A) and pulled gently in traction against the bladder neck to help control venous bleeding (Fig. 15-7, B). The Foley balloon must not be inflated within the prostatic fossa (Fig. 15-37, C), where it may cause excessive bleeding from the resected prostatic capsule. If desired, continuous irrigation with gravity drainage is initiated with normal saline as the bladder irrigant, instead of sorbitol or glycine. A 3- to 4-liter urinary drainage system is suggested to avoid frequent emptying of the drainage bag.

11. When VLAP or TULIP is performed, the surgeon may choose to place a standard 18 Fr Foley with a 5 or 30 ml balloon connected to straight drainage. If irrigation is required postoperatively, it is then performed manually with sterile solution and a Toomey syringe.

Transurethral Incision of the Prostate

Transurethral incision of the prostate (TUIP) is a procedure in which the prostate is incised at the 5 and 7 o'clock positions to provide relief of obstruction with results similar to those provided by a complete transurethral resection, but with a lower incidence of bladder neck contracture and retrograde ejaculation. The shorter operative time inherent with the procedure minimizes fluid absorption and may decrease postoperative pulmonary and cardiovascular complications. The procedure may be performed with cold or hot knives as well as the standard resectoscope, or laser fiber. This procedure is appropriate for sexually active patients with moderate to small obstructive prostates without a significant middle lobe component. One major disadvantage is the potential for missing occult prostatic cancer. Despite this, some clinicians view this as an underused, feasible form of treatment.

Transurethral Incision of the Ejaculatory Ducts

This procedure is performed for the relief of obstructed ejaculatory ducts, a common condition in men with chronic prostatitis and prostatic calculi. Symp-

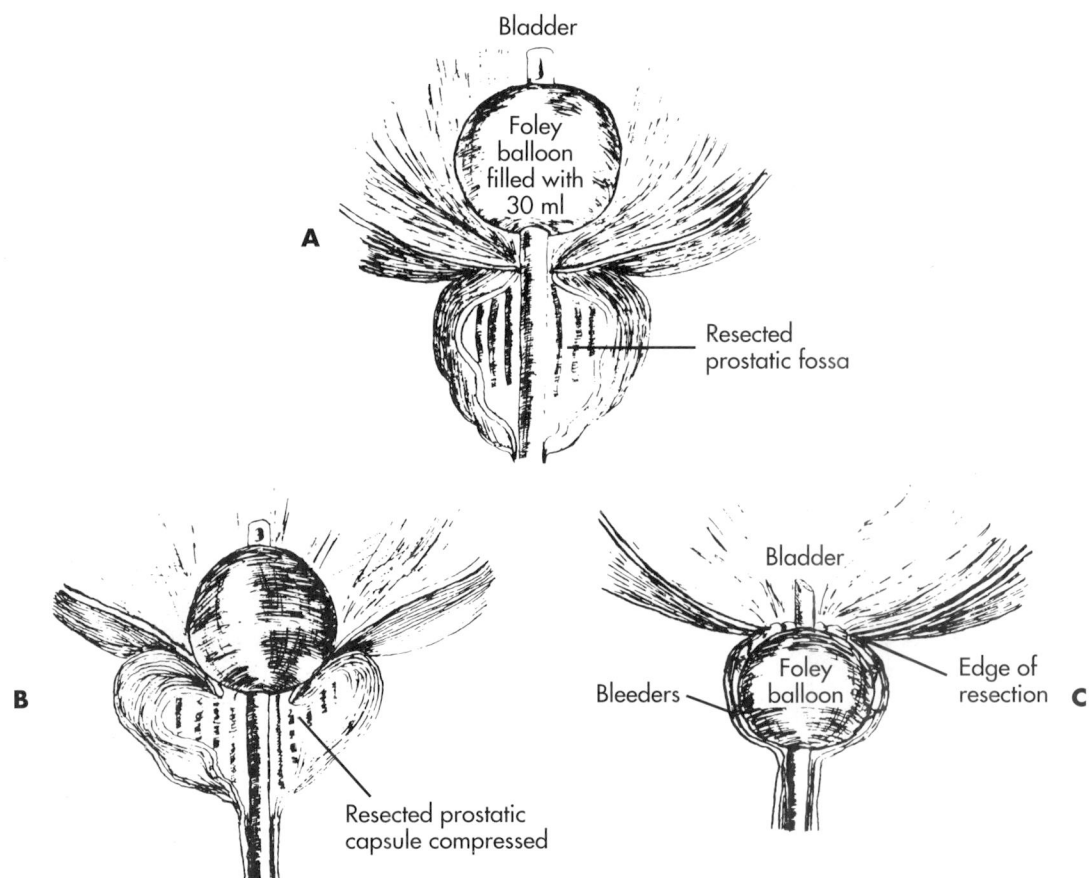

FIGURE 15-37 **A, B,** Proper position for Foley catheter with inflated balloon beyond prostatic capsule. **C,** Improper position.

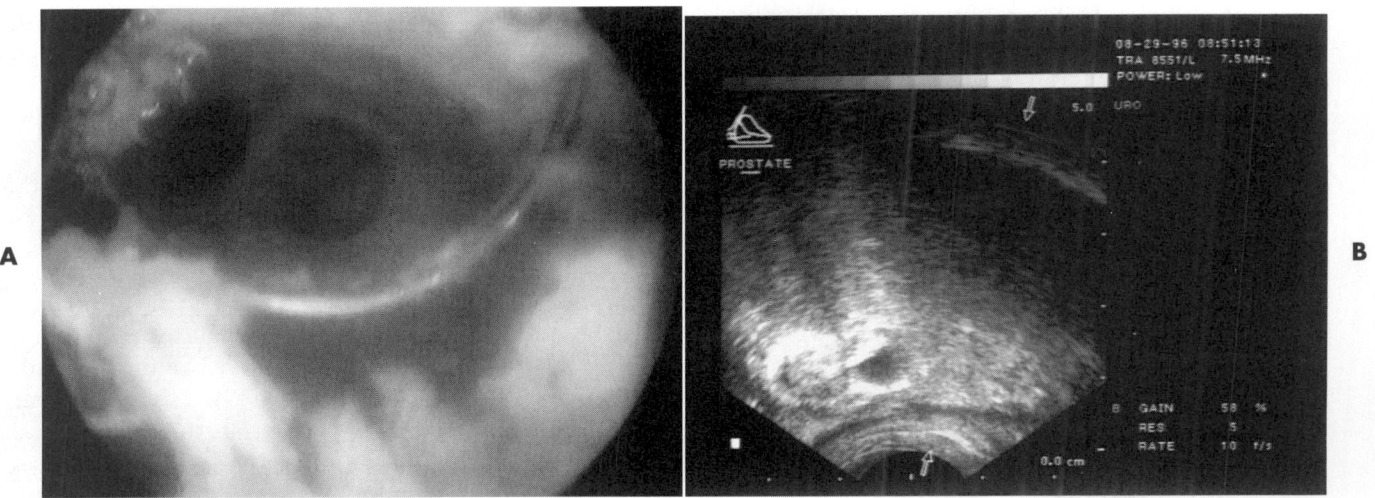

FIGURE 15-38 **A,** Dilated seminal vesicle (ejaculatory duct) with resectoscope loop approaching. **B,** Resectoscope loop entering dilated seminal vesicle (ejaculatory duct).

toms closely mimic prostatodynia and include aching in the perineal and genital areas with no lasting or significant improvement from conservative therapy (antibiotics and analgesics). The resectoscope loop is guided with transrectal ultrasound imaging to the dilated ejaculatory ducts, and the obstructed ducts are resected. Calculi may be fragmented if necessary and removed (Fig. 15-38). A catheter is generally not needed.

Transurethral Microwave Therapy

Transurethral microwave thermotherapy (TUMT) is a minimally invasive method of applying heat to the prostate gland for the relief of the symptoms associated with BPH

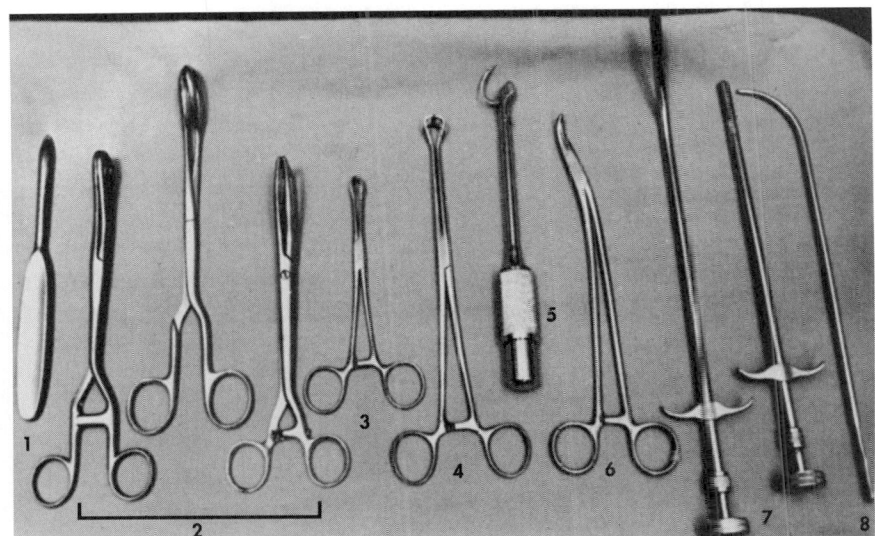

FIGURE 15-39   Prostatic instruments. *1*, Prostatic enucleator; *2*, three prostatic lobe forceps; *3*, Lahey forceps; *4*, long Babcock forceps; *5*, boomerang; *6*, Heaney needle holder; *7*, two Lowsley prostatic tractors; *8*, urethral sound.

and bladder-outlet obstruction. TUMT maintains temperatures in the urethra, sphincter, and rectum at a level that is physiologically safe while heating the tissue deep within the transitional zone of the prostate. A water-cooled catheter is combined with microwave radiation to the lobes of the prostate. The Prostatron received FDA approval in May of 1996.

Procedural considerations

The treatment unit (Prostatron) consists of a microwave generator, a cooling system, a fiberoptic temperature-monitoring system, a technical computer, and a power supply that are built into the treatment module (couch) that the patient lies on during the procedure. A separate control module operates the system. A dual-channel Foley catheter with a built-in microwave antenna and temperature sensor and a rectal probe with three fiberoptic thermal sensors complete the instrumentation.

The patient is placed in the supine position, the perineal area is aseptically prepared, and the urethra is anesthetized. Prophylactic antibiotics are prescribed postoperatively for 5 to 7 days and may be administered intraoperatively. During treatment 20° C water circulates through the catheter maintaining the urethra at a near-normal physiologic temperature and protecting the sphincter and rectum from the heat targeted to the transition zone.

Operative procedure

1. After instillation of the local anesthetic, the treatment catheter is inserted intraurethrally and the balloon is inflated at the bladder neck. Position is confirmed with ultrasound imaging and a multiplane transrectal transducer.
2. The patient may be repositioned to lie on his left side for placement of the rectal probe and measurement of the rectal temperature. The rectal probe is covered with a standard condom and inserted.
3. With the patient in the supine position, treatment

ensues for 60 minutes with a maximum output of 45 W and urethral and rectal temperatures programed to remain below 45° F and 42.5° F respectively.
4. The patient will be discharged once he has demonstrated the ability to void. Those patients that required a catheter preoperatively will commonly have a catheter reinserted for the postoperative recovery period.

Simple Retropubic Prostatectomy

Simple retropubic prostatectomy is the enucleation of hypertrophic prostatic tissue through an incision in the anterior prostatic capsule by an extravesical approach. The retropubic approach offers excellent exposure of the prostate bed and vesical neck and readily controllable intraoperative and postoperative bleeding.

Procedural considerations

The patient is placed in a slight Trendelenburg position with the pelvis elevated and the legs slightly abducted. Routine skin preparation is carried out. Electrocoagulation is usually employed. Although the draping procedure must conform to individual operating room policies, the following procedure is suggested for draping the patient.

The first towel, with a cuff, is placed under the scrotum. The next three towels are placed around the lower abdominal incision site, followed by a sterile laparotomy sheet. A fifth towel, folded in half, is placed over the penis and scrotum below the retropubic incision site and secured with two nonperforating towel clamps.

The instrument setup includes a basic laparotomy set and bladder and prostatic instruments (Figs. 15-39 to 15-41). The following supplies should be readily available: Jackson-Pratt drains, water-soluble lubricant, Toomey and Asepto syringes, a urinary drainage system, a 20 Fr 5 ml Foley catheter, a 22 or 24 Fr 30 ml Foley catheter, 10 and 30 ml syringes, and a self-retaining retractor such as the US200 adjustable urology retractor (Fig. 15-42).

Operative procedure

1. Through a Pfannenstiel or low vertical midline incision the anterior rectus sheath is incised along with portions of the internal and external oblique muscles.
2. The rectus abdominis muscles are retracted laterally to expose the space of Retzius.
3. After placement of traction sutures, the anterior portion of the prostatic capsule is incised transversely (Fig. 15-43, *A*).
4. The prostatic adenoma may be dissected or finger-enucleated from the surgical capsule (Fig. 15-43, *B*).
5. Care is taken to place hemostatic sutures at the 5 and 7 o'clock positions, encompassing the vesical neck and prostatic capsule, to ligate the primary blood supply to the prostate. Other bleeding points within the capsule may be suture ligated with 2-0 absorbable sutures.
6. A Foley catheter is inserted in the urethra and through the bladder neck and inflated within the bladder. Frequently, a three-way catheter is used for continuous bladder irrigation.
7. The prostatic capsule incision is closed with either a continuous or an interrupted 0 absorbable suture (Fig. 15-43, *C*).
8. A drain is placed in the space of Retzius and brought out through the fascia and skin through a separate stab incision.
9. The abdominal incision is then closed in layers, and the wound is dressed.
10. If continuous bladder irrigation is to be used, normal saline solution irrigation is initiated through a 4-liter closed irrigation system.

Suprapubic Prostatectomy

Suprapubic prostatectomy is the removal, through a transvesical approach, of benign periurethral glandular tissue obstructing the outlet of the urinary tract. A low midline, or Pfannenstiel, incision may be used. One advantage of the suprapubic approach is that it allows access for surgical correction of any existing bladder condition such as vesical calculi or vesical diverticula. Control of bleeding is a major consideration in any prostatectomy and is one disadvantage of the suprapubic approach. Because the prostate is located beneath the

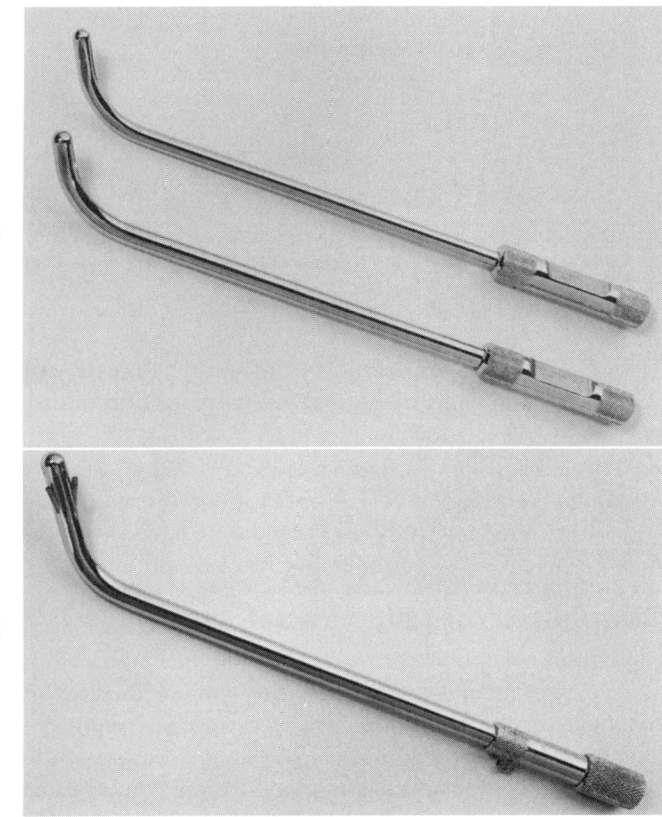

A

B

FIGURE 15-40 **A,** Roth urethral suture guiders, 24 Fr and 28 Fr. **B,** Roth Grip-Tip urethral suture guide, 28 Fr extended.

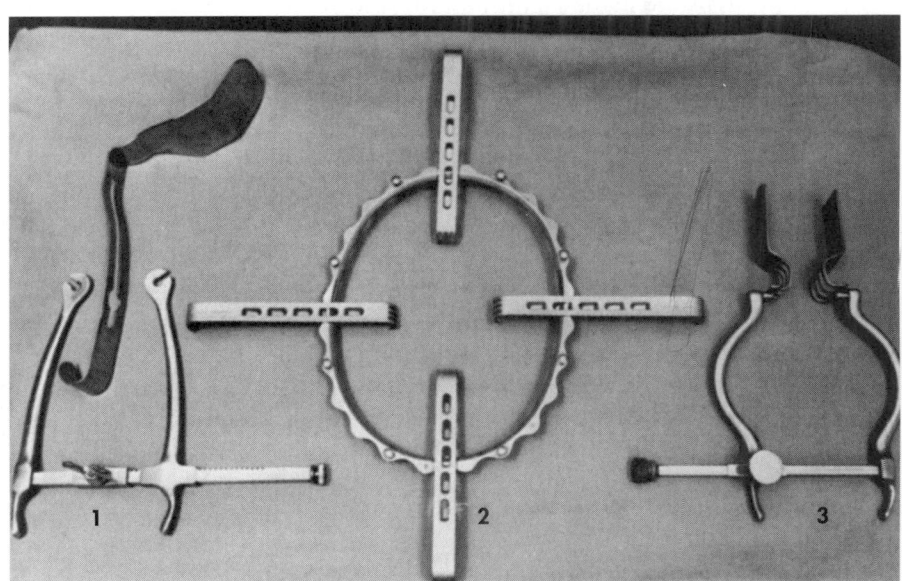

FIGURE 15-41 Retractors for prostatectomy. *1*, Millin retropubic bladder retractor; *2*, Denis-Browne ring retractor (perineal); *3*, Masson-Judd bladder retractor (suprapubic).

symphysis pubis, ligation of bleeding capsular vessels is difficult. However, control of hemorrhage and replacement of blood loss, coupled with skilled perioperative nursing care and early mobilization of the patient, have greatly minimized complications.

Procedural considerations

Spinal, epidural, and general anesthesia may be equally acceptable types of anesthesia for patients having a suprapubic prostatectomy, depending on their medical condition. The patient is placed in a slight Trendelenburg position with the umbilicus elevated and the legs slightly abducted. Skin preparation, draping, and instrumentation are as described for retropubic prostatectomy.

Operative procedure

Bilateral vasectomy may be performed to decrease the postoperative incidence of epididymoorchitis. A meatotomy may also be required if the penile meatus is too small to accommodate a Foley catheter.

1. A Foley catheter is inserted through the urethra into the bladder, and the bladder is inflated with a preferred irrigating fluid. This maneuver facilitates identification of the bladder.
2. A transverse or midline lower abdominal incision is made through the skin and the two layers of superficial fascia (Fig. 15-44, *A*).
3. The external and internal oblique muscles are cut along the lines of the original incision.
4. Bleeding vessels are clamped, coagulated, or tied with fine absorbable ties.
5. The rectus muscles are separated in the midline and retracted laterally.
6. After the placement of traction sutures, the bladder is opened at the dome with a scalpel. Liquid contents are aspirated, and the bladder incision is enlarged.
7. The bladder is visually and manually explored for calculi, a tumor, or diverticula.
8. The tip of the index finger of the operating hand is inserted through the vesical neck into the prostatic urethra, and the adenomatous tissue is enucleated (Fig. 15-44, *B*). If difficulty is experienced with the enucleation, a finger may be placed into the rectum to elevate the prostate gland. Aseptic technique is maintained during enucleation with the use of a sterile second glove on the hand used in the rectum.
9. After enucleation is completed, attention is directed to maintaining good hemostasis by suture ligation of the vesical neck at the 5 and 7 o'clock positions. Other significant bleeding points may also be ligated.
10. A suprapubic catheter of the urologist's choice is placed into the bladder lumen through a small stab incision.
11. A 22 or 24 Fr two- or three-way Foley catheter with a 30 ml balloon is inserted into the urethra, and the

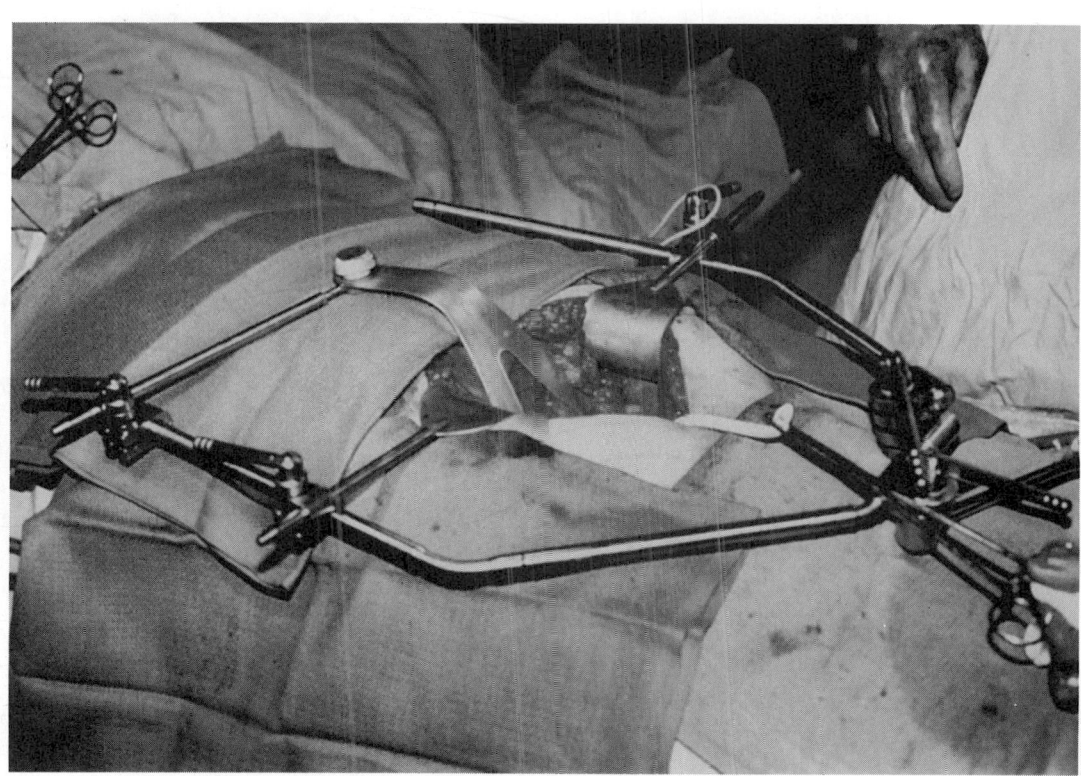

FIGURE 15-42 Omni-Tract adjustable US200 urology retractor system.

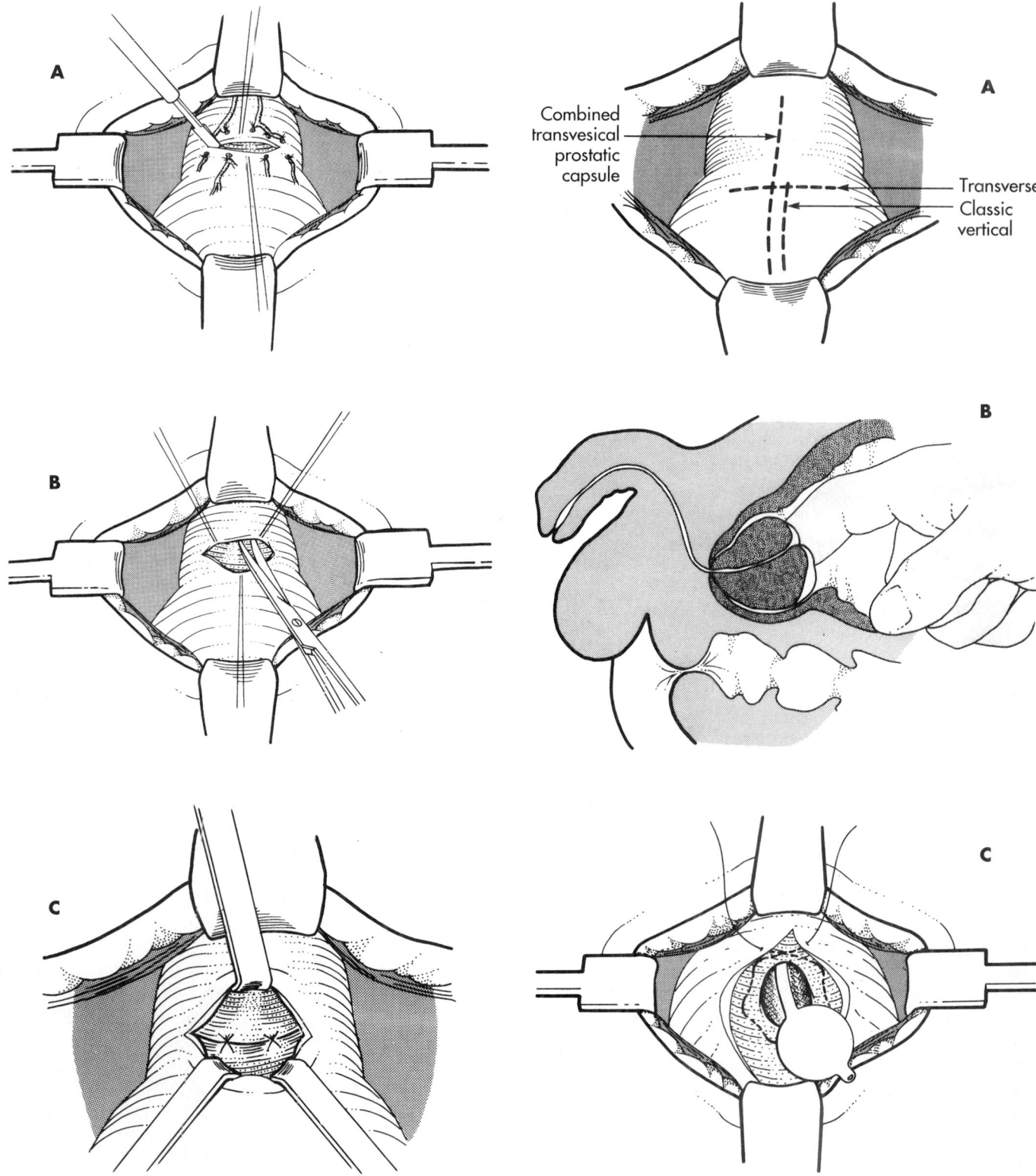

FIGURE 15-43   Retropubic prostatectomy.

FIGURE 15-44   Suprapubic prostatectomy.

balloon is inflated to a size that prevents the catheter from falling or being pulled into the prostatic fossa (Fig. 15-44, *C*).

12. The cystotomy incision is then closed with interrupted 2-0 absorbable sutures.

13. A drain is left along the cystotomy incision, brought out through a separate stab wound, and secured to the skin with a silk suture.

14. The muscles, fascia, and subcutaneous tissues are closed in layers, and a dressing is applied.

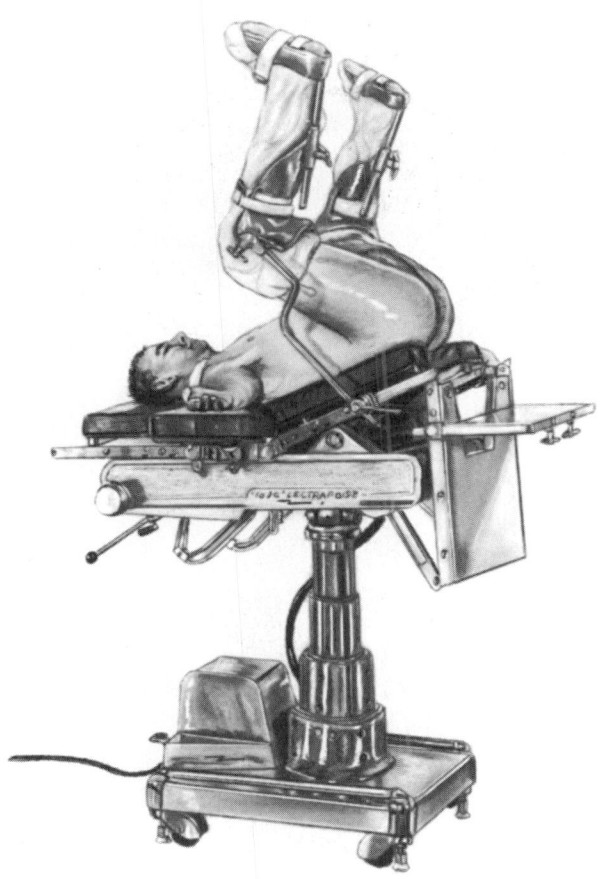

FIGURE 15-45 Exaggerated lithotomy position for perineal prostatectomy.

15. Normal saline irrigation solution may be connected to the Foley catheter to provide continuous irrigation to the bladder to reduce clot formation and maintain catheter patency. Continuous irrigation may be initiated during closure.

Simple Perineal Prostatectomy

Simple perineal prostatectomy is the removal of a prostatic adenoma through a perineal approach. A perineal approach to the prostate gland is most suitable when open prostatic biopsy is desired and, after receipt of pathologic confirmation, radical excision is to follow. Other advantages include preservation of the bladder neck, improved urethrovesical anastomosis, and easier control of bleeding. Some surgical disadvantages are (1) inability to perform biopsy of the iliac and obturator nodes for determining extension of disease and (2) possible formation of urethrorectal fistulas.

Procedural considerations

The patient is placed in an exaggerated lithotomy position with the legs above the level of the pelvis (Fig. 15-45). A bolster beneath the sacrum allows the perineum to be as parallel to the operating room bed as possible, with the buttocks extending several inches over the bed edge. Stirrups should be well padded to protect the

popliteal fossa. Sequential compression stockings are recommended to assist peripheral vascular flow. The patient is often placed in a steep Trendelenburg's position. Well-padded shoulder braces, placed over the acromial processes in a manner to prevent stretch or pressure injury, may be required to prevent the patient from sliding upward on the operating room bed. Routine skin preparation is carried out and includes an interior rectal prep. Special draping is as follows:

A towel folded in half is placed over the pubic area. Two towels with a cuff are placed on either side of the perineum. Two leggings, with points down, are placed over the legs. One impervious drape is placed over the anus. A large sheet fully opened with a large cuff is placed across from one stirrup to the other and secured by towel clamps. A laparotomy sheet follows, with the short end to the floor.

The instrument setup is as described for suprapubic prostatectomy, omitting abdominal self-retaining retractors and adding straight and curved Lowsley tractors (Fig. 15-46), Roux retractors, Jackson retractors with short and long blades, Doyen vaginal retractors, perineal prostatic retractors (Fig. 15-47), Sauerbruch retractors, and a narrow and wide self-retaining perineal retractor such as the UM150 (Fig. 15-48).

Operative procedure

1. A curved Lowsley tractor is placed through the urethra into the bladder and held back by the surgical assistant, causing the prostate to be pushed down toward the perineum.
2. An inverted U-shaped incision is made from one ischial tuberosity to another, curving just anteriorly to the anus (Fig. 15-49, *A*).
3. Three Martius clamps are secured to the posterior edge of the incision and retracted downward, over the anal drape.
4. Subcutaneous bleeders are clamped with straight mosquitoes and coagulated or tied with 3-0 absorbable ligatures.
5. The central tendon is isolated, clamped, and cut distally to the external anal sphincter (Fig. 15-49, *B*).
6. The rectourethral muscle is incised and pushed downward from the central tendon.
7. The levator ani muscle is exposed and retracted laterally (Fig. 15-49, *C*).
8. The prostate gland is exposed. Biopsy of the prostate may be performed for pathologic confirmation. If the results are negative, the prostatic adenoma is removed. If the frozen section reveals malignancy, the urologist may choose to do a radical prostatectomy at this time.
9. If simple enucleation is to be performed, the prostatic capsule is incised, and the Lowsley tractor is removed (Fig. 15-49, *D*).
10. The urethra is divided and the Young prostatic retractor is inserted.
11. The blades are opened, drawing the prostate down,

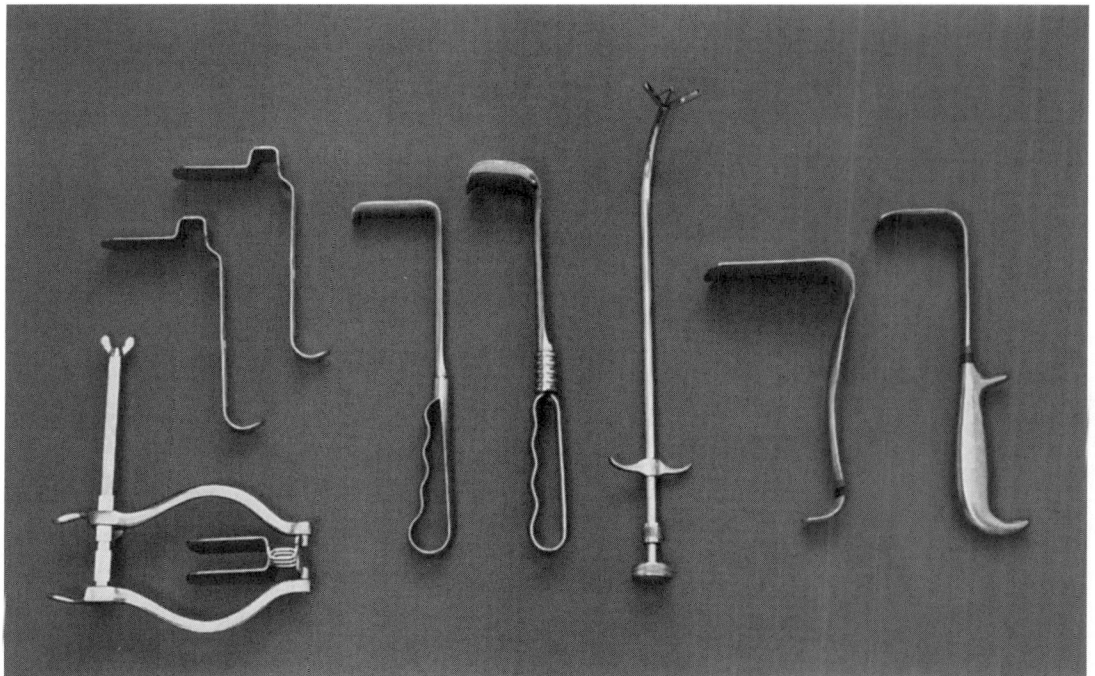

FIGURE 15-46 Perineal and suprapubic prostatectomy instruments, including straight and curved Lowsley retractors.

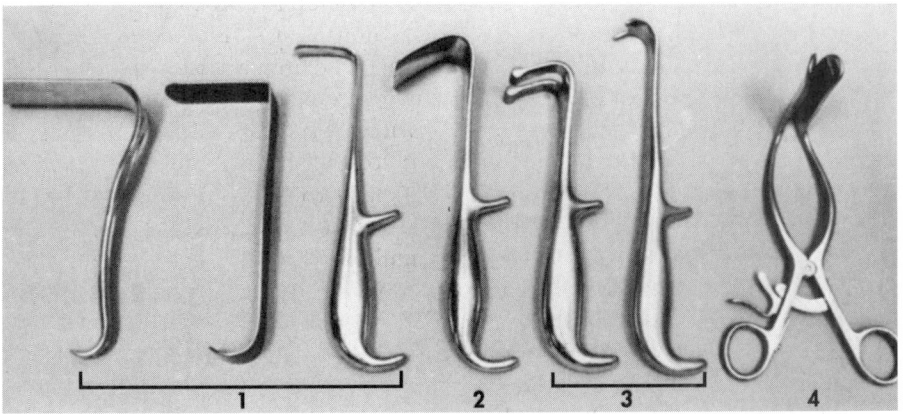

FIGURE 15-47 Perineal prostatectomy retractors. *1,* Three prostatic lateral retractors; *2,* prostatic anterior retractor; *3,* two prostatic bifurcated retractors; *4,* self-retaining retractor.

and the adenoma is manually enucleated from the surgical capsule.

12. A 22 Fr Foley catheter with a 30 ml balloon is inserted through the urethra into the bladder.

13. Bleeding is controlled at the 5 and 7 o'clock positions.

14. The capsulotomy incision is repaired with a continuous 2-0 absorbable suture (Fig. 15-49, *E*).

15. A drain is left in place at the level of the capsulotomy incision.

16. The subcutaneous tissue is reapproximated with 3-0 absorbable suture.

17. The skin incision is reapproximated with 4-0 absorbable subcutaneous sutures.

18. The wound is dressed according to the surgeon's preference and taped or held with a supportive device such as mesh pants. A vasectomy may be performed before the prostatectomy.

Transrectal Seed Implantation (Interstitial Radiotherapy with Brachytherapy)

Brachytherapy of the prostate gland is one procedure that validates the necessity of a collaborative, multidisciplinary approach to patient care. The radiation oncologist and medical physicist, in addition to the urologist, are vital

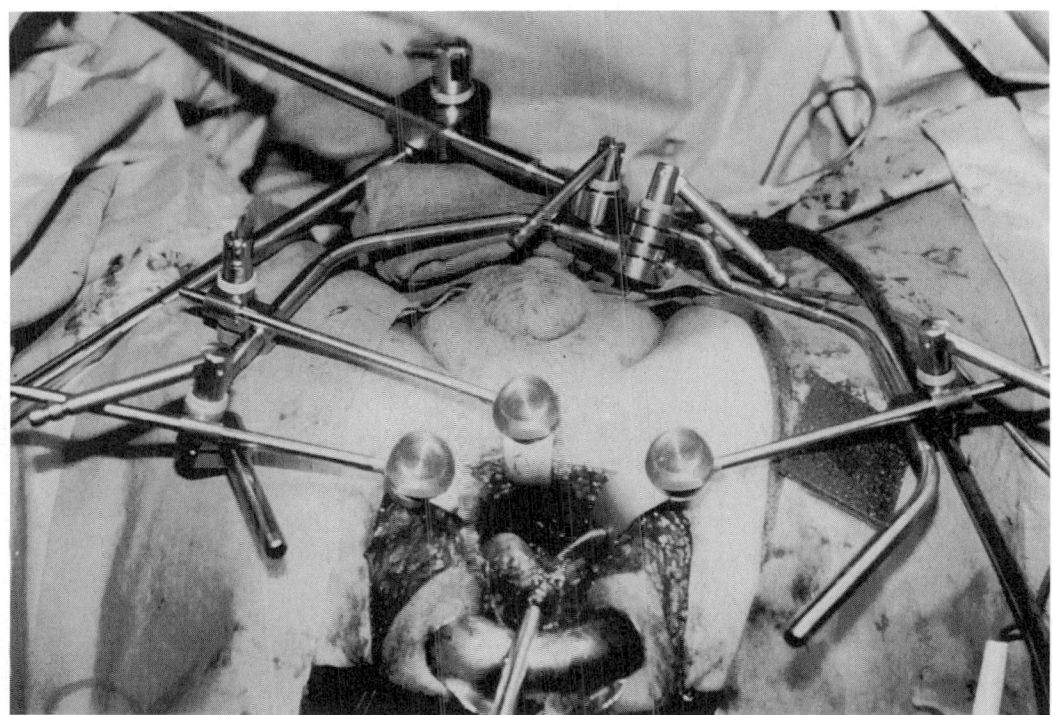

FIGURE 15-48   UM150 Omni-Tact adjustable urology perineal minitractor.

to an optimum outcome from the initial planning stage throughout the postoperative surveillance. Preplanning is required to determine the dose of each seed, the spacing necessary between each seed, and the number of seeds required. A template plan is developed preoperatively by using the ultrasound and the probe-anchoring equipment to measure and map the appropriate seed sites within the prostate. This may be accomplished in the surgeon's office, radiology department, or oncology clinic.

The facility that offers this treatment must be licensed for "Group 6" with the radioactive materials licensing department of their respective state. Six year follow-up examinations from multiple institutions indicate a disease-free interval and survival equivalent to the results of radical prostatectomy. If seed implantation is indicated as an adjunct to radiation therapy, it should be performed 3 to 4 weeks after the radiation treatment.

During percutaneous implantation of iodine 125 or palladium 103 seeds, the patient is positioned in the dorsal lithotomy position. The prostate is visualized with transrectal ultrasonic imaging, and the midportion of the prostate is located on a transverse image. This location becomes an index for positioning the axial ultrasound plane at the base of the prostate. Approximately 2 to 3 hours should be allowed from start to completion. The procedure is amenable to outpatient management utilizing regional or general anesthesia.

Iodine seeds are commercially available in titanium-encased rods that absorb the electrons. These seeds may be obtained embedded in an absorbable suture that allows them to remain positioned appropriately in relation to themselves and their location within the prostate and minimizes the risk of seed migration. Palladium seeds, not presently available prethreaded, are plated onto a graphite pellet. The pellets are loaded into titanium tubes with a lead marker. The half-life of iodine 125 (60 days) is longer than palladium 103 (17 days) and allows the therapy to be delivered over the duration of tumor cell replication, altering the ability of the tumor cells to multiply. Palladium 103 affords a larger dose of radiation in a shorter time interval to more rapidly growing tumors than iodine 125 does.

Procedural considerations

Percutaneous implantation of radioactive seeds allows the delivery of significantly higher doses of radiotherapy to the prostate than external beam therapy does. The radius of penetration around each seed is only 5 mm, sparing adjacent organs. The typical radiation dose that can be delivered by external beam may be 6500 cGy (centigrays), whereas the dose that can be delivered with implantation of seeds alone is in the range of 12,000 to 16,000 cGy. The patient will be receiving hormone therapy, to shrink the prostate gland, for 3 months before implantation, and some will require radiation therapy before implantation. Patients with stage A or stage B prostate cancer are appropriate candidates, and selection is not influenced by a rise in the PSA, biopsy specimens indicative of further involvement, or age.

Intraoperatively there is the danger of implantation into the bladder; implantation too close to the urethra resulting in postoperative urethral stricture; implantation into the

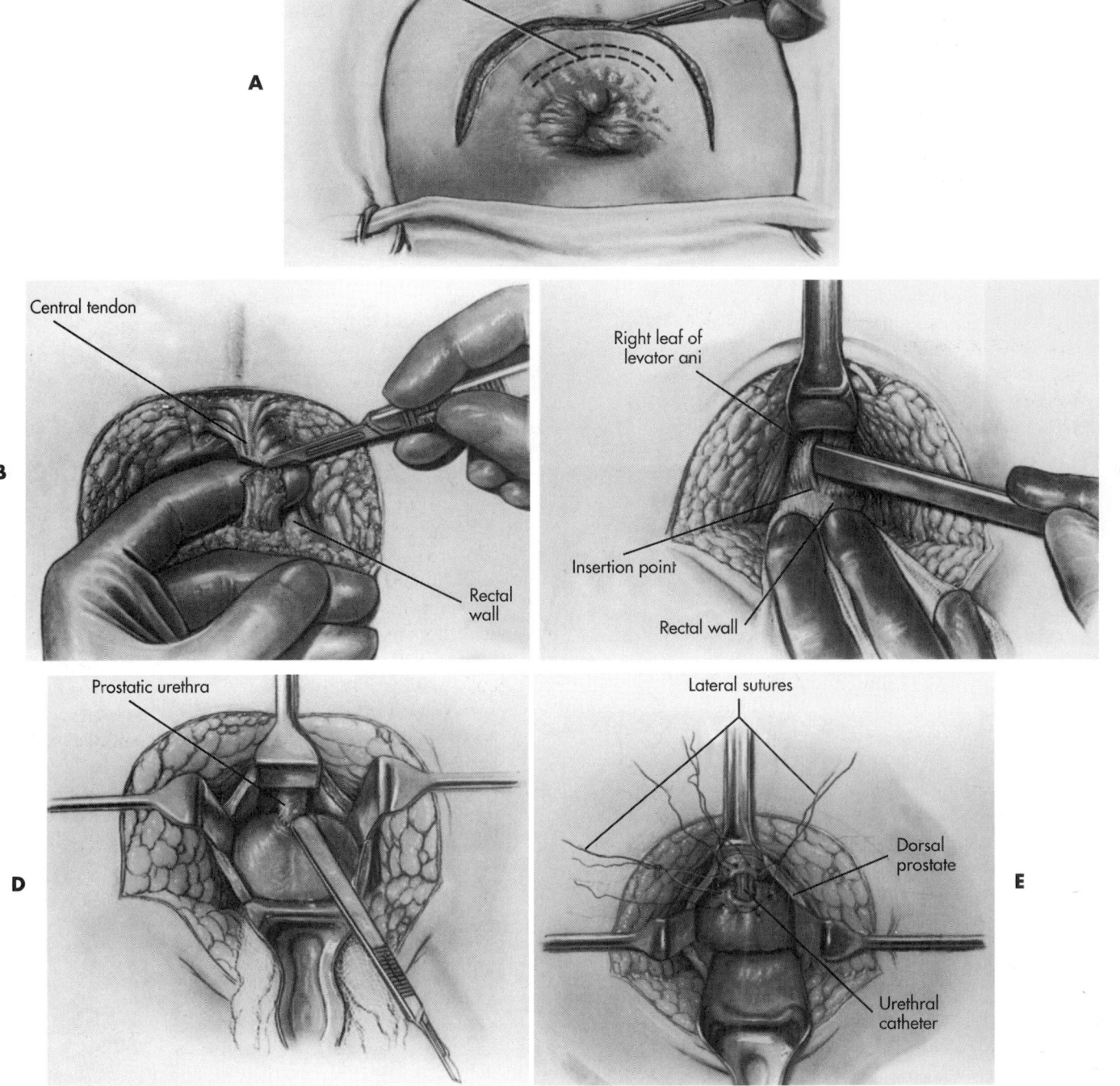

FIGURE 15-49   Perineal prostatectomy.

perineum if the needles are withdrawn too quickly; and implantation into the neurovascular bundle, because the anterior venous plexus is not distinguishable from the prostate on CT scan. There is also the chance of migration of seeds, placed just outside the periphery of the gland and in the periprostatic plexus, to the lung. The patient should be cautioned to avoid extended contact with and keep a 6-foot distance from children and pregnant females for 2 months. Urine must be strained, and any seeds expelled should be retrieved and returned to the oncologist. Bodily wastes are not considered hazardous, however.

Patients with a recent TURP (<60 days), a prostate

gland measuring >60 cc, or a Gleason grade >6 should not be considered for this procedure. One alternative for the patient with a recent TURP is implantation concentrated in the periphery of the gland.

Bleeding from the percutaneous sites is minimal, but postoperative ecchymosis of the perineum is to be expected. Other postoperative complications that may occur in the first 12 months include acute cystitis, prostatitis, and urinary retention. After 12 months, chronic prostatitis with cystitis, urethral stricture with contracture, stress with urge or total incontinence, proctitis, and impotence have been documented. Some patients have required posttreatment TURP, bladder-neck incision, suprapubic catheter insertion, or urethral dilatation to alleviate the above conditions. Less commonly, interventions such as laparotomy, colostomy, and urinary diversion have been necessary. Patients are generally able to void 24 to 48 hours after implantation. The patient is placed in the dorsal lithotomy position and prepped and draped as for cystoscopy. The scrotum must be secured cephalad to allow a clear operating field. This may be accomplished with a traction stitch placed through the lateral edges of the scrotum and anchored to the groin region.

Initially, C-arm fluoroscopy is utilized to judge the position of the needle at the base of the prostate referable to the bladder. After several cases have been performed with fluoroscopy, it may be eliminated, and seeding may then be done with ultrasound imaging only. Throughout the procedure, random room checks with the Geiger counter will be performed to determine radiation levels. All personnel will be scanned before leaving the room at the end of the procedure.

Operative procedure

Before seeding is begun, the ultrasound transducer must be positioned so that the posterior margin of the prostate is parallel to the axis of the ultrasound transducer. The direction of seed insertion and the transverse images of the prostate must have a similar appearance to those on the preoperative volume study. The volume study and implant worksheet are utilized for continual verification of coordinates. A stabilizer bar is attached to the OR bed. This secures the "stepping unit," which allows a 5 mm incremental forward-and-backward motion of the probe. The "sledge," which holds the transducer, is attached to the stepping unit. The probe must be securely anchored so that the position of the prostate relative to the needles used to implant the seeds remains unaltered throughout the procedure. For the needles to be positioned appropriately the template with labeled grid is attached to the transrectal transducer so that the needles placed through the probe grid match the grid locations on the plan. The volume of the apex of the gland is drawn somewhat larger on the plan. The grid is labeled alphabetically *Aa, Bb, Cc,* etc. with the center of the prostate corresponding to *D* on the grid.

1. At the beginning of the procedure a urethral catheter may be inserted to drain the bladder and to refill it with 150 ml of sterile water. Contrast medium for fluoroscopy is then instilled to more clearly delineate the bladder neck. Alternatively a cystoscopy may be performed, the bladder drained, and an open-ended ureteral catheter placed to instill contrast material and then removed. Ureteral catheters may also be inserted and left in situ during the implantation.
2. The urethral catheter is removed during implantation of seeds to avoid placement of seeds close to the urethra. The catheter causes the tissue surrounding the urethra to be compressed, and if attempts are made to implant seeds into this compressed tissue, penetration of the catheter and urethra may occur.
3. The transducer (probe) is covered with a sterile probe cover that is filled with 15 ml of sterile water to remove the artifact. Filling with too much fluid will change the configuration of the prostate and alter the anatomic presentation. The transducer will be aimed with the tip toward the floor at a 20-degree angle. The posterior wall of the prostate must be far enough away from the probe so that the posterior row of seeds is placed just inside the posterior capsule. Seeds are implanted by means of loaded needles placed into the prostate according to the template plan with the midline seeds placed slightly off center to avoid the urethra. The preoperative implantation plan should take into consideration the position of the urethra in the prostate so that it can be avoided during seed implantation. The bladder neck and rectum must be avoided during implantation to prevent urethrorectal fistula formation, irradiation of the bladder, and scarring at the bladder neck level.
4. Stabilization of the prostate may be achieved with stabilization needles placed laterally to the center into the right and left lobes and then moved once the anterior seeds are in place. Another method is to use a Foley catheter as a tractor for implantation of the periphery and until implantation near the urethra occurs. The best method may be to overcompensate for the rotation of the prostate by angling or turning the needle slightly opposite to the direction desired.
5. The most anterior seeds are placed first so that imaging of the anterior portion of the gland is not obscured by the ultrasonic shadows created by seeds placed posteriorly. If single seeds are used, the bevel of the needle should be sealed with bone wax to keep the seed in place until implantation. If strands are utilized, Anusol-HC (hydrocortisone) is used to seal the bevel before implantation. Strands should be cut cleanly with electrosurgery to seal the ends and avoid frayed ends, which may be split further when the stylette is inserted into the needle, adversely affecting seed placement.

6. Contrary to normal needle insertion with the bevel up, these needles are placed into the prostate with the solid, or back side, up. Every effort is extended to avoid implanting seeds into the bladder or too close to the urethra, to prevent necrosis, which causes significant postoperative irritative symptoms.

7. When placing the anterior seeds, the needle may become lodged in the pubic bone. The needle tip is visualized as a bright echo, and the angle may be altered to compensate for the bone. Alternatively the placement of the anterior seeds may be postponed until the end when the template may be dropped down, the probe positioned parallel to the pubic arch, and the needles inserted past the anterior portion into the prostate. During implantation, measurements can be taken from the hub of the needles to the template to check the location of the needle tips, since this distance should not change and assures positioning of the first seeds at the base of the prostate. The distance, in centimeters, from the needle hub to the needle trocar is equal to the number of seeds in each needle.

8. The needle is inserted beyond the desired site and then retracted. The bladder wall can generally be felt with the needle tip, and insertion should just enter the wall but not pass through it. The first seed will then determine where the balance will lie because the seeds will fall into a plane that follows the first seed in a specific needle. The target volume is greater than the actual volume of the prostate so that the capsular edge of the prostate and just beyond are also subjected to seed penetration. These peripherally placed seeds have a higher energy and may also have a greater tendency for migration because the tissue is not dense enough to hold the seed in place.

9. The base of the prostate is also slightly overimplanted.

10. Cystoscopy should be carried out at the end of the treatment so that seeds protruding into the urethra or left in the bladder may be removed.

11. A Foley catheter is placed and left for 24 to 48 hours.

Transrectal Cryosurgical Ablation of the Prostate Gland

Cryoablation of the prostate is a feasible, less invasive option for patients suffering from prostate cancer. The continence rates 1 year postoperatively are over 99% making this an attractive alternative to conventional therapy. Definitive results regarding postcryoablation erectile dysfunction are still not available but may be a significant consideration for the sexually active patient because the recovery rate is anticipated to range between 30% and 50%. Five-year statistics indicate equivalent results compared to surgery. Of 382 patients treated, 80% had normal prostate biopsy specimens, and 50% had PSA levels <1.0 ng/dl. All the other therapeutic options remain open to the patient, including repeat cryosurgery, radiation therapy, hormone therapy, observation, or surgery. Recur-

rence of an elevated PSA and abnormal biopsy specimen after cryosurgery prompt additional therapy. A prior TURP may increase the difficulty but is not a contraindication. Patients with extensive local tumor that does not allow for adequate visualization of disease extension or poses increased risk to the ureters, bladder, or rectum, if fully encompassed by freezing, may not be candidates for cryoablation.

During this procedure five 3 mm probes are inserted percutaneously into the prostate. Liquid nitrogen is then circulated through the probes to freeze the gland. This causes cell destruction and cell membrane rupture during thawing. A suprapubic catheter is inserted to allow urinary drainage and trials of voiding until prostatic swelling has subsided enough to allow micturition to occur (approximately 14 days). The freezing process may be extended beyond the prostatic capsule, potentially eradicating extracapsular extension. The purpose is to eradicate locally recurrent cancer and effect a cure. The procedure may kill diverse populations of cancer cells, including chemoresistant and androgen-resistant forms.

Complications that have been documented include urethrorectal and urethrocutaneous fistula, urethral necrosis, ureteral obstruction, retention as a result of sloughing of prostate tissue, transient renal failure, incontinence as a result of freezing of the external sphincter, impotence (incidence lower than that with other approaches), sepsis, hemorrhage (rare), myoglobinuria, and hemoglobinuria.

Procedural considerations

The patient is positioned in the lithotomy position (low or exaggerated by surgeon preference). The procedure averages about 2 hours. Alternating compression stockings and Allen boot stirrups, or well-padded candy-cane stirrups, are employed. The perineum is shaved, prepped with a povidone-iodine solution, and draped as for cystoscopy. Patients treated with cryosurgery are generally admitted and discharged the following morning unless bleeding, fever, or anesthetic complications prevent their discharge.

Operative procedure

1. A cystoscopic examination is carried out to assess the external sphincter, prostatic urethra, bladder neck, and bladder (trigone in particular).

2. The bladder is filled with sterile irrigant to facilitate percutaneous insertion of a Cope suprapubic catheter.

3. An 18-gauge needle with trocar is inserted suprapubically into the bladder. The trocar is removed allowing passage of the 0.038 guidewire through the needle.

4. The tract is progressively dilated with 6 to 12 Fr fascial dilators.

5. The catheter is placed into the bladder dome to reduce bladder spasms and is connected to drainage.

6. A trocar with cannula is inserted into the bladder through a 1 cm suprapubic incision placed between the pubis and the suprapubic catheter.

7. Cystoscopic evaluation is performed to assess puncture site and bladder integrity, the trocar is removed, and irrigation tubing is passed through the cannula, into the bladder, and out the urethra under cystoscopic guidance. This tubing is attached to sterile water irrigant that is circulated through a solution warmer and irrigation pump system to raise the urethral temperature during the freezing process.

8. The scrotum is tethered to the lower outer abdominal wall using a 3-0 silk stay suture.

9. A Bookwalter retractor is attached to the OR bed with the oval ring extending over the patient's genitalia.

10. Transrectal ultrasonography is carried out, and the volume of the prostate calculated. The anatomy of the bladder neck, trigone, seminal vesicles, and urogenital diaphragm are noted.

11. Five 18-gauge needles with trocar obturators are inserted into the prostate at the 10, 2, 4, 6, and 8 o'clock positions with their tips placed within 5 mm of the upper extent (base) of the prostate.

12. As each needle is inserted, the trocars are removed and 0.038 J tipped guidewires are inserted.

13. Once all wires are in place, fascial sleeved dilators are used to create tracts into the prostate. A stab wound may be necessary initially to allow entrance of the dilators.

14. The dilators are removed, leaving the sleeves in situ for placement of the cryoprobes.

15. Each sleeve is irrigated with saline to confirm their position before placement of the cryoprobes.

16. The cryoprobes are inserted, and the cryotechnician is instructed to "stick all probes." This will adhere the probes to the prostate so that they will be stabilized. Elastic straps (leg straps) should be used to support the probes, attaching them to the ring of the retractor.

17. Freezing is begun through the anterior probes, followed by complete freezing to the prostate-rectal border, to a freeze temperature of −180° C. The freezing process is begun at the anterior aspect of the gland so that the border of the freeze zone may be observed on ultrasonography, as it progresses posteriorly. Care is taken to avoid freezing the rectal wall and bladder neck, and below the pelvic floor. Some surgeons place thermocouples into the prostate to determine the exact freeze temperature.

18. Ultrasound examination is performed on the apex of the gland to assess for residual unfrozen tissue. The probes are thawed and withdrawn 1 to 2 cm.

19. When the probes have been repositioned, the remaining apical tissue should be frozen.

20. After all tissue has been frozen, the procedure is terminated by removing the cryoprobes once they have been "unstuck" (thawed).

21. The warming tubing is removed, and its insertion site and all cryoprobe sites are closed with absorbable 3-0 suture on a cuticular needle.

22. A #18, 5 ml Foley catheter is inserted and connected to straight drainage if the urine is bloody. The catheter may be removed the following morning.

Nerve-sparing Radical Retropubic Prostatectomy with Pelvic Lymphadenectomy

Radical prostatectomy is the treatment preferred for patients with organ-confined carcinoma of the prostate. This procedure involves removal of the entire gland, its capsule, and the seminal vesicles. Until recently the risk of impotence was extremely high after this approach. Now, with careful anatomic consideration, the posterolateral neurovascular bundles, supplying the corpora cavernosa, may be spared for erectile potency in many patients. Urinary incontinence is generally not the threat it used to be. Those with tumors confined in the prostatic capsule are the best candidates. Often, however, in the presence of more advanced tumor extension, one of the bundles may still be spared, allowing the chance for potency.

Procedural considerations

Patient preparation and basic surgical instrumentation are as for the simple retropubic approach. Additional supplies include long-tipped right-angled clamps, urethral suture guides (see Fig. 15-40), a Bookwalter or Wishbone (US200) retractor (see Fig. 15-42), long Martius clamps, straight and right-angled clip appliers and clips, and right-angled scissors.

Operative procedure

1. After insertion of a 20 or 22 Fr Foley catheter, a vertical midline, lower abdominal, extraperitoneal incision is made.

2. A bilateral pelvic lymphadenectomy is performed, removing the external iliac, obturator, and hypogastric nodes en bloc. This is done primarily for tumor staging. Theories differ on whether to proceed with radical surgery if nodal packets reveal metastatic disease.

3. The puboprostatic ligaments are exposed, and the endopelvic fascia is incised on each side of the gland to the puboprostatic ligaments (Fig. 15-50, *A*). Right-angled scissors are employed to divide the puboprostatic ligaments. The dorsal vein complex is easily subject to injury, and excessive venous bleeding may occur during this phase of the procedure. The perioperative nurse needs to be alert to this potential complication.

4. A plane is developed between the lateral prostatic border and the levator ani muscles with sharp and blunt dissection. Once visualized, the muscle is dissected laterally to the urogenital diaphragm.

5. Collateral veins originating from the levator ani muscle and running laterally to the puboprostatic ligaments are ligated and divided to free the apex of

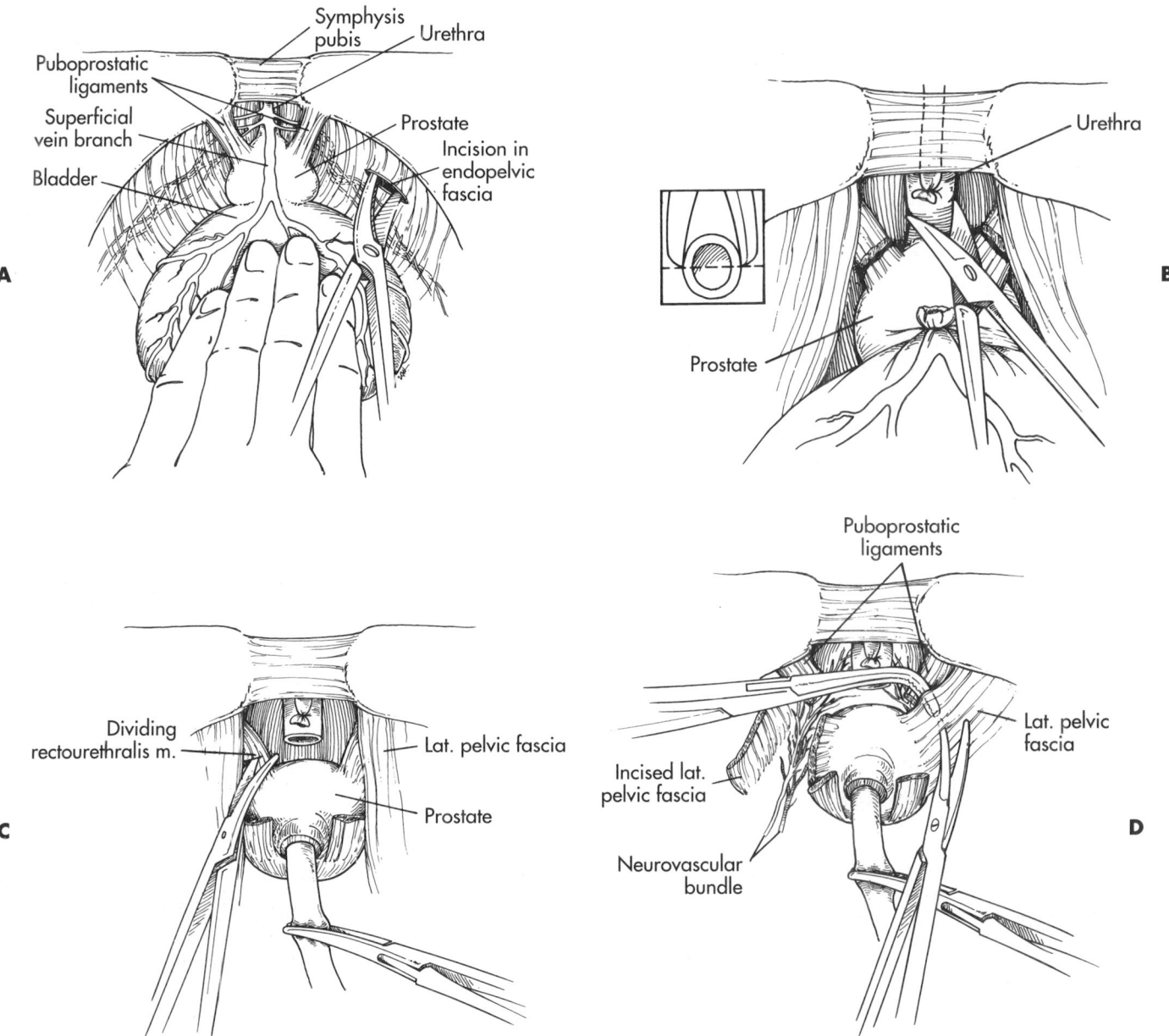

FIGURE 15-50 Radical retropubic prostatectomy.

Continued

the prostate. The perioperative nurse may hear the surgeon refer to these tributaries as the *veins of Kelley*.

6. The dorsal venous complex, supplying the penis, is carefully retracted medially. Once a plane is developed, the venous complex is separated from the urethra with a long-tipped right-angled clamp. The venous complex is tied off with 0 or 2-0 absorbable ligatures. Some surgeons opt to use a stapler designed for this purpose. The complex is then transsected with a #15 scalpel. Backbleeding, from the vessels onto the anterior surface of the prostate, is suture ligated.

7. The right-angled clamp mobilizes the urethra from the rectourethralis muscle between the two neurovascular bundles, avoiding damage to them.

8. A Penrose drain or vessel loop is passed around the urethra, and it is elevated and divided with a long-handled scissors or scalpel (Fig. 15-50, *B*). The catheter is clamped proximally and pulled upward through the urethral incision where it is cut and held cephalad.

9. The posterior urethra is transsected (Fig. 15-50, *B*).

10. The rectourethralis fibers are dissected free from and medial to the neurovascular bundles (Fig. 15-50, *C* and *D*).

11. Enucleation of the prostate, division of the bladder neck, and clip ligation of the seminal vesicles follow (Fig. 15-50, *E* and *F*).

12. Once bleeding is controlled, the urethral suture guide is inserted in place of the Foley and six 2-0 absorbable

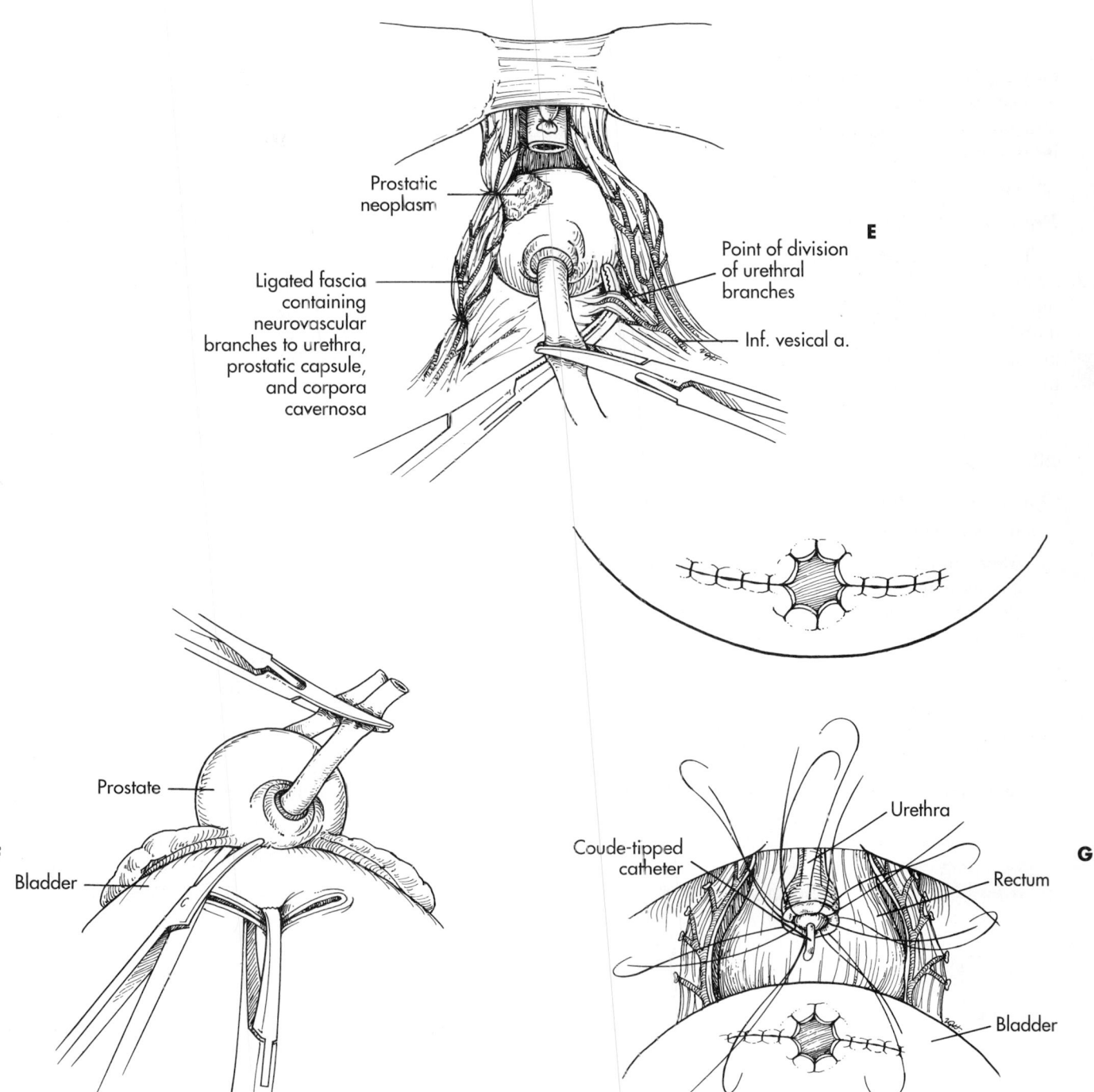

FIGURE 15-50, cont'd Radical retropubic prostatectomy.

sutures on a ⅝ needle are placed inside to outside on the distal urethral segment. These are tagged and left uncut to be anastomosed to the bladder neck (Fig. 15-50, G).

13. The bladder neck is trimmed and everted, and a rosebud stoma is fashioned. The sutures are placed from the urethra to a corresponding position on the bladder neck. When all are placed, they are brought together in single fashion and tied.

14. Closure is as for simple retropubic prostatectomy. Continuous postoperative irrigation is rarely used. A 22 Fr 30 ml Foley catheter is inserted and placed to gentle traction and dressings are applied.

Radical (Total) Perineal Prostatectomy

Patient preparation and instrumentation are identical to simple perineal prostatectomy. Additionally, however, the radical approach is accompanied by laparoscopic or low abdominal lymph node dissection, if not previously performed as a separate procedure. Currently, laparoscopy outweighs the standard incisional approach. Supplies needed for laparoscopy include standard laparoscopic instrumentation, three 10 mm trocars, one 5 mm trocar, an insufflation needle, a video camera unit, and CO_2 insufflation supplies.

Procedural considerations

Two operative setups are necessary. Most commonly, laparoscopy precedes prostatectomy. The patient is in the supine position for the laparoscopy with the area of the umbilicus slightly elevated. Sequential compressive stockings and preoperative Foley catheterization are necessary. Instruments should be available in the operating room to do an open procedure if necessary. Lymph nodes are sent for frozen section, primarily for tumor staging. Theories differ about proceeding if abnormal nodes are discovered.

Operative procedures

Laparoscopic Lymph Node Dissection

1. After initial instillation of CO_2 gas through the umbilical needle, 10 mm trocars are placed at the 12 o'clock (umbilicus), 3 o'clock, and 9 o'clock positions.
2. A 5 mm trocar is placed at the 6 o'clock position.
3. The placement of the last three trocars is observed with the laparoscope.
4. The peritoneum is grasped over the vas deferens, and an incision is made with scissors. The vas is identified, clipped or coagulated, and divided.
5. The peritoneal dissection is continued laterally and cephalad to the sigmoid colon on the left and the ascending colon on the right.
6. After identification of the spermatic cord structures,

iliac vessels, ureters, and psoas muscle, the incision is developed to the pubic ramus.
7. Cloquet's node is identified and freed from under the external iliac vein.
8. Dissection continues until the obturator nerve is isolated.
9. At the level of the bifurcation of the common iliac vein, the large lymph channel is located and removed. Endoclips or scissor-coagulation may be employed. Clips offer a lower risk of postoperative lymphocele.
10. In a similar fashion the tissue overlying the external iliac artery is removed.
11. The procedure is repeated on the opposite side.
12. Trocars are removed once hemostasis has been achieved. Each trocar is removed under direct observation with the laparoscope, to allow for identification of inner abdominal wall bleeding sites.
13. After evacuation of the gas from the abdomen, the fascia layers are closed at the 12, 3, and 9 o'clock positions.
14. The skin is then closed with 4-0 absorbable subcuticular sutures. The wounds are dressed with Steri-Strips, Telfa, and Tegaderm. The patient is then repositioned and prepared for radical perineal prostatectomy.

Radical Perineal Prostatectomy

Surgical approach is as for simple perineal prostatectomy (Fig. 15-51, A and B).

1. A layer of subcutaneous fascia is incised, and a space is developed within the ischial rectal fossa (Fig. 15-51, C).
2. The central tendon is incised, permitting dissection to be carried out beneath the triangle formed by the superficial external anal sphincter (Fig. 15-51, D).

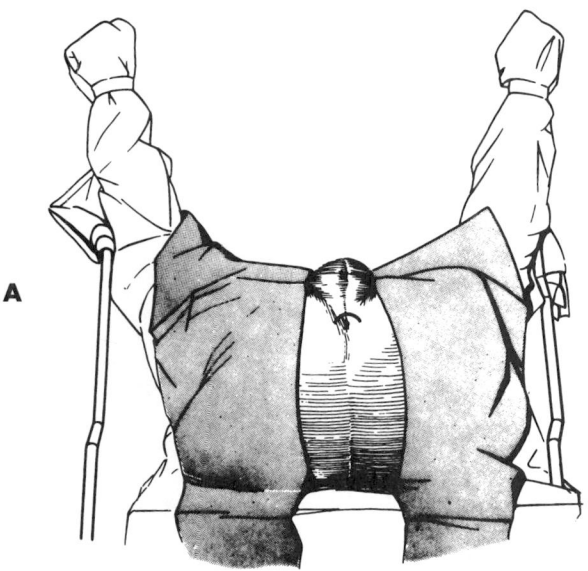

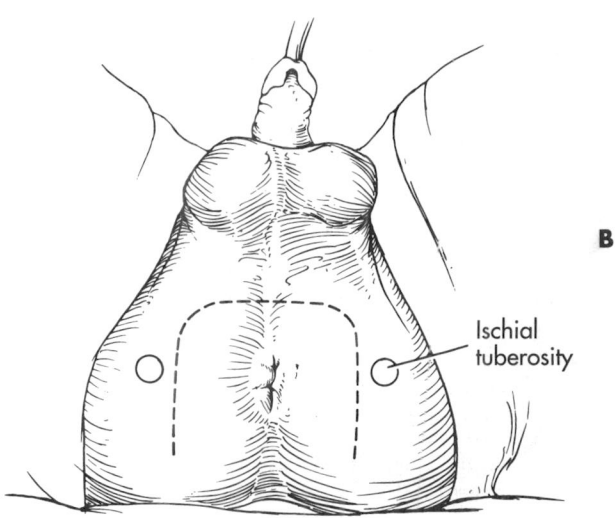

Ischial tuberosity

FIGURE 15-51 Radical perineal prostatectomy.

Continued

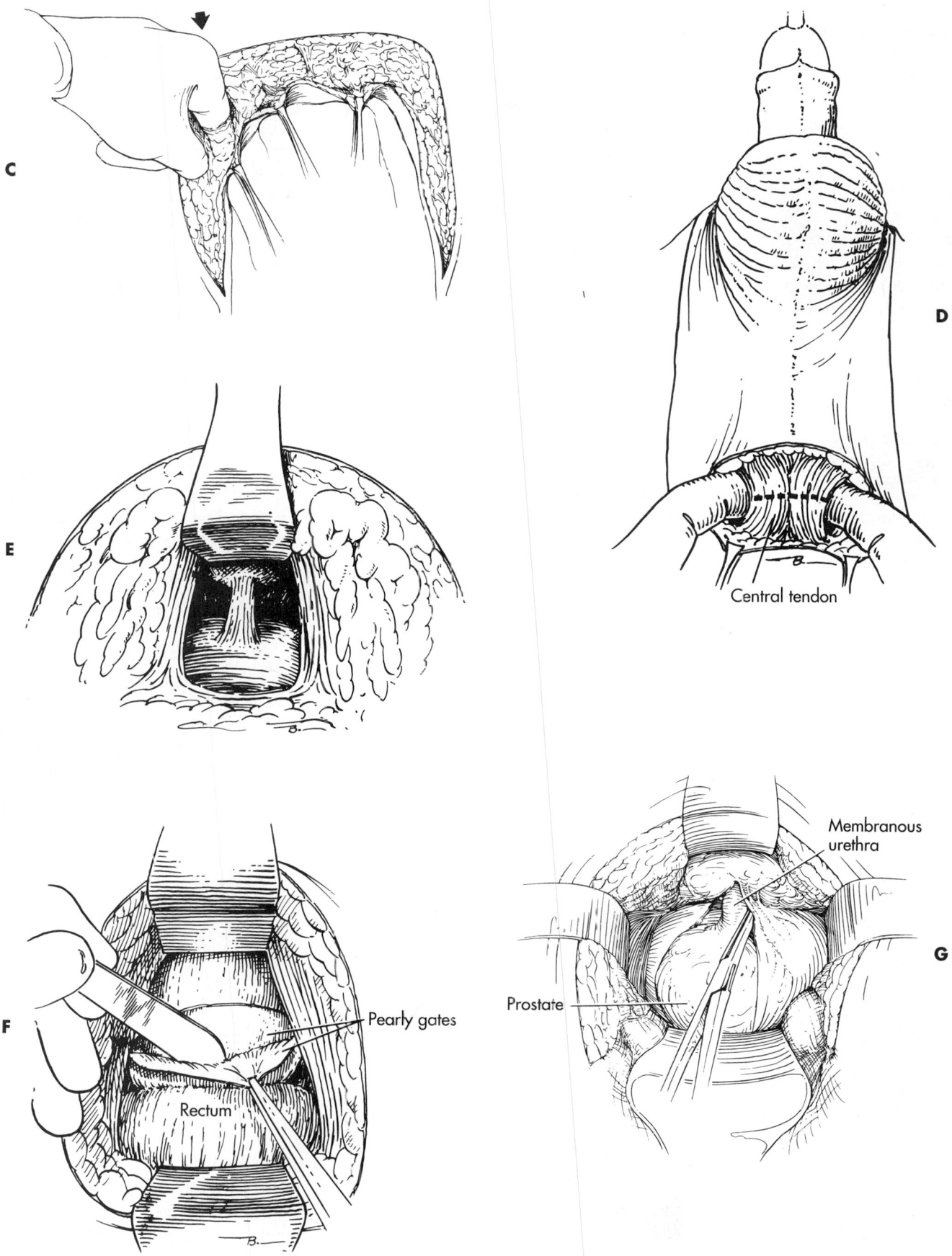

FIGURE 15-51, cont'd   Radical perineal prostatectomy.

Continued

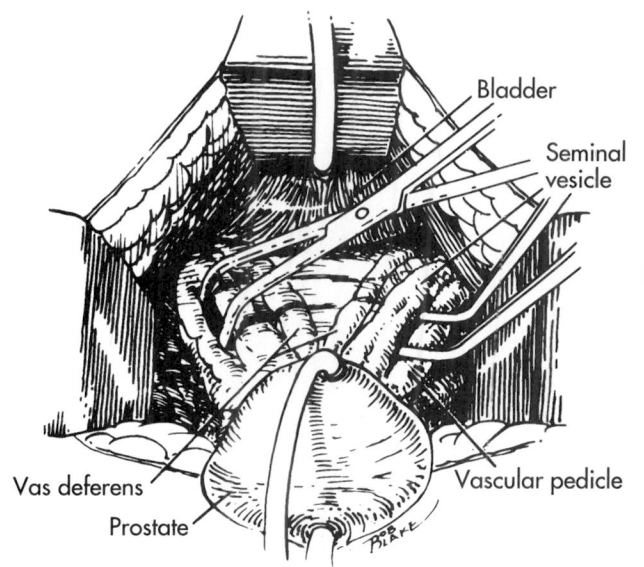

H

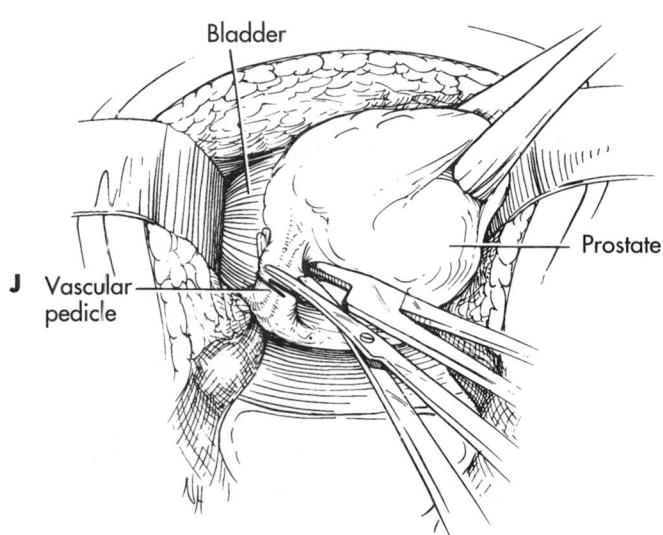

J

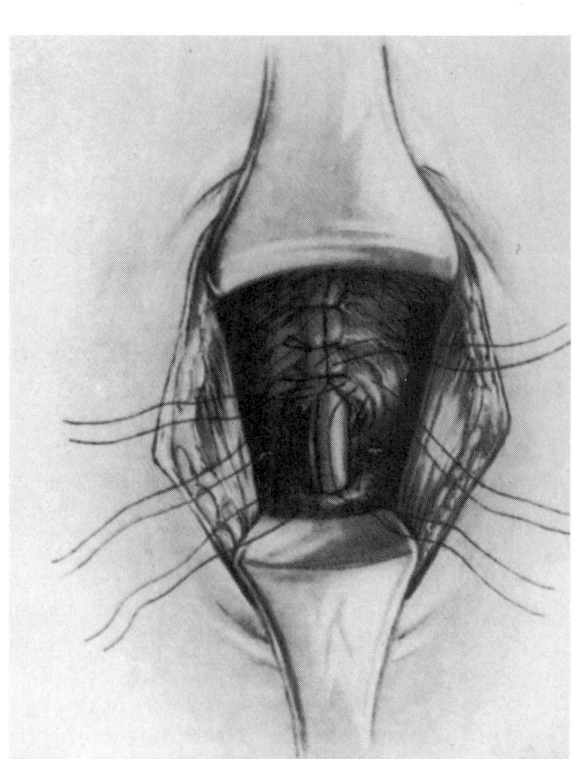

I

K

FIGURE 15-51, cont'd   Radical perineal prostatectomy.

3. The sphincter is retracted cephalad, and the rectoure-thralis is visualized (Fig. 15-51, *E*).
4. The true prostatic capsule is exposed by incision of the overlying fascia (Fig. 15-51, *F*).
5. After dissection of the periprostatic fascia unilaterally, a right-angled clamp is passed around the membranous urethra, and the urethra is sharply incised (Fig. 15-51, *G*).

6. The posterior bladder neck is severed, and the bladder is retracted superiorly (Fig. 15-51, *H*).
7. A plane is then developed between the anterior bladder and the posterior prostate and seminal vesicles (Fig. 15-51, *I*).
8. The vascular pedicles are identified at the 5 and 7 o'clock positions, incised, and divided (Fig. 15-51, *J*).
9. Before closure of the bladder neck, vest sutures of no.

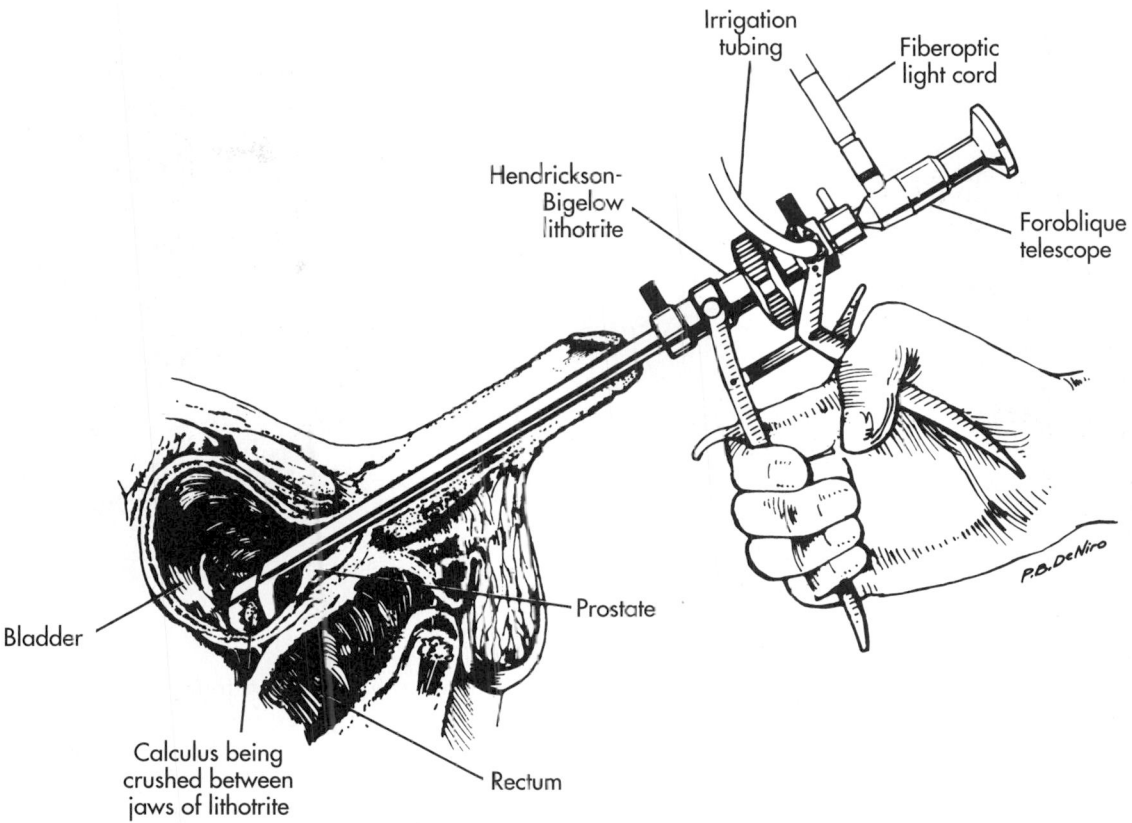

FIGURE 15-52   Hendrickson-Bigelow lithotrite.

0 or 2-0 absorbable material may be placed in a mattress fashion in the open bladder neck at the 2 and 10 o'clock positions and left long for later lateral perineal placement (Fig. 15-51, *K*).

10. Once reanastomosis is accomplished, these vest sutures are crossed and brought through the perineal body laterally and parallel to the urethra, anterior to the incision, and secured just beneath the skin, or to the skin with suture buttons.

11. After placement of the Foley catheter, the urethra is reanastomosed to the bladder neck with four to six 2-0 absorbable sutures and placed at the 2, 4, 8, and 10 o'clock positions. Some surgeons opt to place sutures at the 6 and 12 o'clock positions as well.

12. A drain of the surgeon's preference is placed anteriorly to the rectal surface and drawn out through the incision line or through a separate stab wound.

13. Final closure and dressings are as described in the simple procedure.

SURGERY OF THE BLADDER

Operations on the urinary bladder may be performed through an open abdominal incision or a transurethral route. Special transurethral instruments such as the lithotrite may be used to crush vesical calculi manually (Fig. 15-52). A lithotriptor may be used to fragment the

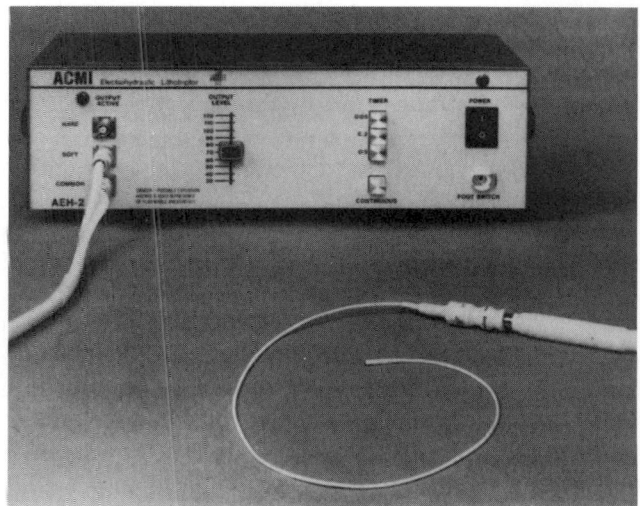

FIGURE 15-53   ACMI electrohydraulic lithotriptor and probe.

stone within the bladder by using an electric current to initiate shock waves (Fig. 15-53).

Ultrasonic lithotripsy is another procedure used in the management of vesical calculi. Ultrasound waves are transmitted through a hollow metal probe (sonotrode), which creates vibration at the tip. When applied to the surface of a calculus, the vibrating tip drills and fragments

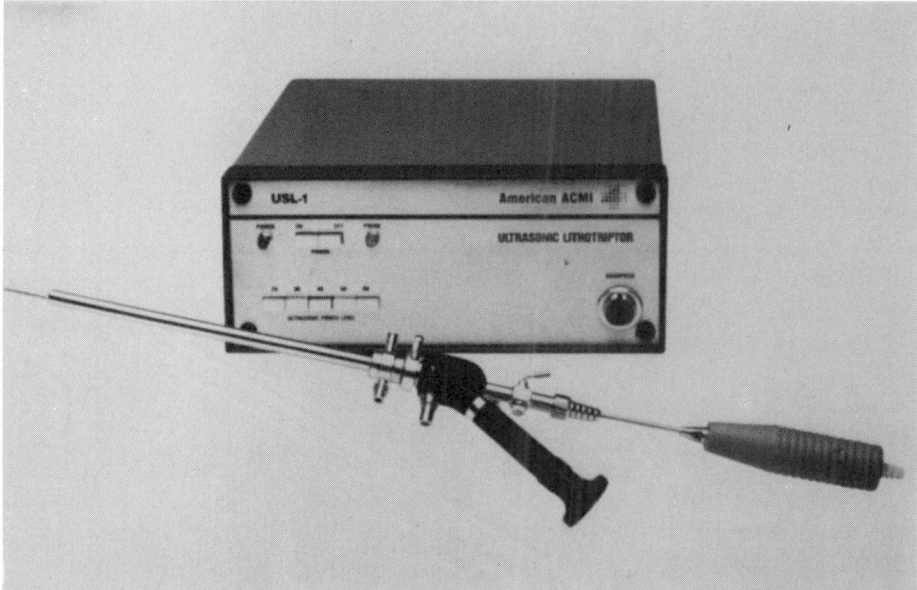

FIGURE 15-54   Ultrasonic lithotriptor with rigid nephroscope.

the calculus. This mechanical disintegration is continued until the stone is reduced to small fragments that are evacuated by suction through the hollow center of the probe (Fig. 15-54).

Stones may also be removed from the bladder through a suprapubic incision (cystolithotomy). Bladder tumors, diverticula, congenital defects, or trauma may necessitate an open abdominal approach. A thorough diagnostic workup and endoscopic examination can help to determine the appropriate surgical approach to be employed. Radical procedures, such as total cystectomy, are performed for the treatment of invasive carcinoma of the bladder and require permanent urinary diversion.

For most open-bladder surgery the patient is placed in the supine position with a bolster under the pelvis. Trendelenburg's position may be desired because this position tilts the head down and allows the viscera to fall cephalad. This allows excellent exposure of the pelvic organs, including the bladder. The patient is draped as described for routine suprapubic prostatectomy, using a disposable impermeable drape that is placed immediately below the bladder incision. A catheter of choice may be inserted into the urethra, and the bladder is distended with sterile saline at the start of surgery for easy identification. The ESU may be required. The instrument setup for open bladder operations requires a basic laparotomy set, plus Mason-Judd bladder retractors, long and short thyroid traction forceps, retropubic needle holders (or other long needle holders as desired), one trocar, vessel loops, a catheter stylette, a closed wound suction system, and assorted Foley, Pezzar, and Malecot catheters

Suprapubic Cystostomy

Cystotomy is an opening made into the urinary bladder through a low abdominal incision. When a drainage tube is inserted into the bladder through an abdominal incision, the procedure is a cystostomy.

Procedural considerations

The patient is in the supine position. A basic laparotomy set is generally sufficient for the procedure. Foley catheters ranging from 22 to 30 Fr should be available as well as Malecot suprapubic catheters and a drainage bag. Anesthesia may be general, spinal, or local with sedation. Frequently the urologist will incorporate a flexible cystoscopy into the procedure.

Operative procedure

1. A vertical or Pfannenstiel incision (transverse) is used. The rectus fascia is divided in the midline (Fig. 15-55, *A*). The surgical approach is as described for suprapubic prostatectomy.
2. The bladder is distended with saline solution that is instilled with an Asepto syringe through a catheter.
3. The dome of the bladder is then dissected free with Metzenbaum scissors and blunt dissection (Fig. 15-55, *B*).
4. The wall of the bladder is grasped on either side of the midline with Martius forceps (Fig. 15-55, *C*).
5. Two traction sutures may be placed through the bladder wall and held with straight hemostats.
6. The bladder is then incised downward with a scalpel. Bleeding vessels in the bladder wall are clamped and ligated.
7. The bladder contents are aspirated with a Poole suction device.
8. The bladder opening may be extended if the bladder is to be explored for diverticula or calculi.
9. A large-sized Malecot or Pezzar catheter is introduced into the bladder (Fig. 15-55, *D*).

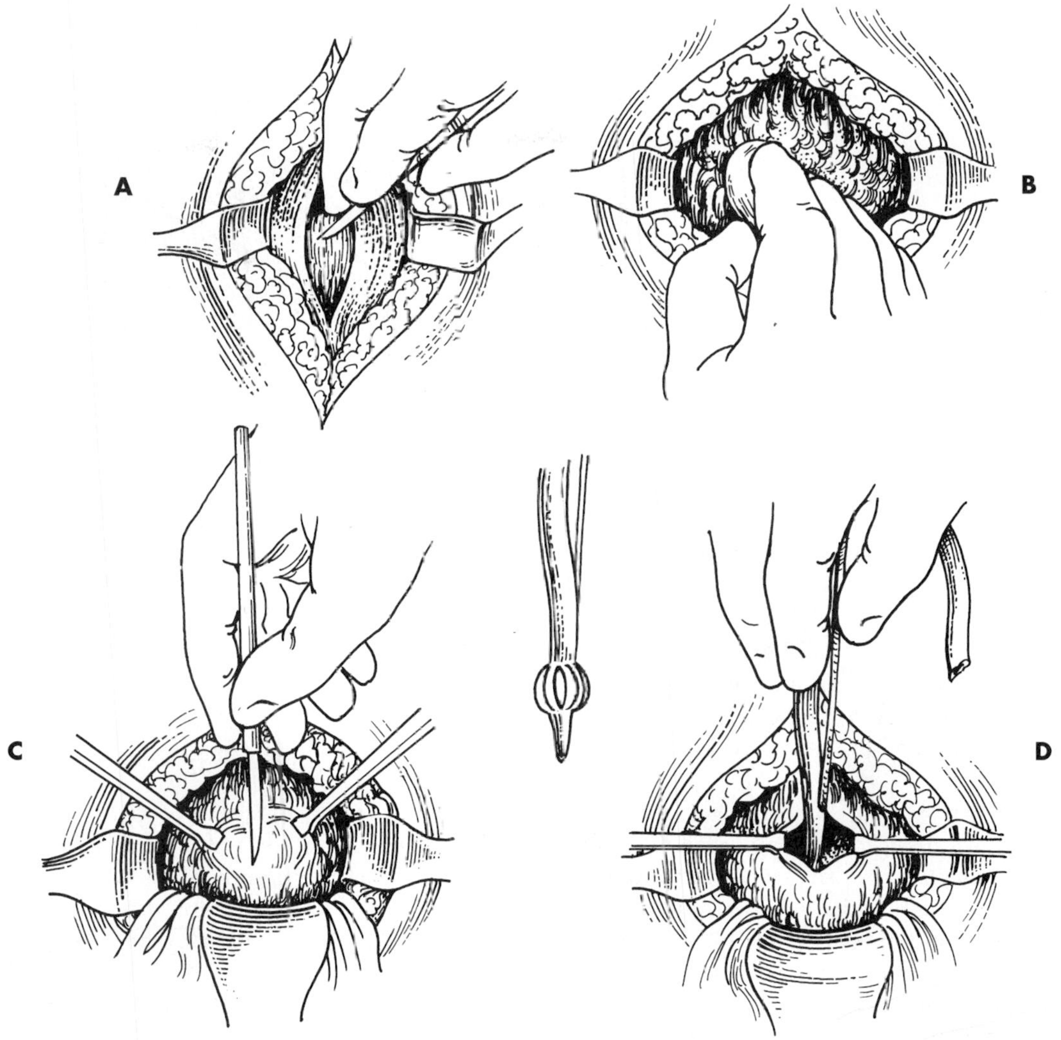

FIGURE 15-55 Suprapubic cystostomy.

10. The incision is closed snugly about the catheter with absorbable sutures to render the closure watertight about the cystostomy tube.

11. The muscle, fascia, and subcutaneous tissue are closed with absorbable suture.

12. The skin is closed with staples or the suture of choice in the manner of preference.

13. The cystostomy tube is secured to the skin with a 0 or 2-0 nonabsorbable suture to prevent it from being inadvertently dislodged from the bladder. A drain such as a Jackson-Pratt may be left in the prevesical space.

14. The wound is dressed, and the cystostomy tube is connected to a straight urinary drainage system.

Transurethral Resection of Bladder Tumors

Bladder lesions may be removed using a standard resectoscope, working element, loop, and a Foroblique telescope, which is passed through the urethra into the bladder. A 24 Fr cystoscope sheath with a catheterizing bridge and biopsy forceps may be used to remove bladder tumors located at the very top or dome of the bladder (Fig. 15-56). Transitional cell carcinoma of the bladder is one of the most difficult lesions to track because it can occur wherever there is transitional cell lining of the urinary tract. Bladder cancer has a tendency to recur in other areas of the bladder even after complete resection of the original lesions.

Usually the surgeon removes not only the bladder lesion but also a portion of the muscle of the bladder underlying the lesion so that the pathologist can determine if any tumor has invaded the muscle. Random biopsy specimens of the normal bladder lining are also taken to ascertain if microscopic transitional cell carcinoma in situ is present.

Lesions that deeply invade the muscle must be treated with an open surgical procedure, such as a partial cystectomy or total cystectomy.

The resection technique, setup, and preparation of the patient are virtually the same as that for transurethral resection of the prostate. A general, spinal, or regional anesthetic is administered. If the surgeon has any questions

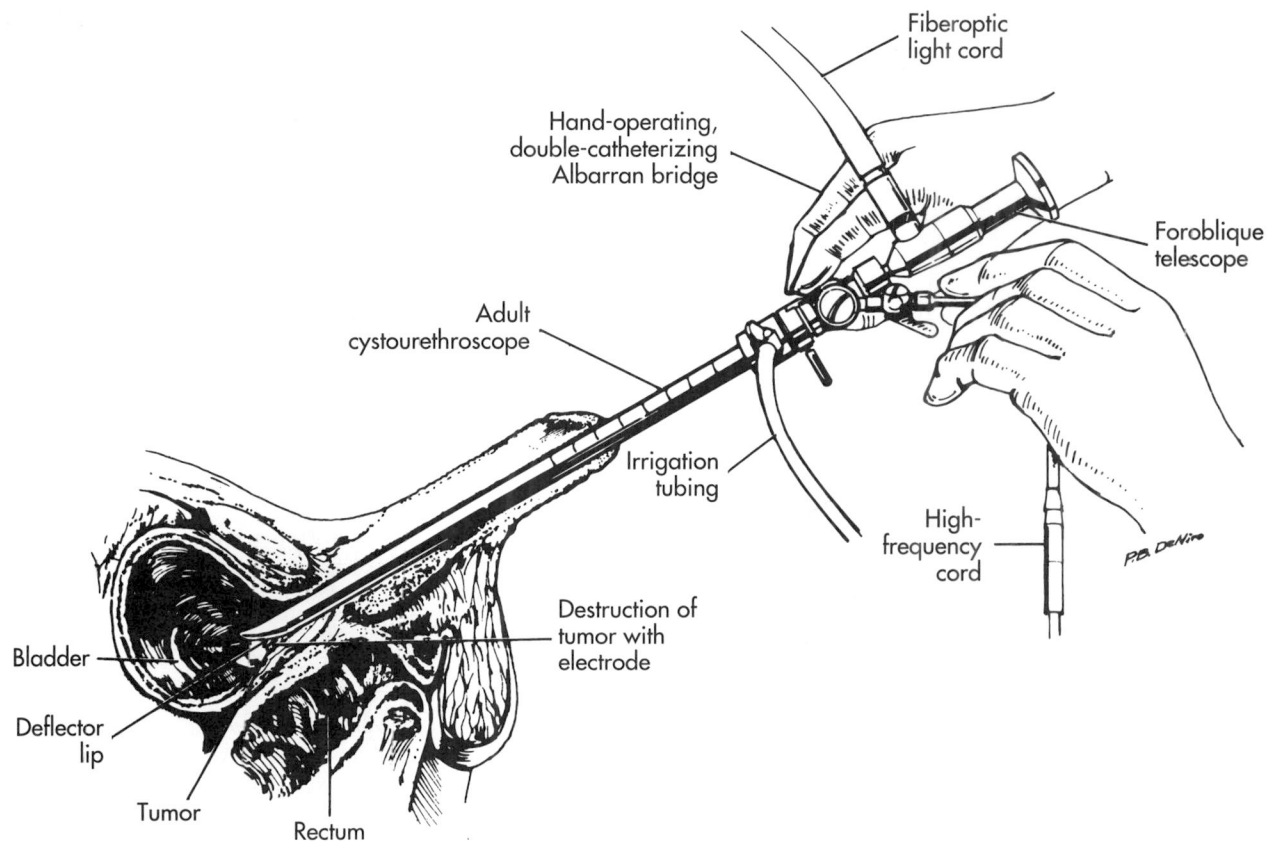

FIGURE 15-56   Bladder fulguration.

about lesions existing in the upper urinary tract, a retrograde pyelogram is done.

Sterile water is recommended as an irrigating solution in transurethral resection of bladder tumors. Because few vessels are uncovered during this short resection procedure, water absorption with hemolysis and systemic complications such as hyponatremia do not occur. In addition, there is a tendency for cancer cells released during the procedure to absorb water, causing them to rupture and lyse rather than remain viable and capable of implanting themselves into the raw surface of the bladder created by the surgery.

On completion of the procedure a large catheter, usually a 24 Fr, is passed into the bladder and connected to drainage.

Transurethral Laser Ablation of Bladder Tumors

The Nd:YAG or holmium:YAG laser may be used to destroy small recurrent bladder tumors and to coagulate the tumor bed of larger bladder tumors resected with an electrosurgical loop. A powerful, highly focused beam of light in the near-infrared range is transmitted to the tumor site through a flexible glass fiber. This laser fiber is passed through the catheter channel of a cystoscope, and the fiber is directed by a deflecting laser bridge (Fig. 15-57). The

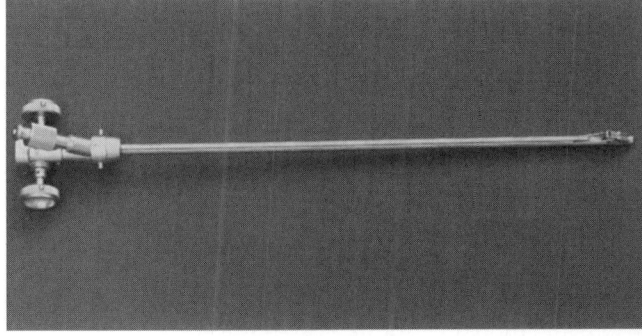

FIGURE 15-57   Laser bridge, laser fiber deflected, Foroblique telescope, 21 Fr cystoscope sheath.

advantages of a laser in the eradication of bladder tumors are that bleeding is minimized, only sedation is required, the operating time is shortened, there is minimal damage to healthy tissue, and there is no need for postoperative drainage of the bladder by a urethral catheter.

Alternatives to Surgery for Superficial Bladder Cancer

Patients with various types of cancer may be treated in the urology office setting with various therapeutic modalities. These measures may be initiated instead of surgery or as an adjunct to surgery.

Patients with bladder cancer that has been staged as Ta, Tis, and T1 are being treated with intravesical, antineoplastic chemotherapy agents such as thiotepa, mitomycin (Mutamycin), doxorubicin (Adriamycin), etoglucid (Epodyl), and bacille Calmette GuJrin (BCG). These medications have been proved effective in both the eradication of obvious tumor and the prevention of recurrence. BCG has been found, through an unknown mechanism, to strengthen the body's immune reaction to cancer and is considered the most effective therapy for recurrent and residual bladder cancer. Currently the complete response rate of BCG is 80%. Other therapies show complete response of 60% with a 30% recurrence, compared to 70% recurrence with no treatment.

Trocar Cystostomy

Trocar cystostomy consists of draining the bladder by puncture with a needle or trocar and inserting a catheter.

Procedural considerations

A minor set of instruments along with a metal probe and grooved director, an Anthony suction tube and tubing, and trocar catheters or a prepackaged cystostomy kit are required. A local anesthesia setup may be used.

Operative procedure

1. The skin at the site of the puncture is nicked with a scalpel, and the trocar is inserted into the bladder.
2. The trocar obturator is withdrawn, the bladder is drained through the trocar by suction, and a catheter is passed through the trocar cannula into the bladder.
3. The cannula is carefully withdrawn, and the catheter is sutured to the wound edges. The wound is dressed.

Suprapubic Cystolithotomy

Suprapubic cystolithotomy is the removal of calculi from the bladder. Obstructions, such as prostatic enlargement or foreign bodies, are common causes of bladder calculi and may be corrected at the time of surgery.

Procedural considerations

The instrument setup for open-bladder operations along with Millin T-shaped stone forceps, Millin capsule forceps, and Lewkowitz lithotomy forceps are required.

Operative procedure

The surgical approach is similar to that described for suprapubic cystotomy. When the bladder is opened, calculi are identified and extracted. If indicated, bladder outlet obstruction is repaired.

Repair of Vesical Fistulas

Vesical fistulas occurring between the bladder and the intestines or vagina may be repaired surgically. Vesicointestinal fistula may be caused by ulcerative colitis, diverticulitis, or neoplasms of the colon or rectum.

Vesicovaginal fistula may be a complication of radiotherapy for cervical cancer or endoscopic procedures involving surgery of the trigone or vesical neck. Such fistulas are also caused by obstetric injuries and hysterectomies.

Procedural considerations

The instrument setup is as described for open-bladder operations. An intestinal resection setup (see Chapter 11) is also necessary for vesicointestinal fistulas. For vesicovaginal fistulas, vaginal preparation and a colporrhaphy set (see Chapter 14) with colostomy or ileostomy instruments are used. Alternating compression stockings are applied.

Vesicointestinal fistulas are more common than vesicovaginal fistulas. Of the intestinal fistulas, the sigmoid colon is most often involved. A colostomy proximal to the fistula may be performed to protect the repaired segment of bowel. The communicating area of bladder and bowel is totally resected. Generally, an end-to-end bowel resection is performed after excision of the involved intestinal segment. The bladder is then repaired in three layers.

If the fistula is at the dome of the bladder, the approach will be transperitoneal, transvesical, or a combination of the two. If the fistula is in the trigone of the bladder, a vaginal approach may be employed. A suprapubic tube is usually left in the bladder.

Operative procedures

Vesicovaginal Fistula Repair with Vaginal Approach

1. With the patient in lithotomy or supine, a suprapubic catheter is inserted, clamped, and connected to closed drainage.
2. The patient is placed in hyperflexed lithotomy position or Kraske's position (prone).
3. The vagina and external genitalia are prepped with povidone-iodine solution.
4. The area is draped with four adherent drape towels and a lithotomy or laparotomy sheet. If the intended position is Kraske, separate draping material and instrumentation are set up for the suprapubic catheter insertion with the patient supine. The catheter is secured, and the patient is turned for the procedure.
5. The labia are sutured to the outer groin or inner thigh for retraction and visualization.
6. A weighted vaginal retractor is placed posteriorly and the defect examined. A relaxing vaginal incision may be necessary at 5 or 7 o'clock position.
7. A 4 Fr ureteral catheter is inserted through the fistula, and the tract is dilated to admit the 8 Fr balloon catheter. The balloon is inflated, and the catheter is used as a tractor.
8. The area is infiltrated with epinephrine solution 1:200,000.
9. The vaginal mucosa and perivesical fascia around the defect is incised, well outside the scarred tissue.

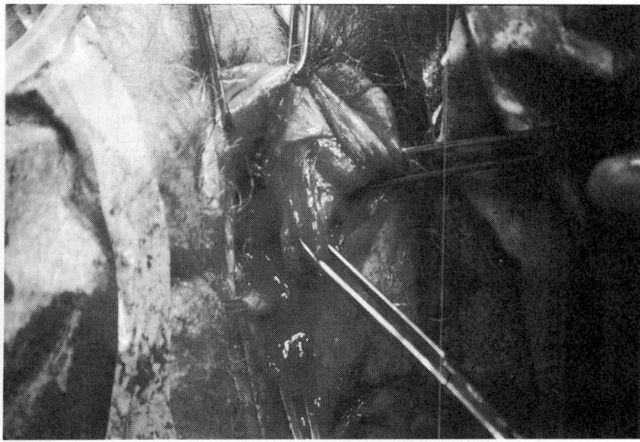

FIGURE 15-58 Labial pedicle or full-thickness flap (Martius flap) being placed between the vesical closure and the vaginal closure to prevent suture-line stress and overlay.

10. Two planes are developed: one between the mucosa and fascia, and one between the fascia and the bladder wall with fine scissors, forceps, and Kittner dissectors.

11. The bladder wall is freed from the vaginal wall.

12. The vesical defect is grasped with Martius clamps, and the scarred edges are everted. It is then closed vertically with interrupted 3-0 absorbable sutures after removal of the catheter previously placed. In some instances, a labial pedicle or full-thickness flap (Martius flap) may be placed between the vesical closure and the vaginal closure (Fig. 15-58). This prevents suture-line stress and overlay and removes the need for a relaxing incision. Larger fistulas that do not adequately reapproximate may necessitate a vascularized muscle flap to reinforce closure.

13. The perivesical fascia and vaginal mucosa are approximated separately with transverse, interrupted 3-0 absorbable sutures. A one-sided ellipse of vaginal mucosa may be excised to offset the closure.

14. Alternatively, an inverted-U incision may provide more exposure than other incisions and result in a posterior flap that completely covers the site of the defect.

15. The suprapubic catheter is unclamped, the labial stitches are removed, and the vagina is loosely packed.

Vesicovaginal Fistula and Transperitoneal (Transvesical) Approach

1. The patient is placed in low lithotomy and moderate Trendelenburg's position. Both the perineum and the abdomen are prepped and draped appropriately. A laparoscopy pack works well for this approach.

2. Ureteral catheters are inserted endoscopically, and a #16 Foley catheter is placed in the bladder and clamped.

3. A rubber ball or tight gauze pack is placed into the vagina.

4. A vertical midline or Pfannenstiel incision is made.

5. The peritoneum is incised and bluntly dissected from the dome of the bladder.

6. The small bowel is packed cephalad.

7. Stay sutures of 2-0 absorbable suture are placed in the bladder dome and the bladder opened.

8. The bladder wall and overlying peritoneum are divided down to the fistula. Stay sutures are placed periodically to serve as tractors for bladder elevation.

9. The peritoneum is incised transversely at the level of the fistula, forming a pedicle flap.

10. The vagina and bladder are separated widely on each side of the fistula. An assistant places upward pressure on the vaginal ball or pack to facilitate dissection.

11. As the fistula is exposed, it is excised until completely removed. A probe may be used to localize it, if small, or the 8 Fr balloon catheter may be inserted and used for traction during dissection.

12. The bladder and vagina are freed from each other until there is enough mobility for separate closures.

13. The vagina is then closed, without tension, with inverting 2-0 or 3-0 interrupted sutures in two layers.

14. The peritoneal flap is swung into the defect and sutured in place for retroperitonealization. A long attached peritoneal or free peritoneal pedicle flap may be needed for reperitonealization. Alternatively, the omentum may be brought from behind the right side of the colon for an omental graft, or a vascularized muscle flap may be placed. Fistulas resulting from radiation necrosis may best be managed with the latter option.

15. A 22 Fr Malecot catheter and a wound drain are inserted and pulled through separate stab wounds in the abdomen.

16. The ureteral catheters are removed, and the bladder mucosa and submucosa are closed in separate layers with 2-0 or 3-0 absorbable suture in a running fashion.

17. The muscularis and adventitia are externally approximated with interrupted 3-0 suture.

18. The wound is closed in layers in the standard fashion with 2-0, 3-0, and 4-0 sutures or skin clips.

19. Dressings are applied, the Foley is unclamped, the rubber ball or gauze roll are removed, and the vagina is loosely repacked.

Vesicosigmoid Fistula Repair by Abdominal Approach

1. With the patient in supine and Trendelenburg's position a #20 or #22 5 ml Foley cather is inserted into the bladder, and the bladder is filled with 100 ml of sterile water. Once prepped and draped as for laparotomy, a midline, or paramedian, and transperitoneal incisions are made.

2. The abdomen is explored, and contents are examined.
3. The descending and sigmoid colon are mobilized by incising along the fascia fusion line of Toldt.
4. The involved loop of colon is identified. If a walled-off inflammatory mass is found, a transverse colostomy should be performed and a two-stage intervention considered.
5. The fistulous tract is separated by blunt finger dissection.
6. A probe is inserted to determine the extent of involvement.
7. The defects in the bladder and bowel are debrided to obtain healthy tissue. Large inflammatory masses require a colon resection.
8. The bladder is closed in two layers with a 3-0 absorbable, submucosal running stitch, and a 2-0 absorbable, interrupted muscularis and adventitial stitch.
9. The edges of the bowel defect are trimmed to reach normal tissue, and stay sutures are placed on each side.
10. The cavity is pulled transversely, and the mucosa and submucosa are closed in one pass with a Connell stitch of 3-0 chromic catgut.
11. The muscularis and serosa are approximated and closed in one pass with 4-0 silk Lembert sutures.
12. The abdomen is irrigated with 2000 ml of sterile saline with an attempt to reach all areas.
13. A sump style of drain is placed intraperitoneally and a Penrose or small Jackson-Pratt drain is placed suprapubically, exiting through separate stab wounds.
14. The abdomen is closed in layers in the conventional manner. If a colostomy was performed, it is opened for fecal diversion and the appropriate appliance is applied.
15. Gauze and bulky absorbable dressings are applied and secured with Montgomery straps.

Vesicourethral Suspension (Marshall–Marchetti–Krantz)

A Marshall–Marchetti suspension is performed for the correction of stress incontinence caused by an abnormal urethrovesical angle. The intent of the Marshall-Marchetti-Krantz operation is to bring the bladder and urethra into the pelvis by suturing paraurethral vaginal tissue to the back of the symphysis pubis. A recent modification of this technique is the Burch procedure. The approach mimics the Marshall-Marchetti until placement of the buttressing sutures. Instead of attempting difficult periosteal sutures the surgeon places nonabsorbable size 0 sutures into Cooper's ligament from each side of the bladder neck. The Burch is technically easier, and long-term results are fairly equivalent.

A large percentage of patients with stress incontinence suffer from obesity and diabetes. It is important to evaluate for these conditions and prepare for proper patient management (that is, positioning concerns relating to peripheral vascular circulation and pressure points, skin breakdown, risk for infection, wound healing).

Procedural considerations

The patient is usually placed in a moderate Trendelenburg's position, frog-legged, with supports under each knee to allow for intraoperative vaginal manipulation. Abdominal and vaginal preps are required. A Foley catheter is inserted into the urethra at the beginning of surgery. This procedure is combined with an abdominal hysterectomy. Surgeon and assistant double-glove for vaginal manipulation. The basic laparotomy set and abdominal hysterectomy instruments (see Chapter 14), if needed, are used. The patient will commonly have a vaginal pack and a urethral catheter with or without a suprapubic catheter and possibly a wound drain postoperatively.

Operative procedure

1. A Foley catheter is inserted into the bladder through the urethra.
2. A suprapubic transverse incision is made to expose the prevesical space of Retzius.
3. The bladder retractor is positioned with small, moist laparotomy pads in place.
4. The bladder and urethra are freed from the posterior surface of the rectus muscle and symphysis pubis by gentle blunt manipulation.
5. The assistant places two fingers into the vagina, lifting the urethra upward against the symphysis pubis to facilitate ease of repair of the periurethral musculofascial structures.
6. A heavy, nonabsorbable atraumatic suture on a Heaney needle holder is placed through the supporting fascia of the vaginal wall on each side of the urethra. The suture is passed through the symphysis pubis, providing support to the urethra and bladder neck. Generally a row of three heavy, nonabsorbable sutures is placed on each side of the urethra, the most proximal being located just at the vesical neck.
7. The area is drained, and the wound is closed in layers and dressed.
8. The vagina may be packed with 2-inch packing, which should be removed after 24 to 36 hours.
9. The Foley catheter is connected to a closed urinary drainage system.

Transvaginal Bladder Neck Suspension

Vesical neck suspensions have distinct advantages over traditional open retropubic urethrovesical suspensions. The incision is superficial, the bladder and bladder neck are not dissected, and the paraurethral tissues that suspend the vesical neck are buttressed vaginally.

The original vesical neck suspension for urinary stress incontinence was developed by Pereyra. This method involved insertion of the Pereyra needle (Fig. 15-59) blindly through a small suprapubic stab wound.

The paraurethral tissues were suspended with 30 stainless steel wire.

Stamey modified this technique and developed the first endoscopic vesical neck suspension by using the cystoscope to place heavy nonabsorbable sutures, buttressed by GoreTex or Dacron bolsters, exactly at the vesical neck. Raz modified the Stamey method by placing sutures laterally to the urethra and bladder neck, lowering the risk of postoperative bladder neck obstruction. The Raz procedure has become the most popular technique for simple bladder neck suspension. Other urethrovesical suspensions for stress incontinence, without an accompanying cystocele, include the Winter procedure and the Gittes procedure. Variations of these techniques for the patient with an accompanying cystocele include the Raz sling procedure (vaginal wall sling) and the pubovaginal sling procedure.

Procedural considerations

The patient is placed in the lithotomy position. Although the procedure is not lengthy, care must be taken to ensure proper body alignment and avoid pressure areas when positioning the patient. The legs, positioned in stirrups, are extended to promote a flat lower abdomen. The buttocks must be at the edge of the lower hinge of the OR bed for placement of the weighted vaginal retractor. A lumbar support may help alleviate undue stress on the lower back and sacrum. After preoperative hair removal, the entire perineum, vagina, and suprapubic area are prepped. A drape is placed across the rectum to isolate it from the surgical field. Depending on the technique chosen Pereyra or Stamey needles (Fig. 15-59), double-prong ligature carriers, or the In-Tac bone anchor system may be employed. Instrumentation includes a vaginal instrument set and cystoscopy setup, #7 Martin

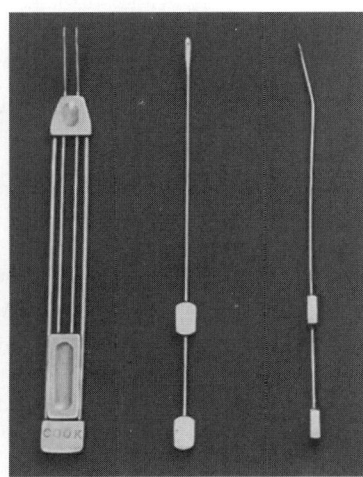

FIGURE 15-59 *Left,* Litvak Pereyra ligature needle, 28 cm long. *Middle and right,* Stamey needles. Used in the treatment of female urinary incontinence.

needles, a 14 Fr, 5 ml Foley catheter or Stamey-Malecot suprapubic catheter, an Asepto syringe, vaginal packing, nonabsorbable monofilament suture ties, 4 mm GoreTex bolsters, antibiotic irrigation (often gentamicin), indigo carmine (for IV administration), and triple sulfonamide or antibiotic vaginal cream.

Operative procedures

Two-Incision Approach

1. The labia minora may be sutured laterally to expose the vaginal introitus.
2. The weighted speculum is placed into the vagina.
3. A suprapubic catheter is generally placed through a stab wound in the usual manner.
4. A Foley catheter is placed intraurethrally and the bladder drained.
5. With gentle traction on the intraurethral Foley, the anterior vaginal wall is palpated to locate the bladder neck.
6. Often a local anesthetic and vasopressin (Pitressin) are injected into the anterior vaginal wall for bleeding and pain management and to aid in tissue dissection.
7. An inverted-U incision is made with the legs of the U distal to the bladder neck and the base of the U midway between the bladder neck and the external urethral meatus.
8. The vaginal tissue is dissected laterally from the legs of the U toward the pubic bone over the periurethral fascia.
9. Using sharp dissection with scissors, the surgeon opens the retropubic space. All adhesions within the space and along the urethral length are released with blunt finger dissection.
10. Bilaterally, helical stitches of heavy nonabsorbable monofilament suture material, on a Mayo needle, are placed vaginally to incorporate the urethropelvic fascia (at the medial edge of the retropubic space) with the pubocervical fascia and anterior vaginal wall.
11. A 3 cm transverse suprapubic incision is made above the superior margin of the pubic bone to the level of the rectus fascia.
12. The Pereyra or Stamey needle of choice or a double-prong ligature carrier is inserted into the suprapubic incision and through the rectus fascia just above the symphysis pubis.
13. The needle is guided through the rectus fascia into the vaginal incision to meet the surgeon's index finger in the retropubic vaginal space. The ligatures are transferred to the suprapubic wound with the ligature carrier and pulled upward.
14. The Foley is removed, and the cystoscope is inserted to determine bladder patency.
15. The vaginal incision is closed with a continuous locking stitch of 2-0 absorbable suture.
16. A vaginal packing impregnated with a triple sulfonamide cream is placed.

17. The suspension sutures are tied separately with multiple knots and are then brought across the midline and tied together.
18. The skin is closed, after irrigation, with 4-0 subcuticular absorbable suture. Steri-Strips and a small gauze dressing are placed over the abdominal wound, and the catheter is secured and connected to drainage.

Incisionless Approach

1. The labia minora may be sutured laterally to expose the vaginal introitus.
2. The weighted speculum is placed into the vagina.
3. A suprapubic catheter may be placed through a stab wound in the usual manner.
4. A Foley catheter is placed intraurethrally and the bladder drained. With gentle traction on the intraurethral Foley, the anterior vaginal wall is palpated to locate the bladder neck.
5. Often a local anesthetic and vasopressin (Pitressin) are injected into the anterior vaginal wall for bleeding and pain management and to aid in tissue dissection.
6. The inserter for the In-Tac bone anchor is placed into the vagina and pressed against the anterior vaginal wall, below the bladder neck and 2 cm lateral to the urethra. It is pulled upward to lie perpendicularly to the pubic bone (Fig. 15-60).
7. A total of four anchors or screws are driven into the pubic bone, two on each side of the urethra. Four threads will protrude from the vaginal wall.
8. One thread is placed into the Martin needle, and the

needle is passed submucosally from the entry point of the first anchor or screw to the entry point of the ipsilateral thread.

9. Cystoscopy is performed to confirm bladder and urethral integrity.
10. The threads are tied together on each side, and the knot is buried beneath the vaginal mucosa.
11. A Foley catheter may be placed for the immediate postoperative period. A vaginal packing coated with triple sulfonamide cream may be placed.

Suburethral Sling

The suburethral (pubovaginal or pubofascial) sling procedure utilizes an autograft strip of fascia lata, synthetic material, or a strip of cadaver fascia lata. The graft is placed between the urethra and anterior vaginal wall and anchored to the anterior rectus fascia or pectineal ligament.

When the allograft material is used, the procedure lends itself to the ambulatory surgery setting. If an autograft is chosen, an overnight stay might be more advisable because of the potential for increased postoperative pain.

Some women display severe stress incontinence with little or no urethral mobility as intraabdominal pressures change. Frequently they have had prior corrective surgery, neurologic injury, radiation therapy, poor urethral resistance, or pelvic trauma. Urine is lost with minimal exertion, and low urethral closing pressures are apparent during diagnostic examination. They have what is termed *type III stress incontinence with a partially or totally opened urethral sphincter at rest.* The suburethral sling approach is indicated when it is believed that simple elevation and stabilization will not improve continence. It has not been general practice to use this technique as the primary form of treatment. Some practitioners advocate that patients with resting urethral closing pressures <20 cm H_2O are candidates. Others considered as candidates are patients with chronic pulmonary disease, obesity, athleticism, and congenital tissue weakness.

Procedural considerations

Under general or regional anesthesia, the patient is placed in lithotomy position, prepped, and draped. Alternating compression stockings and Allen stirrups are employed. A Foley catheter is placed after cystoscopy. The labia minora are sutured back laterally. The vaginal speculum is placed, and local anesthetic with epinephrine or vasopressin (Pitressin) is instilled into the vaginal mucosa to aid hemostasis. Local anesthetic is injected deeply and laterally into the suprapubic incision site. A transverse midline abdominal incision is made at the upper border of the symphysis pubis. When rectus fascia is used, a Pfannensteil incision is made, extending from one iliac crest to the other, exposing the anterior abdominal wall rectus fascia. The bone anchor may be employed for an incisionless approach.

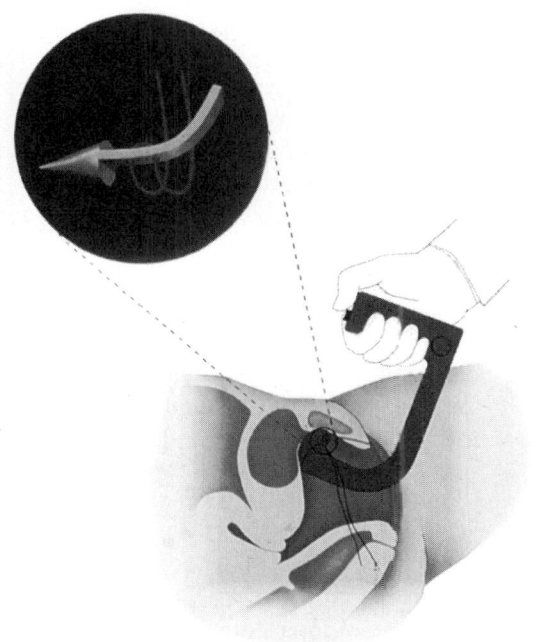

FIGURE 15-60 In-Tac bone anchor system for bladder neck suspension.

Operative procedures
Autograft Harvest

1. Two incisions are made in the fascia, and it is dissected free. Each end is oversewn with 2 nylon suture.
2. The margins from the excised graft are closed with interrupted absorbable 2-0 sutures.
3. Fascia lata from the lateral thigh is retrieved through 2 vertical incisions, one in the midthigh and one approximately 3 cm above the knee.
4. The fascia is incised twice at 3 cm intervals proximally.
5. Dissection is carried bilaterally in a tunnel fashion to the knee wound.
6. A Penrose drain is placed under the fascia at the knee wound and is detached, passed to the thigh wound, and removed.
7. The graft margins are closed with interrupted 2-0 absorbable sutures.
8. A drain is inserted, and the leg wound is closed in layers.
9. A compression dressing is applied.
10. The tissue is spread bluntly to the anterior rectus muscle. Antibiotic-soaked gauze sponges are packed into the incision while the vaginal portion of the procedure is carried out.

Two-Incision Approach

1. The urethral length is measured with a Foley catheter by placing the inflated balloon at the internal vesical neck.
2. The point of the urethral meatus is marked on the catheter, and the Foley is deflated and withdrawn. The catheter is then reinflated, and the length from meatal mark to the balloon is measured.
3. The Foley catheter is reinserted, the weighted speculum is placed into the vagina, and the anterior vaginal mucosa is incised bilaterally to the urethra. The traditional approach utilizes an inverted-U incision approximately 2 to 2.5 cm in length.
4. An anterior vaginal wall flap is raised, and dissection is carried to the pubic bone bilaterally.
5. The endopelvic fascia is perforated, and the retropubic space is entered.
6. Dissection is carried across the urethra, beneath the anterior vaginal mucosa, to create a space for the sling.
7. Dissection is carried laterally to the pubic bone, the endopelvic fascia perforated, and the retropubic space entered.
8. A power drill is used to create bilateral small defects in the pubic bone. The Mitek suture is anchored in the defect immediately after each one is established.
9. A Stamey needle is passed cephalad from one of the vaginal incisions to the ipsilateral pubic bone, and the free end of the Mitek suture is threaded through the eye of the needle.
10. The superior edge of the symphysis is probed with the needle tip, and the needle is passed 1 to 2 cm parallel

to the posterior symphysis. One index finger is inserted into the vagina at the bladder neck as in the other maneuvers with the needle along the bladder neck and through the fascia and periurethral tissues.
11. The Foley catheter is removed and the cystoscope inserted to check the needle position. The Foley catheter is reinserted.
12. Steps 9 to 11 are repeated on the opposite side.
13. The free end of the Mitek is sutured and tied, but not cut, to the graft at one end.
14. The graft is passed to the pubic site by threading the free end through the Stamey needle and passing the needle cephalad.
15. The Stamey needle is removed and the graft retained by placing a hemostat on the suture.
16. The second Mitek suture is threaded into the free end of the graft.
17. Cystoscopic examination is again performed.
18. The traditional approach sutures the graft on each end and passes a long curved clamp proximally to distally to grasp the sutured tissue. The graft is sutured in place to the pubic tubercle or paraurethral fascia after each pass.
19. The free end of the graft is passed between the urethra and the vaginal mucosa (Fig. 15-61).
20. Length is measured by having the assistant secure the abdominal end of the graft as the surgeon temporarily places the free end into the opposite vaginal wound. Excess graft material is excised and step 13 is repeated.
21. Tension is checked before suturing the sling in place.
22. The cystoscope is reinserted and the bladder filled. Under direct visualization, the sutures are pulled upward so that the flow of fluid is alternately released and stopped.
23. One side of the graft is sutured in place suprapubically with a free Mayo needle. Position and tension are again checked cystoscopically, and the second side is secured. The sutures are then cut.
24. The Foley catheter is reinserted, and the incisions are closed with absorbable sutures.
25. The vaginal mucosa is closed with 3-0 absorbable suture, and a sulfonamide cream–coated vaginal pack is inserted.
26. The Foley catheter may be removed. A stab wound can be made in the lower abdomen for placement of a suprapubic catheter while the bladder is still full. A small gauze dressing is placed over the abdominal wounds, and the catheter is secured and connected to drainage.

Incisionless Approach

1. A Foley catheter is inserted into the bladder and the balloon inflated.
2. The catheter is pulled gently with one hand as two fingers of the other hand locate the balloon at the bladder neck.

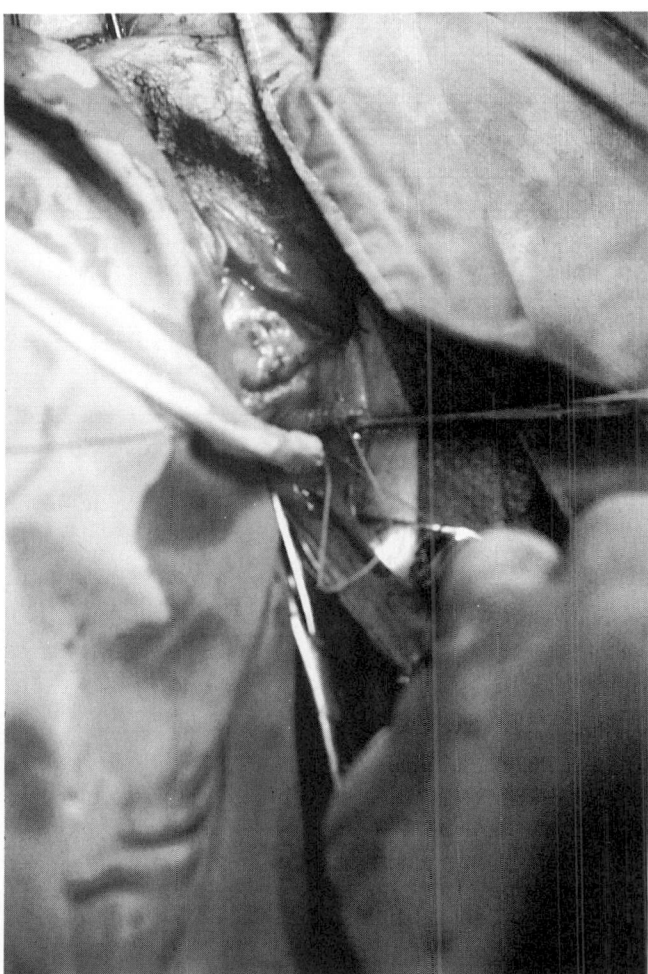

FIGURE 15-61 Fascia lata graft being placed for suburethral sling procedure.

3. The index and middle finger push up and forward, pressing the anterior vaginal wall against the posterior surface of the pubic bone, with the catheter positioned between them and the finger tips touching the balloon.

4. The inserter is placed into the vagina, just below the bladder neck, 2 cm laterally to the urethra.

5. The instrument is pulled upward, perpendicularly to the pubic bone surface, and the anchor or screw is released into the pubic bone.

6. A second anchor or screw is placed on the contralateral side of the urethra.

7. The channels created by the bone anchor sutures are dilated with a right-angled clamp.

8. A right-angled clamp is passed submucosally below the bladder neck from one vaginal mucosal opening to the other, creating a tunnel.

9. The sling material is passed through the submucosal tunnel.

10. One end of the sling is attached to one of the pair of threads with a Mayo needle and tied to the remaining thread.

11. Cystoscopy verifies bladder and urethral integrity.

12. The cystoscope is held in position at a 90-degree angle to the surface of the pubic bone as the contralateral threads are attached to the free end of the sling and tied together. This causes elevation of the sling extremity below the cystoscope and toward the posterior surface of the pubic bone.

13. The threads are cut, and the vaginal openings are sutured closed with absorbable material.

14. A Foley catheter is placed intraurethrally for the immediate postoperative period. A suprapubic catheter may be placed instead of or in addition to the Foley catheter.

15. A vaginal pack coated with triple sulfonamide cream is placed.

Bladder Augmentation

Augmentation enterocystoplasty is the procedure employed to surgically enlarge the bladder capacity. The segment of bowel used is reformed into a semispherical shape to decrease peristaltic contractions and anastomosed to the opened bladder dome. The result is a low-pressure reservoir that provides improved bladder capacity and urinary compliance. Almost all segments of bowel as well as the stomach have been employed for bladder augmentation. Selection depends on anatomic factors, functional characteristics, and the surgeon's preference. In some cases, ureteral reimplantation or associated bladder-outlet procedures are deemed necessary. They should be incorporated to achieve a one-stage procedure.

Intermittent catheterization and bladder irrigations will be necessary postoperatively. The patient must be able and willing to learn and perform these and accepting of this alteration in life-style.

A wide range of conditions that were previously treated with urinary diversion may now be successfully managed with this technique. Indications include reflex incontinence unresponsive to medical management, detrusor hyperactivity with compromised bladder function, chronically contracted bladder as results from radiation or repeated infections, and neuropathic bladder combined with recurrent urinary tract infections or compromised renal function.

Procedural considerations

The patient is in the supine position and under general anesthesia. The female patient may be in a frog-leg or lithotomy position, particularly if an outlet procedure is to be performed. A nasogastric tube is inserted after induction. The entire abdomen and genitalia are prepped and draped. A Foley catheter is inserted into the sterile field, and the bladder is filled to capacity once the abdomen has been entered. Basic laparotomy and intestinal instruments are required.

Operative procedure

1. A supraumbilical to symphysis midline abdominal incision is made.

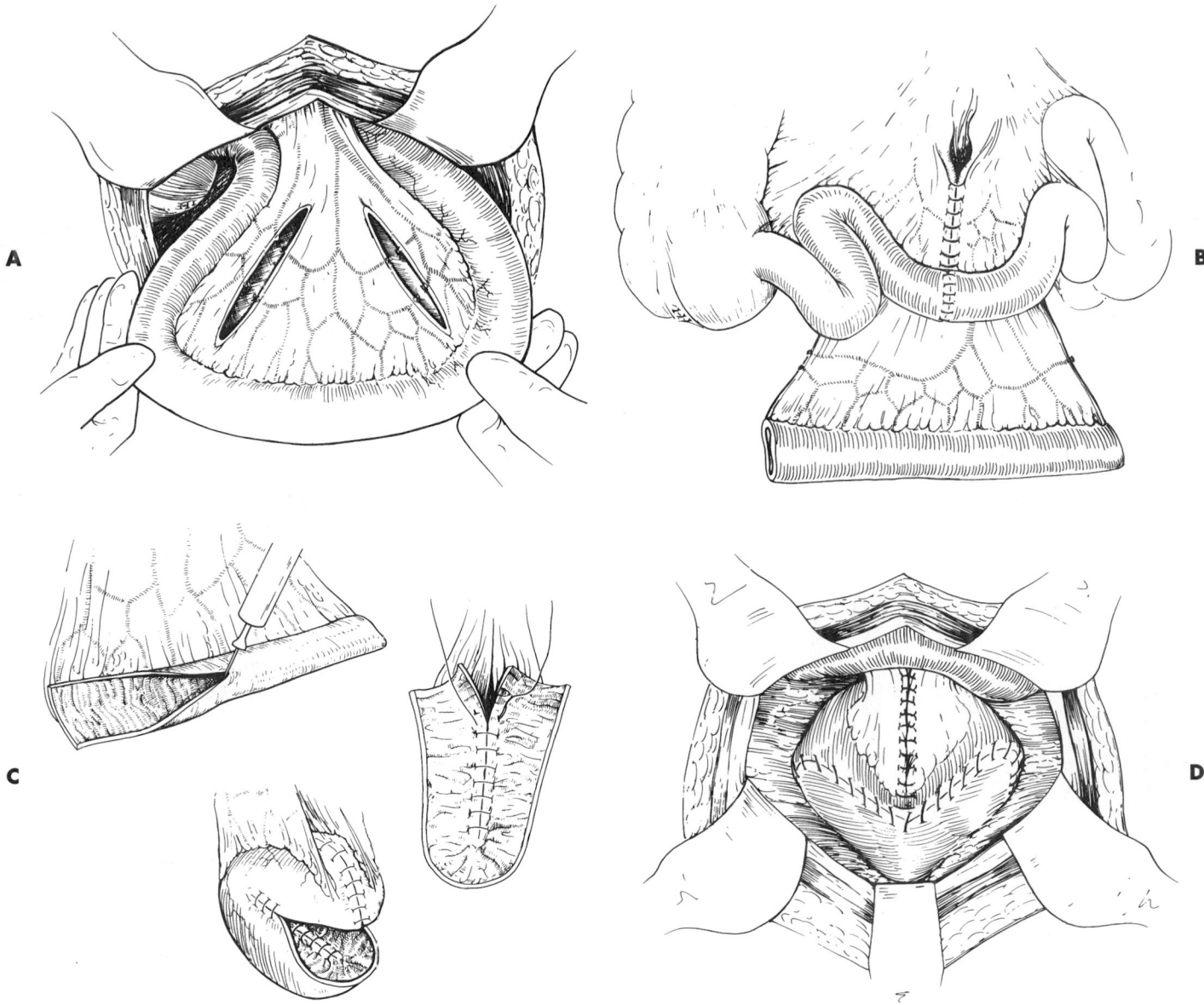

FIGURE 15-62 Ileocystoplasty for bladder augmentation.

2. The peritoneal cavity is exposed using a Bookwalter or similar retractor.

3. The intestines and stomach are examined, and the appropriate segment for reconstruction is chosen (Fig. 15-62, *A*).

4. A sagittal bladder incision is made from 2 cm cephalad to the bladder neck anteriorly across the anterior bladder wall, the peritonealized dome surface, and the posterior bladder wall to 2 cm above the posterior interureteric ridge. This causes the bladder to be bivalved in a clam-shaped design.

5. Traction sutures are placed bilaterally along the bladder incision.

6. The length of the incision is measured to correlate with the corresponding segment of bowel or stomach. Average length required is 25 cm.

7. The segment to be used is mobilized, and the mesentery is closed cephalad so that the segment is on the retroperitoneum. The segment is left attached to its mesentery to maintain blood supply (Fig. 15-62, *B*).

8. The isolated segment is opened, trimmed, and detubularized. It is then doubly folded and sutured to form a cup patch (Fig. 15-62, *C*).

9. Anastomosis is accomplished with a running, intermittent locking, absorbable suture, beginning at the posterior apex and running up each side.

10. With one third of the attachment complete, sutures are then placed at the anterior apex and run bilaterally to meet cephalad (Fig. 15-62, *D*).

11. Integrity of the anastomosis is checked by again filling the bladder and observing for leaks.

12. A routine abdominal closure is performed, and dressings are applied. The nasogastric tube stays in place for 3 postoperative days. The Foley catheter will remain for 7 to 14 days. Some surgeons may choose to place a suprapubic catheter instead of a Foley.

Implantation of Prosthetic Urethral Sphincter

This procedure is usually done as a last measure for patients with stress incontinence where other modalities have failed. Problems with the device have included foreign-body reaction, persistent urethral pressure causing urethral erosion, and fluid hydraulic failure. The artificial sphincter unit has an abdominally placed, pressure-regulated reservoir that maintains a constant predetermined pressure on the periurethral cuff. Because of the connection between the reservoir and cuff, any increase in intraabdominal pressure transmits more fluid into the cuff. This connection allows for a compensatory increase in urethral resistance during coughing or straining.

The scrotal or labial pump shifts the fluid into the cuff to the reservoir to allow bladder emptying. The fluid reenters the cuff through a resistor in about 60 to 120 seconds. The locking button in the AMS 800 artificial sphincter unit traps fluid in the reservoir to allow activation of the cuff.

Procedural considerations

Standard laparotomy and lithotomy setups are required, as well as the sphincter components, contrast material diluted according to the manufacturer's recommendations, and an antibiotic solution. The patient is placed in a modified lithotomy position.

Stricture disease is more commonly found in the male population, and the most common cuff placement is around the bulbous urethra. Bladder neck placement of the cuff is generally reserved only for females.

Operative procedure
Bulbous Urethral Cuff

1. Perineal and transverse suprapubic incisions are made.
2. The bulbous urethra is mobilized through a midline perineal incision (Fig. 15-63, A).
3. A 2 cm space is created beneath the bulbocavernous muscle and around the bulbous urethra.
4. The cuff, tab end first, is placed around the bulbous urethra (Fig. 15-63, B).
5. The reservoir is placed beneath the rectus muscle through the suprapubic incision (Fig. 15-63, C).
6. The pump is introduced through the suprapubic incision and transferred to the scrotum through a subcutaneous tunnel created between the two incisions.
7. The reservoir, cuff, and pump are connected and filled with contrast material or injectable saline to the appropriate volume (Fig. 15-64).

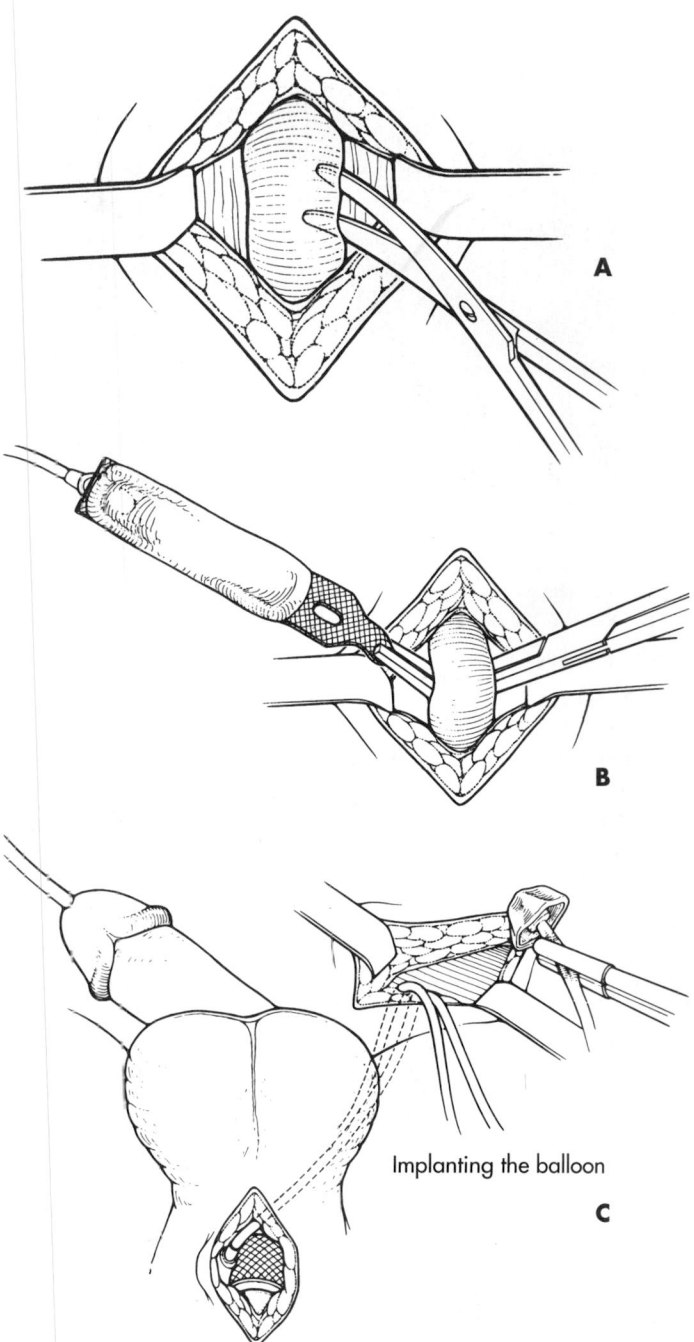

FIGURE 15-63   Implantation of artificial urinary sphincter.

8. The wound is closed and dressed with gauze sponges. A urethral catheter is usually not inserted.

Radical Cystectomy with Pelvic Lymphadenectomy

Cystectomy is the total excision of the urinary bladder and adjacent structures along with pelvic lymph nodes. Cystectomy is a surgical consideration when a vesical malignancy has invaded the muscular wall of the bladder or

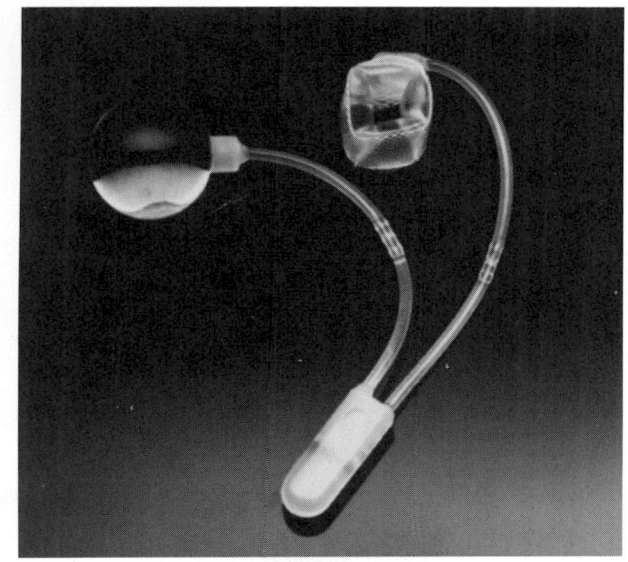

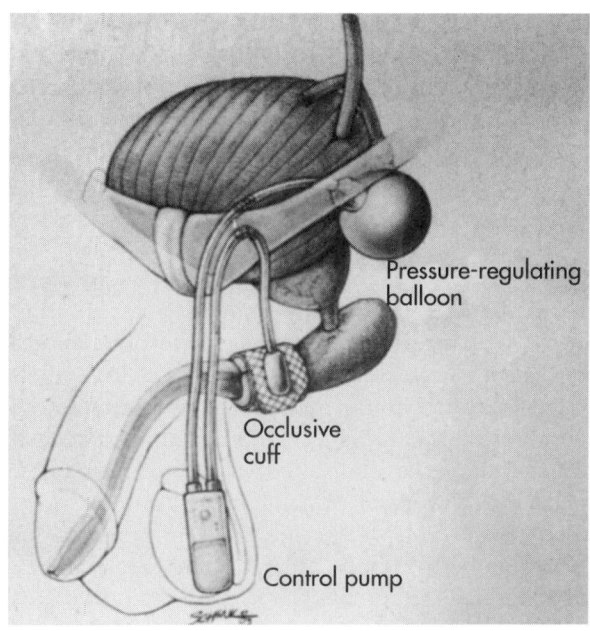

FIGURE 15-64   **A,** AMS Sphincter 800. **B,** Final placement of artificial urinary sphincter.

when frequent recurrences of widespread papillary tumors do not respond to endoscopic or chemotherapeutic management. The patient should be medically able to withstand surgery with the expectation of reasonable longevity. Total cystectomy necessitates permanent urinary diversion into an ileal or colonic conduit. Conservative measures such as radiotherapy or chemotherapy may be used when the neoplasm is far advanced.

In a male patient the prostate gland, seminal vesicles, and distal ureters are removed with the bladder and its peritoneal surface. In a female patient the bladder, urethra, distal urethra, uterus, cervix, and proximal third of the vagina are removed.

Procedural considerations

The patient is placed in the supine position. Instruments are as described for major abdominal procedures. For a male patient, if the prostate and seminal vesicles are to be removed, prostatectomy instruments should be added. For a female, vaginal and abdominal hysterectomy as well as plastic surgery instruments should be added (see Chapters 14 and 24).

Operative procedure

1. A midline incision from the epigastrium to the symphysis pubis, curving to the left of the umbilicus, is generally preferred.
2. The peritoneal cavity is entered above the umbilicus. The entire urachal remnant is clamped, divided, and tied off with heavy silk ligatures (Fig. 15-65, *A*). It will be removed en bloc with the bladder.
3. The bladder dome is lifted at its peritoneal surface, and dissection proceeds laterally on either side with

ligation of the major vesical arteries to the level of the vas deferens or round ligament (Fig. 15-65, *B*).
4. The vas deferens is divided, and the urethra is cut at the level of the pelvic diaphragm.
5. The ureters are identified and traced to the bladder. Care is taken to preserve the adventitial tissue (Fig. 15-65, *C*).
6. Abdominal exploration and pelvic lymphadenectomy with frozen sections are performed to rule out metastatic disease.
7. In the *male* patient the bladder is then retracted to expose the endopelvic fascia and puboprostatic ligaments. The prostate, dorsal venous complex, and seminal vesicles are dissected free, as described for a radical retropubic prostatectomy (Fig. 15-65, *D*). These will be removed in continuity with the bladder.
8. In the *female* patient the broad ligament is bilaterally incised posterior to the fallopian tube and ovary to the level of the posterior vagina to be removed en bloc with the bladder (Fig. 15-65, *E*). The endopelvic fascia is incised at the bladder neck to expose the proximal urethra. The vagina is then incised along the lateral walls to the level of the proximal urethra and bladder neck. The anterior vaginal wall is incised in a U fashion to circumscribe the urethra (Fig. 15-65, *F*). The vagina is reconstructed.
9. The surgical specimen consists of the bladder, distal ureters, prostate, seminal vesicles, and distal vas in the male and the uterus, fallopian tubes, and ovaries in the female and is removed en bloc.
10. The urethra is ligated with absorbable suture. If urethrectomy is indicated, this is done en bloc with the bladder.

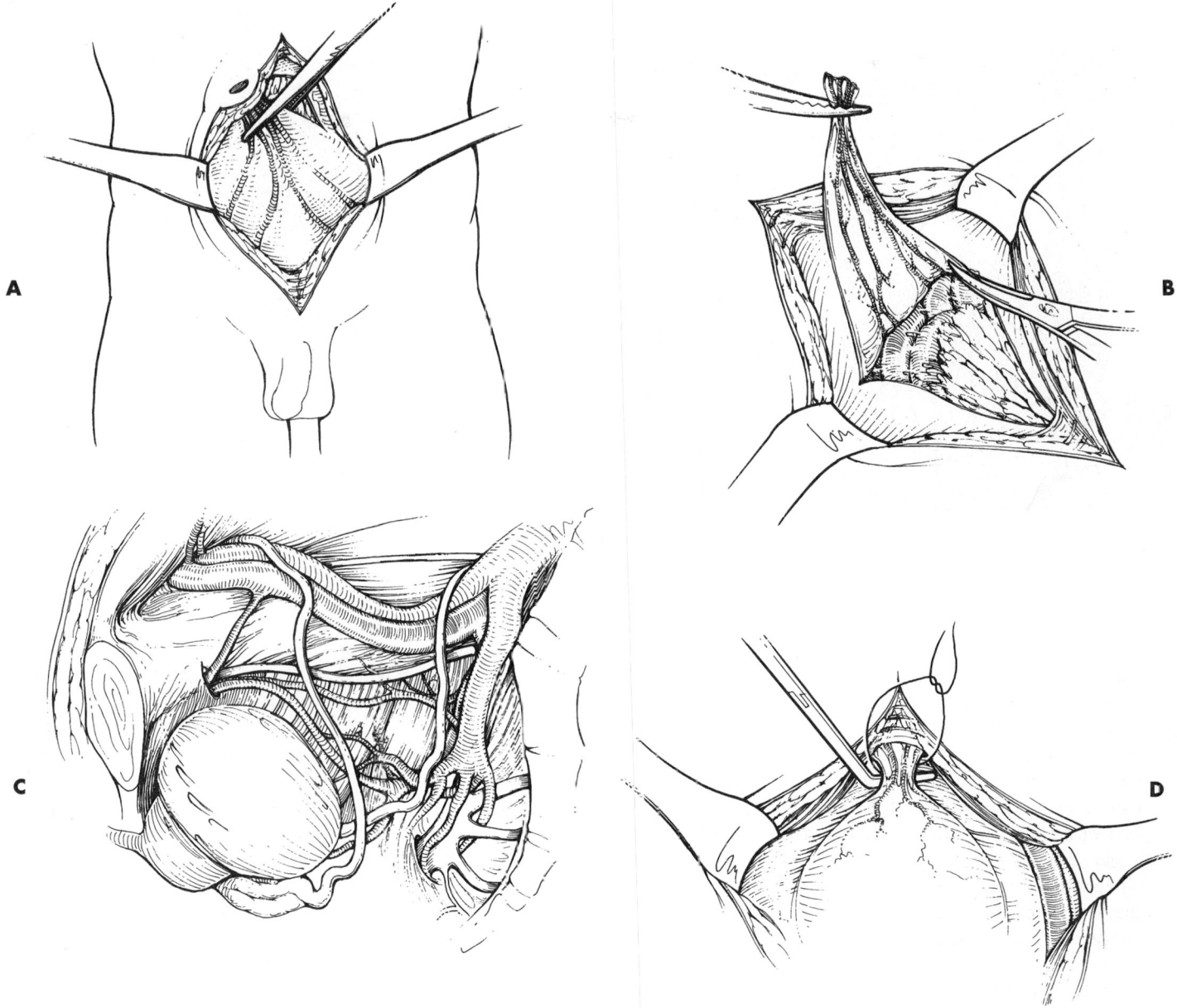

FIGURE 15-65 **A**, The urachal remnant is identified and divided just below the umbilicus. **B**, The peritoneum is divided laterally to the umbilical ligaments to the level of the vas deferens or round ligament. **C**, The ureter crossing the bifurcation of the iliac vessels is identified. **D**, Right-angled clamp is passed beneath the dorsal venous complex, anterior to the membranous urethra.

Continued

11. Lap pads are placed in the denuded pelvis, and pressure is applied to reduce blood loss from oozing.
12. Urinary diversion is accomplished by means of an isolated ileal or colonic conduit, an orthotopic diversion, or a continent urinary diversion.

Bladder Substitution (Substitution Cystoplasty)

Techniques to create a neobladder have utilized various segments of the intestinal tract. The ideal candidate for a bladder replacement after cystectomy for carcinoma is a patient with a normal urethra, a proximally located, well-differentiated bladder tumor, absence of carcinoma in situ, and proof, in the male patient, that the prostatic urethra is free of disease. High-dose radiation offers appreciable risks for postoperative complications and is contraindicated with enterourethral anastomosis. Techniques to create a neobladder include the following:

Right colocystoplasty

Depending on the extent of involvement, the right side of the colon may be used to replace the bladder, the bladder and prostatic urethra, or the bladder and prostate

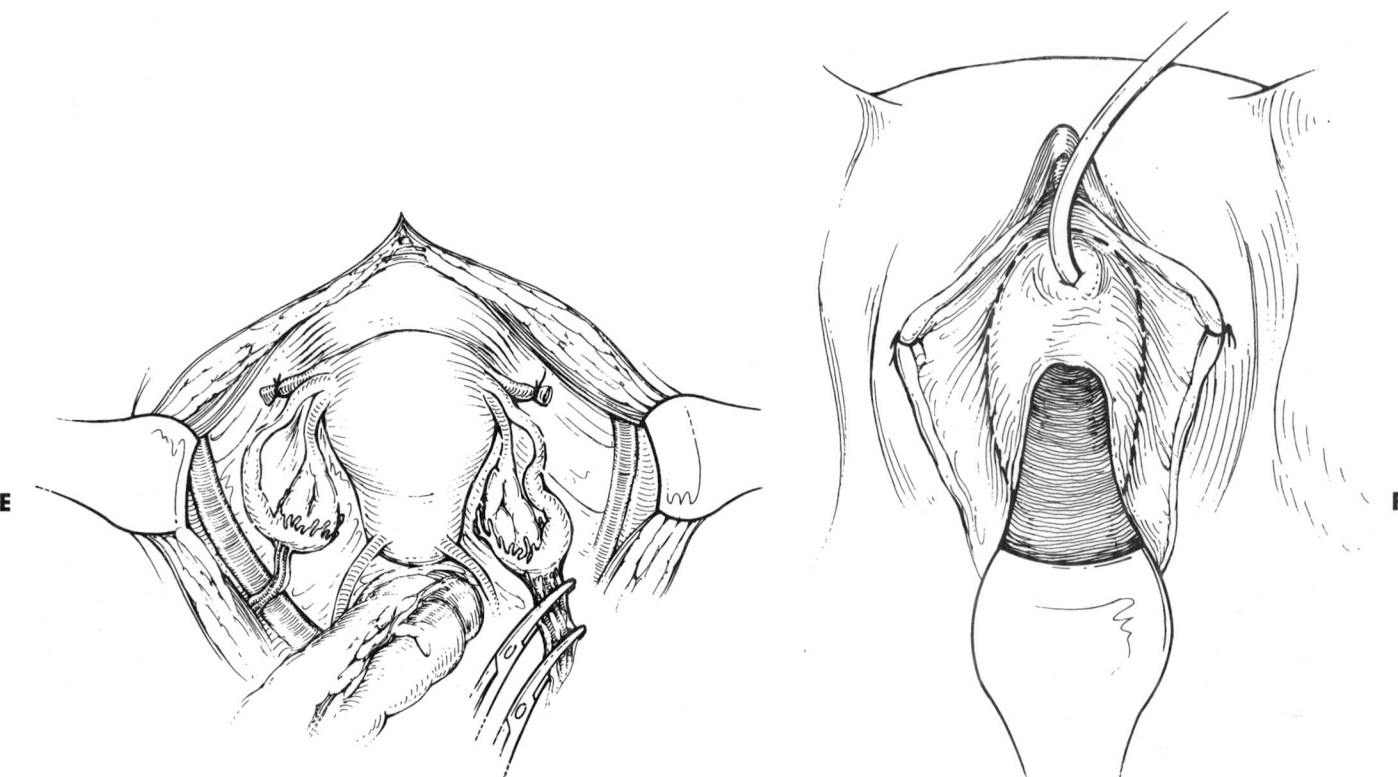

FIGURE 15-65, cont'd   **E**, In female patients the ovaries, fallopian tubes, and uterus are removed en bloc with the bladder and anterior vaginal wall. **F**, U-shaped incision is made on the anterior vagina to circumscribe the urethra.

with a direct enteric-to-proximal bulbar urethral anastomosis. The ideal candidate for a right colocystoplasty after cystectomy for carcinoma is a male with a normal urethra, a proximally located, well-differentiated bladder tumor, absence of carcinoma in situ, and proof that the prostatic urethra is free from disease. High-dose radiation offers appreciable risks for postoperative complications and is contraindicated with enterourethral anastomosis. This procedure has become more functionally effective with the use of intermittent self-catheterization and selective implantation of a prosthetic urinary sphincter.

Ileocecal bladder substitution

The ileum has been used as a reservoir to restore urinary continuity because it possesses a low intraluminal pressure. However, the short mesentery does not always permit the bowel to reach the urethra, and the results with the current antireflux techniques are not consistently successful. There have been significant incidences of recurrent carcinoma, renal damage, incontinence, postoperative strictures, fistula, hypokalemia, anemia, suture-line breakdown, and stone formation. Although most patients attain daytime urinary control, approximately 30% still have problems with enuresis. Deterioration of the upper urinary tract as a result of infection and obstruction has historically been a significant risk with this procedure, and therefore ileocecal substitution is met with mixed reactions and recommendations.

Sigmoidocystoplasty

Because of its ease of construction, bladder proximity, decreased obstruction from mucus, and large capacity, the sigmoid colon has been more appealing to many surgeons in their attempt to create a new bladder. More efficient emptying with a larger reservoir capacity seems to occur with a sigmoid replacement. Results yield higher intraluminal pressures, more effective urinary flow rates, and less nocturnal incontinence than with ileal segments.

Ileoascending bladder substitution

In an effort to improve the intestinal reservoir's capacity and antirefluxing effectiveness, the use of the ascending colon as a continent reservoir was introduced. This technique has several anatomic advantages over other methods of bladder replacement. The segment used can include the hepatic flexure and proximal transverse colon. A large-capacity reservoir is obtained, and colonic incision or tailoring is not required to achieve an appropriate shape. It easily reaches any site within the pelvis and can be anastomosed directly to the urethra without tension.

Orthotopic Ileocolic Neobladder

A bladder substitution utilizing the right colon and ileum has shown remarkable results in the last decade. "Le bag" continent diversion technique was developed specifically for orthotopic bladder replacement. Bladder substitution relies on meticulous dissection of the prostatic apex with preservation of the urinary sphincter and neurovascular bundles, as well as a water tight urethral anastomosis. Most patients have achieved a high degree of daytime continence and a minimum of nocturnal enuresis. Short-term complications encountered include bleeding, infection, urinary extravasation, bladder perforation, urethral stricture, fistula formation, urinoma, and small bowel obstruction. Long-term problems include chronic constipation or diarrhea, compromised enterohepatic circulation, vitamin B_{12} deficiency, and urinary incontinence in a small percentage of patients.

Considerations influencing patient selection include age, general health, and fitness for extensive, complicated surgery. Contraindications include previous radiation therapy, bowel disease (diverticulosis, Crohn's disease, colitis), and other major medical problems that might jeopardize the patient or procedure. Preoperative urethral biopsy specimens are frequently performed to rule out tumor or cellular atypia in the urethra, which would prevent this particular intervention.

Procedural considerations

The patient is placed in the supine position. Alternating compression stockings are applied before the induction of anesthesia. A cystectomy and prostatectomy or hysterectomy is performed. Major, deep, intestinal, bladder, and prostate or hysterectomy instruments, as well as a large self-retaining retractor are needed.

Operative procedure

1. After cystoprostatectomy, the right side of the colon is reflected medially along the mesentery to the hepatic flexure. The distal ileum is inspected to be used in the neobladder. The appendix may be used to catheterize the reservoir.
2. The small bowel is divided and laid in an S shape, and stay sutures of 2-0 or 3-0 absorbable material are placed.
3. The posterior walls are sewn from inside to outside with running 3-0 absorbable suture.
4. A seromuscular wedge of the dependent cecum is excised, and the mucosa is everted with 4-0 absorbable sutures to form a bladder neck.
5. The left ureter is brought retroperitoneally under the sigmoid mesentery, a submucosal tunnel is created, and the ureters are reimplanted through the colonic wall. Anastomosis is done from the interior of the pouch.
6. Anchor sutures of 3-0 or 4-0 silk are placed at the outer entry point. The wall of the colon is anchored to the psoas muscle with 3-0 or 4-0 silk to prevent migration of the neobladder.
7. Ureteral stents are placed and brought out through the colonic segment and a separate abdominal stab wound, along with a catheter to serve as a suprapubic tube.

8. Sutures of 2-0 absorbable material are placed around the urethral stump and tagged.
9. A Foley catheter is inserted into the urethra in a retrograde manner, and the urethra is anastomosed to the neobladder at the point of the new bladder neck.
10. The neobladder is closed in an intestinal fashion or with gastrointestinal staples in a side-to-side anastomosis. Wound drains are place to the outside. The bladder is filled to test for leaks. The wound is closed in a conventional manner.

Cutaneous Urinary Diversions
Ileal conduit

The ileal conduit is the classic method by which the urine flow is diverted to an isolated loop of bowel. One end of the isolated loop is brought out through the skin so that the urine can be collected in a drainage bag, which is intermittently emptied. The stoma sites should be carefully selected preoperatively by the surgeon and enterostomal therapist. The selected site, usually in the right lower quadrant of the abdomen, above the beltline, is marked with a fine needle dipped in methylene blue to prevent erasure during skin preparation. The goal is to create a round, protruding stoma without wrinkles in the skin, to prevent urine leakage under the collecting device. Puckering of the skin around the stoma is minimized by using a subcuticular technique when the surgeon is suturing the stoma in place. The candidate for ileal diversion must have a retrievable ureter at least 1 cm in diameter with a thick, well vascularized wall. The patient must be able to care for the appliance. Conditions amenable to diversion include neurogenic bladder, interstitial cystitis, and bladder carcinoma. Cystectomy may be performed before or after this procedure, depending on the patient's condition and diagnosis. In cases that do not involve bladder cancer, a surgeon may choose to leave the bladder in situ rather than subject a debilitated patient to further surgery. In certain cases of extensive bladder carcinoma, the surgeon may elect to treat the patient with radiation in an attempt to decrease the size of the tumor and "sterilize" the regional lymph nodes before performing a cystectomy.

Procedural Considerations

The patient is placed in the supine position. Abdominal and gastrointestinal instruments are required. A cystectomy, prostatectomy, or hysterectomy may also be done at the time of the surgery. The advent of stapling devices has allowed a modification of the standard intestinal anastomosis. Stapling devices, with absorbable staples, are available for use in ureterointestinal procedures.

Operative Procedure

1. The bladder is decompressed with a catheter.
2. The abdomen is entered through a midline abdominal incision. A self-retaining abdominal retractor is placed so that the viscera are excluded from the region of dissection.

3. The ureters are identified and mobilized by severing them 1 to ½ inch from the bladder.

4. A retroperitoneal tunnel is made so that the left ureter lies close to the right ureter.

5. The distal ileum and mesentery are inspected to identify the bowel's blood supply.

6. A drain is passed through the mesentery, midway between the two main arterial arcades adjacent to the ileum at the proximal and distal ends of the selected segment. This segment usually comprises 15 to 20 cm of the terminal ileum, a few centimeters from the ileocecal valve. Care is exercised to preserve the ileocecal artery and maintain adequate circulation to the isolated ileal segment.

7. The peritoneum is incised over the proposed line of division of the mesentery.

8. Intestinal clamps are placed across the ileum, and the bowel is divided flush with the clamps.

9. By use of gastrointestinal technique (see Chapter 11), the proximal end of the isolated ileal segment is closed first with a layer of absorbable sutures and then with a second layer of interrupted 2-0 nonabsorbable sutures.

10. The proximal and distal segments of ileum are reanastomosed end-to-end in two layers.

11. The mesenteric incision is closed with interrupted nonabsorbable sutures.

12. The closed proximal end of the conduit segment is fixed to the posterior peritoneum.

13. The ureters are implanted in the ileal segment by use of fine instruments and 4-0 absorbable ureteral sutures on atraumatic needles.

14. The peritoneum and muscle of the abdominal wall lateral to the original incision are separated by blunt dissection.

15. The abdominal opening for the stoma is made, and the distal opening of the ileal conduit is then drawn through a fenestration in the muscle, fascia, and skin.

16. The ileum is fixed to the fascia with 2-0 quadrant sutures. A rosebud stoma is constructed at the same time the ileum is sutured to the skin with subcuticular suture (Fig. 15-66).

17. Ureteral stents are usually left in the stoma, and a urinary collecting pouch is placed over the rosebud stoma to collect urine.

18. The wound is drained with two Jackson-Pratt drains. The abdominal incision is closed with 0 nonabsorbable suture. The skin is reapproximated with skin staples.

Continent Urinary Diversions

The Kock pouch, the right colocystoplasty, and the Camey version of the ileocystoplasty have been modified for anastomosis to a urethral stump, or the prostatic capsule, resulting in effective continent bladder replacement.

All continent urinary diversions provide an easily

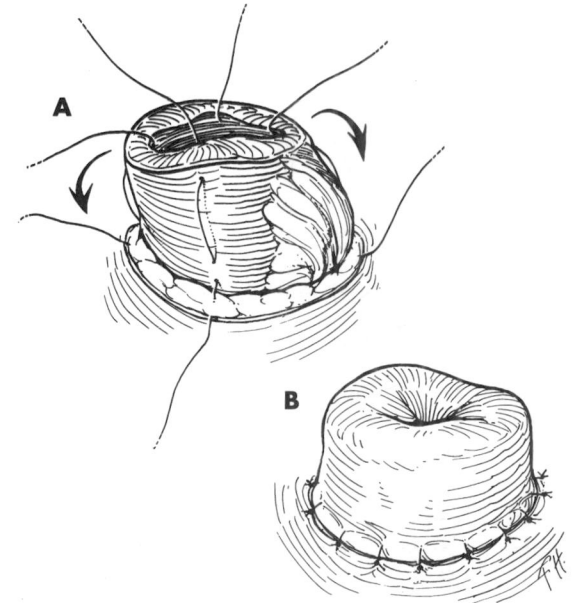

FIGURE 15-66   Rosebud suture technique for stoma.

catheterized stoma and a nonrefluxing ureteral anastomosis and require a reservoir, an antireflux mechanism, and a catheterizable stoma that will not leak. Different parts of the bowel and the stomach have been used as continent reservoirs. The choice of the antireflux mechanism is dependent on the implantation site. The stoma does not require an appliance; therefore the site may be placed below the beltline or bikini line, making them catheterizable when the patient is sitting. They may potentially be anastomosed to the proximal urethra, thus forming an orthotopic bladder.

If the patient is dexterous and able to intubate the pouch and shows no psychologic or medical contraindications, that person is a candidate. Patients with insufficient bowel because of adhesions, previous resection, or disease (colitis); patients who have had radiation to the intestines; patients with limited life expectancy because of age, infirmity, or malignancy; and patients without the proper motivation to perform the care necessary are not good candidates for this procedure.

Ileal reservoir (Kock pouch)
Procedural Considerations

A continent reservoir formed into a U configuration is constructed of a section of ileum proximal to the ileocecal valve. The legs of the U are sewn together at the antimesenteric border. The intestine is opened adjacent to the serosal suture at the antimesenteric border, and the back wall of the pouch is reinforced with absorbable suture.

Continence is achieved by the valve mechanism within the construction of the nipple valve attached to the skin. Nipple valves are created proximally and distally by intussusception of the bowel into the reservoir cavity. Once the nipples are fixed to the sidewall of the reservoir with absorbable suture or polyglycolic staples, the anterior wall is closed. The ureters are anastomosed to the afferent limb of the pouch, preventing reflux. The efferent limb is drawn through the stoma site and anchored to the abdominal wall fascia.

Operative Procedure

1. The mesentery is divided and suture or staple ligated along the avascular plane between the superior mesenteric artery and the ileocolic artery.
2. The bowel is divided, and four segments are measured and marked with silk suture tags. These segments will serve as the efferent conduit, the pouch, and the afferent limb.
3. A portion of the proximal ileum is resected and discarded along with a wedge of mesentery. Suction is passed down the lumen to clear any fecal material or mucus.
4. The proximal end is closed in an intestinal manner or stapled.
5. The segment to be employed is spread out in a U-shaped fashion. The sides are sewn together with 3-0 absorbable suture in a running fashion, or connected with gastrointestinal staples.
6. The bowel is incised with electrosurgery laterally to the suture into the two loops. The medial edges are oversewn with 3-0 or 4-0 silk.
7. The mesentery is cleared on the limb segments, and the lumens are intussuscepted into the open pouch.
8. Marlex mesh is used to serve as a strut to prevent parastomal herniation and to fix the base of the efferent nipple to the abdominal wall, facilitating catheterization. The TA or similar stapler is used to form each nipple and to attach the nipples to the back wall of the pouch.
9. An 8 Fr stenting catheter is placed inside the nipple of the efferent conduit to prevent making the collar too tight.
10. The limbs are secured with 3-0 or 4-0 silk suture.
11. The pouch is closed in a gastrointestinal manner with sutures or staples.
12. The ureters are anastomosed, as described under ileal conduit, to the afferent limb.
13. A small stoma site is prepared as described under ileal conduit. A catheter of choice is placed in the stoma for postoperative care. Stents may be placed in the ureters for the immediate postoperative period. This will necessitate initial placement of an ileostomy appliance until all systems are functioning.
14. A drain is placed, leaving through a separate stab wound.
15. Closure is in the standard manner for laparotomy. Retention sutures may be employed. Bulky absorbent dressings and Montgomery straps are applied.

Indiana pouch
Procedural Considerations

This technique is a modification of the original ileocecal diversion. A continent reservoir is constructed of the right side of the colon, which may include the ileum and cecum, the ileocecal valve, and ascending colon. Surgery proceeds as for any diversionary procedure. The ileocecal valve is reinforced with nonabsorbable suture. Two rows of nonabsorbable suture are used to then imbricate the ileal segment, which serves as a catheterizable limb once it is brought to the skin level as a stoma. The cecal segment is detubularized by incising along the taenia and anastomosing the distal edge horizontally to the proximal portion. Intussusception of the ileocecal valve into the cecum and narrowing of the ileal segment attached to the skin allow for continence.

Operative Procedure

1. The large bowel is split down the antimesenteric border for approximately three fourths its length.
2. The U-shaped defect is closed in an intestinal manner.
3. The terminal ileum is sutured along its length over a small Robinson catheter in an intestinal fashion.
4. The pouch is filled with 400 ml of saline, and a larger catheter is placed to determine catheterizability.
5. The ureters are tunneled into the cecum through its taenia. They are then tacked to the outer bowel wall, and the cecum is secured to the pelvic wall. Ureteral stents may be placed.
6. The pouch is secured to the abdominal wall.
7. The stomal site is prepared as described in ileal conduit.
8. A 22 Fr Malecot drain is placed in the reservoir to drain the cecostomy, leaving through a separate stab wound.

SURGERY OF THE URETERS AND KIDNEYS

Stones, infections, and tumors are the most common causes of urinary tract obstruction necessitating surgery to prevent renal obstruction and subsequent failure. Obstruction may also result from congenital malformations or previous operations on the urinary tract (Fig. 15-67).

Although the causes of many kidney stones are obscure, certain conditions such as obstruction, stasis, and imbalance of metabolism predispose to their formation. Stones consist of various elements: calcium oxalate, calcium phosphate, magnesium ammonium phosphate, uric acid, calcium carbonate, and cystine. An increase in the concentration of any of these can cause tiny crystals to form; as these clump together, they begin to form a stone.[10] Stones removed during surgery are subjected to chemical analysis. These specimens should be submitted in a dry jar. Fixative agents such as formalin invalidate the results of the analysis.

Stones in the renal pelvis may fall into the ureteropelvic junction and obstruct the flow of urine. However, calculi

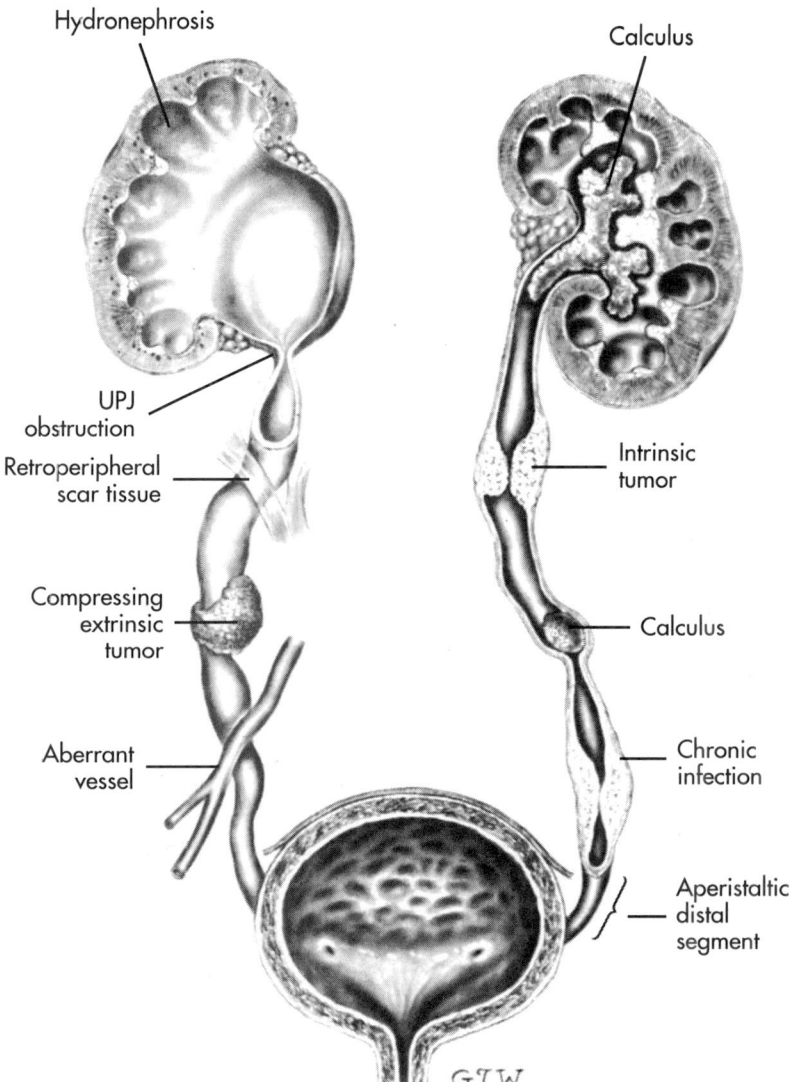

FIGURE 15-67 Some common causes of urinary tract obstruction.

less than 1 cm in diameter may pass down the ureter and lodge at a more distal location, such as where the ureter crosses the iliac vessels or at the ureterovesical junction. A stone may remain in a renal calyx and continue to enlarge, eventually filling the entire renal collecting system (staghorn calculus). Hydroureteronephrosis, infection, and destruction of renal parenchyma frequently result from unrelieved obstruction.

Hypothermia is useful in renal stone surgery as a means of prolonging the safe period of renal ischemia during extensive parenchymal manipulation. This method is also employed for surgery of the renal artery. Several methods enable renal cooling: ice slush or cold saline solution, surface cooling coils, perfusion of cold solutions through the renal artery, or a variation of these basic techniques, such as perfusion of the renal pelvis with saline that has been cooled by a coil immersed in ice slush.

A refrigeration unit "slush machine" that produces sterile slush provides a cost-effective, time-saving alterna-

tive to the other methods of slush preparation. Commercially synthesized ultrafiltrate of sterile plasma in liter bottles is also available for use as the slush. Saline slush for renal surgery may also be manually prepared in several ways. Sterile Mason jars are filled with sterile normal saline solution and double wrapped in sterile plastic bags. Each bag is individually wrapped and secured with a twist tie. The Mason jars are placed in a bucket of ice, to which 2 pints of isopropyl alcohol (isopropanol) and two boxes of salt are added and mixed, for 2 to 3 hours. When the saline is ready for use, the circulating nurse removes the wrapped Mason jar from the ice, opens the plastic bags by sterile technique, and presents the Mason jar to the scrub nurse. The scrub nurse shakes the contents of the Mason jar to cause crystallization of the saline. The slush is removed from the Mason jar with a sterile spoon. Alternatively a rigid plastic container of 1000 ml of normal saline or lactated Ringer's solution may be placed on its side in a freezer several hours before surgery. To prevent the

A Flank approach   **B** Lumbar approach   **C** Thoracoabdominal approach

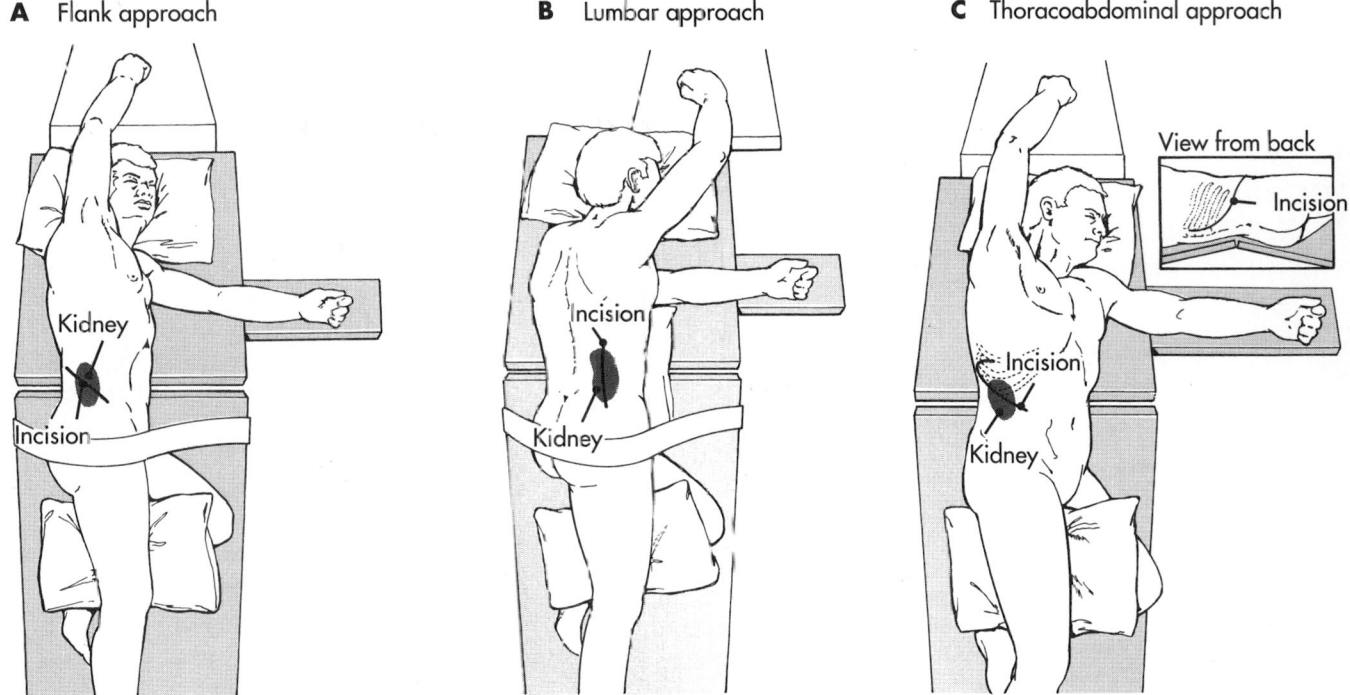

FIGURE 15-68   Principal surgical approaches to the kidney.

solution from solidifying, the container should be rotated one half turn every 20 to 30 minutes. Sterile slush may then be poured directly into a sterile basin as required.

The surgical approach in renal surgery depends on the patient's condition, the amount of exposure needed, and the surgical procedure to be performed. For renal masses attention is directed toward control of the vascular pedicle. For this reason patient position and surgical exposure are of prime consideration. There are three principal surgical approaches to the kidney. The simple *flank*, or *transabdominal*, incision is most frequently used and may include removal of the eleventh or twelfth rib. The incision begins at the posterior axillary line and parallels the course of the twelfth rib. It extends forward and slightly downward between the iliac crest and the thorax (Fig. 15-68, *A*). For the *lumbar* incision, the patient may be initially placed in the supine position, then rotated to lateral and slightly forward over protective bolsters with the operative side up (Fig. 15-68, *B*). This effectively places the flank in an oblique position, causing the abdominal viscera to fall away from the operative incision, and affords an excellent approach to the renal pedicle. Alternatively, the patient may be placed prone with bolsters under the affected side to provide elevation. The *thoracoabdominal* exposure is employed primarily for large upper-pole renal neoplasms. The tenth and eleventh ribs are usually removed, and the chest cavity is opened, collapsing the lung. The leaves of the diaphragm are separated to expose the kidney. A large retractor, such as a Finochietto, and chest drains are required (Fig. 15-68, *C*).

Surgery of the Ureter

Ureterostomy (ureterotomy) is opening the ureter for continued drainage from it into another body part. Cutaneous ureterostomy is diversion of the flow of urine from the kidney, through the ureter, away from the bladder, and onto the skin of the lower abdomen (Fig. 15-69). A suitable urinary collecting device is then placed over the ureteral stoma.

Ureterectomy is complete removal of the ureter. This procedure is generally employed in collecting system tumors and includes nephrectomy and the excision of a cuff of bladder.

Ureteroureterostomy is segmental resection of a diseased portion of the ureter and reconstruction in continuity of the two normal segments.

Ureteroenterostomy is diversion of the ureter into a segment of the ileum (ureteroileostomy, or more commonly ileal urinary conduit) or into the sigmoid colon (ureterosigmoidostomy). Ureteroneocystostomy (ureterovesical anastomosis) is division of the distal ureter from the bladder and reimplantation of the ureter into the bladder with a submucosal tunnel.

Reconstructive operations may be indicated because of a pathologic condition of the bladder or lower ureter that interferes with normal drainage. Conditions requiring urinary diversion or reconstruction of the urinary tract include malignancy, cystitis, stricture, trauma, and congenital ureterovesical reflux. Invasive vesical malignancy requiring surgical removal of the bladder necessitates urinary diversion.

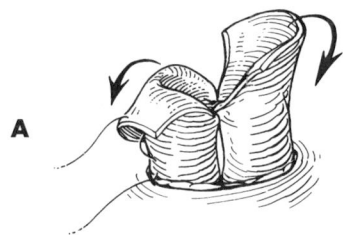

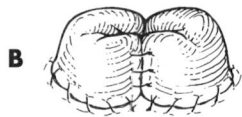

FIGURE 15-69   Double-barreled cutaneous ureterostomy stoma.

Ureterocutaneous transplant, ureterosigmoid anastomosis, and ileal conduit are urinary diversionary procedures performed when the bladder is no longer functioning as a proper urine reservoir. Etiologic factors causing irreparable vesical dysfunction are chronic inflammation, interstitial cystitis, neurogenic bladder, exstrophy, trauma, tumor, and infiltrative disease (amyloidosis). Ureterolithotomy is incision into the ureter and removal of an obstructing calculus.

Procedural considerations

The site of the incision and position of the patient depend on the nature of the proposed surgery. The patient may be placed in the supine position for abdominal surgery, in modified Trendelenburg's position for low abdominal or pelvic surgery, or in the lateral position for high or midureteral obstructing calculi.

Instruments include the nephrectomy set, plus plastic instrumentation for pyeloplasty. Additional instruments may be required, depending on the type of operation and the surgical approach used.

Operative procedures
Ureteral Reimplantation

1. The ureter is exposed through the desired incision, which is determined by the location of the pathologic condition. A ureteral catheter, passed retrograde, may be used to facilitate identification and isolation of the ureter.
2. The ureter is identified and dissected free with long forceps and scissors. The ureter is picked up with the fine traction sutures, freed from the surrounding tissues, and severed at the desired level.
3. The distal end of the ureter is ligated, and the proximal stoma is transferred to the site of anastomosis. The anastomosis is accomplished with fine dissection instruments and fine atraumatic sutures.
4. A soft splinting stent is usually left in place until healing

has taken place and free drainage is ensured. The wound is closed in layers and dressed in the routine manner.

Ureterocutaneous Transplant (Anastomosis)

The surgical approach is the same as that for a low ureterolithotomy.

1. The ureter is divided as far distally as possible.
2. The severed ureter is passed retroperitoneally through the lower abdominal wall and is sutured to the skin with an absorbable, everting suture of 4-0 on an atraumatic needle to form a stoma. The ureter is handled gently with plastic instruments, fixation forceps, and iris scissors.
3. A small Silastic stenting catheter is passed up into the ureter and is left in situ for 48 to 72 hours, during which time ureteral edema subsides. The patient will require a urine-collecting device after surgery.

Ureterosigmoid Anastomosis

1. The peritoneal cavity is entered in the routine manner through a lower left paramedian incision.
2. The major portion of the large bowel is protected with moist packs.
3. Deep retractors are placed, and with long forceps and scissors the posterior peritoneum is incised.
4. The ureters are identified, divided close to the bladder, mobilized, and brought through the posterior peritoneal incision to lie near the sigmoid. Traction sutures and smooth tissue forceps are used to handle the ureters.
5. The sigmoid colon is mobilized to prevent tension on the ureteroenteric anastomosis.
6. The sigmoid colon is sutured with 3-0 nonabsorbable material to the pelvic peritoneum at a point where the ureter falls easily on the bowel.
7. Using a scalpel with a #15 blade, the surgeon makes an incision into the taenia of the sigmoid down to the mucosal layer. The edges of the taenia are undermined to create two parallel flaps.
8. The ureter is laid on the bowel mucosa, and a small slit is made through the mucosa into the lumen of the colon.
9. With fixation forceps and iris scissors the ureter is beveled to lie flat in the tunical incision.
10. The distal ureter is anchored to the bowel mucosa with 4-0 absorbable ureteral sutures on atraumatic needles. The other ureter is anastomosed in the same manner in a position slightly above the first.
11. The tunicae are then loosely reapproximated over the ureter with 4-0 absorbable sutures, creating an antireflux anastomosis.
12. The posterior peritoneum is closed with absorbable sutures. Drains are brought out retroperitoneally. The incision is closed, and the wound is dressed.

Ureterolithotomy
Procedural Considerations

An x-ray examination of the kidney, ureter, and bladder (KUB) should be done immediately before surgery to determine the exact location of the stone. The surgeon may also schedule a cystoscopic examination preoperatively and may attempt to remove the calculus endoscopically if the stone is in the most distal portion of the ureter. The location of the calculus determines the surgical approach. A calculus high in the ureter requires a flank incision with possible removal of the twelfth rib; a more distal ureteral calculus requires a lower abdominal incision.

Operative Procedure

1. After exposure of the ureter, the calculus may be kept stationary with Babcock clamps or vessel loops applied above and below the calculus.
2. With a #15 blade, the incision in the ureter is made directly over the calculus. The calculus may then be easily removed with a Randall stone forceps.
3. A 10 Fr catheter is passed proximally up and distally down the ureter while irrigating with saline to check for ureteral patency and to dislodge any remaining fragments of calculus.
4. The ureter is closed with 4-0 or 5-0 absorbable sutures. All urologic stones should be placed in dry receptacles and sent to the chemistry laboratory for analysis.

Surgery of the Kidney (Box 15-3)
Procedural considerations

Patient preparation and instrument setup are as described for ureteral surgery.

Operative procedures
Pyelotomy and Pyelostomy

1. The pelvis of the kidney is incised with a small scalpel blade. Fine traction sutures may be placed at the edges of the incision for gentle retraction while the pelvis and calyces are explored.
2. In pyelostomy a small Malecot or Foley catheter is placed through the incision into the renal pelvis. Pyelotomy should be used only for very short periods of renal drainage because tubes tend to be dislodged easily from the renal pelvis.

Nephrostomy

1. A curved clamp or stone forceps is passed through a pyelotomy incision into the renal pelvis and then out through the substance of the renal parenchyma through a lower pole minor calyx.
2. The tip of a Malecot, Foley, or Pezzar catheter is drawn into the renal pelvis, and the pyelotomy incision is sutured closed.
3. The distal end of the nephrostomy tube is brought out through a separate stab incision in the flank.

BOX 15-3 | **Terms Pertaining to Kidney Surgery**

nephrostomy Creation of an opening into the kidney to maintain temporary or permanent urinary drainage. A nephrostomy is used to correct an obstruction of the urinary tract and to conserve and permit physiologic functioning of renal tissue. It is also used to provide permanent urinary drainage when a ureter is obstructed or for temporary urinary drainage immediately after a plastic repair on the kidney or renal pelvis.
nephrotomy Incision into the kidney, usually over a collecting system containing a calculus.
pyelolithotomy Removal of a calculus through an opening in the renal pelvis.
pyelostomy Making an opening in the renal pelvis for temporarily or permanently diverting the flow of urine.
pyelotomy Incision into the renal pelvis used as an access to stones in the renal pelvis or collecting system.

---

4. A drain is placed at the level of the pyelotomy incision, and all layers are closed in the regular manner.

Pyelolithotomy and Nephrolithotomy

1. The renal pelvis is opened (Fig. 15-70, A), and the pelvic calculus is gently removed.
2. The pelvis and collecting systems are thoroughly irrigated with saline using an Asepto syringe to dislodge any small remaining calculi and remove them from the kidney.
3. Nephrolithotomy or extended pyelolithotomy is employed when calculi are locked in the calyceal system and cannot be removed through a pyelotomy incision. In such cases the renal parenchyma above the calculus is incised and the calculus removed. In many instances such a situation is associated with a calyceal diverticulum (Fig. 15-70, B).
4. After removal of the calculus the collecting system is closed and the renal cortex reapproximated with deep hemostatic 2-0 absorbable sutures.
5. A nephroscope is sometimes used to localize and remove calyceal calculi (Fig. 15-71). It is also useful in staghorn calculi nephroscopy to remove residual fragments in the pelvic portion of the calculus.
6. An incision in the renal pelvis may be closed with 4-0 absorbable atraumatic sutures.
7. The renal fossa is drained and closed, as for nephrectomy. Reinforced absorbent dressings are useful because some urinary leakage occurs for 3 to 4 days after surgery

Percutaneous nephrolithotomy and litholapaxy

Percutaneous nephrolithotomy and litholapaxy facilitate the removal or disintegration of renal stones using a rigid or flexible nephroscope (see Fig. 15-71) passed through a percutaneous nephrostomy tract. Accessory

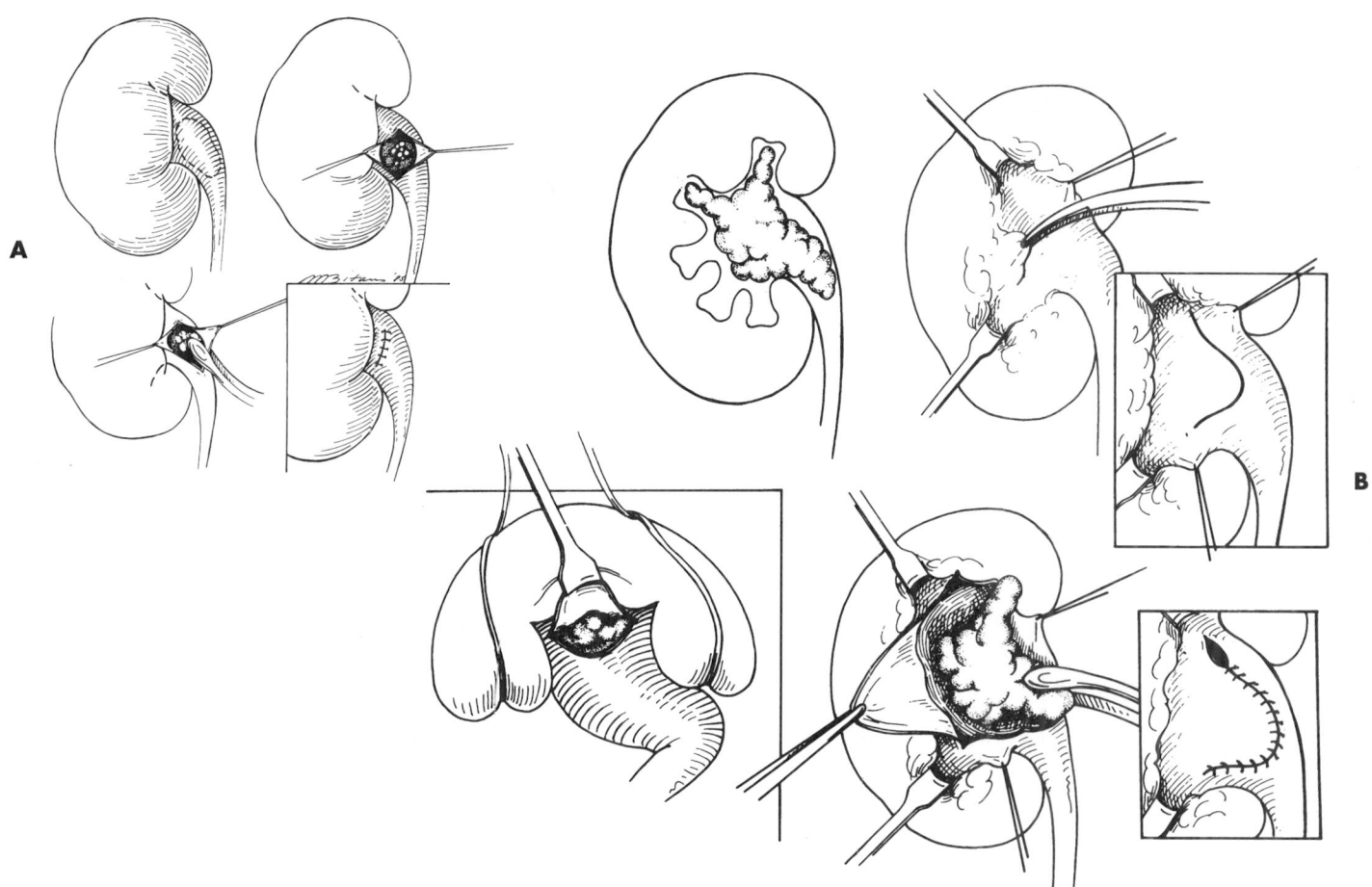

FIGURE 15-70   Pyelolithotomy. **A,** Technique of simple pyelolithotomy. **B,** Technique of extended pyelolithotomy.

instrumentation, such as the ultrasound wand (sonotrode), electrohydraulic lithotriptor probe, laser fiber, stone basket, and stone grasper, is passed through the lumen of the nephroscope to achieve the desired result.

Ideally the patient is in good health and nonobese, and the calculus is no larger than 1 cm in diameter, free floating, radiopaque, and solitary. However, advances in technology complemented by the experience gained by the uroradiology team have allowed patients with more complex problems to be managed in this manner. The patient may or may not have had previous renal surgery or stone recurrence and may have an established nephrostomy tract.

Creation of the nephrostomy tract and removal of the stone can be accomplished by three different methods. Proper placement of the nephrostomy wire can decrease the operating time significantly. In the one-step procedure, creation of the nephrostomy tract, tract dilatation, and stone removal are completed in a single session. This method is generally preferred unless there are contraindications.

In the immediate two-step procedure the radiologist places the nephrostomy tube under radiographic guidance and the urologist removes the stone later the same day or the next morning. The second step is usually done in the operating room with the patient under general anesthesia.

In the delayed two-step procedure the nephrostomy tract is established with the patient under local anesthesia. The patient is discharged the following day with a 22 or 24 Fr nephrostomy tube connected to drainage. The patient is readmitted to the hospital 5 to 7 days later for the percutaneous removal of the calculus under general anesthesia.

Of basic concern during the operative phase are the patient's position and body temperature, the potential for sudden and rapid blood loss, the type of anesthesia to be given, medications required during surgery, and catheter management during and after the procedure. The patient's position, which may be prone or up to 30 degrees prone-oblique, and the draping procedure depend on whether the surgery is done in the radiology department or the operating room and the type of x-ray equipment that will be used.

Extracorporeal shock–wave lithotripsy

The risk of AIDS being spread through the water and the perfection of third- and fourth-generation extracorporeal shock-wave lithotripsy (ESWL) machines have caused

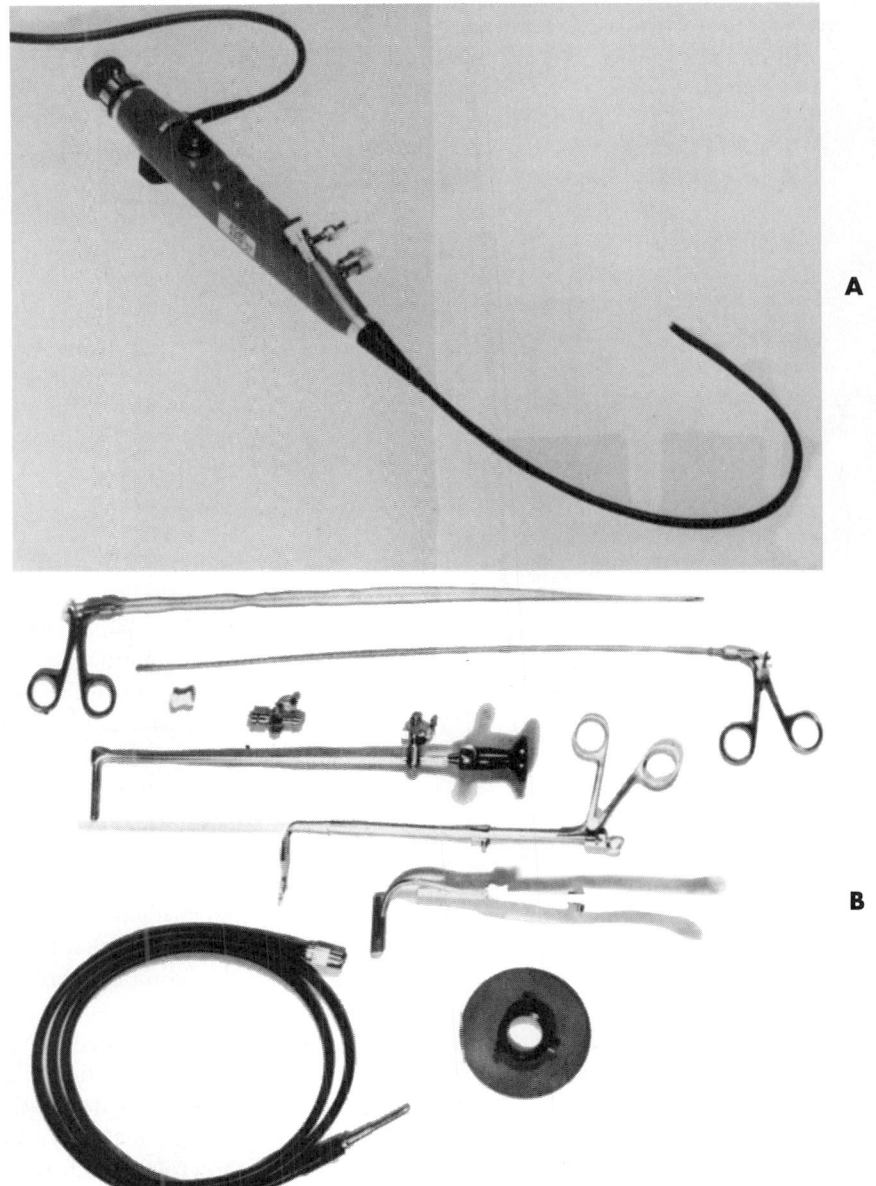

FIGURE 15-71 **A,** Flexible percutaneous nephroscope. **B,** Rigid nephroscope and accessories.

first-generation water tubs to be little used. Third-generation ESWL units use water-filled cushions adjacent to the kidney area (Fig. 15-72, *A*). An x-ray image intensifier with two monitors is used to visualize the kidney stone at the focal point of the shock wave (Fig. 15-72, B). After every 100 shocks, fluoroscopy is used to locate remaining stone particles. Adjustments are made, and the patient is repositioned before further treatments. ESWL is often used with percutaneous nephrolithotomy, surgery, and transurethral ureteropyeloscopy if the patient does not pass the gravel.

Calculi that are treated with ESWL are fragmented by the energy focused on the stone with the lithotriptor. Shock waves may range from 500 to 2000 and are administered over a time that can vary from 30 minutes to 2 hours. Shock waves reverberate inside the calculus causing fragmentation, initially at the front and back of the shock-wave path, with ultimate complete or partial destruction of the calculus. The amount of destruction is dependent on the number and energy of the shock waves delivered and the hardness of the stone. This technique is effective because shock waves can be transmitted and focused through tissue, without loss of energy. A loud reverberating popping sound occurs each time a wave pulse is activated. It is advisable that ear plugs be worn by all.

The requirement for anesthesia is determined by the power of the shock wave, the area of shock-wave entry at the skin level, and the size of the shock-wave focal point. The summation of shock waves used during the procedure can cause pain at the skin level. Typically, general, spinal or

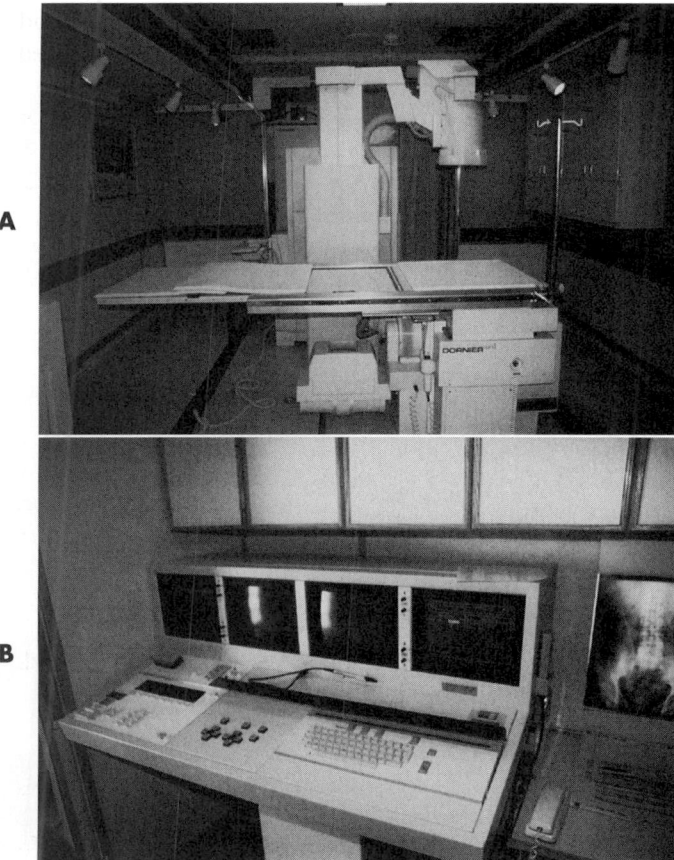

FIGURE 15-72 **A**, Third-generation extracorporeal shock-wave litho-tripsy (ESWL) unit. **B**, X-ray image intensifier with double monitor for ESWL.

local anesthesia is used with the first-generation lithotrip-tors, such as the HM-3. Later versions that allow for lithotripsy with only intravenous sedation, oral sedation, or a transcutaneous electrical nerve stimulator (TENS unit) have been developed.

The need for ancillary procedures such as ureteral stenting (stones >1.5 cm) or percutaneous nephrostomy (that is, staghorn calculi where a large volume of stone fragments will cause obstruction or where percutaneous stone extraction is contemplated for the complex calculi in a "full kidney") must be evaluated. The incidence of renal infection attributable to stone disease rises relative to the length of time the calculus has been present and the increase in the size of the calculus during that time. It is important to assess for and eliminate urinary tract infection, determine renal function, and review the results of coagulation studies. The patient must be informed of alternative therapies and potential complications, includ-ing the potential necessity of repeat treatments or auxiliary procedures to remove fragments. Stones >1.5 cm may require more than one treatment to render the kidney stone free in 90% of patients. Stones larger than this may require additional procedures such as percutaneous or ureteroscopic approaches to achieve complete elimination

of calculus material. Patients with stones >1.5 cm, or who require hospitalization because of renal colic are more likely to benefit from the placement of a ureteral stent before the procedure.

Patients presenting with a large obstructing stone (>3 cm) may have a diminished effect from treatment as a result of the lack of available expansion space in the kidney. A large calculus may cause particle shielding or not allow room in the kidney for the full effect of cavitation, resulting in less effective fragmentation of the stone. The accumulation of these stone fragments (*Steinstrasse*, or 'street of stones') in the ureter occurs in <5% of lithotripsy cases and is located in the upper ureter 18% and lower ureter 75% of the time. Intervention for steinstrasse is required in 35% of these patients because of a solitary kidney, pain, total obstruction, or a 3 cm length of ureter full of fragments.

A staghorn calculus is a complex branching calculus, carrying a high morbidity, that involves most of the renal pelvis and at least two major calyces. If the renal system is "overdilated," the propulsion of fragments is less effective because they settle into the dilated sections and are distanced from the peristaltic action that aids expulsion. If the stone burden created by a staghorn calculus exceeds a surface area of 500 mm or if a large calculus exists (>3 cm), it may best be treated with anatrophic nephrolithotomy or percutaneous nephrostolithotomy.

The use of a stent before ESWL is dependent on the patient and the character of the calculus or calculi. It should be predetermined that the urine culture is normal. Studies show that complication rates decrease if a stent is utilized with a stone >1.5 cm. A stent placed before ESWL tends to decrease the need for ancillary interventions, reduces overall complications, and assists in proper positioning for ESWL by delineating the ureteral anatomy and the precise stone location. On the other hand, those patients who tend to readily form stones may demonstrate calcification of the ureteral stent in a relatively short time. Without a stent the risk of silent renal obstruction resulting in loss of kidney function, obstruction of the ureter, nephritis, and sepsis is increased.

Complications related to ESWL are attributable to the cavitation effects of treatment and are proportional to the number of shocks. The ability of the kidney's tubular cells to survive shock waves is related to the number of shock waves to which the kidney is exposed and not to the energy level. The overall mortality for ESWL is 0.02%. Gross hematuria is seen almost universally, resolves in 12 to 48 hours, and is believed to be attributable to parenchymal edema that spontaneously heals within 1 week. Subcapsu-lar or perirenal hematoma caused by perinephric fluid collections are seen in 15% to 30% of cases. The incidence appears to be higher in the hypertensive patient. Subcap-sular hematoma may resolve in 6 weeks or may take up to 6 months, whereas perirenal hematoma will usually be relieved in a matter of days. Less than 1% of patients have demonstrated cardiac dysrhythmias, myocardial infarction, pulmonary contusion, pancreatitis, or splenic rupture. Renal colic has been exhibited in <25% of patients, obstructive pyelonephritis in 2% to 6%, and sepsis in 0.5%. Impairment of renal function may be seen in patients with solitary kidneys. Iliac artery and vein thrombosis have been reported with lithotripsy for ureteral stones. The majority of lithotripsy patients will demonstrate little or no long-term morbidity.

Laser lithotripsy

Laser lithotripsy has become an exciting alternative to ESWL and EHL. The holmium:YAG and tunable pulse-dyed laser systems have the ability to disintegrate stones without damaging soft tissue. The technique may be used during a ureteropyeloscopy or nephroscopy.

It may also be employed to manage ureteral calculi instead of ureterolithotomy. When the laser probe is discharged in direct contact with the calculus, a plasma (ionized gas) coats the stone's surface. This plasma expands with repeated firings, creating a shock wave that fractures the stone. Normal saline is used for continuous irrigation throughout the procedure. It is not necessary to immobilize the calculus. All persons in the room wear laser goggles, and all laser precautions apply (see Chapter 3).

Dismembered pyeloplasty

Pyeloplasty is revision or plastic reconstruction of the renal pelvis. Pyeloplasty is performed to create a better anatomic relationship between the renal pelvis and the proximal ureter and to allow proper urinary drainage from the kidney to the bladder. A temporary nephrostomy is usually included in such surgery to protect the plastic reconstruction of the ureteropelvic junction (UPJ). Tissue healing usually occurs in 10 to 12 days, and the nephrostomy tube is removed once ureteral patency is demonstrated. *Ureteroplasty* is reconstruction of the ureter distal to the ureteropelvic junction. A *dismembered pyeloplasty* is the combined correction of the redundant renal pelvis and resection of a stenotic portion of the ureteropelvic junction.

Procedural Considerations

The instrument setup is as described for nephrectomy, plus fine plastic and vascular instrumentation and Randall stone forceps. A ureteral stent and red rubber catheters will also be employed. The patient will generally be in the lateral position.

Operative Procedure

1. The kidney and upper ureter are exposed through a supracostal flank incision.
2. Gerota's fascia is entered, and the renal pelvis and ureter are freed while the kidney is rotated medially.
3. The ureter is freed and stabilized with a vessel loop below the level of the UPJ.
4. A 4-0 stay suture is placed in the tip of the ureter, and the ureter is incised, trimmed, and shaped to the desired contour with fine forceps and scissors.
5. Anchoring sutures of 4-0 material are placed for traction during reconstruction of the renal pelvis. A diamond-shaped incision is made into the renal pelvis, and the tissue is removed. The Foley Y-V-plasty technique may be followed. It converts a Y-shaped surgical incision of the renal pelvis into a V by drawing the apex of the arms of the Y to the foot of the Y with absorbable sutures.
6. Sutures are placed at each end of the refashioned renal pelvis, passed to the ureteral stoma and tagged. The pelvis is irrigated free of clots. The sutures are run in a continuous manner, creating the anastomosis.
7. A Silastic tubing may be used to stent the repaired pelvis until adequate healing has occurred. A nephrostomy tube is also placed within the pelvis to divert urine safely while the edema in the area of the repair resolves.
8. Gerota's fascia is closed over the repair.
9. A drain is placed where the pelvis was reconstructed, and the surgical incision is closed in layers.

Nephroureterectomy

Nephroureterectomy is removal of a kidney and its entire ureter. This procedure is indicated for hydroureteronephrosis of such a degree that reconstructive repair is impossible. It is also employed for collecting system tumors of the kidney and ureter.

Procedural Considerations

This procedure requires an extension of the incision anteriorly with the patient positioned semilaterally and fully prepped and draped for the surgeon to access the flank and lower abdomen. Only one instrument set is required, but a second skin-preparation setup and set of sterile drapes may be necessary.

An alternative to open nephroureterectomy is laparoscopic nephroureterectomy.

Operative Procedure

1. The patient is placed in a lateral position.
2. The kidney and upper ureter are exposed, and nephrectomy is performed as described below. The kidney may be placed in a plastic bag to prevent possible spillage of tumor cells.
3. The ureter is not cut at this time but is mobilized as far distally as possible. The operating room bed is adjusted so that surgery on the lower ureter may proceed. The lower ureter and bladder are identified and mobilized.
4. The ureter and a small cuff of the bladder are removed in continuity, and the bladder is repaired with a single layer of 2-0 absorbable interrupted sutures. The ureter and cuff of bladder are pulled superiorly, and the intact kidney and ureter are removed from the surgical field.
5. An 18 or 20 Fr Foley catheter is left in the bladder, and

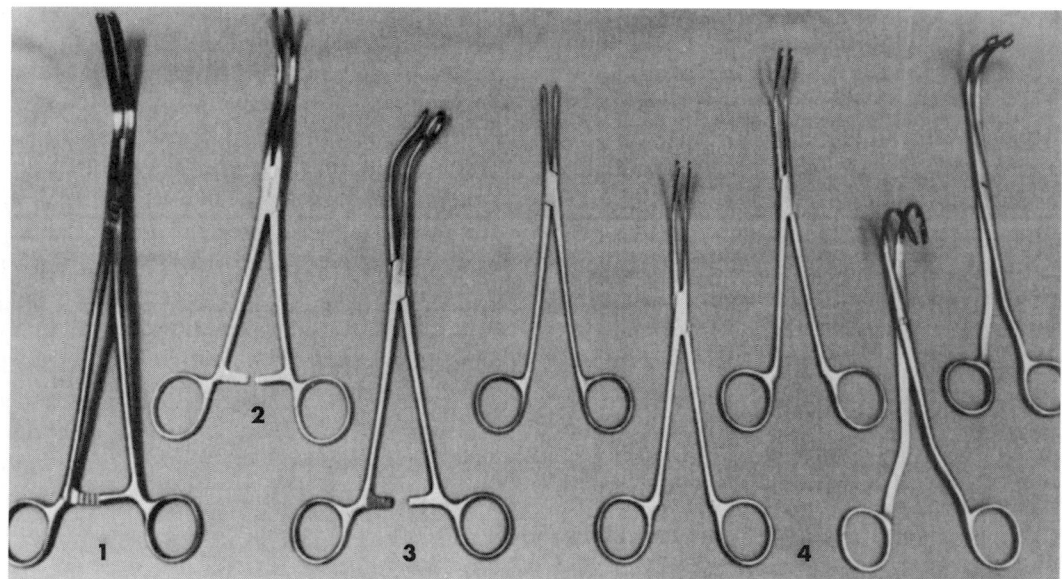

FIGURE 15-73   Kidney instruments. *1*, Statinsky pedicle clamp; *2*, Mayo pedicle clamp; *3*, Lewkowitz lithotomy forceps; *4*, set of five Randall stone forceps.

a drain is placed behind the bladder. The incision is closed in layers.

Nephrectomy

Nephrectomy is the surgical removal of a kidney. It is performed as a means of definitive therapy for many renal problems, such as congenital ureteropelvic junction obstruction with severe hydronephrosis, renal tumors, renal trauma, calculus disease with infection, cortical abscess, pyelonephrosis, and renovascular hypertension.

The advent of innovative technology in the 1990s now allows a unique approach to nephrectomy—laparoscopic nephrectomy.

Procedural Considerations

In routine renal surgery the patient is placed in the lateral position with the loin directly over the kidney rest. The operative flank is uppermost, with the patient's back brought to the edge of the OR bed. The upper arm is supported on an overhead arm support, and the lower arm is flexed at the elbow so that the hand rests on or under the head pillow. The patient's legs are positioned by placing a pillow between them and flexing the lower leg at the knee. The upper leg remains extended. The kidney rest is then raised, and when the desired bed flexion is achieved, 3-inch adhesive tape is used to stabilize the patient throughout surgery. Routine skin preparation and draping procedures are carried out.

The nephrectomy setup includes routine laparotomy setup, kidney instruments (Fig. 15-73), a variety of red rubber, Malecot, or Pezzar catheters, a wound drainage system, and vessel loops.

In certain nephrectomies the chest or the gastrointestinal tract may be opened. If the chest is opened, appropriate instruments and postoperative chest drains are needed.

When the gastrointestinal tract is opened, precautions must be taken in the anastomosis and closure techniques. Rib resection requires the addition of a Finochietto rib retractor, a large Matson costal periosteotome, the Alexander costal periosteotome, right and left Doyen rib raspatories, a Bethune rib cutter, a double-action duckbill rongeur, the Bailey rib approximator, and a Langenbeck periosteal elevator.

Operative Procedure

1. The incision is carried through the skin, fat, and fascia. Bleeding vessels are clamped with hemostats and ligated.
2. The external oblique, internal oblique, and transversalis muscles are sequentially exposed and incised in the direction of the initial skin incision.
3. If necessary, a rib or ribs (eleventh or twelfth) may be resected to provide better access to the kidney. The periosteum is stripped with an Alexander costal periosteotome and Doyen rib raspatory. A scalpel and heavy scissors may be used to cut through the lumbocostal ligaments. The rib is grasped with an Ochsner clamp and cut with rib shears, so that the portion necessary to expose the kidney is removed. Gerota's fascia is identified and incised with Metzenbaum scissors.
4. The incision is extended, and the kidney and perirenal fat are exposed by blunt and sharp dissection. All perirenal fat that is removed during surgery may be saved in a small basin of normal saline. Perirenal fat may be used later as a bolster to stop bleeding.
5. The ureter is identified, separated from its adjacent structures, doubly clamped, divided, and ligated with absorbable 0 material.
6. The kidney pedicle containing the major blood vessels is isolated and doubly clamped; each vessel is triply

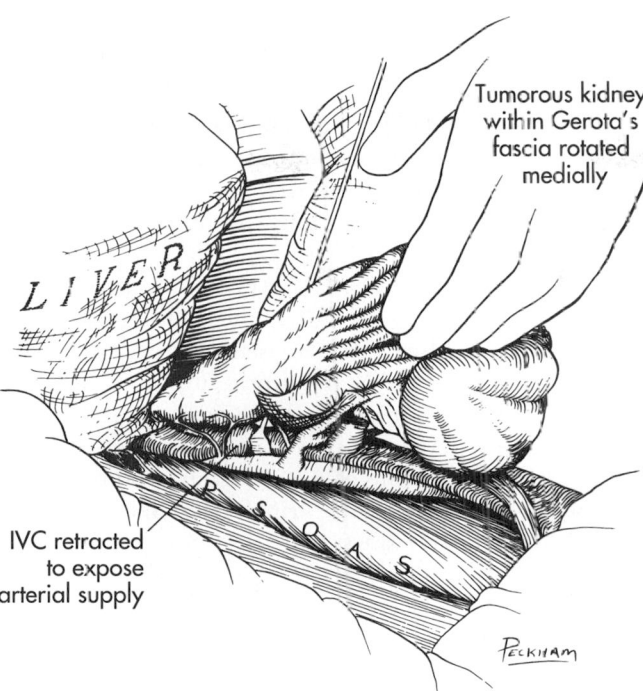

Tumorous kidney
within Gerota's
fascia rotated
medially

LIVER

PSOAS

IVC retracted
to expose
arterial supply

PECKHAM

FIGURE 15-74 Nephrectomy.

ligated with heavy nonabsorbable ties. Each vessel is then severed, leaving two ligatures on the pedicle, and the kidney is removed (Fig. 15-74).

7. The renal fossa is explored for bleeding, and necessary hemostasis is achieved. The fossa is then irrigated with normal saline, and the irrigant is removed by suction.

8. The fascia and muscles are closed in layers with interrupted, absorbable sutures. If necessary, retention sutures may be used in obese or chronically ill individuals in whom wound healing may be a problem.

9. The skin edges are approximated with sutures or skin staples, and the dressing is applied.

Laparoscopic nephrectomy

The approach for laparoscopic nephrectomy may be transabdominal or retroperitoneal. Transabdominal is the most common approach. Indications for laparoscopy are generally for benign disease, although more radical surgeries have been accomplished in this manner. Preoperative workup is similar to any renal surgery with the addition of a full mechanical antibiotic bowel prep. Although surgery time is lengthier (an average of 3½ to 5 hours), postoperative recovery, analgesia requirements, and total hospital stay have lessened dramatically. The procedure always includes cystoscopy with placement of a renal balloon catheter, a ureteral catheter, and a Foley urethral catheter under C-arm fluoroscopy. Indigo carmine may be injected into the skin overlying the renal pelvis.

There should always be an open setup available in the event laparoscopy is unsuccessful. The patient is initially placed on a beanbag in the supine position. A standard laparoscopy instrument and equipment setup that includes three 5 mm trocars, an insufflation needle, and two 10 to

12 mm trocars is used. Cystoscopic and ureteroscopic supplies will be needed as well as an 0.035 Bentson guidewire, an occlusion balloon catheter, an 0.035 Amplatz stiff guidewire, a 16 Fr Foley catheter and drainage bag, Indigo carmine, an irrigator/aspirator, a 1-liter bag of saline with 5000 units of heparin and 500 mg of cefazolin sodium (Ancef), a 1-liter pressure bag to pressurize the irrigant to 250 mm Hg, a #12 or #11 knife blade, 10 mm clip appliers, the entrapment sack, and tissue morcellator.

Procedural Considerations

After endotracheal intubation and placement of pneumatic compression stockings, a nasogastric tube and electrosurgical dispersive pad are placed. The patient is prepped and draped as for laparotomy. Use of a draping pack with four large adherent drape sheets, instead of a standard laparotomy sheet, affords better access for the port sites.

The technique of placing the patient in supine position to initiate the procedure is the method used when laparoscopic nephrectomy was new. Many surgeons still use this approach. Others place the patient in lateral decubitus position on a deflated beanbag positioner at the outset, or turn the patient after endoscopic intervention. Assuring that the patient is adequately secured to the bed is critical. Before prepping, the OR bed is tilted laterally to afford a central abdominal access. The patient is prepped and draped, and access of the first three ports is achieved as described. Before insertion of the remaining trocars, the bed is returned to its normal configuration so that the patient is again in lateral decubitus position. The kidney rest is then elevated. The operation then continues as described.

If the procedure is to begin with the patient supine, the contralateral arm is padded with thick foam from the shoulder to the fingertips. The patient is prepped and draped in the usual manner for thoracoabdominal surgery. Extra draping materials are utilized when the patient is repositioned.

The nasogastric tube is removed in the operating room, and the Foley catheter is removed on the first postoperative day. Oral intake may begin 6 hours postoperatively. The compression stockings are removed when the patient is ambulatory. Most patients leave the hospital in 4 days, return to work in approximately 2 weeks, and achieve full convalescence in 3 weeks.

Operative Procedure

1. Access is gained to the peritoneal cavity through a 1 cm transverse subumbilical stab-wound incision, with the blade of choice. After elevating the anterior abdominal wall with towel clips, the insufflation needle is inserted with the stopcock valve control in the closed position.

2. Once the insufflation needle is in place, sterile saline is dropped into the lumen of the needle, and the valve of

the needle is opened. If the saline enters freely (a successful test), the abdominal cavity is inflated with CO_2 until a pressure of 15 to 20 mm of Hg is obtained. If saline does not enter freely, it indicates improper placement of the needle.

3. A nick is made in the rectus fascia with the chosen blade, and the 10 mm trocar replaces the insufflation needle. Towel clips are again used on each side of the incision to stabilize the abdominal wall during insertion.

4. The 10 mm laparoscope is inserted.

5. A second incision is made immediately below the costal margin in the midclavicular line, and a 10 to 12 mm trocar is inserted.

6. The third trocar, 5 mm, is inserted through a small incision 2 cm below the umbilicus in the midclavicular line.

7. The last two 5 mm trocars are placed, one in the anterior axillary line at a level with the umbilicus and one immediately subcostal in the anterior axillary line. All trocars are then withdrawn until 2 to 3 cm of each sheath protrude into the abdomen. Polypropylene (Prolene) suture may be used to secure the side arm ports to the patient's skin. Each trocar site is laparoscopically inspected after trocar insertion to identify any bleeding or perforation. It may be necessary on occasion to extend the incision to allow trocar insertion.

8. The ascending or descending colon is completely mobilized with electrosurgical scissors and deflected medially. The retroperitoneum is opened.

9. Through gentle motion of the ureteral catheter the ureter is identified and dissected. A Babcock forceps is clamped around the dissected ureter for retraction.

10. The ureter is dissected until the lower pole of the kidney is visualized. Any veins encountered are clipped twice proximally and twice distally. The kidney is cleared of surrounding tissue and freed laterally and superiorly. Gerota's fascia is entered to free the adrenal gland and exclude it from the dissection.

11. The renal artery and vein are identified and cleared to create a 360-degree window around each vessel. The clip applier is inserted through the 10 to 12 mm port. Two clips are placed on the specimen side, and three clips are clamped to the stump side of both vessels. The vessels are then sharply incised.

12. Two pairs of clips are placed proximally and distally on the ureter, and it is sharply incised. The specimen end is grasped, and the kidney is moved into the upper abdominal quadrant.

13. The entrapment sac is introduced through the 10 to 12 mm port. The bottom of the sac is pulled into the abdomen with graspers until the neck of the sac clears the end of the port and is then unfurled.

14. The sac is opened, and the ureteral stump with attached kidney are placed inside. The drawstrings are pulled tight, closing the mouth of the sac.

15. The patient is returned to the supine position, by tilting the OR bed, and the sac strings are extracted through the umbilical port. Under laparoscopic observation, the port is removed and the neck of the sac is brought to lie on the abdominal surface. The tissue morcellator is inserted into the sac, and the kidney is morcellated under suction in a clockwise fashion.

16. The abdominal cavity is exited with laparoscopic observation of each trocar site, during and after removal, to assure that hemostasis has been achieved. Fascial layers at the 12 mm trocar sites are closed with 2-0 or 3-0 absorbable suture in a figure-of-eight pattern.

17. Subcuticular closure of 4-0 absorbable suture is done on all port sites. Steri-Strips, Telfa, and Tegaderm complete the dressings.

Heminephrectomy

Heminephrectomy is removal of a portion of the kidney. It is usually indicated for conditions involving the lower or upper pole of the kidney, such as calculus disease, or trauma limited to one pole of a kidney. In rare instances in which a patient has only one kidney, such surgery may be used for renal neoplasms to avoid the need for dialysis and subsequent renal transplantation.

Procedural Considerations

The setup is as described for nephrectomy with the addition of vascular and bulldog clamps.

Operative Procedure

1. The kidney and its pedicle should be completely mobilized as described for nephrectomy. The main vessels may be temporarily occluded for only 20 to 30 minutes, after which progressive renal damage may occur. Local hypothermia may be indicated to prolong ischemic operating time.

2. The renal capsule is incised and stripped back.

3. A wedge of kidney tissue containing the diseased or damaged cortex is excised. Interlobar fat or arcuate and interlobular arteries are clamped with Hopkins clamps and suture ligated with 4-0 absorbable suture on urologic needles.

4. The open collecting system is reapproximated with a continuous 4-0 suture.

5. Perirenal fat is placed in the area in which tissue was excised, and the renal parenchyma is reapproximated with horizontal mattress sutures.

6. If possible, the renal capsule is reapproximated with a continuous 2-0 suture.

Radical nephrectomy

Radical nephrectomy is excision of kidney, perirenal fat, adrenal gland, Gerota's capsule (fascia), and contiguous periaortic lymph nodes. This procedure is performed for parenchymal renal neoplasms. A lumbar, transthoracic, or transabdominal approach to the kidney is performed depending on the size and location of the lesion. The transthoracic or transabdominal approach is preferred because the blood vessels of the kidney can be more easily reached and ligated before the tumor is mobilized, thus decreasing the possibility of tumor embolization into the bloodstream.

Procedural Considerations

The setup is as described for nephrectomy.

Operative Procedure

In general, the procedure is as described for nephrectomy with two exceptions: (1) the renal pedicle is ligated before the kidney is mobilized, and (2) Gerota's capsule is not incised but is removed en bloc with the kidney. Involved lymph nodes surrounding the renal pedicle are excised. A chest tube is inserted if the transthoracic approach is used.

Kidney transplant

Kidney transplant entails transplantation of a living-related or cadaveric donor kidney into the recipient's iliac fossa (Fig. 15-75). It is performed in an effort to restore renal function and thus maintain life in a patient who has end-stage renal disease.

Transplant from a Living Donor

The kidney donor must be in perfect health. ABO (blood typing) and histocompatibility (HLA tissue typing) along with a negative white cell (lymphocyte) crossmatch determine donor-recipient compatibility. It is not necessary to match the Rh factor. Once the donor has been chosen, a complete workup that includes history and physical examination as well as chest x-ray examination,

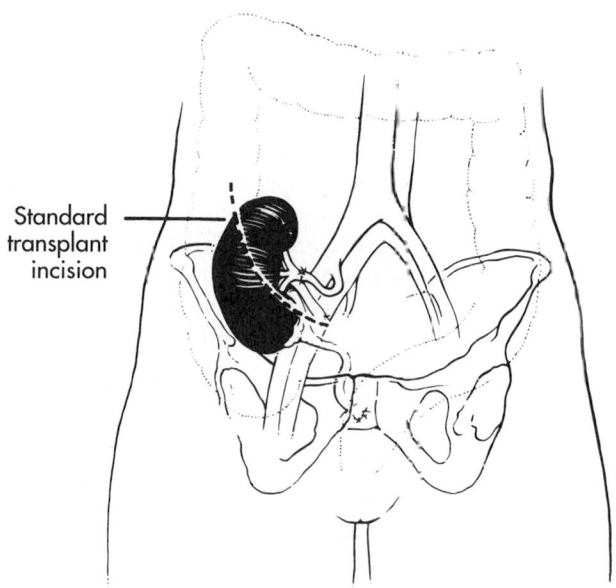

Standard transplant incision

FIGURE 15-75   Transplanted kidney in recipient's iliac fossa.

ECG, CBC, BUN and creatinine values, blood chemistry profiles, coagulation studies, and viral titers is done. Renal function is assessed with three creatinine clearances, urinalysis, and urine cultures followed by IVPs and excretory urography. A flush aortogram assesses the vascular anatomy, and renal angiography pinpoints the kidney of choice while ruling out the presence of renal lesions. A kidney with a single renal artery is preferred, but kidneys with double and triple arteries may be used if necessary. If there is a family history of diabetes, a 5-hour glucose tolerance test is also performed.

The ideal living donor is an identical twin, although any immediate family member (usually a sibling or parent) may be a donor if the person is medically acceptable. The donor is given an intravenous solution of 1000 ml of 5% dextrose in lactated Ringer's on the evening before nephrectomy. This is followed with 500 ml of 5% dextrose in water over the next 10 to 12 hours. The morning of surgery, about 45 minutes before transport to the operating room, 12.5 g of mannitol is administered to ensure diuresis during the induction of anesthesia.

Procedural considerations

Two adjacent operating rooms are prepared for the procedures; surgery on the donor and recipient proceeds simultaneously.

A Foley catheter is inserted and left in the donor's bladder to measure urinary output and prevent bladder distention from the increased urine production induced by diuretics. The donor is placed in the lateral position, prepared from midchest to midthigh, and draped in the usual manner, exposing the flank area.

Required instruments and equipment are identical to those for the nephrectomy setup plus the supplies for the sterile perfusion table and include an IV pole, electrolyte solution (in iced basin until needed), 2 intravenous extension tubes, a kidney basin with cold (4° C) intravenous saline solution, a three-way stopcock, an 18-gauge needle catheter, mosquito hemostats, vascular forceps, Metzenbaum scissors, suture scissors, and Kelly hemostats.

An electrolyte solution of Ringer's lactate that contains procaine and heparin is commonly used to perfuse the harvested kidney. Collins's or Sachs's solution may be used to perfuse cadaveric kidneys after harvest but should never be used to perfuse a kidney from a living donor because of the potential effect of elevated potassium in the recipient attributable to residual perfusate in the kidney.

Operative procedure

1. The donor nephrectomy procedure is as described for nephrectomy; however, the ureter and renal vein and artery require meticulous dissection.
2. Maximum length of the ureter is achieved by dividing it at or below the pelvic rim if possible. To preserve adequate ureteral vascularization, the surgeon is cautious not to skeletonize the ureter.
3. Particular care is taken to remove the maximum

length of the renal vein and artery. To obtain the maximum length of the right renal vein sometimes requires partial occlusion of the inferior vena cava with a Statinsky clamp and dissection of a portion of the inferior vena cava. This is best done after the ureter has been freed.

4. Repair of the inferior vena cava is made with a continuous 4-0 or 5-0 vascular suture.
5. Five minutes before the surgeon clamps the renal vessels, 5000 units of heparin sodium and 12.5 g of mannitol are systemically administered to the patient to prevent intravascular clotting and maximize diuresis.
6. Immediately after the kidney is removed from the donor, 50 mg of protamine sulfate is given intravenously to reverse the heparinization.
7. Furosemide, mannitol, and intravenous fluids are administered to the donor to maintain adequate urinary output from the donor's remaining kidney.
8. Gentle handling of the kidney is essential. Team members must prevent undue traction on the vascular pedicle, which may induce vasospasm and reduce perfusion of the kidney.
9. To reduce warm ischemia time, the surgeon double-clamps the vein and the artery, excises the kidney, and immediately places it in cold saline solution on a sterile back table where the kidney is flushed with the designated electrolyte solution. Warm ischemia time (from the clamping of renal vessels to a point at which the kidney is perfused with cold electrolyte solution) should be kept to a minimum to prevent acute tubular necrosis and to maintain maximum renal function after transplantation.
10. Mosquito clamps and fine vascular forceps are used to expose the renal artery to permit insertion of a needle catheter, such as a Medicut. The cold electrolyte solution passes through the intravenous tubing and the needle catheter, flushing any remaining donor's blood from the kidney. This also decreases the kidney's metabolic rate by lowering its temperature. Flushing time is usually 2 to 5 minutes.
11. After flushing, trimming the vessels of adventitia may be necessary to facilitate the vascular anastomosis to the recipient's iliac vessels.
12. The kidney, in cold saline solution, is covered with sterile drapes and taken by the surgeon to the room in which the recipient's iliac vessels have been exposed.
13. Wound closure for the donor is as described for nephrectomy.

Transplant from a Cadaveric Donor

The ideal cadaveric donor is young, free from infection and cancer, normotensive until a short time before death, and under hospital observation several hours before death. Permission to harvest the donor kidney must be obtained from the family and the medical examiner after brain death

has been unequivocally established. Awareness of existing state legislation in this complex area is advisable.

The donor goes through a complete evaluation including physician consultations and lab studies. The medical history is reviewed for any possible contraindications such as chronic organ-donor disease, ongoing systemic infection, intravenous drug abuse, malignancy, heart or lung disease, trauma to the donor organ, and the presence of HIV. Laboratory studies include blood typing, urinalysis, urine and blood cultures, BUN, serum creatinine, CBC, hepatitis B antigen evaluation, venereal disease, and HIV. Evaluation of arterial blood gases, electrolyte values, and liver enzymes is also necessary. Because of improvements in medical therapy the only absolute contraindications to organ donation is HIV and metastasis.

Preoperative management of the cadaver donor is vital to the success of the transplant. Organ perfusion, oxygenation, and hydration must be maintained. Arterial blood-gas evaluation determines ventilatory support, and dopamine may be administered if fluids alone are not able to maintain an adequate systolic blood pressure. Urine output is monitored, and antibiotics may be administered to combat and prevent infection.

Procedural considerations

After brain death has been established, the donor is taken to the surgical suite with respiratory and cardiac function maintained mechanically. The donor is placed in the supine position and is prepared for a laparotomy. Anticoagulant and alpha-adrenergic receptor blocking agents are administered systemically during the procedure. Adequate renal perfusion and function are maintained with intravenous fluids and diuretics.

Instruments and equipment are the same as for the nephrectomy setup, with exclusion of the rib instruments and the addition of Metzenbaum scissors, suture scissors, vascular forceps, DeBakey forceps, Dean hemostatic forceps, mosquito hemostats, DeBakey clamps, angled clip appliers with medium and large clips, bulldog clamps, vascular clamps, Deaver retractors, Harrington splanchnic retractors, vascular needle holders, a sternal saw or Lepshey knife and mallet, umbilical tapes, electrolyte solution (lactated Ringer's, Sachs, or Collins), cold packing in an iced basin until needed, an IV pole, intravenous extension tubes, a kidney basin with cold (4° C) intravenous saline solution, a three-way stopcock, an 18-gauge needle catheter, a centimeter ruler, the perfusion machine or kidney transplantation equipment, and ice.

Operative procedure

1. A midline incision is made from the xiphoid process to the symphysis pubis with bilateral supraumbilical transverse extensions through the skin, subcutaneous layer, fascia, and muscle.
2. Hemostasis is obtained with clamps, ties, suture ligatures, and electrocoagulation.

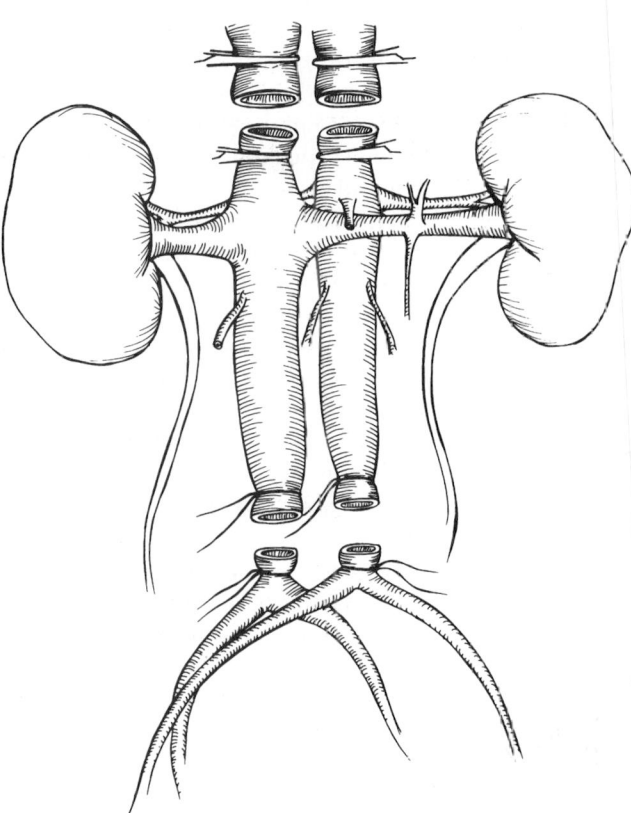

FIGURE 15-76   En bloc resection.

3. The kidney, renal vessels, and ureter are carefully dissected with Metzenbaum scissors, DeBakey forceps, and Dean hemostatic forceps.

4. Heparin sodium, 15,000 units, is given intravenously 5 to 10 minutes before the renal vessels are clamped.

5. The usual method of resection is en bloc resection (harvesting of donor kidneys) (Fig. 15-76), which involves the removal of sections of the inferior vena cava and aorta with both kidneys in continuity.

6. An incision is made along the route of the small bowel mesentery up to the esophageal hiatus.

7. The entire gastrointestinal tract, spleen, and inferior portion of the pancreas are mobilized by dividing the celiac axis and the superior mesenteric artery, exposing the entire retroperitoneal region.

8. The inferior vena cava and aorta are clamped below the renal vessels with vascular clamps, and the vessels are divided.

9. Lumbar tributaries are secured with metal clips and are divided.

10. The kidneys and ureters are freed from their surrounding soft tissues.

11. The ureters are divided distally at the pelvic brim.

12. The suprarenal aorta and inferior vena cava are clamped and divided at the level of the diaphragm, close to the bifurcation.

13. The vessels and kidney are severed from the surgical field, and the aorta and vena cava are ligated.

14. After removal of the kidneys, immediate perfusion with cold (4° C) electrolyte solution is carried out as in step 9 for a donor kidney. The kidneys are placed in a container of cold saline solution and surrounded by saline slush in an insulated carrier or placed on a hypothermic pulsatile perfusion machine for transport. A new preservative solution developed at the University of Wisconsin is being used in many institutions. It contains hydroxyethyl starch, providing a better metabolic substrate for organ metabolism. The cold ischemia time has been dramatically increased with this solution, allowing more time for transport.

15. While kidney perfusion is begun, the abdominal lymph nodes and spleen are removed for use in tissue typing.

16. The incision is closed with interrupted sutures and artificial life-support systems are terminated. The perioperative nurse cares for the patient's body, preserving privacy, dignity, and humanity at the patient's death.

Transplant Recipient

Each potential recipient is judged individually in regard to kidney transplantation. Most persons below 55 years of age are acceptable; older patients are less tolerant of postoperative complications. Contraindications for renal transplantation include (1) systemic disease that precludes major surgery, (2) oxalosis (a metabolic disorder), (3) a positive HLA cytotoxic antibody screen, and (4) active cancer. If required, a patient may need to undergo bilateral nephrectomy before renal transplantation for uncontrollable hypertension or kidney infections and for reflux when there is a significant history of infections. Occasionally a large polycystic kidney may need to be removed to create a space for the new kidney. Splenectomy may be performed at this time to improve leukopenia and enhance the effects of myelosuppressive and immunosuppressive drugs.

The transplant recipient requires optimal nutritional support and adequate dialysis. All potential sources of infection must be treated. Most commonly these include teeth, bladder, nasal sinuses, and skin. The patient may need a short hemodialysis to control fluid overload or electrolyte imbalances. A repeat cytotoxic crossmatch with fresh serum specimens should follow hemodialysis. Preoperative antibiotics are commonly administered. Other important diagnostic tools for preoperative evaluation are chest x-ray examination, abdominal ultrasonography, voiding cystourethrography, liver function studies, hematologic assays, and serum values for screening hepatitis, HIV, and viral diseases.

Procedural considerations

The patient is placed in the supine position. A Foley catheter with an attached Silastic stenting catheter is inserted into the bladder by sterile technique. From 50 to 75 ml of antibiotic solution is instilled in the bladder through a sterile catheter-tipped syringe, allowed to remain for 20 minutes, and drained. The patient is prepped from nipples to knees and is draped in the routine manner.

Operative procedure

1. A curved right lower quadrant incision is made through the skin, subcutaneous layer, fascia, and muscle.
2. Bleeding is controlled with clamps, ties, and electrocoagulation.
3. The inferior epigastric vessels are divided between suture ligatures.
4. A retroperitoneal dissection is performed by mobilizing the peritoneum superiorly and medially.
5. A Balfour self-retaining retractor is placed in the wound for exposure, and a wide Deaver retractor is inserted to reflect the peritoneum superiorly and medially.
6. With the use of the 9¼-inch Metzenbaum scissors and DeBakey forceps, dissection is made along the entire length of the hypogastric artery and the external and common iliac arteries to the bifurcation of the aorta, continuing down the internal iliac artery.
7. The internal iliac artery is ligated distally and divided, with proximal control maintained by a vascular clamp.
8. The iliac vein may be dissected free by ligating and dividing the internal iliac venous branches with 3-0 nonabsorbable sutures or ligating clips. In more recent years there has been a tendency to dissect only the hypogastric artery and that portion of iliac vein to be anastomosed.
9. The donor kidney is brought into the operative field and placed in cold (4° C) intravenous saline solution.
10. Mosquito hemostats, 4-inch DeBakey forceps, and curved and straight fine scissors are used to make the necessary alterations on the donor kidney vessels to facilitate the anastomoses.
11. The donor kidney is returned to the cold intravenous saline solution until the time of the anastomosis.
12. Two angled DeBakey vascular clamps are placed on the internal iliac vein.
13. A #11 blade is used to make a 1 cm incision in the iliac vein between the clamps.
14. The vessel is rinsed with heparin sodium solution (10 U/ml) in the Asepto syringe.
15. Angled Potts scissors are used to extend the incision to accommodate the donor renal vein.
16. The donor kidney is placed in a 3- by 10-inch, cold saline–soaked stockinette, with the renal vessels leaving from a hole in the side. Use of the stockinette prevents direct contact with the kidney and therefore trauma.

17. The renal vein is anastomosed to the side of the recipient's iliac vein with 5-0, double-armed, vascular sutures.
18. In like manner the renal artery is anastomosed end to end with the proximal portion of the internal iliac artery using 5-0 vascular sutures.
19. The vessels are irrigated proximally and distally with heparin sodium solution by using the 10 ml syringe attached to the Medicut catheter before placing the final sutures.
20. The stockinette is removed for adequate visualization of the entire kidney. The angled DeBakey clamps are removed from the venous vessels, and the anastomosis is checked for leakage.
21. Immediately afterward, the clamps on the internal iliac artery are released, and the anastomosis is checked.
22. Meticulous inspection is made of the hilum and surface of the kidney for bleeding and infarction.
23. Diuretics are administered intravenously as needed.
24. Attention is then directed to the ureter and bladder.
25. Two long Martius forceps are used to grasp the anterior bladder wall.
26. Using a scalpel with a #10 knife blade, a 4 cm incision is made anteriorly.
27. Two narrow Harrington retractors and one narrow Deaver retractor are inserted into the bladder for exposure.
28. The ureter is passed through the bladder wall and tunneled suburothelially for 2 to 2.5 cm.
29. The spatulated end of the ureter is then sutured into the bladder urothelium with four to six 4-0 or 5-0 atraumatic absorbable sutures, creating a ureteroneocystostomy.
30. A 5 Fr pediatric infant feeding tube is passed through the ureteroneocystostomy, up to the renal pelvis, and out through the urethra with the Foley catheter. This stenting catheter will remain in place for 36 to 48 hours to ensure ureteral patency during a period in which ureteral edema may occur.
31. Retractors are removed, and the bladder is closed in three layers.
32. Continuous 4-0 absorbable suture is used for urothelial closure and interrupted 2-0 absorbable suture for closure of bladder muscles.
33. An imbricating layer of 2-0 nonabsorbable material is used to bury the suture line.
34. The bladder is irrigated with an antibiotic solution to check for leaks.
35. The renal anastomoses are again checked for bleeding.
36. Three metal clips are placed on the superior, inferior, and lateral aspects of the kidney to radiographically measure renal size and determine postoperative swelling.
37. Retractors are removed from the incision.

38. Closed wound suction drains are inserted into the wound, brought through the skin laterally, and secured with 2-0 nonabsorbable suture on a cutting needle.
39. Muscle and fascial layers are closed with a single layer of 0 nonabsorbable sutures on a large atraumatic needle.
40. The subcutaneous layer is closed with 3-0 absorbable sutures on an atraumatic needle.
41. Skin closure is accomplished with skin staples, and dressings are applied.
42. The bladder is irrigated with 50 to 75 ml of antibiotic solution to prevent infection and free any blood clots.

Adrenalectomy

Adrenalectomy is partial or total excision of one or both adrenal glands. It may be performed for several reasons: hypersecretion of adrenal hormones, neoplasms of the adrenal gland, secondary treatment of neoplasms elsewhere in the body that depend on adrenal hormonal secretions, such as carcinoma of the prostate and breast, and pheochromocytoma.

Care of the patient with pheochromocytoma carries with it particular concerns for the perioperative nurse. These patients are subject to extreme elevations in blood pressure, often accompanied by tachycardia, and hypovolemic states that can induce vascular collapse. If an adrenal tumor is being excised, early ligation of the adrenal vein is crucial in avoiding a sudden blood pressure elevation from the manipulation of the gland. After tumor removal there will be a rapid drop in blood pressure that can be minimized by maintenance of blood volume and administration of norepinephrine. With bilateral adrenalectomy, cortisone replacement will be instituted.

Procedural Considerations

For unilateral adrenalectomy, the patient may be placed in the lateral or supine position. More often, however, both glands are explored, and the supine or prone position is selected. The prone position is especially useful for a known disorder, such as aldosteronism, localized benign lesions, and solitary adenomas of Cushing's disease, and debilitated patients with an advanced neoplasm.

The setup for a lateral approach is like that described for nephrectomy, including rib-resection instruments, vascular instruments, and vessel clips and appliers. The setup for an abdominal approach is like that described for laparotomy, including vascular instruments, extra-long scissors, tissue forceps, Rochester-Pean forceps, Mixter forceps, and needle holders. Penrose tubing is needed for retraction. Vessel clips and appliers may also be needed as well as various sizes of nonabsorbable braided sutures. The setup for the posterior approach is like that described for the lateral approach. The patient is placed prone in a 35-degree jackknife position with the kidney rest under the inferior margin of the anterior rib cage. Both arms should be carefully extended cephalad with adequate support under each shoulder.

Operative Procedures
Lateral approach

1. A flank, thoracolumbar, or transthoracic incision is performed as described for nephrectomy.
2. The rib underlying the chosen approach is resected or deflected for optimum exposure of the upper pole of the kidney.
3. Entry is between the eleventh and twelfth ribs in a flank approach, the tenth and eleventh ribs in a thoracolumbar approach, and the ninth and tenth ribs in a transthoracic approach.
4. An opening is made through the transverse fascia with scissors.
5. The pleura and diaphragm are protected with moist packs, and Gerota's capsule is incised to expose the kidney and adrenal gland.
6. The gland is identified and dissected free from the upper pole of the kidney by scissors and Babcock forceps.
7. The blood supply of the gland is identified, clamped or clipped, and divided. Bleeding vessels are ligated.
8. To release the gland, the left adrenal vein, a branch of the left renal vein, is separated by clamping and cutting. The right adrenal vein, a tributary of the vena cava, is also divided. Fine vascular sutures may be required to repair inadvertent injury to the vena cava.
9. When hemostasis has been ensured, the wound is closed sequentially in layers: muscle, fascia, subcutaneous tissue, and skin.

Abdominal approach

1. The abdominal wall is incised with an upper abdominal incision, and the peritoneal cavity is opened and explored.
2. Bleeding vessels are clamped and ligated.
3. The abdominal wound is retracted, and the surrounding organs are protected with moist laparotomy packs.
4. The retroperitoneal area near the diaphragm is opened on the left side, exposing the renal fascia.
5. The renal fascia is opened to reveal the left kidney and adrenal gland.
6. The adrenal gland is freed from the kidney by sharp and blunt dissection, and all bleeding vessels are clamped and ligated with 3-0 nonabsorbable sutures.
7. After all bleeding is controlled, the kidney is gently replaced in the renal fascia, which is closed with interrupted 0 absorbable sutures.
8. The peritoneum is closed over the left kidney and renal fascia.
9. The abdominal retractors are rearranged to give access to the peritoneum over the right kidney and adrenal

gland. Care must be taken to prevent trauma to the liver.

10. The same procedure is repeated on the right side, taking care to clamp and ligate the short adrenal vein.

11. The abdomen is inspected for bleeding vessels, which are clamped and ligated.

12. The wound is closed as in laparotomy.

Posterior approach

1. An incision is made over the eleventh or twelfth rib.

2. The periosteum is elevated, avoiding the nerve and vessels on the inferior margin.

3. The diaphragm and pleura are displaced superiorly, and the appropriate rib is resected.

4. Hemostasis is maintained with electrocoagulation.

5. Gerota's fascia is incised, and through sharp and blunt dissection the posterior aspect of the upper pole of the kidney is exposed.

6. The upper pole is mobilized, and a padded retractor is placed to deflect the kidney downward for the approach to the adrenal gland.

7. The suprarenal fat is meticulously dissected.

8. Vessel clips are utilized for control of smaller vessels.

9. Dissection continues superiorly, laterally, and inferiorly while the integrity of the hilum of the adrenal is maintained.

10. With right-angled clamps, the adrenal vein and artery are freed, divided, and ligated with 0 or 2-0 braided nonabsorbable ties.

11. Babcock clamps are employed for manipulation and removal of the adrenal gland.

12. Bleeding is controlled, and the wound is inspected for injury to renal structures.

13. Gerota's fascia is closed with interrupted absorbable sutures.

14. The wound is closed, and dressings are applied.

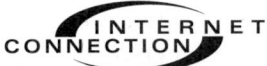

American Nephrology Nurses' Association:
http://www.inurse.com/~anna

Society of Urological Nurses and Associates (SUNA):
email suna@mail.ajj.com

Prostate Cancer Infolink: http://www.comed.com/Prostate/

Impotence: http://www2.impotent.com/whatis.html

Renal Diseases Electronic Journal: http://www.hden.com/

Digital Urology Journal: http://www.duj.com

Nephrolithiasis:
http://uhs.bsd.uchicago.edu/uhs/topics/nephro.htm

REFERENCES

1. Association of Operating Room Nurses recommended practices for electrosurgery. (1998). In *AORN Standards, recommended practices and guidelines.* Denver: the Association, pp. 187-196.

2. Bostrom, J. (1998). Employee competency programs: how computer technology can help. *Surgical Services Management, 4*(2), 8-11.

3. Dahl, S. (1998). Navigating clinical pathways. *Surgical Services Management, 4*(1), 10-11.

4. Fogg, D.M. (1998). Glutaraldehyde sterilization. In Clinical Issues, *AORN Journal, 67*(4), 870-871.

5. Frank, S.M. (Feb. 7, 1998). Body temperature and clinical outcome in the perioperative period. Paper presented at Consensus Conference on Perioperative Thermoregulation, Bethesda, Md.

6. Frizzel, J. (1998). The PSA test. *American Journal of Nursing, 98*(4), 14-15.

7. Gardner, T.A., & Theodorescu, D. (1997). Diagnosis and treatment of prostate cancer, *Surgical Services Management, 3*(12), 20-28.

8. Goodwin, S.A. (1998). A review of preemptive analgesia, *Journal of Perianesthesia Nursing, 13*(2), 109-114.

9. Johnson, J.E., Fieler, V.K., Jones, L.S., et al. (1997). *Self-regulation theory: applying theory to your practice,* Pittsburgh, PA: Oncology Nursing Press.

10. Lipman, M.M. (1998). Kidney stones, *Consumer Reports on Health, 10*(4), 11.

11. Marchiondo, K. (1998). A new look at urinary tract infection. *American Journal of Nursing, 98*(3), 34-39.

12. Mitchell, P.H., Ferketich, S., & Jennings, B.M. (1998). Quality health outcomes model, *Image, 30*(1), 43-46.

13. Walker, S. (1998). Two new germicides offer more reprocessing choices, *OR Manager, 14*(3), 6.

14. Wilson, M. (1997). Care of the patient undergoing transurethral resection of the prostate. *Journal of Perianesthesia Nursing, 12*(5), 341-351.

CHAPTER SIXTEEN

Thyroid and Parathyroid Surgery

Anna H. Burns

THE THYROID GLAND is the largest endocrine organ in the body, weighing approximately 20 grams in an adult.[4] The thyroid gland produces three hormones: thyroxine (T_4) and triiodothyronine (T_3), two iodine-containing amine hormones together known as the *thyroid hormones* (TH), and calcitonin, a peptide hormone.[25] The thyroid hormones' primary function is to regulate energy metabolism; they also play an important role in growth and development. Calcitonin is involved with the regulation of calcium homeostasis. Thyroid-stimulating hormone (TSH) is synthesized by the anterior pituitary which stimulates the production and release of thyroid hormones and the uptake of iodide. The hypothalamus secretes thyrotropin-releasing hormone (TRH), which controls synthesis and release of the TSH in the anterior pituitary.

Thyroid hormones cannot be synthesized without iodine.[13] Postprandial absorption of iodides is through the small intestines into the circulatory system, from which they are sequestered by the thyroid gland. Iodides are converted into thyroid hormones, some of which are stored in the gland as thyroglobulin or are secreted into the blood as thyroid hormone. After removal or ablation of the thyroid gland, a normal metabolic process may be maintained through oral administration of synthetic thyroxine.

In 1646 the thyroid gland was referred to as the *laryngeal gland* by Wharton. It was over 200 years later that Billroth and his group performed several successful thyroidectomies. Despite Billroth's earlier success with thyroidectomies, Theodor Kocher is regarded as the father of thyroid surgery. Kocher performed over 2000 thyroid surgeries in the late 1800s with only a 4.5% mortality, receiving the Nobel prize in 1909 for advances in this field. In 1914 the isolation of the hormone thyroxine (T_4) was accomplished by Kendall.[8] Since 1941, thyroidectomy as treatment of thyroid mass (goiter) has become less frequent because of the use of radioactive iodine and antithyroid drugs, which reduce the activity of the thyroid gland. Surgical intervention for diseases of the thyroid is performed on primary nodules of the thyroid and diffuse toxic goiters associated with hyperthyroidism.

Benign thyroid anomalies include functioning and nonfunctioning thyroid adenomas, cysts, multinodular goiter, and inflammatory lesions such as Hashimoto's thyroiditis.[27] Approximately 14,000 cases of thyroid cancer are diagnosed each year in the United States, representing 1% of all cancers. Classification of thyroid malignancies are as follows: (1) carcinomas: papillary, follicular, oncocytic (Hürthle cell), poorly differentiated, undifferentiated (anaplastic), medullary thyroid carcinoma, and rare epithelial tumors and (2) others: lymphoma and sarcoma. The most common thyroid malignancy in adults and children is papillary thyroid carcinoma. Papillary carcinoma accounts for 55% to 80% of all thyroid malignancies.[27] An estimated 50% of solitary tumors found in children are malignant. Thyroid disease and thyroid malignancy is generally more common in females than in males. A solitary thyroid nodule found in a male is likely to be malignant. Most reviews of thyroid malignancy indicate that the highest incidence occurs in patients younger than 20 years of age.[21] Patients who received low-dose external radiation to the neck area as a child or who have a family history of medullary cancer of the thyroid are at risk for developing thyroid cancer.

Diseases of the thyroid are usually manifested by alterations in hormonal secretion, enlargement of the thyroid, or both. Three forms of treatment are available: antithyroid drugs, radioactive iodine, and surgery. Before undergoing surgery, patients usually have their hyperthyroid state controlled with antithyroid drugs. Patients thus treated are restored to a euthyroid state and do not exhibit the common symptoms of rapid pulse, tremors, and nervous symptoms often associated with hyperthyroidism (Box 16-1).

The parathyroid gland secretes parathyroid hormone (PTH), which is an antagonist to calcitonin.[24] PTH and vitamin D are responsible for regulating calcium and phosphorus concentrations. Removal of all parathyroid tissue can result in severe tetany or death. The primary disease attributed to the parathyroid glands is hyperparathyroidism, which results in elevation of serum calcium. Primary hyperparathyroidism seems to be the most common cause of hypercalcemia in nonhospitalized patients, occurring in about 1 in every 500 women over 40 years of age and in about 1 in every 2000 men. The most common cause of hypercalcemia in hospitalized patients is carcinoma metastatic to the bone, with primary hyperparathyroidism being the second most common cause.[8] Symptoms of hyperparathyroidism include bone disease, renal calculi, pancreatitis, peptic ulcer, listlessness, weakness, and depression. Surgical intervention is indicated when symptoms occur, calcium levels are greater than 11.0 mg/dl, or renal function is impaired.

Hyperparathyroidism is being diagnosed more frequently with the increased use of tests that include multiphasic screening of blood calcium. Manifestations may be quite subtle; many patients with mild hypercalcemia (serum calcium levels 10.5 to 11 mg/dl) are without any apparent symptoms (Box 16-2).

SURGICAL ANATOMY

Thyroid Gland

The thyroid gland is a highly vascular organ situated in the anterior portion of the neck. It consists of right and left lobes united by a middle portion, the isthmus. The isthmus is situated near the base of the neck, and the lobes lie below the larynx and beside the trachea. The pyramidal lobe, a long thin projection of thyroid tissue protruding cranially from the isthmus, is found in about 80% of patients at surgery; it is the vestige of the embryonic thyroglossal duct.[8] The upper pole of the gland is hidden beneath the upper end of the sternothyroid muscle. The lower pole extends to about the level of the sixth tracheal ring. The posterior surface of the isthmus is adherent to the anterior surface of the tracheal rings, and the gland is enclosed by the pretracheal fascia (Fig. 16-1).

Blood supply to the thyroid is from the external carotid arteries via the superior thyroid arteries and from the subclavian arteries via the inferior thyroid arteries. Occasionally (10% of cases) a single thyroid artery (thyroidea ima) may arise from the brachiocephalic artery or from the arch of the aorta.[26] The thyroid gland is drained by three pairs of veins (superior, middle, and inferior thyroid veins) that extend from a plexus formed on the surface of the gland and on the front of the trachea. The capillaries form a dense plexus in the connective tissue around the follicles.

The nerve supply to the thyroid gland is derived from the cervical sympathetic trunk. On each side the superior laryngeal nerve lies in proximity to the superior thyroid artery. The recurrent laryngeal nerve that supplies the vocal cord ascends from the mediastinum and is in close association with the tracheoesophageal sulcus and the inferior thyroid artery. Sympathetic and parasympathetic nerves enter the gland, probably exerting their influence primarily on blood flow.

Lymphatic drainage of the thyroid gland is usually to the prelaryngeal (delphian), bifurcation, omohyoid, pretracheal, paratracheal, and supraclavicular nodes but may also drain directly into the deep cervical nodes, the thoracic duct, or the right lymph duct.

Parathyroid Gland

The parathyroid glands usually consist of four small, red-brown to yellow-tan, ovoid masses of tissue lying behind or, rarely, within the thyroid gland inside the pretracheal fascia. The upper pair of glands lies behind the superior pole of the thyroid; the lower pair lies near the lower pole of the thyroid (Fig.16-2, A). Aberrant nodules of parathyroid tissue may be found outside the pretracheal fascia as low as the superior mediastinum, especially within the thymus (Fig.16-2, B). Each parathyroid gland measures 5 to 7 mm by 3 to 4 mm by 0.5 to 2 mm and weighs an average of 30 to 40 mg. The upper glands are generally smaller than the lower ones.

Upper, or superior, parathyroid glands receive blood from a branch of the superior thyroid artery. Lower or inferior parathyroid glands receive blood from a branch of the inferior thyroid artery in approximately 90% of the cases.[8] Venous blood returns through tributaries of the thyroid veins. Lymphatic drainage of the parathyroid glands is the same as that for the thyroid gland. The nerve supply of the parathyroid glands is from the cervical sympathetic trunks.

PERIOPERATIVE NURSING CONSIDERATIONS

Assessment

An understanding of the potential complications after thyroid surgery can guide the perioperative nurse with the initial nursing assessment as well as with postoperative patient assessment.[14] Preoperatively the patient with hyperthyroidism most likely has undergone appropriate drug therapy that has returned the thyroid hormone levels and metabolic state to normal. Nonetheless, the perioper-

BOX 16-1	Overview and Signs and Symptoms of Hyperthyroidism

Hyperthyroidism A clinical syndrome that causes tissues to be exposed to overproduction of thyroid hormones. The excessive production of thyroid hormones produces a state of hypermetabolism that is responsible for the symptoms. There are several varieties of hyperthyroidism, ranging in seriousness from mild to severe. Graves' disease (toxic diffuse goiter), the most common form, is more frequently seen in women than in men during the third and fourth decades. The exact cause of Graves' disease is unknown, but it is believed to be an autoimmune disorder resulting from thyroid-stimulating immunoglobulins. Thyrotoxic crisis, or thyroid storm, is an acute manifestation of hyperthyroidism that is life threatening. Precipitating factors include stressful events such as surgery, trauma, and infection.

Signs and Symptoms

- Lid retraction and lag
- Proptosis
- Conjunctival irritation; lacrimation
- Characteristic bright-eyed, frightened, or startled look
- Increased systolic blood pressure, widening pulse pressure
- Increased body temperature and sweating
- Tachycardia
- Palpitations
- Weight loss
- Increased appetite
- Diarrhea
- Generalized muscle wasting and weakness
- Hyperactive deep tendon reflexes
- Tremors
- Restlessness, irritability
- Decreased concentration, decreased memory
- Insomnia
- Labile emotions and manic behavior

From Canobbio, M.M. (1996). *Mosby's handbook of patient teaching.* St. Louis: Mosby, pp. 387–388.

BOX 16-2	Overview and Signs and Symptoms of Hyperparathyroidism

Hyperparathyroidism Overactivity of one or more of the parathyroid glands. Excessive secretion of parathyroid hormone causes an increase of calcium that cannot be controlled by renal excretion or uptake in soft tissue or bones. Hyperparathyroidism is common in postmenopausal women and is classified as a primary or secondary disorder.

Causes and Contributing Factors

- Primary hyperparathyroidism
  - Parathyroid adenoma
  - Cell hyperplasia
- Secondary hyperparathyroidism
  - Rickets
  - Chronic renal failure
  - Osteomalacia
  - Excessive intake of drugs: thiazide diuretics, calcium supplements.

Signs and Symptoms

- Polyuria, polydipsia, kidney stones
- Abdominal pain, constipation, nausea, anorexia
- Fractures of ribs, spine
- Joint or back pain
- Depression, paranoia, mood swings
- Muscular weakness and atrophy

From Canobbio, M.M. (1996). *Mosby's handbook of patient teaching.* St. Louis: Mosby, pp. 380–381.

ative nurse should assess the patient for the presence of any symptoms that may relate to accelerated metabolism. They include irritability, hyperexcitability and exaggerated emotional responses, an abnormally elevated resting pulse, weight loss with fatigue and weakness, elevated systolic blood pressure, and cardiac symptoms such as palpitations or atrial fibrillation. The patient's cardiac and respiratory rate, muscle strength, elimination patterns, history of weight loss and heat intolerance, and emotional status should be noted. The patient may be anxious about the disease state and the success of surgery and may express concern regarding surgery in the area of the neck and its cosmetic results. Patients who are concerned about body image should have the opportunity to discuss these issues with the perioperative nurse. Skin integrity should be determined; patients with hyperthyroidism may have finely textured skin and edema in the lower extremities,

placing them at risk for skin breakdown. The most common complications specific to thyroid surgery are hypoparathyroidism and injury to the recurrent laryngeal nerve.[22] Preoperative assessment of the patient's voice quality should also be observed.

In addition to clinical signs and symptoms, results of diagnostic tests should be reviewed. Tests performed most commonly before thyroid surgery include measurements of T_3 and T_4, radioisotope or ultrasonic scans, as well as a current electrocardiogram (ECG). Thyroid function tests are interpreted in light of the patient's clinical presentation. They compliment the findings of the physical examination. The single best test to measure the thyroid status in a given person is a serum TSH concentration.[12] The most sensitive TSH tests of all are the "third-generation" chemoluminescent assays (ICMA).[16] Common laboratory tests and their normal adult ranges are found in Table 16-1. Thyrotropin–releasing hormone (TRH) testing is no longer needed because of the availability of sensitive "third-generation" TSH assays.

Assessment of thyroid anatomy

In addition to palpation of the thyroid gland for size, contour, consistency, nodes, and fixation, scans are used to elucidate thyroid anatomy.

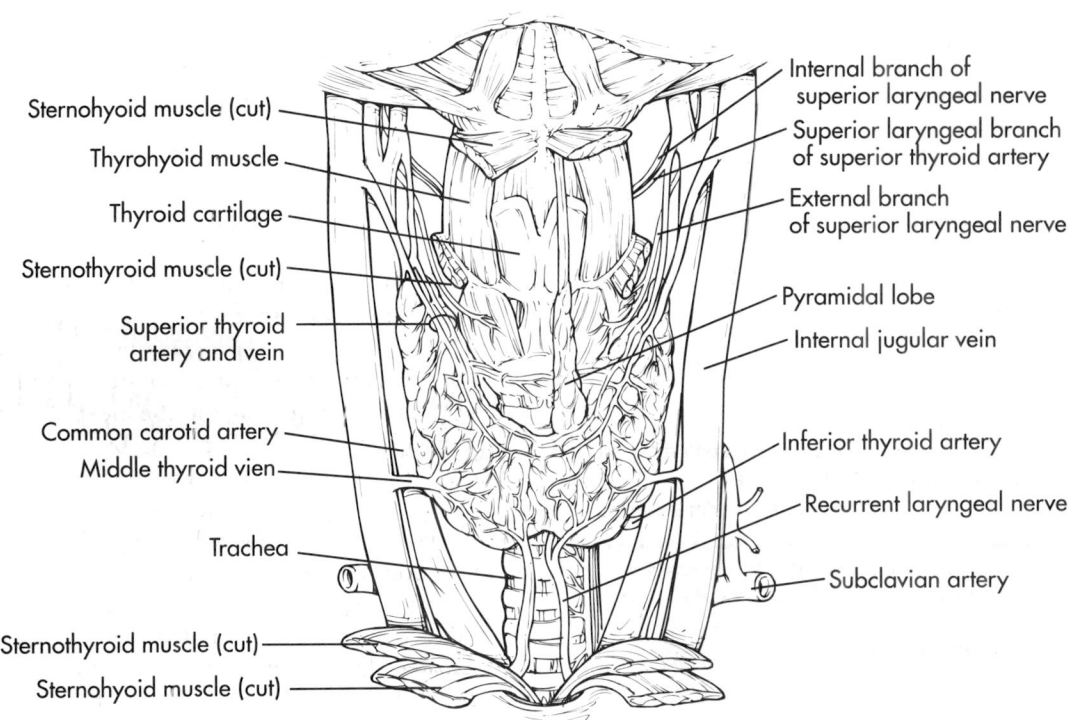

Sternohyoid muscle (cut)
Thyrohyoid muscle
Thyroid cartilage
Sternothyroid muscle (cut)
Superior thyroid artery and vein
Common carotid artery
Middle thyroid vien
Trachea
Sternothyroid muscle (cut)
Sternohyoid muscle (cut)

Internal branch of superior laryngeal nerve
Superior laryngeal branch of superior thyroid artery
External branch of superior laryngeal nerve
Pyramidal lobe
Internal jugular vein
Inferior thyroid artery
Recurrent laryngeal nerve
Subclavian artery

FIGURE 16–1   The thyroid gland.

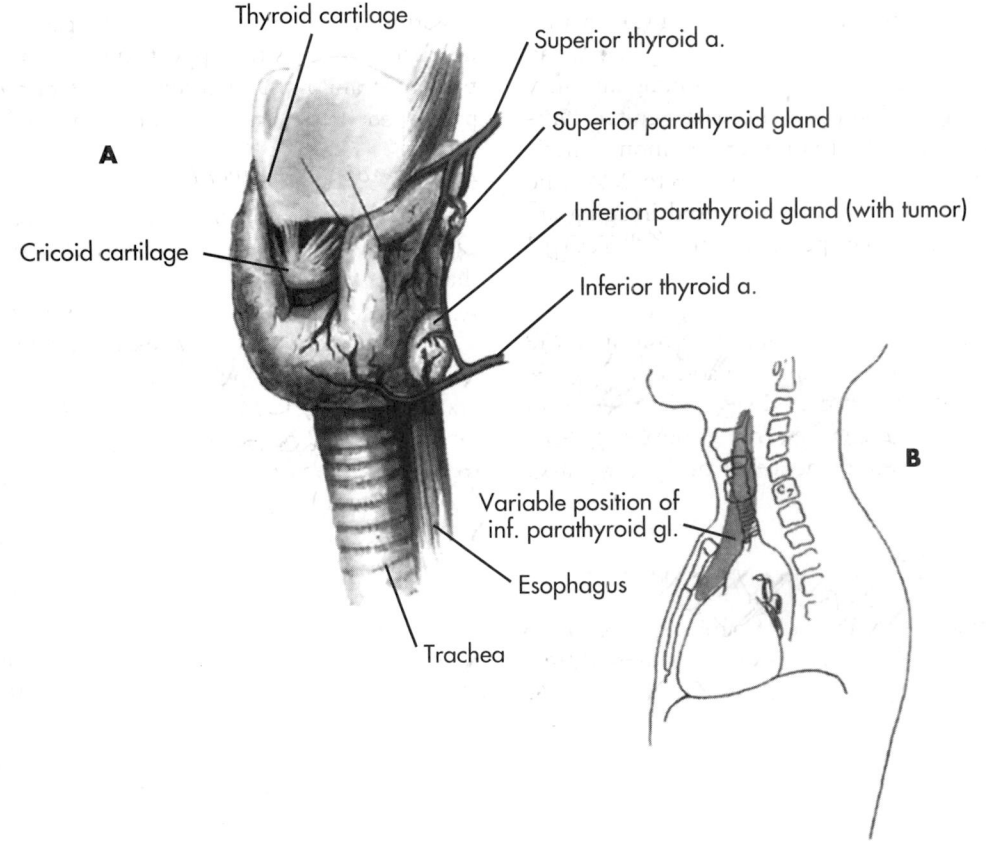

Thyroid cartilage
Superior thyroid a.
Superior parathyroid gland
Inferior parathyroid gland (with tumor)
Inferior thyroid a.
Cricoid cartilage
A
Variable position of inf. parathyroid gl.
Esophagus
Trachea
B

FIGURE 16–2   **A**, Thyroid and parathyroid glands. Notice their relation to each other and to the trachea. **B**, Notice the shaded area for varied locations of inferior parathyroid glands.

TABLE 16-1	Common Laboratory Tests	
TEST	**NORMAL RANGE**
Serum thyroid-stimulating hormone (TSH)	0-5 to 3.8 µU/ml
Chemoluminescent assay (ICMA)	Many labs list 6.5 as the upper limits for normal; most of the patients with levels of 3.9 and above are hypothyroid
Serum triiodothyronine (T$_3$)	110 to 230 ng/dl
Resin T$_3$ uptake (RT$_3$u)	24% to 34% Variations with different labs
Serum thyroxine (T$_4$)	4 to 11 µg/dl
Free thyroxine index (FTI, FT$_4$)	0.8 to 2.4 ng/dl Variations with different labs
Radioactive iodine uptake (RAIU)	24 hours: 8% to 30% absorbed Variations with different labs

Data from Moore, W.T., & Eastman, R.C (1996). Laboratory evaluation of diseases of the thyroid. In Moore, W.T., & Eastman, R.C. (Eds.). *Diagnostic endocrinology* (ed. 2). St. Louis: Mosby; Pagana, K.D., & Pagana, T.J. (1997). *Mosby's diagnostic and laboratory test reference* (ed. 3). St. Louis: Mosby.

Thyroid Isotope Scan for Thyroid Scintigraphy

Imaging of the normal thyroid with radionuclide agents shows normal size, shape, position, and function of the thyroid, with no areas of decreased or increased uptake. Nodules that are warm or hot are functioning and may indicate a benign adenoma or localized toxic goiter. Cold nodules are hypofunctioning or nonfunctioning and may indicate a cyst, nonfunctioning adenoma or goiter, lymphoma, localized area of thyroiditis or carcinoma. Incidence of malignancy in a cold nodule is 15% to 20%. The two most commonly used agents in thyroid imaging are radioactive iodine and $^{99m}Tc^-$ pertechnetate ($^{99m}TcO_4^-$).[4]

Ultrasonic Scan

Ultrasonic scans indicate size, shape, and position of the thyroid gland. The ultrasonic scan is valuable in differentiating cystic from solid thyroid nodules and in identifying nonpalpable multiple nodules (multinodular goiter), which have a much lower incidence of malignancy than the solitary nodule has.[6]

Fine needle aspiration

Palpation, thyroid scintigraphy, and ultrasonography do not determine whether a thyroid nodule is benign or malignant.[18] Performing a preoperative fine needle aspiration (FNA) of the nodule, combined with cytologic examination of the aspirate, can provide a definite diagnosis of cancer. FNA should not be confused with core-needle biopsy, which takes a core of tissue that can be examined microscopically. The disadvantage of the core-needle biopsy is that it may cause bleeding and other morbidity in some patients.[9]

Patient education for the FNA should include the following. The patient will be lying down for the procedure and may expect coldness on the neck from the prepping solution. Local anesthesia may or may not be used. Once the prick of the needle is felt, no talking, swallowing, or moving is allowed. FNA may be an emotionally stressful procedure for the patient. Vials of ammonia should be kept in the room in case the patient feels faint.[18] Lowering the head (as in Trendelenburg's position or sitting with the head down) is also important in treating vasovagal syncope. Postprocedure education should include the need to refrain from using aspirin or aspirin-containing medications or nonsteroidal antiinflammatory drugs (NSAIDs) for the next 24 hours and to expect to have a half-dollar–sized bruise at the FNA site. There are no restrictions on food or activity.[23]

Preoperative patient education for patients undergoing a partial or total thyroidectomy should include an explanation of perioperative events, discussion of the incision site, type of dressing to be used, and explanation of the closed-wound suction drainage system if its use is anticipated. Discussion of pain and pain relief should also be covered. Patients may also be told that there are various ways of protecting their eyesight during surgery, and if ointment is used, they can expect temporary blurred vision when they first open their eyes. If sequential compression stockings are to be used for prophylaxis of deep vein thrombosis (DVT), an explanation of their use and sensation should be described. The patient should also be instructed in ways to support the neck postoperatively to prevent strain on the incision line. (A further discussion of patient education can be found on p. 610.)

Parathyroid assessment

An elevation of serum PTH in association with hypercalcemia is diagnostic of hyperparathyroidism in more than 90% of cases.[4] PTH normal levels are <2000 pg/ml (the value varies with laboratory); serum calcium (9 to 10.5 mg/dl) is usually measured at the same time.[19] The causes of primary hyperparathyroidism are single adenoma (85%), hyperplasia of the glands (10% to 15%), and rarely (<1%) parathyroid carcinoma.[11] Ultrasonography, thallium-technetium scan, or sestamibi scan (Fig. 16-3) of the parathyroids can indicate the presence of one or more adenomas or hyperplasia. The sestamibi scan seems to be an improvement over the thallium-technetium scan[5] (Research Highlight 16-1).

Hyperparathyroidism causes an imbalance in the level of serum calcium and a decrease in the level of serum phosphate. Nursing diagnoses and care planning will be based on these imbalances and on the severity of the associated symptoms. Some patients are asymptomatic; others have symptoms that manifest themselves as disturbances in the renal, gastrointestinal, cardiovascular, musculoskeletal or central nervous system.

Assessment should include determining whether the patient is apathetic or emotionally irritable; whether there

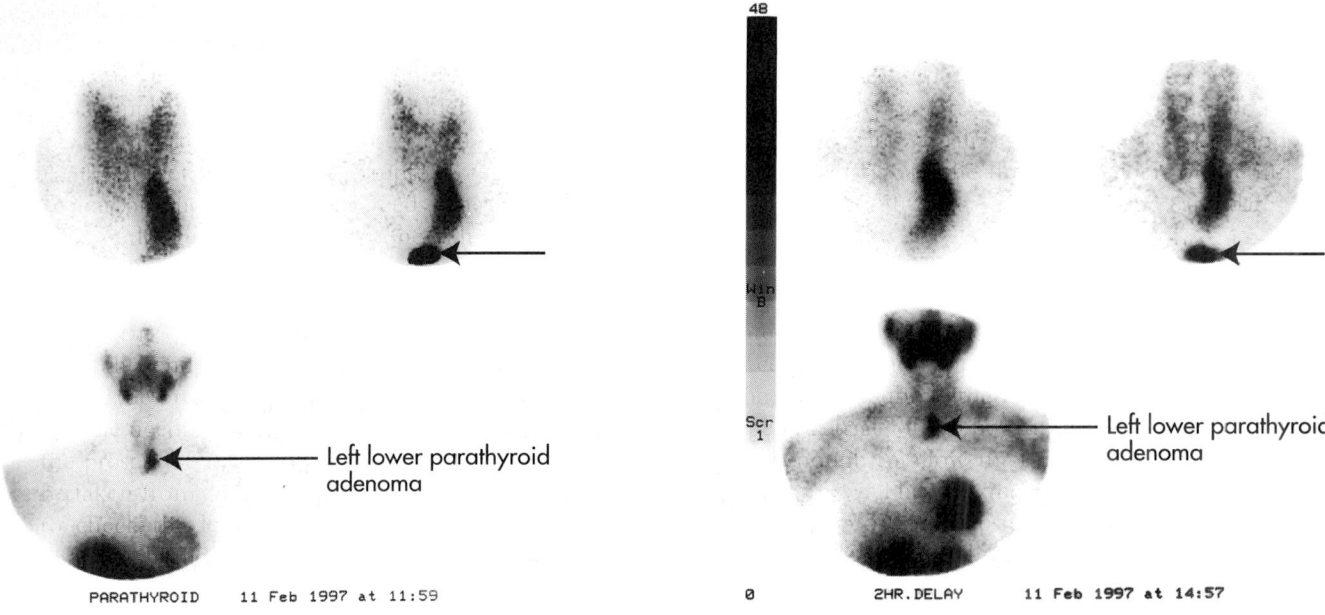

FIGURE 16-3 Sestamibi scan, showing a left lower adenoma at *arrow*. (Courtesy White Plains Hospital Center, White Plains, New York.)

16-1 RESEARCH HIGHLIGHT

The dispute among surgeons as to the value of preoperative localization studies before parathyroid surgery is being settled as reliable noninvasive procedures have became accessible. Without localization studies, the success rate in initial parathyroid surgery performed by an experienced surgeon approximates 95%. However, occasionally failures occur, commonly because of ectopic or supernumerary abnormal glands. Malhotra and colleagues point out that "an unsuccessful exploration performed without preoperative localization, after which scintigraphy reveals a lesion that could have been removed if its location had been known, is an unsatisfactory outcome that does not meet current standards of care."

These researchers reported the results of noninvasive preoperative parathyroid localization with technetium 99m–labeled sestamibi in a series of 51 patients who had surgery between November 1993 and September 1995. Retrospective analyses of these patients were utilized to determine the usefulness of ^{99m}Tc-sestamibi scanning. Forty-four of the 51 patients were surgically treated for hyperparathyroidism for the first time, and 7 patients underwent reexploration for recurrent or persistent hyperparathyroidism. Of the 44 who had hyperparathyroid surgery for the first time, 26 had solitary adenomas and 18 had multiple lesions. For those with solitary tumors, all 26 were localized preoperatively by the sestamibi scan. The sensitivity in this study group was 100%. Of the 18 patients with a multiglandular disorder, 8 scans showed either a single lesion or no uptake, yielding a 56% sensitivity. Of the patients who were evaluated by sestamibi scan for recurrent hyperparathyroidism or failed exploration, 5 of the 7 patients had parathyroid lesions correctly localized, yielding a sensitivity of 71%.

In a comparison of the sensitivity of the sestamibi scan to the sensitivity to other noninvasive means of localization, sensitivity ranged from approximately 35% for sonography to 67% for thallium scintigraphy.

The researchers concluded that sestamibi scanning is superior to other means of noninvasive localization of hyperfunctioning parathyroids. The scan is extremely useful for parathyroid reexploration and accurate in detecting ectopic lesions, leading to the recommendation of the sestamibi scan before initial exploration in all cases.

From Malhotra, A., Silver, C.E., Deshpande, V., & Freeman, L. (1996). Preoperative parathyroid localization with sestamibi. *American Journal of Surgery, 172,* 637-639.

is muscle weakness and fatigue; skeletal pain or tenderness; nausea; vomiting; constipation; peptic ulcer disease; cardiac dysrhythmia; or renal damage, stones, or disease. If any of these signs or symptoms are present, the plan of care should be adjusted. Otherwise, perioperative patient education and nursing management of the patient undergoing parathyroidectomy is essentially the same as that for thyroidectomy. In the early postoperative period for both thyroidectomy and parathyroidectomy the patient should be closely observed for any signs of hypocalcemia. Serum

16-2 RESEARCH HIGHLIGHT

Reducing the cost of health care without sacrificing quality is part of balancing the ethics of safety and economy. With this in mind, Mowschenson and Hodin carried out a prospective study of the feasibility, safety, and cost savings of outpatient thyroid and parathyroid surgery. The study population included all patients ($N = 100$) who were undergoing thyroidectomy or parathyroidectomy over a 10-month period in 1994-95. Before surgery, patients were told that they would be allowed to go home, provided that both the surgeon and the patient felt at ease with this decision. Patients with comorbid conditions or social circumstances not favorable to outpatient surgery were told they would require admission and were also included in the study. General endotracheal anesthesia was used. To allow for maximum observation time, the surgical procedures were scheduled as early in the day as possible. For prophylaxis against deep vein thrombosis (DVT), calf-compression boots were used. None of the patients had drains. Before discharge (6 to 8 hours after the procedure), patients were carefully examined for any signs of neck swelling or other difficulties. Each patient was seen between 2 and 6 weeks for a postoperative visit. Both inpatients and outpatients were mailed written questionnaires to assess satisfaction with time spent in the hospital. Comparisons were made with a control group of 30 consecutive patients undergoing laparoscopic cholecystectomy. Of the 100 patients in the study, 61 were outpatients and 39 were inpatients. The average age of the inpatient was slightly older than that of the outpatient. The reasons for and frequency of admission were as follows: extent of surgery (6), nausea (5), oversedation (4), urinary retention (2), inadequate home help (6), long travel time (2), comorbid disease (5), and strong patient preference (9).

Questionnaires were returned by 73% of the patients who underwent thyroid and parathyroid surgery and 70% of the patients who underwent laparoscopic cholecystectomy. Sixty-five of the outpatients who underwent thyroidectomy or parathyroidectomy stated that they were satisfied with outpatient surgery; 35% stated that in hindsight they would have preferred to be admitted overnight. Of the patients who underwent outpatient laparoscopic cholecystectomy, 68% were satisfied and 32% would have preferred to be admitted to the hospital. This difference was not significant.

The average cost for outpatients ranged from $1594 to $2783, and for inpatients the range was $2031 to $4216. Outpatient surgery on average resulted in a 30% cost savings.

Based on these results, the study authors expect to be able to perform 80% of thyroid and parathyroid surgery on an outpatient basis.

From Mowschenson, P.M., & Hodin, R.A. (1995, Dec.). Outpatient thyroid and parathyroid surgery: a prospective study of feasibility, safety and costs, *Surgery*, 1051-1053.

---

calcium levels of less than 8 mg/dl indicate hypocalcemia. Symptoms include numbness and tingling of extremities and around the lips. Hyperactive tendon reflexes and a positive Chvostek's sign (tapping on the facial nerve elicits spasm or irritability) can be demonstrated before the progression of spontaneous tetany.[15]

Nursing Diagnosis

Nursing diagnoses related to the care of patients undergoing thyroid and parathyroid surgery might include the following:

- Impaired swallowing related to mechanical obstruction (enlarged thyroid preoperatively; edema postoperatively).
- Ineffective thermoregulation related to altered metabolic rate.
- Body image disturbance related to surgical scar in prominent location.
- Ineffective airway clearance related to obstruction (enlarged thyroid preoperatively; edema postoperatively; or bilateral recurrent laryngeal nerve injury.
- Impaired gas exchange related to postoperative bleeding or swelling or inability to move secretions.
- Impaired verbal communication related to recurrent laryngeal nerve injury.
- Tactile sensory alterations related to postoperative hypocalcemia.

Outcome Identification

Outcomes identified for the selected nursing diagnoses could be stated as follows:

- Patient will maintain normal swallowing.
- Patient will maintain normal body temperature.
- Patient will verbalize decreased disturbance in feelings related to body image.
- Patient will maintain a patent airway.
- Patient will maintain effective gas exchange.
- Patient will maintain preoperative voice quality.
- Patient will verbalize absence of numbness and tingling around lips and extremities.

In the 1990s, clinical paths emerged as a mechanism to streamline and standardize patient care and control resource utilization[1] (Research Highlight 16-2). Most clinical paths begin with assessment. Although each institution often develops its own terms, common elements in clinical paths include a timeline and the

INDEPENDENT ACTIONS BASED ON THE HUMAN RESPONSE TO ACTUAL OR POTENTIAL PROBLEMS

HOSPITAL DAY	CONSULTATIONS	TESTS	ACTIVITY/REST	MEDICAL INTERVENTIONS	MEDICATIONS	NUTRITION
PTA or Day of admission Date: _____			Up ad lib		Own, if any	NPO
Surgery Date: _____		Calcium phosphate stat every day for 2 days Day of surgery POD #1	Head of bed elevated 15 degrees, and when stable and able, ambulate Ambulate	IV to heparin well with good oral intake JP empty every 4 hours and PRN Check Chvostek's with vital signs	With doctor's order resume usual meds postop when able to tolerate oral intake IV/IM/PO analgesics Call for antiemetic if nausea and vomiting and one not ordered	Usual diet
Day 1 Date: _____		Calcium, phosphate stat. every day for 2 days	Head of bed elevated 15 degrees, and when stable and able Ambulate	IV to heparin well with good oral intake JP empty every 4 hours and PRN D/C JP (MD) Check Chvostek's sign Change original dressing, monitor incision, and drain site	With doctor's order resume usual meds postop when able to tolerate oral intake IV/IM/PO analgesics Call for antiemetic if nausea and vomiting and one not ordered	Usual diet

Key: ad lib, ad libitum; *ADL,* activities of daily living; *D/C,* discontinue; *DRG,* diagnosis related group; *IM,* intramuscular; *IV,* intravenous; *JP,* Jackson-Pratt; *LOS,* length of stay; *MAP,* mean arterial pressure; *MD,* physician; *NPO,* nothing by mouth; *PO,* by mouth; *POD,* postoperative day; *PRN,* as needed; *PTA,* prior to admission.

FIGURE 16-4 Thyroid and parathyroid clinical pathway.

clinical pathway through which care regimens (tests, education, activities, treatments, medications, diet, and so forth) are sequenced. A clinical pathway for a thyroid patient follows (Fig. 16-4). When institutions analyze variance in their clinical paths, quality improvement results.

Planning

Intraoperatively warm saline should be provided for irrigation. Studies have indicated that intraoperative hypothermia of the parathyroids is a cause for temporary hypoparathyroidism postoperatively.[7] Because a potential problem for patients with hyperthyroidism is thyroid storm

ASSESSMENT	DISCHARGE PLANNING	TEACHING	PSYCHOSOCIAL	SELF-CARE	NURSES' SIGNATURES
Lung status	Assess "at home needs"	Reinforce preoperative teaching	Assess anxiety level	ADLs	_____ (7-3) _____ (3-11) _____ (11-7)
Airway integrity Lung status Bowel sounds Vital signs with Chvostek's, as ordered Call positive Chvostek's or any variations from normal vital signs as ordered Notify doctor if bleeding, increased edema at incision	Assess "at home needs"	Head of bed elevated to 15 degrees Postop teaching Scar maturation secondary to location on more obvious body location Chvostek's sign explanation	Assess anxiety level	Assisted ADLs	_____ (7-3) _____ (3-11) _____ (11-7)
Airway integrity Lung status Bowel sounds Vital signs with Chvostek's, as ordered Call positive Chvostek's or any variations from normal vital signs as ordered Notify doctor if bleeding, increased edema at incision	Assess "at home needs" Incisional line care	Head of bed elevated to 15 degrees Postop teaching Scar maturation secondary to location on more obvious body location Chvostek's sign monitoring	Assess anxiety level	Assisted ADLs	_____ (7-3) _____ (3-11) _____ (11-7)

FIGURE 16-4, cont'd   For legend see opposite page.   *Continued*

(thyrotoxic crisis), the perioperative nurse must be prepared to respond quickly. Thyroid storm can occur in patients who have been partially controlled or who are untreated for their hyperthyroidism. Thyrotoxic crisis can be precipitated by a stressful event such as surgery. By planning a quiet, calm atmosphere and helping the patient relax, the perioperative nurse can reduce the risk of thyroid storm. Collaborating with the surgical and anesthesia team, the perioperative nurse can plan for appropriate interventions to assist in reducing body temperature and heart rate, provide oxygen and intravenous solutions, and administer medications as prescribed in the event thyrotoxic crisis occurs.

A Sample Care Plan for a patient undergoing thyroid and parathyroid surgery follows.

Implementation
Positioning

Proper patient positioning on the operating bed is crucial for optimal exposure of the thyroid gland. Hyperextension of the neck moves the thyroid from under the manubrium, allowing it to assume a more anterior

MAP reviewed by:

Date: _____

Nurse case manager:

_____

Date: _____

Associate case manager:

_____

Date: _____

Associate case manager:

_____

Date: _____

Date	Individualization/variation	Cause	Action taken	Signature

All items not provided as planned
Enter explanation in the individualization/variance section on the last page

DRG Number: 290 NRA-17899 07/97 (modified)
Expected LOS: 2 days
Developed by Gail Greene, RN
Updated by Patti Drake, RN

TUCSON MEDICAL CENTER
DIVISION OF NURSING
Thyroid and Parathyroid
CarePlan MAP

FIGURE 16-4, cont'd   Thyroid and parathyroid clinical pathway.

position.[10] After the patient is properly anesthetized, the position is changed to a modified dorsal recumbent one, with an inflatable pillow or rolled sheet placed between the scapulas to extend the neck and raise the shoulders. The head is stabilized by placement on a foam pillow. If an inflatable pillow is used, it should be placed (uninflated) before the patient is anesthetized and then inflated. Some surgeons prefer to keep the legs level and elevate the back of the OR bed until distended neck veins disappear. Others position the patient in slight (about 20-degree) reverse Trendelenburg's position. The latter position necessitates the use of a padded footboard to keep the feet in proper alignment and prevent the patient from sliding down on the bed. The arms are positioned at the sides with the elbows adequately protected by the lift sheet or elbow guards.

Skin preparation

The operative area, including the chin and anterior neck region, lateral surfaces of the neck, from the earlobes down to the outer aspects of the shoulder, and the upper anterior chest region to the nipples, is prepared with an

SAMPLE CARE PLAN

Nursing Diagnosis: Impaired swallowing, related to mechanical obstruction (enlarged thyroid preoperatively; edema postoperatively)

Outcome: Patient will maintain normal swallowing.

Interventions:

Keep suction line and suction catheter ready until patient is discharged from OR.

Monitor for and report difficulty in swallowing.

Gently suction oropharyngeal secretions as required.

Keep vein open postoperatively until patient can swallow without difficulty.

Nursing Diagnosis: Ineffective thermoregulation related to altered metabolic rate

Outcome: Patient's body temperature will be maintained within normal range.

Interventions:

Monitor patient's temperature; report abnormalities.

Provide light covers if temperature is elevated or patient states that he or she is warm.

Change linens preoperatively and postoperatively if wet from perspiration.

Avoid using plasticized drapes.

Nursing Diagnosis: Body image disturbance related to surgical scar

Outcome: Patient will verbalize decreased disturbance in feelings related to body image.

Interventions:

Explain that incision is made in natural fold of skin.

Explain how techniques used for surgical closure minimize scarring.

Instruct patient in postoperative turning measures that decrease strain on suture line. Suggest that jewelry, scarves, and certain necklines can be used to cover scar until normal fading occurs.

Nursing Diagnosis: High risk for ineffective airway clearance related to obstruction secondary to enlarged thyroid (preoperatively), edema (postoperatively), or bilateral recurrent laryngeal nerve surgical injury.

Outcome: Patient's airway will remain patent.

Interventions:

Position patient so that enlarged gland does not obstruct airway. Head of transport vehicle may need to be elevated preoperatively.

Assist anesthesia personnel during induction.

Monitor respiratory rate and signs of respiratory distress (stridor, wheezing, dyspnea, labored respirations).

If distress occurs because of recurrent laryngeal nerve injury, a tracheostomy may be required. Have a trach tray available.

Observe dressing and neck area (front, sides, and back) for signs of edema or bleeding (postoperatively).

Nursing Diagnosis: High risk for impaired gas exchange related to postoperative bleeding or swelling, bilateral recurrent laryngeal nerve surgical injury, or inability to move secretions

Outcome: Patient's gas exchange will remain effective.

Interventions:

Monitor respiratory status and results of pulse oximetry.

If patient is extubated in OR, be prepared to assist anesthesia personnel; closely observe for respiratory stridor or respiratory obstruction (recurrent laryngeal nerve injury). Tracheostomy may be required; trach tray should be available.

Assess color of nailbeds.

Monitor surgical site for swelling and bleeding.

Suction patient as required to remove secretions.

Monitor patency of surgical drain.

Nursing Diagnosis: Impaired verbal communication related to recurrent laryngeal nerve injury

Outcome: Patient will maintain preoperative voice quality.

Interventions:

Position patient on operative bed to enhance gland exposure.

Have headlights available.

Observe quality of voice postoperatively.

Immediately report any changes in voice quality such as hoarseness or "breathy" voice.

Nursing Diagnosis: Tactile sensory alterations related to postoperative hypocalcemia

Outcome: Patient will verbalize absence of numbness and tingling of extremities and around lips.

Interventions:

Intraoperatively provide warm saline for irrigation.

Educate patient to report any numbness or tingling of extremities or around lips.

---

antimicrobial solution. Appropriate precautions must be taken to prevent the solution from pooling under the neck or in the axillary area. The patient is draped with sterile towels and a fenestrated sheet. A sterile towel or lap sponge may be placed on each side of the neck to prevent pooling of blood under the neck during surgery.

The surgeon marks the incision site with a marking pen or with the pressure of a full-length fine silk tie to help ensure a wound line that blends with the patient's neck creases and skin lines.

Evaluation

Evaluation of intraoperative interventions determines effectiveness of positioning aids and pressure-relief devices, drip towels to collect excess prep solutions, and other interventions based on the patient's special needs. The report to PACU personnel includes the surgical procedure, anesthesia given, location of drain if any, dressing used, condition of skin postoperatively, and any other information specific to the patient's nursing diagnoses. Documentation is according to hospital protocol. It should reflect achievement of patient outcomes related to planned interventions; these should also be included in the nursing report to PACU personnel. For the nursing diagnoses selected for the patient undergoing thyroid or parathyroid surgery the following outcomes would be communicated:

- Patient maintained normal swallowing.
- Patient maintained normal body temperature.
- Patient verbalized decreased disturbance in feelings related to body image.
- Patient maintained a patent airway; there was no edema at the surgical site or signs of respiratory distress.
- Patient maintained adequate gas exchange; O_2 saturation remained normal. The patient was extubated without incident.
- Patient maintained preoperative voice quality.
- Patient verbalizes absence of numbness and tingling around lips and extremities.

Patient and Family Education and Discharge Planning

Patient education and discharge planning should include any family members, significant others, or even friends who will be helping the patient at home. Written discharge instructions should be provided (Box 16-3) and orally reviewed, with clarification of information and correction of misperceptions. The name and telephone number of the physician or nurse to call with questions should be included, as should information regarding a follow-up office appointment (if that is available). General information, such as the thyroid or parathyroid procedure and any changes that will occur as a result of the surgery, should be explained. Included with signs and symptoms to report are those of hypocalcemia. If this occurs, it usually manifests itself 24 to 72 hours after surgery.[14] The patient should notice and report any numbness or tingling around the lips or extremities, twitching, or spasms. Time should also be spent in discovering the patient's concerns, anxieties, thoughts, and feelings. This concern assists the perioperative nurse in finding the meaning in the patient's expressed or unexpressed "What does this mean for me, for getting well, and for my family/job/loved ones?" Education begins with the perioperative nursing assessment and continues through discharge and perhaps even home care. If the patient voices concern related to the surgical scar or has a history of hypertrophic scarring, the perioperative nurse may want to discuss the use of paper tape with the surgeon.[20] Suggesting the use of scarves, high-necked blouses, loosely buttoned collars, or jewelry at the neckline may be helpful for this patient.

SURGICAL INTERVENTIONS UNILATERAL THYROID LOBECTOMY, SUBTOTAL LOBECTOMY, BILATERAL SUBTOTAL LOBECTOMY, NEAR-TOTAL THYROIDECTOMY, AND TOTAL THYROIDECTOMY

Unilateral thyroid lobectomy is removal of one thyroid lobe with division at the isthmus. *Subtotal lobectomy* is a lobectomy that spares the posterior capsule and may or may not spare a portion of the adjacent thyroid tissue. *Bilateral subtotal thyroidectomy* is removal of both lobes of the thyroid in the fashion stated for subtotal thyroidectomy. *Near-total thyroidectomy* is a total lobectomy with contralateral subtotal thyroidectomy. *Total thyroidectomy* is removal of both lobes of the thyroid and attempted removal of all thyroid tissue present.[2] The purpose of the surgical intervention relates to the patient's medical diagnosis.

Hyperthyroidism (Graves' disease) is associated with diffuse, bilateral enlargement of the thyroid gland. Hashimoto's thyroiditis is believed to be an autoimmune disease, and nontender enlargement of the gland occurs. Surgery is performed to relieve tracheal obstruction. Nontoxic nodular goiter does not produce an excess of hormones and is noninflammatory in character; thyroid tissue proliferates in an apparent attempt to produce the minimal hormonal requirement. Surgery may be indicated to relieve tracheal or esophageal obstruction or to rule out a malignant nodule of the thyroid gland. Total thyroidectomy may be done for malignant tumors.

Procedural considerations

These patients need an environment that is calm and quiet to reduce the risk of overstimulation, which could result in thyroid crisis, as well to make the overall experience more tolerable.

Operative procedure

1. A transverse incision parallel to the normal skin lines of the neck is made through the skin and first layer of the cervical fascia and platysma muscle, approximately 2 cm above the sternoclavicular junction (Fig. 16-5).
2. An upper skin flap is undermined to the level of the cricoid cartilage; straight clamps are placed on the dermis and retracted anteriorly and superiorly to facilitate dissection. A lower flap is then undermined to the sternoclavicular joint. A knife, fine curved scissors, tissue forceps, and gauze sponges are used to undermine the flaps. Bleeding vessels are clamped with hemostats and ligated with fine, nonabsorbable sutures. Lateral retraction with a vein retractor or Army-Navy retractor helps identify the plane for dissection.

BOX 16-3 | Home Care After a Thyroidectomy

A surgical procedure called a thyroidectomy has been performed on you. The surgeon has removed all or part of your thyroid gland. You should expect to experience discomfort in your neck for the next several days. You may also experience hoarseness for the first few days following the procedure.

Medications

Depending on the amount of thyroid tissue that was removed, you may need to take a thyroid hormone. The thyroid hormone is necessary for body function; it should not be stopped and doses should not be skipped. You have been advised to take the following medication and dose for thyroid replacement:

_____

Medication

_____   _____

Dose   Frequency

The amount of medication you take may change after 3 or 4 weeks. It is important that you take your thyroid medication at the same time every day. Most people take the medication in the morning to prevent sleeping problems. Some of the side effects you may experience include the following: nervousness, tremors or muscle twitching, fast heart beat, palpitations (feeling that your heart beat is jumping), nausea, diarrhea, weight loss, and excessive sweating. All of these should be reported to your health care provider.

Caring for the Surgical Incision

You will have an incision that runs across your neck. The incision will probably have sutures (stitches), staples, or tape holding the edges of the wound together. By the time you go home, you will not require a dressing on this unless otherwise directed by your physician. If you have staples or sutures, these will be removed when you have a follow-up appointment. If you have tape (Steri-Strips) on your incision, do not pull it off. If the ends are loose, you may cut off the ends with scissors.

Basic wound care guidelines for the surgical incision include the following:

1. *Keep the incision clean and dry*
   - Avoid wearing clothing that will rub against the incision until it has healed.
   - Avoid touching the incision with your fingers.
   - Do not apply makeup, body lotion, or body cream to the incision.
     Some people use lanolin cream on the incision after it has healed to soften the scar.
   - If at all possible, do not get your incision wet for the first 5 to 7 days following your surgery. If your incision does get wet, be sure to dry it immediately.
2. *Watch for signs of infection*
   Call your health care provider if you:
   - See redness, swelling, or drainage at the incision site.
   - Experience increased pain at the incision site.
   - Notice the incision has become hot.
   - Think you have a fever.

Neck Exercises

On the third or fourth day after the surgery to your neck, it is very important that you perform exercises to maintain optimal movement in your neck. Some of the exercises you should complete include the following:
- Touch chin to chest.
- Lift chin up as high as you can.
- Turn head and touch chin to left shoulder.
- Turn head and touch chin to right shoulder.
- Rotate head around in circular motion.

General Care and Information

You should regain strength without any problems. Several warning signs that may indicate that something is not right include the following: increased sweating, tremors, restlessness, difficulty sleeping, increased weakness, increased fatigue, agitation, depression, or changes in how your eyes look. If you begin to have any of these signs or symptoms, you should contact your health care provider.

Summary

As time goes on, your surgical scar will fade and will be difficult to see. For now, it is important that you provide care for your wound so that healing will occur without complication. Take your medications as prescribed, rest so that you may regain your strength, and report any problems to your health care provider.

From Mosby. (1998). *Mosby's Patient Teaching Guides*. St. Louis: Mosby, p. 232A.

---

3. Flaps may be held away from the wound with stay sutures inserted through the cervical fascia and platysma muscle or by one of the various self-retaining retractors.
4. The fascia in the midline is incised between the strap (sternohyoid and sternothyroid) muscles with a knife (Fig. 16-6, *A*). The sternocleidomastoid muscle may be retracted with a loop retractor. Ordinarily it is not necessary to divide the strap muscles; however, the strap muscles may be divided between clamps should additional exposure be required as with a very large gland, using Mastin muscle clamps, Kocher clamps, or hemostats and a knife. The divided muscles are retracted from the operative site with retractors, thereby exposing the diseased lobe.
5. The inferior and middle thyroid veins are clamped, divided with Metzenbaum scissors, and ligated with fine nonabsorbable sutures (Fig. 16-6, *B*).
6. The lobe is rotated medially, and loose areolar tissue is divided posteriorly and medially toward the tracheoesophageal sulcus with hemostats and Metzenbaum scissors. Small sponges are used for blunt dissection.

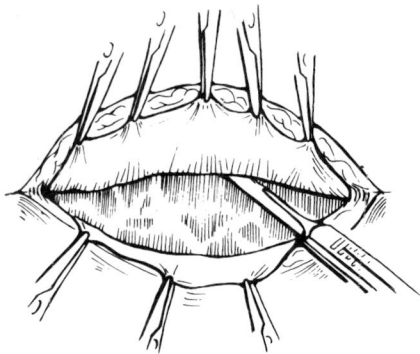

FIGURE 16-5   Beginning of thyroidectomy. Skin flaps are created by dissection deep to platysma muscle and cervical fascia. Clamps are placed on the dermis and then retracted to facilitate dissection.

Bleeding is controlled by hemostats and ligatures, as well as by electrosurgery; the bipolar electrosurgical unit (ESU) may be used. The recurrent laryngeal nerve, which enters the cricothyroid muscle at the level of the cricoid cartilage, is identified and carefully preserved (Fig. 16-7). Electrocoagulation should not be used in the vicinity of the recurrent or superior laryngeal nerve because the spread of the current could damage the nerve.

7. The thyroid lobe is pulled downward, a Lahey goiter or polar retractor is inserted as necessary, and the avascular tissue between the trachea and upper pole of the thyroid is dissected by means of Metzenbaum scissors.

8. The superior thyroid artery is secured with two or three curved hemostats or right-angled clamps; the artery is ligated, divided, and then transfixed with nonabsorbable sutures. Care is taken here to not injure the superior laryngeal nerve. The upper parathyroid gland is often identified at this time.

9. The inferior thyroid artery is identified and ligated by means of fine forceps, sutures, and scissors (see Fig. 16-7). The lower parathyroid is identified. The thyroid lobe is then dissected away from the recurrent nerve with Metzenbaum scissors and hemostats. Bleeding vessels are clamped with hemostats and ligated with fine nonabsorbable sutures.

10. The lobe is elevated with Lahey vulsellum clamps; it is freed from the trachea with fine scissors, forceps, knife, and hemostats. The fibrous bands attached to the trachea and cricoid cartilage are divided.

11. The isthmus of the gland is elevated with fine forceps and divided between hemostats with scissors, removing the lobe and isthmus. If a pyramidal lobe is present, it is removed from its attachment to the gland to its termination in the neck, which may reach the hyoid bone. If it is necessary to transect the hyoid bone, a small bone cutter is used.

12. The cut surface of the opposite lobe requires careful hemostasis. A running suture may be utilized for this purpose as well as to reapproximate it to the pretracheal fascia.

13. The strap muscles, if severed, are approximated with fine interrupted absorbable or nonabsorbable sutures. If necessary, a drain may be inserted into the thyroid bed and brought out between the strap muscles and sternocleidomastoid muscle. Many surgeons prefer to drain the wound laterally through the sternocleidomastoid muscle and the lateral extremity of the incision in the belief that this produces better healing and cosmetic results.

14. The edges of the platysma muscle are approximated. The skin edges are then approximated with subcuticular, fine absorbable sutures.

15. Wound closure tapes (such as Steri-Strips) are applied to the wound edges, and gauze dressings are placed on the wound with minimal tape.

SUBSTERNAL OR INTRATHORACIC THYROIDECTOMY

Extensions of enlarging goiters into the substernal and intrathoracic regions may occur. They may cause tracheal and esophageal obstruction, in which case they are usually excised surgically. Longer instruments are sometimes required. Splitting the sternum is rarely necessary because access to the substernal part of the gland is usually satisfactory through the standard collar incision.

THYROGLOSSAL DUCT CYSTECTOMY

The thyroglossal duct cyst is the most common congenital cyst found in the neck. Persistent remnants of the thyroglossal duct may be found in an estimated 7% of the overall population. Although a thyroglossal duct cyst may be found in patients of any age, 50% usually occur before 20 years of age, and about 70% are seen by 30 years of age.[17] The thyroglossal duct is an embryonic structure present during the descent of the thyroid gland into the anterior portion of the neck. When present in an adult, it exists as a pretracheal cystic pouch attached to the hyoid bone, with or without a sinus tract to the base of the tongue at the foramen cecum (Fig. 16-8). Thyroglossal duct cystectomy requires complete excision of all portions of the cyst and duct and a portion of the hyoid bone, which contains the duct, to avoid recurrent cystic formation and to prevent infections.

Procedural considerations

The perioperative nursing assessment should be appropriate to the patient's age because the patient is frequently a child or teenager (see Chapter 29 for a detailed discussion of the younger patient's needs). Reassurance and information regarding the procedure should be given.

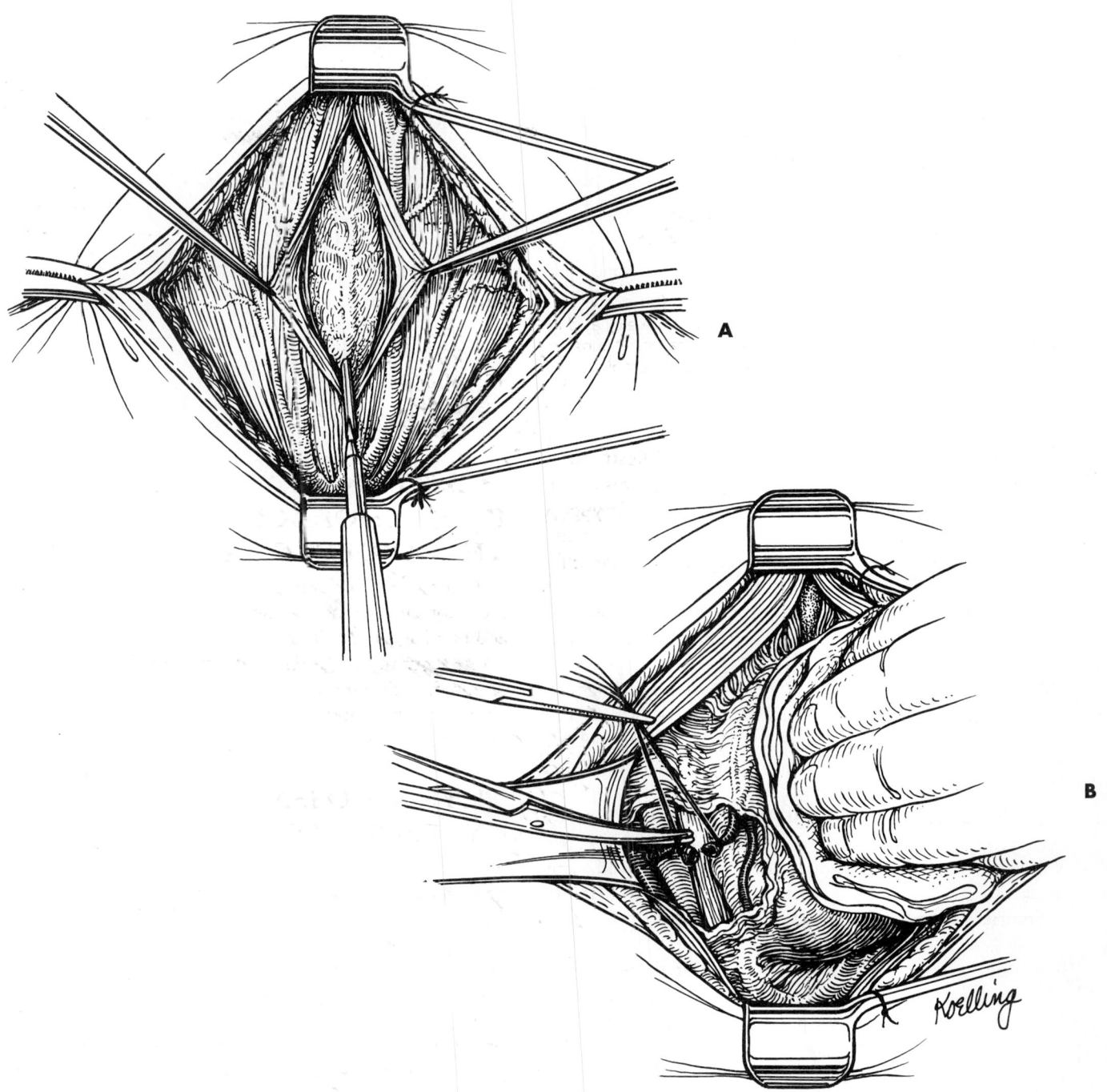

FIGURE 16-6   **A**, Fascia in the midline is incised **B**. Division of the middle thyroid vein.

Operative procedure

1. After the head is extended and the chin is elevated, a transverse incision is made between the hyoid bone and the thyroid cartilage through the subcutaneous tissue.
2. The platysma muscle is incised, and the flaps are raised as described previously.
3. The strap (sternohyoid and sternothyroid) muscles are separated in the midline.
4. Sharp and blunt dissection is used to mobilize the cyst and duct, up to the attachment to the hyoid bone. The hyoid bone is transsected twice, removing the center section with bone-cutting forceps, and the segment of bone and cyst is freed from adjacent structures.
5. The cephalic part of the duct is identified, a transfixion suture is passed through it, and the duct is transsected. (Methylene blue dye injection is used occasionally to visualize the whole tract.)
6. The cyst is removed. The strap muscles are closed with interrupted, fine nonabsorbable sutures. A drain may be placed. The skin is closed with subcuticular, fine absorbable sutures.

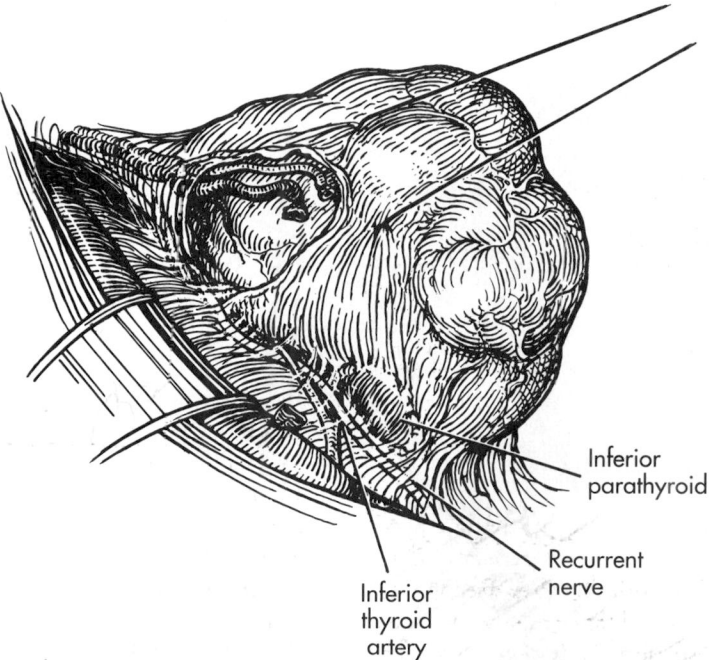

FIGURE 16-7   Identification of nerve and parathyroids.

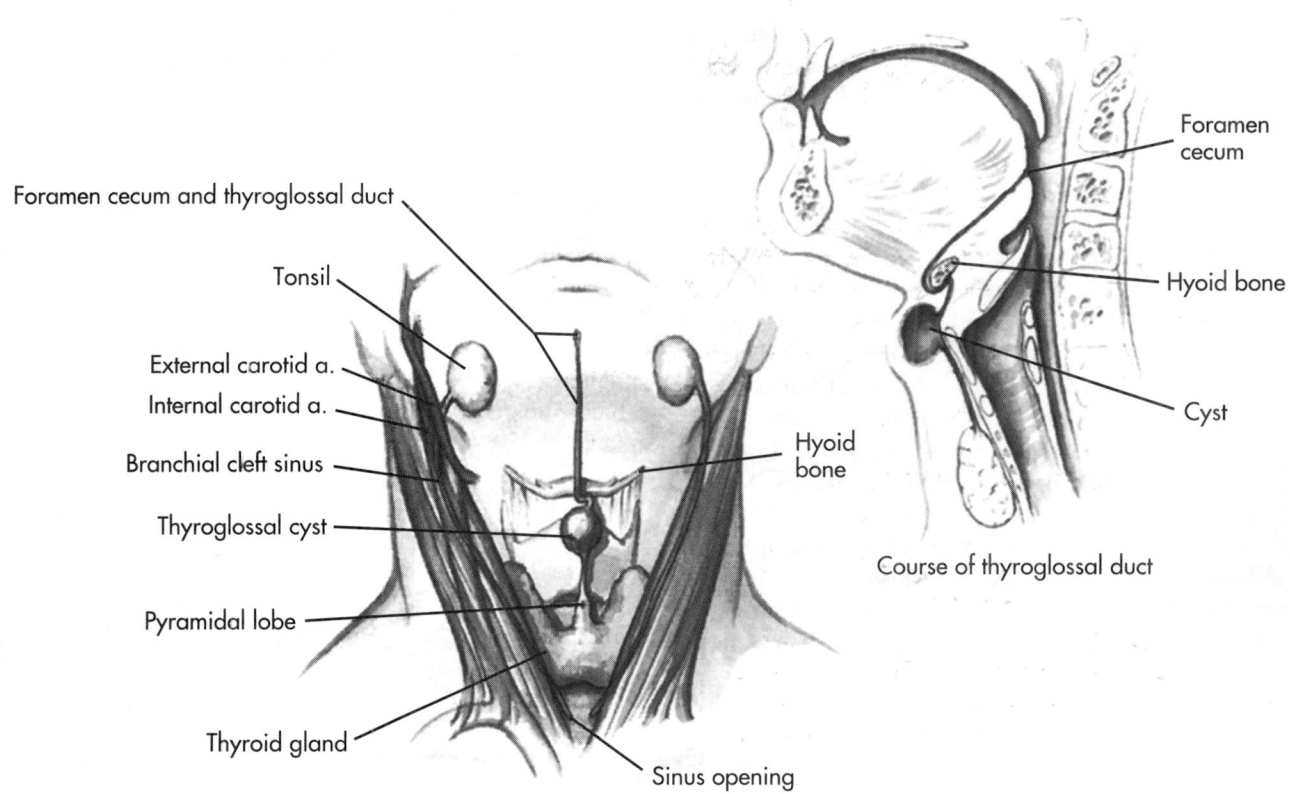

FIGURE 16-8   Thyroglossal cyst showing both anterior and lateral views.

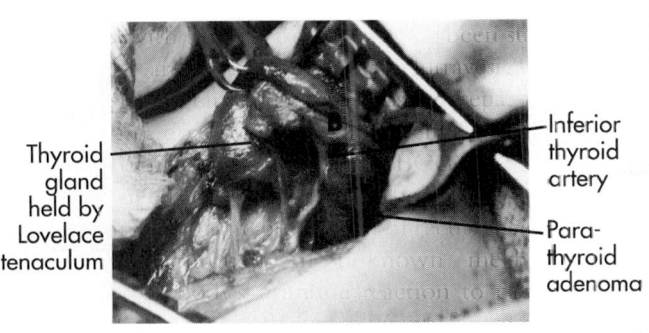

Thyroid gland held by Lovelace tenaculum

Inferior thyroid artery

Para-thyroid adenoma

FIGURE 16-9   Left lower parathyroid adenoma. Notice the relationship between the adenoma (**A**) and the inferior thyroid artery (**B**). (Courtesy Josefina D. Reyes, RN, MS, CNOR, White Plains Hospital, New York.)

PARATHYROIDECTOMY

Parathyroidectomy is excision of one or more parathyroid glands. Normal or atrophic glands are generally not removed. The presence of adenomas (hypersecreting neoplasms), hyperplasia, or carcinomas requires surgical excision. In the last case, resection of lymph nodes is essential, although metastasis may also occur by way of the bloodstream. After local excision, a cut metastatic site may secrete parathormone, causing hypercalcemia and its attendant problems.

Procedural considerations

Because multiple biopsies are often performed to determine the presence or absence of parathyroid tissue, numerous specimen containers may be necessary. Check with the surgeon in regard to any preoperative localization studies and the possibility of a mediastinotomy. Have mediastinotomy instruments available if necessary (see Chapter 25).

Operative procedure

1. See approach to the thyroid gland, described on p. 610.
2. With the thyroid gland visible, a thorough exploration of the "normal" locations of the four parathyroid glands is conducted. Meticulous hemostasis by means of mosquito hemostats and fine ligatures is a prerequisite to location and identification of these small glands.
3. The thyroid gland is gently rotated anteriorly to provide access to the posterior thyroid sulcus, where the parathyroid glands are almost always found. Identification of the parathyroid vascular pedicle as it leaves the superior thyroid artery is an excellent means of locating the upper glands. Metzenbaum scissors, mosquito hemostats, and Kitner (peanut) sponges are used in the dissection.
4. Attention is directed toward the posterior lateral surface of the thyroid lobe or just beneath the lower thyroid pole, where the lower parathyroid glands are frequently found. Finding the vascular pedicle from the inferior thyroid artery may aid in identification (Fig. 16-9). Occasionally the lower pair is found in the thymic

capsule or tissue, in which case a portion of the thymus is resected. In only 1% of patients is a mediastinotomy indicated.[5] It has been reported that thoracoscopy is a successful minimally invasive technique to remove parathyroid tumors situated deep in the mediastinum.[3]

5. Should one of the parathyroid glands show evidence of disease, the surgeon resects it by clamping the vascular pedicle with mosquito hemostats, dividing with small scissors or knife, and ligating with a fine nonabsorbable suture. The question of how much parathyroid tissue to remove is controversial and relates to whether single or multiple glands are involved, regardless of their size and appearance. A portion of one gland must remain to prevent hypocalcemia and its complications. NOTE: A current concept or alternative for multiple gland involvement is to excise all four glands, transplanting a portion of one in an accessible site such as the neck or forearm for later removal if hypercalcemia recurs. This eliminates reexploration and potential injury to the recurrent laryngeal nerve.
6. The neck region is explored for aberrant parathyroid tissue, which is also resected (see Fig.16-2, *B*).
7. The remainder of the operation is the same as that described for the thyroid gland.

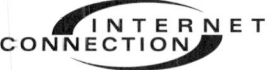

INTERNET CONNECTION

National Institutes of Health: http://www.niddk.nih.gov
http://thyroid.miningco.com/

Endocrine Society Diseases Fact Sheets:
http://www.endosociety.org/pubaffai/factshee.htm

REFERENCES

1. Barnette, J.E., & Clendenen, F. (1996). Making the transition to clinical pathways: a community behavioral health centers approach. *Best Practices and Benchmarking in Health Care, 1*(3), 147-156.
2. Birkin, E.A., Falk, S.A., & Feins, R.H. (1997). The technique of thyroidectomy by cervical and thoracic approaches. In Falk, S.A. (Ed.), *Thyroid disease, endocrinology, surgery, nuclear medicine, and radiotherapy* (ed. 2). Philadelphia: Lippincott-Raven.
3. Bonjer, H.J., & Bruinin, H.A. (1997). Technique of parathyroidectomy. In Clark, O.H., & Quan-Yang, D (Eds.), *Textbook of endocrine surgery* (ed. 1). Philadelphia: W.B. Saunders.
4. Brunt, L.M., & Halverson, J.D. (1996). The endocrine system. In O'Leary, J.P. (Ed.), *The physiologic basis of surgery* (ed. 2). Baltimore: Williams & Wilkins.
5. Doherty, G.M., & Wells, S.A. (1997). The parathyroid glands. In Sabiston, D.C. (Ed.), *Textbook of surgery: the biological basis of modern surgical practice* (ed. 15). Philadelphia: W.B. Saunders.
6. Dudley, N. (1994). The thyroid gland. In Morris, P.J., & Malt, R.A. (Eds.), *Oxford textbook of surgery*. New York: Oxford University Press.
7. Falk, S.A. (1997). Metabolic complications of thyroid surgery: hypocalcemia and hypoparathyroidism; hypocalcitonemia; hypothyroidism and hyperthyroidism. In Falk, S.A. (Ed.), *Thyroid disease, endocrinology, surgery, nuclear medicine, and radiotherapy* (ed. 2). Philadelphia: Lippincott-Raven.

8. Kaplan, E.L. (1994). Thyroid and parathyroid. In Schwartz, S.I., Shires, G.T., & Spencer, F.C. (Eds.), *Principles of surgery* (ed. 6). New York: McGraw-Hill.

9. Kaplan, E.L., & Tanaka, R. (1995). Surgical endocrinology. In Polk, H.C., Gardner, B., & Stone, H.H. (Eds.), *Basic surgery*, (ed. 5). St. Louis: Quality Medical.

10. Leight, G.S. (1994). Subtotal and total thyroidectomy. In Sabiston, D.S. (Ed.), *Atlas of general surgery* (ed. 1). Philadelphia: W.B. Saunders.

11. Levin, M.A. (1996). Laboratory evaluation of calciotropic hormones and minerals. In Moore, W.T., & Eastman, R.C. (Eds.), *Diagnostic endocrinology* (ed. 2). St. Louis: Mosby.

12. LoPresti, J.S. (1996). Laboratory tests for thyroid disorders, *Otolaryngologic Clinics of North America, 29*(4), 557-575.

13. Marieb, E.N. (1994). *Essentials of human anatomy and physiology* (ed. 4). Redwood City, Calif: Benjamin/Cummings.

14. McKennis, A., & Waddington, C. (1997). Nursing interventions for potential complications after thyroidectomy, *ORL—Head and Neck Nursing, 15*(1), 27-35.

15. Millikan, W.J., & Shires, G.T. (1995). Parenteral fluid and electrolyte therapy. In Polk, H.C., Gardner, B., & Stone, H.H. (Eds.), *Basic surgery* (ed. 5). St. Louis: Quality Medical.

16. Moore, W.T., & Eastman, R.C. (1996). Laboratory evaluation of diseases of the thyroid. In Moore, W.T., & Eastman, R.C. (Eds.), *Diagnostic endocrinology* (ed. 2). St. Louis: Mosby.

17. Myer, C.M., & Cotton, R.T. (1997). Congenital thyroid cysts and ectopic thyroid. In Falk, S.A. (Ed.), *Thyroid disease, endocrinology, surgery, nuclear medicine, and radiotherapy* (ed. 2). Philadelphia: Lippincott-Raven.

18. Oertel, Y.C. (1996). Fine-needle aspiration of the thyroid. In Moore, W.T., & Eastman, R.C. (Eds.), *Diagnostic endocrinology* (ed. 2). St. Louis: Mosby.

19. Pagana, K.D., & Pagana, T.J. (1997). *Mosby's diagnostic and laboratory test reference* (ed. 3). St. Louis: Mosby.

20. Reiffel, R.S. (1995). Prevention of hypertrophic scars by long-term paper tape application, *Plastic and Reconstructive Surgery, 96*(7), 1715-1718.

21. Schuller, D.E., & Schleuning, A.J. (1994). *DeWeese and Saunders' otolaryngology head and neck surgery* (ed. 8). St. Louis: Mosby.

22. Shah, J.P. (1996). *Head and neck surgery* (ed. 2). St. Louis: Mosby.

23. Streff, M.M., & Pachucki-Hyde, L.C. (1996). Management of the patient with thyroid disease, *Nursing Clinics of North America, 31*(4), 779-796.

24. Thibodeau, G.A., & Patton, K.T. (1996). *Anatomy and physiology* (ed. 3). St. Louis: Mosby.

25. Vander, A.J., Sherman, J.H., & Luciano, D.S. (1994). *Human anatomy: the mechanism of body function* (ed. 6). New York: McGraw-Hill.

26. Woodburne, R.T., & Burkel, W.E. (1994). *Essentials of human anatomy* (ed. 9). New York: Oxford University Press.

27. Yousem, D.M., & Scheff, A.M. (1996). Thyroid and parathyroid. In Som, P.M., & Curtin, A.D. (Eds.), *Head and neck imaging* (ed. 3). St. Louis: Mosby.

CHAPTER SEVENTEEN

Rosemary Ann Roth

Breast Surgery

SURGICAL PROCEDURES ON the breast are commonly performed in numerous hospitals and free-standing surgical centers. Most procedures are performed to establish a definitive diagnosis when cancer is a possibility or to treat a breast cancer.

The possibility of and actual occurrence of breast changes, either benign or malignant, are some of the most emotionally upsetting health problems confronting women. Breast cancer is the most common cancer in women. The probability of developing breast cancer increases with age. Estimates predict that 1 in 8 women in the United States will develop breast cancer during her life. This risk is increased if a woman's mother, sister, or daughter has had breast cancer, especially if the cancer developed before menopause. An early menarche before 12 years of age and a late natural menopause after 50 years of age are associated with a slight increased risk for developing breast cancer. Further, a woman who has had cancer in one breast is at increased risk for another cancer in the other breast. Heightened public awareness, an increased number of women practicing self-examination, and the early detection of breast masses by mammography may have started to slow the annual increase in breast cancer mortality.

Changing hormone levels from puberty throughout the remainder of life affect breast tissue in its physical and microscopic characteristics. In association with these changes, numerous aberrations and tumors can occur.

Operative procedures on the breast may be indicated in the presence of disease or as a result of other physical or psychologic patient considerations. Reconstructive surgery of the breast is discussed in Chapter 24.

SURGICAL ANATOMY

The breasts are bilateral mammary glands that lie on the pectoralis major fascia of the anterior chest wall. They are surrounded by a layer of fat and are encased in an envelope of skin. The breasts extend from the second to the sixth rib and horizontally from the lateral edge of the sternum to the anterior axillary line. The largest part of the mammary gland rests on the connective tissue of the pectoralis major muscle and laterally on the serratus anterior (upper outer quadrant of the breast), with a normal globular contour occurring as a result of the fascial support (Cooper's ligaments). An elongation of mammary tissue normally extends laterally on the pectoralis major toward the axilla and is known as the *tail of Spence* (Fig. 17-1).

Each breast is made up of 12 to 20 glandular lobes that are separated by connective tissue. Each lobe drains by a single lactiferous duct that opens on the nipple. The nipple, located at about the fourth intercostal space,

forms a conical projection into which the ducts open independently of each other on the surface. A pigmented circular area called the *areola* surrounds the nipple. Smooth muscle fibers of the areola contract to allow for nipple projection.

Three major arterial systems (Fig. 17-2) generously supply the mammary glands with blood. The main sources are branches of the internal mammary and the lateral branches of the anterior aortic intercostal arteries, all of which form an extensive network of anastomoses over the breast. A third source is the pectoral branch, deriving from a branch of the axillary artery. The veins that mainly drain the breasts follow the course of the arteries. The superficial veins frequently become dilated during pregnancy.

The lymph-drainage system generally follows the course of the vessels. The lymphatics drain into two main areas represented by the axillary nodes and the internal thoracic chain of nodes (Fig. 17-3). The internal thoracic

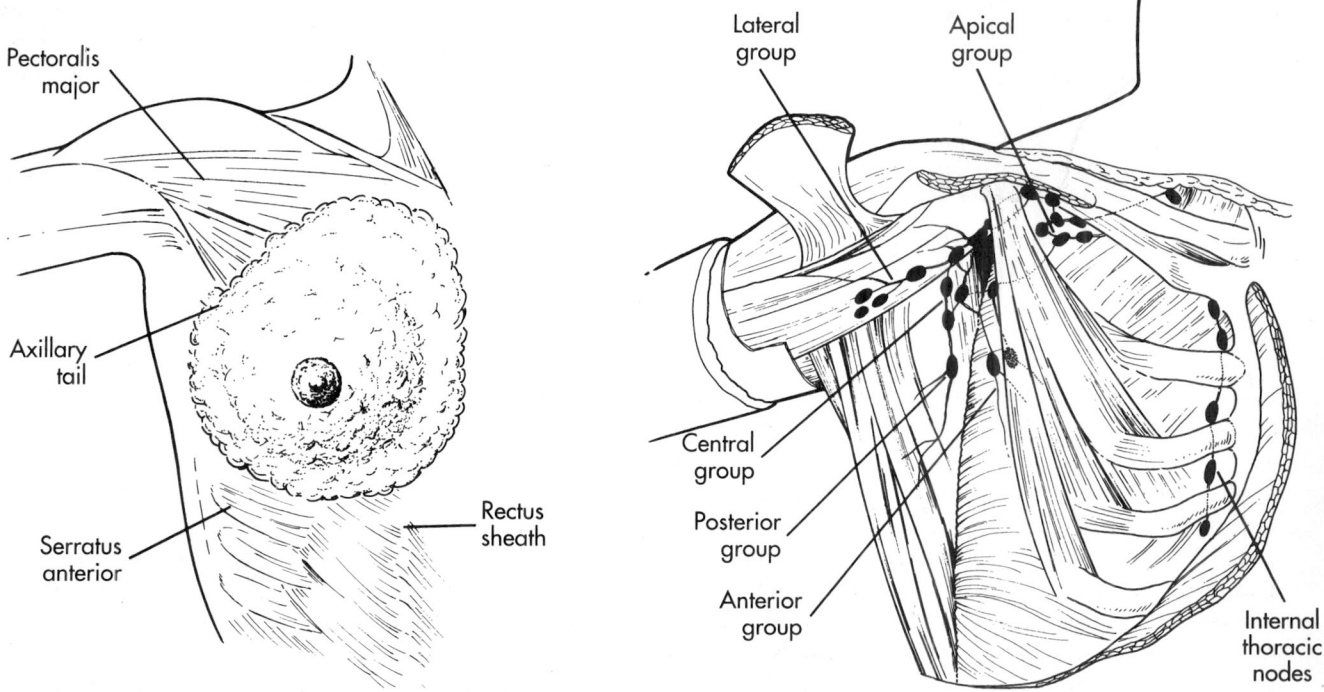

FIGURE 17–1 Normal distribution of mammary tissue of adult female breast.

FIGURE 17–3 Distribution of axillary and thoracic lymph nodes.

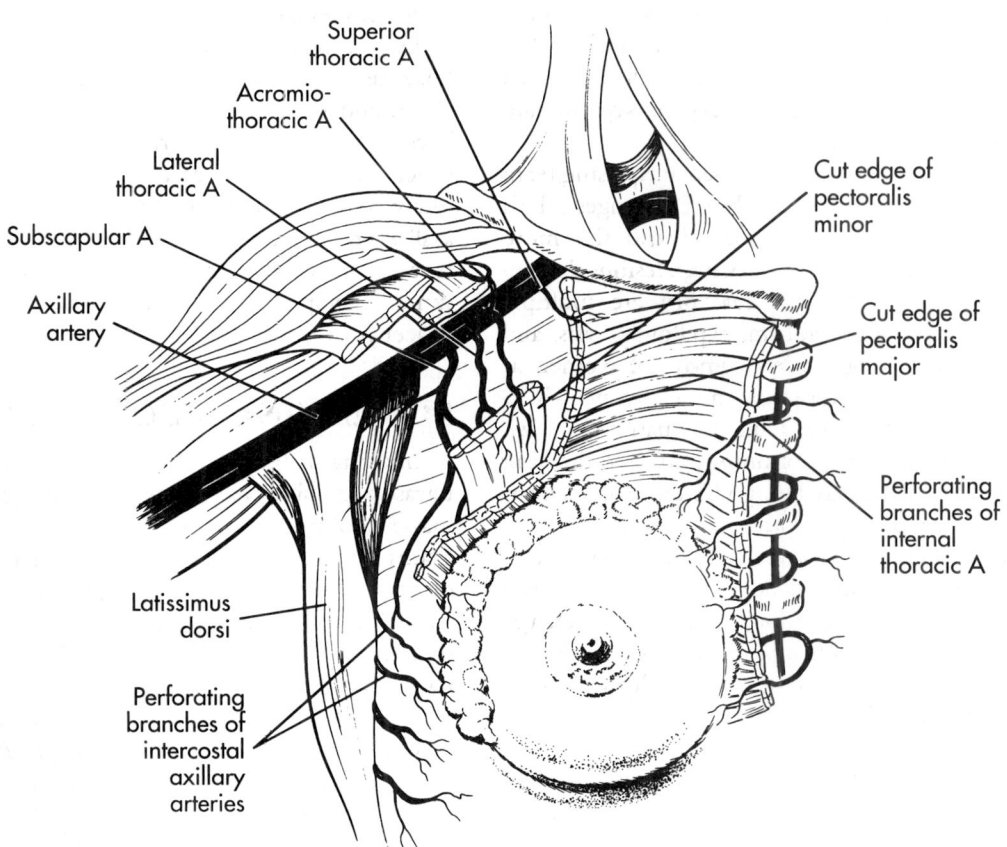

FIGURE 17–2 Normal arterial blood supply of the breast.

nodes are few but are responsible for most of the lymph drainage from the inner half of the breast. Thus one can see how the lymph system could be a channel for the spread of malignant disease from the breast to associated areas of the chest wall or to the axilla.

The sensory nerve supply is mainly from the anterior cutaneous branches of the upper intercostal nerves, the third and fourth branches of the cervical plexus, and the lateral cutaneous branches of the intercostal nerves.

Occasionally, developmental errors of the breast occur. Additional nipples or extramammary tissue in the axilla or over the upper abdomen may be present. The preferred treatment of these supernumerary structures is excision. Absence of one or both nipples may also occur and may be associated with absence of the underlying pectoral muscle and chest wall. The mammary glands are affected by three types of physiologic changes: (1) those related to growth and development, (2) those related to the menstrual cycle, and (3) those related to pregnancy and lactation. The mammary glands are present at birth in both males and females. Hormonal stimulation, however, produces the development and function of these glands in females. Estrogen promotes growth of the ductal structures, whereas progesterone promotes lobular development.

BENIGN LESIONS OF THE BREAST

A fibroadenoma, affecting primarily young women under 30 years of age, is usually a solitary nodule. These masses are small, painless lesions that are well delineated and relatively mobile. They grow very slowly and are generally discovered by accident.

Fibrocystic change in the breast is an all-encompassing term used to describe many different breast changes. This descriptive term should be discouraged and the more specific diagnosis used. Examples of benign lesions that are generally considered under this category are multiple lesions of fibrous disease, intraductal papilloma, cysts, and solid masses. These changes affect almost all women at some time in their lives. Frequently pain is present, which calls attention to the problem. Pain, fluctuations in size, and multiplicity of lesions are common features in helping to differentiate these generally benign lesions from cancer.

Nipple discharge is more commonly associated with benign lesions than with cancer. A postmenopausal woman who has some duct ectasia or who has borne children can manually produce nipple discharge. Discharge is usually significant only if it is spontaneous and persistent. Chronic unilateral nipple discharge, especially if bloody, should prompt an investigation for occult carcinoma.

BREAST CANCER

Breast cancer primarily affects women. Until it can be prevented, early detection is the greatest hope for cure. All women should practice monthly self-examination to detect palpable lesions and immediately report any changes or masses to a physician. External physical changes, such as dimpling of the skin, can also indicate the presence of a benign or malignant pathologic process.

Benign breast lesions, such as fibrocystic changes and fibroadenomas, are the most common lesions excised. The older the patient, the more likely it is that a mass is malignant. The most common form of breast cancer is infiltrating ductal carcinoma.

The cause of breast cancer is still unknown. Many factors, including environmental, dietary, and familial influences, have been suggested as contributors to its development. Whatever the cause, its incidence is definitely increasing. The previously held belief that breast cancer spreads by direct extension from the initial site in the breast to adjacent lymph nodes may not always be correct. Breast cancer may be a systemic condition at the time of diagnosis. Distant metastases may have already occurred without adjacent lymph node involvement at the time of its palpable detection. This theory could explain why the radical breast surgery of the past, which involved removal of all axillary and thoracic lymph nodes, did not greatly lower mortality. Survival from breast cancer is best when detected early, reducing axillary lymph node involvement and improving long-term survival. Tumor size can usually be correlated with involvement of lymph nodes. The larger the tumor, the more likely it is that lymph nodes are involved.

Less radical surgery is the treatment of choice today. Surgical excision of the tumor, the use of radiation therapy alone, and a combination of surgery and radiation therapy have become feasible alternatives to more radical surgical procedures. The use of adjuvant chemotherapy is definitely recommended for premenopausal women with axillary-node metastasis. There have been studies and a recommendation by the National Institutes of Health that similar therapy can be beneficial in node-negative breast cancer patients.

SCREENING TECHNOLOGIES

Imaging methodologies, such as mammography and ultrasonography, have helped in the detection of breast masses too small for clinical detection. Screening mammograms are definitely indicated for women 50 years of age or older. There is a lack of agreement regarding the value of annual screening mammograms in women under 50 years of age without the evidence of definite risk factors or family history of breast cancer (Research Highlight 17-1).

The best available screening mechanism for occult and palpable lesions is x-ray mammography (Fig. 17-4). Mammograms can detect abnormal-appearing densities, irregular or spiculated margins, microcalcifications, and clusters of calcium deposits that are clinically nonpalpable (Fig. 17-5). These masses may be only 3 to 10 mm in

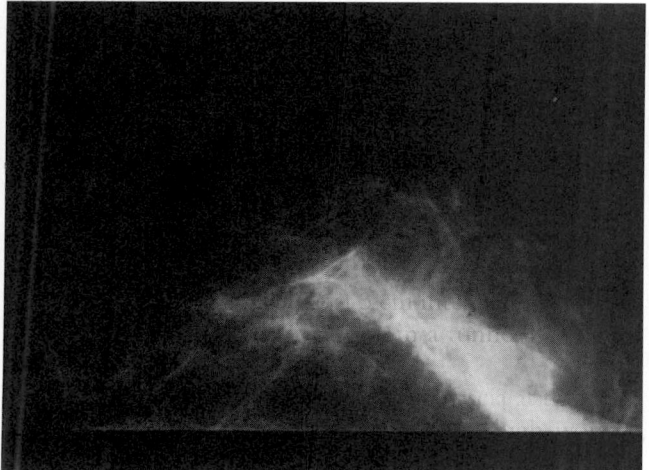

FIGURE 17-4 Mammogram. Craniocaudad view of normal breast.

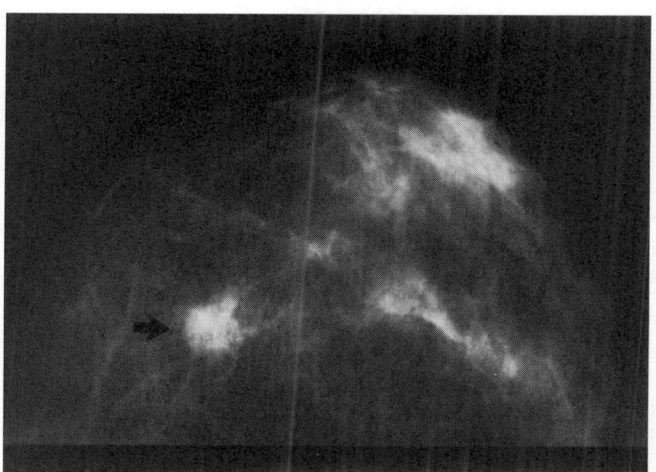

FIGURE 17-5 Mammogram. Craniocaudad view of breast. *Arrow* indicates nonpalpable lesion of about 1.5 cm.

17-1 RESEARCH HIGHLIGHT

This study investigated the controversy of screening mammograms in women 40 to 50 years of age. The survival benefits of mammograms after 50 years of age is easy to demonstrate because the incidence of breast cancer increases significantly with age. The controversy centers on the benefits of this test before 50 years of age.

In this study the results of needle-localized breast biopsies were retrospectively reviewed over a 6½-year period to determine the age at the time of biopsy. Eight hundred nine charts of women were reviewed with an age range from 27 to 91 years (with a mean of 56). Two hundred nineteen biopsies demonstrated malignancy: 3 patients were under 40 years; 32 patients between 40 and 49 years; and 184 patients were 50 years and older. Thirty-three percent of the patients reviewed were under 50 years of age. The study concluded that without the screening mammography 32 patients between 40 and 49 years of age would have had their diagnosis delayed. The authors recommended the use of the screening mammography for this specific age range.

From Lein, B., Alex, W.R., Zebley, D.M., & Pezzi, C.M. (1996). Results of needle localized breast biopsy in women under age 50. *American Journal of Surgery, 171,* 356-359.

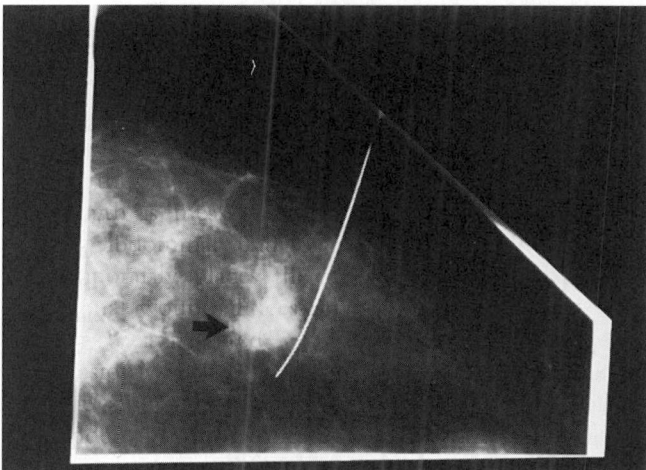

FIGURE 17-6 Mammogram section. Craniocaudad view of breast. *Arrow* indicates breast lesion localized by wire before surgical excision.

diameter. Often, previous mammograms are used for comparison.

In mammography the entire breast is visualized when x-ray beams are directed in several planes through the breast, yielding craniocaudad and other views (see Fig. 17-4). Mammograms should be analyzed by a trained radiologist, who sends the report to the referring physician. In some instances, as when the lesion is too small to palpate, mammograms are done immediately before surgery. The lesions, previously detected by mammogram, are localized by the insertion of a needle or needles or a wire within a needle. The needles may be left in place or removed after insertion of the wire (Fig. 17-6). Once the suspect area is identified, the needle or wire is taped in place, and the patient is sent to the operating room for surgical biopsy. After the biopsy, the specimen can be sent to the radiology department for mammography validation of the correct surgical excision of the questionable breast tissue before the pathologic examination.

The accuracy of mammography depends on careful x-ray technique and breast size, structure, and density. Radiation dosage varies with individuals and techniques. As a result of improvement in radiologic techniques, the radiation exposure in a mammogram is very low. The benefits of this screening mechanism far outweigh the minute risks of radiation exposure.

Ultrasonography differentiates between solid and cystic lesions. As a screening methodology, its sensitivity and specificity are less definitive than mammography is. This technique can be useful with dense or dysplastic breasts and in pregnant or lactating women. An alternative approach to determine if a mass is solid or cystic is the use of fine-needle aspiration (FNA).

Magnetic resonance imaging (MRI) is another technique that is showing promise as an adjunct to mammography in the detection of breast lesions.

DIAGNOSTIC TECHNIQUES

Once a mass has been identified the physician has a variety of techniques available to establish a diagnosis (Research Highlight 17-2). During a fine-needle aspiration, the physician anesthetizes a small area of the breast with lidocaine. A 22- or 25-gauge needle attached to a 20 ml syringe is inserted into the mass, and a small amount of the contents is aspirated. Cytologic examination of the aspirate can assist in microscopic evaluation of the mass.

New instrumentation advances now allow for the biopsy and removal of mammographic densities that are up to 20 mm in size. This new system combines digital stereotactic imaging and minimally invasive instruments to locate and remove tissues for diagnosis. The patient is assessed preoperatively for neck or back problems. In addition, the patient should not be receiving anticoagulant therapy. Masses located near the patient's areola, high in the axilla, or near the chest wall are not appropriate for this technique.

The patient is placed upon a specially designed table (Fig. 17-7) in the prone position with the affected breast through the table's 10-inch aperture to the work area below. The patient's head is turned away from the physician. Padding is placed under the patient's bony prominences to improve the patient's comfort. When the suspicious area in the breast is located through stereotactic imaging, its coordinates are transferred to the table's automated instrument (Fig. 17-8). After preparing the skin with povidone-iodine complex solution while the patient is under local anesthesia, the physician makes a small incision in the breast. The disposable biopsy device is available in a variety of sizes and consists of a localization needle, cannula, blade, and cautery adapter. The physician positions the disposable device to remove the identified tissue. Additional biopsies can be made if indicated and cautery can be used if necessary. A titanium vessel clip can be placed at the base of the biopsy specimen as a point of reference for future evaluations. A postoperative dressing is then applied to the area. The benefits to the patient include small incisions for cosmetic results and decreased disfigurement, shortened time between detection and diagnosis, and elimination of the need for more involved surgical intervention.

17-2 RESEARCH HIGHLIGHT

In this prospective study, patients with a nonpalpable mammographic breast abnormality were offered the following: open-wire localization biopsy, stereotactic core needle biopsy, or a random assignment to one of the two options. Patients were then contacted 1 to 2 weeks after the biopsy and telephone interviewed about the pain encountered during the biopsy, the length of time to return to normal activities, and the degree that their expectations compared to the actual biopsy experience. The women were then instructed to return for a follow-up mammogram within 6 months.

Fifty-one women had open biopsy, and 52 women had stereotactic biopsy. The average age of the women was 60 years. Pathologic results and complications were approximately the same for both groups. The average cost of the open biopsy was $2,400 and $650 for the stereotactic biopsy, and such costs were statistically significant ($p < 0.01$). The telephone interview revealed no significant difference in patient satisfaction between the two types of procedures. Only two patients required open biopsy after the follow-up mammogram because of the progression of the mammographic findings or a missed lesion. The conclusion was that there was no difference between open-wire localization and stereotactic biopsies except for the differences in the costs.

From Frazee, R.C., Roberts, J.W., Symmonds, R.E., et al. (1996). Open versus stereotactic breast biopsy. *American Journal of Surgery, 172,* 491-495.

SURGICAL TREATMENT OPTIONS

Surgical treatment ranges from breast-conserving surgeries, such as lumpectomy or the wide excision of the tumor mass, to modified radical mastectomy involving the breast and axillary lymph nodes. The choice of operation depends on the size and site of the mass, the stage of the disease, and the patient's choice. The goal of breast-conserving surgery is the removal of the cancerous mass with a margin of normal tissue and a good cosmetic result. Radiation therapy, chemotherapy, or hormonal therapy may be used with surgery or as alternative treatment methods.

Techniques have been developed to determine the ability of breast cancer to bind with estrogen and progestins. This positive binding capability identifies the patient with a hormone-dependent tumor. It is estimated that about two thirds of all breast cancers are positive for estrogen binding, and the majority of these tumors are also positive for progestins. The presence of these receptor sites is conducive to hormone manipulation. The use of antiestrogen tamoxifen, in addition to surgery and chemotherapy, increases disease-free survival in premeno-

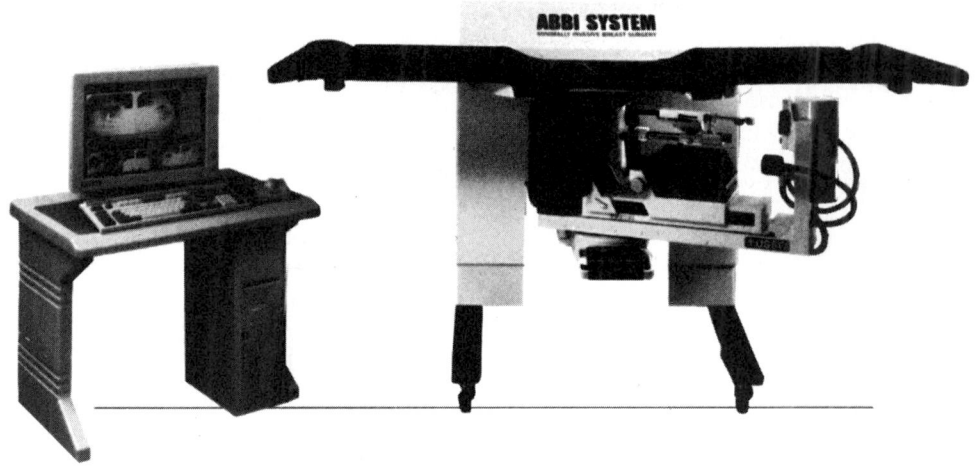

FIGURE 17-7   USSC ABBI System stereotactic table and computer system.

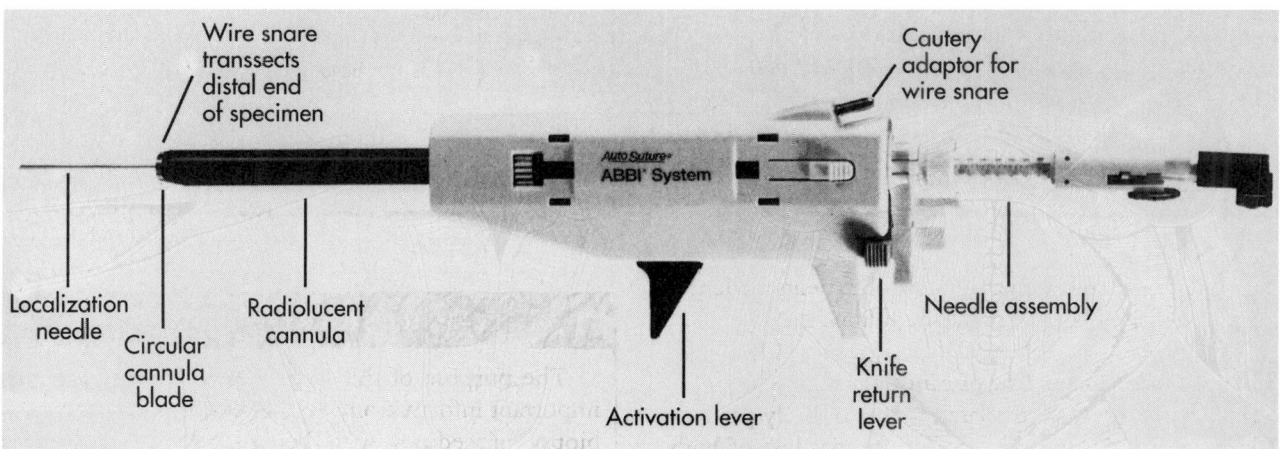

FIGURE 17-8   USSC ABBI System disposable instrument.

pausal and postmenopausal women with positive binding for estrogen. Tumors excised at surgery are evaluated for their estrogen and progestin-binding abilities.

A breast cancer diagnosis is usually staged to measure the extent of the disease and to classify patients for possible treatment modalities. The TNM classification has been adopted as a mechanism to clinically stage this disease (Box 17-1). The results of staging are used in designing a specific treatment plan.

PERIOPERATIVE NURSING CONSIDERATIONS

Assessment

A patient undergoing breast surgery can be extremely apprehensive about the possibilities of having a malignancy, losing a body part, facing a negative reaction from her spouse and family, and experiencing a change in self-image. During a preoperative interview the perioperative nurse should assess the patient's level of anxiety and possible causes, such as the possibility of the diagnosis of cancer. Identification of the patient's fears and concerns helps the nurse in planning appropriate nursing interventions. The patient should identify the breast that is affected and, if possible, the quadrant of the breast mass. The nurse should assess the patient's understanding of the proposed surgical procedure. Reinforcement of knowledge or correction of misunderstandings is possible only if the nurse identifies the patient's current level of knowledge. Identifying the patient's psychological supports will help manage anxiety during the patient's stay and enhance the discharge planning process (Research Highlight 17-3). If the patient has lost a relative or close friend to breast cancer, her coping mechanisms may be affected because of memories of that loss.

Nursing Diagnosis

Based on the nursing assessment, the perioperative nurse uses nursing diagnoses to develop a plan of care.

| BOX 17-1 | The TNM Staging System for Breast Cancer |

Stage 1

$T^1N^0M^0$

Tumor size less than 2 cm

May extend into pectoral fascia or muscle

No distant metastasis

No positive nodes

Stage II

$T^2N^0M^0$ or $T^1N^1M^0$ or $T^2N^1M^0$

Tumor size 2 to 5 cm

May or may not extend into pectoral fascia or muscle

No distant metastasis

Mobile axillary nodes

Stage III

$T^1N^1M^0$ or $T^2N^1M^0$ or $T^{1-3}N^2M^0$ or $T^3N^0M^0$

Tumor size greater than 5 cm

May or may not extend into pectoral fascia and muscle

Skin edema, infiltration, or ulceration may be present

Nodes fixed to skin, deeper structures, supraclavicular nodes

No distant metastasis

Stage IV

Any TN^2 any M or T^1 any N any M

Any TN plus M^1

Definitions

T = primary tumor

T^1 = tumor extension to the chest wall or skin

N = regional lymph nodes

N^0 = no growth

N^1 = movable nodes with tumor growth

N^2 = homolateral axillary nodes fixed to one another or other structures and containing growth

N^3 = homolateral infraclavicular or supraclavicular nodes containing growth

M = distant metastasis

M^0 = absent

M^1 = present, includes skin beyond the breast

Modified from Stein, P., & Zera, R. (1991). *AORN Journal, 53*, 4.

Nursing diagnoses related to the care of patients undergoing breast surgery might include the following:

- Anxiety related to the fear of cancer.
- Body image disturbance related to loss of body part.
- Anticipatory grieving related to potential loss of body part.
- Risk for injury related to use of electrosurgery.
- Knowledge deficit related to unfamiliarity with perioperative routines.

Outcome Identification

Outcomes identified for the selected nursing diagnoses could be stated as the following:

- Patient will verbalize and exhibit decreased anxiety.
- Patient will discuss feelings regarding the possible adverse outcome of the surgical procedure.
- Patient will experience no untoward injury from electrosurgery.
- Patient will verbalize understanding of perioperative procedures.

Planning

Using nursing diagnoses, the perioperative nurse can individualize the plan of care for each patient and allow for communication with other colleagues on the patient care team. The plan of care for a patient undergoing breast surgery can include nursing interventions that allow the

---

17-3 RESEARCH HIGHLIGHT

The purpose of this study was to identify the most important information needs of women who had breast biopsy procedures with benign results. Ten women were recruited from a Canadian hospital breast clinic for a focus group representing three age categories: younger than 40 years, 40 to 60 years, and older than 60 years. These age ranges were selected to represent premenopausal, perimenopausal, and postmenopausal women. Only nine women were able to attend the actual focus group session. During the first part of the session, the individuals completed a Likert scale information needs questionnaire. The second part involved having the participants identify the nine most important information needs of women undergoing breast biopsy. The results indicated that these women require information on the type of benign breast disease, the meaning of risk associated with benign breast disease, and diagnostic tests associated with the evaluation of a breast lump. Adequate and timely information on these subjects was helpful in reducing the womens' anxiety and assisted with their coping mechanisms.

From Deane, K., & Degner, L. (1997). Determining the information needs of women after breast biopsy procedures. *AORN Journal, 65* 767-776.

S A M P L E   C A R E   P L A N

Nursing Diagnosis: Anxiety related to fear of cancer or surgical intervention
Outcome: Patient will verbalize and exhibit decreased anxiety.
Interventions:
Allow time for patient's questions.
Assess verbal and nonverbal signs of anxiety.
Encourage ventilation of concerns and fears.
Provide emotional support and comfort measures (warm blankets, touch as appropriate).
Maintain quiet environment.
Demonstrate warmth, calmness, and acceptance of the patient's anxiety.
Instruct the patient in relaxation techniques such as rhythmic breathing or guided imagery.
Record patient's reactions.
Nursing Diagnosis: Body image disturbance related to loss of body part
Outcome: Patient will discuss feelings regarding possible adverse outcome of the surgical procedure.
Interventions:
Allow patient to discuss concerns about her sexual attractiveness and perceived loss of femininity.
Discuss available resources and options (external prosthesis, alternatives in garments and dress, reconstructive surgery, as appropriate). Make referrals to nurse on discharge unit as indicated.
Maintain the patient's privacy.
Nursing Diagnosis: Anticipatory grieving related to potential loss of body part
Outcome: Patient will discuss feelings regarding the possible adverse outcome of the surgical procedure.
Interventions:
Allow ventilation of feelings.
Clarify misconceptions.

Promote an environment of support, respect, and comfort.
Refer to other professionals as appropriate.
Explore realistic alternatives and breast reconstruction.
Nursing Diagnosis: Risk for injury related to use of electrosurgery
Outcome: Patient will experience no untoward injury from electrosurgery.
Interventions:
Position the dispersive pad as close to the operative site as possible.
Select a site that is clean and dry, with good muscle mass; notice the condition of the skin.
Protect pad from fluids and contact with metal objects.
Turn electrosurgical unit on after dispersive pad and active electrode are connected.
Set power setting as low as possible to achieve desired effect.
Use holster for active electrode on the sterile field.
Check dispersive pad contact and all connections after changes in position or requests to increase power.
Evaluate the condition of the skin upon removal of the dispersive pad.
Nursing Diagnosis: Knowledge deficit related to unfamiliarity with perioperative routines
Outcome: Patient will verbalize understanding of perioperative procedures.
Interventions:
Assess the patient's experience with previous surgical procedures.
Provide clear and concise explanations of all nursing interventions.
Explain roles of the health care team members.
Encourage questions.

patient freedom to express concerns, have specific questions answered, and discuss breast reconstruction options, as appropriate. The Sample Care Plan shows some examples.

The perioperative nurse needs to develop criteria to measure achievement of the outcomes. A patient experiencing decreased or relief from anxiety would be evidenced by verbalization of her specific anxieties, relaxed facial and body structures, and vital signs within the normal range for the patient.

Implementation

Before surgery the perioperative nurse should procure the necessary medical and surgical supplies, instruments, and equipment for the intended operation. Mammogram films should be available in the OR for the surgeon's review. A breast biopsy done under local anesthesia will require local anesthetics, adjunct sedation, and monitoring equipment (ECG, pulse oximeter, blood pressure apparatus). Patient allergies should again be reviewed and the patient closely observed for allergic or toxic reactions to local anesthetics. For a mastectomy, extra sponges and instrumentation are often needed. An electrosurgical unit (ESU) or a surgical laser is used to provide both hemostasis and tissue dissection. The incision site is usually drained postoperatively with a closed-wound suction device. Ensuring the availability of supplies before the procedure allows the nurse to remain with, provide support to, monitor, and observe the patient.

During the intraoperative phase the patient is placed on the OR bed in a supine position with the operative side near the edge of the bed. The arm on the involved side is carefully extended on a padded armboard at no greater than 90 degrees to prevent brachial plexus injury. Depending on the location of the lesion and the planned surgery, a small pad can be placed under the operative side to facilitate exposure of the incision area. Positioning the OR bed in slight Fowler's position with a lateral tilt away from the surgeon can also facilitate exposure.

Skin preparation depends on the location of the lesion and the surgery intended. Skin prep solutions vary, depending on the surgeon's preference. For a breast biopsy the area prepped is usually the affected breast and the immediate surrounding skin. For a mastectomy the area prepped can extend from above the clavicle to the umbilicus and from the opposite nipple to the bedline of the operative side, including the axilla, and possibly the upper arm on the operative side. Some surgeons caution against vigorous scrubbing of the surgical site to prevent possible seeding of cancer cells from the main mass. The surgeon may request that only an antiseptic solution be applied to the breast.

Surgical draping should allow exposure of the affected breast. For a mastectomy the arm on the operative side should be draped free using a stockinette and drapes that allow free movement of the associated arm to facilitate access to the axilla. If a breast biopsy is to be immediately followed by a modified radical mastectomy, the surgeon may prefer to repeat the skin prep and surgical draping before proceeding with the definitive surgery.

During implementation of the plan of care, the perioperative nurse continues to collect data, continuously reassesses the patient's needs and the needs of the surgical team, initiates nursing interventions, and documents all care delivered. Formats for documenting perioperative patient care vary from institution to institution. However, documentation of patient problems and nursing interventions addressing these problems is essential. For the patient undergoing breast surgery, consideration should be given to documenting the patient's level of anxiety, the surgical position and accessory positioning devices used, the location of the electrosurgical dispersive pad, unit settings and identification number, results of perioperative monitoring, medications administered by the perioperative nurse or from the sterile field, and any drains inserted into the surgical wound.

Evaluation

Evaluation of the patient before discharge from the operating room includes both general observation parameters important for every surgical patient and specific evaluation of the goals of the plan of care. The patient's skin at dependent pressure sites, skin preparation sites, and the dispersive pad placement site should be assessed and any change in skin integrity documented. Whether the dressing is intact and the wound suction device is properly functioning should also be noted. The report to the nurse in the PACU should include any unusual events or patient problems during surgery, the incorporation of any drains in the wound, and the achievement of identified patient outcomes. These outcomes, based on the nursing diagnoses selected, should be a part of documentation as well as the nursing report.

Patient and Family Education and Discharge Planning

Discharge planning should begin as soon as the patient is informed of the necessity for surgery or when the nurse first meets the patient. Dependent upon the extent of the anticipated surgery, information about appropriate exercises to enhance recovery, prosthetic devices, reconstruction options, and available community support groups should be explained to the patient. The perioperative nurse provides or reinforces information based on clinical nursing judgment and the patient's desire for information, readiness to learn, and anxiety level.

The patient is often discharged within hours or the day after the surgery. The patient and other care givers need to be instructed regarding aseptic wound care and how to care for the closed-wound suction drain. Possible signs of complications should be included along with instructions regarding when and how to notify the physician. Postoperative exercises need to be taught to the patient to facilitate her return to normal activities and to minimize lymphedema. Home care may be necessary and should be coordinated with the physician and the patient. A follow-up telephone call to the patient can help the nurse assess the patient's ability to cope with her diagnosis and surgery.

SURGICAL INTERVENTIONS
BIOPSY OF BREAST TISSUE

Biopsy of breast tissue is removal of suspicious tissue for pathologic examination. In a needle biopsy, a disposable cutting type of needle is introduced and advanced into the breast mass to entrap a core or plug of tissue. The needle is withdrawn, and the tissue specimen is sent to a pathologist for diagnostic examination. In an incisional biopsy, a portion of the mass is surgically excised using a curved incision line. The tissue is sent for pathologic examination. In an excisional biopsy the entire tumor mass is excised from adjacent tissue for examination as with incisional biopsy.

Biopsy is indicated in the presence of a tumor mass detected by palpation, mammography, nipple discharge, or skin changes. Fibroadenoma, an isolated cyst, or intraductal papilloma may be encountered. Definitive surgical treatment is contraindicated in the absence of a formal biopsy.

Procedural considerations

The biopsy procedure incurs little risk and is usually performed with the patient under local anesthesia. A minor instrument set is used. The short delay between biopsy and further treatment has not been shown to adversly affect survival. However, when an extensive surgical procedure is anticipated in conjunction with the biopsy, general anesthesia is preferred. In these instances the patient has preoperatively given informed consent to proceed with the more definitive surgery.

Operative procedure

1. An incision in the direction of the skin lines or along the border of the areola is made over the tumor mass. The circumareolar incision gives the best cosmetic effect.
2. Gentle traction is applied to the mass with holding forceps. If the lesion is small, the entire mass and an edge of normal tissue are removed by sharp dissection. If a large lesion is present, a small incisional biopsy of the main mass is done. The specimen should not be placed into a formalin solution if a frozen section is to be done at the time of surgery. Exposure to formalin prevents this type of pathologic examination. The tissue specimen is examined by a frozen section to determine immediate diagnosis while the patient is still anesthetized. If a 48-hour permanent section is required for a definitive diagnosis, the patient must be scheduled at a later time for any further surgery that may be necessary.
3a. If the lesion is benign, the subcutaneous breast tissue of the wound is approximated with an absorbable suture. The skin is closed with fine sutures or skin staples, and a firm pressure dressing is applied.
3b. If the lesion is malignant, the incision is tightly closed with a continuous locking suture on a cutting needle.
4. If a more extensive operation is required, it may be performed immediately. The team members regown and glove; the operative site is again prepped and draped. A separate sterile setup and set of instruments for a more radical procedure are then used.

INCISION AND DRAINAGE FOR ABSCESS

Incision of an inflamed and suppurative area of the breast is performed for drainage of abscess. Breast abscesses occur most frequently during the first 4 weeks of breastfeeding. Staphylococcal or streptococcal organisms enter the breast through abraded or lacerated nipple surfaces or through the lactiferous ducts. Chronic abscesses are rare. Free drainage is required with the association of an abscess around the nipple or in breast tissue.

Procedural considerations

The condition is very painful and may require surgery under general anesthesia. Instruments are the same as those for a biopsy.

Operative procedure

1. Generally, a radial incision extending outward from the nipple or a circumareolar incision is preferred. A short incision into the thoracomammary fold may be used for deep breast abscesses in the lower or outer quadrant.
2. After skin incision, the wound is deepened until pus is encountered.
3. A curved hemostat is directed into the cavity to determine the extent of the abscess. Culture specimens for aerobic and anaerobic organisms are usually taken.
4. Loculations are broken up by exploring the cavity with the index finger.
5. The opening is enlarged to ensure adequate drainage, the cavity is irrigated with warm saline solution, and bleeding vessels are ligated with absorbable sutures or coagulated.
6. The wound is drained or loosely packed with gauze. Healing occurs by granulation.

SEGMENTAL RESECTION (LUMPECTOMY, QUADRANT RESECTION, WEDGE RESECTION)

Segmental resection is removal of the tumor mass with at least a 1-inch margin of surrounding tissue. A segmental resection combined with an axillary node dissection and irradiation in stage I and stage II breast cancer appears to provide results equal to a more radical procedure. If one or more axillary nodes are involved, chemotherapy is also recommended.

Procedural considerations

In patients with large breasts, increased bleeding may occur, requiring additional hemostatic clamps.

Operative procedure

The procedure is as described for excisional biopsy.

SENTINEL NODE BIOPSY

Identification and microscopic examination of the sentinel nodes, the first lymph nodes along the lymphatic channel from the primary tumor site, will help in determining the need for additional or more extensive surgeries and treatments and potentially adverse outcomes for the patient. The sentinel node is not located in the same site in every patient. This procedure helps to focus pathologic attention in more detail on a small amount of tissue to determine the evidence of micrometastatic disease. Patients with histogically negative lymph nodes can have a greater likelihood of survival than patients with metastatic lymph nodes. Evidence of a positive node results in an axillary node dissection and adjunct therapy.

Procedural considerations

This procedure is similar to that for a breast biopsy. Sentinel node identification is accomplished by an injection of either isosulfan blue dye or metastable technetium 99 (^{99m}Tc), a radioactive material. The procedure is coordinated with the staff of the nuclear medicine department and requires the use of a hand-held detector like a geiger counter if technetium is used.

Operative procedure

1. With isosulfan blue dye:
   a. The area of the breast mass is exposed as part of a breast biopsy. After identification of the tumor mass, the surgeon injects the dye directly into the tumor mass or the previous biopsy site.
   b. The sentinel nodes stained with the blue dye are identified and excised. The node is sent to the pathology department for examination. Based upon the results, the surgeon proceeds with the planned surgery or may elect breast conservation.
2. With technetium:
   a. The patient's tumor or previous biopsy site is injected with a small amount of radioactive material in the nuclear medicine department on the morning of surgery.
   b. A hand-held detector is passed over the top of the patient's chest to identify the area of the sentinel node through a positive reading.
   c. The surgeon marks the skin with a skin scribe to indicate the reactive area. The area is prepped and

the surgeon proceeds with the planned procedure for excisional biopsy.

AXILLARY NODE DISSECTION

Axillary node dissection (Fig. 17-9) is the removal of the axillary nodes through an incision in the axilla. An axillary dissection is usually done through an incision separate from that for other breast operations. The removal and examination of the axillary nodes allow staging (see Box 17-1) of the disease. Adjunct treatment can be more accurately planned when the pathologic stage is determined.

Procedural considerations

The patient is placed supine on the OR bed with the operative side near the bed edge. The arm on the operative side is extended to less than 90 degrees on an armboard. The skin is prepped and draped as previously described.

Operative procedure

1. An incision is made slightly posterior and parallel to the upper lateral border of the pectoralis major muscle, or transversely across the axilla.
2. The fascia is incised over the pectoralis muscle. The pectoralis minor muscle is exposed. Major blood and

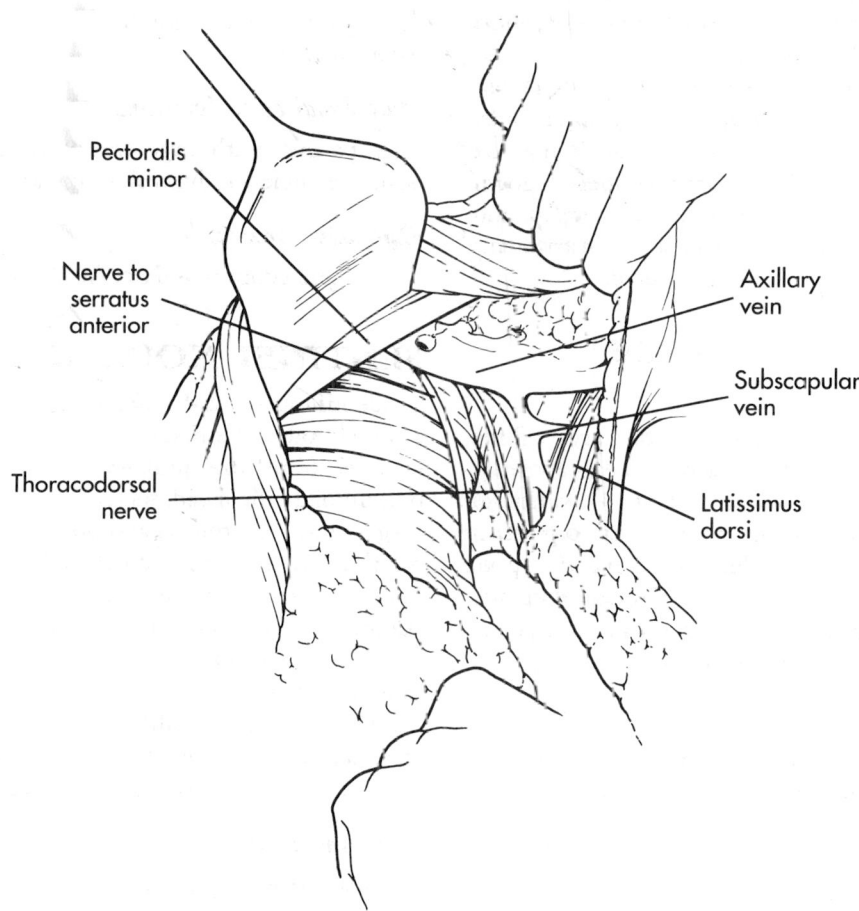

FIGURE 17-9   Axillary dissection.

lymphatic vessels are clamped and ligated. The use of electrosurgery is avoided around the axillary vessels and nerves to reduce the risk of inadvertent injury and subsequent impaired muscle function.

3. The tissue over the axillary vein is incised.
4. The lymph nodes between the pectoralis major and pectoralis minor muscles are removed. Care is taken not to injure the medial and lateral nerves of the pectoralis major muscle.
5. The axillary fat and lymph nodes are freed from the axillary vein and chest wall. The long thoracic nerve is identified along the chest wall near the axillary vein, and the thoracodorsal nerve posteriorly is dissected free from the specimen.
6. The fat and nodes are removed. The incision is closed with sutures and staples, and a dressing is applied. A suction drain is usually placed through a separate stab incision for lymphatic drainage.

SUBCUTANEOUS MASTECTOMY (ADENOMAMMECTOMY)

Subcutaneous mastectomy is removal of all breast tissue with the overlying skin and nipple left intact. This procedure is recommended for patients who have central tumors of noninvasive origin, chronic cystic mastitis, hyperplastic duct changes, or multiple fibroadenomas, or who have undergone several previous biopsies. Breast reconstruction may be undertaken at the time of mastectomy or at a later date if desired.

Procedural considerations

The patient is positioned as for a biopsy. If reconstruction is to be undertaken, appropriate equipment and supplies (see Chapter 24) are also required.

Operative procedure

1. An incision is usually begun in the inframammary crease and may be made on the medial or the lateral aspect of the breast. Some surgeons initially remove and preserve the nipple areola complex by employing lateral extensions of wide circumareolar incisions.
2. Blunt dissection is performed to elevate the breast from the pectoral fascia.
3. The breast tissue is separated from the skin with an attempt made to remain in a plane between the subcutaneous tissue and the breast. Dissection is carried out toward the axilla. With care, 90% or more of the breast tissue, including the tail of Spence, can be removed. Some lymph nodes in the axillary area also may be removed. Bleeding vessels are clamped and ligated.
4. If a preoperative decision was made for immediate reconstruction, that procedure follows at this time. Provided that the subareolar tissue shows no signs of tumor, as verified by a pathologist, the salvaged areolar complex is placed on a deepithelialized dermal bed.

5. A closed-wound suction catheter typically is inserted. The wound is closed, and a light pressure dressing is applied.

SIMPLE MASTECTOMY (TOTAL MASTECTOMY)

Simple mastectomy is removal of the entire involved breast without lymph node dissection. A simple mastectomy is performed to remove extensive benign disease, if malignancy is believed to be confined only to the breast tissue, or as a palliative measure to remove an ulcerated advanced malignancy.

Procedural considerations

The patient is positioned as for a biopsy.

Operative procedure

1. Through a transverse elliptical incision (see Fig. 17-11, *A* on p. 630), using a knife and curved scissors, the skin edges are freed from the fascia. Bleeding vessels are clamped with hemostats and ligated with sutures or electrocoagulated.
2. The skin edges of the wound can be protected with warm, moist laparotomy pads; the breast tissue is grasped with Allis forceps and is dissected free from the underlying pectoral fascia with curved scissors and a knife.
3. The tumor and all breast tissue are removed. Bleeding vessels are clamped and ligated or electrocoagulated.
4. A closed-wound drainage catheter is inserted and anchored to the skin with a fine suture. The wound is closed with fine sutures or staples; a dressing is applied.

MODIFIED RADICAL MASTECTOMY

Modified radical mastectomy is performed after a tissue biopsy with a positive diagnosis of malignancy and involves removal of the involved breast and all axillary contents (all three levels of nodes—axillary, pectoral, and superior apical). The underlying pectoral muscles are not removed before or after removal of axillary nodes. A modified radical mastectomy is done to remove the involved area with the hope of decreasing the spread of the malignancy. This surgery's elliptic incision with lateral extension toward the axilla gives a good cosmetic result for plastic surgery reconstruction (see Chapter 24), provides good arm movement because the pectoralis muscles are not removed, and usually does not require a skin graft. A clinical pathway for modified radical mastectomy is shown in Fig. 17-10.

Procedural considerations

The patient is placed supine on the operating room bed with the operative side near the bed edge. The arm on the operative side is extended to less than 90 degrees on a

Mastectomy: Modified Radical

DRG Number: _____

ELOS: _____

	Pre Op (Outpatient)	Day of Operation (Holding Room) 1 hr	Day of Operation (OR → close) 2 hr 15 min	Day of Surgery PACU (2 hr)	Day of Operation (9 S)	POD 1 (9S)	POD 2 (9S/Day of Discharge)
Goals	Pre-op testing complete and data available for review 1-4 days pre-op / Pre-op testing results WNL for surgery / Pt/family teaching complete / Consent signed	Pre-op checklist completed / Support to family / Support to patient / Permit signed	Pt. safety maintained → / Sterile tech maintained → / Pt. positioned correctly → / Initial counts documented / Final counts correct	Pain controlled / VSS, Lung CTA / Normothermia achieved / SaO$_2$ ≥ 90%	Voids w/o difficulty / Temp < 100° / Drsg dry & intact / Incision w/o S/Sx infection / Drains patent & functioning / Tol reg diet w/o difficulty	Reach to Recovery referral made / Demonstrates drain care	Home care teaching complete / Drains patent and functioning till return to clinic / F/U appointment scheduled
Treatments		Shave/prep	Correct position / Pad extremities and bony prominence → / Warm blanket / Pt. prep / Bovie pad / Counts x 3 if applicable	Standard PACU care / Monitor drainage in hemovac / Check dsg q 1 hr	No needle sticks, BP to ___ arm / JP drains x 2		MD remove dressing / → Till RTC
Activity	Ad lib	Bedrest / Check bony prominence →		Progress as tolerated	OOB to chair in p.m.	OOB to chair / Ambulate halls TID	
Diet	NPO at MN night before surg	NPO →		Sips and chips if tolerated	Clear liquids → advance to regular as tolerated		
Labs	SMA6 / SMA12 / CBC with plts / PT, PTT / UA } → Pre-op value on charts		Specimen to Surgical Path.		PCV		
Tests	History & physical / CXR / EKG if > 50 yrs or indicated by history } Test results on chart						
Consults	Anesthesia	Surgical Resident / Anes. Resident / Circulator for the case	Core Staff → / PCM (prn) / PACU Notified / Pathologist	Surgeon	→	Reach to Recovery (call early w/ bra size) / Assess need for HIR	
Meds/IV		IV access / Pre-op meds	Anesthesia drugs → / Ancef 1 gm	Pain meds prn IV / Antibiotic IV (if requested) / May D/C IV (if ordered)	Analgesic (IV, IM or PO)	PO analgesic	
Teaching/ D/C Plan	Procedure / Plan of care / VUMC orientation / Consent signed	Reinforce pre-op teaching / Support to family • waiting room infor. • update phone call / Support to pt. • answer questions • comfort		Volurex →	TCDB / Request pain med if not PCA / Assess home situation/primary care giver	Drain care (empty, reactivate, record output & change dressing q d) / Request pain med	Post mastectomy teaching / Exercises / How to take care of arm / F/U Reach to Recovery / Review drain care, meds, activity, reportable S/Sx, precautions / Complete "patient discharge list" sheet
Patient Flow	H&P MD office / Labs: Pre adm testing / CXR: Radiology / EKG: Heart Station	HR → To OR suite →		→ PACU	9S		
Equipment & Supplies		IV start kit / Anes. supplies / X-ray folder on bed	Case cart / Bovie / Padded armboard / OR supplies / JP drains x 2 / PACU stretcher	Respirator equipment	IMED		Schedule F/U 5-7 days post op to remove drains

Mastectomy Modified Radical
6/3/94
General Surgery 1

© 1994 Vanderbilt University Medical Center. All rights reserved.

FIGURE 17–10 Clinical pathway for modified radical mastectomy.

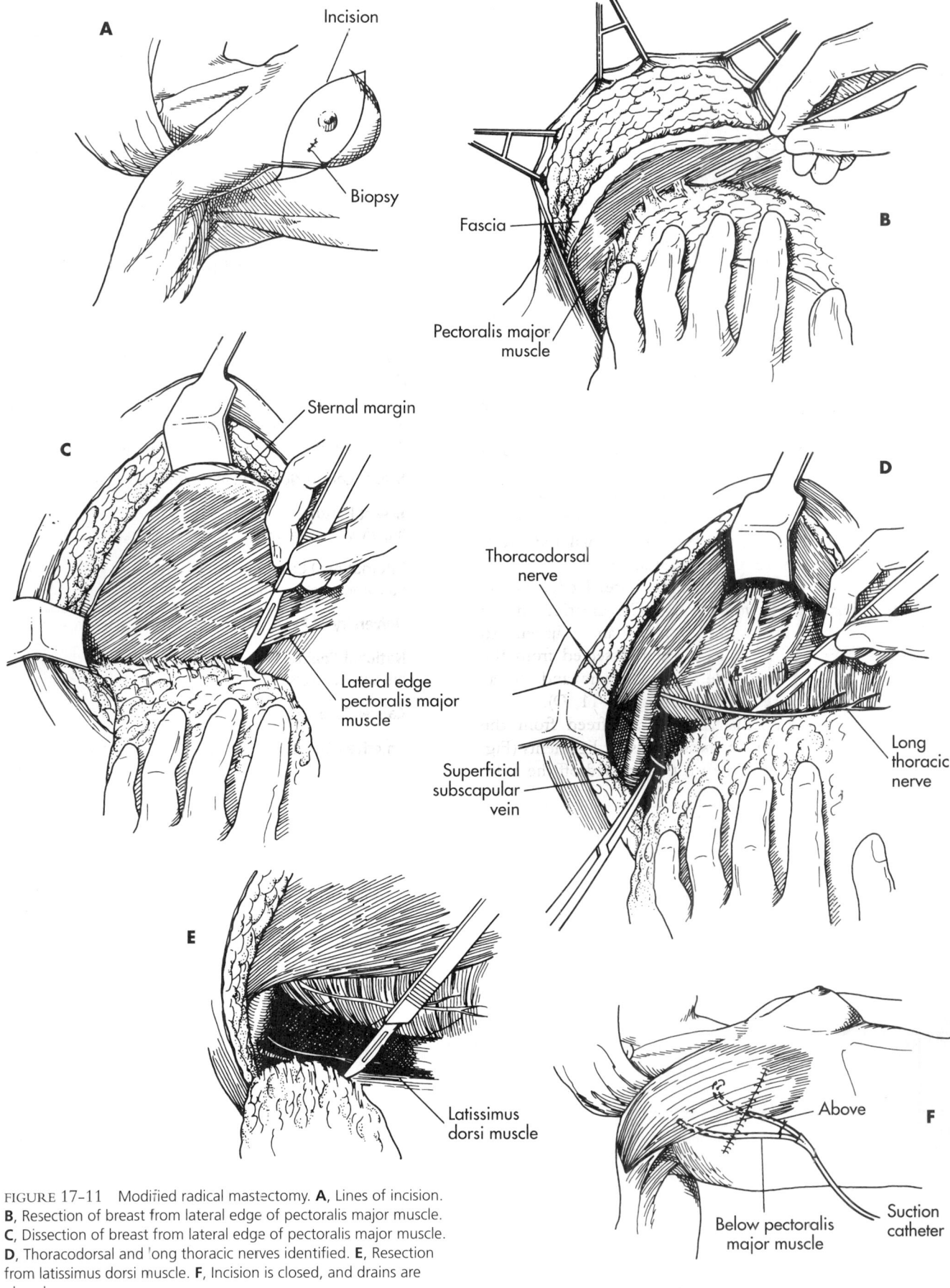

FIGURE 17-11 Modified radical mastectomy. **A,** Lines of incision. **B,** Resection of breast from lateral edge of pectoralis major muscle. **C,** Dissection of breast from lateral edge of pectoralis major muscle. **D,** Thoracodorsal and long thoracic nerves identified. **E,** Resection from latissimus dorsi muscle. **F,** Incision is closed, and drains are placed.

padded armboard. The skin is prepped and draped as previously described.

Operative procedure

1. An oblique elliptic incision with a lateral extension toward the axilla is made through the subcutaneous tissue (see Fig. 17-11, *A*). The bleeding points are controlled with hemostats and ligatures or electrocoagulation.
2. The skin is undercut in all directions to the limits of the dissection by means of a #3 knife handle with a #10 blade and curved scissors. Knife blades need to be changed frequently to ensure precise dissection.
3. The margins of the skin flaps are covered with warm, moist laparotomy pads and held away with retractors. The fascia and breast are resected from the pectoralis major muscle (Fig. 17-11, *B*) starting near the clavicle and extending down to the midportion of the sternum. The pectoralis muscle is left intact.
4. The intercostal arteries and veins are clamped and ligated.
5. The axillary flap is retracted for a complete dissection of the axilla. Careful attention is directed to preventing injury to the axillary vein and medial and lateral nerves of the pectoralis major muscle.
6. The fascia is dissected from the lateral edge of the pectoralis muscle (Fig. 17-11, *C*). Ligation of the vessels is preferred in the axilla and adjacent to the sternum. The fascia is then dissected from the serratus anterior muscle. The thoracic and thoracodorsal nerves are preserved (Fig. 17-11, *D*).
7. The breast and axillary fascia are freed from the latissimus dorsi muscle and suspensory ligaments (Fig. 17-11, *E*). The specimen is then passed off the field.

8. The surgical area is inspected for bleeding sites, which are ligated and electrocoagulated. The wound is irrigated with normal saline. Closed-wound suction catheters are inserted into the wound through stab wounds and secured to the skin with a nonabsorbable suture on a cutting needle (Fig. 17-11, *F*).
9. A few absorbable sutures may be used in the subcutaneous tissue to approximate the skin edges. The incision is closed with interrupted nonabsorbable sutures or staples.
10. The dressing can be a simple gauze dressing, a bulky dressing held in place by a Surgi-Bra, or a gauze or elastic bandage wrap.

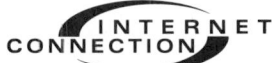

Komen Breast Cancer Foundation:
http://www.breastcancerinfo.com

Breast Cancer Network: http://www.cancer.orgbcn/bcn.html

Breast Lecture:
http://www.biostat.wisc.edu/surgery/wolberg/breast.html

International Cancer Information Center:
http://cancernet.nci.nih.gov

University of Pennsylvania: http://oncolink.upenn.edu/

National Coalition for Cancer Survivorship:
http://www.access.digex.net/~mkragen/

Cancer Care, Inc.: http://www.cancercareinc.org/

American Cancer Society: http://www.cancer.org

CHAPTER EIGHTEEN

Ophthalmic Surgery

Maryann Skasko Mawhinney

FIFTY YEARS AGO ophthalmic surgery was confined mainly to the eyelids and intracapsular cataract extraction that required bedrest, a prolonged hospital stay, and thick "cataract" glasses. During the last decade ophthalmic surgery, like other surgical specialties, has expanded its horizons dramatically. Today innovative developments use laser applications to reshape the cornea, endoscopy for oculoplastic procedures, topical anesthesia and no-stitch techniques with foldable intraocular lenses for cataract extraction, and fiberoptics and microsurgical technology for vitreoretinal procedures. These advances in surgical techniques and improved anesthetics, along with increasing pressures to contain healthcare costs, have created another major change in the management of patients who undergo ophthalmic surgery. Except for a small percentage of patients who have complex procedures or medical problems that contraindicate early discharge, patients today who have eye surgery do so on an ambulatory basis.

The perioperative nurse who assists in the care of the ophthalmic patient must combine the art and science of nursing with up-to-date knowledge and finely tuned, highly technologic skills. Therefore preoperative preparation and, in most cases, discharge teaching occur in a limited period and is coordinated by the perioperative nursing team. The success of the surgical intervention depends, to a degree, on the knowledge and skill of that team as they develop and implement a perioperative plan of care. Recent studies examined during the development of Clinical Practice Guidelines for Cataract in Adults[2] support the important role the surgical team plays in positive outcome attainment. The increasing emphasis on shorter stays even in the ambulatory setting has increased the need for patient and family education and the demand for providing quality care with a more cost–effective approach to using resources. Some ambulatory surgery settings have implemented primary nursing[5] and case management through the use of clinical pathways.[12]

SURGICAL ANATOMY

A working knowledge of the anatomic structures involved in ophthalmic surgery is necessary to facilitate selection of instrumentation and equipment for the procedure. The surgical team must also use this knowledge to understand the surgeon's plan of treatment and prepare the patient appropriately.

Bony Orbit

The two orbital cavities are situated on either side of the midvertical line of the skull between the cranium and the skeleton of the face. Above each orbit are the anterior cranial fossa and the frontal sinus; medially, the nasal cavity; below, the maxillary sinus; and laterally, from behind forward, the middle cranial and temporal fossae.

The seven bones that form the orbit are the maxilla, palatine, frontal, sphenoid, zygomatic, ethmoid, and lacrimal bones (Fig. 18-1). The margins of the bony orbit may be divided into four continuous parts: supraorbital, lateral, infraorbital, and medial.

The orbit can be considered a four-sided pyramid, with its base directed forward, laterally, and slightly downward and its apex facing posterior. The periosteum of the orbital walls is continuous with the dura mater. The orbit is essentially a socket for the eyeball and the muscles, nerves, and vessels necessary for proper functioning of the eye.

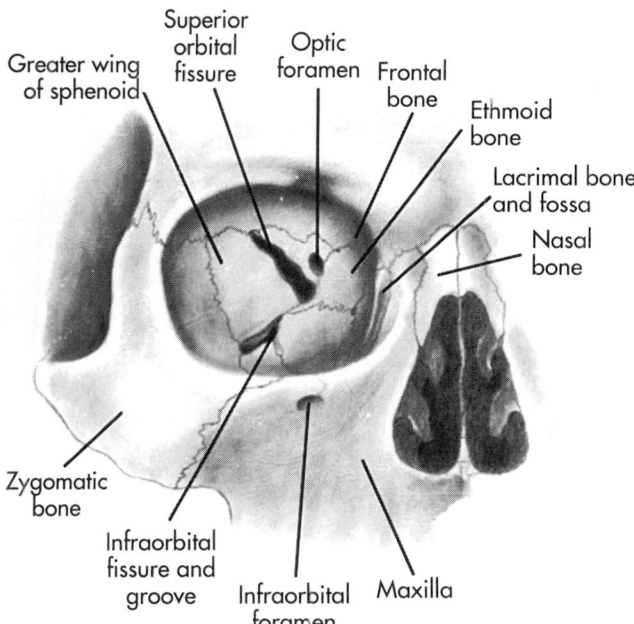

FIGURE 18-1 Bony orbital cavity.

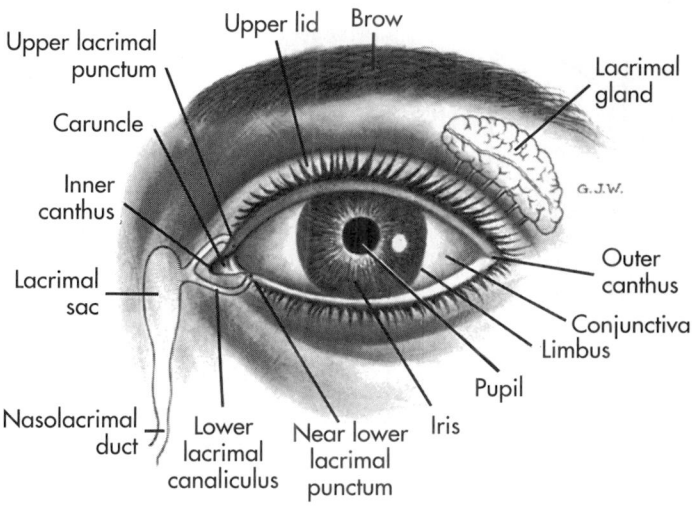

FIGURE 18-2 Lacrimal apparatus, external view.

The orbit is also a distribution center for certain vessels and nerves that supply the facial areas around the orbital aperture.

Lacrimal Apparatus

The lacrimal apparatus consists of the lacrimal gland and its ducts, the lacrimal passages, the lacrimal canaliculi and sac, and the nasolacrimal duct. The lacrimal gland produces tears and secretes them through a series of ducts into the conjunctival sac. The tears then make their way inward to the puncta, from which they are conducted by the canaliculi to the lacrimal sac and finally pass into the nasolacrimal duct. When the lacrimal glands secrete too profusely, the normal drainage process becomes insufficient and overflow tearing results (Fig. 18-2).

Conjunctiva and Eyelids

The conjunctiva is a thin, transparent mucous membrane divided into a palpebral and a bulbar part (Fig. 18-3). The palpebral portion lines the back surface of the eyelids and contains the openings (puncta) of the lacrimal canaliculi, which establish a passageway between the conjunctival sac and the inferior meatus of the nose. The bulbar part of the conjunctiva lines the front surface of the globe, allowing the sclera, or white of the eye, to show through. The central portion of the bulbar conjunctiva is continuous at the limbus with the anterior epithelium of the cornea.

The conjunctiva forms a sac (conjunctival sac) that is open in front. The opening is called the *palpebral fissure* and is located between the margins of the two eyelids. When the eye is closed, the fissure becomes a mere slit, and the cornea is completely covered by the upper eyelid.

The eyelids are two movable musculofibrous folds in front of each orbit that protect the globe and the eye from light. The upper eyelid is more mobile and larger than the lower. The upper and lower lids meet at the medial and lateral angles (canthi) of the eye. The eyelids are closed by the orbicularis oculi muscle, which is a circular muscle that acts as a sphincter. When the fibers contract, the eyes close. The upper lid is opened by the levator muscle, which is innervated by the third cranial nerve, as well as by relaxation of the orbicular muscle.

Each eyelid consists of several layers. From front to back these are the skin, subcutaneous tissue that contains the lymphatics, and muscles. Dense fibrous tissue, called *tarsal cartilage*, forms the framework of the lids. The tarsus is anchored to the walls of the orbit by the medial and lateral palpebral ligaments.

The free margins of each eyelid possess two or three rows of hairs called *cilia*, or *eyelashes*. Posterior to the lashes is a row of glandular orifices of the meibomian glands. Near the medial edges the free margin of each eyelid presents an opening called the *punctum lacrimale*. The eyelids distribute all lacrimal secretions, thereby keeping the cornea moist and washing away any dust.

Muscles

The extrinsic ocular muscles of the eyeball are the four rectus and two oblique muscles. These six striated muscles are inserted into the sclera by tendons. Except for the inferior oblique muscle, they arise from the back of the orbit. All the muscles are supplied by cranial nerves: third (oculomotor), fourth (trochlear), and sixth (abducens). The muscles work in pairs. Movements of the eyes are brought about by an increase in the tone of one set of muscles and a decrease in the tone of the antagonistic muscles. According to the position of the rectus muscles on the eyes, they are referred to as the superior rectus, inferior rectus, medial rectus, and lateral rectus. The oblique muscles insert on the back of the eye and are designated the superior oblique and inferior oblique (see Fig. 18-3).

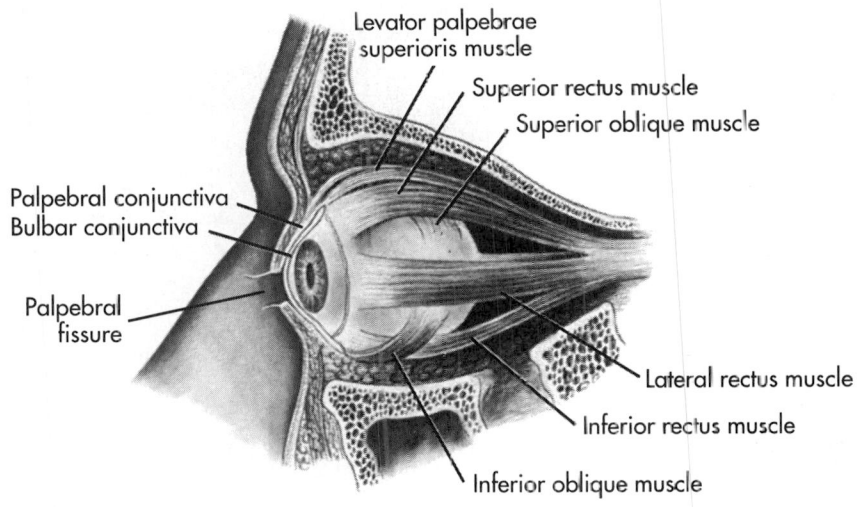

FIGURE 18-3 Diagrammatic section of orbit. Medial rectus muscle is located on nasal side of globe.

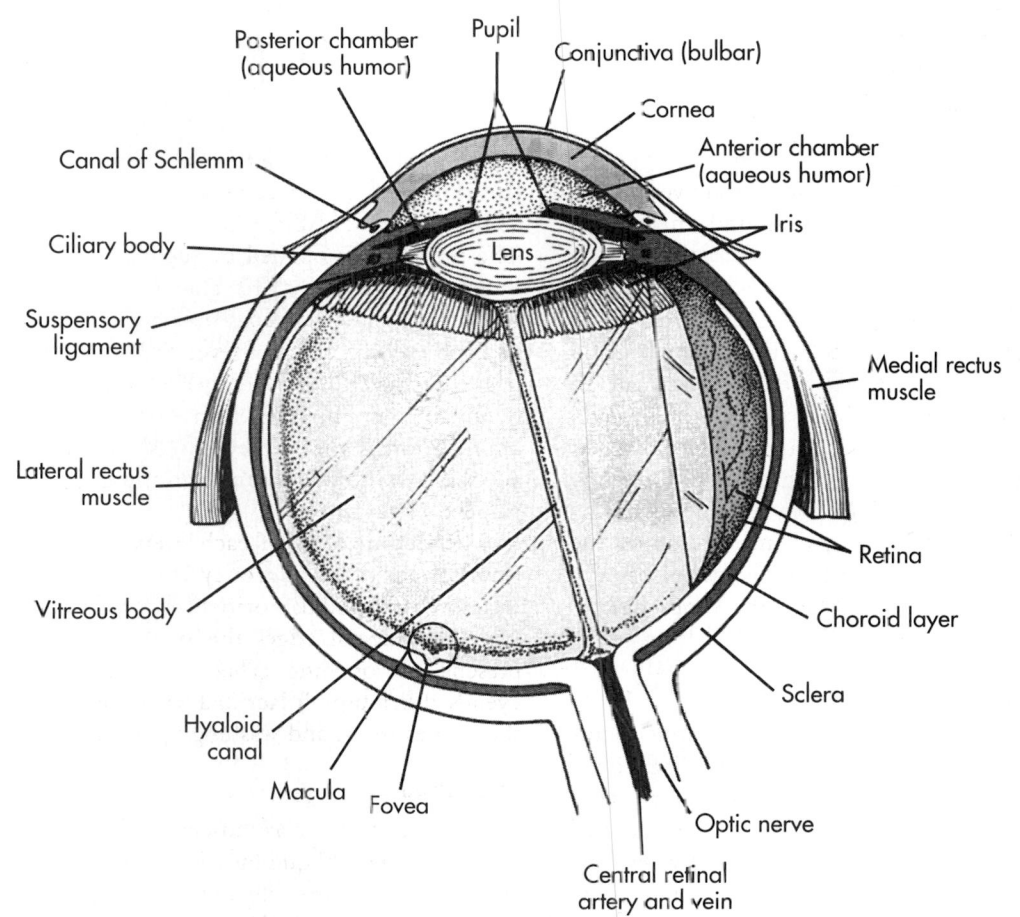

FIGURE 18-4 Horizontal section through left globe.

Globe

The eyeball (globe) is supported in the orbital cavity on a cushion of fat and fascia. It is composed of three layers surrounding a fluid-filled center and occupies less than one third of the orbit. The external, corneoscleral layer is fibrous and protects the other two; the middle, vascular, pigmented layer comprises the iris, ciliary body, and choroid; and the internal layer is the sensory retina. The fluid contents, which give the eye its globular shape, are aqueous humor (anterior) and vitreous humor (posterior to the lens). The lens, suspended behind the pupillary opening of the iris, and the cornea, combined with the aqueous and vitreous, form the refractive media of the eye (Fig. 18-4).

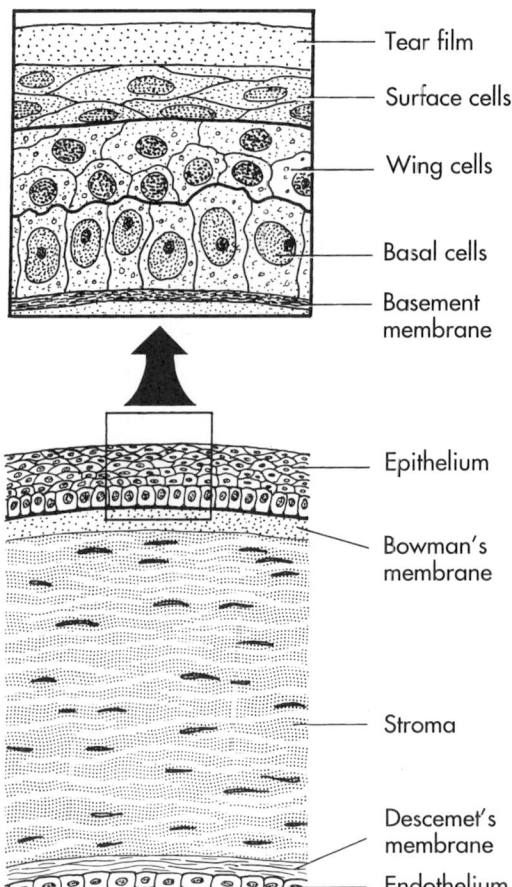

Tear film
Surface cells
Wing cells
Basal cells
Basement membrane
Epithelium
Bowman's membrane
Stroma
Descemet's membrane
Endothelium

FIGURE 18-5 Cornea is composed of five layers: the epithelium, Bowman's membrane, stroma, Descemet's membrane, and endothelium. *Small inset*, Layers of epithelium.

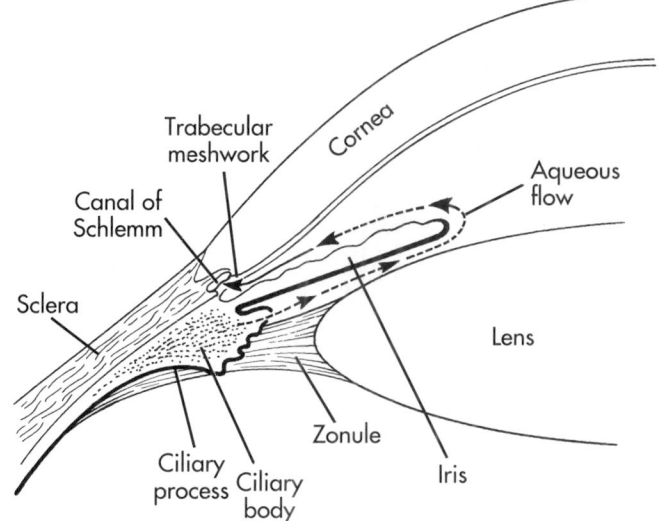

Trabecular meshwork
Cornea
Canal of Schlemm
Aqueous flow
Sclera
Lens
Ciliary process
Ciliary body
Zonule
Iris

FIGURE 18-6 Diagrammatic section of anterior chamber, ciliary body, and aqueous circulation.

External layer (corneoscleral)

The *cornea* is the anterior, transparent, avascular part of the external layer. It is crescent shaped and joins the sclera at a transitional zone called the *limbus*. The cornea serves as a window through which light rays pass to the retina. The branches of the ophthalmic division of the fifth cranial nerve supply the cornea.

The cornea is composed of five layers: the epithelium, Bowman's membrane, stroma, Descemet's membrane, and endothelium (Fig. 18-5). The epithelium consists of five constantly renewing cell layers and many nerve endings, which account for corneal sensitivity. Bowman's membrane is composed of connective tissue fibers and forms a barrier to trauma and infection. If damaged, it does not regenerate, and a permanent scar is left. The stroma accounts for 90% of the corneal thickness and is composed of multiple lamellar fibers. Descemet's membrane is a thin layer between the endothelial layer of the cornea and the substantia propria. This membrane may become inflamed (descemetitis) or may protrude (descemetocele). The endothelium is a single layer of hexagonal cells that do not regenerate. These cells are responsible for the proper state of dehydration (deturgescence) that keeps the cornea clear. Damage to these cells causes corneal edema and loss of transparency.

The *sclera* is the posterior opaque part of the external layer. A portion of the sclera can be seen through the conjunctiva as the white of the eye. The sclera is made up of collagenous fibers loosely connected with fascia, which receives the tendons of the muscles of the globe. The sclera is pierced by the ciliary arteries and nerves and posteriorly by the optic nerve (see Fig. 18-4).

Middle layer

The middle covering of the eye comprises the choroid, ciliary body, and iris from behind forward. The choroid contains many blood vessels and is the main source of nourishment of the receptor cell and pigment epithelial layer of the retina (see Fig. 18-4).

The *ciliary body* consists of an extension of the choroidal blood vessels, a mass of muscle tissue, and an extension of the neuroepithelium of the retina (Fig. 18-6). It extends 6 to 6.5 mm from the root of the iris to the ora serrata. The anterior 2 mm of the ciliary body is called the *pars plicata*, and the posterior 4 to 5 mm is the *pars plana* (Fig. 18-7). The ciliary muscle effects accommodation. The neuroepithelium is secretory in nature and is responsible for the formation of the aqueous humor.

The *iris*, a thin membrane, is the anterior portion of the middle layer and is situated in front of the lens. The peripheral border of the iris is attached to the ciliary body, whereas its central border is free. The iris aperture is located slightly nasal to its center, known as the *pupil* (see Fig. 18-4). The iris divides the space between the cornea and the lens into an anterior and a posterior chamber. Both chambers are filled with aqueous humor.

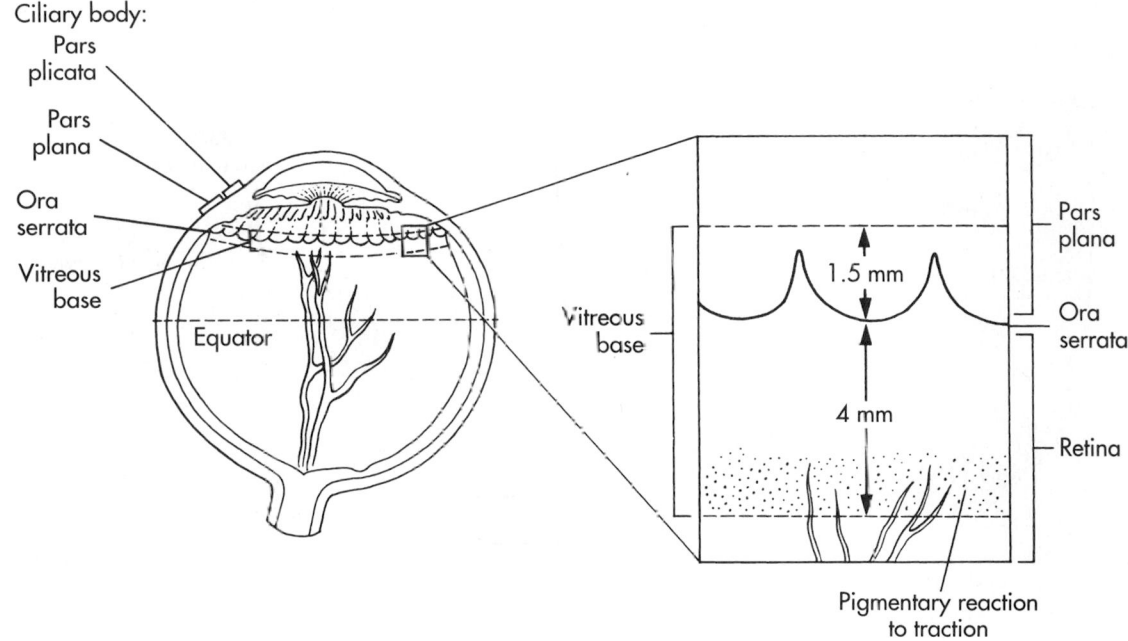

FIGURE 18-7   Location of the pars plicata, the pars plana, and the ora serrata.

The iris with its many striations regulates the amount of light entering the eye and assists in obtaining clear images. The iris moves by means of smooth muscle fibers within the connective tissue. The sphincter pupillae muscle contracts the pupil, and the dilator pupillae dilates it. As more light strikes the eye, the sphincter constricts the pupil.

Internal layer

The innermost layer, sometimes called the *nervous covering*, is the retina, a thin transparent membrane extending from the ora serrata to the optic disk (see Figs. 18-7 and 18-8). This network of nerve cells and fibers receives images of external objects and transfers the impression through the optic nerve, optic tracts, lateral geniculate body, and optic radiations to the occipital lobe of the cerebrum. The nerve fibers from the retina converge to become the optic nerve, which enters the eyeball almost at its posterior point, slightly to the inner side. The point at which the nerve enters the eyeball is called the *optic disk*. In field testing this is the anatomic blind spot.

The retina is composed of many layers. The pigment epithelium is a single layer of epithelial cells on the external side of the retina through which oxygen and other nutrients are diffused from the choroid. The other nine layers of the retina consist of photoreceptor cells (rods and cones) and sensory neurons (bipolar cells and ganglion cells) (Fig. 18-9). The photoreceptors within the retina respond to light energy and initiate the neural response, which is eventually interpreted in the occipital cortex.

The macula lutea shows as a yellow spot in the center of

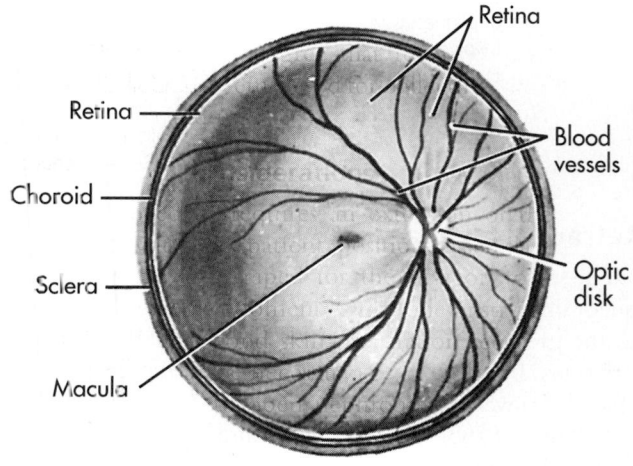

FIGURE 18-8   Normal fundus of eye seen through ophthalmoscope.

the retina located 2 mm from the optic disk. The foveal centralis, which is a pit consisting of a layer of closely packed cone cells in the center of the macula, is responsible for the highest resolution and central vision.

An inverted image of the object being viewed is focused on the retina. The nerve fibers leaving the retina by the way of the optic nerve travel to the lateral geniculate body of the thalamus. The fibers nasal to the foveal pit cross in the optic chiasma to go to the contralateral geniculate body. Thus all fibers composing the same half of the visual field project to the same geniculate body, from which fibers project to the ipsilateral occipital cortex for interpretation (Fig. 18-10).

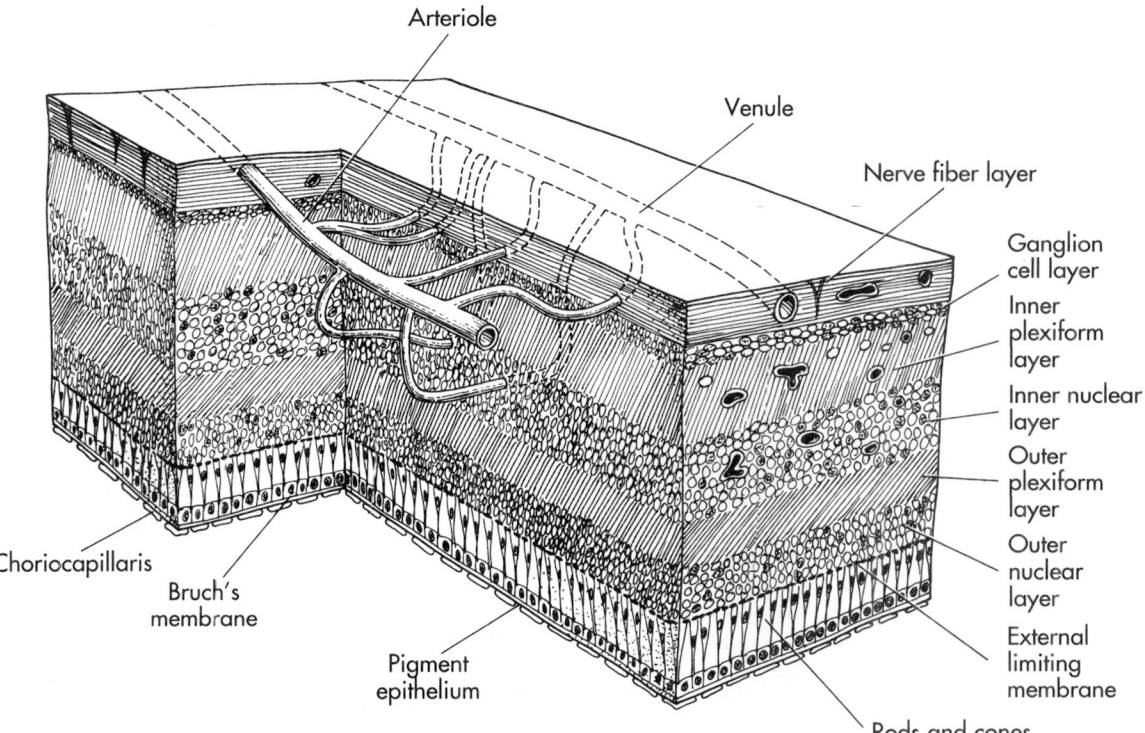

FIGURE 18-9   Retinal layers. Retinal arterioles provide two major capillary layers in retina: one in nerve fiber layer and one in inner nuclear layer. In general, diseases affecting primarily arteries, such as vascular hypertension, involve capillary network in nerve fiber layer, whereas predominantly venous diseases, such as diabetes mellitus, involve layer of capillaries in inner nuclear layer. Outer receptors, together with their cell bodies in outer nuclear layer and portion of outer plexiform layer, are nurtured by choriocapillaris of the choroid. Both systems are necessary to function of retina.

Refractive Apparatus

The refractive apparatus consists of the cornea, the aqueous humor, the lens, and the vitreous body. The *cornea* has the greatest refractive power of the ocular structures. Variations in the curvature of the cornea change its refractive power (Fig. 18-11).

The *lens* of the eye is biconvex and has a diameter of 1 cm. It is suspended behind the iris and connected to the ciliary body by zonular fibers (see Fig. 18-6). Its anterior and posterior surfaces are separated by a rounded border, the equator. The crystalline lens does not shed cells. As it grows, the cells are compressed and harden. The lens can expand and retract by means of the zonular fibers (accommodation); this accommodative power is lost with the aging process, as the lens loses its elasticity when the cells harden. This visual defect, known as *presbyopia*, usually occurs between ages 40 and 45 and is corrected with bifocals. Eventually the hardening causes opacity of the lens—a cataract.

The *vitreous body* is a glasslike, transparent, gelatinous mass composed of 99% water and 1% collagen and hyaluronic acid. It fills the posterior four fifths of the eyeball and is adherent to the retina at the vitreous base.

The central components of a light wave enter the eyes perpendicularly, and a light wave enters at the sides obliquely. For clear vision the oblique rays must converge and come to a focus with the central rays on the retina. Light rays from an object pass through the system of refractory devices—the cornea, aqueous humor, lens, and vitreous—and are refracted so that the rays strike the macular area.

Nerve and Blood Supply

The optic nerve (second cranial nerve) extends between the posterior eyeball and the optic chiasma. This nerve carries visual impulses, as well as the sensations of pain, touch, and temperature, from the eye and its surrounding structures to the brain. The third cranial nerve (oculomotor) is the primary motor nerve to all rectus muscles except the lateral rectus, which is innervated by the sixth cranial nerve (abducens). The fourth cranial nerve (trochlear) innervates the superior oblique muscle.

The ophthalmic artery, the main arterial supply to the orbit and globe, is a branch of the internal carotid artery. It divides into branches supplying the globe, muscles, and eyelids. The central retinal artery and central retinal vein travel through the optic nerve and provide an independent circulation for the inner retina.

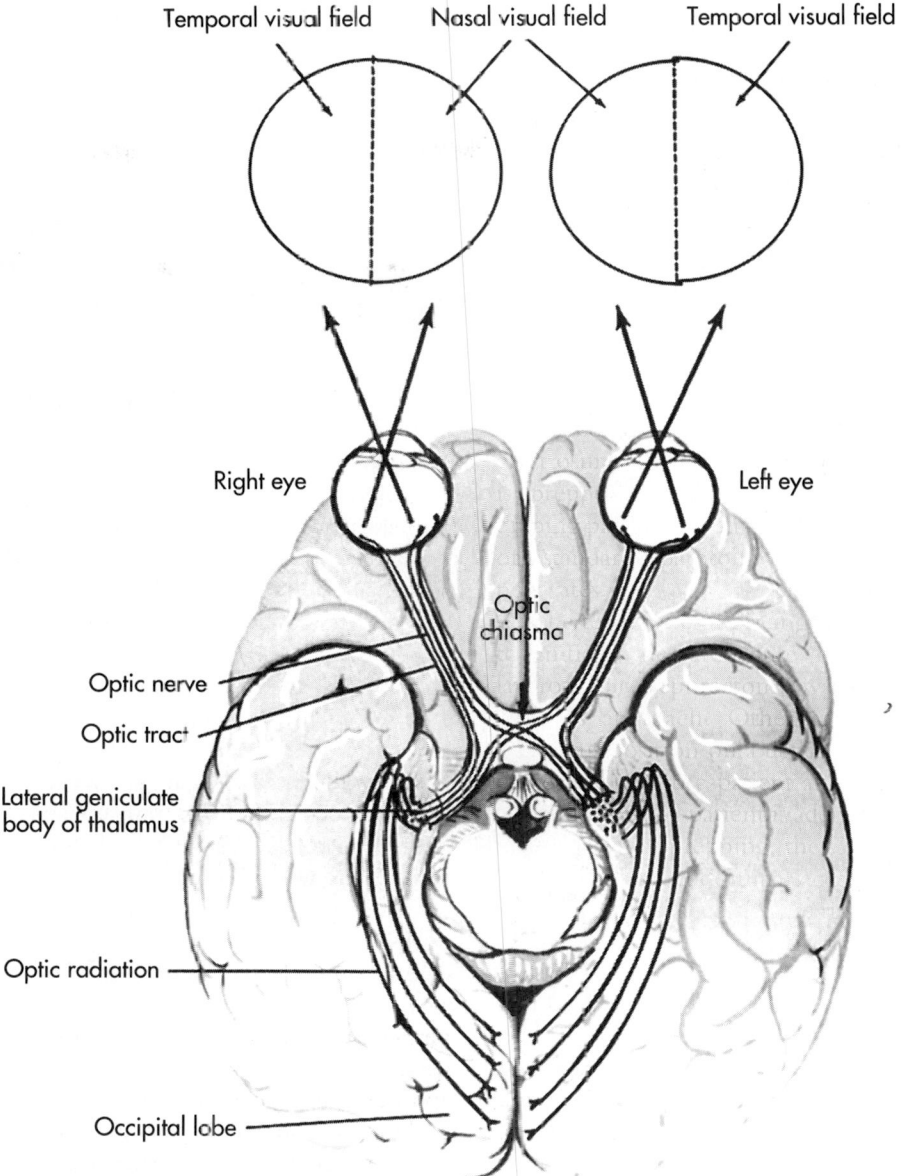

Temporal visual field   Nasal visual field   Temporal visual field

Right eye

Left eye

Optic chiasma

Optic nerve

Optic tract

Lateral geniculate body of thalamus

Optic radiation

Occipital lobe

FIGURE 18-10 Visual pathways. Notice structures that compose each pathway: optic nerve, optic chiasma, lateral geniculate body of thalamus, optic radiations, and visual cortex of occipital lobe. Fibers from nasal portion of each retina cross over to opposite side at optic chiasma, hence terminating in lateral geniculate body of opposite side. Location of lesion in visual pathway determines resulting visual defect. For example, destruction of an optic nerve produces permanent blindness in same eye, and pressure on optic chiasma (by pituitary tumor, for example) produces bitemporal hemianopsia, or, more simply, blindness in both temporal visual fields because it destroys fibers from nasal sides of both retinas.

PERIOPERATIVE NURSING CONSIDERATIONS

Assessment

Patients entering the hospital or ambulatory surgery center for eye surgery exhibit many emotions and reactions, such as hostility, anger, fear, grief, and helplessness. Of prime concern to most is the success of the surgical procedure. Patients undergoing eye surgery vary from infants with congenital conditions to geriatric patients whose conditions are a result of the aging process. With the increase in ambulatory surgery, the perioperative nursing staff must be prepared to not only meet the specific needs of each patient when providing care but also prepare the patient for home care.

Preparation is begun in the physician's office or clinic. Communication with the physician's office to coordinate patient preparation and teaching increases the efficiency and effectiveness of preoperative procedures.

On the patient's admission to the ambulatory surgery

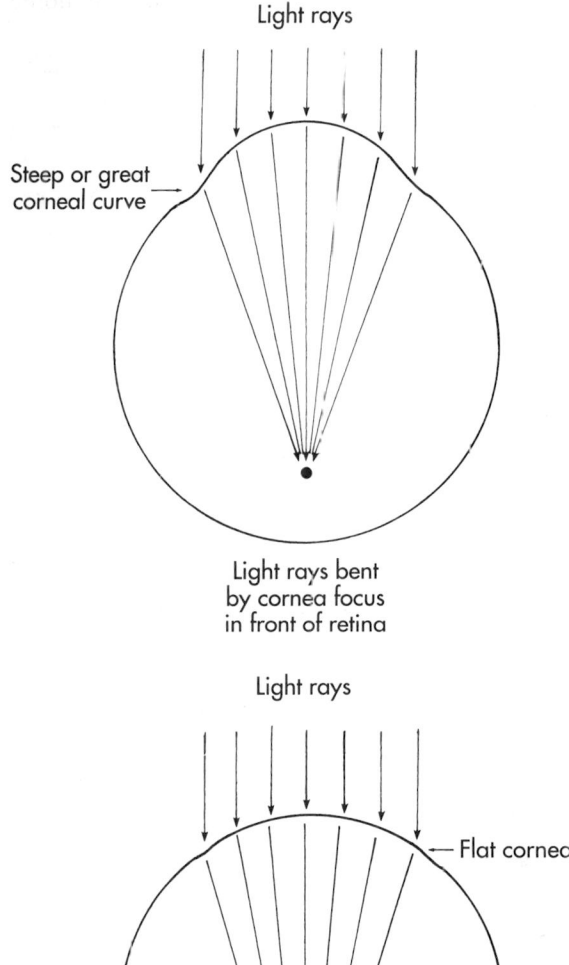

Light rays

Steep or great corneal curve →

Light rays bent by cornea focus in front of retina

Light rays

← Flat cornea

Light rays do not bend as much with flat cornea, therefore focus on retina

FIGURE 18-11 Variations in the curvature of the cornea change its refractive power.

unit or to the preoperative area, a staff member should fully orient the patient to the physical surroundings. Constant description and reinforcement are important to the visually impaired. Approaching the patient from the nonaffected side increases the patient's independence, facilitates care, and decreases the possibility of startling the patient. Most patients are no longer admitted to an inpatient nursing unit but are admitted through an ambulatory admission area adjacent to the surgical suites. This presents a challenge to all involved staff to collaborate and communicate effectively so that continuity of patient care is not jeopardized.

The nursing assessment is designed to collect and disseminate pertinent information and must be carried out in a comprehensive, yet efficient, manner. A standard set of parameters should provide enough information to facilitate appropriate care in the event of an emergency. The priority of data collection depends on the patient's condition. Biophysical information, including height, weight, and vital signs; biopsychosocial factors, which include support systems, fears, and anxiety; along with environmental, education, and self-care needs are assessed. The general health history includes current medication therapy and whether the patient has brought medications along. Because ocular problems may be directly related to other diseases, the medical history is very important. Additional discharge planning factors are also explored.

Data may be collected from family or significant others, or directly from physicians or their office staff. All information should be documented so that it is readily available to others. An ocular history, which includes the patient's primary problem, history of the present condition, nature of symptoms, and visual limitations imposed on the patient by the disease or condition, is collected. An external examination of the eye, including lids, lashes, conjunctiva, and lacrimal apparatus, should be performed to detect any deviations from normal. The corneal reflex should be tested and the cornea inspected for superficial irregularities. Pupil size and contour, as well as pupillary reaction, both direct and consensual, should be noted. Anterior chamber depth should be checked with oblique illumination to alert staff members to the potential for angle closure with dilatation of the pupil. When a light is shined from the side of the pupil, normal anterior chamber depth is determined if the entire iris is illuminated and the shallow anterior chamber is determined when half of the iris is in shadow.

The function of the extraocular muscles should be determined. Movement should be synchronous, and visual lines should meet on a fixed object. Documentation of this examination must be descriptive, accurate, and concise. It is of value later in assessing the outcome of the procedure. The following observations should be obtained or confirmed and recorded during perioperative nursing assessment:

- General appearance of the eye (edema, asymmetry, redness, condition of conjunctiva, sclera, and skin around eyes)
- Symptoms of irritation (itching, burning)
- Position of eyelids (opened and closed), condition of upper and lower lid surfaces, eyelid spasm
- Visual acuity, pupillary dilatation (notice whether pupils are equal, round, reactive to light, and accommodative), visual fields
- Extraocular muscle movement
- Drainage from eye
- Vital signs

- Restlessness, discomfort, anxiety
- Limitations in mobility, prosthesis
- Current and significant past medical problems (eye disease, diabetes, cardiovascular disease, hypertension, allergies)
- Current medication history

Laboratory studies

The results of laboratory studies, as applicable to the individual patient, should be reviewed during perioperative nursing assessment. Deviations from normal should be noted and recorded.

- Blood glucose (80 to 110 mg/dl) may be higher or lower depending on intake; critical levels are <50 or >400 mg/dl in adult males, and <40 or >400 mg/dl in adult females
- Serum potassium (adults and elderly: 3.5 to 5 mEq/L) and other electrolytes (calcium: total 9 to 10.5 mg/dl, ionized 4.5 to 5.6 mg/dl; sodium: 136 to 145 mEq/L)
- Serum enzymes and other blood work (CBC, coagulation studies)

Electrocardiogram and chest x-ray examination

In older adults, reports of prescribed chest x-ray examination and an ECG should be on the patient record. The older adult is more predisposed to respiratory infection from less elastic alveoli, decreased heart size unless there is enlargement associated with hypertension or heart disease, and ECG changes secondary to cellular alteration, conduction system fibrosis, and neurogenic changes.

After the assessment information has been compiled, nursing diagnoses are identified and the plan of care for the entire perioperative period is developed.

Nursing Diagnosis

Nursing diagnoses related to the care of patients undergoing ophthalmic surgery might include the following:

- Knowledge deficit related to diagnosis, surgical intervention, and home care management
- Anxiety related to vision loss, surgical intervention, awake status during surgical intervention, and surgical outcome
- Sensory and perceptual alteration related to visual impairment, surgical intervention, and patching of operative eye or both eyes
- Pain related to increased intraocular pressure, visual impairment, and surgical intervention
- Risk for infection related to surgical intervention

Outcome Identification

Outcomes identified for the selected nursing diagnoses could be stated as follows:

- Patient, family, or significant other will verbalize knowledge of the diagnosis, planned surgical intervention,

medication management, and requirements for home care maintenance before discharge.
- Patient will verbalize concerns and fears and utilize coping mechanisms.
- Patient will demonstrate ability to cope with visual sensory and perceptual alteration safely.
- Patient will remain comfortable during surgical intervention and will identify activities that increase intraocular pressure to be avoided during postoperative period
- Patient will be free from signs and symptoms of postoperative infection.

Planning

Care plans are the framework for organizing activities in the perioperative period. Although ophthalmic surgery is often perceived as minor because of the small incision site and because many procedures generally are not lengthy, the perioperative nurse must be fully prepared for potential complications or emergencies. Patients who are admitted for ophthalmic surgery often have complex medical histories. After a review of the patient record, supplemented by a patient or family interview or collaboration with colleagues, data collected are incorporated into a perioperative plan for patient care. A Sample Care Plan for the patient undergoing ophthalmic surgery is on p. 642.

Implementation

Managing and monitoring patient safety needs

Since many ophthalmic procedures are performed under local anesthesia, the circulating nurse or an additional perioperative nurse must be prepared to monitor the patient and provide supportive care. Reassurance is especially important for patients whose eyes will be patched postoperatively. Ophthalmic patients, like other surgical patients, have increased sensitivity to noise and activities within the room. The room should be kept quiet and peaceful to decrease anxiety and increase cooperation, thereby reducing the need for heavy sedation.

Additional patient safety needs must also be managed by both scrub nurse and circulating nurse. Foreign substances must not be introduced intraocularly. Lint-free barriers should be used to create the sterile field on the instrument table. Gloved hands must be wiped with moistened gauze sponges to remove starch powder particles before the procedure begins. The portion of an instrument used in an intraocular wound should not be touched by gloved hands and debris should be cleansed from instruments with cellulose sponges. The entire surgical team must be knowledgeable about their roles and be prepared to function quickly in the event of a complication.

Members of the perioperative nursing team have several important responsibilities in the admission of the patient to the operating room and in the preparation of the room and the equipment. Technologic advances in ophthalmic surgery require that perioperative nurses have familiarity with equipment and check each piece carefully before the patient arrives in the operating room. The availability of

S A M P L E   C A R E   P L A N

Nursing Diagnosis: Knowledge deficit related to diagnosis, surgical intervention, and home care management

Outcome: Patient, family or significant other will verbalize knowledge of the diagnosis, planned surgical intervention, medication management, and requirements for home care maintenance before discharge.

Interventions:

Determine the patient's understanding of the diagnosis, the planned intervention, and the type of anesthesia to be administered.

Clarify misconceptions and provide additional explanations (or refer to appropriate member of health care team).

Explain sequence of perioperative events and what to expect in the operating room in terms that the patient can understand.

Review postoperative limitations to self-care activities.

Provide and review written instructions (in large letters) regarding medications, including specific techniques for instilling eyedrops and ophthalmic medications, applying compresses (as necessary), and applying appropriate eye dressing or protective shield.

Supervise patient practice with prescribed self-care activities (such as instillation of medications).

Nursing Diagnosis: Anxiety related to vision loss, surgical intervention, awake status during surgical intervention, and surgical outcome

Outcome: Patient will verbalize concerns and fears and utilize coping mechanisms.

Interventions:

Allow patient time to verbalize concerns.

Assist patient to identify sources of anxiety.

Help the patient identify existing personal strengths and external resources.

Encourage independence by allowing patient to assist with plan of care; involve patient in identifying diversional activities.

Observe the patient's facial expressions, body posture, and vital signs.

Broadly classify the patient's level of anxiety based on nursing observation (low, moderate, high).

Offer comfort measures (such as warm blankets).

Provide emotional support; reinforce information the patient has been previously given.

Use touch (as appropriate) to communicate reassurance.

Control environmental stimuli in the operating room.

Nursing Diagnosis: Sensory and perceptual alteration related to visual impairment, surgical intervention, and patching of operative eye or both eyes

Outcome: Patient will demonstrate ability to cope with visual sensory and perceptual alteration safely.

Interventions:

Introduce self and other team members so that patient can recognize voices.

Familiarize and orient patient to immediate surroundings; continuously reorient patient.

Approach patient from unaffected side.

Offer reassurance, explanations, and understanding.

Before discharge, review and have patient list safety measures to prevent falls and other injuries.

Refer patient to appropriate agency if home assistance is required.

Nursing Diagnosis: Pain related to increased intraocular pressure, visual impairment, and surgical intervention

Outcome: Patient will remain comfortable during surgical intervention and will identify activities that increase intraocular pressure to be avoided during postoperative period.

Interventions:

Instruct patient to verbalize pain during procedure under local anesthesia or sedation.

Monitor the presence of or an increase in eye pain, pain around orbit, blurred vision, reddened eye, abdominal pain, nausea, vomiting, neurologic changes, and changes in visual fields; initiate appropriate action.

Instruct the patient to refrain from excessive exertion, such as crying, coughing, straining, overlifting, bending, rubbing the eyes, and blowing the nose.

Discuss methods to facilitate bowel elimination (diet, appropriate exercise, stool softeners if prescribed).

Nursing Diagnosis: Risk for infection related to surgical intervention

Outcome: Patient will be free from signs and symptoms of postoperative infection.

Interventions:

Preoperatively notice whether the patient has a preexisting infection, is immunocompromised, or has other conditions that compromise resistance to infection.

Maintain an aseptic perioperative environment.

Adhere to good handwashing practices.

Determine and record the wound classification.

Postoperatively monitor vital signs, fluid balance, and presence of pain.

Instruct the patient in self-care, including postoperative antibiotic therapy, if prescribed.

Teach the patient to wash hands before the instillation of any ophthalmic medications.

Instruct the patient to watch for redness, pain, swelling, drainage, and changes in visual acuity postoperatively and to report these problems promptly to the physician.

specially ordered implants or prostheses needs to be checked to prevent delay or cancelation of the procedure.

Scrupulous attention to aseptic technique and perioperative nursing measures designed for safety and comfort of the patient are of prime importance. The duties of the perioperative nursing team include the following:

1. Identifying the patient by name, seeking patient cooperation and confidence by speaking softly, distinctly, and confidently, and endeavoring to keep the patient quiet and relaxed by staying close by and establishing contact by touch

2. Checking the patient's name on the wristband with the name on the chart and surgical schedule and orally confirming it with the patient

3. Reviewing the surgical consent, surgeon's preoperative orders, and nurses' notes to determine if the correct operative eye has been prepared (including verification of operative eye and dilatation, if appropriate) and other procedures have been carried out according to facility policies

4. Preparing the operating room bed and making sure all the necessary attachments are in readiness. Since patients may receive hyperosmotic drugs, which induce diuresis, have urinals, bedpans, and sterile urethral catheters available.

5. Starting an intravenous drip, placing the blood pressure cuff and pulse oximeter, recording the baseline blood pressure and heart rate, and attaching the cardiac monitor according to facility policy. When the patient is not managed with monitored anesthesia care (MAC), an oxygen cannula should be available for administration of oxygen if needed.

6. Observing laser safety precautions.

7. Documentation of care including recording of implants and lot numbers

Safety measures in administering medications

Medications used in the perioperative period are extremely important to the outcome of the procedure and the safety of the patient. Drugs for diagnosing and treating eye disorders are potent. One error could result in total, irreversible blindness.

The patient's medical and ocular histories determine the selection of an appropriate ophthalmic agent. This information should be included in the patient's initial nursing assessment. The perioperative nurse needs to be aware that mydriatic and cycloplegic eye drops are contraindicated in narrow-angle glaucoma.

The following established protocols for medication administration greatly reduce the possibility of medication errors:

1. The perioperative nurse must be knowledgeable about the specific medication ordered, including purpose, strength, action, duration, adverse reactions, route of administration, and contraindications.

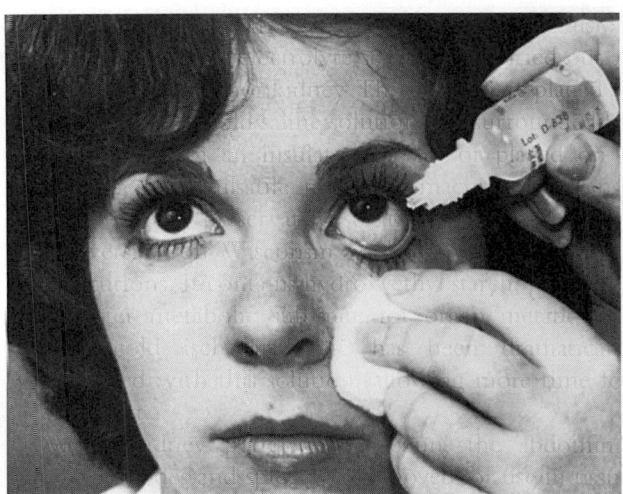

FIGURE 18-12   Proper position of head for installation of eyedrops. Gentle retraction of lower lid is necessary for drop to be placed in lower cul-de-sac.

2. The medication label must be checked for name, strength, and expiration date during preparation and before medication administration. This precaution is especially important because many ophthalmic drugs are distributed in single-dose units that closely resemble one another.

3. The patient must be positively identified, and the site of the administration must be clearly translated from the physician's orders. The abbreviations OD, OS, and OU indicate 'right eye', 'left eye', and 'both eyes' respectively.

4. The precise dosage of medication must be given at its scheduled time to enhance its effectiveness.

5. Hand washing between patients when administering eye drops is imperative, and standard precautions should be followed.

6. All solutions on the sterile field must be clearly labeled, and intraocular solutions must be separated from those not used intraocularly.

Instillation of eye drops

With the patient's face tilted upward and gentle retraction of the lower lid, the first drop is placed into the lower cul-de-sac (Fig. 18-12). The tip of any drug applicator must not touch the patient's skin or any part of the eye. The succeeding drops (prescribed number depends on the type of operation to be performed) may be placed from above, with the patient looking downward and the upper lid raised. Care should be taken to avoid placing eyedrops directly onto the cornea. The natural blinking of the lids distributes the drug evenly onto the eye surface, regardless of where the drop is placed.

After instillation of a systemic drug, such as atropine, hold light finger pressure over the lacrimal duct for 1 minute to prevent absorption into circulatory system. When a toxic drug is instilled, the inner corner of the eyelids should be dried of excessive fluid with a tissue or clean cotton ball after each drop to minimize systemic absorption of the drug.

The patient should be made aware of the expected effect of each medication to be able to evaluate its effectiveness, detect signs and symptoms of adverse reactions, and know when to notify the physician concerning problems. The patient should also be well informed of the special considerations associated with specific medications so that appropriate safety precautions can be taken. An example is protection of the cornea after application of a topical anesthetic. Selection of specific medication is influenced by the physician's education and experience and the patient's disease condition.

Ophthalmic pharmacology

Numerous medications are used during ophthalmic surgery. See Table 18-1 for the purpose and description of each.

Anesthesia

General Anesthesia

Youth, deafness, language barriers, dementia, severe anxiety, specific systemic diseases, known sensitivity to local anesthetics, and long duration of the operative procedure are among the conditions that may dictate use of general anesthesia.

Local Anesthesia

Local or local standby (MAC) anesthesia is preferred for most eye surgery. Consideration must be given to the patient's age, systemic condition, and discharge plan in determining whether to use preoperative sedation. Intraoperative sedation, when indicated, may be prescribed and managed by either the surgeon or the anesthesiologist. The perioperative nurse, however, is often accountable for monitoring the patient's response to the sedation and the local anesthetic in the perioperative period.

The circulating nurse assembles the sterile local anesthesia setup as required by the surgeon before the patient enters the operating room, checking to ensure correct medications, proper concentrations and dosages, and needles and syringes of appropriate sizes and gauges. Local anesthetics should not be mixed far in advance of the time of intended use because they may become deteriorated, and the reduced effect could result in discomfort for the patient. Epinephrine prolongs the duration of action of most local anesthetics.

Administration methods of local anesthesia

TOPICAL. The topical method is recently regaining popularity especially for cataract-extraction procedures. Combination of anesthetic drops are instilled into the eye and may be supplemented with infiltration anesthetic into the anterior chamber.

INFILTRATION. The surgeon injects the anesthetic solution beneath the skin, beneath the conjunctiva (subconjuncti-val), or into Tenon's capsule, depending on the type of surgery.

PERIBULBAR. Peribulbar anesthesia has replaced retrobulbar anesthesia as the preferred method. The anesthetic is injected around the soft tissue of the globe after the needle is directed to the floor (inferior) or roof (superior) of the orbit (Fig. 18-13).

RETROBULBAR. Retrobulbar block is injection of anesthetic solution into the base of the eyelids at the level of the orbital margins or behind the eyeball to block the ciliary ganglion and nerves (Fig. 18-14). For eyelid repairs the solution is injected through the upper or lower lid. For operations on the lacrimal apparatus the anesthetic is injected at the level of the anterior ethmoidal foramen to anesthetize the internal and external nasal nerves. Retrobulbar injection is usually performed 10 to 15 minutes before surgery to produce temporary paralysis of the extraocular muscles.

Positioning

Positioning the patient for ophthalmic surgery generally requires additional devices for stabilizing the head, protecting bony prominences, and providing appropriate alignment to prevent peripheral neurovascular injury. The safety needs of the patient are related to age, size, and risk factors for discomfort. If the patient is to be sedated, ask him if he is comfortable and reassure him that there are ways to make him more comfortable. Some elderly patients prefer to not discuss their discomfort for fear of being bothersome.[15]

In addition, since most ocular surgery is carried out with the use of a microscope, a special wrist rest is used to stabilize the surgeon's hands (Fig. 18-15) and may include a perforated tubing or bar to provide oxygen under the drapes. This should be attached to the bed and secured approximately 2.5 cm below the lateral canthus before the patient is draped. The wrist rest may be placed unilaterally or may encircle the head. A 1-inch strip of nonallergic tape may be placed over the patient's forehead and secured to the operative bed to prevent movement of the head.

Prepping

The operative site is prepared under aseptic conditions usually after the anesthetic is administered. A sterile prep tray containing sterile normal saline solution, irrigation bulb, basins, gauze sponges, cotton-tipped applicators, towels, and antimicrobial skin disinfectant is prepared.

The clipping of eyelashes or shaving of eyebrows is not usually done. When eyelashes are clipped, it is done before the skin preparation. A thin film of water-soluble lubricant is smoothed over the cutting surfaces of a curved eyelash scissors so that the free lashes adhere to the blades rather than fall into the eyes or onto the face.

Some surgeons now use drops of 5% povidone-iodine complex solution on the conjunctiva as part of the prep to remove surface microbes. One to two drops of the 5% povidone-iodine solution is placed onto the eye surface

TABLE 18-1 | Medications Used During Ophthalmic Surgery

DRUG/NAME	PURPOSE/DESCRIPTION
Mydriatic	
Phenylephrine (Neo-Synephrine, Mydfrin), 2.5%, 10%	Mydriasis (dilates the pupil but permits focusing), used for objective examination of the retina, testing of refraction, easier removal of lens; used alone or with a cycloplegic
Cycloplegics	
Tropicamide (Mydriacyl), 1%	Cycloplegia (paralysis of accommodation; inhibits focusing); dilates the pupil; anticholinergic, used for examination of fundus, refraction
Atropine, 1%	Anticholinergic, dilates pupil, inhibits focusing; potent, long duration (7 to 14 days)
Cyclopentolate (Cyclogyl), 1%, 2%	Anticholinergic, dilates pupil, inhibits focusing
Scopolamine hydrobromide, (Isopto-Hyoscine) 0.25%	Anticholinergic, dilates pupil, inhibits focusing
Homatropine hydrobromide (Isopto Homatropine), 2%, 5%	Anticholinergic, dilates pupil, inhibits focusing
Epinephrine (1:1000) preservative free (PF)	Dilates the pupil; added to bottles of balanced salt solution for irrigation to maintain pupil dilatation during cataract or vitrectomy procedure
Miotics	
Carbachol (Miostat), 0.01%	Potent cholinergic, constricts pupil, used intraocularly during anterior segment surgery
Carbachol (Isopto Carbachol), 0.75%, 1 5%, 2.25%, 3%	Potent cholinergic, constricts pupil, used topically for lowering intraocular pressure in glaucoma
Acetylcholine chloride (Miochol-E), 1%	Cholinergic, rapidly constricts pupil, used intraocularly during anterior-segment surgery, reconstitute immediately before using
Pilocarpine hydrochloride, 1%, 4%	Cholinergic, constricts pupil, used topically for lowering intraocular pressure in glaucoma
Topical Anesthetics	
Tetracaine hydrochloride (Pontocaine), 0.5%	*Onset:* 5-20 seconds; *duration of action:* 10-20 minutes
Proparacaine hydrochloride (Ophthaine), 0.5%	*Onset:* 5-20 seconds; *duration of action:* 10-20 minutes
Injectable Anesthetics	
Lidocaine (Xylocaine), 1%, 2%, 4%	*Onset:* 4-6 minutes; *duration of action:* 40-60 minutes, 120 minutes with epinephrine
Methylparaben free (MPF)	Preservative free; adjunct to topical anesthesia
Bupivacaine (Marcaine, Sensorcaine), 0.25%, 0.50%	*Onset:* 5-11 minutes; *duration of action:* 480-720 minutes with epinephrine; often used in 0.75% combination with lidocaine for blocks
Mepivacaine (Carbocaine), 1%, 2%	*Onset:* 3-5 minutes; *duration of action:* 120 minutes; duration of action greater without epinephrine
Etidocaine (Duranest), 1%	*Onset:* 3 minutes; *duration of action:* 300-600 minutes
Additives to Local Anesthetics:	
Epinephrine 1:50,000 to 200,000	Combined with injectable local anesthetics to prolong anesthesia and reduce bleeding
Hyaluronidase (Wydase)	Enzyme mixed with anesthetics (75 units per 10 ml) to increase diffusion of anesthetic through tissue, improving the effectiveness of the block; contraindicated if skin inflammation or malignancy present
Viscoelastics	
Sodium hyaluronate (Healon, Amvisc, Provisc, Vitrax) in a sterile syringe assembly with blunt-tipped cannula	Lubricant and support; maintains separation between tissues to protect the endothelium and maintain the anterior chamber intraocularly; removed from anterior chamber to prevent postoperative increase in pressure; should be refrigerated (except Vitrax); allow 30 minutes to warm to room temperature
Sodium chondroitin–sodium hyaluronate (Viscoat) in a sterile syringe assembly with blunt-tipped cannula	Maintains a deep chamber for anterior-segment procedures, protects epithelium of cornea, and enhances visualization; may be used to coat intraocular lens before implantation; should be refrigerated
Viscoadherent	
Hydroxypropyl methyl cellulose (Ocucoat) in a sterile syringe assembly with blunt-tipped cannula	Maintains a deep chamber for anterior-segment procedures, protects epithelium of cornea and may be used to coat intraocular lens before implantation; removed from anterior chamber at end of procedure; stored at room temperature

Continued

TABLE 18-1 | Medications Used During Ophthalmic Surgery—cont'd

DRUG/NAME	PURPOSE/DESCRIPTION
Irrigant	
Balanced Salt Solution (BSS, Endosol)	Used to keep cornea moist during surgery; also used as internal irrigant into anterior or posterior segment
Balanced Salt Solution enriched with Bicarbonate, Dextrose, and Glutathione (BSS Plus, Endosol Extra)	Used as internal irrigant into anterior or posterior segment; need to reconstitute immediately before use by addition of Part I to Part II with transfer device
Hyperosmotic Agents	
Mannitol (Osmitrol)	Intravenous osmotic diuretic; increases the osmolarity of the plasma, causing osmotic pressure gradient to pull free fluid from the eye to the plasma and reduces the intraocular pressure
Glycerin (Osmoglyn, Glyrol)	Oral osmotic diuretic given in chilled juice or cola; increases the osmolarity of the plasma, causing osmotic pressure gradient to pull free fluid from the eye to the plasma and reduces the intraocular pressure
Antiinflammatory Agents	
Betamethasone sodium phosphate and betamethasone acetate suspension (Celestone)	Glucocorticoid; injected subconjunctivally after surgery for prophylaxis; also used to treat severe allergic and inflammatory conditions
Dexamethasone (Decadron)	Adrenocortical steroid; inject subconjunctivally after surgery for prophylaxis; also used to treat severe allergic and inflammatory conditions and intraocularly for endophthalmitis
Methylprednisolone acetate suspension (Depo-Medrol)	Glucocorticoid; inject subconjunctivally after surgery for prophylaxis; also used to treat severe allergic and inflammatory conditions
Antiinfectives	
Polymyxin B/bacitracin (Polysporin ointment)	Topically to treat superficial ocular infections of the conjunctiva or cornea; prophylactically after surgery
Polymyxin B/neomycin/bacitracin (Neosporin ointment)	Topical treatment of superficial infections of the external eye; prophylactically after surgery
Tobramycin/dexamethasone (TobraDex)	Topical treatment or prevention of superficial infections of the external part of eye; also has antiinflammatory properties
Cefazolin (Ancef, Kefzol)	Prophylactically injected subconjunctivally after procedure; also topically, intraocularly, and systemically for endophthalmitis
Gentamicin sulfate (Garamycin)	Prophylactically injected subconjunctivally after procedure; also topically, subconjunctivally, and intraocularly for endophthalmitis
Ceftazidime (Fortaz, Tazicef, Tazadime)	Injected subconjunctivally and intraocularly for treatment of endophthalmitis
Miscellaneous	
Cocaine, 1% to 4%	Topical use, never injected; used on cornea to loosen epithelium before debridement and on nasal packing to reduce congestion of mucosa
5-Fluorouracil (5-FU)	Antimetabolite used topically to inhibit scar formation in glaucoma-filtering procedures; handle and discard in compliance with OSHA and facility policies for safe use of antineoplastics
Mitomycin (Mutamycin)	Antimetabolite used topically to inhibit scar formation in glaucoma-filtering procedures; handle and discard in compliance with OSHA and facility policies for safe use of antineoplastics
Tissue plasminogen activator (TPA) (Activase)	Thrombolytic agent; to treat fibrin formation in postvitrectomy patients; lysis of clots on retina
Fluorescein	Yellowish green fluorescence of this intravenous diagnostic aid is used in fluorescein angiography to diagnose retinal disorder
	Topical stain; fluorescein strip temporarily stains the cornea yellow-green in areas of denuded corneal epithelium
Timolol maleate (Timoptic)	Beta-adrenergic receptor blocking agent; treatment of elevated intraocular pressure in ocular hypertension or open-angle glaucoma
Acetazolamide sodium (Diamox)	Carbonic anhydrase inhibitor; given IV to decrease the secretion of aqueous humor and results in a drop in intraocular pressure; diuretic effect
Dextrose, 50%	Added to BSS Plus or Endosol Extra for diabetic patients during intraocular procedures

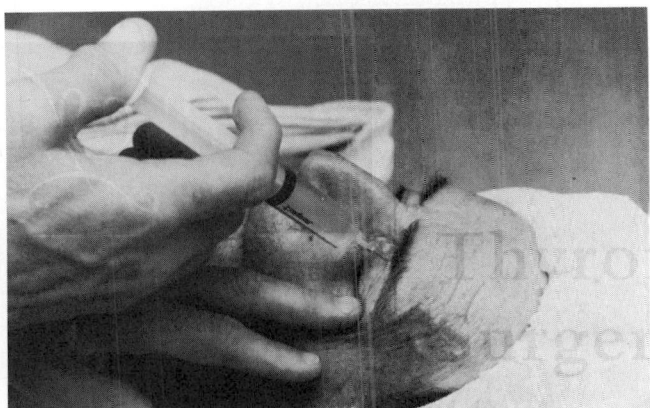

FIGURE 18-13   Peribulbar anesthesia.

before the prep of the face and eyelids. This 5% povidone-iodine solution is rinsed from the eye with normal saline.

Eye preparation includes cleansing the eyelids of the operative eye or eyes, lid margins, lashes, eyebrows, and surrounding skin with an appropriate antimicrobial solution. To clean the lid margins, evert the lids and clean with cotton-tipped applicators moistened with antimicrobial skin disinfectant (Fig. 18-16, *A*). Care is taken to prevent the solution from entering the patient's eyes and ears (Fig. 18-16, *B*). The eye or eyes are then irrigated with normal saline solution using an irrigating bulb (Fig. 18-16, *C*). When toxic chemicals or small particles of foreign matter must be removed, the eyes are irrigated with tepid sterile physiologic saline solution. The conjunctival sac is thoroughly flushed using an irrigation bulb or an Asepto syringe.

Draping

Special concerns for eye surgery draping include eliminating lint and fiber particles, water repellency, and providing adequate air exchange for patients receiving local anesthetics. To avoid placing handpieces on top of patients, a Mayo stand may be placed above the patient and incorporated into the draping process. The use of a one-piece disposable drape, with self-adherent, fenestrated plastic section for the eye, eliminates the need to lift the patient's head during draping and facilitates drape removal at the end of the procedure (see Fig. 18-15).

In an alternative method, (1) the head is draped with a double-thickness half-sheet and two towels, (2) a large sheet is used to cover the patient and operating room bed, and (3) a fenestrated plastic eye sheet is placed over the operative site (Fig. 18-17). A fluid drainage bag with wicking strip may also be adhered to the plastic eye sheet.

Instrumentation

Rapid progress in ophthalmic surgical techniques and instrumentation has contributed to almost unbelievable results for eye patients. Exacting performance of eye instruments is crucial to the success of operations.

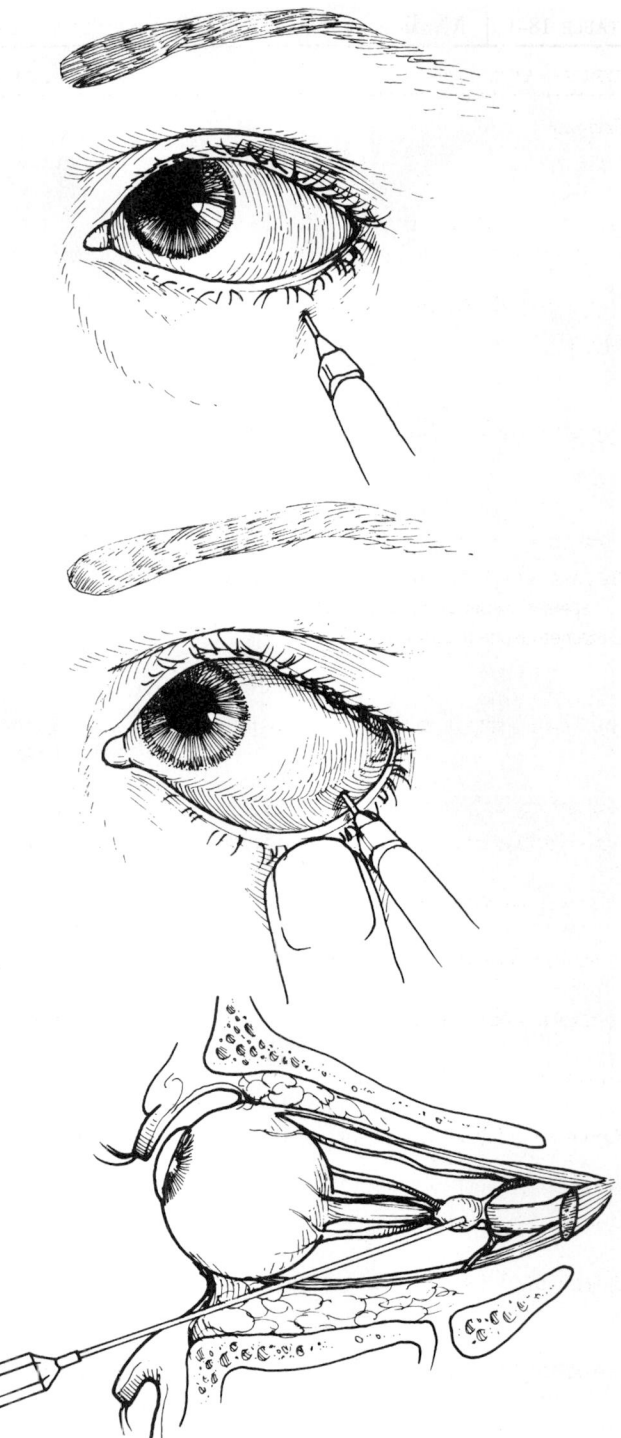

FIGURE 18-14   Retrobulbar block.

Basic eye instruments are shown in Fig. 18-18. Additional instruments, depending on the type of procedure, can be added to the basic instrument set. Special surface finishes are used to reduce light reflection. Instruments are designed with round handles for smoother motion and rotation under the microscope. Instruments routinely needed for the type of operation and each

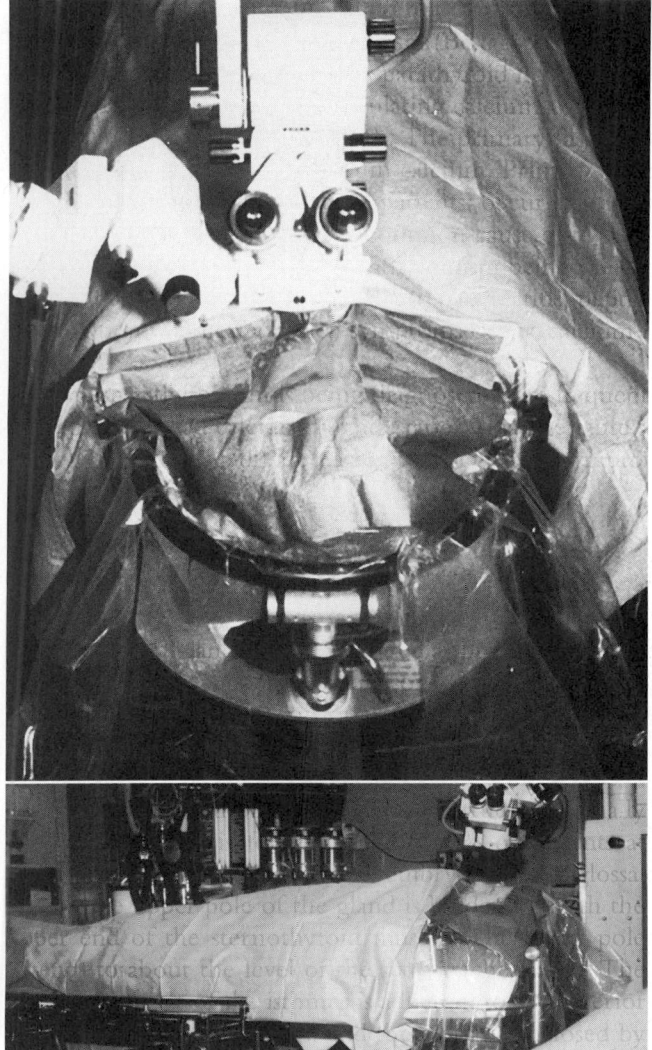

FIGURE 18-15 One-piece disposable drape with Chan wrist rest in place.

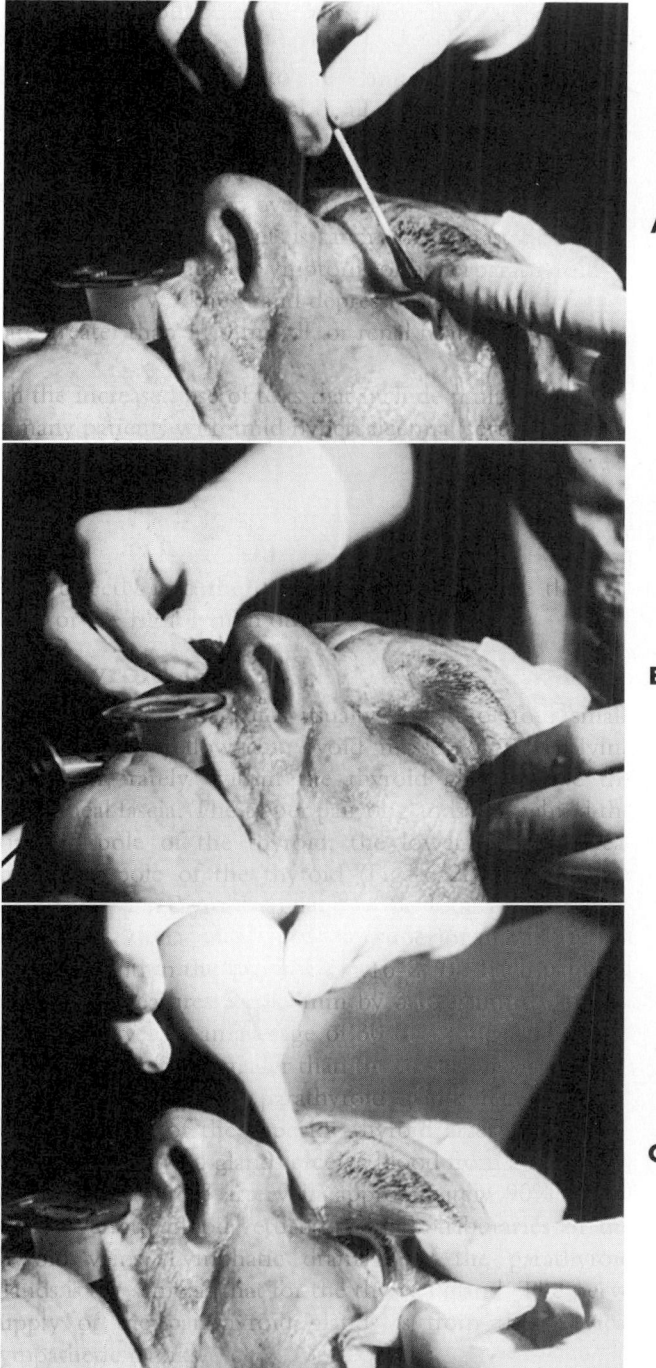

FIGURE 18-16 **A**, Eyelid is everted when lid margins are cleaned. **B**, Prepping procedure for eye surgery. **C**, Bulb syringe and normal saline solution are used to irrigate eye during prepping procedure. Direction of solution flow is always to outer side of face.

surgeon's preferences should be kept in a computer file. The instruments to be placed on the Mayo stand and the order of their use can also be listed on the preference card or computerized picklist.

A variety of ophthalmic forceps are designed for specific use with different tissues of the eye. Fixation forceps, used to hold tissue firmly in place or provide traction before incision, have an angled tooth that overlaps for secure fixation. Suturing forceps, used to pick up wound edges for dissection or suturing, are single-toothed forceps with the tooth at a right angle to the shank of the forceps. Tying forceps have a flat platform for holding suture as it is tied. The tips of those most commonly used forceps are illustrated in Fig. 18-19.

Care and Handling

To maintain the quality and precision of all ophthalmic instruments, including microsurgical instruments, strict criteria for care and handling must be followed. Storage cases protect instrument tips and cutting surfaces. The instruments should be inspected under magnification

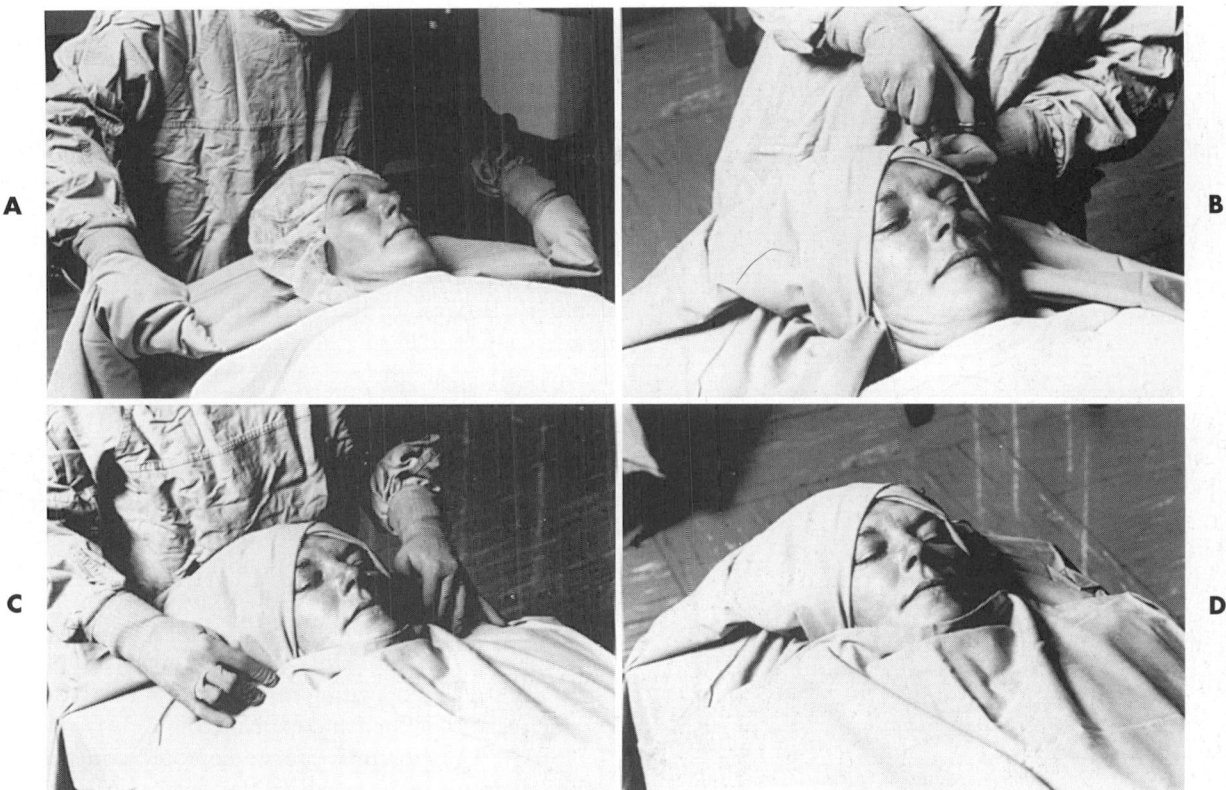

FIGURE 18–17   Alternative method of draping eye surgery patient. **A**, Double-thickness half-sheet and two towels are placed under head. **B**, Towel is secured around head, covering ears and hair. **C**, Patient and operating room bed are covered with large folded sheet. **D**, Patient under local anesthetic is now ready for fenestrated plastic drape, completing procedure.

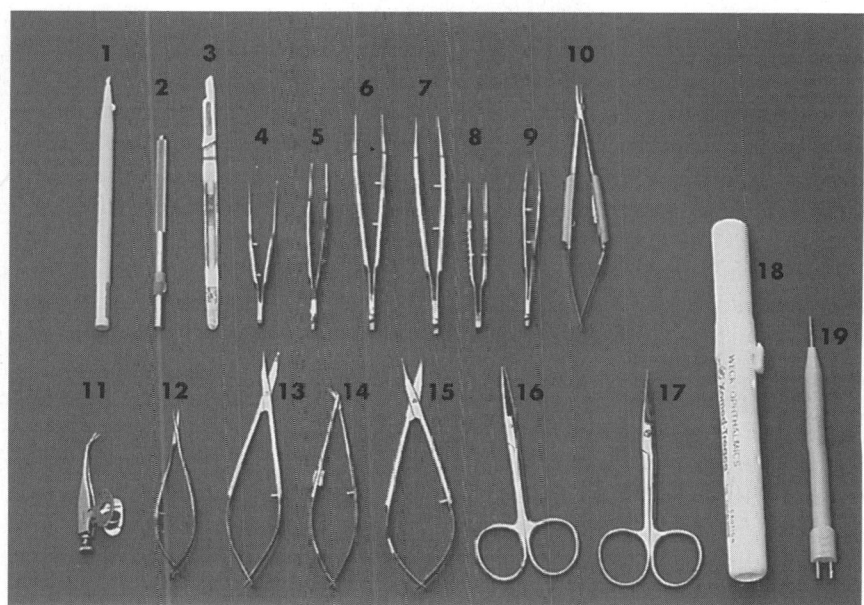

FIGURE 18–18   Basic eye instrument setup. *1*, Super blade (disposable); *2*, Beaver knife handle; *3*, #9 Bard-Parker knife handle; *4*, Colibri corneal forceps; *5*, Bishop-Harmon suturing forceps; *6*, Castroviejo suturing forceps, 0.5 mm; *7*, Castroviejo suturing forceps, 0.12 mm; *8*, Castroviejo tying forceps; *9*, Kelman-McPherson suturing forceps; *10*, Harper needle holder; *11*, Barraquer iris scissors; *12*, Vannas iridocapsulotomy scissors; *13*, Westcott tenotomy scissors; *14*, Castroviejo corneal scissors; *15*, Westcott stitch scissors; *16*, Knapp strabismus scissors; *17*, iris scissors; *18*, eye cautery, disposable; *19*, bipolar eraser-tip eye cautery, disposable.

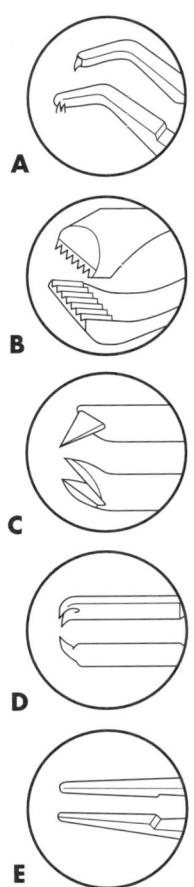

FIGURE 18-19 Close-up view of tips of forceps. **A,** Colibri forceps. **B** and **C,** Fixation forceps. **D,** Suturing forceps. **E,** Tying forceps.

when purchased and before and after each use, observing for burrs on tips, nicks on cutting surfaces, and alignment of jaws. Eye instruments should be cleaned during use with nonfibrous sponges to avoid damaging delicate instrument tips. Personnel handling instruments should know the name and purpose of each instrument. Tissue can be damaged by the use of an inappropriate instrument, and instruments can be damaged by inappropriate use. After use, the instruments should be cleaned and thoroughly dried before storage.

It is recommended that microsurgical instruments undergo ultrasonic cleaning with distilled water and an appropriate cleansing agent. They can be individually hand held or immersed together in the ultrasonic cleaner as long as they are not touching each other. Instruments should be rinsed with distilled water and thoroughly dried. A hot air blower (never a towel) should be used for drying instruments. Instrument lubricant should not be used on irrigating cannulas because residue can be introduced into the eye and cause damage.

In addition to basic care and handling, a routine preventive maintenance program should be established for sharpening, realigning, and adjusting the precision eye instruments. Keeping an instrument in good repair is much less expensive than buying a new one.

Operating microscope

During the past 10 years there has been a dramatic increase in the number of microsurgical procedures in various surgical disciplines. The operating or surgical microscope is employed in many types of surgical procedures. For ophthalmology it is an integral part of the surgery. Because of the demand for use of the operating microscope and its special adaptations, perioperative nurses must understand the basic principles of operation and care of this important piece of surgical equipment.

Microscope Components

Generally speaking, the surgical microscope comprises two parts, the microscope and the suspension system. The principal part of the microscope is the optical system, which has several subparts: the eyepieces, binocular tube, magnification changer, objective lens, and illumination system (Fig. 18-20). To facilitate understanding of the functions of the operating microscope, a few basic optical principles are defined and explained.

Surgical microscopes are stereoscopic and feature the ability for the user to adjust the level of magnification. Viewing the surgical image starts with the binoculars. Binoculars are two telescopes mounted side by side that give stereoscopic vision (three dimensional). The length of the binoculars is condensed by the use of prisms.

The eyepieces, or oculars, which fit into the binocular tubes, are the lens combinations through which a surgeon views the microsurgical field. Eyepieces are interchangeable and are available in different magnifying powers, such as 10X, 12.5X, 16X, and 20X. To focus the microscope, the user sets the spherical diopter adjustment on the oculars to correspond to his or her individual eyeglass correction and works without eyeglasses. Users who have astigmatism should wear their eyeglasses and set the oculars at zero.

The binocular tubes permit the distance between the oculars to be adjusted to fit the pupillary distance of the user (the distance between the pupils of the user's eyes), ensuring stereoscopic vision.

The objective lens is attached to the bottom of the microscope, usually by a threaded mount, and the working distance is the distance between the objective lens and the operative field. The working distance determines the focal length of the objective. Longer focal lengths, such as 400 mm, are commonly employed in neurosurgery. Procedures with shorter working distances and needing less magnification for a relatively large surgical field, such as an ophthalmic procedure, might require a 12.5X eyepiece and a 175 mm or 200 mm objective lens.

Illumination is the source of light used to view an object. The microscope illuminator is the light source used to throw light downward to illuminate the surgical area.

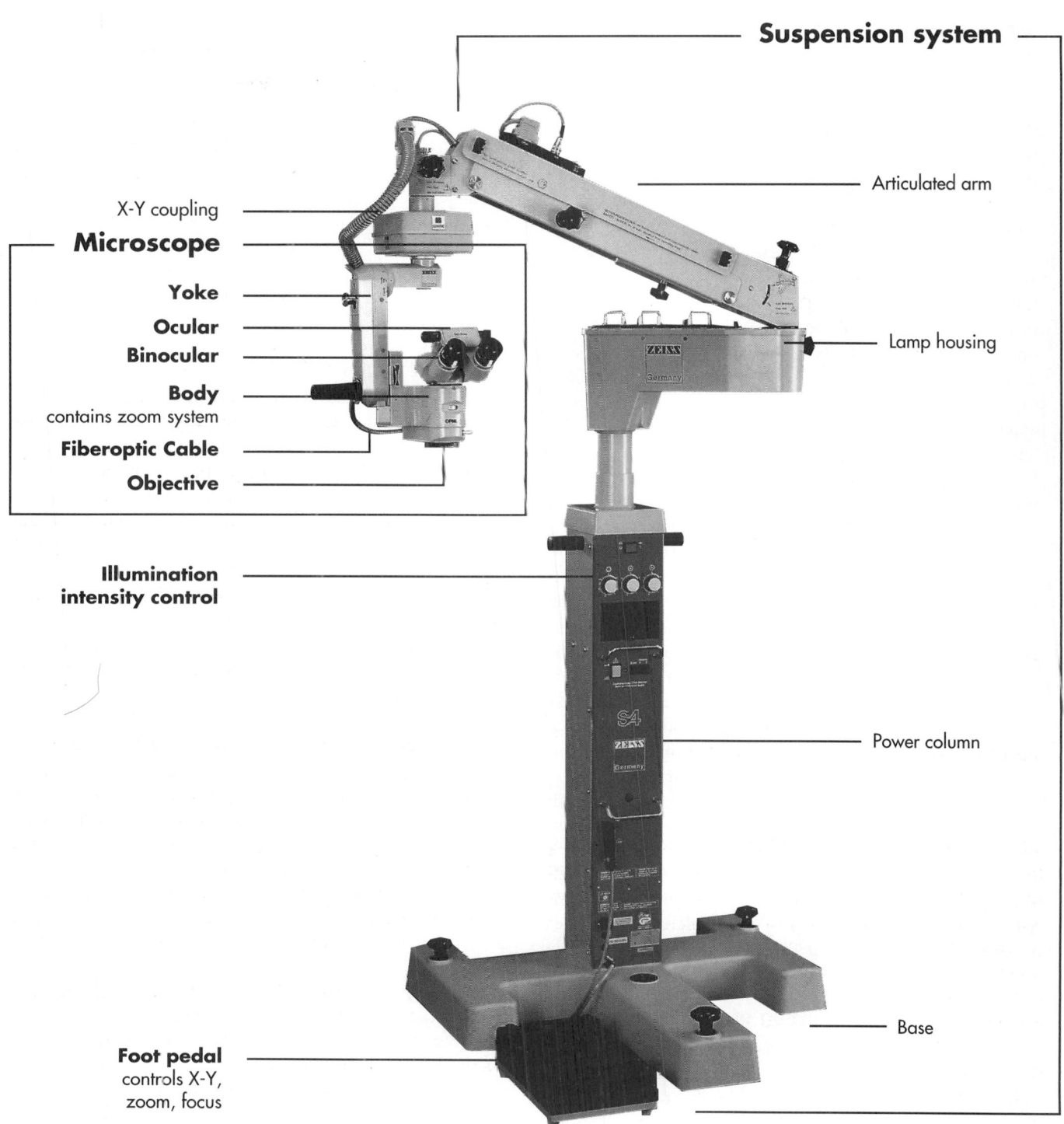

Suspension system

X-Y coupling

Microscope

Yoke

Ocular

Binocular

Body
contains zoom system

Fiberoptic Cable

Objective

Illumination intensity control

Foot pedal
controls X-Y,
zoom, focus

Articulated arm

Lamp housing

Power column

Base

Carl Zeiss Surgical Microscope (OPMI® CS/XY2 on S4 Floorstand)

FIGURE 18–20   Surgical microscope.

The most common type of microscope illumination used today is coaxial illumination. Light from the illuminator bulb is routed near the viewing axis of the microscope and projected down through the objective lens. This type of illumination provides a bright circular spot that is uniformly illuminated, often referred to as *homogeneous*, even in deep and narrow wounds. Coaxial light can be transferred through a fiberoptic cable or from an incandescent bulb housed near the objective lens of the microscope. The big advantage of fiberoptic illumination is the ability to place the light source and generated heat away from the surgical field. The light that is transmitted through the fiberoptics is then a so-called *cold light*.

Magnification is the process by which the apparent size of an image is increased. Magnification of an image is increased when the object is moved closer to the eye or optical aids such as telescopes, binoculars, or microscopes are used to increase the image size on the retina without reducing the eye-to-object distance. The amount of image increase becomes the magnification value of the optical aid. The objective lens, magnification changer, binocular tube length, and eyepieces influence the microscope's magnification. Two types of magnification changers used on surgical microscopes are the revolving telescope type, in which miniature telescopes of differing powers are rotated into position by means of knobs on the microscope body, and the zoom type, which is a motorized system of shifting lens elements to vary the magnification, operated with a hand switch or foot control. These principal parts are integrated in or attached to the microscope body.

Microscope Accessories

The use of microscope accessories varies according to requirements of the procedure and the surgeon's preferences. On the upper portion of the microscope body is a ring-dovetail receptacle for attaching accessories. One of the most common accessories is a beam splitter, which fits into the receptacle, permitting the attachment of binocular and monocular observation tubes and documentation accessories such as cameras and video equipment. A beam splitter has two-way mirrors or prisms that divert or split the optical image in several directions. With use of a beam splitter 50% or less of available light is usually diverted away from the surgeon's oculars. However, the human eye is usually versatile enough to adjust to lower light levels. Adequate lighting is essential for photographic systems, which may in some instances of older microscope systems require a beam splitter that diverts as much as 70% of the available light.

Movement and Mounting of the Microscope

The X-Y coupling, located above the entire optical system and usually contained in a square casing, enables the operator to move the microscope body horizontally and accurately over the operative field. The microscope body is mounted onto the yoke, the connecting carrier arm, which in most cases, attaches to the X-Y coupling and then to the articulated arm. The articulated arm is part of the suspension system, which can be either a floor stand or ceiling mounted. Each suspension system can offer manual or motorized features for various functions such as gross positioning, focus, and magnification (zoom).

Care and Maintenance

Proper care and maintenance of the operating microscope are essential to ensure optimal function and durability of this sophisticated, expensive piece of equipment. The procedures are as follows:

1. Inspection and cleaning of all external lens surfaces before use
2. Checking all power controls including illumination intensity, magnification changer, focus, and X-Y coupling to ensure proper functioning before use
3. Determining the particular procedure in advance and checking the needed accessories such as the correct objective lens, beam splitter, cameras, observer tubes, and filters
4. Cleaning and covering after use

Care of Optics

Before and after each procedure all external lens surfaces should be cleaned and inspected for damage. The objective lens frequently needs cleaning as a result of dried splash marks of balanced salt solution (BSS). Scratched or damaged optical systems must be repaired or replaced.

The following procedure is used for cleaning lens surfaces:

1. Loose particles (lint or dust) are removed with a soft, clean camera lens brush or with a rubber bulb syringe. When a bulb syringe is used, the bulb is held about 1 cm from the surface and squeezed briskly, directing the air toward the lens surface.
2. Blood, water, and irrigating solutions are removed with a cotton-tipped applicator or cotton ball moistened with distilled water. A circular motion is used, beginning at the center of the optic and working toward the outer edge (lens paper may also be used). The surface is dried with a cotton-tipped applicator or cotton ball in the same manner.
3. Oil or fingerprints are removed with a cleaning solvent of commercially prepared lens-cleaning solution or with 50% denatured alcohol. The lens is wiped with a lightly moistened cotton-tipped applicator or cotton ball in a circular motion. The process is repeated until the surface is clean and free from streaks.

Solvents should be used sparingly. Excessive fluid may destroy the cemented surfaces of the lens or plastic mounts if used.

Cleaning

The external surfaces of the microscope should be cleansed after use and before storage. The cleaning procedures are as follows:

1. The external surfaces are washed with a clean, damp cloth moistened with a mild soap or disinfecting solution.
2. The surfaces are wiped dry with a lint-free cloth.
3. The function of each moving part is inspected during

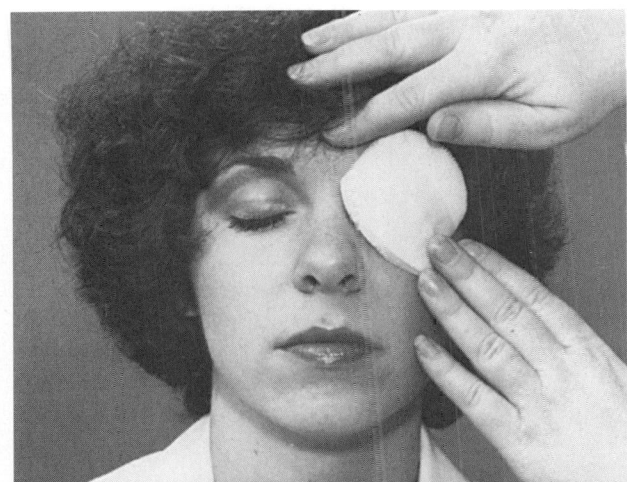
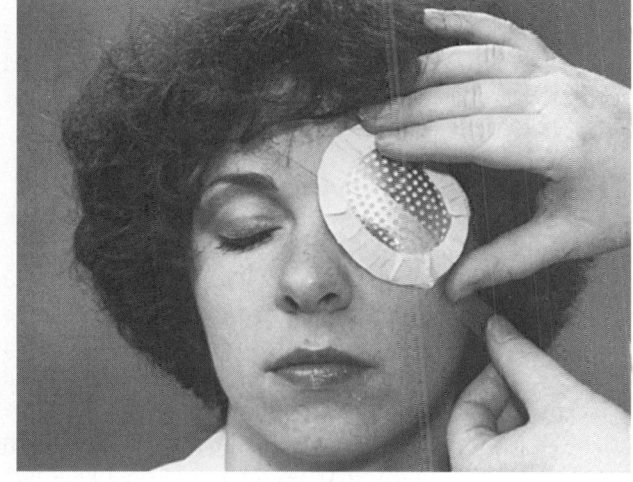

FIGURE 18-21   **A,** Eye dressing is held in place by plastic, paper, or cellophane strips. Lids are gently closed before patch is applied. **B,** Protection of wound is provided by application of metal shield over dressing.

the cleaning process. The coupling joints can be greased with petrolatum jelly if necessary. The lamp cable should be free from kinks. A new bulb should be used for each procedure expected to be over 4 hours in duration. It is good practice to have a spare bulb on hand at all times. Fiberoptic cables are cleaned with cotton-tipped applicators.

4. The microscope arms are moved to lowest position. The locks on the arm are loosened, and the ocular systems are moved in toward the base.
5. Dust caps are placed over the eyepieces and a dust cover over the microscope head. The microscope is ready for storage.

Proper care and preventive maintenance add years of service to an operating microscope. Checking the microscope before use and being knowledgeable about proper function of the microscope and its accessories are responsibilities of the perioperative nurse.

Ophthalmic sutures

Sutures used in ophthalmic surgery are very fine and range in size from 4-0 to 10-0. Handling and arming these sutures can be a challenge for the perioperative nurse with uncorrected presbyopia. Fine eye sutures produce minimum reaction and discomfort for the patient. They should be handled as little as possible to avoid weakening and fraying. Surgical gut and collagen suture, which is packaged in solution, should be rinsed before use to prevent introducing irritants into the eye. Ophthalmic needles are also very delicate and must be handled with extreme care. Before use, needles must be inspected for evidence of burrs.

Ophthalmic dressings

Dressings are applied to prevent palpebral movements, protect the operative wound from dust and external contaminants, and absorb any blood and tears produced. The presence and type of dressing depends on the procedure.

At the completion of the operation the operative eye area is cleansed with saline sponges. After plastic procedures on the lids or lacrimal ducts, antibiotic ointment may be thinly spread over the skin and eyelashes to prevent adhesion of the bandage.

The initial dressing is a sterile eye pad secured with nonallergenic tape (Fig. 18-21, *A*). After intraocular operations, when external pressure on the eyes might be harmful, the initial dressing is covered with a protecting, perforated aluminum plate or other varieties of Fox shields (Fig. 18-21, *B*).

A pressure bandage may be used when a compression affect is desired. A gauze roller bandage is applied over the initial dressing, encircling the head.

Advancements in cataract procedures have altered the usually postoperative dressing of ophthalmic ointment, an eye pad, and a protective shield. Collagen corneal shields that are rehydrated in an antiinfective-antiinflammatory solution may be all that is used as a dressing. With some of the latest topical anesthetics and clear corneal incisions, no dressings are needed.

Evaluation

Before the patient is transported to the PACU or observation unit, his or her general condition is evaluated. The general appearance of the skin is assessed, with areas around the face and bony prominences being noted for redness and other changes from the preoperative condition.

If the procedure was lengthy and osmotics were given, the patient may be catheterized while still anesthetized or given a bedpan if awake. A report to the receiving nurse in the PACU or observation area should include postoperative positioning requirements, potential problems specific to the patient, and preoperative anxiety level and utilization of coping mechanisms. Most patients have one

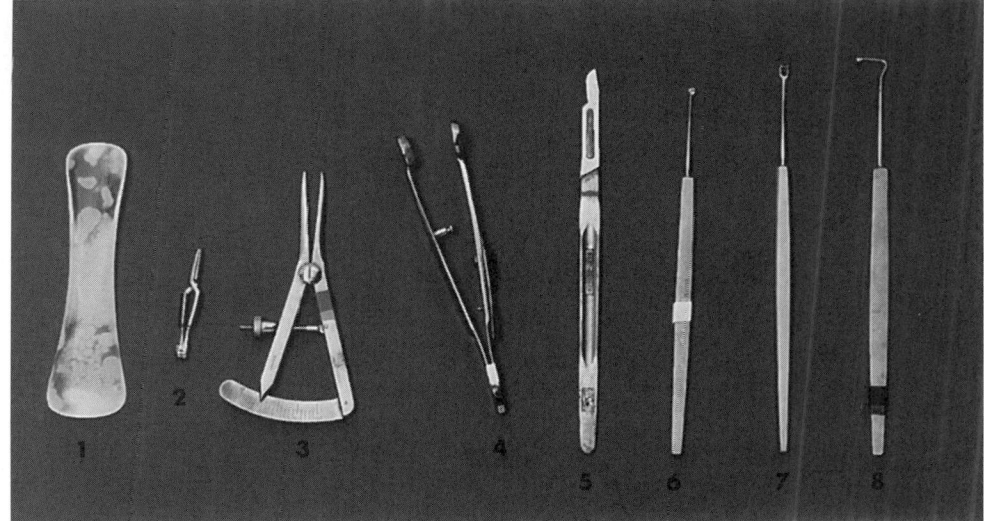

FIGURE 18-22   Instruments for surgery of the eyelids and conjunctiva. *1*, Jaeger lid plate; *2*, serrefine; *3*, caliper; *4*, Green chalazion clamp; *5*, #9 Bard-Parker knife handle with #15 blade; *6*, chalazion curette; *7*, retractor; *8*, muscle hook.

or both eyes patched, and the sensory deficit should be noted. Documentation of all postoperative observations is important.

Evaluation should address whether the patient met the desired perioperative nursing outcomes; the patient's responses may be documented as outcome statements. The following examples are based on the nursing diagnoses identified in the care plan on p. 642.

- The patient, family, or significant other verbalized knowledge regarding the diagnosis, planned intervention, medication management, and requirements for home care maintenance.
- The patient verbalized concerns and fears and utilized coping mechanisms.
- The patient safely coped with visual sensory and perceptual alterations.
- The patient remained comfortable during intervention and identified activities that may increase intraocular pressure.
- The patient will remain free from signs and symptoms of postoperative infection.

Patient and Family Education and Discharge Planning

Implementation of the care plan actually begins during the patient interview. Planning to meet the patient's educational needs should play an equal role with meeting other needs. Review and reinforcement of information initially provided in the physician's office ensure consistency in teaching. Written material and audiovisual media (closed circuit television, videocassettes, photos, and patient information internet websites) may be used to enhance patient education programs but do not eliminate the need for direct interchange with patients and feedback from them.

Family members or friends should be included to add support and increase understanding of the planned surgery. The loss of sight produces the same staged coping behaviors of grieving that move the individual from denial to acceptance. Thorough preoperative preparation of the patient and in most cases the family, who will assist with care at home in the postoperative period, plays a vital role in the successful outcome of the surgical procedure.

Patient and family education for the patient undergoing ophthalmic surgery should include the following:

- Purpose and desired results of preoperative eye drops and sedation
- Explanation of what to expect from the anesthetic
- Activities and routines of the intraoperative period.
- What to expect immediately after surgery
- Verbal and written instructions for use of eye drops and other medication
- Any limitations on activities
- Wound care
- Signs and symptoms of complications
- Who to call with questions or concerns
- Clinical appointments

SURGICAL INTERVENTIONS
SURGERY OF THE EYELIDS

The oculoplastic procedures most commonly performed on the eyelids are for treatment of chalazion, entropion, ectropion, dermatochalasis, excisional biopsy, and repair of traumatic injuries. Additional instruments for procedures of the eyelids and conjunctiva are shown in Fig. 18-22.

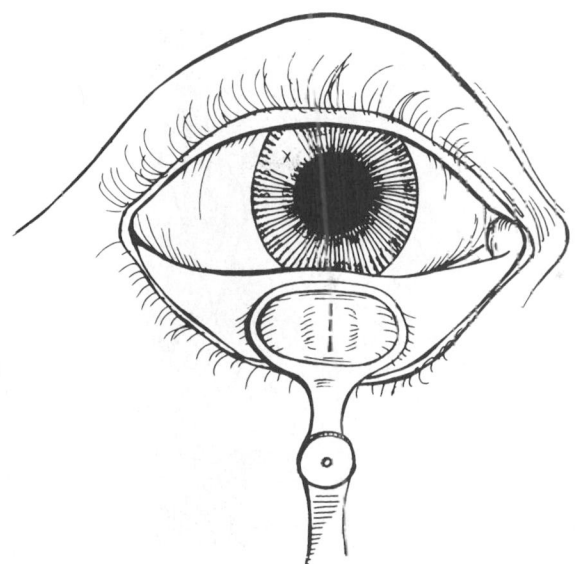

FIGURE 18-23 Transconjunctival approach. Clamp everts eyelid during surgery for chalazion. Viscous contents of chalazion will be removed with curette.

Removal of Chalazion

Removal of a chalazion is the incision and curettage of a chronic granulomatous inflammation of one or more of the meibomian glands in the tarsal plate of the eyelid.

Procedural considerations

This procedure is most commonly done with local anesthesia. The incisional approach depends on the location of the major portion of the chalazion. If the chalazion is located anterior to the tarsal plate, an external or transcutaneous incision is used. If the majority of the chalazion is located on the conjunctival side of the tarsal plate, the transconjunctival approach is used (Fig. 18-23).

Operative procedure (transconjunctival approach)

1. The affected lid is everted with a chalazion clamp to expose the chalazion.
2. A cruciate incision is made on the inner lid surface with a sharp knife; a small triangular flap of tarsal plate and conjunctiva is resected.
3. The contents of the chalazion are removed with a chalazion curette. The wound is left open for drainage. The eye is dressed and patched.

Repair of Entropion

Entropion (turning inward of the lower lid margin) seldom occurs in persons under 40 years of age. The inturned eyelashes and skin of the lower lid rub against the corneal surface and cause irritation, which leads to breaks in the integrity of the corneal surface. The most common type is involutional entropion resulting from degeneration of facial attachments between the pretarsal muscle and the tarsus, which permits the pretarsal muscle to override the lid margin during contraction. Cicatricial entropion is attributable to contraction of either the upper or lower tarsus and its conjunctiva, turning in the lashes (trichiasis) so that they rub on the cornea.

Procedural considerations

The causes of entropion vary, and corrective procedures also vary depending on the pathologic process. Local anesthetic is typically used and antiinfective ointment is applied postoperatively.

Operative procedures
Blepharoplasty of Lower Lid for Involutional Entropion

1. Local anesthetic is injected into the lower lid through the conjunctiva using an angled needle.
2. Skin is marked, and an incision is made in lateral canthus.
3. Orbicularis is dissected off the orbital septum.
4. Skin excision is extended across lower lid.
5. Orbital septum is incised to expose fat pockets.
6. Extra fat is removed, and hemostasis is achieved with disposable cautery.
7. An incision is made into the lateral canthus, and the lower lid is pulled laterally and shortened to correct entropion.
8. Using 7-0 absorbable suture, the tarsus is reattached to the lateral canthal tendon, and the lower lid fascia is reattached to the orbicularis.
9. The excess skin is pulled up, marked, and excised.
10. Skin incisions are closed with a continuous absorbable 6-0 suture.

Wies Procedure for Cicatricial Entropion (Fig. 18-24)

1. A marking pen is used to draw a parallel line 4 mm below the lower lid margin before local anesthetic is injected.
2. A double-armed 4-0 nonabsorbable retraction suture is passed through the conjunctiva and lower lid 4 mm from the lateral canthus and 4 mm from the medial canthus.
3. A lid plate retractor is placed behind the lower lid as it is pulled up with the traction suture. Using a #15 blade the skin incision is made on the marked line.
4. The lid plate retractor is placed in front of the lid, and the lower lid is everted using the traction suture. The conjunctiva is incised with the #15 blade.
5. A full-thickness blepharotomy is extended laterally and medially with scissors.
6. One end of the 4-0 double-armed suture is passed through the conjunctiva and lower lid tendons and between the orbicularis and tarsus on the medial aspect of the lower lid, and the other end of the 4-0 suture repeats this process approximately 4 mm laterally.

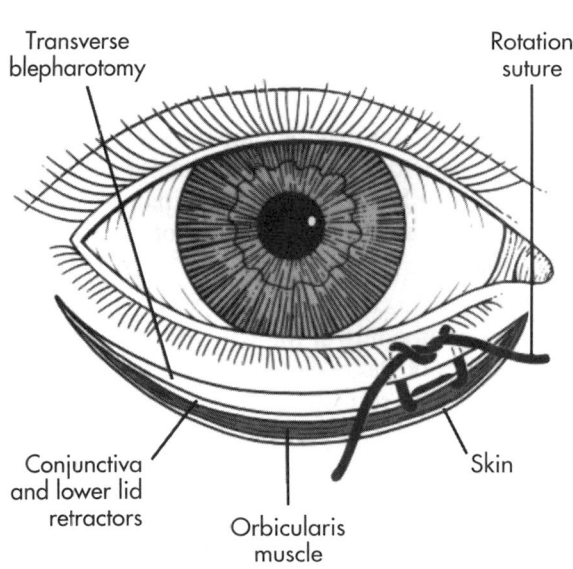

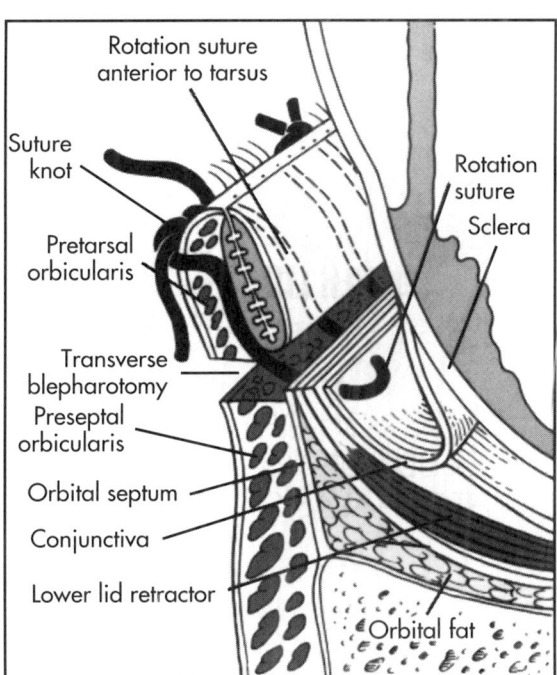

FIGURE 18-24   Wies procedure for entropion. Placement of an everting mattress suture across a transverse blepharotomy.

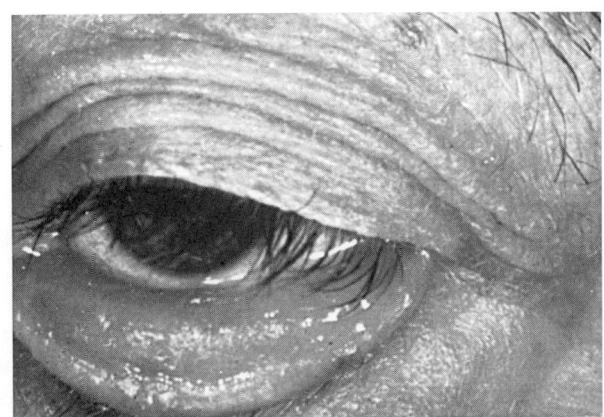

FIGURE 18-25   Ectropion, or turning out of lid, is most commonly caused by senile relaxation of eyelid framework.

7. Six mattress sutures are placed and tied to evert the lower lid (see Fig. 18-24).
8. Excess skin is excised, and the skin incision is closed with 7-0 nonabsorbable sutures.

Repair of Ectropion

Ectropion (sagging and eversion of the lower lid), usually bilateral, is common in older persons (Fig. 18-25). Ectropion may be caused by the relaxation of the orbicular muscle. Symptoms are tearing, conjunctival infection and irritation, and inadequate corneal protection leading to injury to the cornea. Surgery is indicated when facial paralysis is permanent or when scarring follows lacerations, lesions, or penetrating injuries, and the cornea becomes exposed, resulting in ulceration and photophobia.

Procedural considerations

The causes of ectropion vary, and corrective procedures also vary depending on the pathologic process. Local anesthetic is typically used, and antiinfective ointment and ice compresses are applied postoperatively.

Operative procedure
Lateral Canthal Sling Procedure

One method of correction for ectropion is the lateral canthal sling procedure (Fig. 18-26), which repositions and tightens the lower lid in a horizontal direction.

1. The lateral canthus is incised and a strip of tarsus is isolated.
2. The lower lid is stretched horizontally and held against the lower surface of the eye, and a nonabsorbable suture is placed through the strip of tarsus.
3. Loose tissue and orbicularis are pushed laterally.
4. The lid is repositioned with a 4-0 nonabsorbable suture that is placed at the rim and through the strip of tarsus.
5. This suture is tightened and tied.

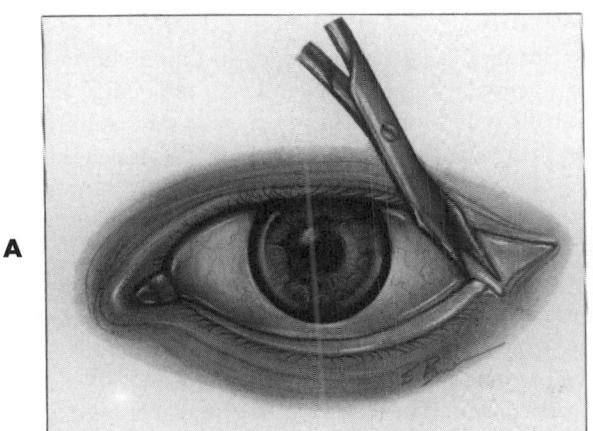

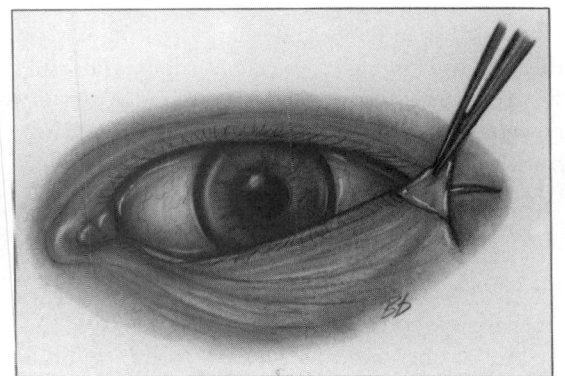

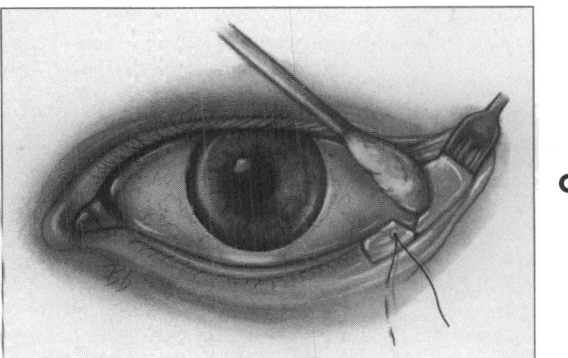

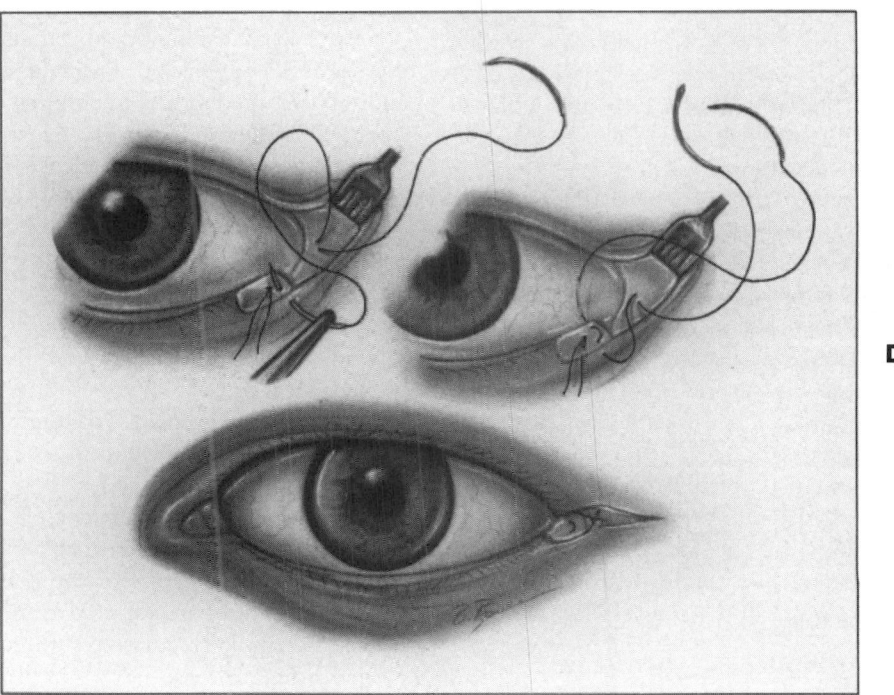

FIGURE 18-26   Lateral canthal sing procedure for ectropion. **A**, A cantholysis of the lower arm of the lateral canthal tendon is performed. **B**, Horizontal laxity of the lid is relieved by stretching the lid temporally until it fits tightly against the globe. A tarsal strip is isolated. **C**, A nonabsorbable suture is placed through the tarsal strip. Using a cotton applicator, the loose tissue and orbicularis muscle are cleaned from the orbital rim. **D**, A 4-0 nonabsorbable suture is placed through the tarsal strip, tightened, and tied.

Plastic Repair for Dermatochalasis

Dermatochalasis is a condition of drooping skin and herniated fat of upper and lower lids that causes the skin of the upper eyelids to hang down over the palpebral fissure, sometimes obscuring vision. It may occur in older persons who have lost normal elasticity of the skin of the upper lids or in persons who have suffered from persistent angioneurotic edema with stretching of the skin of the eyelids. If ptosis is present, it accentuates the condition.

Procedural considerations

Dermatochalasis is corrected with blepharoplasty of the redundant skin of the upper or lower eyelid or both eyelids. A segment of skin and fat is removed. A transconjunctival excision that leaves no external incision may be performed. Brow droop, or ptosis, may also be corrected alone or in combination with blepharoplasty to correct dermatochalasis. Procedures for correcting brow ptosis include direct brow lift, coronal brow lift, and endoscopic brow lift.

Operative procedures
Blepharoplasty of Upper Lid for Dermatochalasis

1. The upper lid is marked at the temporal and nasal crease, and local anesthetic is injected.
2. With a constant stretch applied to the skin of the upper lid, the incision is made from the lateral aspect to the nasal aspect.
3. The skin between the marked lines is excised, and the orbicularis between the incision edges is excised. Hemostasis is obtained with cautery.
4. The septum is incised in a buttonhole fashion, finger pressure is applied posteriorly, and bulging white fat is clamped, cut, and cauterized.
5. If fat is found in the temporal pocket, it may contain a prolapsed lacrimal gland. The lacrimal gland should be resuspended with 5-0 nonabsorbable suture.
6. Three 9-0 nonabsorbable sutures are placed through the levator aponeurosis and subcuticular tissue to reform the lid crease.
7. The skin is closed with 6-0 nonabsorbable suture using a continuous subcuticular suture that is changed to an over-and-over suture near the lateral canthus. Small squares of latex are attached to the ends of the tied suture to facilitate removal of the sutures.[14]

Transconjunctival Blepharoplasty of Lower Lid

1. Local anesthetic is injected into the lower lid through the conjunctiva using an angled needle.
2. Finger pressure is placed on the upper lid while the lower lid is being retracted to elevate the conjunctiva.
3. The conjunctiva is incised to expose fat pockets. Prolapsed fat is clamped and removed, and hemostasis is achieved with disposable cautery.
4. Conjunctival incision is closed with interrupted 6-0 clear or white absorbable suture.

Surgery for Unilateral or Bilateral Ptosis

Ptosis is true drooping of the upper lid and may be congenital, acquired, or senile. In congenital ptosis there usually is developmental weakness of the levator muscle. In 69% of cases the condition occurs unilaterally, and 30% of cases may also have weakness of the superior rectus muscle.[6] The child may compensate by raising the eyebrow or tilting the head upward.

Acquired ptosis can be (1) neurogenic related to third cranial nerve (oculomotor) palsy where there often is complete ptosis or (2) involutional, which is manifested by a gradual weakness or dehiscence of the levator aponeurosis. The eyelid crease may be high or absent. Senile ptosis is the result of stretching of the levator aponeurosis.

Procedural considerations

The objective of ptosis surgery is to achieve a good cosmetic result and restore function by creating a good upper lid fold with elevation of the lid. The many surgical procedures that have been devised are directed at the levator aponeurosis, the frontalis muscles, or the levator–Müller's muscle complex. These muscles are the elevating forces of the upper lids. Some of the commonly used procedures are levator aponeurosis repair, frontalis suspension, and posterior Müller's muscle–conjunctival resection. Local or general anesthesia can be used. Local may be preferred so that required adjustments can be made with the patient's cooperation. Frontalis suspension uses autogenous fascia, used mostly in children over 3 years of age, or synthetic materials, often used in adults or in local anesthetic procedures. Excising of fascia lata requires general anesthesia and an additional incision in the leg.

Operative procedures
Levator Aponeurosis Repair (Fig. 18-27)

1. The existing or potential eyelid crease is marked, and with the skin of the upper lid held taut, the skin incision is made.
2. An incision is made through the orbicularis and through the orbital septum to expose the aponeurosis and the tarsus.
3. The aponeurosis is reattached to the tarsus with interrupted 6-0 nonabsorbable suture.
4. If patient is awake, he or she is asked to look forward, and the sutures are adjusted as needed.
5. The pretarsal orbicularis is sutured to the aponeurosis to make the lid crease.
6. The skin incision is closed with a running 6-0 nonabsorbable suture.

Frontalis Suspension

1. The upper lid is marked, one incision is made in the lid crease, and two incisions are made above the eyebrow (Fig. 18-28, *A* and *B*).
2. A lid plate is placed behind the upper lid, the tarsus is exposed, and the suspension material (fascia graft or a

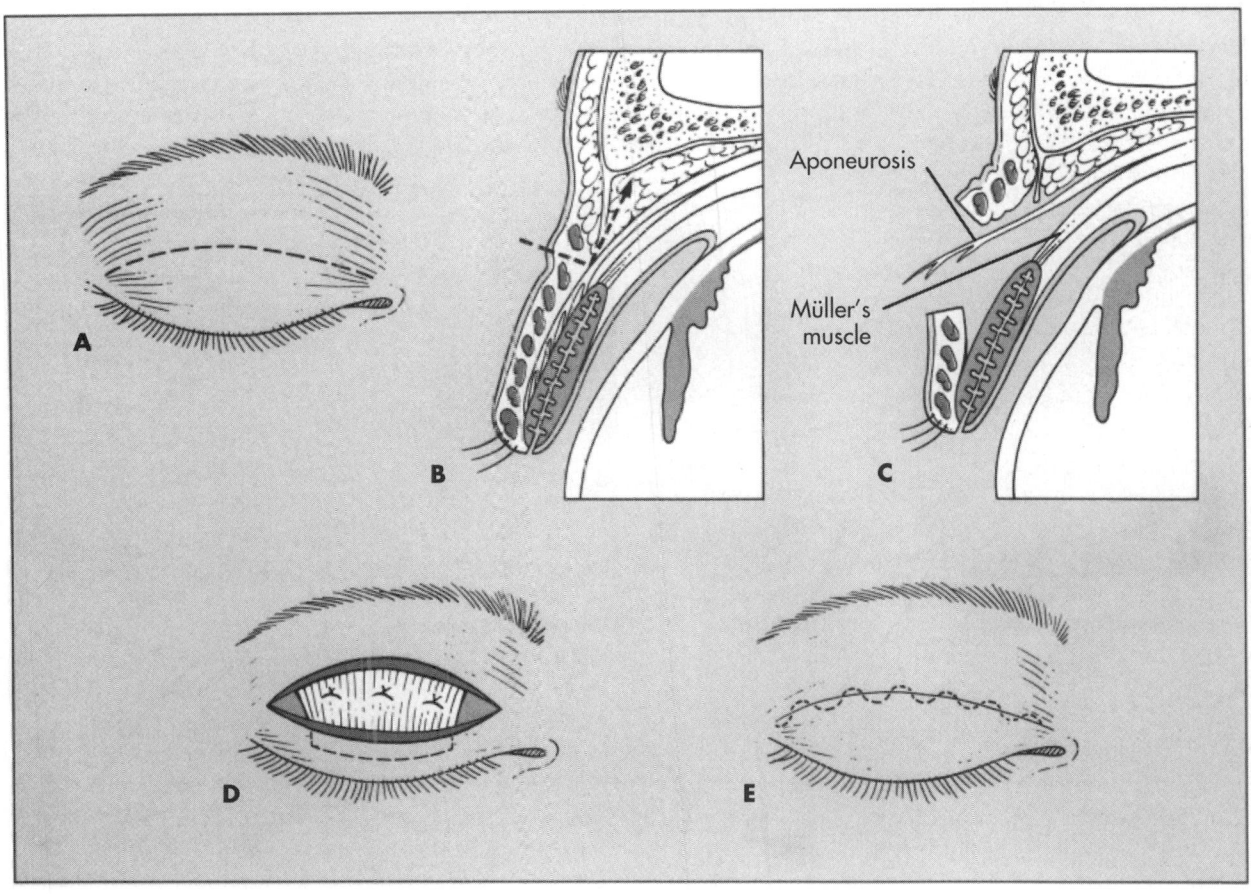

FIGURE 18-27   Levator aponeurosis repair for ptosis. **A**, Eyelid crease is marked. **B**, Skin incision is made, and the orbicularis and orbital septum are divided while dissection proceeds toward the orbital rim. **C**, The anterior surface of the tarsus is exposed, and the aponeurosis is separated from Müller's muscle. **D**, The aponeurosis is reattached to the tarsus with partial-thickness permanent sutures. Lid contour and position are adjusted. **E**, The eyelid crease is created by suturing the pretarsal orbicularis muscle to the aponeurosis, and the skin is closed.

synthetic implant) is secured to the tarsus with nonabsorbable sutures (Fig. 18-28, *C*).

3. Using a Wright needle the suspension material is passed away from the globe deeply into the orbital septum and out through one eyebrow incision (Fig. 18-28, *D*).
4. The remaining end of the suspension material is passed in the same manner.
5. The pretarsal orbicularis is sutured to the tarsus to form the lid crease (Fig. 18-28, *E*).
6. The lid incision is closed with a running 6-0 nonabsorbable suture (Fig. 18-28, *F*).
7. The long end of the suspension material is passed under the skin between the brow incisions to complete the loop, and the ends of the material are sutured together.
8. The brow incisions are closed with interrupted 6-0 nonabsorbable suture.

Excisional Biopsy

Excisional biopsy is removal of lesions, either neoplastic (benign or malignant) or viral in nature, for diagnostic examination. Basal cell carcinomas account for 95% of neoplastic lesions of the lid; the treatment of choice is excisional biopsy.

Operative procedure

Through-and-through excision of skin, muscle, tarsus, and conjunctiva is followed by careful structural closure of anatomic spaces. Depending on the type, extent, and location of the lesion, rotation flaps or free grafts may be necessary.

Plastic Repair for Traumatic Injuries

Lacerations of the lids, including damage to the inferior canaliculus, are repaired surgically. Paramount for success is the careful approximation of the borders of the lid margin and the ends of a torn canaliculus.

Operative procedure

Lacerations of the lid margin are closed with a 5-0 nonabsorbable suture to align the gray line of the lid that

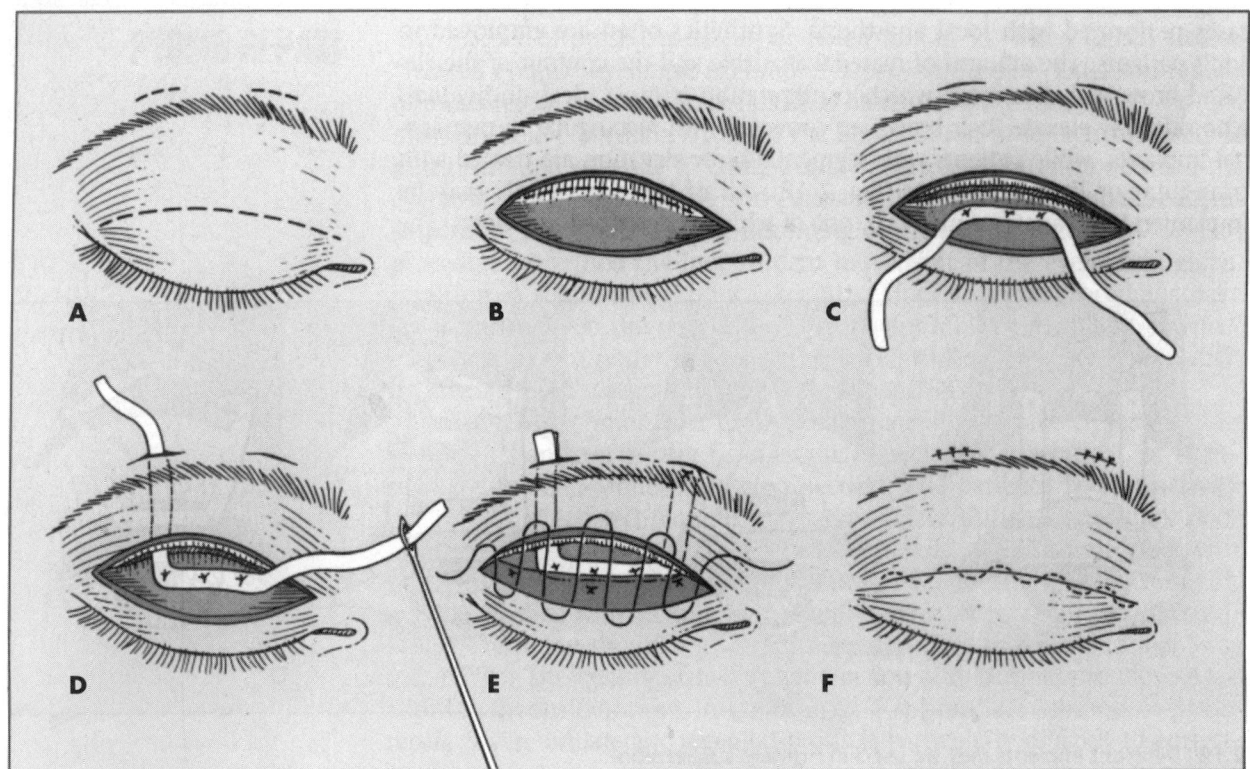

FIGURE 18-28 Frontalis suspension for ptosis. One method used to suspend the eyelid from the brow.

lies between the lash follicles and the orifices of the meibomian glands. Once this anatomic line has been approximated, all other sutures are placed, maintaining the approximation.

If the canaliculus has been lacerated, a pigtail probe is passed through the uninvolved punctum, through the sac, and carefully through the proximal and distal ends of the lacerated structure to emerge from the involved punctum. A 4-0 nonabsorbable suture is hooked onto the probe and, by reversing the previous procedure, is pulled out of the uninvolved punctum, thus establishing continuity of the system. Accurate plastic closure of the lid defect is then carried out.

SURGERY OF THE LACRIMAL GLAND AND APPARATUS

Surgery of the lacrimal gland and apparatus is usually performed for treatment or diagnosis of tumors of the lacrimal fossa or to correct epiphora, which is abnormal overflow of tears related to obstruction of the lacrimal drainage system. Additional instrumentation for procedures of the lacrimal system is shown in Fig. 18-29.

Surgery of the Lacrimal Fossa

Surgery of the lacrimal fossa is performed for biopsy of any structure in the lacrimal fossa and possible removal of the lacrimal gland (extirpation) to eliminate excessive tearing.

Operative procedure

The lacrimal fossa, which is in the upper temporal quadrant of the orbit, may be approached directly through the lid or through the conjunctiva by everting the upper lid. The lacrimal gland is divided into a palpebral and an orbital part by the orbital septum. All drainage ducts go through the palpebral portion; surgery on this part alone affects tearing because, although the orbital part is intact, no access to the eye is available. Routine surgical closure procedures are followed.

Probing of Tear Duct

Congenital obstruction of the nasolacrimal drainage system occurs in 2% to 4% of newborns usually because there is no perforation at Hasner's membrane.[7] In 80% to 90% of cases, the membrane opens spontaneously or with directed gentle massage within the first 6 to 8 months of life. When the lacrimal drainage system does not open spontaneously, an acute infectious process involving the lacrimal drainage system becomes obvious. The infectious process is treated with antibiotics, followed by probing under general anesthesia. The probing procedure is done between 8 and 12 months of age with a 90% to 95% success rate, which decreases after 1 year of age.

Operative procedure

1. The punctum is dilated with a punctum dilator.
2. With a blunt lacrimal needle, a fluorescein solution is irrigated through the punctum to determine the

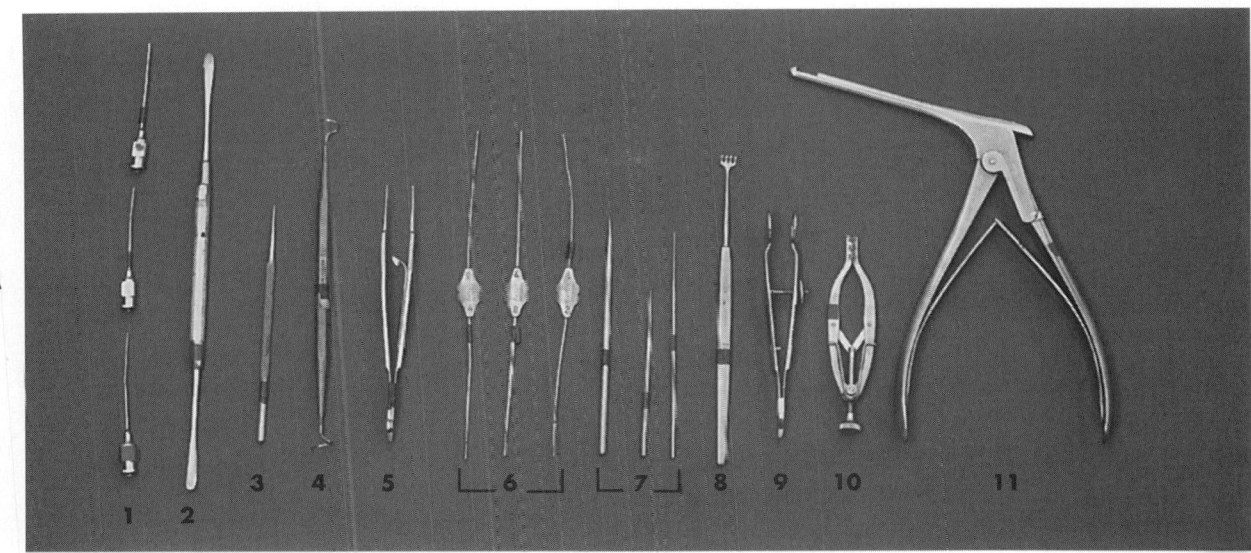

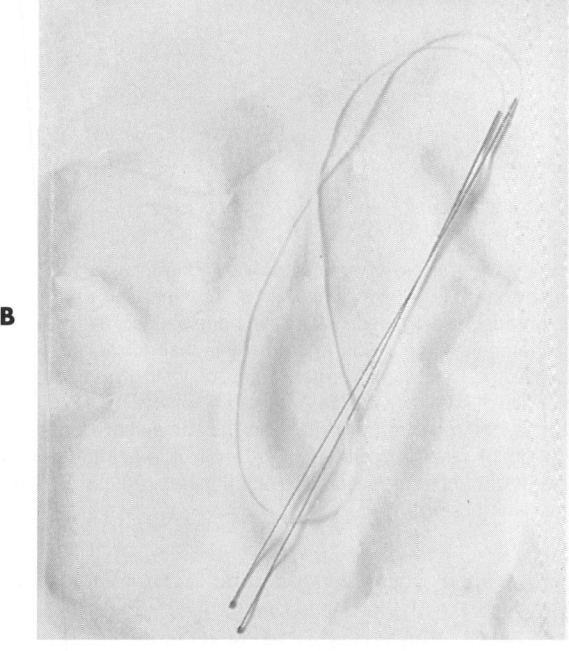

FIGURE 18-29 **A**, Instruments for surgery of the lacrimal system. *1*, Lacrimal cannulas; *2*, Freer elevator; *3*, Muldoon dilator; *4*, Worst pigtail probe; *5*, Castroviejo suturing forceps; *6*, Bowman lacrimal probes; *7*, Nettleship-Wilder lacrimal dilators; *8*, lacrimal sac retractor; *9*, Erhardt lid clamp; *10*, lacrimal sac retractor; *11*, small Kerrison rongeur. **B**, Lacrimal duct intubation set.

patency of the system. Nasopharyngeal suction is readily available. If no yellowish green dye appears in the nose, the probing is performed.

3. A lacrimal probe is then passed (1 mm) through the punctum. The lid is pulled laterally as the probe is passed through the canaliculus into the sac, where resistance is met from the lacrimal bone.

4. The probe is rotated 90 degrees, passed through the bony canal, and forced through the imperforate opening into the nose. A small amount of blood may be regurgitated at this time. Irrigation and suction are repeated.

Dacryocystorhinostomy

Dacryocystorhinostomy (DCR) is the establishment of a new tear passageway for drainage directly into the nasal cavity. Recent developments of a minimally invasive approach to DCR surgery include the use of a transcon-junctival incision, lasers, and endoscopic techniques (Research Highlight 18-1).

Dacryocystitis (Fig. 18-30) is an infection in the lacrimal sac and its mucous membranes that extends to the surrounding connective tissue and results in a localized cellulitis. Chronic dacryocystitis in adults requires dacryo-cystorhinostomy (DCR) because of resistant obstruction of the nasolacrimal duct related to infection, dacryolith (calculus in the duct), or trauma.[13]

Dacryocystorhinostomy is also performed when the lower canaliculus is patent but the tear duct is blocked, causing epiphora (abnormal overflow of tears) that the patient cannot tolerate. This deformity frequently follows a malunited fracture of the medial wall of the orbit.

Procedural considerations

The nasal cavity is anesthetized topically with cocaine just before surgery, and a general anesthetic is administered

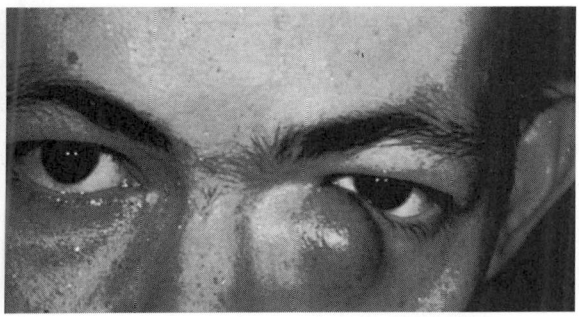

FIGURE 18-30 Chronic infection of lacrimal sac (dacryocystitis) causes swelling of inner lower corner of eye socket.

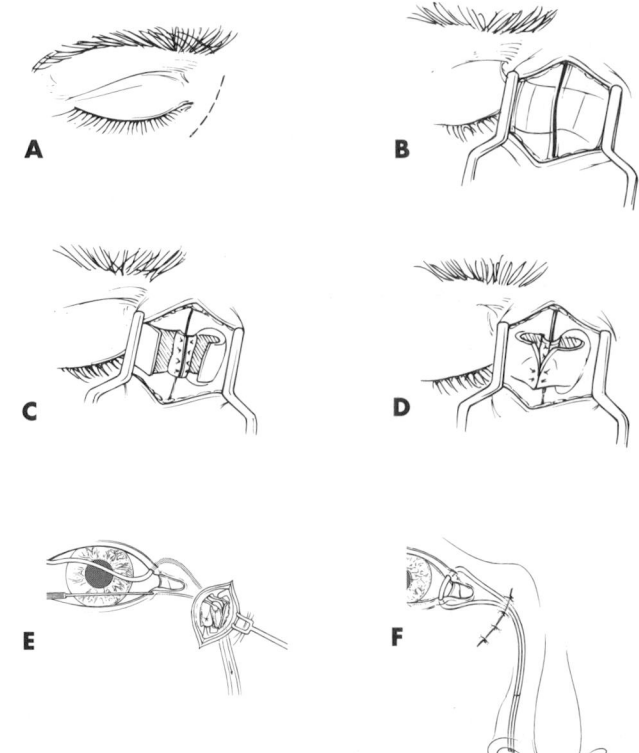

FIGURE 18-31 Dacryocystorhinostomy. **A,** Skin incision for dacryocystorhinostomy or dacryocystectomy. **B,** Lacrimal sac and lacrimal bone exposed. Opening made in lacrimal bone and lacrimal crest, with *dotted lines* indicating incision to be made in wall of sac and in nasal periosteum and mucosa. **C,** Posterior flap of wall of sac sutured to posterior flap of nasal mucosa. **D,** Anterior flap of wall of sac sutured to anterior flap of nasal mucosa. (Drawing is somewhat distorted for visualization of relative positions.) **E,** Canaliculi are intubated with Silastic tubes. **F,** Tubes are secured to lateral nasal wall and allowed to slide back into nose.

18-1 RESEARCH HIGHLIGHT

External dacryocystorhinostomy (DCR) is the standard treatment of nasolacrimal duct obstruction, and the primary procedure has a success rate of greater than 90% and an 85% success rate for external revision DCR. The evolution and refinement of endoscopy and lasers has led to the development of endonasal laser-assisted dacryocystorhinostomy (ENLDCR). Primary ENLDCR has a success rate ranging from 68% to 100%, which includes patients with short follow-up data and cases with silicone stents in place. Since the common cause of failure of external DCR is canalicular scarring or granulation overgrowth of the ostium and a disadvantage of primary laser-assisted DCR is removal of bone, it would appear that laser-assisted DCR would be ideal for revision of failed external DCR because the bony opening has already been achieved. Patel and colleagues conducted a study to determine the efficacy of transcanalicular laser-assisted revision dacryocystorhinostomy (TCLARDCR). Nd:YAG laser was used for TCLARDCR of 24 failed DCRs (previous external DCRs 1 [$n = 15$], 2 [$n = 7$], and 3 [$n = 2$]). Success rate was 46% with a mean follow-up time of 20 months, and three of the failures underwent further unsuccessful TCLARDCR. The researchers concluded that TCLARDCR success rate of 46% compares poorly with revision DCR success rate of 85%, laser lacrimal surgery is more costly than external DCR, and TCLARDCR cannot be recommended for revision DCR using the Nd:YAG laser.

From Patel, B., Phillips, B., McLeish, W., et al. (1997). Transcanalicular neodymium:YAG laser revision of dacryocystorhinostomy. *Ophthalmology, 104,*(7), 1191-1197.

---

in the operating room. The patient is prepared as described for eye surgery.

Operative procedure (Fig. 18-31)

1. An incision is made in the medial canthal area.
2. Blunt dissection is carried through the orbicularis down to the nasal bone. The orbicularis is separated from the bone with a freer elevator. The lacrimal fossa sac is exposed.
3. The nasal packing is removed, and a hemostat is used to press an opening through the lacrimal bone. If this is unsuccessful, the anterior lacrimal crest is perforated with a power burr or mallet and chisel. The opening is enlarged to a 10 mm circle with a Kerrison rongeur, and hemostasis is obtained with bone wax if necessary.
4. The inferior punctum is dilated, and a probe is passed into the lacrimal sac.
5. The lacrimal sac and nasal mucosa are incised with H flaps. The posterior nasal mucous membrane flap is sutured to the posterior lacrimal sac flap with 4-0 absorbable sutures.
6. The first end of the wire stylette of a Silastic lacrimal duct intubation set is passed through the upper canaliculus, through the opening, and out through the nose. The other end is passed in the same fashion through the lower canaliculus.
7. The anterior nasal mucous membrane flap is sutured to the anterior lacrimal sac flap with 4-0 absorbable sutures to create a bridge over the Silastic tubing. The

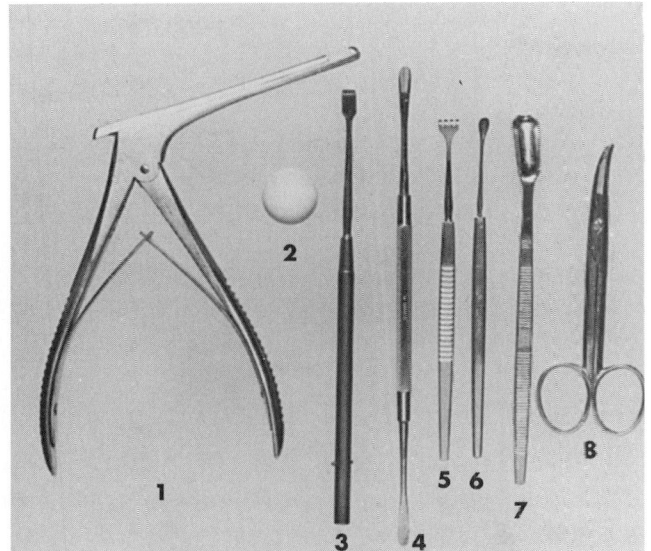

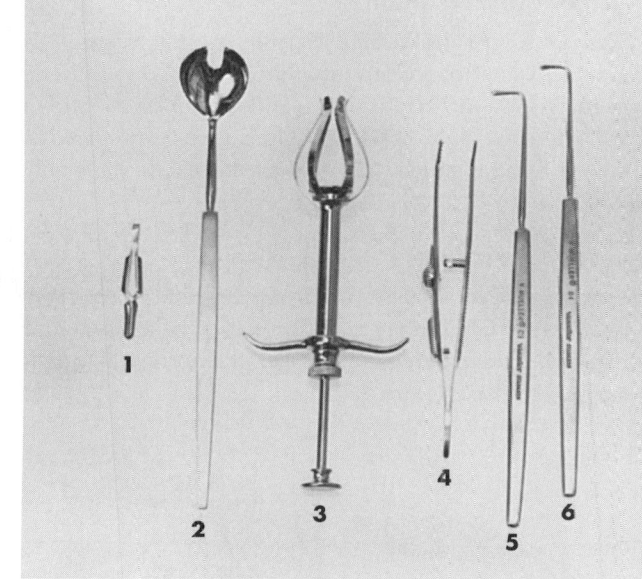

FIGURE 18-32 Instruments for surgery of globe or orbit. **A**, *1*, Kerrison rongeur; *2*, orbital implant or sphere; *3*, lacrimal chisel; *4*, Freer elevator; *5*, Lacrimal sac retractor; *6*, exenteration spoon; *7*, Arruga orbital retractor; *8*, enucleation scissors. **B**, *1*, Serrefine; *2*, Wells evisceration spoon; *3*, sphere introducer and holder; *4*, Jameson recession forceps; *5* and *6*, von Graefe muscle hooks.

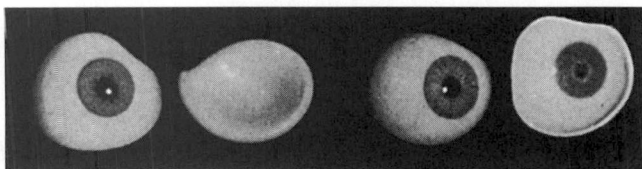

FIGURE 18-33 Artificial eyes. Shell prosthesis is seen at right.

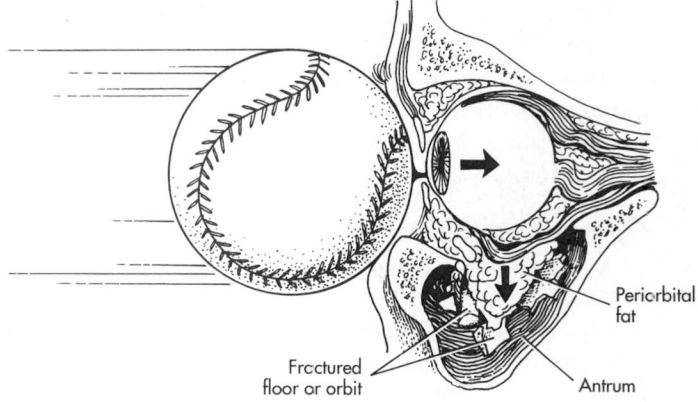

FIGURE 18-34 Orbital fracture. Ball has struck rim of orbit and has pressed orbital contents backward, displacing fragments of bone into maxillary sinus. Inferior rectus muscle is incarcerated in fracture. Inferior oblique muscle may also be involved.

nostril. An absorbent sponge may be taped under the nostrils.

SURGERY OF THE GLOBE AND ORBIT

Surgery of the globe (eyeball) and orbit is usually performed because of trauma. Additional instruments for procedures of the globe or orbit are shown in Fig. 18-32.

Rupture of the eyeball may be direct at the site of injury or, more frequently, indirect from an increase in intraocular pressure that causes the wall of the eyeball to tear at weaker points such as the limbus. When the intraocular contents have become so deranged that useful function is prohibited or the blind eye becomes painful, removal of the eye contents (evisceration procedure) or of the entire eyeball (enucleation) is indicated. If either procedure is required, an inert globe or a coralline hydroxyapatite (coral) implant may be implanted as a space filler and to aid in the movement of a prosthesis (artificial eye) (Fig. 18-33).

Fractures of the walls of the orbit may be caused by direct blows or by extension of a fracture line from adjacent bones. Isolated orbital floor, or blowout, fractures usually occur after injury to the region of the eye by an object the size of an apple or an adult's fist. Orbital contents herniate into the maxillary sinus, and the inferior rectus or inferior oblique muscle may become incarcerated at the fracture site (Fig. 18-34). A Caldwell-Luc antrostomy may be done with reduction of the fracture from below, or the fracture site may be approached directly through the lower lid along the orbital floor and the

tubing remains in place until the sutures become absorbed, thereby acting as a stent about which epithelial union between the lacrimal and nasal mucosa can occur.

8. The orbicularis is closed with 6-0 absorbable sutures. Skin margins are approximated and closed with nonabsorbable 6-0 sutures. Antiinfective ointment is applied to the incision.

9. The wire stylettes are cut off the Silastic tubing, and the ends of the tubing are tied together. The tubing is sutured to the lateral nasal wall with 6-0 nonabsorbable suture. The tubing is cut so that it retracts into the

prolapsed tissue reduced, the orbital floor reduced, and the orbital floor defect bridged with bone grafts, molded metal implants, or plastic material.

Enucleation

Enucleation is removal of the entire eyeball usually with the insertion of a round implant into the socket to replace the globe. The coral implant is an ideal foundation for a prosthetic eye because it allows for normal movement and can be infused with blood to prevent foreign-body reaction.[10] Coralline hydroxyapatite sphere implants are gaining popularity and will probably replace methyl methacrylate as the sphere of choice after enucleation and evisceration.

Operative procedure

1. A speculum retractor is introduced into the palpebral fissure.
2. The conjunctiva is divided around the cornea with sharp and blunt dissection.
3. The medial, lateral, inferior, and superior rectus muscles are divided, leaving a stump of medial rectus muscle. If a coralline hydroxyapatite implant with donor sclera will be used, the four rectus muscles and two oblique muscles are identified and secured with 6-0 nonabsorbable suture (to be used to reattach muscles to cut-out areas in donor sclera) before the muscles are divided.
4. The globe is separated from Tenon's capsule with blunt-pointed curved scissors, retractors, hemostats, and forceps. The eye is rotated laterally by grasping the stump of the medial rectus muscle.
5. A large, curved hemostat is passed behind the globe, and the optic nerve is clamped for 60 seconds. The hemostat is removed, the enucleation scissors are passed posteriorly, and the optic nerve is transected. The oblique muscles are severed as the eye is lifted out of the socket by the stump of the medial rectus muscle.
6. The muscle cone is packed with saline-soaked sponges to obtain hemostasis.
7. The muscle cone is filled with an implant, and Tenon's capsule and conjunctiva are carefully closed. Hydroxyapatite spheres, with donor sclera to reattach the muscles, are frequently placed for later use, which will allow synchronous movement.
8. A socket conformer is placed into the cul-de-sac.
9. A pressure dressing is applied.

Evisceration

Evisceration is removal of the contents of the eye, leaving intact the sclera and the attached muscles.

Operative procedure

1. The conjunctiva is not separated from the sclera as it is for enucleation. A sharp-pointed knife is inserted through the limbus anterior to the iris.

2. The contents of the eye (iris, vitreous, lens) are removed.
3. The choroid adhering to the sclera is removed with curettes.
4. Bleeding is controlled with delicate hemostatic forceps, electrocoagulation, and sutures.
5. A plastic or coral implant is placed within the empty shell.
6. The conjunctival and scleral edges are brought together with nonabsorbable 4-0 or 5-0 sutures, and a pressure dressing is applied.

Repair of Fracture of the Orbit (Blowout)

A fractured orbit (Fig. 18-35) is repaired by means of graft or realignment of contents of the orbit.

Procedural considerations

The setup is as for dacryocystorhinostomy, plus a graft set (for implantation of an autogenous graft or synthetic graft materials of various sizes and thicknesses) and a flexible, narrow-width retractor. The patient is prepared as described for eye surgery. A general anesthetic is usually administered.

Operative procedure

1. The maximum ocular rotation is tested by exerting traction with a forceps on the tendon of the inferior rectus muscle to determine if the inferior muscle sling is trapped in the fracture.

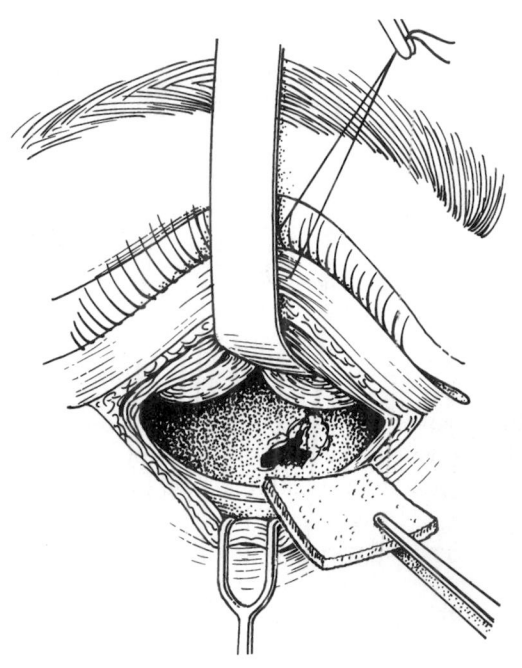

FIGURE 18-35 *Stippled area* shows blowout fracture site. Autogenous graft from iliac crest is held by forceps ready to be placed over fractured site. Graft usually does not require suturing.

2. To distribute tension over the lower lid and stretch the orbicular muscle, a traction suture is inserted through the lower lid margin.
3. With a #3 knife handle and #15 blade the lower lid is incised in the lid fold above the orbital rim.
4. The skin is separated from the orbicular muscle, and the orbital septum is identified by blunt dissection. Dissection is continued down to the periosteum of the orbital rim by means of scissors, loop retractors, elevators, and forceps.
5. The periosteum of the orbital rim is incised with a #15 blade. With periosteal elevators the floor of the orbit is exposed and explored. When the fracture site is identified, bone spicules (needle-shaped bone fragments) are removed, and the herniated contents are freed from the maxillary antrum. The contents of the orbit are elevated by means of narrow-width, flexible retractors. A 4-0 traction suture is placed around the tendon of the inferior rectus muscle.
6. An autogenous graft is taken from the iliac crest, or an alloplastic material of proper size is used to repair the bony defect. The material may or may not be anchored to the orbital rim by wire sutures.
7. The periosteum is carefully closed with 4-0 absorbable sutures.
8. The skin is closed with 6-0 nonabsorbable sutures, and a pressure dressing is applied. Interosseous wiring may be carried out for fractures of the frontozygomatic junction. In addition, oculoplastic surgery has been greatly enhanced by the use of microplates and screws to stabilize fractures involving the fragile facial and orbital bones.

Exenteration

Exenteration is removal of the entire orbital contents, including periosteum, for certain malignancies of the globe or orbit. The procedure may also include removal of the external structures of the eyelids.

Procedural considerations

Considerations are as described for fracture of the orbit. General anesthesia is usually administered.

Operative procedure

1. Depending on circumstances, exenteration of the eye may or may not include the removal of the lids. An incision is made down to the orbital rim, through the periosteum, and around the entire orbit.
2. With periosteal elevators the periosteum is freed from the orbital walls and the apex of the orbit.
3. The optic nerve is clamped, and the entire contents of the orbit are removed en bloc.
4. Hemostasis is obtained by the use of electrosurgery and bone wax.
5. A skin graft or temporal muscle implant may be used to fill the orbital cavity, or the patient may be fitted with an oculofacial prosthesis 2 months postoperatively. If a graft emplacement is not done, iodoform gauze is used to fill the cavity, a pressure dressing is put in place, and the cavity is allowed to granulate.

SURGERY FOR STRABISMUS

Strabismus (squint) is the inability to direct the two eyes at the same object because of lack of coordination of the extraocular muscles. Corrective surgery is performed to change the relative strength of individual muscles and therefore improve coordination. Additional instruments needed for procedures on the eye muscles are shown in Fig. 18-36.

The deviation of the eye may be inward, outward, upward, or downward, and the amount of deviation is a

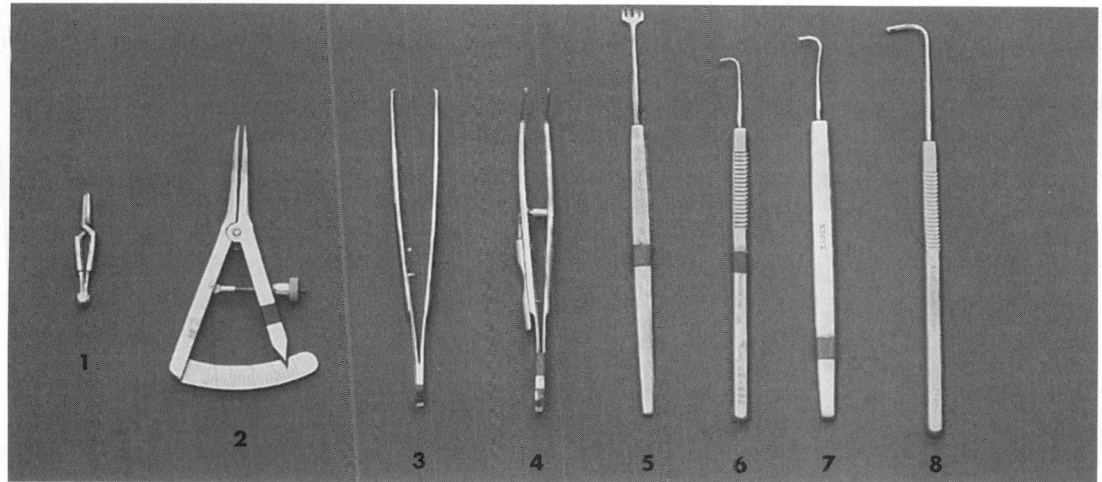

FIGURE 18-36 Instruments for surgery of eye muscles. *1*, Serrefine; *2*, Castroviejo caliper; *3*, O'Brien fixation forceps; *4*, Jameson recession forceps; *5*, lacrimal sac retractor; *6 to 8*, von Graefe strabismus hooks, small, medium, and large.

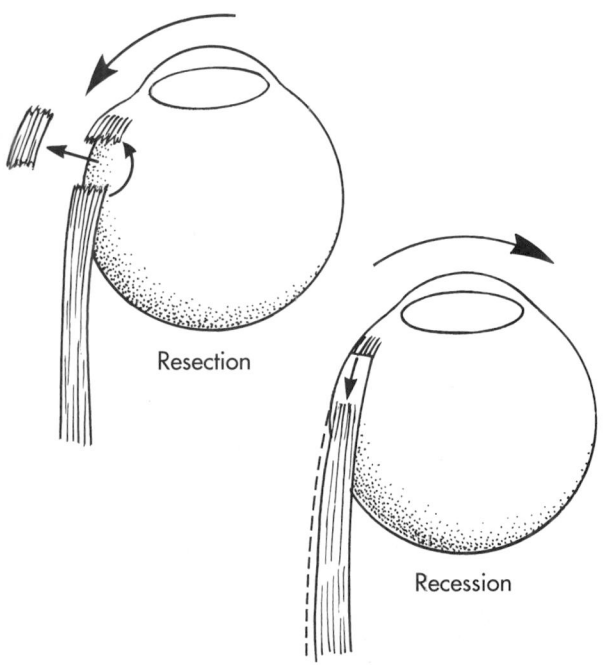

FIGURE 18-37   In surgery for strabismus, *resection* of part of ocular muscle tendon rotates eye toward operated muscle, whereas *recession* moves muscle tendon backward on eye, permitting eye to rotate away from operated muscle.

measurement of the angle formed by the visual axis of the two eyes. The lateral rectus muscle abducts the eye, the medial rectus muscle adducts it, and the other ocular muscles have both primary and secondary functions in elevation, depression, intorsion, and extorsion, according to the position of the eye. Two basic surgical approaches are used to correct strabismus: strengthening is usually accomplished by a resection procedure, and weakening is usually done with a recession procedure (Fig. 18-37). Operating on three or more muscles, in two stages, may be necessary. To some extent the type of strabismus influences the type of surgery.

Resection

Resection is removal of a portion of muscle and attachment of cut ends (see Fig. 18-37) to strengthen the pull of the muscle.

Procedural considerations

Suture material varies according to the surgeon's preference, but usually the suture is on a spatula needle. The patient is prepared as described previously for eye surgery; local or general anesthesia is used. Perioperative nurses should be aware that tension or traction on ocular muscles can precipitate bradycardia.

Operative procedure

1. A speculum is inserted, and the conjunctiva is incised to expose the muscle to be resected.

2. Conjunctival tissue is cleaned from muscle, and a Jameson hook is placed under muscle and lifted up to form a tunnel under muscle. Vessels of muscle and sclera are cauterized.
3. A second muscle hook is inserted opposite the first to pull the muscle taut to expose the area to be resected.
4. The area to be resected is measured and marked. A double-armed absorbable suture is passed through the muscle belly at the desired position of shortening and the muscle is incised anterior to this suture.
5. The stump of the muscle is excised from the insertion, and the muscle is then sutured to the insertion using the double-armed suture.
6. The conjunctiva is closed with an absorbable suture.

Recession

Recession is severance of the muscle from its original insertion with reattachment more posteriorly on the sclera (see Fig. 18-37) to weaken the pull of the muscle.

Operative procedure

1. A speculum is inserted, and the conjunctiva is incised to expose the muscle to be recessed.
2. Conjunctival tissue is cleaned from muscle, a Jameson hook is placed under muscle and lifted up to form a tunnel under muscle. Vessels of muscle and sclera are cauterized.
3. Sutures are passed through the tendinous part of the muscle at its insertion site, and the sutures are knotted near the muscle edge. The tendon is severed distal to the suture.
4. With calipers, marks are made on the globe at the desired distance behind the insertion, and the muscle is anchored to the globe at that point.
5. The conjunctiva is closed with absorbable suture.

Myectomy

Myectomy is a method of weakening the action of a muscle for V-pattern strabismus or superior oblique palsy. This may be done as a recession of the inferior oblique muscle or as a complete severance of a muscle, such as an inferior oblique myectomy.

Operative procedure

1. A traction suture is placed at the limbus, and the globe is pulled upward to expose the muscle site.
2. An opening is made into the conjunctiva and Tenon's capsule, and the involved muscle is isolated, lifted, and spread with two muscle hooks.
3. Myectomy of the inferior oblique muscle is performed by placing two straight hemostats across the muscle belly and excising the isolated strip of muscle close to the hemostats. The ends of the muscle are cauterized and released. Because of the peculiar anatomy of this muscle, lateral discontinuity weakens but does not paralyze it.

4. The edges of the conjunctiva are lifted with forceps, and the incision is closed with interrupted absorbable sutures.

Tuck

A tuck is a method of shortening a muscle and thus strengthening it for superior oblique palsy and torsional diplopia. Tucking is performed primarily on the superior oblique muscle tendon.

Operative procedure

1. A traction suture is placed at the limbus, and the globe is pulled downward to expose the tendon site. An opening is made in the conjunctiva and Tenon's capsule, medial to the superior rectus muscle.
2. A lid retractor in inserted into the incision to hold back the conjunctiva and Tenon's capsule. The superior rectus muscle is retracted out of the way with muscle hooks.
3. The Jameson muscle hook is passed posteriorly into the orbit, and the superior oblique muscle tendon is hooked and brought into the incision.
4. The tendon is elevated and doubled, like looping a rope, and a double-armed nonabsorbable suture is passed through the base of the loop, effectively shortening the muscle.
5. The tip of the loop is sutured to the sclera, laterally to the superior rectus muscle.
6. The edges of the conjunctiva are lifted with forceps, and the incision is closed with interrupted absorbable sutures.

SURGERY OF THE CONJUNCTIVA

The conjunctiva of the eye is a transparent and elastic membrane that lines the inner surface of the eyelids and covers the sclera. Lacerations caused by injury as well as deficits resulting from excision of tumors, cysts, nevi, or pterygiums can usually be repaired by simple undermining and suturing.

Pterygium Excision

A pterygium is a fleshy, triangular encroachment of conjunctiva onto the peripheral area of the cornea. Since pterygiums tend to reoccur, surgery is delayed until vision is affected by encroachment on the visual axis.

Operative procedure

The major steps in the McReynolds technique are illustrated in Fig. 18-38. A pterygium can also be excised totally and the limbus treated with an eye cautery or electrocoagulation. The conjunctiva can then be closed, or the sclera can be left bare.

Surgery may be combined with beta-radiation, application of mitomycin, conjunctiva autologous grafts, and lamellar corneal grafts.[4]

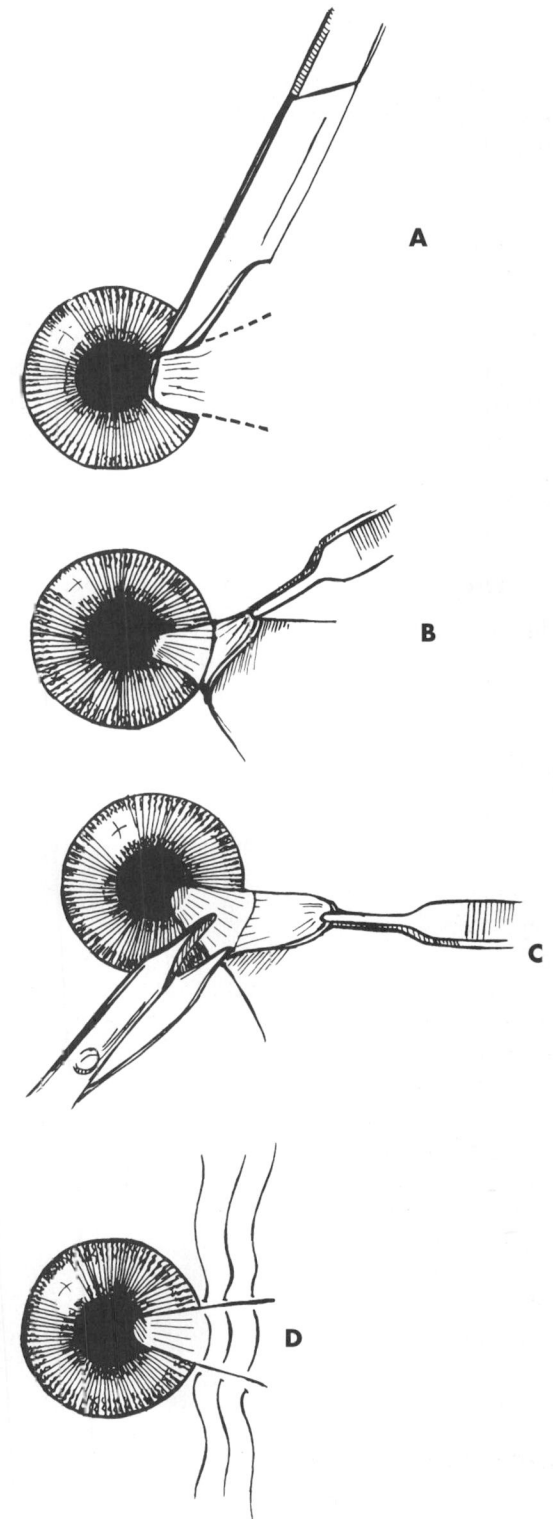

FIGURE 18-38   McReynolds technique for pterygium repair. **A,** Cornea around head of pterygium is incised. **B,** Pterygium flap is dissected upward, leaving clear cornea. **C,** Lower margin of pterygium is dissected, and whole pterygium is freed from sclera. **D,** Sutures are placed for closure of conjunctiva.

Excisional Biopsy

Any suspect lesion of the conjunctiva can be removed by simple elliptic excision and sent for pathologic examination. The conjunctiva may or may not be closed, depending on the surgeon's particular technique.

SURGERY OF THE CORNEA

Surgery of the cornea is indicated for a variety of conditions in which cosmetic, therapeutic, restorative, and refractive outcomes are desired. New technology and the development of the eximer laser has been responsible for the introduction of procedures that offer more choices for restoration of vision. Additional instrumentation for corneal transplants (lamellar and penetrating) as well as for repair of lacerations and removal of foreign bodies of the cornea is shown in Fig. 18-39.

Phototherapeutic Keratectomy

The FDA recently approved the 193 nm excimer laser for phototherapeutic keratectomy (PTK) procedures that utilize laser ablation to remove superficial corneal lesions and smooth the corneal surface. PTK can be used on conditions that would require corneal transplant and may delay or replace the occurrence of penetrating keratoplasty in some cases.[9]

Repair of Lacerations

The preferred method of closing corneal lacerations is with direct appositional suturing with 10-0 suture viewed through an operating microscope.

Tissue adhesives, that is, cyanoacrylate monomers, are being used experimentally. The tissue adhesive is applied to well-dried tissue that has been properly oriented anatomically. It polymerizes and seals the wound on contact with the tissue. The tissue adhesive is supplied in packaged sterile vials (Co-Apt).

Culture specimens are usually obtained at the time of surgery. Antibiotics are injected subconjunctivally before the dressing is applied.

Corneal Transplantation (Keratoplasty)

Corneal transplantation is a grafting of corneal tissue from one human eye to another. Since the cornea is tissue that lacks blood vessels, it can be transplanted with less rejection and at a 90% success rate. Keratoplasty may be

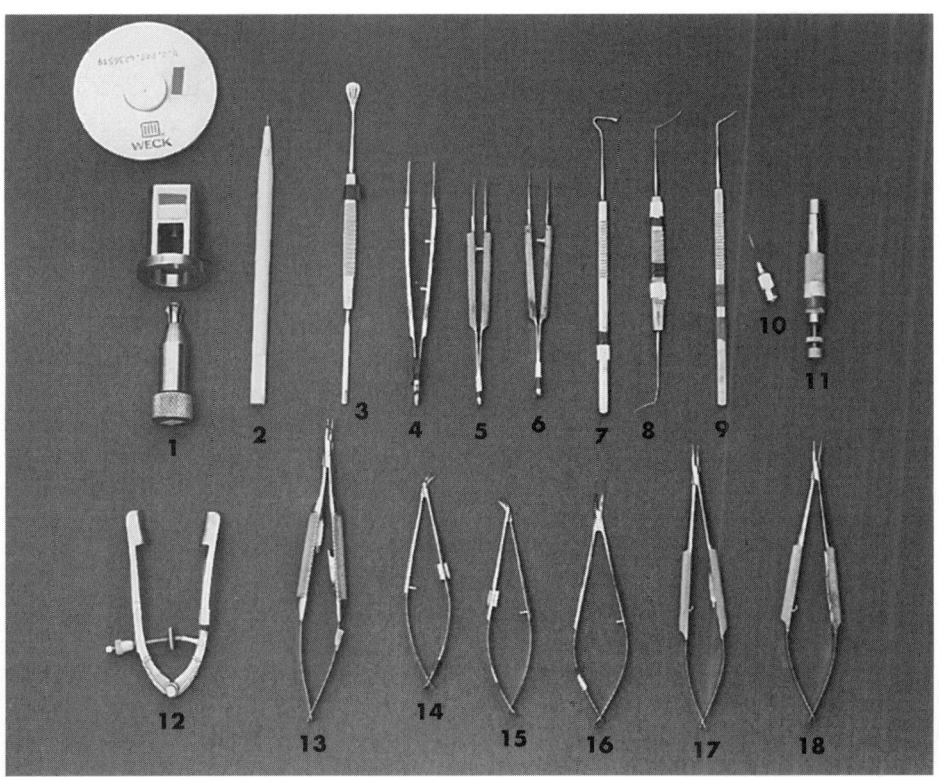

FIGURE 18-39 Instruments for corneal transplant and other procedures on the cornea. *1*, Universal trephine handle with Cottingham punch; *2*, Super blade; *3*, Paton spatula; *4*, Castroviejo suturing forceps, 0.12 mm; *5*, Bishop-Harmon forceps; *6*, Colibri corneal forceps; *7*, Green strabismus hook; *8*, Castroviejo cyclodialysis spatula; *9*, Troutman corneal dissector; *10*, air cannula, 27 gauge; *11*, Castroviejo trephine; *12*, Lancaster eye speculum; *13*, Barraquer curved microneedle holder; *14* and *15*, Troutman-Castroviejo corneal scissors, right and left; *16*, Castroviejo corneal scissors; *17*, straight microneedle holder; *18*, corneal scleral scissors.

performed as lamellar (partial-thickness) graft or penetrating (full-thickness) graft. A corneal transplantation is performed when the patient's cornea is thickened and opacified by disease and degeneration. The transparency of the cornea may be impaired as a result of scars, infection (bacterial, fungal, or viral), thermal or chemical burns, Fuchs's dystrophy, or keratoconus (abnormal steepening). A corneal transplantation is done to improve vision when the retina and optic nerve are functioning properly.

Procurement of corneas

The eye bank may be a central community agency or may be owned and operated by a hospital. Eye banks help coordinate the procurement of eyes from recently deceased persons under the Eye Bank Association of America (EBAA) guidelines. Persons 2 to 70 years of age can be eye donors, and poor eyesight or cataracts does not matter. The donor's family, medical, and social history is reviewed. It is not necessary to do antigen matching as with other tissue or organ transplants, but blood serum tests for human immunodeficiency virus (HIV) and hepatitis B virus are performed on the donor. Donor eyes are removed within 6 hours of death in accordance with legal regulations. If the donor eye is unsuitable for the cornea to be transplanted, the eye can be used for research or education.

Many individuals have signed donor cards or eye-donor designation on their driver licenses. A special consent form is required and should be signed by the authorized next of kin and by a hospital representative designated by institutional policy.

The enucleations may be done in the hospital morgue or emergency department under aseptic conditions. The procured cornea is placed in Optisol GS sterile buffered tissue culture medium within 12 hours of death and transplanted within 3 to 7 days. Optisol GS sterile buffered tissue culture medium contains polypeptides, dextran, and antibiotics (gentamicin and streptomycin) and can preserve a donor cornea for 14 days under refrigeration. It is best if corneal transplantation is performed in 2 or 3 days because the cornea may become boggy from constant exposure to the tissue culture solution.

Procedural considerations

The eyes are washed and irrigated in the routine manner of preparation for eye surgery. The sterile field, drapes, and instruments are essentially the same as those for an enucleation on a living patient.

Operative procedures

1. Eye specimen bottles are labeled for right and left eyes.
2. The speculum is inserted, and after routine enucleation the donated eye is placed with the cornea up on a saline-soaked sponge in the sterile specimen bottle.
3. The eye sockets are packed with cotton, and the lids are closed.

4. Specimen bottles are sealed with tape and labeled with the donor's name, time of death, time of enucleation, and date.

Penetrating Keratoplasty (Fig. 18-40)

1. The eye speculum is put in place, and superior rectus and inferior rectus bridle sutures are placed if a Flieringa ring is not to be used. If a ring is used, it is sutured in place with four 5-0 sutures.
2. A corneoscleral button that has been refrigerated and stored in tissue culture medium (Optisol GS) is removed from its container.
3. The corneoscleral button is placed epithelial (outside) surface down on a sterile Teflon block. The corneal trephine is then used as a punch, and the donor button is pressed out centrally. A drop of balanced salt solution may be used to cover the donor button until it is implanted.
4. The section of cornea removed from the recipient's eye may be the same size as the graft taken from the donor's eye or may as much as 0.5 mm smaller. The button is excised with a hand-held trephine or a disposable suction trephine.

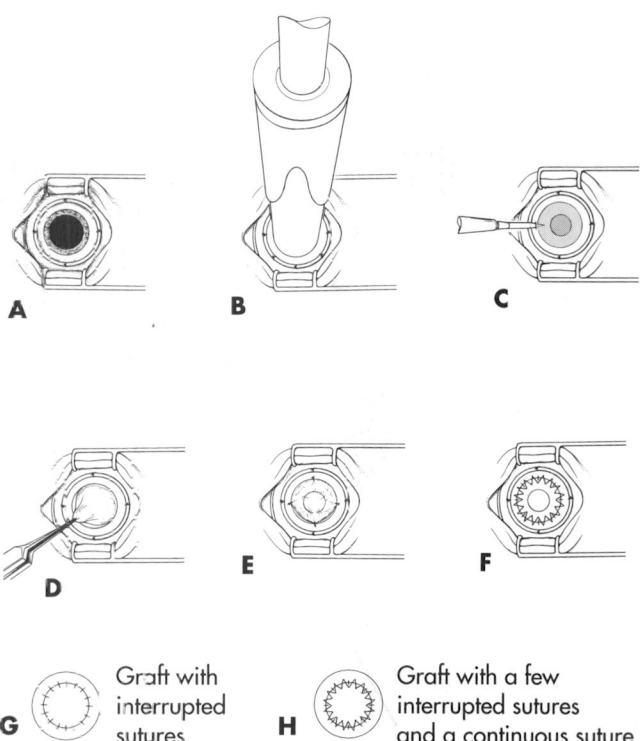

FIGURE 18-40 A, Eye of patient who will undergo corneal transplantation. A Flieringa fixation ring is sutured in place with 5-0 nonabsorbable sutures. B, Corneal trephine is placed on patient's cornea, and partial penetration is made approximately three fourths through stroma. C, Anterior chamber is entered with a blade and the remainder of button is excised with right and left corneal microscissors. D, Patient's corneal button is removed. E, Donor cornea graft is sutured in place with four sutures. F, Donor cornea graft is sutured in place with interrupted or continuous 10-0 non-absorbable suture (G and H).

5. Peripheral iridectomies or iridotomies may be performed at this time at the surgeon's discretion, or a cataract extraction with intraocular lens (IOL) implantation may also be performed if the lens is opaque.

6. The graft is placed into the opening of the recipient's eye and anchored in place by means of four single-armed sutures placed at the four cardinal meridians, viewed through an operating microscope. Some surgeons preplace sutures in the graft. The graft is sutured to the host with either continuous or interrupted 10-0 nonabsorbable sutures.

7. Air or sodium hyaluronate (Healon) may be injected into the anterior chamber of the recipient's eye to keep the iris from adhering to the suture line. Mydriatic or miotic solutions are used at the surgeon's discretion.

8. A subconjunctival injection of antibiotic solution or a topical application of antibiotic drops may be used at the completion of the procedure. Antibiotic ointment is applied, followed by an eye pad and a protective shield.

Lamellar Keratoplasty

1. The eye speculum and superior rectus and inferior rectus bridle sutures are placed if needed.
2. The eye from the eye bank is removed from its container and washed in balanced salt solution.
3. The eye is wrapped in a surgical dressing. A groove is made at the desired depth in the cornea with the trephine. The Castroviejo keratome is set at the desired depth, and the lamellar sheet of cornea is removed and placed into a Petri dish.
4. The recipient cornea is grooved with the same trephine to the appropriate depth. Using the operating microscope, the surgeon performs a lamellar resection, that is, removes the anterior part of the cornea at a predetermined depth with a Gill knife, Beaver knife blade #64, or other corneal splitter.
5. The donor tissue is sutured in place with a continuous 10-0 nonabsorbable nylon suture.
6. A mydriatic agent and subconjunctival or topical antibiotics may be used.
7. The eye is patched.

Keratorefractive Procedures

Keratorefractive procedures are corneal procedures designed to correct myopia, astigmatism, and aphakia. They include radial keratotomy, keratomileusis, and keratophakia. These procedures require reshaping the cornea with relaxing incisions or cryolathing corneal tissue to change the refractive power of the cornea. Newer procedures utilizing various technologies include photorefractive keratectomy (PRK), which uses the excimer laser to treat myopia (nearsightedness), and laser in situ keratomileusis (LASIK), which uses the excimer to shape the corneal stroma bed. LASIK has been reported to

18-2 RESEARCH HIGHLIGHT

With the use of topical anesthesia for cataract removal, clear cornea incisions provide the opportunity for correction of refractive errors. Clinical study of 690 consecutive cataract surgeries using topical anesthesia, clear cornea incision, phacoemulsification, and microinjection of an elastic IOL was conducted between March 1993 and March 1995. The purpose of the study was to assess the effectiveness of keratolenticuloplasty (KLP), the simultaneous modification of the cornea at cataract removal to correct refractive errors. Length and location of the corneal incisions were varied depending on absence of astigmatism, preoperative astigmatism of 1.00 diopters (D) or less, 1.00 D to 2.00 D, and greater than 2.00 D. Results demonstrated that patients can be free of glasses after clear corneal cataract surgery with proper selection of IOL power and surgical correction of astigmatism with keratolenticuloplasty.

From Kershner, R.M. (1997). Clear cornea cataract surgery and the correction of myopia, hyperopia, and astigmatism. *Ophthalmology, 104*(3), 381-389.

achieve postoperative visual acuity of 20/40 or better in over 80% of eyes including those that are highly myopic.[8]

Clinical trials have been conducted using holmium: YAG laser thermokeratoplasty to correct hyperopia (far-sightedness). The holmium:YAG laser causes shrinkage of cornea collagen, thus creating central corneal steepening at the treated sites.[3] The recent advancements in cataract surgery with clear cornea microincisions have created the opportunity for full correction of refractive errors during the surgical procedure (Research Highlight 18-2).

Radial keratotomy

Radial keratotomy is a series of precise, partial-thickness radial incisions in the cornea from a 3 mm or larger central optical zone to the limbus. These incisions result in a flattening of the cornea, which reduces the refractive error. Radial keratotomy was first performed in the United States in 1978. Since then, modifications in the procedure have improved the predictability of results. Studies to ascertain the long-term results continue.

Radial keratotomy is a procedure for an adult who has at least -1 D of myopia and whose eyes are otherwise healthy. Preoperative measurement of corneal curvature (keratometry), corneal thickness (ultrasonic pachymetry), and refractive error is required to assist in the determination of optical-zone diameter and depth of incisions.

Procedural Considerations

The surgery is performed as an ambulatory procedure with local and topical anesthetics. Instruments for radial keratotomy are shown in Fig. 18-41.

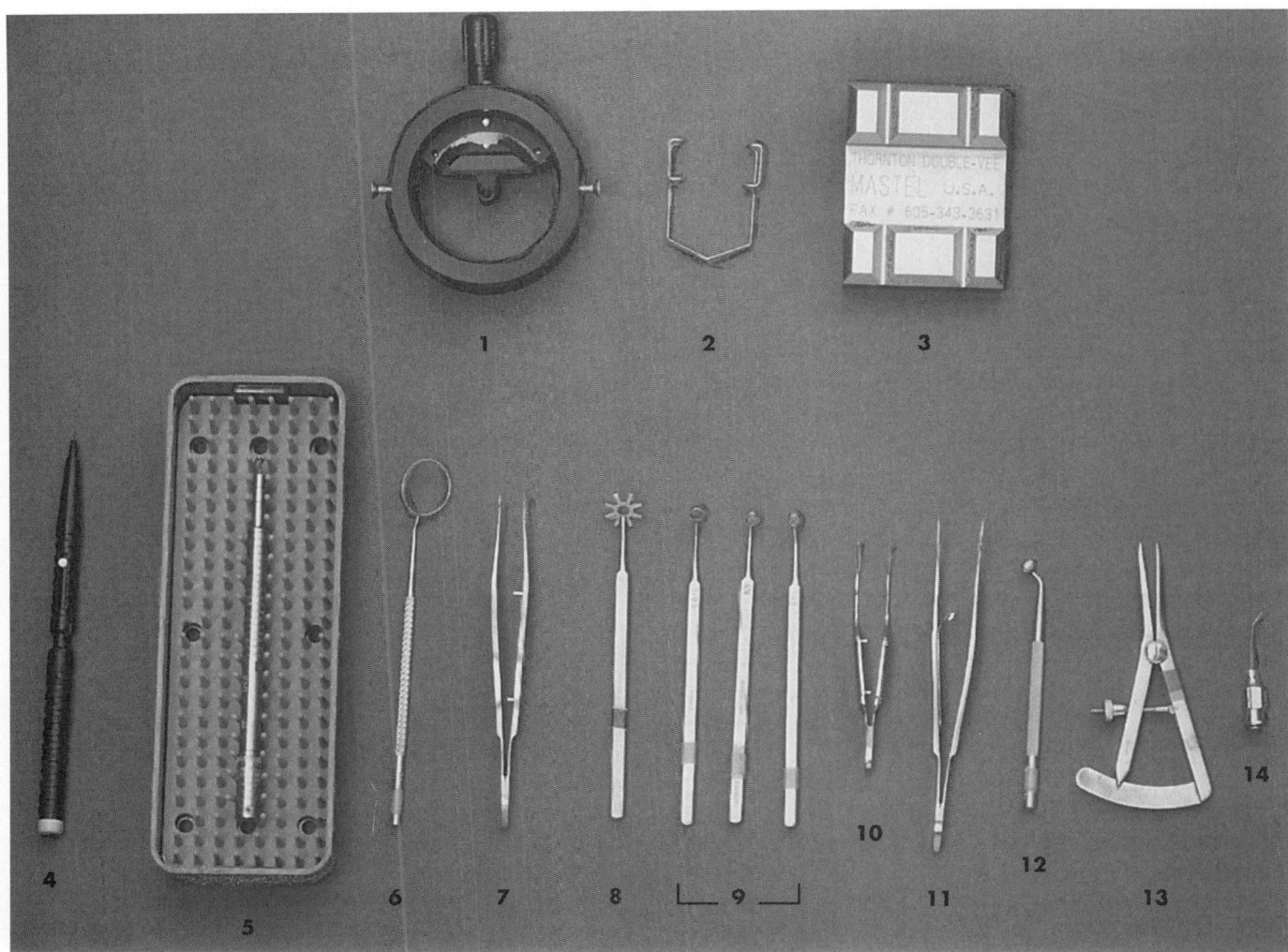

FIGURE 18-41   Radial keratotomy instrumentation. *1*, Fixation device (to be attached to microscope) for patient to focus to mark optical zone; *2*, Barraquer wire speculum; *3*, Bores corneal knife gauge; *4*, Katena micrometer XTAL sapphire knife; *5*, Storz micrometer diamond knife; *6*, incision-depth gauge; *7*, Rubman-Bores corneal fixation forceps; *8*, Bores corneal marker for eight radial incisions; *9*, Hoffer corneal markers with cross-hairs; *10*, Castroviejo-Colibri very delicate forceps, 0.12 mm; *11*, Bores incision-spreading forceps; *12*, elliptical optic center marker; *13*, Castroviejo caliper; *14*, air cannula, 27 gauge.

Operative Procedure

1. As the patient focuses on the fixation device attached to the objective lens of the operating microscope, the visual axis is marked.
2. The blade depth is set on the micrometer of the surgical knife (diamond, sapphire, or steel) and double-checked against a micrometer gauge.
3. The surgeon fixates the globe with double-toothed Bores fixation forceps to decrease rotation.
4. Radial incisions are made from the margin of the optical zone to the limbus (Fig. 18-42). The numbers and depth are determined by the amount of correction desired.
5. The depth of the incisions is checked to verify uniformity.
6. The incisions are irrigated with balanced salt solution

(BSS). An antibiotic solution is instilled and an eye patch applied.

SURGERY OF THE LENS

Cataract Extraction

A cataract extraction is removal of the opaque lens from the interior of the eye. The lens consists of 65% water, 35% protein, and a trace of other body minerals. The disorders of the lens are opacification and dislocation, resulting in blurred vision without pain or inflammation. Cataracts (opacification) vary in degree of density, size, and location and are usually caused by aging or trauma.

The intracapsular cataract extraction (ICCE) method of cataract removal consists of removing the lens within its capsule with a cryoprobe and is rarely performed to-

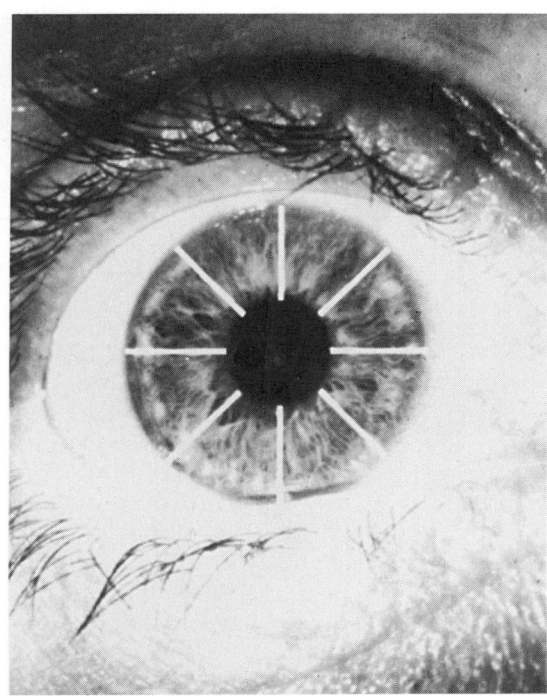

FIGURE 18-42   Location of incisions in radial keratotomy. Central 3 to 4 mm optical zone of cornea is not incised, and incisions do not extend beyond corneoscleral limbus. Four, eight, or 16 radial incisions are made.

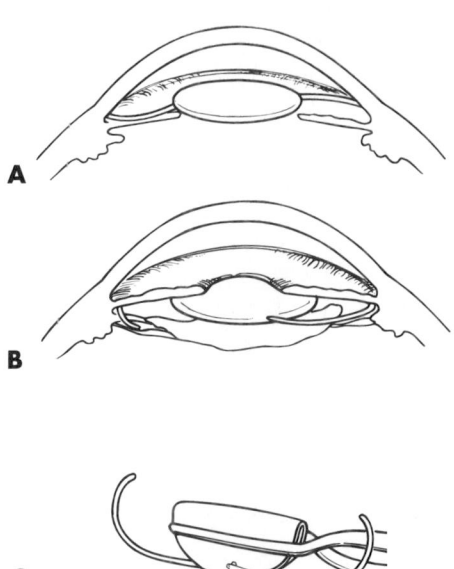

FIGURE 18-43   **A,** Anterior chamber intraocular lens that is held in position with loop of nylon (haptics) placed in anterior chamber angle. **B,** Posterior chamber lens placed in lens capsule from which most of anterior portion has been excised. **C,** Foldable posterior chamber lens.

day except in the event of a dislocated lens. Since ICCE is not frequently used, the medication alpha-chymotrypsin (Zolase, Catarase, Chymar), which is an enzyme that acts on the zonules of the lens, will not be immediately available. If an ICCE is scheduled, the medication and a cataract cryoprobe need to be procured.

In the extracapsular method the anterior portion of the capsule is first ruptured and removed, and the lens cortex and nucleus are expressed from the eye, leaving the posterior capsule behind. Restoration of functional vision is necessary after removal of the crystalline lens (aphakia). Contact lenses can be used to correct aphakia. They offer an excellent option for visual correction and can be used for monocular aphakia.

Intraocular lens

The most commonly used option for visual correction after lens removal is the implantation of an intraocular lens (IOL) during the surgical procedure. IOLs offer many advantages to patients. They are used for monocular aphakic correction. Rehabilitation times for patients are shortened.

IOLs are made of polymethyl methacrylate (PMMA), silicone, or acrylic resin (Fig. 18-43). New foldable and injectable designs and new implantation techniques challenge perioperative nursing personnel to keep abreast of constant changes in techniques for IOL implantations. Posterior chamber lenses (PCL) can be implanted only when the cataract was removed by extracapsular lens

extraction (ECCE). This is the most physiologic position for an artificial lens and is now the most common method of lens extraction. Anterior chamber lenses (ACL) are used after intracapsular lens extraction (ICCE) and for secondary lens implantation.

IOLs are available in various diopter powers. The necessary power is determined by measuring the curvature of the patient's cornea (keratometry) and the axial length (length from cornea to retina). A mathematical formula is then used to calculate the correct lens power.

In recent years sutureless cataract techniques have become increasingly popular because of rapid visual rehabilitation. Clear cornea microincisions with the use of topical anesthesia and insertion of foldable IOLs have produced even better visual results with the opportunity to fully correct refractive errors. A clinical pathway for cataract surgery is shown in Fig. 18-44.

Procedural considerations

Instrumentation varies with surgeon's preference but usually includes forceps to insert the lens and lens haptics and a hook to aid in rotating and positioning the lens (Fig. 18-45). Perioperative nursing personnel must be familiar with institutional policies pertaining to IOLs and their use.

Extracapsular Method with Phacoemulsification

Over the past years numerous microsurgical techniques have been developed for lens removal through a small self-sealing incision and most recently through a clear

DRG/ASC # GRP 9 66884	LOS 3-4.5 hours	Reimbursement _____
Pt. ID _____	Date _____	

	Preop (60 min)	Intraop (90 min)	PACU/postop (120 min)
Tests/lab	Preop CBC, EKG Chest X-ray	Pulse oximeter ---------------------------> EKG -------------------------------------->	D/C oximeter D/C EKG
Diet/fluids	NPO--> IV fluids --->		as tolerated D/C IV fluids
Mobility	Ambulate/ up in chair -> stretcher	Immobile	Ambulate with assistance ---> ambulate alone
Treatment	Monitor vital signs -->	Surgical procedure	DC
Medication	Eyedrops	Anesthesia Analgesia --->	DC Discharge meds
Teaching	Preop activities Surgical info Postop activities Discharge teaching		Verbal & written instructions Clinic appointment instructions
Key nursing actions	Anxiety assessment, History & PE assm't. Create therapeutic environment Assess knowledge level Check permits Eyedrops Vital signs	Position, prep, Monitor physiologic status, Prevent movement during surgery --> Prevent nausea & --> vomiting, Assure safety --> Monitor physical status	Assess self-care ability Ensure understanding of discharge instructions
Key patient outcomes	Tolerable anxiety level Knowledge about procedure and self-care.	Free from injury due to positioning, movement, chemicals, electrical sources	Knows discharge meds Able to care for self, can ambulate safely Able to eat and drink Knows signs & symptoms of complications Can care for eye

Sources: Hampton, 1993; Bower, 1992; Zander, 1991; Guiliano & Poirier, 1991; Cronin & Maklebust, 1989; Etheridge, 1986.

FIGURE 18-44   Clinical pathway for cataract surgery.

cornea incision. Extracapsular cataract extraction (ECCE) with phacoemulsification is still performed especially with very mature or hard cataracts and may be done in combination with trabeculectomy for patients with glaucoma.

Basically each technique involves opening the lens capsule and using a phacoemulsification unit with irriga-tion and aspiration (I/A) (Fig. 18-46). The ultrasonic energy of phacoemulsification fragments the hard lens material, which can then be aspirated from the eye. All perioperative personnel using specialized instruments and equipment must have thorough knowledge of the operation as well as problems that may be encountered and actions to correct them.

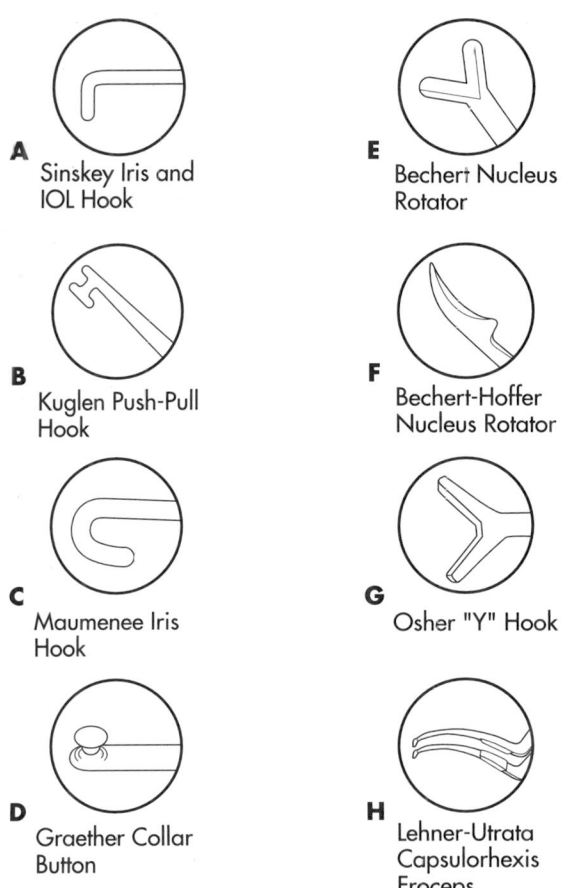

A Sinskey Iris and IOL Hook

B Kuglen Push-Pull Hook

C Maumenee Iris Hook

D Graether Collar Button

E Bechert Nucleus Rotator

F Bechert-Hoffer Nucleus Rotator

G Osher "Y" Hook

H Lehner-Utrata Capsulorhexis Froceps

FIGURE 18-45 Close-up view of tips of microinstruments used in phacoemulsification procedures and for inserting IOLs.

Operative procedure (Fig. 18-47)

1. After a superior rectus bridle suture is placed, a small limbus-based flap is dissected superiorly.
2. The surgical limbus is cleaned by sharp dissection with a Beaver knife blade. Hemostasis is obtained with cautery.
3. A 3 mm incision is made into the eye with either a keratome or a sharp microknife.
4. The lens capsule is opened with capsulorhexis forceps or a cystotome. The anterior chamber may be kept formed with air or an irrigating solution.
5. The lens nucleus is loosened from the cortex with the cystotome or a blunt cyclodialysis spatula.
6. The ultrasonic handpiece is checked by the physician for appropriate vacuum control. *This check should be made before any handpiece is introduced into the eye.*
7. The ultrasonic handpiece is introduced into the eye. The following modes are operational with the foot pedal under the surgeon's control: irrigation alone; irrigation and aspiration; phacoemulsification; and irrigation, aspiration, and phacoemulsification. Some machines also have an anterior vitrector. As the surgeon manipulates the handpiece and operates the foot

pedal to emulsify the lens nucleus, the perioperative nurse is responsible for operating the console controls and monitoring the function of the instrument.

8. When the lens nucleus has been emulsified and removed, the lens cortex is removed with the irrigation-aspiration handpiece.
9. If a foldable IOL is to be implanted, a keratome is used to widen the incision to 3.2 mm, and the lens is folded and inserted. If rigid IOL is to be implanted, the wound is extended to 5.1 mm to accommodate the lens diameter. Acetylcholine may be introduced to constrict the pupil.
10. A peripheral iridectomy may be performed.
11. The corneoscleral wound is closed with a 10-0 nonabsorbable suture.
12. The conjunctival flap is closed with a suture or using bipolar cautery.
13. An eye pad and shield are applied.

Topical Clear Corneal Cataract Procedure

Recent developments with the use of topical anesthetics, new materials for foldable IOLs, and diamond knives for self-sealing or no stitch wounds have led to clear cornea incisions and new techniques for phacoemulsification and lens implantation for cataracts.

Topical anesthesia replaces retrobulbar anesthesia for cataract surgery, and since the patient can fixate, this allows for refractive surgical techniques. Patients must be able to hear and follow directions in order to cooperate with verbal reassurance and instructions to fixate on the microscope light. Various medications and protocols are used for administering topical anesthesia before cataract surgery.

A typical protocol is as follows:

A drop of topical tetracaine 0.5% is placed into the operative eye before the patient enters the operating room. The patient is instructed to keep this eye closed to prevent the cornea from drying out. As the patient is being positioned, another drop of tetracaine is given. An armrest is positioned on the operative side, and the patient's head and microscope are adjusted. The patient is instructed to look at the light of the microscope and told where to fixate. If the patient cannot open his or her eye, consideration should be given to a facial nerve block. If the patient can't fixate on the light at all, consideration should be given to a retrobulbar block.

Operative procedure. (Fig. 18-48)

1. A speculum that sits over the nose and has no attachment temporally is placed in the eye.
2. A stab incision is made at 5 o'clock in a left eye and at 11 o'clock in a right eye into the anterior chamber. A 1 mm wide incision is desirable.
3. One ml of unpreserved lidocaine (Xylocaine) is slowly injected into the anterior chamber through a 30-gauge cannula using a tuberculin syringe.

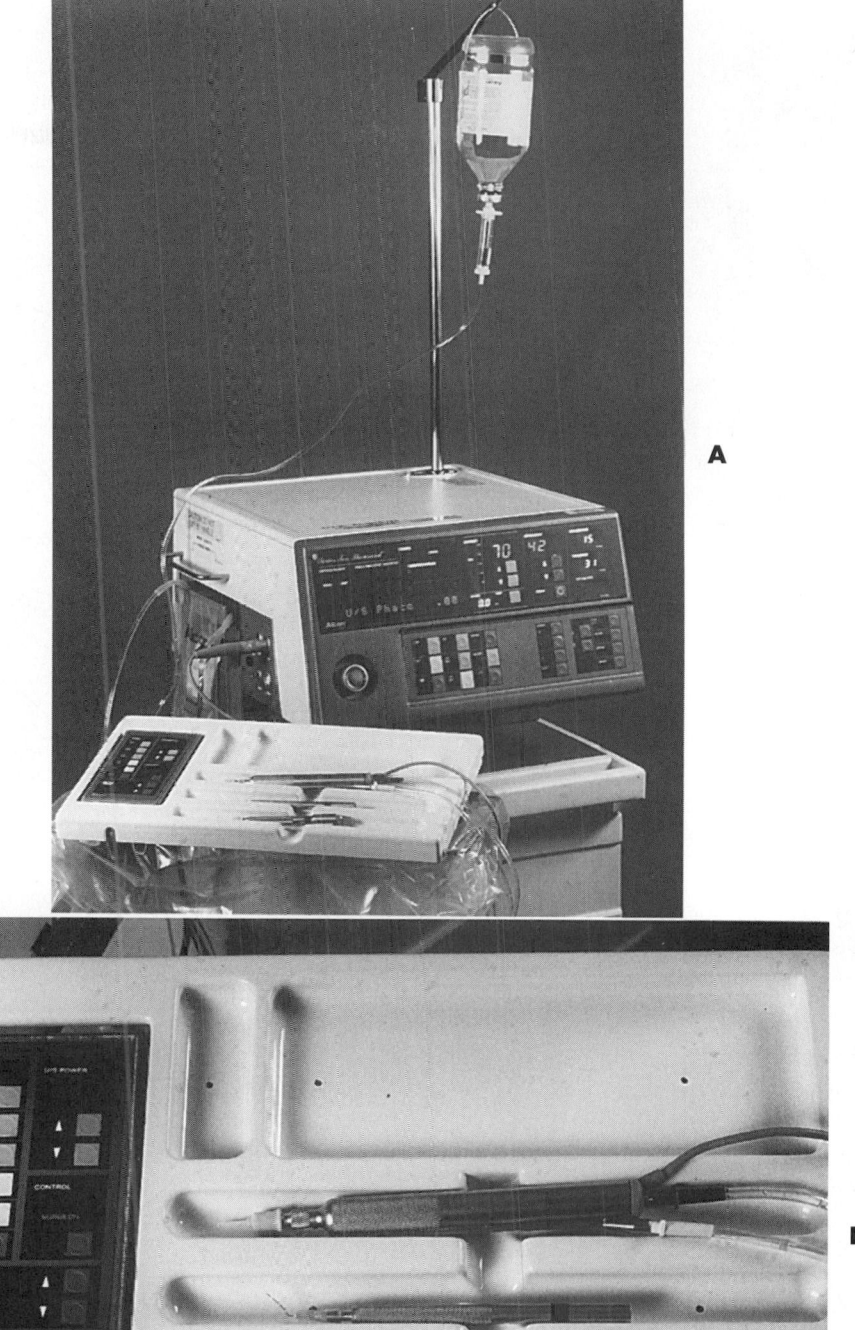

FIGURE 18-46   **A**, Alcon Phaco Emulsifier Aspirator Series 10,000. **B**, Instrument tray shows Phaco handpiece, cystotome handle, irrigation and aspiration (I&A) handpiece, and remote control.

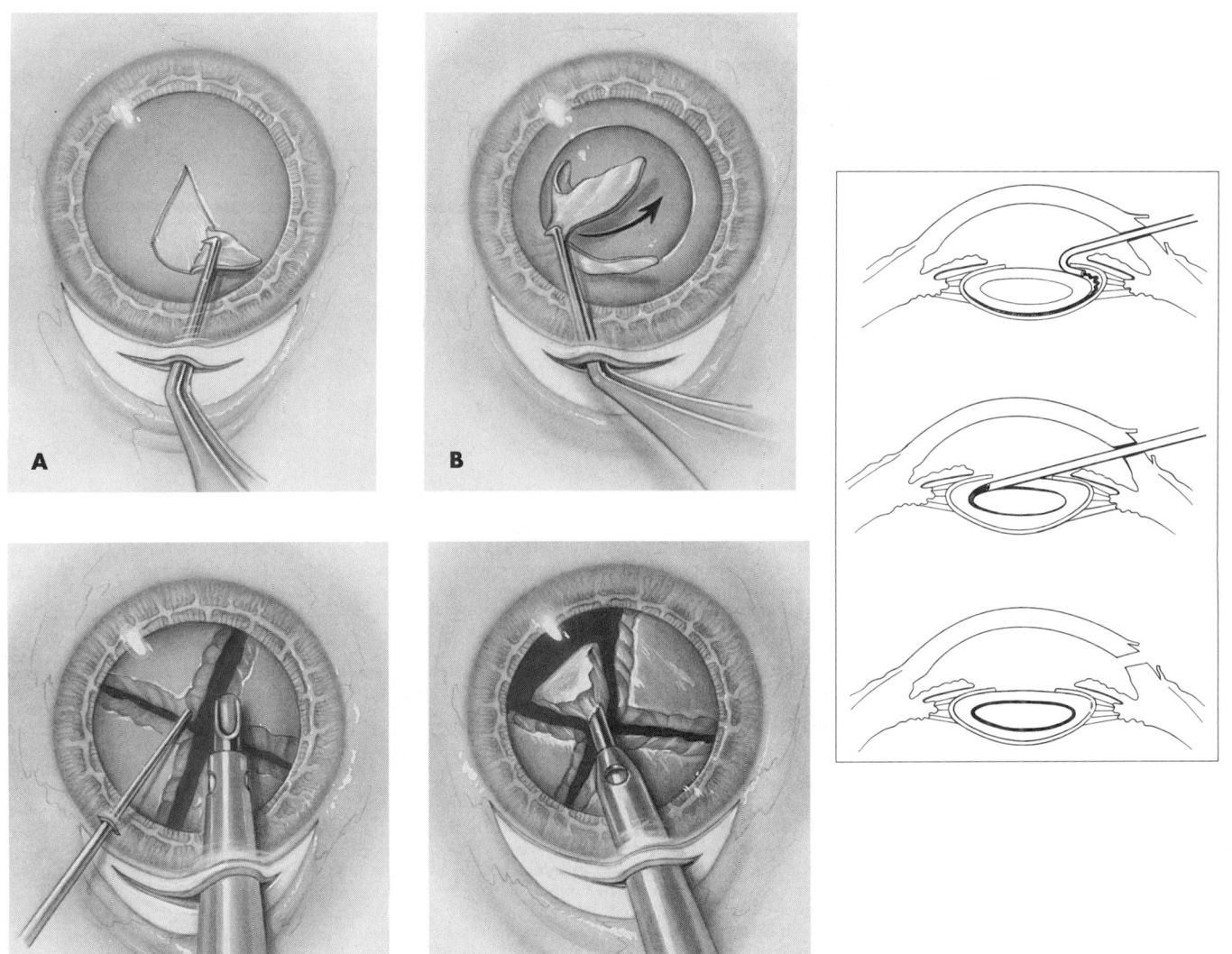

FIGURE 18-47 Cataract extraction with phacoemulsification. **A** and **B**, Capsulorhexis is performed on anterior capsule of lens. **C**, The nucleus of the lens is loosened by hydrodissection. **D**, The nucleus of the lens is "cracked" into four quadrants and **E**, removed with phacoemulsification. *Continued*

4. A viscoelastic material is injected into the anterior chamber to deepen the chamber and widen the pupil.

5. A space of 3 mm is marked on the cornea temporally with a caliper. A vertical incision of 0.3 to 4.0 mm depth is made with a trifacet diamond knife.

6. A diamond keratome is used to make a stepped incision into the anterior chamber 2.6 mm in length on the endothelial surface of the cornea (Fig. 18-48, *A*).

7. A capsulotomy and capsulorhexis are performed with a capsulorhexis forceps (Fig. 18-48, *B*).

8. Hydrodissection and hydrodelineation are carried out with a 30-gauge cannula and saline (Fig. 18-48, *C*).

9. A phacoemulsification tip is placed into the eye and used to sculpt the nucleus.

10. Using a cyclodialysis spatula at 5 o'clock in the left eye and 11 o'clock in the right eye, the nucleus is divided

into quadrants with the phacoemulsification tip and removed from the eye (Fig. 18-48, *D*).

11. An irrigation-aspiration tip is placed into the eye and used to remove the remaining cortical material (Fig. 18-48, *E*).

12. A Kratz scratcher is used to polish the posterior capsule.

13. A viscoelastic material is placed into the capsular bag to inflate the it.

14. A steel keratome is used to widen the incision to 3.2 mm.

15. A posterior chamber IOL is folded and placed into the eye and into the capsular bag (Figs. 18-48, *F* and *G*). The IOL is positioned with a Sinsky hook.

16. An irrigating-aspirating tip is used to remove the remaining viscoelastic material. Using saline through a 30-gauge cannula, the anterior chamber is repressur-

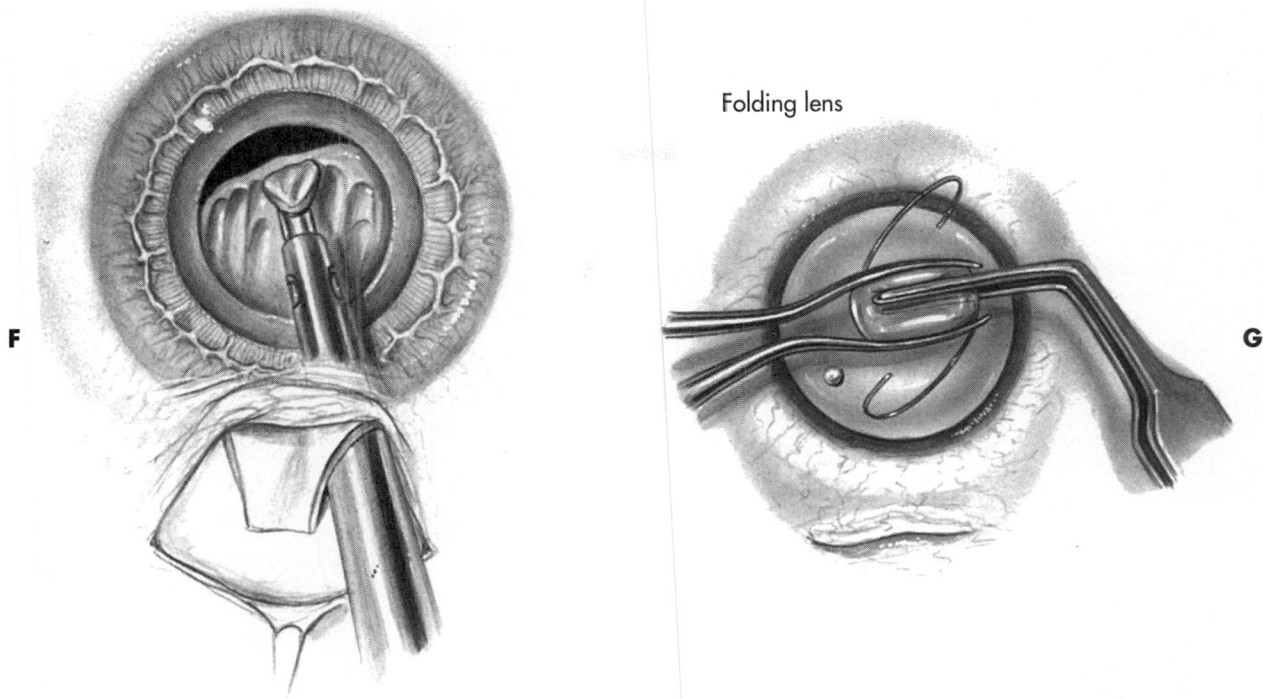

Folding lens

F

G

Placement of haptics into capsular bag

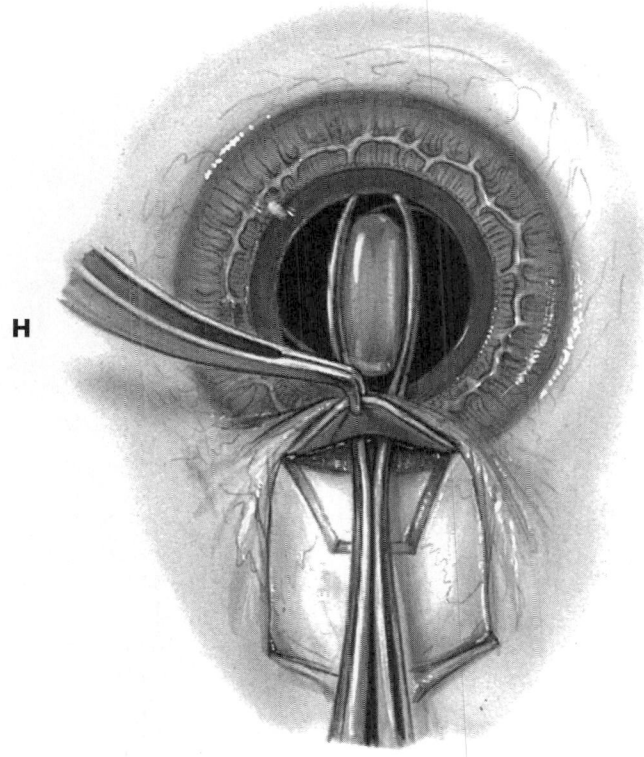

H

FIGURE 18-47, cont'd   Cataract extraction with phacoemulsification. **F,** The irrigation and aspiration (I&A) handpiece is used to strip the remaining cortex from the capsule. **G,** The IOL is folded. **H,** The IOL is placed into the capsular bag.

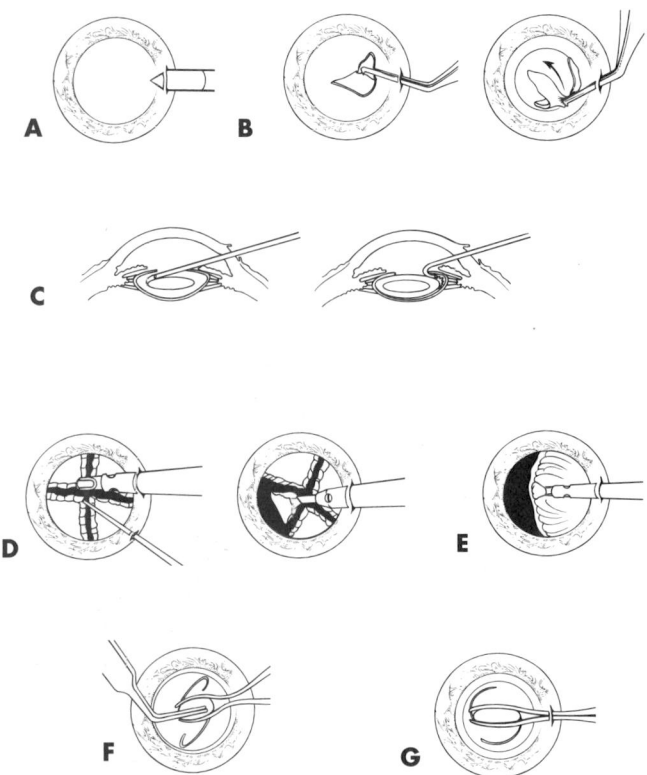

FIGURE 18-48 Clear cornea cataract extraction. **A,** A 2.6 mm incision is made into the cornea. **B,** Capsulorhexis is performed on anterior capsule of lens. **C,** Nucleus of lens is loosened by hydrodissection. **D,** Nucleus of lens is "cracked" into four quadrants and removed with phacoemulsification. **E,** I/A handpiece is used to strip the remaining cortex from the capsule. **F,** IOL is folded. **G,** IOL is placed into the capsular bag.

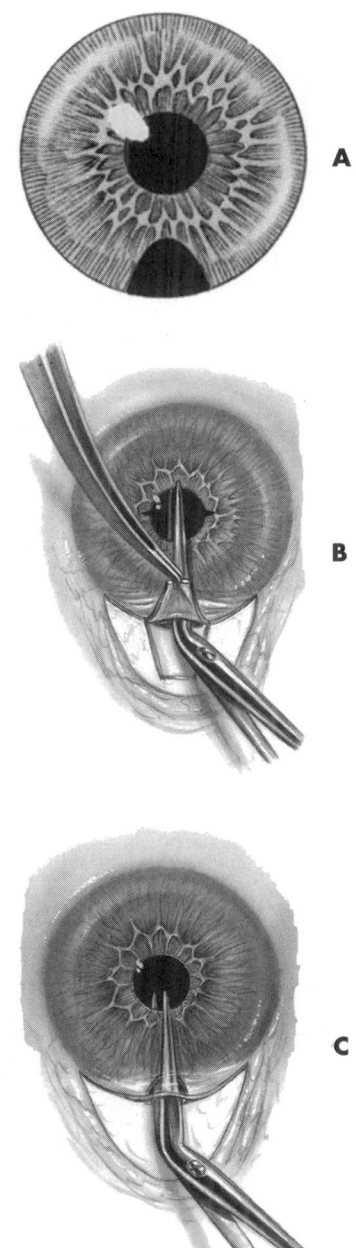

FIGURE 18-49 Types of iridectomies. **A,** Peripheral. **B,** Radial. **C,** Sector.

ized. Leaking of the wound can be stopped by hydrating the wound edges. Occasionally a 10-0 nylon suture is necessary.

17. Timoptic (timolol) 0.5% drops and Tobradex (tobramycin and dexamethasone) drops or Ocuflox (ofloxacin) drops are placed into the eye. The eye is not patched.

SURGERY FOR GLAUCOMA

Iridectomy

Iridectomy is removal of a section of iris tissue. Types of iridectomies are peripheral, sector, and radial (Fig. 18-49). Iridectomy is usually performed as part of a trabeculectomy procedure or may be performed when laser iridectomy is not feasible because of cloudy cornea or uveitis. Peripheral iridectomy is done in the treatment of acute, subacute, or chronic angle-closure glaucoma when extensive peripheral anterior synechiae have not formed. This operation is performed to reestablish communication between the posterior and anterior chambers, thus relieving pupillary block and permitting the iris root to

drop away from the trabecular meshwork to reestablish the outflow of aqueous fluid through Schlemn's canal.

Operative procedure

1. The speculum is introduced. The globe is fixed with a 4-0 traction suture passed under the superior rectus and fastened to the drape with a hemostat.
2. A small beveled incision is made at the superior limbus, or a perpendicular incision is made in the clear cornea.
3. The peripheral iris is grasped with forceps, pulled through the incision, and excised.

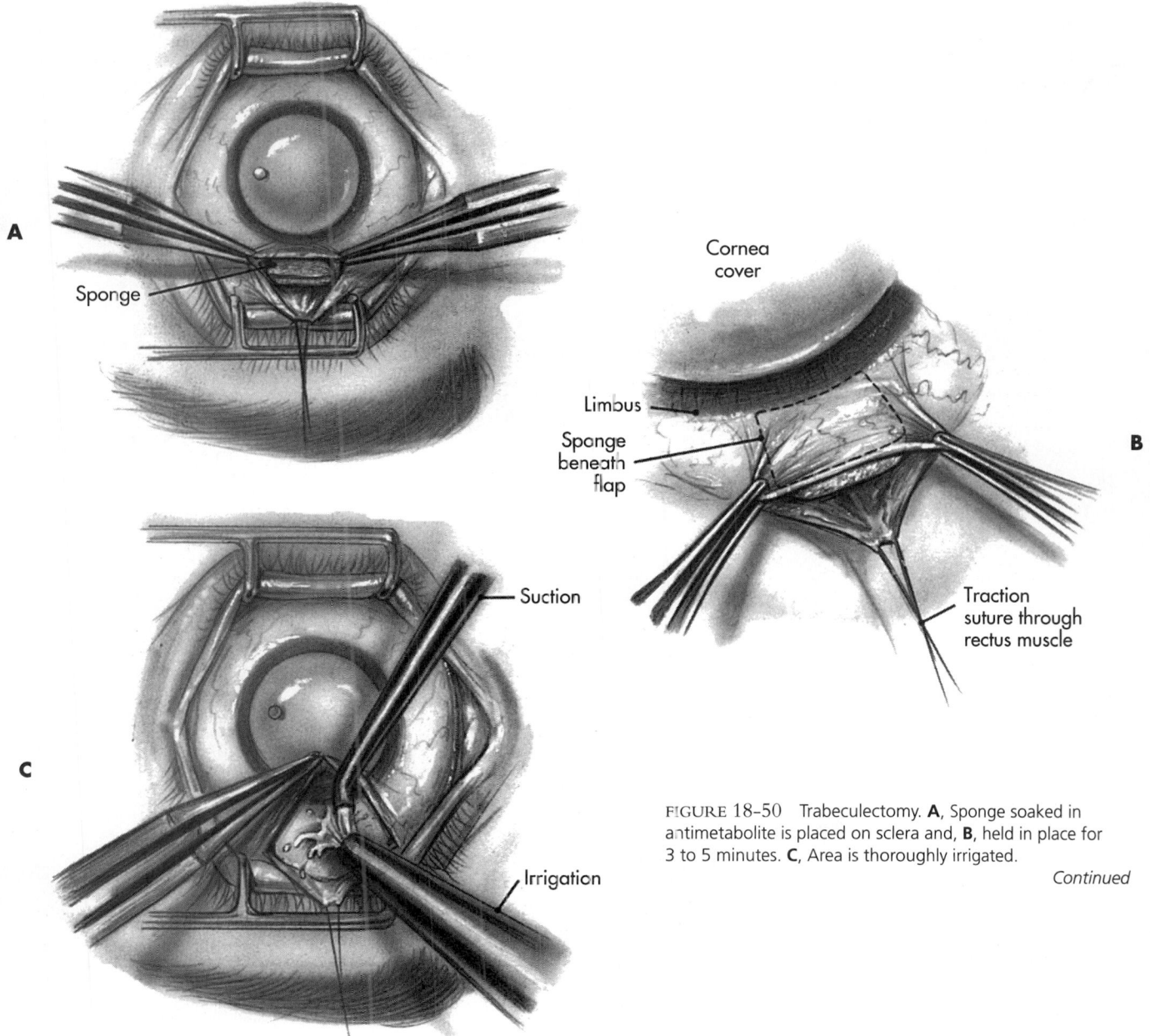

FIGURE 18-50   Trabeculectomy. **A**, Sponge soaked in antimetabolite is placed on sclera and, **B**, held in place for 3 to 5 minutes. **C**, Area is thoroughly irrigated.

Continued

4. The iris is repositioned by gently stroking the cornea with a blunt spatula or muscle hook. The iris can also be repositioned by irrigating with balanced salt solution.
5. A clear corneal incision is closed with 10-0 nonabsorbable suture, and a limbal incision is closed with absorbable suture. Subconjunctival antibiotics may be administered, and an eye pad is applied.

Trabeculectomy

The term *trabeculectomy* is a misnomer because it implies that part of the trabecular meshwork is removed during surgery. Trabeculectomy is a filtering procedure accom-plished by incising a conjunctival flap and a scleral flap, creating of a fistula, performing an iridectomy, and creating the filtering bleb. Trabeculectomy is often combined with cataract removal (phacoemulsification) and insertion of an IOL.

Procedural considerations

Adjunctive medical therapy to decrease postoperative fibrosis includes application of an antimetabolite-soaked sponge (5-fluorouracil [5-FU] or mitomycin) placed under the conjunctival flap. Because 5-FU and mitomycin are antimetabolites, nursing precautions for handling hazard-ous waste must be carried out. The circulating nurse must

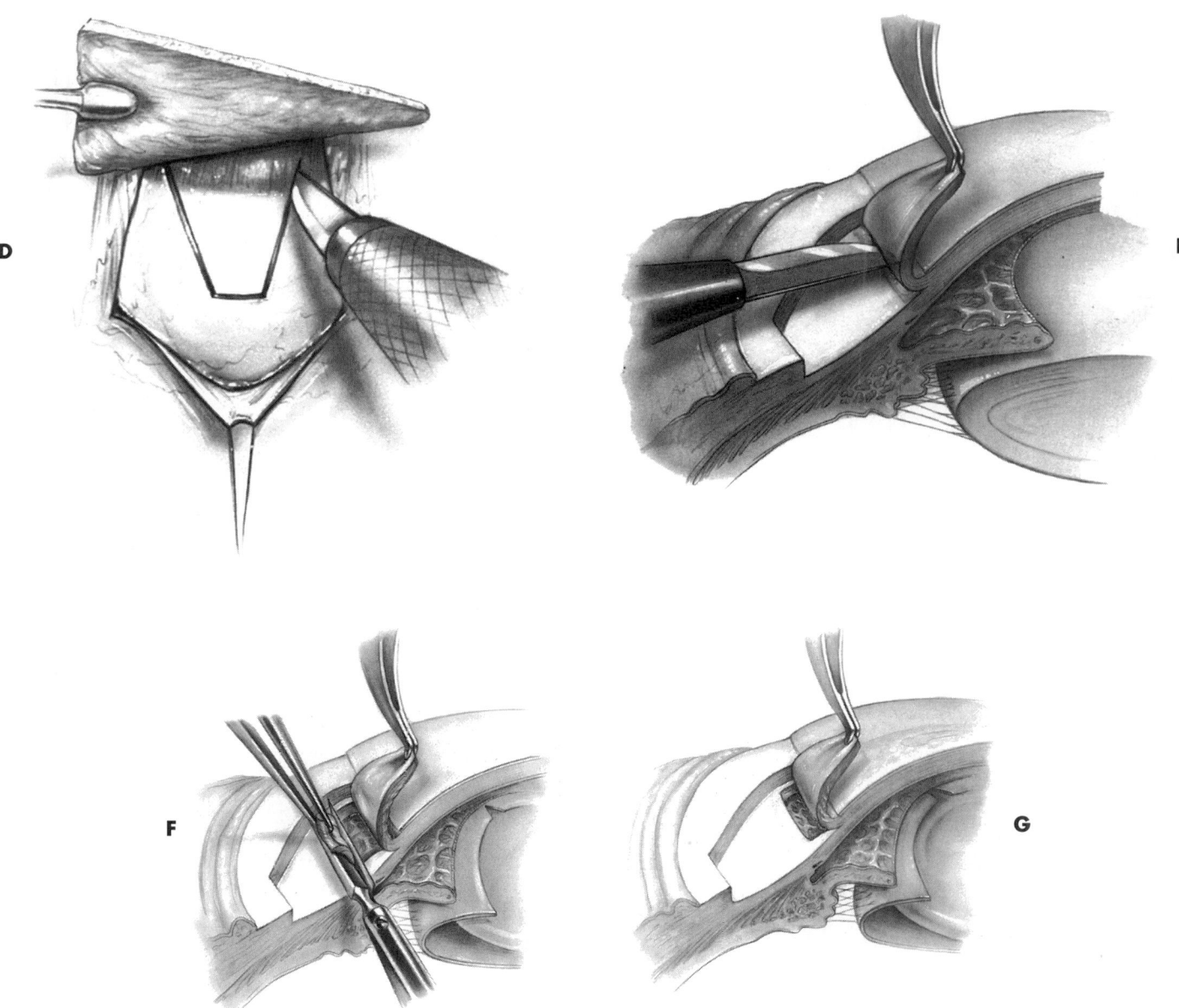

FIGURE 18-50, cont'd　Trabeculectomy. **D**, Scleral flap is formed. **E**, Incision is made into anterior chamber. **F** and **G**, Fistula is created by removing a flap of limbal tissue.

wear gloves while drawing up the antimetabolite from the vial to transfer to the operative field. All items used with the medication should be disposed of as hazardous waste. Instruments that come into contact with antimetabolites should be washed separately.[11]

Operative procedure (Fig. 18-50)

1. Incisions are made into the conjunctiva and Tenon's capsule, dissection is done, and a conjunctival-Tenon's flap is created. Hemostasis is obtained with bipolar cautery.

2. If antimetabolite is to be used, it is applied to the sclera before any incision into the sclera. The tip of a spear sponge is saturated in the antimetabolite (5-FU or mitomycin C) and placed between the conjunctival-Tenon's flap and the sclera. The sponge is left in place for 3 to 5 minutes, and then the site is irrigated vigorously with copious amounts of BSS.

3. A partial-thickness scleral flap is incised. The flap can be square or triangular.

4. The scleral flap is retracted, and an incision is made into and through the limbus into the anterior chamber with

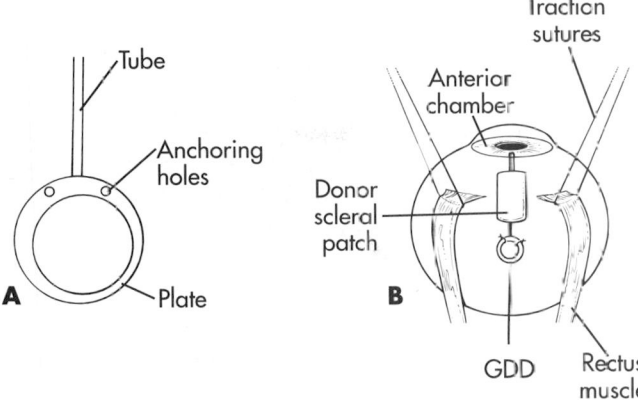

FIGURE 18-51 Glaucoma drainage devices. **A,** Components of glaucoma drainage device (GDD). **B,** Glaucoma drainage device (GDD) in place. Tip of drainage tube in anterior chamber. Donor sclera patch covering tube from plate to limbus.

the tip of the blade. The limbal incision is extended to a rectangular flap of deep limbal tissue, which is then excised to create the fistula.

5. An iridectomy is performed. Cautery is applied to bleeding sites and to the ciliary processes.
6. The scleral flap is replaced and sutured with interrupted 10-0 nonabsorbable sutures. The conjunctival-Tenon's flap is closed with a running suture, and the conjunctiva is closed.
7. BSS is injected through a cannula into the anterior chamber to deepen the anterior chamber and elevate the conjunctival bleb.
8. An eye pad and shield are applied.

Glaucoma Drainage Devices (Fig. 18-51)

In recent years several types of drainage devices have been implanted into the posterior subconjunctival space with varying success when filtering procedures have been unsuccessful. These include the Molteno implant, Krupin valve, Ahmed device, and Baerveldt device. Complications have been reduced through modifications in design and technique.

Operative procedure

1. The conjunctiva is incised to expose the sclera.
2. Two rectus muscles are isolated using silk ties as traction sutures.
3. Measurements are made for placement of plate of the device. The plate is sutured to the sclera.
4. After the patency of the device is checked, an occluding suture is inserted into drainage tube.
5. With a needle, a tunnel is created into the anterior chamber for the tube and paracentesis tract.
6. The tube is trimmed and inserted into the anterior chamber. The tube is sutured to the sclera with 5-0 nonabsorbable suture.

7. The tube is covered with patch graft of donor sclera or pericardium.
8. An occluding suture is passed through Tenon's capsule and conjunctiva into the inferior cul-de-sac and trimmed.
9. Traction sutures are removed from around the rectus muscles, and the conjunctiva is closed with a continuous 10-0 absorbable suture.
10. Antiinfective agents are injected subconjunctivally. The eye is dressed with an eye pad and shield.

Goniotomy

Goniotomy is the opening of a congenital membrane from the iris surface to Schwalbe's line, allowing aqueous humor to reach the trabecular meshwork in cases of congenital glaucoma.

Operative procedure

1. The patient is anesthetized without intubation.
2. An examination is performed. Corneal clarity and size, intraocular pressure, microscopic examination of the anterior segment (including gonioscopy), and examination of the posterior pole of the eye (especially the optic disk) are recorded.
3. The patient is intubated, if indicated, and prepped and draped.
4. A pediatric eye speculum and superior and inferior rectus bridle sutures are placed.
5. Under microscopic control with an appropriate goniotomy lens (gonioprism) in place, the goniotomy knife is introduced through the temporal limbus. The anterior chamber is maintained with viscoelastic material. The membrane covering the iris and angle structures is cut without damaging the trabecular meshwork. The knife is removed.
6. BSS may be used to reform the anterior chamber, and a suture may be used to close the incision.
7. A miotic (pilocarpine) may be used topically. Antiinfective-antiinflammatory ointment is used.
8. The eye is dressed with an eye pad and protective shield.

Laser Therapy

Argon or Nd:YAG laser therapy is being used to treat acute (angle-closure) glaucoma and open-angle glaucoma. Laser therapy is a fairly uncomplicated ambulatory procedure in which a slitlamp is used for delivery of the laser beam. Laser treatment of glaucoma is a noninvasive procedure and, if successful, may eliminate the need for more invasive surgical procedures.

Laser Trabeculoplasty

Laser trabeculoplasty is treatment for open-angle glaucoma by the placement of laser burns in the posterior part of the trabeculum, anterior to the scleral spur, to cause the surface of the trabecular meshwork to contract. This

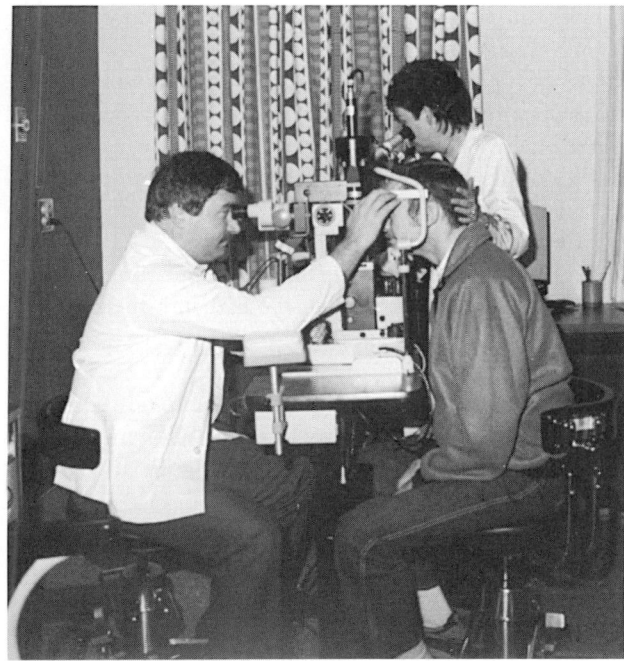

FIGURE 18-52 Patient positioned at argon laser slitlamp for treatment of glaucoma.

theoretically pulls open the adjacent intertrabecular spaces, resulting in increased aqueous outflow.

Procedural considerations

Preoperative sedation is usually unnecessary. A topical anesthetic such as proparacaine is used. Intraocular pressure is measured preoperatively. Laser safety precautions are initiated.

Operative procedure

1. One or two proparacaine (Ophthaine) drops are instilled in the operative eye.
2. The patient is positioned at the laser slitlamp (Fig. 18-52).
3. A three-mirror Goldmann lens is placed, allowing visualization of the chamber angle and retraction of the eye lid. The perioperative nurse assists in this placement.
4. A landmark is selected as a starting point, and laser treatment is begun, with a 50 mm spot size applied for 0.1 second at 850 mW power. Light-pigmented tissue requires more power, whereas dark-pigmented tissue requires less power. The laser "burns" are placed into the anterior portion of the functional trabecular meshwork, pigmented zone, to yield about 20 burns in each quadrant for a total of 70 to 90 burns. The power should be titrated to the threshold of whitening or tiny bubble formation.
5. One hour after completion of the treatment the intra-ocular pressure should be measured, and topical prednisolone or dexamethasone drops should be instilled.

6. The procedure may be performed in two treatment segments rather than completed in one.

Argon Laser Iridotomy

Argon laser iridotomy is the placement of penetrating argon laser burns in the peripheral part of the iris to create an opening, allowing aqueous humor to flow from the posterior chamber into the anterior chamber and out through Schlemm's canal to treat angle-closure glaucoma.

Procedural considerations

The operative considerations are as for laser trabeculoplasty. The duration of exposure will need to be adjusted depending on the color of the iris (0.5 second for blue, 0.1 second for medium brown, and 0.05 second for dark brown).[1]

Operative procedure

1. Topical anesthetic drops of proparacaine or an equivalent are instilled.
2. The patient is positioned at the laser slitlamp.
3. The Abraham lens is placed into the operative eye.
4. An iris crypt or "thin" area of iris is selected.
5. Initial burns are placed in a circle to put the iris on a stretch using 200 mm spot size for 0.1 second at 200 to 300 mW power. (Usually six to eight burns accomplish this.)
6. Penetrating burns are placed as needed to make an adequate opening (usually 10 to 30 applications) using 50 mm spot size for 0.1 to 0.2 second at 600 to 1000 mW power.
7. Prednisolone or dexamethasone eyedrops are instilled into the operative eye.

SURGERY FOR RETINAL DETACHMENT

Retinal detachment is a separation of the neural retinal layer from the pigmented epithelium layer of the retina. Retinal detachment may occur because of the presence of intraocular neoplasms originating in the retina or choroid (exudative type) or, more commonly, as a result of retinal tears or holes associated with injury, degeneration, or rhegmatogenous detachment.

Retinal detachment usually causes the sudden onset of the appearance of floating spots before the eye, resulting from freeing of pigment or blood cells in the vitreous. The vitreous humor of the eye is a gelatinous liquid possessing an ultrastructure of fine protein fibers in a network arrangement, with some attachment to the retina. Fluid from the vitreous cavity seeps through the retinal tears and progressively detaches the retinal components. The part of the retina that has separated from its nutritional source becomes damaged and relatively nonfunctional. Prompt treatment of retinal detachment is aimed at preventing permanent loss of central vision.

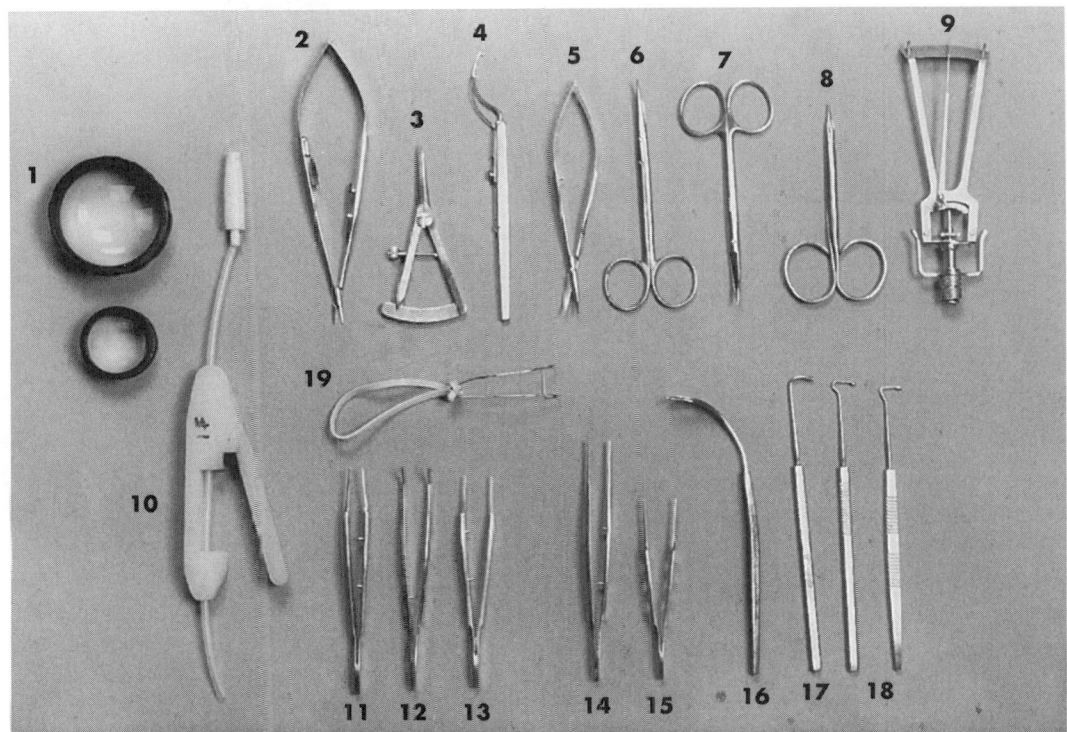

FIGURE 18-53   Instruments for retinal surgery. *1*, 20 D and 30 D Nikon lenses; *2*, Castroviejo needle holder; *3*, Castroviejo caliper; *4*, Gonian marker. *5*, Westcott blunt scissors; *6*, tenotomy scissors; *7*, utility scissors; *8*, straight Stevens scissors; *9*, Schiotz tonometer; *10*, irrigating tip (Baylor); *11*, 0.5 forceps; *12*, angled Nugent forceps; *13*, tying forceps; *14*, smooth Bonaccolto forceps; *15*, Bishop forceps with teeth; *16*, Schepens retractor; *17*, cannulated muscle hook; *18*, muscle hooks; *19*, lid retractor.

Scleral Buckling
Procedural considerations

In the treatment of retinal detachment the aim is to return the retina to its normal anatomic position. Repair is done from outside the globe. The purpose of the scleral buckling procedure for retinal detachment is to cause an intrusion or push into the eye at the site of the pathologic cause. Treatment by diathermy or cryotherapy causes an inflammatory reaction that leads to a permanent adhesion between the detached retina and underlying structures. The surgery also involves sealing off the area in which the tear or hole is located and may include drainage of the subretinal fluid.

The procedure may be performed under general anesthesia or monitored anesthesia care (MAC) with local blocks. The scleral buckling may be done using episcleral (working on outside of sclera) technique or by scleral dissection (making a partial-thickness incision into the sclera and creating flaps to expose the underlying tissue). Both techniques may use drainage of subretinal fluid, encircling bands, diathermy, light coagulation, or cryotherapy. Cryosurgery or light coagulation may be used alone or in combination with a buckling procedure. Instrumentation for retinal surgery is shown in Fig. 18-53.

Operative procedures (Fig. 18-54)

A detailed drawing of the retina is made before surgery and is displayed in the operating suite. On the basis of this drawing, the conjunctiva is opened to a previously determined extent, that is, 90 degrees for a simple horseshoe tear or 360 degrees for an aphakic detachment.

The four rectus muscles are isolated using 0 silk ties as traction sutures. With the indirect ophthalmoscope the detachment and tear are located under direct visualization, and the site is marked with nonpenetrating diathermy by indentation or with a methylene blue marking pen.

Episcleral Technique

1. Under direct visualization, the retinal cryoprobe is applied to the external surface of the globe in the area of the pathologic condition, and the area is treated. An iceball is seen to form in the proper areas until all of the lesion has been treated.
2. The buckling component of the procedure secures explants (for example, silicone bands, sponges, plates, tires) to the sclera. 4-0 or 5-0 nonabsorbable sutures are set into the sclera surrounding the lesion and tied over silicone sponges, causing the outer shell of the eye to be pushed toward the elevated retina. If an encircling

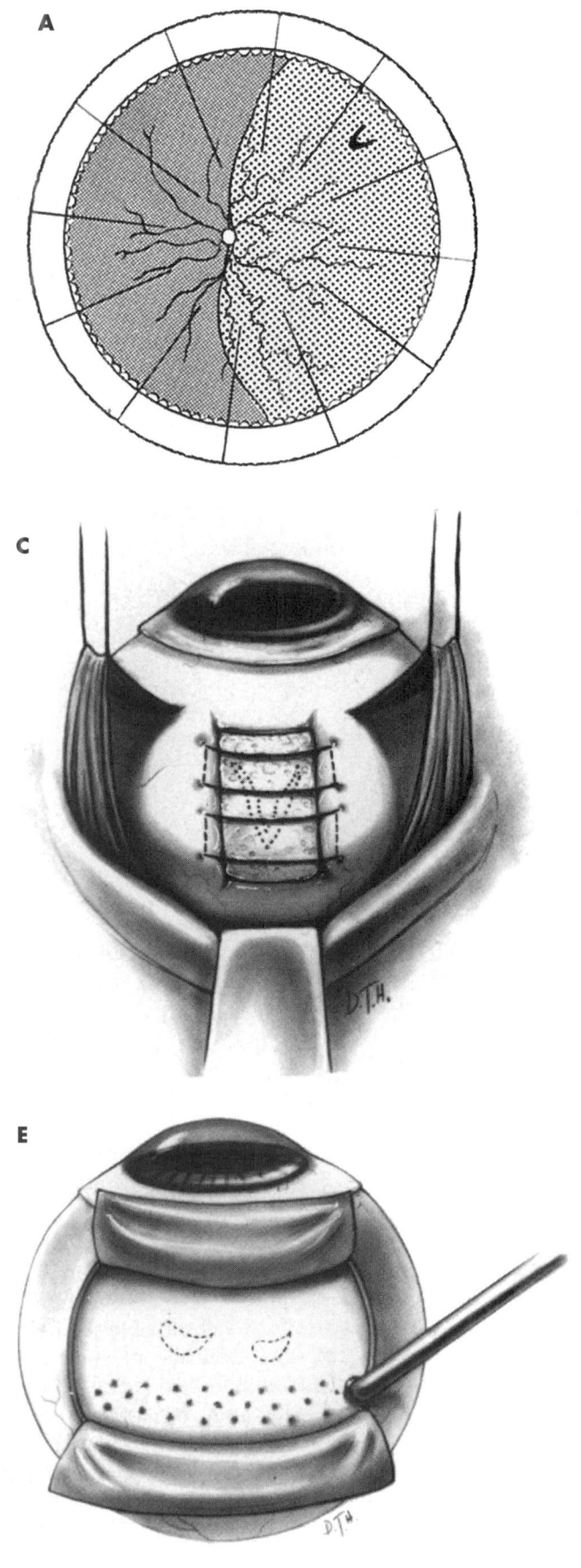

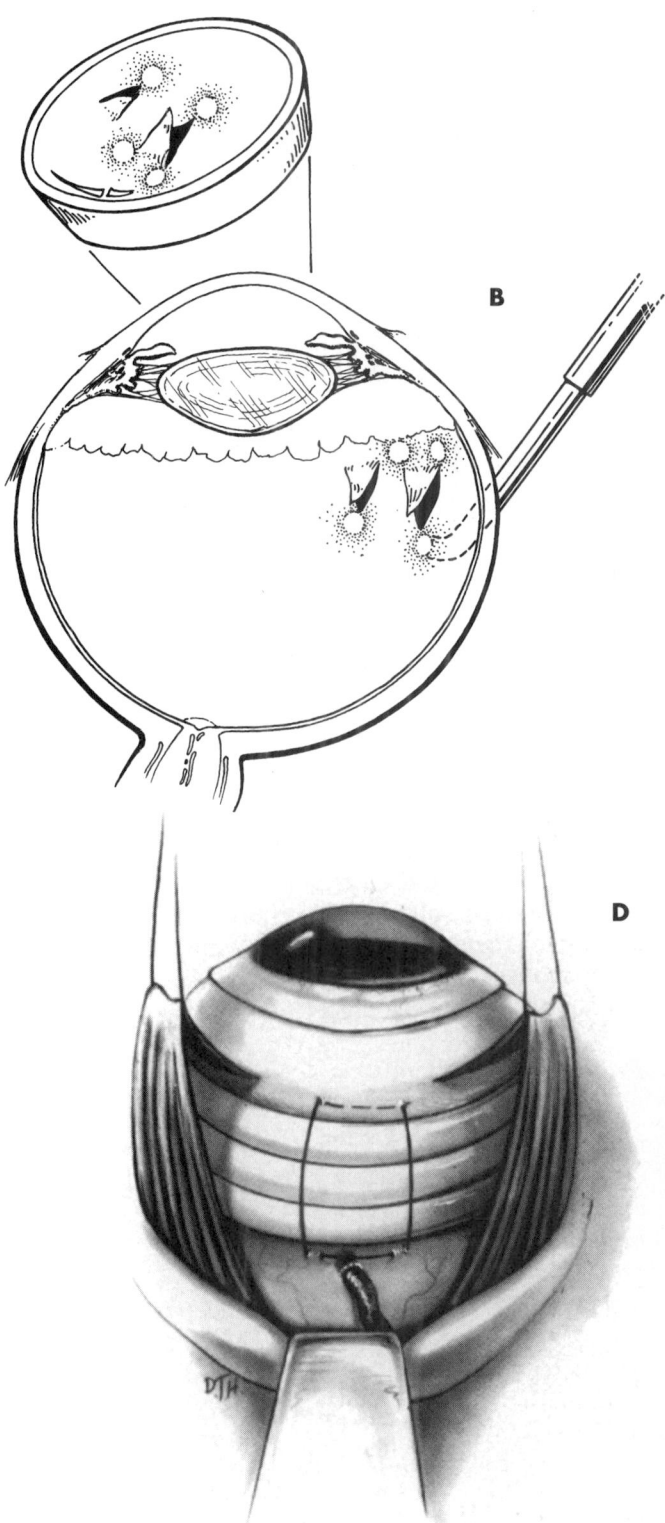

FIGURE 18-54   Scleral buckling operation for treatment of retinal detachment. **A**, Diagram of retina showing detachment of retina of temporal half of left eye, with retinal tear at equator of globe at 1:30 o'clock position. **B**, Examination of fundus by means of ophthalmoscope and hand-held lens and depression of sclera with diathermy electrode. Surgeon visualizes field and places electrode beneath retinal tear; burn mark is made on sclera at site of retinal tear with diathermy electrode. **C**, A sponge is sutured in place over treated site of retinal tear. **D**, Band and tire are used to encircle the eye. **E**, Scleral dissection method: flaps are made and diathermy used on sclera.

Continued

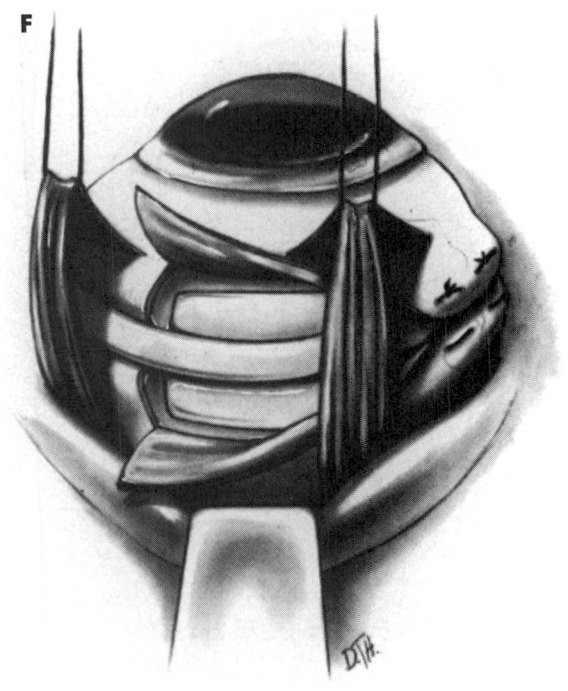

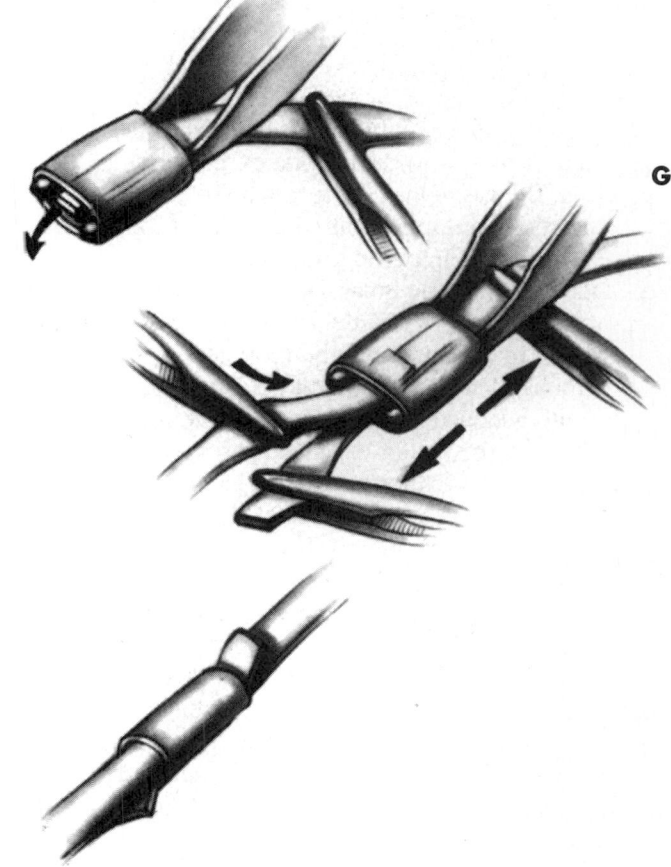

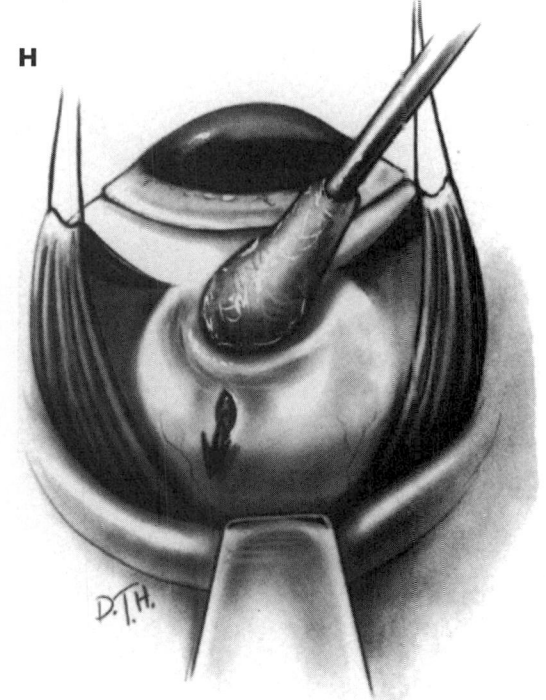

FIGURE 18-54, cont'd   Scleral buckling operation for treatment of retinal detachment. **F,** Silicone band is laid in scleral bed. Edges of scleral flaps are closed over silicone band. **G,** Placement of Watzke silicone sleeve is one method to secure edges of encircling band. **H,** Small incision is made through sclera, and choroid is finely incised to allow subretinal fluid to drain.

band is to be used, mattress sutures are placed into the sclera in four quadrants. A silicone band is passed 360 degrees around the eye under the sutures and the rectus muscles. The sutures are tied and a self-holding Watzke sleeve is applied to the band to maintain a predetermined circumference. This causes a 360-degree constriction of the outer coats into the eye.

3. If drainage of subretinal fluid is desired, under direct visualization an area is chosen in which a significant fluid level exists under the retina, and a diathermy mark is made on the sclera. A 6-0 or 7-0 absorbable suture is placed at the proposed drainage site. The sclera is split to the choroid, and a small amount of diathermy is applied to the choroid bed. A needle or blade is then used to puncture the choroid into the subretinal space to permit drainage of fluid. The preplaced suture is tied.

Scleral Dissection

1. Same as that for episcleral technique.
2. An incision is made into the sclera, and a scleral flap is dissected both anteriorly and posteriorly from the original incision. Diathermy can be used in this thinned scleral bed, or cryotherapy can be used under direct visualization. A scleral sponge may be sutured into the bed, using 4-0 or 5-0 nonabsorbable sutures with or without an encircling band as previously described.
3. Drainage of subretinal fluid may be accomplished as previously described.
4. The scleral flaps are approximated and closed.

Air or other replacement or ballast fluids may be introduced into the eye after the drainage of subretinal fluid. This is usually done through the pars plana under direct visualization. The traction sutures are removed from around the muscles. The conjunctiva is closed with a 7-0 absorbable suture. A subconjunctival injection of an antibiotic, steroid, or both may be given, and an eye pad is applied.

Retinopexy (Fig. 18-55)

Pneumatic retinopexy is the intraocular injection of a bubble of air or therapeutic gases to press against retinal breaks and allow the detached retinal breaks to approximate each other. Retinopexy may be used in combination with scleral buckling and posterior vitrectomy and is gaining popularity as part of an ambulatory procedure for

treatment of certain retinal detachments using laser photocoagulation with injection of the gas bubble followed by specific postoperative positioning. The gases are drawn through a Millipore 0.22-micron filter and may be mixed with filtered air so that the concentration may be varied.

Sulfur hexafluoride gas (SF_6) is colorless, odorless, and nontoxic. It doubles its volume within 24 to 36 hours after injection by drawing other gases from the surrounding tissues. A 1 mm bubble will diffuse from the eye in 7 to 10 days.

Perfluoropropane gas (C_3F_8) is colorless, odorless, and nontoxic. It quadruples its volume within 24 hours after injection. A 1 mm bubble will diffuse from the eye in 30 to 50 days.

VITRECTOMY

Vitrectomy is narrowly defined as removal of all or part of the vitreous gel (body). In the broader clinical sense of the term it also includes the cutting and removal of fibrotic membranes, removal of epiretinal membranes, and electrocoagulation of bleeding vessels. In its normal state the vitreous gel of the eye is transparent. In certain disease states bleeding from damaged or newly formed vessels may cause the vitreous to become opaque, which may severely decrease vision. In addition to the patient's inability to see, the ophthalmologist is unable to visualize the retina and therefore treat the underlying pathologic condition before

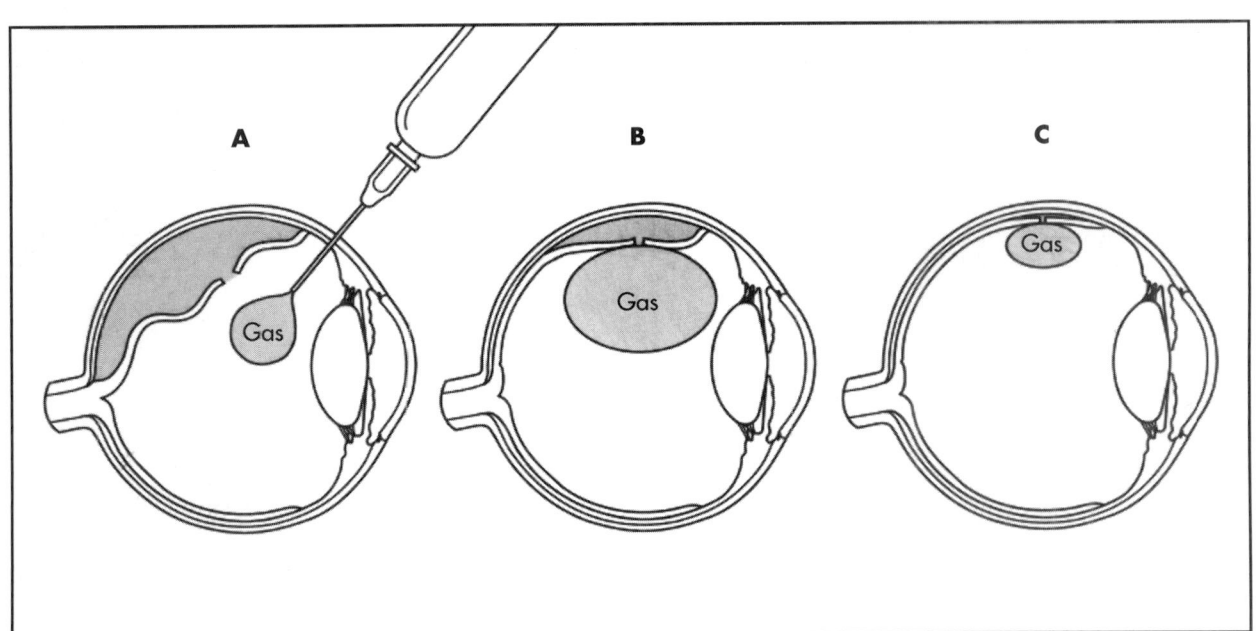

FIGURE 18-55   Pneumatic retinopexy. **A**, Gas bubble is injected through the pars plana. **B** and **C**, The bubble closes and supports the retinal break. After a 7- to 10-day healing period and the retina is back in place, laser surgery or cryotherapy can be performed to seal the break.

permanent damage can occur. In these cases vitrectomy is indicated to allow the patient to see and the surgeon to institute treatment if indicated.

Certain ophthalmic diseases are associated with the formation of membranes, which may block the visual axis and cause decreased vision. Contraction of these membranes may produce traction-type or rhegmatogenous retinal detachment. In these cases vitrectomy is indicated to relieve the underlying pathologic processes leading to decreased vision.

Anterior Segment Vitrectomy

The main indications for vitrectomy in the anterior segment are as follows:

1. Vitreous loss during cataract extraction
2. Opacities in the anterior segment
3. Complications associated with vitreous in the anterior chamber
4. Miscellaneous causes, such as hyphema, pupillary membranes, and residual soft lens material

Procedural considerations

The procedure varies according to the location of the pathologic condition (anterior or posterior segments), the instrumentation available, and the surgeon's preference. A pathologic condition in the anterior segment can be approached through a limbal incision, as in lens extraction with vitreous loss; through "open sky," after trephine incision for penetrating keratoplasty; or through the pars plana. Most phacoemulsification equipment has a vitrector that can be quickly attached if needed.

Operative procedures

Anterior Vitrectomy for Accidental Vitreous Loss During Cataract Extraction (Fig. 18-56, *A*)

1. A vitreous cutter is placed into the eye through the cataract wound. Infusion may be through the handpiece or a separate cannula and infusion line.
2. The cutter is placed in the middle of the pupil, posterior to the iris, and enough vitreous is removed to ensure that no vitreous remains in the anterior chamber and that the iris has fallen back into its normal position.
3. The pupil is constricted with acetylcholine. The anterior chamber may be reformed with BSS.
4. The procedure is completed as for a lens extraction.

Anterior Vitrectomy for Anterior Segment Opacities, Hyphema, Pupillary Membranes, and Residual Soft Lens Material (Fig. 18-56, *B*)

1. Appropriate fixation sutures or a lid speculum is placed.
2. An incision is made at the limbus either through clear cornea or under a conjunctival flap. One to three incisions are made, depending on the vitreous cutter chosen and the technique.

3. If a multifunction probe is not used, an infusion cannula is placed into one incision and the vitreous cutter into another. A third incision may be used for an accessory instrument. The vitreous, blood, or other material is removed.
4. The incisions are closed, and the eye is patched.

Posterior Segment Vitrectomy

A pathologic condition in the posterior segment is usually approached through the pars plana. The main indications for posterior segment vitrectomy through the pars plana are as follows:

1. Vitreous opacities of long standing
2. Advanced diabetic eye disease
3. Severe intraocular trauma
4. Retained foreign bodies
5. Proliferative vitreoretinopathy
6. Retinal detachment from giant tears
7. Endophthalmitis
8. Diagnostic vitreous biopsy

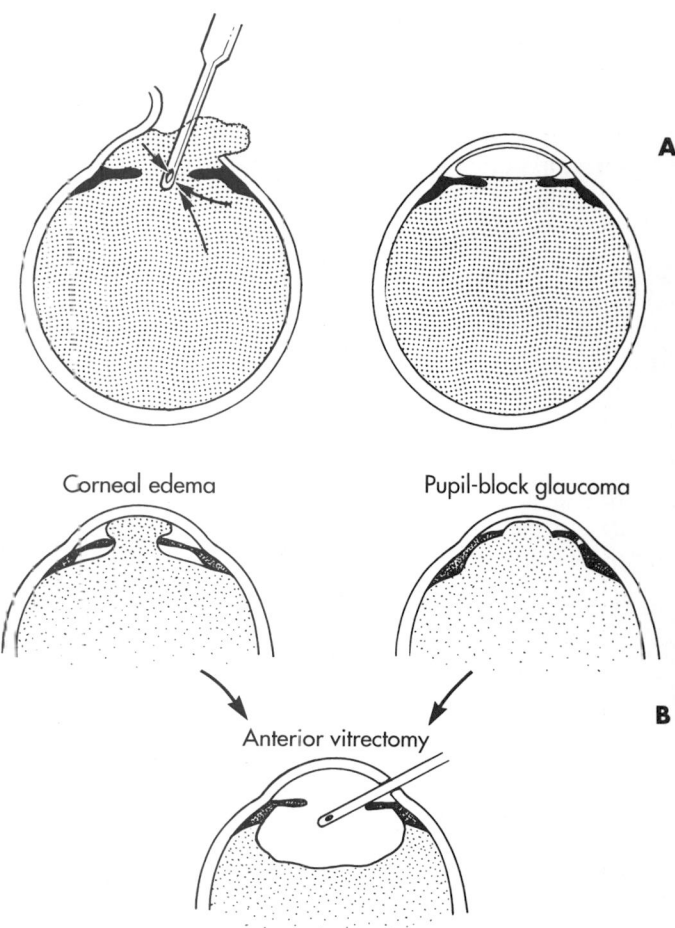

Corneal edema   Pupil-block glaucoma

Anterior vitrectomy

FIGURE 18-56   **A,** Diagram of management of vitreous loss at time of cataract extraction. **B,** Anterior vitrectomy procedure for complications of vitreous in anterior chamber.

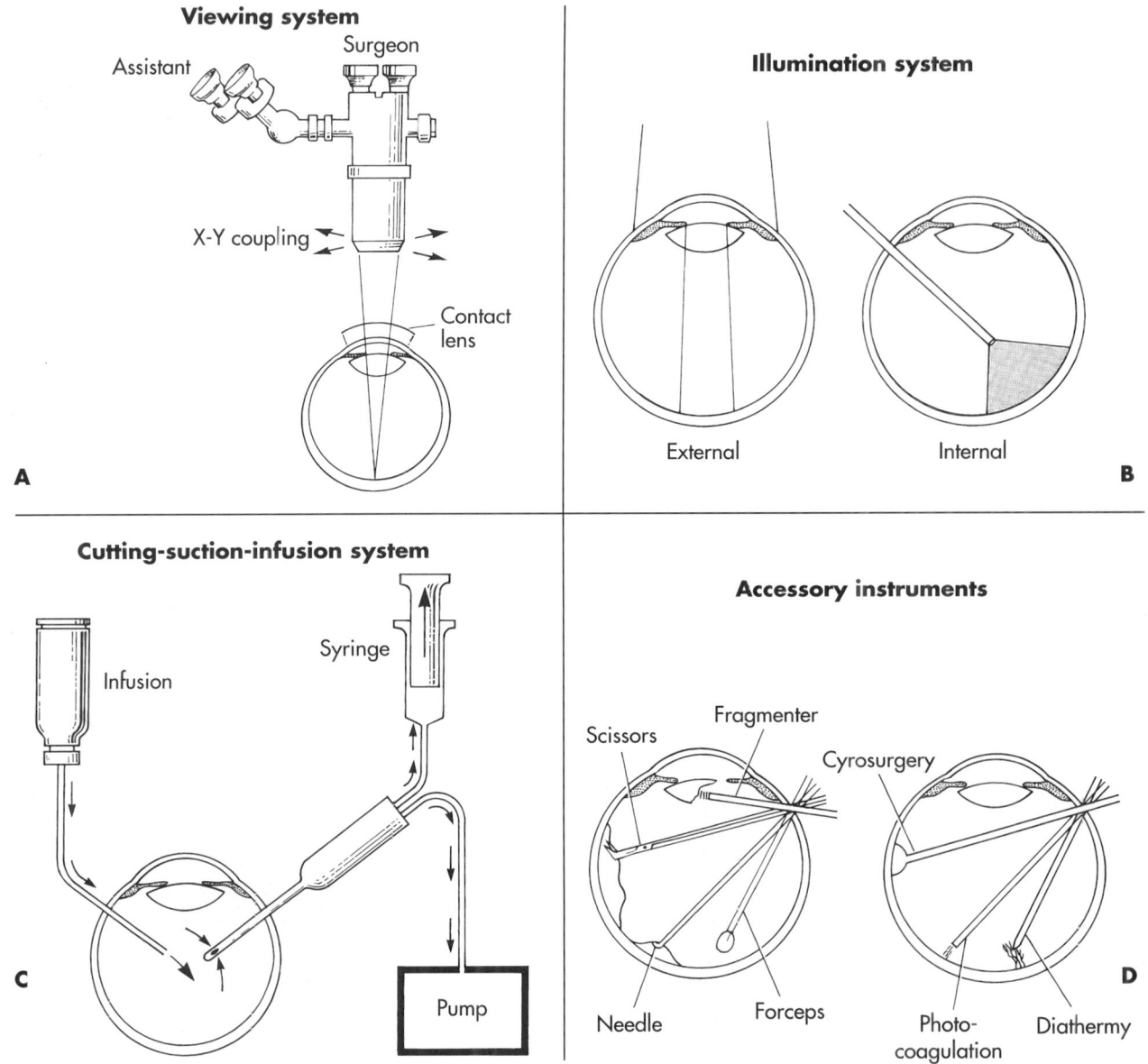

FIGURE 18-57 Vitrectomy procedures require the following: **A**, viewing system with X-Y coupling. **B**, Illumination system. **C**, Cutting-suction-infusion system. **D**, Accessory instruments.

Procedural consideration

Vitrectomy of the posterior segment is a microsurgical procedure requiring a viewing system (operating microscope with an X-Y coupling, zoom lens, and fine focus), an illumination system, a cutting-suction-infusion system, and accessory instruments (Fig. 18-57).

The infusion system consists of a 500 ml bottle of buffered BSS, such as BSS Plus or Endosol Extra, a standard intravenous administration set, and an infusion needle or sleeve. The level of intraocular pressure can be varied by elevating or lowering the infusion bottle in relation to the patient's eye.

The suction and cutting systems vary in sophistication, but all cutters engage tissue into a port and then cut it by the shearing action between the edges of a moving and a nonmoving part. Guillotine cutters have a linear, to-and-fro action, whereas reciprocating or oscillating cutters rotate in a clockwise-counterclockwise fashion. Suction is operated with a pump controlled by a foot switch to maintain the level of aspiration. The cutter may be part of a single-use multifunction handpiece (Fig. 18-58).

An endolaser or indirect laser delivery system is usually available for photocoagulation (Fig. 18-59). Illumination for vitrectomy is external, using the operating microscope for anterior segment vitrectomy, and internal, using a fiberoptic light pipe (endoilluminator) for posterior segment vitrectomy (see Figs. 18-58 and 18-60). Replacement of the vitreous with air is facilitated with a special air-exchange unit (see Fig. 18-58). Other substances for intraocular tamponade are perfluoropropane gas (C_3F_8),

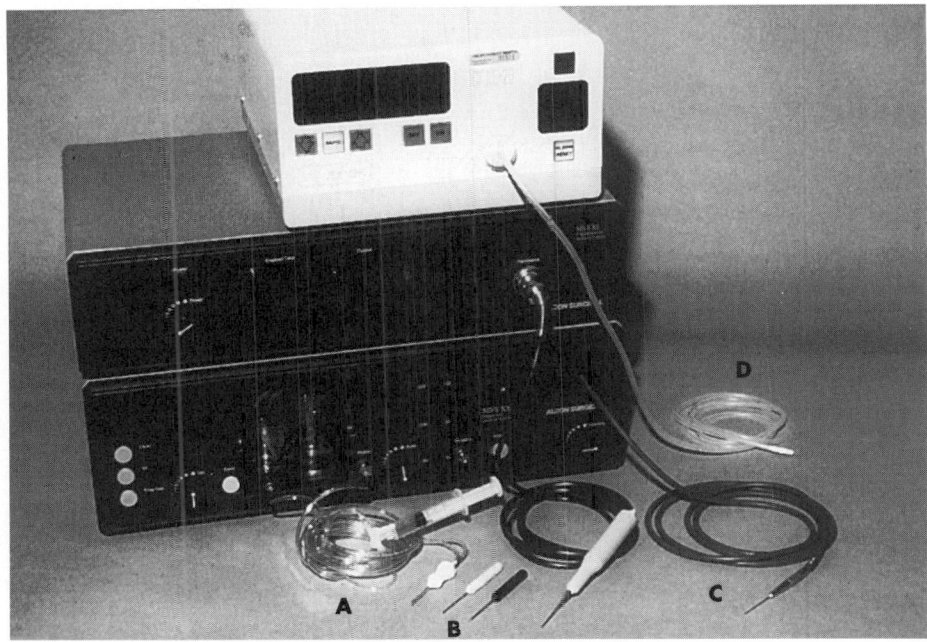

FIGURE 18-58   *Top*, Trek air-exchange unit and tubing. *Bottom*, Alcon surgical vitrectomy and fragmentation units showing accessories from *left to right*: *A*, vitrectomy tubing with disposable handpiece; *B*, extrusion handpieces; *C*, fragmentor handpiece; *D*, fiberoptic light pipe (endoilluminator).

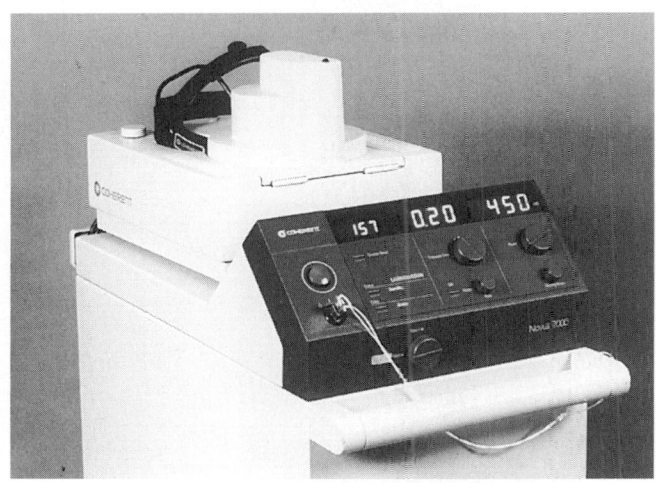

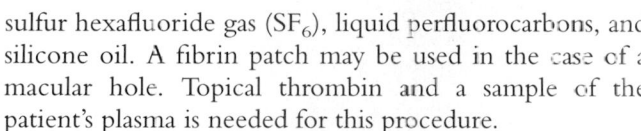

FIGURE 18-59   Argon laser with indirect ophthalmoscope.

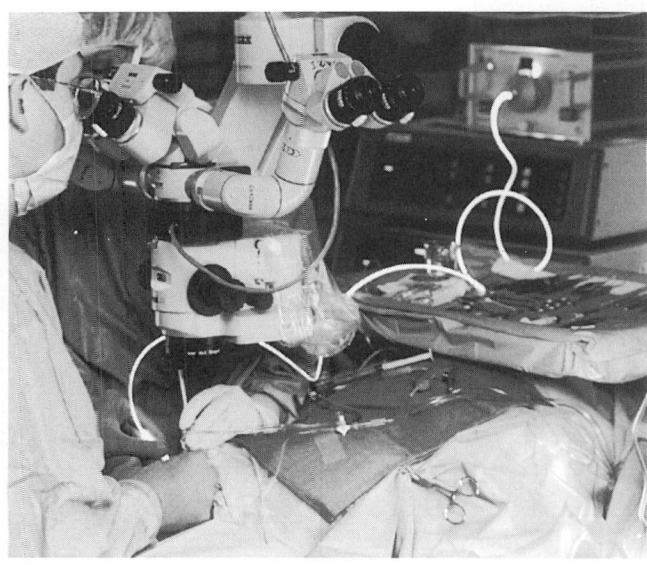

sulfur hexafluoride gas (SF_6), liquid perfluorocarbons, and silicone oil. A fibrin patch may be used in the case of a macular hole. Topical thrombin and a sample of the patient's plasma is needed for this procedure.

Accessory instruments (Figs. 18-61 and 18-62) usually have a 20-gauge diameter so that they can be interchanged throughout the procedure. There are several accessory instruments that may be used for pars plana vitrectomy depending on the extent of the procedure. Microhooks, picks, and subretinal forceps and scissors (Fig. 18-63) are used for dissection, peeling, and removal of membranes. These instruments can be manually operated with a thumb control or run with compressed air from the automated vitrectomy console.

FIGURE 18-60   Surgical field during vitrectomy procedure showing position of instrumentation: surgeon looks through the operating microscope while illuminating the retinal layer and vitreous with a fiberoptic light pipe. When the microscope is not draped, sterile plastic bags are used to adjust the lenses. The scrubbed personnel and surgeon must be especially vigilant to avoid contamination.

Foreign-body microforceps and various magnetic devices are used to retrieve foreign objects of glass, metal, or other substances. Intraocular cryoprobe for cryocoagulation directly on the retina surface can be attached to the cryotherapy device. Flute needles or disposable soft-tipped cannulas are handheld or attached to an extrusion or

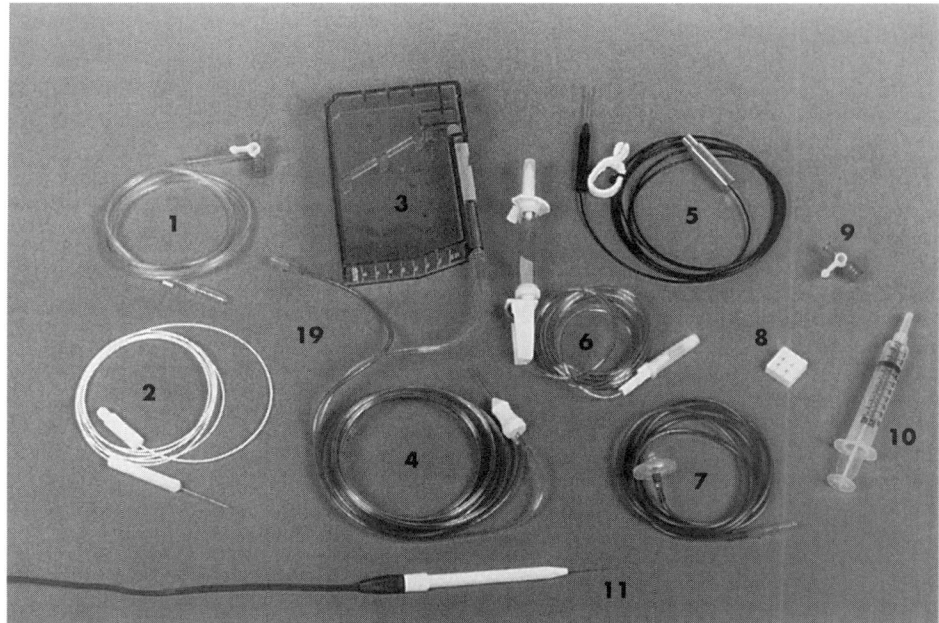

FIGURE 18–61   Disposable vitrectomy accessories: *1*, Tubing with three-way stopcock for fragmentor extrusion; *2*, fiberoptic light pipe; *3*, collection cassette connected to vitrectomy tubing and probe (*4*); *5*, endolaser probe; *6*, infusion tubing; *7*, air pump tubing; *8*, scleral plugs; *9*, three-way stopcock; *10*, syringe; *11*, wet-field cord with hemostatic eraser.

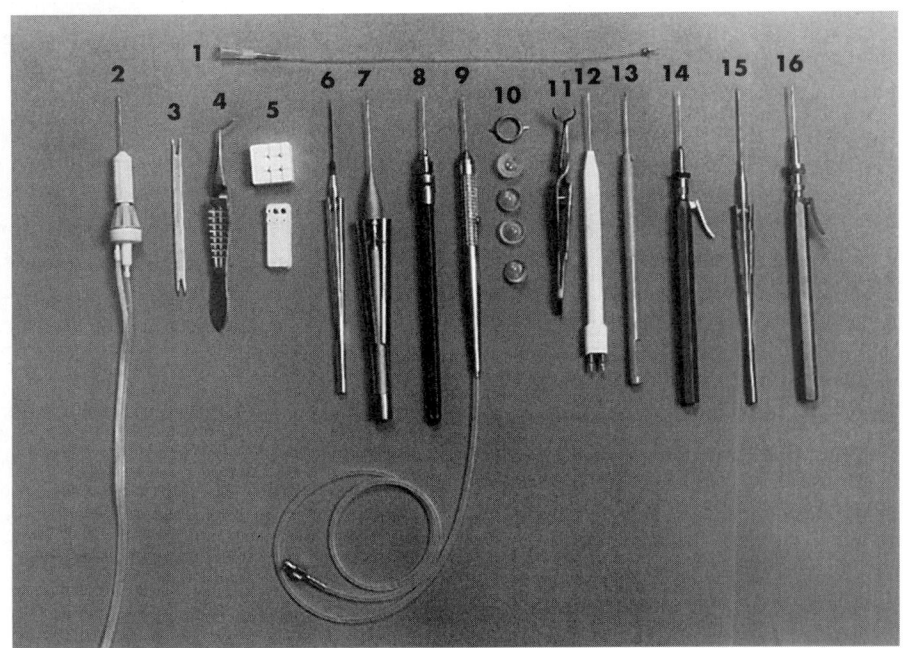

FIGURE 18–62   Accessory instruments for vitrectomy. *1*, 4 mm infusion cannula; *2*, variable port vitrector *3*, 3.5 and 4 mm premeasured calipers; *4*, scleral plug holder; *5*, scleral plugs in tablets; *6*, Lambert subretinal forceps; *7*, Thomas subretinal handle; *8*, Charles vacuum cannula; *9*, Flynn needle; *10*, lens set with sew-on ring; *11*, Landers lens holder; *12*. wet-field endocautery; *13*, MVR blade; *14*, Grieshaber side-gripping forceps; *15*, DORC end-gripping forceps; *16*, Grieshaber vertical cutting scissors.

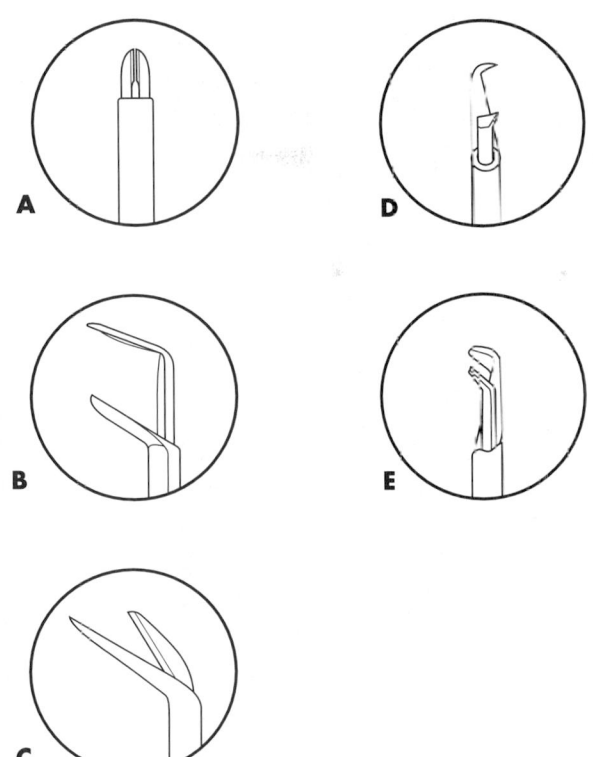

FIGURE 18-63 Tips of microinstruments used in vitrectomy procedures. **A** and **B**, Peeling forceps. **C**, Horizontal scissors. **D**, Vertical scissors. **E**, Membrane peeler and cutter.

aspiration line for evacuating pools of blood or for fluid-gas exchange.

To prepare for a vitrectomy procedure, the perioperative nurse must know the location of the problem, how the surgeon plans to address the problem (route of entry into the eye—anterior or posterior, "open sky," or closed), instrumentation to be used, and anticipated extent and length of the procedure. Instrument and equipment functioning should be thoroughly checked before the patient is brought into the operating room. When a lens extraction procedure is planned, vitrectomy instrumentation should be ready in the event of accidental vitreous loss. When preparing for pars plana vitrectomy in the posterior segment, the perioperative nurse must be aware that a combined scleral buckling procedure may be necessary.

In the case of giant retinal tears, C_3F_8, SF_6, liquid perfluorocarbons, and silicone oil are now used to provide retinal tamponade. These techniques allow repositioning and tamponade of the retina without the need for extremely awkward and uncomfortable positioning that was previously mandated.

Silicone oil and liquid perfluorocarbons such as perfluorooctane (PFO), being heavier than vitreous and BSS, will allow the tears to sink and so are used as a tamponade to reduce a giant retinal tear. Both are then removed from the posterior segment. Silicone oil may be left in place, but it is recommended that it be removed within 1 year if the retina is reattached and stable.

Vitrectomy procedures vary in length from less than 1 hour to over 6 hours. When a long procedure is anticipated, care must be taken to protect the patient's skin and reduce pressure areas. A foam mattress pad, heel and elbow protectors, and elasticized stockings may be used. When the patient is positioned for vitrectomy, the head should be higher than the heart, the cheeks higher than the forehead, and the neck extended. A wrist support may be placed around the patient's head to support the surgeon's wrist during manipulation of the intraocular instruments.

While draping, the perioperative nurse should provide for removal of infusion fluid from the operative field and should take care to protect electrical foot switches from fluid damage.

Operative procedure
Pars Plana Vitrectomy (Fig. 18-64)

1. A lid speculum is placed, and the conjunctiva is incised. The rectus muscles may be isolated, and 0 silk fixation sutures are placed.
2. The infusion line is sutured in place with a purse-string suture. The line is checked to ensure proper placement.
3. Three incisions are made through the pars plana: one for infusion, one for endoillumination, and one for a vitreous cutter or other instrumentation (for example, pick, forceps, scissors, laser probe, extrusion needle).
4. The operating microscope is aligned, and a fundus lens is fixed on the anterior surface of the cornea.
5. The infusion rate, cutting rate, and aspiration rate are set on the machine console. If a dense cataract or retained lens material blocks the view of the retina, a lensectomy may be performed with a fragmatome or other ultrasonic handpiece at this time.
6. The vitreous is removed under direct visualization. Once the medium has been removed and the retinal condition visualized, the necessary injections or treatments (endolaser photocoagulation, repair of macular pucker, insertion of silicone oil, gas-fluid exchange) (Fig. 18-65) are completed. A scleral buckling procedure may also be performed.
7. The pars plana incisions are closed, and the conjunctival incision is sutured. Cultures from the vitreous washings are taken if necessary.
8. Subconjunctival injections of steroids or antibiotics are given. An eye pad and shield may be applied, but there is a trend not to patch or shield.

LASER PHOTOCOAGULATION

In addition to intraocular photocoagulation with argon laser or cryocoagulation used during vitrectomy procedures, argon laser photocoagulation can be delivered through a slitlamp to the retina as a noninvasive, ambula-

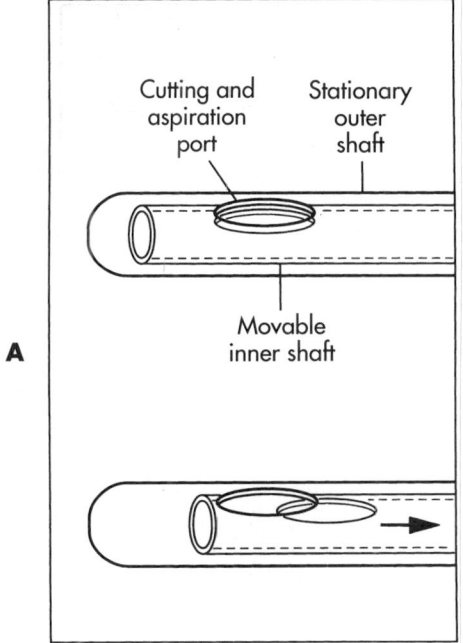

A

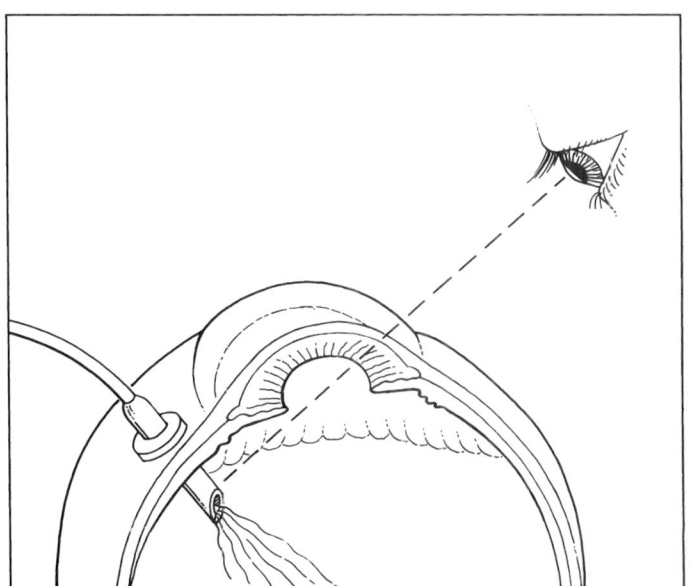

B

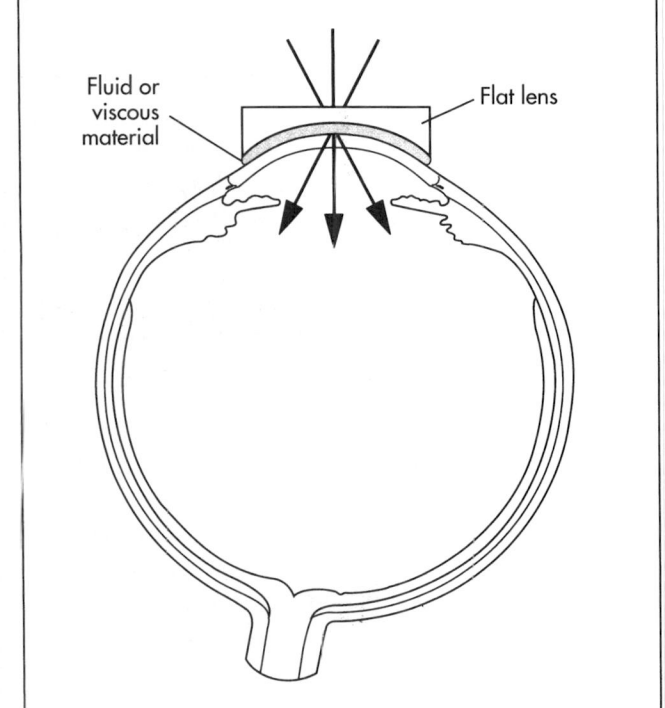

C

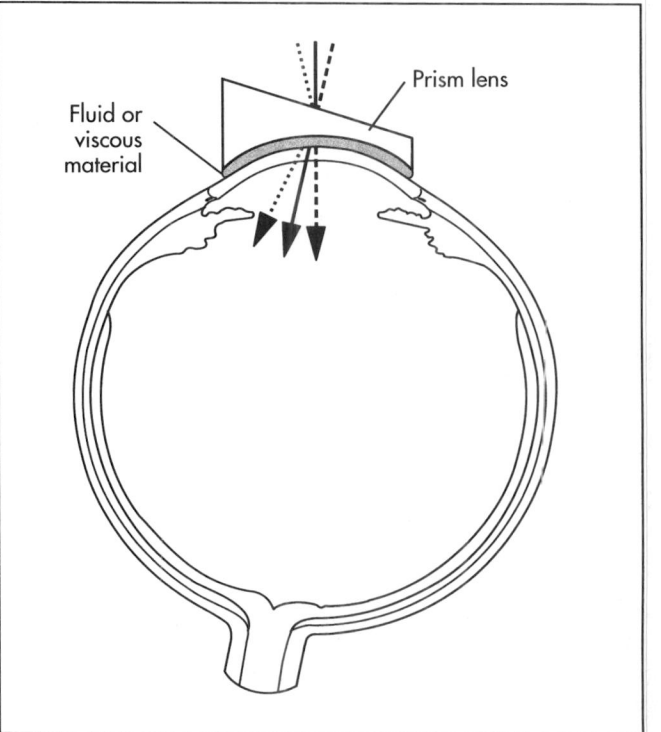

D

FIGURE 18-64   Essential compcnents for vitrectomy. **A**, Vitrector probe with its cutting and aspirating port close to the tip of the intraocular portion of the handpiece. **B**, Infusion cannula, placed in the pars plana, is viewed for correct position. **C**, Flat contact lens, resting on cushion of fluid or viscoelastic material on the cornea, is used for viewing posterior half of the vitreous cavity and retina. **D**, Prism contact lens used for viewing anterior structures in the vitreous cavity.

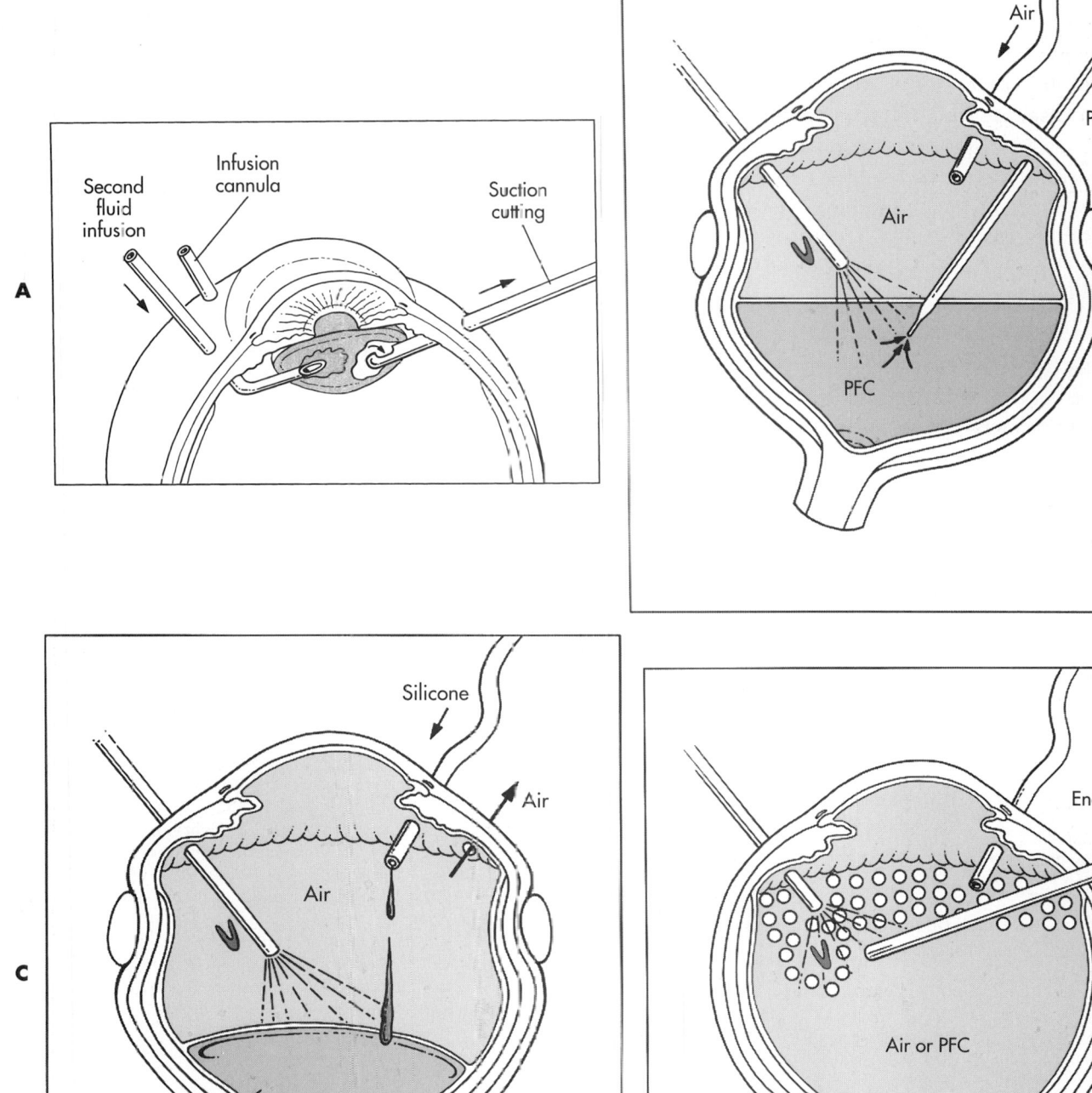

FIGURE 18–65   Procedures done with vitrectomy. **A**, Pars plana lensectomy performed with a second infusion line. **B,** Air-perfluorocarbon (PFC) exchange. The PFC has been placed in the vitreous cavity for removal of subretinal fluid and anatomic reattachment of the retina. Air under positive pressure is then placed through the infusion cannula as the PFC is simultaneously extruded through the tapered needle. **C**, Silicone-air exchange. Silicone is inserted through the infusion cannula as a temporary intraocular tamponade. Silicone is heavier than air and fills the globe from the bottom up, and the air escapes through the sclerotomy site. In silicone-fluid exchange the silicone floats on the fluid, and the fluid is removed with an extrusion needle. **D**, Endolaser photocoagulation is performed after the retina is back in place.

tory procedure to treat flat retinal holes or tears, sites of potential pathologic conditions, and vascular proliferative diseases, such as diabetic retinopathy and the "wet" form of macular degeneration.

Operative procedures

Argon Laser Treatment

1. The patient's pupil is dilated, and a retrobulbar anesthetic may be used.
2. Proparacaine drops are instilled into the operative eye.
3. A three-mirror Goldmann or similar lens, which has been lubricated, is placed on the cornea, and the patient is positioned at the laser slitlamp.
4. The proper spot size, power setting, and duration of exposure are set.
5. Laser burns are placed in the prescribed areas.
6. The patient's eye is irrigated with physiologic saline solution to remove the viscous lens lubricant.
7. The eye is patched as necessary.

Nd:YAG Laser Treatment

An Nd:YAG laser is also used for lysis of vitreous strands or bands and to open opaque posterior capsules. The procedure is similar to argon laser treatment in its delivery through a slitlamp. A Peyman lens for a specific depth is selected and used in place of the Goldmann lens when cutting vitreous strands. No lens or anesthetic is needed to open posterior capsules. The patient is positioned at the laser slitlamp, and pulsed laser applications using 1 to 3 millijoules of power are used to open the posterior capsule.

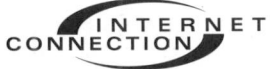

Cyberspace Hospital Ophthalmology Department:
http://ch.nus.sg/CH/ch.html

Digital Journal of Ophthalmology:
http://www.djo.harvard.edu/

National Eye Institute: http://www.nei.nih.gov/

Wilmer Eye Institute: http://www.wilmer.jhu.edu/

American Academy of Ophthalmology:
http://www.eyenet.org/

A Site for Sore Eyes: http://www.eye2eye.com

REFERENCES

1. Buckley, E.G., et al. (1995). *Atlas of ophthalmic surgery*, Vol. 3: *Strabismus and glaucoma*. St. Louis: Mosby.
2. Cataract Management Guideline Panel. (1993). *Cataract in adults: management of functional impairment* (Clinical Practice Guideline, No. 4). Rockville, Md.: U.S. Department of Health and Human Services, Public Health Service, Agency for Health Care Policy and Research. (AHCPR Pub. No. 93-0542. Feb. 1993, pp. 40-43.)
3. Cavanaugh, T.B., & Durrie, D.S. (1994). Holmium YAG laser thermokeratoplasty: synopsis of clinical experience. *Seminars in Ophthalmology, 9*, 110-116.
4. Chandler, J.W., Sugar, J., & Edelhauser, H.F. (1994). *External diseases: cornea, conjunctiva, sclera, eyelids, lacrimal system*. St. Louis: Mosby.
5. Covell, C.A., & Walton, R.P. (1994). "AMB-Track": development of a surgicenter model within a main operating room. *AORN Journal, 59*, 1257-1265.
6. Custer, P.L. (1993). Ptosis. In Tenzel, R.R. (Assoc. Ed.). *Textbook of ophthalmology*, Vol. 4: *Orbit and oculoplastics*. New York: Gower.
7. Dutton, J.J. (1992). *Atlas of ophthalmic surgery*, Vol. 2: *Oculoplastic, lacrimal, and orbital surgery*. St. Louis: Mosby.
8. Fiander, D.C., & Tayfour, F. (1995). Excimer laser in situ keratomileusis in 124 myopic eyes. *Journal of Refractive Surgery, 11*(suppl.), S234-S238.
9. Gill, K.S., Sitbon, J.R., & Trocme, S.D. (1997). Phototherapeutic keratectomy. *AORN Journal, 66*, 242-252.
10. Harkness, B.S. (1996). Hydroxyapatite eye implant. *Today's Surgical Nurse*, May/June, 16-20.
11. Langseth, F. (1993). The use of 5-fluorouracil in glaucoma filtration surgery. *Journal of the American Society of Ophthalmic Registered Nurses, 23*(20), 11-13.
12. MacKenzie, M., & Waterman, M. (1995). Utilization of a clinical pathway in the care of the ambulatory cataract surgical patient. *Journal of the American Society of Ophthalmic Registered Nurses, 20*(6), 6-11.
13. McEwen, D.R. (1997). Surgical treatment of dacryocystitis. *AORN Journal, 66*, 268-280.
14. Tenzel, R.R. (1993). *Textbook of ophthalmology*, Vol. 4: *Orbit and oculoplastics*. New York: Gower.
15. Yamada, S., et al. (1993). An eye on comfort: positioning a patient for ophthalmic surgery. *Journal of Ophthalmic Nursing Technology, 12*(2), 75-78.

CHAPTER NINETEEN

Otologic Surgery

Carol Richard

HEARING IS THE sense by which sounds are appreciated. Referred to as the watchdog of the senses, hearing is the last sense to disappear when one falls asleep and the first to return when one awakens. *Position sense* refers to the orientation of the head in space and the movement of the body through space, its balance and equilibrium.[3]

The word *auditory* refers to the sense of hearing and comes from the Latin word *audíre*, which means 'to hear'. The physical nature of sound results from the compression and rarefaction of pressure waves and moving molecules, but the sensations humans actually experience are the product of complex mechanical, electrical, and psychologic interactions in the ear and central nervous system. The study of the ear and its diseases is known as *otology*, derived from Greek word *ótos*, meaning 'ear'.

The basic principles applied to all operations on the ear and temporal bone include the necessity for maintaining aseptic technique, the use of the operating microscope, the development of improved instrumentation, and the use of preoperative sedation, anesthesia, and antibiotic therapy.

The success of surgical restoration of useful hearing is attributed to new concepts and techniques, the types of approaches to gain access to the temporal region, and improvements in the design and materials used in implantable prosthetic devices. Better understanding of the anatomy and physiology of the ear has allowed the surgeon to perform reconstructive surgeries to improve the patient's hearing and equilibrium and to have greater control of diseases in the middle ear and mastoid. Procedures to correct conductive hearing loss resulting from conductive apparatus abnormalities may include a stapedectomy and partial or total ossicular replacement surgery. Surgical treatment for sensorineural hearing loss, or Meniere's disease, can be offered to patients suffering from intolerable tinnitus or the disabling effects of vertigo. Cochlear implants and implantable hearing aids have brought new hope for deaf patients.

New monitoring techniques have proved to be beneficial in the preservation of the facial nerve by minimizing trauma during reconstructive surgery. New diagnostic techniques on the horizon will enable the surgeon to identify anatomic areas that may present a surgical challenge and to plan the best approach to the target tissue. This same methodology will also help patients to better understand their disease process. These technologic advancements contribute to decreased otologic complications, shortened hospital stays, and improved outcomes for patients.

SURGICAL ANATOMY

External, Middle, and Inner Ear

The ear is a sensory organ that functions in the identification, localization, and interpretation of sound as well as in the maintenance of equilibrium. Anatomically, it is divided into the external ear, middle ear, and inner ear (Fig. 19-1).

The *external ear*, including the auricle (or pinna) and external auditory canal, is composed of cartilage covered with skin. The auricles, which are fixed in position and lie close to the head, are responsible for concentrating sound waves and conducting them into the external auditory canal. Both ears provide stereophonic hearing for judging the direction of sound, whereas the shape of the auricles helps to differentiate sounds coming from directly behind from those sounds arriving directly in front.[12]

The external auditory canal, an S-shaped pathway leading to the middle ear, is approximately 2.5 cm in length in adults and shelters the tympanic membrane (see Fig. 19-1). Its skeleton of bone and cartilage is covered

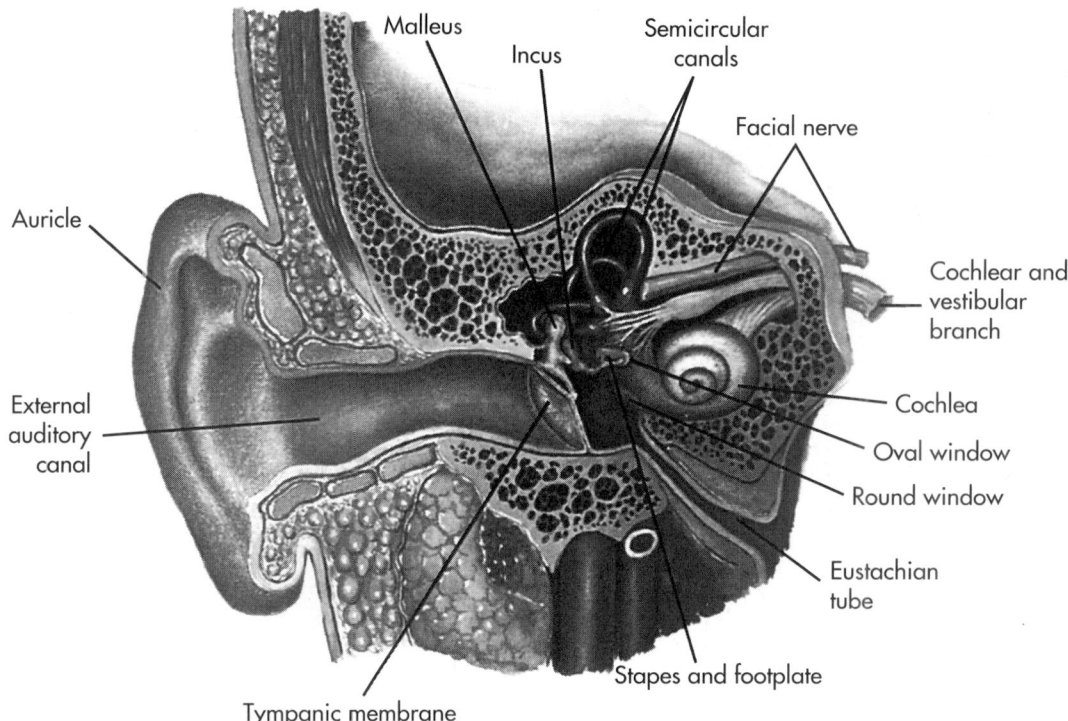

FIGURE 19-1   Schema of external ear, middle ear, and inner ear.

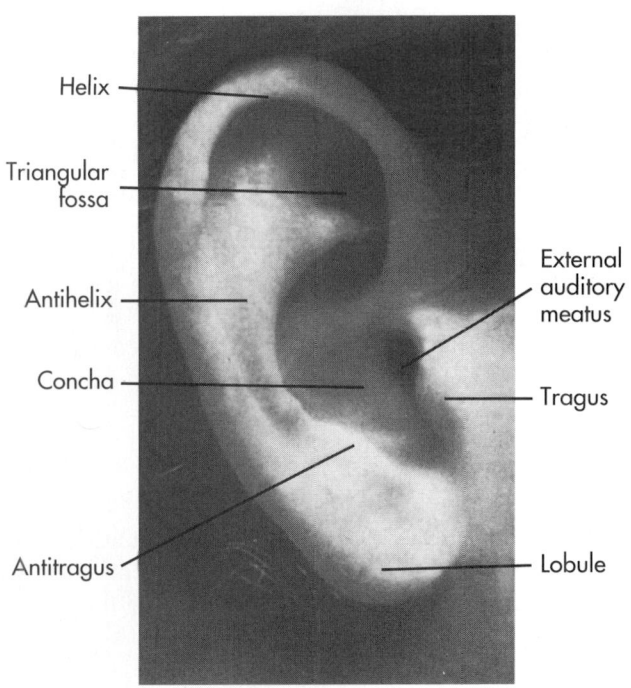

FIGURE 19-2   Anatomic structures of auricle. Helix is prominent outer rim, whereas antihelix is area parallel and anterior to helix. Concha is deep cavity containing the auditory canal meatus. Tragus is protuberance on antihelix opposite tragus. Lobule is soft lobe on bottom of auricle.

with very thin, sensitive skin. The canal lining is protected and lubricated with cerumen, a waxy substance secreted by sebaceous glands in the distal third of the canal. Cerumen helps to trap foreign material and reduces bacterial levels in the outer ear. Notice the structural landmarks in Fig. 19-2.

Located at the end of the external auditory canal is the *tympanic membrane* (eardrum). It is a thin fibrous membrane covered with skin on its lateral aspect and medially is covered with mucous membrane that is continuous with the lining of the middle ear.

The *middle ear* is filled with air, which comes from the nasopharynx through the eustachian tube. Posteriorly the middle ear communicates with the mastoid air cells of the temporal bone. The mucous membrane of the middle ear is continuous with that of the pharynx and the mastoid cells, making it possible for infection to travel to the middle ear (otitis media) and mastoid cells (mastoiditis). The eustachian tube serves to aerate the air-filled spaces of the temporal bone and to equalize pressure in the middle ear with atmospheric pressure. It will open during yawning, sneezing, or swallowing and remains closed when the pressure is greater outside.

A chain of three tiny movable bones (ossicles) extends across the middle ear cavity and conducts vibrations (airborne sound waves) from the tympanic membrane across the middle ear into the oval window and the fluid-filled inner ear.

The *malleus* (hammer) consists of a head, neck, handle, and short process (Fig.19-3). The handle and short process

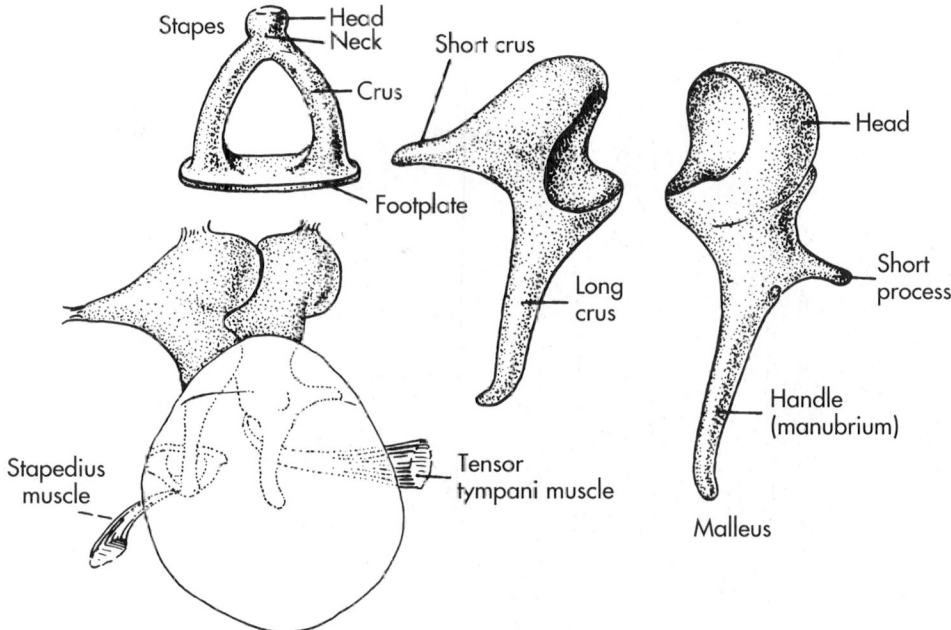

FIGURE 19-3   Articulated ossicles of right middle ear.

are attached to the undersurface of the eardrum and join it to the incus. The *incus* (anvil) consists of a body and long and short processes (see Fig. 19-3). The long crus of the incus is attached to the stapes, which is the third, innermost bone. The *stapes* (stirrup) consists of a head, neck, anterior and posterior crura, and a footplate that fits into the oval window (see Fig. 19-3). The movable joints between these bones contribute to a lever system converting the transmission of vibrations from air to the fluid of the inner ear.

The inner ear is protected from loud noise by two small muscles. The *tensor tympani* muscle draws the drum inward to increase tension, thus restricting its ability to vibrate. The *stapedius* muscle pulls the stapes away from the oval window reducing the intensity and potentially damaging vibrations passing through the ossicles into the inner ear. The middle ear and mastoid are supplied with blood from the branches of the internal and external carotid artery systems.

The *inner* ear is a membranous curved cavity located in the petrous portion of the temporal bone and contains receptors for hearing and balance. It consists of a bony labyrinth filled with a watery fluid (perilymph) that surrounds and bathes a membranous labyrinth. Perilymph serves as a protective cushion to the end organ of hearing. There are three divisions of the bony labyrinth: the cochlea, the vestibule, and the semicircular canals.

Within the membranous labyrinth lies four structures: the cochlear duct, the utricle, the saccule, and the semicircular ducts. A second fluid (endolymph) bathes and nourishes the sensory cells contained within the membranous labyrinth.

Cochlea

The cochlea has a tubular shape resembling a snail shell. It is divided into three compartments: the scala vestibuli, which is associated with the oval window; the scala tympani, which is associated with the round window; and the cochlear duct. Both the scala vestibuli and scala tympani are filled with perilymph, whereas the cochlear duct contains endolymph. On the vestibular surface of the basilar membrane of the cochlea lies the organ of Corti, the neural end organ for hearing. From its neuroepithelium project thousands of hair cells that are set into motion by vibrations passing through the ossicles and oval window to the perilymph. The hair cells convert mechanical energy of wave movement from vibration in the perilymph into electrochemical impulses. The inner ear is connected to the brain through the acoustic nerve (eighth cranial nerve).

Vestibular Labyrinth

The vestibular labyrinth is composed of the utricle, the saccule, and three semicircular canals referred to as the *lateral, superior* and *posterior canals*. They are positioned at right angles to one another so that any movement of the head will excite at least one of the semicircular canals. The maculae of the utricle and saccule of the vestibular labyrinth are gravity oriented and are concerned with static equilibrium. The internal auditory branches of the basilar artery supplies the inner ear.

Hearing

Hearing is an interpretation of sound waves by the brain. The auricle serves as a sound-localizing device and

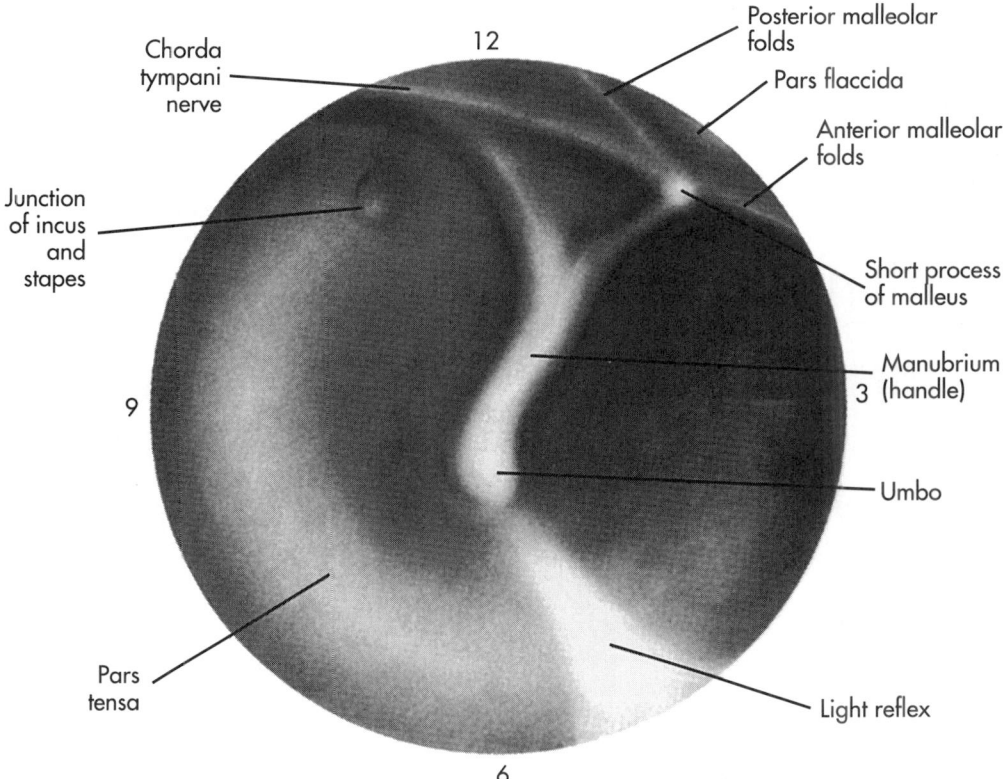

FIGURE 19-4　Structural landmarks of tympanic membrane.

functions as a conduit by transmitting sound waves traveling through the external auditory canal to the tympanic membrane. This vibration initiates ossicular motion. The malleus, attached to the tympanic membrane, begins vibrating, as do the incus and stapes, which are attached to the malleus on the other side (Fig. 19-4). The vibrations are passed to the oval window of the inner ear in which the stapes is inserted. From here they travel through the fluid of the cochlea to the round window, where they are dissipated. Vibrations in the membrane cause the delicate hair cells of the organ of Corti to strike against the membrane of Corti, stimulating impulses in the sensory endings of the auditory division of the eighth cranial nerve. These impulses are transmitted to the temporal lobe of the brain for interpretation. Sound vibrations may also be transmitted by bone directly to the inner ear. A cross-section of the external, middle, and inner ear in relation to other structures of the head and face are shown in Fig. 19-5.

Equilibrium

The three semicircular canals each contain a sense organ (crista). These sense organs are responsive to fluid movement in the endolymph, which sets up impulses in the vestibular branch of the acoustic nerve. Cristae are stimulated by sudden movements or by changes in rate (acceleration and deceleration) or direction of movement.

Facial Nerve

The facial nerve is encased in the temporal bone and is the longest bony enclosure of a nerve in the human body. Its path through the bone and its intracranial and extracranial relationship determines its vulnerability to disease and the particular symptoms of whatever segment of the nerve is involved.[7] This bony enclosure also subjects the facial nerve to injury from swelling and injury to the temporal bone.

The facial nerve enters the internal auditory meatus above the cochlear nerve and travels through the internal auditory canal passing through the labyrinthine portion of the temporal bone to the geniculate ganglion where it turns sharply and passes superior to the oval window. It then turns inferiorly through the mastoid and exits through the stylomastoid foramen. There are three primary branches of the facial nerve in the temporal bone: The greater superficial petrosal nerve controls lacrimation; the stapedial branch controls the stapedius muscle and the chorda tympani nerve, which carries taste to the anterior two thirds of the tongue.[13]

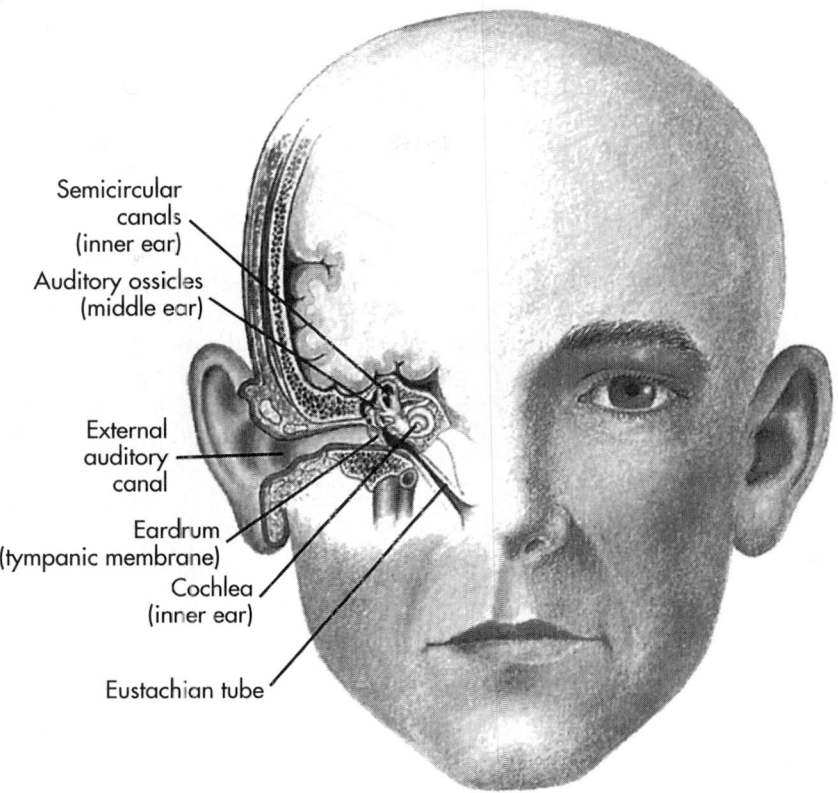

FIGURE 19-5   Cross-section of external, middle, and inner ear in relation to other structures of head and face.

PERIOPERATIVE NURSING CONSIDERATIONS

Assessment

Assessment is a systematic and intentional process of collecting and interpreting data concerning a patient's health history and status with otologic dysfunctions. Information obtained helps the nurse to develop a nursing diagnosis that directs nursing plans, interventions, and evaluation. The assessment should include a review of the following:

1. The presenting complaint (Hearing what brings the patient to the hospital often provides clues to fears and psychological factors that will need attention.)
2. Symptoms for vertigo or dizziness
   a. Description of the attack, its time of onset, frequency, and duration, and its relation to a positional change of the head and neck. To and fro movements versus rotary motion—a room spinning around the patient or the patient rotating.
   b. Associated symptoms—the presence of ataxia, nausea, and vomiting with or without tinnitus, hearing loss, distortion of hearing, fullness or pressure in the ear, visual changes, unsteadiness, loss of balance or falling.

3. Symptoms for impaired hearing (in one or both ears)
   a. Mode of onset—instant (may indicate a vascular disruption); over a few hours or days (may indicate viral infection); and progression—slow or gradual, fluctuations of hearing, influenced by illnesses.
   b. Behavioral changes—no reaction to loud noises, inattention and reliance on gestures.
   c. Adaptive responses—lip reading, sign language, written communication, physical disability that interferes with adaptation such as difficulty operating a hearing aid.
   d. Speech preference—soft or loud, monotonous tone or erratic volume.
   e. Optimal hearing—on the telephone, in quiet or noisy environment, use of hearing aid.
   f. Effect of hearing loss on daily life—inability to hear traffic, alarms, telephone, conversation, television.
4. History of earache
   a. Onset, duration, pain, fever, discharge (serous, mucoid, purulent, sanguinous).
   b. Concurrent upper respiratory tract infection, frequent swimming, head trauma, related complaints in the mouth, teeth, sinuses, or throat.
   c. Associated symptoms—reduced hearing, ringing in the ear, vertigo.
   d. Method of ear cleaning.

5. Medical history, age, frequency of ear problems during childhood, previous medical or surgical therapy, trauma to head, physical limitations such as arthritis, neck, and back problems

6. Ototoxic drugs taken including salicylates, aminoglycosides, furosemide, streptomycin, quinine, and ethacrynic acid.

7. Family history—hearing problems or hearing loss or Meniere's disease.

8. Environmental factors and exposure to loud continuous noise (factory, airport, loud music, power equipment, machinery).

9. External ear examination, including size, shape, symmetry, landmarks, color, position, and presence of deformities, lesions, and nodules.

10. Facial or abducens nerve involvement—inability to look downward, nystagmus, facial asymmetry, and facial paresis.

In addition to standard office diagnostic procedures performed by the surgeon, several other tests may be performed on the patient before arrival in the operating room. Studies of greatest significance to the perioperative team and those that the nurse should be responsible for having in the operating room before the procedure may include the following:

Audiogram

The audiogram determines whether the patient has normal hearing, conductive hearing loss, or sensorineural hearing loss. Two types of audiometric testing are performed on patients with suspected hearing loss:

Pure-tone audiometry is a technique that presents a single-frequency tone to patients through a headphone and is performed in each ear. The intensity of the tone is then varied until the lowest audible intensity in decibels (dB) is measured. It determines the degree of hearing impairment by evaluating air-conduction and bone-conduction thresholds. Air-conduction thresholds are a measure of the entire auditory system, whereas bone-conduction thresholds are a measure of the preceptive mechanism of the ear (cochlea and auditory nerve). In normal hearing and in pure sensorineural hearing loss, air- and bone-conduction thresholds are equal. In conductive hearing loss, bone-conduction scores are essentially normal and slightly better than air-conduction scores. In mixed-hearing loss, air- and bone-conduction scores are lower but with less bone-conduction loss.[7]

Speech audiometry evaluates the patient's ability to hear, understand and distinguish phonetic elements of speech. Higher scores (90% to 100%) reflect excellent speech-discrimination ability and is seen in normal hearing, pure conductive loss, and some cochlear losses. Scores lower than than 90% indicate an impaired ability to discriminate speech and are seen in patients with cochlear and retrocochlear lesions.

Pure-tone and speech audiometry testing is done on patients preoperatively and up to 6 weeks postoperatively.

Magnetic resonance imaging

Magnetic resonance imaging (MRI) is an imaging modality using powerful magnetic and radio frequency waves to reproduce cross-sectional images of the human body without exposing the patient to ionizing radiation. On an MRI scan, fat and fluid produce high-intensity signals and appear as bright areas, whereas bone and air (as in the normal mastoid) emit weak signals and appear as darkened areas on the scan. Abnormal tissue and fluid caused by infection, trauma and tumors within the external auditory canal, middle ear, and mastoid are identified by abnormally high-intensity signals.

MRI is more sensitive than computerized tomography (CT) for early identification of changes in pathology of the temporal bone; however, it is unable to detect the exact location and extent of the abnormality and involvement of bony structures (such as the ossicles).[11]

MRI may be contraindicated for patients with implantable metal objects such as inner ear implants, since the magnet could move the implant causing injury to the patient. Today, most middle ear prostheses are manufactured using nonmagnetic materials, which include different grades of stainless steel. If in doubt as to the material used in the implanted device, check with the physician.

Computerized tomography (CT)

CT scans are x-ray studies that visualize structures by producing serial sections in various planes. It uses computers to measure small x-ray absorption differentials not recognizable by direct recording on x-ray films and enables the radiologist to manipulate factors that produce the image to optimize visualization of bone, soft tissue, and adjacent intracranial and extracranial pathologic conditions. Intravenous injection of iodine contrast agents produces visual enhancement of some anatomic structures and pathologic tissues including highly vascularized tumors. CT is the study of choice to access intratemporal bone pathology by showing the relationship of mass to ossicles and other bony structures of the ear and for postoperative evaluation of the ear. However, if a lesion extends outside the confines of the temporal bone, MRI will define involvement of intracranial and extracranial spaces more precisely than CT would.[11]

Virtual otoscopy

Endoscopic, CT, and MRI image techniques assist in diagnosing disease and in surgical planning. Endoscopy is an invasive procedure and limits visualization to the lumen. CT and MRI scans allow the surgeon to view tissue beyond an exposed surface but are only two-dimensional images. Both require a mental reconstruction of the anatomy, which is often difficult because of the small complex structures housed in the temporal bone. Virtual

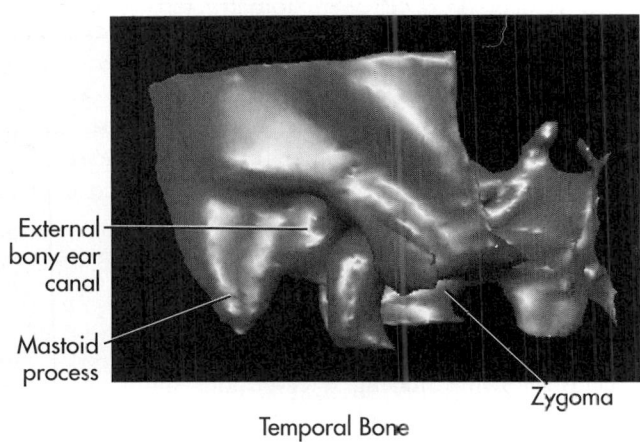

FIGURE 19-6 Virtual otoscopic 3-D image of the temporal bone denoting the mastoid process, zygoma, and external bony ear canal.

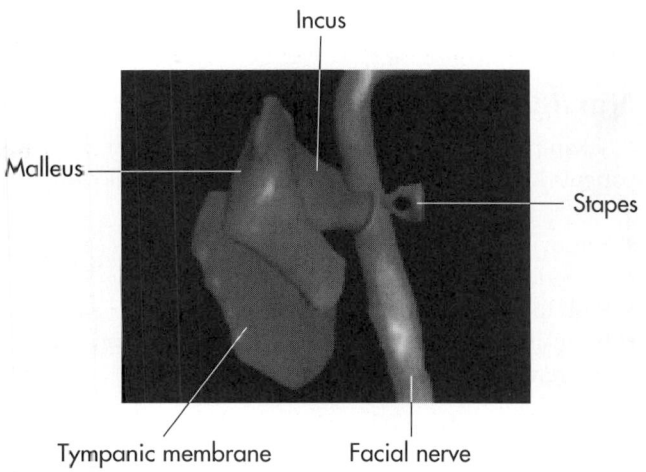

FIGURE 19-7 Virtual otoscopy 3D visualization of the ossicular chain in the middle ear. Note its relationship to the facial nerve and tympanic membrane.

otoscopy combines the benefits of these imaging techniques and, at the same time, decreases their disadvantages.

Virtual endoscopy consists of a computer-assisted three-dimensional (3-D) image of a patient's anatomy and pathologic condition. Registration (or alignment) is completed by transferring the patient's CT and MRI images onto the computer. Various anatomic structures undergo segmentation (identification and isolation). They include the temporal bone (Fig. 19-6), ossicular chain, internal auditory canal and its structures, internal carotid artery, facial nerve, stapedius muscle, and eustachian tube. 3-D reconstruction of the segmented structures is performed and integrated into a complete model, which is used for virtual otoscopy.

Currently surgeons have to perform surgery to visualize the middle and inner ear. Virtual otoscopy allows the surgeon to visualize this same anatomy in a 3-D format. The virtual camera can be navigated through the ear by two methods: manually by using a mouse to change the camera position and field of view and automatic path finding, which uses the camera as a point robot. The animation process begins when the external auditory canal is approached. The camera passes through the eardrum and backs into a recess of the middle ear cavity to view the incus, malleus, and stapes and stapedius muscle (Fig. 19-7). It then glides along the middle ear cavity until the cavity wall dissolves, revealing the inner ear structures including the facial nerve, carotid artery, internal auditory canal, cochlea, and semicircular canals (Fig. 19-8). The camera is able to move in such a way as to view inside the skull where the carotid artery and facial nerve entry points are visible. All anatomic structures visible on the computer screen (display) are identified by different colors.

Computer screen capabilities include the simultaneous display of three different views: the virtual endoscopic camera view, an external (global) view, and a display of the nearest CT or MRI slice.

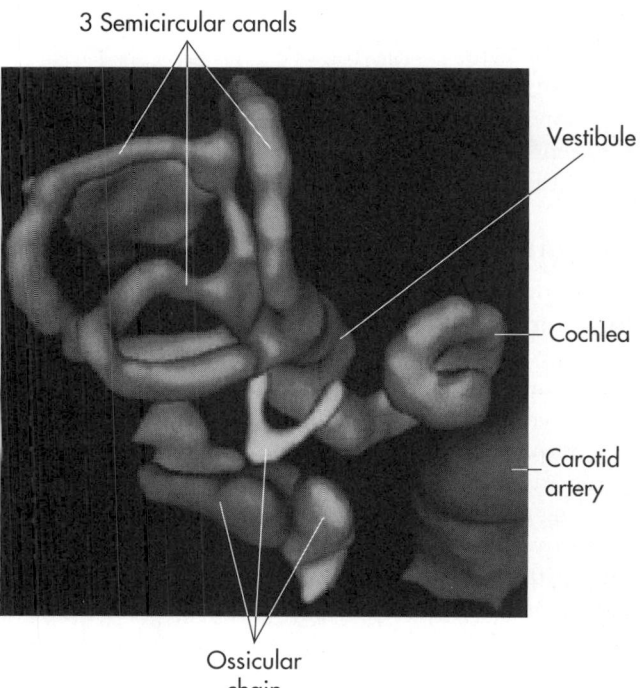

FIGURE 19-8 Virtual otoscopy 3D image of the inner ear including Cochlea, Vestibule, and three semicircular canals which are at right angles to each other. The ossicular chain and carotid artery are also displayed.

Advantages of virtual otoscopy include enabling the surgeon to better anticipate areas that may present an intraoperative challenge and to plan the best trajectory to target tissue. It provides a tremendous potential in education of staff, students, and residents, and it facilitates a patient's understanding of the disease process.

At this time, virtual otoscopy does not help if the surgeon wants to acquire a biopsy specimen, if a patient needs interventional treatment (such as cauterization of bleeding), or in emergency situations.[5]

Nursing Diagnosis

Examples of nursing diagnoses that pertain to many patients having otologic surgery include the following:

- Sensory and perceptual alteration (auditory)
- Powerlessness as a result of a hearing deficit
- Risk for injury, related to sensory deficit
- Body-image disturbance related to neurologic deficit and removal of hair

Outcome Identification

Outcomes identified for the selected nursing diagnoses for patients undergoing otologic surgery could be stated as:

- Patient will demonstrate improved self-expression and decreased frustration with communication.
- Patient will be able to identify factors that can be controlled personally or by family, nursing staff, or surgical team.
- Patient will be free from injury at completion of perioperative experience.
- Patient will discuss feelings regarding outcome of the surgical procedure.

Planning

The development of a perioperative nursing care plan is based on the preoperative assessment, nursing diagnosis, and expected outcomes in addition to a general knowledge of the surgery. Appropriate planning should focus on patient education, positioning, and room environment.

Hearing deficits may increase patient anxiety. Thus, effective communication techniques are essential when teaching the patient. The nurse should determine the best way to communicate with the patient and, if necessary, utilize the institution's hearing-impaired services for patients requiring assistance. Speak slowly and clearly and confirm that the information is heard and understood. Procedures should be explained in a language that the patient understands. This helps to create confidence and alleviate any apprehension. Preoperative instructions and information given to the patient will be reinforced as needed throughout the perioperative experience. Visual teaching aids, teaching brochures, and written discharge instructions provide the patient with knowledge of the surgery and what to expect during the postoperative period.

Proper patient positioning is important to the success of the procedure and in maintaining skin integrity. Positioning accessories such as foam head supports, gel mattress pads, and heel and elbow padding will contribute to patient comfort. Patients receiving local anesthesia are reminded of the need to remain still during the procedure.

The operating room environment must be quiet and free of any loud noise. Intraoperative noises generated from suction, electrocautery, and other equipment should be explained to the patient before use, thus avoiding startling the patient and adversely affecting the success of the surgery. The room temperature should be set at a comfortable setting and the patient adequately covered to maintain normal body temperature.

A Sample Care Plan for the patient undergoing otologic surgery is on p. 703.

Implementation

The following nursing interventions should be instituted for the otologic patient:

1. Verify the operative side with the patient and confirm by review of informed consent and diagnostic test reports.
2. Verify that the patient has maintained an NPO status.
3. When in the operating room, provide calm, careful, and comforting nursing measures to reduce patient's anxiety. The sequence of perioperative events should be explained. It is important, at the outset, to inform the patient that hearing acuity may not return immediately.
4. If the patient uses a hearing aid, it should be worn to surgery and may be properly removed at the time of or after anesthesia induction. Likewise, prescription eyewear should be brought into the operating room because patients may require them to assist in lip reading when instructions and procedures are explained. If local anesthesia is used, the hearing aid in the unaffected ear should remain in place. Documentation of the hearing aid disposition is essential.
5. Patients with impaired hearing acuity need to be protected from injury. The environment should be controlled, because excess stimulation, loud conversations, and use of the intercom interfere with the patient's ability to hear and comply with instructions and explanations. If hearing loss is uncompensated, a pad of paper and pencil may be used as a means of communication.
6. For the patient receiving a local anesthetic, carefully review the patient's need to remain immobile during the procedure. Explain perioperative monitoring devices and accessories (electrosurgical unit, drills) that may be used if the patient will be awake.
7. Patient monitoring during local anesthesia may be performed by the perioperative nurse for stapedectomy or tympanoplasty procedures and should follow institutional protocol.
8. Remain with the patient throughout the induction phase of anesthesia.
9. Hair should be secured with a shower cap; shaving may be indicated, depending on the surgical approach.

S A M P L E   C A R E   P L A N

Nursing Diagnosis: Sensory and perceptual alteration (auditory)

Outcome: Patient will demonstrate improved self-expression and decreased frustration with communication.

Interventions:

Identify a method by which patient can communicate basic needs.

Promote continuity of care to reduce frustration.

Identify factors that promote communication.

Allow patient to wear hearing aid to the OR.

Speak slowly and deliberately into the dominant ear.

Nursing Diagnosis: Powerlessness from hearing deficit

Outcome: Patient will be able to identify factors that can be controlled personally or by family, nursing staff, or surgical team.

Interventions:

Increase effective communication between patient and healthcare personnel regarding the surgical intervention.

Allow patient to assume position of comfort.

Offer emotional support.

Ensure privacy.

Provide patient and family opportunities to express their feelings.

Provide and reinforce information given to patient.

Keep needed items within reach during postoperative period.

Nursing Diagnosis: Risk for injury related to sensory deficit

Outcome: Patient will be free from injury at completion of perioperative experience.

Interventions:

Speak clearly and deliberately to patient and confirm that patient has heard and understood communications.

Provide adequate assistance during movement onto OR bed and positioning.

Complete all transfer and positioning maneuvers slowly.

Identify physical limitations and position or support patient accordingly to provide optimal comfort during the procedure.

Control excess stimulation and noise level in OR.

Nursing Diagnosis: Body-image disturbance related to neurologic deficits and removal of hair

Outcome: Patient will discuss feelings regarding outcome of the surgical procedure.

Interventions:

Allow patient to discuss concerns about removal of hair and potential for facial weakness or paralysis.

Discuss available resources and options (use of wig, wearing of head scarf, acoustic neuroma support group, as appropriate). Make referrals to nurse on discharge unit as indicated.

Skin preparation should be carried out carefully to protect the eyes and prevent pooling of solution.

10. Thermal warming blankets and warm intravenous and irrigating solutions assist in maintaining normothermia. Warm irrigation is essential during local procedures to reduce the risk of inducing dizziness.

11. Sequential compression stockings may be utilized per physician request to decrease the risk of deep venous thrombosis and pulmonary embolism during long surgical procedures such as acoustic neuroma resection.

12. Document the serial number and lot numbers of otologic implants according to institutional policy.

13. If a laser is used, initiate and document laser safety precautions (see Chapter 3).

14. Discharge teaching and planning may be initiated by the perioperative nurse. Precautions and restrictions in ear and dressing care, nutritional, fluid, and activity needs, signs and symptoms to report to the physician (elevated temperature, pain, drainage, loss of hearing acuity), and medications (antibiotics, antiemetics, analgesics) should be reviewed.

Preoperative room preparation

Before the patient enters the operating room suite, equipment and supplies for the scheduled procedure should be gathered. A well-organized room can significantly reduce anesthesia time and enables the circulating nurse to spend more time attending to the preoperative and intraoperative needs of the patient. Preoperative room planning includes identifying the necessary equipment, instrumentation, furniture, and positioning accessories necessary to perform the surgery. Such equipment may include the operating microscope, video system, electrosurgical and bipolar units, suction, nerve-integrity monitors, specialty instrument kits, prosthetic devices, drill and irrigation accessories, and the laser. An otologic specialty storage cart centrally houses assorted prostheses, drill burrs and accessories, backup ear instrumentation, ear drapes, and dressing and packing materials.

The nursing team should check the functioning of all equipment and arrange the equipment and furniture in an efficient manner. These preoperative measures will save time and facilitate the ease of the operation. It also provides a calm, quiet environment conducive to the induction of anesthesia and to performing otologic surgery.[8] The patient is now transferred into the suite.

Positioning

Proper patient positioning is essential for adequate surgical exposure during otologic surgery. Based on the design of microscope and OR bed used, the patient may be placed on the bed in the reverse position with the patient's head at the foot of the bed. This position facilitates proper placement of a microscope mounted on a floor stand as well as allowing adequate space for the surgeon and assistant to be positioned on sitting stools near the surgical site. Before transferring the patient to the OR bed, the bed should be prepared with the mattress and sheets taped securely to its frame to prevent the patient and mattress from sliding during lateral rotation of the bed.

The patient should be in a supine position with the operative side as close to the edge of the OR bed as possible with the head turned and the operative ear upward. This positioning gives the surgeon access in viewing all areas of the middle ear and mastoid. Using one or more belts, secure the patient on the OR bed to ensure safety when turning or rotating the bed. During some procedures, such as myringotomy with the patient under local anesthesia, the patient's head may be secured in position by placing tape across the head and attaching it to the frame of the OR bed or by an attendant holding the patient's head firmly in position. For other procedures, the patient's head may be immobilized and supported on a foam headrest. A doughnut-shaped foam head support will help to immobilize the head and permit easy adjustment of the angle while the operating microscope is being used.[7]

To protect the nonoperative ear, the nurse should ensure that it is in the center of the doughnut hole and that the headrest does not cause any pressure on the ear. Special consideration must be given when the patient's head is positioned for surgery, especially under general anesthesia. Extremes in neck extension and head torsion can cause injury to the brachial plexus or cervical spine. Patients with limited carotid artery blood flow are vulnerable to further decrease in blood flow.[4] If the patient has a neck or back disorder caused by arthritis or other conditions, special padding or supports must be provided. Other options to assist in patient positioning are determined by the otologic procedure to be performed and by surgeon preference. They may include ophthalmic headrests with a cresent-shaped pad, a padded horseshoe-shaped headrest, and a headrest with skull pins such as the Mayfield, which is used in certain neurotology procedures.

Positioning of the surgeon is equally important to the success of the surgery. The surgeon's chair should be positioned at a height and distance that allows comfortable access to the operative field. The use of hydraulic or electric chairs enables the surgeon to adjust the position to meet these needs.

Anesthesia

The infiltration of a local anesthetic agent (local anesthesia) and general anesthesia have advantages during ear surgery. Local anesthesia will allow hearing to be tested on the adult patient and may result in slightly less bleeding with some procedures. General anesthesia provides better airway control and allows the patient to remain still throughout the procedure thereby making it technically easier to perform.

Local anesthesia along with closely monitored sedation is a preferred method for surgery in the premeatal region and for stapedectomy and uncomplicated middle ear procedures of less than 2 hours' duration. Preoperative sedation should render the patient calm, comfortable and cooperative, and able to understand and communicate. Patients should remain still and not be overmedicated to the point of demonstrating obtunded reflexes or being out of touch with their surroundings.[4] General anesthesia requires particular attention to preserving the facial nerve, extremes in head positioning, possible air emboli, the control of bleeding, and the effects of nitrous oxide in the middle ear.

Nitrous Oxide and the Middle Ear

The middle ear and paranasal sinuses are normal body air cavities and consist of open nonventilated spaces. The middle ear cavity is vented periodically when the eustachian tube opens. During general anesthesia, inhaled nitrous oxide enters the middle ear space through the eustachian tube and replaces the cavity's nitrogen. High concentrations of inhaled nitrous oxide enter the air cavity faster than the nitrogen can leave. This results in increased middle ear pressure. Rapid increases in middle ear pressure proportional to inhaled levels of nitrous oxide and abnormal eustachian tube function may cause nausea, vomiting, and rupture of the tympanic membrane in susceptible patients. This includes patients having previous ear surgery, otitis media, sinusitis, upper respiratory infections, enlarged adenoids, or other disorders of the nasopharynx.

When nitrous oxide is discontinued, the gas is rapidly reabsorbed, and strong negative pressure in the middle ear may occur. This negative pressure may result in serous otitis, disarticulation of the stapes, and impaired hearing. Some practitioners believe the use of nitrous oxide as an anesthetic inhalation agent is hazardous to hearing in patients who have undergone previous reconstructive middle ear surgery.[4]

Monitoring aseptic technique

Many procedures in otolaryngology are performed in a clean rather than sterile environment or field. Surgeons are accustomed to operating in such unsterile areas as the nose, nasopharynx, sinus cavities, mouth, and larynx. However, this "clean" technique cannot be carried over into surgeries to restore hearing without risking wound infection and failure to improve hearing.[7] All surgical team members must remain alert to possible breaks of aseptic technique. Auxillary and assistive personnel and visitors to the surgical suite should be properly attired and well informed of the boundaries of the sterile field.

Preparation of the operative site

Many otologic procedures require hair removal and skin to be clipped or shaved. Clipping is preferred because shaving may injure the skin and increase the risk of infection. Proper skin preparation combined with adequate isolation draping techniques help to lower infection rates and facilitate postoperative dressing of the ear. Postaural and endaural incisions extending upward from the meatus require hair to be clipped 2 inches in front, above, and behind the ear. Underhair may be clipped, whereas the top hair is maintained for postoperative cosmetic esthetic image enhancement. Plastic drapes may be applied to the clipped area to ensure that the surgical field is free from hair.

A povidone-iodine solution is used (unless the patient is allergic to iodine) to prep the exposed auricle and the periauricular skin. The meatus is cleansed with cotton

---

19-1 RESEARCH HIGHLIGHT

During chronic ear surgery, it is difficult to differentiate granulation tissue from nerve tissue. A prospective study of 250 procedures was conducted to evaluate the benefits of intraoperative nerve monitoring during routine chronic ear surgery in an academic resident teaching program. Procedures included tympanoplasties, some with mastoidectomies (canal wall-up technique), and tympanoplasties with canal wall-down technique performed by surgical resident staff with faculty participation.

The use of a facial nerve monitor during chronic ear surgery has sparked some debate as to its necessity versus its being simply a research tool. Electrophysiologic monitoring is neither a substitute for anatomic knowledge nor good technical and clinical skills. It does affect the ability to identify the facial nerve and to perform safe dissection techniques. When a nerve is exposed and surrounded by diseased tissue, the monitor will provide early feedback that will allow a modification of dissection and exposure techniques. This process along with detailed anatomic knowledge builds resident confidence, ensures the development of competent surgeons, and benefits both the resident surgeons and their patients.

From Pensak, M.L., Willging, J.P., & Keith, R.W. (1994). Intraoperative facial nerve monitoring in chronic ear surgery: a resident training experience, *American Journal of Otology, 15*(1), 108-110.

---

applicators if there is no hole in the eardrum. If requested by the surgeon, a syringe containing the prepping solution is placed into the external ear canal. A skin degreaser may be used to dry the ear canal. The face may be prepped on the operative side to permit observation of facial nerve stimulation.

Facial nerve monitoring

Audible facial nerve monitors are used intraoperatively during procedures in which the facial nerve is at risk. The purpose of this monitoring technique is to assist in the early identification of the nerve, to increase the possibility of its preservation by minimizing trauma, and to assess its integrity after dissection.[8] The validity and benefits of intraoperative facial nerve monitoring were studied in an academic resident teaching program (Research Highlight 19-1).

Electrodes are placed into the facial muscles before draping the patient. Consultation and communication with the anesthesia provider are essential because the use of muscle relaxants and long-term paralyzing agents must be avoided.

During some procedures, intraoperative hearing assessment may be necessary. This may be performed using a conventional audiometer if the patient is awake (under local anesthesia). If the patient is under general anesthesia, hearing may be assessed using auditory brainstem response (ABR), which will require an intraoperative neurophysiology technician or audiologist to assist in the monitoring.

Facial nerve monitoring is used during acoustic neuroma and mastoid surgery (Fig. 19-9).

Draping

Barrier draping minimizes the risk of postoperative infection. Draping technique is based on surgeon preference. For major otologic procedures, plastic adhesive drapes are applied around the ear to keep the patient's hair out of the surgical field. Sterile plastic aperture drapes may be placed over the surgical site with the ear exposed through the opening. The surgeon may elect to expose a portion of the face on the affected side to observe facial movement.

Three to four towels are draped over the aperture drape around the ear and may be secured with towel clips. A fenestrated drape is unfolded over the patient with the opening centered over the operative site. An alternative method is the use of a split sheet with the split end secured at the base of the ear and the open flaps wrapped around the patient's head. Disposable drapes with adhesive backing may be used to secure the sheet to the patient.

During mastoid surgery and for resections of acoustic tumors, fluid collection pouches may be attached to the drape. This pouch will catch fluid runoff when drilling and irrigation are planned.

Special consideration must be given to the selection of draping material used during ear surgery and to the

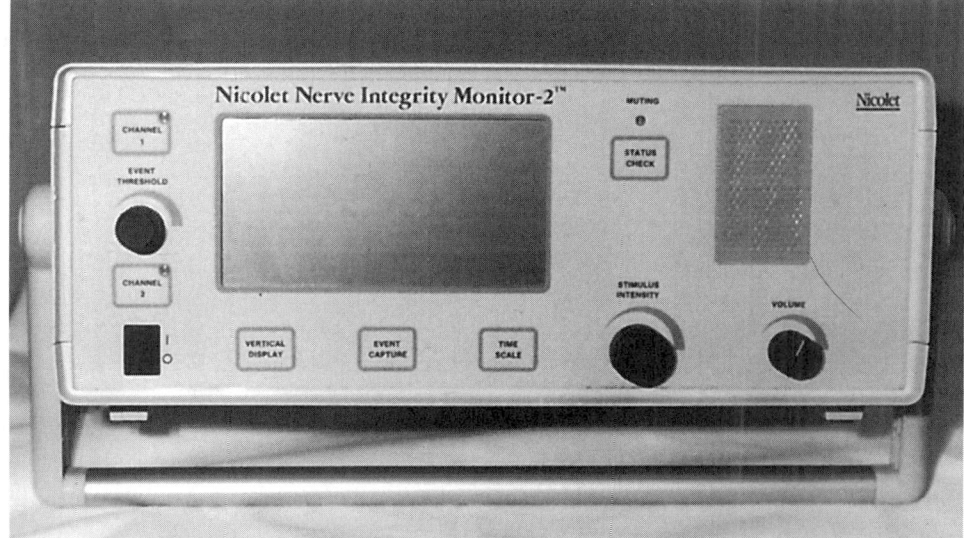

FIGURE 19-9 Nerve integrity monitor system for intraoperative facial nerve monitoring.

technique for removing powder from surgical gloves. Powder and lint cling to unwashed gloves and can be transferred to instruments and introduced into the ear. They act as a foreign body in the wound causing the formation of granulomas in the middle and inner ear and may contribute to irreversible hearing loss. It is imperative that gloves worn by the surgical team be washed, thus making them free from powder and lint. Lint-free drapes should be used.

A draped Mayo stand with sterile instruments and the draped operating microscope are positioned over the patient (Fig. 19-10).

Operating microscope

The complexity of ear surgery is partly attributable to the location of the delicate, bony anatomic structures contained within a confined operative area. Approaching the operative field is best accomplished by the use of the operative microscope, which provides illumination and magnification. Several kinds of operating microscopes (Fig. 19-11) with different attachments are available for otologic surgery. The microscope may be a floor- or ceiling-mounted model. Optimal light for an otologic microscope is provided by a xenon or halogen light source. Numerous types of monocular and binocular heads are available for the microscope. These heads may be fixed in a straight or angled plane, or they may be designed to be adjustable in an inclinable plane. For operations through an ear speculum the microscope provides direct light and permits the surgeon to select a magnification of 6, 10, 16, 25, or 40. A common eyepiece magnification for an otologic microscope is 12.5, and a usual objective (lens) is a 250f or 300f. The total magnification is determined by multiplying the magnification of the eyepiece times that of the microscope body times that of the objective. The type of head and objective selected is based on surgeon preference. Video equipment may be attached to the microscope, which allows other team members to follow the procedure and to anticipate the necessary instrumentation. Before lenses are put into the microscope, they should be checked to ensure that they are free from lint, dust, fingerprints, and soil. The surgeon adjusts the microscope before it is draped for surgery and manipulates it during the procedure. The microscope is draped with a sterile cover. It is necessary to keep the drape material away from the light fan of the microscope. Doing so will allow cool air to continue to circulate and will avoid overheating of the fan, which could prematurely burn out the lamp and possibly cause a fire as well. When micromanipulators are secured to transmit laser energy to tissue through the operating microscope, special microscope laser drapes must be used. These drapes have an opening in the plastic at the base of the micromanipulator covering the objective allowing laser energy to pass through the opening of the drape without risk of burning the drape.

Care should be taken when removing the drapes from the microscope to avoid discarding the eyepieces with the drapes or dropping them on the floor. Eyepieces have been lost or damaged in this manner, necessitating costly repair or replacement.

When the microscope is not in use, it should be kept in a locked, upright position and stored in an area that is away from traffic, free from dust, and properly ventilated. Ideally, a set of eyepieces should be left in the scope to prevent the inside of the scope from becoming dusty. The microscope may also be covered with either a protective cover or a plastic bag.

Care and handling of otologic instruments

The basic principles of care, handling, and sterilization of instruments are discussed in Chapter 4. To prevent damage, delicate microinstruments should be handled

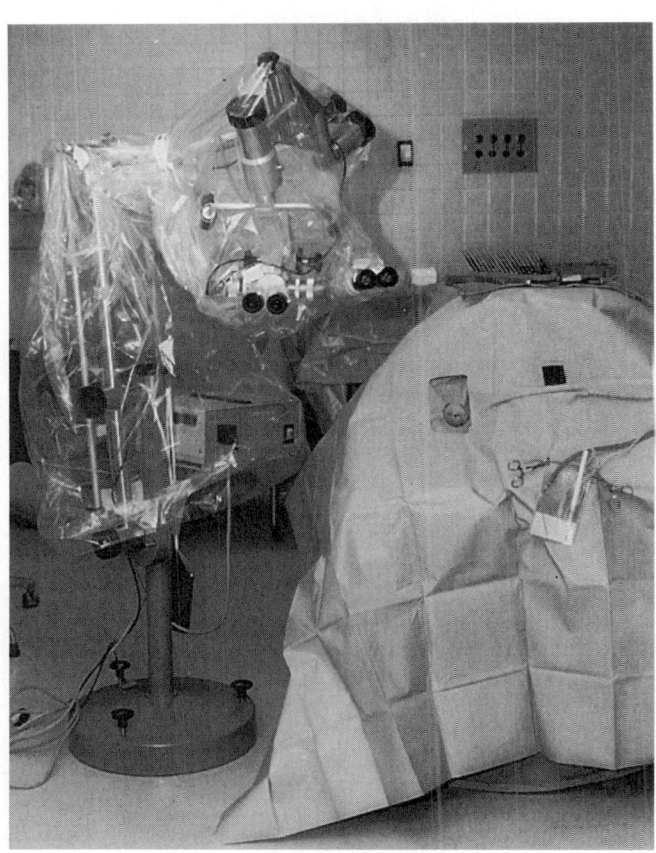

FIGURE 19-10   Draped microscope in place over patient in preparation for stapedectomy. Suction, tubing, and drill are assembled in position ready for use.

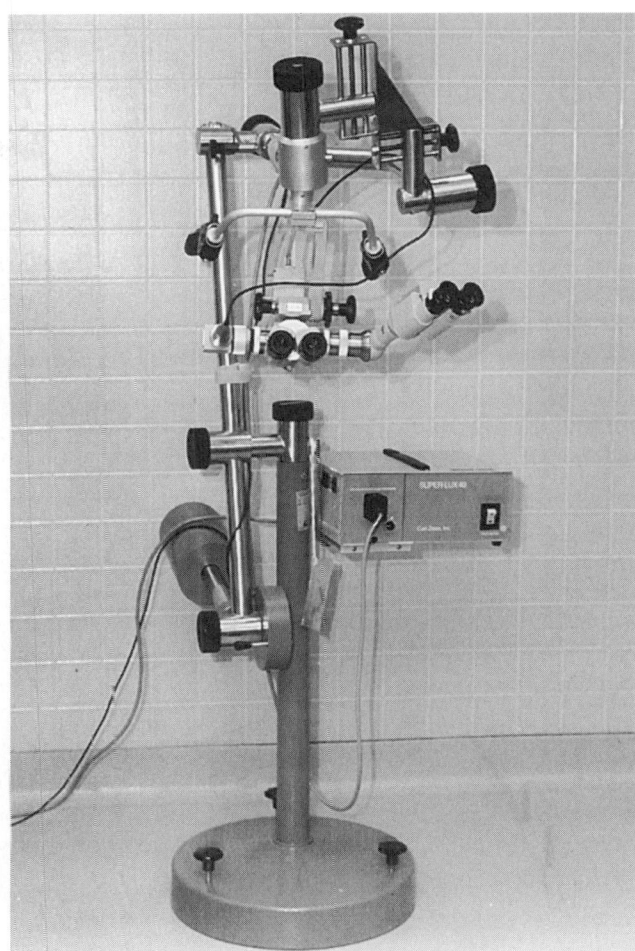

FIGURE 19-11   Operating microscope used during various otologic procedures. Lens system allows magnification of 6 to 40 without change in distance between microscope and ear. Xenon light provides excellent visualization.

individually and should not be allowed to come into contact with each other. They should be washed, rinsed, and dried individually. Soft-bristled brushes can be used to clean the instruments, and care should be given to prevent damage to their delicate tips. Preoperatively instruments should be closely inspected to ensure that they are in good working order. Fine tympanoplasty and stapedectomy instrumentation should be kept in special storage and sterilization trays (Fig. 19-12). These trays help to separate instruments, aid in quick identification, protect the instruments from damage, and facilitate handling during surgery (Fig. 19-13). When arranging instruments in the trays, one should consider grouping like items together, such as knives, elevators, hoes, and hooks. Color-coded taping of the instruments and the tray is helpful in maintaining the order of the instruments and helps the scrub nurse to quickly identify and deliver the instrument to the surgeon.

Drills and burrs

A power drill and assorted rotating burrs are essential for middle ear surgery. They are used exclusively for the removal of cortical, or hard cellular, bone. Many drills are comercially available that are pneumatically or electrically driven. Pneumatic drills must have high torque (power) and greater then 20,000 rpm (speed). Electrically powered drills are believed by some surgeons to offer equal torque but better control of the drill tip. There are two types of electric drills, those with the motor in the handpiece and others with a separate power supply. The drill may be fitted with either a straight or angled handpiece. A selection of burrs including assorted sizes of round cutting burrs and diamond polishing burrs should be available (Fig. 19-14). When drilling, the surgeon holds the handpiece similar to the way one holds a pen and uses the side of the burr as the cutting edge. Larger sized burrs decrease the risk of injury to the dura, sigmoid sinus, and facial nerve. Overheating and local devitalizing of bone may occur with continuous pressure on one spot. Overheating near the facial nerve may result in facial paralysis. When the drill is used, light intermittent pressure with continuous irrigation is recommended.

A diamond burr cuts slowly and pushes soft tissue away

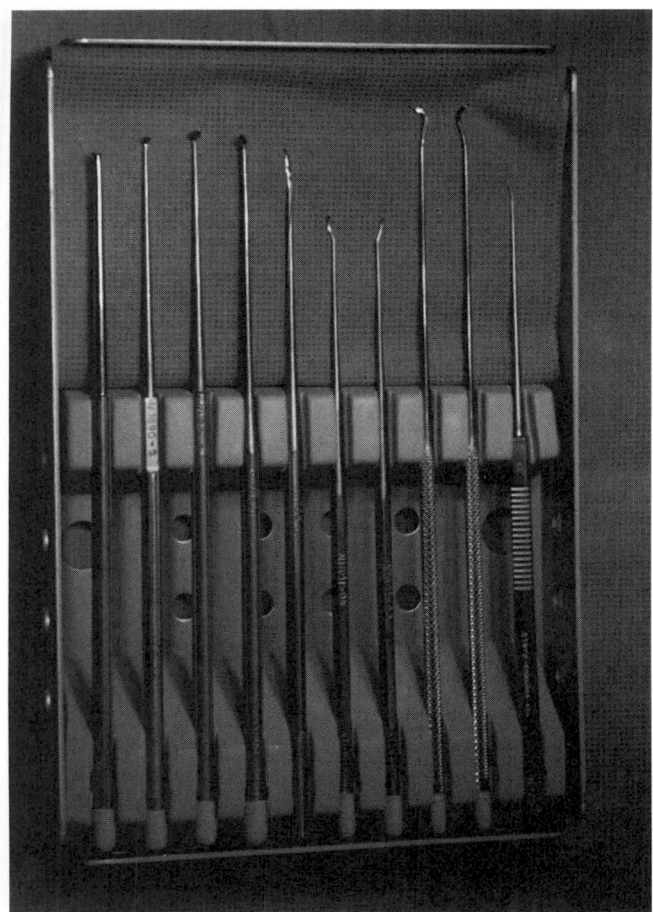

FIGURE 19-12 Microsurgical middle ear instruments (illustrating assorted knives) in protective rack, which separates the instruments from one another. The delicacy of these instruments requires protection of tips.

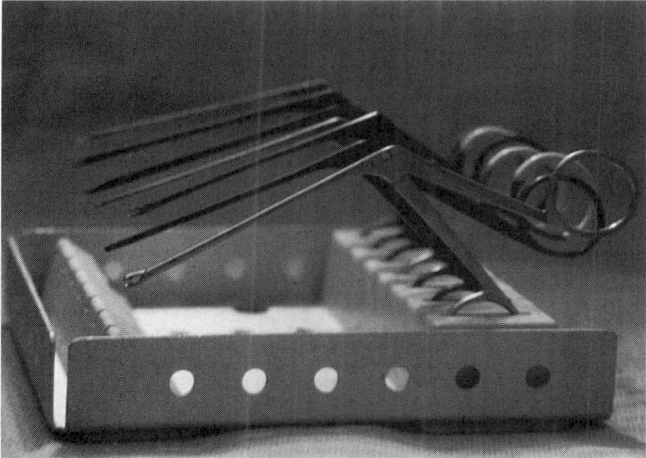

FIGURE 19-13 Microsurgical middle ear forceps, including various sizes of cup forceps and alligator forceps. Storage rack allows like items to be grouped together. Instruments are angled upright to allow for quick, easy identification.

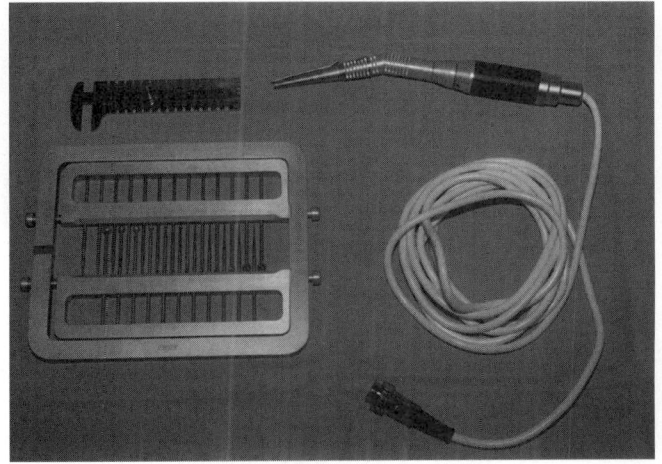

FIGURE 19-14 Surgical drill system with angled handpiece; the burr rack contains a variety of burrs of different sizes and shapes with carbide and diamond cutting surfaces. Caliper verifies size of of burr.

rather then tearing into it and is commonly used around vital structures. It has been known to help control bleeding from bone by pushing the vessel down into its channel and filling the channel with bone dust.

Cutting burrs assist in quickly removing bone from areas not close to vital structures. The grooves or teeth of burrs must be clean of bone dust. Bone cutting burrs tend to clog more easily than coarse-toothed burrs. A sterile wire brush may be used to keep burrs clean intraoperatively. Because of its potent osteogenic properties, bone dust must be prevented from settling in potentially problematic osteogenic areas such as that in stapedectomy, tympanoplasty, endolymphatic sac, or fenestration surgery.[7] A sterile field continuously flooded with irrigation solution helps to lessen clogging of the burr and washes away bone dust.

Irrigation and suctioning of the operative field

Adequate irrigation and suction ensures visibility of the operative field while clearing it of bone dust, blood, and bacteria from chronically infected ears. Irrigation solutions include warm saline, Tis-U-Sol, or lactated Ringer's solution and may be delivered to the sterile field by means of bulb syringes or suction irrigators or through sterile IV tubing connected to irrigation ports on the handpiece of selected drill systems. Some surgeons prefer to have the scrub nurse irrigate as they suction and drill; others choose a suction irrigator, allowing them to control the flow and direction of the irrigation as they drill and suction away debris.

Multiple suction tips must be available in a range of sizes including 18 gauge through 26 gauge. They are designed to allow the operator's thumb to control and vary the degree of suction. Small-gauge suction tips clog frequently, especially during drilling of bone, and must be routinely flushed throughout the procedure to ensure patency.

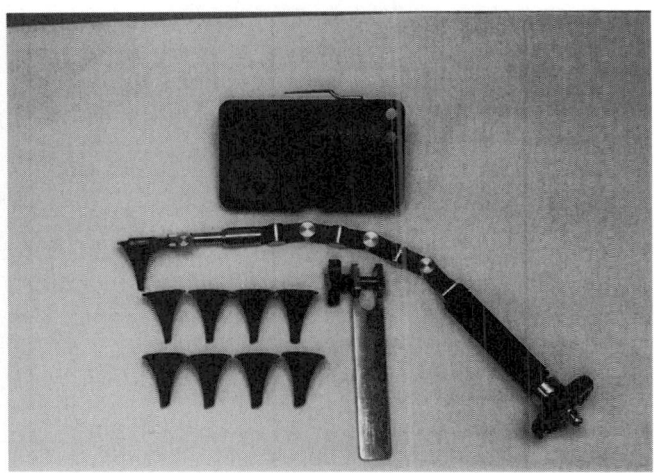

FIGURE 19-15   Universal ear speculum holder and assorted specula. Work table can be mounted to the holder and used to secure implants, ossicles, and ear packing.

Bone curettes

Bone curettes are used for the removal of soft cellular bone. Whenever possible, larger curettes are preferred because they decrease the risk to dura, sinus wall, and facial nerve. Sharp curettes are safer, cut with less pressure, and are more effective than dull curettes. They should be held so that the cutting edge is in full view and not obscured by the hand. The side of the curette should be used as the cutting edge rather than its tip.[7]

Specula and holder

A universal ear speculum holder fits into the sliding bar clamp of the OR bed and remains adjustable and flexible until locked in a semirigid position. This allows the surgeon's hands to remain free. A work table containing several wells with a transparent wheel-like cover may be used to safely store prosthesis, ossicles, and ear packing. The work table may be secured to the lower portion of the speculum holder or used separately (Fig. 19-15).

Ear specula are designed with a nonreflective finish to reduce glare generated by the operating microscope's bright halogen lamp. This finish minimizes eye fatigue during surgery and reduces reflection of laser beams during laser-assisted procedures. The design of the distal tip of the ear speculum may be oval and beveled or round and nonbeveled and is a matter of surgeon of preference. The largest speculum that fits comfortably into the ear should be used to achieve the greatest area of visualization. It should not cause pain or pressure in the bony canal.

Needles and syringes for local anesthesia

Local anesthesia is preferred for selected patients and procedures. In the absence of inflammation, the mastoid bone lacks sensation except for the outer periosteum and to a lesser extent within the tympanus and antrum.[7] A local anesthetic consisting of lidocaine with epinephrine may be used for the infiltration of the skin and periostium to block the sensory nerve supply. A 27-gauge, 1½-inch needle secured to a 3 ml Luer-Lok syringe may be used to administer the block injection.

Knives

Myringotomy procedures require a sharp knife for making incisions into the tympanic membrane. Sterile, disposable single-use blades are supplied with integrated handles or as single blades that may be secured into reusable handles. Myringotomy blades are spear, lancet, and sickle shaped and are a matter of surgeon preference. Disposable myringotomy kits containing a speculum, blade, suction tip, and ventilation-tube inserter are available from several manufacturers. For stapes surgery, right and left circumferential knives are designed for various uses including making the primary incision, elevating the periosteum and the fibrous annulus, separating the incudostapedial joint, and dissecting or resecting scar tissue or the stapedial tendon.

Scissors

In addition to Mayo and Metzenbaum scissors, which may be used for general dissection purposes, delicate fingerloop scissors with angular blades or crossover blades (Bellucci or Jacobsen type) are used in middle ear operations to incise and divide the stapedial tendon or scar tissue bands.

Dissecting forceps

In radical mastoidectomy and tympanoplasty several types of smooth and serrated alligator forceps are needed for manipulation within the canal and the middle ear.

Instrumentation features

Like ear specula, instruments used in the path of the operating microscope may have an ebony glare-reducing finish. Handles of assorted knives and dissectors may be flat, hexagonal, or round for better gripping or handling during surgery. The shaft of these instruments may be straight, angled, or bayonet (Fig. 19-16). Some surgeons believe that angled shafts offer a better view into the operative site, but others believe that bayonet shafts offer the best view.

Sterile instruments should be passed in a manner that allows the surgeon to remain focused on the operative site and not forced to turn away from the microscope. Middle ear instruments should be passed with the tips pointing downward. Slight pressure is used when the nurse is placing it into the web of the surgeon's hand between the thumb and index finger (as one would place a pencil ready for use). The surgeon senses the instrument and is able to close the fingertips on the instrument without needing to visualize it. The nurse passes the middle ear forceps (scissors and crimpers) by holding onto the shaft of the instrument just above the fingerloops and delivers the

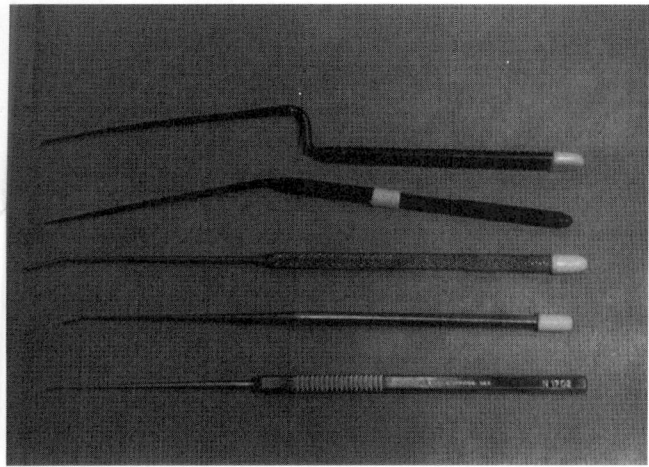

FIGURE 19-16 Types of handles and tip design for typical ear microinstrumentation. Angled instruments offer better views of the operative area than nonangled ones do and are a matter of surgeon preference.

forceps by providing slight pressure of the fingerloops against the palmar surface of the surgeon's hand. The scrub nurse should hold the instrument in this position and allow the surgeon to adjust the index finger and thumb into the fingerloops of the instrument. Microsurgical instruments should be handed on an exchange basis thereby preventing costly damage to instruments from inadvertent falls. After each use, all microsurgical instruments should be wiped clean of debris using a commercially available foam-rubber sponge wipe.

Suction tips are passed in the same fashion as the middle ear instruments and should be irrigated clean after each use with a control syringe filled with water.

A universal set of ear surgery instruments can be used for all middle ear procedures. When an endaural approach is required, only endaural retractors must be added to the universal set.

Hemostasis

Intraoperative management of bleeding is critical so as not to compromise the surgical exposure. Methods may include the infiltration of the skin and underlying soft tissue with lidocaine containing epinephrine. For transcanal approaches, slow ooze can be controlled with small cotton, pledget, or Gelfoam material soaked in epinephrine and left in place. To control bleeding from bony surfaces as in mastoid surgery, the application of bone wax may be necessary. However, bone wax is considered to be a foreign body, and absorbable substances are preferred. Synthetic collagen sponges moistened with thrombin will stop venous bleeding and can be left in the wound. Blood vessels in the skin, subcutaneous tissue, and lateral wall should be cauterized with a monopolar cautery, but deeper vessels especially those adjacent to the facial nerve should be cauterized using a bipolar unit.[11]

Lasers

The laser energy's ability to precisely vaporize tissue without vibratory movements leading to better results makes microscopic laser surgery an attractive modality for otologic surgery. Lasers assist in vaporization of scar tissue, granulomas, and cholesteatomas without damaging surrounding tissue.[2] They have also been used to divide the vestibular nerve on patients with severe vertigo. During acoustic tumor surgery, CO_2 laser offers a significant advantage in debulking of tumors. The surgery is less traumatic because laser vaporization eliminates much of the tugging and pulling necessary with conventional techniques.

During stapedectomy, laser energy may be used to create (drill) a hole in the footplate of the stapes for insertion of a prosthesis or to vaporize the stapedial tendon. Ideal laser energy should be completely absorbed by the footplate and should not heat the perilymph or damage the inner ear.[10] The CO_2 laser has ideal tissue properties for stapedectomy and its revision. It has limited tissue penetration and is completely absorbed by the stapes footplate without significant scatter. The laser stapedotomy offers improved postoperative hearing results, while reducing postoperative dizziness and sensorineural hearing loss.

CO_2 and potassium titanyl phosphate (KTP) lasers can be secured to the operating microscope and laser energy delivered to the tissue by means of a micromanipulator. Laser energy is delivered directly to tissue by the use of fiberoptic probes, which can be navigated around obstructing structures.

KTP lasers have ideal optical properties and provide precise focus, whereas the optical properties of the CO_2 laser must be routinely aligned and preoperative "test firing" must be performed before every case to ensure that the beam is coaxial and parfocal.

Laser safety in otologic laser surgery includes draping wet towels around the surgical field and having a basin of sterile water and a syringe on the field to extinguish a possible fire. Smoke evacuation must be employed to remove vaporized tissue because the plume can scatter subsequent laser beams.[15] The laser should be placed in a standby mode when not in use. Documentation of laser settings as well as patient and personnel safety measures is recorded per institution standards (see Chapter 3).

Evaluation

Perioperative nursing care should be closely monitored and evaluated at the completion of the procedure before the patient is transported to the postanesthesia care unit (PACU) or ambulatory recovery area. If the patient has had a local anesthetic, the nurse will have had the opportunity to evaluate care because the patient is able to communicate any discomfort throughout the procedure.

Potential surgical complications include hearing loss, a change in taste, and injury to the facial nerve. Evaluation of facial nerve function is routinely performed and requires the patient's cooperation in smiling, closing the eye, and wrinkling the nose on the operative side. If facial palsy is observed and not resolved within 2 hours of the procedure, it may be caused by surgical trauma.

During evaluation, the perioperative nurse determines if the patient met the outcomes in the nursing care plan. Some outcomes can be reached during the preoperative and intraoperative phases of care; they are evaluated before the patient's discharge from the operating room. Others require ongoing monitoring and measurement in the postoperative phase. Part of the nursing report to the PACU or nursing unit should include the outcomes of care provided:

- The patient will express himself or herself effectively and with minimal frustration.
- The patient will identify factors that can be controlled personally or by family, nursing staff, or surgical team.
- The patient is free from injury.
- The patient will discuss feelings regarding outcome of the surgical procedure.

Patient and Family Teaching and Discharge Planning

Patient and family teaching should be begun before the day of surgery if possible. It may include the recommendation that the hair be shampooed the night before surgery. By the day of discharge, patients and family members should have a thorough knowledge and understanding of what to expect during the postoperative recuperation period. Specific instructions based on the type of surgery performed must be reviewed with the patient and must focus on pain and discomfort, restricted activity levels, and observing for signs of infection. Patient teaching and discharge planning may include the following:

- The ear canal should be kept dry for 10 days to 3 weeks postoperatively for all stapes and middle ear surgery and for up to 3 months after mastoid surgery.
- Patients are cautioned to not lie on the operative side for the first 24 hours postoperatively.
- The head of the bed should be elevated 30 degrees for the first 24 hours.
- Antibiotics, analgesics, and antiemetics may be prescribed for the postoperative period.
- Hearing may be diminished during the immediate postoperative period. It is temporary and usually hearing improves gradually. This may be attributable to full packing of the ear at the completion of surgery.
- Vertigo may occur postoperatively. Therefore the patient may need assistance to get out of bed. Moving slowly and smoothly may alleviate these sensations. If symptoms persist or are severe, the physician should be notified, and antimotion medication may be prescribed.

- To prevent possible dislodgment of a graft or prosthesis, the patient should be advised as follows:
  - Refrain from heavy lifting, straining, or strenuous exercise.
  - Exercise caution against coughing or nose blowing.
  - Open both the nose and mouth if sneezing is unavoidable.
- Restricted activities include the following:
  - No driving for the first postoperative week
  - No swimming or diving for the first month after surgery
  - Air travel is not advised for 1 to 4 weeks postoperatively. This is dependent on the type of surgery performed and surgeon preference.
- The physician should be immediately consulted if the patient experiences any of the following symptoms:
  - An upper respiratory tract infection
  - Any other change in physical status
  - Foul smelling drainage from the affected ear
  - Increasing pain from the affected ear
  - Fever
  - Bleeding or a discharge of clear fluid from the ear or nose
  - Vertigo

Follow-up telephone calls within 48 hours of discharge enables the nurse to assess the patient's progress and level of understanding of instructions and allows the patient to ask pertinent questions.

SURGICAL INTERVENTIONS
INCISIONAL APPROACHES

The majority of otologic procedures are performed either through the ear canal or from behind the ear. Incisions through the ear canal include endaural and transcanal approaches. The postauricular approach is made through an incision from behind the ear.

Endaural

The *endaural* incision is made in two steps using a Lempert triangular knife or a #15 blade. With the patient in an upright position, the first incision is made from the superior meatal wall about 1 cm in from the outer edge of the meatus and extends down the posterior meatal wall to the edge of the conchal cartilage. The second incision on the superior meatal wall extends upward to a point halfway between the meatus and upper edge of the auricle. This approach offers direct access to the external auditory meatus and tympanic membrane and may be used for meatoplasty, canalplasty, and selected tympanic membrane perforations and stapes surgery.

Transcanal

The *transcanal* approach is used for those procedures that are limited to the mesotympanum, hypotympanum, and tympanic membrane. The incision involves a superiorly based tympanomeatal flap through the ear canal and involves making a semilunar canal skin incision just lateral to the tympanic membrane. For exposure, the skin, fibrous annulus, and tympanic membrane are elevated as a unit. Posterior tympanomeatal flaps may be used in stapedectomy, labyrinthectomy, myringoplasty, tumor biopsy, ossiculoplasty, and removal of glomus tympanicum tumors. Congenital cholesteatomas are best approached by superior tympanomeatal flaps, whereas perforations of the tympanic membrane may be accessed through an inferior tympanomeatal flap.[11]

Postauricular

The *postauricular* incision is made behind the ear as the surgeon follows the curve of the posterior auricular fold. It provides wide-field exposure and is a versatile and adaptable incision. This approach is used to expose the mastoid process for simple mastoidectomy and for surgery on the endolymphatic sac, internal auditory meatus, and, on occasion, tympanoplasty and radical mastoid procedures.

The *middle fossa* approach represents a neurosurgical incision for access to the middle cranial region. Above the ear and at the level of the zygomatic arch, skin and subcutaneous tissue incisions are made, and bleeding is controlled with electrocautery. The temporalis fascia and muscle are incised and retracted using self-retaining retractors. After the squamous portion of the temporal bone is exposed, a standard craniectomy is performed. The middle fossa approach may be used for small acoustic tumor excision and vestibular nerve sections.

A postaural incision may be used to expose the mastoid process. It follows the curve of the postaural fold, beginning at the upper attachment of the auricle and continuing behind the postaural fold downward to the tip of the mastoid process.

For stapes surgery a circumferential incision is made in the posterior half of the canal, starting at the inferior aspect of the annulus and ending posterior to the short process of the malleus.

For myringotomy a circumferential (posteroinferior) incision is made. It provides for wide drainage and removal of pus or fluid under pressure from the middle ear.

OTOLOGIC PROCEDURES

Myringotomy

Myringotomy is the incision of the pars tensa of the tympanic membrane, the aspiration of fluid under pressure in the tympanum, and often the subsequent placement of small hollow tympanostomy (myringotomy) tubes. It is indicated for acute otitis media in the presence of an exudate that has not responded to antibiotic therapy.

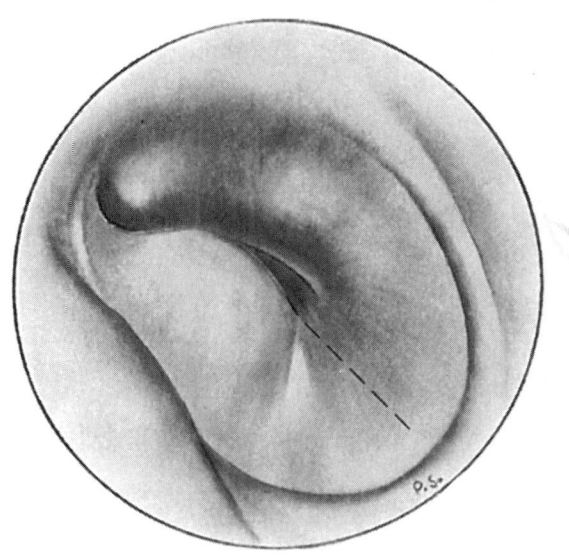

FIGURE 19-17   In purulent otitis media, pus under pressure pushes eardrum outward, resulting in bulging tympanic membrane. *Dotted line,* Radial myringotomy incision.

Serous otitis media can be difficult to diagnose because it is asymptomatic in pediatric patients. The only symptom may be conductive hearing loss. Negative pressure secondary to a blocked eustachian tube causes middle ear effusion.

Serous otitis media is very common in children between 6 months and 3 years of age. About 50% to 60% of children in this age group have effusion in the middle ear. Serous otitis media may peak again between 4 and 6 years of age; 30% of children in this age group have fluid in the middle ear with hearing loss at some time. The majority of children with serous otitis media have spontaneous resolution. Hearing loss is the main concern when fluid is present in the middle ear. If left untreated, hearing loss could affect language development and IQ level. If the fluid persists more than 8 to 12 weeks and is accompanied by hearing loss, the removal of the fluid and placement of ventilating tubes in the eardrum are necessary.

Otitis media, although primarily a pediatric problem, may be seen in adults. Tympanic fibrosis is common in adults and is a result of repeated infections that have occurred in childhood. Acute otitis media is a collection of infected pus in the middle ear. The patient may have severe pain and bulging of the tympanic membrane (Fig. 19-17). Failure to respond to oral antibiotics and analgesics or other complications such as facial nerve paralysis or labyrinthitis may require a myringotomy. By release of the pus or fluid, hearing is restored, and the infection can be controlled. The procedure may be performed for chronic serous otitis media in which the presence of fluid in the middle ear produces a hearing loss. Frequently tubes are inserted into the tympanic membrane (Fig. 19-18) to allow ventilation of the middle ear. Myringotomy tubes may be used for the treatment of colds and fluid in the ear

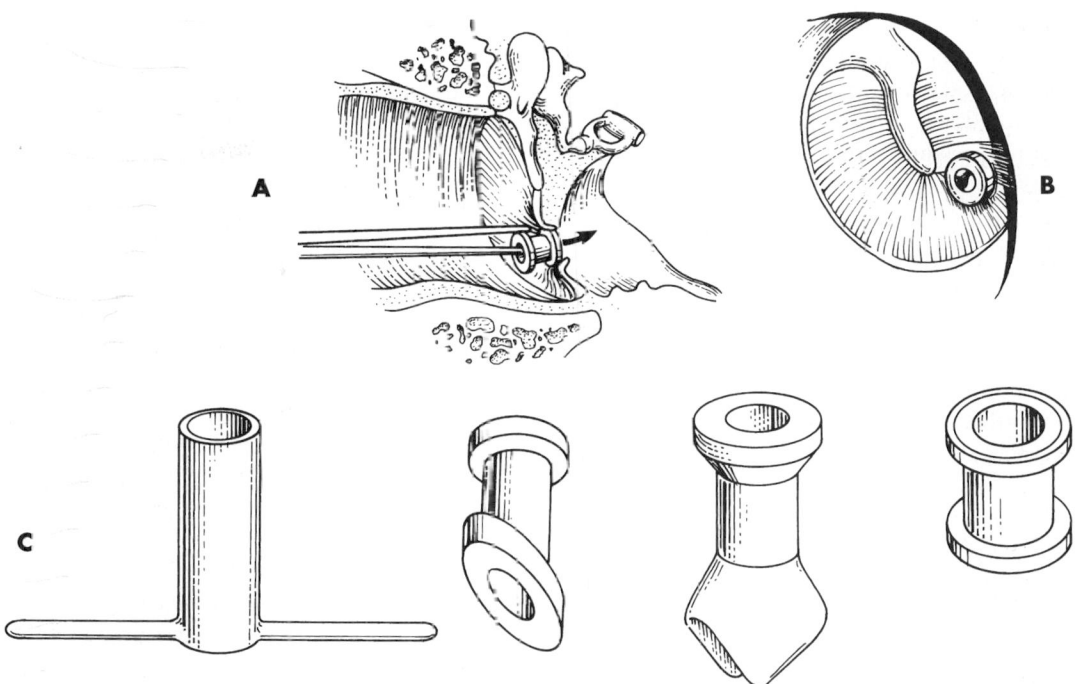

FIGURE 19-18   **A**, Tube (placed on end of alligator forceps) being inserted into tympanic membrane. **B**, Tube in place. **C**, Several types of plastic tubes that may be inserted into tympanic membrane. Purpose of tubes is to aerate middle ear and reduce middle ear infections.

on a short-term basis (a few months), on an intermediate basis (6 months to 18 months), and in long-term treatment (years) for chronic situations. Care must be taken to avoid getting water in the ears while the tubes are in place. Myringotomy is usually performed on an ambulatory surgery basis.

Procedural considerations

Myringotomy is considered a clean procedure. The patient is usually not prepped or draped. The surgeon may wear gown and gloves or gloves only, depending on the policy related to universal precautions at the institution in which the procedure is performed. The instrument setup includes a myringotomy knife and disposable blade, assorted sizes of aural specula, ear curettes, suction tip and tubing, a delicate Hartmann forceps, metal aural applicators, a Rosen needle, and a culture tube if cultures are to be taken.

Operative procedure

1. With the head and microscope in position, the aural speculum is inserted into the ear canal. The external canal is cleaned of excess cerumen using a wire loop curette. With a sharp myringotomy knife a small, curved or radial incision is made in the anterior inferior quadrant of the pars tensa (see Fig. 19-17).
2. A culture may be taken to determine the type of organism present. Pus and fluid are suctioned from the middle ear.
3. A tube may be inserted into the incision with alligator forceps or a tube inserter.

4. Antibiotic drops may be instilled after the positioning of the tube.

Several types of disposable myringotomy tubes are available for implantation, depending on the length of time the surgeon wishes the tube to remain in place (see Fig. 19-18). Once the tube falls out, the tympanic membrane incision usually heals.

Tympanoplasty

Tympanoplasty is the surgical repair of the tympanic membrane, the tympanum, and the reconstruction of the ossicular chain. It is indicated for conductive hearing losses caused by perforation of the tympanic membrane as a result of trauma or infection, for ossicular discontinuity, chronic or recurrent otitis media, and progressive hearing losses, and for the inability to safely bathe or participate in water activities as a result of perforation of the tympanic membrane with or without hearing loss.[1]

Perforation of the eardrum (tympanic membrane) is the most common serious ear injury necessitating surgical intervention. Perforations may result from (1) direct injury (such as cotton applicators or a pencil), (2) blow to the ear, (3) tears from temporal bone fractures, and (4) lightning injury. Early diagnosis is the key to proper management.

Conductive hearing loss is caused by an obstruction in the external canal or middle ear, which impedes the passage of sound waves to the inner ear. It may be attributable to disease of the middle ear or tympanic membrane. Occasionally the tympanic membrane does not heal after myringotomy.

Ossicular discontinuity may result from chronic otitis media, trauma, or cholesteatoma, a skin cyst that erodes bone. Various methods and materials are being used in constructing a closed, air-contained middle ear cavity and restoring a sound-pressure transforming action. Among these materials are homografts and Teflon, Plasti-Pore, silicone, hydroxyapatite, and metal prostheses.

There are five types of tympanoplasties:

1. Repair of the tympanic membrane by covering the perforation in the eardrum with a graft; reconstruction extends to the malleus
2. Closing the perforation with a graft and building the eardrum onto the body of the incus
3. Positioning the graft against the head of the stapes when the malleus and incus are missing
4. Securing the graft to the mobile footplate of the stapes when all ossicles are missing
5. Securing the graft to the oval window when the footplate of the stapes is immobile

A clinical pathway for tympanoplasty is shown in Fig. 19-19.

Procedural considerations

The ear is prepped and draped as previously described. An endaural or postauricular approach may be used. Both these approaches provide similar functional results. The procedure is most often performed with the patient under local anesthesia.

Operative procedure

1a. When an endaural approach is used, the ear speculum is introduced into the external meatus of the ear canal, and the microscope is brought into place. The surgeon injects local anesthetic into the external meatus and external auditory canal and postauricularly, using a 1 or 3 ml syringe. Lidocaine (Xylocaine) with epinephrine is generally used unless the patient's general medical condition necessitates a substitute. The purpose of the injection of local anesthetic is twofold: to make the operation painless and to reduce the amount of bleeding. A tympanomeatal incision is then made using a sharp round knife.

1b. When a postauricular approach is used, the surgeon injects local anesthetic (lidocaine with epinephrine) postauricularly using a 3 ml or 5 ml syringe. An ear speculum is introduced, and the microscope is brought into place. The surgeon injects local anesthetic into the external auditory canal using a 1 ml syringe. The microscope head is moved from directly over the patient's ear. The skin incision is made behind the fold of the ear with a #15 knife blade. The bleeding vessels are coagulated. An incision is made into the periosteum down to the bone, and the periosteum is elevated from behind the incision with a Lempert elevator.

1c. During the transcanal approach, the surgeon uses a 27-gauge angled needle to inject the four quadrants of the fibrocartilaginous canal with a 1% or 2% lidocaine solution with 1:100,000 epinephrine. An endaural speculum gently compresses the tissue edema resulting from the injection and assists in the placement of a speculum within the confines of the bony canal. A 30-gauge needle is used to inject the skin of the bony canal. Two canal incisions are made with a roller knife or other sharp knife. The posterior tympanomeatal flap is made superior and posterior to the lateral process of the malleus and ends laterally on the midpoint of the posterior canal wall. The inferior incision extends from the inferior canal wall to the superior incision. The skin is elevated to the tympanic annulus, subcutaneous tissue at the tympanomastoid suture is dissected, and bleeding is controlled before the middle ear is reached.[11]

2. At this point the temporalis fascia is usually harvested to provide the graft material for the repair of the tympanic membrane. Lidocaine with epinephrine may be injected under the fascia to separate it from the temporalis muscle. A narrow Shambaugh elevator or duckbill elevator is used to separate the fascia. Small, sharp scissors or a knife blade serves to remove the amount of fascia needed. The fascia is trimmed of excess tissue with small, sharp scissors and either laid flat or molded onto an ear speculum. Some surgeons prefer to thin the fascia by using a House Gelfoam press. The fascia is then set aside to dry while the tympanic membrane is prepared.

3. The canal skin may be elevated from the canal with a duckbill elevator, Rosen needle, gimmick, or similar microinstrument, or it may be removed, depending on the size and location of the tympanic membrane perforation.

4. The edges of the tympanic membrane are prepared for the graft by removing all epithelium from the drum surrounding the perforation, usually with a sickle knife, Rosen needle, 45- or 90-degree pick, or cup forceps.

5. If an edge of the perforation or tympanic membrane cannot be visualized because of the bony canal, the surgeon uses a microcurette or drill to remove the overhang of bone.

6. The middle ear is explored with a pick or similar instrument, and any epithelium present is removed with an alligator, or cup, forceps. The ossicular chain is tested for mobility. Each ossicle is inspected to ensure that it is intact and mobile.

7. If the malleus or incus is diseased or eroded, it may be removed and replaced with a partial ossicular replacement prosthesis (PORP). Ossicles that are removed may be reshaped with the aid of a drill and small burr and replaced. If all ossicles are diseased or eroded, they may be removed and replaced with a total ossicular

Tympanoplasty

Clinic	→	MCE	→	Clinic
Evaluation		Operation		F/U

DRG Number: _____

ELOS: ___Outpatient—SAS_____

	Preop (Clinic/Pre-admission)	Day of Operation (HR → Intra-Op)	Day of Operation (PACU → HR)	Follow-up: Clinic Home/2 Week follow up	Follow-up: Clinic 4 Weeks Postop
Goals	Evaluation completed Patient/family education completed Patient/family tour of MCE completed- PATCH Visit	Informed consent process completed → form signed	Patient tolerates operation without complications D/C from MCE when meet criteria: • VSS • Awake • Tolerating po	No complications from procedure	No complications from procedure
Evaluation & Assessment	H + P Audio evaluation	Nursing assessment Anesthesia evaluation H + P per MD Informed consent per ENT		Repeat evaluation and assessment ———→ Interval History ———→ Physical Exam ———→ Débridement of external canal as tolerated	Audio evaluation
Tests & Labs	CBC with diff Gravida index for females > 12 years				
Activity			Ad lib No strenuous physical activity x 7-14 days ——→ Do not blow nose, if must sneeze, sneeze with mouth open		
Diet	NPO after 12 MN, night before surgery	NPO	Sips → progress as tolerated		
Consult-ations	Child Life - age appropriate	Anesthesia			
Meds/IV		Premed per anesthesia IV - D$_5$LR at maintenance + deficit replacement per anesthesia ———→ Lidocaine with epinephrine intraop	Maintenance rate after deficit replacement → D/C IV when taking PO well Tylenol q 4-6° x 5-7 days	Cortisporin (otic suspension) 3 gtts tid x 5 days	
Teaching/ D/C Plan	Per MD: Procedure Risks/benefits Postop care Follow-up care Per surgery scheduler: Precertification completed Surgery date set Call family two days preop to review plan		Postop care When/how to call MD Follow-up appointment Give family home care instruction sheet	Postop phone call	
Equipment & Supplies		O$_2$ tank Ambu bag OR supplies per Surgeon's preference card		Pediatric ENT Issues 1) Paths to develop • Endoscopy/DL/B with laser • Mastoidectomy (23°) • Functional sinus surgery • LTP 2) How to get Child Life/preop tour done for EMA children 3) Review home care instruction sheet	

© 1996 Vanderbilt University Medical Center. All Rights Reserved.

Tympanoplasty
8/13/96
Peds/Otolaryngology

FIGURE 19-19   Clinical pathway for tympanoplasty.

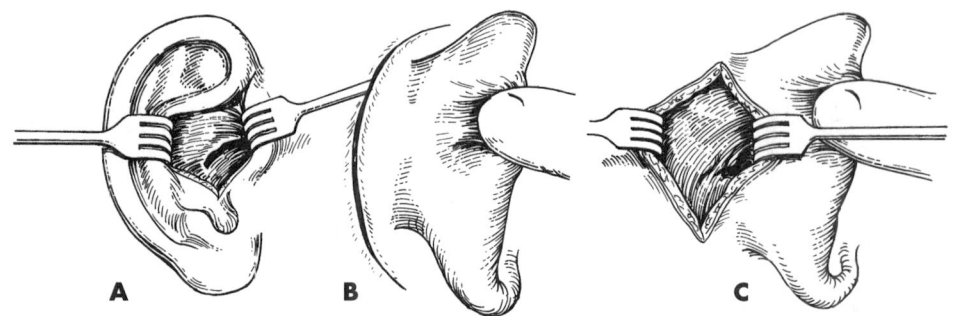

FIGURE 19-20   Mastoidectomy incision. **A**, Endaural. **B**, Postauricular. **C**, Postauricular incision retracted.

replacement prosthesis (TORP). This step is accomplished with microinstrumentation such as Bellucci scissors, cup forceps, malleus nipper, incudostapedial joint knife, sickle knife, picks, and Rosen needle.

8. Once confident that the middle ear has been explored and corrected, the surgeon prepares the graft for insertion. The edges are trimmed with a #15 knife blade or sharp scissors. The surgical site is suctioned with a microsuction. Hemostasis may be achieved by applying very small, epinephrine-soaked Gelfoam balls with an alligator forceps. Radiopaque microcottonoids are available for use in hemostasis if necessary.

9. Different tissues, such as temporalis fascia, or loose connective tissue, tragus perichondrium, and vein grafts, have been used for a tympanoplasty procedure. The most common tissue used is temporalis fascia. Most surgeons prefer to use autograft tissue, although homograft tympanic membranes have also been used. The risk of transmission of infectious disease has reduced homograft use. For easier manipulation, the graft may be dipped in water, saline, or a Tis-U-Sol solution before its insertion with alligator forceps. A gimmick, sickle knife, pick, Rosen needle, or similar microinstrument is used to position the graft into place. Small pledgets of absorbable gelatin sponge may be packed around the graft to ensure support and position. Some surgeons prefer to pack the middle ear before the graft insertion to provide support.

10. The external ear canal is packed with moistened absorbable gelatin sponge pledgets or antibiotic ointment.

11. The incision is closed with suture of the surgeon's preference.

12. A pressure dressing may be applied for the first 24 hours to prevent dislodgment of the new graft. This dressing usually consists of fluffed gauze placed around the ear and an elastic gauze wrapped around the affected ear and the head.

Mastoidectomy

Mastoidectomy is the removal of the diseased bone of the mastoid process, along with the cholesteatoma present in the middle ear and mastoid. Cholesteatoma is the result of accumulation of squamous epithelium and its products

in the middle ear and mastoid. It occasionally forms a cystlike mass. As it expands, it is destructive to the middle ear and mastoid. As a result, the diseased bone (ossicles and mastoid bone) must be removed to prevent recurrence of the cholesteatoma.

There are three types of mastoidectomy. A *simple mastoidectomy* is removal of the diseased bone of the mastoid while the ossicles, eardrum, and canal wall are left intact. The simple mastoid procedure is performed to eradicate chronic infections unresponsive to antibiotics or for removal of cholesteatoma. The surgeon must use caution to prevent any injury to the facial nerve. Facial nerve monitoring must be performed to preserve the facial nerve. Other complications include injury to the sigmoid sinus, inner ear balance or hearing mechanisms, and dura.

A *modified radical mastoidectomy* is removal of the diseased bone of the mastoid along with some of the ossicles and the canal wall. The eardrum and some of the ossicles remain, thus leaving a mechanism for the patient to hear. A canal wall-up mastoidectomy is similar to the modified mastoidectomy without taking down the canal wall. A *radical mastoidectomy* is the removal of the canal wall along with the ossicles and tympanic membrane. The radical mastoidectomy is rarely performed today except for unresectable disease. With either the modified radical or radical mastoidectomy a meatoplasty is performed to enlarge the ear canal opening. This facilitates cleaning the mastoid bowl that has been created.

Procedural considerations

General anesthesia is usually selected, but local anesthesia can be used. The patient is prepped and draped as for a tympanoplasty. An endaural or postauricular incision may be used (Fig. 19-20), but most surgeons believe that the postauricular incision offers better exposure to all areas of the mastoid and middle ear. A drill is used to remove diseased bone and tissue while the surgeon continually observes for anatomic structures, such as the facial nerve, within the mastoid.

Operative procedure

1 to 6. These steps are as for tympanoplasty.

7. The mastoid bone is drilled initially with a large cutting burr, usually under direct vision. As the

mastoid cavity is created, the scrub nurse should be able to anticipate changes needed in burr size. Once the vital structures have been identified, diseased bone is usually removed from them by use of diamond burrs of the appropriate size. The surgeon may interrupt drilling to explore areas of the mastoid with a pick, Rosen needle, mastoid searcher, or other microinstrument to identify surrounding structures.

8. On completion of the mastoidectomy the surgeon focuses on the middle ear. Diseased ossicles are removed, middle ear mucosa is inspected and removed if necessary, and all evidence of cholesteatoma is removed. Depending on the extent of the disease and the reliability that the patient will be available for follow-up study, the surgeon then reconstructs the ossicular chain or prepares the cavity created by a radical mastoidectomy. Some surgeons do not reconstruct at the time of mastoidectomy but follow the patient for a specified time. If cholesteatoma does not recur during that period, the patient receives a reconstructive procedure to restore hearing.

9. The mastoid cavity and middle ear may be packed with absorbable gelatin sponge. The external auditory canal may be packed with absorbable gelatin sponge or antibiotic ointment.

10. The incision is closed with suture of the surgeon's preference. A pressure dressing is applied and kept in place for the first 24 hours. This dressing usually consists of fluffed gauze around the ear and plain or elastic gauze wrapped around the head and affected ear. A commercially available product known as a *Glasscock dressing* may be used for this purpose (Fig. 19-21).

11. Currently the use of rigid endoscopes is being evaluated in several otologic and neuro-otologic procedures with the prospect of improving and possibly replacing more traditional approaches. In selected procedures, rigid endoscopes may eliminate some open, extensive surgeries (Research Highlight 19-2).

Stapedectomy

Stapedectomy is removal of the stapes for treatment of otosclerosis and replacement with a prosthesis to restore ossicular continuity and alleviate conductive hearing loss. Otosclerosis is the overgrowth of bone around the stapes footplate, resulting in immobility of the footplate. Sound waves cannot be transmitted adequately through the oval window and round window to be changed into electrochemical impulses in the cochlea.

There are two types of procedures for replacing the immobile stapes. In *stapedotomy* the footplate of the stapes is not removed; only the superstructure is removed. A hole is made in the stapes footplate, and the prosthesis is secured laterally to the long process of the incus and positioned medially over the hole created in the footplate. In *stapedectomy* the entire stapes (superstructure and footplate) is removed, a graft is placed over the oval window, and a

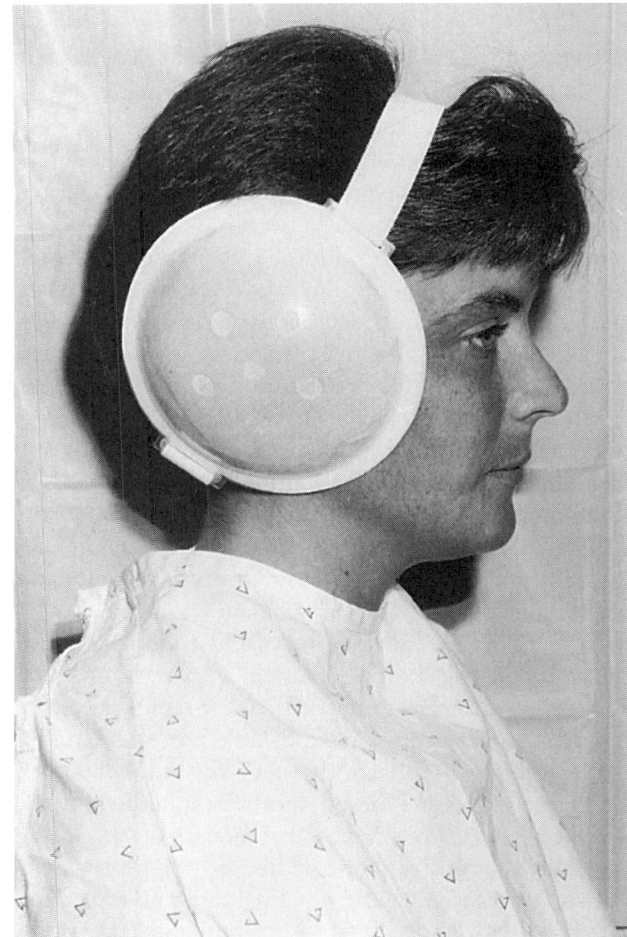

FIGURE 19-21 Completed Glasscock dressing after mastoidectomy. Telfa and fluffed gauze bandage constitute the primary dressing. Rigid ear cup and Velcro adjustable nonelastic strap constitute the protective exterior dressing.

prosthesis is attached laterally to the long process of the incus and positioned medially on the graft over the oval window.

Procedural considerations

Various materials are used as the prosthesis for the stapes; the most common are stainless steel and Teflon (Fig. 19-22). The types of prosthesis include the following:

- *The Robinson (bucket-handle) type of prosthesis* (see Fig. 19-22), *which has a metal stem designed to fit under the lenticular process of the incus.* The footplate must be removed and the oval window sealed with a tissue graft before the implant can be inserted. Advantages of this design include easy insertion with no required crimping. It is self-centered and sits in the center of the oval window after insertion.

- *The Shea Teflon prosthesis* (see Fig. 19-22), *which attaches to the long process of the incus.* It can be used with total footplate removal or small fenestra techniques. The prosthesis measures from the undersurface of the long process of the incus to the footplate, plus 0.5 mm. The Teflon ring is opened and secured on to the incus.

19-2 RESEARCH HIGHLIGHT

The use of rigid endoscopes has been evaluated as an adjunct to several otologic and neuro-otologic surgeries. A study was conducted to assess the validity of endoscopes and to determine whether their use could improve or replace traditional otologic and neuro-otologic procedures. Surgical procedures included second-look mastoidectomy, middle ear exploration, vestibular neurectomy, and acoustic neuroma surgery.

Through a myringotomy incision, the endoscope aided in the diagnostic evaluation of the middle ear and ossicular chain for purposes of identifying cholesteatomas and ruling out perilymphatic fistulas. During acoustic neuroma surgery, endoscopes were used to examine the lateral aspect of the internal auditory canal (IAC). During vestibular neurectomy, endoscopes helped to visualize the IAC and assisted in identifying the cochlear vestibular cleavage plane.

The findings confirmed that rigid endoscopes have been useful for locating residual cholesteatoma and visualizing anatomy often difficult to see using the operating microscope. Second-look procedures using endoscopes may alleviate the need for an open, more extensive procedure. Endoscopes assist in inspecting the lateral aspect of the IAC for residual tumor during acoustic neuroma surgery. Endoscopic vestibular neurectomy, however, has the potential for brain injury and bleeding with poor access for control and far exceeds the extremely low morbidity during an open vestibular neurectomy.

From Rosenberg, S.I., Silverstein, H., Willcox, T.O., & Gordon, M.A. (1994). Endoscopy in otology and neurotology, *American Journal of Otology, 15*(2), 168-172.

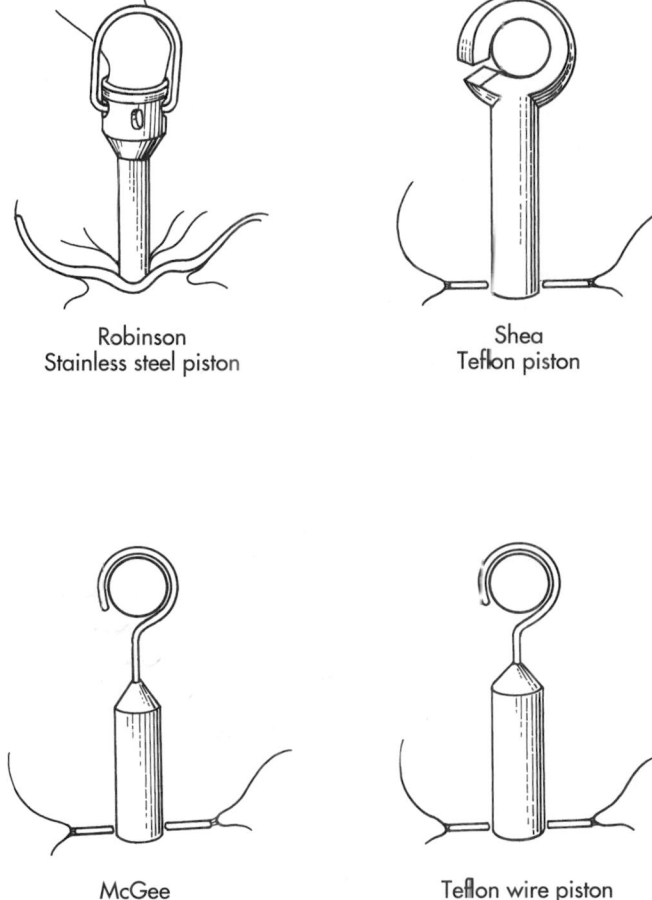

Robinson
Stainless steel piston

Shea
Teflon piston

McGee
Stainless steel piston

Teflon wire piston

FIGURE 19-22 Stapedectomy prostheses. *Top left,* Prostheses used after the footplate has been removed. *Top right and bottom,* Footplate had been "drilled" to accept a prefabricated piston precisely.

Because of the memory of Teflon, the prosthesis is said to be self-crimping (the ring closes without crimping). The position of the prosthesis is adjustable.

- *The Fisch-McGee type of stainless steel and Teflon pistons having a malleable ribbon crook connected to a metal or teflon stem.* The crook is secured to the long process of the incus and crimped into position. It is measured from the undersurface of the incus to the footplate and is easy to attach and crimp into position.

The prosthesis of choice is determined by the surgeon. The scrub nurse must be aware of each step in the procedure and hand the instruments to the surgeon expediently. Because the oval window is left uncovered, some perilymph may leak from the inner ear into the middle ear. This leak subjects the patient to the possible complication of a sensorineural hearing loss postoperatively or, more seriously, a "dead ear."

Microsuctions (18 to 26 gauge) are used in this procedure because large suction tips may suction perilymph from the oval window as well as promote bleeding in the middle ear. After the incision and reflection of the flap, footplate hooks are used because the tips on picks are too large and long and may cause damage rather than assist in the procedure.

Operative procedures
Stapedectomy

1. A temporalis fascia, fat, perichondrium, or vein graft may be harvested before the procedure. This graft is used to cover the oval window. Depending on the surgeon's graft preference, the ear, hand, or a portion of the abdomen may be prepped for the graft.
2. The ear speculum is introduced, and the microscope is brought into position. The ear canal is cleansed of wax and debris and may be gently washed with Tis-U-Sol and suctioned with a Baron or microsuction tip.
3. The surgeon injects lidocaine with epinephrine into the ear canal.

4. An ear speculum is inserted, the tympanomeatal flap is created (using a flap knife, roller knife, or sickle knife), and the tympanic membrane is reflected forward (using duckbill elevators or a drum elevator), exposing the middle ear.

5. If visualization of the ossicles is inadequate because of the overhang of bone, the surgeon may use micro-curettes or a drill to remove enough bone to allow proper visualization. Attempts to save the chorda tympani nerve are made because it controls taste from the anterior two thirds of the tongue. If this nerve obstructs the view of the stapes, it may on rare occasion be sacrificed for exposure.

6. The surgeon may measure the distance from the incus to the stapes footplate at this time or after the removal of the stapes. It is accomplished with a depth gauge and done to ensure the proper fit of the prosthesis.

7. The incudostapedial joint is disarticulated to allow fracture and subsequent removal of the stapes, usually accomplished through the use of a House or Guilford-Wright joint knife or by a laser (CO$_2$ or KTP).

8. Both crura of the stapes are lasered or fractured laterally, usually with a footplate pick or Rosen needle, and the superstructure is removed with alligator forceps. The surgeon may take this opportunity to ensure hemostasis using tiny sponges soaked in epinephrine along with a microsuction tip. The laser helps coagulate middle ear vessels, thus improving hemostasis.

9. An opening is created in the footplate with a laser or a sharp footplate pick. If the footplate is extremely thick, the laser or a microdrill may be used. If a stapedectomy is to be carried out, each half of the footplate is then removed using a Hough hoe, footplate pick, or footplate hook.

10. The oval window is then inspected, and the graft is placed over the oval window with alligator forceps or a pick. The edges of the graft are smoothed and positioned with a Hough hoe, pick, or gimmick.

11. The prosthesis is passed on alligator forceps to the surgeon, who introduces it into the middle ear with the shaft of the prosthesis resting against the oval window graft.

12. The wire is positioned over the long process of the incus (Fig. 19-23) by using picks, Hough hoes, or footplate hooks. Once it is in proper position, the surgeon crimps the wire onto the long process of the incus and thus ensures its attachment.

13. The surgeon may test the patient's hearing by softly whispering to the patient (if the procedure is performed under local anesthesia) or by touching the malleus with a pick and observing for mobility of the malleus, incus, and stapes prosthesis (if performed under general anesthesia).

14. Tiny squares of moistened, compressed, gelatin

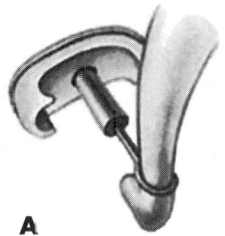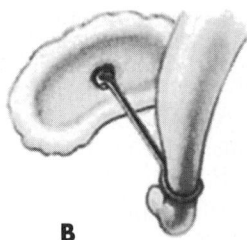

A   **B**

FIGURE 19-23 **A,** Placement of wire piston firmly crimped about incus. **B,** Total stapedectomy after placement of perichondrium over oval window. Wire loop prosthesis is crimped and placed against oval window membrane.

sponge may then be placed around the base of the prosthesis to ensure its stability. Alligator forceps, picks, a gimmick, and similar instruments may be used for this step in the procedure.

15. The tympanomeatal flap is returned to its original location, using a drum elevator, duckbill elevator, or Rosen needle, and the external ear canal may be packed with an antibiotic gel or ointment or a moistened compressed gelatin sponge.

16. Cotton is placed in the concha of the ear and a Band-Aid or small dressing is usually applied to the graft site.

Stapedotomy

The stapedotomy procedure is similar to stapedectomy but has these differences:

1. No graft is taken before the procedure.
2. The footplate is not removed. A hole is made in the footplate, using the CO$_2$ or KTP or drill bits of increasing size. The prosthesis is inserted when the perforation in the footplate is the appropriate size.
3. After positioning and crimping of the prosthesis, either a moistened, compressed, gelatin sponge or a few drops of the patient's blood may be placed around the junction of the prosthesis and the footplate to ensure stability of the prosthesis.

The scrub and circulating nurses must be knowledgeable in the operation, safety, and procedure for use of the laser if the surgeon elects to perform stapedotomy with a laser (see Chapter 3).

Ossicular Chain Reconstruction

Ossicular reconstruction may be required for the ear with long-standing recurrent ear infections. It is commonly performed for the replacement of the incus portion of the ossicular chain. There are many surgical techniques for ossicular reconstruction.

Natural and synthetic prosthetic materials are available for ossicular reconstruction or replacement. The autologous ossicle (incus or head of malleus) taken from the patient's ear is the prosthesis of choice. Preserved homologous ossicles are less popular than in the past because patients are refusing to even consider these grafts as a result of the risk (albeit very low) of transmission of infectious disease.

A partial ossicular replacement prosthesis (PORP) is indicated if an ossicle is not available. A TORP is indicated for difficult major columella reconstruction.

Alloplastic materials used in the manufacturing of partial and total ossicular reconstruction prostheses have been produced and improved upon for use in ossicular reconstruction. Hydroxyapatite is currently utilized in many prostheses because its mineral content is very similar to that of bone and it is well tolerated by the middle ear, thereby decreasing extrusion rates over other materials. Because it is brittle, it is often combined with other materials to make it more easily trimmed for a precise fit in the middle ear. Regardless of the type of prosthesis used, the surgeon must sculpt it to bridge the ossicular gap by simulating the ossicular configuration and preserving the lever mechanism of the middle ear.[11]

About 50% to 60% of ossicular problems are related to the incus, and 10% affect the stapes as a result of otosclerosis. Malleus dysfunction accounts for 10% of ossicular problems and is mainly attributable to the formation of cholesteatoma. The balance of ossicular problems may be a combination of the above.

Procedural considerations

Minor columella is a term that refers to an ossiculoplasty with a strut from the head of the stapes to the tympanic membrane (or graft) or manubrium. Major columella refers to a strut extending from the footplate to the tympanic membrane (or graft) or manubrium. The patient is prepped and draped as for stapedectomy.

Operative procedure

The procedural steps are similar to those for stapedectomy except that the stapes footplate is not removed or opened.

Endolymphatic Sac Decompression or Shunt

An endolymphatic shunt procedure is the creation of an opening into the endolymphatic sac and the insertion of a shunt to allow drainage of excess endolymph into the cerebrospinal fluid or into the mastoid cavity. In Meniere's disease the endolymphatic sac cannot resorb endolymph, resulting in an overaccumulation. This surplus leads to vertigo, in which patients feel a spinning sensation. Movement usually increases the vertigo, which may be accompanied by severe nausea and vomiting. The vertigo attacks occur unpredictably and may last from several minutes to several hours. Most patients with Meniere's disease complain of tinnitus, pressure or fullness in the affected ear, and a fluctuating hearing loss that begins in the lower frequencies. Diagnostic audiometry reveals the hearing loss to be sensorineural. The vertigo may be so severe that it

disrupts the patient's lifestyle. On a medical regimen of tranquilizers, diuretics, vasodilators, and a low-sodium diet, approximately 85% of patients are able to adequately control their symptoms. For those whose symptoms persist, surgical intervention is recommended.

Procedural considerations

Preoperative assessment by the perioperative nurse confirms that the patient's electrolyte levels (especially potassium) are adequate and provides a basis for the support system to be carried out intraoperatively and postoperatively. Because Meniere's disease may develop bilaterally in 20% of patients, conservative therapy is often employed. The patient is prepped and draped as for a mastoidectomy.

Operative procedure

1 to 7. These steps are as for mastoidectomy.
8. Drilling with a diamond burr over the posterior fossa dura is continued until the endolymphatic sac is identified.
9. An incision is made into the lateral wall of the sac with a microknife such as a sickle, Beaver blade, or Ziegler. An incision is then made through the medial wall, exposing the subarachnoid space.
10. A shunt (commercially prepared tube, Silastic tubing, or Silastic sheeting) is inserted with microforceps and is manipulated into place, usually with microinstruments such as a Rosen needle, fine pick, or gimmick. When the shunt is designed to drain into the mastoid, only the lateral wall of the sac is incised.
11. The incision is closed with suture of the surgeon's preference.
12. A pressure dressing is applied to the affected ear.

Labyrinthectomy

Labyrinthectomy is a procedure that destroys the vestibular and auditory function of the labyrinth to relieve the patient of severe vertigo. The procedure is usually performed when the disease is unilateral, a shunt has been ineffective, and the affected ear has severe or total loss of hearing. Because the inner ear is destroyed, the patient may be very dizzy for several days until the brainstem begins to compensate for the destroyed labyrinth. The operation also leaves the ear deaf.

Procedural considerations

This procedure may be performed on the patient by means of the transcanal or transmastoid approach. The patient is prepped and draped as described for tympanoplasty.

Operative procedures
Transcanal Approach

1. Through a tympanomeatal flap, with the chorda tympani nerve preserved, the incudostapedial joint is separated, and the stapedial tendon is sectioned.

2. The incus and stapes are disarticulated and removed.
3. A right-angled hook is inserted into the vestibule, and all neuroepithelium (the contents) is removed.
4. The open vestibule is filled with Gelfoam soaked in streptomycin to ensure destruction of all nerve elements. The tympanomeatal flap is returned to its original position. A pressure dressing is applied.[1]

Transmastoid Approach

1. Through a postauricular incision, a simple mastoidectomy is performed.
2. The vertical segment of the facial nerve is identified, and the incus is disarticulated and removed.
3. The horizontal, posterior, and superior semicircular canals are drilled away. The neuroepithelium is completely removed from the ampullae of the three semicircular canals.
4. The external auditory canal may be packed with absorbable gelatin sponge or a rosebud pack as described for the tympanoplasty procedure.
5. The incision is closed in layers. An external pressure dressing of elastic gauze is applied.

Vestibular Neurectomy

Vestibular neurectomy is the cutting of the vestibular portion of the eighth cranial nerve (acoustic nerve) with the cochlear portion being left intact. It may be performed for a unilateral ear disorder including classic Meniere's disease, recurrent vestibular neuronitis, traumatic labyrinthitis, or vestibular Meniere's disease. It may also be performed when attacks of vertigo severely affect a patient's lifestyle. Vestibular neurectomy is performed when a patient has adequate hearing and a labyrinthectomy is not indicated.

A vestibular neurectomy may be done through multiple approaches: transcochlear, translabyrinthine, middle fossa, retrolabyrinthine, or retrosigmoid.

Procedural considerations

The patient's abdomen or lateral aspect of the thigh is prepped and draped for the purpose of obtaining fat or a segment of muscle and fascia to be used for obliteration of the mastoid cavity at the end of the procedure. If the abdomen is used, most surgeons prefer to take fat from the left side to avoid future confusion with an appendectomy scar. Setups for the graft and neurectomy procedure are separate to avoid cross-contamination. The graft may be taken before the procedure or after the vestibular nerve has been transected, depending on the surgeon's preference. The patient is prepped and draped as for tympanoplasty.

Operative procedures
Transcochlear Approach

1. A postauricular incision is made and the posterior external auditory canal is incised. A large tympanomeatal flap is elevated to expose the middle ear structures.

2. A bony canaloplasty is created, and the round window and facial nerve are identified. The incus, stapes, and promontory bone are removed. The utricle is removed using a 3 mm right-angled pick.
3. The posteroinferior aspect of the internal auditory canal is skeletonized (the process of removing soft tissue to clearly define the bony or skeletal anatomy), the transverse crest is removed, and the superior vestibular nerve is identified.
4. The middle turn of the cochlea is opened anteriorly to assist with cochlear nerve identification.
5. The modiolus is opened, and cerebrospinal fluid (CSF) flows freely and provides irrigation during the drilling. Bone is removed to expose the superior vestibular nerve before it enters the internal auditory canal.
6. The dura is opened, and the cochlear nerve is transected at the modiolus. The facial nerve lies anterior, superior, and beneath the vestibular nerve and is identified by electrical stimulation.
7. After a cleavage plane is found between the facial and superior vestibular nerve, the vestibular fibers are transected, using caution to avoid stretching the facial nerve.
8. A free temporalis muscle and fascia graft obliterates the opening in the internal auditory canal.
9. The flap is returned to its position over the muscle and secured in place by packing the ear for 2 weeks.[1]

Translabyrinthine Approach

1. A postauricular incision is made, and a simple mastoidectomy is performed.
2. The sigmoid sinus is identified and skeletonized.
3. The attic is opened and the incus extracted. The bone over the posterior fossa and endolymphatic sac is removed. The vertical portion of facial nerve is identified.
4. A bony labyrinthectomy is performed, and the semicircular canals are removed. The endolymphatic duct is followed into the vestibule of the internal auditory canal.
5. The bone is removed, skeletonizing the dura of the internal auditory canal from the vestibule to the porus acusticus. Half of the circumference of the internal auditory canal provides good exposure to perform the eighth-nerve section safely.
6. The petrosal facial nerve, superior vestibular nerve, and the vertical crest (Bill's bar) are identified at the superior aspect of the internal auditory canal. The superior vestibular nerve lies more superficially and distally in the bone than the facial nerve does.
7. A sharp sickle knife is used to incise the dura of the internal auditory canal, and the superior vestibular nerve is transected in its bony canal and dissected from the facial nerve. The inferior vestibular nerve and cochlear nerve are bisected.
8. Harvested abdominal adipose tissue is used to obliterate the mastoid defect.

9. The attic and the antrum are sealed with bone wax. The wound is closed, and a mastoid dressing is applied and remains intact for 48 hours.[1]

Retrolabyrinthine Approach

1. Lidocaine with or without epinephrine is injected subcutaneously using a 3 or 5 ml syringe.
2. A retrolabyrinthine U-shaped incision is made slightly posterior to the area of the postauricular incision used in other otologic surgery.
3. An incision is made in the mastoid muscles with a #10 or #15 blade. These muscles are elevated with a Lempert, Joseph, or similar elevator.
4. A self-retaining retractor is inserted after the muscles and periosteum are elevated.
5. The surgeon begins drilling, usually with a large cutting burr, and continues until a complete mastoidectomy is performed. The sigmoid sinus and posterior and inferior semicircular canals are skeletonized with a diamond burr. The posterior fossa bone is removed to expose the posterior fossa dura. During the drilling process burr sizes and types (cutting and diamond) may be changed as vital structures are identified. The scrub nurse must ensure that irrigation and suction are adequate. The surgeon may pause during the drilling to verify vital structures with a microinstrument such as a Rosen needle, gimmick, pick, or searcher.
6. The posterior fossa dura is incised with a sickle or Ziegler microknife. Hemostasis may be achieved by the use of bipolar forceps, a moistened absorbable gelatin sponge covered by a cottonoid or Surgicel. Cottonoids, Surgicel, and gelatin sponge may be loaded onto bayonet forceps before the forceps are placed into the surgeon's hand or may be introduced into the field by the scrub nurse with the use of bayonet forceps while the surgeon controls another bayonet forceps.
7. As exploration and dissection of the cochleovestibular nerve are carried out, cottonoids may be used to cover vital structures and thus maintain orientation. The vestibular portion of the eighth cranial (acoustic) nerve is identified by the surgeon and transsected with microscissors or a microknife.
8. Hemostasis is achieved by the methods mentioned in step 6.
9. The dural incision is closed with suture of the surgeon's preference, usually 4-0 silk or nylon on a very small needle.
10. Fat from the abdomen or fascia and muscle from the lateral aspect of the thigh are packed over the closed dural incision, and the skin incision is closed.
11. A pressure dressing of elastic gauze is applied.

Facial Nerve Decompression

Facial nerve decompression is a procedure designed to identify and relieve an area of compression of the facial nerve. The most common form of facial paralysis is Bell's palsy. It provokes more controversy regarding proper management than any other disorder of the facial nerve. The cause is unknown, although clinical and laboratory evidence indicates a virus of the herpes simplex group. The patient experiences multiple problems such as decreased tearing, inability to close the affected eye, and drooping of the affected corner of the mouth with pooling of oral secretions. Preoperatively the eye is protected by ointments and the eyelid is taped closed, or an adhesive bubble is placed over the eye to trap moisture. This protection is continued into the postoperative period unless a tarsorrhaphy (suturing the eyelid closed) is performed intraoperatively. The patient is taught to place food at the back of the tongue on the unaffected side to assist in mastication. Tilting the head to the unaffected side while eating decreases the pooling of oral secretions and drooling. The patient must be taught proper mouth care because the pooling of oral secretions may lead to dental caries or gingivitis. This regimen is continued until the nerve manifests its regeneration by the return of facial movement. The facial nerve may be decompressed by a translabyrinthine approach when trauma has destroyed the hearing and caused facial nerve paralysis. The narrowest segment of the bony canal compressing the facial nerve is deep in the temporal bone and may also be approached through the middle cranial fossa approach when hearing is to be preserved. Both approaches may be useful under selected circumstances.

Transmastoid, translabyrinthine approach
Procedural Considerations

The patient is prepped and draped as described for tympanoplasty. Neurologic intensive care is required for the first 24 hours.

Operative Procedure

1 to 7. These steps are as for mastoidectomy.
8. After complete mastoidectomy, the dissection is carried out by the use of cutting and diamond burrs until the internal auditory canal and the posterior fossa bone are removed.
9. The bone immediately over the facial nerve is removed by the use of nerve excavators and picks.
10. The facial nerve sheath is incised with a facial nerve knife, neurectomy knife, sickle knife, neurectomy scissors, or micropicks. The incision and decompression are carried out from the stylomastoid foramen to the brainstem.
11. Hemostasis is achieved by the use of moistened absorbable gelatin sponge, cottonoids, Surgicel, bipolar forceps, or a combination.
12. The incision is closed with suture of the surgeon's preference, and a pressure dressing of elastic gauze is applied.

Middle cranial fossa approach
Procedural Considerations

The patient's hair is shaved almost to the midline on the affected side. Povidone-iodine solution is usually used for the prep, which includes the portion of the head that has been shaved, the affected side of the face, and the neck. Lidocaine with or without epinephrine is usually injected subcutaneously above the ear to assist in hemostasis.

Operative Procedure

1. The temporalis muscle is incised and elevated with a Lempert, Shambaugh, or similar elevator.
2. Hemostasis is achieved by clamping and tying vessels or with electrocoagulation.
3. A square of bone is drilled from the temporal bone to expose the middle cranial fossa dura. (The bone is saved for replacement at the end of the procedure.)
4. A self-retaining retractor with a blade for retraction of the middle fossa (such as a Fisch middle fossa retractor or House–Urban retractor) is inserted.
5. The microscope is brought into place, and the dura is elevated from the floor of the middle fossa with a Freer elevator, a gimmick, or similar instruments.
6. Once hemostasis is achieved and the blade is inserted over the dura to expose the middle fossa, drilling may proceed.
7. When the bone becomes quite thin, the surgeon may remove the remaining bone with excavators to avoid damaging the nerve sheath.
8. The facial nerve sheath is incised with a facial nerve knife, neurectomy knife, neurectomy scissors, or microknife.
9. The retractor is removed when hemostasis is achieved, and the bone flap is replaced.
10. The temporalis muscle is approximated and sutured. The incision is closed with suture of the surgeon's preference. A pressure dressing of elastic gauze is applied.

Damage to the facial nerve from trauma, infection, or tumors may be treated surgically by these approaches. Facial nerve grafting requires the use of a separate setup for obtaining a nerve for grafting and microinstrumentation for handling the nerves as well as suturing them. Microsutures such as sizes 8-0 to 11-0 are used.

Removal of Acoustic Neuroma (Vestibular Schwannoma)

Acoustic neuromas arise from the Schwann cells of the vestibular portion of the eighth cranial (acoustic) nerve and are therefore more appropriately termed *vestibular schwannomas*. These tumors are benign but may grow to a size that produces symptoms of cerebellar and brainstem origin.

Vestibular schwannoma was a rare clinical finding in the past. With the extension of life expectancy and improved diagnostic technology, the diagnosis of these tumors has become more frequent. Brainstem auditory evoked response is a highly sensitive noninvasive test for this tumor. If this test yields suspicious findings, an MRI scan of the brain and internal auditory canals is performed.

Depending on the rate and direction of tumor growth, symptoms may include hearing loss, tinnitus, vertigo, headaches, double vision, diplopia, decreased corneal reflex, decreased blink reflex, impaired taste, reduced lacrimation, facial paralysis, diminished gag reflex, vocal cord paralysis, atrophy or fasciculation of the tongue, weakness of the sternocleidomastoid and trapezius muscles, disturbance in balance and gait, hydrocephalus, lethargy, confusion, drowsiness, and coma. Most patients complain of only a unilateral tinnitus and hearing loss, the main symptoms of a possible acoustic neuroma.

Several centers have developed great expertise in acoustic neuroma surgery, which requires the combined team of an otologist and a neurosurgeon.

Procedural considerations

The translabyrinthine approach for the removal of an acoustic tumor has increased in popularity over the past decade. It reduces mortality and morbidity and offers a good chance of saving the facial nerve if the tumor has not directly invaded it. The patient should be informed preoperatively about the presence of a Foley catheter, arterial line, temperature probe, shaved head, and graft-site incision during the postoperative period. Postoperative complications may include a cerebrospinal fluid leak, vertigo, facial nerve weakness or paralysis, and wound infection. These patients require considerable postoperative teaching in preparation for discharge. Areas addressed in discharge instructions include activity, oral care, diet, medication, return office visit, eye care, and graft-site and suture-line care. Emotional support is vital because of the severity of the disease, the operative procedure, and the altered body image patients experience as a result of removal of their hair and facial weakness or paralysis. Members of the national support group, the Acoustic Neuroma Association, may be of assistance.

The patient's hair is shaved to the midline of the affected side. Some patients prefer to have the entire head shaved to facilitate wearing a wig. The options should be presented preoperatively to enable the patient to make a decision before surgery.

The patient is prepped and draped as described for labyrinthectomy. Lidocaine with or without epinephrine may be injected subcutaneously behind the ear. A facial nerve monitor is routinely utilized in the excision of cerebellopontine angle tumors.

Sequential compression hosiery is used intraoperatively and for the first 24 to 46 hours postoperatively or until the patient is ambulatory to decrease the risk of deep venous thrombosis and pulmonary embolism.

Operative procedure

1. A postauricular incision is made slightly longer and wider than the incision in mastoidectomy. The periosteum is elevated from the mastoid bone with a Lempert, Shambaugh, or similar elevator.
2. Self-retaining retractors are inserted, and the cortical mastoidectomy is begun with a large cutting burr.
3. The microscope is brought into position, and the attic is opened to visualize the ossicles. The sigmoid sinus, middle fossa dura, and superior petrosal sinus are left with a thin covering of bone. The semicircular canals are exposed. The incus is removed with alligator forceps or cup forceps and suction.
4. The semicircular canals are excised with the drill. The utricle and saccule are removed, and the aqueduct of the vestibule is drilled out.
5. On completion of the drilling, the remainder of bone is removed with nerve excavators, Fisch dissectors, or picks from the dura of the internal meatus, posterior fossa, middle fossa, and petrosal angle. The wedge of bone between the facial and superior vestibular nerves (Bill's bar) is removed.
6. The dura is opened with microscissors or a dura knife. Dissection of the tumor ensues with a gimmick, Freer microelevator, microinstrument, and bipolar forceps (with or without suction, depending on the surgeon's preference). Hemostasis is frequently achieved through the use of a moistened absorbable gelatin sponge, cottonoids, Surgicel, and a bipolar coagulator.
7. When the tumor has been removed by the use of pituitary cup forceps, long alligator forceps, and similar instruments, hemostasis is achieved.
8. Graft material is obtained to pack the mastoid cavity created from the drilling. It may be fat, fascia, or muscle. The packing is performed meticulously to avoid a cerebrospinal fluid leak postoperatively.
9. On completion of the packing, the wound is closed with suture of the surgeon's choice.
10. A thick pressure dressing, consisting of gauze for absorbency and elastic gauze for pressure, is applied.

The patient is placed in an intensive care setting for close observation for 24 hours. Initial postoperative nursing care includes monitoring of neurologic and routine vital signs, monitoring of facial nerve function on the affected side, observation of the dressing for drainage, close monitoring of temperature, monitoring of intake and output, observation and testing of nasal drainage to determine cerebrospinal fluid leak, positioning, deep breathing by the patient (coughing is discouraged because of the possibility of dislodging the graft), administering medications for pain and nausea, antibiotics, and stool softeners (to prevent straining, which might dislodge the graft), and providing emotional support to the patient. Early ambulation is advised to maintain proper circulation and avoid pulmonary complications, which could lead to coughing and subsequent dislodgment of the graft. Although the patient's opposite vestibular system is compensating for the removed system, the patient needs assistance in moving and ambulating. The family is advised to help as needed, while allowing the patient to move at his or her pace to avoid sudden vertigo and nausea.

If facial function is altered on the affected side because of manipulation, edema, or surgical excision, the patient must use supportive measures until adequate function returns. These include lubrication, covering, and inspection of the eye to avoid corneal injury, frequent brushing and rinsing of the oral cavity to prevent dental caries from the pooling of secretions on the affected side, a semisoft to soft diet to allow the patient more ease in directing the food toward the back of the unaffected side of the mouth, and tilting the head toward the unaffected side. The soft diet and head tilting are designed to decrease the collection of food and the spillage of food from the affected side yet allow the patient to maintain dignity while eating.

Cochlear Implantation

Cochlear implants are electrical devices that convert mechanical sound energy into electric signals. Implantation involves the placement of an electrode into the snail-shaped cochlea of the inner ear for stimulation of remaining nerves in the otherwise profoundly deaf patient. Cochlear implants are appropriate for patients with profound bilateral sensorineural hearing loss. Approximately half a million people in the United States have complete deafness. Cochlear implantation seems to be beneficial for a certain segment of that group. The most important prerequisite for candidacy is of little or no benefit from the use of conventional hearing aids. Adults who become profoundly deaf after acquiring language skills are candidates. Children who are either congenitally deaf or acquire deafness before 18 years of age are cochlear implant candidates. The acquisition of language skills before deafness is not a necessary requirement for children to be candidates. Appropriate auditory training and psychologic counseling are needed after appropriate selection of candidates.

Technologic advancements have given the deaf patient new hope in the area of cochlear implantation. The device is implanted in the cochlea, with the receiver resting in the mastoid. As the device receives sound through the receiver, it emits electrical impulses through the transmitter into the cochlea and along the acoustic nerve (Fig. 19-24). These impulses are interpreted as sound in the temporal cortex of the cerebrum. The patient must be taught to interpret these sounds through extensive training.

Risk of meningitis or infection is rare, but these patients should be followed closely postoperatively.

Operative procedure

1. A U-shaped incision is made, creating a skin flap well behind the mastoid. The flap, including the temporalis

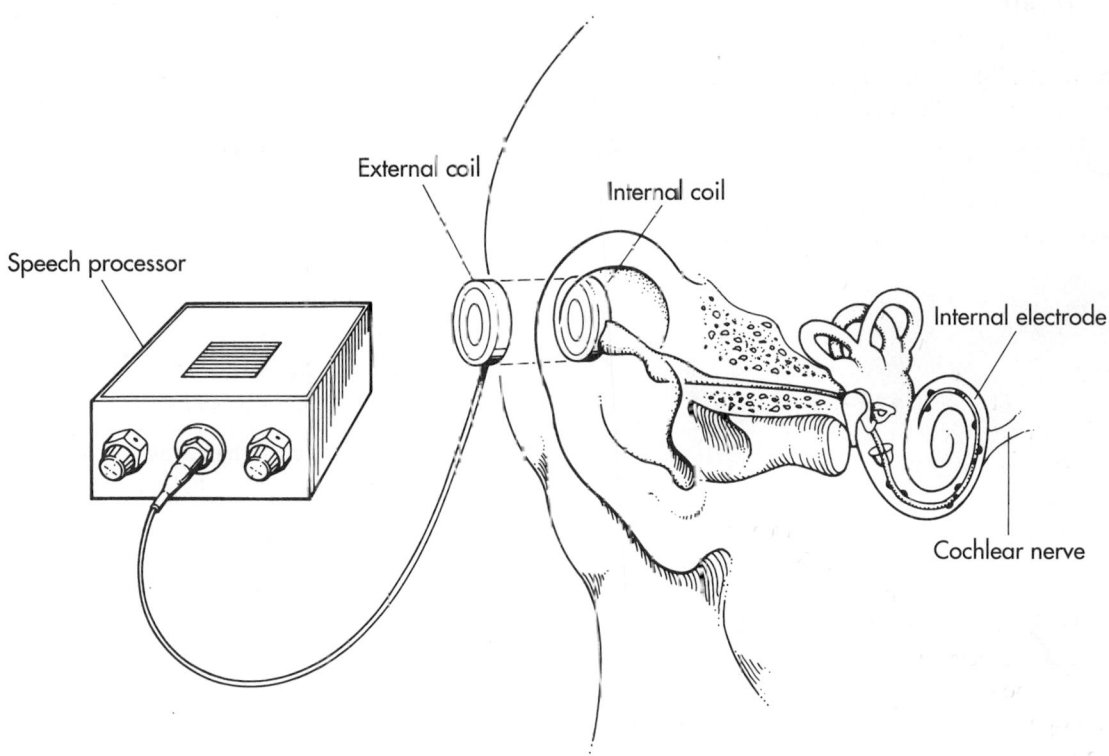

FIGURE 19-24   Cochlear implant system. Sound is transformed into electrical signal in speech processor. Signal is transmitted from external to internal induction coil, which is connected to electrode implanted near cochlear nerve.

muscle, is elevated, exposing the underlying bone. The site of the internal coil is identified, and with a special drill a circular depression in the squamous portion of the temporal bone is made to house the internal coil.
2. A mastoidectomy is accomplished with preservation of the bony ear canal and opening of the facial recess.
3. The coil is secured in the depressed area in the temporal bone, and the electrode is introduced through the facial recess and through a cochleostomy into the cochlea. It is secured in place with a piece of temporalis fascia.
4. The wound is closed. The patient is observed for 6 to 8 weeks until complete wound healing has occurred. Then the external device is applied over the internal coil. This allows transmission of an electrical signal, picked up at an ear-level microphone and processed in a microprocessor worn on the body.

Computerized Facial Nerve Monitoring

Technology enables the surgeon to monitor movement and function of the facial nerve intraoperatively. This monitoring decreases trauma to the facial nerve during tumor dissection and assists the surgeon in determining the point of surgical intervention in idiopathic facial nerve palsy.

The mechanism of hearing can also be tested during surgical intervention to determine the effectiveness of a procedure and thus predict the patient's postoperative result.

Implantable Hearing Aids

Soundwaves are received in two ways: by air conduction through the ear canal and by bone conduction through the bones of the jaw and skull. Conventional hearing aids transmit sound using both methods. Air-conduction devices uses an ear mold that fits into the ear canal. The design of conventional bone-conduction hearing aids makes them uncomfortable and obtrusive, causing headaches and skin abrasions. The quality of sound is inferior, and they often require a higher battery consumption.

Bone-conduction hearing devices

Hearing by bone-conducted sound is a natural way of hearing. When conventional bone-conduction hearing aids are in use, hearing is accomplished when bone-conducted sound bypasses a diseased or impaired external or middle ear.[14]

Implantable hearing devices are designed for patients with moderate to severe conductive hearing loss (unilateral or bilateral) caused by congenital malformations but who maintain good cochlear function. These devices are indicated for patients with draining mastoid cavities or chronic external otitis who are not surgical candidates or patients who are unable to benefit from conventional hearing aids. Ideally, implantable hearing devices should improve sound quality, provide comfort, improve appearance, and reduce the risk of chronic ear infections.

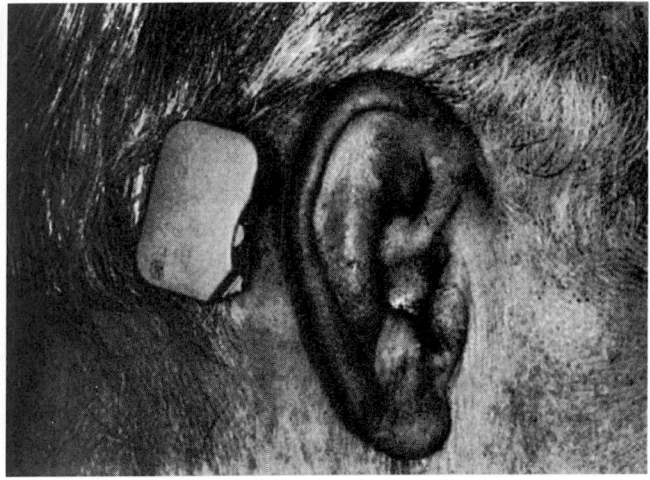

FIGURE 19-25   Patient with implanted bone-anchored hearing aid. The implant is positioned to avoid contact with the pinna, which could cause acoustic feedback should the device be driven at maximum output.

Currently there are two types of bone-conduction hearing devices. The first type has a transducer consisting of two magnetic parts. A postauricular semilunar incision is made, and a flap is raised to expose the temporal bone. A double-tapping orthopedic technique is performed to create threads in the bone into which a magnetic implant is firmly secured. Specialty instrumentation is provided in the implant instrument set. The incision is closed in two layers, and a pressure dressing is applied. The external magnetic processor is not fitted until osseointegration occurs, usually 8 to 12 weeks. The gap between the two magnetic parts of the transducer is filled with soft tissue. The two magnets serve to reduce distortion and firmly secure the device over the intact skin and soft tissue. This type of bond conduction is called "transcutaneous direct bone conduction." There is no permanent skin penetration.[1]

The second type of bone-conduction hearing device is the bone-anchored hearing aid (BAHA™ by Nobel Biocare, Westmont, Ill.). The area behind the ear is prepped and draped, and the implant site is marked. It is important to assure that the hearing aid does not touch the pinna (Fig. 19-25), which may cause acoustic feedback. A semicircular incision is made around the proposed fixture site. A titanium fixture is permanently implanted (tapped) into the mastoid bone, and a permanent skin penetration is made with a titanium abutment. A percutaneous transducer is attached. The air-filled gap of the transducer may be adjusted for length. A hearing aid is fitted and adjusted to the patient's hearing loss 6 to 8 weeks postoperatively.[14]

Surgical implantation of hearing devices may be performed on an outpatient basis and under local anesthesia or local with general anesthesia. It is recommended that the device be implanted in the ear with the best cochlear function.

Research continues on implantable hearing aids for sensorineural hearing loss.

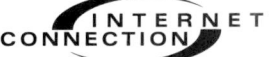

Society of Otorhinolaryngology and Head-Neck Nurses:
http://www.entnet.org

Society of Otorhinolaryngology:
http://www.bcm.tmc.edu/oto/SOHN

ENT Grand Rounds:
http://www.bcm.tmc.edu/oto/grand/grand.html

Association for Research in Otolaryngology:
http://www.aro.org/showcase/aro/

National Information Center on Deafness:
http://www.gallaudet.edu:80/~nicd/

JHU Center for Hearing and Balance:
http://www.bme.jhu.edu//labs/chb/

Otology Online: http://www.ears.com/

REFERENCES

1. Bailey, B.J., Calhoun, K.H., Coffey, A.R., & Neely, J.G. (1996). *Atlas of head and neck surgery—Otolaryngology*. Philadelphia: Lippincott-Raven.
2. Ball, K.A. (1995). *Lasers—the perioperative challenge* (ed. 2). St. Louis: Mosby.
3. Chaffee, E.E., & Lytle, I.M. (1980). *Basic physiology and anatomy* (ed. 4). Philadelphia: J.B. Lippincott.
4. Donlon, J.V., Jr. Anesthesia and eye, ear, nose and throat surgery. In Miller, R.D. (1994). *Anesthesia* (ed. 4). New York: Churchill Livingstone.
5. Frankenthaler, R. (1998). Virtual otoscopy. *Otolaryngologic Clinics of North America, 31*(2), 383-392.
6. Fried, M.P., Kelly, J.H., & Strome, M. (1986). *Complications of laser surgery of the head and neck*. St. Louis: Mosby.
7. Glasscock, M.E., III, & Shambaugh, G.E., Jr. (1990). *Surgery of the ear* (ed. 4). Philadelphia: W.B. Saunders.
8. Janecka, I., Guest Editor. (1993). Principles in cranial base surgery. In Serafin, D., (Ed.). *Problems in Plastic and Reconstructive Surgery, 3*(2). Philadelphia: J.B. Lippincott.
9. Janecka, I., & Tiedmann, K. (1997). *Skull base surgery, anatomy, biology and technology*. Philadelphia: J.B. Lippincott.
10. Lesinski, S.G. (1990). Lasers in otosclerosis—which one if any and why. *Lasers in Surgery and Medicine, 10*, 448-467.
11. Nadol, J.B., Jr., & Schuknecht, H.F. (1993). *Surgery of the ear and temporal bone*. New York: Raven.
12. Silverstein, H., Wolfson, R.J., & Rosenberg, S. (1992). Diagnosis and management of hearing loss. *Clinical Symposia, 44*, 3. Summit, N.J.: Ciba-Geigy.
13. Strome, M., Kelly, J.H., & Fried, M.P. (1992). *Manual of otolaryngology diagnosis and therapy*. Boston: Little, Brown.
14. Tjellström, H., & Håkansson, B. (1995). The bone-anchored hearing aid. *Otolaryngologic Clinics of North America, 28*(1), 53-72.
15. Vernick, D.M. Otologic complications of laser surgery. In Fried, M.P., Kelly, J.H., & Strome, M. (Eds.). (1986). *Complications of laser surgery of the head and neck*. St. Louis: Mosby.

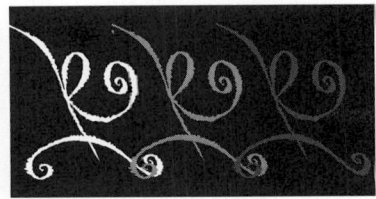

CHAPTER TWENTY

Rhinologic and Sinus Surgery

Charlotte Guglielmi
Theresa Jasset

RHINOLOGIC SURGERY IS performed to treat internal and external malformations and injuries to the nose. Sinus procedures are performed to treat disease processes of the sinuses. The surgical outcome goals of these types of procedures ensure effective functioning of the respiratory system.

Sinus surgery has changed significantly during the past several decades primarily because of the evolution and refinement of endoscopic sinus surgery. As with other surgical procedures that are now being done endoscopically, successful sinus surgery can be accomplished in a less invasive manner in an ambulatory setting. The continued advances in radiologic techniques, especially tomography, allow for the identification of even subtle pathophysiologic changes that can be safely addressed in a surgical setting. Sinus endoscopy has moved from a once diagnostic procedure to a surgical intervention that can be offered to patient's suffering from sinus disease.

SURGICAL ANATOMY

The nose is covered with skin and is supported internally by bone and cartilage. The two external nares provide openings through which air can enter and leave the nasal cavity. These openings contain internal hairs that help prevent coarse particles sometimes carried by air from entering the nose.

The nose is divided into the prominent external portion and the internal portion known as the *nasal cavity* (Fig. 20-1). The chief purpose of the nose is the preparation of air for use in the lungs.

The external nose projects from the face. The upper portion of the external nose is formed by the nasal bones and the frontal process of the maxillae, and the lower portion is formed by a group of nasal cartilages and connective tissue covered with skin (Fig. 20-2). The nostrils and the tip of the nose are shaped by the major alar cartilages. The nares are separated by the columella, which is formed by the lower margin of the septal cartilage, the medial parts of the major alar cartilages, and the anterior nasal spine, all of which are covered by skin. The nasal

cavity is a hollow space behind the nose that is divided medially into right and left portions by the nasal septum.

The nasal septum is composed of three structures: the nasal cartilage, the vomer bone, and the perpendicular plate of the ethmoid bone. The septum is covered by mucous membrane on either side. A deviated or fractured septum may be repaired surgically by mobilization of the fracture or removal of the deformed cartilage or bone.

The internal portion, or nasal cavity, is divided by the nasal septum into two parts at its midline. The nasal cavity communicates with the outside by its external openings, called the *nares*. The nares open into the nasopharynx through the choanae. The nasal cavity is also associated with each ear by means of the eustachian tube and with the paranasal sinuses (frontal, maxillary, ethmoidal, and sphenoidal) through their respective orifices (meatuses). The nasal cavity also communicates with the conjunctivae through the nasolacrimal duct. The nasal cavity is separated from the lingual cavity by the hard and soft palates (see Fig. 20-1) and from the cranial cavity by the ethmoid bone. It is held together by periosteal covering over bone

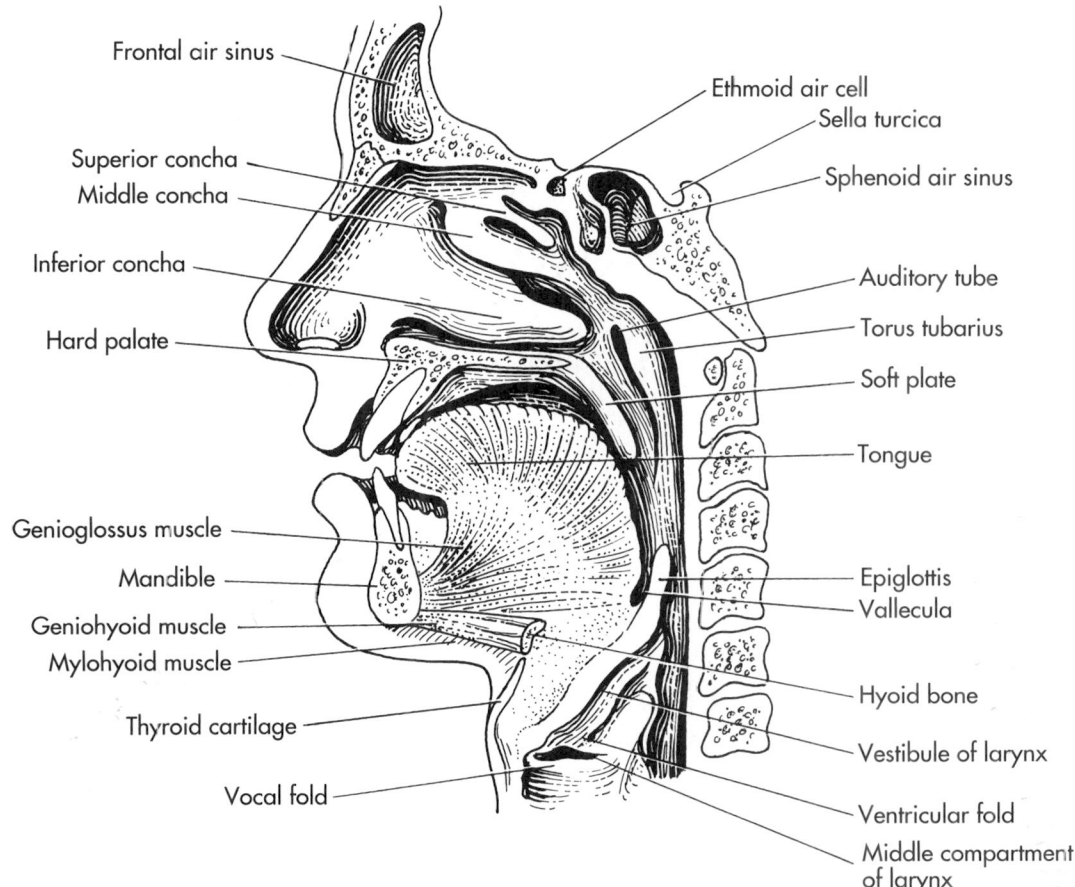

Frontal air sinus

Superior concha
Middle concha

Inferior concha

Hard palate

Genioglossus muscle

Mandible

Geniohyoid muscle

Mylohyoid muscle

Thyroid cartilage

Vocal fold

Ethmoid air cell
Sella turcica

Sphenoid air sinus

Auditory tube

Torus tubarius

Soft plate

Tongue

Epiglottis
Vallecula

Hyoid bone

Vestibule of larynx

Ventricular fold

Middle compartment
of larynx

FIGURE 20–1   Sagittal section of face and neck.

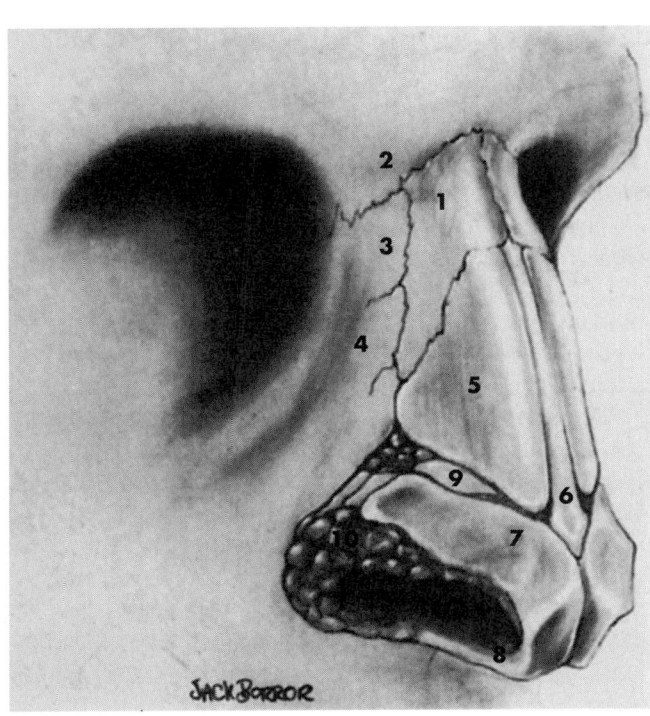

FIGURE 20–2   Nasal bony framework *1*, Nasal bone; *2*, frontal bone; *3*, lacrimal bone; *4*, maxillary bone; *5*, upper lateral cartilage; *6*, nasal septum; *7*, lower lateral cartilage, lateral crus; *8*, lower lateral cartilage, medial crus; *9*, sesamoid cartilage; *10*, fibrofatty tissue.

and by perichondrium, which extends over the cartilages. The turbinate bones of the nasal structure are arranged one above the other, separated by grooves and meatuses. These act as drainage passages of the accessory sinuses and are known as the sphenoethmoidal recesses and the superior, middle, and inferior meatuses respectively (Fig. 20-3).

The nasal sinuses serve as air spaces and communicate with the nasal cavity through the meatuses. Anteriorly, on each side of the skull, the frontal sinus, the anterior ethmoidal sinus, and the maxillary sinus (antrum of Highmore) drain into the middle meatus; posteriorly the ethmoidal and the sphenoidal sinuses drain into the superior meatus and the sphenoethmoidal recess. A passageway for the flow of air is provided by the irregular air spaces between these structures. Because of their shape, the air is forced to flow in thin air waves.

The sensory nerve supply of the nasal cavity is derived from the trigeminal nerve. The nose and sinuses receive their blood supply (Fig. 20-4) from the branches of the internal maxillary, anterior ethmoid, sphenopalatine, naso-palatine, pharyngeal, and posterior ethmoid arteries. Masses of communicating veins lie below the epithelial layer of the turbinate bones, and the veins just beneath the skin anastomose freely. Dilatation of the superficial veins may cause the turbinate bones to swell, whereas contraction of these vessels may cause the bones to shrink.

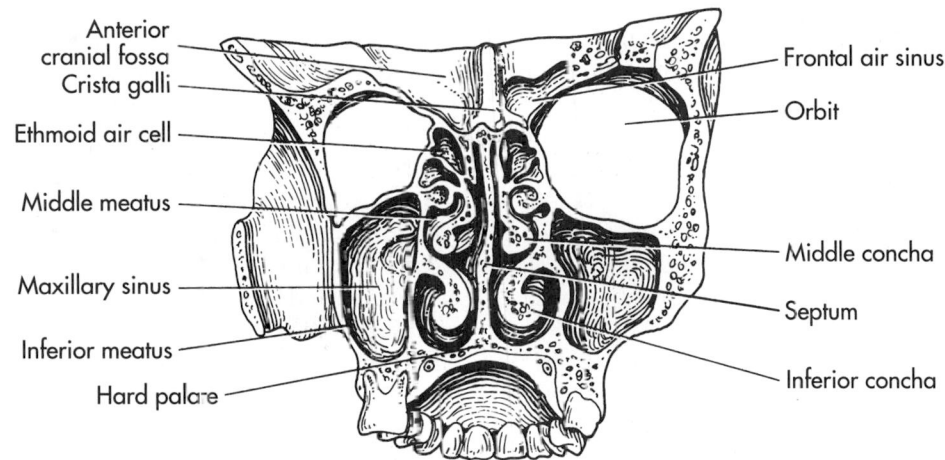

Anterior cranial fossa
Crista galli
Ethmoid air cell
Middle meatus
Maxillary sinus
Inferior meatus
Hard palate

Frontal air sinus
Orbit
Middle concha
Septum
Inferior concha

FIGURE 20-3   Vertical section through nose. Plane of section passes slightly obliquely through left first molar tooth and behind second right premolar tooth. Posterior wall of right frontal sinus removed.

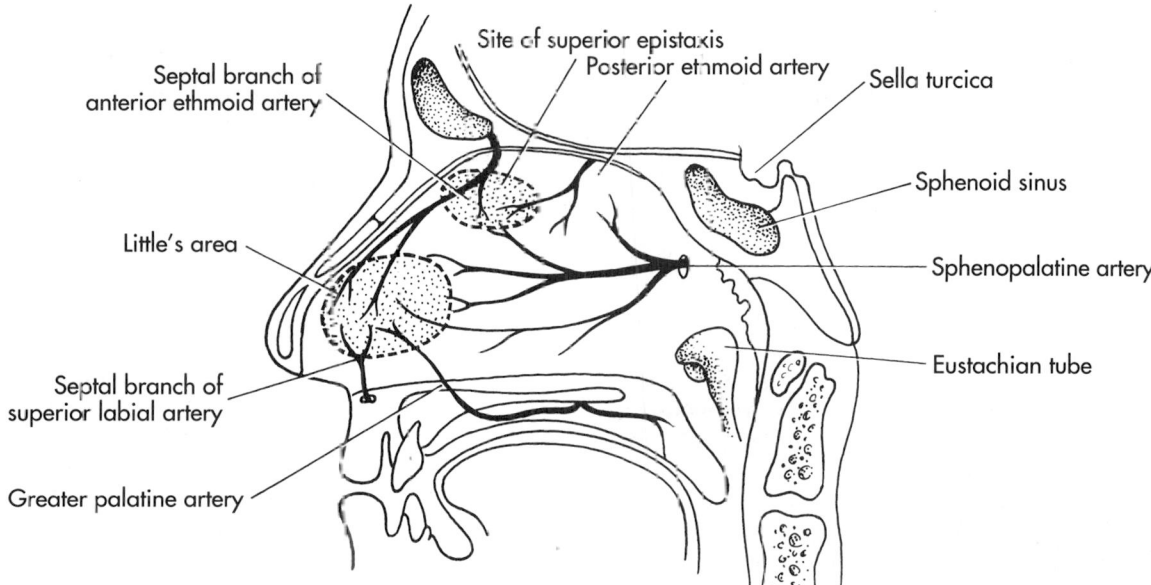

Site of superior epistaxis
Posterior ethmoid artery
Septal branch of anterior ethmoid artery
Sella turcica
Little's area
Sphenoid sinus
Sphenopalatine artery
Septal branch of superior labial artery
Eustachian tube
Greater palatine artery

FIGURE 20-4   Arteries of nasal septum.

PERIOPERATIVE NURSING CONSIDERATIONS

Assessment

As with any surgical procedure performed especially in light of today's healthcare environment, the patient and family's understanding and cooperation are important. The purpose and nature of the nasal and sinus procedures must be explained in a manner that is understandable. The plan of care for the patient is tailored to the local practice that has been established within the surgical team. Practice related to anesthetic considerations is determined between the surgeon, anesthesia provider, and perioperative nurse. Once established the plan is designed to meet institutional policies and JCAHO standards. Anesthetic choices include local anesthetics administered by the surgeon with a nurse

monitor who is trained in airway management and the safe administration of drugs, monitored anesthesia care (MAC) delivered by an anesthesia provider, or general anesthesia. The evolution of new short-acting anesthetic agents employed in the ambulatory setting has increased the safe and efficient care of patients undergoing procedures with general anesthesia who are returning home on the day of surgery.

Before the day of surgery the patient's physician will have discussed the indications, purpose, sequence, and risks of the proposed procedure. In anticipation of the fact that in many situations the patient is a conscious participant in the procedure, he or she should also be informed about the sedative effects of the premedications. Although drowsy, patients will still be aware that their nose is being operated upon but will not feel pain. They should also be educated to know that they will be awake enough to expectorate if necessary and to indicate to the surgical team if they do not feel well, are experiencing pain, or become nauseated. The surgeon's postoperative protocol should be explained to the patient to lay the groundwork for future patient education and a positive experience on the day of surgery. At the conclusion of the surgeon's preoperative visit the operative consents may be signed depending on institutional policy, and the physician should be confident that he or she has obtained informed consent.

A preoperative assessment should be completed by a perioperative nurse either in person or by telephone before the day of surgery. The perioperative nurse caring for the patient should review this assessment as well as the physician's in preparation for caring for the patient. The assessment immediately preceding the procedure should include vital signs, allergies, NPO status, skin condition, sensory deficits, central nervous system problems, and the mental status of the patient. Close attention should be paid to any past drug reactions experienced by the patient, especially if related to administration of local anesthetics. The patient's account of previous dental experiences with local anesthetics can provide a clue to how the patient will respond to the anesthetic agents. Cardiac status should be noted because many surgeons use epinephrine as an additive to the local anesthetic. The epinephrine acts as a vasoconstrictor and reduces the blood loss, which should be minimal, during surgery. The epinephrine effect may contribute to cardiac dysrhythmias and an increased potential for cardiac arrest. In addition, cocaine is often administered topically intranasally to achieve vasoconstriction and to afford the awake patient more comfort during the injection of local anesthesia. Respiratory patterns and any respiratory conditions, such as asthma, should also be noted.

Nursing Diagnosis

Nursing diagnoses appropriate to patients undergoing rhinologic or sinus surgery are as follows:

- Breathing pattern ineffective
- Sensory and perceptual alterations (olfactory and gustatory) related to nasal packing postoperatively
- Anxiety related to fear of the unknown
- Pain related to local anesthesia in the awake patient

Outcome Identification

Outcomes identified for the selected nursing diagnoses could be stated as follows:

- The patient will demonstrate effective breathing patterns.
- The patient will verbalize understanding of the anticipated postoperative alteration in the senses of smell and taste.

- The patient's anxiety will be reduced or controlled.
- The patient will demonstrate effective coping with the physical and psychologic effects of pain.

Planning

Planning of the patient's care is based on the preoperative assessment, application of critical thinking skills, identified nursing diagnoses, and expected outcomes as well as the nurse's knowledge of the scheduled surgical procedure and associated events. Development of a meaningful care plan enables the perioperative nurse to effectively meet the patient's needs during the surgical intervention. Supplies necessary to ensure comfort of the patient in a supine position should be obtained. These usually include a foam headrest, a pillow for under the knees, and warm blankets. Foam padding should be available to assist in positioning the arms if they are going to placed at the side. Care should taken to avoid the placement of intravenous lines in the arm that is to be tucked at the side, but in cases where this in not avoidable careful attention should be made to maintain patency of those lines. Specific equipment needs for endoscopic procedures are discussed later in this chapter.

Preparation of the operating room includes checking the availability and functional capacity of suction, the surgeon's headlight and light source, and the electrosurgical unit (ESU). It is essential that the x-ray viewbox is in working order and appropriately located so that scans may be easily viewed by the surgeon during the procedure. In video-assisted cases the camera should be checked, the printer should be set up as preferred by the surgeon, and an adequate supply of paper should be available. In procedures in which the nurse will function as the primary patient monitor, equipment such as oxygen-saturation monitors, blood pressure monitors, ECG monitor, and oxygen delivery systems should be checked before the procedure.

Because local anesthesia is frequently used for nasal surgical procedures, the nurse must be prepared to react quickly to signs of allergic reactions or toxic symptoms. Symptoms of adverse drug reactions include changes in skin such as rash or itching, restlessness, unexplained anxiety or fearfulness, diaphoresis, complaints of blurred vision, tinnitus, dizziness, nausea, palpitations, disturbed respiration, pallor or flushing, and syncope. Emergency drugs, suction apparatus, and resuscitation equipment including a defibrillator should be readily available. In the awake patient introperative pain can serve an important warning function that contributes greatly to the avoidance of injury to the roof of the ethmoid, the orbit, and the optic nerve.

The Sample Care Plan on p. 731 addresses the needs of patients undergoing rhinologic or sinus surgery.

Several principles of nursing care are basic to all types of nasal surgery. The following information should be given to all patients and their families:

SAMPLE CARE PLAN

Nursing Diagnosis: Breathing pattern ineffective

Outcome: The patient demonstrates effective breathing patterns.

Interventions:

1. Elevate head of the bed (for decreasing the edema, which can interfere with breathing).
2. Apply ice compresses (to increase vasoconstriction, thereby decreasing the edema).
3. Increase humidification with a bedside humidifier or a humidified face mask.
4. Monitor respiratory rate, rhythm, and pulse oximetry. Maintain pulse oximetry greater than 90%.
5. Explain to the patient and his or her family that packing will interfere with ability to breathe through the nose.
6. Review mouth breathing with patient and his or her family.
7. Routine mouth care is reviewed with patient and his or her family.

Nursing Diagnosis: Sensory and perceptual alterations (olfactory and gustatory) related to nasal packing postoperatively

Outcome: The patient verbalizes understanding of the anticipated alteration in the senses of smell and taste.

Interventions:

1. Explain to the patient and his or her family that a "moustache" dressing and packing will be in place postoperatively and will interfere with the sense of smell.
2. Inform the patient and his or her family that the sense of taste will also be altered, as with having a head cold.
3. Assure the patient and his or her family that these alterations are usually temporary.
4. Encourage the patient to maintain proper dietary intake even if the food does not smell or taste as it should.
5. Provide frequent mouthcare, rinse with water or half hydrogen peroxide and half normal saline.

Nursing Diagnosis: Anxiety related to fear of the unknown

Outcome: The patient verbalizes knowledge of the steps of the perioperative process.

Interventions:

1. Following the protocol in place, inform the patient and his or her family what to expect on the day of surgery.
2. Explain all activities performed by the nursing staff and provide the rationale for each.
3. Assure the patient that he or she will be informed before any procedure is done.
4. Provide time for the patient and his or her family to express fears and concerns.

Nursing Diagnosis: Pain related to local anesthesia in the awake patient

Outcome: The patient demonstrates effective coping with the physical and psychologic effects of pain.

Interventions:

1. Explain to the patient that some initial discomfort (such as pinprick followed by slight burning and then numbness) may be felt during the administration of local anesthetic.
2. Inform the patient before the injection of local anesthetic; provide support and reassurance.
3. Describe the sequence of events to the patient to prevent unrealistic expectation.
4. Observe for, document, and report any changes in the patient's vital signs (blood pressure, heart rate and rhythm, respiratory rate, and oxygen saturation), skin condition, and mental status.
5. Be aware of the maximum recommended dosage of local anesthetics (see Chapter 7) and be alert for signs of allergic reactions or toxic responses.
6. Ask the patient whether he or she is experiencing any pain; communicate the presence of pain sensation to the surgeon.
7. Administer sedation or analgesics as ordered by the surgeon.

---

1. Some discomfort may occur during the initial administration of a local anesthetic. If the surgeon uses a topical anesthetic (usually cocaine as the first phase of anesthesia), it is applied to the nose with cottonoids or applicators. The patient may find the applicators or packing uncomfortable or may have the urge to sneeze. These sensations will disappear as the anesthetic takes effect. The needle may cause momentary discomfort, and a burning sensation may occur as the anesthetic is injected. If the patient expresses difficulty in breathing, the nurse should encourage slow deep breaths through the mouth and continually provide reassurance to allay the patient's anxiety. If the surgeon uses epinephrine with the local agent, the resulting weak quivering feeling and increased heart rate are effects of the epinephrine and disappear after a few minutes. The nurse may liken this to the experiences a patient may have had in the dentist's office to prepare the patient in advance. The patient's cardiac status should be noted at this time.

2. Certain procedures may be performed on entry to the preoperative holding area or the operating room in

accordance with institutional policies, such as insertion of intravenous lines and application of monitoring devices. Attempts should be made to allow the patient to continue to be supported by his or her family or significant other as long as possible before the patient is admitted to the operating room.

3. During the surgical procedure the awake patient feels the surgeon working and may feel pressure at some point but should not feel pain. The patient should let the surgeon know if any discomfort is felt during the procedure, and more anesthetic can be given.

4. After surgery the head of the bed is elevated to facilitate breathing and drainage.

5. A nasal pack will probably be inserted, and there may be some difficulty in swallowing. When the patient attempts to swallow, a sucking action occurs in the throat because the packing does not allow air passage through the nose, thereby creating a partial vacuum.

6. Some bruising and swelling can be expected after surgery, but it will gradually subside.

7. Forceful nose blowing must be avoided for a time to prevent movement of the rearranged nasal structures. If necessary to clear nasal passages, the patient should sniff inwardly.

8. The sense of smell is diminished for a time after surgery but gradually returns.

9. Some numbness may be noticed postoperatively but gradually disappears.

10. A moderate amount of discomfort should be expected after surgery; medication is prescribed, and the patient should be encouraged to take it.

11. The procedure for changing the moustache dressing that is in place postoperatively to absorb any drainage should be reviewed with the patient and his or her family. Blood-tinged secretions in the nasopharynx are normal in the first few hours after the procedure.

12. Potential complications of bleeding, cerebrospinal fluid leak, and visual or tear duct problems should be reviewed with the patient or his or her family.

Implementation

Patient positioning for nasal cases is supine. A standard head rest may be used to maintain the head in normal position. The head of the bed is turned 90 degrees in the room to allow the surgeon to work from the patient's right side, and the right arm is tucked in at the patient's side. The arm should be padded as necessary when tucked to prevent nerve injury. The left arm is maintained by anesthesia and usually has the IV line placed in it for easier access. The anesthesia provider and equipment will be to the patient's left as well. Alternatively a modified "beach chair" position can also be used for these procedures. The scrub person may stand at the patient's head or down near the patient's waist next to the surgeon's right arm. A Mayo stand can be set up either at the head of the bed off to the side or positioned over the patient's chest depending on where the scrub person is standing. Video equipment should be set up at the patient's head if applicable. Safety straps should always be used.

Local anesthesia

As discussed in the assessment section, rhinologic and sinus surgery can be done with various routes of anesthetic delivery. There are two types of medications that will be used by the surgeon regardless of which route is chosen. The first is a local anesthetic that is almost always used to block the patient's pain and temperature fibers. Lidocaine is also an excellent medium to which to add epinephrine. A concentration of 1:200,000 will provide maximum vasoconstriction, but some surgeons prefer a concentration of 1:100,000. Cocaine 4% topical solution is the second medication that is used consistently. It too is a good vasoconstrictor but has the added benefit of anesthetic properties as well. Many surgeons will use a nasal decongestant instead of cocaine for nasal vasoconstriction. These decongestants do not produce some of the cardiac effects seen with cocaine. Because nasal and sinus surgery are performed in such a confined space, vasoconstriction becomes crucial for appropriate visualization of the surgical field. Hypertension can also increase bleeding despite vasonconstrictive agents used and often may need to be managed medically by the anesthesia provider intraoperatively if the visual field becomes compromised and surgery is impaired (Research Highlight 20-1).

It is almost uniform that surgeons will pack the nose with the vasoconstrictive solution before prepping and draping to allow time for the vasoconstrictive properties to work. A separate prep table, which includes a container of the vasoconstrictor solution, x-ray detectable cottonoids, usually ½ by 3 inches with attached strings, bayonet forceps, and a small nasal speculum, should be prepared for this purpose. These cottonoids should always be counted before and at the end of the procedure. (If a cottonoid is placed extremely posterior along the nasal floor, it can slide past the palate and be swallowed by the patient.) The cottonoids are left in place. Some surgeons

---

20-1 RESEARCH HIGHLIGHT

A technique that utilized topical and regional anesthesia of a 25% cocaine paste combined with intravenous midazolam hydrochloride was used in a study of 554 patients undergoing functional endoscopic surgery. Appropriate visualization of the operative fields was maintained, and the patients were comfortable. Postoperatively, patients achieved discharge criteria rapidly and were discharged on the same day.

From Lee, W.C., Kapur, T.R., & Ramsden, W.N. (1997). Local and regional anesthesia for functional endoscopic sinus surgery. *Annals of Otology, Rhinology and Laryngology, 106*(9), 767-769.

will also inject local anesthetic at this time, but others may wait to inject on the operative field. Maximum vasoconstriction occurs in approximately 10 to 12 minutes after the administration of epinephrine. If a local anesthetic is to be injected next, the prep table should also include a 10 ml Luer-Lok syringe, appropriate-sized needle (usually 25 gauge, 1½ inches), and lidocaine (either 0.5% or 1% or even 2%) according to surgeon's preference. Additional syringes, needles, and local anesthetic solution should be available on the sterile field for additional administration intraoperatively. All containers of local anesthetic solutions must be clearly labeled. Additional cocaine solution and cottonoids should be available on the sterile field as well. The circulating nurse, nurse monitor, or the anesthesia provider should observe any changes in the vital signs of the patient. Documentation should include both topical and injectable agents as with all perioperative cases.

Prepping and draping

Prepping of the nose and face is considered optional for the surgical team. The intranasal area is considered dirty and not possible to prep effectively. Some surgeons may cleanse the nose and face with povidone-iodine solution or other topical antiinfective solution such as hexylresorcinol 1%. The surgical field is maintained in sterile fashion, and most surgeons will scrub before donning gloves and gowns, but these cases have a "clean-contaminated" wound classification.

Draping is done as for most head and neck cases. A small sheet with a towel on top of it is placed under the patient's head, and the towel is secured around the hairline with a towel clip. A split sheet is then placed around the head. It is good practice to place a towel over the endotracheal (ET) tube if one is in place to prevent the adhesive portion of the split sheet from sticking to the ET tube and causing inadvertent pulling on the tube once the procedure is completed and drapes are removed. The patient's eyes should be covered with moist gauze or towels if the patient is awake or taped closed if the patent is under general anesthesia to be protected from nasal drainage or injury from instruments except during certain endoscopic procedures.

Instrumentation and equipment

A headlight will always be worn for local and topical administration of medications before draping. If the procedure is planned for all endoscopic work, the headlight will not be necessary after that point. Headlights will be required for septoplasty and rhinoplasty procedures. A standard electrosurgical unit (ESU) should be available but is usually not required in a straight endoscopic case. If the use of a turbinate needle is planned, the patient will require grounding.

Specimen cups, labels, and a marking pen should be available on the sterile field because often several specimens are obtained.

The operative instruments necessary for rhinologic surgery can be seen in Figs. 20-5 to 20-8.

Postoperative care of the instruments used in nasal surgery follows the general care regimens of all other surgical instruments. Chisels, gouges, and other cutting instruments should be inspected carefully for any nicks and for dullness and repaired as needed. Rasps and files should be thoroughly cleaned and all bone debris removed. Special attention should be given to suction tips. Sinus endoscopes should be cared for as any endoscope and cleaned and sterilized according to institutional policies. Sinus instruments should be handled carefully because of their delicate nature. They should be in good working order and able to be opened and closed easily to grasp and release delicate nasal and sinus tissue. Lenses on headlights used during the procedure should be checked for cleanliness and cleaned according to the manufacturer's instructions.

Evaluation

The patient should be assessed postoperatively for any difficulties in breathing. Nasal packing inhibits breathing; however, the patient should be able to breathe normally through the mouth. Skin integrity related to positioning and ESU dispersive electrode should be documented, and intervention, if any, should be instituted immediately. The amount of drainage present on the moustache dressing should be noted. The head of the PACU bed should be elevated before transport to the unit. Report of the patient's status and special needs should be given to the PACU by institutional policy, and any variances should be clearly communicated. Goals of the nursing care plan are reviewed and an evaluation of outcomes as identified in the assessment phase may be communicated and documented as follows:

- The patient demonstrated effective breathing patterns.
- The patient verbalized understanding of anticipated postoperative alteration in the senses of smell and taste.
- The patient's anxiety was reduced or controlled.
- The patient demonstrated effective coping with the physical and psychologic effects of pain.

Patient and Family Education and Discharge Planning

Discharge teaching and planning for postdischarge activities and needs are essential for the patient and family to successfully cope with the postoperative recovery period. These may be initiated by the perioperative nurse. Patients and families should be made aware of the following activities, restrictions, and precautions as they relate to rhinologic or sinus surgery:

1. The head of the bed may be elevated to facilitate breathing and drainage.

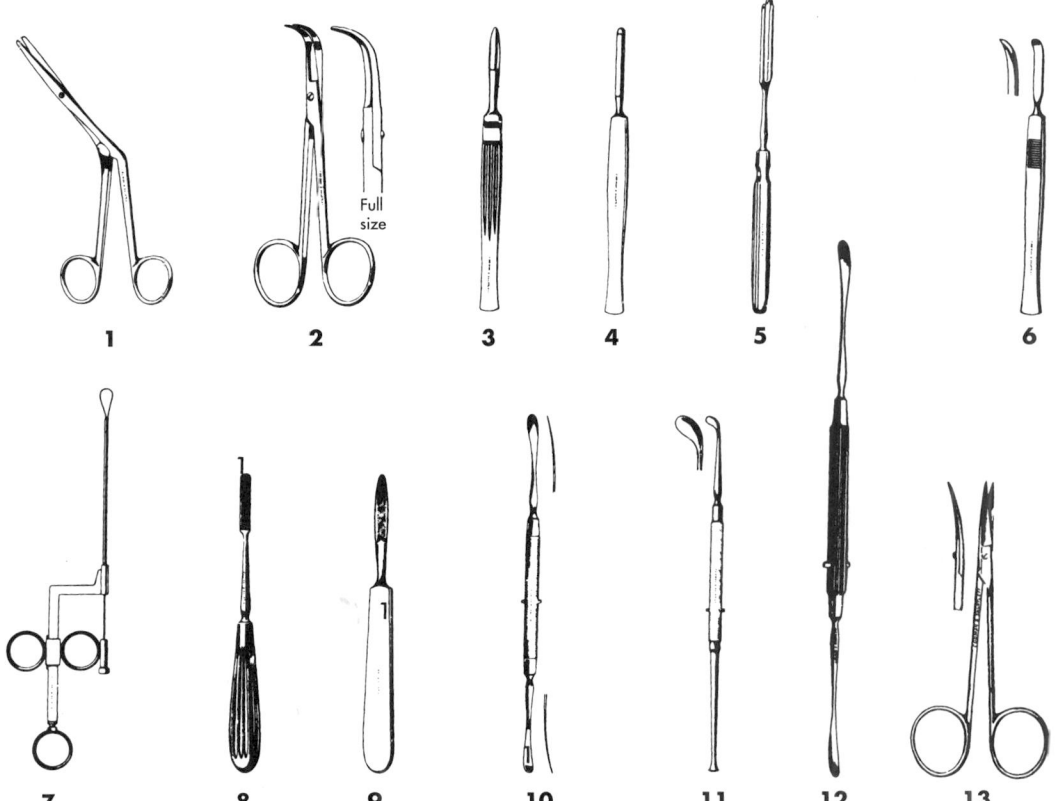

FIGURE 20-5   Cutting instruments for operations on external nose and nasal cavity. *1*, Nasal scissors, angled; *2*, Fomon upper lateral scissors; *3*, cartilage knife, beveled blade; *4*, cartilage knife, straight; *5*, cartilage knife, swivel blade; *6*, cartilage nasal knife, curved; *7*, nasal snare; *8*, nasal rasp, narrow; *9*, nasal rasp; *10*, double-ended elevator; *11*, golf-stick elevator-dissector; *12*, Freer dissecting elevator; *13*, iris scissors, straight and curved.

2. If a nasal pack is in place, the patient may have some difficulty in swallowing. When the patient attempts to swallow, a sucking action occurs in the throat because the packing does not allow air to pass through the nose, thereby creating a partial vacuum.

3. The patient should be encouraged to breathe through the mouth until the packing is removed. Frequent oral hygiene measures should be offered and encouraged.

4. The patient should be made aware of the temporary nature of nasal and eye edema and discoloration and numbness in the nasal tip and upper lip.[4]

5. Forceful nose blowing must be avoided to prevent movement of the rearranged nasal structures. If necessary to clear nasal passages, the patient should sniff inwardly. If a sneeze is unavoidable, the mouth should be opened.

6. The sense of smell is diminished for a time after surgery but gradually returns.

7. A moderate amount of discomfort should be expected after surgery; medication is prescribed, and the patient should be encouraged to take it.

8. The procedure for changing the moustache dressing that may be in place postoperatively to absorb any drainage should be reviewed with the patient and family. Blood-tinged secretions in the nasopharynx are normal during the first few hours after surgery.

9. Signs and symptoms such as bleeding, visual or tear duct problems, respiratory difficulty, or vertigo should be reported to the doctor.

10. Patients should avoid smoking or exposure to other noxious fumes that could irritate the nasal passages or nasal mucosa.

11. Use of a humidifier or normal saline nasal spray may help keep nasal passages and mucosa moist.

12. Lifting heavy objects and excessive straining should be avoided.

SURGICAL INTERVENTIONS
RHINOLOGIC SURGERY

Procedures that involve both internal and external nasal reconstruction can be done with local anesthesia, usually supplemented with IV sedation and analgesia (MAC). If the patient is particularly apprehensive or anxious, general anesthesia may be more appropriate. In most cases, the surgeon will opt to wear a headlight to improve visualization of the intranasal structures.

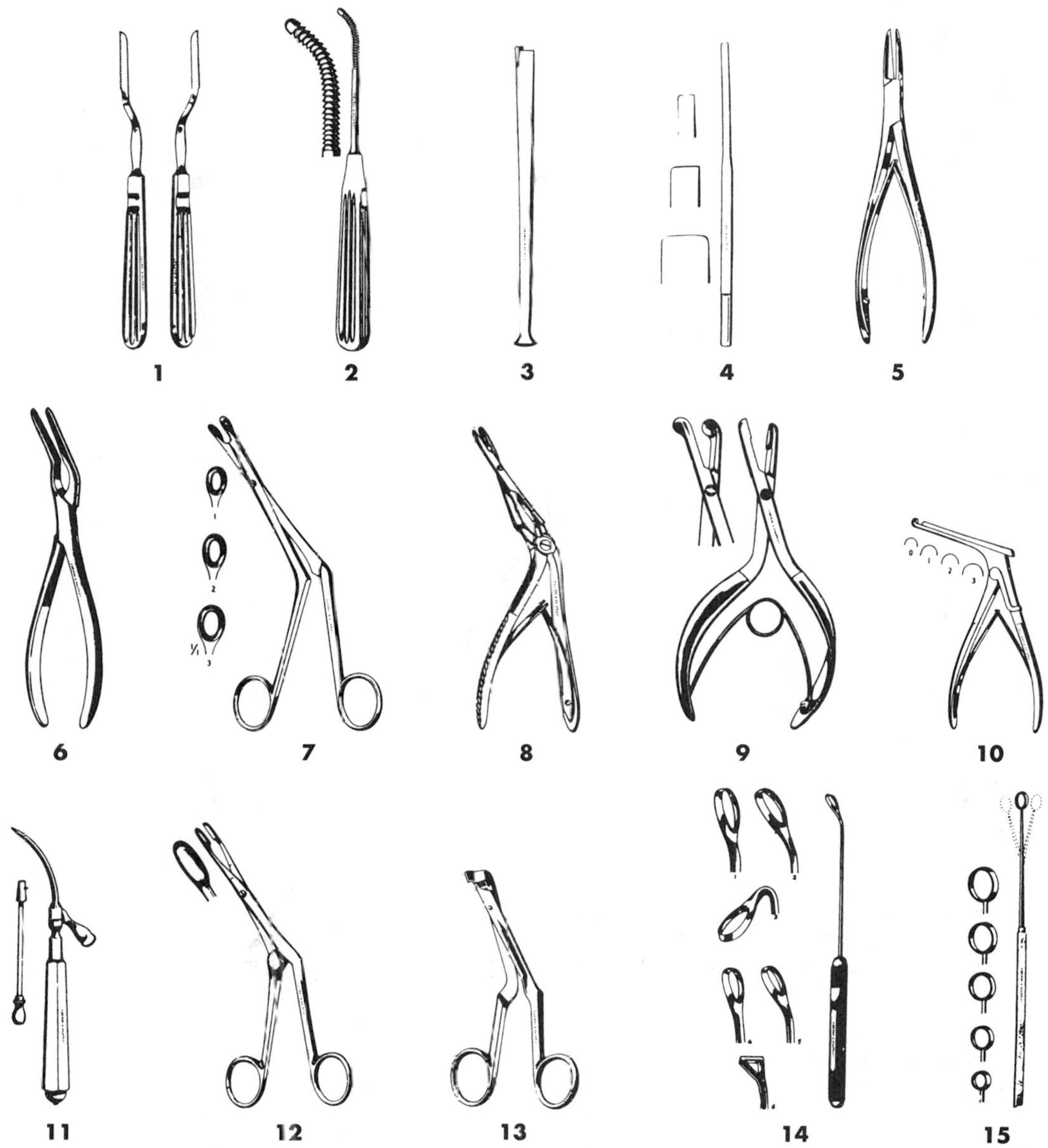

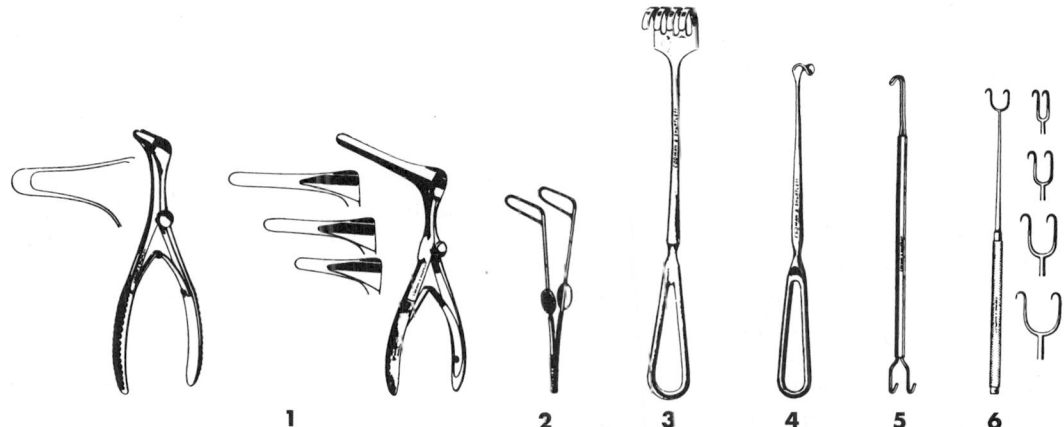

FIGURE 20–6 Cutting instruments for operations on external nose and nasal cavity, continued. *1*, Freer nasal saws, right and left; *2*, reamer; *3*, nasal chisel with guard; *4*, osteotome, narrow widths; *5*, nasal bone cutter; *6*, Asch septum forceps; *7*, Bruening septum forceps; *8*, double-action nasal rongeur; *9*, McCoy septum forceps; *10*, Kerrison rongeur; *11*, antrum trocar and stylette; *12*, septum-cutting forceps; *13*, septal ridge-cutting forceps; *14*, Coakley ethmoidal sinus curettes; *15*, Myles antrum ring curettes.

FIGURE 20–7 Exposing instruments for operations on external nose, nasal cavity, and sinuses. *1*, Vienna and Killian nasal specula; *2*, Bosworth nasal wire speculum; *3*, Volkmann rake retractor; *4*, Cushing vein retractor; *5*, one-and two-pronged retractor, double-ended; *6*, two-pronged retractors, sharp, various sizes.

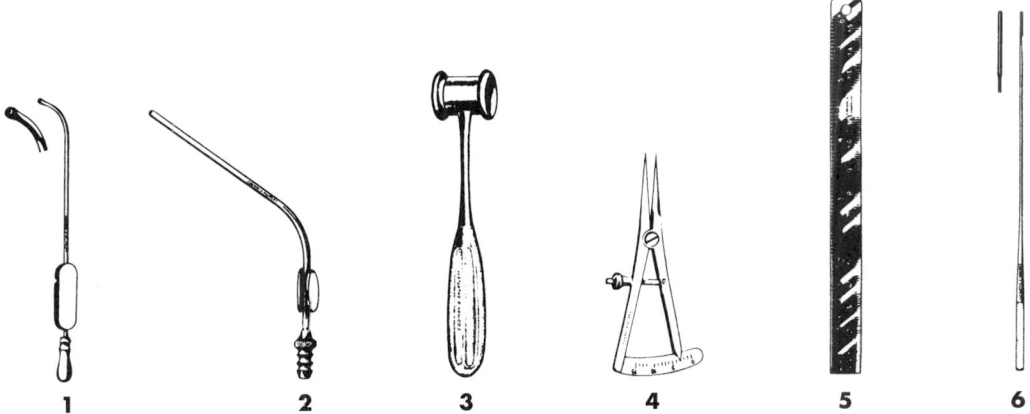

FIGURE 20-8   Accessory instruments for operations on external nose and nasal cavity. *1*, Antrum suction tip; *2*, Frazier suction tip; *3*, metal mallet; *4*, caliper; *5*, ruler; *6*, nasal applicator.

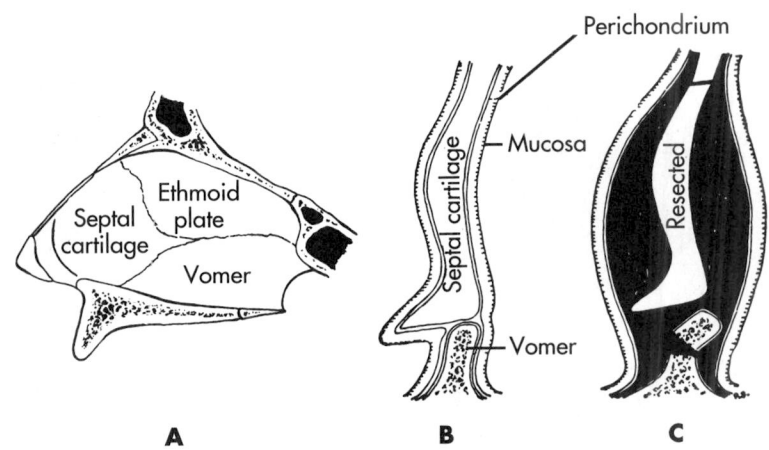

FIGURE 20-9   **A**, Primary components of septum. Incision line is for Killian type of submucous resection. **B**, Septum with deviated cartilage and spur at junction of vomer and septal cartilage. **C**, Resection of obstructive parts after careful elevation of mucoperichondrium and mucoperiosteum.

Septoplasty or Submucous Resection of the Septum (SMR)

A septoplasty is straightening of either the cartilaginous or osseous portions of the septum that lie between the flaps of the mucous membrane and the perichondrium. When the nasal septum is deformed, fractured, or injured, normal respiratory and nasal function may be impaired. Deviations of the septum involving cartilage, bony parts (spurs), or both, may block the meatus and compress the middle turbinate on that side, thereby resulting in an obstruction of the sinus opening. Septal deviations tend to produce sinus disease and nasal polyps.

The objective of the septoplasty is to establish an adequate partition between the left and right nasal cavities, thereby providing a clear airway through both the internal and external cavities of the nose.

Procedural considerations

The setup is as described in the general preparation for nasal surgery.

Operative procedure

1. The nostril is opened with a nasal speculum. An incision is made through the mucoperichondrium of the septum with a knife having a #15 blade. The tissues are separated and elevated with a Freer elevator (Fig. 20-9).
2. The cartilage is incised with a knife, and the mucous membrane is elevated with a septal elevator; deviated cartilage and bony thickened structures are trimmed or removed with a septum punch and a nasal cutting forceps.
3. The bony septal spurs are trimmed by means of a chisel, gouge, and mallet, or punch forceps. Suction is used to expose the field. Bleeding is controlled by insertion of additional cottonoids soaked with a topical hemostatic agent.
4. The perpendicular plate of the ethmoid as well as the vomer may be removed by means of a suitable septum-cutting forceps (see Fig. 20-6).
5. The incision may be sutured with 4-0 absorbable atraumatic suture on a small straight needle.

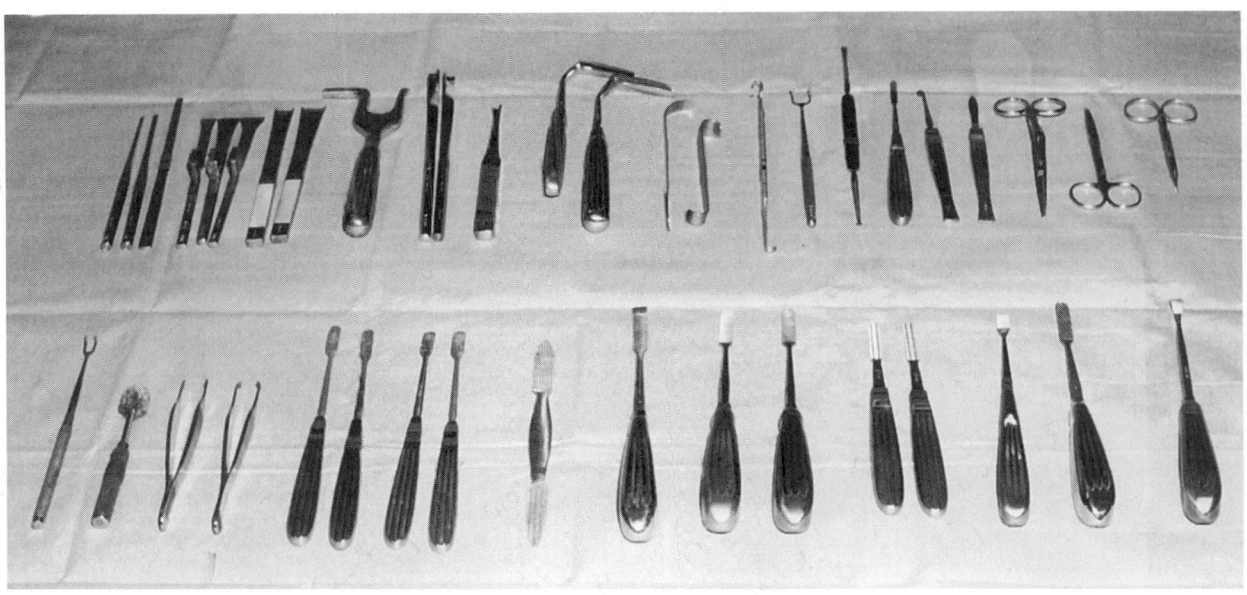

FIGURE 20-10   Rhinoplasty instruments. *Top row,* 2 mm osteotome; 3 mm osteotome; 4 mm Cottle osteotome; 10 mm Rubin osteotome; 14 mm Rubin osteotome; 16 mm Rubin osteotome; 10 mm Cinelli osteotome; 14 mm Cinelli osteotome; Rubin nasofrontal osteotome; right-curved guarded chisel; left-curved guarded chisel; Parkes lateral osteotome chisel; two Aufricht nasal retractors (long and short); Parkes nasal retractor; S-shaped blade retractor; Cottle knife guard and retractor; Fomon ball retractor; Cottle elevator; Joseph periosteal elevator; Freer septum knife; Joseph nasal scissors; Fomon dorsal scissors; Stevens tenotomy scissors. *Bottom row,* Double-pronged skin hook; wire brush; Adson-Brown tissue forceps, Beasley-Babcock tissue forceps; four diamond rasps (two straight, two curved); converse rasp; Aufricht glabellar rasp; Parkes rasp (one fine, one medium); two Maltz rasps; Lewis rasp; rasp, straight fine; Glabella rasp.

6. Nostrils are packed with gauze impregnated with antibiotic ointment to keep the septal flaps in a midline position. Nasal splints made of plastic or Silastic may also be used to prevent adhesions and maintain the septum. Some surgeons use mattress sutures to provide a patent airway while maintaining support for the septum. The face is cleansed and a moustache dressing (that is, a 2 X 2–inch gauze folded and secured with tape across the face or bridge of the nose) may be applied. A small ice bag (which can be made out of a surgical glove filled with ice) may be applied to the nose.

Corrective Rhinoplasty

A corrective rhinoplasty is removal of the hump, narrowing and shortening of the nose, and reconstruction of the tip of the nose. It is considered an elective cosmetic procedure. Often it is done in combination with a septoplasty so that there is only one anesthetic and recovery period for the patient. Cases may be scheduled so that a plastic surgeon performs the rhinoplasty after the otolaryngologist completes the septoplasty, but many otolaryngologists are trained to perform the rhinoplasty procedure as well.

Procedural considerations

The patient is prepped and positioned for nasal surgery. The rhinoplasty and nasal instruments are shown in Figs.

20-10 and 20-11. Rhinoplasty can be performed as an internal rhinoplasty where all the incisions are within the nasal cavity. It can also be done as an external procedure where the incision is on the skin across the bases of the nasal columella (Fig. 20-12). This incision allows for the reflection of the columellar nasal tip flap, providing exposure of the underlying bony and cartilaginous structures.

Operative procedure

1. A hemitransfixion incision is made through the skin of one nostril with a knife having a #15 blade. A nasal speculum, sponges, and skin hooks can be used for exposure.
2. The skin of the nose is undermined by elevators, knives, and scissors. The periosteum and periochondrium are freed with elevators and a periosteal dissector.
3. The nasal bones may be fractured with a straight or curved osteotome or a saw. The upper lateral cartilage may be trimmed with a #15 blade or a small plastic scissors. The dorsal hump can be taken down with an osteotome. A cartilaginous hump can be taken down with a #15 blade. The septal cartilage may be removed by a cutting forceps such as the Jansen-Middleton. Bony spurs can be taken down with a mallet and osteotome. The field is cleared by suctioning.
4. The edges of the cartilage are trimmed with scissors or a #15 blade.

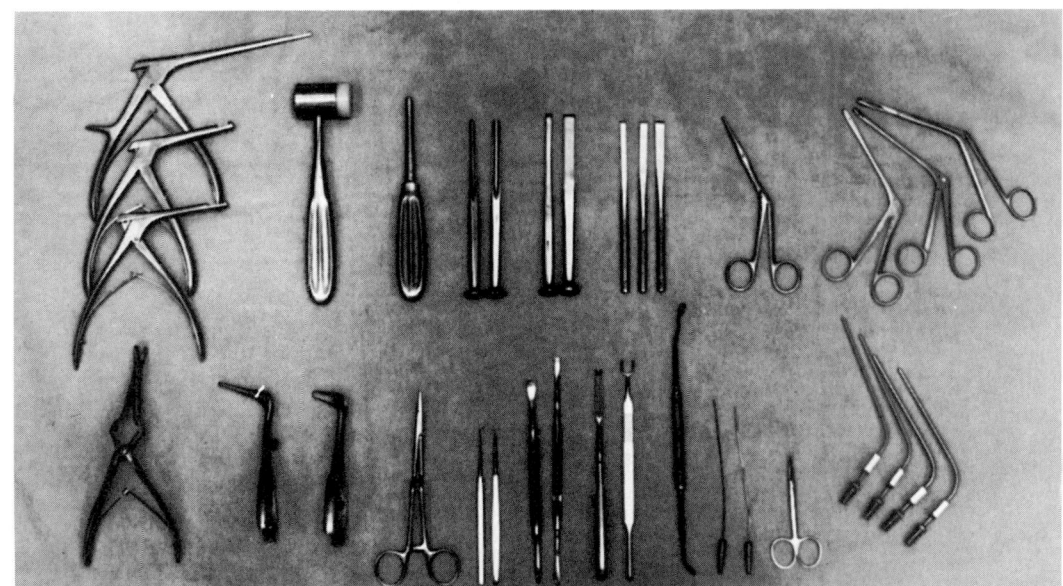

FIGURE 20–11   Nasal instruments. *Top row, left to right,* Kerrison rongeurs, 2, 4, and 6 mm; mallet; septal displacer; gouges; small chisels; small osteotomes; Knight nasal scissors; Knight polyp forceps, small, medium, and large. *Bottom row, left to right,* Jansen-Middleton forceps; medium and short nasal specula; Jacobson bayonet needle holder; single skin hooks; Alberg periosteal elevator; Freer elevator; Ballenger swivel knife; Cottle knife guard and retractor; Faulkner antrum curette (double ended); University of Iowa cotton applicators; Knapp scissors, light curve; Frazier suction tips, sizes 1, 2, 3, and 4.

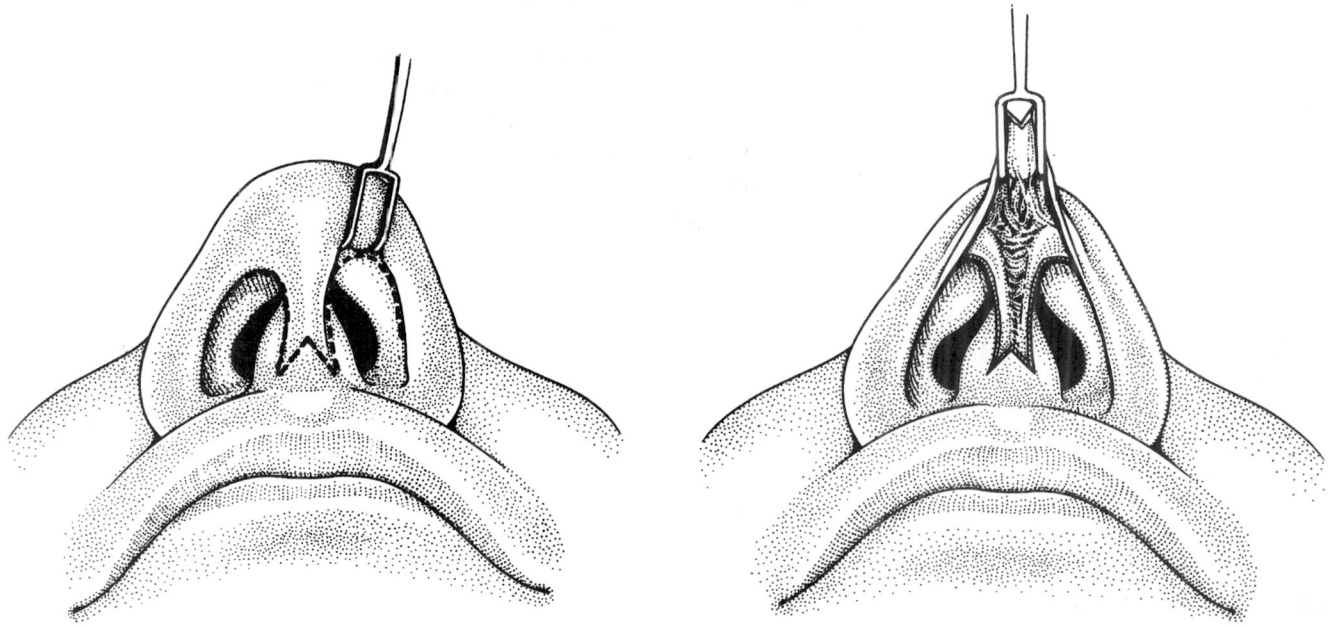

FIGURE 20–12   Surgical technique of external rhinoplasty.

5. To prevent or control infection or the formation of a hematoma, blood is suctioned from the nose, and the wound is cleansed. A drainage port is often made in the mucoperichondrial flap to allow for drainage.
6. The cartilage and bones are molded into proper position. The hemitransfixion incision is sutured with absorbable suture. Dressings with a pressure splint are applied. A moustache dressing and ice packs to the nose may be applied as previously described. The head of the

bed should be elevated postoperatively. Iced gauze may be applied to the eyes to reduce postoperative bruising and swelling according to the surgeon's preference.

Repair of Nasal Fracture

The nose is the structure most susceptible to trauma because it is seated midface. The paired nasal bones are thin and project like a tent on the frontal process of the maxilla. If the trauma is caused by a direct frontal blow, usually both

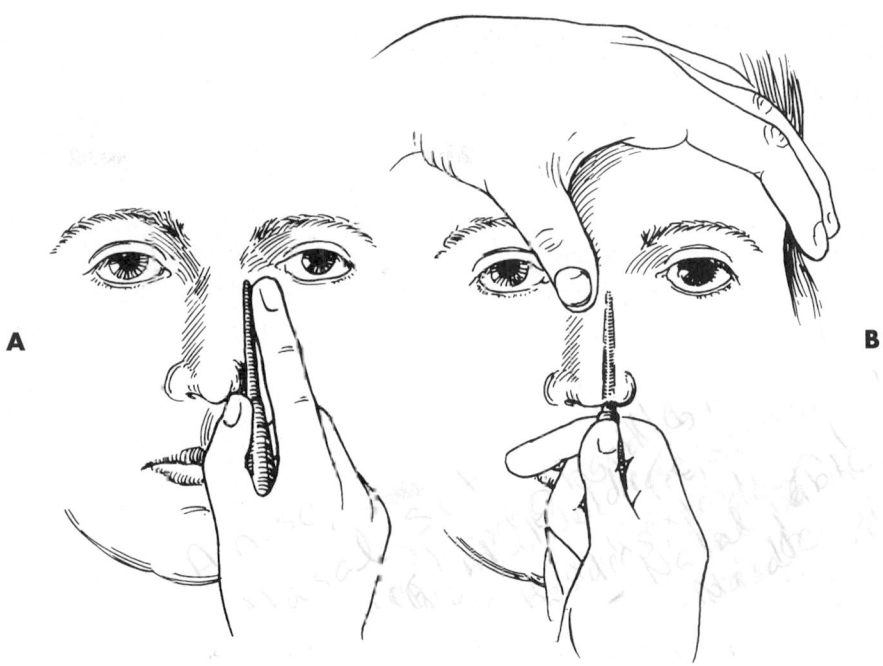

FIGURE 20-13   Reduction of nasal fracture. **A,** Boies elevator is placed along lateral wall of nose to point below nasofrontal angle. Distance to ala is marked with thumb. **B,** Elevator is then placed under depressed nasal bone, lifting it into position; opposite thumb carefully exerts downward pressure on elevated contralateral bone.

nasal bones are fractured, displaced outward, and depressed into the ethmoid sinus (see Fig. 20-3). The septal cartilages are displaced.[1]

Procedural considerations

Repair of nasal fractures can be performed in either an outpatient or inpatient setting. Simple nasal fractures can be managed with topical and local anesthesia (see pp. 732-733). However, as with most nasal procedures, if the patient has significant anxiety, general anesthesia may be necessary. Topical and local anesthetics should be used even with a general anesthetic to provide vasoconstriction and enhance visualization for the procedure. The patient is prepped and positioned for nasal surgery.

Operative procedure

1. The nose is packed with nasal cottonoids saturated with a hemostatic agent, and then a local anesthetic may be injected. When epinephrine is used, 10 minutes is the optimum time to wait for the effects of the hemostatic agent. This period of time will vary with other agents.
2. A Boies elevator is inserted into the nostril, and the nasal bones are elevated and molded into place by external manipulation (Fig. 20-13).
3. Nasal packing or intranasal splints may be used to stabilize the reduction because sometimes the bony fragments tend to return to a depressed status.

Treatment of Epistaxis

Patients with nasal bleeding usually control the problem themselves with direct pressure application. When their own efforts fail, they seek help from their own physician or an emergency department. When more conservative measures taken in the emergency department fail (which involve vasoconstrictive agents and nasal packing), it becomes necessary for surgical intervention. Most epistaxis can be treated with cautery or packing, but occasionally ligation of the ethmoid, carotid, or maxillary artery is necessary. Each patient's case must be considered individually when choosing a treatment plan.[1]

The basic actions to achieve proper visualization apply: the use of a headlight by the surgeon, suction to clear the operative field, and nasal specula to facilitate the initial examination. The application of a hemostatic agent is valuable because cautery is often used to coagulate the problematic vessel. The vasoconstrictive properties of hemostatic agents diminish blood flow and make the cautery more effective. A topical agent should be considered depending on the anesthetic choice. Various types of packing can be used according to the surgeon's preference. The packing may be 1-inch gauze impregnated with antibiotic ointment, commercially manufactured nasal packing, or Foley catheters with the balloon inflated. The packing is placed directly against the bleeding site. Posterior nasal packing is accomplished when a red rubber catheter is pulled through the oral cavity with a Kelly clamp. The strings of the posterior pack, which has been coated with antibiotic ointment, are attached to the catheter. The catheter is withdrawn through the nose to position the pack in the nasal pharynx. Anterior nasal packing is placed into both nares. The posterior plug is untied from the catheter and tied over a tonsil sponge to secure the packing.[5]

20-2   RESEARCH HIGHLIGHT

This prospective clinical study conducted at Harvard Medical School in Boston, Massachusetts, looked at pain in patients who had endoscopic sinus surgery for sinusitis. It looked at relief of preoperative pain and new pain in the postoperative period. Two hundred fifty-two patients who underwent endoscopic sinus surgery presenting with inflammatory disorders and meeting specific criteria were studied at 6- and 12-month intervals. The results indicated that the application of consistent definitions and clinical criteria for various forms of surgically treatable sinusitis will more likely allow prediction of improvement of pain and discomfort after surgical treatment. The study speaks to the negligible risk of developing new pain after surgery. The future implications from this study include improved and more predictable pain management in patients with sinus disease.

From Acquadro, M.A., Salman, S.D., & Joseph, M.P. (1997). Analysis of pain and endoscopic sinus surgery. *Annals of Otology, Rhinology, and Laryngology, 106*(4), 305-309.

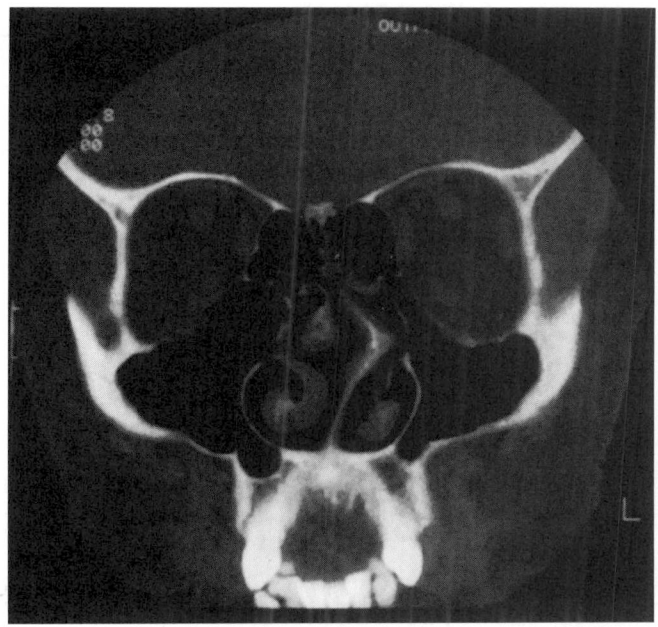

FIGURE 20-14   CT scan of maxillary and ethmoid sinuses. Notice septal deviation, maxillary sinus ostia, turbinates, and ocular muscles.

SINUS SURGERY

Medical management of acute sinusitis involves a course of appropriate antibiotic therapy. If a patient does not respond to medical treatment and the symptoms persist, surgical drainage of the sinuses is necessary. Sinus procedures can be performed intranasally with or without the aid of endoscopes and video or through an open approach determined by which sinus cavity is involved.

The field of endoscopic sinus surgery is expanding as surgeons' experience with it increases along with improvement in technology and instrumentation available. Procedures performed endoscopically decrease trauma to normal structures and reduce morbidity. Less trauma means a reduced healing process for the patient. Many procedures once done with an open approach can now be performed endoscopically and are considered safer because they are performed under direct visualization by means of an endoscope (Research Highlight 20-2).

The following sections will be discussed with the understanding that they are more commonly performed endoscopically but may be done with an open approach as necessary.

Endoscopic Sinus Surgery

Endoscopic sinus surgery involves the endoscopic resection of inflammatory and anatomic defects of the sinuses. It is considered to be technically demanding surgery, and these techniques vary significantly.[1] It is also referred to as *functional endoscopic sinus surgery* (FESS) because it provides a more physiologically type of drainage by reducing trauma to normal tissues. It is performed using direct endoscopic visualization. Many surgeons prefer the endoscope to be attached to a video monitor as in many other endoscopic procedures, but some may still prefer to look directly through the eyepiece. The operative instruments are introduced into the nose alongside the endoscope.

The purpose of endoscopic sinus surgery is to ensure adequate ventilation and restore mucociliary clearance in the sinuses. If there is contact between the mucosa and the sinus, mucociliary clearance is inhibited and secretions are retained in the sinus. This predisposes the patient to sinus infections.

Sinusitis can be either recurrent acute or chronic. Chronic sinusitis can be caused by anatomic deformities that require correction. Often the patient will first require a septoplasty to correct a deviated septum and allow access to the sinuses. Chronic sinusitis can also be caused by an allergy history, and contributing factors may include immunologic abnormalities, fluctuations in hormones, and environmental factors. Patients who are considered candidates for endoscopic sinus surgery undergo an office endoscopic examination preoperatively when none of the sinus cavities is opened. Patients also must have a preoperative CT scan to determine the areas affected by the sinusitis. These CT scans should be available in the OR and will be referred to by the surgeon during the surgery (Fig. 20-14). A clinical pathway and a patient handout for endoscopic sinus surgery are found in Figs. 20-15 and 20-16.

VANDERBILT UNIVERSITY MEDICAL CENTER

Endoscopic Sinus Surgery
(Pediatric and Adult)

Includes:
- Spheniodotomy
- Ethmoidectomy
- Polypectomy
- Sphenoid-ethmoidectomy
- Nasopharynx Biopsy
- Frontal Sinus Trephination
- Antrostomy
- Septoplasty
- Caldwell Luc
- Endoscopic Frontal Sinusotomy
- Turbinectomy

DRG Number: _____

ELOS: ___SAS or ERR___

	Preop	Day of Operation (HR → OR)	Day of Operation (PACU/ERR)	Follow-up Clinic POD #1	Follow-up Clinic 1-2 Weeks Postop
Goals:	Preop evaluation completed Pt. teaching completed Pt./family know where to go for surgery Signed consent form in preop packet	Lab results in chart Pt to holding room on time CT w/MD to OR PT tolerates operation w/o complications	D/C from VUH in <24° when meet criteria: • Taking PO well • No fever • Stable vital signs • Minimal bleeding • No other complications • Follow-up appointment scheduled • Home care instructions complete	No complications from procedure	No complications from procedure Improved sleeping and breathing patterns
Assessment and Evaluation	Ck for ASA and Ibuprofen use Ck for H/O easy bruising/bleeding	Nursing assessment Preop H&P reviewed by surgeon/resident; attending note completed		Interval history	Interval history Physical exam
Treatments		IV ————————————→	VS per routine Change drip pad prn Vision √, pupil √, q hr. × 4, then q4° √ for periorbital swelling/edema q1° × 4, then q4° Elevate HOB 45-60° Ice pack to cheeks (Caldwell Luc)	Remove nasal packing	Week #1 Remove frontal sinus stent Week #1 & #2 Cleanse sinus openings
Activity	Ad lib				
Diet	NPO after MN night before surgery (adults and children); infants - per MD	NPO	Sips → Full liquids as tolerated		
Tests & Labs:	Per anesthesia: • lab work • ECG • CKR Sinus CT: coronal or axial	Bacterial and/or fungal culture			Week #1 CK pathology reports CK culture reports

Meds/IV		In Holding Room:
		• Premed per anesthesia
		• IV D5LR (adult)
		• Order perioperative medications
		• Afrin (generic) nasal spray
		–2 sprays in each nostril
		→ to go home with patient/family
		In OR post induction:
		• IV (pediatric)
		at maintenance + deficit replacement per anesthesia
		• Decadron 20 mg IV (outpt only)
		• Cocaine (adults):
		Dilute 5 cc 4% with 5 ml of NS
		→ topical administration per MD
		• Neo-Synephrine (Pediatrics) ½% nasal spray
		• 1% lidocaine w/ Epi: 1:100,000- DO NOT OPEN UNTIL SURGEON IN ROOM
		• Ancef (IV) or Cleocin if PCN allergic
		• Bactroban topical ointment
			If ERP:
			PCA analgesia
			Home medications:
			Afrin spray (same bottle used in HR)
			Prescription for:
			- Pain med (PO) × 2
			  - 1 for severe pain
			  - 1 for moderate pain
			- Antibiotic (PO) × 10 days ——→
					Adjust antibiotic according to culture report

Consultations	Anesthesia				
Teaching/ D/C Plan	Per physician: Procedure Risks/benefits Postop care Follow-up care Per surgery schedule: Precertification complete Surgery date set Call family 2 days preop to review plan Per clinic nurse: Give patient: • Procedure specific information sheet • "After endoscopic surgery" sheet • List of aspirin products to avoid		Schedule RTC appointment for packing remove (if pt. is SAS) Give pt. procedure specific F/U sheet Verify w/pt. previously scheduled F/U clinic appointments for wks 1 & 2	Review discharge instructions	Copy of operative report given to & reviewed with patient
Equipment and Supplies		Endoscopic sinus surgery preference card			

Discharge Instructions
1. Elevate HOB
2. Use humidifier or NaCl spray
3. Change drip pad prn
4. Avoid blowing nose-sniff instead
5. Sneeze with mouth open
6. Presence of packing 24-48°
7. Avoid straining, lifting, strenuous exercise × 1 week
8. Avoid ASA & NSAIDS 2 weeks Postop
9. Take pain med before packing removal
10. Avoid smoking and noxious fumes
11. May have temporary fatigue after surgery
12. Avoid nasal trauma
Notify physician of:
- Temp. >101
- Severe pain not relieved by medication
- Large amount of bleeding

© 1996 Vanderbilt University Medical Center. All Rights Reserved.

FIGURE 20-15   Clinical pathway for endoscopic sinus surgery (adult and pediatric).

Notice to Patient:
Keep in mind that each person undergoing surgery may have different outcomes. This plan is modeled after an "average" case with cost efficiency and quality of care as a priority. Your actual length-of-stay or progress may vary.

VANDERBILT UNIVERSITY MEDICAL CENTER

Patient Handout

Path Name: Endoscopic Sinus Surgery (Pediatric and Adult)

Includes:
- Sphenoidectomy
- Ethmoidectomy
- Polypectomy
- Sphenoid-ethmoidectomy
- Nasopharynx Biopsy
- Frontal Sinus Trephination
- Antrostomy

Expected length of stay: __24 hours__

	Before Operation	Day of Operation	After Operation Until Next Morning	Follow-up at Clinic	Follow-up at Clinic
Goals:	Complete questionnaire Complete all labs & tests within 30 days of operation Find out when & where to go for surgery	Consent given & form signed All lab work done Operation done w/o complications	Drinking plenty of fluids Very little bleeding All teaching completed & understood	Return to clinic in a couple of days	Return to clinic in a couple of weeks Improved breathing and sleeping pattern
Tests & Labs:	Blood drawn for essential elements such as potassium Glucose tests, blood count, bleeding times Chest X-ray & ECG (heart tracing) CAT scan-sinus	During surgery, samples taken from nose to check for infection			
Treatments	Sign consent form	IV started	Your vital signs will be monitored Pad on nose changed as needed Nurse will check vision & pupils often	Nasal packing removed	Doctor will check your nose
Diet	As desired - nothing to eat past midnight	After you awaken, start with sips	Clear (broth, Jell-O) and progress as tolerated		
Activity	As desired		Head of bed raised high You can get up and move around as tolerated		
Consultations	Anesthesia dept. will check your heart & lungs				
Meds/IV		IV fluids IV antibiotics } → IV removed Pain medication → Antibiotic ointment Afrin nasal spray → You may take home Ocean spray → Take home and use for humidity			
Teaching/ D/C Plan	Doctor will talk with you about operation Clinic RN will give you handout & talk with you about precautions		Nurses will give you a handout: "Home Care Instructions Following Sinus Surgery"		

Discharge Instructions:
1. Elevate head of bed
2. Use humidifier or salt water spray
3. Change drip pad as needed
4. Avoid blowing nose-sniff instead
5. Sneeze with mouth open
6. Avoid straining, lifting, strenuous exercise for 1 week, sexual activity for 72 hrs
7. Avoid aspirin, Advil, Motrin, Ibuprofen 2 weeks after surgery
8. Take pain med before packing removal
9. Avoid smoking and noxious fumes
10. May have temporary tiredness after surgery
11. Avoid nasal injury

Notify Physician of:
- Temp. greater than 101 degrees F
- Severe pain not relieved by medication
- Large amount of bleeding (more than 30 min)

© 1996 Vanderbilt University Medical Center. All rights reserved.

FIGURE 20–16   Patient handout for endoscopic sinus surgery (adult and pediatric).

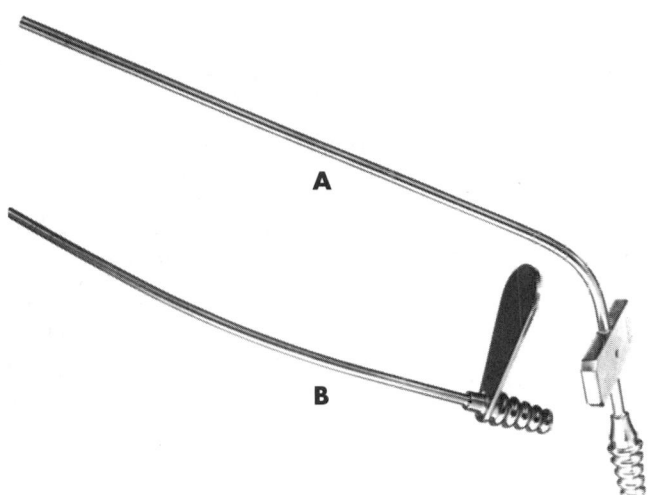

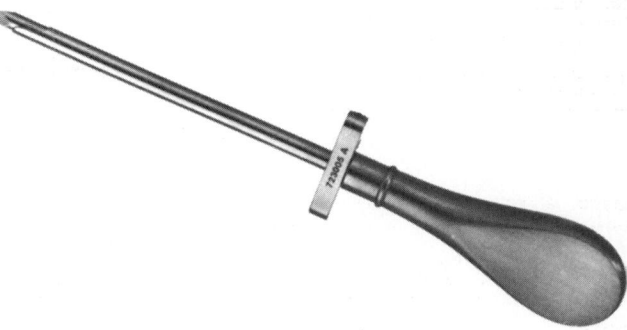

FIGURE 20-19 Maxillary sinus trocar used for performing maxillary sinus endoscopy through canine fossa (and in exceptional cases through inferior meatus).

FIGURE 20-17 Most commonly used suction tips. **A**, Angled surgical suction tip with small hole in handle so that surgeon can control force of suction with fingertip. Its primary use is in diagnostic and surgical sinus procedures. Newer suction tips have centimeter scale etched along shaft, so that approximate position of tip can be estimated, as from anterior nasal spine. **B**, Bent nasal suction tip is used primarily to remove secretions and crusts postoperatively.

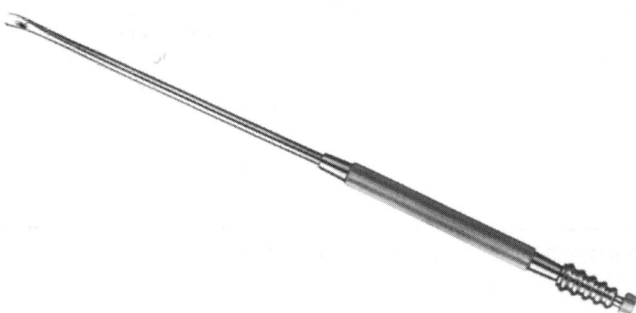

FIGURE 20-20 Freer type of suction elevator. It is most commonly used in diagnostic endoscopy for careful displacement of middle turbinate, when endoscope must be introduced into nasal passages. Suction hole in tip of this elevator permits simultaneous removal of secretions and thus eliminates need to switch back and forth between Freer elevator and suction tip.

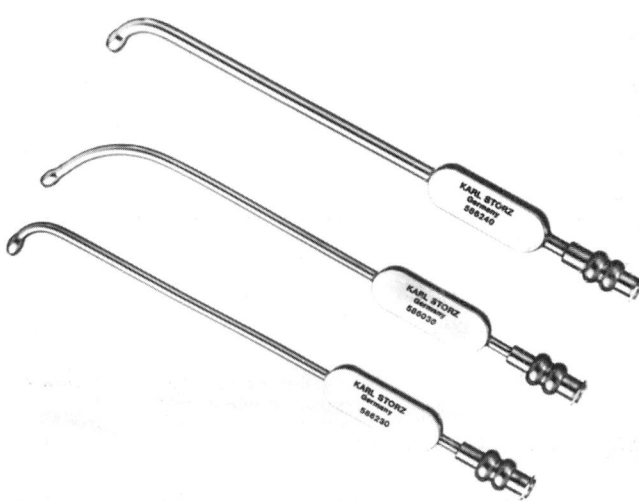

FIGURE 20-18 Set of angled suction tips of different sizes and shapes. These suction tips are used primarily for removing secretions form maxillary sinus and from middle meatus. Frequently fungal masses can also be removed by suction. Thin instruments are useful primarily when frontal recess must be entered from below far anterior insertion of middle turbinate.

Procedural considerations

The endoscopic sinus surgery instruments enable the physician to view the patient's anatomy as well as to remove diseased or problematic tissues that are interfering with the sinus cavity functioning and drainage processes. The surgery can be performed under general anesthesia or

MAC as with other nasal procedures, depending on the surgeon and patient's preference.

The endoscopes used in sinus surgery are much like endoscopes used in other procedures and have different directions of view that vary between 0, 30, 70, 90, and 120 degrees. Depending on which sinus the surgeon is planning on working in, the appropriate lens will be requested. Often if there is work to be done in several sinus cavities, the surgeon may change lenses intraoperatively.

The setup for endoscopic sinus surgery is the same as the setup for nasal surgery in terms of prepping, draping, and positioning. The instruments required are the basic nasal set (that is, septoplasty kit), video equipment including monitor, and light source with the appropriate light cord adapted to the type of endoscope used. In addition to endoscopes, other instruments that may be used in endoscopic sinus surgery are represented in Figs. 20-17 to 20-33 along with a description of their use.

The room setup is like that for any nasal case and includes the video equipment, which is located at the head

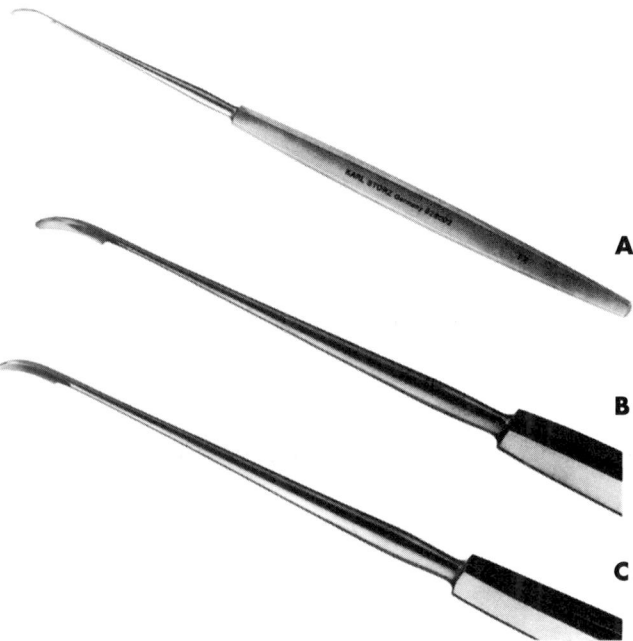

FIGURE 20-21   **A**, Sickle scalpel (curved blade); available in rounded (**B**) and pointed (**C**) forms. Sickle-shaped scalpel is used for initial resection of uncinate process, opening of concha bullosa, and for splitting mucosa for removal of septal spurs or ridges.

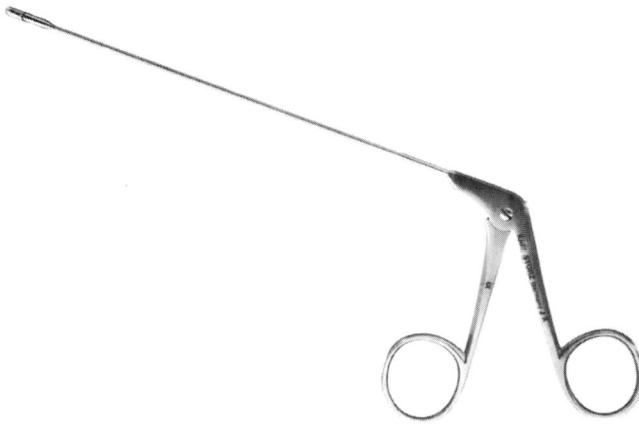

FIGURE 20-22   Delicate biopsy forceps used in removal of small cysts or polyps and for biopsy through trocar sheath from maxillary sinus.

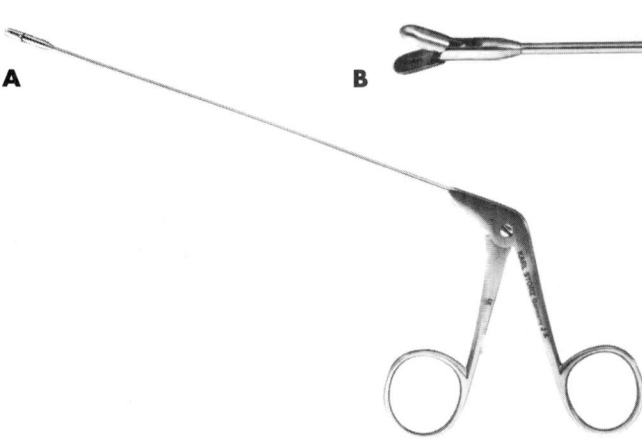

FIGURE 20-23   **A**, Biopsy forceps to be used through trocar sheath. **B**, Close-up view of forceps mouth.

of the bed. The surgeon operates from the right side of the patient and may sit during the procedure. If so, the surgeon's legs must be able to fit under the OR bed at the level of the patient's neck. He or she may rest his or her elbows on the armrest of the chair or on a table placed nearby to prevent fatigue.

Instruments should be passed to the surgeon in the closed position and never over the patient's face to avoid possible injury. They should be passed smoothly and carefully so that the surgeon's eyes do not leave the endoscope or video monitor and to limit distractions.[6] Some surgeons will request to perform this surgery with a suction-irrigation device that provides visualization of the sinus recesses.

An antifog solution is used to treat the lens as in other endoscopic procedures. The solution should not be wiped off the lens but left on in a thin layer.

Another consideration that is crucial to a successful outcome in endoscopic sinus surgery is to maintain the integrity of the patient's periorbital cavities. Especially if the procedure is performed under general anesthesia, the patient's eyes must be visible to the surgeon at all times to allow for the recognition of injury to the orbit. A lubricant is placed in the patient's eyes to protect the corneas. The surgeon will monitor for movement of the eyeball or appearance of an intraorbital hematoma. If the patient is awake, pain will be experienced in the eye region.

Encroachment of the orbit can be recognized when any tissue that is yellow can be identified because orbital fat is yellow in color. This finding should be communicated immediately to the surgeon. Another good technique is for the scrub person to place all tissue removed by the surgeon into a small container of normal saline or lactated Ringer's solution on the surgical field. If any of the tissue "floats," the surgeon should be notified immediately. The surgeon will check to see if a small air bubble is caught in the tissue causing it to float by pushing it with an instrument and turning it over a few times to release any air and allowing it to sink to the bottom of the container. Any tissue that floats naturally is fat or brain tissue.[6]

Operative procedure

1. The surgeon will apply topical anesthetics and hemostatic agents as with any nasal surgery.
2. The lens of the endoscope requested by the surgeon is treated with antifog solution before the endoscope is introduced into the nose.

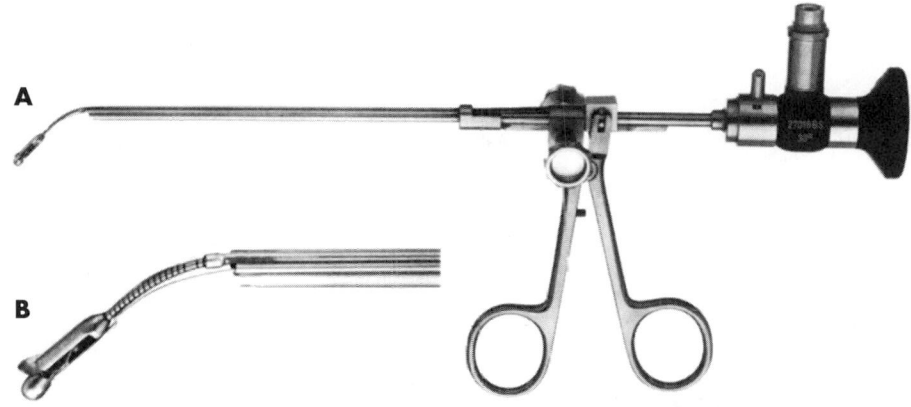

FIGURE 20–24 **A**, Optical biopsy forceps with 2.7 mm, 30-degree endoscope, with larger view (**B**). For insertion through trocar sheath, flexible part of forceps is maximally retracted. After insertion, flexible forceps can be advanced gradually downward into visual field of 30-degree lens.

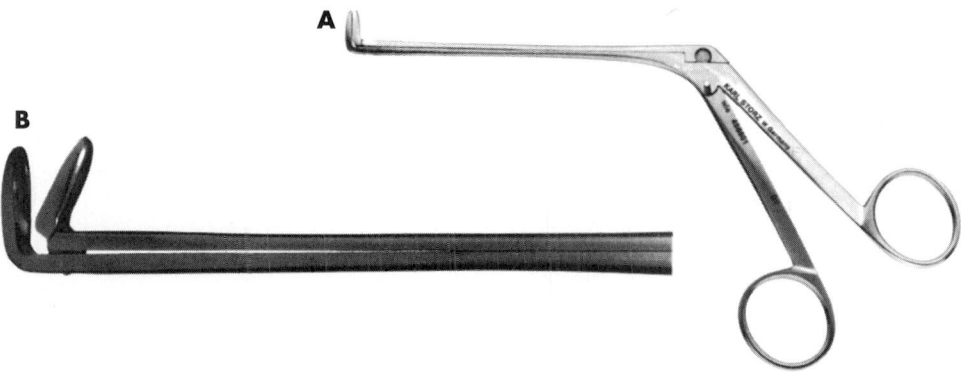

FIGURE 20–25 **A**, Blakesley-Weil forceps. Jaws flex at right angle. **B**, Jaws, which are shown in detail, are also available in 4 mm longer version. Forceps are used to prepare roof of ethmoid or for work in frontal recess and in maxillary sinus, through enlarged ostium.

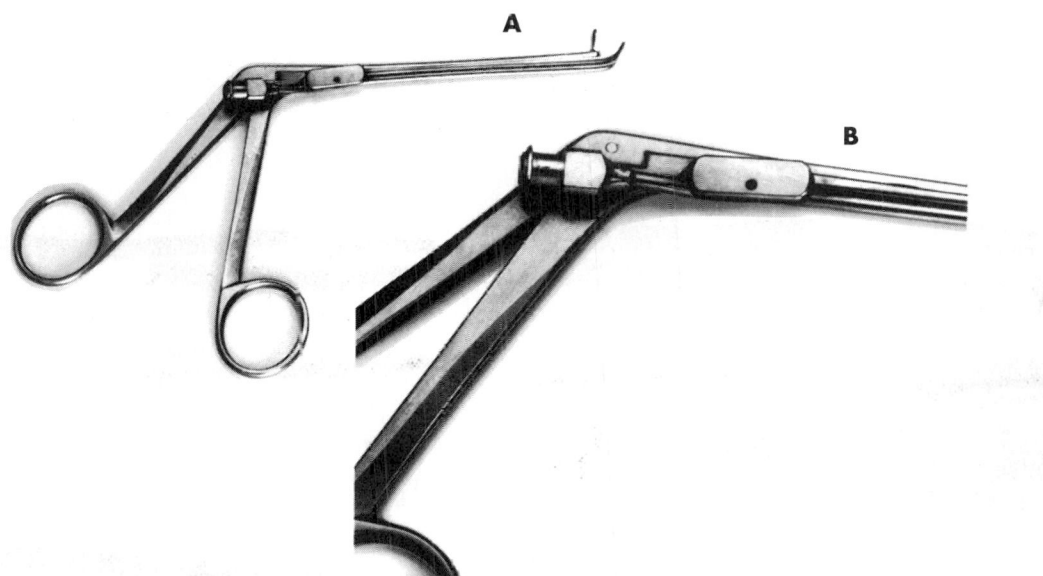

FIGURE 20–26 **A**, Flexed Blakesley-Weil forceps with built-in suction channel. Suction can be regulated with finger. **B**, Close-up view.

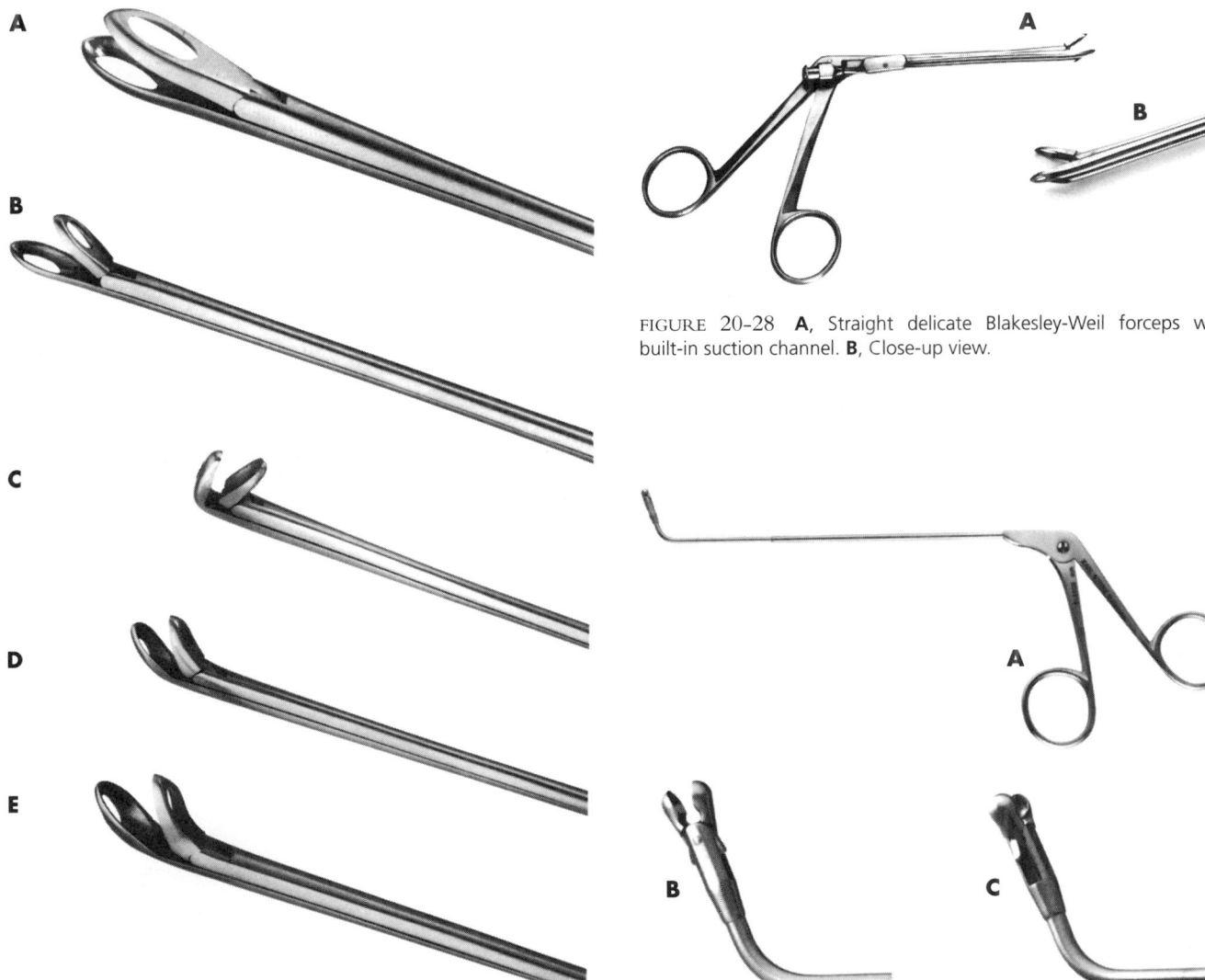

FIGURE 20-28 **A**, Straight delicate Blakesley-Weil forceps with built-in suction channel. **B**, Close-up view.

FIGURE 20-27 Blakesley-Weil forceps (**A**) is available in variety of sizes and shapes. Most procedures are performed with delicate Blakesley-Weil forceps in its straight form (**B**) and in its flexed form (**D** and **E**). Large form (**C**) is used very rarely, as in cases of excessive polyposis, when all finer bony structures have been destroyed by chronic inflammation or by pressure from polyps. This instrument is too large for most other purposes.

FIGURE 20-29 **A**, Upward bent, delicate forceps. **B**, Jaws close longitudinally. **C**, Jaws close crosswise. These forceps are useful for manipulations in frontal recess in combination with 30- or 70-degree lenses. They are also suitable for manipulations in maxillary sinus, such as removal of small polyps or opening of cysts through natural ostium.

3. The natural ostium of the maxillary sinus is enlarged to provide physiologic drainage through the middle meatus (see Fig. 20-3).
4. The diseased tissue is visualized through the endoscope. Straight or angled forceps may be used to remove only the diseased tissue (Fig. 20-34).
5. If an anterior ethmoidectomy is indicated, the endoscope is inserted through the middle meatus and into the frontal recess, and the ethmoidectomy is performed.
6. Because of the small incision made, no sutures are required.
7. Absorbable gelatin film splints may be placed into the patient's middle meatus to maintain patency and reduce

stenosis. It is rolled into a cylindrical splint and set in place with bayonet forceps. An antibiotic ointment may be applied to the splint first according to the surgeon's preference.
8. A moustache dressing is applied.

Computer-Assisted Endoscopic Sinus Surgery

Before the introduction of computer-assisted endoscopic sinus surgery, surgeons could rely only on direct visualization of the actual operative field, which they must combine with their previous surgical experience and their own ability to mentally translate data from the patient's

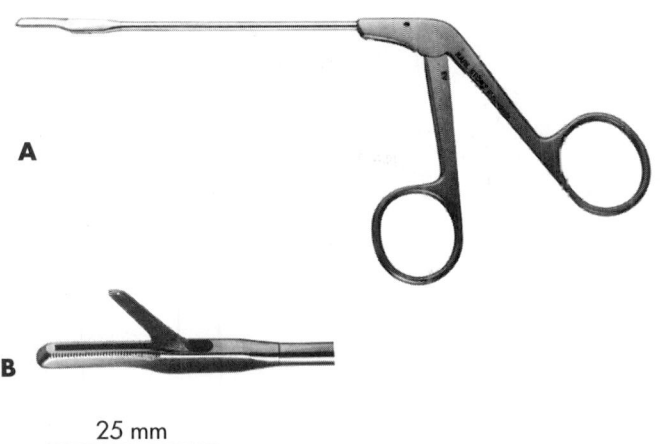

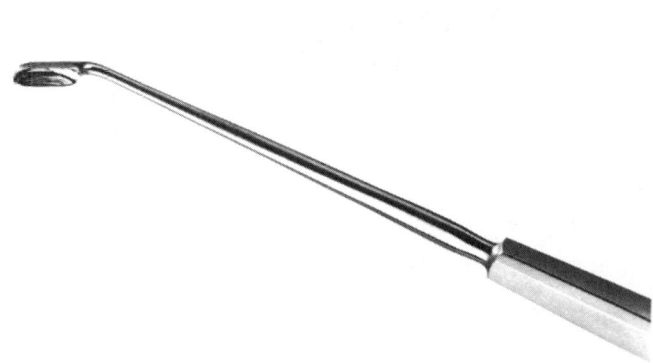

FIGURE 20-30 **A,** Struycken modified nasal cutting forceps. Jaws are considerably more delicate than those in Struycken's original model but still strong. They are useful for opening concha bullosa, cutting fibrous bands, septal spurs, and ridges. **B,** Close-up view of jaws.

FIGURE 20-32 Bent spoon is instrument of general usefulness available in two sizes. Not only is it used for locating and enlarging ostium of maxillary sinus, but it is also excellent in palpating resistances. It is also used for carefully removing fine bony lamellae in search of ostium of frontal sinus and for perforating anterior wall of sphenoid sinus.

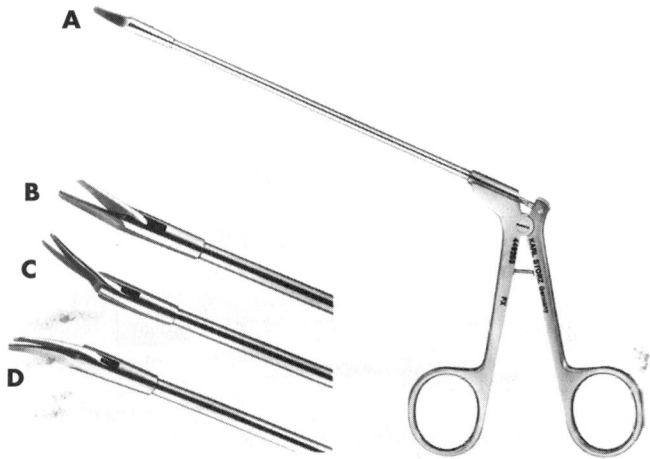

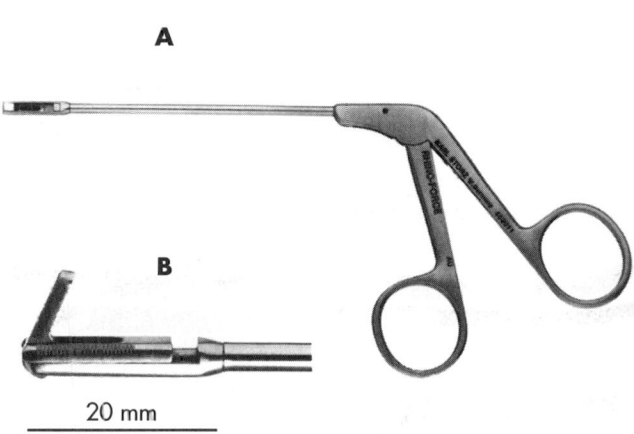

FIGURE 20-31 **A,** Set of scissors for endoscopic use. **B,** Straight jaws angled to right (**C**) and to left (**D**). This set of scissors is useful for opening concha bullosa, resecting stalks of coarse single or recurrent polyps, and cutting fibrous strands and synechiae.

FIGURE 20-33 **A,** Stammberger-Ostrum backward-cutting antrum punch. **B,** Close-up view of jaws. These back-biting forceps are available in two models (sideward cutting to right and left). They are used for enlargement of ostium of maxillary sinus at expense of anterior fontaneiles and for retrograde resection of uncinate process.

two-dimensional CT scan to determine their location in the patient's sinuses.[7] Computer-assisted endoscopic sinus surgery combines the use of computerized planning tools and intraoperative navigation systems with endoscopic techniques to ensure the goal of safe surgery for patients.[3] The operative field is more clearly defined and the patient's risk of surgical complications is reduced compared with such surgery without a computer. It is especially useful in revision sinus surgery where the familiar anatomy of the sinuses has been altered by previous surgery.

Microdebriders

The recent introduction of powered instrumentation in functional endoscopic sinus surgery has further enhanced this highly effective surgical treatment of chronic sinusitis. The microdebrider is a powered instrument that functions much like an arthroscopic joint shaver but is smaller.[2] It consists of a powered rotary shaving device whose mechanism is to pull tissue (whether it be blood, bone, soft tissue, or irrigation) through a small window by means of suction and then remove the tissue with internal rotating blades. The tissue is removed through the suction tubing;

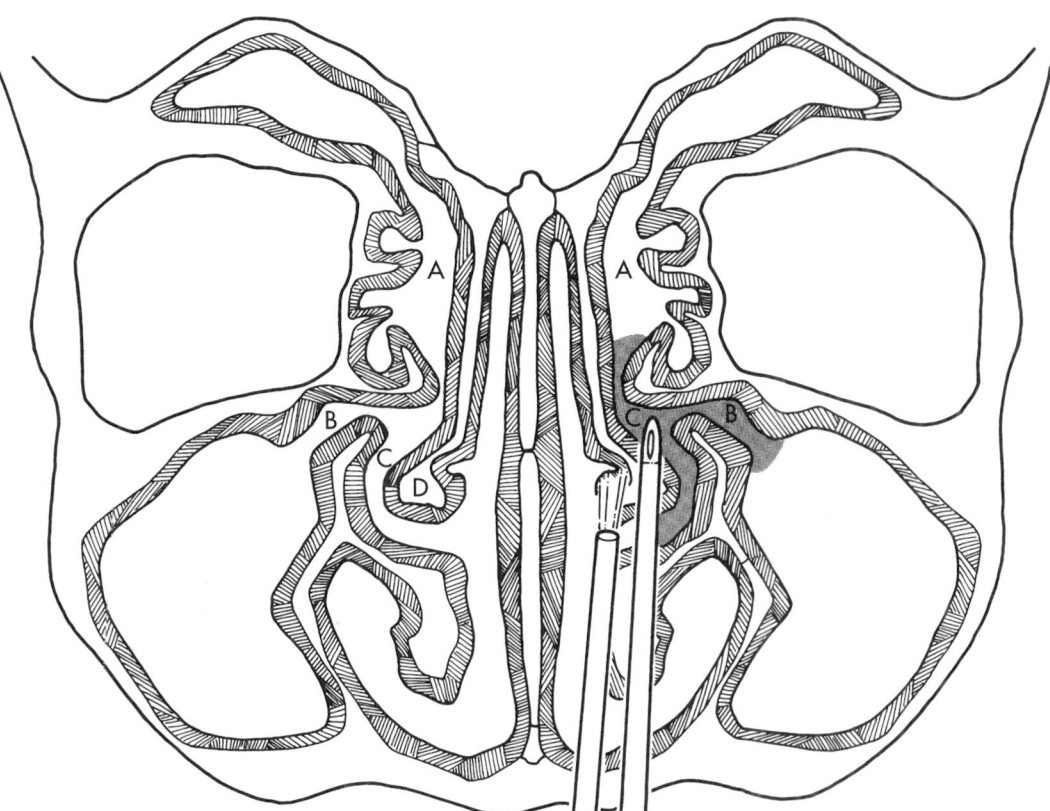

FIGURE 20–34   Surgery is performed using endoscope and forceps by intranasal approach. Diseased tissue is being removed from shaded areas depicting ethmoid sinus area (**A**), maxillary sinus ostia (**B**), and middle meatus (**C**). **D**, Middle turbinate is unaffected.

therefore the working instrument does not have to be removed from the operative field to clear the tissue. Many models of microdebriders have continuous irrigation lines that help decrease clogging of the lines.

Microdebriders facilitate greater precision of the surgeon by increasing the visual field. The patient's postoperative recovery time is shortened because there is decreased trauma to the tissues because bleeding is reduced.[7]

Powered instrumentation was initially developed for soft-tissue resection and polypectomies, but as otolaryngologists increase their experience with them, their use is broadening. Microdebriders can now be used in extensive bony dissection of the sinuses. They can be used in various sinus procedures including ethmoidectomy, maxillary antrostomy, sphenoidotomy, and frontal recess dissections.[7]

Several rhinologic and sinus procedures may be accomplished by either internal (with or without endoscopic assistance) or external approaches. The following procedures fit into this category.

Frontal Sinus Trephination

Frontal sinus trephination is the creation of a hole in the frontal sinus to drain pus or fluid accumulation. It is performed to treat the symptoms of frontal sinusitis, which may include fever and headaches. A catheter may be surgically sewn into place at the incision site of the opening made into the affected frontal sinus to act as a drain and medium with which to irrigate the sinus until the disease resolves.[1]

Procedural considerations

The patient's face is prepped according to surgeon's preference. The head is draped as in nasal procedures. Local anesthesia may be injected in the skin under the eyebrow.

Operative procedure

1. The incision is made medially below the eyebrow, along the same contour of the brow (Fig. 20-35).
2. The periosteum is elevated from the bone, and a small diamond or cutting burr is used to drill a hole into the sinus.
3. Cultures may be taken of any pus present in the sinus followed by irrigation.
4. A large Silastic or Teflon tube or appropriate-sized catheter may be placed through the incision into the sinus.

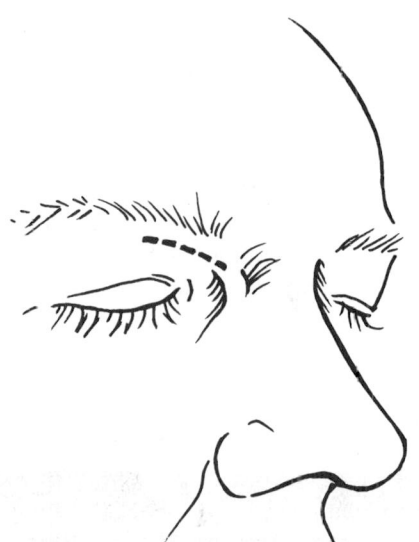

FIGURE 20-35 Incision to expose ethmoidal and frontal sinuses. Resulting scar is almost invisible.

5. The incision is closed with suture of the surgeon's preference.
6. A small dressing is usually applied to absorb drainage from the incision and catheter.

Frontal Sinus Operation (External Approach)

A frontal sinus operation involves the making of an incision through the anterior wall of the floor of the frontal sinus for removal of diseased tissue, cleansing of the sinus cavity, and drainage. In acute frontal sinusitis, patients suffer from persistent headaches and edema of the upper eyelid. As with other types of sinus problems, when medical management of these symptoms fails, surgical treatment may be indicated. Drainage of the frontal sinus may be achieved through a simple frontal sinus trephination alone. If chronic suppuration with repeated acute attacks of frontal sinusitis persist, further surgery may be performed to remove the diseased lining of the sinus and reconstruct the nasofrontal duct to provide the necessary drainage.

Procedural considerations

The setup is as for nasal surgery and includes some additional items such as a power saw with oscillating blade, frontal rasps, blunt nerve hook, straight fine Cushing forceps, Adson tissue forceps, dural hooks, and Raney clip appliers and clips.

The patient is given a general anesthetic. The surgical approach depends on the preference of the surgeon and the patient. If a coronal incision is to be made, the hair should be shaved from the hairline to slightly past the crown of the head. If a brow incision is to be made, no shaving is necessary. Fat may be harvested from the abdomen for subsequent use in obliterating the sinus space.

The patient's eyes are protected during the procedure, and the head and face are prepped according to the surgeon's preference.

Operative procedure

1a. When a coronal approach is used, the incision is made in the scalp skin from ear to ear, well behind the hairline. The edges of the skin are compressed by the application of Raney clips. The flap is reflected to expose the upper portion of the nose, thus exposing the anterior sinus.
1b. When a brow approach is used, the incision is made in the superior margin of the eyebrow or eyebrows, hemostasis is obtained, and the flap is elevated to expose the anterior sinus wall.
2. A template (steam-sterilized radiologic outline of the frontal sinus) is placed over the sinus and marked on the pericranium with a marking pen.
3. The pericranium is elevated.
4. An oscillating saw is used to cut through the overlying frontal sinus. An elevator may be used to free the bone from the sinus.
5. The mucosa of the sinus is removed in its entirety through the use of elevators and a drill.
6. Absorbable gelatin sponge or a fat graft taken from the abdomen is placed in the sinus to obliterate the space.
7. The bone flap is replaced, and the pericranium is repositioned and sutured.
8. The skin incision is closed with suture of the surgeon's preference.
9. A pressure dressing of elastic gauze is applied for 48 to 72 hours

Potential postoperative complications include osteomyelitis, meningitis, cerebrospinal fluid leak, abscess, and stenosis of the nasofrontal duct.

Ethmoidectomy

Ethmoid sinus surgery is usually performed to treat chronic inflammatory sinus disease or polyps that are caused by allergies. An ethmoidectomy is the removal of the diseased portion of the middle turbinate, ethmoid cells, and diseased tissue in the nasal fossa. It can be done by three approaches: intranasally, externally, or transantrally. As the field of endoscopic sinus surgery continues to advance, most surgeons will choose the endoscopic intranasal approach for reasons previously discussed. The purpose of an ethmoidectomy is to reduce the many-celled ethmoid labyrinth into one large cavity to ensure adequate drainage and aeration.

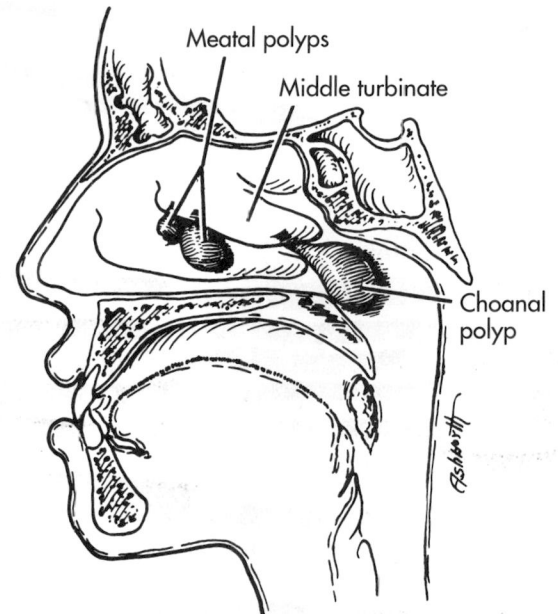

FIGURE 20-36 Nasal polyps. A choanal polyp is usually single and originates in maxillary sinus; however, most polyps are found in middle meatus.

Procedural considerations and operative procedure

The setup for the intranasal approach is the same as that for a nasal setup, which will most likely include endoscopic sinus equipment. The external approach is as described in frontal sinus trephination. The transantral approach is referenced in the Caldwell-Luc procedure.

Sphenoidotomy

A sphenoidotomy is the creation of an opening into one or both of the sphenoidal sinuses. It can be performed by either the intranasal route or through an external approach as described in the frontal sinus operation. Sphenoidotomies are often done with ethmoidectomies because once the ethmoid labyrinth is removed, the surgeon has excellent access to the sphenoids. Again, these procedures are now typically done endoscopically.

Procedural considerations and operative procedure

For the intranasal route the setup and operative procedure is as described for intranasal surgery often with endoscopic sinus equipment. Additional instruments that may be required are long sphenoid curettes, antrum rasps, and antrum punches. The external approach is as described for frontal sinus surgery.

Nasal Polypectomy

A nasal polypectomy is the removal of polyps from the nasal cavity (Fig. 20-36). The tissues become edematous, resulting in the formation of polyps that obstruct the free passage of air and make breathing difficult. Nasal polypectomies are often performed with other sinus procedures that also require removal of diseased tissue and particularly are done endoscopically.

Procedural considerations and operative procedure

Nasal polypectomy setup is as for any intranasal procedure, and the operative procedure is the same and often includes endoscopic equipment. Additional instruments may include a nasal polyp snare. Packing is according to the surgeon's preference.

Turbinectomy and Outfracture Cautery of Turbinates

Anterior inferior turbinectomy is removal of the anterior end of the inferior turbinate. *Inferior turbinectomy* is removal of the greater part of the lower border of the hypertrophied inferior turbinate. *Anterior middle turbinectomy* is removal of the anterior end of the middle turbinate body. In all cases turbinectomy may include removal of any existing nasal polyps. Turbinectomies are more often performed endoscopically with other sinus procedures.

Outfracture of the turbinates is similar to turbinectomy except that the turbinate is infractured and then outfractured by the use of a septal displacer or Boies elevator. A turbinate needle designed to deliver unipolar cautery may be used on the turbinate to reduce the potential for recurring hypertrophy. These procedures are performed to provide adequate ventilation and drainage as well as to relieve pressure against the floor of the nose.

Procedural considerations and operative procedure

Turbinectomies and outfracture cautery of turbinates require a nasal setup. The problematic portion of the turbinate is amputated and removed, polyps are removed as indicated, and cautery is applied to the turbinates after fracturing is completed.

Caldwell-Luc with Radical Antrostomy

The purpose of a radical antrostomy is to establish a large opening into the wall of the inferior meatus, which ensures adequate gravity drainage and aeration. This large opening allows removal of the diseased tissues in the sinuses under direct vision. This procedure requires an incision into the canine fossa of the upper jaw and exposure of the antrum for removal of bony diseased portions of the antral wall and contents of the sinus (Fig. 20-37).

As otolaryngologists increase their experience and skill level with endoscopic sinus surgery along with continued improvement in equipment and technologic advances, more radical procedures such as this are being replaced. Endoscopic sinus surgery can be used to treat patients suffering from chronic sinusitis with a decreased morbidity and a more physiologic type of drainage.

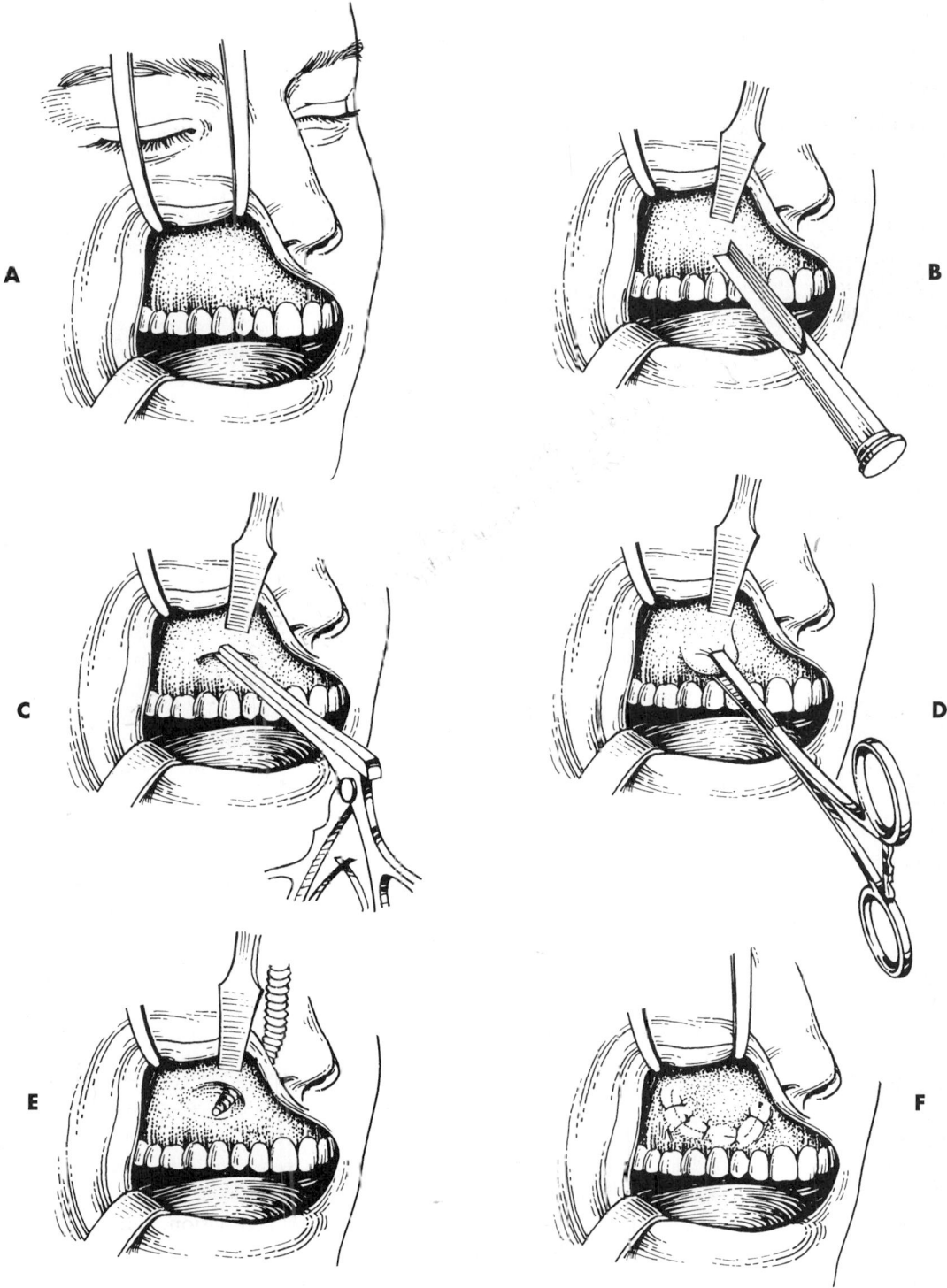

FIGURE 20-37   Caldwell-Luc operation. **A,** Incision. **B,** Flap retracted and perforation made in canine fossa. **C,** Perforation enlarged with Kerrison rongeur. **D,** Removal of diseased antral membrane. **E,** Rasp used to make nasoantral window. **F,** Incision closed.

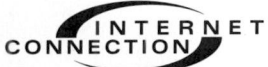

Society of Otorhinolaryngology and Head-Neck Nurses:
http://www.entnet.org

Society of Otorhinolaryngology:
http://www.bcm.tmc.edu/oto/SOHN

ENT Grand Rounds:
http://www.bcm.tmc.edu/cto/grand/grand.html

REFERENCES

1. Cummings, C.W., Frederickson, J.M., Harker, L.A., et al. (1997). *Otolaryngology head and neck surgery.* St. Louis: Mosby.

2. Krouse, H.J., Parker, C.M., Purcell, R., et al. (1997). Powered functional endoscopic sinus surgery. *AORN Journal, 66*(3), 405.

3. Petroff, P.F. (1997). Computer-assisted endoscopic sinus surgery. *AORN Journal, 66*(3), 416-420.

4. Rothrock, J.C. (1996). *Perioperative nursing care planning* (ed. 2). St. Louis: Mosby.

5. Sigler, B., & Schuring, L. (1993). *Ear, nose and throat disorders.* St. Louis: Mosby.

6. Stammberger, H., & Hawke, M. (1993). *Essentials of functional endoscopic sinus surgery.* St. Louis: Mosby.

7. Stankiewicz, J.A. (1996). *Advanced endoscopic sinus surgery.* St. Louis: Mosby.

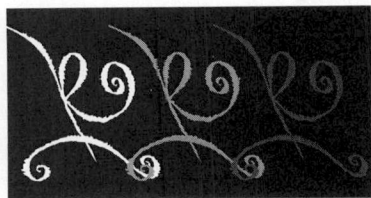

CHAPTER TWENTY ONE

Laryngologic and Head and Neck Surgery

Laurie A. Saletnik

PATIENTS UNDERGOING LARYNGOLOGIC or head and neck surgical procedures present a challenge to the perioperative nurse. These patients have physical as well as psychosocial needs. They may be experiencing upper airway insufficiency upon arrival in the operating room or have an altered airway postoperatively. Head and neck surgery patients must cope with an altered body image. Body image is associated with appearance and positive self-concept.[1,2] Postoperative bleeding can create feelings of panic and suffocation. The perioperative nurse must quickly assess, plan, and implement actions to ensure an adequate airway as well as reassure the patient, explain patient care interventions and expected outcomes, and assist patients and their families in identifying coping strategies.

These patients range from pediatric to geriatric; thus imagination and creativity are vital components of the perioperative nurse's armamentarium in assessing the patient's comprehension of the anticipated surgical procedure. Special considerations for pediatric patients are discussed in Chapter 29; the elderly surgical patient is discussed in Chapter 30.

SURGICAL ANATOMY

The throat includes the structures of the neck in front of the vertebral column; these are the mouth, tongue, pharynx, tonsils, larynx, and trachea.

Oral Cavity

The mouth is formed by the cheeks, hard and soft palates, and the tongue. It extends from the lips to the anterior pillars of the throat. The portion of the mouth outside the teeth is the buccal cavity, and that on the inner side of the teeth is the lingual cavity. The hard and soft palates form the upper and posterior boundaries of the oral cavity. The hard palate is formed by the maxilla and palatine bones. The soft palate is an arch-shaped muscular partition between the oropharynx and the nasopharynx. The soft palate emerges from the posterior border of the hard palate to form the uvula, a fingerlike movable projection. The uvula joins the base of the tongue anteriorly and the pharynx posteriorly.

Pharynx

The pharynx, extending from the posterior portion of the nose to the esophagus and larynx, serves as a channel for both the digestive and respiratory systems. Approximately 13 cm long, it lies anterior to the cervical vertebrae and posterior to the nasal and oral cavities. The food and air passages cross each other in the pharynx, a funnel-shaped structure, wider above and narrower below. It is composed of muscular and fibrous layers and is lined with mucous membrane. It is associated above with the sphenoidal sinus and the basilar part of the occipital bone, and it joins the esophagus below. Seven cavities communicate with the pharynx: the two nasal cavities, the two tympanic cavities, the mouth, the larynx, and the esophagus. Infection can spread from the pharynx to the middle ear through the eustachian tube. The pharynx comprises three groups of constrictor muscles (Fig. 21-1). Each muscle fits within the one below, and each inserts posteriorly in the median line with its mate from the opposite side. The constrictor muscles provide constriction of the pharynx for swallowing. Between the origins of the constrictor muscle groups are so-called intervals through which ligaments, nerves, and arteries pass. The recurrent laryngeal nerve is closely associated with the lower portion of the pharynx. The pharynx is divided anatomically into three sections: the nasopharynx, oropharynx, and hypopharynx.

Nasopharynx

The nasopharynx lies posterior to the nasal cavity and extends over the soft palate. It communicates with the oropharynx through the pharyngeal isthmus, which is closed by muscular action during swallowing.

Oropharynx

The oropharynx lies posterior to the oral cavity extending from the soft palate to the level of the hyoid bone.

Hypopharynx

The hypopharynx extends from the hyoid bone and empties into the esophagus posteriorly and the larynx anteriorly.

The tonsils are situated one on each side of the oropharynx, lodged in a tonsillar fossa that is attached to folds of membrane-containing muscle. One pair, the palatine tonsils (a pair of oval structures), are the only lymphatic organs covered with stratified squamous epithelium. These tonsils may become inflamed (tonsillitis). The lateral surface of each tonsil is usually covered with a fibrous capsule. The anterior and posterior tonsillar pillars join to form a triangular fossa, with the posterior lateral aspects of the tongue at its base. The lingual tonsils are lodged in each fossa. The adenoids or pharyngeal tonsils are suspended from the roof of the nasopharynx and consist of an accumulation of lymphoid tissue.

The arteries of the tonsils enter the upper and lower poles. The tonsils are supplied with blood by tonsillar branches of the ascending palatine branch of the facial artery (branch of the external carotid artery). The external carotid artery on each side lies behind and lateral to each tonsil. The nerves supplying the tonsils are derived from the middle and posterior palatine branches of the maxillary and glossopharyngeal nerves.

Larynx and Associated Structures

Larynx

The larynx lies in the midline of the neck and is supported by cartilage. It is situated between the trachea and the root of the tongue, at the upper front part of the neck. The location of the larynx between the GI and respiratory systems is strategic in protecting the airway during swallowing and breathing. The larynx has three main functions: as a passageway for air, as a valve for closing off air passages from the digestive system and the pharynx, and as a voice box on which sound and speech depend to a degree.

The larynx is a cartilaginous box situated in front of the fourth, fifth, and sixth cervical vertebrae. The upper portion of the larynx is continuous with the pharynx above, and its lower portion joins the trachea. The skeletal structure provides for patency of the enclosed airway. The complex muscle action and arrangement of tissues within

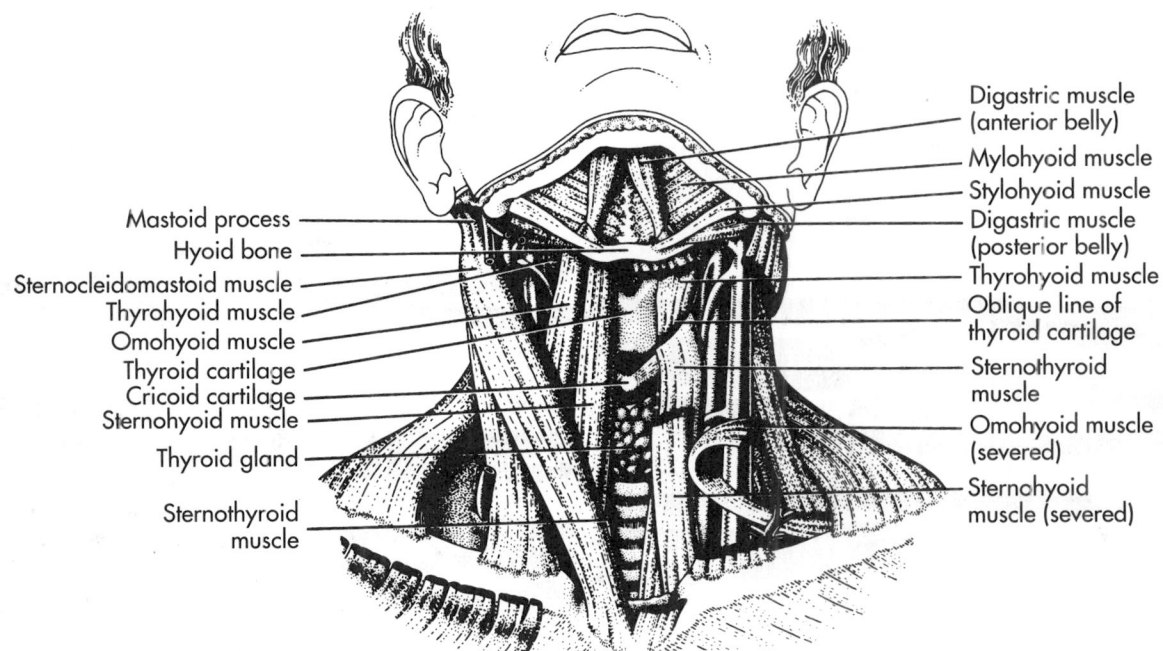

Mastoid process
Hyoid bone
Sternocleidomastoid muscle
Thyrohyoid muscle
Omohyoid muscle
Thyroid cartilage
Cricoid cartilage
Sternohyoid muscle
Thyroid gland
Sternothyroid muscle

Digastric muscle (anterior belly)
Mylohyoid muscle
Stylohyoid muscle
Digastric muscle (posterior belly)
Thyrohyoid muscle
Oblique line of thyroid cartilage
Sternothyroid muscle
Omohyoid muscle (severed)
Sternohyoid muscle (severed)

FIGURE 21-1 Extrinsic muscles of the larynx.

the structure provide for closure of the lumen for protection against trauma and entrance of foreign bodies and for speech.

Cartilages

The skeletal framework of the larynx consists of cartilages and membranes. Of the nine separate cartilages, three are single and six are arranged in pairs. The main cartilages of the larynx include the thyroid, cricoid, epiglottis, two arytenoid, two corniculate, and two cuneiform. The thyroid cartilage, or Adam's apple, forms the anterior portion of the voice box. The cricoid cartilage is a complete cartilaginous ring that resembles a signet ring and rests beneath the thyroid cartilage and supports the airway (Fig. 21-2). The epiglottis is a slightly curled, leaf-shaped, elastic fibrous membrane. It is prolonged below into a slender process, attached in the midline to the upper border of the thyroid cartilage. The epiglottis helps to protect the larynx during deglutition. When the cricothyroid muscle contracts, it pulls the thyroid cartilage and the cricoid cartilage, thereby tightening the vocal cords and, if unopposed, closing the glottis. The arytenoid cartilages, which rest above the signet-ring portion of the cricoid cartilage, support the posterior portion of the true vocal cords.

Laryngeal ligaments

The extrinsic ligaments of the larynx are those connecting the thyroid cartilage and epiglottis with the hyoid bone and the cricoid cartilage with the trachea (Fig. 21-3). The intrinsic ligaments of the larynx are those connecting several cartilages of the organ to each other. They are considered the elastic membrane of the larynx.

The mucous lining of the larynx blends with the fibrous tissue to form two folds on each side of the larynx. The upper set is known as the *false cords*. The lower set is called the *true vocal cords* because they are primarily concerned with the speaking voice and protection of the lower respiratory channels against the invasion of food and foreign bodies. The region of the larynx at the true vocal cord level is called the *glottis*, a triangular space between the vocal cords. During swallowing, the rising action of the muscular larynx, the closure of the glottis, and the doorlike action of the epiglottis all serve to guide food and fluid into the esophagus.

Laryngeal muscles

The laryngeal muscles perform two distinct functions: the extrinsic muscles regulate the degree of tension on the vocal cords and the intrinsic muscles open and close the glottis. The spoken voice also depends on the sphincter action of the soft palate, tongue, and lips. The muscle action of the larynx permits the glottis to close either voluntarily or involuntarily by reflex action. The closure of the inlet by this mechanism protects the respiratory passages. The closure of the glottis and the action of the vocal cords are precisely coordinated to produce the voice. The recurrent laryngeal nerve branch of the vagus is the important motor nerve of the intrinsic muscles of the larynx. The sensory nerve, which is derived from the branches of the superior laryngeal nerve, supplies the mucous membrane of the larynx. The larynx derives its blood supply from the branches of the external carotid and the subclavian arteries.

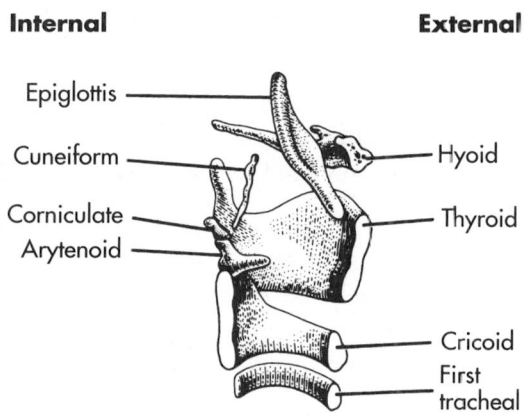

Internal

- Epiglottis
- Cuneiform
- Corniculate
- Arytenoid

External

- Hyoid
- Thyroid
- Cricoid
- First tracheal

FIGURE 21-2 Skeletal framework.

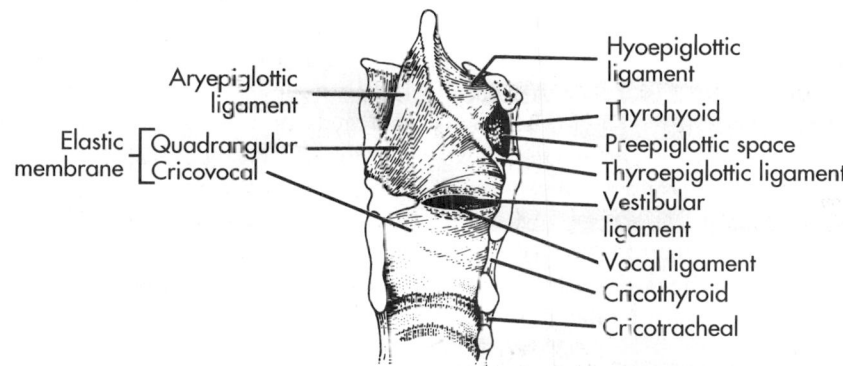

- Aryepiglottic ligament
- Elastic membrane
  - Quadrangular
  - Cricovocal
- Hyoepiglottic ligament
- Thyrohyoid
- Preepiglottic space
- Thyroepiglottic ligament
- Vestibular ligament
- Vocal ligament
- Cricothyroid
- Cricotracheal

FIGURE 21-3 Ligaments of larynx.

Trachea

The trachea, a cartilaginous tube about 15 cm in length and 2 to 2.5 cm in diameter, begins in the neck and extends from the lower part of the larynx, on a level with the sixth cervical vertebra, to the upper border of the fifth thoracic vertebra. The tube descends anteriorly to the esophagus, enters the superior mediastinum, and divides into right and left main bronchi. The trachea is composed of a series of C-shaped rings of hyaline cartilage. The posterior surface of the trachea is flattened rather than round because the cartilaginous rings are incomplete. The carina is a ridge on the inside of the bifurcation of the trachea. It is a landmark during bronchoscopy and separates the upper end of the right main branches from the upper end of the left main branches of the bronchi. The carina is heavily innervated and can produce severe bronchospasm and coughing when stimulated. Branches given off from the arch of the aorta—the brachiocephalic (innominate) and left common carotid arteries—are in close relation to the trachea. The cervical portion of the trachea is related anteriorly to the sternohyoid and sternothyroid muscles and to the isthmus of the thyroid gland.

Salivary Glands

The salivary glands consist of three paired glands: the sublingual, submandibular, and parotid. They communicate with the mouth and produce saliva, which serves to moisten the mouth and initiate digestion of carbohydrates. The salivary glands consist of tissues found in the mucosa of the cheeks, tongue, palates, floor of the mouth, pharynx, lips, and paranasal sinuses. Tumors can occur in any of these structures.

The external carotid artery supplies the salivary glands and divides into its terminal branches: the internal maxillary and the superficial temporal. The superficial temporal and internal maxillary veins unite to form the posterior facial vein.

The sublingual gland lies on the undersurface of the tongue beneath the mucous membrane in the floor of the mouth at the side of the tongue, on the inner surface of the mandible. It is supplied with blood from the submental arteries, and its nerves are derived from the sympathetic nerves. The many tiny ducts of each gland separately enter the oral cavity on the sublingual fold.

The submandibular gland lies partly above and partly below the posterior half of the base of the mandible and on the mylohyoid and hyoglossus muscles. This gland is closely associated with the lingual veins and the lingual and hypoglossal nerves. The facial artery lies on the posterior border of the gland. Its duct (Wharton's duct) runs superficially beneath the mucosa of the floor of the mouth and enters the oral cavity behind the central incisors.

The parotid gland, the largest of the salivary glands, lies below the zygomatic arch in front of the mastoid process and behind the ramus of the mandible. This gland is enclosed in fascia, attached to surrounding muscles, and is divided into two parts—a superficial and a deep portion—by means of the facial nerve. The parotid duct (Stensen's duct) pierces the buccal pad of fat and the buccinator muscle, finally opening into the oral cavity opposite the crown of the upper second molar tooth. The superficial temporal artery and small branches of the external carotid artery arise in the parotid gland behind the neck of the mandible. Because of its location, injury to the facial nerve is a risk from any surgical procedure involving the parotid gland area.

General Structures of the Neck

A layer of deep cervical fascia surrounds the neck like a collar and is attached to the trapezius and sternocleidomastoid muscles. The sternocleidomastoid muscle extends from the upper part of the sternum and medial third of the clavicle to the mastoid process. The trapezius muscle extends from the scapula, the lateral third of the clavicle, and the vertebrae to the occipital prominence. The relationship of these muscles to each other and to the adjacent bone creates triangles used as anatomic landmarks.

The pretracheal fascia of the neck lies deep in the strap muscles (sternothyroid, sternohyoid, and omohyoid) and partially encloses the thyroid gland, trachea, and larynx. The pretracheal fascia is pierced by the thyroid vessels. It fuses with the front of the carotid sheath on the deep surface of the sternocleidomastoid muscle. The carotid sheath consists of a network of areolar tissue surrounding the carotid arteries and vagus nerve.

Laterally the carotid sheath is fused with the fascia on the deep surface of the sternocleidomastoid muscle; anteriorly it is fused with the middle cervical fascia along the lateral border of the sternothyroid muscle. Lying between the floor and roof of this triangular formation of muscles are the lymph glands and the accessory nerve. Arteries and nerves traverse and pierce this triangle.

Lymphatic System of the Neck

The lymphatic system serves both immunologic and circulatory functions. Interstitial fluid, which may contain bacteria, viruses, or tumor cells, is returned to the blood circulation through the lymphatic channels. As the lymph nodes trap the foreign matter, they may become enlarged, infected, or the focus of metastatic cancer.[8] The lymphatic drainage of the neck can be divided into superficial and deep nodes (Fig. 21-4). The nasal cavity, paranasal sinuses, and the pharynx drain into the retropharyngeal nodes. The mouth, lips, and external nose are drained by the submandibular nodes. The lymphatics of the tip and lateral aspects of the tongue drain to the submental nodes, and the posterior tongue lymphatics drain to cervical nodes.

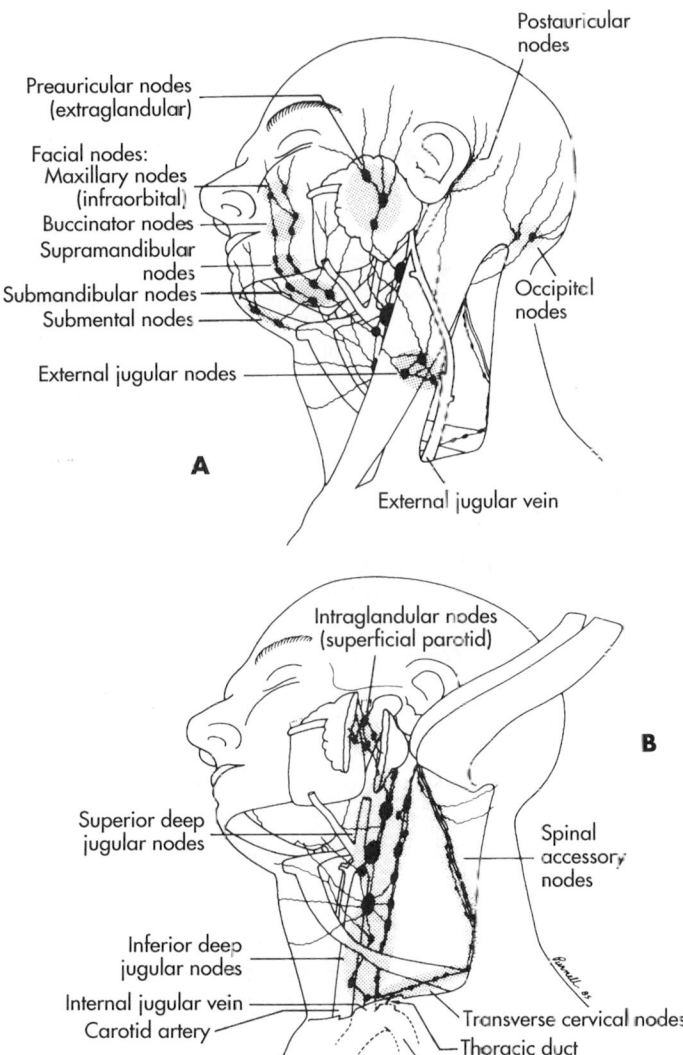

Postauricular nodes

Preauricular nodes (extraglandular)

Facial nodes:
 Maxillary nodes (infraorbital)
 Buccinator nodes
 Supramandibular nodes
Submandibular nodes
 Submental nodes

External jugular nodes

Occipital nodes

A

External jugular vein

Intraglandular nodes (superficial parotid)

B

Superior deep jugular nodes

Spinal accessory nodes

Inferior deep jugular nodes

Internal jugular vein
Carotid artery

Transverse cervical nodes
Thoracic duct
Subclavian vein

FIGURE 21-4 **A**, Superficial cervical and facial nodal drainage patterns. **B**, Deep cervical lymphatic drainage patterns. Notice that sternocleidomastoid muscle is reflected.

PERIOPERATIVE NURSING CONSIDERATIONS

Assessment

The nursing history must be thorough, including the patient's symptoms, health history, and definite and questionable risk factors, such as sun exposure, tobacco use, ethanol use, previous radiation therapy, family history of carcinoma, and the patient's dental history. In addition to the physical assessment of the neck (Box 21-1), specific factors that should be assessed include the following:

- *Respiratory status*. Observe and note the quality and character of respirations; observe and note the quality

and character of the voice, hoarseness, "hot potato" voice, or hyponasal speech; inspiratory stridor, expiratory stridor, hemoptysis, or dyspnea; a lesion in the oral cavity, nasopharynx, or larynx; bleeding from the oral cavity or nasopharynx. Note any history of chronic obstructive pulmonary disease (COPD).

- *Nutritional status*. Note weight loss and length of time; dysphagia. The patient may be nutritionally depleted from dysphagia, tumor, chemotherapy, or radiation therapy.

- *Circulatory status*. Observe and note pedal pulses and color of the nailbeds, especially in children, elderly patients, and patients in respiratory distress. Note preoperative vital signs compared with vital signs on admission to the patient care unit; note the presence of antiembolism stockings (the perioperative nurse should ensure proper fit of these stockings when checking pedal pulses).

- *Infection*. Note the temperature, color, and turgor of the skin over the affected site; note any lesions and their characteristics.

- *Dentition*. Observe dentures and their fit, lesions, loose teeth, persistent bad breath, and poor oral hygiene.

- *Emotional status and anxiety level*. Observe for restlessness, poor eye contact, facial tension, increased perspiration. Notice the area around the patient's eyes for signs of crying (edema, redness).

- *Pain*. Observe location and character, odynophagia, sore throat, facial pain, otalgia; note preoperative medications and the time they were administered.

- *Musculoskeletal system*. Observe problems in range of motion in all four extremities; note joint replacements, back or neck stiffness or pain, trismus.

- *Allergies*.

- *Patient's knowledge and understanding of the surgical procedure*. Note questions and give answers or ask surgeon to clarify information for the patient. Review equipment and care (such as suctioning) that will be part of the postoperative regimen.

- *Presence of a mass*. Note the length of time the mass has been evident; note if decrease in size of the mass occurred after antibiotic therapy; note a fixed mass versus a mobile mass; note cranial nerve palsies involving VII, IX, X, XI, and XII.

- *Availability of replacement blood*. Note if the patient has designated donor units (the patient's blood usually will have been typed and the blood samples held, or typed and cross-matched for two units, minimally, depending on the anticipated extent of the procedure).

- *Patient's support system*. Note family members' names and their location during the surgical procedure, introduce the family to the nurse who will be in contact with them during the procedure, and establish initial communication and the intervals between which the nurse will be in contact with them regarding the patient.

BOX 21-1 | **Physical Assessment of the Neck**

Inspection

Inspect the neck in the usual anatomic position, in slight hyperextension, and as the patient swallows. Look for bilateral symmetry of the sternocleidomastoid and trapezius muscles, alignment of the trachea, the landmarks of the anterior and posterior triangles, and any subtle fullness at the base of the neck. Notice any apparent masses, webbing, excess skin folds, unusual shortness, or asymmetry. Observe for any distention of the jugular vein or prominence of the carotid arteries.

Webbing, excessive posterior cervical skin, and an unusually short neck may be associated with chromosomal anomalies. The transverse portion of the omohyoid muscle in the posterior triangle can sometimes be mistaken for a mass. Noticeable edema of the neck is associated with local infections. A mass filling the base of the neck or visible thyroid tissue that glides upward when the patient swallows may indicate an enlarged thyroid.

Evaluate range of motion by asking the patient to flex, extend, rotate, and laterally turn the head and neck. Movement should be smooth and painless and should not cause dizziness.

Palpation

The ability to palpate and identify structures in the neck will vary with the patient's habitus. It will be more difficult to examine a short, thick muscular neck than a long slender one.

Palpate the trachea for midline position. Place a thumb along each side of the trachea in the lower portion of the neck. Compare the space between the trachea and the sternocleidomastoid muscle on each side. An unequal space indicates displacement of the trachea from the midline and may be associated with a mass or pathologic condition in the chest.

Identify the hyoid bone and the thyroid and cricoid cartilages. They should be smooth and nontender and should move under your finger when the patient swallows. On palpation, the cartilaginous rings of the trachea in the lower portion of the neck should be distinct and nontender.

With the patient's neck extended, position the index finger and thumb of one hand on each side of the trachea below the thyroid isthmus. A downward tugging sensation, synchronous with the pulse, is evidence of tracheal tugging, suggestive of the presence of an aortic aneurysm.

Lymph Nodes

Palpate the entire neck lightly for nodes. The anterior border of the sternocleidomastoid muscle is the dividing line for the anterior and posterior triangles of the neck and serves as a useful landmark in describing location. Bending the patient's head slightly forward or to the side will ease taut tissues and allow better accessibility to palpation.

Feel for nodes in the following six-step sequence:

1. The occipital nodes at the base of the skull
2. The postauricular nodes located superficially over the mastoid process
3. The preauricular nodes just in front of the ear
4. The parotid and retropharyngeal (tonsillar) nodes at the angle of the mandible
5. The submaxillary nodes halfway between the angle and the tip of the mandible
6. The submental nodes in the midline behind the tip of the mandible

Then move down to the neck, palpating in this four-step sequence:

1. The superficial cervical nodes at the sternocleidomastoid muscle
2. The posterior cervical nodes along the anterior border of the trapezius muscle
3. The cervical nodes deep to the sternocleidomastoid (The deep cervical nodes may be difficult to feel if you press too vigorously. Probe gently with your thumb and fingers around the muscle.)
4. The supraclavicular areas, probing deeply in the angle formed by the clavicle and the sternocleidomastoid muscle, the area of Virchow's nodes. (Detection of these nodes should always be considered a cause for concern.)

From Seidel, H.M., Dains, J.E., Ball, J.W., & Benedict, W. (1995). *Mosby's guide to physical examination.* (ed. 3). St Louis: Mosby, pp. 197-198, 218-219.

- *Laboratory and diagnostic studies.*
  - Chest radiograph (to rule out mediastinal or pulmonary involvement and tracheal compression and to assess the patient's pulmonary status)
  - CT or MRI of neck (to delineate normal and abnormal soft-tissue structures)
  - Ultrasonography of mass (to determine solid versus cystic mass)
  - ECG
  - Complete blood count
  - RBC (may be increased with dehydration or decreased with dietary deficiencies)

  Male. 4.7 to 6.1 million/mm^3
  Female. 4.2 to 5.4 million/mm^3
  Child. 3.8 to 5.5 million/mm^3
  - Hemoglobin (elderly values slightly decreased; may be increased with dehydration, congestive heart failure (CHF), or COPD; may be decreased with cancer, nutritional deficiency, or severe hemorrhage)
  Male. 14 to 18 g/dl
  Female. 12 to 16 g/dl
  Child. 11 to 16 g/dl
  - Hematocrit (may be increased with trauma or dehydration; may be decreased with hyperthyroidism,

cirrhosis, hemorrhage, malnutrition, dietary deficiency, or in the elderly)

Male. 42% to 52%

Female. 37% to 47%

Child. 31% to 43%

- WBC (may be increased with infection, trauma, stress, tissue necrosis, and inflammatory process; may be decreased with dietary disease, autoimmune disease, and overwhelming infections)

  Adult. 5000 to 10,000/mm^3

  Child 2 years old and younger. 6200 to 17,000/mm^3

- Platelet count. 150,000 to 400,000/mm^3 (may be increased with malignant disorders, cirrhosis, and trauma; may be decreased with hemorrhage, liver disease, kidney disease, or systemic lupus erythematosus [SLE])[9]

- Urinalysis (observe glucose level; if not negative, check blood glucose level)

- Prothrombin time (PT), partial thromboplastin time (PTT), and activated partial thromboplastin time (APTT)

  PT. 11 to 12.5 seconds (may be increased with cirrhosis, hepatitis, vitamin K deficiency, salicylate intoxication, or disseminated intravascular coagulation [DIC])

  PTT. 60 to 70 seconds

  APTT. 30 to 40 seconds (may be increased with clotting factor deficiencies, biliary obstruction, hepatocellular diseases, vitamin K deficiency, or DIC; may be decreased with early stages of DIC or extensive cancer)[9]

- *Blood chemistry analysis.*

  - Chloride—adults and elderly. 90 to 110 mEq/L (may be increased with dehydration, kidney dysfunction, or anemia; may be decreased with CHF, diuretic therapy, or hypokalemia)

  - Potassium—adults and elderly. 3.5 to 5 mEq/L (may be increased with acute or chronic renal failure; may be decreased with diuretic therapy, diarrhea, vomiting, or insulin, glucose, or calcium administration)

  - Blood urea nitrogen (BUN)—adults. 10 to 20 mg/dl (elderly may be slightly higher); may be increased with renal disease, CHF, or dehydration; may be decreased with liver failure, overhydration, or malnutrition)[9]

If the thyroid gland is suspect, the following tests may be indicated:

- Serum calcium levels (to determine parathyroid function—adults: 9 to 10.5 mg/dl

- Serum calcitonin (to assess potential for medullary carcinoma)

- Thyroid scan (to assess presence of "cold" nodule, which is often indicative of carcinoma)

- Thyroid antibody tests (may show decreased levels in carcinoma): titer less than 1:100

- Serum thyroxine (T^4): 4 to 11 mg/dl

- TSH: 2 to 10 mU/ml

- T^3 resin uptake: 25% to 35%[9]

The patient should be given explanations about the operating room environment and perioperative routines and their sequence to decrease apprehension. Warm blankets, thermadrapes, reassurance, and a quiet environment should be provided to ensure that the patient is comfortable, calm, and warm before the surgical experience. Keeping the patient warm is both part of the "caring" of perioperative nursing as well as a physiologic intervention to prevent hypothermia after surgery.[5]

Nursing Diagnosis

Nursing diagnoses related to the care of patients undergoing laryngologic or head and neck surgery might include the following:

- Impaired gas exchange caused by airway obstruction
- Anxiety related to impending surgery
- Risk for infection
- Body-image disturbance
- Altered nutrition, less than body requirements
- Impaired verbal communication

Outcome Identification

The decade of the 1990s has been characterized by an emphasis on the evaluation and management of healthcare quality and outcomes research.[7] Both outcomes of treatment and health-related quality are gaining respect as measures of equal importance. By including patient-perceived dimensions, such as physical, social, and role function, mental health, coping ability, satisfaction with care, and overall perceptions of health, perioperative nurses are more likely to capture the contributions of their nursing interventions, analyze them, and subsequently improve them.

Outcomes identified for the selected nursing diagnoses could be stated as follows:

- The patient will experience adequate gas exchange.
- The patient will demonstrate effective coping skills and a decreased level of anxiety.
- The patient will be free from infection at the surgical site.
- The patient will experience a sense of self-worth and self-respect.
- The patient will maintain weight within 10 pounds of admission weight.
- The patient will establish an effective communication method with staff and family.

SAMPLE CARE PLAN

Nursing Diagnosis: Impaired gas exchange caused by airway obstruction, glottic resection, secretions, and edema

Outcome: The patient will experience adequate gas exchange.

Interventions:

Check BP, rate and quality of respirations, rate and quality of pulse, and apical pulse preoperatively.

Auscultate chest for breath sounds preoperatively.

Elevate head of bed 30 degrees or higher as tolerated preoperatively and intraoperatively.

Check arterial blood gases if obtained.

Monitor oxygen saturation perioperatively.

Administer steroids as ordered.

Monitor preoperatively for and report signs of impaired gas exchange, such as stridor, confusion, hypoxia, restlessness, and irritability.

Provide equipment, instruments, and supplies for a tracheotomy and tracheostomy.

Nursing Diagnosis: Anxiety related to impending surgery

Outcome: The patient will demonstrate effective coping skills and a decreased level of anxiety.

Interventions:

Assess patient's level of anxiety (alertness, ability to comprehend, ability to perform ADL).

Maintain calm and safe environment.

Assist patient in identifying possible sources of stress.

Allow patient to ventilate and ask questions. Assess patient for desire of preoperative visit by patients with altered communication methods.

Nursing Diagnosis: Altered nutrition: less than body requirements

Outcome: The patient will maintain weight within 10 pounds of admission weight.

Interventions:

Weigh daily and record.

Monitor I&0.

Consult dietitian about formula or food selection.

Encourage full consumption of prescribed diet.

Initiate protective measures during surgical positioning.

Consult with surgeon regarding occupational therapy referral to assist with instruction for swallowing.

Nursing Diagnosis: Risk for infection

Outcome: The patient will not exhibit signs of infection.

Interventions:

Check temperature and WBC preoperatively.

Check temperature, color, and turgor of skin at operative site.

Check lesions in proximity to surgical site.

Check patient's nutritional status.

Ensure sterile environment during surgical procedure.

Monitor traffic patterns during surgical procedure.

Monitor blood loss and fluid replacement during surgical procedure.

Check patient's temperature during surgical procedure.

Ensure that initial dressing is dry and clean.

Administer antibiotics as prescribed.

Nursing Diagnosis: Body-image disturbance

Outcome: The patient will experience a sense of self-worth and self-respect.

Interventions:

Encourage patient to verbalize feelings and self-perceived changes related to health status and surgical procedure.

Involve family or significant others in initial communication with patient.

Encourage patient to ask questions.

Discuss referrals for support groups.

Nursing Diagnosis: Impaired verbal communication

Outcome: The patient will establish an effective communication method with staff and family.

Interventions:

Agree upon a method of communication preoperatively to be used postoperatively. Suggestions include:

1. Writing with a pen or pencil and paper, or using an erasable slate
2. Hand signals or signs, body expressions
3. Picture board

Provide assurance and support postoperatively as speech pathologist initiates speech training.

Collaborate with surgeon in determining patient's ability to learn esophageal speech.

Consult with surgeon regarding prosthetic voice restoration.

Place IV lines in nondominant hand.

Planning

Development of a meaningful perioperative nursing care plan is essential in meeting the needs of patients undergoing laryngologic or head and neck surgery. A Sample Care Plan for a patient undergoing laryngologic and head and neck surgery is shown above.

Implementation

The patient with a malignant neck mass seldom undergoes surgical excision of the neck mass as a primary procedure. Endoscopic evaluation may be the initial surgical procedure, unless the primary lesion is clearly delineated.

Positioning

Routine positioning of the laryngologic or head and neck surgical patient involves placement of the patient in a supine position on the operating room bed. A shoulder roll may be utilized for hyperextension of the neck, depending on the surgeon's preference. The headrest should allow easy movement of the head from side to side yet maintain support. The extremities are well padded at pressure points and at major nerves. A pillow should be placed under the thighs and the legs slightly frogged to decrease pressure on the patient's back; this positioning should be carried out before the patient is anesthetized to ensure comfort, with the exceptions of placement of the shoulder roll and hyperextension of the neck.

Prepping

Removal of hair intraoperatively depends on the site of surgery and the anticipated extensiveness of the surgical intervention. Parotid surgery may require shaving the patient's hair from just below the temple to a line even with or slightly behind the pinna of the ear. Head and neck surgery often requires removal of hair on the chest to the nipple area on both sides.

Laryngeal procedures for benign lesions do not usually involve preparation of the skin because of the intraoral approach. Head and neck procedures may involve extensive skin preparation and usually include the entire area from the chin to the nipples. Some surgeons prefer the patient's face to be included in the prep, depending on the type of surgery anticipated and the site of the lesion. Povidone-iodine scrub and solution are generally preferred for preparation of the skin. If a flap may be raised to reconstruct a defect, saline should be available to remove the discoloration from the skin to allow the surgeon to check for flap viability.

Draping

As with prepping, draping of the patient for a laryngeal procedure for a benign lesion (intraoral approach) is minimal, with the primary focus being protection of the patient's eyes and face. This may be accomplished by (1) placing ointment in the patient's eyes, (2) taping the eyelids closed with a nonabrasive, nonirritating tape, (3) applying moist padding over the tape (if use of a laser is anticipated), and (4) placing self-adhering eyepads over the moistened pads. A head drape may be placed over the patient's face to expose only the lips and chin.

Draping for head and neck procedures often varies according to surgeon preference. If the preference is to have the patient's face exposed, a commercially prepared head drape may be used. If unavailable, a head drape can be made by using a sterile sheet folded in half with a sterile towel on the innermost side to wrap the patient's hair. A towel clamp or sterile tape can secure the head drape in place. If using penetrating towel clamps, care must be taken not to pierce the skin of the patient. Towels can be opened fully, crushed, and placed into the space at both sides of the patient's neck and shoulder area to prevent contact with the unsterile operating room bed linen during the procedure. The area of the endotracheal tube may be isolated by a self-adherent, clear drape. Sterile towels are utilized to drape the neck, shoulder, and chest areas. An impervious drape is used to cover the patient from the chest to the foot of the operating room bed. A split sheet may then be used to drape over the towels and body drape. Commercially prepared split sheets have adhesive backing along the split that facilitates adherence to the area to be draped out and decreases slippage with subsequent contamination resulting from manipulation of the head during the surgical procedure.

Instrumentation

The instrumentation used in laryngologic surgery is quite specific and is discussed with each surgical intervention. Head and neck instrumentation consists in general surgical instruments and procedure-specific instruments.

Intraoral, laryngeal, and mandibular procedures require the addition of periosteal elevators (such as Joseph, Freer, Cleoid), cartilage scissors, bone cutter, rongeurs (such as Lempert, Adson), oral or mouth retractors, tracheal hooks, tracheal spreader, and saws. Although a Gigli saw and handles may be used on rare occasions, technology has made the sagittal saw standard in the operating room armamentarium. Saws are either nitrogen or battery powered, or electric. The choice of power source should be a collaborative effort among the perioperative nursing staff and surgeon. A dermatome may be used if skin grafting of surgical defects or flap reconstruction is anticipated. In the case of large reconstructive surfaces, a skin mesher may be used to extend the skin graft.

Equipment

Equipment that may be utilized in head and neck surgery includes an electrosurgical unit (both monopolar and bipolar), a forced-air warming unit or other device to maintain normothermia, headlights (both fiberoptic and nonfiberoptic), pulse oximeter, blood warmer, temperature recorder, and humidifier. Although the last four items of equipment are primarily the responsibility of anesthesia personnel, the circulating nurse collaborates in providing access to electrical outlets to power the equipment and participates in interventions based on the results of patient monitoring.

Lasers used in head and neck and laryngeal surgery include the carbon dioxide (CO_2) and Nd:YAG lasers, depending on the location and type of lesion.

The evolution of microvascular free flap surgery for head and neck reconstruction has added a host of equipment to ensure the success of the surgical procedure and the safety of the patient (Research Highlight 21-1). This equipment includes a surgical microscope (where the assistant may work at a 180-degree angle from the

21-1 RESEARCH HIGHLIGHT

Technologic advancements with surgical applications have continued to offer enhancements to various surgical interventions. Robotics, with orthopedic applications (Robodoc) and Robosurgeon, a voice-controlled robot to manipulate the thoracoscope, have already been used in the United States and Japan. Stereotactic-guided breast biopsies may become obsolete with the use of a 3-D technique that adapts digital technology already in place with stereotactic systems; 3-D images have a 77% accuracy rate compared with surgical biopsy.

Such developments are not isolated to the actual performance of a procedure but have become of interest in teaching the procedure. Simulators for airway management are used in some schools of anesthesia and computer simulations of the human body have been available for medical and nursing education for a few years.

Large-scale flight simulation was pioneered in the 1940s to help meet the training requirements and demand for pilots in World War II. Flight simulators have been effective for training, evaluating, and certifying military and commercial pilots. Accurate scenarios have been developed that allow pilots in training to gain experience without risk and expense of learning while in flight. Because of the successful use of flight simulation as a training technique, computer-based simulators are now used in a variety of domains.

Within the otolaryngology–head and neck surgery specialty, surgical simulators will be useful to master the complex anatomical structures of the head and neck to learn common techniques with potentially high morbidity. Currently, temporal bone dissection, skull base surgery, and endoscopic sinus surgery simulators are under development at several institutions.

From Kuppersmith, R.B., Johnston, R., Jones, S.B., & Jenkins, H.A. (1996). Virtual reality surgical simulation and otolaryngology, *Archives of Otolaryngology—Head and Neck Surgery, 122,* 1297-1298.

surgeon), a Doppler unit (to determine the viability of blood vessels), an electromyographic nerve monitor (to determine the location and quality of nerves), and a demagnetizer (to treat microsurgical instruments).

Safety in head and neck surgery is primarily patient related, except for lasers, which warrant both patient and staff safety precautions (see Chapter 3). All equipment should be checked before use to ensure that it is in proper working condition. Visual inspection should ensure that all equipment is clean. Headlights, in particular, should be inspected for blood before and after each use. Guidelines for between-use processing of the various endoscopes used is essential in preventing inadequate disinfection. Guidelines established by the Association for Practitioners in Infection Control (APIC) recommend immediate, thorough manual cleaning with an enzymatic cleaner followed by complete immersion in a high-level disinfectant or use of an automated system.[3]

Medications

Medications used in laryngeal surgery are targeted at decreasing bleeding and edema in the airway. Typical medications include the following:

- Steroids are sometimes given intraoperatively and postoperatively but may be given preoperatively in the presence of edema or airway obstruction.
- Epinephrine, phenylephrine hydrochloride, or cocaine may be placed topically when vocal cord lesions are excised manually or biopsy specimens are taken to identify a primary tumor site.
- Lidocaine (Xylocaine) is often instilled into the trachea to decrease coughing immediately before insertion of a tracheostomy tube.

Medications used in head and neck surgery include antibiotics and steroids. They are primarily given intravenously; however, an antibiotic may also be added to irrigating solutions. Chemotherapeutic agents are often an important aspect of adjuvant therapy for the head and neck cancer patient. The perioperative nurse should be familiar with the chemotherapeutic agents prescribed for the patient.

Monitoring considerations

Intraoperative monitoring of the patient includes assessment of the circulatory, metabolic, urinary, respiratory, and musculoskeletal systems at regular intervals. Assessment of fluid volume is a collaborative effort. Blood loss and urinary output are communicated to anesthesia personnel. The perioperative nurse participates in the administration of fluid replacement therapy, assists in maintaining patency of lines, provides in-line blood and solution warmers, and notes the patient's response. Pedal pulses and pressure points should be checked without disturbing the surgical field or team. The scrub person and circulating nurses must be aware of significant findings during the surgical procedure to anticipate changes or additional supplies and equipment needed. Communication with the patient's family or support persons is vital during the surgical procedure to decrease their anxiety.

Additional methods of monitoring the laryngologic or head and neck surgical patient include pulse oximetry and blood pressure readings, as well as the following:

- *Arterial line.* Detects sudden changes in BP and serves as a vehicle to obtain P_{O_2} and P_{CO_2} levels
- *Foley catheter.* Monitors the patient's urinary function, especially important for the elderly or debilitated patient

- *Temperature monitoring.* Usually by a rectal probe or an endotracheal tube probe to maintain core normothermia
- *Esophageal stethoscope.* Usually contraindicated in laryngeal procedures because of the interruption of the esophagus or structures adjacent to the esophagus, but it may be used in other head and neck procedures
- *Computerized anesthesia monitoring system.* Standardized method of ensuring the safety of the patient while the anesthetic is being administered.

Accurate and thorough monitoring is critical to safe and effective patient outcomes. Perioperative nurses should be familiar with monitoring equipment, able to interpret results, and remain responsive to implementing collaborative interventions based on those results.

Evaluation

Postoperative evaluation includes reassessing potential patient problems identified in the preoperative assessment as well as assessing the electrosurgical dispersive pad site, surgical incision, dressing, drains, respiratory status, skin turgor, core temperature, and color of the head and extremities. Preoperative assessment findings, intraoperative changes in the patient's condition, and the postoperative evaluation must be documented and communicated to ensure continuity of care and patient safety. The report should also include relevant nursing diagnoses and outcomes of care. Some nursing diagnoses may have already been resolved; others are ongoing and require continued planning and intervention during the patient's recovery from anesthesia and postoperative rehabilitation. A complete nursing report allows the PACU or ICU nurse to detect significant changes in the patient's condition in an early stage. Special considerations should also be reported, such as the necessity for flexion of the neck to avoid disruption of the suture line of the trachea in a patient who has undergone tracheal resection. Documentation should include the postoperative report given and the name of the RN to whom that report is given before the patient is discharged from the operating room. Based on the nursing diagnoses selected for the patient undergoing laryngologic or head and neck surgery, the nursing report might include the following outcome statements:

- The patient's gas exchange remained normal; respiratory rate and skin color were satisfactory.
- The patient demonstrated effective coping skills and a decreased level of anxiety and communicated needs and concerns.
- The patient will not exhibit signs of infection (ongoing); temperature will remain normal and the surgical incision will heal without erythema, odor, or drainage at the site.
- The patient verbalized feelings regarding disturbances in body image, interacted positively with perioperative

staff, maintained eye contact, and identified personally effective coping strategies.
- The patient's nutritional status will be maintained (ongoing).
- The patient is able to communicate effectively (ongoing) and use alternative method (specify) of communication.

Patient and Family Education and Discharge Planning

Standards of care describe competent levels of nursing practice and nursing responsibilities for all patients. As developed by the American Nurses Association,[1] they reflect the need for nurses to provide age-appropriate, culturally and ethnically sensitive care. Nurses are expected to educate patients about healthful practices and treatment modalities provided by the nurse. Part of patient education is assuring continuity of care by means of reports and referrals, coordinating the patient's care across settings and among various care givers, managing information, and communicating effectively with colleagues, patients, and their families. As perioperative nurses design preoperative and postoperative educational content and strategies, they incorporate theory into their practice. A relevant theory for patient and family education and discharge planning for laryngologic and head and neck surgical patients is that of self-regulation. This theory postulates that the perioperative nurse involve the patient as an active participant in the healthcare process, recognizing the functional and emotional outcomes of coping with a surgical event. One of the assumptions of this theory is that goal-oriented perioperative patient care seeks to minimize the influence of the surgical experience on the patient's usual activities and assists the patient in becoming emotionally comfortable. Using self-regulation theory guides the perioperative nurse in selecting content of information for patient and family education and discharge planning in order for the patient to be able to predict and understand the surgical experience and recovery and rehabilitation from it.[4]

Preoperative patient education includes preparing the patient for alterations in body image and function. Altered methods of communication must be discussed before disruption of oral or laryngeal function, allowing the patient the opportunity to practice before the disruption of speech. The presence of edema, drains, nasogastric tube, Foley catheter, dressings, and altered mobility must be discussed. The operating room environment and presence of equipment should be described to the patient preoperatively to keep anxiety at a minimum. Dietary preferences and eating habits should be discussed to effectively develop a postoperative nutritional plan. Any special considerations for surgical positioning should be discussed before surgery to prevent injury or postoperative discomfort.

Postoperative patient education for laryngologic and head and neck surgery includes interventions to keep the airway clear and patent (turning, coughing, and deep

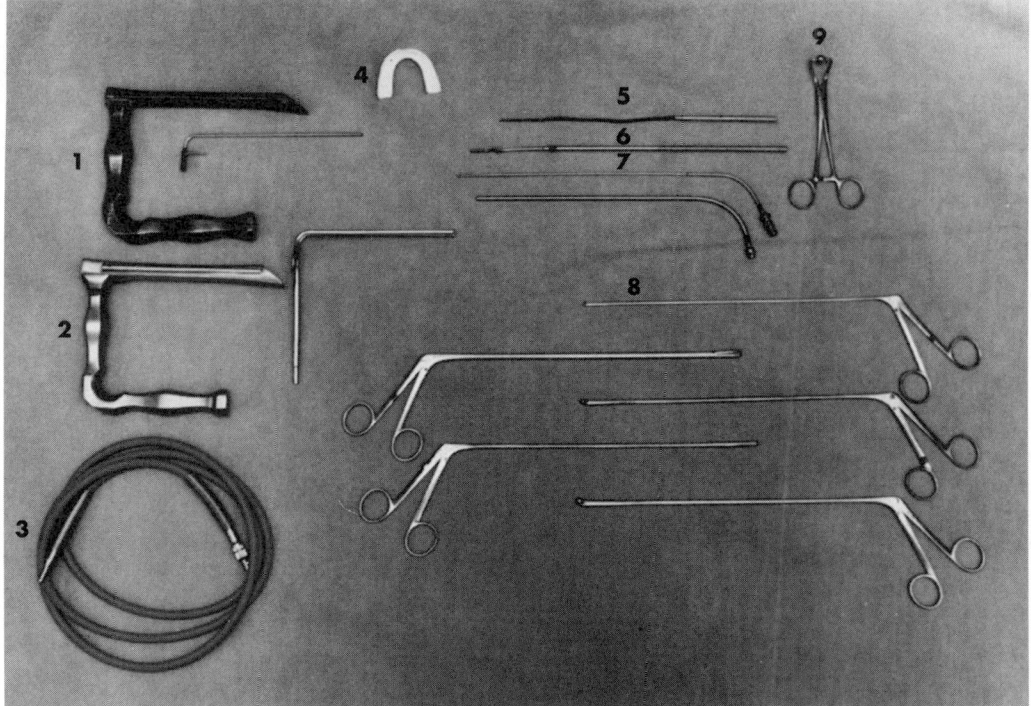

FIGURE 21-5   Laryngoscopy instruments. *1*, Anterior commissure laryngoscope and light carrier; *2*, Dedo-Pilling laryngoscope and light carrier; *3*, fiberoptic light cord; *4*, tooth guard; *5*, laryngeal pigtail applicator; *6*, long knife handle; *7*, laryngeal suction tubes, small and medium; *8*, assorted laryngeal cup forceps and laryngeal alligator forceps; *9*, nonperforating towel clamp.

breathing; providing a humidified environment; monitoring sputum; tracheostomy care), maintenance of adequate nutritional status to promote healing (dietary consultation; monitoring intake and weight; eating small, multiple meals and snacks), wound care (incision site care, oral hygiene, symptoms indicative of infection or potential wound breakdown), medications, pain managemnt, activity limitations, potential complications, postoperative course, additional therapies and coping mechanisms to avoid alcohol and tobacco use, as well as the patient's altered body image. Recommended content for patient and family education and discharge planning are included under procedural considerations for select surgical interventions on pp. 774, 778, and 788.

SURGICAL INTERVENTIONS
LARYNGOSCOPY

Laryngoscopy is direct visual examination of the interior of the larynx by means of a lighted speculum known as a *laryngoscope* (Fig. 21-5) to obtain a specimen of tissue or secretions for pathologic examination.

Procedural considerations

To facilitate this examination, the patient should be sufficiently relaxed by reassurance and by pharmacologic preparation if the procedure is performed under local anesthesia. Sedatives may be administered before surgery. Immediate preoperative assessment should include the presence of any dental appliances and condition of dental work and loose teeth. Any stiffness or immobility of the neck or shoulders should be evaluated. Respiratory problems such as asthma must receive careful attention. The patient should be cautioned about not eating or drinking after surgery until the gag reflex has returned and swallowing occurs without difficulty. Most laryngoscopies are performed with the patient under general anesthesia. If an adult cannot tolerate a general anesthetic, the patient must be well prepared preoperatively, and the application of a local or topical anesthetic of lidocaine (Xylocaine), tetracaine (Pontocaine), cocaine, or cetacaine will be performed immediately before the procedure.

The setup includes the following:

- Local anesthesia setup
- Gauze sponges, 4 X 4 inches
- Laryngeal mirror
- Cotton balls
- Small cup of hot water (to warm the laryngeal mirror so that it does not fog when inserted into the mouth to view the vocal cords) or an antifog solution
- Emesis basin
- Syringe, 5 ml, and Abraham cannula
- Medication cup

- Jackson laryngeal applicating forceps
- Cetacaine spray, with angulated tip, or other topical anesthetic for the oral mucosa
- Instrument setup
  - 1 laryngoscope (surgeon's choice)
  - 2 laryngeal suction tubes
  - 1 light carrier, fiberoptic
  - 2 laryngeal biopsy forceps, 1 straight and 1 upbiting
  - 2 sponge-carrier forceps with extra sponges
  - 1 tooth guard
  - 1 fiberoptic light cord
  - Zero-degree telescope may be requested for close visualization or attached to the camera for photographs of specific areas
  - 1 laryngeal probe; may be used to retract tissue or assess mobility of tissue

Accessory items include suction tubing, a specimen container, a basin with sterile saline, gauze sponges, sterile towels, and gloves.

If the surgeon wishes to perform a suspension laryngoscopy, a self-retaining laryngoscope holder is added to the instrument table, as well as microlaryngeal instruments, which include scissors, cup forceps, and alligator forceps. A special platform may be mounted onto the operating room bed, or a Mayo stand may be placed above the patient's chest and over the operating room bed to provide a place for the laryngoscope holder to rest. The surgeon normally uses the operating microscope with a 400 mm lens during suspension laryngoscopy. The patient is placed in a supine position to facilitate visualization of the vocal cords. A shoulder roll should be immediately available if slight hyperextension of the neck is necessary to assist in visualization of the larynx.

Operative procedure

1. Moist gauze pads or tape should be put over the patient's eyes to protect them from the instrumentation and to prevent injury and irritation from secretions during the procedure. The head may also be wrapped in a sterile towel. A sterile drape may be used to cover the patient. A tooth guard or moist 4 X 4–inch gauze sponge is placed to protect the patient's teeth.
2. The spatula end of the laryngoscope is introduced into the right side of the patient's mouth and directed toward the midline; then the dorsum of the tongue is elevated, so that the epiglottis is exposed.
3. The patient's head is first tipped backward and then lifted upward as the laryngoscope is advanced into the larynx.
4. The larynx is examined, a biopsy is taken, secretions are aspirated, and bleeding is controlled.
5. The patient's face is cleansed. The patient is then taken to the PACU.

Laryngoscopy instrumentation should remain set up in the room until the patient is transferred because the equipment may be needed if the patient experiences laryngospasm postoperatively.

MICROLARYNGOSCOPY

Microlaryngoscopy facilitates improved diagnosis and allows the laryngologist to view with relative ease areas that were previously inaccessible or difficult to visualize. It may also be used for minor surgery of the larynx, especially for the removal of polyps or nodules on the vocal cords. Intralaryngeal surgery using the laryngoscope is often referred to as *phonosurgery*. Instrumentation may vary according to surgeon preference.

Procedural considerations

If the procedure is done to remove polyps or nodules from the vocal cords, the patient must be cautioned to observe complete voice rest or to whisper postoperatively. The patient should be provided with a pencil and paper or erasable slate to aid in communication. The patient's restriction on speaking should be noted on the nursing care plan and on the front of the chart.

The basic instrument setup for laryngoscopy is used. Microlaryngeal instruments are added to the setup and include the following (Fig. 21-6):

- Self-retaining laryngoscope holder
- Jako microlaryngeal grasping forceps
- Jako microlaryngeal cup forceps, straight and upbiting cups
- Jako microlaryngeal scissors, straight, angled, and upbiting
- Jako microlaryngeal knives, straight and curved
- Laryngeal probe
- Microlaryngeal mirror
- Open-ended microlaryngeal suction tube
- Laryngoscope (dual light channel)

The aforementioned instruments have a length of 22 cm to allow use with the microscope, being long enough to keep the surgeon's hands out of the visual field. The microscope is used. The head is adjusted to allow visualization of the larynx. The surgeon usually adjusts the microscope. The microscope lens should have a 400 mm focal length. Focal length is the distance from the lens to the operative area and is the point at which the field can be clearly viewed through the microscope. Beyond this point the field becomes fuzzy. The 400 mm lens gives the surgeon a 40 cm focal length, or working distance.

Care of Endoscopic Equipment

Endoscopic equipment is fragile and should be handled carefully. Rigid endoscopes should be thoroughly cleaned in accordance with the APIC guidelines, and lumens checked for cleanliness. Long, narrow brushes and long pipe cleaners are available for cleaning the lumen and suction and light channels. The scopes should be dried carefully before sterilization. The light carriers are stored

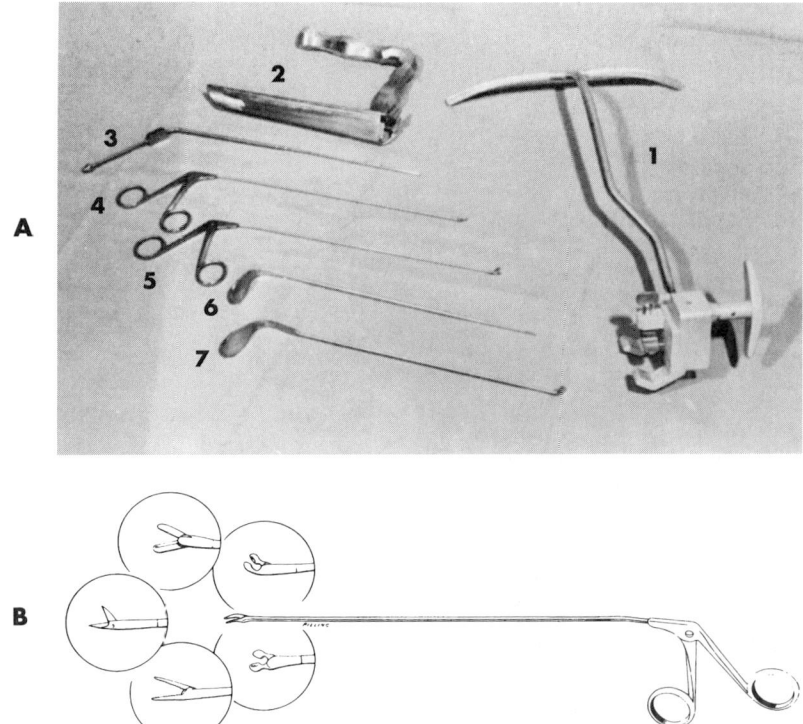

FIGURE 21-6   Jako microlaryngeal instrumentation. **A**, Basic setup for microlaryngoscopy. *1*, Lewy self-retaining laryngoscope holder; *2*, Jako laryngoscope; *3*, suction tube; *4*, grasping forceps; *5*, cup forceps; *6*, probe; *7*, mirror. **B**, Close-up view of working ends of instruments.

in the endoscopes. The endoscope should be checked for any dents, roughened edges, or deep scratches on the surface. Any of these can cause tissue damage or lead to corrosion of the instrument. Endoscopes should be handled individually.

Fiberoptic equipment is also fragile. The light cables should be handled with care and not allowed to drop or swing free while being carried. This can break the filaments inside the cords, rendering them unusable. Most cables can be autoclaved but according to manufacturer's instructions only. They should be coiled loosely when not in use, and care should be taken not to put anything heavy on top of the cables. Kinking and sharp bending of the cables must be avoided.

The main advantage of fiberoptics is that the light, although very bright, remains cool when used for a relatively long time. A simple test for the integrity of the cable is to hold one end of the cable to a bright light and inspect the opposite end. Dark spots are an indication that some of the fibers are broken. If more than 25% of the fibers are broken, the cable should be sent for repair, or replacement should be considered.

Telescopes for rigid equipment, as used for bronchoscopy, should also be handled carefully to prevent damage. The telescope should be cleaned carefully, dried thoroughly, and returned to its case for protection during storage. Telescopes may be sterilized, but strict adherence to manufacturer's instructions must be followed. If a telescope is dropped or hit against another object, it should be sent to the manufacturer for examination and repaired if required. Suction tips should be flushed thoroughly with running water. An instrument-cleaning solution may also be used for this purpose. The lumen should be cleaned with a long pipe cleaner to remove remaining debris, rinsed again, and then dried with a clean, dry pipe cleaner. Suction tips should be inspected for dents or nicks, especially on the end, to prevent damage to delicate tissues.

Biopsy forceps should be thoroughly cleaned, and the edges of the cups inspected for chips or nicks. They should also be checked periodically for sharpness. If the forceps are dull, nicked, or chipped, tissue will be torn or ripped instead of cut cleanly when a specimen is taken, resulting in more bleeding than usual. It is a good practice to rotate the use of biopsy forceps regularly depending on the frequency of use. All forceps should be thoroughly cleaned, dried, and inspected for damage after use and should be sent for repair if necessary.

Proper care of endoscopic equipment can extend the service life of these instruments indefinitely.

CARBON DIOXIDE LASER SURGERY OF THE LARYNX

The advent of the CO_2 laser added a new dimension to the laryngologist's treatment of lesions of the larynx and vocal cords. This laser is efficient and has a high power

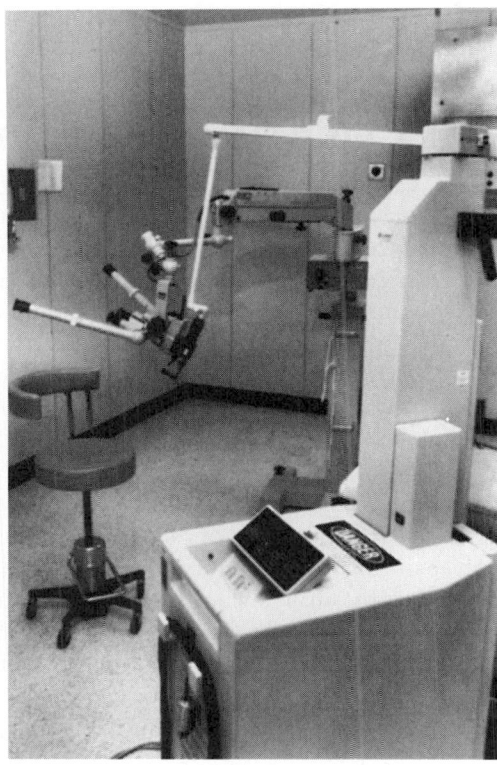

FIGURE 21-7 Operating microscope with laser micromanipulator attached.

output. It uses a combination of carbon dioxide, nitrogen, and helium gases that becomes energized to a high degree by an electric current. As the energy level subsides, light beams are produced and are reflected off the mirror-lined walls of the laser tube. These beams eventually form a single beam of light that has a high intensity in the ultraviolet range and is therefore invisible to the eye. For this reason a red beam from a helium-neon laser is added to the CO_2 beam so that it can be properly aimed at the affected tissue. The beam destroys tissue at a precise point with minimal destruction of the surrounding tissue. It is especially useful in surgeries such as removal of webs in the larynx, vocal cord papillomas, and carcinoma in situ of the larynx, as well as benign endobronchial lesions.

Procedural considerations

The basic setup for laryngoscopy and microlaryngoscopy is used. All instrumentation used for laser laryngoscopy should be ebonized. General anesthesia is usually given. The operating microscope with a 400 mm lens is used, with the laser micromanipulator attached to the microscope head (Fig. 21-7). The manufacturer's instructions for attaching it must be followed. The beam should also be tested for proper working order before use on the patient. Signal lights on the console become illuminated if any malfunction occurs in the equipment or if the gas supply is low. Extreme care should be used when handling this delicate piece of equipment. A smoke evacuator should be used to remove the laser plume, a smokelike

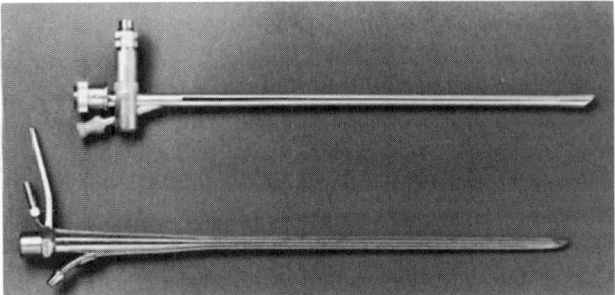

FIGURE 21-8 Pediatric and adult esophagoscopes.

steam rising from the impact site; high-filtration laser masks should be worn by personnel. Where minimal plume is generated, a central wall suction with an in-line filter may be used for plume evacuation.[2] All other laser precautions apply (see Chapter 3).

BRONCHOSCOPY

The trachea, bronchi, and lungs are visualized directly with a rigid or flexible bronchoscope that has a fiberoptic lighting system. A rigid scope gives a larger viewing area, whereas a flexible scope is easily inserted into the patient and manipulated. Bronchoscopy is fully described in Chapter 25. The Nd:YAG laser may be utilized for lesions of the trachea or bronchi, depending on the type of lesion. Most diagnostic bronchoscopies are performed with use of topical anesthesia and conscious sedation, requiring careful patient monitoring by the postoperative nurse.

ESOPHAGOSCOPY

Esophagoscopy is the direct visualization of the esophagus and the cardia of the stomach. This procedure is utilized to observe the area for extension of tumor, remove tissue and secretions for study, or observe for primary tumor site.

Procedural considerations

Esophagoscopy facilitates the diagnosis of esophageal carcinoma, diverticula, hiatal hernia, stricture, benign stenosis, or varices. Patients with suspected obstruction, symptoms of bleeding, or regurgitation may require endoscopy. The Nd:YAG laser may be utilized in the treatment of some of these lesions. Esophagoscopy may also be used for therapeutic manipulations, such as removal of a foreign body or insertion of an esophageal bougie.

The setup includes the following:

- Esophagoscopes, desired type, size and length (Figs. 21-8 and 21-9)
- Suction tubing
- Fiberoptic light source and light cords
- Bougies, if desired
- Forceps, desired type and length

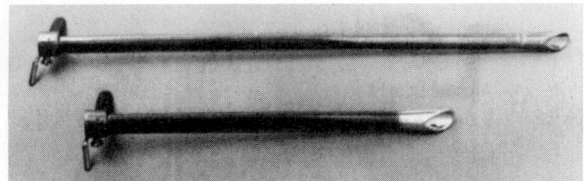

FIGURE 21-9   Jesberg adult esophagoscopes.

- Specimen containers
- Water-soluble lubricating jelly
- Gauze sponges
- Basin with sterile saline
- Suction tips (with velvet-eyed tips to avoid suctioning the mucosa of the esophagus into the tip)

Operative procedure

1. The fiberoptic light carrier is inserted into the esophagoscope, and a fiberoptic light cord is attached. A thin layer of lubricant is applied to the scope. The scope is passed into the mouth. The tongue, epiglottis, laryngeal inlet, and cricopharyngeal lumen are identified. If necessary, a person holding the patient's head may be required to tip the head backward while extending the neck anteriorly. Usually the esophagoscope is passed to the right side of the tongue, and the patient's head is turned slightly to the left.
2. When the scope has passed the inferior constrictors, the patient's head is moved in various directions so that all areas of the esophageal wall may be examined.
3. Specimens of secretions from the esophageal lumen may be obtained with an aspirating tube and suctioning apparatus. In some cases saline may be injected through the esophagoscope's aspirating channel and the fluid is withdrawn immediately for histologic study. A biopsy of tissue may be taken using forceps of the surgeon's preference. After biopsy, the area is assessed for bleeding, and the esophagoscope is then removed.

TRIPLE ENDOSCOPY

When laryngoscopy, bronchoscopy, and esophagoscopy are performed on a patient, the procedure is termed *triple endoscopy*. The order in which the procedures are performed depends on the surgeon's preference. The purpose of triple endoscopy is usually diagnostic. While inspecting for a malignancy, the surgeon views the structures, takes specimens for biopsy, and possibly makes smears or washings of the suspect areas. For any of the aforementioned endoscopy procedures, all equipment or instrumentation should be set up and be in working order, that is, light carriers in place and light cables connected and working, before use on the patient. Instrumentation to be used through the various scopes, that is, suction tips, telescopes, and biopsy forceps, should be checked for appropriate length. Specimens taken during endoscopic procedures should be labeled and removed from the table as soon as possible. In some instances, it may be helpful to indicate that the specimens are microscopic on the specimen label.

SURGERY OF THE ORAL CAVITY

The oral cavity is susceptible to both benign and malignant lesions, in part because of environmental risk factors. As early as 1941, a two-stage mechanism for the development of cancer was proposed—the *initiation stage,* induced by a mutagen, followed by the *promotion stage,* mediated by another agent (Fig. 21-10, Research Highlight 21-2). Oral malignancies may be initiated after exposure to a carcinogen, the most important one being tobacco use. In 1993, there were an estimated 29,800 new cases of oral cancer, ranking it as the sixth type of cancer out of 20 specified sites.[6]

Benign or malignant lesions of the tongue, floor of the mouth, alveolar ridge, buccal mucosa, or tonsillar area are excised. Benign or small malignant tumors of the oral cavity may be excised without neck dissection. In the presence of tongue cancer without evidence of metastasis, a prophylactic neck dissection may be performed in an effort to control a cancerous growth in the upper jugular chain of the neck.

In the treatment of carcinoma of the floor of the mouth with involvement of the mandible, a portion of the tongue is removed in a combined operation—a radical neck dissection and a composite resection of both the mandible and the tongue. When the primary intraoral lesion is confined to the tongue, a neck dissection and a hemiglossectomy are performed without resection of the mandible. In the presence of a lesion of the tonsil or an extensive lesion at the base of the tongue with pharyngeal wall involvement, a resection of the ascending ramus of the mandible is necessary, and portions of the base of the tongue, pharyngeal wall, and soft palate are removed to secure an adequate margin of normal tissue around the lesion.

Psychologic preparation of the patient is extremely important because these procedures may be done for a minor lesion in the oral cavity or may be the first part of much more extensive surgery in the head and neck area. A supportive and accepting family is most important to the patient at this time because of the possibility of disfigurement after surgery.

Procedural considerations

The patient is placed in a supine position with shoulders elevated. Generally, endotracheal anesthesia is used, and a pharyngeal pack of moist gauze may be inserted in the mouth. Instruments and supplies vary depending on the surgical intervention.

Operative procedure

Although the procedure may be scheduled as a local excision, frequently lesions of the oral cavity require more extensive excision. The setup should be designed to

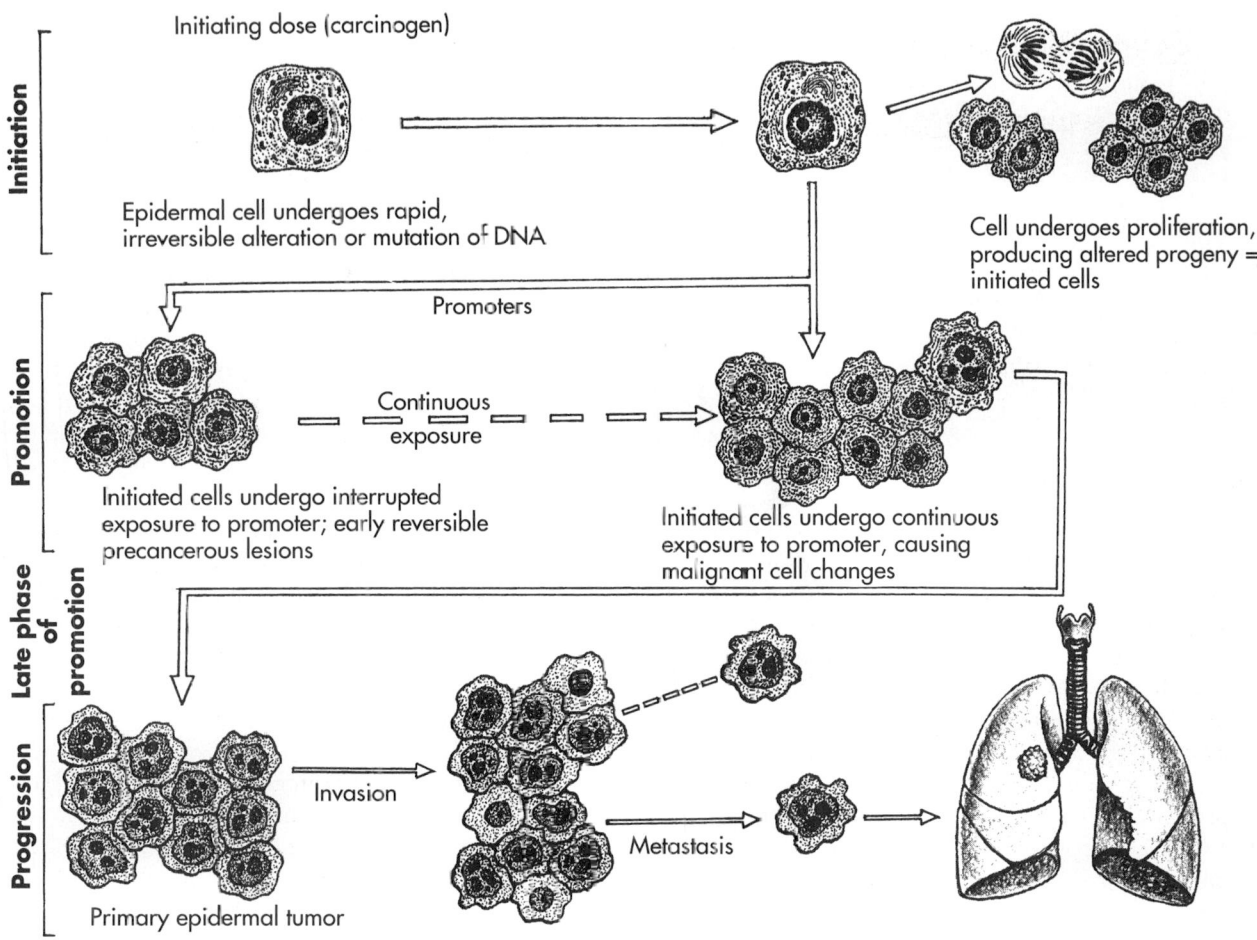

FIGURE 21-10 Multistage theory. Tumor development according to the multistage theory: initiation, promotion, progression.

21-2 RESEARCH HIGHLIGHT

Cancer gene-therapy is accomplished by transferral of nucleic acids onto tumor or normal cells to reduce or eliminate tumor burden by direct killing of cells, immunomodulation, or correcting of genetic errors to reverse a malignant state. DNA can be introduced into target cells directly (in vivo) or indirectly (ex vivo) and placed back into the host. Vectors are agents that facilitate the transfer of genes to the recipient cells. Viral vectors with promoter elements to mediate tissue-specific gene-expression have been identified in the liver for hepatomas and in breast cancer cells. Transduction of tumor cells with a gene that encodes an enzyme is under investigation for herpes simplex virus (HSV).

In head and neck cancer, directly transferring genes to a microscopic residual carcinoma may not be technically difficult. When the primary malignant neoplasms are removed, the tumor milieu is readily accessible for molecular therapy. Regional lymphatic dissections also provide access to the site most likely to harbor residual or occult disease. Therefore, new means of addressing microscopic residual disease that use direct transfer of genes capable of specifically promoting tumor cell death and sparing nonmalignant cells may provide desperately needed improvement in local and regional control of these cancers. The importance of developing such strategies is emphasized by the fact that the overall survival rate in patients with SCCHN (squamous cell carcinoma of the head and neck) has remained essentially unchanged during the past 30 years. Other solid malignant neoplasms pose a similar treatment dilemma, and SCCHN may serve as a model, providing valuable information that can be translated to different systems.

From Clayman, G.L., Liu, T.J., Overholt, S.M., et al. (1996). Gene Therapy for Head and Neck Cancer. *Archives of Otolaryngology—Head and Neck Surgery, 122,* 489-490, and Weichselbaum, R.R., & Kufe, D., (1997). Gene therapy of cancer. *Lancet, 349* (suppl. II), 10-12.

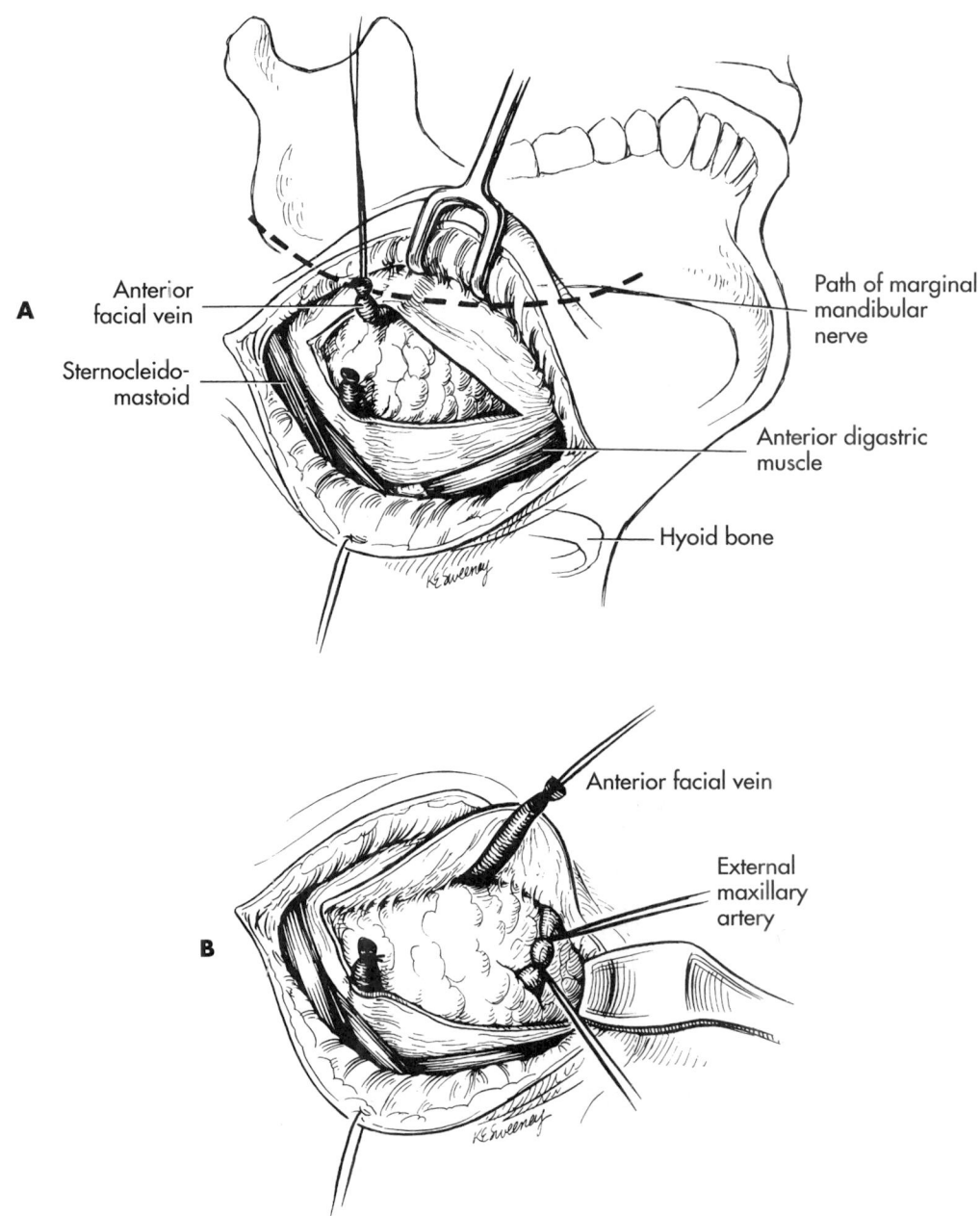

A

Anterior facial vein

Sternocleido-mastoid

Path of marginal mandibular nerve

Anterior digastric muscle

Hyoid bone

B

Anterior facial vein

External maxillary artery

FIGURE 21-11   Excision of submandibular gland. **A**, Submandibular incision, made in a natural skin crease 3 to 4 cm inferior to mandible. Marginal mandibular nerve generally lies just superficial to anterior facial vein. **B**, External maxillary artery is identified on submandibular gland (*continued*).

include the instruments for a neck dissection, or they should be readily available. For some tumors of the oral cavity a tracheostomy is performed to ensure a patent airway after surgery. A laser may be used to excise locally confined lesions of the oral cavity.

EXCISION OF THE SUBMANDIBULAR GLAND

Excision of the submandibular gland is performed to remove mixed tumors and multiple calculi associated with extensive chronic inflammation. An incision is made

below and parallel to the mandible extending to beneath the chin to remove the gland and tumor.

Procedural considerations

The patient is placed on the operating room bed in a supine position, with the affected side uppermost, and prepped as for neck surgery. The instruments include a minor neck dissection setup. A set of lacrimal probes should also be added to the instrument setup if exploration of the submandibular (Wharton's) duct is necessary during surgery. The circulating nurse must ensure that no local anesthetic is delivered to the sterile field if identification of

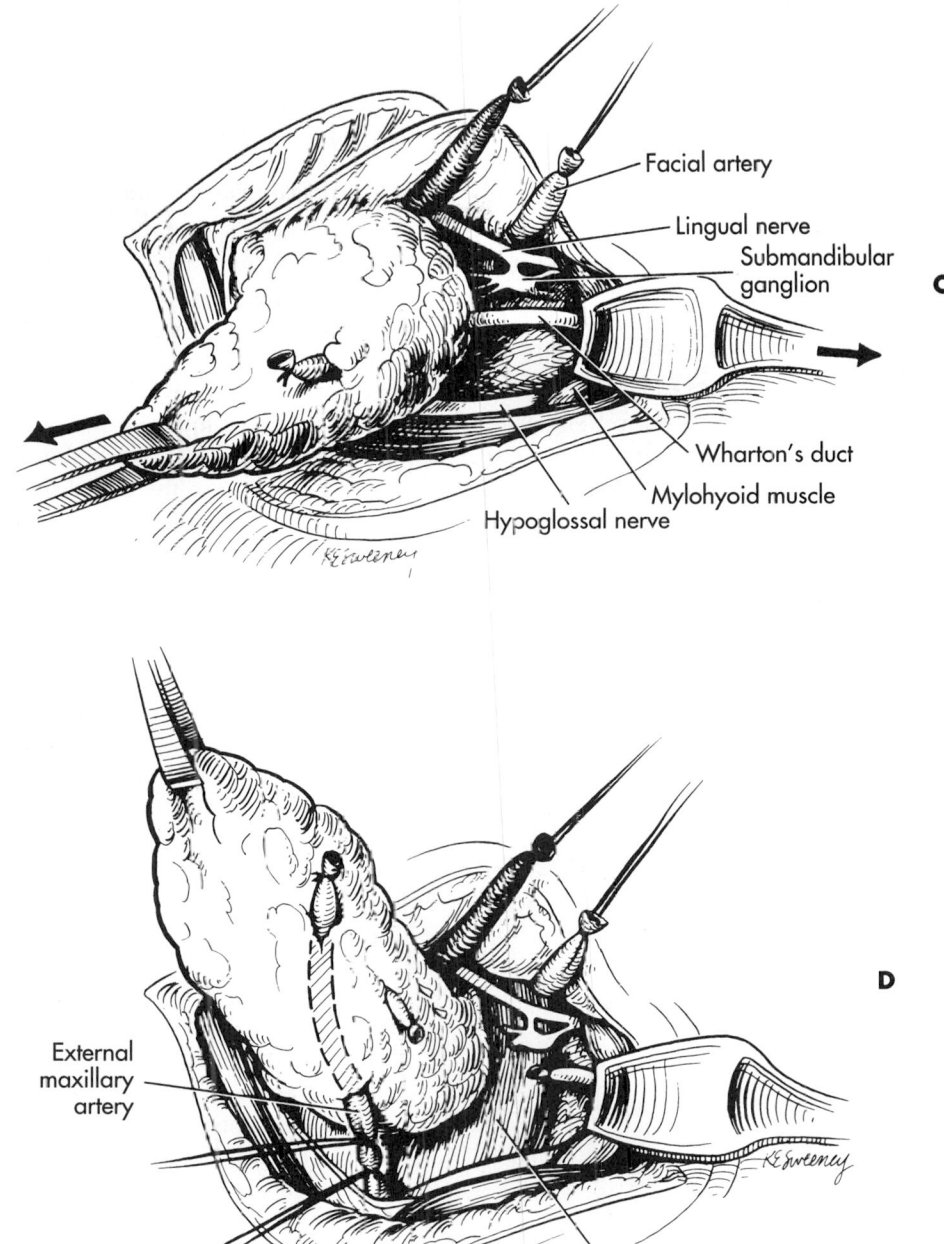

FIGURE 21-11, cont'd Excision of submandibular gland **C**, Mylohyoid is retracted anteriorly and gland posteriorly. This exposes lingual nerve, submandibular ganglion, and Wharton's duct. **D**, Hypoglossal nerve, running between hypoglossus and mylohyoid muscles. External maxillary artery must be divided a second time.

major nerves is anticipated. A nerve stimulator and bipolar ESU may be requested.

Operative procedure

1. A small skin incision is made below and parallel to the mandible, extending forward to beneath the chin (Fig. 21-11, *A*). The platysma is incised with scissors; the skin flaps and undersurface of the platysma and cervical fascia covering the gland are undermined with fine hooks, tissue forceps, and Metzenbaum scissors (Fig. 21-11, *B*).

2. The mandibular branch of the facial nerve is retracted away with a small loop retractor or nerve hook.

3. The submandibular gland is elevated from the mylohyoid muscle (Fig. 21-11, *C*). The edge of the muscle is retracted anteriorly to expose the lingual veins and nerve and the hypoglossal nerve, which is identified and preserved.

4. The gland is freed by blunt dissection, and the submandibular duct is clamped, ligated, and divided, with care to prevent injury to the lingual nerve.
5. The facial artery is clamped, ligated, and divided. The submandibular gland is removed (Fig. 21-11, *D*).
6. The wound is closed with interrupted absorbable sutures. The skin edges are approximated with nonabsorbable sutures. A drain is inserted into the submandibular bed and secured to the skin. Dressings are applied.

PAROTIDECTOMY

Approximately 80% of masses in the parotid gland are benign and 20% malignant.[10] In parotidectomy, the tumor and a portion of or the entire parotid gland are removed through a curved incision in the upper neck, in front of the ear lobe, or through a Y type of incision on both sides of the ear and below the angle of the mandible. Even when a mass in the parotid gland is benign, the closeness of the facial nerve makes removing the entire mass surgically challenging (Fig. 21-12). The facial nerve exits the stylomastoid foramen, enters the substance of the salivary gland, and then bifurcates into the temporofacial and cervicofacial branches, variably communicating with the gland. These branches then further divide into the temporal, zygomatic, buccal, and marginal mandibular and cervical branches near the edge of the parotid. The gland is divided artificially into a *superficial* and a *deep* lobe according to its relationship to the facial nerve. Preopera-

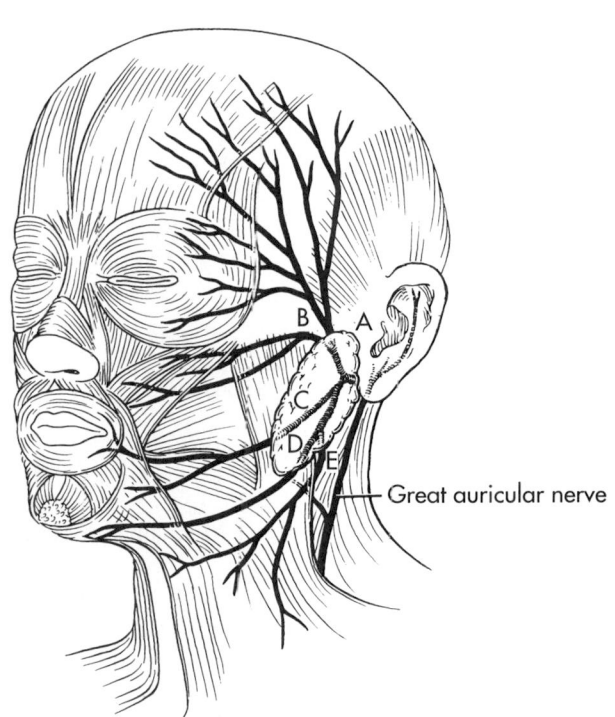

FIGURE 21-12 Branches of facial nerve. **A**, Temporal. **B**, Zygomatic. **C**, Buccal. **D**, Mandibular. **E**, Cervical.

Great auricular nerve

tively, patients should have an understanding of the possible complication of facial nerve weakness or paralysis. Additionally, they should understand that a more radical procedure might be required if a malignant tumor is discovered to involve adjacent structures.

Procedural considerations

The patient is placed on the operating room bed in a supine position with the entire affected side of the face uppermost. The entire side of the face, the mouth, the outer canthus of the eye, the ear, and the forehead are prepped and left exposed.

The instrument setup is a neck dissection set. A nerve stimulator or nerve integrity monitor should be available for use. A set of lacrimal probes should be included in the setup if exploration of the ductal system of the parotid is necessary during the course of surgery. Bipolar electrosurgery may also be required.

Operative procedure (Fig. 21-13)

1. The incision may extend from the posterior angle of the zygoma downward in front of the tragus of the ear and behind the lobule of the ear backward over the mastoid process and then downward and forward on the neck parallel to and below the body of the mandible. (A chin incision may also be used.) Bleeding vessels are controlled by hemostats and fine ligatures, or by electrocoagulation.
2. With fine-toothed tissue forceps and scissors the skin flaps are elevated as described for thyroidectomy (see Chapter 16). The skin wound edges are retracted by means of silk sutures fastened to clamps.
3. The upper portion of the sternocleidomastoid muscle is exposed and retracted, the auricular nerve is identified, and the lower part of the parotid gland is elevated with curved hemostats.
4. The superficial temporal artery and vein and external jugular vein are identified by means of blunt dissection. The parotid tissue is dissected from the cartilage of the ear and the tympanic plate of the temporal bone. The temporal, zygomatic, and mandibular and cervical branches of the facial nerve are identified and preserved.
5a. The *superficial portion* of the parotid gland containing the tumor is removed. In some cases the entire superficial portion is removed, followed by ligation and division of the parotid duct.
5b. When the *deep portion* of the parotid gland must be removed, the facial nerve is retracted upward and outward, and then the parotid tissue is removed from beneath the nerve. Kocher retractors are used to retract the mandible. The external carotid artery is identified. In many cases the internal maxillary and superficial temporal arteries are clamped, ligated, and divided.
6. The wound is closed in layers with absorbable suture. A small drain is inserted, the skin is closed with fine nonabsorbable suture, and a pressure dressing is applied.

TRACHEOSTOMY

Tracheostomy is the opening of the trachea and the insertion of a cannula through a midline incision in the neck, below the cricoid cartilage. A tracheostomy may be permanent or temporary. It is used as an emergency procedure to treat upper respiratory tract obstruction, which can be caused by bilateral vocal cord paralysis, inflammatory swelling, or edema caused by trauma or allergic reaction or neoplasms and as a prophylactic measure in the presence of chronic lung disease, in extensive composite resections where massive upper airway edema is anticipated, or for sleep apnea in which an obstruction could occur. A prophylactic tracheostomy is performed at the time of surgery to permit easy and frequent aspiration of the tracheobronchial tree secretions and diminish the dead space that exists from the opening of the mouth down to the supraclavicular region. The creation of a new clearance (tracheostomy) nearer to the functional areas in the lung provides for a greater volume of air for the patient with a partly destroyed lung. Anesthesia may be maintained through a prophylactic tracheostomy.

The patient's psychologic status should be carefully evaluated because of the altered body image, which may be either temporary or permanent, depending on the disease entity involved. Tracheostomy care should be explained carefully and thoroughly so that the patient will understand why it must be done so frequently, especially the suctioning of the tube. Reinforcement should be given about the ability to communicate with others by means of a pencil and paper or message board. As recovery progresses, the patient can be shown how to occlude the opening of the tube for brief periods to be able to speak a few words and learn and master tracheostomy self-care (Box 21-2). If a tracheostomy tube with a disposable inner cannula is inserted, the circulating nurse must ensure that the patient has replacement cannulas in the event occlusion or blockage occurs in the immediate postoperative period.

Procedural considerations

Tracheostomy tube cuffs should be tested for air leaks before insertion by inflating and then deflating the balloon. The patient is placed in a supine position, with the shoulders raised by a small rolled sheet to slightly hyperextend the neck and head. The neck is prepped, and sterile drapes are applied. A soft suction catheter should be available on the sterile field for suctioning after the tube is inserted.

Operative procedure

1. A local anesthetic may be injected into the tracheotomy site before the incision is made. A vertical or transverse incision may be used. A vertical incision is made with a #10, #15, or #11 blade in the midline about midway between the cricoid cartilage and the suprasternal notch. With this incision there is less risk of damage to nerves and vessels and less bleeding. When a

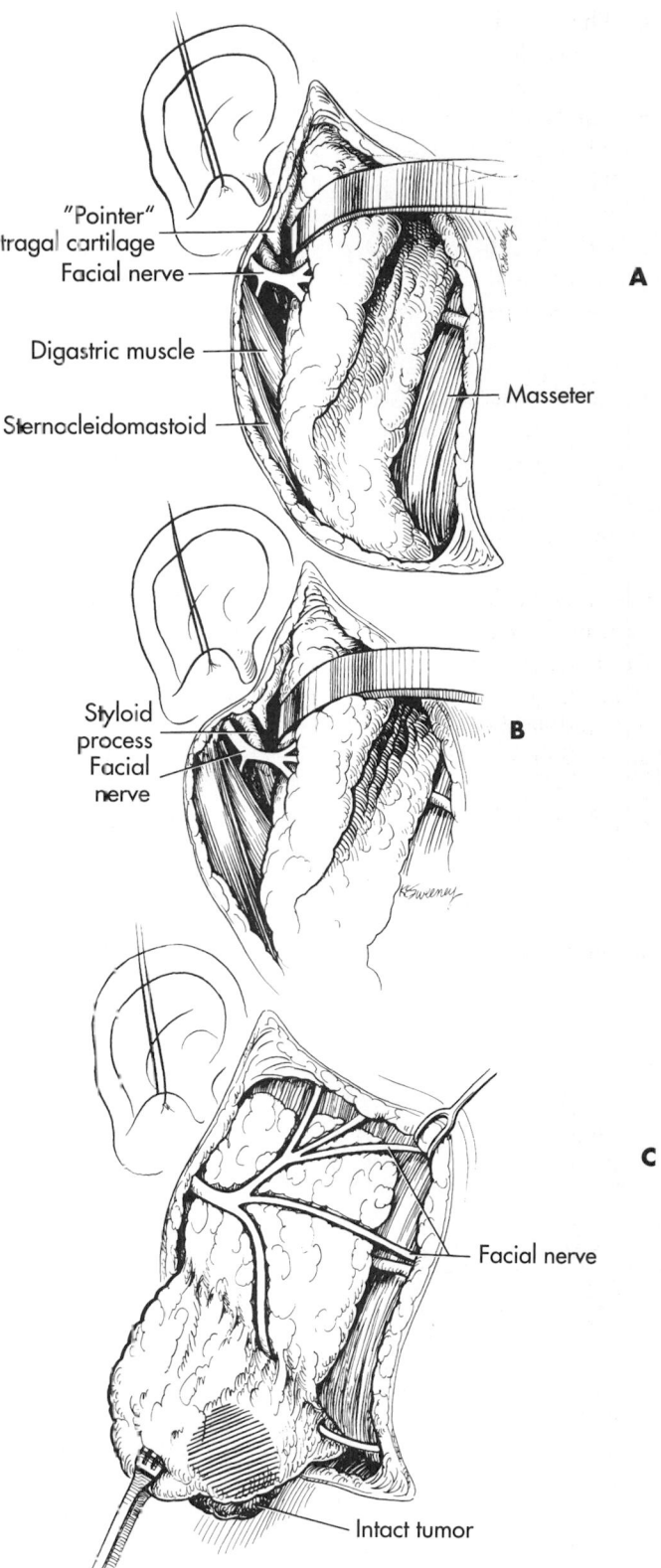

FIGURE 21-13 **A**, Blunt dissection of parotid gland from external auditory canal cartilage exposes tragal pointer. Facial nerve lies approximately 1 cm deep and slightly anteroinferior to pointer and 6 to 8 mm deep to tympanomastoid suture line. **B**, Facial nerve exits stylomastoid foramen to run anteriorly between styloid process and attachment of digastric muscle to digastric ridge. **C**, Nearly completed process with tumor within intact superficial parotidectomy specimen.

BOX 21-2 | **Patient Education Guide Tracheostomy**

The nurse should provide the patient with the following instructions:

1. Bacteria can easily enter the tracheostomy. To avoid infection, always wash your hands before touching your tracheostomy.
2. Observe the stoma daily for any signs of redness, swelling, or drainage.
3. Clean the stoma twice a day using a clean, damp face cloth; do not use soap.
4. A thin coat of petrolatum may be applied to the skin around the stoma; be careful not to let any enter the stoma.
5. Avoid dust, smoke, aerosol sprays, perfumes, car exhaust, powder, and raking leaves. Particles from any of these may enter directly into your tracheostomy. If you must be exposed to any of these agents, cover your tracheostomy with a piece of cotton cloth.
6. Vacuum instead of sweeping. Dust and mop with damp cloths or mops rather than dry ones.
7. Wear a stoma covering to warm and filter the inspired air, especially in cold weather. A variety of clothing and accessories can be worn by men and women over the stoma covering. High-neck sweaters, turtlenecks, and scarves work well. They should fit loosely around the neck, so that there is always easy access to the stoma and breathing is not obstructed.
8. Cover your tracheostomy, not your nose and mouth, when coughing or sneezing.
9. Do not use tissues or cotton-tipped applicators near the stoma because pieces of these materials may break off and enter the tracheostomy. Use a handkerchief when coughing.
10. Additional humidification of the air, especially during the winter when rooms are heated, will help keep secretions moist enough to be removed by coughing. Commercially available vaporizers or humidifiers may be used. The water (H_2O) in the vaporizer should be changed daily, and the vaporizer cleaned with soapy water at least twice a week. Alternatively, a pan

of water can be kept on the stove or radiator. The water should be changed daily. Moist gauze may be used for a stoma cover, rather than the piece of cotton cloth.
11. When taking a bath or shower, stand on a nonslip bath mat because a fall could cause water to be splashed into your tracheostomy; showers are preferred.
12. When showering, adjust the shower head so that the water is directed to a level on your body below your tracheostomy. A well-wrung towel can be draped around the neck, over the tracheostomy for further protection.
13. Be sure to cover your tracheostomy with your hand or with a commercially available shower guard while rinsing your head.
14. While shaving or having a haircut, wear a protective covering and a towel over the stoma to prevent dust and hair particles from entering.
15. Avoid wearing clothing with small ornaments, such as sequins or small buttons, near the neckline. Women should avoid wearing necklaces with small individual parts (i.e., pearls).
16. Clean mouth and teeth at least three times a day. Use mouthwash often because the ability to detect mouth odor is lessened.
17. Purchase and wear a medic alert tag indicating that you have a tracheostomy and with instructions should the tracheostomy become obstructed or in the event of a cardiopulmonary arrest.
18. No change in sleep habits is required. You will be able to breathe easily, even with blankets covering your tracheostomy.
19. If your tracheostomy tube has an inner cannula, clean it daily and PRN with a solution of equal parts of hydrogen peroxide and water. Rinse the cannula thoroughly under running water before reinserting it.
20. Change the twill tape holding your tracheostomy in place when needed. Secure the new tape in place before removing the old tape.
21. Suction the tracheostomy using clean technique as needed.

From Beare, P.G., & Myers, J.L. (1994). *Principles and practice of adult health nursing* (ed. 2). St. Louis: Mosby.

---

transverse incision is made, it extends approximately one fingerbreadth above the suprasternal notch parallel to it and from the anterior border of one sternocleidomastoid muscle to the opposite side. Soft tissues and muscle are divided using blunt and sharp dissection. The isthmus of the thyroid gland that joins both lobes of the gland in the midline over the trachea is retracted cephalad or caudad, or divided, resulting in exposure of the underlying tracheal rings, usually the second and third (Fig. 21-14, *A*). In some cases two curved clamps may be inserted through this incision across the isthmus and the isthmus transsected (Fig. 21-14, *B*). The transsected ends of the isthmus are oversewn or suture ligated with absorbable sutures.

2. Lidocaine 4% may be instilled into the trachea to reduce the coughing reflex when the tube is inserted. Air is first drawn into a syringe to ensure that the needle

point is located in the lumen. With a knife and #15 blade or a tracheal punch, a transverse incision is made in the trachea directly across the two tracheal rings. (Some surgeons prefer to make an H-shaped or T-shaped cut.) The cricoid cartilage is elevated with a hook (Fig. 21-14, *C*) or 2-0 monofilament retraction suture.

3. With the stoma spread, a tracheostomy tube with the obturator in place is inserted into the trachea (Fig. 21-14, *D*), the obturator is quickly removed, and the trachea is suctioned with a soft catheter to remove blood and mucus from the airway.

4. The wound edges are lightly approximated with nonabsorbable no. 2-0 sutures, or the wound edges are allowed to fall together around the tube. One or two skin sutures are inserted above the tube. The lower angle of the wound may be left open for drainage.

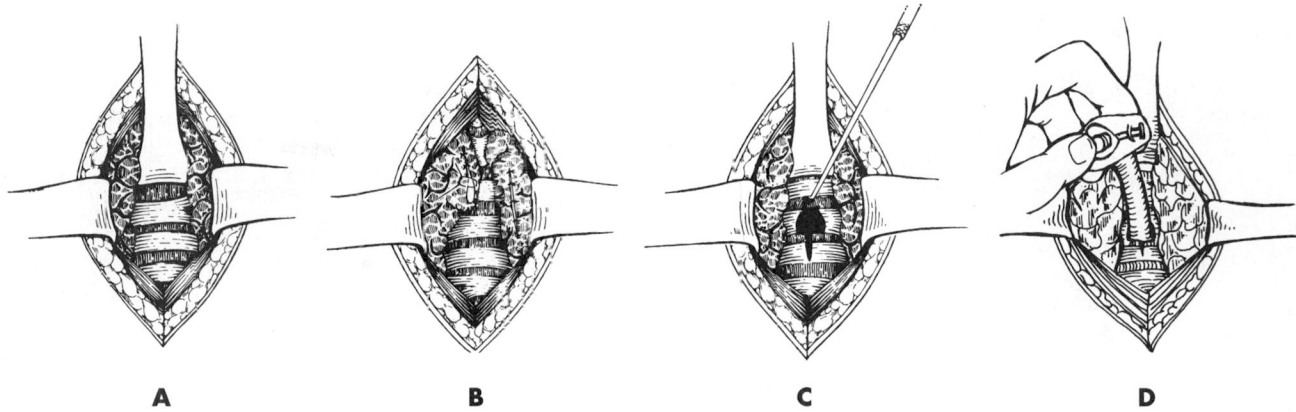

A **B** **C** **D**

FIGURE 21-14 Operative technique for elective tracheostomy. **A,** Retractor exposing trachea by drawing isthmus of thyroid upward. **B,** Alternative method to that shown in **A.** Isthmus of thyroid is divided to expose trachea. **C,** Two tracheal rings are cut, and upper ring is partially resected. Tracheal hook pulls trachea from depth of wound nearer surface. **D,** Insertion of tube.

5. The tracheostomy tube is held in place with tapes tied with a square knot to the side of the neck. The inner cannula is then inserted. A gauze dressing split around the tube is applied to the wound.

6. An additional tracheostomy tube of the same size and the obturator should be kept with the patient at all times, in the event the tube becomes dislodged or plugged with secretions. This practice expedites changing the tracheostomy tube with minimal potential for complications to the patient.

UVULOPALATOPHARYNGOPLASTY

Uvulopalatopharyngoplasty (UPPP) is primarily performed to relieve obstructive sleep apnea and snoring (Fig. 21-15). Two or more of the following indications are reason to perform the operation:

- An O_2 saturation that drops below 80
- Apnea index worse than 20
- Significant daytime sleepiness
- Heroic snoring, producing social or marital problems
- Cardiac dysrhythmias, other than tachycardia, or bradycardia during sleep

Procedural considerations

A tracheostomy may be performed with UPPP because of postoperative edema with subsequent airway obstruction. The tracheostomy tube is removed and the incision is closed when the danger of postoperative edema and bleeding has passed (if the surgical procedure is successful). Because some of these patients are obese (causing the tissue of the pharynx to sag during sleep), preoperative planning should include obtaining an assortment of tracheostomy tubes, including extralong tubes, before the start of the procedure. Care must be taken in positioning the obese patient to ensure proper body alignment. Emergency

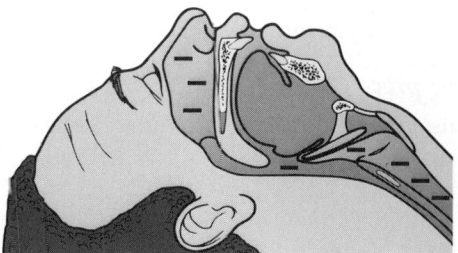

Patient predisposed to OSA

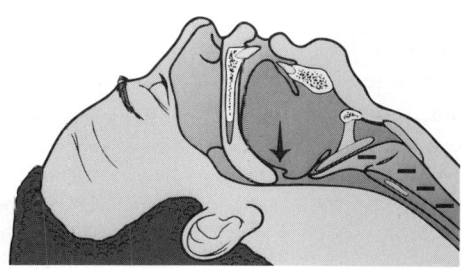

Apneic episode

FIGURE 21-15 Sleep apnea syndrome is a condition in which airflow is temporarily obstructed during sleep. Airflow obstruction occurs when the tongue and the soft palate fall backward and partially or completely obstruct the pharynx. The obstruction may last from 10 seconds to as long as 2 minutes. During the apneic period, the client experiences severe hypoxemia (decreased Pao_2), hypercapnia (increased $Paco_2$), and acidosis. These changes interrupt sleep and cause the client to partially awaken. When the client begins to awaken, the tone of the muscles of the upper airway increases. The tongue and soft palate move forward and the airway opens. Apnea and arousals occur repeatedly during the night separated by several normal breaths. The cause of sleep apnea is not definitely known. However, three factors appear to be involved: (1) shape of the upper airway, (2) neural control of the respiratory muscles, and (3) hormonal balance.

tracheostomy or bronchoscopy should be anticipated, in the event of airway obstruction after anesthetic induction. The surgeon may choose to administer local anesthesia with anesthesia personnel monitoring the patient and then induce general anesthesia after an adequate airway is

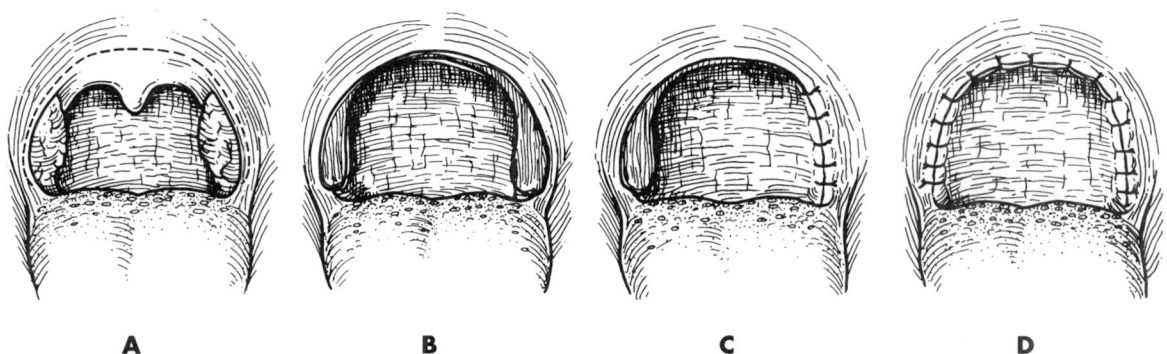

A   **B**   **C**   **D**

FIGURE 21-16   Technique of palatopharyngoplasty as advocated by Simmons et al.

established. A tonsillectomy is performed (if the tonsils are present) along with the UPPP. Instrumentation and positioning are similar to those discussed under tracheostomy and tonsillectomy, with the exception noted previously of the need to properly position the obese patient.

Operative procedure

1. The mouth gag (usually self-retaining) is inserted.
2. The tissue to be resected may be outlined by an electrosurgical blade. A #3 knife handle with #15 blade or a #7 knife handle with a #12 blade may be used to make the incision in the soft palate and anteriorly to the tonsillar pillar (if the patient has not previously had a tonsillectomy), or posteriorly to the tonsillar pillars if the patient has had a tonsillectomy (Fig. 21-16).
3. The tissue is resected by means of Metzenbaum scissors and long forceps with teeth or by a hand-controlled electrosurgical pencil.
4. Larger blood vessels may be clamped until the tissue is removed, or a suction coagulator or hand-controlled electrosurgical pencil may be used to obtain hemostasis as the tissue is excised.
5. Once the tissue is removed and hemostasis is obtained, absorbable sutures are used to approximate the edges of the mucosa. Depending on the surgeon's preference, 2-0 and 3-0 absorbable suture should be available. Needle holders should be long enough to allow the surgeon ease in delivering the atraumatic needle to the edges of the mucosa.
6. The oral cavity should be rinsed of blood and debris and the incision inspected before the patient is discharged from the operating room.

Care should be taken when inspecting the incision in the postoperative period not to disturb the incision with a tongue blade, if one is used to provide access for inspection. The patient must not be provided with a straw for fluid intake because it might disturb the suture line. Gentle oral cavity rinsing is recommended several times daily to decrease the chance of postoperative infection and to increase patient comfort.

LARYNGOFISSURE

Laryngofissure is an opening of the larynx for exploratory, excisional, or reconstructive procedures that cannot be accomplished endoscopically.

Procedural considerations

A laryngofissure may be performed when access to the intrinsic larynx is necessary. The thyroid cartilages are split in the midline, and the true vocal cords and false vocal cords are incised at the midline anteriorly. A neck dissection instrument set is required, plus an oscillating power saw.

Operative procedure

1. A tracheotomy is performed, and an endotracheal tube inserted. A general anesthetic is administered.
2. A transverse incision is made through the skin and first layer of the cervical fascia and platysma muscles, approximately 2 cm above the sternoclavicular junction or in the normal skin crease. The upper skin flap is undermined to the level of the cricoid cartilage, and the lower flap is undermined to the sternoclavicular joint.
3. Bleeding vessels are clamped with mosquito hemostats and ligated. The strap muscles are elevated and incised in the midline.
4. The thyroid cartilages are cut with an oscillating saw, and the true vocal cords are visualized through an incision into the cricothyroid membrane. The true vocal cords are divided in the midline (anterior commissure), and the interior of the larynx is exposed.
5. The tracheostomy tube must be left in place after surgery to ensure an airway.

LARYNGEAL FRAMEWORK SURGERY

Laryngeal framework surgery, such as type 1 thyroplasty, is used to change or improve the voice. Thyroplasty types II and III are used to alter vocal cord tension and voice pitch.

Thyroplasty

Type I thyroplasty is a form of laryngeal framework surgery for the treatment of unilateral vocal cord paralysis, which may be caused by trauma, neoplasms, paralysis from thyroidectomy, paralysis after extensive aortic and mediastinal vascular surgery, and mechanical and central nervous system dysfunction. A window is created surgically in the thyroid cartilage into which a silicone implant is placed. The implant pushes the paralyzed cord medially, which allows the moving cord to touch the paralyzed cord and close the opening.

Procedural considerations

As the preoperative assessment is being done, the circulating nurse can explain to the patient that his or her voice will need to be rested postoperatively in an effort to minimize edema and stress of the vocal cords. An alternative method of communicating can be determined, such as writing.

The procedure is done under monitored local anesthesia to allow the patient to phonate during surgery. This allows the surgeon to evaluate the quality of the patient's voice in an effort to attain the best result.

Operative procedure

1. The patient is positioned supine on the OR bed in a semisitting position. A flexible laryngoscopy will be done by means of a flexible, fiberoptic laryngoscope.
2. As the patient is asked to phonate, the surgeon is determining the extent of approximation of the vocal cords as well as the patient's breath control. After a thorough evaluation, the patient is then prepped and draped.
3. A local anesthetic is injected into the surgical site. A horizontal incision is made at the middle level of the thyroid ala. Gelpi retractors are used to maintain exposure, as dissection to the thyroid cartilage is completed. Measurements for the placement of the window are taken and marked with a marking pencil. A #15 blade is used to create a window in the thyroid cartilage. In some cases, a power drill with a cutting burr may be used. A periosteal elevator may be used to displace the vocal cords during phonation in an effort to determine voice quality.
4. When satisfaction has been reached, the implant is placed into the window. Final laryngoscopy is done to view approximation of the vocal cords with the implant in place. The incision is then closed, and a dressing is placed.

PARTIAL LARYNGECTOMY

Partial laryngectomy is removal of a portion of the larynx. It is done to remove superficial neoplasms that are confined to one vocal cord or to remove a tumor extending up into the ventricle on the anterior commis-

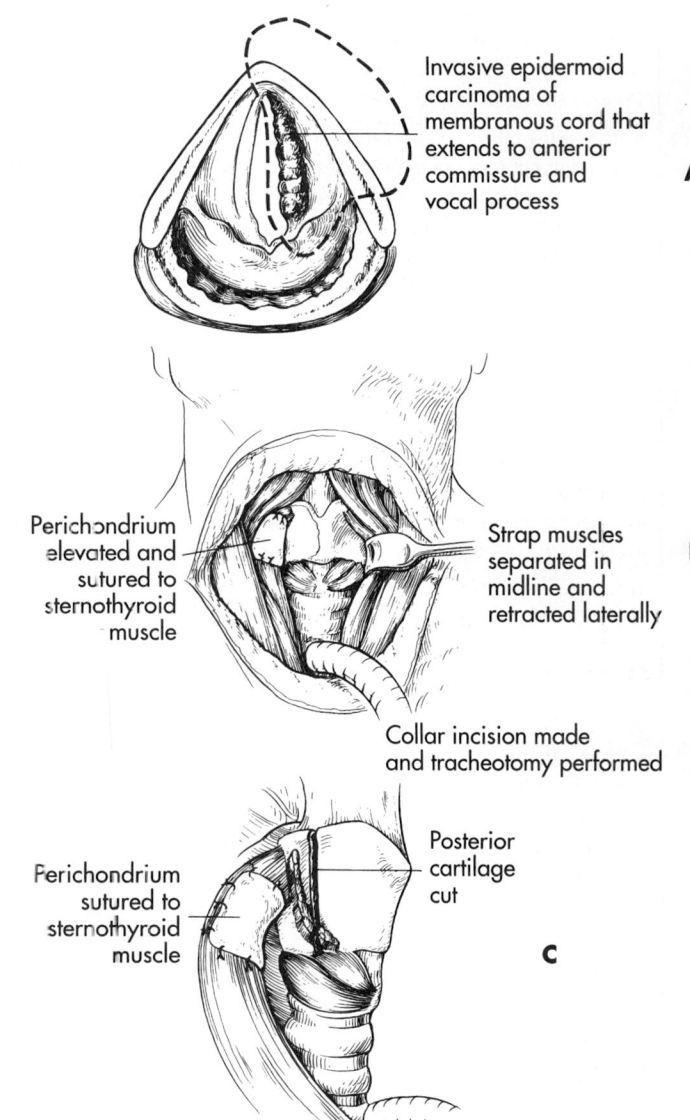

FIGURE 21-17 Standard hemilaryngectomy. **A,** Broken lines outline full extent of resection in standard hemilaryngectomy for invasive epidermoid carcinoma of membranous cord that extends to anterior commissure and vocal process. **B,** Neck flap is elevated after collar incision is made and tracheotomy is performed. Strap muscles are separated in midline and retracted laterally. On side of lesion, perichondrium is elevated, and its attachment to sternothyroid muscle maintained. **C,** External perichondrium is sutured to overlying sternothyroid muscle and is retracted laterally to expose posterior border of thyroid cartilage so that posterior cartilage cut can be made approximately 5 mm from edge.

sure or a short distance below the cord. Cancers confined to the intrinsic larynx (Fig. 21-17, *A*) are generally a low-grade malignancy and tend to remain localized for long periods. The patient should be prepared for an altered voice quality postoperatively as well as for the possibility of total laryngectomy if the tumor proves too extensive for partial resection. General guidelines for patient education

BOX 21-3	Patient Education and Home Care Teaching for Partial and Total Laryngectomy

Preprocedural Teaching

- Review the physician's explanation of the procedure and the reason for it; encourage the patient to ask questions and to discuss any fears or anxieties. Discuss the need for informed consent for surgery and anesthesia.

Review of preprocedural care

- Inform the patient that the skin will be cleansed with bactericidal soap or antiseptic solutions to remove bacteria.
- Discuss preprocedural tests: complete blood count and urinalysis to check for infection and bleeding.
- Tell the patient that NPO status must be maintained from midnight of the night before surgery.
- Provide preparatory instruction in suctioning (oral and tracheal) and wound care.
- Teach the patient to do own tube feedings.
- Review the use of a magic slate or paper and pencil, flash cards, or a communication board.
- Prepare the patient for permanent loss of speech if total laryngectomy is to be performed.
- Have a speech therapist visit the patient to discuss and plan for alternative means of speech.

Review of postprocedural care

- Explain that the patient will be in the high Fowler's position to lessen edema, increase coughing and deep breathing, ease suctioning, and provide comfort.
- Explain that the patient will be given mechanical ventilation by a tracheostomy tube and that suctioning will be done frequently to maintain a clear airway for breathing.
- Discuss the importance of frequent deep breathing and coughing.
- Demonstrate the use of intermittent positive-pressure breathing devices and ultrasonic nebulization treatments.
- Explain the presence of pressure dressings and neck drainage tubes. Discuss the use of a nasogastric tube to assist with feedings (bolus or continuous drip based on patient tolerance).
- Explain that swallowing and speech rehabilitation will begin soon after surgery, with the need based on the type and extent of surgery.

Side Effects and Complications

- Hemorrhage
- Airway obstruction
- Infection
- Thoracic duct leakage
- Nerve injury

Home Care

- Give both the patient and the caregiver *oral* and *written* instructions. Provide them with the name and telephone number of a physician or nurse to call if questions arise. Use visual aids to assist in instruction.

- *General information*
  — Review any explanation about the procedure and any specific follow-up care.
- *Wound or incision care*
  — Instruct the patient and caregiver to inspect the incision site daily and to change the dressing using sterile supplies as demonstrated by the nurse.
- *Warning signs*
  — Review the signs and symptoms that should be reported to a physician or nurse.
    Infection of the stoma or incision: redness, drainage, pain, warm to touch, fever
    Dyspnea without exertion
    Difficulty swallowing
- *Special instructions*
  — Teach the patient to avoid voice strain and to whisper or use alternative methods of communication when the voice needs rest. If the voice is gone (total laryngectomy), have the patient work with a speech therapist to develop an alternative method of communicating.
- *Medications*
  — Provide pain management, encouraging the patient to use mild analgesics when possible.
- *Activity*
  — Remind the patient to plan frequent rest periods to avoid shortness of breath.
  — Assist the patient to begin self-care as soon as possible, including tracheostomy care and taking food and fluids by mouth.
- *Diet*
  — Plan a diet with the patient and caregivers that will avoid the possibility of choking or aspirating. For example, the patient may initially receive tube feedings and progress to soft foods and liquids as the swallowing reflex returns.

Follow-up Care

- Stress the importance of regular follow-up visits. Make sure the patient has the necessary names and telephone numbers.

Psychosocial Care

- Encourage questions and verbalization of fear and anxieties regarding possible loss of the voice.

Referrals

- Assist the patient to obtain referral services, supplies, and information about support groups from the Lost Cord Club/International Association of Laryngectomees, sponsored by the American Cancer Society.
- Arrange a reconstructive surgery consultation as needed.

From Canobbio, M.M. (1996). *Mosby's handbook of patient teaching.* St. Louis: Mosby.

and home-care teaching for laryngectomy patients is presented in Box 21-3.

Procedural considerations

The patient is placed in the supine position. The operative site is prepped and draped as described for thyroidectomy (see Chapter 16), or for the head and neck procedure. The setup for partial laryngectomy includes a neck dissection setup, Freer or Cottle periosteal elevator, oscillating saw, tracheostomy tubes, and an electrosurgical unit.

Operative procedure

1. A tracheostomy is performed as previously described, and an endotracheal tube is inserted.
2. A vertical incision or a thyroid incision with elevation of a flap may be employed (Fig. 21-17, B).
3. The sternothyroid muscles are separated in the midline and retracted by means of Green retractors.
4. The fascial covering over the thyroid cartilage is incised with a knife, and with a Freer periosteal elevator the perichondrium is elevated from the cartilage on the side of the tumor.
5. The thyroid cartilage is divided longitudinally in the midline by means of an oscillating saw.
6. The cartilages are retracted, and the cricothyroid membrane is incised with a knife. A blunt-nosed laryngeal scissors is introduced between the vocal cords to divide the mucosa of the anterior wall of the glottis.
7. The divided cartilages are retracted with Kocher retractors to expose the interior of the larynx. A small, moist gauze pack may be placed in the trachea to prevent aspiration of blood or mucus. A small amount of a topical anesthetic may be applied to the larynx to prevent laryngeal muscular spasm. The extent of the intrinsic laryngeal tumor is determined.
8. With a small periosteal elevator, the mucosa on the involved side of the larynx is freed; the false cord and mucosal layer of the region are lifted by means of a periosteal elevator and hooks. The involved cord is excised with straight scissors (Fig. 21-17, C).
9. In some cases the thyroid cartilage may be removed with a knife and straight scissors. Bleeding is controlled with hemostats, fine absorbable ligatures and sutures, and electrocoagulation.
10. The gauze pack is removed from the trachea. The perichondrium is approximated with 2-0 absorbable sutures. The strap muscles are approximated in the midline with 2-0 absorbable sutures. The platysma and the skin edges are approximated separately with fine nonabsorbable sutures.
11. Dressings are applied to the wound and around the tube. A tracheolaryngeal tube is left in place and removed at a later date when the airway is adequate.

SUPRAGLOTTIC LARYNGECTOMY (Fig. 21-18)

Supraglottic laryngectomy is excision of the laryngeal structures above the true vocal cords, hyoid bone, epiglottis, and false vocal cords.

Procedural considerations

Supraglottic laryngectomy is indicated in cancer of the epiglottis and false vocal cords. It is designed to remove the cancer yet preserve the phonatory, respiratory, and sphincteric functions of the larynx. A neck dissection is almost always performed. The patient will have to undergo swallowing therapy postoperatively to learn how to decrease the incidence of aspiration. The instrument setup is as described for neck dissection.

Operative procedure

The procedure is similar to that described for partial laryngectomy, except for the use of an oscillating saw.

TOTAL LARYNGECTOMY

Total laryngectomy is complete removal of the cartilaginous larynx, the hyoid bone, and the strap muscles connected to the larynx and possible removal of the preepiglottic space with the lesion. A wide-field laryngectomy is done when there is a loss of mobility of the cords and to treat cancer of the extrinsic larynx and hypopharynx (Fig. 21-19). Malignant tumors of the extrinsic larynx are more anaplastic and tend to metastasize. When laryngeal carcinoma involves more than the true cords, a prophylactic (preventive) radical neck dissection is done to remove the lymphatics.

Laryngectomy presents many psychologic problems. The loss of voice that follows total laryngectomy is traumatic for the patient and family. The patient may be taught to talk either by using his or her esophageal voice or with an artificial larynx. The esophageal voice is produced by the air contained in the esophagus rather than by that in the trachea. Speech requires a sounding air column. With instruction and practice, the patient is able to control the swallowing of air into the esophagus and reintroduction of this air into the mouth with phonation. The sounding air column is then transformed into speech by means of the lips, tongue, and teeth. A tracheoesophageal fistula facilitates insertion of a Blom-Singer duckbill prosthesis for purpose of speech (Fig. 21-20, A). This fistula may be created during the initial surgical procedure or at a later date when healing has occurred (Fig. 21-20, B).

Because the stump of the trachea is brought out to the skin of the neck to form a permanent stoma, all the patient's breathing is done directly into the trachea and no longer through the nose and mouth. This air is no longer moistened by the nose. Drying and crusting of the tracheal secretions occur. Humidification may be provided when

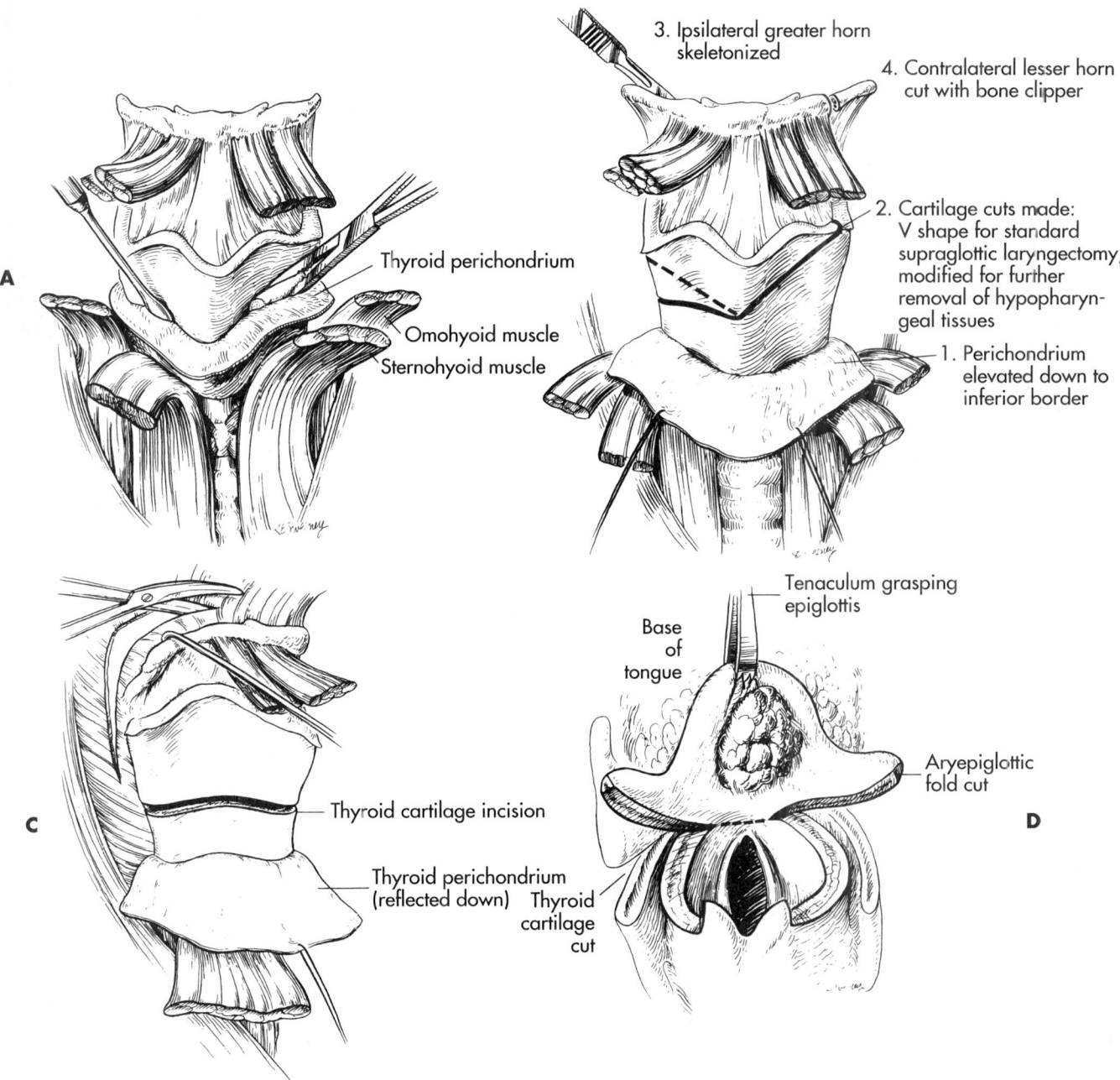

FIGURE 21-18 Supraglottic laryngectomy. **A,** Strap muscles are cut just above thyroid cartilage, and thyroid perichondrium is incised along superior border of thyroid cartilage. Thyroid cartilage perichondrium is carefully elevated and dissected inferiorly by first using "peanut" and then Freer elevator. **B,** Thyroid cartilage perichondrium elevation is completed down to inferior border, and then cartilage cuts are made. V shape is outlined for standard supraglottic laryngectomy. This may be modified for further removal of hypopharyngeal tissues according to size of lesion. Ipsilateral greater horn is skeletonized, and contralateral lesser horn is cut with bone clipper. **C,** Piriform fossa and vallecula are then entered on side of lesion, while greater horn of hyoid bone is retracted for exposure. **D,** Epiglottis is grasped with tenaculum, and scissors are used to cut through aryepiglottic fold in front of arytenoid and down into ventricle. Once both supraglottic cuts have been made through aryepiglottic folds, intervening tissues are cut to join up with thyroid cartilage cuts.

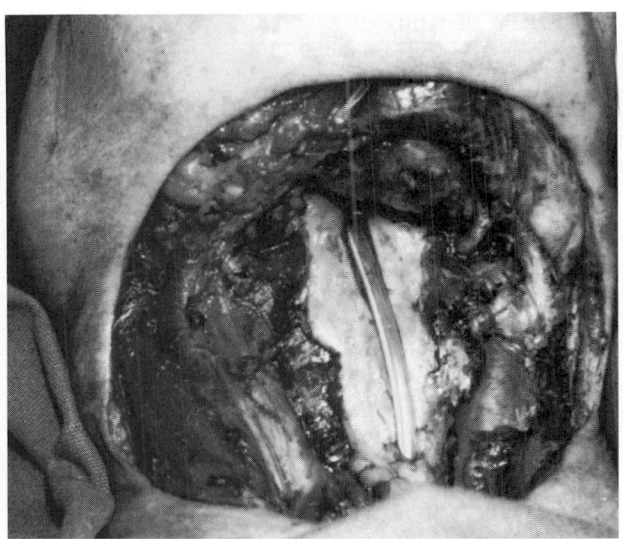

FIGURE 21-19 Wide-field laryngectomy defect for radiation recurrent tumor, including anterior neck skin, thyroid, sternomastoid, and selective neck node resection.

the opening is covered with a moist gauze compress. The patient will be anxious to know about postoperative voice quality, which depends on the specific procedure performed. Table 21-1 lists surgical procedures and associated predictions of postoperative voice qualities. Fig. 21-21 shows a clinical pathway for total laryngectomy.

Procedural considerations

The patient is placed on the operating room bed in a supine position with neck extended and shoulders elevated by a shoulder roll or folded sheet. A general anesthetic is administered. An effective suction apparatus is essential. The proposed operative site, including the anterior neck region, the lateral surfaces of the neck down to the outer aspects of the shoulders, and the upper anterior chest region, is prepped and draped in the usual manner. The instrument setup is a neck dissection set.

Operative procedure

1. A tracheostomy may be performed initially to control the airway, or it may be incorporated into the procedure, depending on surgeon preference. If performed initially, a cuffed, wire-reinforced, flexible endotracheal tube will ensure effective delivery of the anesthetic and give the surgical team flexibility as the larynx and trachea are manipulated during the surgical procedure.
2. A midline incision is made from the suprasternal notch to just above the hyoid bone. Skin flaps are undermined on each side. The sternothyroid, sternohyoid, and omohyoid muscles (strap muscles) on each side are divided by means of curved hemostats and a knife.
3. The suprahyoid muscles are severed from the portion of the hyoid to be divided. The hyoid bone is divided

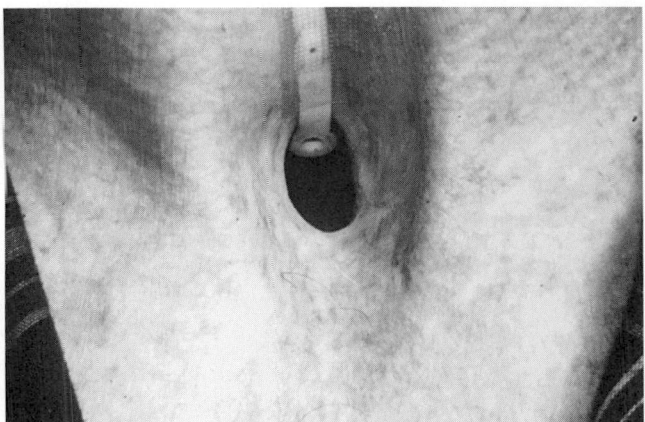
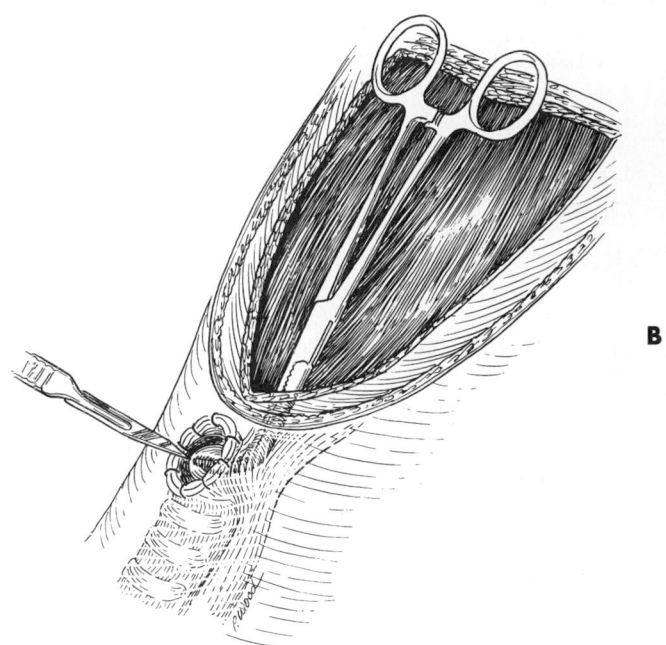

FIGURE 21-20 **A**, Speech valve in place. **B**, Primary tracheoesophageal puncture technique. Notice preliminary repair of stoma to allow accurate positioning of puncture site before pharyngeal closure. Feeding tube (14 French) is inserted through puncture down esophagus to the stomach.

at the junction of its middle and lateral thirds with heavy scissors or bone-cutting forceps. Bleeding vessels are clamped and ligated.
4. The superior laryngeal nerve and vessels are exposed and ligated on each side with long curved fine hemostats and fine ligatures.
5. The isthmus of the thyroid gland is divided between hemostats. Each portion of the thyroid gland is dissected from the trachea with Metzenbaum scissors and fine tissue forceps. The superior pole of the thyroid is retracted. The superior thyroid vessels are freed from the larynx by sharp dissection.
6. The larynx is rotated. The inferior pharyngeal constrictor muscle is severed from its attachment to the thyroid cartilage on each side.

TABLE 21-1 | **Surgical Procedures for Laryngeal Carcinomas and Predictions of Vocal Quality after Surgery**

STRUCTURES REMOVED	STRUCTURES LEFT	POSTOPERATIVE CONDITION
Total Laryngectomy		
Hyoid bone	Tongue	Loses voice
Entire larynx (epiglottis, false cords, true cords)	Pharyngeal walls	Breathes through tracheostoma
Cricoid cartilage	Lower trachea	No problem swallowing
Two or three rings of trachea		
Supraglottic or Horizontal Laryngectomy		
Hyoid bone	True vocal cords	Normal voice
Epiglottis	Cricoid cartilage	May aspirate occasionally, especially liquids
False vocal cords	Trachea	Normal airway
Vertical Laryngectomy (or Hemilaryngectomy)		
One true vocal cord	Epiglottis	Hoarse but serviceable voice
One false cord	One false cord	Normal airway
Arytenoid	One true vocal cord	No problem swallowing
Half thyroid cartilage	Cricoid	
Laryngofissure and Partial Laryngectomy		
One vocal cord	All other structures	Hoarse but serviceable voice; occasionally almost normal voice
		No airway problem
		No swallowing problem
Endoscopic Removal of Early Carcinoma		
Part of one vocal cord	All other structures	May have a normal voice
		No other problems

From Saunders, W.H., Havener, W.H., Fair, C.J., & Hickey, J.T. (1979). *Nursing care in eye, ear, nose, and throat disorders* (ed. 4). St. Louis: Mosby.

7. The endotracheal tube is removed. The trachea is transsected just below the cricoid cartilage over a Kelly or Crile hemostat previously inserted between the trachea and esophagus. The upper resected portion of the trachea and the cricoid cartilage are held upward with Lahey forceps. A balloon-cuffed wire-reinforced endotracheal tube with a Murphy eye is inserted into the distal portion of the trachea.

8. The larynx is freed from the cervical esophagus and attachments by sharp and blunt dissection. A moist pack is placed around the endotracheal tube to help prevent leakage of blood into the trachea.

9. The pharynx is entered. In most cancers of the intrinsic larynx the pharynx is entered above the epiglottis. The mucous membrane incision is extended along either side of the epiglottis; the remaining portion of the pharynx and cervical esophagus is dissected well away from the tumor by means of fine-toothed tissue forceps, Metzenbaum scissors, knife, and fine hemostats. The specimen is removed en bloc.

10. A nasal feeding tube is inserted through one naris into the esophagus; closure of the hypopharyngeal and esophageal defect is begun with continuous, inverting fine 3-0 absorbable sutures. The nasal tube is guided down past the pharyngeal suture line.

11. The pharyngeal suture line is reinforced with interrupted sutures; the suprahyoid muscles are approximated to the cut edges of the inferior constrictor muscles.

12. The diameter of the tracheal stoma is increased by means of a knife and heavy scissors. The two portions of the thyroid behind the tracheal opening are approximated with interrupted nonabsorbable sutures, thereby obliterating dead space posterior to the upper portion of the trachea.

13. A closed wound drainage system is used, and the suction drains are appropriately placed.

14. The edges of the deep cervical fascia and the platysma are closed separately.

15. A laryngectomy tube of desired size is inserted into the tracheal stoma; a pressure dressing may be applied to the wound and neck, although some surgeons prefer leaving the wound without dressings to observe the skin flaps. (A cuffed tracheostomy tube may be inserted for 24 to 48 hours postoperatively until edema subsides; then it is replaced with a laryngectomy tube.)

Text continued on p. 787

THE JOHNS HOPKINS HOSPITAL
OPERATING ROOM CRITICAL PATH

Diagnosis: Laryngeal Cancer   **Procedure:** Total laryngectomy   **Physician:**

	Preoperative	Induction	Postinduction	Intraoperative	Postoperative
Consultations	• Consent • Speech therapy • Surgeon preference sheets • Consult surgeon if questions • Anesthesiologist consults with surgeon regarding airway • Anesthesiologist - call blood bank and review lab results			• Pathology for specimens/cytopathology (3-4 Frozen sections/case)	
Labs	• Blood bank—type & crossmatch 2 units • LFTs • Hg • M_7, M_{12}		• ABG • Na^+/K^+ • Hct or Hem-cue	• ABG • Na^+/K^+ • Hct or Hem-cue • Glucose, Ca^{++}	• Permanent SPEC to pathology dept.
Tests	• CXR • EKG				
Activity • **Mobility** • **Positioning**	• Geomatt on bed • Shoulder roll made • 2 arm boards on bed, padded <90° • Sleds prn • Head and foot on bed, head at proper end toward anesthesiologist • Teds on patient • Assist from wheelchair or stretcher onto bed supine • Warm blankets and safety strap on patient	• Recheck positioning and padding (feet not crossed)	• Assist tucking arms at side with bubble wrap, towels, sled prn • Shoulder roll in place • Turn bed per surgeon's preference	• Remove shoulder roll and turn patient with head toward anesthesiologist at end of case.	• Safe transfer to unit bed supine with HOB elevated • Clean warm blankets and gown • Accompany patient to unit • Head flexed

Continued

FIGURE 21-21   Clinical pathway for total laryngectomy.

Page 2	Preoperative	Induction	Postinduction	Intraoperative	Postoperative
Treatments	• Placement of 2 large PL IV's, central line • Prep and topical anesthetic for awake management (probably FOB) of airway • A-line	• Cricoid pressure PRN • A-line insertion PRN • Possible long arm CVP line • Delivery of anesthetic agents	• Insert rectal temperature probe • Insert Foley catheter • Perform endoscopy PRN • Prep surgical site • Shave • Tape eyes closed after applying Lacrilube	• Supplies onto sterile field PRN • Blood transfusions • Placement of Keo-feed NGT at end of case • Insert Shiley at end PRN • Attach JP drains to bulb suction, note drainage and empty PRN • Anode tube	• Bacitracin to SL PRN • Apply TC for O_2
Equipment and Supplies	• Teds • SCD and stockings • Head and neck and basic basin sterile concept packs • Head and neck linen pack • Long circuit tubing • 2 IV's on blood warmers • 2 transducers and pressure bag • Humidifier for circuit • Available setup FOB and cart with light source • Jet ventilator setup • OR bed with 2 arm boards • Bubble wrap padding • Anesthesia monitors and cart	• 2 suction canisters with suction tubing • Shields or goggles • Salem sump OG tube	• Cautery machine • Headlight box and headpiece • Electrical island • Bipolar and cord • Basic neck set • Anode tube • Jolly tube • 2 light handles • Razor • Prep set • Foley kit	• JP drains - at least 2 • Staples • Shiley trach. tube PRN • Disposable nerve stimulator • Ties, sutures • Sponges	• Ambu-Bag, O_2 tank with adapter and PSI >500, +ECG monitor on bed • ICU bed • Roller for transfer of heavy patient
Medications	• LR (IV solutions) • Reglan (GI Reflux Medications) • Sorbitol • Decadron • Preop Abx - Ancef 1 g - Flagyl 500 mg • "Critical care" bag of medications • "Local anesthesia" bag of medications • Controlled substances • Nebulizer for topicalization • Warm saline if fiberoptic intubation	• O_2 • Inhalation agent - isoflurane • IV anesthetics - pentothal, fentanyl, MSO_4, midazolam	• Lacrilube • 1% lidocaine with epinephrine 1:100,000 • O_2	• Ancef 1 g (if not allergic) • Flagyl 500 mg • Decadron 8 mg • Biobiotic irrigation • NSS irrigation • O_2 • Bacitracin • Maintenance anesthetics and IV solutions	• O_2 • "Critical care" bag of medications on bed during transfer to unit • LR (IV solutions)

FIGURE 21-21, cont'd Clinical pathway for total laryngectomy.

Page 3	Preoperative	Induction	Postinduction	Intraoperative	Postoperative
Discharge planning	• Nursing preop visit SDCC, units, or induction room • Nursing - assure family knows postop destination • Surgeon - answer any questions patient may have • Anesthesiologist - Airway assessment/concerns, talk with surgeon • Discuss postop effects of anesthesia, i.e. N&V • Inform patient re in-hospital airway registry and Medic Alert Airway Project			• Confirm patient's postop destination • Call report to receiving unit nurse ½ hour before arrival to unit—T-piece, ventilator needs • Complete and send bed slip to receiving unit with nursing assistant to get bed • Check O₂, Ambu-Bag, and ECG on bed and call nursing assistant/anesthesia technician if missing	• Call any change in patient status to receiving unit nurse • If patient breathing spontaneously, then T-piece setup in ICU • If patient with controlled ventilation → ventilator needed in ICU

Anesthesia activities	• Anesthesia evaluation
	• Setup for OR:
	  – Long circuit tubing for 2 IV's on blood warmers
	  – 2 transducers and pressure bag
	  – Humidifier for circuit Medications
	  – Fiberoptic bronchoscope and cart with light source
	  – Jet ventilator
	  – Bed and padding
	  – Routine monitors
	• Review chart and check labs in SDCC
	• Check availability of blood products
	• Start PL IV's, CVP, arterial line
	• Prep and topicalization for awake airway management
		• Induction of anesthesia - inhalation and IV
		• Temp. probe
		• Place OG tube PRN
			• Draw ABG, Na⁺, K⁺, Hct. or Hem-cue
			• Tape and lubricate eyes
				• Maintain anesthesia
				• Administer Abx., steroids
				• Draw blood ave. × 2 of each Na⁺, K⁺ ABG, Hct or heme-cue for entire case if ≤4 hours
				• Anode ETT to surgeon
				• Check Ambu-Bag, O₂, + ECG on bed for transport to unit
				• Secure airway for transport (Shley with TC or Ambu-Bag)
				• Connect patient to portable monitor before disconnecting OR monitors
				• Continue ambuing patient
				• Check pulse oximetry
				• Transfer to unit bed
					• Remove IV's from blood warmers and throw out disposables
					• Assure Meds/supplies for transport on bed
					• Place all anesthesia equipment on anesthesia machine
					• Complete QA/QI scan card for Dr. S./ACCM
					• Assist monitor exchange in unit
					• Get green bracelet for in-house airway registry
					• Chart label and Medic Alert form from ACCM
					• Return monitor to work room
					• Return ADR and controlled substances
					• Check out medications for next case
					• Report to receiving unit nurse and bed fellow

FIGURE 21-21, cont'd   Clinical pathway for total laryngectomy.

Continued

Page 4	Preoperative	Induction	Postinduction	Intraoperative	Postoperative

Nursing activity and teaching	• Control count
	• Preop Assessment—on unit, SDCC, or induction room
	• Standard admission protocol
	  – Preop checklist
	  – Consent
	  – Arm band
	  – Allergies - meds/latex
	  – NPO status
	  – Medical/surgical history
	  – Medications
	• Assess anxiety level and relay to anesthesiologist
	• Instruct patient on OR environment and answer questions re procedure
	• Gather instrumentation and supplies, Foley, Geomatt
	• Set up sterile field
	• Apply SCD stockings and start
	• Assist patient into room and onto bed
	• Apply safety strap and warm blanket
	• Pour solutions and meds onto sterile field
	• Obtain Abx/steroids and give to anesthesiologist
		• Stand at patient's side during induction
		• Obtain emergency equipment as needed
		• Keep room noise level down, room warm
		• Assist with padding and positioning of patient.
			• Assist with tucking of arms/sleds PRN
			• Check alignment/feet not crossed
			• Maintain patient dignity
			• Have Foley and prep setup/razor
			• Apply cautery pad
			• Place Chux under prep area
			• Draping (scrub)
				• Counts
				• Draping
				• Instrumentation
				• Maintain sterile field
				• Autoclave items PRN
				• Monitor room temperature for patient and team
				• Provide supplies and equipment and add to sterile field PRN
				• Complete charting
				• Weigh sponges PRN for EBL
				• Send specimen and call pathology
				• At patient's side for extubation
				• Complete bed slip and call nursing assistant to obtain ICU bed.
					• Wash prep solution off patient
					• Assess skin condition
					• Assist with transfer of patient to unit bed
					• Warm blankets
					• Complete charting
					• Accompany patient to ICU
					• Clean instruments and take to instrument room
					• Wipe all equipment with Wescodyne and return to proper place
					• Take specimen to pathology
					• Give paperwork to desk
					• Return radiographs to desk

Patient outcomes	• Will demonstrate low level of anxiety • Will have questions regarding procedure answered	• Maintain adequate body temperature • Uneventful induction	• Free of injury during positioning • Proper alignment • Maintain body temperature • Sustain no skin irritation	• Remain free of injury from equipment, foreign objects, or contamination • Uneventful extubation • Hemostasis	• Maintain skin integrity • Uneventful transfer to ICU
Potential complications	• Noncompliant with NPO • Extreme anxiety impeding IV start/induction, understanding of procedure	• Hypothermia, laryngeal spasm, aspiration, respiratory arrest	• Allergic reaction to meds.	• Hyperthermia, hypoglossal nerve injury, peripheral nerve injury related to positioning • Thrombosis • Hemorrhage • Cautery burn • Loss of airway	• Hemorrhage • Infection • Airway distress—stridor

FIGURE 21-21, cont'd Clinical pathway for total laryngectomy.

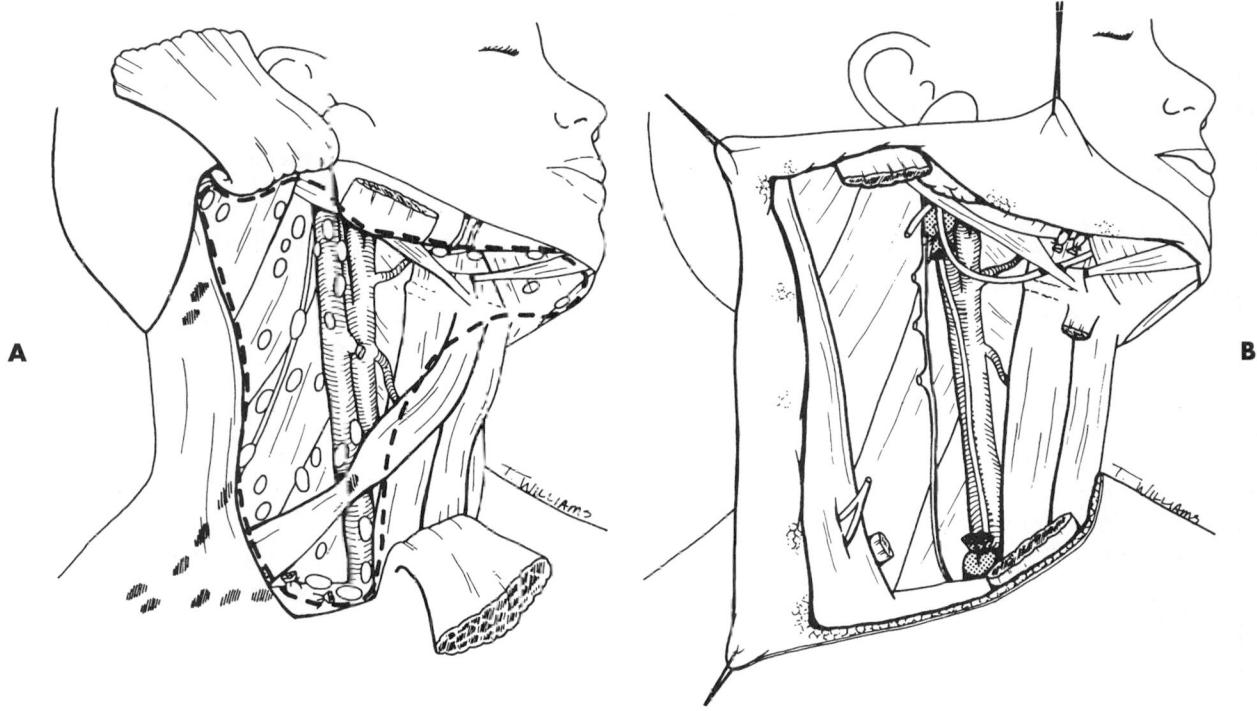

FIGURE 21-22   Radical neck dissection. **A**, Diagram of extent of operation. **B**, Diagram of operation.

RADICAL NECK DISSECTION

In a radical neck dissection the tumor, all soft tissue from the inferior aspect of the mandible to the midline of the neck to the clavicle end posterior to the trapezius muscle, and lymph nodes are removed en bloc in the affected side of the neck.[11] This procedure is done to remove the tumor and metastatic cervical nodes present in malignant lesions as well as all nonvital structures of the neck (Fig. 21-22, *A*). Metastasis occurs through the lymphatic channels by way of the bloodstream. Diseases of the oral cavity, lips, and thyroid gland may spread slowly to the neck. Radical neck surgery is done in the presence of cervical node metastasis from a cancer of the head and neck that has a reasonable chance of being controlled.

A prophylactic neck dissection implies elective radical neck surgery when there is no clinical evidence of metastatic cervical cancer.

Procedural considerations

The patient is placed on the OR bed in a supine position. General endotracheal anesthesia is administered before the patient is positioned for surgery. A shoulder roll may be placed to slightly hyperextend the neck with the head slightly turned to the contralateral side. The head of the bed may be slightly elevated to reduce venous bleeding.

During the operation the anesthesia provider works behind a sterile barrier at the patient's unaffected side. The preoperative skin prep is extensive, including the neck, lower face, and upper chest. The patient's neck is draped so as to leave a wide operative field. For the rare occasion when a dermal graft is to be harvested to cover and protect the carotid artery (as when a patient has received extensive previous radiation therapy), the thigh area is also prepped and draped with sterile towels in readiness for obtaining a dermal graft before closure of the neck wound. It is usually more convenient to use the thigh on the same side as the neck dissection. Patient and family education includes tracheostomy care (if applicable), pain management, care of the surgical incision, reportable signs and symptoms, healthful behaviors, and review of physical therapy exercises. These include range-of-motion exercises for the neck, shoulder, and arm muscles on the affected side (Box 21-4).

Operative procedure

1. One of several types of incisions may be used, including the Y-shaped, H-shaped, or trifurcate incision (Fig. 21-23), all of which aim for complete lymphadenectomy while preserving good, viable skin flaps.
2. The upper curved incision is made through the skin and platysma with a knife, tissue forceps, and fine hemostats; ligatures are used for bleeding vessels. The upper flap is retracted; then the vertical portion of the incision is made, and the skin flaps are retracted anteriorly and posteriorly with retractors. The anterior margin of the trapezius muscle is exposed by

BOX 21-4 | Exercises after Neck Dissection

The following exercises have been developed to increase the movement and strength in your neck, arms, and shoulders.

Neck Range of Motion

1. Bring chin to chest in a relaxed way and then let it fall gently backwards so that a stretch on the neck muscles is felt.
2. Slowly turn head as far as possible to one side as if attempting to look over that shoulder. Do the same to the other side.
3. Bend the head toward the shoulder on the unaffected side. A stretching will be felt on the operated side.

Shoulder Mobility

1. Standing with shoulders relaxed and head facing forward, let arm on the affected side hang freely. Make circles with the shoulder by moving it:
   a. forward
   b. upward
   c. backward
   d. downward
2. With a wand or cane in front of body and shoulders and arms relaxed, raise wand as high as possible keeping elbows extended. After you are able to raise it directly overhead, slowly lower it behind the neck. Raise wand overhead and return it to starting position.
3. Stand facing a wall with your feet a few inches from it. Slide the hand on your affected side up the wall as far as possible, using the wall for support. Perform the same exercise with your affected side facing the wall. Repeat the motion of sliding your hand up the wall but do not turn your body when doing this exercise.

This guide may be copied for free distribution to patients and families. All rights reserved.

From *Mosby's patient teaching guides,* Update II, St. Louis, 1997, Mosby.

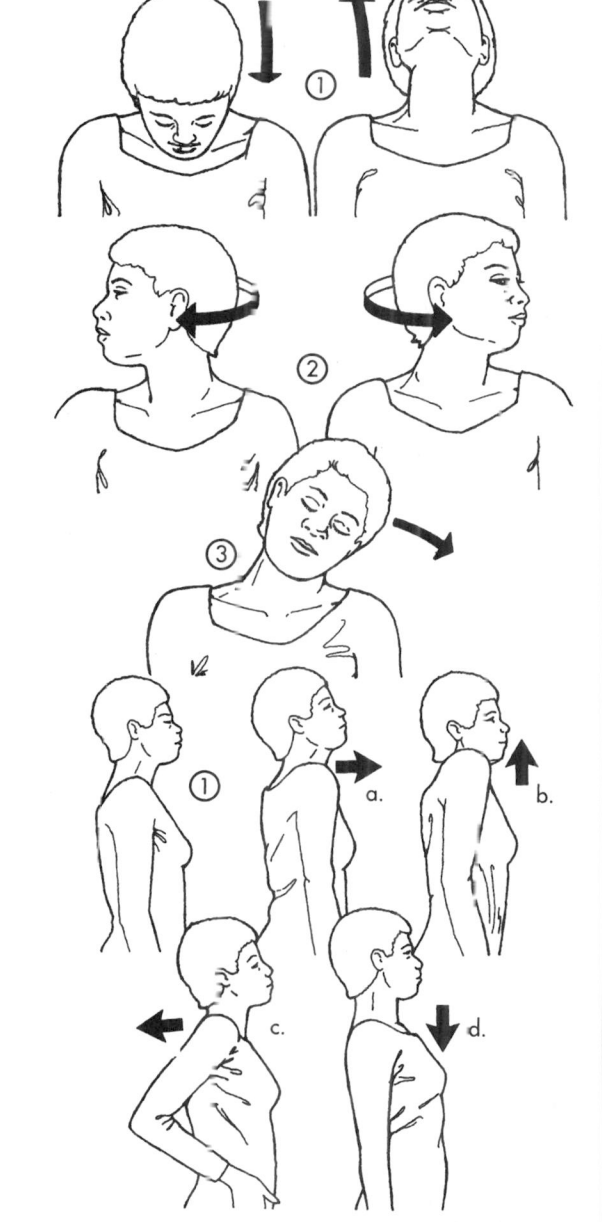

means of curved scissors. The flaps are retracted to expose the entire lateral aspect of the neck. Branches of the jugular veins are clamped, ligated, and divided.

3. The sternal and clavicular attachments of the sterno-cleidomastoid muscle are clamped with curved Pean forceps and then divided with a knife. The superficial layer of deep fascia is incised. The omohyoid muscle is severed between clamps just above its scapular attachment.

4. By sharp and blunt dissection, the carotid sheath is opened. The internal jugular vein is isolated by blunt dissection and then doubly clamped, doubly ligated with medium silk, and divided with Metzenbaum scissors. A transfixion suture is placed on the lower end of the vein.

5. The common carotid artery and vagus nerve are identified and protected. The fatty areolar tissue and fascia are dissected away using Metzenbaum scissors and fine tissue forceps. Branches of the thyrocervical artery are clamped, divided, and ligated.

6. The tissues and fascia of the posterior triangle are dissected, beginning at the anterior margin of the trapezius muscle and continuing near the brachial plexus and the levator scapulae and the scalene muscles. During the dissection, branches of the cervical and suprascapular arteries are clamped, ligated, and divided.

7. The anterior portion of the block dissection is completed. The omohyoid muscle is severed at its attachment to the hyoid bone. Bleeding is controlled.

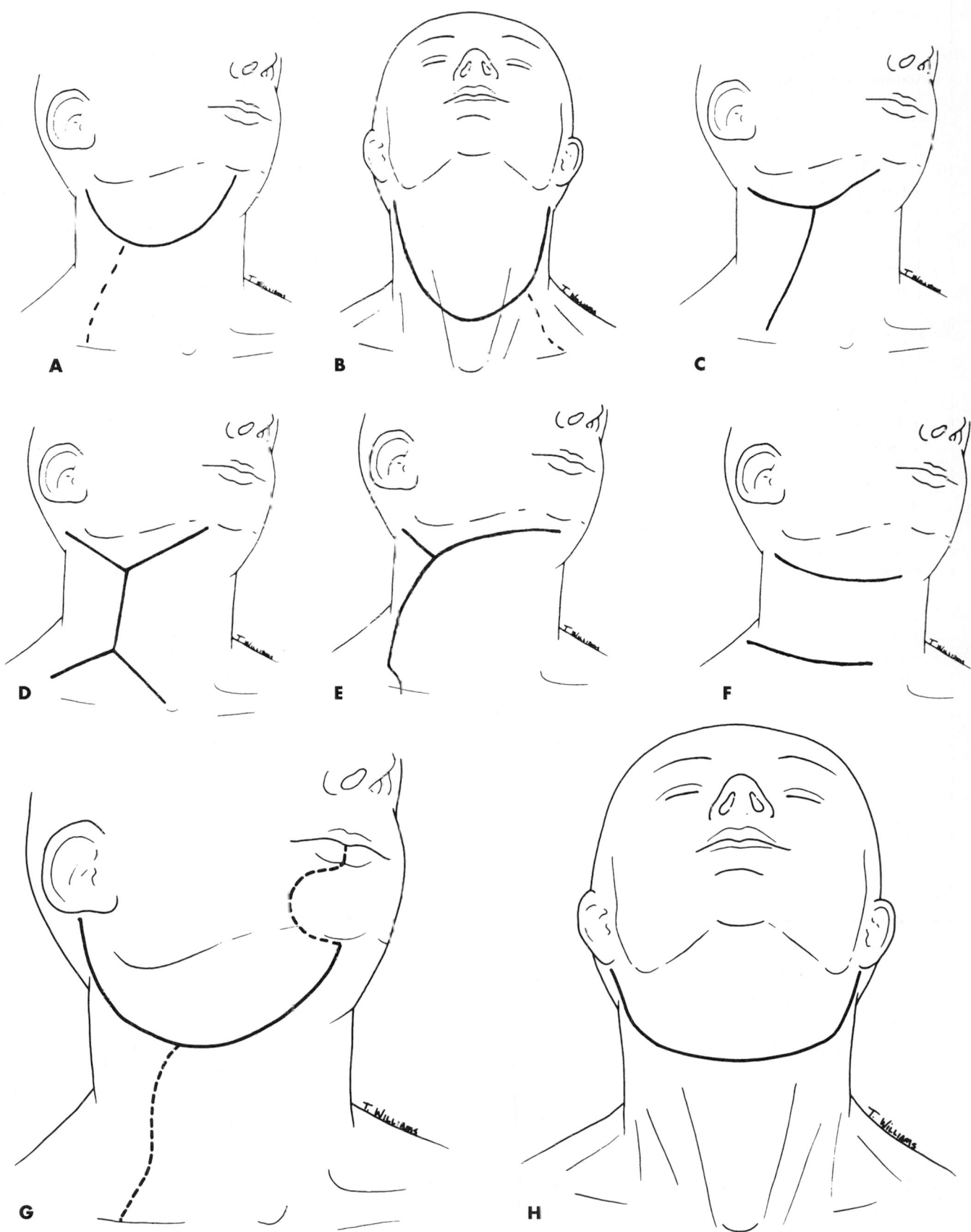

FIGURE 21-23   Neck dissection incisions. **A**, Latyschevsky and Freund. **B**, Freund. **C**, Crile. **D**, Martin. **E**, Babcock and Conley. **F**, MacFee. **G**, Incision used for unilateral supraomohyoid neck dissection. **H**, Incision used for bilateral supraomohyoid neck dissection.

All hemostats are removed, and the operative site may be covered with warm, moist laparotomy packs.

8. The sternocleidomastoid muscle is severed and retracted. The submental space is dissected free of fatty areolar tissue and lymph nodes from above downward.

9. The deep fascia on the lower edge of the mandible is incised; the facial vessels are divided and ligated.

10. The submandibular triangle is entered. The submandibular duct is divided and ligated. The submandibular glands with surrounding fatty areolar tissue and lymph nodes are dissected toward the digastric muscle. The facial branch of the external carotid artery is divided. Portions of the digastric and stylohyoid muscles are severed from their attachments to the hyoid bone and on the mastoid. The upper end of the internal jugular vein is elevated and divided. The surgical specimen is removed (see Fig. 21-22, *B*).

11. The entire field is examined for bleeding and then irrigated with warm saline solution. Although rarely necessary, a skin graft may be placed to cover the bifurcation of the carotid artery, extending down

approximately 4 inches, and sutured with 4-0 absorbable suture on a very small cutting needle.

12. Closed wound suction drains are placed into the wound.

13. The flaps are carefully approximated with interrupted, fine nonabsorbable sutures or with skin staples. A bulky pressure dressing may be applied to the neck, depending on surgeon preference.

MODIFIED NECK DISSECTION (Fig. 21-24)

Modified neck dissection is removal of neck contents, except for the sternocleidomastoid muscle, internal jugular vein, and eleventh cranial nerve.

Procedural considerations

This modified type of neck dissection facilitates removal of a tumor and lymph nodes suspected of metastases and allows the patient a minimal defect and minimally impaired shoulder function. With radical and modified

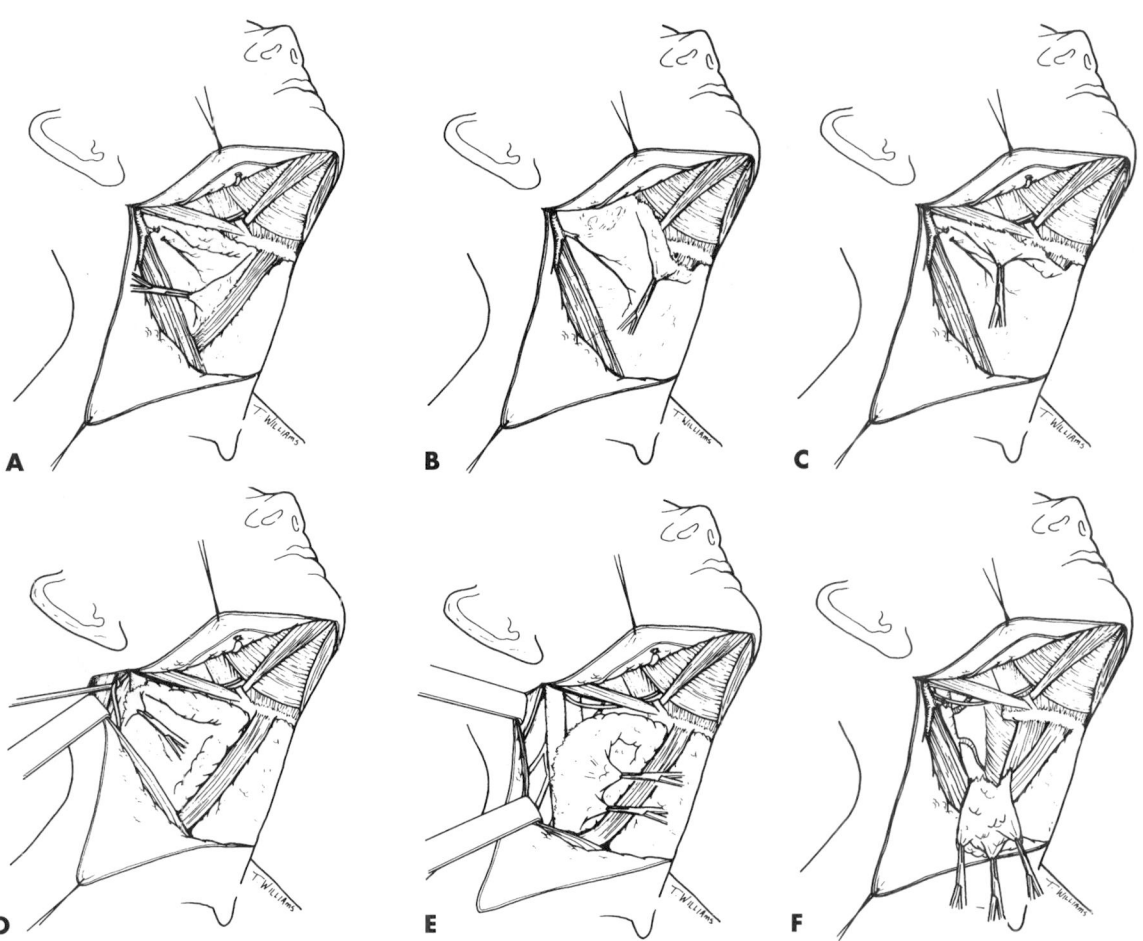

FIGURE 21-24 Steps of modified radical neck dissection with preservation of spinal accessory nerve, internal jugular vein, and sternocleidomastoid muscle.

neck dissection, the surgeon and radiologist may decide on a course of postoperative radiation therapy or chemotherapy. The decision depends on the type and location of tumor, stage of disease, and condition of the patient

RECONSTRUCTIVE PROCEDURES

Head and neck surgical procedures to remove malignant tumors are reconstructed depending on the surgical defect. The wound may be closed primarily or local flaps and split-thickness skin grafts (as with facial and intraoral defects) or full-thickness skin grafts (as in nasal and facial defects) may be used. Regional flaps (such as the pectoralis major musculocutaneous flap), microvascular tissue transfer (such as the radial forearm flap, free jejunal flap, and rectus abdominis flap), or microvascular osteocutaneous flaps (such as the iliac crest flap) may be utilized to restore function as well as cover defects. Combinations of the above grafts and flaps are often necessary when large defects are created. Skin grafts and flaps are discussed in detail in Chapter 24.

Microvascular flaps extend surgical and anesthetic time significantly; since veins and arteries are microscopically connected, nerve grafts may be used, and bone must be connected with the use of plates and screws.

The use of a Doppler unit (intraoperatively and postoperatively) and thorough nursing assessment skills are paramount in detecting occlusions or spasms of the vessels and subsequent survival of the transplanted flap.

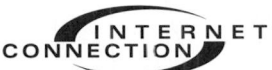

Society of Otorhinolaryngology and Head-Neck Nurses:
http://www.entnet.org

Society of Otorhinolaryngology:
http://www.bcm.tmc.edu/oto/SOHN

ENT Grand Rounds:
http://www.bcm.tmc.edu/oto/grand/grand.html

American Association of Oral and Maxillofacial Surgeons:
http://www.aaoms.org

Pain Net: http://painnet.com/

Dysphagia Resource Center:
http://www.dysphagia.com/

REFERENCES

1. *American Nurses Association standards for clinical practice.* (1998). Washington, D.C.: The Association.
2. AORN recommended practices for laser safety in practice settings, (1998). Denver: Association of Operating Room Nurses, pp. 243-248.
3. Infection control: TB and the link to bronchoscopes. (1998). *American Journal of Nursing, 98*(4), 9.
4. Johnson, J.E., et al. (1997). *Self-regulation theory: applying theory to your practice.* Pittsburgh: Oncology Nursing Press.
5. Mathias, J.M. (1998). What's best method for warming patients? *OR Manager, 14*(3), 10, 12.
6. McCance, K.L., & Huether, S.E. (1994). *Pathophysiology: the biologic basis for disease in adults and children* (ed. 2). St. Louis: Mosby.
7. Mitchell, P.H., Ferketich, S., & Jennings, B.M. (1998). Quality health outcomes model. *Image: the Journal of Nursing Scholarship, 30*(1), 43-46.
8. Meyerhoff, W.L., & Rice, D.H. (1992). *Otolaryngology—head and neck surgery,* Philadelphia: Saunders.
9. Pagana, K.D., & Pagana, T.J. (1995). *Mosby's diagnostic and laboratory test reference* (ed. 2). St. Louis: Mosby.
10. Ritchey, W.P., Steele, G., & Dean, R.H. (1995). *General surgery,* Philadelphia: Lippincott.
11. Scott-Conner, C., & Dawson, D.L. (1993). *Operative anatomy,* Philadelphia: Lippincott.
12. Stuart, G.W., & Laraia, M.T. (1998). *Stuart and Sundeen's principles and practices of psychiatric nursing* (ed. 6). St. Louis: Mosby.

CHAPTER TWENTY TWO

Orthopedic Surgery

Porter Layne

THE WORD *ORTHOPÉDIE*, derived from the Greek *orthos*, meaning 'straight' and *paideia*, meaning 'rearing of children,' was first used by Nicholas Andry in 1741 in the title for a book dealing with the prevention and correction of skeletal deformities in children. Orthopedic surgery has been defined by the American Board of Orthopaedic Surgery (1997)[3] as "the medical specialty that includes the investigation, preservation and restoration of the form and function of the extremities, the spine, and associated musculoskeletal structures by medical, surgical and physical means."

Orthopedic surgery is an ever-changing field that is a challenge for the perioperative nurse. Technologic advances in the multitude of systems and hardware used have resulted in improved treatment of orthopedic disorders. In addition to understanding anatomic and physiologic responses, the perioperative nurse should have a general understanding of the concepts of these systems and the purpose they serve to provide the most safe and efficient care. A knowledge of the principles of bone fixation and healing and the relationship of bone and soft tissues will provide a strong basis to ensure continued understanding of the care required for the orthopedic patient. Using the nursing process provides a systematic approach when providing the unique care required in orthopedics.

SURGICAL ANATOMY

Anatomic Structures

The 206 bones of the body form the appendicular or axial framework that supports soft tissues, provides storage areas and reservoirs for minerals, and serves as a site for formation of blood cells (Fig. 22-1). The skeletal system is composed of varied elements including bone, muscle, and associated structures.

Bone remains in a constant state of formation and resorption, preventing development of excessive thickness or thinness. These processes are related to individual metabolism and absorption of calcium, vitamin D, and phosphorus. Levels of minerals affect disease processes, causing bone changes. A layer of connective tissue called *periosteum* covers all bone.

Muscles are masses of tissue that cover bones and provide movement to the skeletal system. Muscles interact with nerves, minerals, skin, and other connective tissue to contract and extend. Individual muscles are short or long and vary in diameter, depending on their position on a specific bone.

Ligaments, tendons, and cartilage also form the skeletal structures. Ligaments are bands of dense connective tissue that hold bone to bone. They provide stability to a joint by encircling or holding ends of bone in place. Tendons are tough, long strands of fibers that form the ends of muscles. They transmit forces to bone or cartilage without being damaged. Cartilage is a layer of elastic, resilient supporting tissue found at the ends of the bones. It forms a cap over the bone end to protect and support the bone during weight-bearing activities and provides a smooth gliding surface for joint movement. Cartilage is aneural, alymphatic (without nerves or lymph tissue respectively), avascular, and high in water content.[27] The lack of vascularity and loss of water from cartilage during a lifetime are causes of resulting degenerative disease such as arthritis. Weight bearing and joint movements keep cartilage from becoming thin or damaged and help prevent degenerative conditions.[35]

Joints are articulations where bones are joined to one another or where two surfaces of bones come together. Joints are classified by the type of material between them

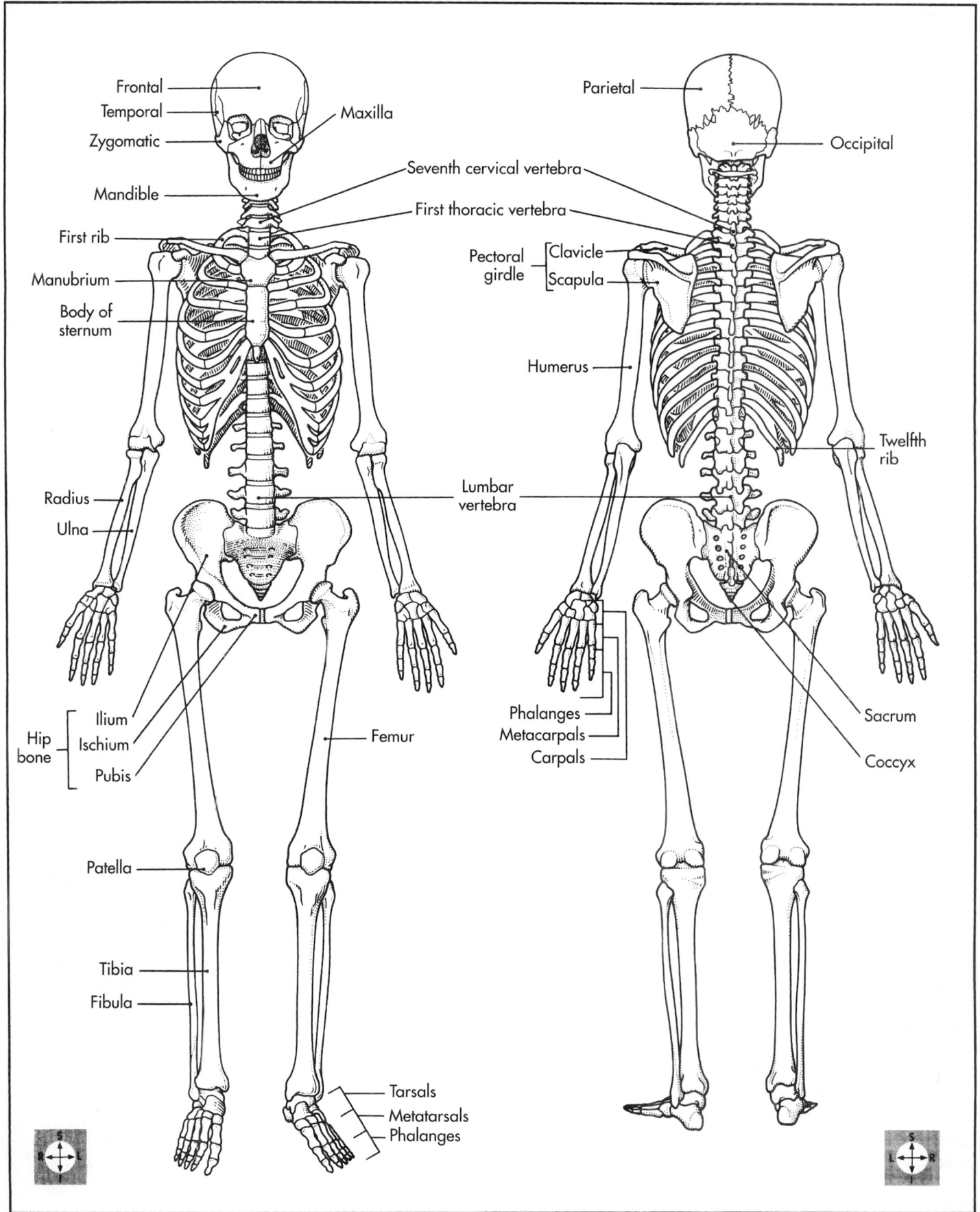

FIGURE 22-1 Anterior and posterior views of the skeleton.

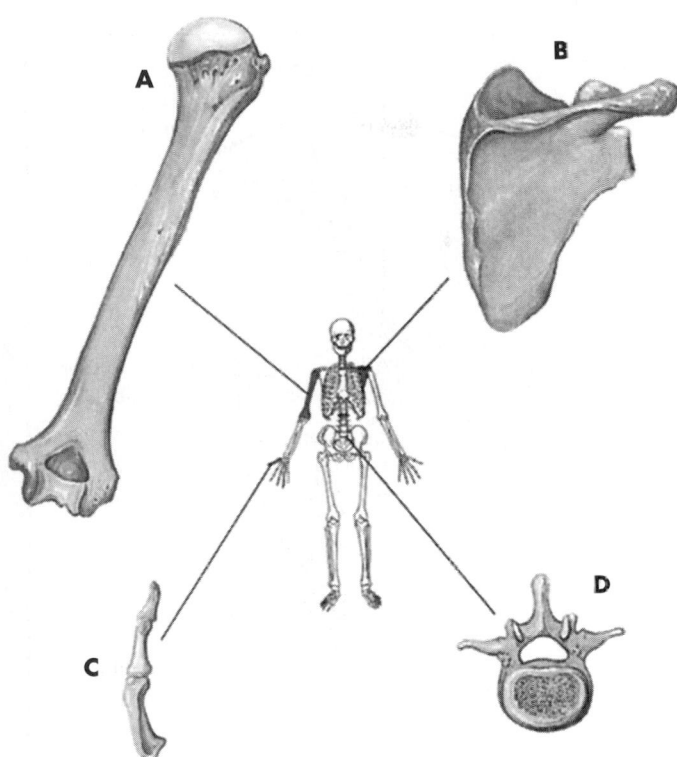

FIGURE 22-2   Types of bones, as examples. **A,** Long bones (humerus). **B,** Flat bones (scapula). **C,** Short bones (phalanx). **D,** Irregular bones (vertebra).

or according to movement. Material between joints is fibrous, cartilaginous, or synovial. The type of movement is synarthrotic (immovable), amphiarthrotic (slightly movable), or diarthrotic (freely movable). Synarthrotic joints are connected by fibrous tissue or ligaments, such as the suture type of joints holding the bones of the skull, and connections between two bones such as the radius and ulna. Amphiarthrotic joints are connected by cartilage. Joints of this type include the symphysis pubis, intervertebral joints, and manubriosternal joint. The majority of joints are diarthrotic; these are the only joints with one or more ranges of motion. These joints are lined with a synovial membrane and are called *synovial joints.* Examples include the knee, cervical vertebrae 1 and 2, the radius articulating on the wrist bones, the hip, and the shoulder.

There are two types of bone tissue: cortical and cancellous. Cortical bone is the hard bone forming the outer shell—the main supporting tissue. Cancellous bone is soft and spongy, located at the iliac crest, tibia, sternum, and ends of long bones. It contains the red bone marrow for hematopoesis.

Bones are divided according to their shape: long, short, flat, irregular, and round (Fig. 22-2). Long bones are present in the limbs and consist of a shaft and two ends; the ends generally flare out, are covered with articular cartilage, and provide a surface for articulation and musculotendinous attachment. Short bones, such as the carpals and tarsals (in the wrist and midfoot area), are

present when the structure is strong but limited movement is required. Flat bones are scapula, sternum, and pelvic girdle. Irregular bones are found in the skull and vertebral column. Round, or sesamoid, bones (resembling a sesame seed) are found within tendons. The patella is a large sesamoid bone, although most are small, such as the two found on the head of the first metatarsal, forming the "ball" of the foot.

Long bones consist of a shaft, or diaphysis, and two ends, or epiphyses. The shaft is composed of compact bone. The epiphyses flare out and consist of cancellous bone. They are covered by cartilage, which provides a cushion and offers protection during weight bearing and movement. Until skeletal maturity, a line of cartilage called the *epiphyseal plate* separates the epiphysis from the diaphysis. Fractures in this region suffered by children can be devastating because they often lead to malformation and permanent limb shortening.

Trabeculae are located within cancellous bone and consist of an interconnecting network of bone oriented along the lines of stress. These structures are important for weight bearing, providing strength to withstand stress placed upon the bone. The periosteum is a thin outer covering of bone containing nutrient arteries for nourishment of bone cells. Disruption of these periosteal vessels after bone trauma can influence the ability of bone to heal. The haversian system consists of thousands of microscopic units found in the cortical bone. These units of matrix cells, canals, and conduits allow flow of nutrients and facilitate calcium absorption.

Vertebrae

Vertebrae form the longitudinal axis of the skeleton. The vertebral bodies are connected by several cartilaginous joints, which enable the vertebrae to flex, extend, or rotate while being held together. The bodies of adjacent vertebrae are connected by intervertebral disks and ligaments. The ligamenta flava bind the laminae of adjacent vertebrae together. Other ligaments connect the spinous processes and vertebral bodies.

Seven cervical vertebrae form the skeletal framework of the neck. Twelve thoracic vertebrae support the thoracic region, and five lumbar vertebrae support the small of the back. Below the lumbar vertebrae lie the sacrum and coccyx. Each of these bones is composed of fused vertebrae, five for the sacrum and four for the coccyx.

The vertebral column is curved. After birth, there is a continuous posterior convexity. As development occurs, secondary posterior concavities develop in the cervical and lumbar regions, resulting in improved balance.

Each area of the vertebral column has specific bony structures. General features include a body (except the first two cervical vertebrae) on the anterior part. The posterior portion of the vertebrae consists of a neural arch formed by pedicles and laminae and the spinous or transverse processes.

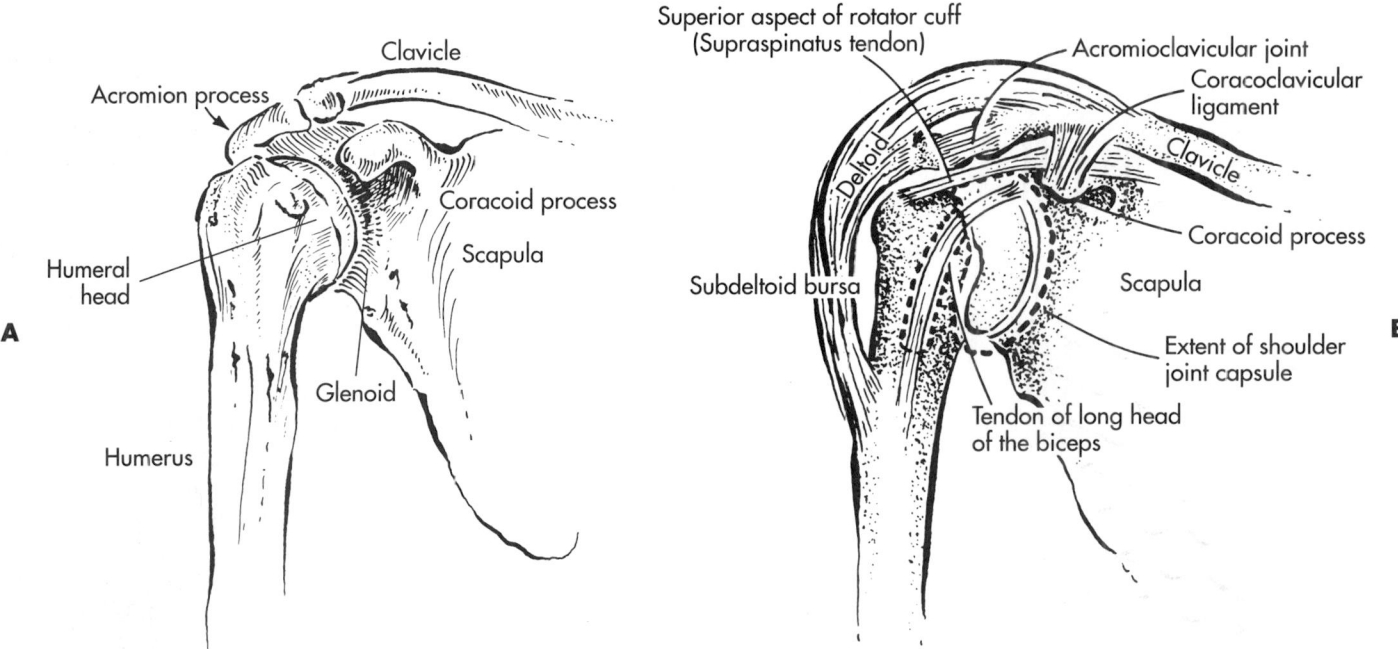

FIGURE 22-3 Shoulder. **A,** Joint showing anterior view. **B,** Girdle showing articulations.

Shoulder and Upper Extremity

The clavicle, which is a long, doubly curved bone, serves as a prop for the shoulder and holds it away from the chest wall. The clavicle rests almost horizontally at the upper and anterior part of the thorax, above the first rib. It articulates medially with the manubrium of the sternum and laterally with the acromion of the scapula and is tethered to the underlying coracoid process of the scapula by the coracoclavicular ligaments.

The scapula (shoulder blade) is a flat, triangular bone that forms the posterior part of the shoulder girdle, lying superior and posterior to the upper chest. The glenoid cavity on the lateral side of the scapula provides a socket for the humerus (the bone of the upper arm). The acromion process articulates with the clavicle medially. The scapula is attached to the thorax by muscles.

The shoulder (pectoral) girdle consists of the gleno-humeral, sternoclavicular, and acromioclavicular (AC) joints (Fig. 22-3). The glenohumeral joint has a multidirectional range of motion, whereas the latter two joints have limited motion. The acromioclavicular joint, located at the top of the shoulder, is the articulation between the outer end of the clavicle and a flattened articular facet situated on the inner border of the acromion. The muscles immediately surrounding the shoulder joint are the supraspinatus, infraspinatus, teres minor, and subscapularis muscles; together they are referred to as the *rotator cuff*. These muscles stabilize the shoulder joint while the entire arm is moved by the powerful deltoid, pectoralis major, teres major, and latissimus dorsi muscles. Shoulder girdle strength and stability is maintained by the soft-tissue integrity, not the bony structures. A pathologic condition

in this area can be the result of bone, soft tissue, or combined injury.

The humerus is the longest and largest bone of the upper extremity. It is composed of a shaft and two ends. The proximal end, or head, has two projections, the greater and lesser tuberosities (Fig. 22-4). The circumference of the articular surface of the humerus is constricted and is termed the *anatomic neck*. The anatomic neck marks the attachment to the capsule of the shoulder joint. The constriction below the tuberosities is called the *surgical neck* and is the site of most fractures.

The greater tuberosity is situated at the lateral aspect of the humeral head. Its upper surface has three impressions where the supraspinous, infraspinous, and teres minor tendons insert. The lesser tuberosity is situated in the anterior neck and has an impression for the insertion of the tendon of the subscapular muscle. The attachment sites for the rotator cuff, the tuberosities, are separated from each other by a deep groove (bicipital groove) in which lies the tendon of the long head of the biceps muscle of the arm. The tendon of the pectoralis major inserts on the lateral margin of the bicipital groove, and the latissimus dorsi and teres major insert on the medial margin.

The distal humerus flattens and ends in a broad articular surface. The surface is divided into the medial and lateral condyles, which are separated by a slight ridge. On the lateral condyle the rounded articular surface is called the *capitulum* and articulates with the head of the radius. On the medial condyle the articular surface is termed the *trochlea*, which articulates with the ulna.

The ulna is located medial to the radius. The proximal portion of the ulna, the olecranon, articulates with the

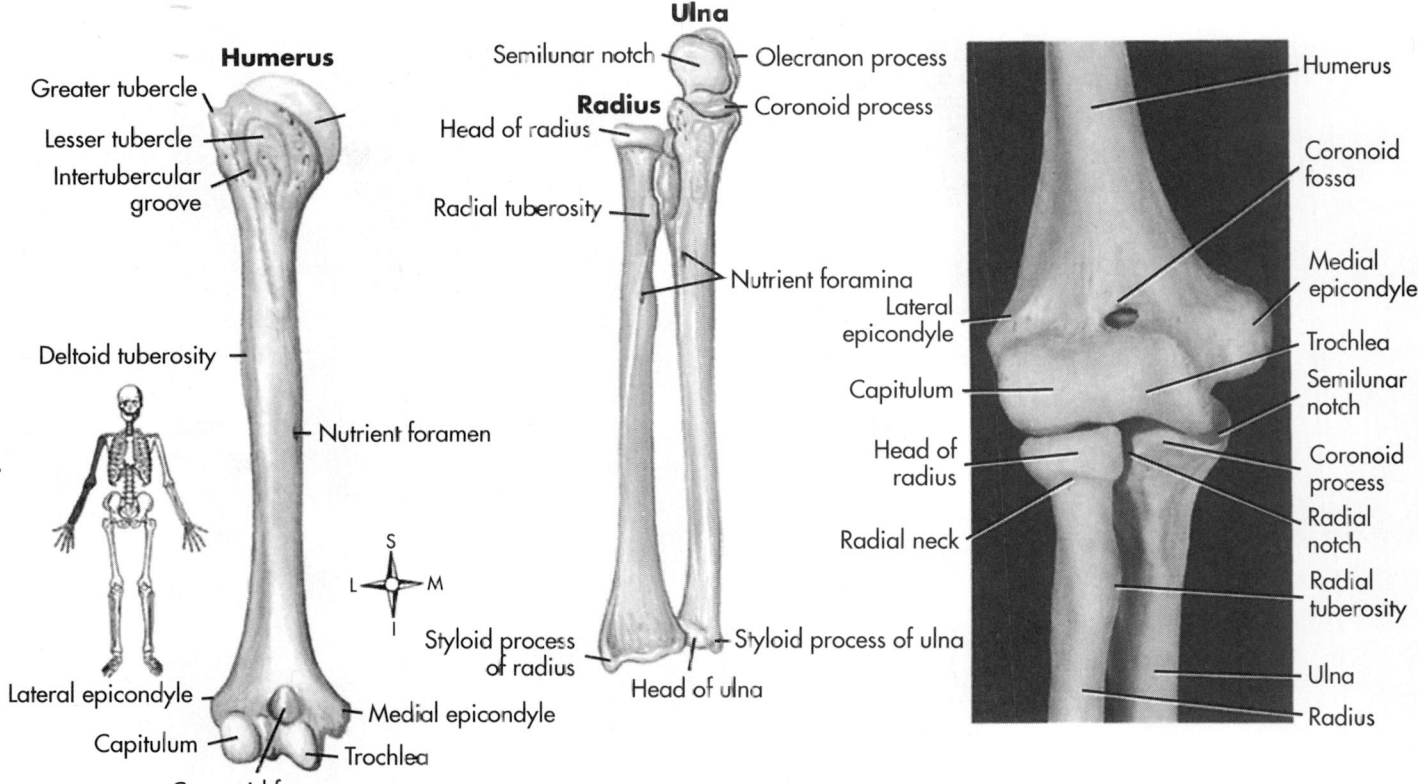

FIGURE 22-4   Bones of the arm anterior view showing the humerus, radius, and ulna.

trochlea of the humerus at the elbow. The radius rotates around the ulna. At the proximal end is the head, which articulates with the capitulum of the humerus and the radial notch of the ulna. The tendon of the biceps muscle is attached to the tuberosity just below the radial head. The distal end of the radius is divided into two articular surfaces. The distal surface articulates with the carpal bones of the wrist, and the surface on the medial side articulates with the distal end of the ulna.

Wrist and Hand

The skeletal bones of the wrist and hand consist of three distinct parts: (1) the carpals, or wrist bones; (2) the metacarpals, or bones of the palm; and (3) the phalanges, or bones of the digits (Fig. 22-5).

There are eight carpal bones arranged in two rows. The distal row, proceeding from the radial to the ulnar side, includes the trapezium, trapezoid, capitate, and hamate; the proximal row consists of the scaphoid (also called the navicular), lunate, triquetrum, and pisiform. Functionally, the scaphoid links the rows as it stabilizes and coordinates the movement of the proximal and distal rows. Each carpal bone consists of several smooth articular surfaces for contact with the adjacent bones, as well as rough surfaces for the attachment of ligaments. The five metacarpal bones (long bones) are situated in the palm. Proximally they articulate with the distal row of carpal bones, and distally the head of each metacarpal articulates with its proper

phalanx. The heads of the metacarpals form the knuckles. The phalanges, or fingers, consist of 14 bones in each hand, two in the thumb and three in each finger. Each phalanx consists of a shaft and two ends.

Pelvis, Hip, and Femur

The pelvis (Fig. 22-6) is a stable circular base that supports the trunk and forms an attachment for the lower extremities. It is a massive irregular bone created by the fusion of three separate bones. The largest and uppermost of the three bones is the ilium, the strongest and lowermost is the ischium, and the anteriormost is the pubis. Together these are termed the *os coxae*, or innominate bone.

The hip, a ball and socket joint, is formed by the acetabular portion of the innominate bone and the proximal end of the femur (Fig. 22-7). The hip joint is surrounded by a capsule, ligaments, and muscles, to provide stability. The iliofemoral ligament connects the ilium with the femur anteriorly and superiorly, and the ischiofemoral and pubofemoral ligaments attach ischium and pubis to the femur respectively. The acetabulum is a deep, round cavity that articulates with the head of the femur. The proximal end of the femur consists of the femoral head and neck, the upper portion of the shaft, and the greater and lesser trochanters (Fig. 22-8).

The greater trochanter is a broad process that protrudes from the outer upper portion of the shaft and projects upward from the junction of the superior border of the

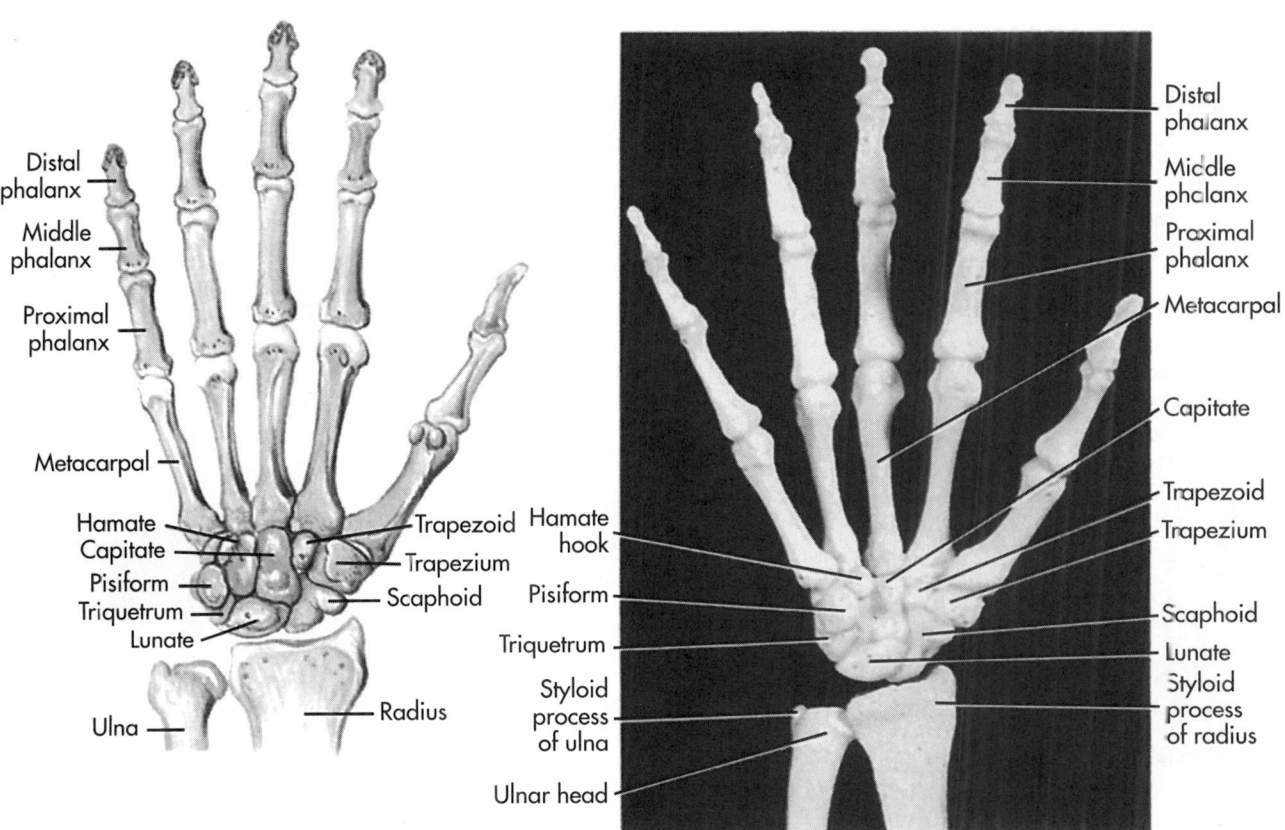

Distal phalanx

Middle phalanx

Proximal phalanx

Metacarpal

Hamate
Capitate
Pisiform
Triquetrum
Lunate

Trapezoid
Trapezium
Scaphoid

Ulna

Radius

Distal phalanx

Middle phalanx

Proximal phalanx

Metacarpal

Capitate

Trapezoid
Trapezium

Scaphoid

Lunate

Styloid process of radius

Hamate hook

Pisiform

Triquetrum

Styloid process of ulna

Ulnar head

FIGURE 22-5   Bones of the wrist and hand, palmar view.

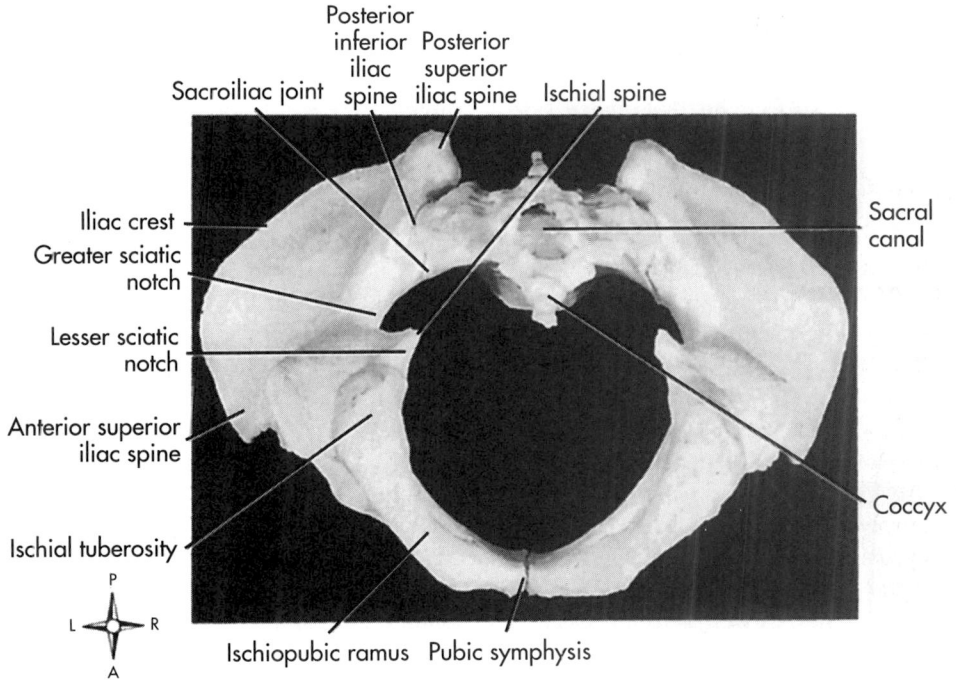

Sacroiliac joint

Posterior inferior iliac spine

Posterior superior iliac spine

Ischial spine

Iliac crest

Greater sciatic notch

Lesser sciatic notch

Anterior superior iliac spine

Ischial tuberosity

Sacral canal

Coccyx

Ischiopubic ramus   Pubic symphysis

FIGURE 22-6   Pelvis, superior view.

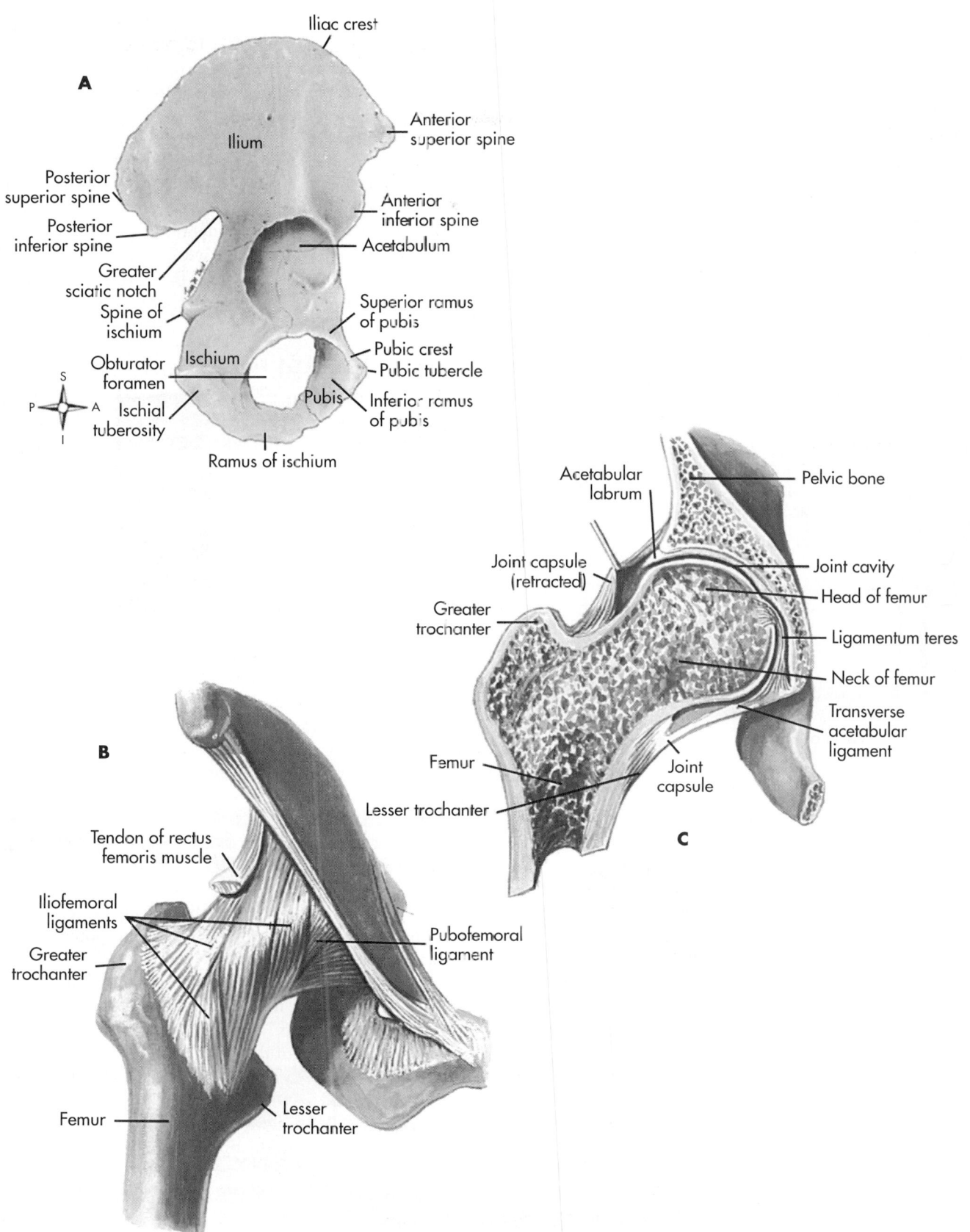

FIGURE 22-7   Hip joint. **A,** Coxal bone disarticulated from the skeleton. **B,** Ligamentous structure. **C,** Bone structure.

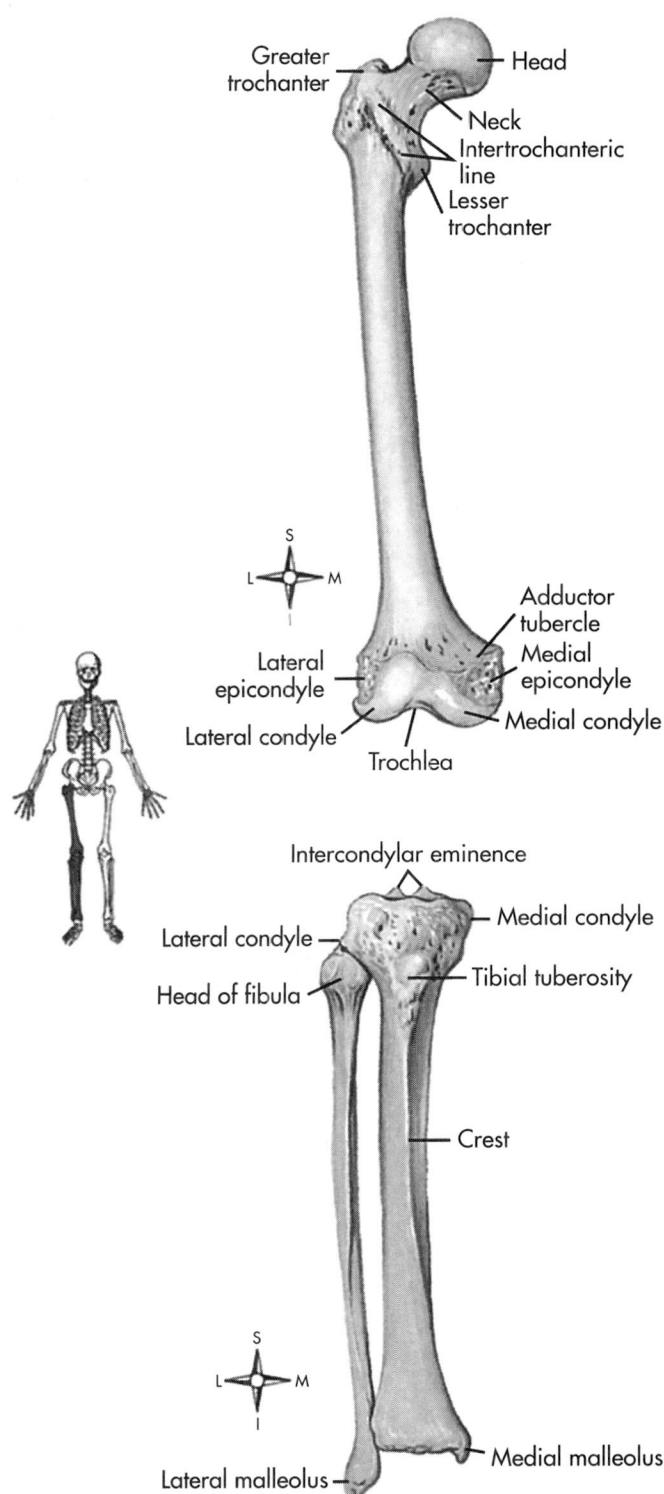

FIGURE 22-8   Bones of the upper and lower leg.

neck with the outer surface of the shaft. It serves as a point of insertion for the abductor and short rotator muscles of the hip.

The lesser trochanter is a conical process projecting from the posterior and inferior portion of the base of the neck of the femur at its junction with the shaft. It serves as a point of insertion for the iliopsoas muscle. The lower end of the femur terminates in the two condyles. Anteriorly the condyles are separated from one another by a smooth depression, called the *intercondylar, or patellar, groove,* forming an articulating surface for the patella. Posteriorly they project slightly, and the space between them forms the intercondylar fossa, a supporting structure for neurovascular structures.

The upper or condylar end of the tibia presents an articular surface corresponding with those of the femoral condyles. The articular surface of the two tibial condyles forms two facets, which are deepened by the semilunar cartilage into fossae for the femoral condyles.

Knee, Tibia, and Fibula

The knee joint (Fig. 22-9) consists of two articulations. One articulation is between each condyle of the femur and the tibial plateau; the second is between the patella and femur. These areas are subject to degenerative changes, often requiring reconstructive surgery. The bones of the knee joint are connected by extraarticular and intraarticular structures. The extraarticular attachments consist of the joint capsule, multiple muscular attachments, and two collateral ligaments. The intraarticular ligaments consist of the two cruciate ligaments and the attachments of the menisci.

The patella, or kneecap, is anterior to the knee joint in the intercondylar groove, or trochlea, of the distal femur. It is a sesamoid bone contained within the quadriceps tendon. The anterior surface of the patella is united with the patellar tendon as the tendon originates and inserts above and below the knee joint. The posterior surface of the patella articulates with the femur.

The capsule of the knee joint is attached proximally to the femoral condyles, and it is attached distally to the condyles of the tibia and to the upper end of the fibula. The capsule is reinforced in front by the patellar and quadriceps tendon, on the sides by the medial and lateral collateral ligaments, and posteriorly by the popliteus and gastrocnemius muscles.

The cruciate ligaments (Fig. 22-10), consisting of two fibrous bands, extend from the intercondylar fossa of the femur to attachments anterior and posterior on the intercondylar surface of the tibia.

The menisci are interposed between the condyles of the femur and those of the tibia (see Fig. 22-10). Each meniscus is attached to the joint capsule. The ends of the cartilage are attached to the tibia in the middle of its upper articular surface. These structures are almost totally avascular, and degenerative changes are usually permanent.

Synovial membrane lines the capsule of the joint and covers the infrapatellar fat pad, parts of the cruciate ligaments, and portions of the bone. The portion of the knee joint cavity that extends upward in front of the femur is called the *suprapatellar pouch,* or *bursa.*

A

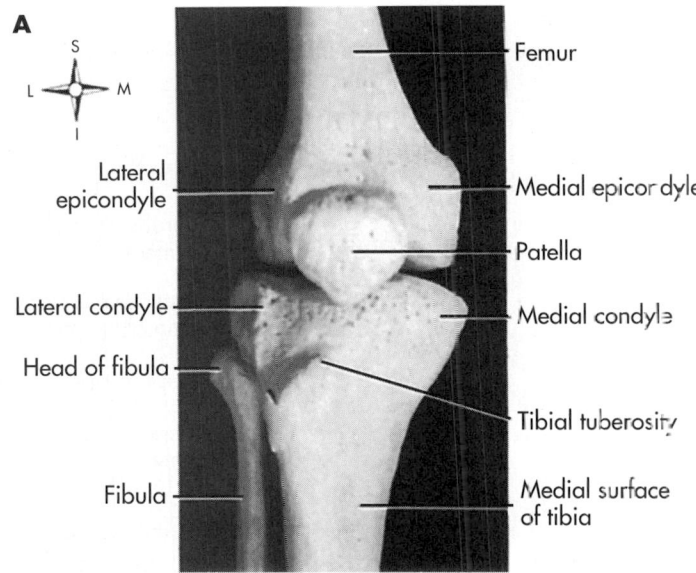

B

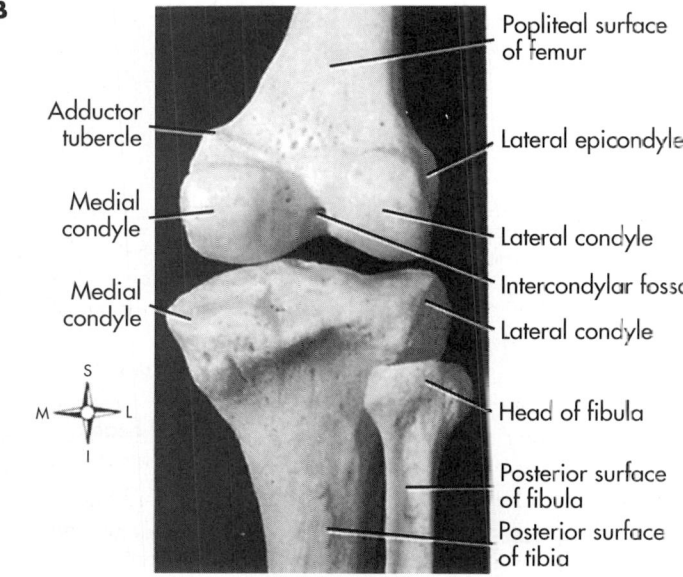

FIGURE 22-9 Bones of the knee showing the tibia and fibula. **A,** Anterior aspect, **B,** Posterior aspect.

The tibia is the larger and stronger of the lower leg bones. The fibula is smaller and located more laterally, articulating at the proximal end with the lateral condyle of the tibia. The proximal end of the tibia articulates with the femur to form the knee joint. Distally the tibia articulates with the fibula and with the talus, forming the ankle joint.

Ankle and Foot

The ankle is a hinge joint, formed by the distal end of the tibia and fibula and the proximal end of the talus. The tibia (medial and posterior malleoli) and fibula (lateral malleolus) form a mortise (notch) for the reception of the upper surface of the talus and its facets. The talus is an irregular bone consisting of a body, neck, and head. The bones are connected by ligaments, which spread out from the malleoli to attach to the talus, calcaneus, and navicular bones (Fig. 22-11). A thin capsule surrounds the joint.

The bony framework of the foot (Fig. 22-12) comprises seven tarsal bones, five metatarsal bones, and 14 phalanges. The calcaneus forms the heel and gives support to the talus. The cuboid bone articulates proximally and posteriorly with the calcaneus and distally with the fourth and fifth metatarsals and the third cuneiform bones.

The navicular bone articulates with the cuneiform bones, which lie side by side just anterior to it. The metatarsal bones articulate proximally with the tarsal bones and distally with the bases of the first phalanges of the corresponding toes. There are two phalanges for the great toe and three for each of the other toes.

PERIOPERATIVE NURSING CONSIDERATIONS

Assessment

Assessment of the orthopedic patient is ongoing, beginning with initial patient contact. Familiarity with orthopedic procedures and anticipated patient outcomes improves the ability to gather appropriate information and complete the nursing process. Obtaining patient-specific information from the physician also enhances the perioperative nursing assessment. The informed consent provides information to confirm the scheduled procedure or procedures and verify the operative site and side. The consent is usually obtained before admission to the surgery suite and should be reviewed for accuracy and completeness.

The patient record is reviewed, noting relevant aspects of the history and physical examination, the nature of the problem and its onset, and results of radiographic studies, laboratory data, and other findings. The nursing history is obtained by observation and interview to determine physical, psychosocial, cultural, spiritual, and other needs. The patient should be assessed for range of motion, neurovascular status, and general condition. The patient's understanding of the surgical procedure and postoperative rehabilitation is determined and patient education begun.

Assessment information helps determine specific needs related to surgical positioning, skin preparation, equipment, instrumentation, and supplies. Environmental safety is also considered, including room temperature, traffic flow, lighting, and personnel attire.

Information should be communicated with surgical and anesthesia team members and persons in other disciplines. The information collected helps the perioperative nurse plan and coordinate activities, facilitate a smooth transition, and reduce operative time.

A

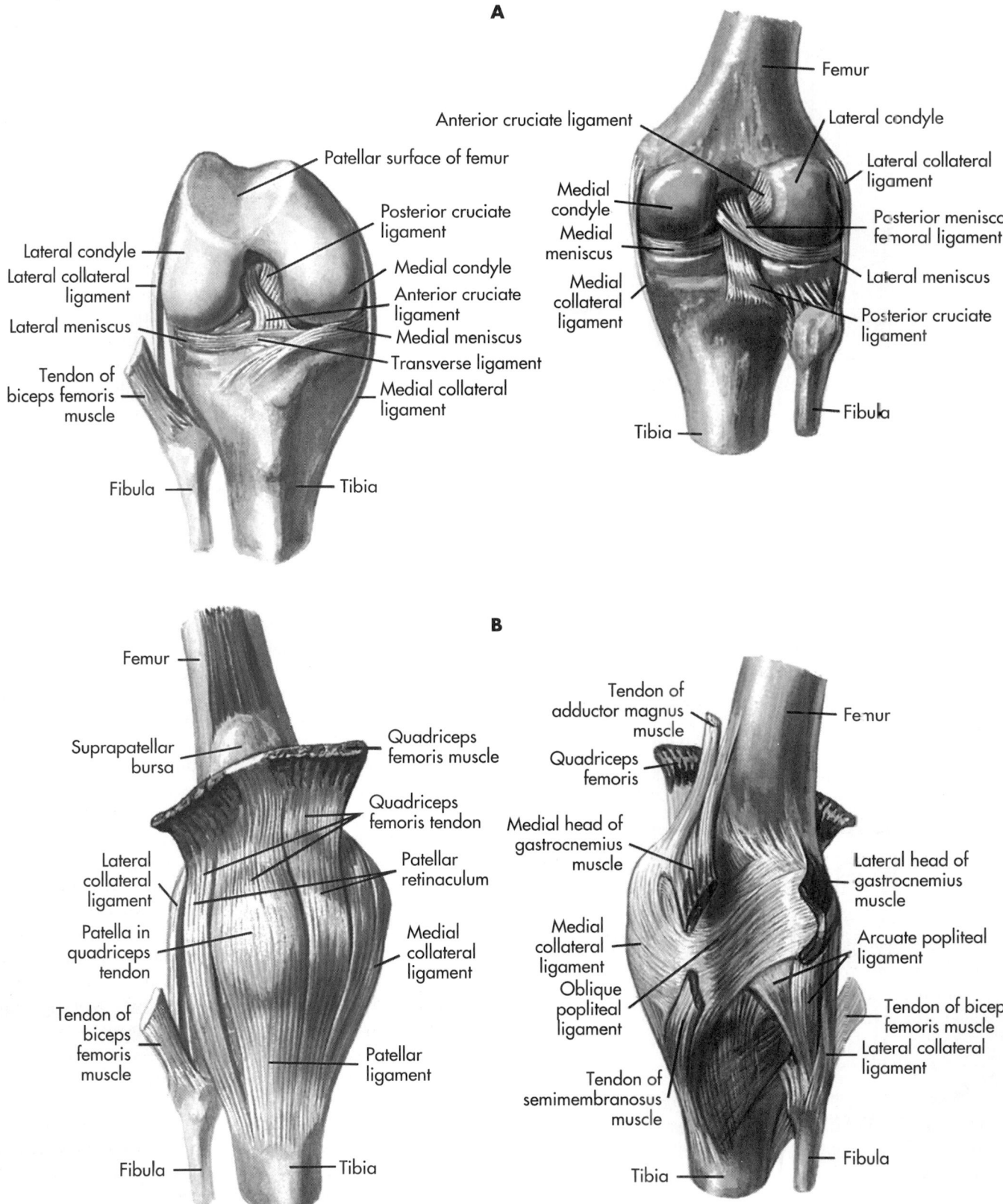

FIGURE 22–10   Knee joint. **A,** Bony structure. **B,** Superficial aspect.

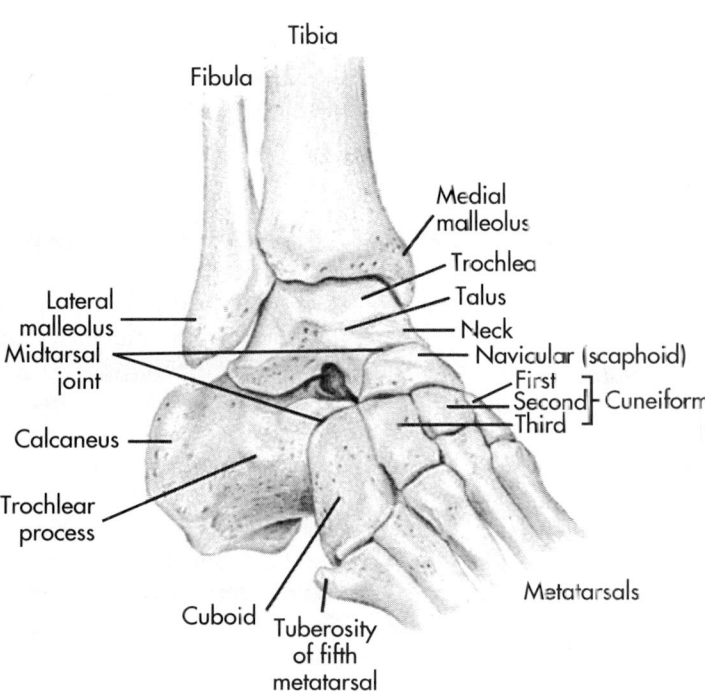

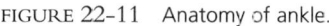

FIGURE 22-11 Anatomy of ankle.

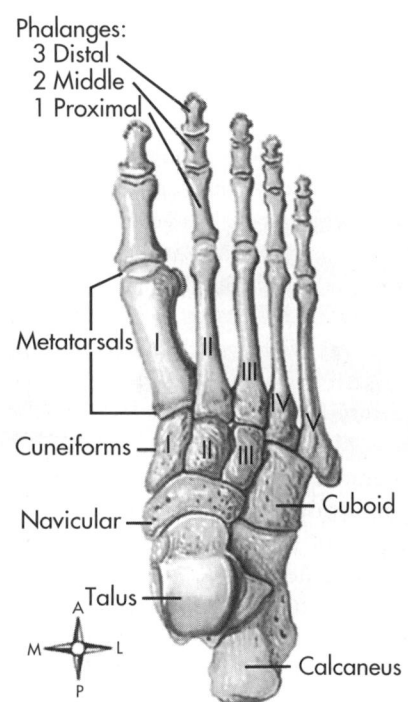

FIGURE 22-12 Bones of the foot viewed from above.

Nursing Diagnosis

Nursing diagnoses related to the care of patients undergoing orthopedic surgery might include the following:

- Anxiety
- Risk for peripheral neurovascular impairment
- Risk for injury
- Impaired gas exchange
- Risk for infection

Outcome Identification

Outcomes identified for the orthopedic patient undergoing surgical repair include the following:

- The patient will verbalize concerns and apprehension related to surgery and recovery.
- The patient will be free from peripheral neurovascular impairment.
- The patient will be free from injury related to surgical positioning.
- The patient will maintain adequate ventilation and oxygen exchange.
- The patient will be free of postoperative surgical site infection.

Planning

The care of surgical patients undergoing any type of surgery requires planning for routine procedures that are always followed as well as anticipating the unexpected. The perioperative nurse should be consistent and systematic in the planning process to expedite actual steps required to facilitate the surgical procedure. Care of the orthopedic patient presents unique challenges because of the psychosocial, physical, and technical aspects of patient care. Planning includes attention to environmental factors, positioning, transfusion supplies, equipment, and instrument needs in addition to practices that will prevent complications.[4,9,11]

The optimal environment is comfortable for the patient and surgical team. The patient should feel relaxed and secure enough to allow the surgical team to become his or her advocates during the procedure. Physical preparation of the environment changes with individual patients. At the time the procedure is posted in the operating room, traffic flow is considered to determine room location. The temperature is selected for the procedure with consideration given to patient age and general health, attire worn by the operative personnel (body exhaust suits), or use of polymethyl methacrylate (PMMA) or bone cement. Temperature monitoring should be performed for all but very brief surgical procedures, such as those lasting less than 30 minutes. To maintain normothermia, the perioperative nurse might consider using warm cotton blankets preoperatively, intraoperative options such as warming the ambient room temperature, intravenous fluid warming, and skin-surface warming, with circulating water mattresses or forced-air warming devices[15] and reapplication of warm cotton blankets at the end of the surgical procedure.

Equipment and instrumentation needed for the procedure are planned before patient arrival in the operating room; orthopedic procedures may vary significantly because of the patient's physical condition or age. It may be necessary to communicate with the manufacturer's representative to facilitate obtaining items needed for the procedure.

Procedural information should be reviewed to plan positioning and protective measures. Aseptic technique is a routine in the perioperative environment and should be considered a priority when caring for the orthopedic patient. Osteomyelitis is an infection of the bone that can go unrecognized for a long time and requires expensive, intensive treatment. Osteomyelitis can lead to severe bone loss and possible loss of a limb. Preventive measures, including administration of antibiotics upon induction of anesthesia or within 10 minutes of inflating a tourniquet, have been demonstrated to be efficacious in preventing surgical site infection.[29]

Operating room equipment such as defibrillators and resuscitative equipment must always be available, functional, and familiar to staff. This includes supplies needed for emergency treatment of a patient condition, such as malignant hyperthermia or unanticipated blood loss. Orthopedic procedures may also require a change in the plan of care in the event of a fracture, damage to vascular integrity, or changes in the patient condition, requiring an understanding of methods and equipment needed to manage these situations.

One method of planning the overall care from preadmission to discharge is to place a patient in a clinical pathway, a multidisciplinary case management tool. Clinical pathways define the expected processes of care and are, in essence, strategies of care to encourage physicians and other health providers who care for the same surgical patient population to agree with each other on a sequence of common interventions. Fig. 22-13 demonstrates a typical clinical path for DRG 209, total knee replacement. Included with this on the patient's chart is a set of orders, which mirrors this path and allows the physician to make minor changes to the protocol. All patients are moved from their acute bed on postoperative day 3 to a rehabilitation or skilled nursing bed or are discharged to home if their medical status warrants. Receiving feedback from all disciplines involved in the patient's care reaps benefits in the form of reduced variance and improved efficiency, outcomes and costs.[21]

The nursing process requires continual reassessment and modifications. An effective plan entails communication, safety, creation of an optimal environment, and effective use of human and physical resources. A Sample Care Plan for the patient undergoing orthopedic surgery is on p. 807.

Implementation

Implementing care for the orthopedic surgical patient requires an understanding of anatomic, physiologic, psychologic, cultural, spiritual, and technical patient needs. Orthopedic surgical procedures demand special equipment, instruments, and psychomotor skills that are different from those required by other specialties. Implementation includes an understanding of the procedures, patient needs, perioperative practices, and perioperative nursing interventions to protect the patient while delivering care.

Patient education

Patient education begins with the first patient contact, usually during the visit to the surgeon, nurse practitioner, or registered nurse first assistant (RNFA). Preoperative patient education requires innovative techniques including videotapes, patient brochures, and other teaching aids. This information is reinforced immediately before surgery. The trend toward same-day surgery and "A.M. admits" further challenges the perioperative skills required to complete a patient assessment and preoperative teaching. Assessment of the patient's level of understanding enhances the ability to reinforce teaching appropriately and address any unresolved issues. Patients must be provided with the opportunity to ask questions and demonstrate psychomotor skills required for their rehabilitation process.

Explanations about the intraoperative phase, including the anticipated sequence of events, personnel, the environment, positioning required, and procedures such as regional anesthesia or application of the tourniquet, should be reviewed with the patient. The patient may be alert during the procedure; therefore noise from power equipment and activities that will occur should be explained. Immobilization devices such as splints, casts, braces, and drains are demonstrated and explained. Pain management techniques should also be discussed.[10]

Positioning and positioning aids

The orthopedic patient requires proper positioning on the OR bed or specialty bed to provide adequate exposure of the operative area, maintain body alignment, minimize strain or pressure on nerves and muscles, allow for optimal respiratory and circulatory functions, and provide adequate stabilization of the body. Selection of position depends on several factors, including the type of procedure, location of the injury or lesion, and surgeon preference. Guidelines for placing the patient in the supine or recumbent position are followed (see Chapter 5), with modifications to facilitate the specific orthopedic procedure.

Procedures performed in lateral, prone, or modified positions require use of positioning aids and devices to support these positions. Patients undergoing surgical procedures risk neuromuscular and skin injury. Preoperative assessment should be thorough to plan the position, taking into consideration the prevention of neurovascular compromise, impaired chest excursion, and the danger of falls. The safety strap does not always provide adequate security, and other methods of securing the patient on the OR bed may need to be implemented. The surgeon is responsible for selecting the position and ensuring that adequate exposure can be obtained. The perioperative staff

DRG 209 KNEE	PRE-OP DATE:	DAY 1 - ADMISSION/OR DATE:

ASSESSMENT & EVALUATION	Admission assessment completed
	Baseline vital signs
	Obtain old chart
		VS q4 × 48 hrs. then q shift; neuro and circ. checks
		   q2 × 12 hrs. then routine
		I & O
		Bowel Sounds assessment
		Observe dressing and hemovac q 2°
		   empty q shift

DIAGNOSTICS	Hemogram; X-ray op site EKG over 50° or Hx of cardiac problem CXR if Hx resp. problems or smokes U/A Chem 7 Coag profile	H & H this evening X-Ray operative knee in PACU - AP & lateral
CONSULTS	Instruction in exercises, ambulation, transfers In home PT evaluation by home health Review clinical path with patient in PAT	Bedside PT exercises per protocol as tolerated Progression to dangle
TREATMENTS		Consider CPM TED Hose/Pneumo boots to unaffected leg prior surgery - bilaterally following surgery Incentive Spirometer q 1° during day --------------------> Cold Therapy to knee Auto - infusion Straight Cath if unable to void - foley if needed

MEDICATIONS	Inform patient to stop all anti inflammatory meds
	   for four (4) days before surgery including
	   ASA
		Other medications: (Address home meds)
		Cefazolin 1gm IVPB 1° pre-op then q 8 × 24° or 48°
		   or until drain out
		Cepastat Lozenges prn
		Colace 100mg every day
		FeSO$_4$ 325mg tid with meals
		Tylenol gx × prn
		Epidural, PCA or IM narcotic
		Anticoagulation medications as ordered

NUTRITION		NPO until post-op, then diet as tolerated if bowel sounds present
ACTIVITY		No pillow behind knee. Elevate operated extremity Instruct in use of overhead trapeze Call light in reach Provide walker to patient room Dangle, stand as tolerated ----------------------------------> Use walker - ambulate at bedside (WBAT) -------------> Up to chair --->
PATIENT/FAMILY TEACHING	Pre-op teaching PCA or epidural Pneumo boots Incentive Spirometer; Hemovac Explain treatment plan Share plan with patient and/or family Explain blood salvage	Review use PCA pain management Incentive spirometry Ankle pumps and movement unaffected extremities
SPIRITUAL/PSYCHOSOCIAL	Assess emotional status of patient & family Assessment of spiritual needs/wishes	---> --->
DISCHARGE PLANNING	Assessment of home situation by home health	Review at D/C rounds any possible needs

EXPECTED OUTCOMES	Patient/family verbalizes understanding pre-op
	   instructions
		Patient verbalizes acceptable pain control ------------->
		Demonstrates hourly use of Incentive Spirometer
		   during day.
		Remains free of CHF, pulmonary edema, or
		   pulmonary embolus. ---------------------------------->

FIGURE 22-13   Clinical pathway for total knee replacement.

Continued

DRG 209 KNEE	DRG 209 KNEE POST OP DAY 1 DATE:	POST OP DAY 2 DATE:	POST OP DAY 3 DATE:
ASSESSMENT & EVALUATION	Routine post-op V.S. Measure hemovac output q shift Assessment continues	Continue assessment Observe incision	Continue assessment
DIAGNOSTICS	H & H in a.m. Consider PT/PTT, Platelets		
CONSULTS	To OT - for evaluation, transfer and equip training To PT via wheelchair for ambulation Order home equipment as needed Consider evaluation for Skilled Unit Food & Nutrition to screen patient	PT - continue exercises and ambulate per protocol Ambulate on stairs if stable Car transfer Schedule OP therapy as appropriate OT - ADL Training	Continue PT & OT
TREATMENTS	D/C foley - straight cath PRN Remove & reapply TED Hose every shift D/C Hemovac with MD order --> Knee exerciser from SPD if ordered	Change dressing Immobilizer only when up or for transfers Remove and reapply TEDS every shift Ice prn D/C hemovac with MD order	Continue pneumo boots and TEDS Change dressing every day and prn Remove & reapply TEDS every shift
MEDICATIONS	D/C PCA basal rate if applicable Laxative of choice PCA D/C IV when taking fluids well and connect to prn adaptor as appropriate	D/C PCA if applicable with MD order --> D/C prn adaptor as appropriate	PO pain med with MD order -->
NUTRITION	Diet as tolerated		Instruct on importance of diet as it relates to healing
ACTIVITY	--> --> --> -->	--> --> --> -->	--> --> --> -->
PATIENT/FAMILY TEACHING	Teach transfer techniques - continue other exercises Teach knee exerciser if ordered	Review home situation - possible needs if not completed pre-op by home health	Review meds Wound care Signs & Symptoms infection Activity limitations Follow up appoint with MD Follow up appoint with PT PT/OT review home exercise program/home health
SPIRITUAL/PSYCHOSOCIAL	--> -->	--> -->	--> -->
DISCHARGE PLANNING	Case Manager: Assess home needs vs. Skilled Unit needs	Consider evaluation for Skilled Unit	Transfer to Skilled or Discharge as appropriate
EXPECTED OUTCOMES	--> Verbalizes or demonstrates hourly use of incentive spirometer. Transfers to chair -->	--> Ambulates minimum of 15 feet. -->	Patient verbalizes understanding of pain management. Ambulates minimum of 35 feet if returning home. Demonstrates home exercise program.

FIGURE 22-13, cont'd   Clinical pathway for total knee replacement.

SAMPLE CARE PLAN

Nursing Diagnosis: Anxiety

Outcome: The patient will verbalize concerns and apprehension related to pending surgery and recovery.

Interventions:

Encourage verbalization of feelings, expression of fear, and questions about procedure, anticipated outcome, postoperative rehabilitation, pain management, and home care/self-care requirements.

Explain anticipated routine activities (diagnostic studies, OR environment, preoperative holding area, PACU) and encourage questions.

Encourage patient and family participation in decision-making activities related to discharge planning.

Demonstrate respect and attend to patient's individual needs and those of the family or significant others.

Remain with patient; ensure other personnel are introduced.

Provide comforting and caring through the use of warm blankets, touch, handholding, etc.

Discuss any other concerns with the patient and family and initiate appropriate referrals.

Nursing Diagnosis: Risk for peripheral neurovascular impairment.

Outcome: The patient will be free from peripheral neurovascular impairment related to positioning, use of equipment, or prolonged surgical time.

Interventions:

Complete a preoperative neurovascular assessment including skin color and temperature, pulses, motor strength and movement, and sensation; reassess at procedure conclusion.

Position in proper body alignment in consideration of range of motion and any limitations in mobility.

Protect vulnerable neurovascular structures and prevent pressure by properly padding bony prominences and pressure points.

Apply pneumatic tourniquet correctly, observing and verifying pressure settings and tourniquet inflation time.

Provide padding (air mattress or gel pads) when long surgical times are expected or patients are predisposed to peripheral vascular compromise.

Anticipate patient and surgical team needs to minimize surgical time.

Nursing Diagnosis: Risk for injury

Outcome: The patient will be free from injury related to the surgical position.

Interventions:

Assess range of motion; identify joints at risk for injury caused by immobilization, pain, trauma, or arthritic or other disease processes.

Observe condition of patient's skin before transfer to the OR bed and again at conclusion of procedure.

Use proper lifting and transfer techniques when transferring the patient to and from the OR bed.

Keep sheets on OR bed dry and wrinkle free.

Ensure that personnel with knowledge of the patient's condition and equipment are available to supervise and assist with transfer of the patient.

Use proper restraint devices to protect patients from falls or movement of the extremities.

Avoid extending or flexing extremities beyond range of motion when there is resistance.

Protect skin in dependent areas from pooling of solutions.

Use positioning devices, such as pillows, to maintain position.

Pad all dependent pressure sites.

Protect vulnerable neurovascular areas from compression.

Nursing Diagnosis: Impaired gas exchange

Outcome: The patient will maintain optimal ventilation and oxygen exchange.

Interventions:

Review preoperative evaluation of the patient's pulmonary status.

Assist anesthesia provider in airway management.

Ensure full chest excursion when positioning, particularly in the lateral and prone positions.

Monitor vital signs, pulse oximetry, and blood loss.

Complete a vascular assessment (pulse, sensation, movement, temperature, and color check) preoperatively and compare to postoperative status.

Nursing Diagnosis: Risk for infection

Outcome: The patient will be free from surgical-site infection.

Interventions:

Modify the plan of care for high-risk patients as determined by assessment results.

Confirm that patient has complied with preoperative skin cleansing (as appropriate).

Implement aseptic practices for skin preparation, draping the patient and equipment, opening supplies and equipment for the procedure, removing hair (as necessary), and controlling traffic patterns in the operating room.

Prepare for pulsatile lavage or irrigation (as needed).

Initiate antibiotic therapy preoperatively or intraoperatively per physician orders.

Implement procedure-specific activities such as using body exhaust systems and pulsatile lavage.

Anticipate equipment needs and check equipment function; implement safety precautions when using equipment.

Sterilize instruments according to policy and procedure and the manufacturer guidelines.

Handle implants cautiously.

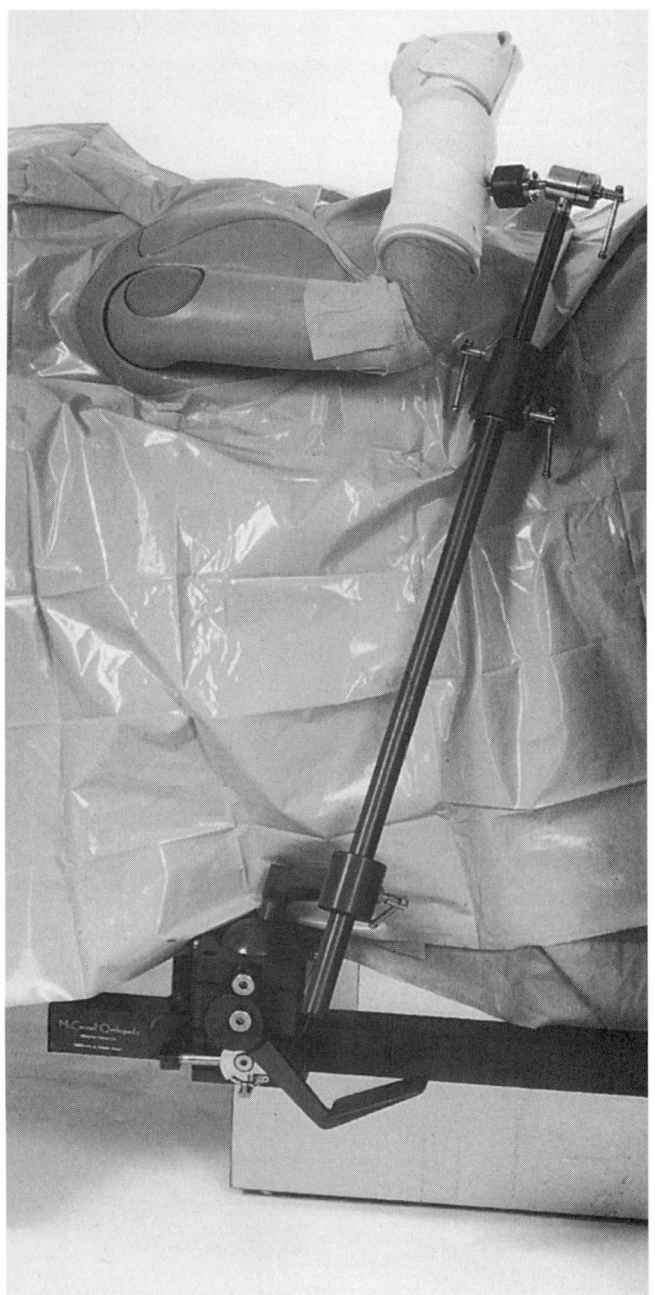

FIGURE 22-14 Shoulder positioner, attached to the bed, allows distraction of the joint for visualization.

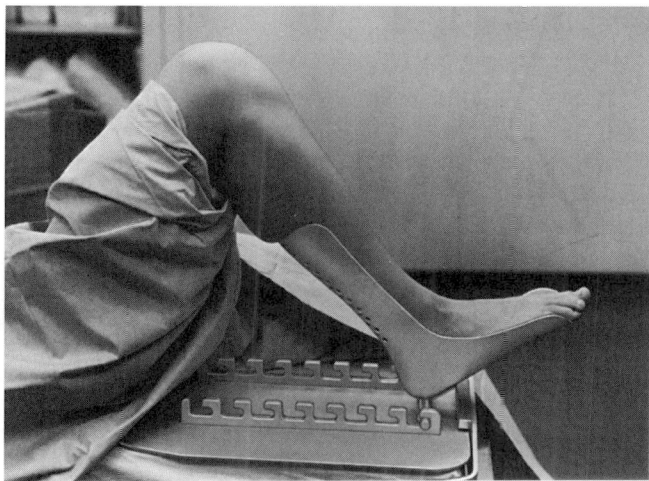

FIGURE 22-15 Alvarado foot holder used during total joint procedures to position the extremity for exposure.

must understand the meaning of terms such as *flexion*, *extension*, *abduction*, and *adduction* when positioning the patient and be thoroughly familiar with the function of the orthopedic surgical bed and its various attachments, such as the leg attachment for arthroscopy, three-point positioner for lateral position, and positioning devices for shoulder procedures.

Many orthopedic operations require a device for holding the extremities. Various holders are available for both upper and lower extremities. Positioners used intraoperatively can be sterilized for the procedure, resulting in the ability to reposition as needed throughout the procedure. These types of positioners include the McConnell shoulder positioner (Fig. 22-14), Alvarado foot holder (Fig. 22-15), and ankle distractor (Fig. 22-16). Many other orthopedic positioning devices are available.

The lateral position is sometimes used for a total hip arthroplasty. Padded anterior and posterior supports may be positioned at the umbilicus and lumbar region, respectively, to hold the patient in the lateral position. A vacuum beanbag can also achieve this position. Pressure points on the lateral area of the skull, ear, axilla, hip, knee, and ankle should be adequately padded. The feet are placed in the neutral position to prevent excessive plantar flexion or dorsiflexion. A conscientious effort should be made by the surgical team to avoid leaning on the patient during the procedure.

The patient is positioned prone for surgery on the posterior aspect of the body, including the back; posterior portion of the shoulder, arms, or legs; and Achilles tendon and for posterior iliac bone graft harvesting. This position presents a challenge for the anesthesia team to monitor and manage the airway because of the potential for impaired chest excursion and gas exchange. Extremities need to be brought through a normal range of motion when transferring and positioning into the prone position. Vascular integrity is always assessed before the patient is moved into position and repeated after the patient is positioned; the quality of pulses, extremity warmth, and capillary refill should be noted.

The prone position is often attained with the use of adjunctive frames, such as the Wilson, Hastings, Canadian, Relton-Hall, Cloward saddle, Andrews frames, or the Andrews bed (Fig. 22-17). Each frame has qualities that meet patient or physician needs. The Hastings and Andrews frames and Andrews bed maintain the patient in a modified knee-chest position. The frames require assembly and are labor intensive when positioning; some can be

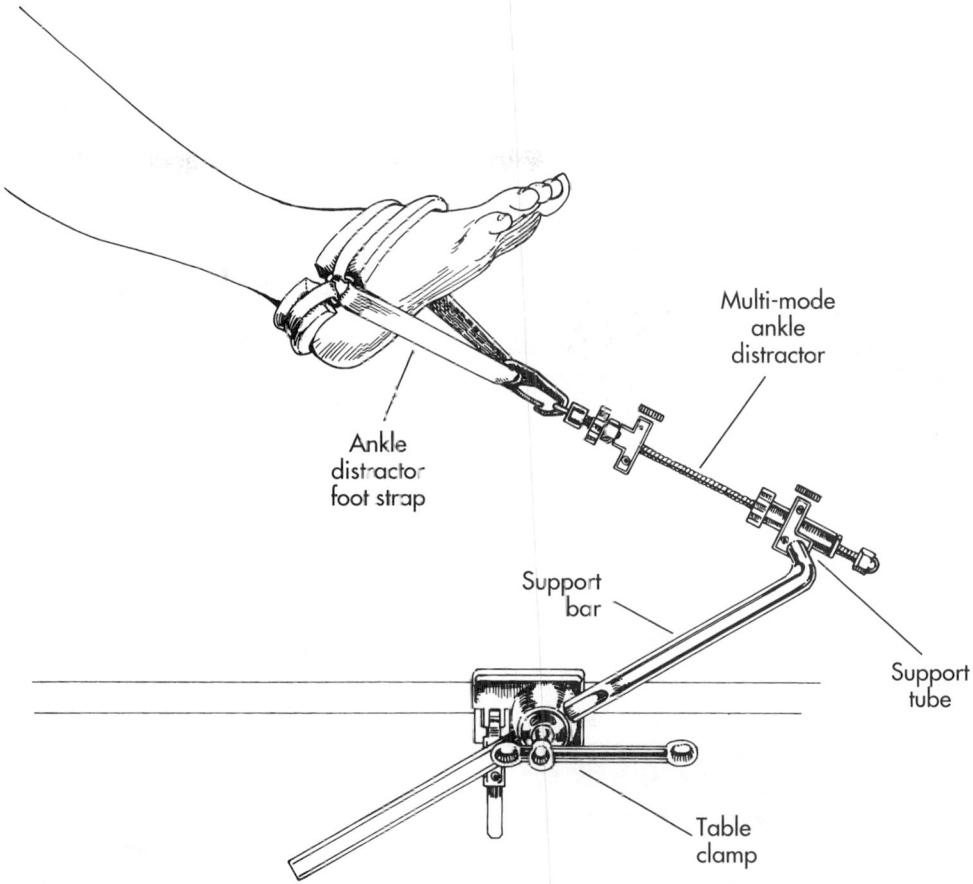

FIGURE 22-16 Ankle distractor, noninvasive, for distraction of the joint and visualization.

used only with certain beds. The Andrews bed is similar to the frame but has the attachments built in and is used exclusively for this position.

On a fracture table (Fig. 22-18), generally used for femoral neck and shaft fixation, the patient is placed in supine or lateral positions to allow exposure of the surgical site while maintaining alignment. The legs are positioned on outriggers, allowing access by the image intensifier to obtain multiple radiographic views. Applying or releasing traction can be done to reduce the fracture or aid in intramedullary surgical techniques. Like all positioning devices, the fracture table must be set up by experienced personnel and padded adequately. There are several moving parts, which can lead to injury if not operated properly.

Surgical prep

A primary concern in orthopedic surgery is the prevention of infection. The orthopedic surgical prep must be meticulously carried out using aseptic technique. Physicians often instruct patients to complete a scrub prep with an antimicrobial cleanser before arrival for surgery. The surgical prep for the orthopedic patient may include preoperative removal of hair from the surgical site (as

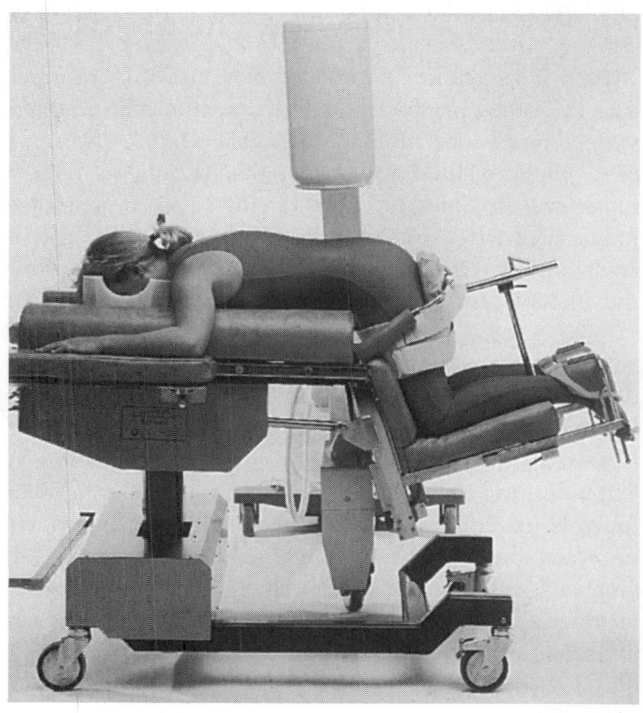

FIGURE 22-17 Andrews' bed used for prone positioning.

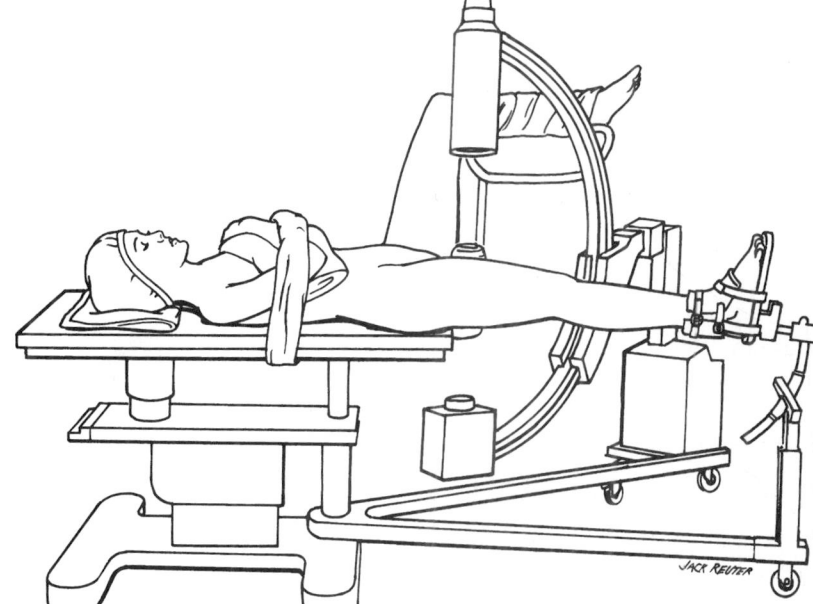

FIGURE 22-18 Patient positioned on the orthopedic fracture bed for femoral neck, femoral shaft fixation, or tibial fixation with image intensifier in position.

necessary) followed by an intraoperative skin prep. Trauma patients require precautions during the skin prep to prevent further injury caused by solution contact with membranes or injury to the bone and soft tissue from movement.

Studies have shown that surgical shave preps contribute to the possibility of infection caused by abrasion and cutting of the skin. If hair removal from the incisional site is necessary, it should occur immediately before surgery, using clippers or a depilatory. If hair removal requires use of a razor, the site can be lubricated with soap before shaving.[6]

Skin preparation is completed to remove microorganisms from the operative site. The site should be prepared with a broad-spectrum antimicrobial agent. The scrub prep might include using soap and water to remove superficial oil and skin debris, followed by a povidone-iodine preparation to scrub the surgical area. The prep is applied using sterile gloves and supplies, proceeding from the incision site to the periphery. Pooling of the prep solution beneath the patient or tourniquet must be avoided.[6] Excess solutions should be allowed to dry before draping. The groin and anal areas should be isolated when the surgical site is on the upper third of the leg.

Devices such as leg stirrups may help in supporting an extremity to complete a circumferential prep. When multiple extremities or other areas, such as a bone graft site, are prepped, cross-contamination of previously prepped areas must be prevented. Knowledge of aseptic technique and the ability to organize the activity are important in proper preparation of the surgical site.

Draping

Application of sterile drapes is the final step in preparing the patient for the operation. Extremities are covered with a cloth or water-impervious stockinette, a cylindrical drape that is rolled up the arm or leg. Strikethrough must be prevented by using impervious sheets when a large amount of fluid is used, as during arthroscopy and wound irrigation. Prefabricated disposable drapes with fenestrations for the upper and lower extremity are available.

Iodophor-impregnated adhesive drapes can be used to isolate the surrounding area from the incisional site. Research indicates that an isopropyl alcohol/iodophor-impregnated adhesive drape prep may be as effective as the iodophor scrub and paint prep/plain adhesive drape method and may be more cost effective when time and materials are compared.[20]

Equipment and supplies

Orthopedic operating rooms require a variety of special equipment and accessories in addition to routine operating room equipment. Nitrogen, battery- and electrically powered equipment, video systems, pneumatic tourniquets, laminar airflow systems, x-ray equipment, lasers, and special orthopedic tables are included in the operative armamentarium. Manufacturers' pamphlets with illustrations and directions on equipment use and sterilization should be readily available for reference. Performance assessment and improvement activities, along with competency-based learning and assessment, should be in place to ensure safety and quality of care. Perioperative nurses should participate in selecting core competencies, performance criteria, and interventions relevant to caring for the perioperative orthopedic patient.[28]

Radiographic Intervention

Radiographic intervention is widely used in orthopedic surgery. Many procedures require portable x-ray or fluoroscopy machines. Fluoroscopy, also known as *image intensification*, allows the team to view the progression of the procedure, confirming fracture reduction or intramedullary reaming of the humerus, femur, or tibia. A technician operates radiographic equipment. An understanding of equipment placement, function, and safety precautions is necessary. The perioperative nurse is responsible for communicating with the radiology personnel concerning the procedure, aseptic technique, and traffic flow in the operating room. X-ray cassettes brought onto the sterile field are draped with a sterile plastic cover. Lead aprons and thyroid shields are to be worn by all personnel in proximity to the x-ray equipment, and personnel should be monitored for exposure to radiation. Patients should be covered with lead aprons or other protective devices.

Pneumatic Tourniquets

Pneumatic tourniquets are frequently used for procedures involving the extremities (Fig. 22-19). A tourniquet is a cylindrical bladder inflated by compressed gas or ambient air. It will produce a relatively bloodless surgical field with circumferential pressure on arterial and venous circulation. The limb is exsanguinated by elevating it or wrapping it, distally to proximally, with an Ace or Esmarch rubber bandage before tourniquet inflation. The majority of tourniquets used today are run by a microprocessor for regulation of pressure and time setting, providing both auditory and visual feedback for the user.

Tourniquet safety should be a priority; the surgical team should understand recommended parameters and precautions. Safety guidelines for the use of tourniquets include preventive measures and evaluation.[6] Preoperative assessment of the patient includes determining contraindications for use, including compartment syndrome, McArdle's syndrome, hypertension, or other vascular problems. If the tourniquet must be used for patients with these conditions, specific guidelines must be observed.

Before application the tourniquet equipment should be checked for proper function. Inflation pressures are established based on the systolic blood pressure, age of the patient, and circumference of the extremity. Tourniquet inflation should be kept to a minimum. It is recommended in the average, healthy 50-year-old person to apply continuous tourniquet pressure less than 1 hour on the upper extremity and 2 hours on the thigh.[14]

The tourniquet should be placed on the extremity without compression on bony structures and superficial neurovascular structures. The cuff should be positioned as high as possible without pinching skin folds. Webril or stockinette is wrapped around the extremity and kept free of wrinkles and gatherings beneath the cuff. Cuffs should overlap a minimum of 3 and a maximum of 6 inches; excess overlap can pinch skin folds. Too short of a tourniquet cuff can loosen after inflation. Care must be taken to ensure that the line from the air supply to the cuff is not kinked.

Tourniquet equipment should be checked periodically

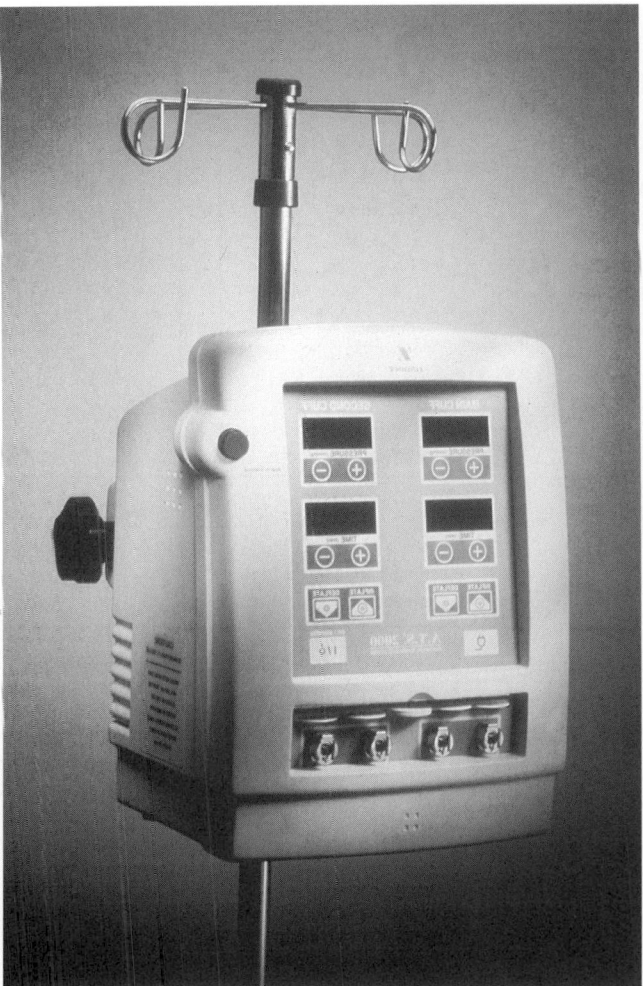

FIGURE 22-19 Pneumatic gauge.

and serviced when problems arise. Injury from tourniquets may result from inadequate precautions, faulty preparation, or use of inaccurate equipment. The gauges and other related equipment can be checked with commercially available test equipment. Patient evaluation requires assessment of the extremity (skin color, temperature, pulses, movement, sensation) after removal of the tourniquet. Abnormal findings need to be reported to the surgeon and documented.

Traction

Traction is used preoperatively, intraoperatively, or postoperatively for prevention or reduction of muscle spasm, immobilization of a joint or body part, reduction of a fracture or dislocation, and treatment of a joint disorder. Traction alignment must be constant.

Various traction techniques can be used, including manual, skin, and skeletal (Fig. 22-20). In manual traction, the hands provide the forces pulling on the bone being realigned. Skin traction uses strips of tape, digital straps, moleskin, or an elastic bandage applied directly to the skin. Common forms of skin traction are Buck's extension and Russell traction. Skeletal traction applies forces directly to

A **B** **C**

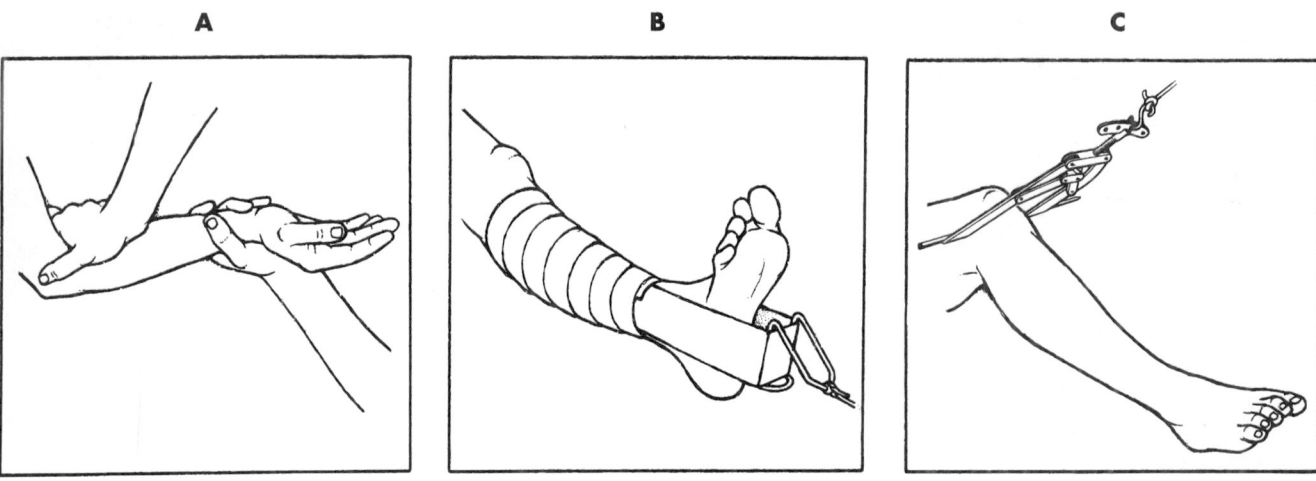

FIGURE 22-20   Traction techniques. **A,** Manual. **B,** Skin. **C,** Skeletal.

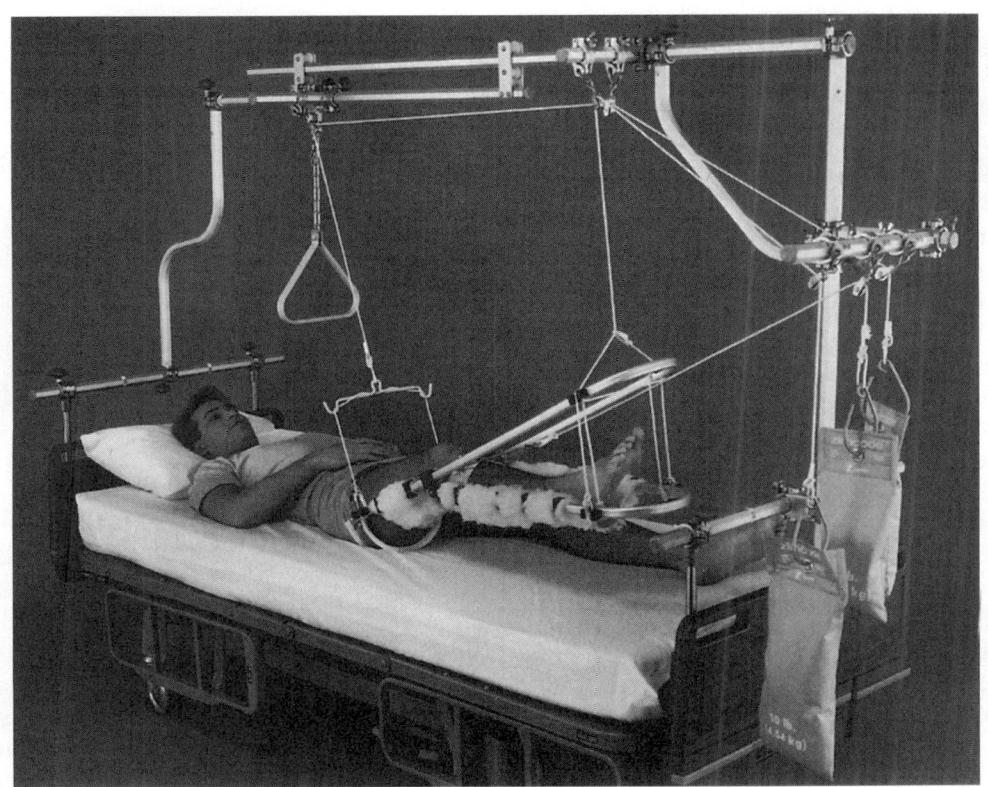

FIGURE 22-21   Thomas splint balanced suspension.

the bone using pins. Manual and skin traction can be applied in the emergency room or patient room, whereas skeletal traction is applied preoperatively in the emergency room or in the operating room.

Skeletal traction is often used in conjunction with the fracture table using the traction attachment to aid in reduction of a long bone fracture. Postoperatively the patient may be confined to bed with balanced skeletal traction using a Thomas splint (Fig. 22-21) and a Pearson attachment. Some cervical spine fractures or injuries may

require Crutchfield or Gardner-Wells tongs inserted directly into the skull to stabilize the vertebrae and reduce spinal cord damage or further injury. Application of skeletal traction requires the use of sterile supplies, including a traction bow, pins, and drill (Fig. 22-22).

Traction frames are placed immediately on the postoperative bed to accommodate traction. Nursing care of the patient in traction should include ensuring that the traction is continuous and skin tapes or skeletal pins are secured. Neurovascular status should be checked routinely,

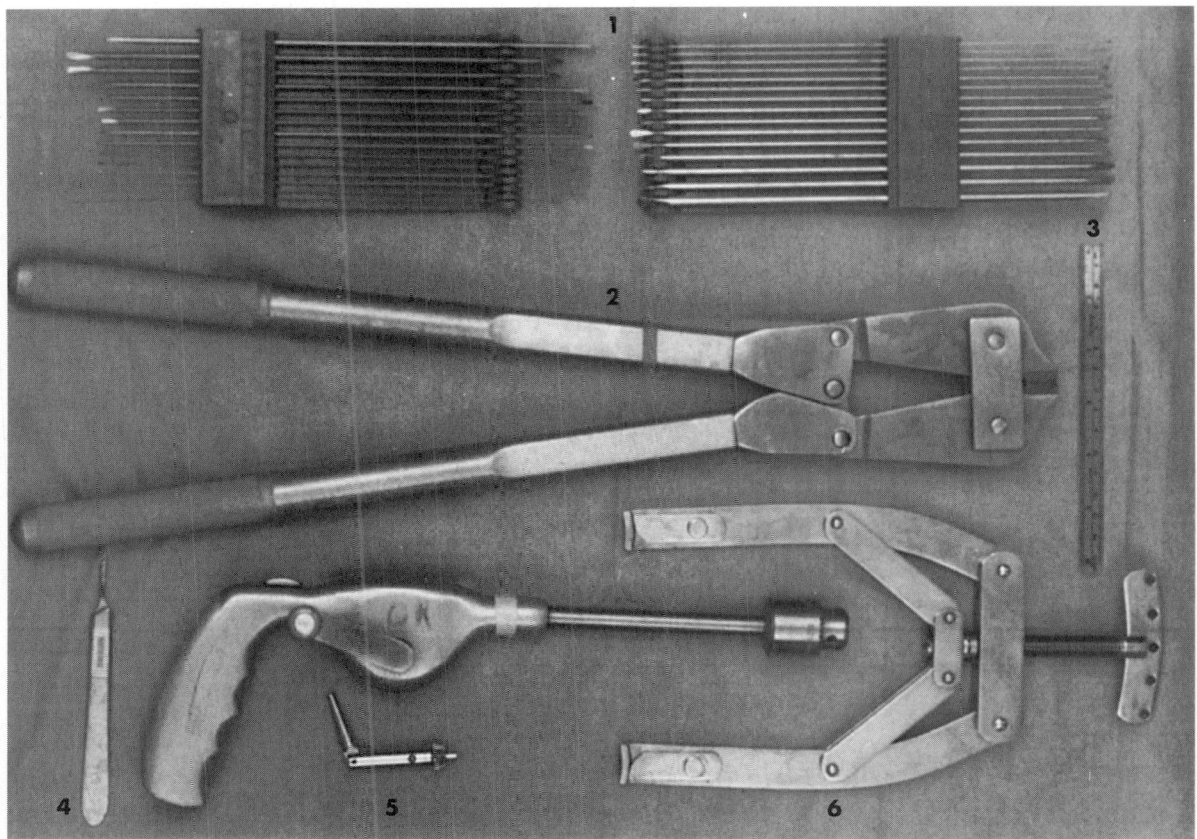

FIGURE 22-22   Instruments for insertion of skeletal traction: *1,* Kirschner wires and Steinman pins; *2,* bolt cutter; *3,* ruler; *4,* knife handle (using no. 15 blade); *5,* hand drill with chuck key, *6,* traction bow.

including skin color, pulse, temperature, and sensation. Changes from baseline or normal value need to be reported. Supplies and frames should be available and assembled before transferring the patient to the postoperative bed.

Postoperative Immobilization

Postoperative immobilization may require use of a cast, splint, or other supplies designed for the specific anatomic part. A cast is a common method of immobilizing a fractured bone during healing. The forces of distraction, rotation, and malalignment can be overcome with the application of a cast. Closed reduction with a cast may be an option, thus minimizing the disadvantages and complications of open reduction, such as infection and tissue damage.

Casting is accomplished primarily with plaster or synthetic materials, such as fiberglass. Plaster is less expensive, with a greater weight-to-strength ratio (it requires a greater weight of plaster to produce the same strength when using fiberglass). Plaster casts may be burdensome to some patients if too heavy. They are routinely used as the primary cast after surgical procedures and are replaced later with a lighter fiberglass cast to promote patient mobility.

Casting material sets up and hardens rapidly once activated with water, and such a property makes it imperative that it be prepared with all necessary materials. Webril or stockinette should be applied to the extremity under the cast to protect the skin from thermal injury while the plaster sets as well as from undue abrasion and pressure. The plaster must be prepared, applied, and handled carefully and safely.

Types of casts are shown in Fig. 22-23. A short arm cast is applied from below the elbow to the metacarpal heads after wrist fractures. A long arm cast is carried from the axilla to the metacarpal heads, immobilizing forearm or elbow fractures. The short leg cast is applied from the tibial tuberosity to the metatarsal heads to immobilize the ankle and foot. The long leg cast is used for fractures involving the femur, tibia, fibula or complicated ankle fractures. The femoral cast brace is used in the treatment of femoral shaft fractures. A snug-fitting thigh cast and short leg cast are hinged at the knee joint. The cast brace is generally used after 4 to 6 weeks of skeletal traction after initiation of callus formation at the fracture site. A cylinder cast incorporates the leg from the groin to the ankle and is applied when complete knee immobilization is required. This is often required after surgery involving soft-tissue reconstruction around the knee.

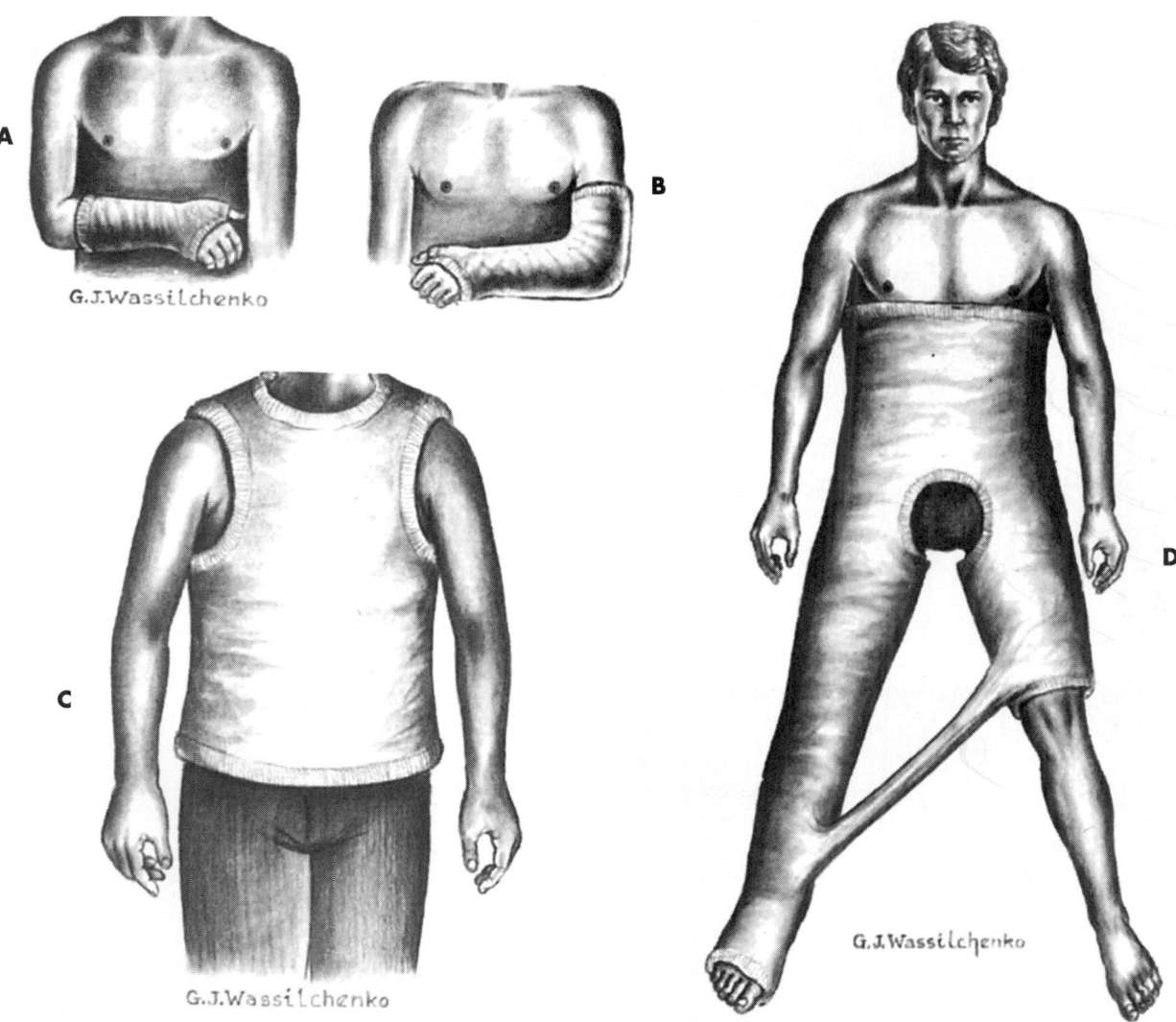

FIGURE 22-23 Types of casts. **A,** Short arm cast. **B,** Long arm cast. **C,** Plaster body jacket cast. **D,** One and one-half hip spica cast.

The hip spica cast is used when complete leg immobilization is desired. The trunk, affected side, and unaffected side may all be incorporated into the cast. Spinal immobilization is accomplished with a body jacket.

Splints are also employed for postoperative immobilization but are not circumferential and allow for swelling and closer observation of the surgical site.

Another immobilization device is the abduction pillow (Fig. 22-24), used after total joint replacement. This prevents leg adduction, internal rotation, and hip flexion, which could cause dislocation of the hip. Further discussion of this and other devices is included in the section on surgical interventions.

Lasers

Laser application has been increasing in the field of orthopedics. Their use mandates safety precautions, certification, patient consent, and protective attire (see

Chapter 3). Laser types include carbon dioxide, holmium:YAG, neodymium:YAG, KTP, erbium, and excimer. Laser technique differs for use on bone, muscle, tendon, and cartilage. Lasers have been used successfully for osteotomy, revision arthroplasty (removal of PMMA), nerve and tendon repair, arthroscopy, and diskectomy.[31]

Airflow Control

Airflow control in the orthopedic operating room is critical to prevent introduction of microorganisms. Surgical site infections may result from airborne bacteria or transient bacteria from the patient or surgical team. Laminar airflow is a system designed to provide highly filtered air and continuous air exchange for reducing airborne bacteria. Body exhaust suits (Fig. 22-25) are also used as a defense against airborne bacteria. Aseptic practices, sterile technique, and conscientious behaviors in operating rooms using conventional airflow can be used to

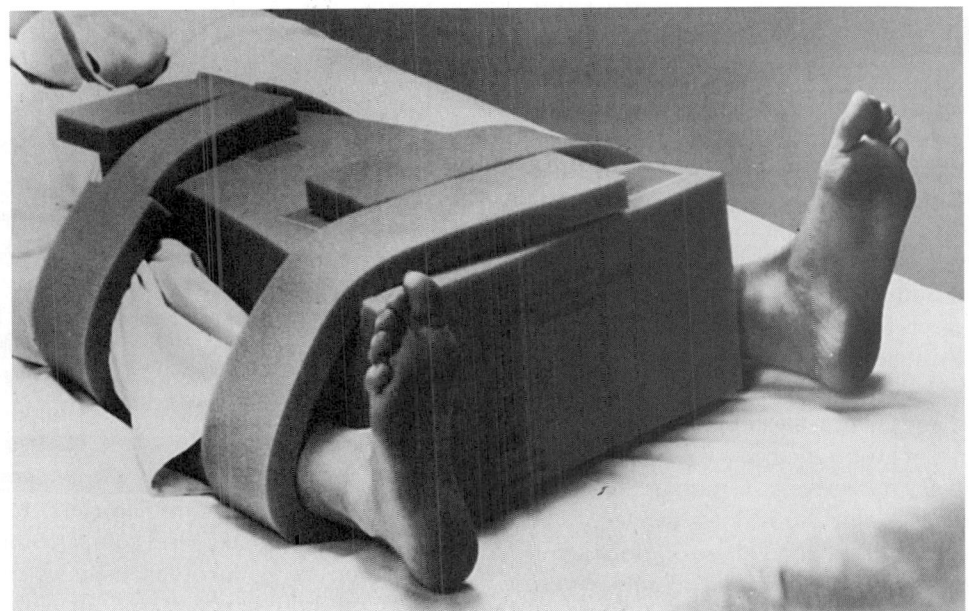

FIGURE 22-24   Abduction pillow aids in immobilizing hip joints after surgery.

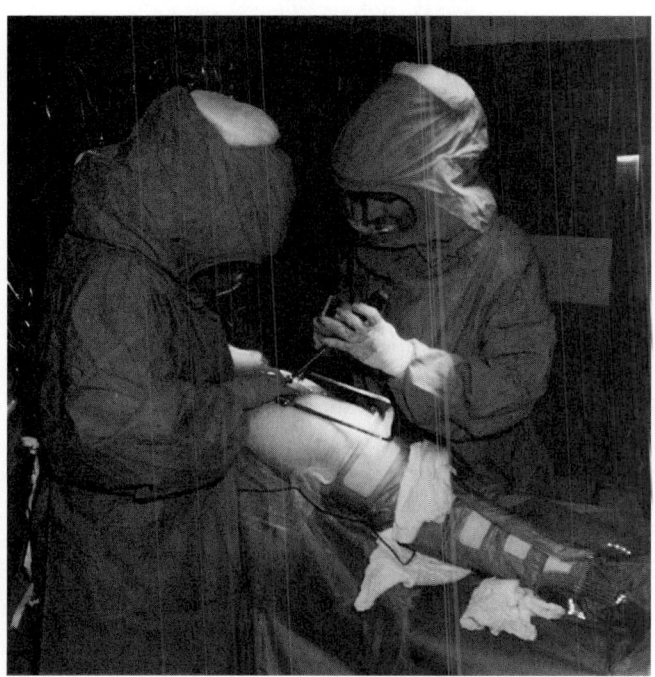

FIGURE 22-25   Body exhaust system.

maintain low rates of surgical site infections. The addition of other protective measures should be weighed to determine the benefit and outcome.[1,4]

Postoperative Management

Postoperative patient management is planned during the preoperative period. Special equipment may include continuous passive range-of-motion (CPM) machines, pain management devices and techniques, compression devices, and blood salvage. CPM machines (Fig. 22-26)

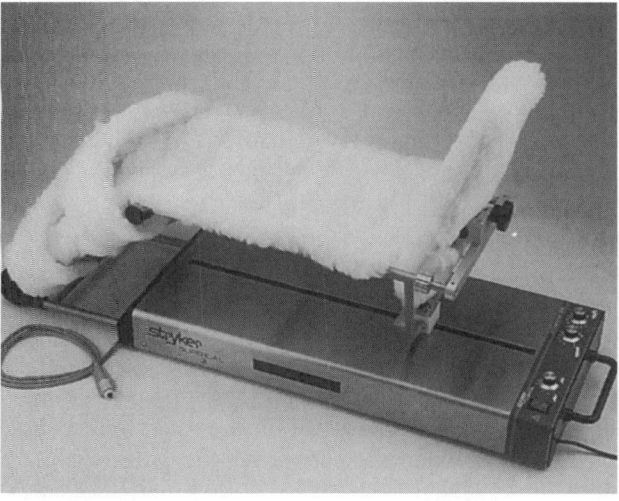

FIGURE 22-26   Continuous passive motion machine used for passive range of motion.

can be used after total knee arthroplasty, knee reconstruction, surgical repair of supracondylar fractures, total elbow arthroplasty, total shoulder arthroplasty, rotator cuff repair, removal of loose bodies, and femoral shaft fracture fixation and, less frequently, in total hip arthroplasty. CPM stimulates the healing effect on articular tissues including cartilage, tendon, and ligaments. The benefits of CPM include inhibition of adhesion formation and joint stiffness, decreased pain and swelling, early functional range of motion, and decreased effects of immobilization.[30,33] It does not interfere with healing incisions over the moving joint. The device is applied early in the postoperative period (Research Highlight 22-1).

Pain management may include insertion of an epidural

22-1 RESEARCH HIGHLIGHT

Forty-six total knee arthroplasties in which a continuous passive range-of-motion (CPM) machine was used were compared with 37 total knees that were rehabilitated with early passive flexion of the knee (called drop-and-dangle protocol). Postoperative physical therapy regimens were otherwise the same for both groups. Surgical technique was the same for both groups except for closure that was performed in the drop-and-dangle group with the knee at 90 to 95 degrees of flexion. Patients in the drop-and-dangle group were discharged from the hospital 1 day earlier than those not in that group and had a statistically better extension range of 2.8 degrees at 6 months. Knees in the drop-and-dangle group also had less drainage. The researchers concluded that a good range of motion and hospital discharge can be achieved in a similar time interval with the drop-and-dangle technique as with using a CPM device and that such a device is not required for postoperative knee rehabilitation. With cost-effectiveness as a consideration, early passive knee flexion by means of the drop-and-dangle technique is a reasonable rehabilitation choice in uncomplicated total knee arthroplasties.

From Kumar, P.J., McPherson, E.J., Dorr, L.D., et al. (1996). Rehabilitation after total knee arthroplasty: a comparison of two rehabilitation techniques. *Clinical Orthopaedics and Related Research, 331,* 93-101.

catheter or use of a patient-controlled analgesia (PCA) pump. The PCA pump administers a predetermined intravenous dose of the prescribed pain medication. It allows continuous infusion of analgesic as well as bolus administration when the patient feels it is necessary. The advantages include rapid pain relief, increased patient satisfaction, and often less use of medication than with traditional intramuscular analgesia.

Management of fluid and electrolyte balance may include use of intraoperative autologous transfusion or postoperative blood salvage. A potential problem with salvage of large amounts of blood is depletion of clotting factors; therefore coagulation problems should be identified. Postoperative blood salvage is accomplished with a closed drainage system. It requires a complete understanding of the system for safe use.

Instruments and accessory items

Orthopedic surgical procedures require an extensive inventory of instruments and implants. Successful management and optimal patient care are dependent on a well-stocked inventory of the specific instruments required to implant and apply hardware. Revision surgery requires that the perioperative staff be prepared with the appropri-

ate tools and extractors needed to remove an old implant and an understanding of equipment use.

Implant Inventories

Implant inventories comprise plates and screws, intramedullary nails and rods, total joint implants, and a host of accessory items. Consideration is given to surgeon preference, patient population, and equipment cost when selecting stock items. These items must be stocked in a timely fashion to prepare for consecutive implant use.

The Food and Drug Administration (FDA) requires strict guidelines in properly documenting and tracking implant devices. Documentation should include but not be limited to the patient's permanent record, the operative record, and an implant registry maintained by the operating room. Many manufacturers now include mailers to return information to the company for data collection. Information to be recorded includes the lot and serial numbers of those implants used, manufacturer, size, type, and anatomic position of the implant.

Many implants are routinely part of modern orthopedic inventory. Inventories should be organized by manufacturer, type of implant (total hip versus knee), and comparative sizes. There are numerous implant systems in stock in operating rooms, but many may be provided on a loaner or consignment basis. Staff must be familiar with the varied types and refer to manufacturer information pertaining to each implant. Practices should ensure that the correct implant is opened on the operative field to prevent unnecessary expense or error in placement.

Many different alloys are used in the manufacturing of implants. However, the implantation of devices with different metallic composition must be avoided to prevent galvanic corrosion; internal fixation implants used during an orthopedic procedure should be of the same metal. Screws, for example, should be of the same composition as the metal plate affixed to the bone. Alloys that are used most frequently include stainless steel, cobalt-chromium, and titanium-vanadium-aluminum.

Internal fixation devices should never be reused. Resulting imperfections, such as abrasions or scratches, increase the potential for corrosion and weakening of the implant.[17] Bending implants to conform to the contour of the bone should be avoided whenever possible to prevent loss of strength. When bending is necessary, the proper bending press should be used. Once an implant is bent, it should not be reshaped or straightened; doing so may weaken the implant.

Orthopedic equipment and implants require special care, storage, and handling. When possible, implants should be individually wrapped and processed. Most implants today, excluding some plates and screws, are separately packaged by the manufacturer. During sterilization, implants should not be placed in a position in which knocking or bumping might occur. Appropriate sterilizing cases and trays should be used, and implants should be sterilized according to the manufacturer's instructions. An internal fixation device that has become damaged as a result of improper storage or handling must be discarded.

The orthopedic perioperative nurse should have a working knowledge of the general types and sizes of implants that might be selected. Radiographs are often templated preoperatively, providing a general idea of the size of the implants needed.

Orthopedic Instrumentation

Orthopedic instrumentation varies from very small to large instruments. Some procedures require multiple instrument containers (sets). Organization of instrument sets for multiple uses prevents the need for duplication and requires thoughtful consideration of anatomic and physiologic needs. When preparing for a procedure, the perioperative nurse should open the minimum of instruments yet be prepared for unexpected or untoward events. Careful planning and preparation of instrumentation ensures efficient utilization of time and equipment.

Instruments that do not function properly (as a result of dullness, poor adjustment, lack of lubrication, damage, improper fit, or incomplete cleaning) are primary sources of complaints and problems in the operating room. Instrument maintenance is vital to ensure availability for the procedure and ease in completion. Instruments should be used for the intended purpose during the procedure. Movable parts should be lubricated after each cleaning and checked for cracks or damage after each use. The perioperative nurse is responsible for instrument maintenance and familiarity with sterilization and packaging procedures.

The following basic bone instrument sets should be available in the orthopedic operating room. Soft-tissue instrument sets appropriate for the size of the anatomic site are used for procedures not requiring bone instruments or in addition to the sets. Additional instruments and special equipment are mentioned in the section on surgical intervention.

- *Incision hip set.* Total hip arthroplasty or fractures of the neck and proximal femur (Fig. 22-27)
- *Total knee set.* Total knee arthroplasty or supracondylar and distal femoral fractures (Fig. 22-28)
- *Shoulder set.* Shoulder arthroplasty and other shoulder procedures (Fig. 22-29)
- *Large bone set.* Bone work on the large bones including hip, knee, upper arm, and elbow (Fig. 22-30)
- *Extremity or small bone set.* Bone work on the hand or foot (Fig. 22-31)
- *Fusion or bone graft instruments.* Additional instruments necessary for an autograft (Fig. 22-32)

Powered Surgical Instruments

Powered surgical instruments (Fig. 22-33) used in the operating room have eliminated the need for many

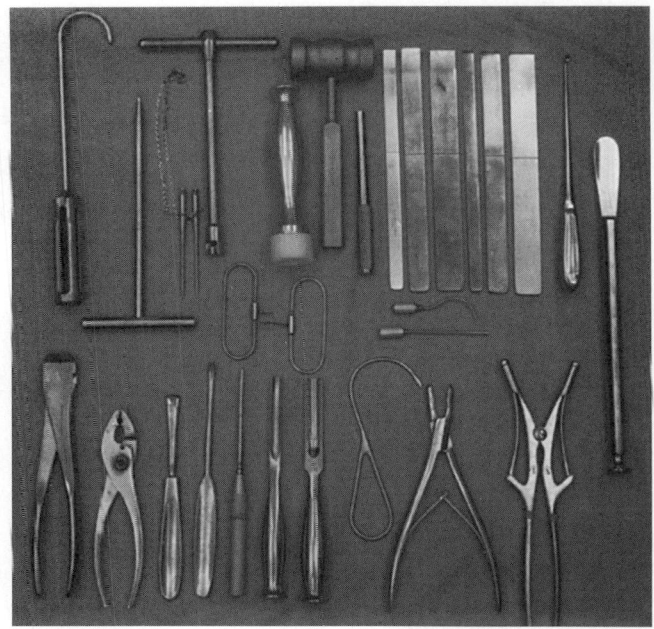

FIGURE 22-27 Instrumentation used for hip procedures, *left to right. Top,* Bone hook, femoral head extractor, pin retractors with T-handle extractor, femoral prosthesis driver, mallet, bone tamp, osteotomes (curved, straight) no. 2 angled Brun curette. *Middle,* Gigli saw handles, small wire passers (curve, straight), Watson-Jones gouge (hip skid). *Bottom,* Pin cutter, pliers, Langenbeck periosteal elevators (wide, narrow), navicular gouge, Smith-Peterson gouge (3/8, 5/8), Charnley trochanteric wire passer, Adson-cranial rongeur, Harris wire tightener.

hand-operated tools, thereby reducing operative time and improving technical results. They are available as air-, battery-, or electrically driven equipment. Fingertip control provides the surgeon speed and power. Variable speed saws, drills, and reamers offer wide flexibility but require an understanding of compatibility between equipment. These instruments are extremely powerful and have high speed. Power equipment has a safety control that prevents inadvertent activation; this should be engaged when passing the instrument to the surgeon or assistant. Powered instruments should not be rested on the patient when not in use.

It is important to follow the manufacturer's recommended cleaning, sterilizing, and lubricating instructions. With proper care, powered surgical instruments have a long life span and many uses.[6]

Suture Material

Suture material requires increased tensile strength and minimal degradability for the select type of tissue. Tendons and ligaments are fibrous, avascular tissues, resulting in a slower healing process than that in tissues rich in blood supply. Absorbable suture may be used for sewing tendon or ligaments to bone. Nonabsorbable suture, including polyester and surgical steel, are also used. For various ligament replacement grafts, a harvested tendon may be customized with multiple strands of suture material,

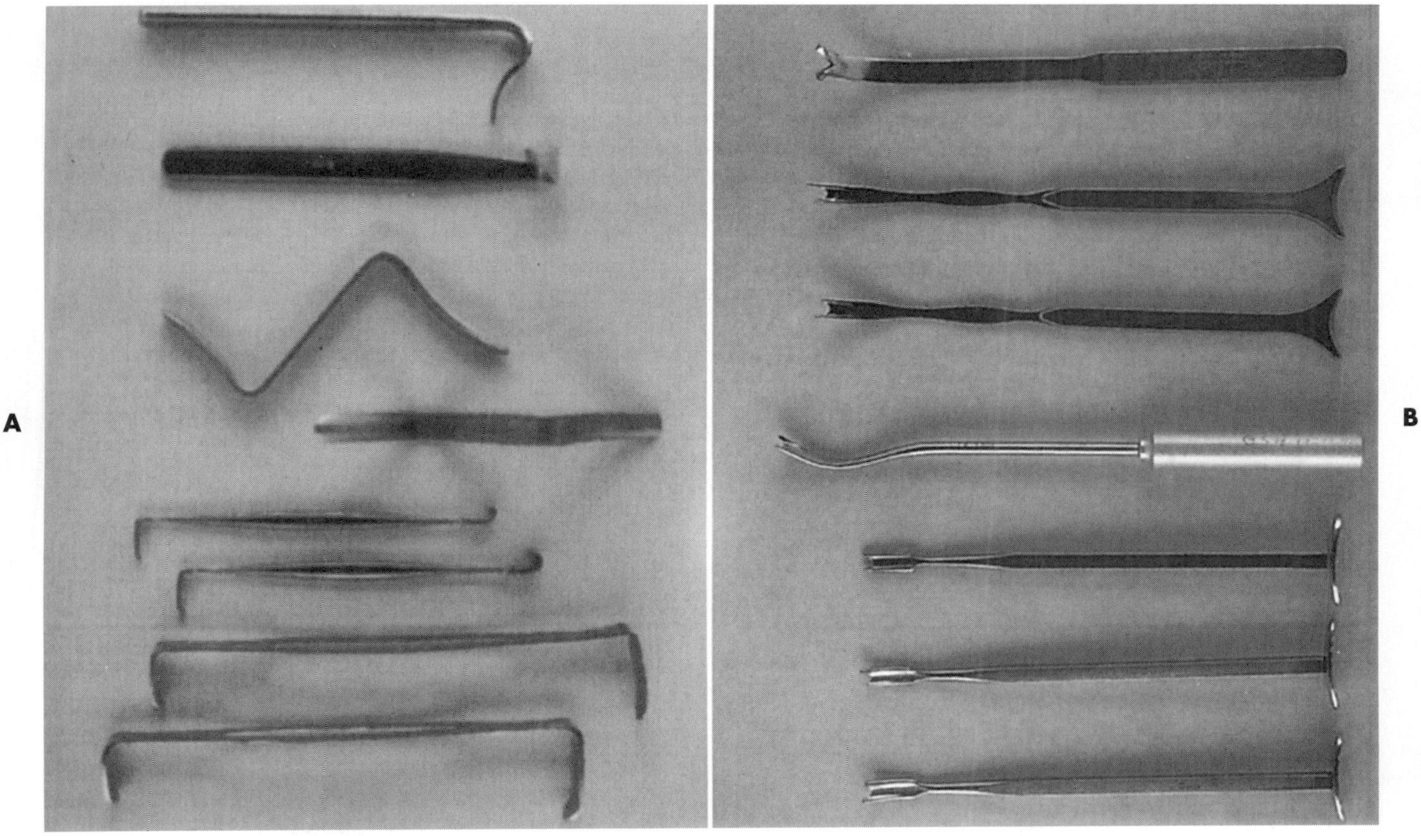

FIGURE 22-28 Instrumentation used for procedures on the knee, *top to bottom.* **A,** 2 Blount knee retractors; 2 Doane knee retractors; 2 Miller-Senn retractors; 2 Army-Navy retractors. **B,** 3 Smillie cartilage knives (left, right, straight); 1 Downing cartilage knife (meniscectomy knife); 2 Smillie cartilage knives (top, bottom); 1 McKeever cartilage knife.

increasing tensile strength and length of time until fibrous union occurs.

Polymethyl methacrylate

PMMA (bone cement) is an acrylic cement–like substance composed of a liquid methyl methacrylate monomer and a powder methyl methacrylate–styrene copolymer. The powder component is 10% barium sulfate, U.S.P., which provides radiopacity to the finished product. The liquid monomer is highly flammable, and the operating room should be properly ventilated. Caution should be exercised during mixing of the two components to prevent excessive exposure of the vapors of the monomer to OR personnel. This exposure can cause irritation of the respiratory tract, eyes, and possibly the liver. It is also recommended that soft contact lenses should not be worn by personnel in a room where methyl methacrylate is being mixed. Many special hoods and mixing devices are available to minimize staff exposure to the fumes.

Adverse patient reactions with PMMA include transitory hypotension, cardiac arrest, cerebral vascular accident, pulmonary embolus, thrombophlebitis, and hypersensitivity reaction.[19,22] Cardiac arrest and death, although uncommon, have resulted after insertion of bone cement. Adverse reactions have been attributed to a combination of factors including a rise in intermedullary canal pressure,[16] causing embolic phenomena, a possible chemical and blood reaction causing sudden hypotension, and certain preexisting patient conditions. Additional research remains to be done to discover the exact cause of adverse reactions. Patient care should include collaboration with the anesthesia care provider before insertion of PMMA and then monitoring for side effects after insertion.

Medications

Medications delivered in the operating room require the same precautions as those in other specialty areas. Antibiotics, hemostatics, and antibacterial agents are used commonly. Antibiotics are delivered both intravenously and locally in irrigation solutions. The intravenous antibiotic of choice is a first-generation cephalosporin. Common antibiotics used in the irrigation include polymixin and bacitracin. Irrigation may also be delivered using pulsatile lavage, with antibiotics added to the solution. Hemostatic agents may include Gelfoam, thrombin, Avitene, and bone wax. Antibacterial ointments are impregnated in gauze dressing (Xeroform) or applied

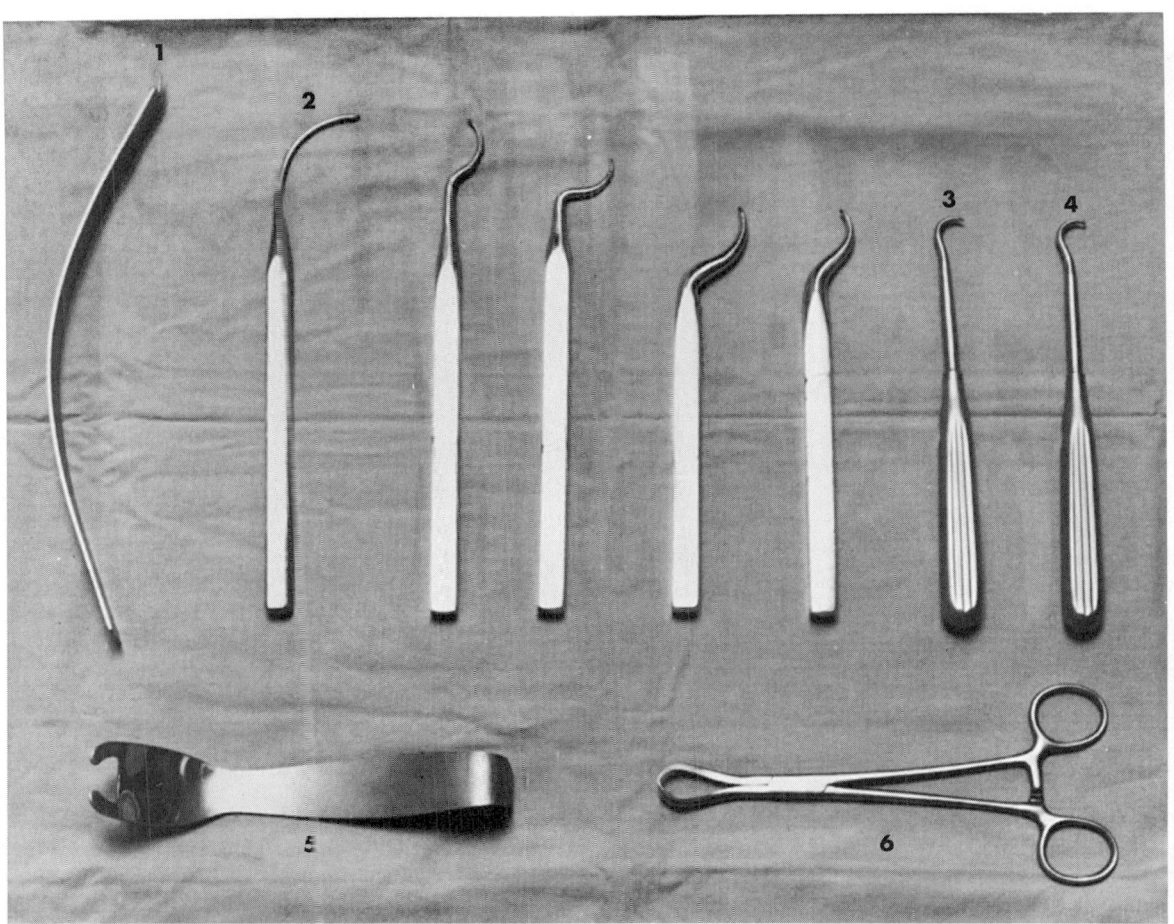

FIGURE 22–29 Bankart instruments. *1,* Rowe capsule retractor (pitch fork); *2,* Five Rowe glenoid punches; *3,* curved awl; *4,* ligature retriever; *5,* humeral head retractor; *6,* glenoid reaming forceps.

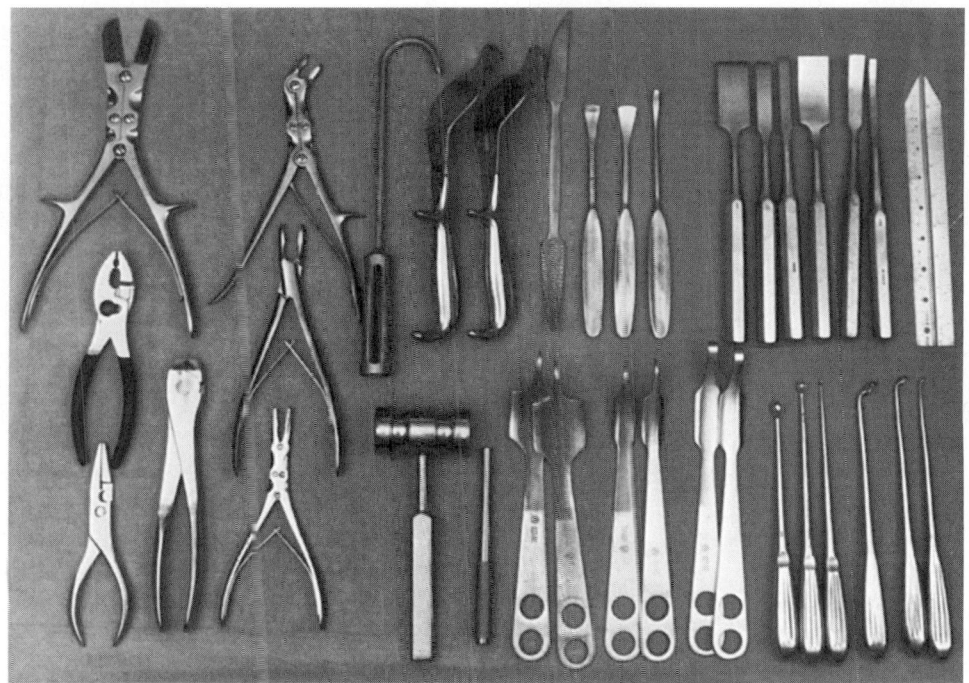

FIGURE 22–30 Large bone set, *left to right. Top,* Stille-Liston bone-cutting forceps, Stille-Luer rongeur, bone hook, Bennett retractors, rasp, Langenbeck periosteal elevators (wide and narrow), Cushing periosteal elevators, osteomes (straight curved) ruler. *Middle,* Pliers, Adson-cranial rongeur. *Bottom,* Needle-nosed pliers, pin cutter, Zaufal-Jansen rongeur, mallet, bone tamp, Hohmann retractors (wide sharp, narrow sharp, and blunt), curettes (straight, curved).

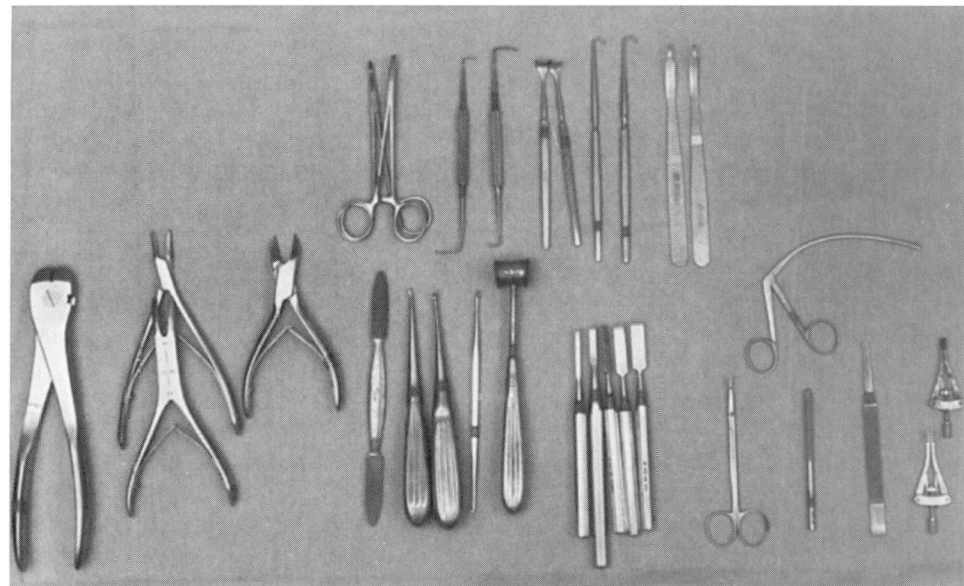

FIGURE 22-31 Extremity or small bone set, *left to right. Top,* Baby Mixters, Ragnell retractors, Alm retractors, Volkman hooks, mini-Hohmann retractors. *Bottom,* Pin cutter, Lempert and Carroll rongeurs, Liston bone cutter, bone rasp, small curettes, fine double-ended curette, small mallet, Hoke osteotomes, Litler scissors, tendon passer, Beaver blade handle, Carroll elevator, Miltex self-retaining retractors.

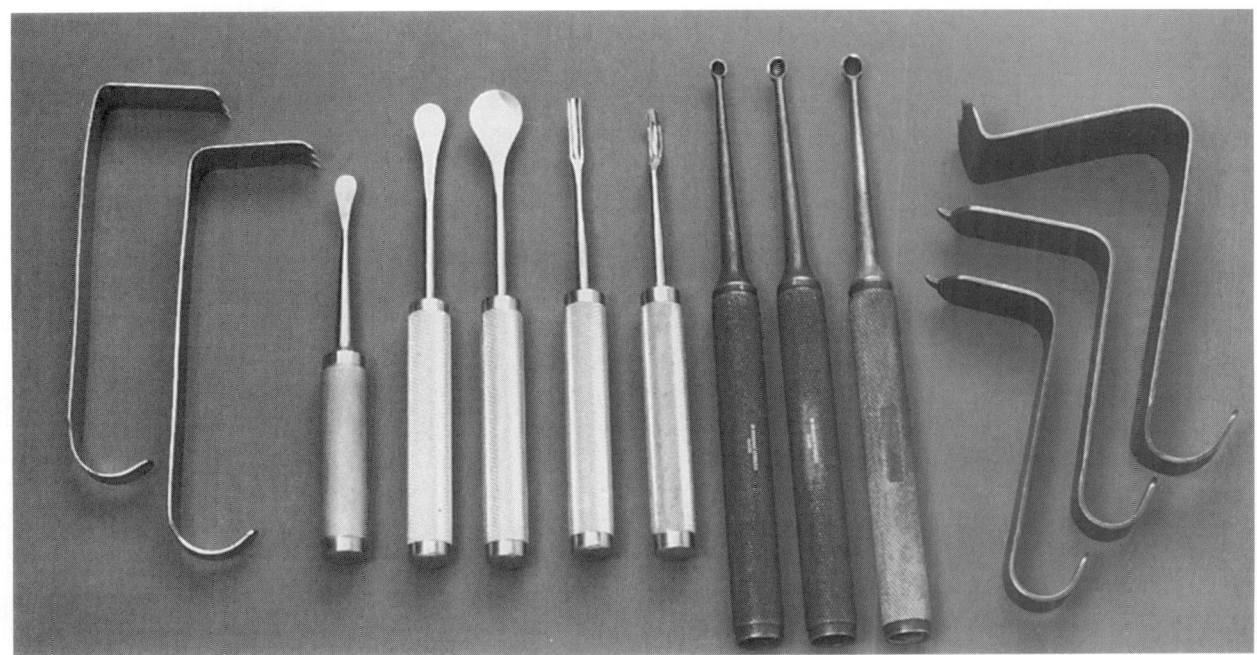

FIGURE 22-32 Fusion and bone graft instruments. *Left to right.* Hibbs retractors, Cobb periosteal elevators, Cobb gouges, McElroy curettes, spinal retractors, and iliac graft retractor.

before the application of the dressing. Other medications used during orthopedic procedures include steroids, local anesthetics, and normal saline.

Protective measures

Protective measures are taken in the perioperative environment during surgical procedures and handling of patient-exposed trash, linen, or instruments. (See Chapter 4 for a thorough discussion of Standard Precautions to reduce the transmission risk of bloodborne and other pathogens.) Orthopedic procedures require caution as a result of the use of fluids for irrigation or bloody procedures. Personnel protective measures include handling items (blades, sharp instruments, and bone) cautiously to prevent inadvertent punctures or cuts and wearing protective masks, eyewear, or a face shield as well

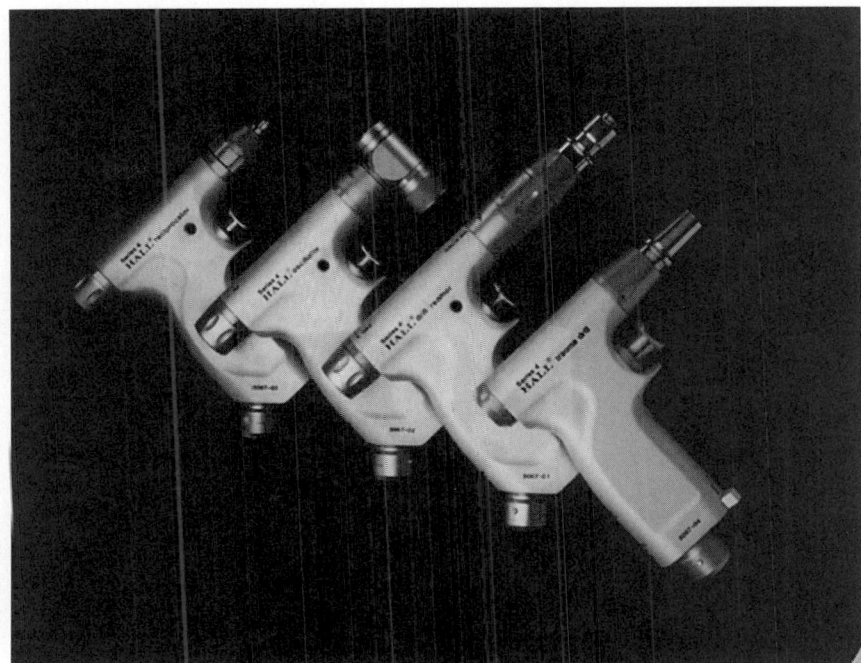

FIGURE 22-33 Pneumatic powered surgical instruments for large bone procedures: reciprocating saw, the oscillating saw, the drill-reamer, and the trauma drill.

as protective attire, including gowns and boots. Sharp bone edges are a hazard and can puncture gloves and skin. Double gloving or use of protective gloves should be employed to protect the patient and personnel. Nonlatex gloves and patient care items are available for personnel or patients with sensitivity to latex.

Bone banking

Programs have developed for acquisition, sterilization, and storage of bone allograft. The American Association of Tissue Banks (AATB) accredits and periodically inspects bone-banking programs to ensure that specific guidelines are followed in the retrieval, processing, storage, and distribution of bone allografts. Accredited programs compose a national tissue network that provides hospitals and surgeons with various types of high-quality allograft tissue. Patients who consent to donate are thoroughly screened. Screening procedures include HIV and hepatitis testing. A detailed medical and social history is obtained. The harvesting process must be completed in accordance with sterile technique. Culture specimens are taken and sent to the institution that performs further testing. Once the tissue is determined acceptable, it is returned to the bone bank for storage. Frozen allografts are stored in plastic or cloth wraps to ensure sterility and prevent grafts from drying out. Allografts are frozen until use. Vacuum-sealed freezers are monitored with an alarm that sounds if the temperature rises above 70° C. Tissue maintained at 70° C or colder may be stored for up to 5 years before expiration.[2] When requested for a procedure, the bone allograft is delivered to the field, slightly thawed, cultured, and washed with an antibiotic solution. Banked bone is

available in many shapes of cortical and cancellous tissue (Fig. 22-34).

Records are maintained on both donors and recipients. Donor records provide the donor identification, medical history (with circumstances of death if applicable), laboratory results, and graft description. Recipient records include recipient identification, surgeon and organization implanting the graft, surgical procedure, culture results, and any adverse reactions. Like other implants, the recipient's operative record should include the name of the bone bank from which the allograft was received, type of allograft, tissue number, and expiration date if applicable.

Bone banking has drastically improved results of reconstruction of the acetabulum or other structures that support implant fixation. Entire segments of bone in the form of the shaft or joint are used when there is great bone loss attributable to trauma and oncologic conditions.[34]

Evaluation

Evaluation is an ongoing process, occurring throughout the procedure. The perioperative nurse evaluates the patient considering the nursing diagnosis and attainment of outcomes. This part of the nursing process provides feedback as to the effectiveness of the plan, its implementation, and alterations needed for improving patient care.

The evaluation process validates nursing care. Was the patient protected from peripheral neurovascular injury? Was he or she free from injury? Was adequate oxygenation maintained? Does the patient have more questions pertaining to the recovery phase? The answers will dictate whether there is a need to maintain or modify the plan. The evaluation information is shared with the nurse

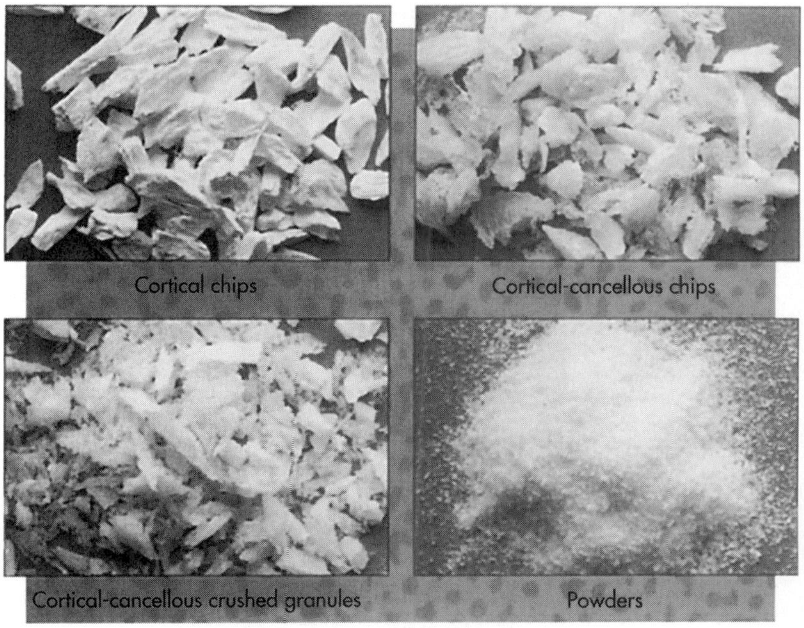

FIGURE 22-34　Demineralized bone showing cortical and cancellous bone in chips, granules, and powder.

caring for this patient postoperatively to provide continuity of care.

The following sample outcome statements apply to evaluating care of the orthopedic patient when using the nursing diagnoses identified earlier in this chapter:

- The patient verbalized fears and feelings and indicated that anxiety and apprehension were lessened.
- The patient was free from peripheral neurovascular compromise on discharge to the postoperative area as evidenced by presence of pulses, warmth of the extremity, good capillary refill, and intact movement and sensation.
- The patient was free from injury related to the surgical position as evidenced by maintenance of skin integrity and absence of reddened areas.
- The patient maintained adequate ventilation and perfusion as evidenced by blood gases, arterial saturation, and vital signs within normal limits.
- The patient was free from surgical site infection as evidenced by temperature within normal limits and an incision site that is clean and dry.

Patient and Family Education and Discharge Planning

As a result of technologic advances and financial constraints, hospital stays have become shorter. Never has planning and patient education been more important for the safety and well being of the patient. Patient education occurs in various settings and is part of the essence of caring in nursing, which aims to help, heal, and improve health. Knowledge and skills to initiate strategies for educating orthopedic surgical patients is critical to the

perioperative nurse's effectiveness in assisting the patient and family as they move through the continuum of an episode of surgery and recovery from it.

Discharge planning and patient education should not be initiated when the patient is 1 or 2 days from leaving the health care facility. Rather, patient and family education and discharge planning begin when that individual first comes into contact with the health care system. It should be complete and, if possible, involve a multidisciplinary approach.[36] Nursing research indicates that, despite discharge planning, 79% of patients, particularly the elderly, experienced problems after discharge from an acute care setting.[25] Another report[26] suggests the development of a discharge planning assessment tool that outlines 10 specific areas to be addressed: treatments, mobility and activities of daily living deficits, sensory impairments, nutrition, psychosocial, home medical equipment, transportation, education, medical diagnosis, and miscellaneous. This tool acts as a roadmap to draw together service providers from nursing, dietary and nutritional services, home care, physical therapy, respiratory therapy, social service, utilization review, and patient financial services. Aside from improved patient care benefits and decreased length of stay, this tool also had the unexpected positive outcome in that issues between departments were addressed and resolved more readily.

For the patient undergoing orthopedic surgery, patient and family education and discharge planning in the following areas is essential: wound care and dressing changes, pain control, wound assessment, physical and occupational therapy, personal care, housekeeping, mobility, nutrition, prescriptions other than pain medication, donning and doffing of orthopedic appliances, and follow-up with a physician. Information concerning these content areas should be described, discussed, and reinforced with written instructions. Perioperative nurses should ensure that the patient and family understand the instructions, have the opportunity to demonstrate a requisite skill if that is part of home care and convalescence, and allow time for questions and concerns. A sample of written educational material that might be provided to the orthopedic surgical patient with a cast is presented in Box 22-1. Relevant content for devising patient and family educational material on pain management at home is presented in Box 22-2.

In Mistiaen's study (1997),[25] patients were interviewed around the seventh postdischarge day and found to have further informational needs concerning recovery time, normal recovery signs, what insurance pays, how much to rest, how to diminish pain, activity level, side effects of medications, when to call the doctor, what to eat, and how to take their medication. This informational deficit does not necessarily mean that the information was not given in the hospital but rather that the patient may have been unprepared for it. Further research is needed on the timing, reinforcement, and effectiveness of informational strategies in relation to postdischarge outcomes.

SURGICAL INTERVENTIONS
BONE GRAFTING

Bone grafting may be used to fill cavities after removal of large amounts of bone that might result in instability, to fill bony defects, and to promote union of fractures at the time of open reduction. The type of graft used depends on the location of the fracture or defect, the condition of the bone, and the amount of bone loss as a result of injury. Bone graft may be used for procedures involving revision of joints if there is significant bone loss caused by resorption or mechanical destruction after removal of bone cement.

The bone graft may be the patient's own bone (autogenous in origin and referred to as *autograft*) or bone obtained from a tissue bank (homogeneous in origin but referred to as *allograft*). Autogenous bone grafts are often harvested from the iliac crest, where there is cortical and cancellous bone. Various harvesting techniques are used. Struts of cortical bone from the iliac crest can be fashioned to the desired shape and used in areas needing structural strength. The amount of cancellous bone is plentiful. It is used to promote bone growth in areas of defect. Local bone graft material may be taken from the site of injury. Homogeneous allografts are used when bone is not available from the patient because of the lack of sufficient quantity or because a secondary procedure is undesirable for the patient.

Procedural considerations

Cancellous grafts may be taken from the ilium, olecranon, or distal radius; cortical grafts may be taken

---

BOX 22-1	Casts

So now you or a member of your family is wearing a cast. The cast is only one of several devices used to promote the healing of broken bones. Doctors also use traction and pins, or a combination of these three, to help heal broken bones. The cast has the advantage of being less expensive, requiring little care on your part, and allowing you to move around. The cast also encloses and immobilizes the broken bone and injured soft tissues to prevent movement that could cause further injury and to keep the bone in place for proper healing.

Your cast may be made of plaster or of a synthetic material such as fiberglass. Although the plaster cast is heavy, the doctor can mold a plaster cast more easily for a close fit over severe injuries. The synthetic cast is lightweight and easier to move around, making it good for elderly patients. Your cast has a name. If it covers your forearm or lower leg, it is a **short arm** or **short leg** cast. A **long leg** cast covers the whole leg, and a **hanging** cast covers the whole arm and forearm. The **body** cast encircles the chest and abdomen, whereas the **Minerva** cast covers the chest, neck, and head with openings for the ears, face, and arms. The cast that covers the hips and one or both legs is the **hip spica** or **spica** cast.

Things to Watch for

Your cast will be warm at first because of the setting process. However, warm areas on the cast later on may indicate infection, and you should notify your doctor at once.

You should watch for increased pain or soreness under the cast, particularly around bony prominences such as the wrist or ankle, that is not relieved by repositioning the body. Check the skin color and temperature periodically. When the tip of a finger or the big toe that protrudes from the cast is squeezed until it is white, the pink color should return within 2 to 4 seconds. If skin color does not return within 4 to 6 seconds or if the skin is red, blue, white, or discolored, notify your doctor. If fingers or toes are cool, cover them. If they do not warm up in 20 minutes, call your doctor. Call your doctor immediately if any of these other symptoms occur:

- An increase in swelling and pain
- A tingling or burning sensation inside the cast
- An inability to move muscles around the cast
- A foul odor detected from the edges of the cast
- Any drainage, which may show through the cast
- Any cracks or breaks in the cast
- Marked loosening of the cast allowing the parts inside the cast to move fairly easily

---

This guide may be copied for free distribution to patients and families. All rights reserved.
From Mosby. (1997). *Mosby's Patient Teaching Guides*, St. Louis: Mosby.

---

from the tibia, fibula, or ribs. When the recipient site of an autogenous graft is diseased, instruments used for the recipient site must be separated from donor graft site instruments. The operating team must change their gowns and gloves to take the bone graft, and again follow the procedure to prevent cross-contamination. The patient is

BOX 22-2	Content for Educating the Patient and Family on Pain Management at Home

- Give both the patient and the caregiver *oral* and *written* instructions. Provide them with the name and telephone number of a physician or nurse to call if questions arise.
- *General information*
— Explain the relationship of pain to the disease process. Assist the patient to understand the source of pain.
- *Special instructions*
— Assist the patient to identify factors or actions that trigger pain, such as activity, movements, and temperature extremes.
— Discuss past effective and ineffective pain relief measures. Explore the past effect of pain relief measures on the patient, such as sleepiness, lethargy, and decreased energy or sexual activity.
— Assist the patient to localize and describe the intensity of pain using a scale (e.g., 0 to 10, with 0 meaning absence of pain and 10 being intense pain).
— Discuss interventions other than taking medications for intractable pain.
  Anesthetic procedures such as nerve blocks, trigger point injections, and use of nitrous oxide
  Neuroablative procedures such as cordotomy
  Physiatric supportive measures such as using a prosthesis, physical therapy, and occupational therapy
— Discuss alternative strategies patients can use to relieve pain without taking prescribed drugs, and explain that these techniques may also augment the effect of pain medication
  Sensory interventions: massage such as back and foot massage: to relax muscular tension and increase local circulation; range-of-motion exercises (passive, assistive, or active): to relax muscles, improve circulation, and prevent pain related to stiffness and immobility; cold application: used initially to decrease tissue injury response (swelling) and decrease pain; heat application: used after cold to aid in clearance of tissue toxins and mobilize fluids; transcutaneous electrical nerve stimulation (TENS): pocket-size battery-operated device used to send mild continuous electrical impulses through the skin by means of electrodes placed on the body (see discussion below)
  Emotional interventions to increase pain threshold by controlling or reducing anxiety, fatigue, or depression: *prevention or control of anxiety:* to reduce muscle tension and increase pain tolerance through relaxation exercises and slow, controlled breathing; *promotion of self-control:* to reduce feelings of helplessness and lack of control that contribute to anxiety and pain; *pacing of activities*
  Cognitive interventions: *distraction:* focus on something unrelated to pain (e.g., conversing, watching television or videos, listening to music); humor; *guided imagery:* use of images to alter a physical or emotional state, promote relaxation, and decrease pain sensation
— Discuss the need to identify body positions of comfort; encourage attention to proper posture and body alignment. Advise the patient to immobilize or rest the affected area.

— Tell the patient to relieve pressure areas by turning or using pressure-reduction devices such as an air-fluidized support system
— Discuss the use of TENS. Explain that the mild electrical current blocks or modifies pain messages before they reach the brain and replaces them with a buzzing or tingling sensation. Inform the patient that TENS may stimulate the body's production of endorphin, a natural pain reliever. Instruct the patient in the use and home care of the TENS unit.
  Apply a thin coat of gel over each entire electrode.
  Place the electrodes securely on the skin with tape.
  Place the electrodes close to the site of pain.
  Turn the intensity knob until a slight tingling or buzzing sensation is felt on the skin. Increase the intensity if the pain is still felt or decrease the intensity if the tingling sensation causes discomfort.
  Turn the TENS unit off before removing it.
  Wipe the electrodes with an alcohol and water mixture after removing them from the skin.
  Do not allow the unit to get wet. If it does get wet, allow it to dry thoroughly before using it again.
  Replace the electrodes if the adhesive surface separates from the backing or if they no longer adhere firmly to the skin.
  Replace the battery pack or recharge as needed. If there is no tingling sensation when the intensity is turned up, the batteries are weakening.
  Use hypoallergenic tape to secure the electrodes to prevent redness or rash, cleanse the skin well after removing the electrodes, and apply lotion to the placement sites.
- *Medications*
— Explain the purpose, dosage, schedule, and route of administration of any prescribed drugs, as well as side effects to report to a physician or nurse.
— Give the patient general guidelines for the use of pain medications.
  Explain that a variety of pain relief measures may be necessary for some types of pain.
  Instruct the patient to use pain relief measures before pain becomes severe. Determine the patient's ability or willingness to participate actively in use of pain relief measures and suggest pain relief measures the patient believes will be helpful.
  Rely on patient behavior that indicates pain severity rather than relying on known physical stimuli.
  Encourage the patient to try a pain relief measure at least twice before abandoning it as ineffective. Instruct the patient to keep an open mind as to what may relieve pain.
  Urge the patient to keep trying to relieve the pain and not to become discouraged.

From Canobbio, M.M. (1996). *Mosby's handbook of patient teaching.* St. Louis: Mosby.

positioned to allow exposure to the surgical site. A sandbag may be placed beneath the area for easier anatomic location and access.

The instrumentation for taking a bone graft includes soft tissue instruments and a bone graft set (see Fig. 22-32). Grafts may be harvested with hand instruments or taken with the use of power tools such as an oscillating saw or high speed tool such as the Midas Rex. Power tools may be necessary if a uniformly shaped graft is needed to fill a defect. Because hemostasis is sometimes difficult to achieve due to the vascular nature of bone, wound drains may be desirable.

Operative procedure
Harvest of Bone Graft

A cancellous bone graft consists of spongy bone usually taken from the anterior or posterior crest of the ilium. A cortical bone graft, consisting of hard, dense bone, is removed from the crest of the ilium or the tibia. The location of the crest of the ilium is subcutaneous, allowing exposure without difficulty.

1. An incision is made along the border of the iliac crest, and the muscles on the outer table of the ilium are stripped, elevated, and retracted.
2. Strips of the iliac crest can be removed with an osteotome or oscillating saw.
3. A cortical window may also be made in the outer table, and the cancellous bone chips are obtained with curettes or gouges.
4. The deep and superficial layers may be drained to evacuate blood and assess any further bleeding.
5. The wound is closed in layers and a pressure dressing applied.

ELECTRICAL STIMULATION

The healing process in bone involves several stages (Fig. 22-35). When a bone is damaged, as during a surgical procedure or fracture, bleeding occurs. The amount of extravasated blood depends on the vascularity of the fracture site. The blood exudate infiltrates the surrounding area, where a clot is formed. Fibroblasts invade the hematoma and form a fibrin meshwork.

As osteoblasts invade the fibrin meshwork, blood vessels develop to build collagen. After several days, calcium deposits may form in the granulation tissue. These deposits eventually form new bone, known as *callus*. Within the callus, cartilage cells develop a temporary semirigid tissue that helps stabilize the bone fragments. The callus is immature bone that is remodeled by new connective tissue cells (osteoblasts) of the periosteum and the inner membrane of the bone cavity. Through this process, mature bone is formed, excess callus is reabsorbed, and trabecular bone is laid down.

After several months, depending on the age and physical condition of the individual, the bone becomes firmly

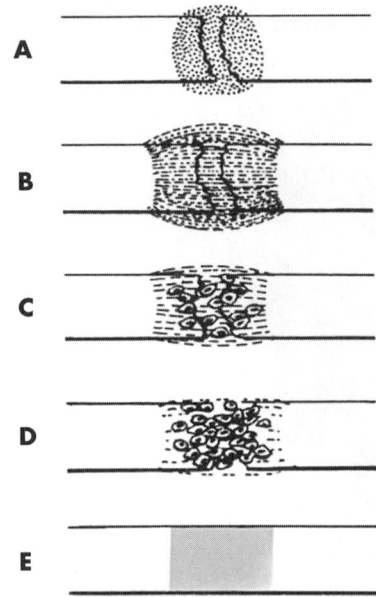

FIGURE 22-35 Bone healing process. **A,** Hematoma formation. **B,** Fibrin network formation. **C,** Invasion of osteoblasts. **D,** Callus formation. **E,** Remodeling.

united, although the ossification process is not yet completed. Complete union of the fractured bone or joint is determined by means of clinical and radiologic examination.

Healing of bone is classified by degree. *Delayed union* signifies that healing has not occurred within the average time. The average time depends on many factors, and delayed unions must not be considered nonunion until the healing process has ceased without bony union. *Malunion* signifies that the fracture has united with deformity sufficient to cause impairment of the function or a significant angulation of the extremity. *Nonunion* signifies that the process of healing has ended without producing bony union; in this case, electrical stimulation may be used.

Electrical stimulation is artificially applied electrical current that induces or influences osteogenesis. Various types of stimulators (Fig. 22-36) are available for treatment of nonunion, including invasive (implantable), semiinvasive (percutaneous), and noninvasive (capacitance coupling). The bone stimulator of choice depends on the patient, pathologic condition, and physician comfort with the device.

The bone growth stimulator is used in patients with high risk of nonunion. It can be used to provide electrical stimulation for treatment of nonunion, delayed union, congenital pseudarthrosis, and bone defects. It may be used with or without internal fixation devices, external fixation devices, or bone grafting. Patients who have undergone previous surgery, who have sustained significant tissue loss, or in whom bone grafting is contraindicated are candidates. Along with their use in accelerating fracture healing, bone growth stimulators have been successfully used in an infected nonunion after débridement because the electrical stimulation retards bacterial growth. The normal range

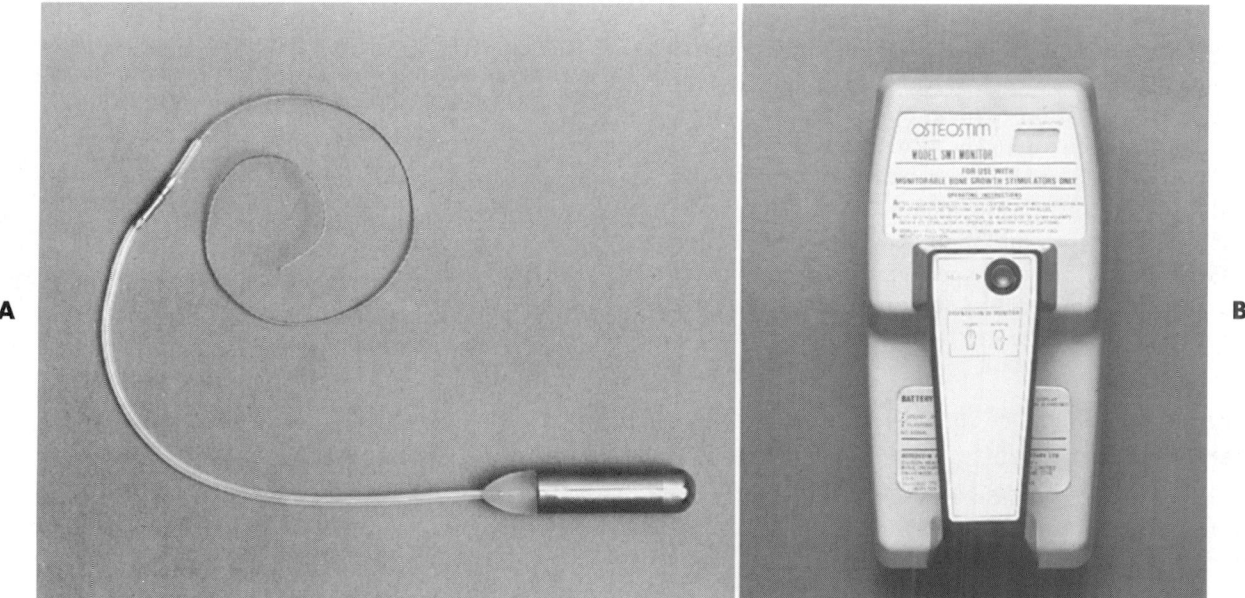

FIGURE 22-36 Bone stimulator used following procedures to induce bone formation. **A,** Bone-growth stimulator cathode and lead. **B,** Monitor for bone-growth stimulator.

of electrical current is 18 to 22 mA. Electrical stimulation requires long periods of immobilization of the site. This prolonged immobilization may impede rehabilitation.

Procedural considerations

Instructions for implanting and components selected vary according to the type. The position of the patient depends on the implant site.

In addition to the implant of the surgeon's choice and the implant-specific instrumentation, a soft-tissue set is used. Curettes, osteotomes, or bone rasps are used for bony débridement and to scarify the donor bed. Power drills with drill bits may be necessary to create access through the bone for the electrical leads.

Operative procedure

1. The surgical site is exposed and debrided as necessary. A stimulator may be implanted after the surgical procedure.
2. A slot is fashioned spanning the nonunion site.
3. A second incision is made about 8 to 10 cm from the first one and dissected. Before implanting the generator, it is imperative that hemostasis be obtained. The use of electrosurgical equipment may interfere with function of the bone-growth stimulator.
4. A subcutaneous channel for the cathode is created, using blunt or mechanical dissection.
5. The long cathode lead is guided through the channel.
6. The generator is carefully implanted near the skin surface. The generator should be inserted into soft tissue, not against bone or metal fixation devices; it should not create a bulge beneath the skin.
7. The electrical coils are placed in the prepared bone slot in equal lengths above and below the fracture site.
8. Cancellous bone grafts are placed between the coils if large bony defects are being treated.
9. Routine closure of the subcutaneous and skin tissue is carried out.
10. Once union has occurred (5 to 6 months), the generator is removed. The stimulator can be removed using local anesthesia with minimal instrumentation.

FRACTURES AND DISLOCATIONS

Bone diseases can be metabolic, infectious, or degenerative. Metabolic diseases are disorders of bone remodeling. The most common are osteoporosis, osteomalacia, and Paget's disease, all of which may result in bone fractures. The most common infectious process is osteomyelitis. Degenerative musculoskeletal conditions are associated with aging. Osteoarthritis is the most common degenerative change.

Osteoporosis is one of the most common and serious of bone diseases. Over a million fractures occurring each year are attributed to osteoporosis; 40% are vertebral fractures, 20% are femoral (hip) fractures, and 15% are distal forearm fractures.[7]

Osteoporosis is characterized by excessive loss of calcified matrix, bone mineral, and collagenous fibers, causing a reduction of total bone mass. Decreasing levels of estrogen and testosterone in the older adult result in reduced new bone growth and maintenance of existing bone. Inadequate intake of calcium or vitamin D; lack of

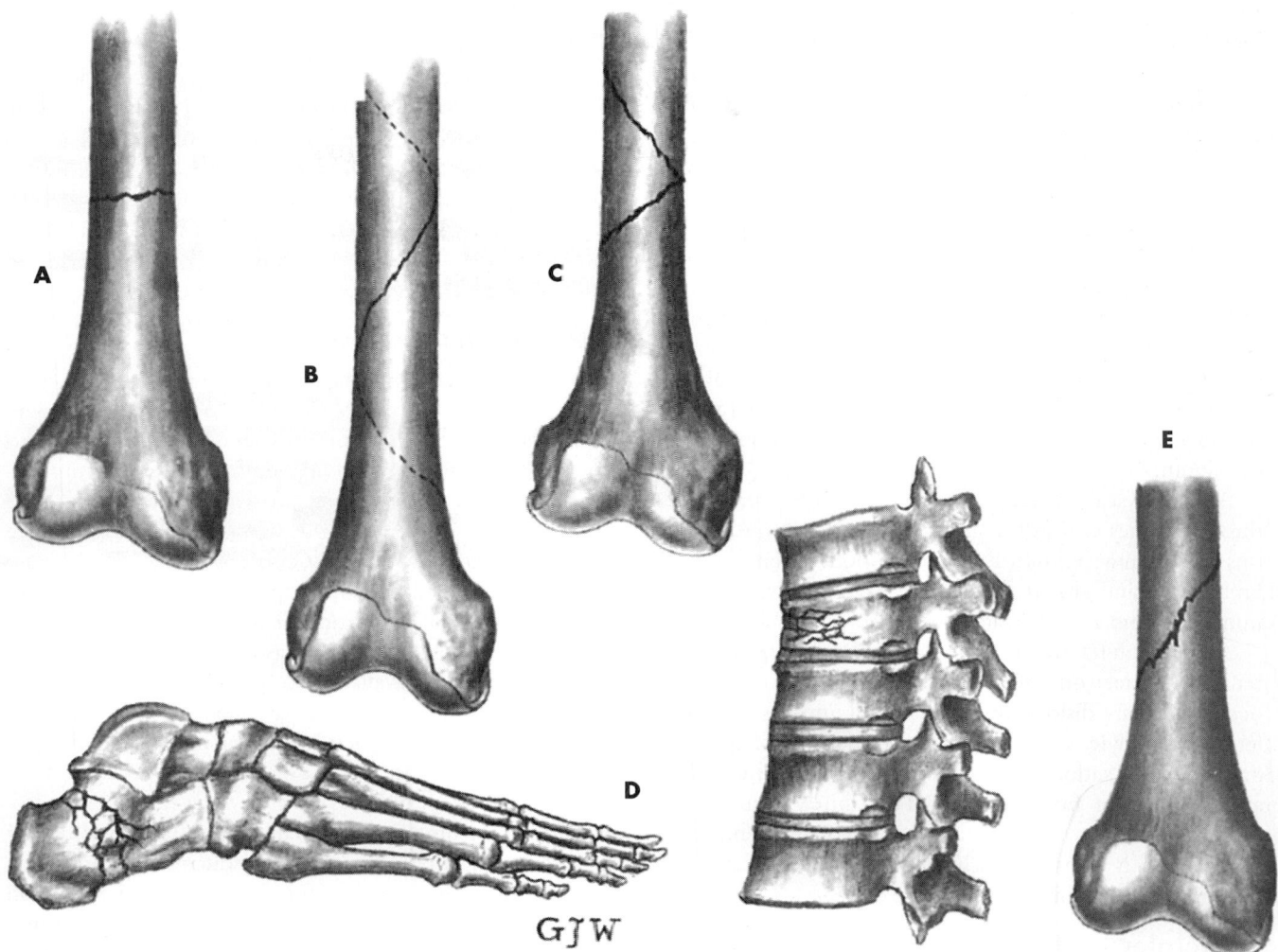

FIGURE 22-37   Fracture types. **A,** Transverse. **B,** Longitudinal or spiral. **C,** Comminuted. **D,** Compression. **E,** Oblique. Fracture types may be open or closed.

weight-bearing activities, exercise, and physical inactivity; smoking; and caffeine intake are other contributing factors. Osteoporotic bone is porous, brittle, and fragile, fracturing easily under stress. This results in susceptibility to spontaneous fractures and pathologic curvature of the spine.

Osteomalacia is a metabolic bone disease characterized by inadequate mineralization of bone as a result of vitamin D deficiency, which leads to reduced absorption of calcium and phosphorus. A large amount of osteoid does not calcify in patients with this disease. Risk factors for development of osteomalacia include malabsorption problems, vitamin D and calcium deficiencies, chronic renal failure, and inadequate exposure to sunlight. Medical treatment includes dietary supplements and exposure to sunlight.

Paget's disease is a disorder affecting older adults. It is characterized by proliferation of osteoclasts and compensatory increased osteoblastic activity, resulting in rapid, disorganized bone remodeling. The bones are weak and poorly constructed.

A fracture is a break in the continuity of a bone. The care of fractured bones or dislocation of a joint is complicated when there is trauma to the soft tissues, including muscles, nerves, ligaments, and blood vessels.

Types

Fractures are classified into two main groups: closed fractures and open or compound fractures. *Closed fractures* are those in which there is no communication between the bone fragments and the skin surface. *Incomplete closed fractures* are those in which the whole thickness of the bone is not broken but is bent or buckled, as in greenstick fractures, which commonly occur in prepubertal children. *Open fractures* exist when the break in the bone communicates with a wound in the skin. These fractures are usually considered contaminated, requiring measures to control potential infection.

There are many varieties of fracture architecture (Fig. 22-37), including (1) transverse fracture, in which the fracture line runs at a right angle to the longitudinal axis of the bone; (2) longitudinal fracture, which runs along the length of the bone; (3) oblique fracture and spiral fracture, in which bone is twisted apart (similar except that oblique is shorter than spiral); (4) comminuted fracture, in which the bone fragments splinter into more than two pieces; (5) compression fracture, in which one fragment is driven into the other end and is relatively fixed in that position; and (6) pathologic fracture in which a bone will fracture easily because it is weakened by disease. A fracture in the shaft of a long bone is described as being in the proximal, middle, or distal third or at the junction of one of these two divisions. A fracture of one of the bony prominences of the end of a long bone is described as a fracture of that prominence by name. Examples include a fracture of the olecranon, medial malleolus, or lateral condyle of the femur.

An epiphyseal separation occurs when a fracture passes through or lies within the growth plate of a bone. When this occurs in a child with immature bone, retardation of limb length and growth may occur. These injuries require immediate and expert treatment.

An avulsion fracture results in a ligamentous attachment remaining intact on a separated bone fragment. This may occur after joint dislocation or rotational injury, such as the femoral condyle separating from the tibial plateau. A dislocation (luxation) is a complete displacement of one articular surface from another. This injury can disrupt neurovascular structures, requiring immediate attention. A subluxation is a partial dislocation, often indicated by ligamentous instability.

Principles of Treatment

The purpose of fracture treatment is to reestablish the length, shape, and alignment of the fractured bones or joints and restore anatomic function. Acute fracture treatment is necessary to alleviate neurovascular compromise. The surgical team should consider the following principles when providing care for the patient: (1) the patient (extremity, fracture site) must be handled gently; (2) initial general medical treatment must be provided; (3) equipment and personnel must be readily available to treat impending or existing shock and control hemorrhage; (4) principles of aseptic technique must be maintained; (5) positioning must allow adequate circulatory and respiratory function with adequate exposure; and (6) patient comfort must be considered.

The primary goal in treatment of an upper extremity fracture is to preserve mobility and restore range of motion, enabling the individual to perform skilled and delicate work. In fractures of a lower extremity the objectives of surgery are to restore alignment and length and provide stability of the extremity for weight bearing. In the presence of open fractures involving soft tissues, several associated conditions may arise, including (1) secondary hemorrhage, (2) infection, (3) severe damage to soft tissues, (4) damage to blood vessels and nerves, and (5) Volkmann's contracture (ischemic paralysis).

Basic Treatment Techniques
Closed reduction

Fractures may be treated by closed reduction, or manipulating the fragments into position without incising the skin. This is the treatment of choice when possible to decrease the opportunity for infection, improve results (including bone union of the fracture), and minimize the recovery period. Significant bone comminution, periosteal damage, or soft tissue entrapped within the fracture site may result in complications.

Procedural Considerations

The choice of anesthesia depends on the site of fracture and patient condition. A closed reduction can be performed with (1) infiltration of local anesthetic agent into the fracture site (hematoma block), (2) intravenous regional anesthesia (Bier block), (3) regional or spinal nerve block, or (4) general anesthesia. Closed reduction may take place before an open procedure to reduce the fracture site. Skeletal traction may also be applied to the fracture site (Fig. 22-38), requiring a surgical skin prep and application of drapes. The appropriate casting or brace materials should be readily available to prevent loss of fracture reduction. Supplies should be available in the event it is necessary to open the fracture site and apply fixation.

Operative Procedure

The fragments are manipulated into alignment by the surgeon, using manual traction. Reduction is confirmed using radiography (x-ray or fluoroscopy). After reduction has been obtained, the fracture is immobilized with casting material or bracing technique.

External fixation

This method of fracture management provides rigid fixation and reduction with the ability to manage severe soft-tissue wounds. Because of the increased chance of infection in patients with an open fracture, external fixation is often the preferred treatment. Advantages of external fixation include the absence of casting material, fracture stabilization at a distance from the injury site, ability to perform subsequent procedures such as skin grafts or vascularized grafts, minimal joint interference, early mobilization, and the ability to use internal fixation or other skeleton-fixation devices at the same time or sequentially.

Indications for external fixation include (1) severe open fractures, (2) highly comminuted closed fractures, (3) arthrodesis, (4) infected joints, (5) infected nonunion, (6) fracture stabilization to protect arterial or nerve anastomoses, (7) major alignment and length deficits, (8) congenital deformities, and (9) static contractures. External fixation provides a bridge between fracture reduction and insertion of an internal fixator such as intramedullary nail, allowing time for vascular recovery. Internal fixation can take place at a later date.

Many improvements have been made in the design and

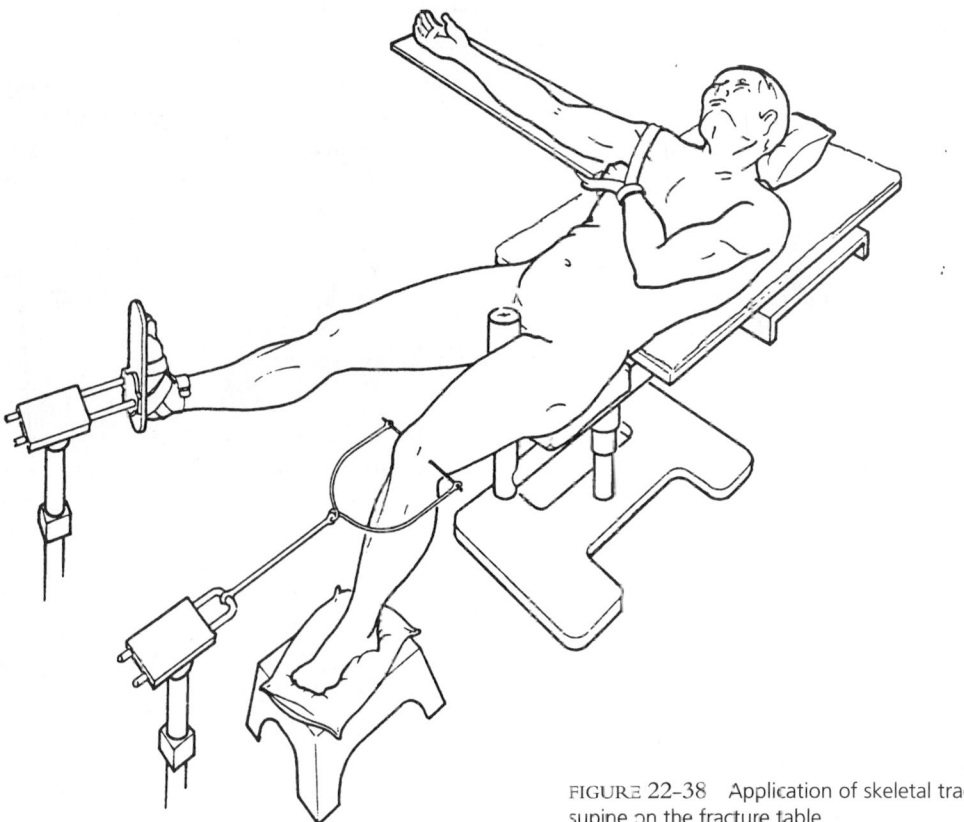

FIGURE 22-38   Application of skeletal traction with the patient positioned supine on the fracture table.

articulations of external fixation devices. The fixators can be applied to most anatomic sites. The available external fixators vary greatly in design; however, all contain three main components: (1) bone-anchoring devices (threaded pins, Kirschner wires), (2) longitudinal supporting devices (threaded or smooth rods), and (3) connecting elements (clamps and partial or full rings). Improvements have resulted in use of lightweight, stronger materials, which are radiopaque, to use as connecting rods. This also prevents postoperative radiographic interference when viewing the fracture site for progress in healing.

The Ilizarov device uses principles of tension-stress and distraction to correct bone defects and limb-length discrepancies. It is not routinely used for acute fracture fixation; however, the principles and technique are similar. Limb length may be adjusted with gradual bone distraction of bone ends, stimulating new bone formation.

Procedural Considerations

External fixators are applied using sterile technique with the patient under general or regional anesthesia. Radiographic imaging ensures fracture reduction after closed manipulation, and proper pin placement. Because the incision site is small to allow introduction of pins, a soft-tissue set appropriate to the site will be necessary. Many different external fixators are available for use. Some examples are shown in Figs. 22-39 to 22-43. Irrigation and débridement at the fracture site and surrounding soft-tissue may be necessary if there is soft tissue damage, so pulsatile

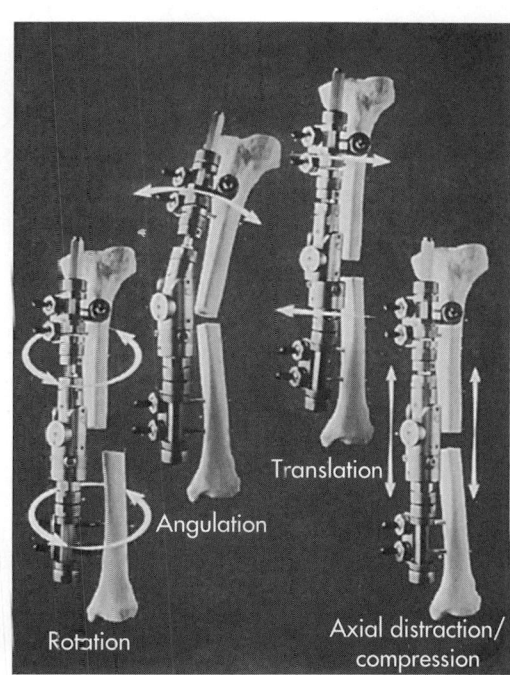

FIGURE 22-39   Torus external fixator positioned on a long bone.

lavage with 3000 ml normal saline solution should be available. A power drill will be used at the pin sites, and a periosteal elevator should be available for blunt or sharp dissection. An appropriate-sized pin cutter should also be available to shorten the pins if the need arises. The dressing

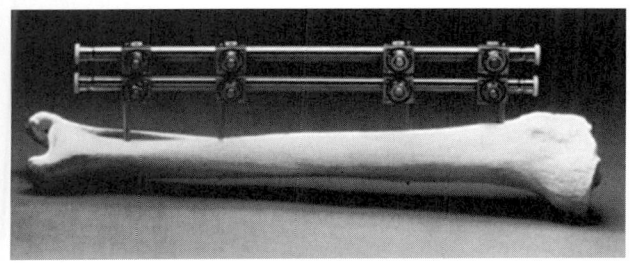

FIGURE 22–40   AO/ASIF fixator tubular external fixation device.

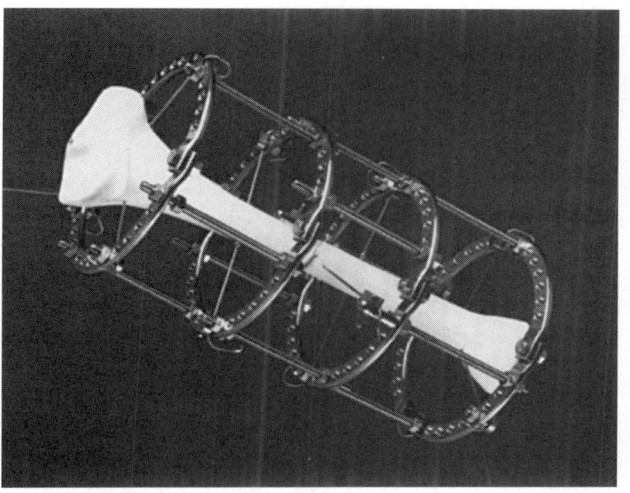

FIGURE 22–41   Ilizarov tibial external fixator.

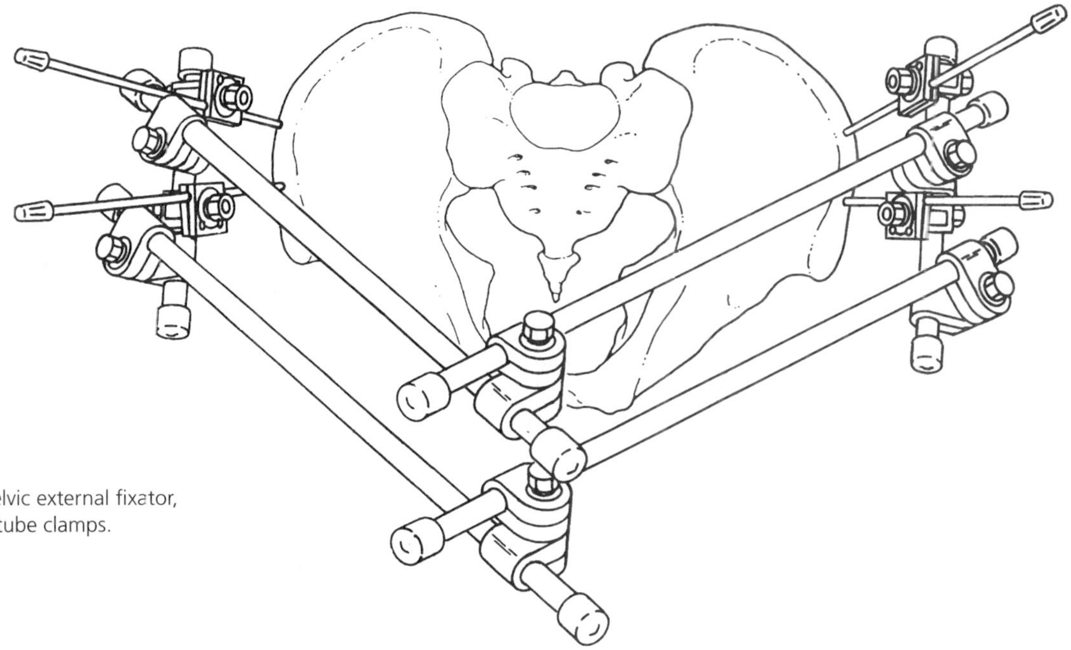

FIGURE 22–42   AO/ASIF pelvic external fixator, double frame using tube-to-tube clamps.

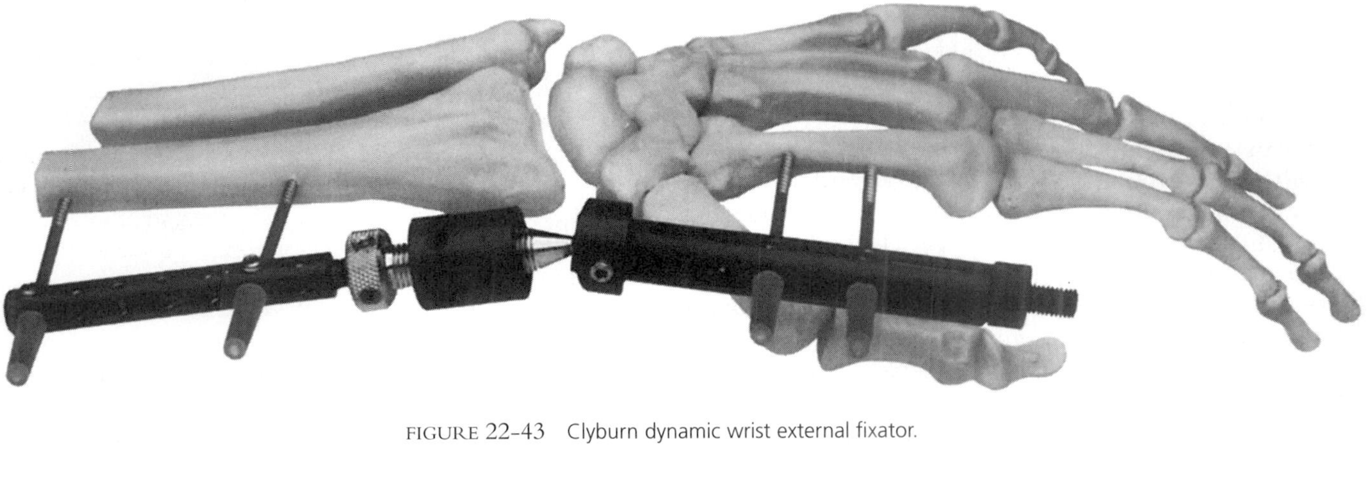

FIGURE 22–43   Clyburn dynamic wrist external fixator.

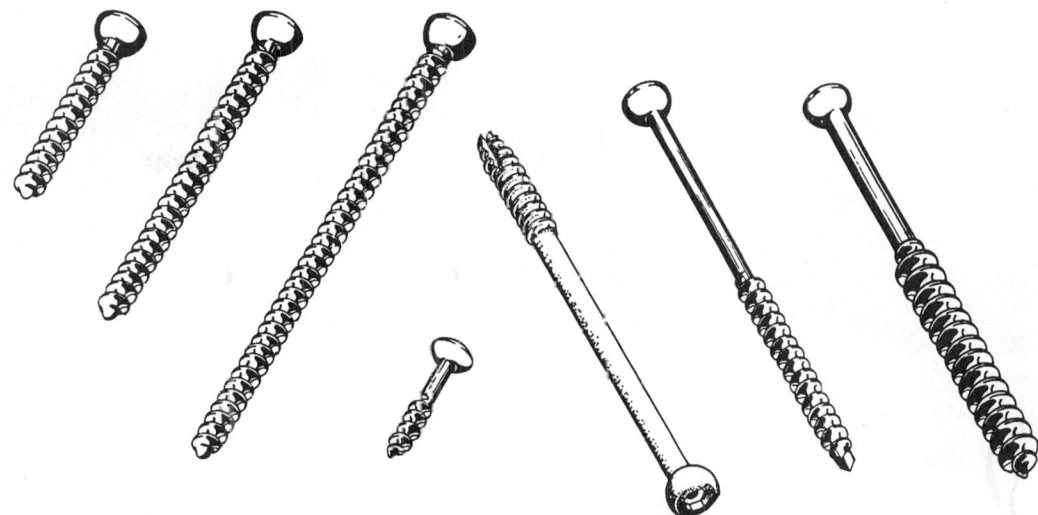

FIGURE 22-44   Types of screws used for fixation with or without plating systems.

consists of povidone-iodine complex ointment, antibiotic impregnated-gauze, or Telfa with a gauze overwrap.

Operative Procedure
Application of a unilateral frame

1. The fracture is reduced manually.
2. The skin is incised over an area free from neurovascular structures.
3. Blunt dissection to the bone or with the elevator may be necessary.
4. A drill sheath is used to protect surrounding soft tissue while predrilling the cortex.
5. Hand or low-speed power drilling is used to insert the half pins above and below the fracture.
6. Universal joints are slipped over the pins and joined with a connecting rod.
7. The frame is tightened using the appropriate wrenches.
8. Radiography or fluoroscopy is used to confirm reduction and alignment.
9. The pin sites are covered with an antibacterial agent and dressed with sterile gauze.

Internal fixation

Internal fixation is often the treatment of choice for correction of fractures of long bones or those in the hip region. Application of compression plates and screws and insertion of pins, intramedullary rods, nails, or wiring are methods of internal fixation. Fractures of most anatomic parts in adults can be repaired using internal fixation.

There are many principles and techniques when using internal fixation of fractures. Types of screws (Fig. 22-44) include cortical, cancellous, lag, pretapped, and self-tapping. Cortical bone screws have threads that are close together and narrower than other types of threads. These threads run along the entire length of the screw and transfix bone, gaining purchase (grab) of bone cortex.

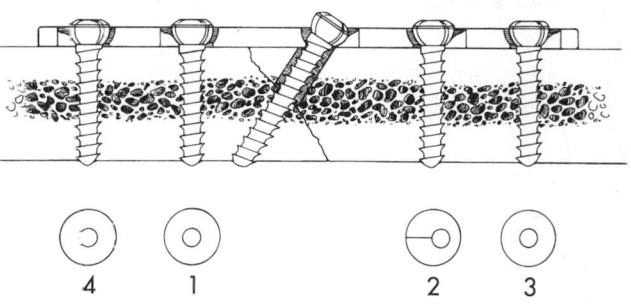

FIGURE 22-45   Plating a closed forearm fracture using dynamic compression showing final position of the screw insertion.

Cancellous bone screws feature threads that are broader and farther apart than those of cortical screws. Cancellous screws are used in cancellous bone, which is less dense than cortical bone; the bone accumulates within the threads to provide the purchase for fixation. Like cortical screws, cancellous screws can traverse fracture sites and hold plates onto bone. The screw threads do not completely traverse the bone through the opposite cortex. Cancellous screws are commonly used when fractures occur at the condylar ends of the shaft.

Plating of a fracture may occur with or without dynamic compression (Fig. 22-45). Dynamic compression uses screw and plate configurations to apply forces through the fracture site. Semitubular plates are less rigid and do not have the ability to produce dynamic compression. This type of plate is used in the forearm and fibula, where weight bearing, which could break the plate, is not a factor.

Closed Method

The fracture is reduced using closed reduction methods of manipulation and traction and then aligned with percutaneous insertion of pins, intramedullary nails, or

A   **B**   **C**

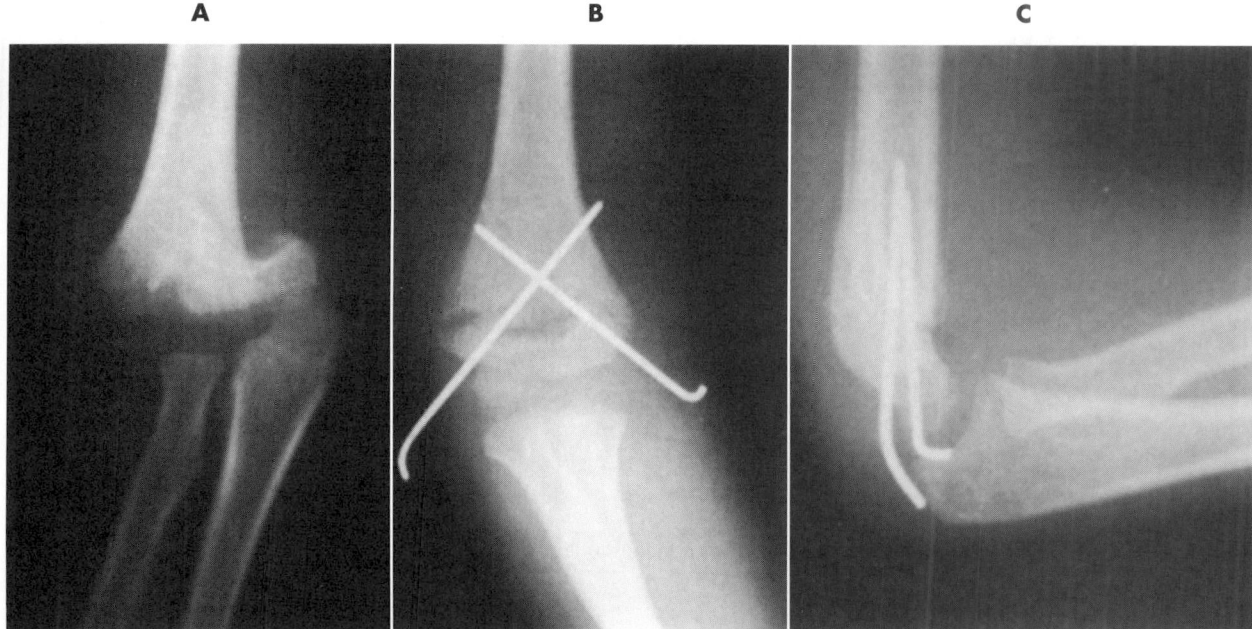

FIGURE 22-46   Percutaneous pinning of a supracondylar fracture. **A,** Severely displaced supracondylar fracture. **B** and **C,** Treated by closed reduction and percutaneous pinning.

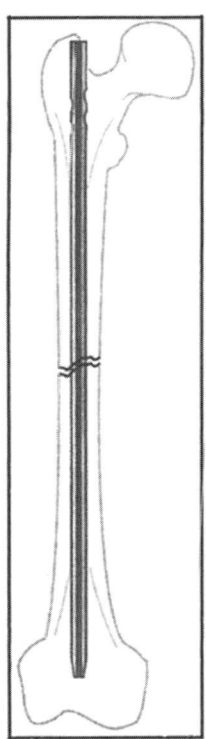

FIGURE 22-47   Rod placement for femoral fracture.

rods. Pins can be placed percutaneously (Fig. 22-46) to fix fractures involving the digits, wrist, elbow, and foot. A rod or nail is placed percutaneously in a large bone such as the humerus or femur (Fig. 22-47). Improved instrumentation and the use of fluoroscopy have made closed reduction with internal fixation a safe and effective practice. Closed

reduction is, however, a misnomer, since small openings in the soft tissue and bone are made to facilitate introduction of the devices. These incisions are considerably smaller than those created when repairing the fracture using open reduction. The advantages of closed reduction over open reduction and internal fixation are (1) a lower incidence of infection and (2) absence of additional soft-tissue or vascular damage.

Open Reduction and Internal Fixation

Open reduction and internal fixation is a method of providing exposure of the fracture site and using pins, wire, screws, a plate and screw combination, rods, or nails to correct the fracture (Fig. 22-48). Open reduction and internal fixation is used when satisfactory reduction of a fracture cannot be obtained or maintained by closed methods, and skeletal traction is not indicated. The advantage is that anatomic alignment of the fracture can usually be obtained and verified through direct observation. Fractures that are comminuted or difficult to reduce can be more effectively treated using this technique. The incidence of infection and nonunion, however, is increased when the wound is opened.

The procedure varies for each anatomic site, using the principles for specific fixation devices. Several procedures described in the text identify steps for completion of open reduction and internal fixation. Reference examples include the following:

- *Pin fixation.* Application of a unilateral frame
- *Wire fixation.* Reduction of patellar fracture, tension banding of the olecranon
- *Screw fixation.* Correction of scaphoid fractures

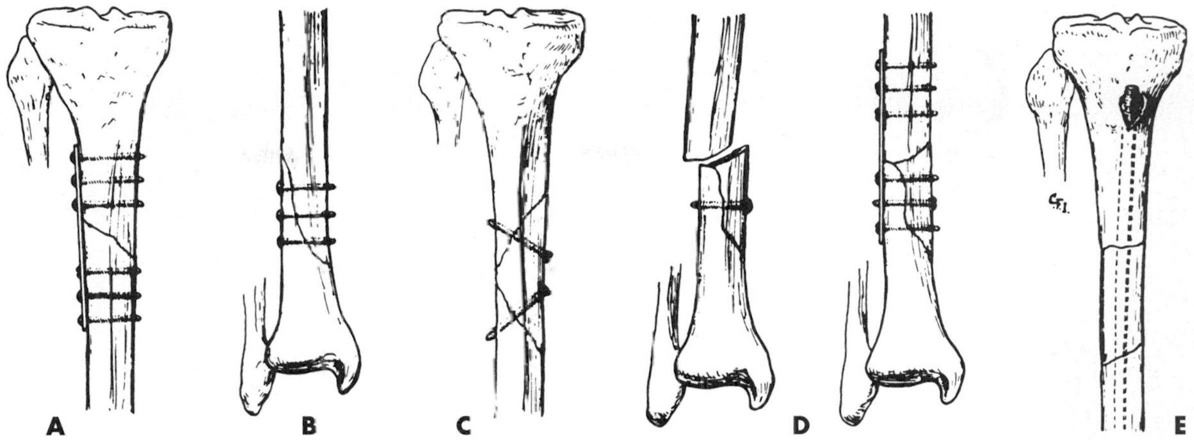

FIGURE 22-48   Types of internal fixation for fracture repair. **A,** Plate and screws for transverse or short oblique fracture. **B,** Transfixion screws for long oblique or spiral fractures. **C,** Transfixion screws for long butterfly fragment. **D,** Fixation for short butterfly fragment. **E,** Medullary fixation.

- *Plate and screw fixation.* Repair of the comminuted distal humeral fracture
- *Rod or nail fixation.* Correction of fractures of the shaft of the humerus, femoral shaft, or tibial shaft

SURGERY OF THE SHOULDER

Correction of Acromioclavicular Joint Separation

Acromioclavicular joint separation (Fig. 22-49), a common occupational and athletic injury, results from a force applied downward, most commonly from a fall directly to the top of the shoulder. The ligamentous support of the distal clavicle in the form of the coracoclavicular, coracoacromial, and acromioclavicular ligaments is disrupted. The result is either a posterior or superior displacement of the lateral end of the clavicle.

The purpose of surgery in an acutely injured patient is to reestablish the proper relationship between the clavicle and the acromion, thereby reducing long-term shoulder pain and increasing function. This is done by replacing the coracoclavicular ligaments with heavy suture or Mersilene tape or by inserting a screw through the clavicle and into the coracoid process. It may also be necessary to stabilize the acromioclavicular joint by placing a smooth Steinman pin across the acromion and into the clavicle. Sometimes the distal end of the clavicle is also resected. If resection of the clavicle is the only treatment required, this may be completed arthroscopically. Shoulder arthroscopy is detailed in the arthroscopic procedures section.

Procedural considerations

The patient is placed in the supine or semisitting position with a sandbag or folded sheet under the affected shoulder. The shoulder is positioned slightly off the operating bed (Fig. 22-50) to allow full range of motion,

or, if mobility of the arm is unnecessary, a shoulder positioner is used (see Fig. 22-14). The head is turned to the opposite side taking care not to apply too much stretch to the nerves of the brachial plexus. The extremity is draped with a stockinette to the midhumeral level.

A soft-tissue set and bone instrumentation specific for the shoulder (Fig. 22-51) is required. Depending on the technique used, bone screws and their instrumentation, free-cutting needles, bone-anchoring devices, and power instruments may be necessary.

Operative procedure
Coracoclavicular Suture Fixation

1. A curved incision is made to expose the acromioclavicular joint, the distal end of the clavicle, and the coracoid process.
2. The acromioclavicular joint is exposed, and any loose fragments or debris is removed.
3. Mattress sutures are placed in the ruptured coracoclavicular ligaments but not tied.
4. Drill holes are made in the clavicle above the coracoid in the anteroposterior (AP) plane.
5. A #5 nonabsorbable suture is placed beneath the base of the coracoid and superiorly through the two holes in the clavicle. With the joint reduced, the sutures are tied.
6. If instability is still a concern, small Kirschner wires can be placed across the acromioclavicular joint, through the lateral border of the acromion. The ends of the wires are bent 90 degrees at the lateral border to prevent proximal migration.
7. The sutures previously placed in the coracoclavicular ligaments are then tied.
8. The acromioclavicular joint capsule and the origins of the deltoid and trapezius muscles are repaired.
9. A sling and swathe bandage is then applied to the extremity.

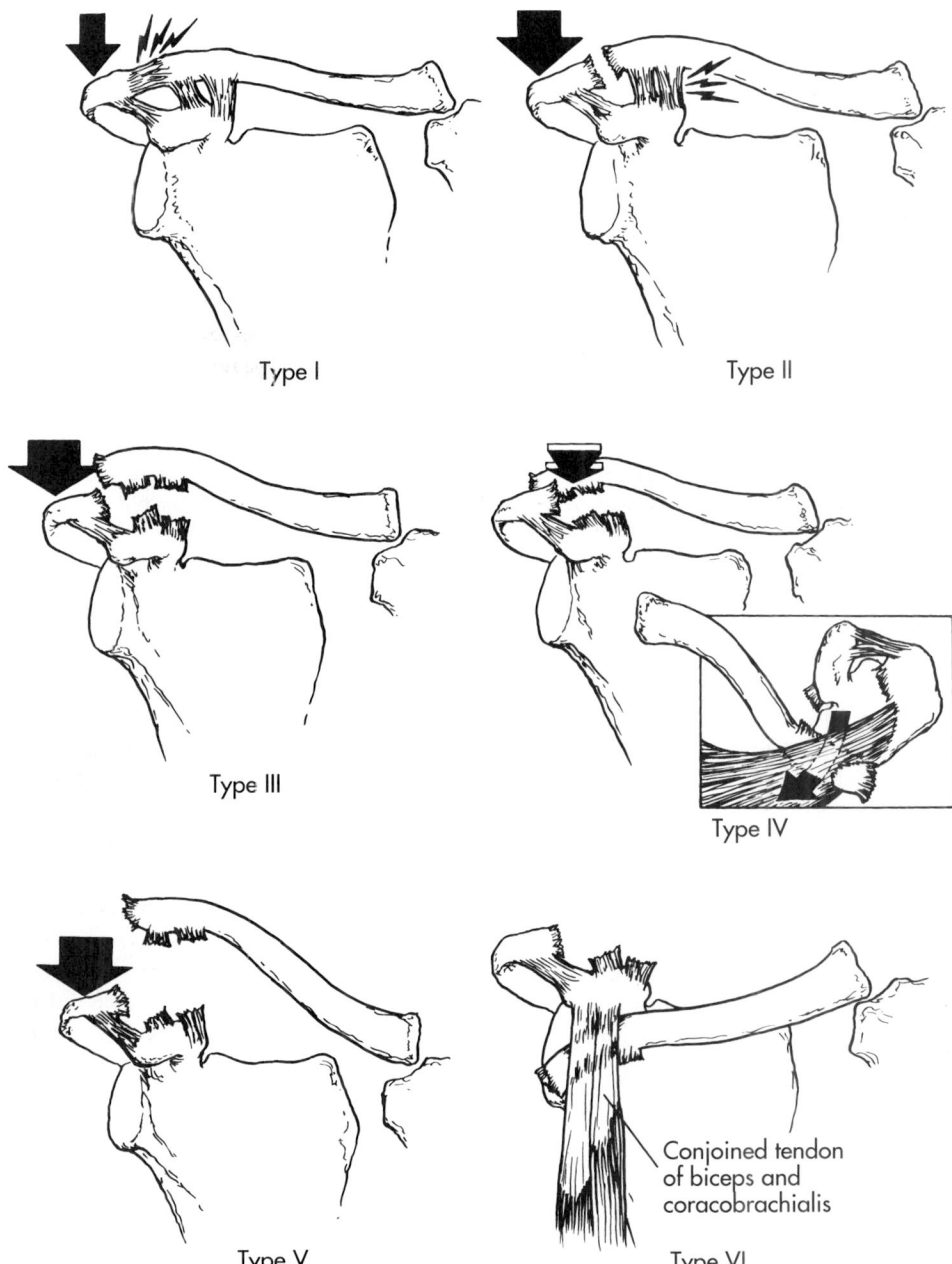

FIGURE 22–49 Classification of acromioclavicular injuries. *Type I,* Neither acromioclavicular nor coracoclavicular ligaments are disrupted. *Type II,* Acromioclavicular ligament is disrupted, and coracoclavicular ligament is intact. *Type III,* Both ligments are disrupted. *Type IV,* Ligaments are disrupted, and distal end of clavicle is displaced posteriorly into or through trapezius muscle. *Type V,* Ligaments and muscle attachments are disrupted, and clavicle and acromion are widely separated. *Type VI,* Ligaments are disrupted, and distal clavicle is dislocated inferior to coracoid process and posterior to biceps and coracobrachialis tendons.

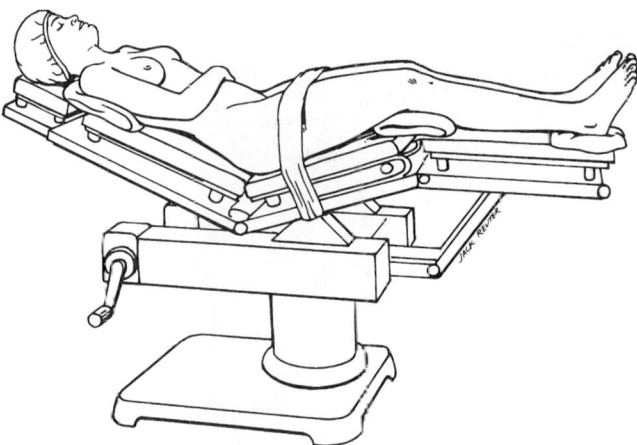

FIGURE 22-50 Positioning for a surgical procedure on the shoulder with the patient in a semisitting position and support beneath the affected shoulder.

Correction of Sternoclavicular Dislocation

Traumatic dislocation of the sternoclavicular joint usually occurs from an indirect blow on the anterior shoulder while the arm is abducted. The clavicle most frequently is displaced anteriorly, but posterior or retrosternal dislocations can occur. Posterior dislocation can be more severe because injury to the trachea, esophagus, thoracic duct, and large vessels of the mediastinum is possible. Except in severe cases, dislocation of the sternoclavicular joint is treated nonoperatively with manual traction and immobilization bandages.

Clavicular Fracture

Fractures of the clavicle are some of the most common bony injuries. These injuries rarely require surgical intervention. Approximately 94% of clavicular fractures are the result of a direct blow on the clavicle. The most common site of clavicular fractures is the middle third portion of the bone, mainly at the middle and outer third junction. Clavicular fractures are usually treated by immobilization in a figure-of-eight splint. The chances of nonunion are greatly increased when open reduction is used for a clavicular fracture. The outcome may result in a bony prominence, which may be disturbing to the patient; the overriding fragments are resorbed with time.

Clavicular fractures may require open reduction and internal fixation after nonunion, neurovascular compromise that cannot be resolved with reduction, distal clavicular fracture with torn coracoclavicular ligaments in an adult, or persistent wide separation of the fragments with soft-tissue entrapment. Surgery is necessary when the fracture is displaced enough to cause underlying damage to the vessels and brachial plexus. Open reduction is accomplished with a tubular plate and screws or intramedullary pin fixation.

Procedural considerations

The patient is placed in the supine or semisitting position with a sandbag or folded sheet under the affected shoulder and the head turned to the opposite side taking care not to apply too much stretch to the nerves of the brachial plexus. The entire extremity is prepped and draped. Soft-tissue and bone instruments are used for dissection. Bone reduction forceps and clamps will be used to gain reduction, and Kirschner wires may be used to temporarily hold the reduction. Permanent reduction will be held with either Steinman pins or plate and screws. A power drill will be necessary to apply these. In the case of a nonunion, bone-grafting instruments will be used.

Operative procedure

1. A 2.5 cm incision is made over the fracture site. The incision may need to be extended for comminuted fractures.
2. Dissection is carried down to the clavicle, taking care not to strip periosteum or disrupt vessels or nerves.
3. The fracture site is exposed and reduced using bone-holding forceps.
4. If pinning the clavicle is to be done, a Steinman pin is passed into the medial fragment medullary canal and removed.
5. The pin is then passed in the same manner into the distal fragment.
6. The fracture is again reduced, and a threaded Steinman pin is transfixed across the fracture site through both fragments.
7. If plating the clavicle is to be done, a small semitubular plate is used with at least two screw holes on each side of the fracture site.
8. The periosteum must be stripped off the clavicle sparingly but sufficiently so that a plate can be applied to the anterior surface.
9. Extreme care must be taken when drilling screw holes to avoid damage to the subclavian vein and thoracic contents.
10. After closure an immobilization sling is applied.

Correction of Rotator Cuff Tear

Most rotator cuff tears occur through the insertion of the tendinous fibers of the supraspinatus muscle that attaches onto the greater tuberosity of the proximal humerus. In severe tears, the remaining tendons of the cuff, the subscapularis, infraspinatus, and teres minor, may also be involved. Supraspinatus syndrome, also known as *impingement syndrome*, can involve multiple pathologic conditions such as calcium deposits, bicipital tendonitis, subacromial bursitis, tenosynovitis, and other nonarticular lesions along with a cuff tear. The approach to diagnosis and treatment is similar for both.

Partial rotator cuff tears and impingement usually affect people in the middle decades of life or later and are

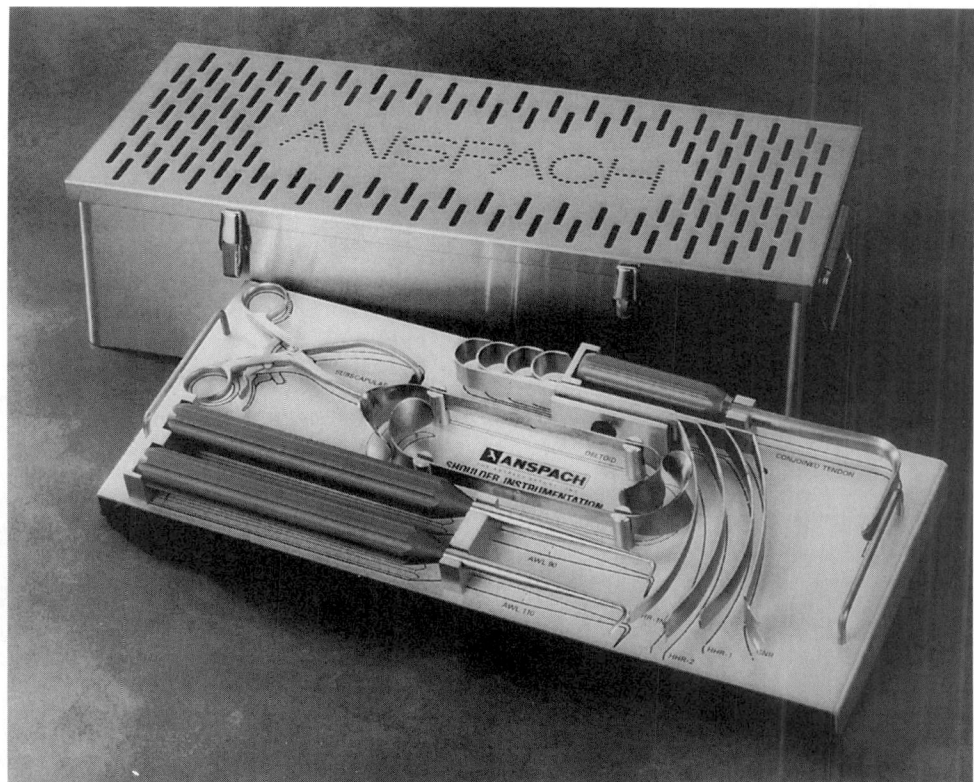

FIGURE 22-51   Shoulder instrumentation set including humeral head retractors, glenoid neck retractor, modified Gelpi retractors, Goulet retractors, conjoined tendon retractor, subscapularis retractor, and glenoid awl.

often attributable to a long-term degenerative process. Complete tears of the rotator cuff occur after accidental injury of younger patients such as pitchers and football quarterbacks. Patients with rotator cuff tears may not be able to initiate abduction of the shoulder because the stabilizing forces of the ruptured tendons on the humeral head are lost. Most rotator cuff tears can be treated conservatively with physical therapy and NSAIDs.

There is a variety of procedures that may be performed for these conditions. Methods of repair depend on the size and shape of the tear. The common goal is to restore joint stability, alleviate pain, and allow the patient to return to normal activities. In some instances a significant reduction in preinjury activity may be permanent.

Procedural considerations

If surgery is necessary, the patient is placed in the supine or semisitting position with a sandbag or folded towel under the affected shoulder. The head is turned to the opposite side, taking care to avoid undue stretch to the brachial plexus. A shoulder positioner can be used if intraoperative mobility of the arm is not a factor. In addition to a bone and soft-tissue set, shoulder instruments will be required. The remaining equipment needs will depend on the severity of the tear. Minor tears may require no more than heavy nonabsorbable suture. Major tears will require a power drill and burr and possibly a microsagittal saw. Fixation may be gained with bone-anchoring devices. Free needles will be necessary if these are used.

Operative procedure

1. An anterosuperior deltoid incision is made.
2. The coracoacromial ligament is divided at the acromial attachment.
3. A subacromioplasty (resection of the undersurface of the acromion) is completed. This is also primary treatment for impingement syndrome.
4. Small, simple tears can be repaired by suturing the torn edges with heavy, nonabsorbable sutures.
5. Massive tears may require attaching the torn edges to the greater tuberosity using bone-anchoring devices.
6. If the defect cannot be bridged, a flap from the subscapularis tendon can be transposed and sutured to the supraspinatus and infraspinatus muscles.
7. If impingement is involved or solely the cause of a rotator pathologic condition, other measures involving the same approach are taken.
8. Calcium deposits encased in tendon are excised to alleviate mechanical obstruction, or acromioplasty is performed.
9. After closure a sling is applied. Patients with small tears may begin motion on the third to fourth postoperative day. Larger tears may be immobilized for 2 to 8 weeks.

Correction of Recurrent Anterior Dislocation of the Shoulder

The anterior fibers of the shoulder capsule are stretched and weakened as a result of frequent dislocations of the shoulder joint. More then 150 operations or modifications have been devised to treat recurrent anterior dislocation. The goals are to (1) prevent recurrence, (2) prevent surgical complications, (3) prevent creation of arthritic changes, (4) maintain joint motion, and (5) correct the problem. The surgeon selects the procedure appropriate for the patient condition that will satisfy the conditions necessary for correction of the problem. A stapling procedure was once common treatment of recurrent dislocation, but it has been replaced by other accepted procedures.

Procedural considerations

The patient is placed in the supine or semisitting position with a sandbag or folded sheet under the shoulder. The arm is draped free so that the extremity can be manipulated. An anterior curved incision or a longitudinal incision in the anterior axillary fold is made over the shoulder joint. A soft-tissue and bone set will be required as well as a set of instruments specific to shoulder surgery (see Fig. 22-51), power drill and burr, bone-anchoring devices, and free needles.

Operative procedures

Bankart Procedure (Fig. 22-52)

For this procedure, the scapula is not elevated with a sandbag or folded sheet. The attenuated anterior capsule is reattached to the rim of the glenoid fossa with heavy sutures. The glenoid fossa rim is decorticated with a curette to provide a raw surface to which the capsule is attached. Special instruments designed for the Bankart procedure, such as the curved awl and humeral head retractor, facilitate the surgery, although the capsule may be attached with bone anchors, obviating the use of the awl. If the coracoid process is to be removed to obtain better operative exposure, a drill, bone screws, and washer should be available for reattachment. Postoperatively the extremity is immobilized in a sling or shoulder immobilizer. Shoulder motion is begun at 3 days postoperatively, and the patient may return to contact sports or heavy labor after approximately 6 months.

Putti-Platt Procedure

The steps of the Putti-Platt are similar to those of the Bankart in that the joint capsule is sutured to the glenoid rim. Additionally, the Putti-Platt procedure requires the lateral advancement of the subscapularis. This produces a barrier against dislocation of the shoulder. This procedure is rarely useful when the anterior capsular mechanism is of poor quality.

The subscapularis tendon is divided 2.5 cm medially to its insertion. The glenoid and humeral head are inspected using palpation to assess osteochondral changes. The lateral

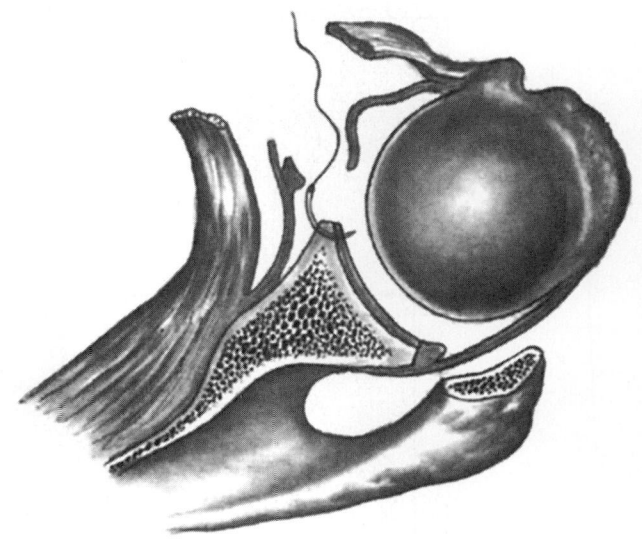

FIGURE 22-52 Bankart procedure for restoration of shoulder stability. Holes are made in the rim of the glenoid, and the free lateral margin of the capsule is sutured to the rim of the glenoid. The medial margin of the capsule is sutured to the lateral surface.

portion of the subscapularis is sutured to the anterior glenoid rim. The medial portion of the subscapularis is sutured to the rotator cuff at the greater tuberosity. The layers of the shoulder joint are imbricated (overlapped), a technique used often in soft-tissue reconstruction. The incision is closed, and a shoulder immobilizer is applied. This is worn for approximately 3 weeks. External rotation of the arm should be avoided immediately after the repair.

Bristow Procedure

In this procedure, the coracoid process, along with the attached muscles, is detached and inserted onto the neck of the glenoid cavity, where it is attached with a screw through the subscapularis muscle. This stabilizes the anterior joint capsule and prevents recurrent dislocation. Disadvantages of this procedure are (1) internal rotation contracture, (2) inattention to labrum or capsule disorders, (3) potential for injury to the musculocutaneous nerve, (4) reduction of internal rotation power by shortening of the subscapularis muscle, (5) possible limitation of external rotation, (6) possible penetration of the screw into the articular surface of the glenoid, and (7) later development of early joint disease of the shoulder. A Bristow procedure is considered an appropriate alternative when the anterior capsular mechanism is of poor quality.[37]

Correction of Humeral Head Fracture

Comminuted fractures of the humeral head (Fig. 22-53) with displacement may require open reduction and internal fixation with screws or pins or closed reduction with a humeral nail or rod. However, if the fracture is badly comminuted, a prosthetic replacement is indicated. Traumatic or degenerative arthritic shoulder joints may be so painful or dysfunctional that a total shoulder joint replacement is necessary.

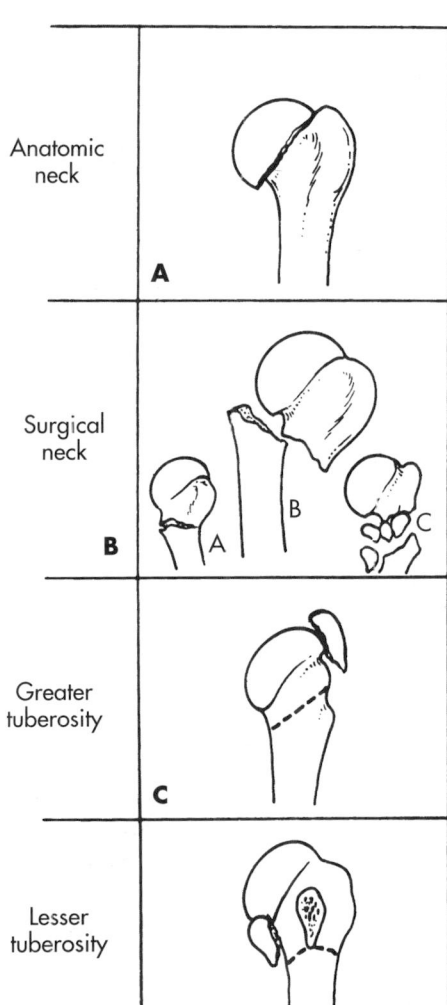

Anatomic neck

A

Surgical neck

A   B   C

B

Greater tuberosity

C

Lesser tuberosity

D

FIGURE 22-53 Fractures and fracture dislocations relate to the pattern of displacement. Fractures can occur in two, three, or four parts.

Extensive rehabilitation for the shoulder is required. Surgery should be performed as soon as possible. Delay can allow time for increasing scar formation, contracture of the muscles, and increasing osteoporosis of the bone fragments. The shoulder is the most difficult joint in the body to rehabilitate because it has (1) the greatest range of motion, (2) a second space beneath the acromion that must be mobilized, and (3) many muscles, weakened by trauma, that enter into complex movements.

SURGERY OF THE HUMERUS, RADIUS, AND ULNA

Fractures of the Humeral Shaft

Closed manipulation and immobilization usually accomplish reduction of a fractured humerus as well as minimizing the risk of nonunion and infection. When closed reduction is impossible or when nonunion of the fracture has occurred, surgery is indicated. The fracture is reduced and held with intramedullary fixation, a compression plate, a lag screw, or a rigid locking nail, with distal and proximal bone screws that will transfix the rod within the canal. This last device can control rotation of the fracture fragments and prevent distraction at the fracture site (Fig. 22-54). Multiple flexible nails may be used if more rigid nails are not available. Bone graft may be used, depending on both the extent of the fracture and the length of time since injury. Compression plating of shaft fractures is usually reserved for when other treatment has failed or with supracondylar involvement.

Procedural considerations

The patient is positioned supine with the body near the edge of the bed to facilitate moving the extremity. The extremity is prepped and draped from the middle of the chest to below the elbow. Fluoroscopy and permanent radiographs are required to ensure proper alignment, reduction, and placement of implants. A radiolucent table improves imaging ability.

Soft-tissue and a large bone set are required. In addition, the intramedullary fixation device of choice and the required instruments for its insertion will be needed. PMMA may be used in the case of pathologic fractures. Instruments required for harvesting bone graft might be needed as well. A traction tray could be used to gain reduction. A power drill will be necessary if screws are used to lock the device. Sterile x-ray cassette covers will be needed for permanent intraoperative films.

Operative procedure
Medullary Fixation: Antegrade Technique

1. Proper length and alignment of the fracture must be attained with traction. Nail length should ensure proximal burying to avoid subacromial impingement and be 1 to 2 cm proximal to the olecranon fossa. A skin incision is made from the lateral point of the acromion over the tip of the greater tuberosity. The fascia is incised and the greater tuberosity palpated.
2. A small awl is inserted to enter medially to the greater tuberosity and confirmed with fluoroscopy in both AP and lateral views.
3. The awl is withdrawn; a ball-nosed reamer guide wire is inserted, advancing down the medullary canal (periodically verified with the fluoroscopy). Confirmation is made with each step to ensure that the wires, reamers, or implant has not fractured through the cortex along the shaft.
4. The guide wire is advanced to within 1 to 2 cm of the olecranon fossa, avoiding distraction or shortening.
5. If Enders nails are being used, each one is advanced in the same fashion as the guide wire.
6. Nail length can be determined by using a second guide wire of the same length held against what remains extended from the humerus. The difference

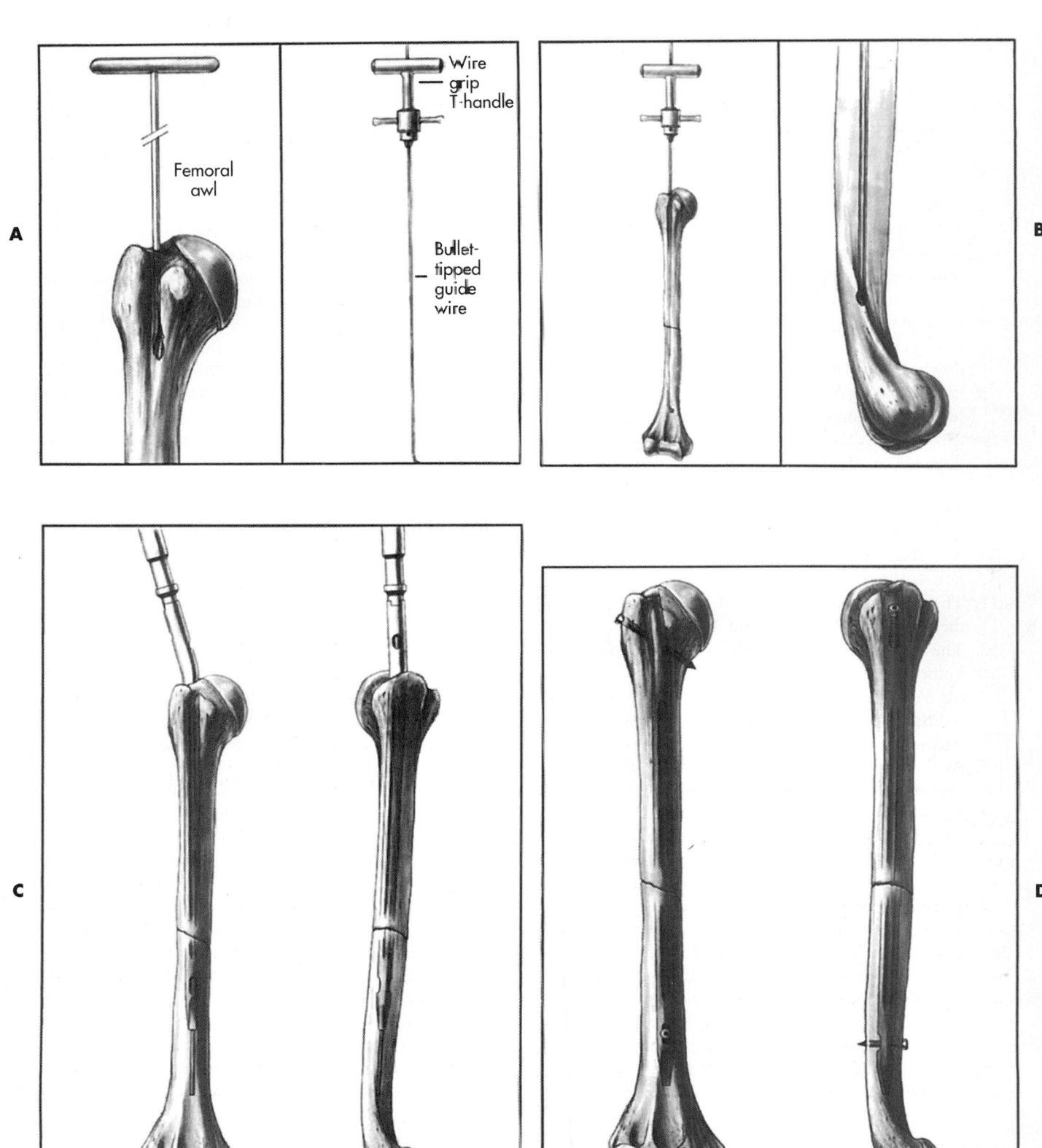

FIGURE 22-54   Placement of the humeral rigid locking nail with distal and proximal screws. **A,** After incision and exposure a femoral awl is used to make an entry portal. **B,** Guide wire is advanced into the center of the epicondylar region. **C,** After reaming, the nail is advanced over the fracture site and seated. **D,** Proximal and distal locking takes place after the correct screw placement is determined.

between the length protruding and the length remaining on the second rod is the approximate length requirement of the humeral nail. Another method uses a nail-length gauge that is held directly against the upper arm, viewed with fluoroscopy, and read directly on the gauge.

7. Enders nails may be held directly against the arm and viewed with fluoroscopy to determine proper length. If Enders nails are used, two or three nails are driven down the shaft, across the fracture site, and into the distal fragment. Fluoroscopy is used to confirm proper placement and reduction.

8. If intramedullary nailing is to be accomplished, the humerus may be reamed with a cannulated reamer down the shaft over the guide wire. Reaming of the canal is completed in 0.5 mm increments. The humerus becomes smaller in diameter. Reaming is gentle to ensure that protrusion through the bone does not occur. The bone is reamed 0.5 to 1 mm larger than the selected nail diameter.

9. The medullary exchange tube is used to maintain fracture reduction.

10. The ball-tipped guide wire is replaced with a non–ball-tipped guide wire.

11. The medullary nail is assembled for impaction with the appropriate outrigger and drill guides.

12. The nail is guided into the proximal end of the humerus and the humeral nail driver is used to impact the nail within the canal. Care must be taken to avoid splitting the humerus or creating a supracondylar fracture by wedging the tip of the nail.

13. As the nail approaches and crosses the fracture site, manual reduction must be maintained.

14. The proximal drill guide is attached to the nail impacter with the nail coupled; a stab wound is made in the skin, and the nail is pushed to reach the bone.

15. An 8 mm drill sleeve is inserted through the drill guide, followed by a 2.7 mm drill guide into the first guide.

16. The cortex is scored with the 2.7 mm trocar, and transfixing of the hole is completed with a 2.7 mm drill from the lateral to distal areas of the cortex.

17. The humeral screw-depth gauge is inserted and read directly to determine the appropriate screw size.

18. A 4 mm fully threaded humeral screw is inserted to the selected length. Screw position can be confirmed by inserting a guide wire down the end of the nail, where it will be impeded by the transfixing screw.

19. Fluoroscopy is used to target the distal humeral locking screw.

20. A second percutaneous access is created to the bone surface of the humerus from the anterior to posterior cortex of the bone.

21. With the free-hand technique, the cortex of the bone is scored followed by the 8 mm hand-held drill sleeve and the 2.7 mm drill bit.

22. The selected size of humeral screw is gauged and inserted. Placement is confirmed with fluoroscopy, and the impacter assembly is removed from the nail.

23. Full-view radiographs are obtained in both dimensions, and the wound is irrigated and closed.

NOTE: This describes a straightforward, uncomplicated procedure. There are many variations of approach and technique used depending on the complexity of the fracture and any associated injury. The fracture site may often have to be opened if it is comminuted or will not reduce properly through closed techniques. The radial nerve or other neurovascular structures may incur entrapment and trauma, requiring exploration and repair.

Although this type of antegrade fixation, using locked rods, is preferred for this type of fracture, it is not the only method. Often a retrograde technique is used, with the patient in the prone or lateral decubitus position. The retrograde technique, used more commonly in the care of femoral shaft fractures, appears later in the chapter.

Distal Humeral Fractures (Supracondylar, Epicondylar, and Intercondylar)

Distal humeral fractures are classified into several types depending on location and the presence or absence of articular involvement (Fig. 22-55). Supracondylar fractures of the humerus do not involve the articular surface and can generally be treated with closed reduction and casting. Transcondylar fractures may or may not have articular involvement, and this will accordingly dictate treatment. Intercondylar fractures involve both condyles with a comminution of injury, are intraarticular, and present the greatest challenge for the surgical team. Fractures of the articular components, the capitulum and trochlea, are usually the result of a fall on an outstretched arm. The force drives the radial head to shear off the capitulum, producing an intraarticular fragment. The lateral or medial condyles and epicondyles are also subject to fracture by various mechanisms.

Patients may present with a single isolated fracture or any combination mentioned above. Neurovascular and other soft-tissue trauma are considered in selecting the type of reduction and fixation. Screws, pins, a variety of different plates, and dynamic compression technique can be used for internal fixation. Certain fixation techniques of the distal portion of the humerus may require an osteotomy of the olecranon (proximal ulna) to properly align and affix hardware (Fig. 22-56). The general goals of treating these injuries are to (1) maintain neurovascular integrity, (2) restore normal joint articulation, (3) preserve motion of the joint, and (4) correct other soft-tissue injuries.

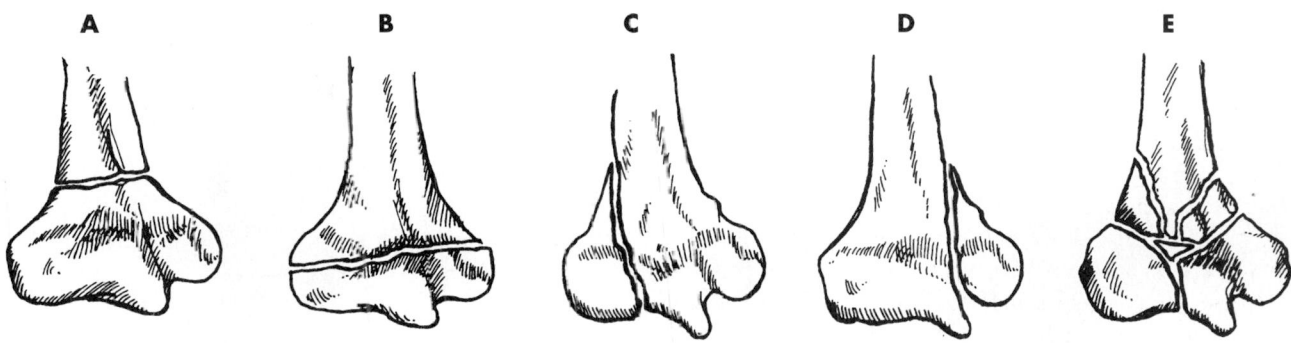

FIGURE 22-55 Classification of distal humeral fractures. **A,** Supracondylar. **B,** Transcondylar. **C,** Lateral condyle with trochlea. **D,** Medial condyle. **E,** Intercondylar with comminution.

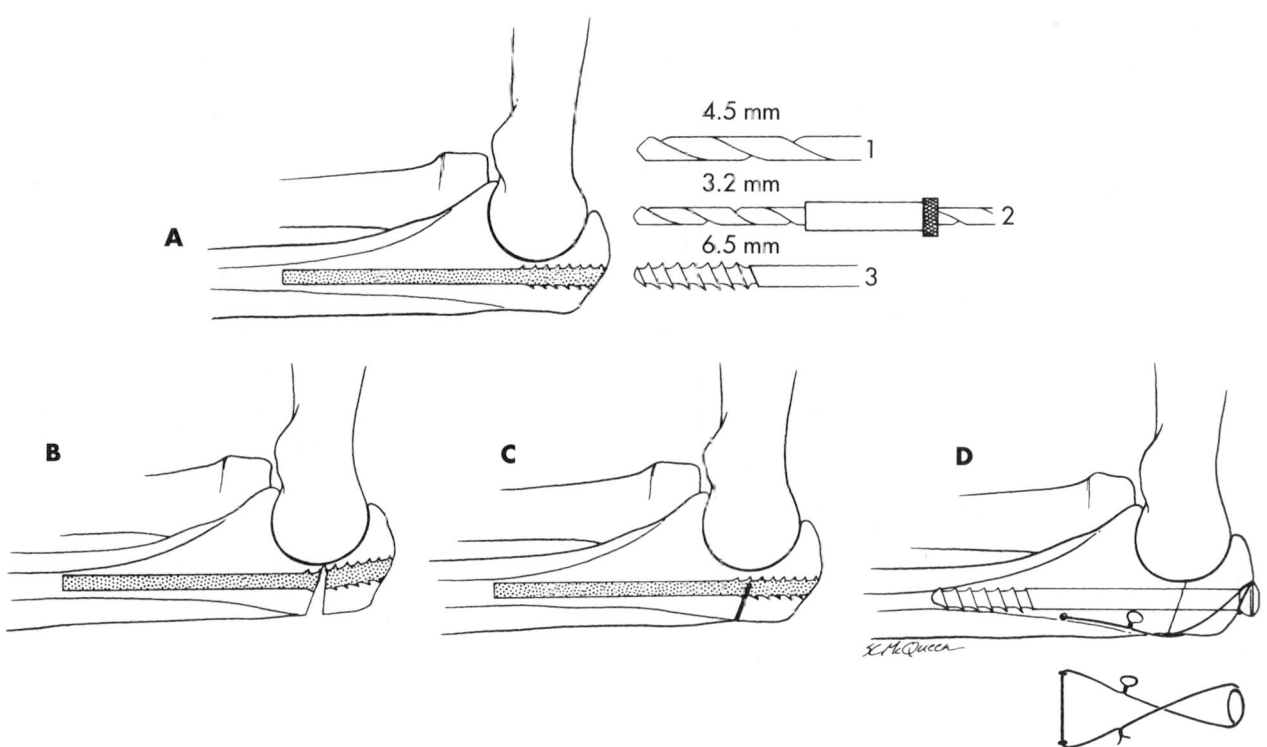

FIGURE 22-56 Osteotomy of the olecranon with placement of a lag screw and tension band wire fixation.

Procedural considerations

Regional anesthesia can be used for procedures on the distal end of the humerus. Bone graft harvesting may require use of general anesthesia. The patient may be prone with the elbow flexed over a small table, supine with the arm over the chest, supine with the arm on a hand table, or in the lateral position. A tourniquet is placed before the surgical prep and may be inflated during surgery as needed.

A soft-tissue set, large bone set, and bone graft set are needed in addition to a compression set (Fig. 22-57), bone-holding clamps (Fig. 22-58), reconstruction plates, and smooth Kirschner wires. A power drill and Kirschner-wire driver will be needed to apply the hardware.

Operative procedure
Comminuted Distal Humeral Fracture (Fig. 22-59)

1. An incision is made over the distal humeral fracture site.
2. The fracture is exposed and reduced using bone reduction clamps and temporary small smooth Kirschner wires, driving them across the fracture sites with the power drill.
3. A cancellous bone screw is placed using drill and tap to transfix from one condyle to the other. Care must be taken not to violate the joint surface with the threads of the screw.
4. Kirschner wires are removed if reduction is maintained.

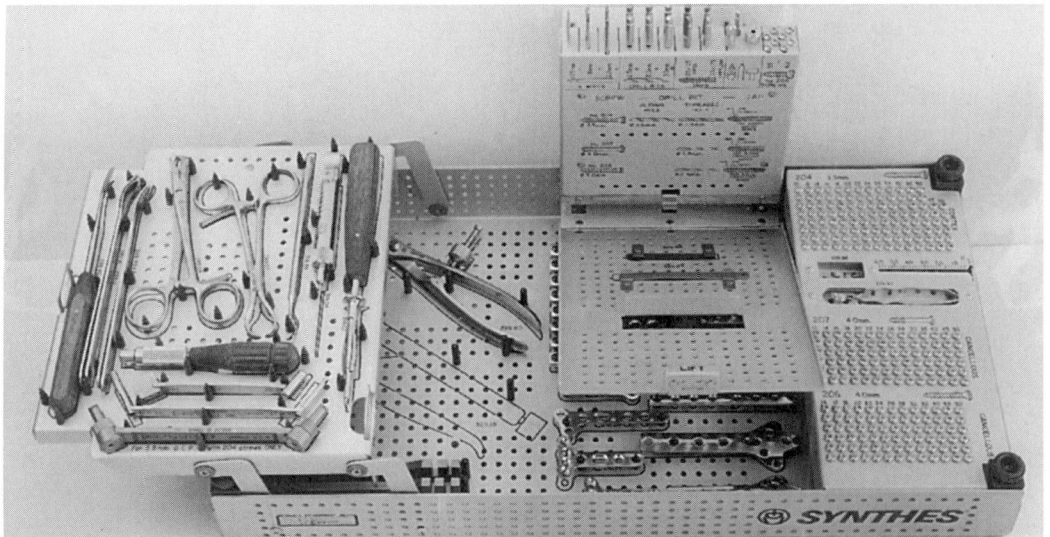

FIGURE 22-57   AO/ASIF compression sets range in size for repair of fractures; small fragment set shown.

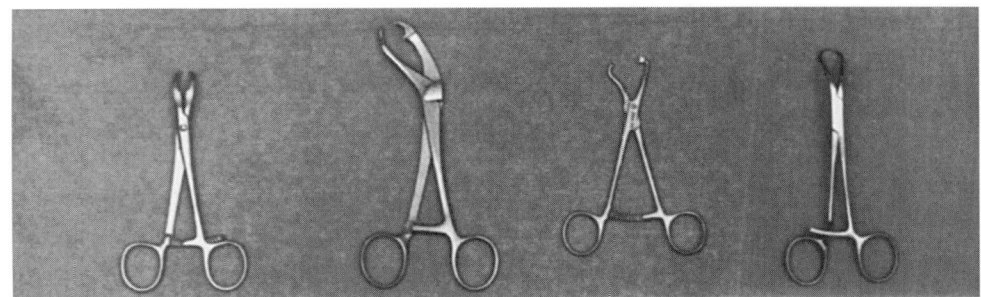

FIGURE 22-58   Small bone clamps. *Left to right,* Reduction, Verbrugge bone holding, plate holding, reduction with points.

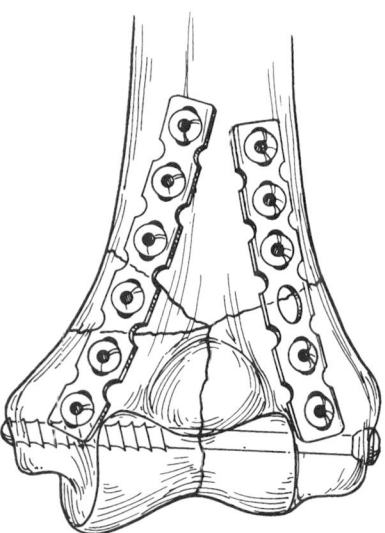

FIGURE 22-59   Repair of the distal comminuted humeral fracture with 3.5 mm reconstruction plates.

5. A one-third semitubular or reconstruction plate is contoured to the shape of the distal humeral fracture and applied to bridge the fracture fragments.

6. Throughout the entire procedure, the articular surface is periodically inspected to ensure integrity. The plates are held in place by hand while the elbow is put through its range of motion. The plates should not encroach upon the olecranon or coronoid fossa (distal end of the ulna), since this will limit flexion and extension of the arm.

7. The bone is drilled and tapped from one cortex to the other with the appropriate drill and tap. The screw is inserted and seated to the bone surface on the plate. This is done for all subsequent screws, observing the fracture site and articular surface.

8. Interfragmentary screws may be used in addition to the cortical screws spanning the condyles. If the olecranon was previously osteotomized for exposure, it is reattached using the tension band technique (Fig. 22-60) with a cancellous bone screw and heavy-gauge (18 or 20) wire.

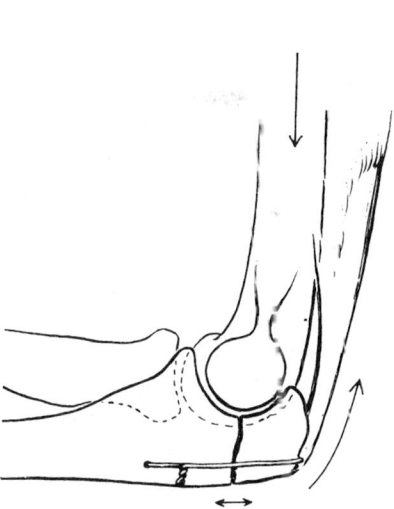

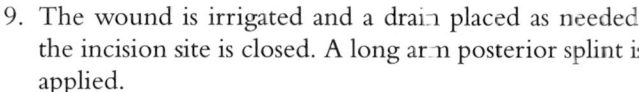

FIGURE 22-60 Tension band technique used for repair of the olecranon.

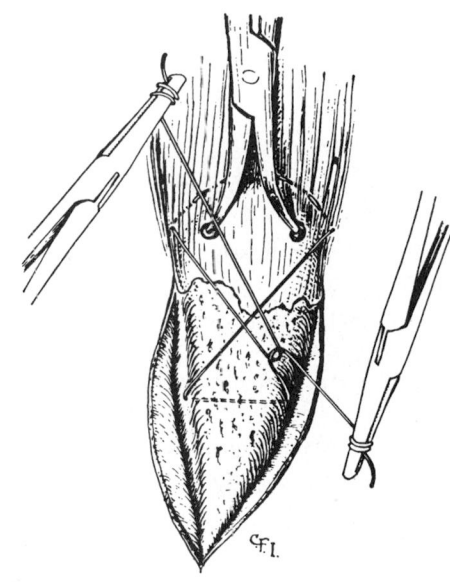

FIGURE 22-61 Operative procedure: tension banding with stainless steel wire passed through drill holes; figure of eight adds stability to the fracture.

9. The wound is irrigated and a drain placed as needed the incision site is closed. A long arm posterior splint is applied.

Olecranon Fracture

If the olecranon fracture fragment is small, it may be excised and the triceps tendon is reattached to the ulnar shaft. This does not result in loss of stability of the elbow joint. However, larger fragments must be reduced and held with internal fixation. The olecranon is often electively osteotomized for surgical exposure (see previous section) and repaired in the same fashion as a traumatic fracture.

Procedural considerations

The patient is placed in the prone position with the arm on an arm board or hand table. A soft-tissue set, bone set, AO/ASIF instrumentation, heavy stainless steel wire (16 and 18 gauge in long lengths), a wire tightener, Kirschner wires, bone-reduction clamps, a power drill, and Kirschner-wire driver will be needed.

Operative procedure
Tension Banding (Fig. 22-61)

1. An incision is made over the olecranon, and the fracture is exposed.
2. A drill hole is made in the distal fragment traversing the bone.
3. Stainless steel wire is passed through the drilled holes, crossed over, and pulled toward the tip of the olecranon.
4. After using the drill and tap, a cancellous bone screw is used to attach the proximal fragment to the distal, stopping short of totally seating the screw.

5. The wire is pulled and looped around the exposed shaft of the screw while reduction is maintained manually or by using a reduction clamp. The wire can be tightened using the wire tightener. The cancellous screws can be substituted by two smooth Steinman pins that are bent over the exposed portion to hook the loop of wire.
6. The remaining screw is threaded into the bone; the fracture site is observed for opposition.
7. The wound is irrigated and closed. Drains are generally not necessary. A long-arm posterior splint is placed.

NOTE: Using this technique requires early active motion of the arm. Compression of the fracture site is achieved by placing the elbow through its range of motion and applying force by the hardware.

Transposition of the Ulnar Nerve

Transposition of the ulnar nerve involves freeing the nerve from a groove at the back of the medial epicondyle of the humerus and bringing it to the front of the condyle. The ulnar nerve is frequently divided or damaged after fracture or wounds to the elbow caused by trauma. Dislocation of the elbow may also cause ulnar nerve damage. Late traumatic neuritis may occur after an old injury resulting in stretching of the ulnar nerve. The hand appears atrophied, and sensory loss is high. In severe cases a claw-hand deformity occurs.

Procedural considerations

The patient is placed in the supine position with the extremity slightly flexed on a hand table or over the chest. A tourniquet is applied to the upper arm, and the entire arm (fingers to tourniquet) is prepped and draped. A soft-tissue set is required. Bone instruments may be required.

Operative procedure

1. An incision is made on the lateral aspect of the elbow near the epicondyle.
2. The fascia and the flexor carpi ulnaris muscle are divided.
3. The ulnar nerve is freed and the medial intermuscular septum is dissected.
4. The nerve is then drawn anteriorly and placed deep into the brachialis flexor muscle origin.
5. The wound is irrigated and closed. A drain is not necessary. A short-arm posterior splint is applied to the elbow postoperatively.

Excision of the Head of the Radius

Fractures of the radial head can be displaced or nondisplaced, segmental, or comminuted. Complications can arise when treatment is delayed, causing limitation of motion, pain, and traumatic arthritis. A congruous radial head is essential for proper rotation of the forearm at the elbow. Consequently, in an adult it is necessary to excise the radial head if a severely comminuted fracture with angulation interferes with rotation. The radial head should never be excised in children. The outcome for the patient undergoing radial head excision may result in some permanent loss of pronation and supination of the forearm. Noncomminuted fractures that are easily reduced can be treated using closed reduction and casting.

Procedural considerations

The patient is supine with the arm over the chest or on a hand table. A tourniquet is applied. A soft-tissue set, small bone set, and oscillating microsaw with blades are needed.

Operative procedure

1. An incision is made on the shaft of the radius from 5 cm distal to the radial head extending proximally over the lateral humeral condyle.
2. Dissection is continued between the extensor carpi ulnaris and extensor digitorum muscles onto the joint capsule.
3. With the head and neck of the radius exposed through the joint capsule, the joint is irrigated to clear bone debris and blood clots.
4. The radial head is then excised just proximally to the radial tuberosity, taking care to remove all periosteum and limit new bone formation. The remaining annular ligament is also excised. The fragments of the radial head should be saved and readily available so that they may be reassembled to ensure that all have been retrieved.
5. The wound is closed, and a long-arm posterior splint is applied with the elbow at 90 degrees.

Fractures of the Proximal Third of the Ulna with Radial Head Dislocation (Monteggia)

The Monteggia type of fracture presents with a proximal ulnar fracture and dislocation of the radial head. The fracture is rarely treated with open reduction in children. The open technique is often used to treat adults. A direct blow to the ulnar aspect or a fall while the arm is hyperextended produces this type of injury. If the open reduction approach is chosen, closed reduction of the radial dislocation is attempted and often successful. At times the annular ligament may prevent reduction of the radial head dislocation, and open reduction becomes necessary. There are various deforming forces of the forearm depending on the location of the fracture in relation to the insertion of muscles. These forces are often encountered when treating forearm injuries.

Procedural considerations

The patient is placed in the supine position with or without a hand table. A tourniquet is applied and inflated as needed. A soft-tissue set and large bone set are required as well as bone-reduction clamps and bone-grasping forceps, AO/ASIF instrumentation, plates, and screws, and a power drill.

Operative procedure
Fixation with Dynamic Compression Plate (Fig. 22-62)

1. The radial head dislocation is reduced using a closed technique.
2. An incision is made; the ulnar fracture site is dissected.
3. The periosteum is stripped, and the fragments are reapproximated using bone-reduction and grasping forceps.
4. The bone is assessed for placement of a small or large fragment dynamic compression plate (DCP), with at least three screw holes proximal and three distal to the fracture site.
5. A concentric (neutral) hole is drilled into the ulna through one of the screw holes on the plate to the opposite cortex.
6. After the hole is gauged, the selected size of screw is inserted, with purchase of the opposite cortex ensured. A second screw is inserted on the opposite fragment in the neutral position.
7. On either side of the fracture site an eccentric (loading) hole is drilled in the same fashion to the opposite cortex. The hole is gauged and tapped, and the screw is inserted.
8. The selected screw is entered eccentrically into the plate. As the screw seeks the center of the screw hole while riding the bevel of the screw hole, it compresses the fracture site. This screw should be tightened down, and the other screws should be slightly loosened.

9. The fracture site is now visualized as the action of the screw in the plate compresses the fracture site.
10. The remaining bone screws are inserted following the same procedure.
11. The wound is irrigated and closed; a drain may or may not be inserted.
12. A long-arm posterior splint is placed with the arm in 110 to 120 degrees of flexion.

NOTE: The dynamic compression technique was developed in Europe, particularly Switzerland and Germany, and is marketed in this country under several different trade names including AO/ASIF group (Synthes) and the European compression technique (Zimmer). Dynamic compression plates are stockier and stronger than the semitubular plates mentioned earlier for distal humeral fractures. They are used to plate shaft fractures where stress forces on the shaft are greater and stronger plates are required. Dynamic compression plating to midshaft fractures of the femur is less common today. The insertion of rods evens the stress load of the bone. Fractures of the radius and ulna may also be treated with Rush rods, a device similar to Enders nails. The technique of dynamic compression plating is generally achieved in the same manner illustrated in the previous procedure when treating all shaft fractures. This technique appears later in the chapter.

Correction of Colles' Fracture with External Fixation

Colles' fracture is a dorsally angulated fracture of the distal end of the radius. Most of these fractures can be managed successfully with closed reduction and immobilization, but external fixation has recently gained wide popularity, especially in the case of a comminuted, intraarticular fracture. Internal fixation is indicated when the distal end of the radius is severely comminuted and displaced. In these cases, Kirschner wires are used for internal fixation.[13]

Procedural considerations

The patient is in the supine position with the arm extended on a hand table and may require traction by means of finger traps. A soft-tissue set and small bone set is required, along with a power drill, small elevator, and the external fixation device of choice. Fluoroscopy will be necessary.

Operative procedure (see application of the unilateral frame)

1. Small incisions are made, and two pins are placed through the second metacarpal, one at the base and the other distalward a distance equal to the span between the openings in the fixator.
2. Two pins are placed in the radius 8 cm from the styloid.

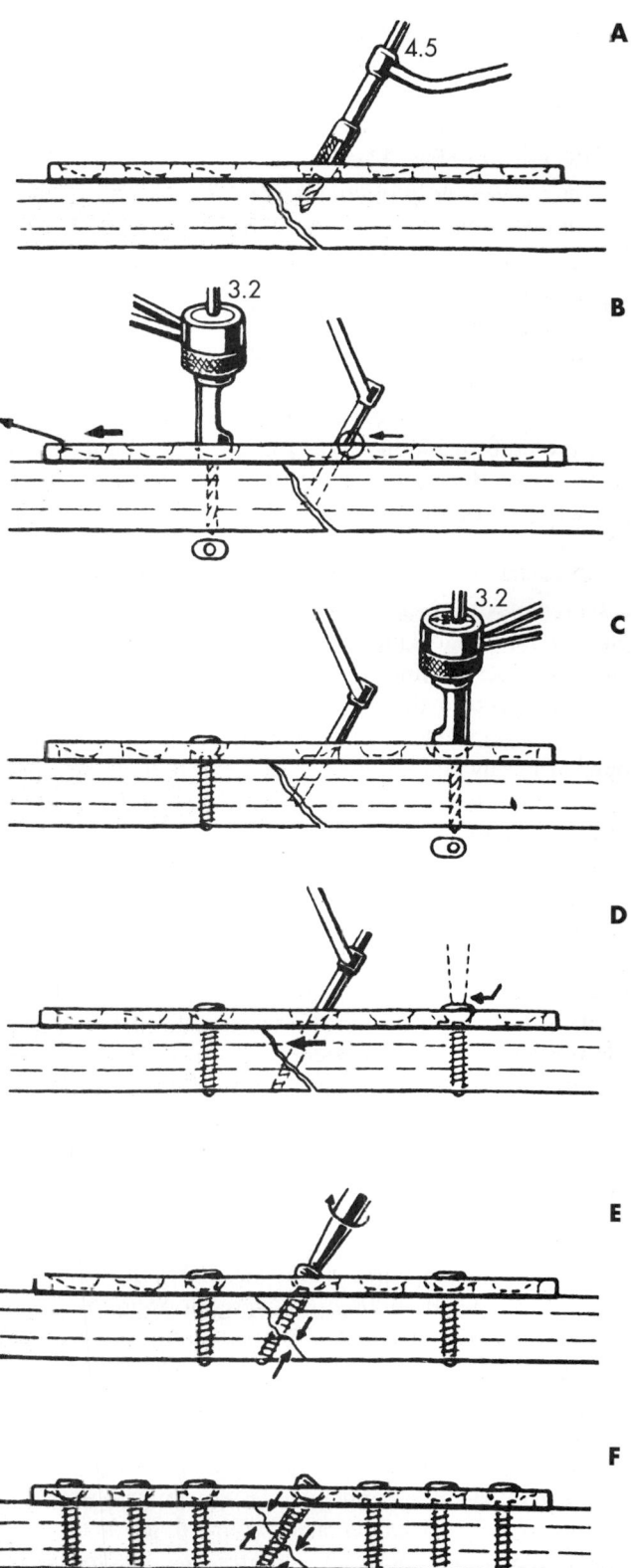

FIGURE 22–62 Fixation with dynamic compression plate. **A,** Gliding hole with drill bit. **B,** Fracture reduced, drill sleeve inserted and the fracture drawn together, a hole drilled and screw inserted in the neutral position to correct the fracture. **C,** and **D,** One screw is inserted in load position (eccentric) into the other fragment; as the screw is tightened, axial compression is generated. **E,** Lag screw inserted across the fracture site. **F,** Remaining screws inserted in the neutral position.

3. Pin placement is confirmed in both the AP and lateral views.
4. A frame is constructed to incorporate all four pins.
5. Reduction of the fracture is obtained, and the frame is secured (see Fig. 22-43).
6. Postreduction films are taken to check alignment and pin position.

SURGERY OF THE HAND

Hand surgery has become highly specialized. There are numerous procedures for treating bone, soft tissue, or both, that the orthopedic perioperative nurse encounters. Many of the techniques and principles applied to large bone are used in the treatment of hand injuries. Hand procedures range from carpal tunnel release to complex digit reimplantation.

Tourniquets are often used for hand surgery, as regional anesthetic techniques are. The operating team usually sits down at a hand table but may move to areas such as the iliac crest for bone grafting. The instruments for hand surgery are common to orthopedics but on a smaller scale. Many instruments and reconstruction systems have been developed primarily for hand surgery. Air or battery power drills and saws are frequently used. The surgery often requires the use of eye loupes (glasses for magnification) or the microscope.

Carpal Tunnel Release

Carpal tunnel syndrome results from entrapment of the median nerve on the volar surface of the wrist caused by thickened synovium, trauma, or aberrant muscles. Carpal tunnel syndrome is frequently seen in patients with rheumatoid synovitis or malaligned Colles' fracture and is associated with obesity, Raynaud's disease, pregnancy, and occupational injuries. The symptoms are pain, numbness, tingling of the fingers, and weakness of the intrinsic thumb muscles. These symptoms are usually reversible after the flexor retinaculum is incised so that the compressed median nerve is relieved. Carpal tunnel release may be completed endoscopically, resulting in the release of the median nerve with minimal trauma, or by open incision.

Procedural considerations

The patient is placed in the supine position with the arm extended on a hand table. A tourniquet is applied to the forearm or upper arm. A hand set is required. The endoscopic approach requires use of specialized equipment.

Operative procedure

1. A curvilinear, longitudinal volar incision is made from the proximal side of the palm, paralleling the thenar crease and extending to the crease of the wrist across the wrist joint.

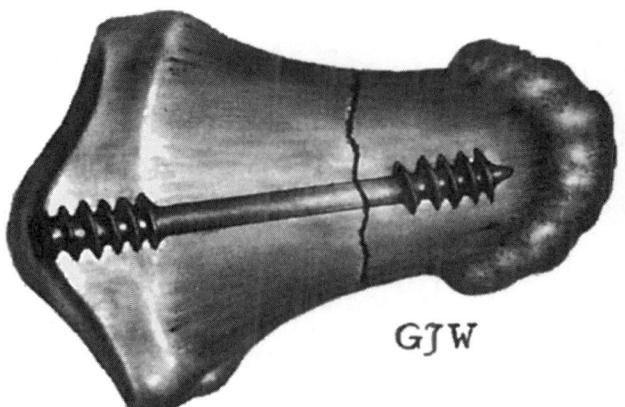

FIGURE 22-63 Herbert bone screw placement.

2. The deep transverse carpal ligament is divided. Care must be taken to avoid damage to the median nerve.
3. At this point the release is completed.
4. If indicated, a tenosynovectomy is completed.
5. The wound is closed, and a compression dressing and volar splint are applied.

Excision of Ganglions

A ganglion is a cystic lesion arising from a joint capsule or tendon sheath and containing glassy, clear fluid. Ganglions are most common on the dorsum of the wrist, palm of the hand, and dorsolateral aspect of the foot. Ganglions appear as firm masses that vary in size. They may resolve spontaneously but occasionally require excision because of discomfort or cosmetic reasons.

Procedural considerations

The patient is supine with the arm extended on a hand table, and a tourniquet is applied to the forearm or upper arm. A hand set is required.

Operative procedure

1. A transverse incision is made over the ganglion.
2. The ganglion is excised with a rim of normal joint capsule or tendon sheath at its base.
3. The wound is irrigated and closed, and a pressure dressing is applied. A plaster splint may also be applied to immobilize the affected joint.

Fractures of Carpal Bones

Most fractures of the carpal bones are treated by closed reduction and immobilization. However, it is occasionally necessary to operate on a fracture because of acute instability, delayed union, or nonunion. The scaphoid is the most commonly fractured carpal bone. Internal fixation is accomplished with Kirschner wires, small compression screws, or minifragment compression plates and screws. A bone graft from the distal end of the radius or olecranon may be taken.

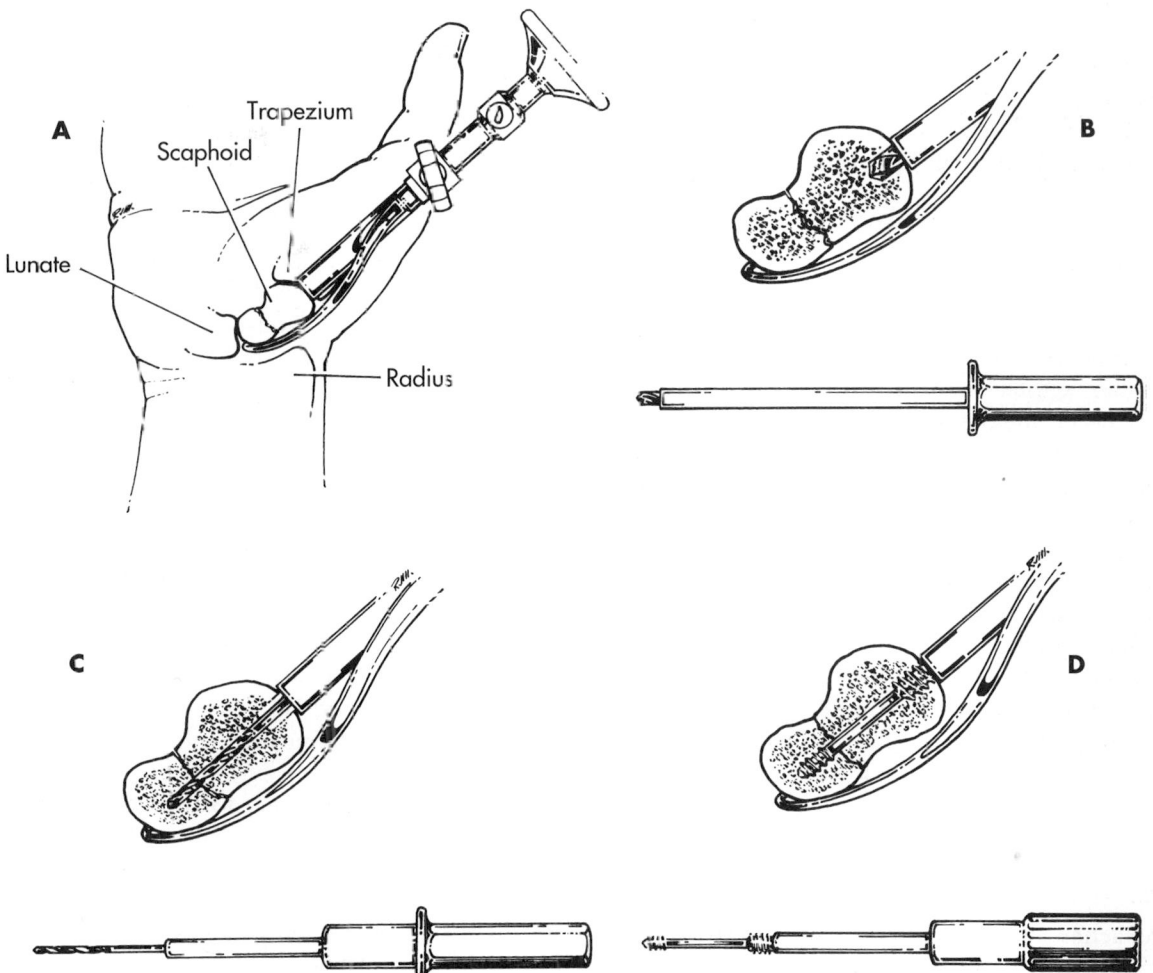

FIGURE 22-64   Repair of the scaphoid. **A,** Fracture site is exposed. **B,** Alignment guide reduces the fracture and guides all subsequent instrumentation. **B,** The screw hole is drilled by hand. **C,** The tap is inserted. **D,** The Herbert bone screw is inserted through the drill guide.

For displaced or unstable scaphoid fractures the Herbert bone screw (Fig. 22-63) has several advantages: (1) strong internal fixation, (2) compression at the fracture site with reversed threads at each end of the screw, and (3) reduced time required for external immobilization.

Procedural considerations

The patient is supine with the arm extended on a hand table. A pneumatic tourniquet is applied to either the forearm or upper arm. Fluoroscopy should be available. A soft-tissue and small bone or hand set are required, in addition to the Herbert screw set. If a minifragment compression set is used, a power drill and smooth Kirschner wires will also be needed. A bone graft set should also be available.

Operative procedure (Fig. 22-64)

1. A longitudinal skin incision is made over the palmar surface of the wrist.

2. The superficial palmar branch of the radial artery is ligated and divided.
3. The flexor carpi radialis tendon sheath is incised and retracted to expose the capsule of the wrist.
4. The capsule is entered, and the scaphoid fracture is identified and inspected to determine the need for bone grafting.
5. The fracture is reduced by manipulation and temporarily held with small Kirschner wires.
6. The scaphoid fracture is reduced and held with the Herbert jig.
7. A short drill bit and then a long drill bit is inserted to create a channel for the screw.
8. The Herbert screw is then inserted and turned until it is seated within the scaphoid.
9. Bone graft is placed around the fracture site if needed. (The loss of significant bone can often be corrected by fashioning a strut of bone from graft.)
10. The wound is irrigated and closed.

11. A splint is applied with thumb spica or long-arm cast incorporating the thumb.

SURGERY OF THE HIP AND LOWER EXTREMITY

Fractures of the Acetabulum

Fractures of the acetabulum usually result from high-energy injuries such as motor vehicle accidents and falls with a landing on the extended extremities. The fracture is directly related to the force transmitted to the femoral head through the greater trochanter or lower extremity. Management of these fractures can often present the orthopedic team with a complex and challenging task. Improvements in implant and instrument design, radiographic technique, and the emergence of magnetic resonance imaging (MRI) and computerized tomography (CT) have revolutionized the management of these fractures. Indications for internal fixation of acetabular fractures include (1) greater than 2 mm of displacement, (2) presence of intraarticular loose bodies, (3) inability to reduce under closed methods, (4) unstable fractures of the posterior acetabular wall, and (5) open fractures. Internal fixation is usually delayed 3 to 10 days to allow time for the patient to be evaluated and clinically stabilized. Until internal fixation is undertaken, the fracture is reduced by means of closed methods and the patient maintained in skeletal traction. General anesthesia may be required for closed reduction and placement of skeletal traction when the acetabular fracture is severely displaced or dislocated. The fractures are divided into five basic groups: fractures of the posterior wall, posterior column, anterior wall, anterior column, and transverse fractures (Fig. 22-65). Internal fixation is accomplished with reconstruction plates and screws, total hip replacement with bone grafting (see total hip replacement, p. 876), or fusion if the fracture cannot be reduced.

Procedural considerations

The surgical approach depends on the type and area of the fracture and the surgeon's preference. The patient is placed on a fracture table or standard OR bed in the lateral or supine position. General anesthesia is generally the anesthetic of choice, but the procedure can be performed solely with a regional block or concurrent epidural infusion. Procedures of this magnitude can be lengthy and involve considerable blood loss. Appropriate measures should be taken to avoid complications attributable to these factors. The room should remain warm, the patient protected from pressure injury, and red blood cell salvaging techniques employed.

A soft-tissue set, large bone, acetabular instruments (Fig. 22-66), pelvic reduction clamps, reconstruction plates and screws (both 3.5 and 4.5 mm), plate-bending irons, and a femoral distractor will be necessary. A total hip set should be available. Also needed are Kirschner wires

and Steinman pins, large fragment bone screws, pulsatile lavage supplies, and power drill and reamer. Fluoroscopy may be used for this procedure.

Operative procedure
Posterolateral Approach

1. A lateral incision is made over the acetabular fracture site.
2. The joint is opened and the femur dislocated from the acetabulum.
3. Self-retaining or hand-held hip retractors are used to maintain exposure of the acetabulum.
4. Measures such as a femoral distraction or osteotomy of the trochanter can be used to improve visualization and access to the fracture.
5. The fracture is reduced using bone clamps, forceps, and a ball spike.
6. Reduction is accomplished in gradual steps using Kirschner wires to hold the fragments temporarily in place.
7. Reconstruction plates are fitted and contoured to the fracture site and secured with screws.
8. Long cancellous lag screw fixation is also used to provide interfragmentary compression, particularly in column fractures.
9. Bone graft may be needed for additional fixation. A femoral head allograft technique is sometimes used, in which the allograft is mushroomed to create a new acetabulum.
10. The wound is irrigated with antibiotic solution delivered by pulsatile lavage, ensuring the articular surfaces are free from loose bodies.
11. The wound is closed, drains are inserted, and pressure dressings are applied.
12. The leg is maintained in abduction and external rotation with traction.

NOTE: If there is associated traumatic dislocation of the hip with the acetabular fracture, prompt treatment should address the dislocation. The dislocation should be reduced as soon as possible and skeletal traction inserted if needed to maintain reduction. Acetabular fractures often accompany femoral shaft fractures, which also need to be treated concurrently with the surgeon's desired method (see femoral shaft fractures).

Hip Fractures

Hip fractures are classified by anatomic location and can be categorized as femoral neck fractures, intertrochanteric fractures and subtrochanteric fractures (Fig. 22-67), and these can each be subclassified. Fracture dislocations also have a classification system and treatment protocol. Fractures of the greater or lesser trochanters alone are less common and can usually be treated nonoperatively.

Femoral neck fractures and intertrochanteric fractures commonly require open reduction and internal fixation. Neck fractures are more common in women because of

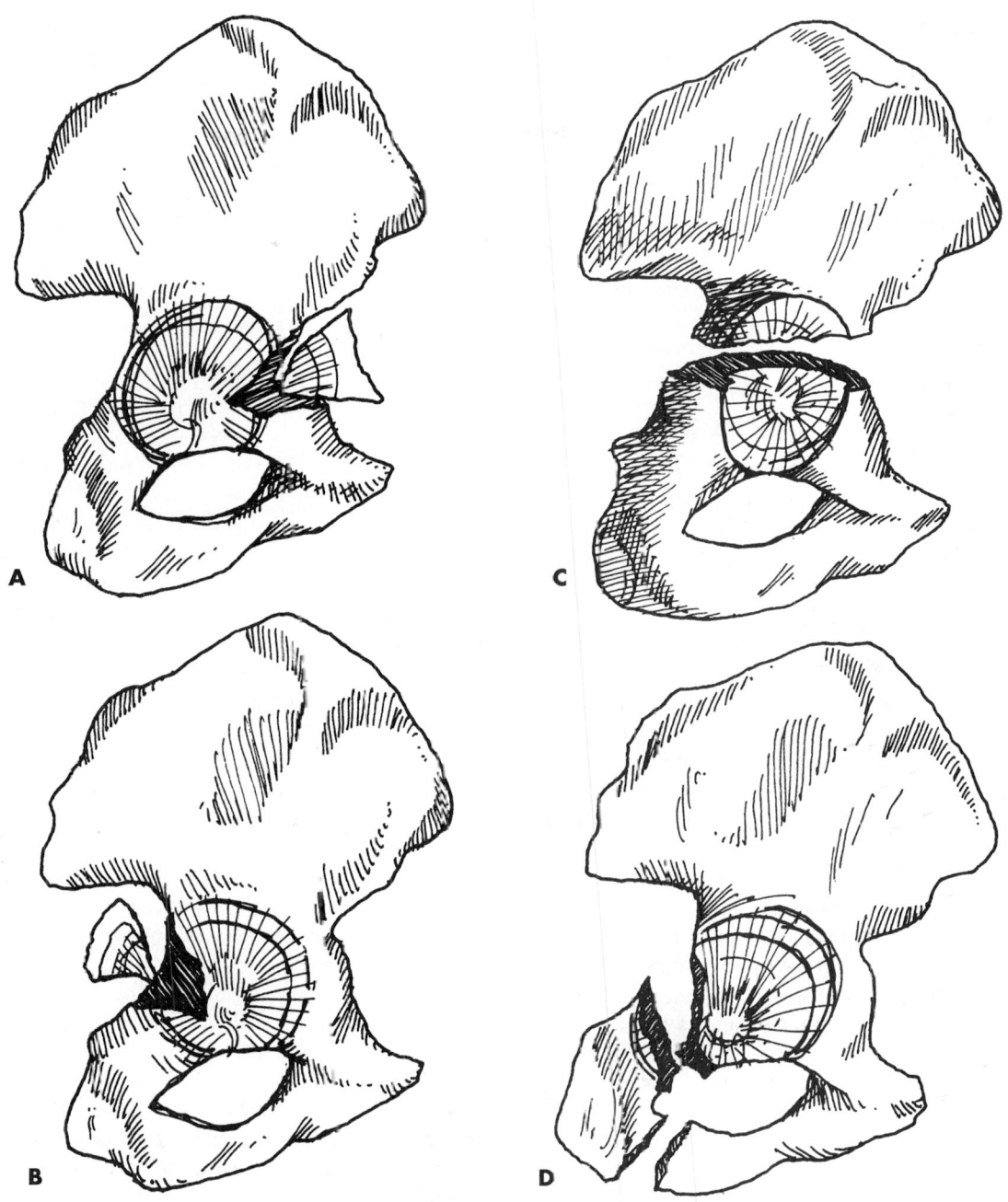

FIGURE 22-65   Acetabular fractures. **A,** Anterior wall. **B,** Posterior wall. **C,** Transverse. **D,** Posterior column.

several factors, including osteoporosis. Most elderly patients require a preoperative medical evaluation to define and treat anesthetic risks. However, effort should be made to correct the fracture as soon as possible to avoid complications related to immobility, skin pressure, pulmonary congestion, and thrombophlebitis. Avascular necrosis and degenerative changes can occur as a result of diminished blood supply to the femoral head, resulting in irreversible changes. Buck's traction may be placed preoperatively to reduce discomfort from muscle spasm caused by overriding of fracture fragments.

Manipulation, reduction, and internal fixation of these fractures is greatly facilitated by use of a fracture table,

which also permits adequate radiographic examination to determine placement of the internal fixation. Subtrochanteric fractures are addressed in a later section on trauma.

Intertrochanteric fractures

Intertrochanteric fractures most frequently occur in older patients. The fractures usually unite without difficulty. However, because the lower extremity is externally rotated at the fracture site, internal fixation is necessary to prevent malunion. Internal fixation allows patients to be mobilized earlier, thereby decreasing mortality and morbidity.

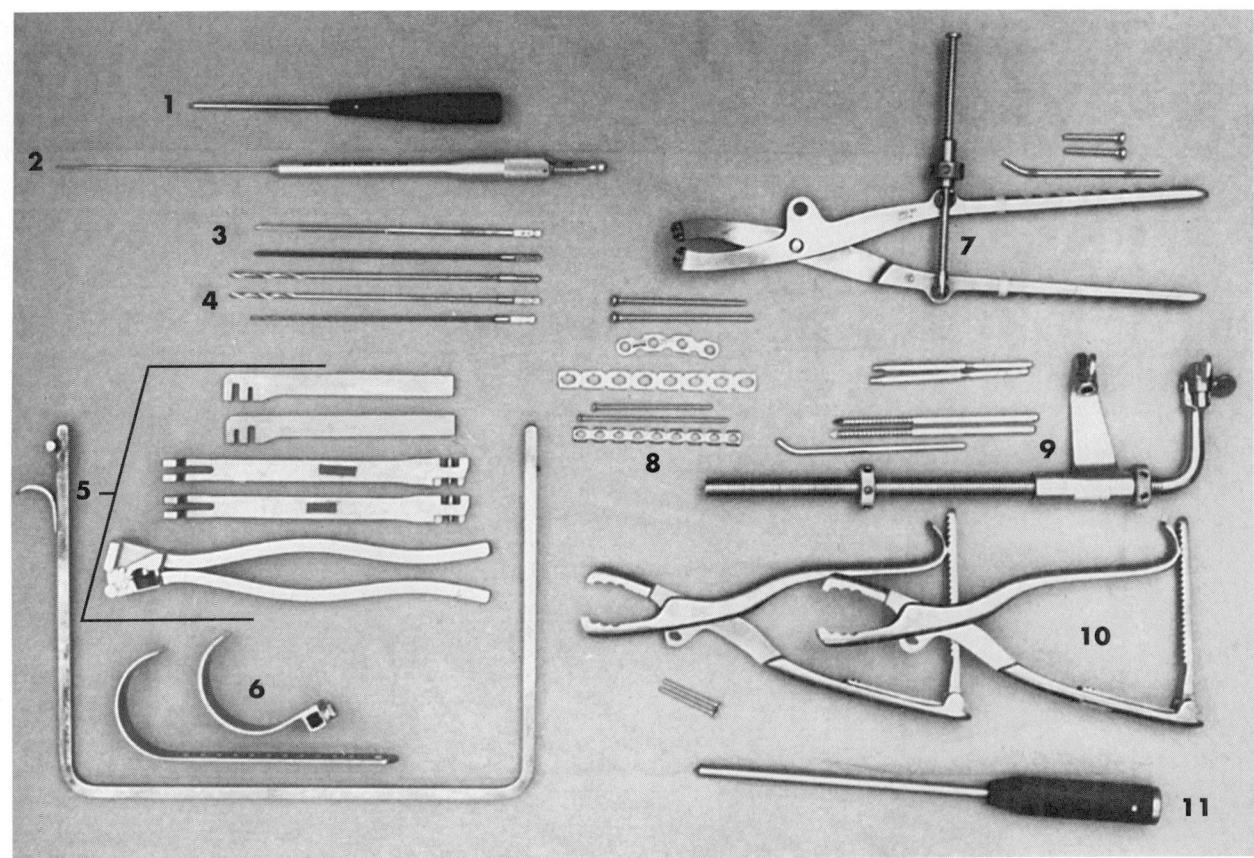

FIGURE 22-66 Acetabular fracture instruments with implants: *1,* Screwdriver, small and large (not shown); *2,* depth gauge; *3,* tap; *4,* drill bits; *5,* plate-bending irons; *6,* initial incision retractor with blades; *7,* pelvic reduction clamp with accessories; *8,* reconstruction plates and screws; *9,* femoral distractor and accessories; *10,* Faraboef forceps with screws; *11,* ball spike.

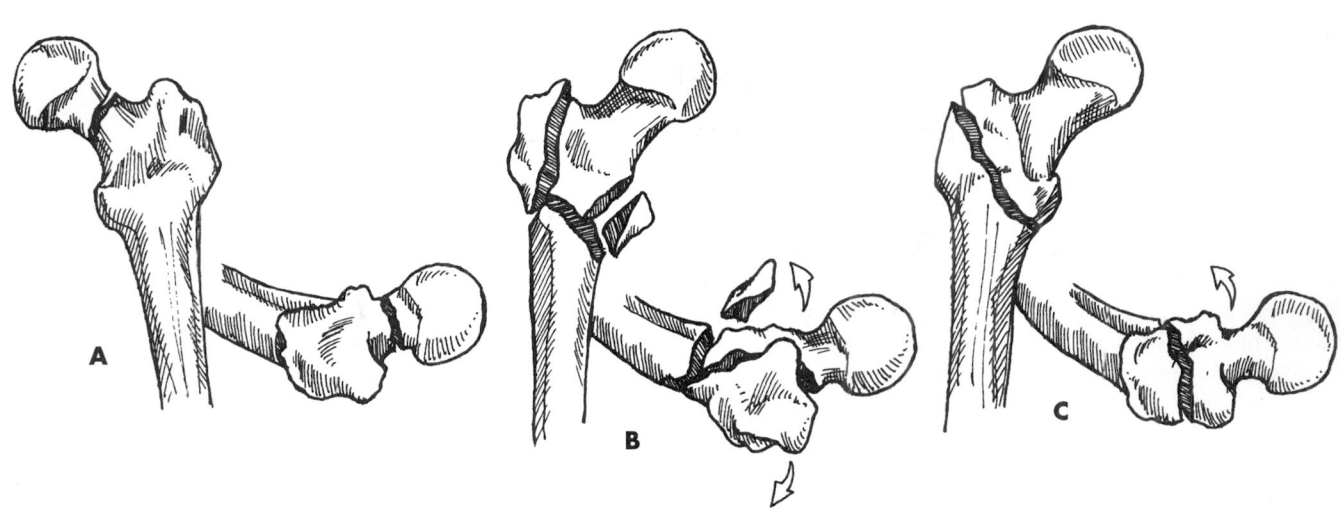

FIGURE 22-67 Proximal femur fractures. **A,** Midcervical. **B,** Comminuted subtrochanteric. **C,** Intertrochanteric.

Procedural Considerations

The patient is placed in the supine position on the fracture table, and the fracture is reduced by manipulating the extremity and confirming with fluoroscopy (see Fig. 22-18). Various internal fixation devices, including Ambi, Freelock, DHS hip screws, and medullary fixation (see section on trauma, p. 860) may be used. Success of the procedure is determined by bone quality, fragment configuration, ability to reduce adequately, implant design, and implant-insertion technique. Intraoperative blood loss is minimized because the hip joint is not opened.

A soft-tissue and large bone set are required, in addition to the compression hip screw instrumentation and implants, bone-reduction and plate-holding clamps, and a power drill and reamer.

Operative Procedure
Freelock compression plate and lag screw
(Fig. 22-68)

1. The fracture is reduced by closed reduction and maintained by adjusting the table traction.
2. Reduction is checked in both the AP and lateral views with fluoroscopy.
3. An incision is made from the greater trochanter distally to accommodate the length of the implant.
4. The dissection is completed through the fascia lata and the vastus lateralis is exposed.
5. The reduction is visually confirmed; the guide pin is inserted after determining the angle of plate to be used. A 135-degree angle plate is commonly used.
6. The pin should be centralized in the femoral head approximately 1 cm short of the femoral articular surface. Care must be taken to not enter the joint space, since this might result in arthritic changes. Further penetration of the pin through the acetabulum and into the pelvis can potentially damage large vessels or bowel. A second pin can be used to control rotation in high neck or unstable fractures.
7. The lateral cortex is opened with the conical cannulated drill bit over the guide pin.
8. The depth gauge is placed over the guide pin. The size of the required lag screw is determined from the guide.
9. A double-barrel reamer is adjusted to correspond to the depth of the guide pin. The cortex is reamed over the guide pin to create a channel for the lag screw and barrel of the compression plate.
10. The lag screw channel is tapped to the full distance of reaming to allow proper seating of the lag screw, particularly in young patients with firm bone.

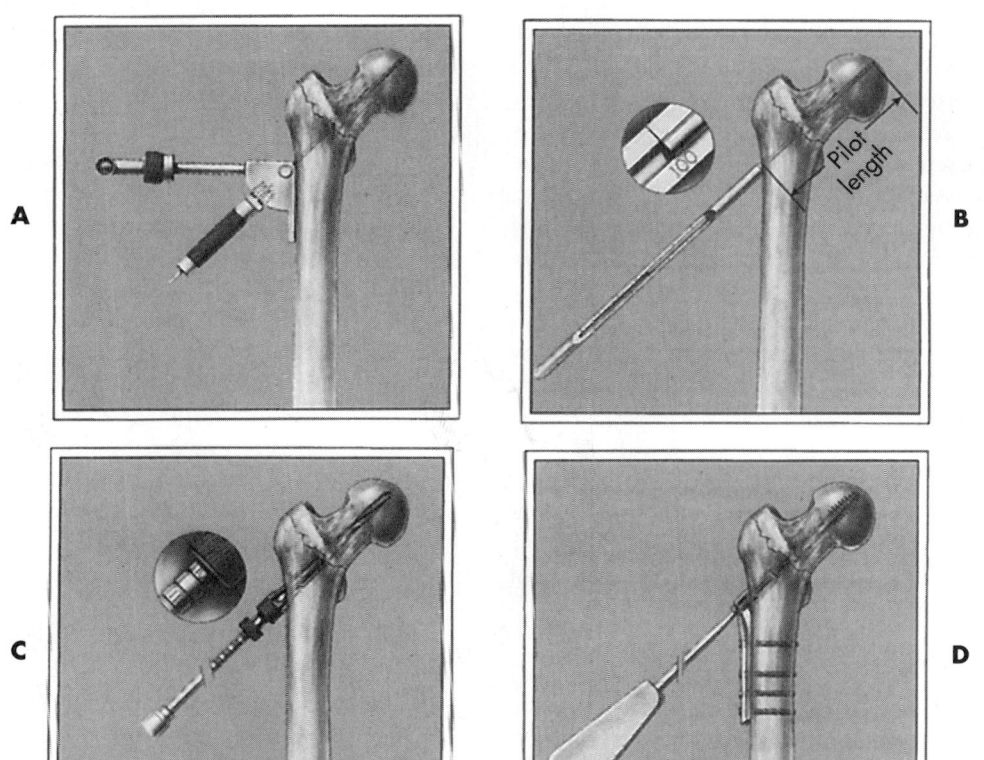

FIGURE 22-68 Intertrochanteric fracture repair with compression plate. **A,** Guide pin is inserted. **B,** Depth of guide pin is obtained. **C,** The lag screw channel is reamed. **D,** The tube/plate is applied and lag screw inserted.

Reaming depth of osteoporotic bone is reduced 5 mm, and the tap depth is reduced approximately 1 to 2 cm to allow sufficient screw purchase.

11. The plate angle can be confirmed with a trial; the implants (plate and lag screw) are then delivered to the back table.

12. The plate, lag screw, and insertion wrench with centering sleeve are assembled. A screw stabilizer is passed through the center of the insertion wrench and threaded into the lag screw.

13. The entire assembly is placed over the guide pin and the lag screw is advanced to the desired depth, with periodic verification with fluoroscopy. Penetration of the lag screw through the femoral articular surface must be avoided.

14. The insertion wrench is disassembled, and the barrel of the compression plate is placed over the lag screw. The barrel of the plate should fully cover the lag screw. The plate is seated on the lateral femoral shaft.

15. The plate is secured to the shaft of the femur with plate-holding forceps. The guide pin is removed. At this point traction can be released to allow compression of the fracture site.

16. Screw holes are made using the drill guide and a 3.5 mm drill bit. The length is determined, and cortical screws are inserted through the screw hole on the plate with sufficient purchase on the opposite cortex of the shaft. The top screw hole on the plate can accept a 6.5 mm cancellous screw, which can be angled for better purchase in comminuted fractures.

17. Traction is released if not done previously. A compression screw is inserted into the barrel of the screw and threaded into the back of the lag screw, compressing the fracture site. The compression screw exerts a powerful force. The amount of compression applied should correlate with the quality of the bone.

18. The wound is irrigated and closed. Two suction drains may be inserted during closure. Weight bearing may begin as early as the first postoperative day depending on reduction and quality of bone.

NOTE: Many of the same techniques and principles of long bone fracture fixation are used in treatment of various types of hip fractures. The different screw types, dynamic compression, and lag screw effect are described throughout the chapter (see ulnar fractures, p. 844).

Femoral neck fractures: internal fixation

Anatomic reduction is necessary before internal fixation of femoral neck fractures because of the high incidence of associated complications, such as nonunion and avascular necrosis of the femoral head. The degree of displacement, tamponade pressure from intracapsular bleeding, and delays in reduction and fixation can affect the blood supply to the femoral head. These factors contribute to death of the femoral head and failed fixation. Growing children

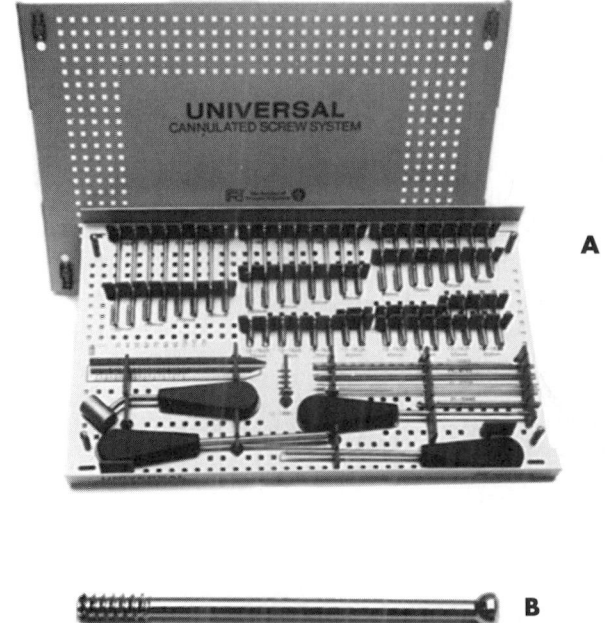

FIGURE 22-69   **A,** Universal cannulated screw system. **B,** Universal cannulated screw.

may sustain fractures through the epiphyseal growth plate (slipped capital femoral epiphysis). These injuries are treated by reduction and internal fixation of the femoral head, similar to the procedures used in the adult. The Garden and AO nomenclature are the most popular classifications for grading the fractures. Pins of various designs, such as Knowles and Hagie pins and universal cannulated screws (Fig. 22-69), are used for fixation (Fig. 22-70). In cases of severe comminution or avascular necrosis of the femoral head the patient may require a prosthetic replacement (see total joint arthroplasty, p. 874).

Procedural Considerations

The patient is placed on a fracture table under general or regional anesthesia (spinal or epidural). Slight traction and external rotation are adjusted on the affected side. A soft-tissue set and large-bone set are required as well as the fixation device of choice with instrumentation, Kirschner wires, Cobra retractors, a power drill, and fluoroscopy.

Operative Procedure
Cannulated screw fixation for nondisplaced femoral neck fractures

1. The fracture is exposed through a 5 cm lateral incision over the greater trochanter.

2. The dissection is carried through the subcutaneous and fascial layers; the vastus lateralis is detached anteriorly and retracted, exposing the femoral neck.

3. Two guide pins are driven into the middle of the femoral head, one anterior and one posterior, within 5 mm of subchondral bone; a third pin is placed

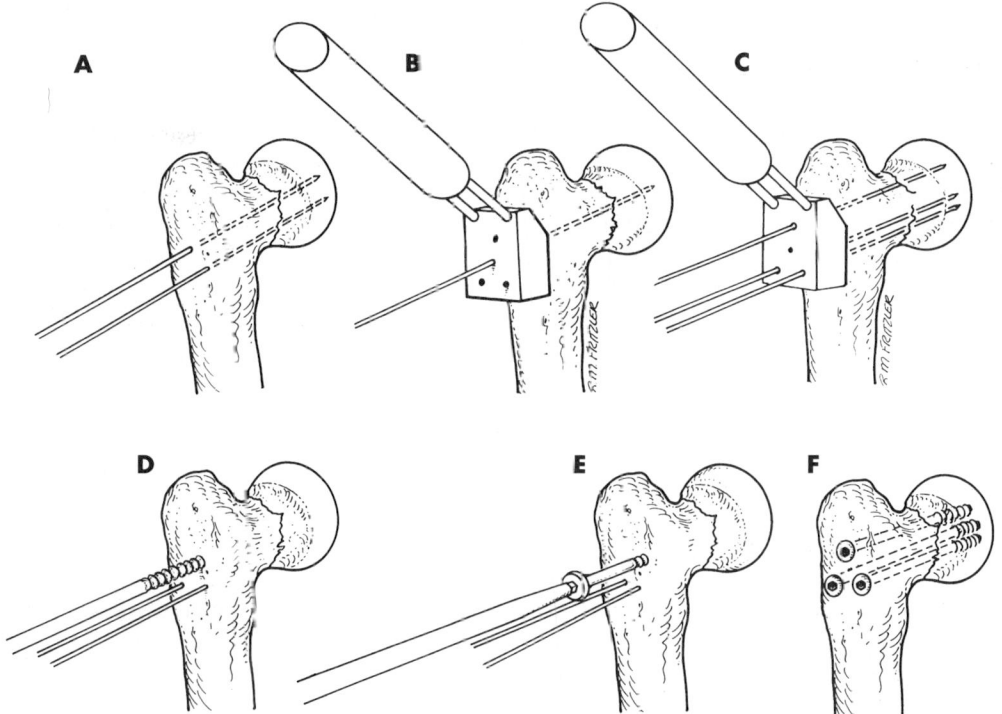

FIGURE 22-70 Internal fixation with cannulated screws (AO technique). **A,** Guide wire parallel to anteversion wire. **B,** Guide wire placed over positioning wire through diamond-patterned positioning holes. **C,** Guide wire placed through each of outer triangle of holes. **D,** Cannulated tap passed over guide wire to tap near cortex. **E,** Large cannulated screw inserted over guide wire. **F,** Remaining screws inserted in same manner.

adjacent to the medial cortex at a 135-degree angle. Care must be taken to not violate the articular surface.

4. The guide pins are measured for correct screw length, and the cannulated screws are inserted over the guide pin without applying compression until all are seated.

5. Compression of the anterior screws is completed first and the posterior screws last to avoid collapse of the posterior aspect of the neck.

6. Traction is released, and the fracture site visualized with fluoroscopy while the hip is rotated through a full range of motion.

7. Radiographs are taken to verify the position of the screws; the wound is irrigated and closed.

NOTE: Screw protrusion into the joint space can be disastrous to the articular surface. Radiopaque dye can be injected to rule out communication with the joint.

Femoral head prosthetic replacement: unipolar and bipolar implants

With the development of current cement fixation techniques and the evolution of the modular bipolar and monopolar design, the use of the fixed endoprosthesis such as the Austin-Moore and Thompson designs (Fig. 22-71) declined. The use of the Austin-Moore has been plagued with complaints of thigh pain and protrusio acetabuli. Revision to a total hip arthroplasty is difficult, and the

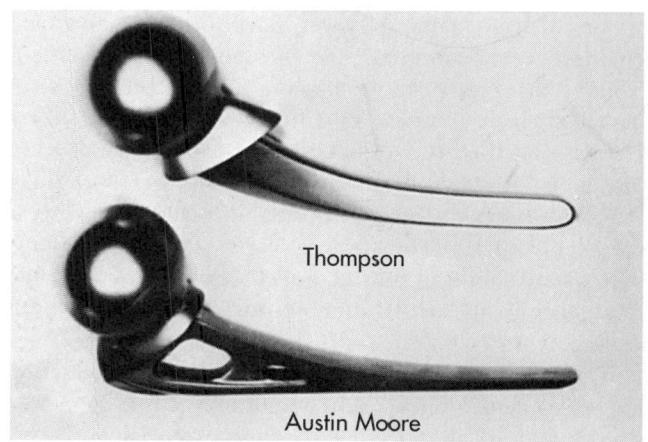

FIGURE 22-71 Femoral endoprosthesis. Austin Moore and Thompson.

complication rate is much higher when the Austin-Moore prosthesis is used. During the early 1980s the bipolar system in conjunction with a cemented femoral stem became popular. Bipolar endoprostheses (Fig. 22-72) were introduced to reduce the shear stresses affecting the acetabular surface, decreasing the motion and friction between the prosthetic head and the acetabulum that is seen with conventional (unipolar) endoprostheses. A femoral head prosthesis is snapped into a rotating

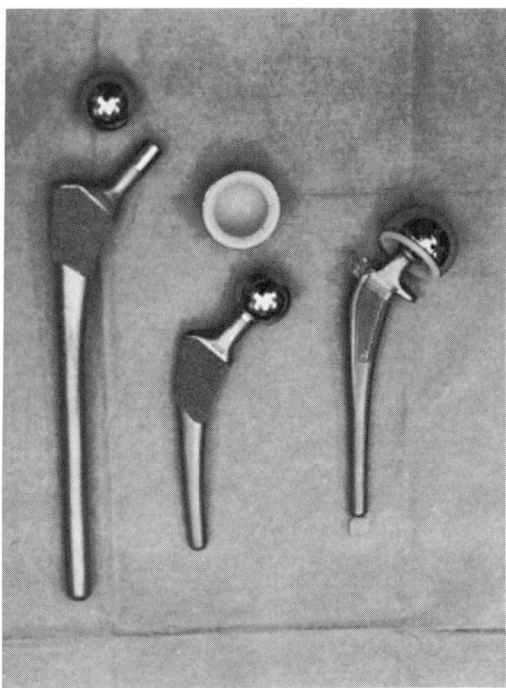

FIGURE 22-72   Modular bipolar endoprosthesis.

polyethylene-lined cup that, when inserted, moves as one unit. Friction occurs between the ball and plastic instead of between the head and the acetabulum. This was a revolutionary design in the mechanics of hip motion and stresses. Current data, however, have some surgeons and engineers reevaluating the use of bipolar prostheses. It is believed that bipolar motion subsides after fibrous growth has taken place, allowing for only unipolar motion. There have also been reports of bone resorption and subsequent prosthetic loosening in cases in which bipolars were used. Researchers are evaluating evidence of metallic head wear of the polyethylene cup creating microscopic debris with a subsequent chemical lysis of bone. Thus, there has been resurgence in the use of unipolar heads for femoral head replacement.

The current trend in health care toward cost reduction has precipitated a further refinement in that prosthesis, the development of the so-called *diagnosis-related group (DRG) prosthesis*. The modular design has been retained allowing for different combinations of head size, neck length, and stem size. Instead of being bipolar, the head is now solid, or unipolar, and the stem is the result of a less costly manufacturing process. The most cost-effective prosthesis is still the original Austin-Moore design, which may be selected for those patients whose life expectancy is short and who have a minimal level of activity. If major deficiencies in the acetabular side of the joint are present a total joint arthroplasty may be performed. In deciding between the hemiarthroplasty and total hip reconstruction, consideration must be given to the patient's medical condition, age, and level of activity.

Current biomaterials, methods of fixation (cemented versus uncemented), prosthetic life, and modular components allow conversion of a hemiarthroplasty (reconstruction of one side of the joint) to a total hip arthroplasty, provided that the femoral component is adequately fixed. Depending on the patient condition, the acetabulum may eventually require arthroplasty as a result of degenerative changes. Improved technology and surgical technique have increased the life span of implanted components. The portion of the implant that articulates within the acetabulum can be removed and replaced with a smaller femoral head. The acetabulum is then prepared for prosthetic implantation by various means of fixation. The ability to convert from hemiarthroplasty to total arthroplasty considerably reduces the amount of surgery required.

Procedural Considerations

The patient is placed in the lateral position after the administration of general or regional anesthesia. A scrub and paint prep is done from the umbilicus down to and including the foot. Instrumentation for total hip replacement should be available but not opened until inspection of the resected joint is completed to determine if a total arthroplasty is required.

The soft-tissue and large-bone sets are required as well as the endoprosthesis instruments, trials, and implants (Fig 22-73). A power reciprocating (Fig 22-74) or sagittal saw may be necessary. Templates or a caliper will be used to measure the size of the femoral head. Bone cement and the supplies for preparing and inserting it should also be available.

Operative Procedure
Modular Austin-Moore endoprosthesis

Both posterior and anterior approaches can be made to the hip to place an endoprosthesis. The posterior approach is quicker and generally involves less blood loss but detractors suggest that there is a higher dislocation rate and a greater chance of infection because of the proximity of the incision to the anus. Although both approaches are widely used, the posterior approach is described as follows:

1. A linear incision is made from 5 cm below the posteroinferior iliac spine toward the posterior aspect of the greater trochanter and distally along the posterior aspect of the proximal femur for 7 mm.
2. The capsule is entered, and the femoral head is removed and gauged with the template. Fragments that may be loose in the acetabulum or attached to the ligamentum teres are removed.
3. A trial cup is inserted into the acetabulum, and axial compression is applied while clearance of lateral motion is checked.
4. The femoral neck is fashioned to achieve an accurate prosthetic fit.
5. A punch is then used to open the medullary canal from

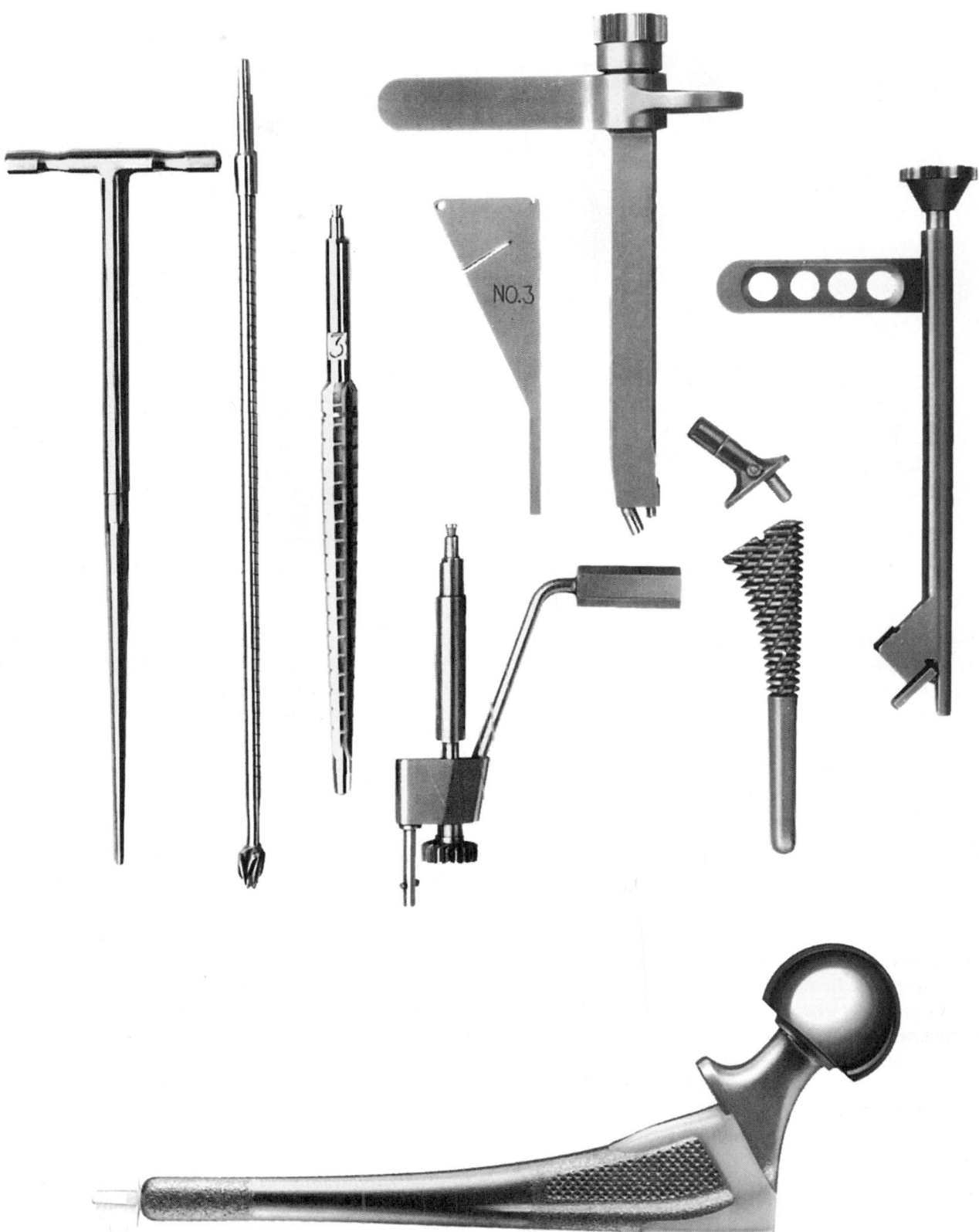

FIGURE 22-73 Instrumentation for endoprosthetic implant.

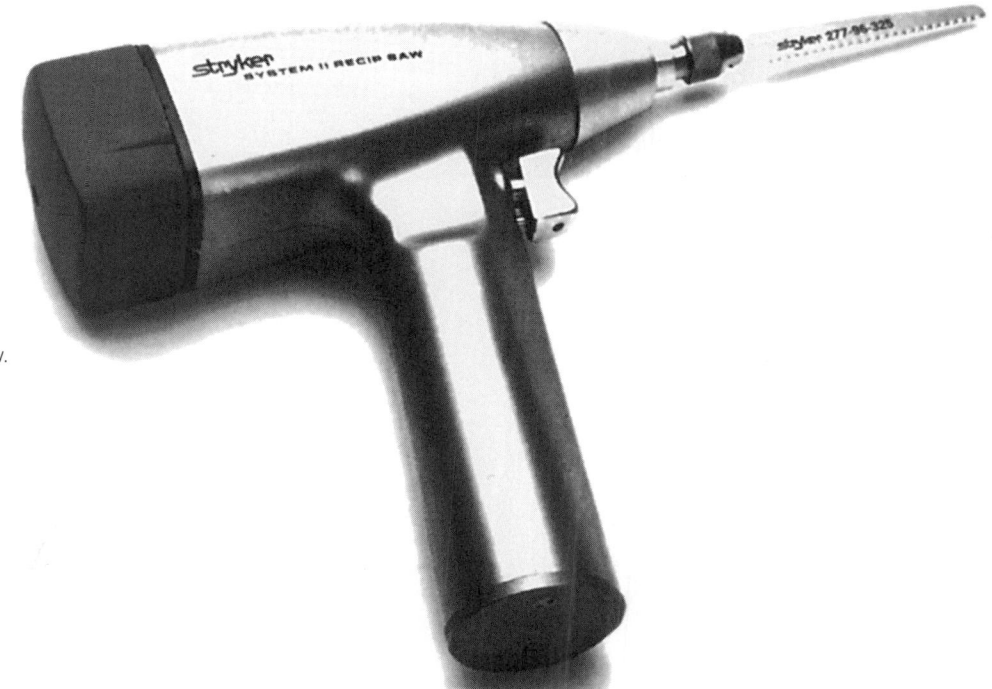

FIGURE 22-74   Reciprocating saw.

the femoral neck. The intramedullary canal is reamed and rasped to accommodate the prosthesis.

6. Once the canal is prepared, the prosthesis of choice is inserted with or without bone cement.

7. A unipolar or bipolar assembly is snapped onto the neck of the femoral stem. The height of the head determines the neck length and is selected after trial reduction.

8. The hip is reduced, and closure is accomplished in layers over suction drains.

Femoral Shaft Fractures: Internal Fixation

Fractures involving the femoral shaft are very common in today's orthopedic operating room. Prolonged immobility, with its attendant complications, and disability can result if femoral shaft fractures are not managed appropriately. The femur is the largest principal load-bearing bone in the body. Fractures of the femoral shaft can be surgically treated with several available techniques. Considerations for treatment are type and location of fracture (location on shaft), the number of segments involved, the degree of comminution (Fig. 22-75), and the activity level of the patient. Femoral shaft fractures are often associated with ipsilateral (same-side) trochanteric or condylar fractures. Pathologic fractures often occur in this region.

Possible treatment methods for femoral shaft fractures are closed reduction, skeletal traction, and femoral cast bracing. External fixation has limited utility when fractures associated with surgical site infection or neurovascular compromise are treated, but it may serve temporarily until

such time that internal fixation can be performed. Although plates and screws are used for femoral shaft fractures, their use is widely disputed and losing popularity. Complications such as bent or broken plates, refractures, and deep surgical site infections have been reported. Intramedullary fixation devices have become the preferred method of treatment. Intramedullary nails and rods increase the load sharing of the bone, making the implant less likely to fracture. Bone healing requires a load across the fracture site to promote osteosynthesis and prevent refracture. The open or closed method of intramedullary nailing can be used with locked and nonlocked nails. Closed methods of intramedullary fixation often minimize exposure of the surgical site and surgical time, resulting in less opportunity for infection.

Intramedullary nail and rod designs vary: (1) flexible nails like the Rusch or Enders type, (2) standard rods such as the Sampson and AO rods, and (3) interlocking nails (see humeral shaft fracture, p. 838) such as the Grosse-Kempf and Russell-Taylor varieties (Fig. 22-76). Closed reduction and intramedullary nailing with or without locking screws has become the method against which other methods are measured. Incidence of scarring, blood loss, and infection are all favorable. Fracture hematoma remains intact at the fracture site, which is important in bone healing, and the rate of bone union is increased.

Procedural considerations

General or epidural anesthetics are used. The patient is placed on the fracture table in the supine position, traction applied, and the fracture manually reduced and confirmed

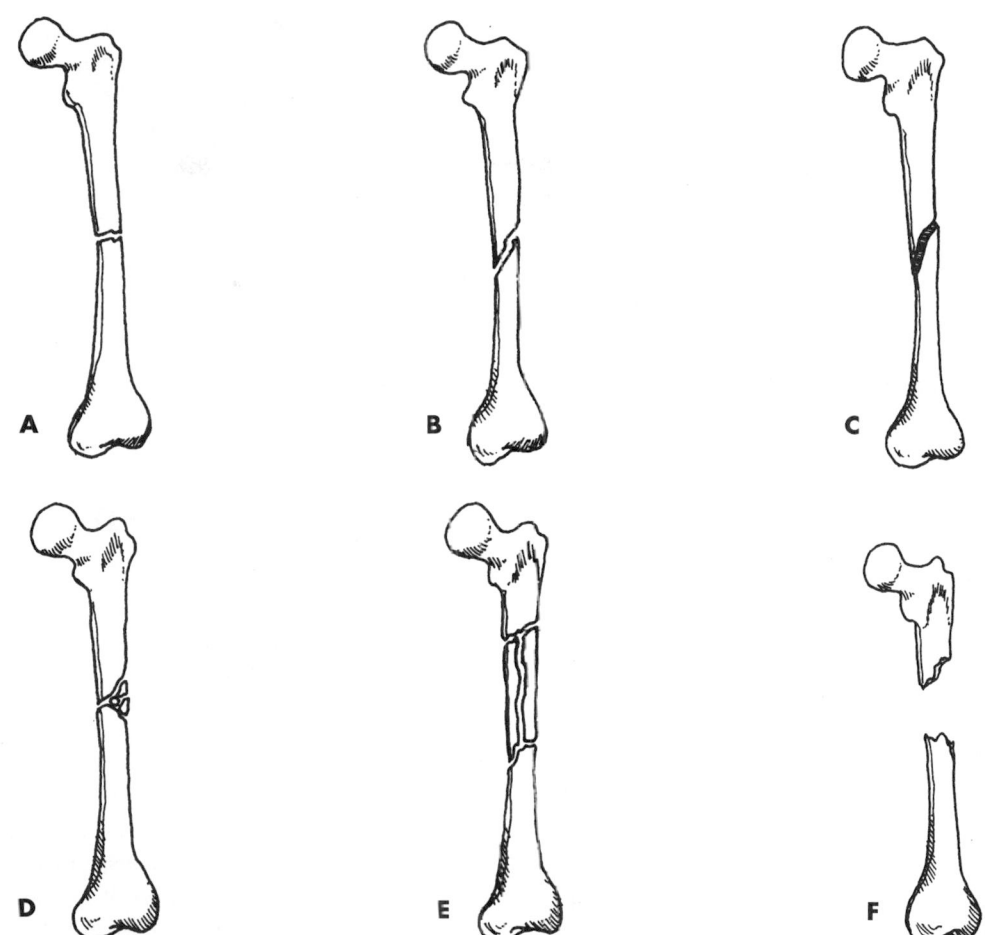

FIGURE 22–75   Femoral shaft fractures. **A,** Transverse. **B,** Oblique. **C,** Spiral. **D,** Comminuted. **E,** Longitudinal split. **F,** Complete bone loss.

with fluoroscopy. If the fracture is profoundly unstable, care must be taken during manipulation to prevent neurovascular complications. For open intramedullary fixation, extra retractors and bone instruments may be required. For a percutaneous reduction, a soft-tissue set and large-bone set are required in addition to the intramedullary nail implants and associated instruments, a power reamer and drill, and long guide wires for reamers. This procedure requires the use of fluoroscopy. A skeletal traction tray (see Fig. 22-22) with Steinman pins may be necessary.

Operative procedure
Russell-Taylor Rod with or without Locking Screws

1. An incision is made over the tip of the greater trochanter and continued proximally and medially for 6 to 8 cm. The fascia of the gluteus is incised, and the piriformis fossa is palpated.

2. With a threaded guide pin followed by cannulated reamers or by use of an awl, the trochanteric fossa is

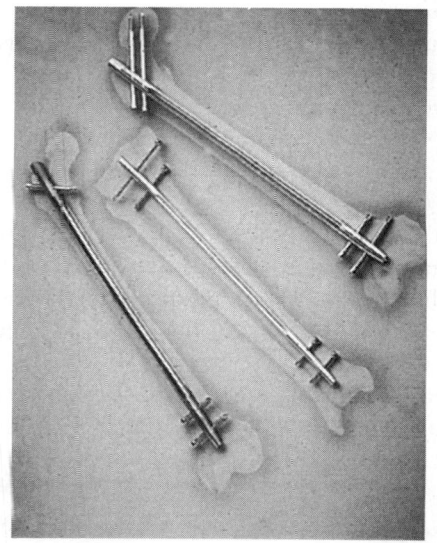

FIGURE 22-76   Interlocking intramedullary nails.

identified, and the cortex is penetrated. A 3.2 mm guide rod is inserted to the level of the fracture. A curved guide pin is available for more severely displaced fractures.

3. Under fluoroscopy, the guide wire is advanced across the fracture site and into the distal fragment until the ball tip of the guide wire reaches the level of the epiphyseal scar. A second guide wire is held against the portion of the guide wire extending out of the proximal femur, and the length is measured. That measurement is subtracted from 900 mm (total guide wire length) to determine the length of the intramedullary nail required.

4. The cannulated reamers are placed sequentially over the guide wire. The entire femur is reamed at 0.5 mm increments. The entire shaft, and especially the fracture site, should be visualized with fluoroscopy as the reamers pass.

5. The final reamer size should be verified with the reamer gauge. The femur is reamed 1 mm over the selected nail diameter. Inserting a nail in an inadequately reamed femur or inserting a nail that is too large can cause severe bone splitting and comminution.

6. The proximal screw guide/slap hammer is assembled onto the nail. The nail is oriented to match the curve of the femur.

7. Using the handle of the inserter, the rotation of the nail is controlled, and the nail is driven into the femur. The nail is fully seated when the proximal screw guide is flush with the greater trochanter. The inserter is disengaged from the slap hammer.

8. Using the power drill and correct drill sleeves, a 4.8 mm hole is drilled through both cortices, and the depth is measured directly off the bit.

9. Through the appropriate drill sleeve, a 6.4 mm self-tapping locking screw is inserted, and the drill sleeve is removed.

10. By fluoroscopy the distal screw holes are confirmed as perfect circles on the screen. The distal targeting device is mounted on the nail followed by the left or right adapter block. The adapter block is adjusted until the calibration reads the length of the nail. The cross hairs are aligned in the adapter to the holes in the distal nail, with confirmation by fluoroscopy.

11. An incision is made through the adapter block over the distal femur to the lateral cortex. After the same steps as those for placing the proximal screw, one or two distal locking screws are inserted. There are various free-hand techniques for inserting distal locking screws.

NOTE: Many errors and complications, some disastrous, can occur when proceeding with intramedullary fixation. Late nailings (12 hours) can lead to complications related to difficulties in reduction. Traction should be used if a delay is expected. Reamers and nail guides can perforate the cortex. Some surgeons may use an unreamed technique in large femoral canals, which alleviates the potential for reaming injuries but increases the chance for femoral fracture. Nails that insert with great difficulty may be too large for the canal and become incarcerated in the bone, requiring bone resection for removal. Nails inserted that are undersized can bend and eventually break with weight-bearing. Infection in the open or closed nailing is a serious complication. The literature reports infection rates from 1.5% to 10% after open reduction and 1% in closed nailings. Safe, efficacious intramedullary nailing requires proper technique and attention to detail.

SURGERY OF THE LOWER LEG (DISTAL FEMUR, TIBIA, AND FIBULA)

Many procedures on the lower leg use the same principles of fracture fixation already mentioned. Meticulous detail is required to ensure proper alignment and optimal surgical results for the patient. As in the hip, fractures around the knee require secure fixation to allow bone healing, preserve motion, and provide joint mobility as early as possible. Fracture treatment for the various described injuries is based upon location and the pattern of fracture. Methods of fixation for the distal end of the femur and proximal end of the tibia include pins, wire, compression plates, intramedullary nails, supracondylar plates, and cannulated screws. Multiple trauma patients with one or a combination of fractures may require more than one method of fixation. Open reduction and internal fixation must ensure anatomic restoration of the joint surface and rigid fixation and allow early motion of the knee joint.

Most operations on the knee are performed with the patient in the supine position and the leg prepped and draped from the groin to the middle of the calf or including the entire foot. It is occasionally necessary for the surgeon to operate with the foot of the OR bed dropped and the patient's knee flexed to 90 degrees. Consequently it is important to position the patient so that the knee is at a break in the bed; if it is necessary, the lower leg can be flexed at the knee during the operation. A tourniquet is often used.

Femoral Condyle and Tibial Plateau Fractures

The joint surfaces are often involved with fractures of the distal end of the femur and proximal end of the tibia. Anatomic alignment of the articular surfaces is necessary to provide joint stability and decrease the chance of posttraumatic arthritis. Nonunion is the most common complication in supracondylar fractures, leading to failure of surgery. As with humeral head and hip fractures, it is

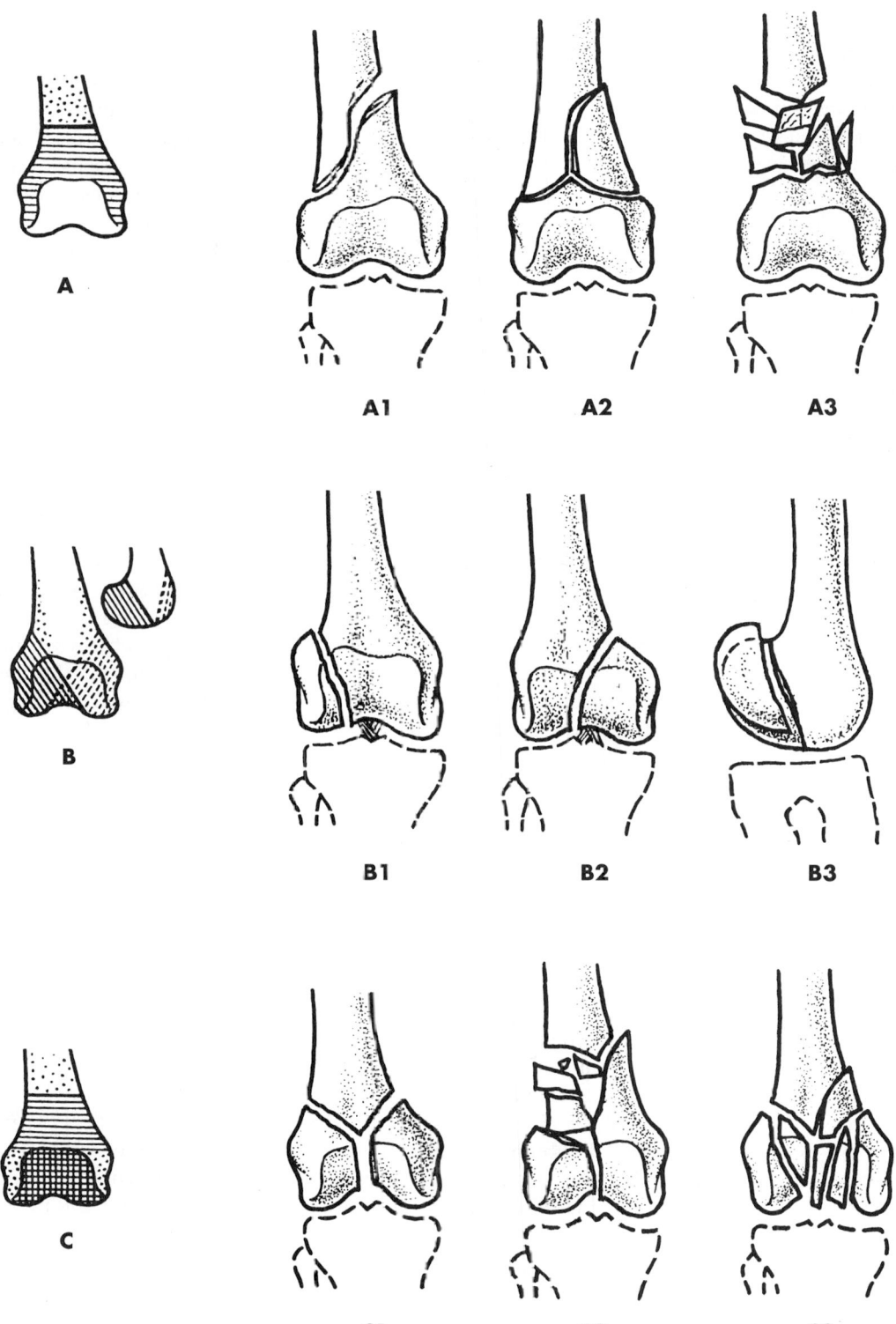

FIGURE 22-77   Classification of fractures of distal femur described by Müller et al.

important that the articular surfaces are reopposed as close as possible to avoid future degenerative changes. Unfortunately, these often cannot be avoided, and patients with this type of injury often face future joint arthroplasty and replacement (see total joint replacement, p. 874).

Distal femoral fractures result in varying degrees of comminution. Condylar fractures can be unicondylar or bicondylar, with separation of both condyles (Fig. 22-77). Type A fractures are extraarticular. Type B are single condyle fractures in the sagittal or coronal planes, whereas type C fractures are T and Y configurations. Type C fractures have varying degrees of shaft and condylar comminution, presenting the greatest challenge to treat.

Simple, undisplaced distal femoral fractures can be treated with closed reduction and immobilization by casting if anatomic reduction is achieved. Nondisplaced extraarticular fractures can be treated with a hinged cast brace. Comminuted fractures in this region can also be treated in this manner if there is minimal shortening and angulation. Traction can be used initially to augment this type of treatment. Distal femoral fractures are treated with open reduction if distal tibial traction and manipulation attempts fail. Flexible nails, locking intramedullary nails, blade plates, condylar compression screws, and condylar buttress plates are accepted methods of treating condylar fractures. Attention must be given to the attachment of the cruciate ligaments, which originate in the condylar notch and may require fixation of a partial or full disruption as a result of the injury (see cruciate deficient reconstruction, p. 865) to the knee.

Tibial plateau fractures historically have been attributed to bumper or fender injuries, but a variety of falls or other trauma frequently is the cause. Compression force of the distal end of the femur upon the tibia produces the varying types of plateau fractures. Commonly this occurs from abduction of the tibia while the foot is planted, driving the lateral femoral condyle into the lateral tibial plateau (also called the condyle). Several authors have developed classification systems based on fracture and dislocation patterns. The general theme of these fracture classifications and examples of their treatment can be summarized by the following types (Fig. 22-78): (1) pure cleavage, unicondylar fracture, (2) cleavage fracture combined with local compression, (3) pure central compression, (4) medial condylar wedge with depression or comminution, (5) bicondylar but with continuity of diaphysis and metaphysis, and 6) comminution with dissociation of metaphysis from diaphysis. Fractures of the tibial plateau are often associated with dislocation, which may spontaneously reduce at the time of trauma.

Special attention must given to the possibility of neurovascular insult, which must be addressed immediately. Elevation and fixation of the depressed fracture is the focus for treatment of plateau fractures. As with distal femoral fractures, the articular surfaces and cruciate insertion require reapproximation and fixation. Repair to the menisci and ligaments should occur simultaneously to prevent knee instability.

Blade plates, buttress plates, and cannulated screws are all methods by which fractures of the tibial plateau are fixed. Severe fractures are treated using multiple buttress plates and screws (Fig. 22-79). Bone graft from the iliac crest and fibular head autograft are often used when there is a significant amount of bone lost to comminution with proximal tibial fractures.

Supracondylar Fractures of the Femur

Fractures of the distal femur in the multiple trauma patient are treated early to promote rapid ambulation, which decreases complications caused by immobility. In an effort to deliver quick fracture reduction and stabilization, many orthopedic trauma systems have been developed. Often these are the same systems used in daily orthopedic procedures with modifications to expedite implantation and fixation. Some of the intramedullary devices do not require reaming.

Procedural considerations

Initial stabilization of the patient may immediately precede the nailing procedure. Often there are other team members attending to treatment of other systems. The perioperative nurse is challenged to control traffic, coordinate team efforts, and protect the patient from increased risk of infection by the inadvertent contamination of instruments and implants. The patient is placed in the supine position under general or regional anesthesia. If possible, the patient is positioned on the fracture table; if not, a radiolucent operating table is used. A pneumatic tourniquet may be applied as high up on the femur as possible, taking care to protect the genitals during placement. The nail can be inserted using the closed or open technique.

The soft-tissue set and large-bone set are required as well as the intramedullary supracondylar nail implant (Fig. 22-80) and the instruments necessary for its insertion. A power drill, guide wires, intramedullary rod set, and fluoroscopy will also be needed. In addition, Steinman pins, Kirschner wires, bone reduction clamps, and a bone graft set should be available. Occasionally a primary total knee arthroplasty will be performed, and the appropriate instruments should be available should that possibility exist.

Operative procedures
Intercondylar Fracture of the Femur, T Type (AIM Supracondylar Intramedullary Nail)

1. A standard midline skin incision with parapatellar arthrotomy is used. Depending on the degree of intraarticular extension, the incision may be as small as 1 inch or involve lateral eversion of the patella to gain visualization of the entire joint.
2. Articular fractures should be anatomically reduced and secured with 6.5 mm or 8.0 mm cannulated screws placed in the anterior and posterior aspect of the condyles to allow adequate space for the placement of the nail.
3. An entry hole is made with an awl into the femoral canal just anterior to the femoral insertion of the posterior cruciate ligament. Care is taken to assure anatomic alignment of the condyles to avoid varus or valgus femoral alignment.

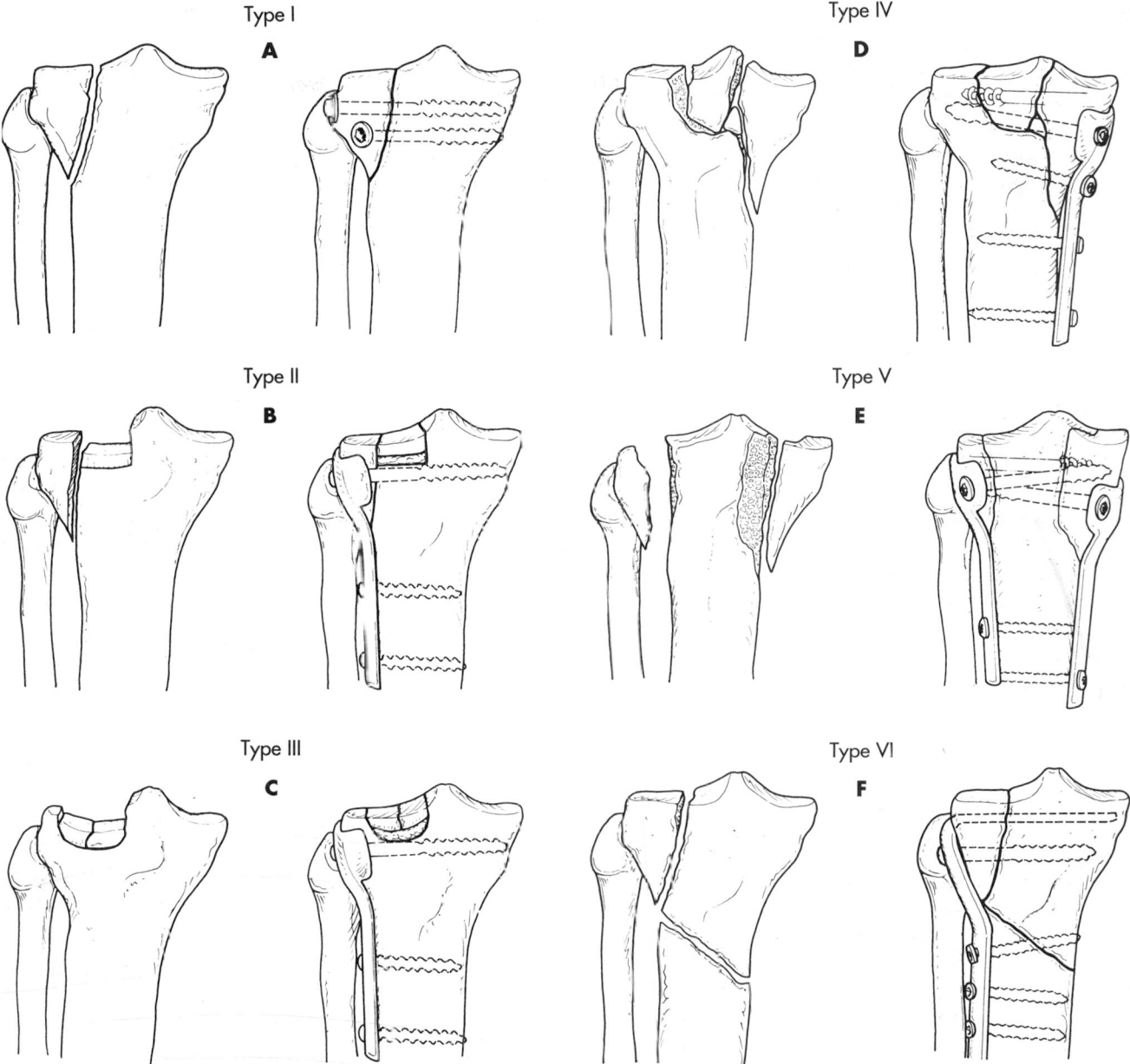

Type I
A

Type II
B

Type III
C

Type IV
D

Type V
E

Type VI
F

FIGURE 22-78 Classification of fractures of the tibia plateau. **A,** Type I, pure cleavage fracture. **B,** Type II, cleavage combined with depression. Reduction requires elevation of fragments with bone grafting of resultant hole in metaphysis. Wedge is lagged on lateral aspect of cortex protected with buttress plate. **C,** Type III, pure central depression. There is no lateral wedge. Depression may also be anterior, posterior, or involve whole plateau. After elevation of depression and bone grafting, lateral apect of cortex is best protected with buttress plate. **D,** Type IV. Medial condyle is either split off as wedge (type A) as illustrated, or it may be crumbled and depressed (type B), which is characteristic of older patients with osteoporosis (not illustrated). **E,** Type V. Notice continuity of metaphysis and diaphysis. In internal fixation both sides must be protected with buttress plates. **F,** Type VI. Essence of this fracture is fracture line that dissociates metaphysis from diaphysis. Fracture pattern of condyles is variable and all types can occur. If both condyles are involved, proximal tibia should be buttressed on both sides.

4. The hole is enlarged with the nonadjustable step reamer to accept the largest diameter of the chosen nail. Further reaming of the canal is necessary only in the case of nonunion, when the canal is reamed 0.5 to 1 mm over the size of the selected nail.

5. The selected nail is attached to the screw-targeting jig, which is then locked into place by the jig adapter. Before insertion of the nail, the alignment of the jig and nail holes is carefully checked by inserting the sheath and trocar through the selected holes by hand.

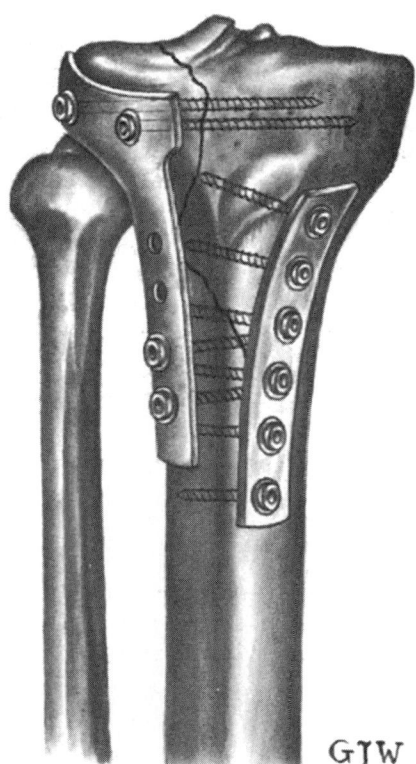

FIGURE 22-79 Severe fractures are treated by use of multiple buttress plates and screws.

6. The nail is placed in the prepared canal and advanced retrogradely either by hand or with gentle blows of a mallet on the jig adapter. The nail should be countersunk approximately 3 to 5 mm below the articular surface.

7. The screws may then be placed using the targeting jig and sheath and trocar assembly. A small lateral incision is made, and the sheath and trocar are advanced to the femoral cortex. A 5.3 mm drill bit is advanced through the medial cortex, and the length is measured from the calibrated drill bit or by use of a depth gauge. The appropriate 6.5 mm cortical screw is inserted, and the process is repeated for placement of the second screw.

8. Proximal locking of the nail is then performed in a similar fashion, taking care to use the appropriate holes in the targeting jig for the length of nail inserted. The 3.8 mm drill bit and 4.5 mm self-tapping screws are used to fill these holes after femoral rotation and alignment are confirmed with fluoroscopy.

9. The jig adapter and screw-targeting jig are removed, and an end cap is placed into the distal end of the nail. The wounds are irrigated and closed in layers. A compressive dressing is applied.

Range-of-motion and muscle-strengthening exercises are begun on the first postoperative day. Care is taken to protect against varus and valgus stresses. Weight bearing is discouraged until there is radiographic evidence of healing.

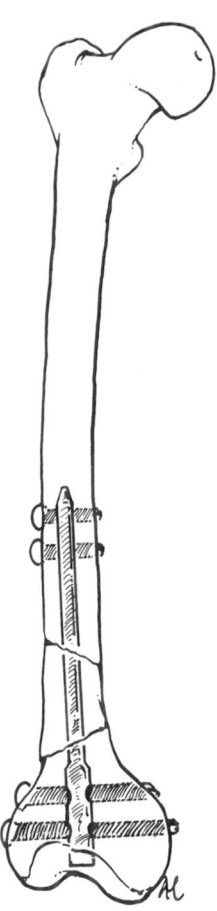

FIGURE 22-80   Supracondylar nail.

Supracondylar Fracture (Compression Plate)

1. The lateral area of the distal end of the femur is exposed above and below the knee joint.

2. The fracture site is reduced, and multiple Kirschner wires are inserted to ensure fixation.

3. A calibrated Steinman pin is placed transversely across the condyles parallel to the joint line. The pin must stop 8 to 10 mm short of the medial cortex.

4. The length of the lag screw is gauged when it is read directly on the calibrated Steinman pin, and adjustable double reamers are used to ream to this depth.

5. A lag screw is inserted across the condyles, followed by the compression screw.

6. The plate is secured and attached to the femoral shaft with cortical bone screws. The repair is visualized by fluoroscopy.

7. The incision site is irrigated and closed. A knee immobilizer is placed.

Medial and Lateral Y-Type Tibial Plateau Fractures

1. A long anterolateral incision, starting 2.5 cm above the superolateral aspect of the patella and tendon and proceeding distally around the patella to the anterior

aspect of the tibia just below the tibial tuberosity, is made. The distal end of the tibial shaft should be exposed.
2. The level of the prepatellar bursa is identified. Blunt dissection beneath the skin is used, and the proximal end of the tibia is retracted to expose it from midline medially to midline laterally.
3. The patellar tendon is detached with a tibial bone plug to expose both the medial and lateral articular surface. The articular surface is reconstructed using temporary Kirschner wires. A contoured T-plate is attached to the medial aspect of the tibia using cancellous screws in the proximal portion and cortical screws in the distal portion. A smaller T-plate is inserted on the lateral side and secured in the same manner. The Kirschner wires are removed. Care should be taken to see that the screws do not interfere with each other as they transverse from opposite sides of the tibia.
4. The patellar tendon is reattached using a 6.5 mm cancellous screw through the bone plug.
5. The wound is closed and immobilized at 30 degrees with a posterior splint.

Patellectomy and reduction of fractures of the patella

Patellectomy was a frequently performed procedure until the early 1970s. It is possible to excise a portion of the patella (for comminuted fracture) or the entire patella (for painful degenerative arthritis) without significantly affecting ordinary activities. However, patellectomy has been shown to significantly reduce power of extension as the joint extends, which is the most important function of the knee. Other complications associated with patellectomy are (1) slow return of quadriceps mechanism strength, (2) quadriceps muscle atrophy, and (3) loss of knee protection from the patella. Removal of the entire patella may result in relative lengthening of the knee extensor mechanism, which necessitates imbrication of the quadriceps tendon at the time of operation to prevent a lag in knee extension. Patellectomy should be performed only when comminution is extensive and reconstruction of the articular surface of the patella is not possible.

If the fracture consists of two large fragments that can be anatomically reduced, fixation is accomplished with a tension band, a circumferential loop technique, or bone screws. Tension band wiring produces compression forces across the fracture site and results in earlier union and immediate mobility of the knee.

Procedural Considerations

The patient is supine. The tourniquet is applied, and the leg is prepped and draped. A soft-tissue set and bone set are required along with a power drill and bits, bone-reduction clamps, 18-gauge wire, heavy needle holders, and a wire tightener.

Operative Procedure

1. A transverse curved incision is made over the patella
2. Dissection is carried down to expose the surface of the patella, the quadriceps, and the patellar tendons.
3. The joint is irrigated, and the fracture is reduced with bone-reduction clamps.
4. One length of wire is passed around the insertion of the patellar tendon and then around the quadriceps tendon. A second wire is passed more superficially through the bone fragments.
5. The fracture is overcorrected, and the wire is tightened with the wire tightener. In flexing the knee or contracting the quadriceps, the condyles press against the patellar fragments, producing compression at the fracture site.

Correction of recurrent dislocation of the patella

Recurrent dislocation of the patella can be the result of violent initial dislocation or more commonly from underlying anatomic abnormalities. The underlying condition causes an abnormal excursion of the extensor mechanism over the femoral condyles. Dynamic forces, such as the vastus lateralis, and static forces, as arising from the shape of the patella, tend to displace the patella laterally. Dislocations occur when there are extreme displacing forces combined with internal rotation of the femur and flexion of the knee. If untreated, patellar dislocations will deteriorate the knee by causing abnormal patellofemoral articulation, chondromalacia, and meniscal tears.

Conservative treatment aimed at quadriceps strengthening may be indicated in some patients. Numerous operations have been designed to realign the knee extensor mechanism. All the procedures include incising the lateral quadriceps tendon and shifting the insertion of the patellar tendon medially or distally to the original insertion of the tibia.

Procedural Considerations

The patient is positioned supine. The tourniquet is applied, and the leg is prepped and draped. A soft-tissue set and bone set are required along with a large-fragment screw set, a power drill, a microsagittal saw (Fig. 22-81), and osteotomes.

Operative Procedure
Patellar realignment (Elmslie-Trillat) (Fig. 22-82)

1. A lateral parapatellar incision is made beginning proximally to the patellar pole, laterally around the patella, and extending to 2 cm distally and just laterally to the tibial tuberosity.
2. A skin flap is developed and retracted medially to expose the capsule. A medial arthrotomy is completed, the joint is inspected, and any pathologic condition is present is repaired.
3. The lateral retinaculum is released from the vastus lateralis proximally and the patellar tendon distally.

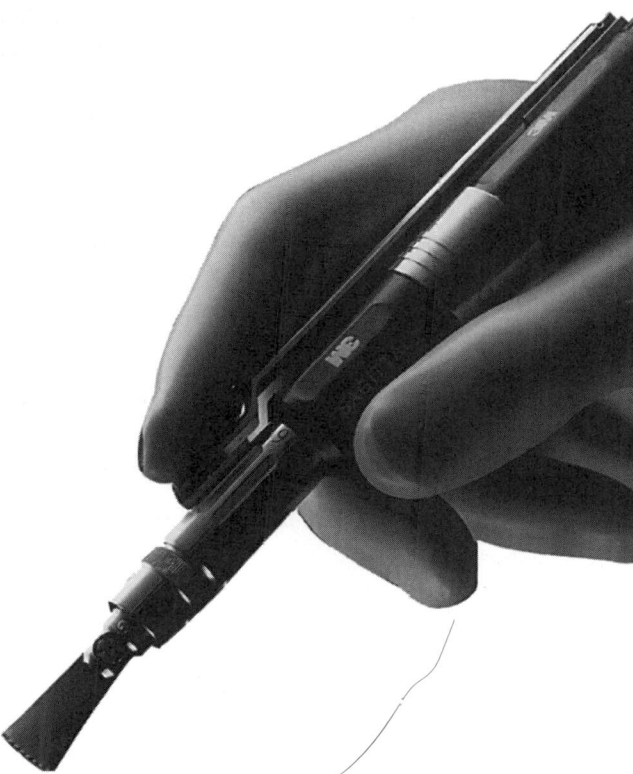

FIGURE 22-81 Sagittal micro saw.

4. With a ½-inch osteotome, the tibial tuberosity is scored medially and laterally, just below the fat pad and under the patella.
5. The osteotomy is continued using a microsagittal saw distally for 4 to 6 cm, leaving the periosteum hinged at the distalmost part of the osteotomy.
6. The entire segment, with patellar tendon attached, is displaced medially and held in place by hand while putting the knee through a range of motion. Tracking of the patella on the femoral groove is completed by systematically moving the knee medially in increments.
7. A cancellous bone bed is prepared at the point of reattachment of the tibial tuberosity.
8. The tuberosity is displaced medially, and a 6.5 mm cancellous bone screw is placed.
9. The wound is irrigated and closed, and a long-leg cylinder cast is applied and bivalved immediately.

Repair of collateral or cruciate ligament tears

The stability of the knee depends on the integrity of the cruciate and collateral ligaments. If any of these supporting structures is damaged, an unstable knee is likely unless properly repaired. Injuries to these supporting structures are usually not isolated. More frequently, several of the ligaments are injured at the same time. For example, the injury commonly referred to as the "terrible triad" includes a torn anterior cruciate ligament, torn medial meniscus, and torn medial collateral ligament.

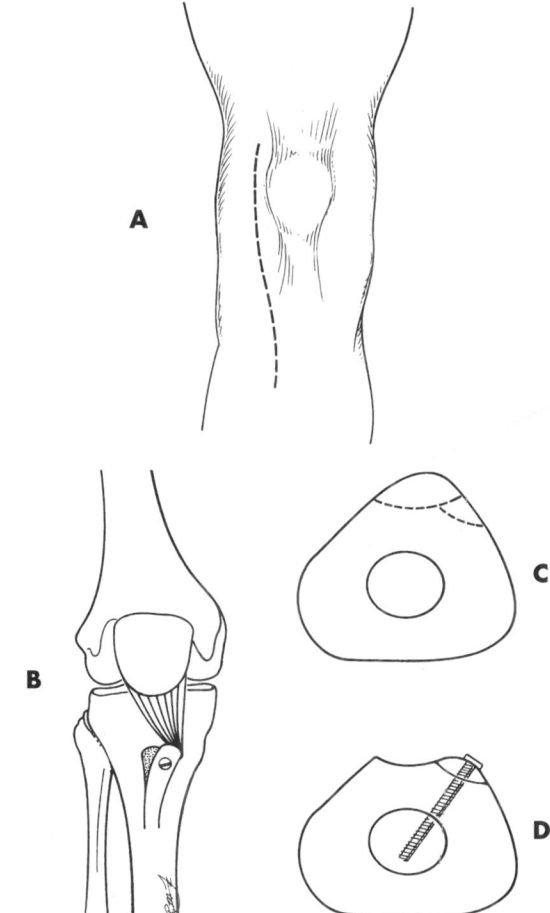

FIGURE 22-82 Elmslie-Trillat procedure as modified by Cox. **A,** Skin incision. **B,** Completed procedure. **C,** Cross section of tibia at level of tibial tuberosity to show bone cuts made to free tuberosity in center and to create new bed for transposed tuberosity to right. **D,** Cross section of tuberosity fixed with screw in new location anteromedially. Screw should not penetrate posterior aspect of cortex.

The knee demonstrates grave disability with major ligamentous disruption. The *collateral ligaments* reinforce the knee capsule medially and laterally. They resist varus and valgus stresses on the knee. The *cruciate ligaments* control AP stability. Along with the ligaments, the muscle groups stabilize the joint and control movement. Because muscle strength is the first line of defense for the knee, damage is repaired to protect the ligaments. For optimum function of the joint, damaged structures should be reconstructed as close as possible to the original anatomic structures. If the knee is left untreated, osteoarthritis will develop.

Injury to a single cruciate ligament may not significantly compromise knee function. When combined with other injuries, surgery may be warranted. Various types of ligament grafts may be used to replace or augment the cruciate ligaments. Autografts, allografts, and artificial substitutes are available. Ligament substitutes act as a scaffold, stent, or augment of the torn cruciate ligaments.

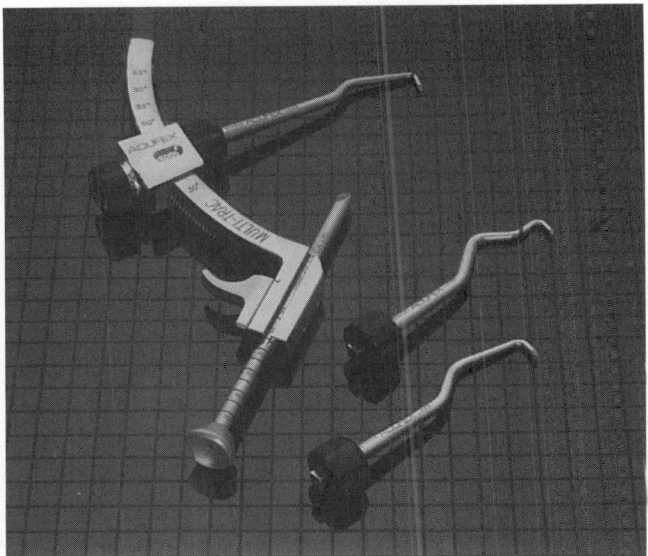

FIGURE 22-83 Reconstruction guide used for ligament repair.

Scaffolds support the soft tissue initially to allow ingrowth of the host tissue. Stents protect the joint from excessive stress while the permanent ligament substitute is healing Augmentation, as by the patient's own iliotibial band, protects the graft initially after repair of a partial tear. Synthetic ligaments, which are less popular and rarely used, include carbon-fiber grafts, polyglycolic acid material, Dacron, polyester, and Gore-Tex. All synthetic grafts are subject to mechanical failure from weakening with fragmentation and synovitis. These are recommended for salvage procedures only when conventional reconstruction has failed and when other autogenous tissue is unavailable for substitution. Biologic materials from animals, such as bovine xenografts, are also available for ligament substitution, although they are subject to increased risk of infection, synovitis, and rejection. Homogeneous allografts are the substitute of choice for knee reconstruction when no autogenous graft is available from the patient. Disadvantages of homogeneous allografts include long-term weakening, possible rejection, and the possibility of infectious disease transfer.

Autogenous tissues are currently the substitute of choice, with the middle third of the patellar tendon and a block of patella being the most reliable. To minimize necrosis and maintain graft strength, the fat pad with its blood supply may be preserved along with the patellar tendon. Using this graft and other soft-tissue autografts, the cruciate-deficient knee is being reconstructed arthroscopically (see arthroscopy section, p. 894). A combination of a torn anterior cruciate ligament, medial meniscus, and medial collateral ligament often indicates the need for an open procedure (arthrotomy). When reconstructing the cruciate ligament, it is important to have the graft biomechanically correct to maintain proper function.

There are many devices and systems used to provide placement assistance and gauge appropriate graft tension. These devices are either used separately or in some combination. Though the variations are many, the principles are the same.[23]

Procedural Considerations

The patient is placed in the supine position with a tourniquet applied to the upper area of the thigh. A surgical prep is done from the upper area of the thigh down to and including the foot. Soft-tissue instruments, arthroscopy instruments (see Figs. 22-111 to 22-116), ACL reconstruction instruments such as Steinman pins and reconstruction guides (Fig 22-83), and a tension isometer are required. A power drill, microsagittal saw, and burrs are essential. The fixation device of choice (Fig. 22-84) should also be available. Meniscal repair instruments should be in the room.

Operative Procedure
Ruptured anterior cruciate repair

An examination under anesthesia (EUA) is performed immediately after induction, when the ligaments are completely lax, to evaluate the severity of the injury.

1. A straight midline or slightly medial incision is made across the knee.
2. Meniscus tears in the vascular zone (peripheral) are repaired with arthroscopic meniscal repair instruments or cutting needles with a heavy absorbable suture to repair the meniscofemoral and meniscotibial ligaments. If the meniscus is not repairable, partial meniscectomy is performed.
3. The middle third of the patellar tendon with patellar and tibial bone plugs is harvested using a power saw and osteotome.
4. A notchplasty is then performed, debriding and smoothing the lateral intercondylar wall with a burr and curette.
5. The femoral and tibial osseous tunnels are developed using the ligament guide to pass guide wires from the lateral area of the femoral condyle and tibial tubercle into the intercondylar notch at isometric points near the anatomic attachment site of the anterior cruciate ligament.
6. The pins are then overdrilled with cannulated drills as close to the size of the patellar tendon graft as possible. The tunnels are smoothed with a curette.
7. Sutures are placed through drill holes at both ends of the graft to pass the graft through the tunnels.
8. Once the graft is passed through the femoral and tibial osseous tunnels, it is fixed at both ends with interference screws, staples, or polyethylene buttons.
9. The medial collateral ligament and posterior oblique ligament are then individually repaired at their insertion sites with bone screws and spiked washers.

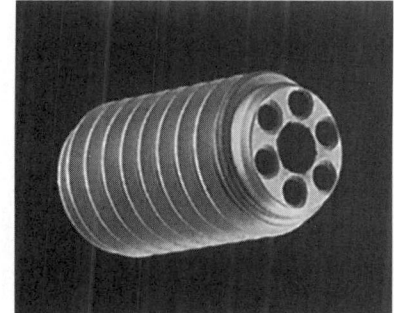

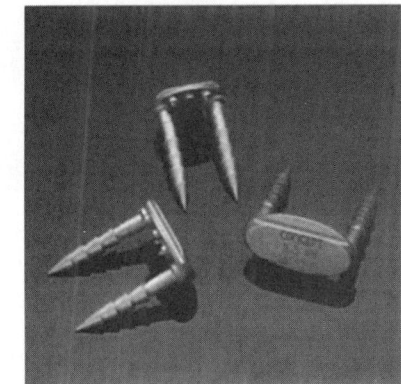

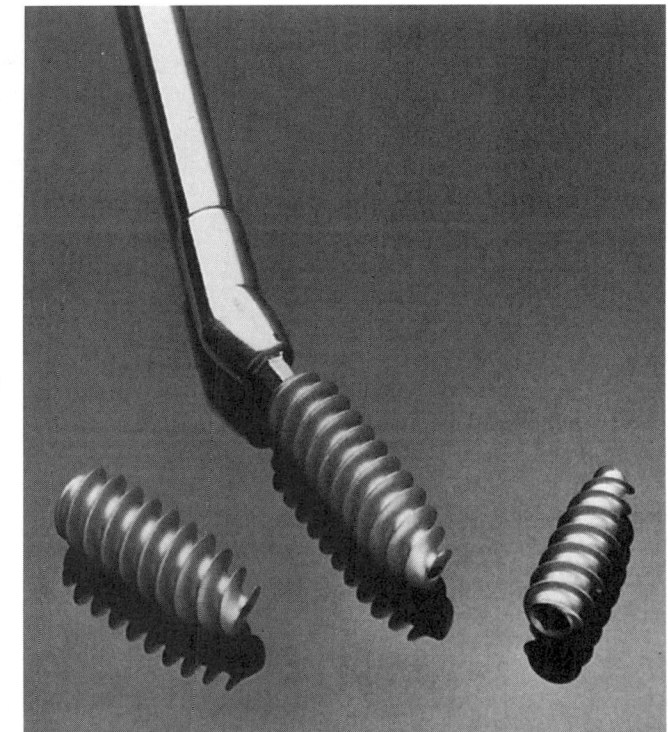

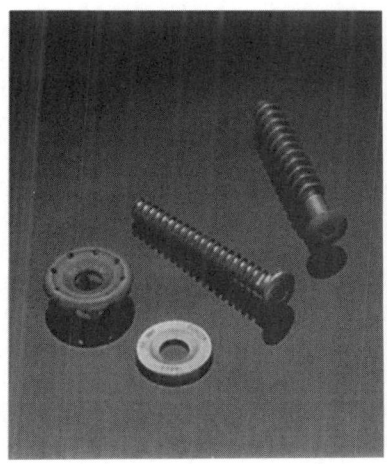

FIGURE 22-84   Fixation devices for ligament repairs. **A,** Interference screws. **B,** Endosteal fixation device. **C,** Soft-tissue fixation staples. **D,** Cortical screws and washers.

10. Additional extraarticular repair is done if necessary.
11. The wound is closed over intraarticular and subcutaneous drains, and a locking knee brace or knee immobilizer is applied.

Popliteal (Baker's) cyst excision

Baker's cysts occur in joints, frequently affecting the popliteal fossa. Baker's cysts are frequently painful and can become very large, especially when associated with rheumatoid arthritis. Cysts in the popliteal fossa occur without a precipitating cause in children; in adults they often indicate an intraarticular disease process, such as rheumatoid arthritis, or a torn meniscus.

Procedural Considerations

In contrast to many other operative procedures on the knee, the patient is placed in the prone position. A soft-tissue set and a bone set are required.

Operative Procedure

1. An oblique incision is made in the popliteal area over the mass.
2. The deep fascia is divided to expose the mass.
3. The cyst is then freed by blunt dissection and clamped at its attachment to the joint capsule.
4. The cyst is divided, and the pedicle is inverted and closed.

5. After the mass has been removed, the wound is irrigated and closed.
6. The knee is immobilized in extension with a posterior splint.

Fractures of the tibial shaft

The location of the tibia results in frequent exposure to injury. Open fractures are more common in the tibia than in other major bones because one third of its surface is subcutaneous. Tibial shaft fractures are difficult to treat. The blood supply to the tibia is more precarious than that of other long bones because of its lack of enclosure by heavy muscle. The presence of hinge joints at the knee and ankle allows no adjustment for rotational deformity after fracture, so special care is required to correct for rotation during reduction and fixation. Rotational deformities are often seen. Delayed union, nonunion, and infection are fairly common complications. Arguments can be made that closed reduction and casting provide excellent healing without significant complications, but this treatment can require casting for 6 months or more. Arguments can also be made for surgical reduction and internal fixation. This treatment pathway generally allows for earlier weight bearing and a shortened period of casting; however, the rate of complications is higher.

In general, torsional fractures seem to heal better and are more amenable to treatment than transverse fractures. It is theorized that twisting injuries cause less damage to endosteal vessels than transverse fractures do, where periosteum and endosteal vessels are torn circumferentially. The important prognostic indicators for tibial fractures are as follows: (1) the amount of initial displacement, (2) the degree of comminution, (3) the presence or absence of infection, and (4) the severity of soft-tissue injury, excluding infection. As a rule, high-energy fractures, such as those caused by auto accidents or crushing injury, have a much worse prognosis than low-energy fractures, such as those caused by falls on ice or skiing accidents.

Because of the increase in intramedullary tibial nailings without a significant increase in infections arising from them, external fixation of open tibial shaft fractures (see Figs. 22-40 and 22-41) is less commonly done. However, in the presence of gross contamination, severe soft-tissue and vascular injury, bone infection, and delayed treatment, external fixation is the treatment of choice. The Ilizarov external fixation device is indicated when there is significant bone loss and limb lengthening is required. Plate and screw fixation is another method in which tibial shaft fractures can be treated, although infection and nonunion of tibial shaft fractures are twice as likely with this method. Plate and screw fixation is indicated when there are intraarticular fragments of the knee and ankle associated with the injury. Closed intramedullary nailing is the treatment of choice in tibial shaft fractures because infection is less likely to occur and the periosteal blood supply is preserved. Static locking nails (locking both proximal and distal ends of the nail) are indicated for fractures with comminution, bone loss, and lengthening osteotomies. Dynamic locking nails (locking the end closest to the fracture site) are indicated for proximal or distal tibial fractures, nonunions, and malunions. Locking tibial nails include the Russell-Taylor and the Grosse-Kempf tibial nail (see Fig. 22-76).

The key to successful treatment of open tibial fractures, as in all open fractures, is meticulous and systematic débridement of all foreign matter and devitalized tissue. Care should be taken to minimize devascularization when reducing and fixing the fracture. Systemic antibiotics and those delivered by pulse lavage help reduce the chance of infection.

Procedural Considerations

The patient is usually given general or regional anesthesia while still on the hospital bed or in the transport vehicle and then transferred to the fracture table. The patient is positioned supine on the fracture table with the affected hip flexed approximately 45 degrees and the knee at 90 degrees. This provides a horizontal orientation of the tibia. Using a calcaneal traction pin or table foot holder, traction is applied and rotational alignment obtained. After rotational alignment is obtained, a tourniquet is applied, and the leg is prepped and draped. Some surgeons prefer to use a standard OR table, breaking the table at the knee. This obviates the need to insert the calcaneal traction pin and allows for easier maneuvering of the tibia during insertion of the locking screws.

A soft-tissue and large-bone set is required in addition to the intramedullary nail and insertion instruments of choice. A power drill and reamer-driver will be needed to use the necessary intramedullary reamers (Fig. 22-85). Fluoroscopy will be needed as well. If an open plating is being considered, the plates of choice and the large-fragment screws need to be available as well as bone-reduction clamps.

Operative Procedures
Closed or open tibial intramedullary nailing (Fig. 22-85)

1. If the open technique is required, the fracture site is exposed, reduced, and irrigated as necessary. Focus is then turned toward the nailing procedure.
2. A 5 cm incision is made medially to the patellar tendon to just below the tibial tuberosity.
3. Using a curved awl, the medullary canal is opened just proximally to the tibial tuberosity.
4. A guide rod (3.2 mm) is inserted into the shaft of the tibia down to the fracture site. The proximal fragment is reduced distally and the guide rod advanced into the distal fragment. Rod types include the straight guide rod for simple fractures, curved for the displaced type, and a cutting tip for an obstructed canal.
5. The length of the required nail is determined by the

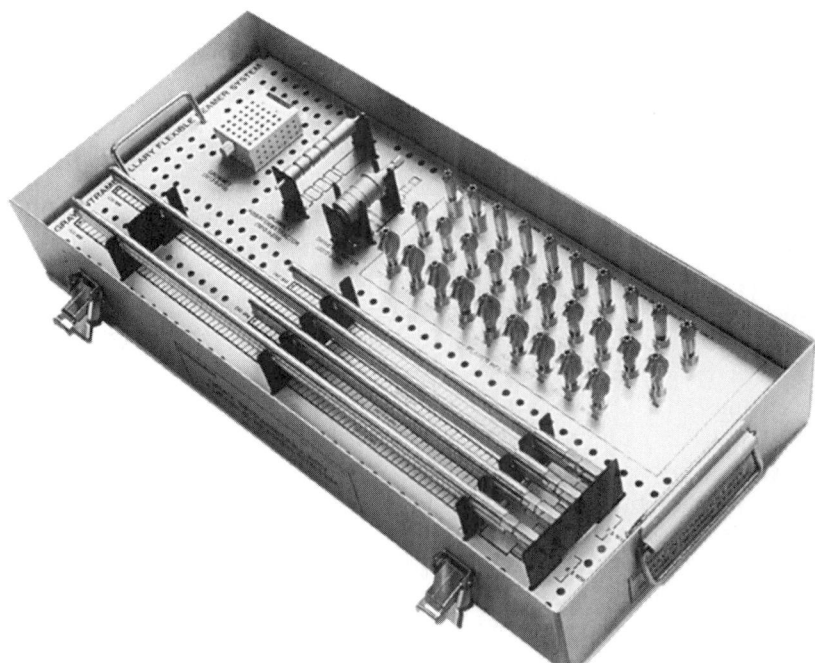

FIGURE 22-85 Intramedullary flexible reamer system.

guide rod method (see the section on femoral nails, p. 857) or by using the nail-length gauge and confirming with fluoroscopy.

6. With cannulated reamers over the guide rods, the entire tibia is reamed 1 mm greater than the nail to be inserted. Inserting a nail too large for the canal can have a detrimental effect.

7. The driver, proximal drill, guide, and hexagonal bolt are assembled onto the tibial nail.

8. The nail is inserted over the guide rod and, with a mallet, driven down the proximal fragment to enter the distal fragment, crossing the fracture site. The nail is not fully seated.

9. The guide rod is removed to prevent incarceration, and complete seating of the nail is performed. The proximal tip of the nail should be flush with the tibial entry site.

10. Proximal locking is accomplished with the corresponding drill and tap through the proximal drill guide for 5 mm cortical bone screws.

11. Distal screws are inserted using the distal targeting device or the freehand technique. The 5 mm cortical bone screws are inserted, traversing the tibia through the tibial nail.

12. The wounds are irrigated. If bone graft is to be used, it is placed around the fracture site, and the layers are closed. Dressings are applied, and cast or splint immobilization is accomplished.

Dynamization, or removal of either the proximal or the distal screws, may take place after 3 months for fractures that are stable but lack callus. Dynamization produces compressive forces at the fracture, thereby promoting osteogenesis.

Tibial dynamic compression plating

1. A longitudinal incision is made (to accommodate the selected plate) laterally to the tibial crest to expose the fracture site.

2. The periosteum is stripped only enough for application of the plate. Circumferential stripping can diminish blood supply.

3. The fracture is reduced, and a plate is placed across the fracture site and secured with bone- and plate-holding forceps. The plate may have to be contoured with a hand-held or plate-bending press.

4. Using the neutral drill guide a 3.2 mm bicortical hole is drilled into the plate screw hole close to the fracture site, gauged, and tapped to 4.5 mm. The first bone screw is inserted, ensuring purchase of the screw on the opposite cortex.

5. Using the load drill guide (eccentric), the second hole is drilled next to the fracture line in the opposite fragment. Drill and tap are accomplished as in the previous step. As the screw enters the bone, it will seek the center of the screw hole (the screw is eccentric and the screw hole is beveled). The fracture site is brought under compression as the screw seats into the hole.

6. The wounds are irrigated. If bone graft is to be used, it is placed around the fracture site and the layers are closed. Dressings are applied, and cast or splint immobilization is completed.

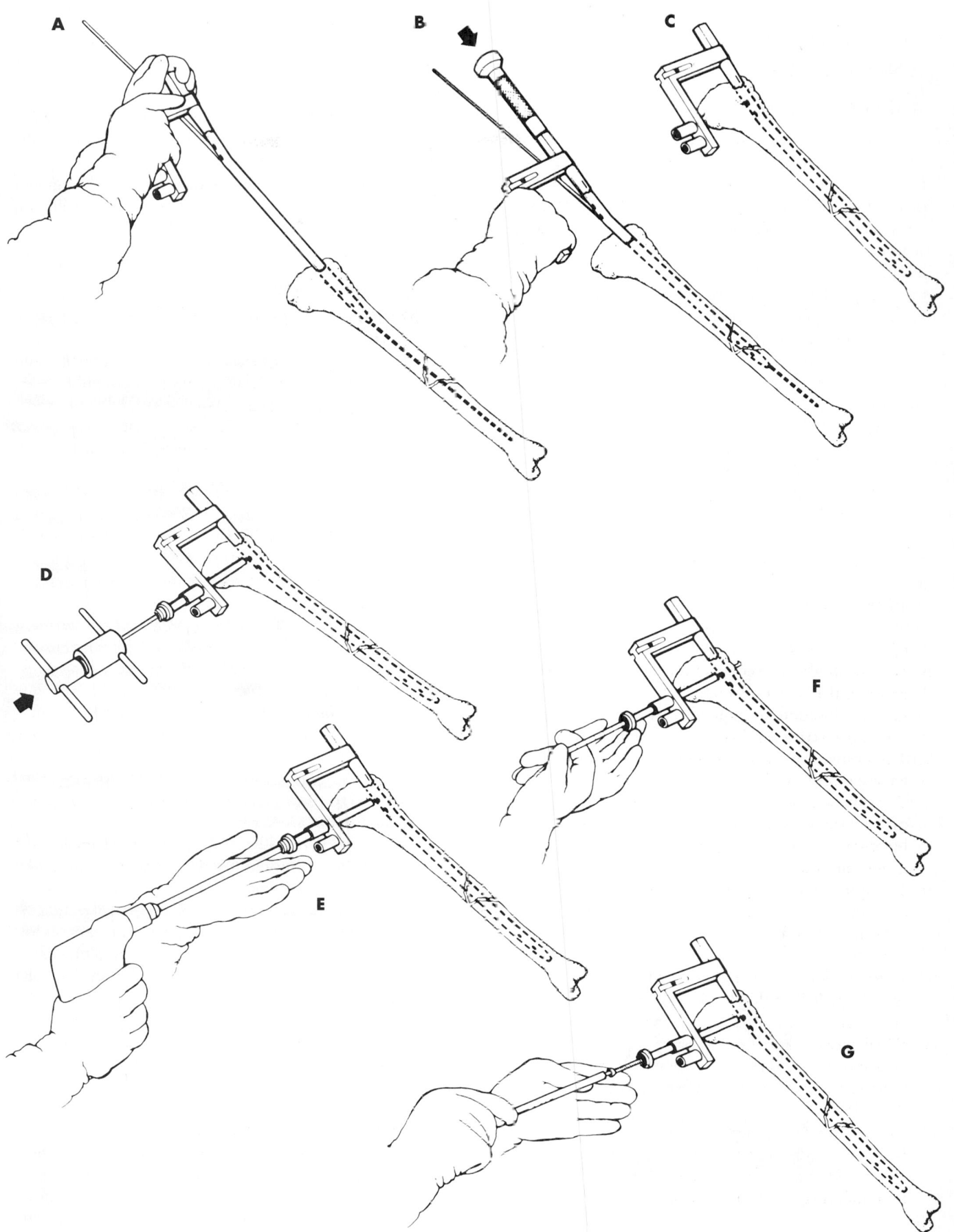

FIGURE 22-86   **A,** Attachment of nail to proximal drill guide. **B,** Driving nail over guide rod. **C,** Final seating of nail with its tip flush with tibial entry portal. **D,** For proximal interlocking, cortex is dimpled. **E,** Depth measurements are made. **F,** Locking screw length is confirmed. **G,** Self-tapping screw is inserted through drill sleeve.

SURGERY OF THE ANKLE AND FOOT

Ankle Fractures

Ankle fractures include fractures of the medial malleolus (tibia), lateral malleolus (fibula), and posterior malleolus (posterior aspect of the articular surface of the distal end of the tibia). They may or may not be associated with ligamentous injury. Ankle fractures can be classified in anatomic lines as monomalleolar, bimalleolar, and trimalleolar. Because medial malleolar and posterior malleolar fractures involve the distal weight-bearing articular surface of the tibia, open reduction and anatomic alignment are necessary. Fixation of the lateral malleolus is also important because it forms the ankle mortise, the socket formed by the distal tibia and fibula into which the body of the talus fits.

Anatomic reduction prevents the occurrence of degenerative joint disease. Displaced fractures are treated with pins, malleolar or bone screws, or plates and screws (Fig. 22-87). Bimalleolar fractures can be treated with closed reduction and casting, but approximately 10% of these develop nonunion. The lateral malleolus (distal end of the fibula) is important for lateral and rotational stability of the joint. Open reduction and internal fixation using Steinman pins or screws placed obliquely into the tibia is a common technique. Lateral or malleolar fractures can be fixed with the cancellous lag technique, overdrilling the first fragment and allowing compression of the fragments. Fracture of the lateral malleolus can also be treated with a Rush rod, inserted through the fragment and into the fibular canal. Trimalleolar fractures require surgery more than the other variety of fractures. The posterior lip of the articulating surface of the tibia is usually involved and needs to be anatomically reduced to minimize degenerative changes. Cannulated screws can provide efficient reduction of a posterior fragment.

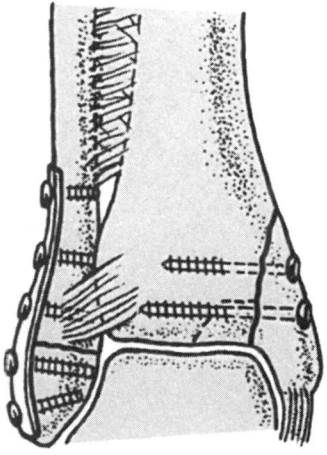

FIGURE 22-87   Plate-screw placement for lateral malleolar fragment repair using one-third tubular plate.

Procedural considerations

The patient is placed in the supine position. The affected leg is prepped and draped after application of a pneumatic tourniquet. If the lateral ankle is involved, a padded sandbag is placed beneath the hip to internally rotate it.

A soft-tissue set; small-bone set; the AO small-fragment set with plates, screws, and pins; a power drill; and bone-reduction clamps are required.

Operative procedure
Trimalleolar Fracture

1. Incisions are made medially and laterally across the ankle.
2. The posterior malleolar fracture is exposed and reduced with bone-holding clamps and manipulation.
3. The fracture is temporarily held in reduction with two Kirschner wires inserted above the anterior tibial lip and directed anteriorly to posteriorly, engaging both fragments.
4. A drill hole is made anteriorly to posteriorly through both fragments. After measuring with a depth gauge, a malleolar, small cancellous, or other preferred screw is inserted through the fracture. The wires are removed.
5. The lateral malleolar fracture is then manipulated into reduction.
6. If the fracture is oblique and not comminuted, it is reduced with one or two lag screws placed anteriorly to posteriorly. If the fracture is transverse, a long screw or medullary pin is inserted across the fracture line into the canal of the proximal fragment. A small semitubular or one-third tubular plate is applied if the fracture occurs above the syndesmosis.
7. Once the posterior and lateral malleolar fractures have been fixed, the medial malleolar fracture is finally reduced using bone clamps.
8. The reduction is held with two Kirschner wires while a hole is drilled through the medial malleolus into the metaphysis of the tibia.
9. Once the appropriate length of screw is determined by a depth gauge, a malleolar screw is inserted across the fracture site. The Kirschner wires are removed.
10. If rotational stability is needed, an additional smaller screw or compression wiring is added.
11. Intraoperative radiographs are taken in AP, lateral, and mortise views.
12. The wounds are irrigated and closed, and a short or long leg cast or splint is applied.

Triple Arthrodesis

The talocalcaneal (subtalar), talonavicular, and calcaneocuboid joints must be fused in patients with pronounced inversion or eversion deformities of the foot. Such deformities occur in clubfoot, poliomyelitis, and rheumatoid arthritis. Occasionally this operation is necessary for patients who have pain resulting from degenerative or traumatic arthritis such as that occurring after intraarticular fractures of the calcaneus. Triple arthrodesis limits motion of the foot and ankle to plantar flexion and dorsiflexion.

Procedural considerations

The patient is placed in the supine position. The surgical prep is carried out from midcalf down to and including the foot. The iliac crest area should also be prepped if bone grafting is anticipated.

A soft-tissue set, small-bone set, a power saw, drill, or rasp, a bone graft set, and the AO compression plates and screws or bone staples to hold the fusion are required. Kirschner wires can be used to provide temporary fixation. A small lamina spreader is helpful in providing exposure.

Operative procedure

1. An anterior or anterolateral approach is used.
2. The subtalar and calcaneocuboid joints are exposed, as well as the lateral portion of the talonavicular joint.
3. The capsules of the talonavicular, calcaneocuboid, and subtalar joints are incised circumferentially to obtain as much mobility as possible. If this release allows the foot to be placed into a normal position, removal of large bony wedges is not required.
4. An osteotome, power saw, or power rasp is used to remove the articular surfaces of the calcaneocuboid joint, the subtalar joint, and the talonavicular joint. The small lamina spreader is used to expose these surfaces. Care is taken to save all bone removed for later use in the fusion.
5. The removed bone is cut into small pieces to be used for bone grafting. If the quantity is insufficient, graft is harvested from the anterior ilium. Most of the bone is placed around the talonavicular joint and in the depth of the sinus tarsi.
6. Smooth Steinman pins, staples, or screws are used for internal fixation.
7. The wound is closed over a suction drain. A short leg cast or splint is applied.

Bunionectomy

A bunion (hallux valgus) is a soft tissue or bony mass at the medial side of the first metatarsal head. It is associated with a valgus deformity of the great toe (Fig. 22-88). A bunion is caused by a basic structural defect of the foot, which predisposes to the development of this deformity. Ill-fitting shoes accentuate the situation and speed the development of bunions. Bunions are 40 times more common in women because of shoe styles, including high heels and pointed toes. Other factors that may contribute to this deformity are heredity, flatfeet, foot pronation, longer first toe, muscle imbalance, and inflammatory disturbances of the feet.

Symptoms include pain on the dorsomedial aspect of the first metatarsal head or directly over the medial exostosis, swelling of the big toe, painful plantar callus, and plantar keratosis. Discomfort to the entire foot occurs as the forefoot becomes more fatigued and symptomatic, with pain radiating to the leg and knee.

Hallux valgus is treated with a variety of surgical procedures (Fig. 22-89). All these procedures remove the exostosis and attempt to realign the great toe by removal of bone transfer of tendons, osteotomy of the first metatarsal shaft, or appropriate imbrication of soft tissue.

The goals of surgery are correction of the deformity (cosmesis), resection of the abnormal bony components (reconstruction), and normal or near-normal range of motion (function).

Procedural considerations

The patient is given general or regional anesthesia, and a tourniquet is applied to the proximal area of the thigh,

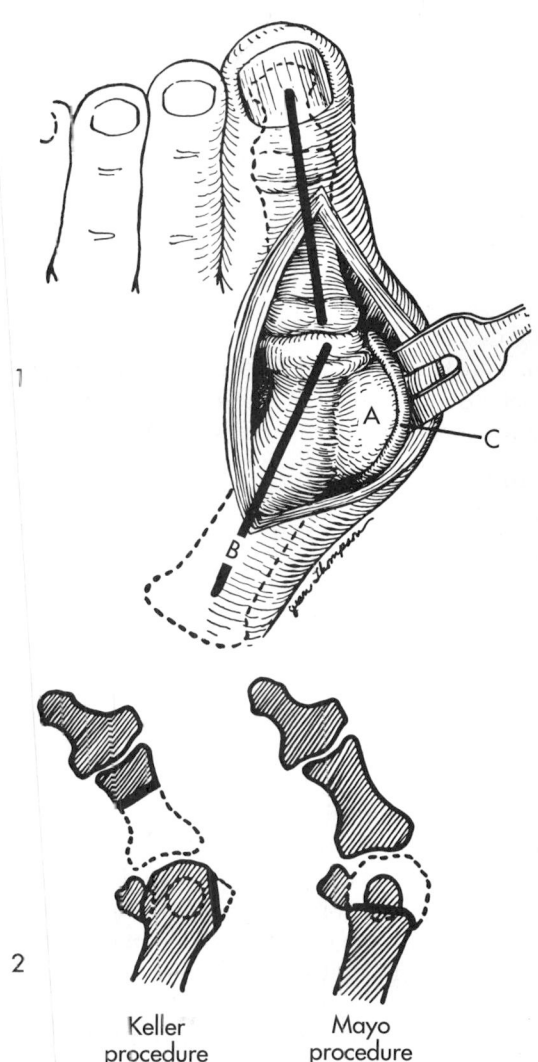

FIGURE 22-88   *1,* Bunion. **A,** Exostosis of metatarsal head; **B,** hallux valgus deformity; **C,** overlying bursa. *2,* Operations for hallux valgus.

Keller procedure   Mayo procedure

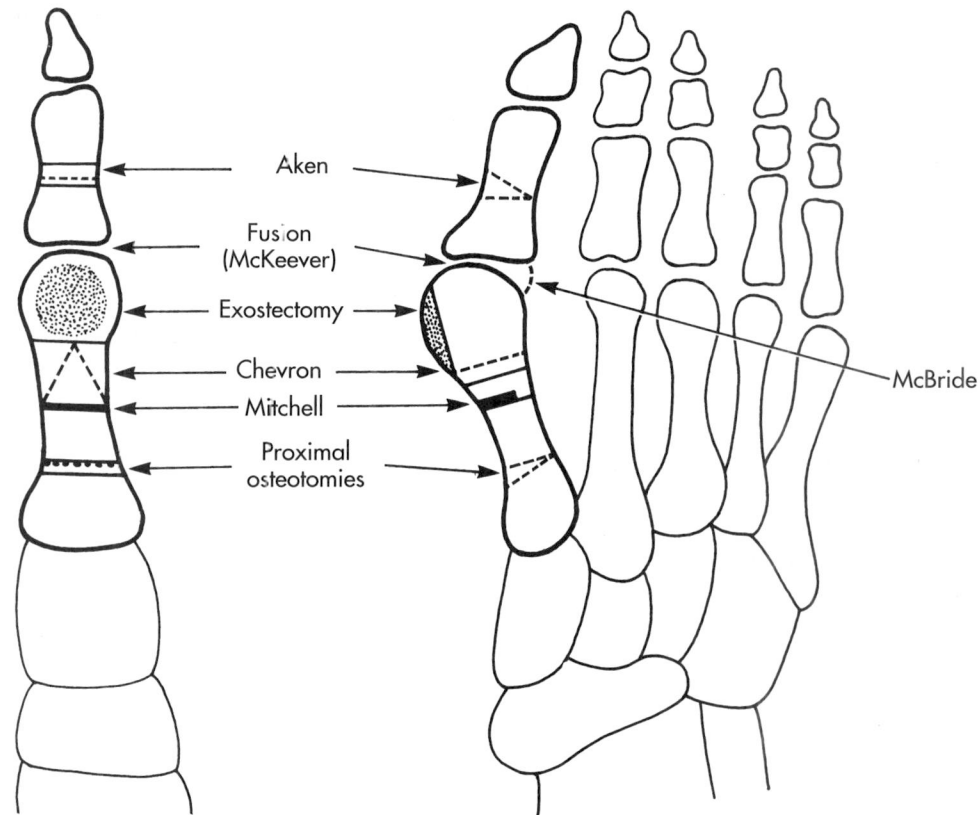

FIGURE 22-89 Types of bunionectomies.

the calf, or around the ankle. The foot and leg are prepped and then draped using a sterile stockinette.

A soft-tissue set, small-bone set, Kirschner wires, a power wire driver, and a microsagittal saw are required.

Operative procedure
Keller Technique

1. A midline, straight, medial incision is made, beginning at the neck of the proximal phalanx and extended in an internervous plane proximally.
2. Dissection is carried down through the joint capsule. A flap incision is made to expose the underlying hypertrophic bone found at the dorsomedial aspect of the first metatarsal head.
3. All soft-tissue attachments are removed from the base of the proximal phalanx.
4. The proximal third of the proximal phalanx is resected with a power-oscillating saw.
5. Proper alignment of the toe is maintained as one or two 0.062-inch Kirschner wires are placed in the center of the medullary canal of the phalanx and then driven into the metatarsal head, neck, and shaft.
6. The wound is then irrigated and closed, and a bandage is applied to maintain the toe in the correct position. Postoperative convalescence requires a minimum of 6 weeks.

Correction of Hammer Toe Deformity

The term *hammer toe* is most often used to describe an abnormal flexion posture of the proximal interphalangeal joint of one of the four lesser toes. This deformity causes painful calluses to develop on the dorsal joints of the four lesser toes, since the cocked-up digits rub against the shoes. The deformity is treated by incising the long extensor tendon to the toes and fusing the proximal interphalangeal joint. A smooth Kirschner wire is frequently used to stabilize the fusion and position the toe properly during the postoperative period.

Procedural considerations

The patient is placed in the supine position, and the tourniquet is applied. The foot is prepped and draped. A soft-tissue set, small-bone set, Kirschner wires, and a power wire driver are required.

Operative procedure

1. An elliptical incision over the proximal interphalangeal joint that measures 5 to 6 mm wide and has a 2 or 3 mm lateral extension on either side is made.
2. The capsular tissue of the distal third of the proximal phalanx and proximal interphalangeal joint is entered to expose the defect completely.
3. A small rongeur or microsaw is used to resect the distal

third portion of the proximal phalanx. Once the capital fragment is excised, the remaining portion of the distal proximal phalanx is debrided with a rongeur or rasp.

4. Digital alignment can be maintained with small Kirschner wires.
5. The wounds are irrigated and closed, and a sterile dressing and orthopedic shoe is applied for postoperative recovery.

Metatarsal Fractures

Metatarsal fractures occur in various sites. These fractures have a reduced healing potential because metatarsals mainly consist of cortical bone, which lacks vascularity. Treatment is determined by the extent of the fracture; the greater the displacement, the greater the need for reduction. In general, transverse and short, oblique midshaft fractures of the metatarsals are internally fixed because of their instability and displacement. Pins, wires, screws, and plates are used for internal fixation of metatarsal fractures. The simplest method is Kirschner wire fixation.

Procedural considerations

The patient is placed in the supine position, a tourniquet is applied, and the foot is prepped and draped. A soft-tissue set, small-bone set, Kirschner wires, and a power wire driver are required.

Operative procedure

1. A small incision is made over the fracture.
2. The distal fragment is identified and retracted.
3. A smooth Kirschner wire is driven distally, exiting the skin.
4. The wire driver is then switched and attached to the end protruding from the skin.
5. The pin is then driven proximally into the canal of the proximal fragment.
6. If the fracture is more complex or comminuted, the fracture site is transfixed by crossing two Kirschner wires through the fracture.
7. The incision is closed, and a postoperative shoe is applied.

Metatarsal Head Resection

Patients with rheumatoid arthritis frequently have dorsally dislocated toes and prominent and painful metatarsal heads on the plantar surfaces of their feet. Excision of all the metatarsal heads commonly relieves the pain and corrects an associated bunion deformity.

Procedural considerations

The patient is placed in a supine position, a tourniquet is applied, and the foot is prepped and draped. A soft-tissue set, small-bone set, Kirschner wires, a power wire driver, and a power microsagittal saw are required.

TYPE A	Stable
	A1-Fractures of the pelvis not involving the ring
	A2-Stable, minimally displaced fractures of the ring
TYPE B	Rotationally unstable, vertically stable
	B1-Open book
	B2-Lateral compression: ipsilateral
	B3-Lateral compression: contralateral (bucket handle)
TYPE C	Rotationally and Vertically unstable
	C1-Unilateral
	C2-Bilateral
	C3-Associated with an acetabular fracture

FIGURE 22-90   Classification of pelvic injuries.

Operative procedure
Clayton Technique

1. A transverse plantar incision is made and tissue dissected to the metatarsal heads.
2. All metatarsal heads and half the proximal phalanges are removed with the microsagittal saw.
3. The extensor tendons are transected and not repaired.
4. The skin is closed, and a dressing and postoperative shoe are applied.

PELVIC FRACTURE AND DISRUPTION

Patients with multiple trauma often present with multiple fractures that can be life threatening. Complications of pelvic fractures include injury not only to major vessels and nerves, but also to major visceral organs, such as the intestines, bladder, and urethra. Factors influencing mortality include associated visceral injury, hemorrhage, and head injury.

Pelvic fracture classification is divided into three main groups (Fig. 22-90). *Type A fractures* are stable, without ring involvement (A1), and minimally displaced fractures of the ring (A2). *Type B fractures* are rotationally unstable and vertically stable and are also subclassified: B1 is an open book fracture, B2 has ipsilateral compression, and B3 has contralateral compression. *Type C fractures* are both rotationally and vertically unstable: C1 is unilateral, C2 bilateral, and C3 is associated with the acetabulum. Roentgenograms, CT scan, and MRI all prove useful in determining the type and appropriate treatment for pelvic trauma.

Treatment is based on classification and may include closed manipulation and reduction or internal and external fixation. Internal and external fixation are also used concurrently in the treatment of some pelvic fractures.

Type A fractures are stable and can be treated nonoperatively. Type B1 fractures may be treated with external fixation or anterior plate fixation. Type C fractures usually require open procedures to fix the fractures with plates and screws and reduce sacral disruptions with transiliac rods or screws. Type C fractures may be treated with external fixation when the patient is hemodynamically unstable, and a quicker, simpler procedure is prudent.

External fixation is the most widely recommended treatment for type B fractures of the pelvis (see Fig. 22-42). A technique similar to that of external fixation of extremity fractures is done in the operating room with anesthesia and sterile conditions. If external fixation is to be used, the earlier it is attempted the greater chance of success.

Procedural considerations

This procedure is often done during other emergent and resuscitative efforts in the operating room. The patient's entire pelvic area is prepped and draped. A pelvic skeleton in the room may help the team visualize maneuvers and pin placement to be attempted to complete the reduction. A soft-tissue set is needed in addition to the external fixator of choice and the instruments for its insertion, including a power drill.

Operative procedure
AO External Fixation

1. The pelvic disruption is reduced manually and confirmed with radiograph. The disruption may not be able to be completely reduced without traction using a distal femoral pin. If required, this is inserted under sterile conditions.
2. Kirschner wires are inserted percutaneously to determine the position of the pin placement, taking into consideration the inward and downward crest slope.
3. Parallel rows of pins are placed into the anterior iliac crest area. This is carried out by drilling the outer cortex and placing 5 mm half pins medially and distally. The pins should enter cancellous bone between the outer and inner table of ilium.
4. Three universal frames are placed over the pins as close to the skin as possible for maximum rigidity.
5. Optimal reduction of the fracture is visualized using radiography. The crossbar is applied, and compression and distraction maneuvers are used to maintain the reduction.
6. The crossbar is removed, and connecting rods are applied with couplers.
7. The crossbar is reattached, and the joints of the frame are tightened.
8. The pin sites of tented skin are released. The wounds are dressed with iodine ointment and gauze.

The frames are generally left in place for 8 to 12 weeks.

TOTAL JOINT ARTHROPLASTY

Arthroplasty of the joints is performed to restore motion of the joint and function to the muscles and ligaments. It is indicated in individuals with a painful, disabling arthritic joint that is no longer responsive to conservative therapy. The procedure is generally reserved for those with a less active lifestyle. The younger patient, very active older person, or laborer may better be served with a reconstructive procedure such as arthrodesis or osteotomy.

Early arthroplasty techniques used interpositional substances from autogenous tissue such as muscle, fat, fascia lata, and skin. These techniques improved results in ankylosed joints but were ineffective in treatment of arthritic joints. Synthetic substances such as Bakelite, glass, and cellulose were used for interposition with the same poor results in the arthritic joint.

The modern age for total joint replacement surgery began in the 1960s with the development by Sir John Charnley of a total hip replacement arthroplasty. The components consisted of a stainless steel femoral head replacement and a polyethylene acetabular component. Fixation of these components was achieved with PMMA cement. Similar components for the knee soon followed as did designs for use in the elbow, wrist, and ankle. Subsequent failure rates have all but eliminated most ankle and wrist replacements, but total hip and knee replacements are done in large numbers each year. Improvements in implant design, materials, and fixation techniques are ongoing.

Although the metals have become stronger and more wear resistant, the classic combination of metal on polyethylene is the mainstay of joint implants. Metals used in hip and knee implants include cobalt-chromium (weight-bearing femoral head) and titanium (stems of hips and tibial components). Femoral heads made of ceramic were developed in an attempt to reduce wear of the polyethylene caused by articulation. The acetabulum and tibial articulating surfaces continue to be substituted with ultrahigh-molecular-weight polyethylene (UHMWPE), which provides superior wear and deforming characteristics.

At one time it was thought that bone cement was the weak link in the longevity of a joint implant because of a relatively high rate of loosening of cement-fixed implants, especially in the younger, more active patient. In response to this belief, alternative methods of fixation have been developed. One method involves the application of a precoat of PMMA to the femoral stem to enhance prosthesis–to–cement-mantle bonding. Another method involves the attachment of a porous metal surface to parts of the femoral stem (Fig. 22-91) and the entire outer surface of the acetabular component. Most of the porous surfaces are composed of multiple layers sintered in place, creating interconnecting, open pores between the various particles. This allows for the ingrowth of bone to occur,

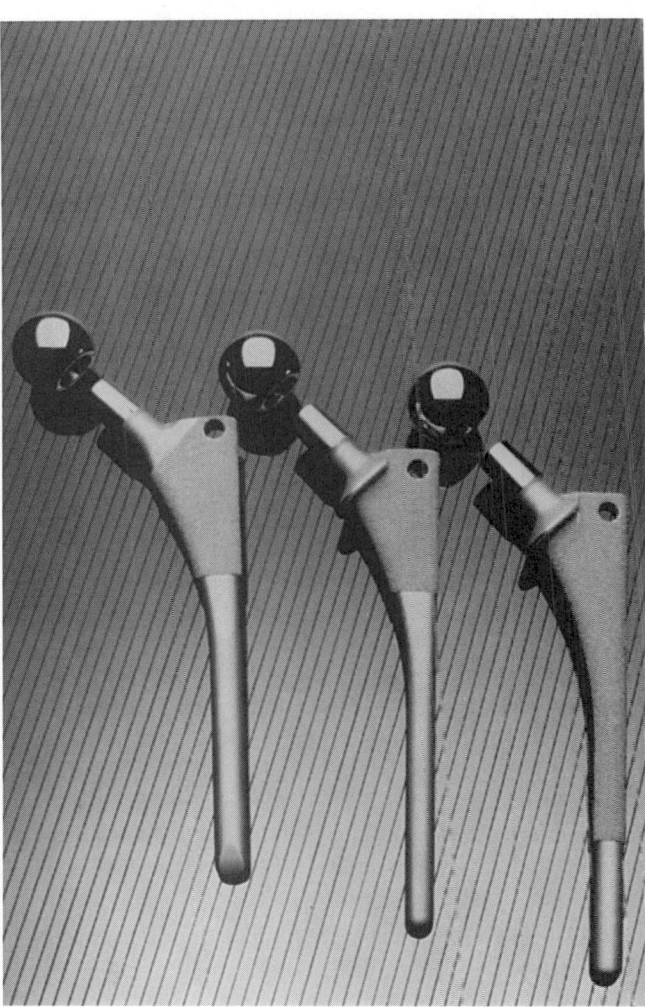

FIGURE 22-91 Porous-coated femoral implants.

22-2 **RESEARCH HIGHLIGHT**

Deep venous thrombosis (DVT) and pulmonary embolism (PE) are serious, potentially fatal complications occurring after total joint arthroplasties. Most practitioners agree that some form of chemical prophylaxis is necessary. But when should it begin, what kind should be used, and how long should it last? Many studies comparing warfarin to low-molecular-weight heparin (LMWH) have been done. One study from the Mayo Clinic examined 680 post-TKA patients in a double-blind, dose-ranging study. They found that although the high-dose LMWH patients had a lower incidence of thrombotic morbidity than the warfarin patients did, they also had a much greater blood loss. Another study compared two different warfarin regimens, one beginning 10 to 14 days preoperatively, the other beginning the night before surgery. The "night-before" group had a similar rate of DVT compared to the other group but experienced fewer postoperative transfusions and a higher postoperative hematocrit. Yet another study from England examined 1162 total hip arthroplasty patients in whom chemical thromboprophylaxis was not routinely used. It was found that the fatal PE rate after thrombosis *without* routine chemical prophylaxis was low; that there was a large discrepancy between the high DVT rate reported in clinical trials using universal screening venography and the symptomatic DVT rate shown in their study, and that there was insufficient evidence to recommend continuing thromboprophylaxis after discharge from the hospital. Additional research is required before perioperative practitioners can conclusively answer questions regarding chemical prophylaxis for their joint arthroplasty patients.

From Heit. J.A., Berkowitz, S.D., Bona, R., et al. (1997). Efficacy and safety of low molecular weight heparin (ardeparin sodium) compared to warfarin for the prevention of venous thromboembolism after total knee replacement surgery; a double-blind, dose-ranging study. *Thrombosis and Haemostasis,* 77(1), 32-38; Francis, C.W., Pellegrini, V.D., Jr., Leibert, K.M. et al. (1997). Comparison of two warfarin regimens in the prevention of venous thrombosis following total knee replacement. *Thrombosis and Haemostasis,* 75(5), 706-711; and Warwick, D., Williams, M.H., & Bannister, G.C. (1995). Death and thromboembolic disease after total hip replacement. *Journal of Bone and Joint Surgery–British volume,* 77(1), 6-10.

ultimately anchoring the prosthesis in place. "Porous coating" was an attempt to eradicate what was termed *cement disease,* a lysis of bone around the prosthesis causing early loosening. It is now believed that this condition is caused by "wear debris," particulate matter being shed from metal-to-polyethylene interfaces and not necessarily from the effects of PMMA.

Bone cement, or PMMA, is an area that has received considerable attention in the search for optimal bone-to-implant fixation. Cement seems to exhibit various degrees of porosity depending on mixing methods and cement pressurization within the canal. Bone cement must prevent motion at the implant interface. Porosity can lead to fatigue and fracture, which ultimately can lead to implant loosening. PMMA, chemically similar to Plexiglas, has barium sulfate added to it to make it possible to assess distribution and changes at a later time. Local tissue effects of PMMA may include (1) tissue protein coagulation caused by polymerization, (2) bone necrosis caused by occlusion of nutrient metaphyseal arteries, and (3) cytotoxic and lipotoxic effects of nonpolymerized monomer.

Despite the high rate of success of total joint implantation over the years, there are numerous potential complications. They are generally divided into medical complications, mechanical complications, and infections. Medical complications include but are not limited to cardiac dysrhythmias, myocardial infarction, hemorrhage, and pulmonary emboli (Research Highlight 22-2). Mechanical complications are implant breakage, loosening,

22-3 RESEARCH HIGHLIGHT

Cemented or noncemented? The debate continues with respect to total hip arthroplasties. One study from Canada found no statistical difference in the radiographic failure rates between cemented and noncemented hip prostheses. Metal-backed cemented acetabular components, however, did have high rates of radiographic failure. Another study from Tulane University focused on a cost-to-benefit analysis. Researchers there examined 50 total hip arthroplasties performed; in 25 cases, the femoral component was implanted with cement, and in the other 25, a cementless stem was implanted. For cemented stems, a third-generation cement technique was used, including centrifugation. The average cost to the hospital for a cementless stem was $900 greater than for a cemented stem. The total cost to the hospital for accessories used to achieve modern cement technique was over $700. The operative time for implanting a cemented stem averaged 20 minutes longer, which resulted in an additional operating time charge of $270 and an additional anesthesia charge of $100. When these charges were added to the cost of cement and accessories, the actual cost to the hospital for implanting a modern cemented stem was greater than the corresponding cementless stem.

From Rorabeck, C.H., Bourne, R.B., Mulliken, B.D., et al. (1996). Comparative results of cemented and cementless total hip arthroplasty. *Clinical Orthopaedics and Related Research, 325,* 330-344; Barrack, R.L., Castro, F., & Guinn, S. (1996). Cost of implanting a cemented versus cementless femoral stem. *Journal of Arthroplasty, 11*(4), 373-376.

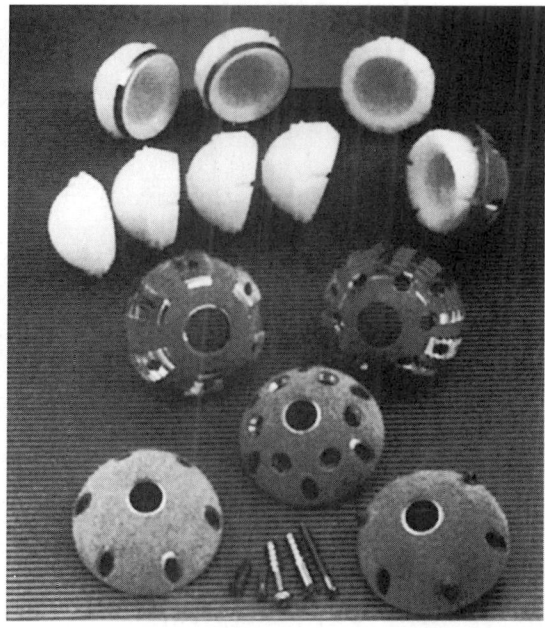

FIGURE 22-92   Press-fit implants. The area is prepared to secure the implant for use without cement.

and wear. Infection in the patient with a total joint implant is a catastrophic complication that usually requires additional surgery, prolonged hospitalization, and a greater economic burden.

Most surgeons recommend the routine use of antibiotics in primary and revision joint arthroplasty. Antibiotic coverage is initiated preoperatively, continued during lengthy procedures, and administered for 24 to 48 hours postoperatively. Pulsatile lavage systems or routine irrigation may be used to keep tissues moist, remove debris, and dilute bacteria, which may be present. Additional antibiotics are added to the physiologic saline solutions used for irrigation and to PMMA; however, data do not conclusively support or dispute this practice. Results of studies vary, due to variables in settings. It is believed that standard measures, appropriate use of perioperative antibiotics, and implementation of techniques recommended in the operating room should result in wound infection rates between 1% and 1.5%.[4]

The operating room and surrounding environment may play a role in the success or failure of total joint implantation. Airborne and contact contamination of a wound may be more significant in this procedure than others and certainly prove more catastrophic. These factors make it imperative that fundamental principles of asepsis and strict sterile technique are observed.

Total Hip Replacement

Total hip replacement (arthroplasty) is a common orthopedic procedure performed on patients with hip pain caused by degenerative joint disease or rheumatoid arthritis. A total hip replacement can be cemented, noncemented, or hybrid (Research Highlight 22-3). Hybrids involve cementing one component, usually the femoral stem, and then inserting a metal-backed, porous-coated acetabular component in a press-fit state (Fig. 22-92). Hybrid arthroplasty was very popular for a time but two factors have made this a controversial procedure. The first relates to research that demonstrates that wear debris is increased with the larger metal to polyethylene interface present in the metal-backed, porous-coated acetabular component. The second relates to cost. The metal-backed, porous-coated acetabular component is significantly more expensive than the all-polyethylene component. Consequently, patient selection is very important in determining which type of component is best.

The primary function of the femoral component is the replacement of the femoral head and femoral neck after resection. The femoral head should ultimately sit where it reproduces the center of rotation of the hip. The neck length is variable and is built into several different heights of femoral heads that are eventually seated onto the Morse

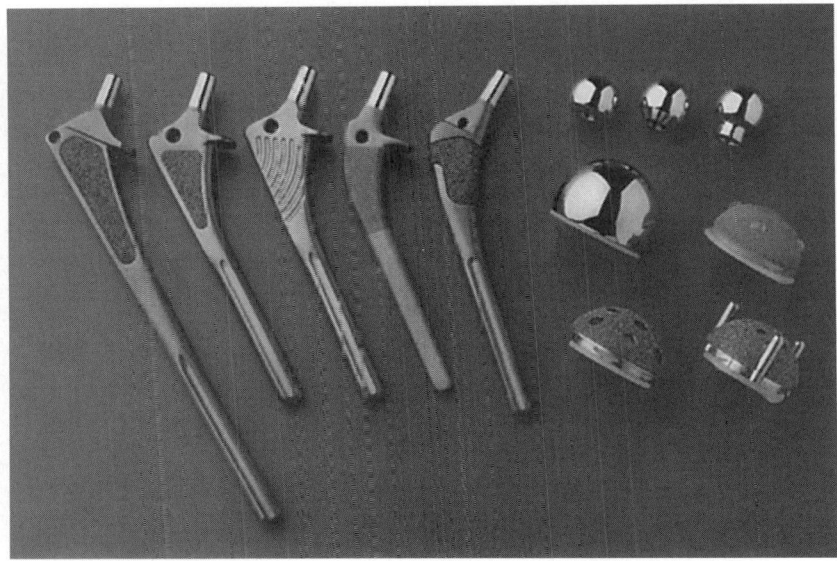

FIGURE 22-93   Modular hip components that can be used independently in the event of need for only one or failure of one component.

taper of the femoral stem. The version (implant rotation within the canal) is very important; too much anteversion or retroversion leaves the hip prone to dislocation. The normal position of the proximal femur is in 10 to 15 degrees of anteversion.

Femoral stems can be collarless or have collars that sit down on the resected femur. Collars will produce forces upon the bone and may be desired in cases of osteoporotic bone, where bone genesis may be diminished because of the disease process.

Acetabular cups have also presented challenges in trying to maintain fixation within the socket. When cement techniques of the 1970s are used, femoral loosening plateaus about 5 years after surgery.[12] Wear properties of the ultrahigh-molecular-weight polyethylene are also a concern. For this and other reasons associated with component failure the idea of modularity was developed. Modular components (Fig. 22-93), such as a polyethylene cup that snaps into a metal acetabular shell, greatly decrease the amount of surgery needed in the case of some revisions. In the case of excessive cup wear or a femoral neck length that is short, surgery is minimized with the ability to exchange the modular components without removing the implants fixed to the bone.

Acetabular cups come with a textured back for cement fixation and may have standoff pegs to allow an appropriate cement mantle. Noncemented cups usually are porous coated and may have screw holes present to aid in anchoring the less than stable cup. The presence of screw holes in an acetabular component is another controversial issue. Some believe that more wear debris is created with micromotion between the screw head and the cup as well as between the uneven surface of the screw and the polyethylene liner. Other methods of anchoring the cup

into the pelvis have been tried. At one time cups with large self-tapping threads circling the outside were screwed into the prepared acetabulum. These failed to gain popularity, however, because of stress placed on bone by the sharp edges of the threads.

No one prosthesis is suitable for every patient's needs. Modular hip systems allow the orthopedic surgeon to choose from an array of interchangeable components that have been developed. Various femoral head sizes (22, 26, 28, and 32 mm) are available to maintain proper center of rotation. Acetabular cups may be snap fit, low profile, or deep profile, which adds additional thickness to the medial wall, where there may be significant bone loss.

With modular systems, unipolar or bipolar cups are also an option when the acetabular articular surface is relatively normal. The unipolar and bipolar cups with appropriate head sizes are designed to fit on various modular system stems.

Custom prostheses or revision and extralong stems are available when there is significant bone loss. These implants are employed in cases of revision where fixation is needed farther down the femoral canal or in oncologic cases where tumor and corresponding bone have been resected.

Young, active individuals with strong healthy bones are ideal candidates for noncemented total hip replacement arthroplasties. Elderly patients with osteoporosis and poor quality bone are usually candidates for cemented components because their bones may lack the compressive strength to support weight-bearing forces.

Hip Reconstruction (Cemented)

There are numerous implants available for total hip implantation. Many of the implants can be used for the

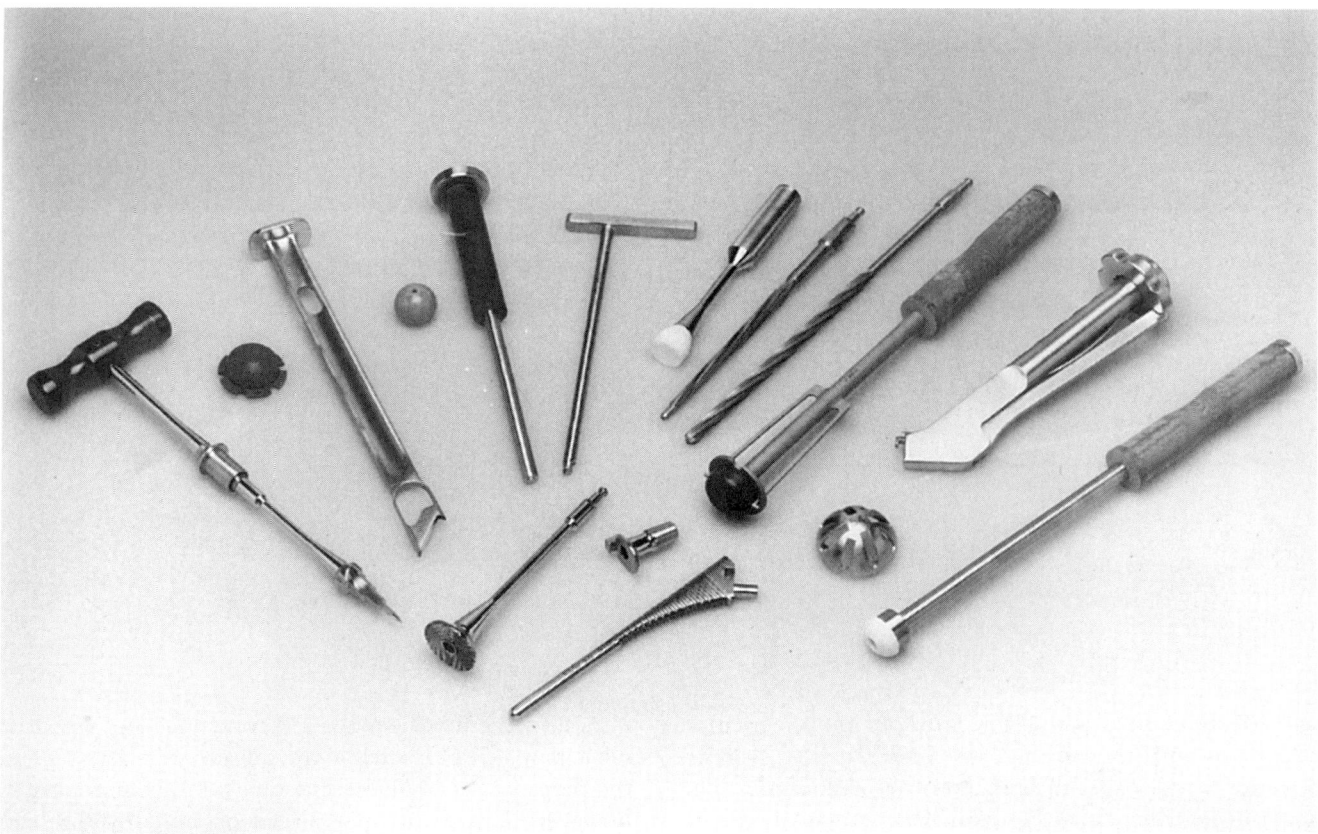

FIGURE 22-94   Anatomical medullary locking (AML) total hip system, used for total hip arthroplasty.

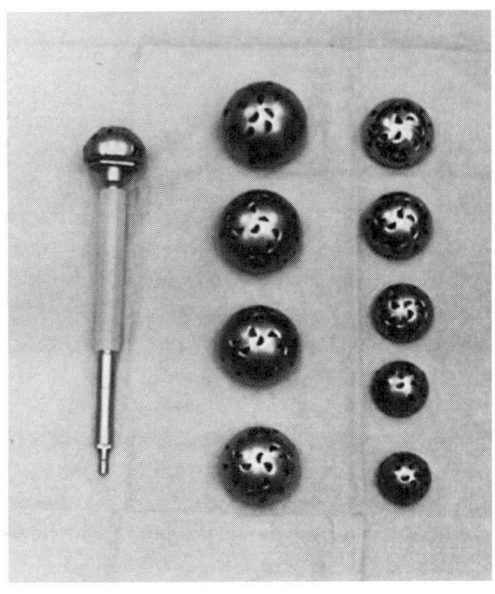

FIGURE 22-95   Acetabular reamers.

instrumentation is available before starting surgery. Furthermore, the surgical effort should be coordinated and without disruption. Once an implant has been inserted with bone cement that has hardened, significant bone resection and loss would result if correction were necessary.

PMMA adheres to the polyethylene and metal but not to the bone. It fills the cavity and interstices of the bone and forms a mechanical bond. PMMA is manufactured as a liquid monomer and a powder and is mixed under sterile conditions by the scrub nurse in the operating room at the time of implantation. It usually takes 10 to 12 minutes to harden. Because of the potentially harmful effects of PMMA fumes to the nasal epithelium, an exhaust system should be used during the mixing process.

Procedural considerations

The patient is positioned in the lateral decubitus position and secured in place with anterior and posterior bolsters. This position is essential to ensure correct anatomic placement of the acetabular cup. Bony prominences should be adequately padded. A surgical preparation is completed from the level of the umbilicus down to and including the foot, and the patient is draped. The radiographs are overlaid with the implant templates.

A soft-tissue set and large-bone set are required. In addition, the total hip implants and corresponding

same surgical indications, and one implant may not function any better then another, provided that all other conditions and techniques are the same. The instruments required to implant any one device cannot be used for another. It is very important to ensure that all the

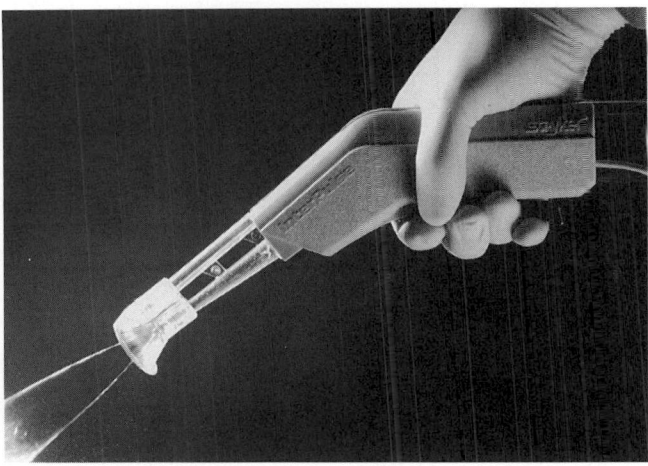

FIGURE 22-96 Pulse lavage used for pressurized irrigation when one is irrigating surgical wounds, debriding bone during a joint replacement, debriding open fractures or physically induced wounds, irrigating soft-tissue injuries, or irrigating contaminated wounds.

instrumentation (Fig. 22-94), acetabular reamers (Fig. 22-95), hip retractor set, power reamer driver and saw, and pulse lavage with a 3-liter bag of NS (Fig. 22-96) will be needed. If PMMA is used, femoral canal suction wicks, a cement restricter and its inserter (Fig. 22-97), and PMMA and supplies used to mix it (Fig. 22-98) will be needed. If a trochanteric osteotomy is performed, the equipment of choice for its reattachment will be needed.

Revision of total hip arthroplasties requires the same instrumentation as cemented total hip in addition to cement removal instrumentation (Fig. 22-99), fluoroscopy, and the revision implants and their corresponding instrumentation.

Operative procedure
Cemented Modular Hip System, Anterior Approach

1. An incision is made 2.5 cm distally and laterally to the anterosuperior iliac spine and curved distally and posteriorly over the lateral aspect of the greater trochanter and lateral surface of the femoral shaft to 5 cm distal to the base of the trochanter.
2. The tensor fasciae latae is divided over the greater trochanter, and this is carried distally to the extent of the incision. Dissection is carried proximally between the interval of the gluteus medius and the tensor fasciae latae muscle.
3. The anterior fibers of the gluteus medius tendon are tagged and detached from the trochanter. The capsule is incised longitudinally along the anterosuperior surface of the femoral neck. In the distal part of the incision the origin of the vastus lateralis may either be reflected distally or split longitudinally to expose the base of the trochanter and proximal part of the femoral shaft.
4. Once a capsulotomy is performed, the hip can be dislocated. Adduction and external rotation will

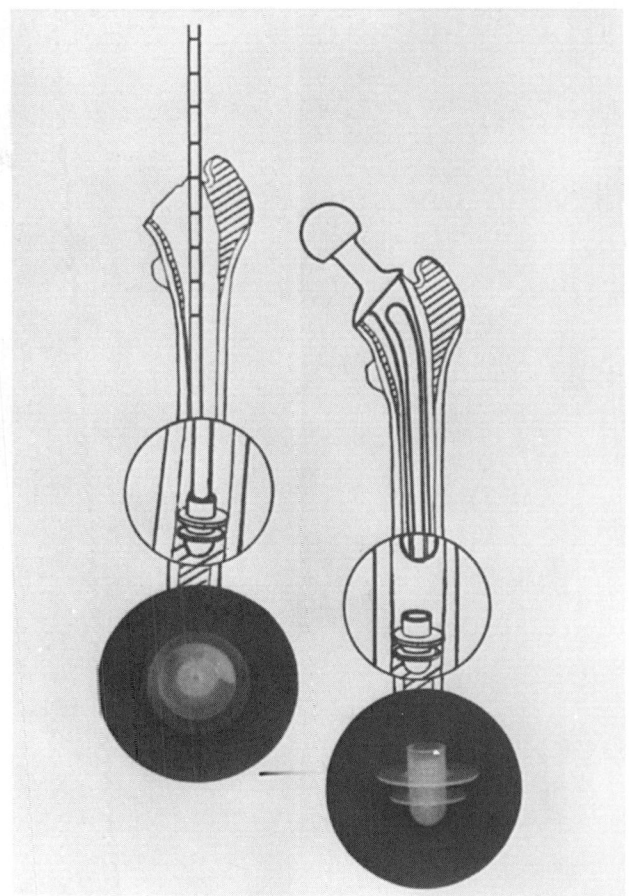

FIGURE 22-97 Cement restrictor and inserter used for occlusion of the medullary canal before delivery of the cement.

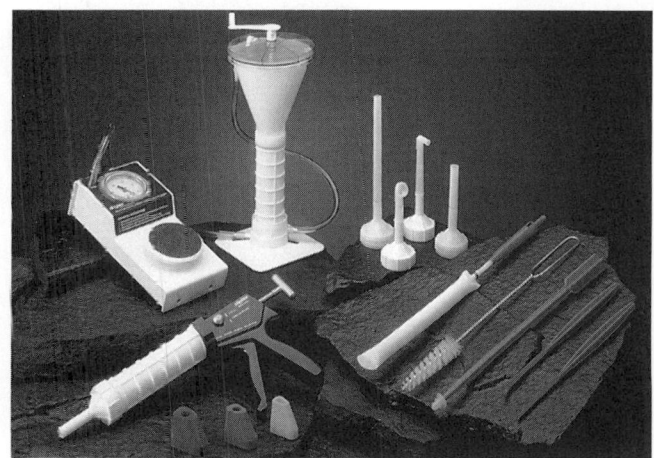

FIGURE 22-98 Polymethyl methacrylate, and supplies for mixing and delivery in the canal.

present the femoral head anteriorly into the surgical site.
5. The femoral osteotomy guide is placed over the lateral femur. This identifies the point on the femoral neck where the osteotomy should be made. Some femoral osteotomy guides will also gauge the neck length

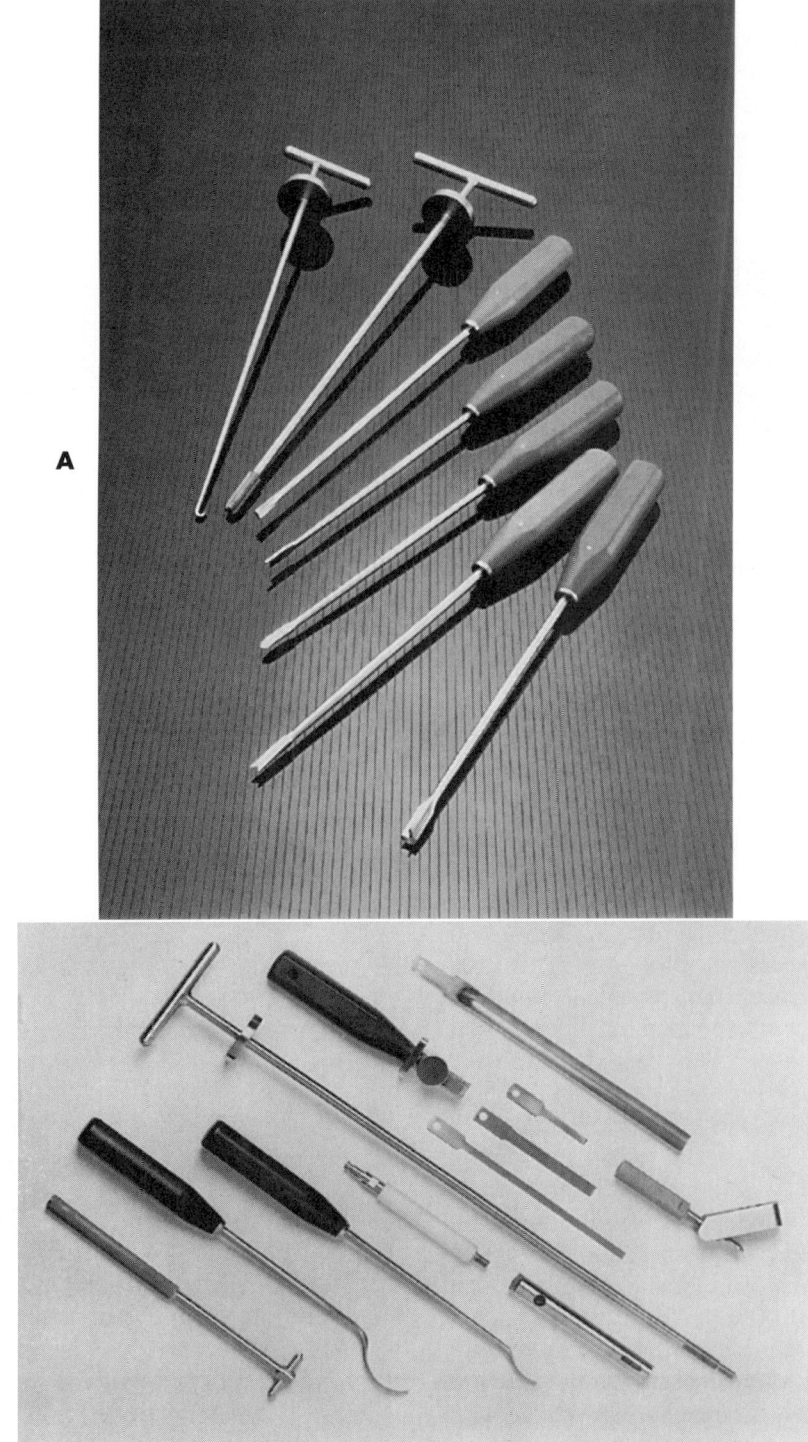

FIGURE 22-99   Implant removal instrumentation for, **A,** cemented or, **B,** noncemented implants.

required. The level is marked, and a femoral osteotomy is carried out with a reciprocating saw.

6. The femur is retracted to expose the acetabulum, allow completion of the capsulotomy, and expose the bony rim of the entire acetabulum.

7. The acetabulum is inspected, any osteophytes are removed, and articular cartilage is reamed with

bone-conserving reamers in a circumferential manner. The smallest reamer is progressed in a graduated method 1 or 2 mm at a time until the cartilage is reamed down to expose osteochondral bone. A hemispheric shape and bleeding bone should result.

8. Remaining soft tissue is curetted from the floor of the acetabulum, and cystic areas are filled with cancellous

bone from the femoral canal and packed with a bone tamp. Any other bone grafting of major bony defects is accomplished using the fixation method of choice (bone screws).

9. Several 6 mm holes are drilled into the floor of the acetabulum, aimed into the ilium, ischium, and pubis. Holes are undercut using curettes. These prepared holes act as anchoring areas for the bone cement.

10. Trial acetabular components are placed on the positioning device and positioned in the socket. The cup is assessed for size, position within the socket, and the relationship of the component compared with the bony margins of the acetabulum.

11. The prepared acetabular socket is given a lavage, dried with wicks, and filled with cement that has been injected and pressurized with an injection gun. The acetabular shell component is positioned and held motionless until the cement polymerizes. Extruded cement is trimmed from around the edge of the component. A polyethylene insert is later snapped into the shell.

12. A sponge is placed in the acetabulum to protect the component from bone debris and subsequent cement as attention is turned to the femur.

13. Dropping the foot toward the floor and internally rotating and pushing the leg proximally exposes the proximal femur. The femoral canal is accessed using a box osteotome or trochanteric reamer followed by the T-handle canal reamer.

14. Beginning with the smallest broach, alternatively impact and extract in the proximal femoral canal. Progressively larger broaches are used to crush and remove cancellous bone until cortical bone is reached. A broach that is not advancing should not be used. This could result in shattering the femur.

15. With the final broach seated to the desired depth in the canal, the neck is prepared with a calcar reamer. The broach remains as the femoral trial component along with the various-sized head, neck, and offset trial components.

16. The trial component is removed, and the canal is given a lavage and brushed to accommodate the PMMA.

17. A cement restricter is inserted into the femoral canal. The femoral components are passed and assembled on the back table.

18. The cement is injected and pressurized within the femoral canal.

19. The femoral component, with the proximal and distal centralizers, is inserted into the canal with or without the femoral head.

20. The appropriate size of femoral head is positioned onto the stem, and reduction is carried out. The joint is taken through a range of motion to check for positioning, stability, and the limit to which dislocation occurs.

21. Depending on the surgeon and the surgical approach, the greater trochanter may or may not have been removed for exposure of the hip joint. If removed, it is reattached with 18-gauge wire or a cable grip system.

22. The wound is closed in layers over suction drains. The skin is closed with staples, and a sterile dressing is applied to provide compression to the wound.

23. An abduction pillow or splint is placed between the patient's legs postoperatively if stability of the joint is of concern.

Hip Reconstruction (Noncemented)

Fixation with a noncemented prosthesis is initially accomplished by a tight fit and intimate contact of the implants within bone of substantial strength. As with all prosthetic designs, it is essential to fill the medullary canal and wedge the prosthesis in as tightly as possible to provide temporary press-fit fixation. These prostheses closely follow normal anatomic shape. Only the instrumentation corresponding to the implant should be used. Precise machining of the femoral canal must be ensured. Acetabular components are usually press fitted, but many systems provide holes for screw fixation if stability of the prosthesis is in doubt. Sufficient time is then allowed for the cancellous bone to heal by growing into the porous portions of the prosthesis.

The healing process requires the same amount of time as a long bone cortical fracture (approximately 3 months). Extreme caution is taken postoperatively to protect the operative hip from excessive compression, rotation, and shear stresses.

Procedural considerations

The position and incision are the same as for the total hip replacement (cemented). The radiographs and implant templates are placed on the view box.

Operative procedure
Noncemented AML Hip System (Fig. 22-100)

1. After the incision is made, the capsule is entered, and the femoral head is dislocated.

2. A pilot hole is established in the trochanteric fossa as an intramedullary reference point.

3. Reaming of the intramedullary canal is then performed in a progressive manner with fully fluted rigid reamers.

4. A femoral neck osteotomy is achieved by positioning an osteotomy template along the axis of the femur and cutting at the level of the collar.

5. Attention is directed to the acetabulum, which is cleared of soft tissue and reamed with hemispheric reamers.

6. Trial acetabular sizers are placed to determine the correct position and size of the prosthetic component.

7. A hollow osteotome is used in the femoral canal to connect the pilot hole to the osteotomy site.

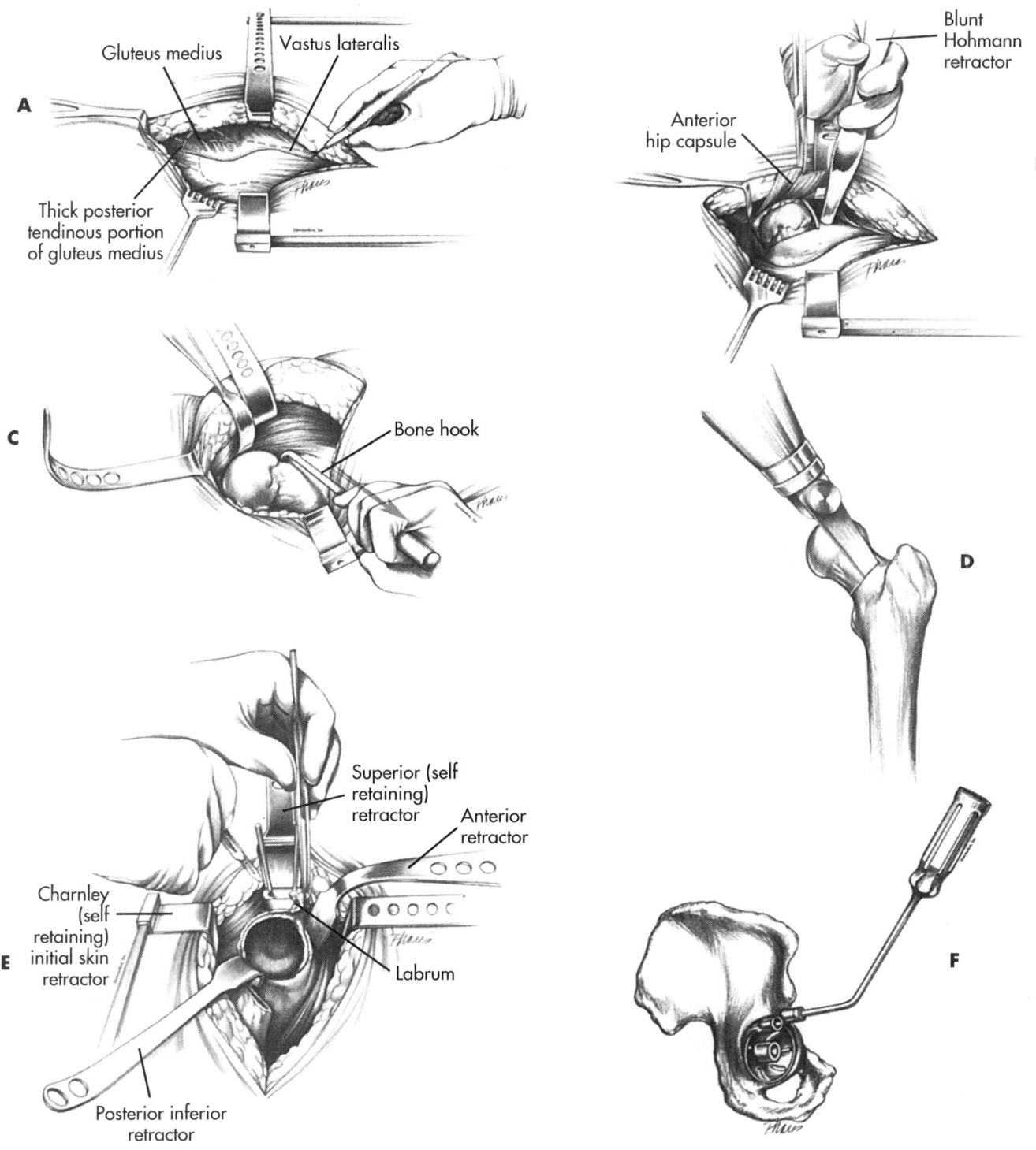

FIGURE 22-100   **A,** After the incision, the Charnley retractor is placed, the fascia lata is incised, and the gluteus minimus is detached. **B,** An anterior capsulotomy is completed. **C,** The hip is flexed, adducted, and externally rotated to dislocate from the acetabulum. **D,** The femoral neck is cut by use of an oscillating saw blade. **E,** The rim of the acetabulum is debrided of labrum, redundant capsule, and marginal osteophytes. **F,** The acetabulum is reamed; after reaming the appropriate drill guide is inserted into the acetabulum.

Continued

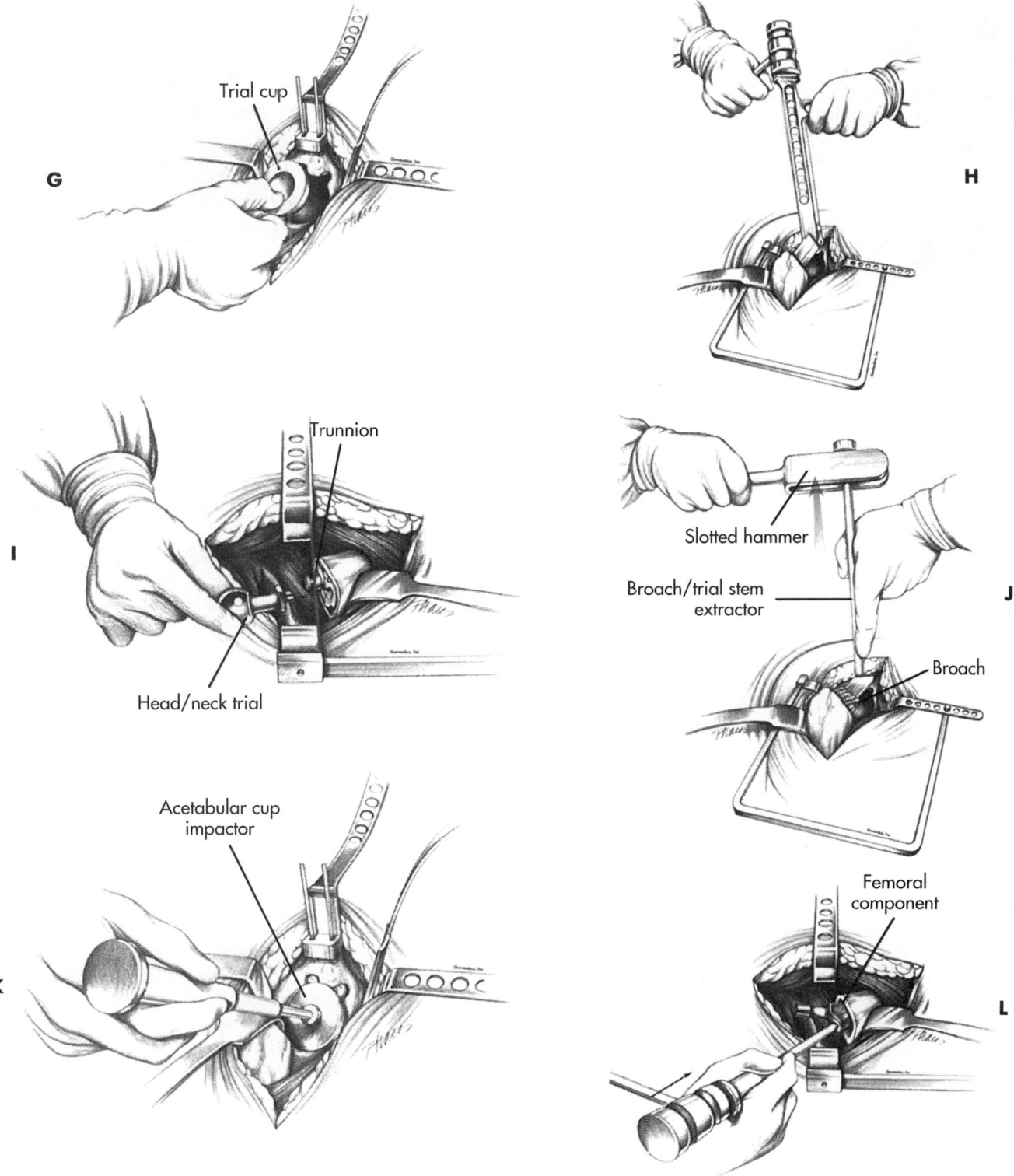

FIGURE 22–100, cont'd   **G,** After drilling of the holes for the acetabular fixation pegs, the trial acetabular cup is inserted. **H,** The proximal wedge of cancellous bone is removed, and the appropriately size femoral broach is introduced down the axis of the femoral canal. **I,** The trial head and neck assembly is placed on the broach trunnion of trial reduction. **J,** With the slotted hammer, the femoral broach is extracted; the trial acetabular cup is removed. **K,** Acetabular fixation pegs are seated, the acetabular cup is introduced, and the component is seated. **L,** The femoral canal is irrigated with pulsatile lavage and dried with suction and gauze sponges; the femoral canal is plugged and filled with methyl methacrylate; the femoral component is inserted.

Continued

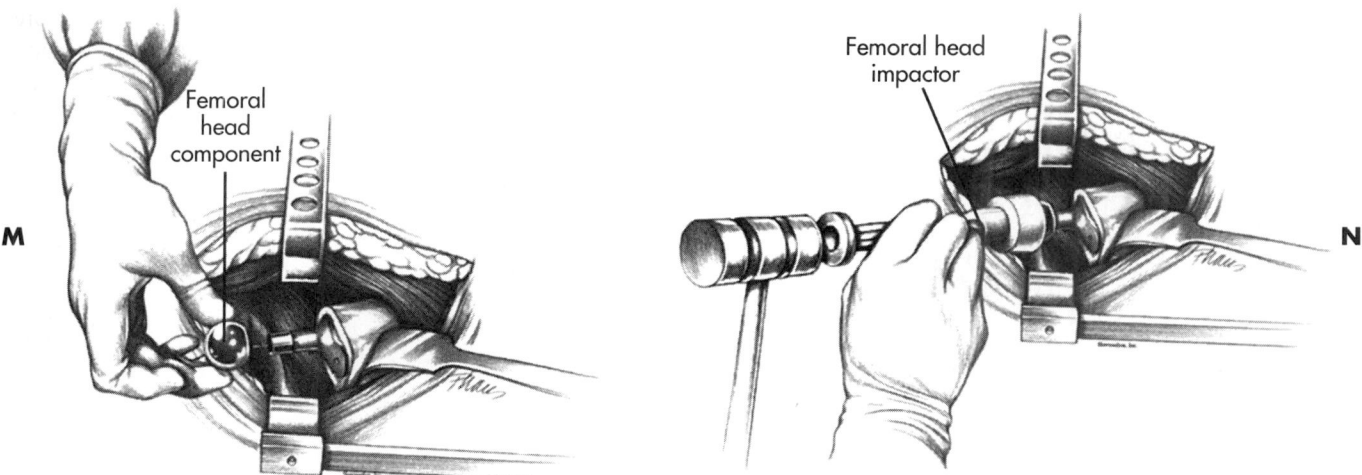

FIGURE 22-100, cont'd   **M,** The femoral head component is placed on the trunnion. **N,** The femoral head is impacted, the femur reduced, and the wound irrigated before closure.

8. Femoral broaches are then inserted to enlarge the intramedullary space for trial insertion.

9. A power calcar planer may be placed over the trunnion of the broach and used to contour the femoral neck.

10. A trial head and neck component is positioned onto the fitted broach, and a trial reduction is carried out.

11. If trial reduction is satisfactory, all trial components are removed.

12. The appropriate-sized acetabular component is inserted into the acetabulum, and a polyethylene insert is locked into place.

13. The femoral component is placed into the canal, and the modular head is seated on the trunnion.

14. Reduction of the hip is followed by standard closure with drains.

15. Abduction of the hip is maintained postoperatively with a foam abduction pillow, if necessary.

Total Knee Replacement

Total knee replacement (arthroplasty) is a surgical procedure designed to replace the worn surfaces of the knee joint. Success depends on patient selection, component design, surgical technique, and rehabilitation.

Patients with severe destruction of the knee joint resulting from degenerative rheumatoid or traumatic arthritis or destruction of only the medial or lateral compartments of the knee joint as a result of extreme varus or valgus deformity complain of pain and instability. Arthroplasty of the knee has been successful in relieving pain and providing stability. Like total hip replacement, knee surface replacement began as interposition of tissue between the resected bone ends to prevent them from fusing. Several substances were used, including skin, muscle, fat, and chromatized pig bladder. In the 1920s and 1930s Campbell used free fascial transplants as interposition material and achieved limited success in ankylosed

(fused) joints but not in the treatment of arthritic joints. After the success with materials for total hip replacement, total knee replacement progressed as a mechanism used to alleviate joint pain and deformity. Most authors believe that the modern age of total knee replacement is as late as 1971, with the development of a minimally constrained prosthesis addressing biomechanical considerations.

Continued clinical analysis of various implant designs and increased knowledge of the biomechanics of the normal knee resulted in the introduction of second-generation implants with improved configuration. Experiences with these second-generation implants led to further refinement of both instrumentation and surgical technique. Both alternative fixation techniques and improvements with the conventional cement methods are areas of current investigational efforts.

The challenge for finding the optimal knee implant is in reproducing the complicated range of motion of the knee. Motion of the knee occurs in three planes: flexion and extension, abduction and adduction, and rotation. Designs of total knees should allow preservation of the normal ligaments whenever possible while providing soft-tissue balance when necessary to maintain stability.

Total knee implants may be classified into three different categories, according to the portions of the knee to be replaced. Unicompartmental implants are used to replace just one opposing articular surface (medial or lateral) of the femur and tibia. These implants, however, lost popularity as a result of biomechanical and technical pitfalls. They account for less than 10% of all total knee replacements performed in the United States.[12] Bicompartmental designs, mentioned only to demonstrate the progression of total knee design, replaced both the medial and lateral surfaces of the femur and tibia. This implant design is almost completely rejected as a technique for knee replacement. Tricompartmental implants replace not only the opposing femorotibial joint, but also the

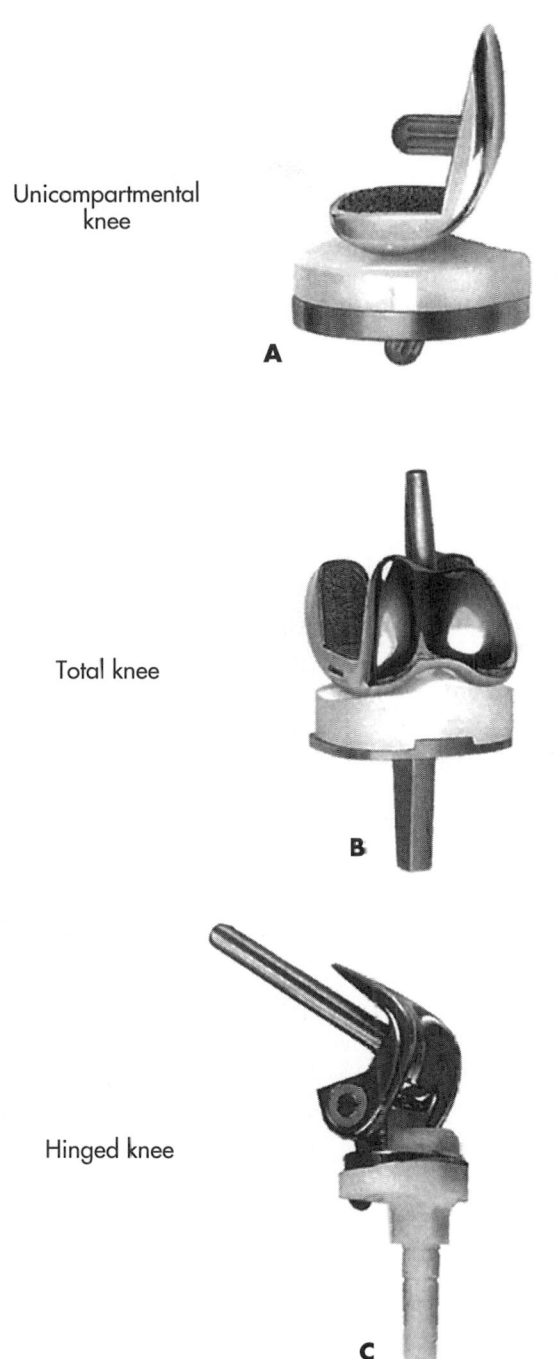

Unicompartmental
knee

A

Total knee

B

Hinged knee

C

FIGURE 22-101 Knee arthroplasty implants. **A,** Unconstrained. **B,** Semiconstrained. **C,** Fully constrained hinge.

semiconstrained prosthesis, which lends itself to more inherent stability necessitated by ligamentous deficiency. *Fully constrained* prostheses are linked together with pure hinges, rotating hinges, and nonhinged designs. They are used in the presence of considerable bone loss, instability, deformity, and revision surgery where there has been significant bone loss. Fully constrained prostheses do not provide a normal range of motion, and such a lack leads to excessive wear and implant loosening and breakage.

Methods of fixation of total knee implants include both cemented and noncemented techniques. The noncemented variety encompasses both porous bony ingrowth and press-fit designs. The choice of implant and method of fixation depend on the predisposition of the bone, patient age and activity level, and surgeon comfort with a particular technique. Previous designs did not allow the retention of the posterior cruciate ligament as it was resected, possibly leading to increased joint instability. Newer designs, however, allow the posterior cruciate to be retained. Some surgeons believe that the retention of the posterior cruciate ligament dictates the need for absolute ligament balancing beyond what may be possible in the reconstructed knee.

In the interest of more cost-effective utilization of medical resources, new designs have been developed for the less active patient with a shorter expected life span. The femoral component design is a symmetric design that can be used on either the left or the right knee. The tibial component is composed entirely of UHMWPE, thereby lowering manufacturing costs. Both components are placed with the use of PMMA.

Procedural considerations

The patient is placed in the supine position. A tourniquet is applied to the upper thigh. The surgical prep is completed. A soft-tissue set, large-bone set, the total knee instruments, trials, and implants of choice, a power drill and saw, PMMA and cement supplies, and a pulse lavage will be required.

Operative procedure
LCS Total Knee Replacement (Fig. 22-102)

1. With the knee slightly flexed, a straight midline incision is made from 3 to 4 inches above the patella, ending at the patellar tubercle.
2. The capsule is entered medially for a neutral or fixed varus knee, or laterally for a valgus knee. After a median parapatellar incision is made, the patella is reflected laterally to expose the entire tibiofemoral joint.
3. Hypertrophic synovium, a portion of the infrapatellar fat pad, and osteophytes are excised to allow easy access to the medial, lateral, and intercondylar spaces and to facilitate soft-tissue releases, should the need arise.
4. The knee is flexed to 90 degrees and retractors are

patellofemoral joint. Most of the total knee replacements completed today are of this variety.

The tricompartmental knees are further divided into three categories (Fig. 22-101). *Unconstrained* prostheses have very little constraint built in between the femoral and tibial components and depend on the integrity of soft tissues to provide stability of the reconstructed joint. Where there is significant deformity and the need for soft-tissue release, the surgeon may decide to use a

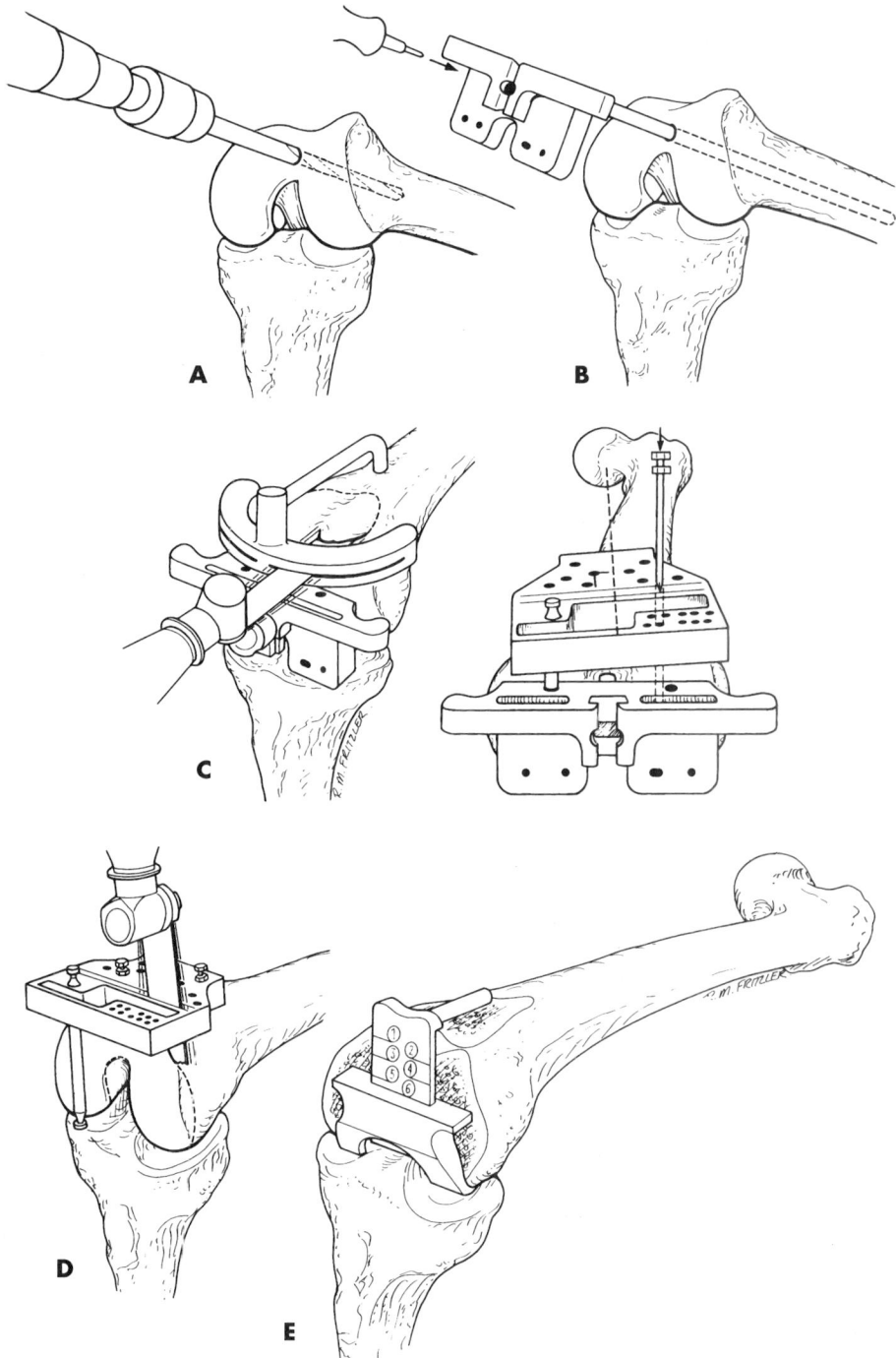

FIGURE 22-102 Total knee implant, instrumentation, and procedure. **A,** After exposure of the intercondylar notch, an 8 mm hole is drilled to the center of the distal end of the femur. **B,** The femoral intramedullary alignment guide is inserted and passed up the medullary canal. **C,** Correct rotational alignment is maintained; the anterior femoral cutting guide is attached to the femoral intramedullary alignment guide. **D,** Femoral cuts are completed. **E,** The anteroposterior measuring guide is placed flat on the cut surface, and the femoral component size is determined. *Continued*

placed deep to the collateral ligaments and anterior to the posterior capsule to protect these structures during resection of the proximal tibia.

5. The long spike of the alignment guide is sunk into the proximal tibial spines. The ankle clamp is attached by wrapping the spring around the ankle. Proper rotational alignment is established by positioning the appropriate malleoli wings parallel to the transmalleolar axis. The alignment rod is proximally placed just slightly medially to the tibial tubercle. When the rod is

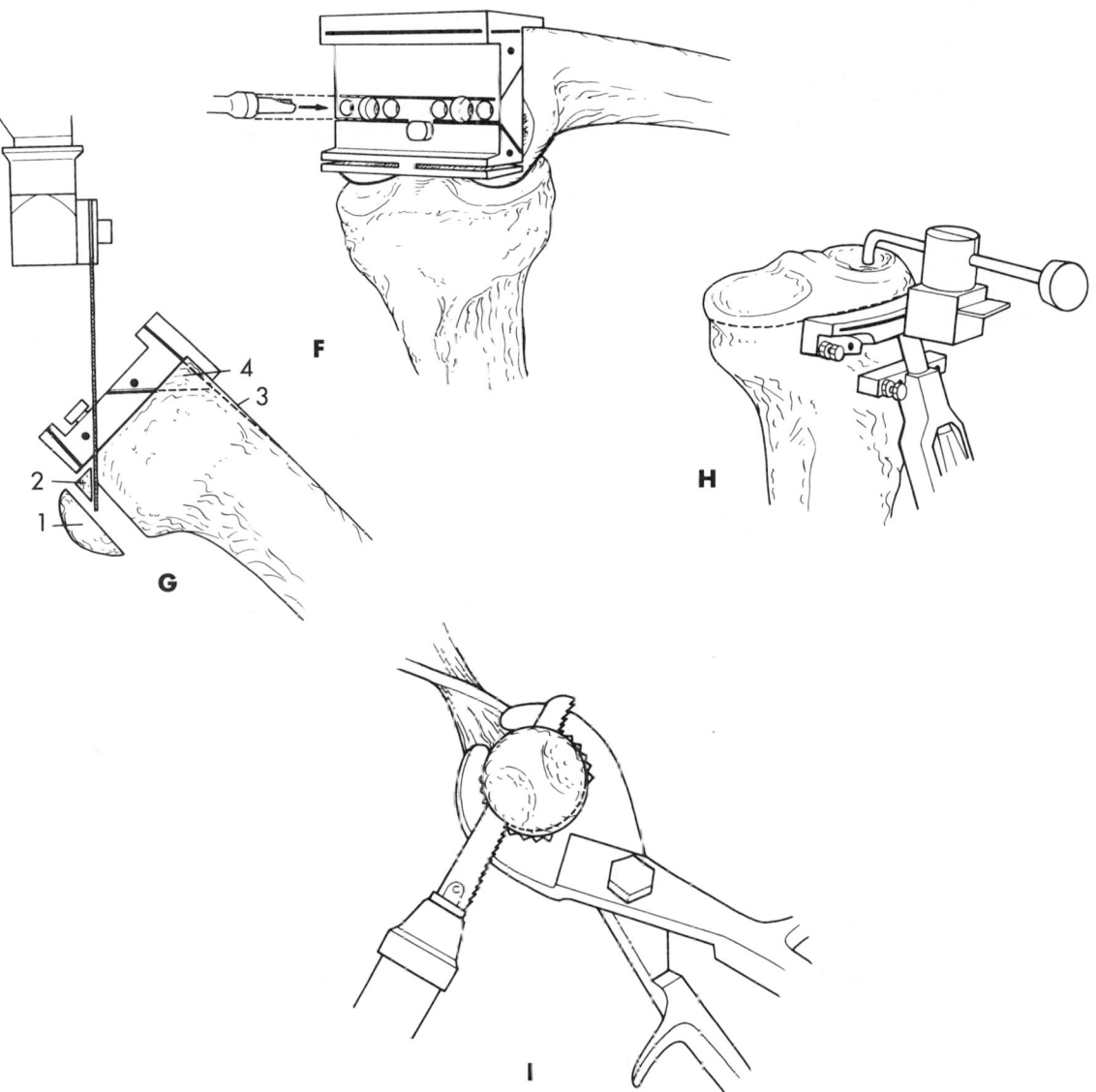

FIGURE 22-102, cont'd Total knee implant, instrumentation, and procedure. **F,** Femoral holes are drilled, and pegs are inserted. **G,** Final femoral cuts are completed. **H,** The tibial cutting guide is selected and positioned, and an oscillating saw is used to resect the tibia. **I,** The patella is grasped with the patellar saw guide, and the reciprocating saw is used to cut the patella. After preparation of the bony surface, a trial reduction is completed, and the component fit is determined; if the implants are to be fixed with poly(methyl methacrylate), surfaces are cleansed with pulsatile lavage; the tibial fixation plate is placed, followed by the femoral and patellar components.

parallel to the intramedullary axis of the tibia as viewed laterally, the second spike is impaled into the proximal end of the tibia.

6. The stylus is attached to the tibial cutting block on the side of the lower tibial compartment. The cutting block and stylus are lowered until the tip of the stylus contacts the tibial plateau. After predrilling, two 3-inch-long ⅛-inch fixation pins are placed in the marked row of holes. The stylus and alignment rod are removed, taking care not to misalign the cutting block. Alignment is checked by attaching the alignment tower and rod to the tibial cutting block. If alignment is found to be in variance, the cutting block

can be removed from the pins, and the special 2-degree varus-valgus block is applied to the pins for correction.

7. The saw capture is applied, and the proximal tibia is resected.

8. Before proceeding further, the surgeon assures that the extremity can be brought into normal mediolateral (ML) alignment in extension. If not, additional soft-tissue balancing is performed until the normal mechanical axis is obtained.

9. A template is made for the femur, and the appropriate AP femoral resection guide is selected. The guide yoke is attached to the AP block and the yoke is

slipped under the muscle anteriorly on the periosteum. The ML centerpoint is found, and a 9 mm hole is drilled into the femoral canal. The yoke is removed and the 7-inch, 9 mm rod is inserted into the femoral canal.

10. The femoral guide positioner is placed into the joint space, engaging the slot of the femoral AP resection guide. Tibial shims are placed to equalize collateral ligament tension, if necessary. The AP resection guide is pinned into place, the femoral guide positioner and intramedullary (IM) rod are removed, and the anterior and posterior femoral cuts are made.

11. A distal femoral cutting block is chosen, based on the patient's height, and it is attached to the distal femoral cutting guide. The 8 mm femoral IM rod is inserted into the distal femoral cutting guide assembly, and that, in turn, is slowly advanced into the femoral canal. The cutting guide should abut the intercondylar notch. The cutting block is pinned into place, the saw capture is applied, and the distal femoral cut is made after removal of the IM rod and cutting guide assembly.

12. The appropriate spacer block is then used to assure equal tension in flexion and extension. If flexion is tighter than extension, additional bone must be resected from the distal femur.

13. The knee is placed in flexion; the femoral finishing guide is centered between the epicondyles and impacted until fully seated. Two anterior fixation pins secure the guide to the femur. Two ¼-inch holes are drilled into the distal end of the femur, and the anterior and posterior chamfers are cut with the oscillating saw. An osteotome is used to make the recessing cut from the proximal end of the finishing guide. A power saw is used to resect the posterior femoral condyle remnants to assure adequate flexion clearance.

14. The tibial size is reassessed using the tibial templates. The selected tibial template is then positioned rotationally, and the appropriate-sized centering punch is used to cut through the subchondral bone. The bone is compressed into the tibia with the tibial impaction punch.

15. The patellar cutting guide is placed onto the patella, and the appropriate resection is performed. The patellar template is placed over the resected surface, and the cruciate channels are created using the patellar burr through the slot in the template.

16. A trial reduction is performed, seating the tibial tray first, the tibial insert, the femoral component, and finally the patella. If this reduction proves satisfactory with regard to alignment and ligament laxity, the trial components are removed, the bone surfaces are irrigated with a pulsatile lavage, and the permanent components are placed. These can be inserted without

bone cement, with bone cement, or a combination of both.

17. Drains are placed in the joint depending on surgeon preference. The joint is closed in the usual fashion, and a compressive dressing is applied to the leg. The tourniquet can be released before closure or after the dressing has been applied. Aftercare consists in rapid mobilization and strengthening, with a target discharge of 3 to 4 days postoperatively.

Total Shoulder Arthroplasty

Physically induced or accidental injury or degenerative arthritis may necessitate prosthetic replacement of the shoulder joint. The procedure may be a hemiarthroplasty with reconstruction of the humeral side, or total with replacement of the humeral head and glenoid (Fig. 22-103).

Shoulder motion is difficult to restore; therefore the need for rehabilitation is vital. A prosthetic implant does not solely ensure return of function, but will offer the anatomy to support exercise for restored function.

Procedural considerations

The patient is placed in a 30-degree, semisitting position with the arm on a padded armboard and draped free and the shoulder hanging slightly off the OR bed to allow movement through the entire range of motion. The head is supported to avoid neck extension. A pad is placed beneath the scapula.

A soft-tissue set, large-bone set, shoulder instruments, PMMA and cement supplies (see Fig. 22-98), the implants with associated instrumentation and trials, a power drill, reamer, and saw, and a pulse lavage system will be needed.

Operative procedure
Neer Total Shoulder Arthroplasty (Fig. 22-104)

1. A 16 cm incision is made from the midacromion distally along the deltopectoral groove.

2. The cephalic vein is identified, and the deltopectoral groove is opened and retracted.

3. The deltoid attachment may be removed if the patient is large or muscular, which may affect rehabilitation.

4. The long head of the biceps is identified as the landmark between the tuberosities and rotator interval.

5. The subscapularis is elevated from the underlying capsule, divided 2 cm medially to the bicipital groove, and a stay suture is placed.

6. The subscapularis is retracted medially with the lesser tuberosity, thereby exposing the joint and associated structures.

7. The capsule is exposed by elevation. An elevator is placed beneath the capsule to protect the axillary nerve. The long head of the biceps is left undisturbed and free in its groove so that it will continue to function as a depressor of the head after surgery.

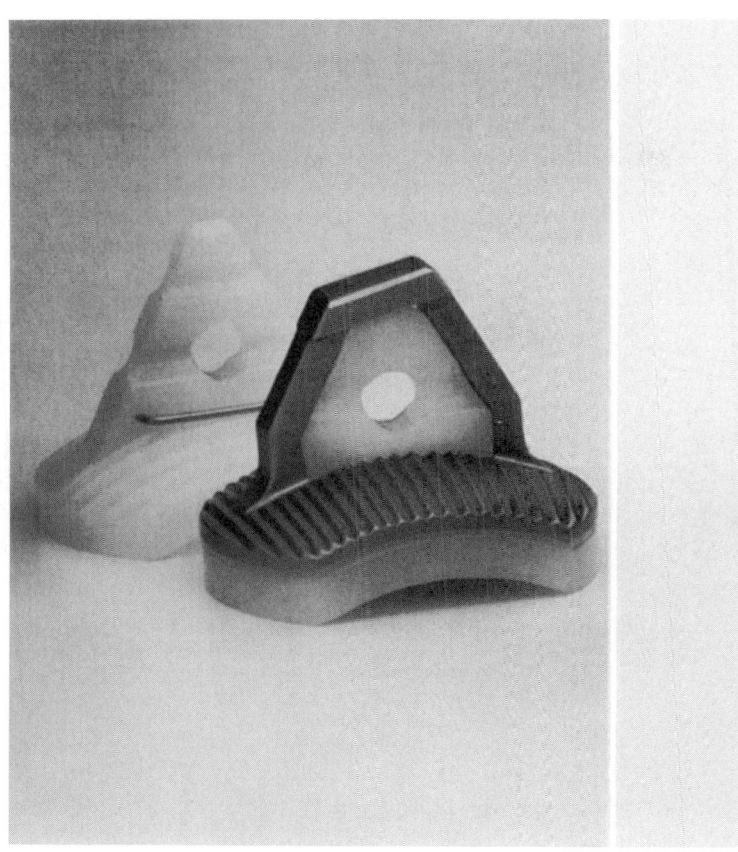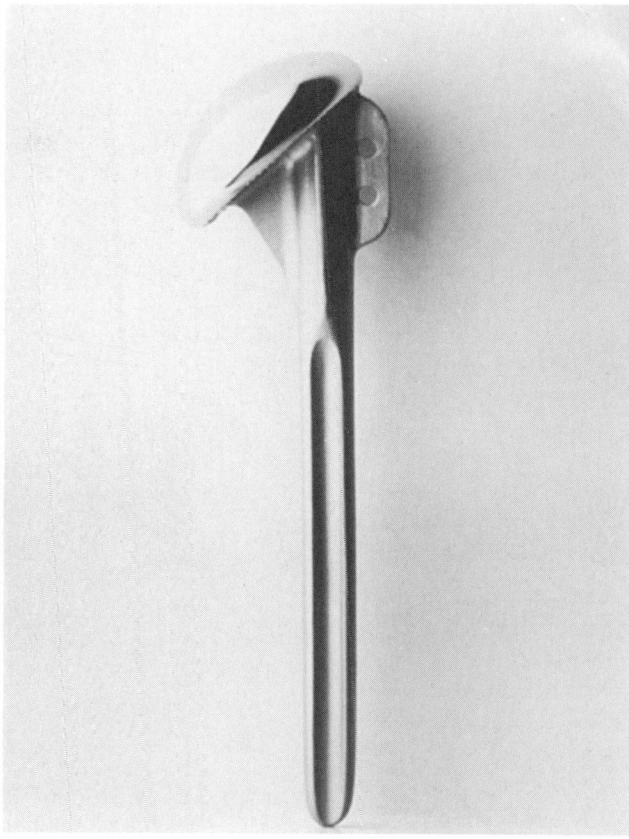

FIGURE 22-103 Neer shoulder prosthesis.

8. After external rotation, the fractured humeral head is removed. The incision site is irrigated to remove blood and clots from the joint.

9. The proximal humeral shaft is examined to select the appropriately sized stem, available in various lengths and diameters.

10. Marginal osteophytes are trimmed.

11. The glenoid is inspected for integrity and sized for a prosthesis if it is to be replaced.

12. A central hole for a prosthesis fit is made into the glenoid with a high-speed burr and curette.

13. Stem diameter and length are estimated to check the prosthesis for fit. The largest stem diameter possible is used.

14. With the shaft held forward and upward, the intramedullary canal is located with a long curette. A ¼-, ⅜-, or ½-inch drill bit is selected to correspond to the diameter of the canal; depending on the prosthesis stem length, 5 or 6 inches down the medullary canal is drilled. Final preparation of the shaft is accomplished with the appropriately sized tapered reamer.

15. A heavy-gauge nonabsorbable suture is passed through holes that have been drilled on the tuberosities. The length of the rotator cuff is checked by pulling the tuberosities distal to the collar of the prosthesis.

16. Neck length and stability of the joint are determined before final impaction of the prosthesis.

17. A check for 35- to 40-degree retroversion is done by palpating the epicondyles at the elbow.

18. The implant is seated on the calcar with a driver and mallet, with its articular surface protected with a moist sponge. Just before final seating, further trimming of high spots with an osteotome or high-speed burr may be required. PMMA is used except in young patients, in whom a firm press-fit can be achieved.

19. Wires or sutures are passed through the holes in the neck of the prosthesis, reducing the tuberosities beneath the collar, and secured. If wires are used, they are buried in drill holes in the bone.

20. The shoulder is reduced. The interval of the rotator cuff is closed and the biceps tendon reattached if previously detached.

21. The joint is irrigated as each compartment and layer is closed.

22. A closed drainage system is inserted between cuff and deltoid, avoiding contact of the drainage tubes with the axillary artery. Routine closure is accomplished.

23. ABD pads are placed between the body and the arm. A shoulder immobilizer is used. Passive range-of-motion machines may be used in patients prone to

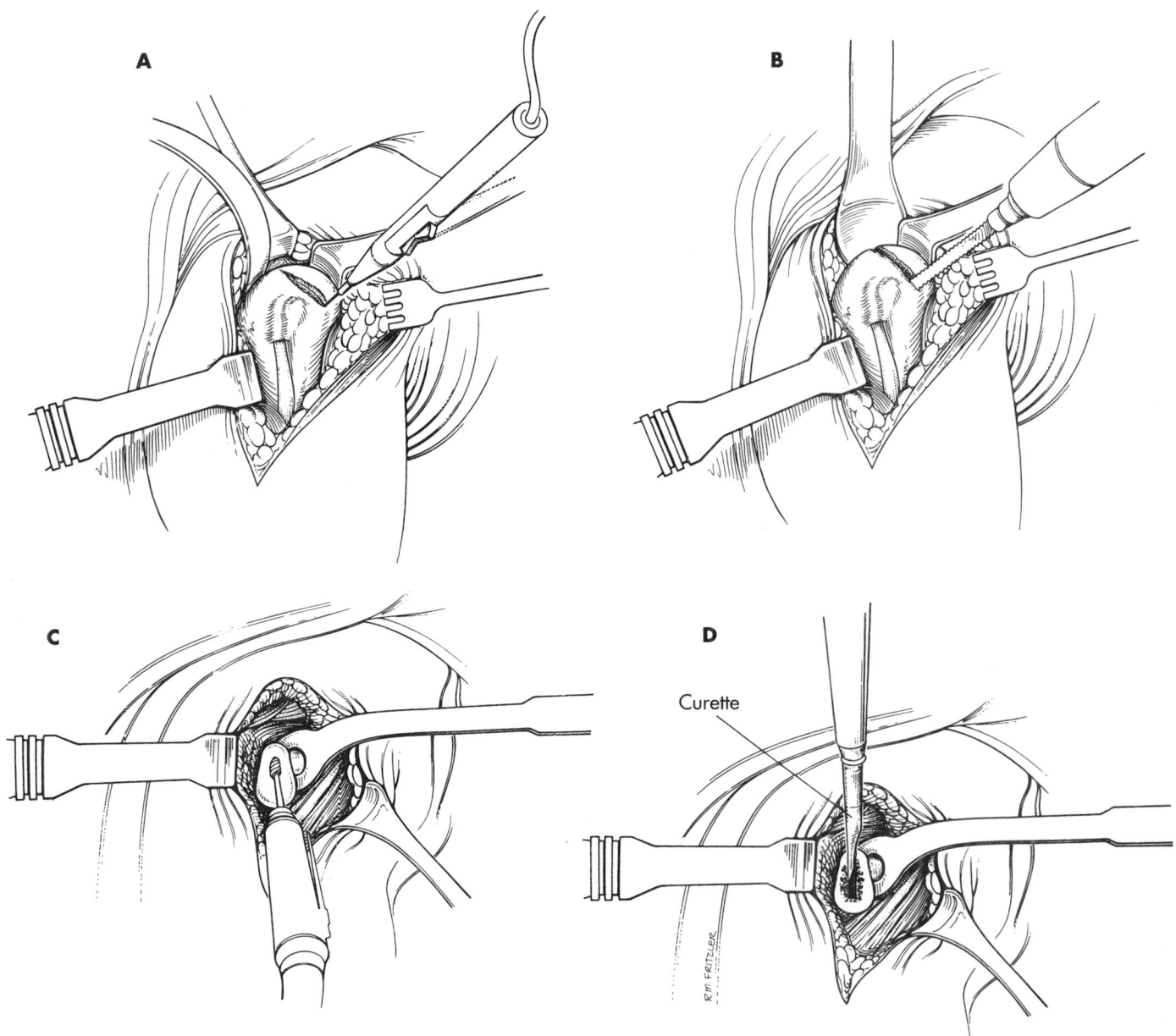

FIGURE 22-104 Total shoulder arthroplasty. **A,** The patient is positioned, and a deltipectoral incision is made to release the capsule. **B,** Humeral head is removed with reciprocating saw. **C,** After exposure of the glenoid, a fenestration for the glenoid component is made. **D,** The glenoid bow is curetted.

Continued

adhesion or contracture. Pendulum and gentle exercise are permitted at 10 days.

Total Elbow Arthroplasty (Fig. 22-105)

Total elbow replacement is indicated for patients with traumatic lesions or excessive bone loss from rheumatic or degenerative arthritis, resulting in elbow instability and pain or bilateral elbow ankylosis. Arthroplasty of the elbow is not as prevalent as arthroplasty of the shoulder, knee, or hip. The design of implants and methods of fixation for postoperative stability have presented challenges that have

been overcome in arthroplasty of other joints but have remained a challenge in elbow arthroplasty. Postoperative stability of the elbow implant depends largely on the soft tissues surrounding the joint. There are devices that provide more constraint for the patient with significant soft-tissue laxity or loss of bone stock. The Coonrad-Morrey, Tri-Axial, and Pritchard-Walker are just a few of the total elbow prostheses available.

The prosthesis may be used with or without PMMA, depending on the quality of the diseased bone and the design of the implant. If PMMA is not employed, bone

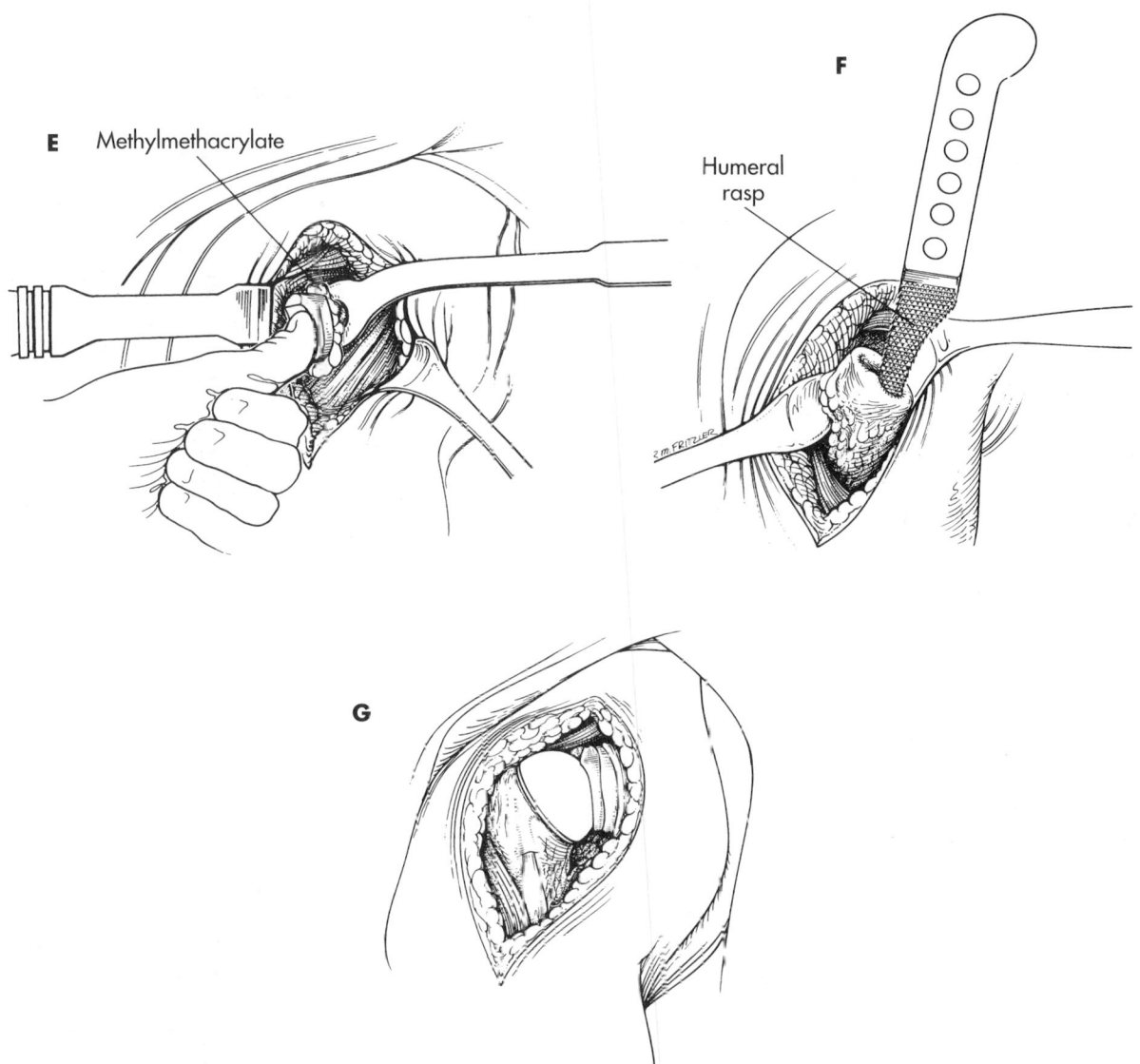

E, Methylmethacrylate

F, Humeral rasp

G

FIGURE 22-104, cont'd   Total shoulder arthroplasty. **E,** Cancellous bone is evacuated and cement impressed. **F,** Humeral shaft is rasped. **G,** Humeral component is inserted.

grafting with local bone that has been resected may be used to help seat the ulnar component snugly and achieve adequate bony contact against the porous coating of the metal ulnar component. Patients with degenerative arthritis generally have better results than those with injury after elbow arthroplasty.

Procedural considerations

The patient is in the supine or semi-Fowler's position with the arm over the chest. A tourniquet is applied and can be inflated if needed. The arm is prepped from shoulder to fingers and draped. A soft-tissue set, small-bone set, the total elbow implants and instruments, a power saw, drill, and burr, an awl, heavy-gauge wire, and a wire tightener will be needed. PMMA and cement

supplies as well as a pulse lavage system are required if the prosthesis is placed with the use of PMMA.

Operative procedure

1. The limb is exsanguinated, and the tourniquet is inflated to the desired pressure.
2. A midline posterior incision is made, protecting the ulnar nerve.
3. The triceps mechanism is elevated in continuity with the periosteum, and the elbow joint is explored.
4. The distal end of the humerus, proximal end of the ulna, and radial head are explored, preserving the collateral ligaments.
5. The midportion of the trochlea is removed to allow access to the distal end of the humerus; the medullary

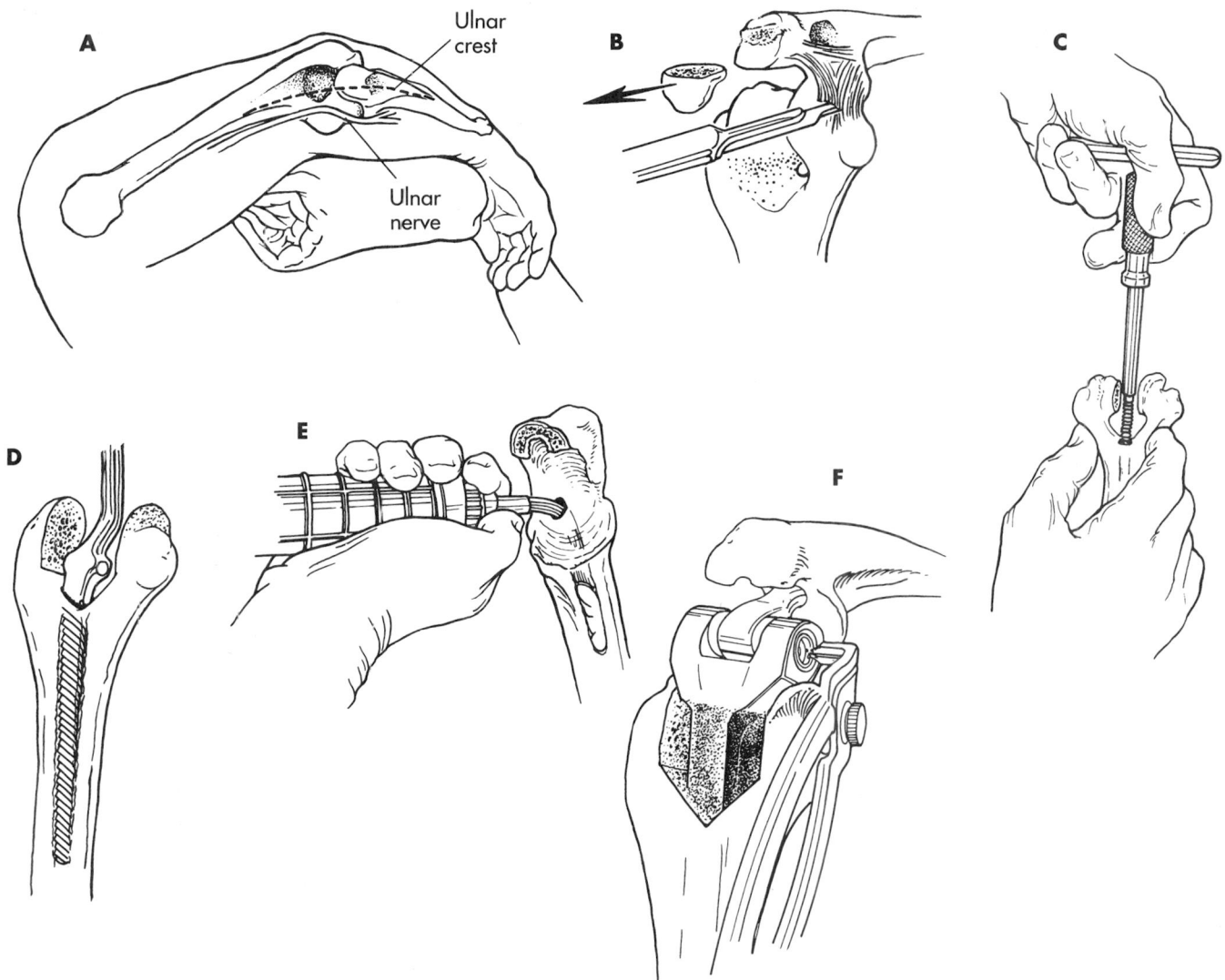

FIGURE 22-105 Total elbow arthroplasty. **A,** The arm is draped free and the incision made. **B,** The tip of the olecranon is excised with an oscillating saw. **C,** The canal is identified with a burr, and the canal is opened with a twist reamer. **D,** The capitellum is measured and cut. **E,** The medullary canal is cleaned and dried, and bone cement is inserted. **F,** Ulnar prosthesis is inserted followed by cementing and inserting of the humeral components.

canal is opened with a high-speed burr and the canal entered with a twist hand reamer.

6. The distal end of the humerus is notched with the appropriate cutting guide.

7. A high-speed burr is used to drill through subchondral bone to allow access to the medullary canal of the ulna and serially ream the canal.

8. After the humerus and ulna have been prepared for insertion of the trial prosthesis, the elbow is evaluated for flexion and extension. Bony adjustments are made where necessary.

9. The canals are cleaned of all bone fragments by irrigating with pulsatile antibiotic lavage.

10. The canal is dried before implant insertion, and the preparation is checked before the cement is mixed to ensure that the correct size component is available.

11. The cement is inserted into the canals followed by the prosthesis. Flexion and extension of the elbow are avoided until the cement has hardened.

12. Any bone graft that may be required is secured with wire or pins.

13. The tourniquet is deflated, and hemostasis is obtained.

14. The triceps mechanism is repaired. The incision site is irrigated and closed. A drain may be inserted.

15. A long-arm posterior splint is applied with the elbow at 90 degrees.

Total Ankle Joint Replacement

Long-term results for total ankle arthroplasty, especially in the young, are extremely poor. The procedure is reserved for older or more sedentary patients, especially those with subtalar or midtarsal arthritis. Ankle arthrodesis

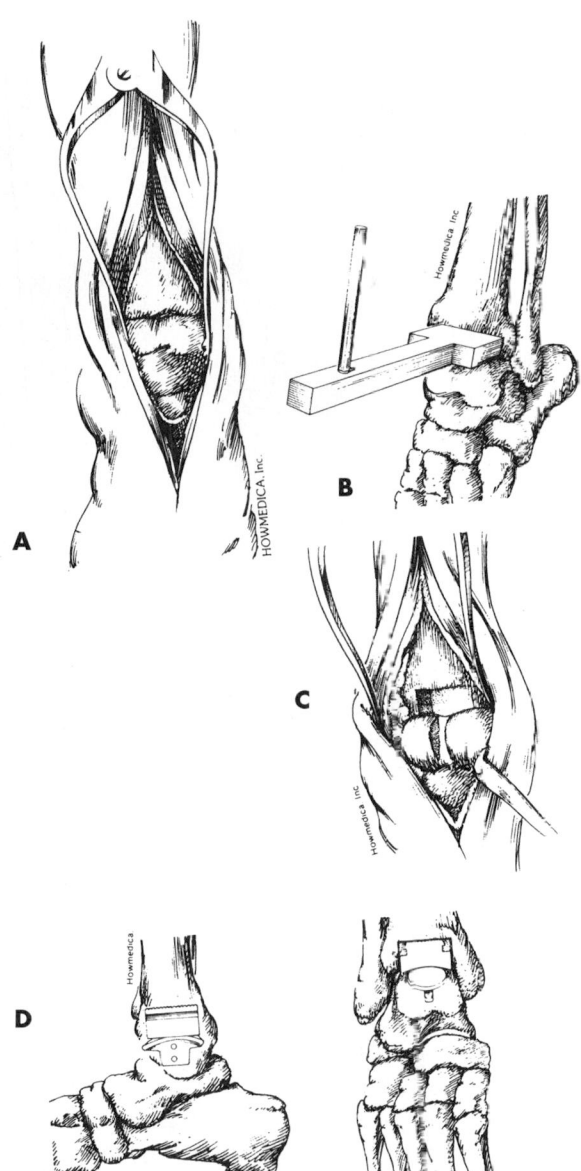

FIGURE 22-106 Total ankle arthroplasty. **A,** An anterior incision is made, and the tibiotalar joint and talus dome are exposed. **B,** The sizing template is used to mark the tibia. **C,** An air drill is used to create a defect, and anchoring holes are prepared. **D,** Trial reduction is completed, and talar and tibial components are cemented into place.

should be considered first in joint reconstruction. Indications for total ankle arthroplasty include (1) failed arthrodesis, (2) bilateral ankle arthritis when arthrodesis has already been performed on one ankle, (3) after talectomy because of avascular necrosis, and (4) revision of a previous arthroplasty. Total ankle replacement prostheses are made of high-density polyethylene and metal components.

Procedural considerations

The patient is positioned supine with the tourniquet placed. The leg is prepped and draped. A soft-tissue set, small-bone set, the total ankle joint replacement instru-

mentation and implants, a power drill and saw, a pulse lavage system, and PMMA cement and supplies will be necessary.

Operative procedure (Fig. 22-106)

1. An anterior incision is made over the ankle joint.
2. Exposure of the tibiotalar joint and talus dome is achieved by dissection.
3. Once the center of the talus is identified and marked, a sizing template is used to mark the tibia.
4. A 1-inch-wide by ⅜-inch-deep defect is made using the air drill. Anchoring holes can be made in the tibia. The template is positioned in the defect while the foot is distracted.
5. The talus is marked, and a ½-inch deep by 3/16-inch groove is made with a reciprocating saw to accommodate the talar component.
6. A trial fit is carried out to ensure that the talar unit is in the center of the talus and that the tibial unit is parallel to the plane of the floor, both centered over the dome of the talus.
7. Once trial reduction is complete, the talar and tibial components are cemented into place.
8. The ankle joint is irrigated and closed, a drain inserted, and a posterior splint applied.

Metacarpal Arthroplasty

Metacarpal joint replacement is most often performed in patients who have pain or a disabling deformity associated with rheumatoid or degenerative arthritis of the metacarpophalangeal or interphalangeal joints. The results of rheumatoid reconstructive surgery are generally good, and pain can be eliminated and joint alignment and joint stability restored in the majority of patients. The greatest problems after surgery are weakness of grasp and pinch and progression of the disease in adjacent joints.

Procedural considerations

The patient is placed in the supine position with the arm extended on a hand table. A tourniquet is applied, and the entire extremity is prepped and draped. A hand set, instrumentation for implants, and implants are required as well as a high-speed burr.

Operative procedure

1. Incisions are made on the dorsum of the appropriate fingers.
2. The proximal and distal portions of the joints are excised, and intramedullary canals are reamed.
3. Sizes are used to facilitate a correct fit of the prosthesis.
4. Once the appropriately sized implant is determined, it is positioned into the canal (Fig. 22-107), and appropriate tendon and ligament repairs are made to improve stability.
5. The joint is irrigated and closed, and a bulky dressing is applied.

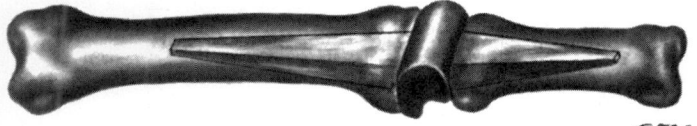

FIGURE 22-107   Metacarpophalangeal implant.

6. A short-arm posterior splint is applied for immobilization.

Metatarsal Arthroplasty

Silastic implantation is indicated in the treatment of deformities associated with rheumatoid arthritis, hallux valgus, hallux rigidus, and a painful or unstable joint.

Procedural considerations

The patient is placed in the supine position. A tourniquet is applied, and the entire extremity is prepped and draped. A small-bone set is required as well as the implant instruments and implants (Fig. 22-108), a power wire driver, and the microsagittal saw.

Operative procedure

1. The incision is made over the appropriate joints.
2. Resection of the proximal phalanx with removal of exostosis of the metatarsal head is carried out.
3. The medullary canal is reamed, and trial implants are fitted.
4. The appropriately sized metatarsal implant is determined and seated.
5. The wound is irrigated and closed.
6. A bulky compression dressing and orthopedic shoe are applied for early ambulation.

ARTHROSCOPY

Progress and development of arthroscopy and arthroscopic procedures have evolved, changing the approach, diagnosis, and treatment to many ailments of the joints. Arthroscopic techniques require skill and accomplishment in identifying three-dimensional relationships.

The advantages of arthroscopic surgery surpass the disadvantages. Among the advantages are (1) decreased recovery and rehabilitation time, (2) smaller incisions, (3) less inflammatory response, (4) less postoperative pain, scar, and extensor disruption, (5) reduced complications, (6) reduced hospital stay and cost, and (7) easier, more rapid surgical procedures.

Disadvantages usually relate to the size and delicacy of the instruments. Maneuverability within a joint may be difficult and produce scuffing and scoring of the articular surfaces.

Improvements in lens systems, fiberoptic cables, and miniaturization have made operative arthroscopy a logical extension of diagnostic arthroscopy. Surgical arthroscopy

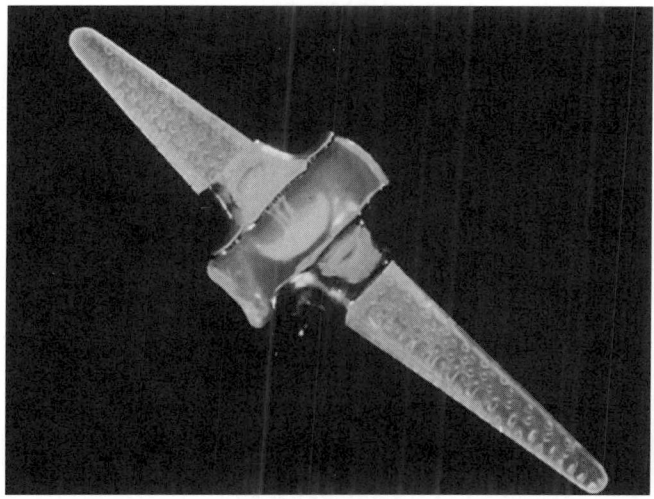

FIGURE 22-108   Silastic implant for finger joint.

has also been aided with development of numerous second puncture instruments and devices to repair and excise defects. There is a multitude of motorized shaving and abrader systems. Irrigation systems provide regulated distention of the knee joint by infusing normal saline or lactated Ringer's solution. These systems may function by gravity flow or are mechanized with microprocessors built in to monitor joint pressures and adjust accordingly. Lasers and electrosurgical units can be used in tandem with arthroscopic equipment. Integrated video systems can record and store still and video images on film, tape, or floppy disk for education and documentation.

Arthroscopy is commonly performed on the knee, shoulder, and wrist. It is used less often in the elbow, hip, and ankle. Many corrective procedures that previously required an arthrotomy or other open procedure can be completed with the assistance of the arthroscope.

Arthroscopic equipment has certain requirements for care and handling. Fiberoptics, lenses, and cameras are heat sensitive, requiring consideration for sterilization. Temperatures and moisture generated by steam autoclaves can damage materials used in video equipment or deteriorate the sealant, making the moisture accessible to the lens. Alternatives to steam sterilization for this equipment are ethylene oxide, cold sterilization, and high-level disinfection. Each requires consideration of patient care options for consistency. Equipment must be soaked according to the manufacturer's instruction, followed by complete rinsing and immersion in sterile water to prevent chemical burns.[6] Cold-water sterilizing machines, which use bactericidal and sporicidal agents, can also be used to sterilize heat-sensitive equipment. The cycle time is approximately 30 minutes, allowing rapid turnover in comparison to the other methods.

Scopes, lenses, and fiberoptic cords used in the surgery should be handled carefully, and cords should never be kinked or twisted. When mishandled, gradual deterioration and fiber breakage occurs in the cables, and light

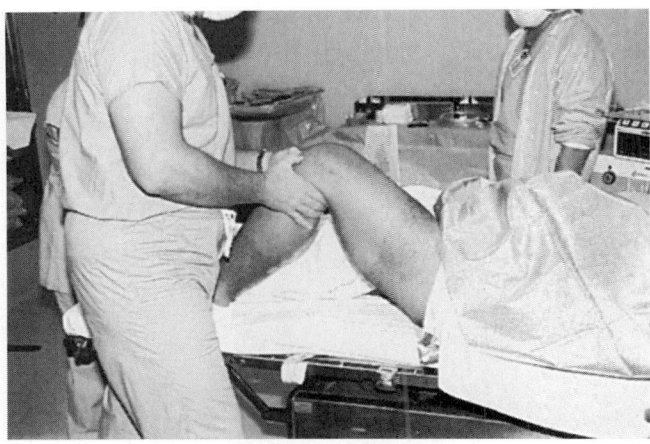

FIGURE 22-109   An examination with the patient under anesthesia may be completed by the surgeon before the patient is positioned.

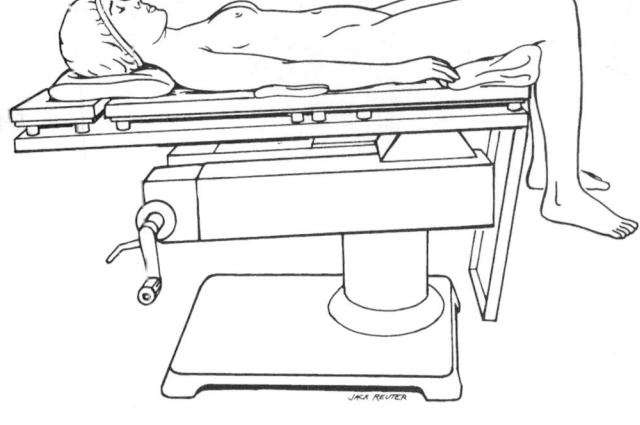

FIGURE 22-110   Positioning for a knee arthroscopy to enhance visualization.

cannot be transmitted. When stored, the cords should be loosely coiled or hung.

Two types of arthroscopy may be performed. Diagnostic arthroscopy is for patients whose diagnosis cannot be determined by history or physical examination or whose CT or MRI findings are insufficient to warrant surgical exploration. Diagnostic arthroscopy may be performed before an anticipated arthrotomy, and surgical treatment may be modified on the basis of the findings of the arthroscopic examination. Operative arthroscopy is for patients presenting with an intraarticular abnormality or ligamentous injury.

Arthroscopy of the Knee

The knee is the joint in which arthroscopy lends itself to the greatest number of diagnostic and surgical procedures. Arthroscopic surgery of the knee is indicated for diagnostic viewing, synovial biopsies, removal of loose bodies, resection of plicae, shaving of the patella, synovectomy, partial meniscectomy, meniscus repair, and anterior cruciate ligament reconstruction.

Arthroscopy may be diagnostic and be the initial step for an arthrotomy. Anesthesia for knee arthroscopy may be general, spinal, or local. Tourniquets are often placed on the thigh but are inflated only if bleeding obscures the view. If there are no contraindications, an epinephrine solution may be injected at the portal sites, or diluted into the distention fluid.

Procedural considerations

The patient is placed in the supine position on a standard OR bed. An EUA may be performed by the surgeon before the patient is placed in position for the arthroscopy (Fig. 22-109). The foot end of the bed may be flexed 90 degrees (Fig. 22-110). A lateral post can be attached to the bed at the level of the midthigh. This post can provide a method of countertraction to open the medial side of the joint, providing better visualization of structures. After the leg is prepped, the entire extremity is

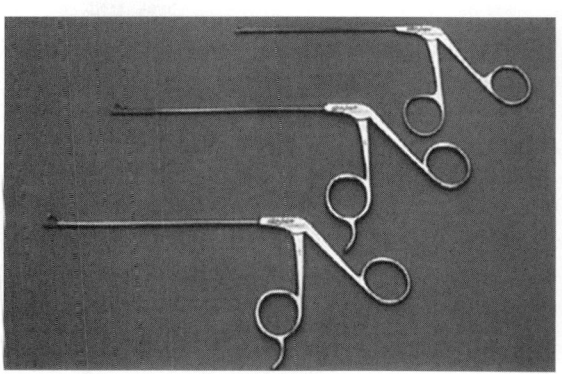

FIGURE 22-111   Arthroscopy instrumentation.

draped to allow complete range of motion and manipulation of the knee joint. The procedure requires specialized equipment for fluid collection and personnel protection.

Instruments and equipment needed for an arthroscopy depend on whether it will be diagnostic or operative. Diagnostic arthroscopy instruments needed include arthroscopy instrumentation (Fig. 22-111), arthroscopes of 30 and 70 degrees (Fig. 22-112), video with camera, light source, and peripheral equipment (Fig. 22-113), an arthroscopy pump and tubing (Fig. 22-114), inflow and egress cannulas (Fig. 22-115), 3-liter bags of normal saline or lactated Ringer's solution, and a spinal needle. Operative arthroscopy instruments depend on the procedure planned. Arthroscopic powered shavers and abraders (Fig. 22-116) are almost universally used. Instruments specific for anterior cruciate ligament reconstruction or meniscal repair will be needed if those procedures are planned.

Operative procedures
Diagnostic Arthroscopy

1. The anteromedial and anterolateral joint lines and portal positions are marked with a skin marker.
2. The skin areas for portal placement are infiltrated with 1% lidocaine with 1:200,000 epinephrine. If the knee

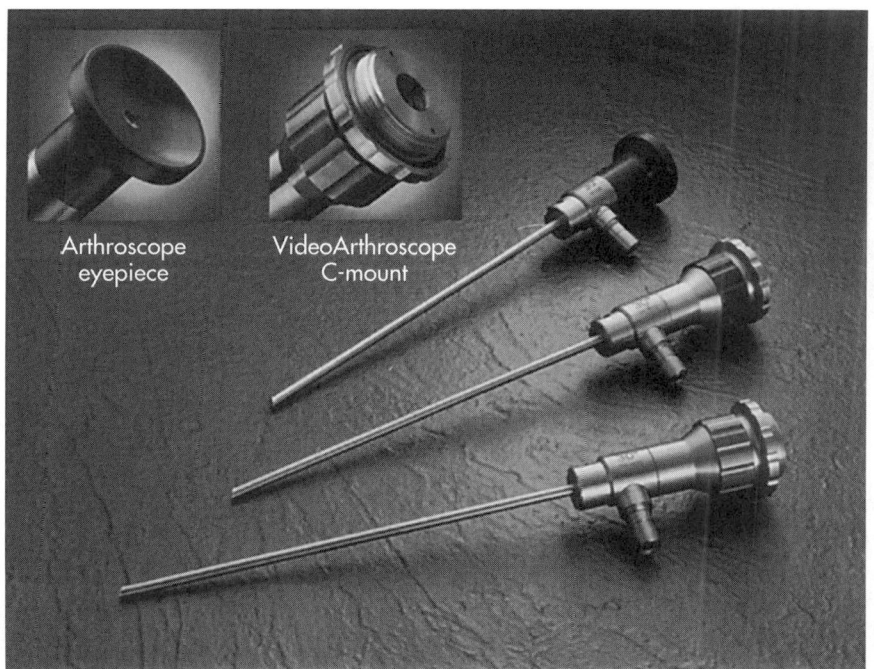

FIGURE 22–112   Arthroscopes, 30 and 70 degrees with camera attachments.

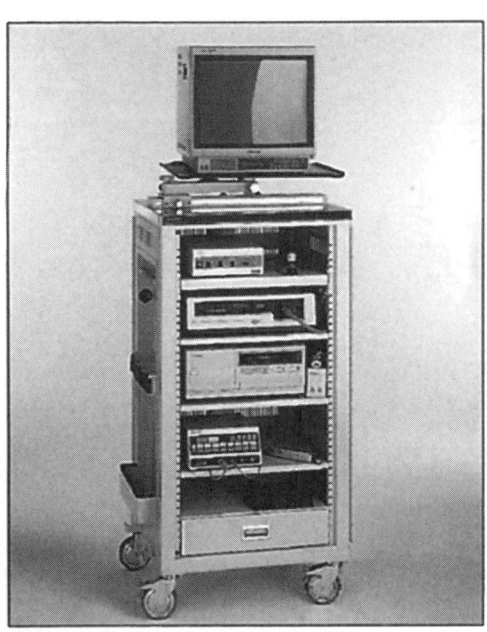

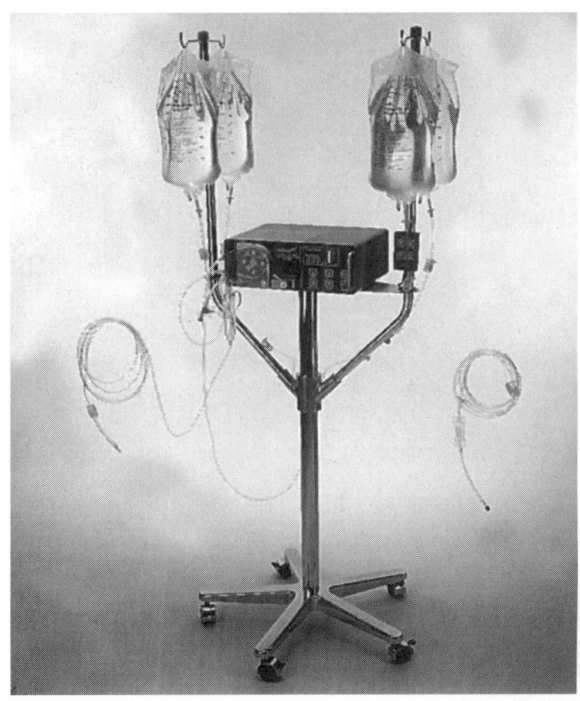

FIGURE 22–113   Arthroscopy tower with video monitor, light source, camera, and shaver system.

FIGURE 22–114   Arthroscopy pump.

has an effusion, this is aspirated with a 16-gauge needle on a 60 ml syringe, followed by a small amount of distending fluid.

3. After a small stab incision with a no. 11 knife blade, the irrigation cannula and trocar are inserted into the lateral suprapatellar pouch near the superior pole of the patella. Lactated Ringer's or normal saline solution

is connected to the cannula, and the joint is distended using gravity or a pressure-sensitive arthroscopy pump.

4. A stab incision is then made anterolaterally or anteromedially 2 to 3 mm above the tibial plateau or patellar tendon at the joint line. A sharp trocar and sheath are inserted through the stab wound and just through the capsule.

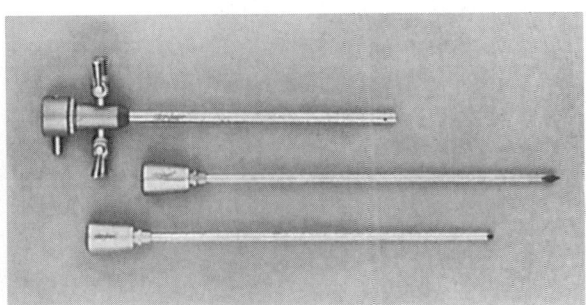

FIGURE 22-115   Cannulas.

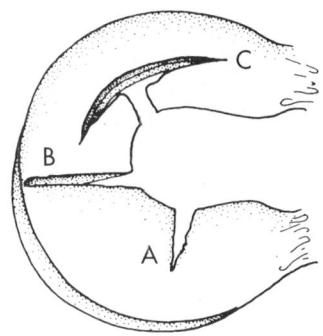

FIGURE 22-117   Meniscal tear. **A,** Incomplete. **B,** Complete. **C,** Incomplete longitudinal.

Operative Arthroscopy

The following is a list of some of the arthroscopic operative procedures:

1. Resection of synovial plica
2. Patellar débridement
3. Excision of meniscal tears
4. Partial or total meniscectomy
5. Lateral retinacular release
6. Removal of loose body
7. Abrasion or drilling of osteochondral defects
8. Synovectomy
9. Treatment of osteochondritis dissecans
10. Meniscal repairs
11. Anterior cruciate ligament reconstruction

Arthroscopic resection and repair of meniscal tear

Menisci are important structures in the knee joint that distribute load across the joint and provide capsular stability. A tear in the meniscus is the most common knee injury requiring arthroscopic surgery (Fig. 22-117). Although both menisci can sustain tears, the medial meniscus is injured much more frequently than the lateral one.

Treatment of meniscus tears is aimed at preserving the structures. Some minor tears heal with cast immobilization, but some persist and cause symptoms. In these more severe cases surgical intervention is necessary. A partial or complete meniscectomy may be necessary to alleviate troublesome symptoms such as locking, pain, and swelling. Partial meniscectomy is preferred, leaving a peripheral rim to share load-bearing and stabilize the knee. Complete meniscectomy removes all of this loadbearing protection and also reduces knee stability. The goal is to leave an intact, balanced rim.

Arthroscopic meniscal repair is widely accepted as the standard of care. Arthroscopy provides better exposure than an arthrotomy does and enables the surgeon to approach the meniscus from the inner margin where most tears begin. Suture repair is appropriate for meniscal tears occurring in the vascular zone (outer 10% to 25%), which heal predictably with repair and immobilization.

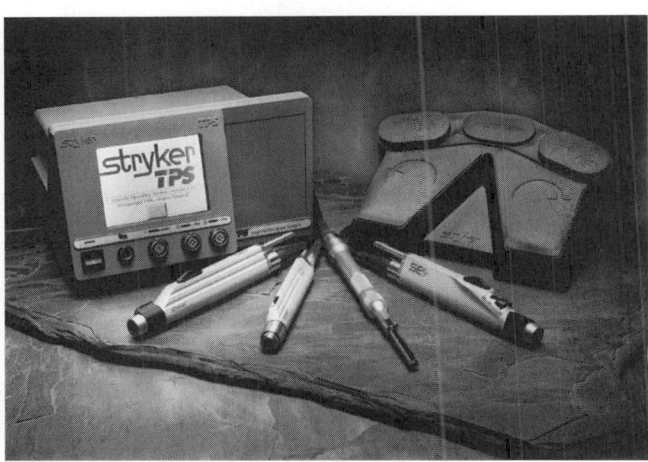

FIGURE 22-116   Arthroscopic shavers.

5. A blunt trocar is used to pass the sheath into the knee joint. The trocar is removed, and a 30-degree scope is inserted into the sheath. The light source and video camera are connected to the scope.
6. The inflow may remain in the suprapatellar area, and the egress tubing is connected to the arthroscope, or the position may be reversed.
7. A spinal needle can be introduced under direct vision to determine the best angle for an opposite portal for insertion of probes and operative instruments. The cruciates and menisci are probed to determine integrity and tears.
8. The scope is moved to the opposite portal to allow a complete examination to be performed.
9. The joint is irrigated periodically and at the end of the procedure to maintain good visualization and clear the joint of blood and tissue fragments.
10. The portals are closed with nylon or undyed Vicryl suture and ½-inch Steri-Strips.
11. Bupivacaine 0.25% (Marcaine), 30 ml, with epinephrine 1:200,000 may be injected intraarticularly to minimize bleeding and postoperative pain.
12. Gauze dressing, Webril, and 4-inch and 6-inch elastic bandages are applied.

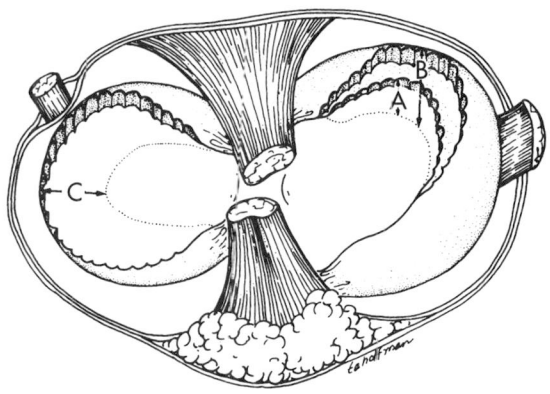

FIGURE 22-118   Lateral and medial meniscal excision.

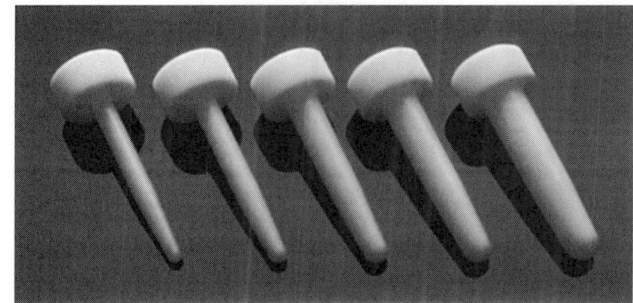

FIGURE 22-119   Bone tunnel plugs.

Operative Procedure (Fig. 22-118)

1. Steps 1 to 9 of the diagnostic arthroscopy procedure are repeated.
2. Working and scope portals are determined. The lateral bucket handle tear is identified, displaced, and reduced with a probe.
3. The attachment of the anterior horn of the meniscus is cut with a hook knife and clamped with a grasper.
4. An accessory portal is determined with a spinal needle.
5. Traction and twisting motion are maintained on the meniscal horn to present a better edge to divide the remainder of the tear. Various scissors or push knives can be used to complete resection.
6. The motorized shaver is used to trim any frayed edges of the meniscus.
7. Limited débridement of chronic tears is completed to clean the edges.
8. When the medial meniscus is to be sutured, a cannula is placed next to the inner edge of the tear. Two long meniscus stitching needles with synthetic absorbable Vicryl or PDS suture are inserted into the cannula, through the meniscus, across the tear, and through the capsule.
9. The needle tips are felt beneath the skin, and a small incision is made to pull the suture out of the joint.
10. The sutures are tied over the capsule. Positioning the cannula enables either horizontal or vertical sutures to be placed.
11. After completing partial meniscectomy or suture repair, the joint is thoroughly irrigated.
12. The incisions are closed, and the knee is lightly dressed and wrapped with Webril and elastic bandages.

Arthroscopic anterior cruciate ligament repair

The anterior cruciate ligament (ACL) is an important stabilizing structure of the knee, and the most frequently torn ligament. Injury is usually a result of simultaneous anterior and rotational stresses. Candidates for ACL reconstruction are active individuals with instability that is sufficient to interfere with their activities and that has failed to respond to bracing, rehabilitation, exercises, and other nonoperative treatment methods. The selected treatment method depends on the classification and severity of the tear, the experience and preference of the surgeon, and whether a previous repair has failed.

ACL reconstruction may be intraarticular, extraarticular, or a combination of both. Arthroscopic repair causes less patellar pain and less disturbance of extensor mechanisms and therefore is becoming the treatment of choice if there is no other significant capsular instability or gross disruption of the knee joint.

ACL repair most often involves replacement of the ligament with a substitute. Substitutes include autografts, allografts, and synthetic ligaments. Autografts are currently the method of choice, with a free central-third patellar tendon graft attached to patellar and tibial bone blocks used most often. The semitendinosus tendon and iliotibial band are sometimes used instead. Autografts may be used alone or augmented, although synthetic augmentation devices have fallen out of favor because of the development of chronic synovitis in these patients.

Procedural Considerations

Instrumentation for an ACL repair includes all instruments required for an operative arthroscopy. In addition, an ACL reconstruction guide system, fixation of choice (bone screws, staples, spiked washers, or interference screws) (see Fig. 22-84), bone tunnel plugs (Fig. 22-119), and a power drill and microsagittal saw will be needed. If the surgeon believes that isometric placement of the graft is important, a tension isometer will be needed as well as a system for finding that intraarticular position.

Operative Procedure
Patellar tendon graft

1. An examination under anesthesia is performed immediately after induction to further evaluate the stability of the knee.
2. A diagnostic arthroscopy is then carried out through the standard anteromedial and anterolateral portals.

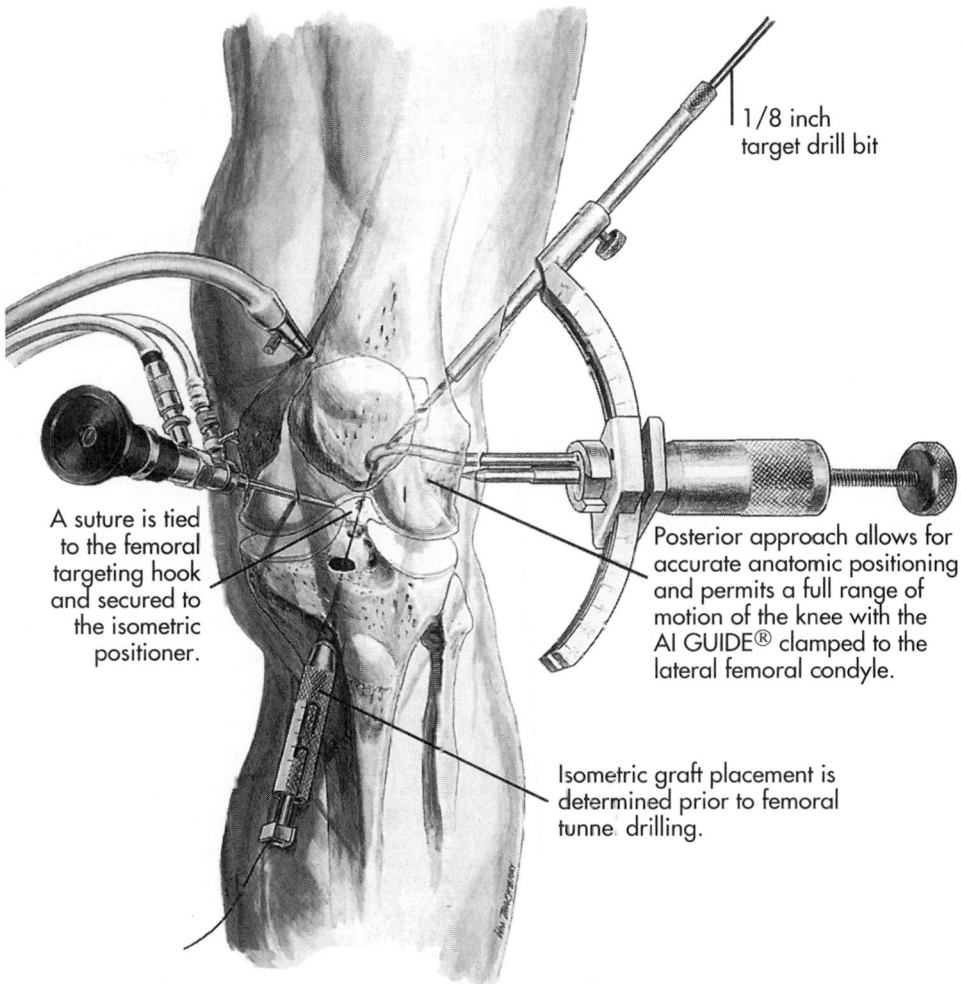

1/8 inch
target drill bit

A suture is tied
to the femoral
targeting hook
and secured to
the isometric
positioner.

Posterior approach allows for
accurate anatomic positioning
and permits a full range of
motion of the knee with the
AI GUIDE® clamped to the
lateral femoral condyle.

Isometric graft placement is
determined prior to femoral
tunnel drilling.

FIGURE 22-120   Femoral aiming device positioned for anterior cruciate ligament reconstruction.

3. Any meniscal tears or other intraarticular injuries are treated before attending to the ligament.

4. The remaining anterior cruciate ligament tissue is debrided with a full-radius resecter.

5. A notchplasty is then performed, widening the intracondylar notch with a 4.5 mm arthroplasty burr, rasp, osteotome, and curettes. Notchplasty aids in arthroscopic visualization and protects the graft from abrasion and amputation.

6. After preparation of the intracondylar area, a small incision is made on the distal lateral aspect of the femur and is carried down to the flare of the lateral femoral aspect of the condyle. A femoral aiming device is positioned, and a guide pin is inserted from the femoral site into the posterosuperior region of the intercondylar notch at an isometric point (Fig. 22-120).

7. Another small incision is made anteriorly, below the knee and medial to the tibial tubercle.

8. The tibial aiming device is positioned, and a guide pin is inserted from the anterior tibial incision into the intercondylar notch, anterior and medial to the center of the tibial anatomic attachment site of the anterior cruciate ligament.

9. The pins are then replaced with a heavy suture passing through the femoral and tibial pin sites.

10. Isometric placement of the guide pins is checked with a tensioning device that is attached to the heavy suture. The knee is put through a range of motion to determine correct isometric measurement.

11. Once isometric positioning is determined, a longitudinal skin incision is made medially to the midline near the patellar tendon.

12. The central-third portion of the patellar tendon with tibial and patellar bone plugs is harvested with a minisaw and osteotome. The graft is sized to the appropriate width, usually 10 to 12 mm, using sizing tubes (Fig. 22-121).

13. Heavy nonabsorbable suture is placed through drill holes made at each end of the graft in the bone plugs (Fig. 22-122).

14. The guide pins are then reinserted and overdrilled with cannulas that are close in width to the prepared graft. Overdrilling establishes the tunnels so that they

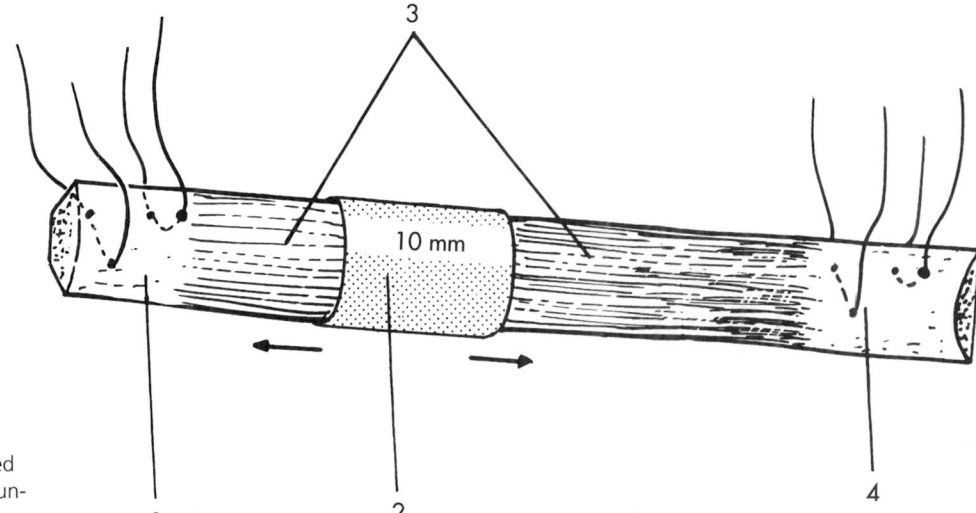

FIGURE 22-121   Sizing tubes are used to determine the minimum-diameter tunnel necessary for passage of the graft.

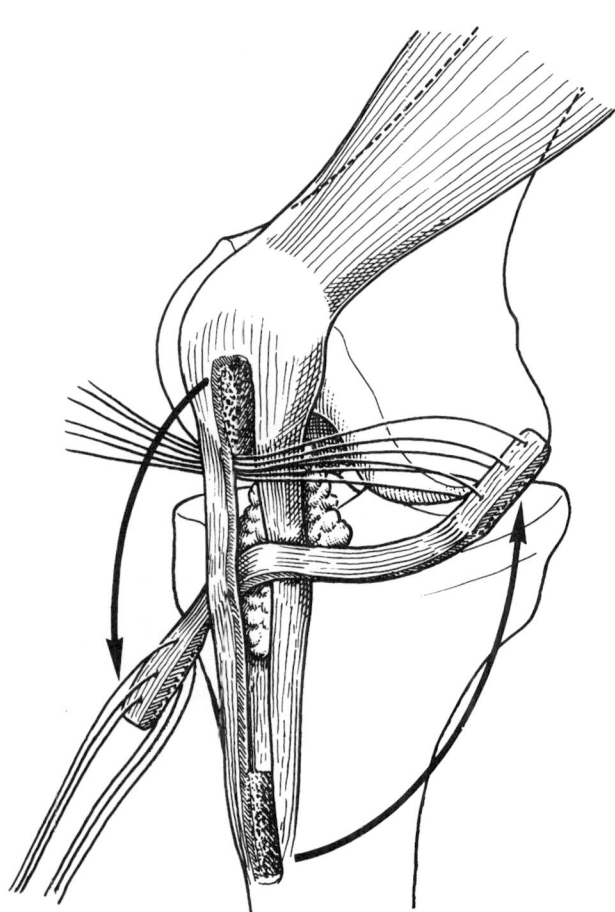

FIGURE 22-122   Three drill holes are placed into each bone block of the patellar graft, and a heavy suture is placed into each drill hole.

are in the center of the previous insertion sites of the anterior cruciate ligament.

15. The femoral and tibial osseous tunnels are smoothed with curettes, a rasp, or an abrader. If the tunnels are made before the graft is harvested, they are temporarily occluded with bone tunnel plugs to minimize fluid extravasation.

16. Both ends of the graft are fixed with a barbed staple, bone screw with washer, interference screw, or ligament button (Fig. 22-123).

17. The incisions and joint are irrigated and closed.

18. A hinged knee brace may be applied over the dressing. The brace allows 10 to 90 degrees of motion (Research Highlight 22-4).

Arthroscopic posterior cruciate ligament repair

Surgical procedures for tears of the posterior cruciate ligament are considered if significant disabling instability has occurred. Patients usually return to adequate function without operative treatment. The arthroscopic procedure for repair of the posterior cruciate ligament is similar to the technique used to repair the anterior cruciate ligament, except that isometric placement is posterior within the joint and the femoral attachment is proximal to the medial epicondyle.

Arthroscopy of the Shoulder

Shoulder arthroscopy is a useful diagnostic and therapeutic tool in the management of shoulder disorders. It is particularly beneficial in the evaluation and management of patients with chronic shoulder problems. Arthroscopy provides extensive visualization of the intraarticular aspect of the shoulder joint. Indications for shoulder arthroscopy include removal of loose bodies, lysis of adhesions, synovial biopsy, synovectomy, bursectomy, stabilization of dislocations, correction of glenoid labrum, biceps tendon and rotator cuff tears, and relief of impingement syndrome.

Procedural considerations

The patient may be placed in the lateral position or in a sitting position using a "beach chair" positioner. The lateral position is maintained using a vacuum beanbag positioning device or lateral rolls with a kidney rest.

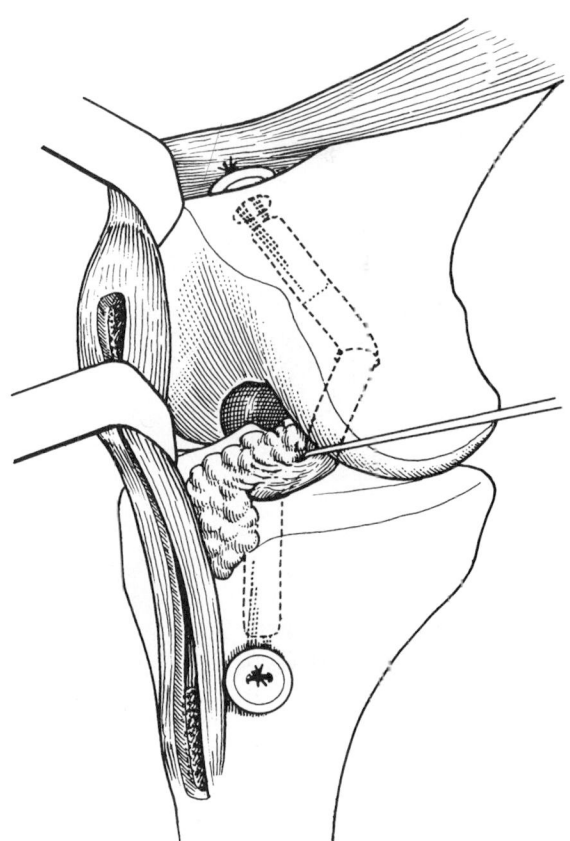

FIGURE 22-123   A patellar tendon graft is affixed by tying of sutures over bone buttons at the tibial and femoral drill holes.

Three-inch adhesive tape is secured across the patient's hips. Proper padding of the uninvolved axilla and lower extremity is important to prevent soft-tissue or neurovascular problems. The affected extremity is placed in a shoulder suspension system, and Buck's traction or a Velcro immobilizer is applied to the forearm to achieve adequate distraction to the glenohumeral joint. The extremity is abducted 40 to 60 degrees and forward flexed 10 to 20 degrees, with 5- to 15-pound weights placed on the pulley system. Weight may be added to further distract the glenohumeral joint, taking care not to overstretch the axillary artery.

The shoulder is prepped and draped free, permitting full range of motion during the procedure.

The operative instruments and arthroscope commonly used for the knee may also be used in the shoulder, plus an 18-gauge needle, switching sticks, and a Wisinger rod. There is a variety of fixation devices (screws and tacks) that can be used to repair bony defects and labral tears.

Operative procedure (Fig. 22-124)

1. An 18-gauge spinal needle is inserted through the posterior soft spot and directed anteriorly toward the coracoid process, where the surgeon's index finger has been positioned.
2. The glenohumeral joint is distended with normal saline or lactated Ringer's solution. This facilitates entry of the arthroscope.
3. Bupivacaine 0.25% (Marcaine), 2 to 3 ml, with epinephrine 1:200,000 is injected along the needle track to minimize bleeding.

22-4 RESEARCH HIGHLIGHT

In the history of anterior cruciate ligament (ACL) reconstruction, aftercare has traditionally consisted in immobilization and non–weight bearing of the operative extremity, typically for 4 to 6 weeks. Shelbourne, in 1990, found that "patient noncompliance to previously established protocols still yielded acceptable results that demanded further investigation." He developed a four-phase aftercare protocol that focused on gaining full extension, full weight bearing, and resumption of activities of daily living by the end of week 4, and a safe return to competitive athletics after 2 to 3 months. He noted that there was a steady decline in the need for postoperative manipulations or scar resections since the initiation of his aggressive rehabilitation program, basing his conclusions on more than 4000 cases of ACL reconstruction between 1983 and 1994.

The initial phase encompasses the preoperative period and emphasizes two important factors. (1) The patient should have a resolution of knee swelling, a return of full range of motion, and a normal gait. (2) The patient should be mentally prepared for the operation and subsequent rehabilitation. Phase 2 encompasses the initial 2 weeks after the operation. The five goals of this phase are to (1) maintain full hyperextension, (2) prevent and control swelling, (3) allow wound healing, (4) achieve and maintain good quadriceps leg control, and (5) obtain at least 90 degrees of flexion. This phase begins on the day of surgery, when the patient is placed in a continuous passive motion (CPM) machine with a Cryo/Cuff. Weight-bearing-as-tolerated ambulation is also allowed at this time, with crutches being used for assistance. In phase 3, from postoperative week 3 to week 5, the emphasis is on flexion (without losing full hyperextension), restoration of a normal gait pattern, and light strength work. Phase 4 begins at 5 weeks. At this stage, most patients should have a range of motion from 5 degrees of hyperextension to 135 degrees of flexion and should be back to full normal daily activities. Once the strength of the repaired knee is at least 70% of the unaffected leg, the patient is allowed a light functional running program. If strength is improved, a return to competitive athletics is anticipated in 2 to 3 months.

From Shelbourne, K.D., & Patel, D.V. (1996). Rehabilitation after autogenous bone–patellar tendon-bone ACL reconstruction, *Instructional Course Lectures, 45,* 263-273.

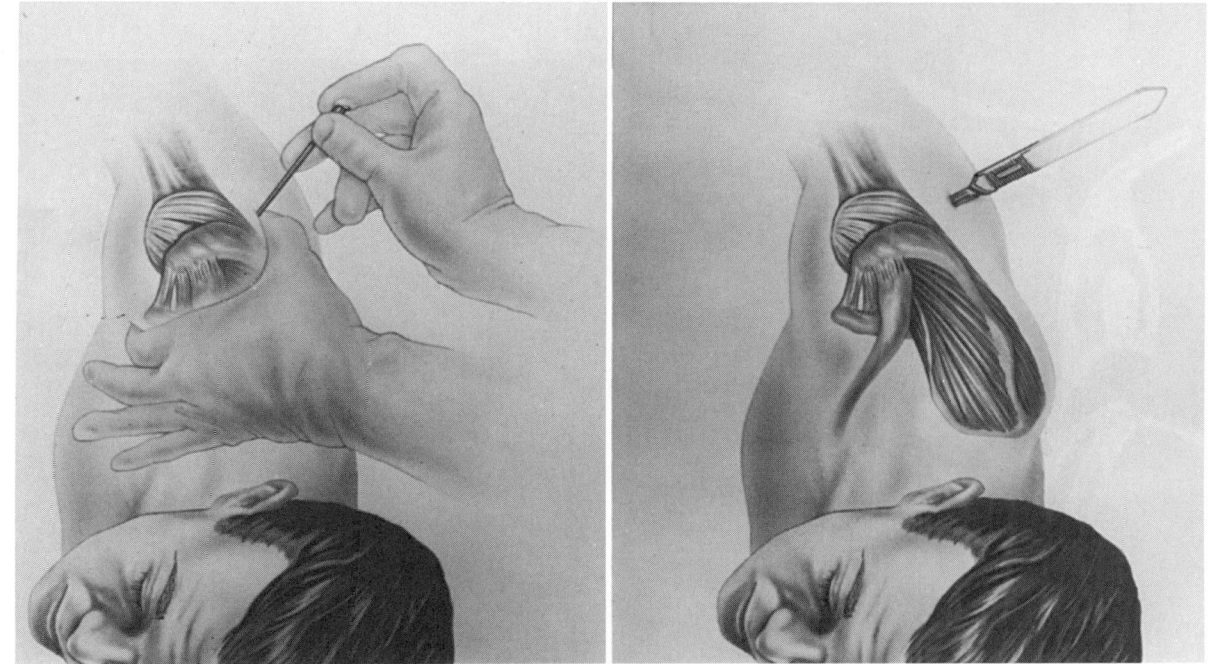

FIGURE 22-124   Shoulder arthroscopy. **A,** The spinal needle is inserted for dilatation of the joint if indicated. **B,** An incision is made over the glenohumeral joint.   *Continued*

4. With the needle removed, a stab incision is made with a #11 blade over the needle site.

5. The arthroscope sleeve and sharp trocar are then introduced through the posterior joint capsule.

6. Once the capsule has been penetrated, a blunt obturator replaces the sharp trocar to enter the joint.

7. The arthroscope is inserted and attached to inflow and outflow tubing, the video camera, and the light source.

8. Operative instruments are placed through an anterior portal that is established laterally to the coracoid process by using a Wisinger rod. A third portal can be established near the anterior portal or supraspinous fossa portal. Switching sticks are used to change portals.

9. The arm is moved and rotated as needed to visualize various structures in and around the joint.

10. Glenoid tears can be repaired with the insertion of an absorbable fixation tack.

11. At the conclusion of the procedure, the joint is irrigated. The surgeon may inject a long-acting local anesthetic into the joint and subacromial space through the portal to minimize postoperative discomfort.

12. The puncture wounds are closed and dressed with a sterile 4 × 4 gauze pad. The patient's arm is placed in a sling for recovery.

Arthroscopy of the Elbow

The elbow joint is accessible to arthroscopic examination, although it requires more attention to detail than the knee because instruments must be placed through deeper muscle layers and close to important neurovascular structures.

Arthroscopy of the elbow, both diagnostic and operative, has become fairly routine. Indications for its use include extraction of loose bodies, evaluation or débridement of osteochondritis dissecans of the capitulum and radial head, partial synovectomy in rheumatoid disease, débridement and lysis of adhesions of posttraumatic or degenerative processes at or near the elbow, diagnosis of a chronically painful elbow when the diagnosis is obscure, and evaluation of fractures of the capitulum, radial head, or olecranon.

Procedural considerations

General anesthesia is preferred to local anesthesia because it affords complete comfort to the patient and provides total muscle relaxation.

The patient is placed either in the supine or prone position. If supine, the forearm is flexed on an armboard or placed in a prefabricated wrist gauntlet connected to an overhead pulley device and tied off at the end of the OR bed. If lifted overhead, the entire arm is allowed to hang free over the side of the bed with the elbow flexed approximately 90 degrees. This provides excellent access to both the medial and lateral aspects of the elbow, allows the forearm to be freely pronated and supinated, and places the important neurovascular structures in the antecubital fossa at maximum relaxation. A tourniquet is routinely used for hemostasis. The entire arm, including the hand, is prepped and draped.

The three portals most commonly used for diagnostic

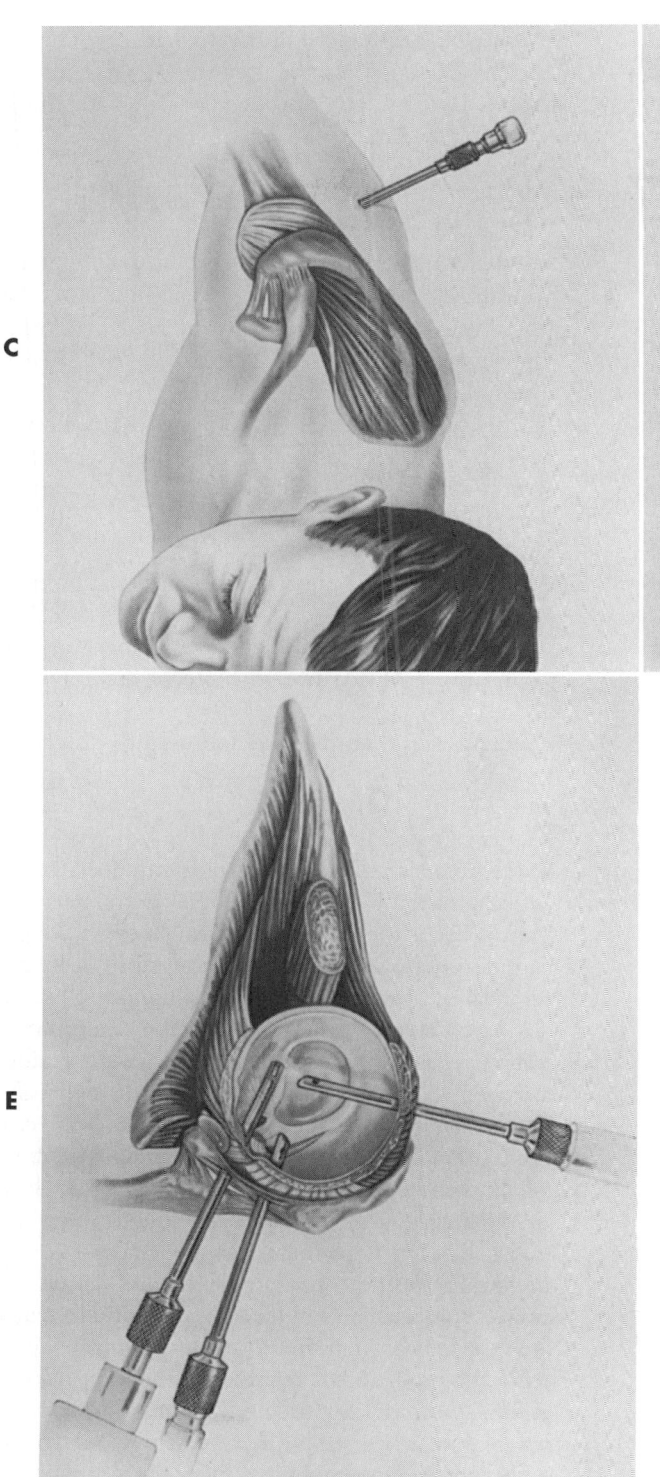

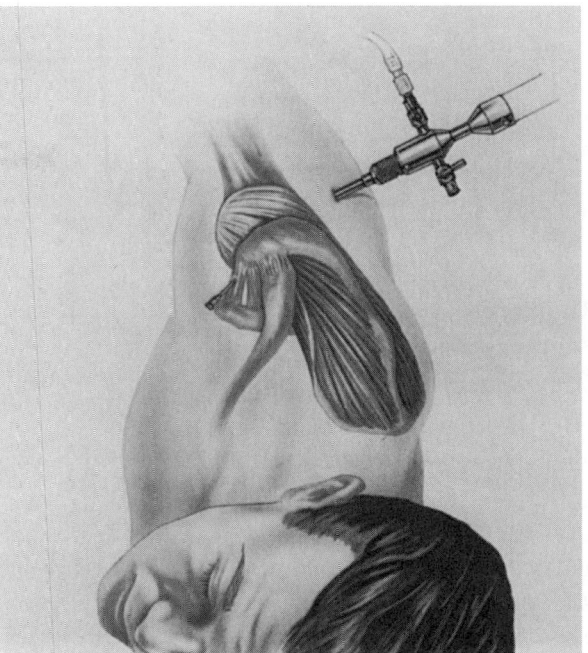

FIGURE 22-124, ccnt'd Shoulder arthroscopy. **C,** The arthroscope sleeve and sharp trocar are inserted. **D,** The arthroscope is inserted and attached to the inflow and outflow tubing, video camera, and light source. **E,** Operative instruments are placed through the portal.

and operative arthroscopy of the elbow are the anterolateral, the anteromedial, and the posterolateral.

Operative arthroscopy instruments commonly used for the knee may also be used in the elbow. However, smaller-diameter scopes and instruments may be desired instead.

Operative procedure

1. The bony anatomic landmarks are outlined with a marking pen before initiation of the procedure. Lateral structures to be marked and identified are the radial head and the lateral epicondyle. The medial epicondyle is also marked.

2. An 18-gauge needle is inserted anteriorly to the radial head from the lateral side, and the joint is distended.

3. Once joint distention has been achieved with approximately 15 to 30 ml of lactated Ringer's or normal saline solution, a stab wound incision is made with a #11 blade, and the sharp trocar with cannula is inserted through the joint capsule.

4. The sharp trocar is replaced with the blunt obturator to provide safe entry of the cannula into the joint.

5. The scope replaces the blunt obturator and is attached to the video and light source.

6. A second and third portal are established anteromedially and posterolaterally for triangulation. With the patient's elbow flexed to 90 degrees and adequate distention maintained at the time of insertion of the instruments, the neurovascular structures are displaced anteriorly. This provides greater area above the medial and lateral humeral epicondyles in which to insert the various instruments.

7. Outflow and inflow are controlled by alternating the valve on the scope or using a separate 18-gauge needle with drainage tubing.

8. After diagnostic and operative procedures have been completed, the joint is irrigated, the puncture sites are sutured, and a compression dressing is applied with Webril and elastic bandages.

Arthroscopy of the Ankle

The talocalcaneal articulations are complex and play an important role in the movements of inversion and eversion of the foot. The subtalar joints function as a single unit, but anatomically they are divided into anterior and posterior joints. The surgeon and perioperative nurse must be familiar with the extraarticular anatomy of the ankle to prevent neural or vascular damage.

Indications for ankle arthroscopy include osteochondral fragments or loose bodies, persistent ankle pain after trauma and despite adequate conservative treatment, biopsy, posttraumatic arthritis of the ankle joint, unstable ankle before lateral ligamentous reconstruction, and osteochondritis dissecans of the talus.

Procedural considerations

General anesthesia is preferable because manipulation and distraction of the joint to obtain adequate arthroscopic viewing require muscle relaxation. The position of the patient is based on the surgeon's preference. The patient may be supine with the knee flexed approximately 70 degrees or supine with a sandbag under the buttock of the operative side. Ankle and thigh holders may be used; when better posterior visualization is necessary, a distracter may be used to increase the space between the tibia and talus (see Fig. 22-16). A tourniquet is placed around the upper thigh but is not used unless excessive bleeding, uncontrolled by irrigation, is encountered. Routine skin prepping and draping are done.

Operative instruments and the arthroscope commonly used for the knee may also be used for the ankle; however, miniaturized instruments and needle scopes for the ankle are becoming available.

Operative procedure

1. The important extraarticular anatomic structures are outlined on the skin using a sterile marking pen.

2. Examination of the ankle joint using the anterolateral portal is then performed. The anteromedial joint line is palpated, and an 18-gauge, 1½-inch needle is inserted into the joint.

3. Sterile plastic extension tubing is attached to the needle, and a 50 ml plastic Luer-Lok syringe filled with normal saline is connected to the tubing to distend the joint. Approximately 15 to 20 ml are needed.

4. After intraarticular injection is confirmed by the ease with which the saline can be injected and by palpation of the joint as it is distended, a small incision is made with a no. 11 blade over the site of the anterolateral portal.

5. A hemostat is then inserted and used to dissect to the capsule.

6. The sheath of the arthroscope and sharp trocar are placed into the incision, angled approximately 30 to 45 degrees laterally, and inserted with a sharp plunge as joint distention is maintained. Entrance into the joint is felt as the sleeve and trocar "pop" through the capsule and is confirmed by the rush of saline on removal of the trocar from the sheath.

7. The arthroscope is inserted into the sheath, the needle is removed, and the plastic tubing and syringe are attached to the stopcock on the arthroscope sleeve. The video camera and light source are connected to the scope. Joint distention must be maintained.

8. Triangulation through other portals is easily done by first inserting the 18-gauge needle for localization while viewing with the arthroscope. Posterior viewing is done in the same fashion except that the patient is usually placed in the prone position and instruments are inserted through the posterior portals.

9. After the procedure is completed, the joint is irrigated and the wounds are closed with Steri-Strips or a single suture and covered with a dressing and short leg compression elastic wrap.

SURGERY OF THE SPINAL COLUMN

Treatment of Back Pain

Back pain is a natural result of degenerative and arthritic change, punctuated by protrusion or rupture of a disk. It gradually progresses but may also disappear gradually. With aging, a degenerative disk-space narrowing or facet arthropathy begins to appear radiologically. The lower lumbar spine carries the burden of the body, holds a person upright, and returns the body to the vertical position from sitting, lying, or a bent-over position. Degenerative changes, ruptured disk, and facet arthropathy develop at the lowest two limb segments, where the greatest weight, torsion, and shearing stress occur. It sometimes extends into the upper and middle spine.

Cervical-spine degenerative disk–narrowing also develops most often at the two lowest cervical spaces, which are also the levels of greatest stress resulting from movement of the head and neck. Sometimes lumbar or cervical degenerative changes develop early from excessive repetitive movements or injury.

Back pain may be treated by injection procedures, electrodes, stimulators, braces, or traction. A natural recovery may result after 6 or 7 days of intense pain, subsiding between 6 weeks and 4 months. Motor and sensory deficits usually disappear with resolution of pain. The ability to recover without surgery depends on fragment size and compression on the nerve root. Neural compression remains the major indication for disk excision.

Spinal fusion is a consideration, usually with demonstrable posttraumatic, postsurgical, rheumatoid, infectious, or neoplastic instability.

Procedural considerations

After assessment, patient-specific care is provided. Radiographs are obtained. Bilateral pulses are assessed in the extremities. Elastic wraps or stockings may be placed. Range of motion is assessed, particularly of the arms, because of the need for the extended prone position. The patient is positioned prone to eliminate lordosis, reduce venous congestion, and keep the abdomen free. A Foley catheter may be placed. The patient is positioned using chest rolls or special frames (see Fig. 22-17) after administration of general anesthesia. Depending on the extent of the procedure, blood availability may be required. The skin is prepped and the area draped. A spinal laminectomy set is used, in addition to a spinal retractor of choice and a bipolar electrosurgical unit. Hemostatic adjuncts such as Gelfoam, Surgicel, thrombin, and bone wax should be available.

Operative procedure
Laminectomy

1. A midline incision is made over the affected disk and carried sharply down to the supraspinous ligament.
2. The supraspinous ligament is incised, and the muscles are dissected subperiosteally from the spines and laminae of the vertebrae. These are retracted with a self-retaining retractor.
3. The laminae and ligamentum flavum are denuded with a curette.
4. A small part of the inferior margin of the lamina is removed with a rongeur.

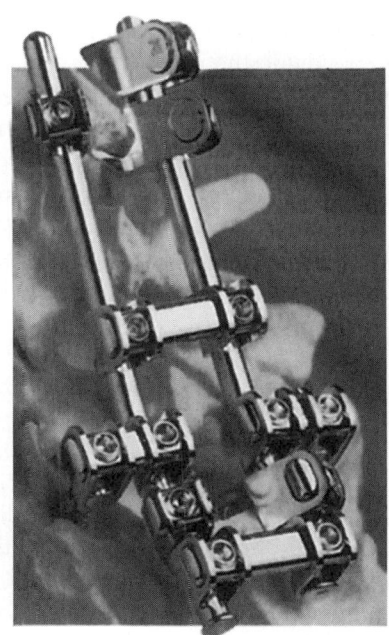

FIGURE 22-125 Pedicle screw placement using the Rogozinski system.

5. The ligamentum flavum is grasped and incised where it fuses with the interspinous ligament, and this flap is then sharply removed to expose the dura.
6. The dura is then retracted medially, and the nerve root is identified.
7. Once identified, the nerve root is retracted medially so that the underlying posterior longitudinal ligament can be exposed.
8. The posterior longitudinal ligament is incised over the intervertebral space in a cruciate fashion, and the disk space is entered with a pituitary grasping forceps.
9. The disk material is systematically removed, taking care not to exceed the distance to the anterior annulus. A complete search for additional fragments of nucleus pulposus, both inside and outside the disk space, is then carried out.
10. All cotton pledgets are removed and counted, and residual bleeding is controlled with bipolar coagulation.
11. The wound is closed routinely with absorbable sutures in the supraspinous ligament and subcutaneous tissue. Various nonabsorbable sutures or staples are used for skin closure.

Pedicle Fixation of the Spine

Pedicle screw fixation (Fig. 22-125) has become an increasingly popular method of surgical fixation of the spinal column. Screw fixation was initially used in an attempt to avoid postoperative external immobilization and prolonged bed rest. Pedicle screw fixation has been used most often in degenerative processes, particularly iatrogenic instability after decompression, degenerative and isthmic spondylolisthesis, and diskogenic disease. It is also indicated for tumor, trauma, degenerative spinal disorders, postoperative hypermobility, and infection.

Three basic approaches for fixation have been described as the procedure has evolved. Each has improved upon the first, based on anatomic placement of the screw. Positioning and placement of the screw within the spine are established after direct visualization of the pedicle.

Procedural considerations

Patient-specific considerations are noted after the assessment (see laminectomy section). The patient is placed under general anesthesia and positioned prone. The skin is prepped, and drapes are applied.

A spinal laminectomy set is used in addition to the instrumentation and implants of choice, a spinal retractor, power equipment such as a high-speed motorized hand tool, and hemostatic adjuncts such as Gelfoam, thrombin, and bone wax. A bone graft set will be needed to harvest graft from the iliac crest.

Operative procedure

1. A standard midline incision is made. The laminectomy procedure is followed.
2. The areas of the pedicles to be fixated are located using external landmarks.
3. The posterior cortical wall at the entrance site is removed using a high-speed burr.
4. A Penfield dissector is used to identify the entrance hole through the pedicle.
5. A gearshift probe is inserted to identify the path into the vertebral body.
6. The hole is tapped (5.5 mm), and the hole is widened.
7. The screw is placed. Guidelines for screw sizes are 7 mm for S1, L5, and L4; 6.25 mm for L3 and L2; 5.5 mm for L1 and T12.
8. A posterolateral graft is performed, using graft strips from the iliac crest.
9. The plate or rod is contoured to approximate the patient's physiologic lordosis. The longitudinal device is locked onto the screws in the appropriate position.
10. A screw-plate system may require use of the oblique and transverse washers between the screw head and plate to provide a flush fit at the screw-plate interface.
11. The foramina are checked for patency before closure. The excess machined portion of the screw is cut close to the upper locking device.
12. A suction drain is placed; the wound is closed in layers.

Treatment of Scoliosis

Scoliosis is a three-dimensional deformity (Fig. 22-126) with lateral deviation of the spinal column from the midline; it may include rotation or deformity of the vertebrae. Types are congenital, juvenile, adolescent, and adult. School screening programs provide quick and simple

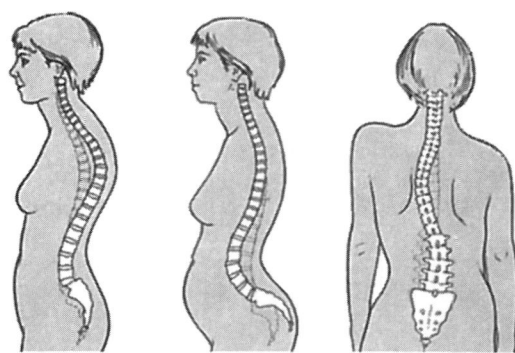

FIGURE 22-126 Scoliotic deformity.

detection. For effective treatment of scoliosis, early detection is critical.

Some form of scoliosis occurs in 1 in 10 people, affecting 1 million people in the United States. Two in 100 require medical treatment. Of all treated patients, 80% are female. Scoliosis can be idiopathic (80% of the time) or congenital and may result from muscular or neurologic diseases or unequal leg lengths.[18] A multitude of posterior and anterior segmental spinal instrumentation systems are now available for the treatment of idiopathic scoliosis. As a consequence, fixation strategies are more complex than they were with Harrington instrumentation. The newer systems provide better sagittal control and more stable fixation, allowing quicker mobilization of the patient. On thin patients, the bulk of these implants may be a problem.[8]

Posterior spinal fusion with Harrington rods

Posterior spinal fusion is most frequently performed in adolescence, when the laterally deviated curve is still flexible. Harrington rods are internal splints that help maintain the spine as straight as possible until the vertebral body fusion has become solid. Distraction rods are placed on the concave side of the curve, and compression rods are placed on the convex side. On the convex side of the curve, three to eight hooks are inserted in the transverse processes of the vertebrae and pulled together with a threaded rod. In this way the scoliotic deformity can be corrected as much as the flexibility of the spine allows.

The posterior elements of the vertebrae are denuded of soft tissue, and the bone graft is added. Blood loss can be expected and an accurate record of the loss must be maintained. After surgery the patient is placed in an immobilizing jacket.

Some disadvantages of the Harrington rod system over other systems are that there is only end-point fixation, rod breakage is increased, fixation is less, sagittal plane curves are difficult to manage, distraction for correction is not always desired, and the patient is required to wear a postoperative cast or brace. Other systems have evolved from the Harrington rods that are used for correction of some scoliotic deformities. It remains a feasible treatment of idiopathic scoliosis.

Procedural Considerations

The patient is placed in the prone position on a frame or with rolls under the chest and abdomen to facilitate respiration. Before the procedure begins, an x-ray cassette is placed under the patient so that a radiograph for accurate identification of the vertebrae to be fused can be taken during the operation. A single straight longitudinal incision is made down the midline of the back. Because of the amount of bleeding, the skin and subcutaneous tissues are often infiltrated with a vasoconstricting solution, such as epinephrine.

Basic spinal instrumentation and bone graft instruments are required, plus the Harrington rod instrumentation. A large pin cutter, designed to cut large pins but provided with a small end so that it will fit in the wound, should be available.

Operative Procedure

1. The appropriate hooks are selected and inserted. A Harrington distraction rod of appropriate length is inserted through the two proximal self-adjusting hooks, which have been placed under the laminae.
2. A rod clamp is clamped onto the Harrington rod just below the hook, and a single regular spreader is used to obtain the first inch of distraction.
3. The Bobechko spreader is used to span over the first hook, closest to the smooth part of the rod, to apply distraction force on the most proximal hook.
4. Two C locking rings are inserted around the first ratchet immediately below the hook to prevent dislodgment of the hooks. The excessive length of protruding rod above the most proximal hook is cut off with a rod cutter. The compression is tightened.

Luque segmental spinal rod procedure

The Luque segmental method employs smooth, L-shaped, stainless steel rods, usually $3/16$ or $1/4$ inch in diameter, with sublaminar wires placed at every level possible (Fig. 22-127). It is more secure and longer than the Harrington rod system and was the first system to employ multiple-point fixation. Luque instrumentation applies corrective forces to the spinal segments at each level, thereby spreading the corrective forces throughout the length of the deformity. Two Luque rods are wired to both sides of the spine. The rods are contoured to achieve no more than 10 degrees of increased correction beyond that exhibited on preoperative x-ray study.

Procedural Considerations

The patient is placed in the prone position on a frame or with rolls under the chest and abdomen to facilitate respiration. Patient care is provided (see section on laminectomy), including assessment of pulses. A straight

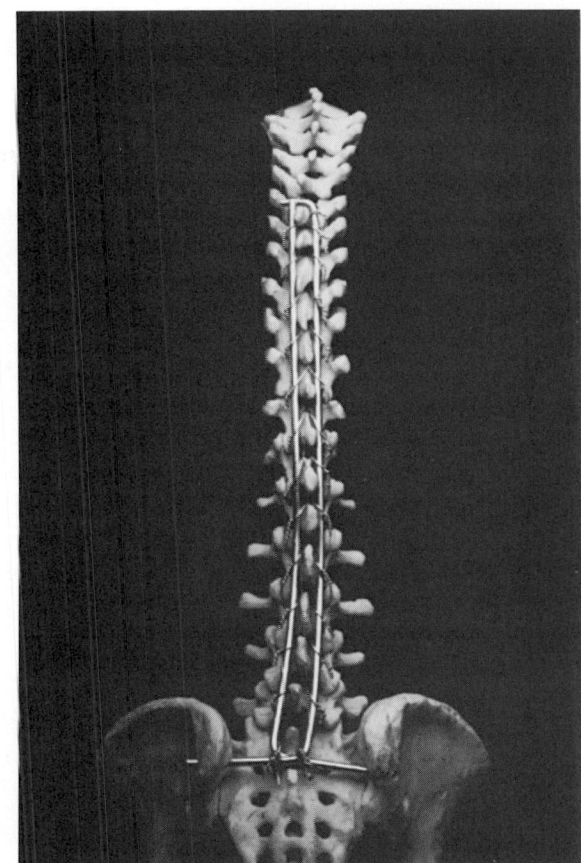

FIGURE 22-127   Luque spinal system in place on a scoliotic spine.

midline incision is made in the back. Because of the amount of bleeding, the skin and subcutaneous tissues are often infiltrated with a vasoconstricting solution such as epinephrine.

Basic spinal instrumentation is required. In addition, Luque rods and instrumentation, a wire tightener and cutter, and bone graft instruments will be needed.

Operative Procedure

1. The ligamentum flavum is detached, exposing the neural canal.
2. Doubled stainless steel suture wire is passed under the lamina. The wire loop is cut later to form two wires at each level.
3. Total bilateral facetectomies are made, forming posterolateral troughs for subsequent bone grafts.
4. Wedge osteotomies may be necessary in severe immobile curves to avoid stretching the spinal cord during correction.
5. The wire loop is cut, resulting in two separate wires at each level.
6. The L bend is secured to the base of the spinous process to prevent rod migration.
7. Initial placement of the convex rod is made.
8. Initial placement of the concave rod is made.

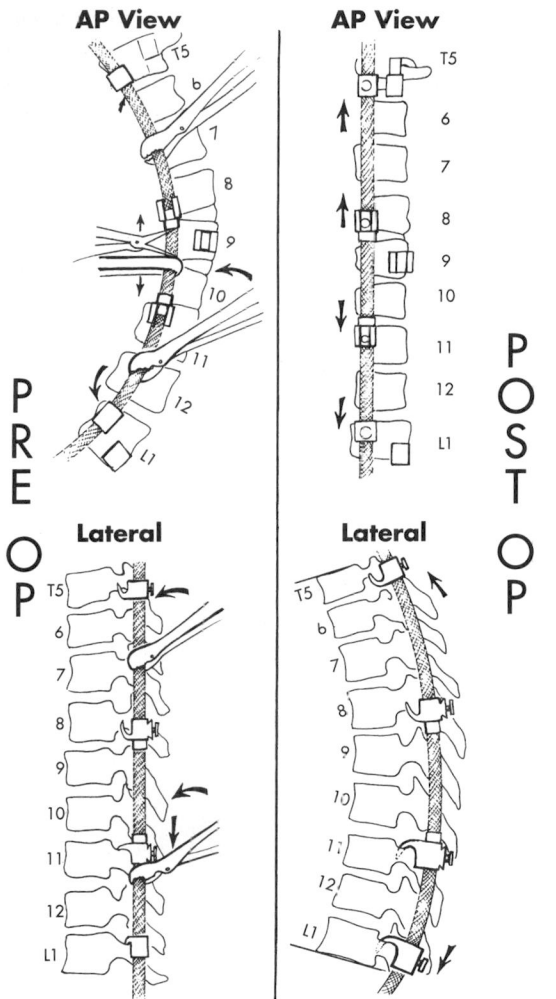

AP View   **AP View**

Lateral   Lateral

FIGURE 22-128 Cotrel-Dubousset system, representing rotation of rods.

9. Transverse wiring is done to add increased stability to the system.
10. Stabilization of the lumbosacral joint is corrected by bending the rods distally to form sacral bars.

Cotrel-Dubousset system procedure

The Cotrel-Dubousset system (Fig. 22-128) provides three-dimensional correction of spinal deformities without sublaminar wiring and neurologic risks. This instrumentation permits distraction, compression, and derotation. The scoliotic curve is corrected by derotation and, at the same time, restores the normal sagittal contours. In addition to correction of scoliosis, the Cotrel-Dubousset system can be applied to correct kyphosis or lordosis and to stabilize and rebuild the spine after tumor resection or after injury. No external support is necessary. The Cotrel-Dubousset system has no ratchets or notches. It consists of metallic rods with diamond crosscut patterns on which hooks and screws can be positioned in any position, level, or degree of rotation. The rod is held in the open hooks with blockers. The rods are then interlocked by means of

devices for transverse traction (DTT). The Cotrel-Dubousset system was the forerunner to the systems used today, such as the Texas Scottish Rite Hospital system, and the Isola system.

Procedural Considerations

The patient is placed in the prone position under general anesthesia. Patient assessment and precautions for the prone position are initiated (see laminectomy section, p. 905). Basic spinal instrumentation is required in addition to the Cotrel-Dubousset system and instrumentation and instruments used for harvesting bone graft.

Operative Procedure

1. Closed hooks are inserted at both ends of the surgical site, and open hooks are inserted at various levels in between.
2. Decortication and facet excision are done at the remaining interposed vertebral levels for rod placement.
3. Bone graft is placed in the areas that will be under the rod.
4. The appropriate concave rod is bent to shape for sagittal-plane correction and manipulated into the end hooks.
5. Stabilization along the length is achieved with blockers that anchor the rod into the open hooks.
6. The spine is then derotated using the rod holders. The frontal-plane scoliosis curve becomes the sagittal-plane kyphosis.
7. Hooks are reseated for secure fixation.
8. To correct kyphosis, the convex rod is then bent to shape and seated.
9. Once the rods have been placed, stabilization is completed by applying the DTT, usually near the ends of the rods.
10. Remaining bone graft is applied to the fusion area.

Texas Scottish Rite Hospital (TSRH) crosslink system

The TSRH crosslink system (Fig. 22-129) is a multicomponent stainless steel implant used to lock spinal rods together rigidly. Locking the rods increases construction stiffness and prevents rod migration. The system was originally designed for the Luque segmental system to prevent migration between the rods and wires before complete fusion occurred. By rigidly crosslinking the rods, loss of scoliotic correction was reduced. This system can also be used with the Harrington and Cotrel-Dubousset systems. Crosslinks are indicated when the rigidity of a spinal system alone is not sufficient to generate fusion in a reasonable amount of time.

Procedural considerations

Patient-specific considerations are implemented after the assessment (see laminectomy section, p. 905). The

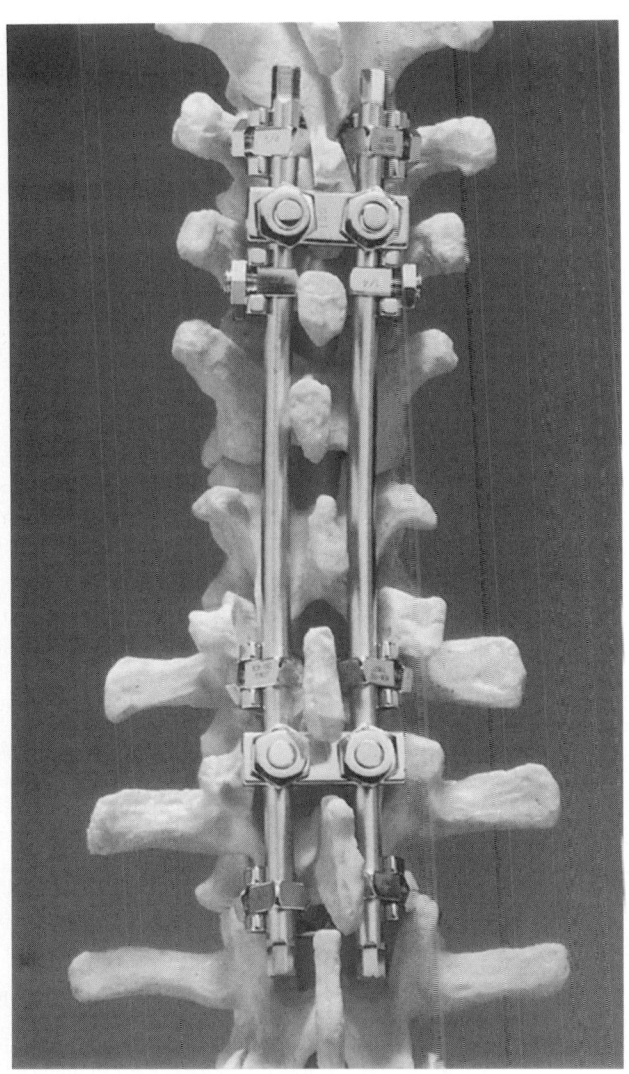

FIGURE 22-129 Texas Scottish Rite system.

patient is placed under general anesthesia and positioned prone. The skin is prepped, and drapes are applied. A spinal laminectomy set is used. Instrumentation and implants of choice, a spinal retractor, and power equipment such as a high-speed hand-held tool will be necessary. Hemostatic adjuncts such as Gelfoam, thrombin, Oxycel, and bone wax should be available.

Operative Procedure

1. Eyebolts are placed on the spinal rods before the rods are implanted.
2. The rods are secured with hooks or wires, depending on the system used.
3. Once the rods are positioned, crossplates of varying widths accommodating different rod-to-rod distances are bolted in placed between the rods and nuts.

Anterior spinal fusion with Isola instrumentation

Isola instrumentation involves screw fixation into each vertebral body, complete disk excision and grafting, and segmental connection of the vertebral bodies. A semirigid rod connects the segments. The Isola anterior instrumentation is indicated in adolescent idiopathic scoliosis patients, approximately 10 to 30 years of age, with thoracolumbar or upper lumbar curves of 40 to 65 degrees.[5]

Procedural Considerations

The patient is positioned in a lateral decubitus position so that posteroanterior and lateral intraoperative radiographs can be taken. The usual anesthetic and positioning precautions are necessary. The anesthetic technique should provide incomplete pharmacologic paralysis, allowing for intraoperative neurophysiologic monitoring. In addition to a major soft-tissue set and laminectomy set, the Isola instrumentation and implants, a vascular set, and power equipment will be needed.

Operative Procedure

1. The spine is approached through a transthoracic retroperitoneal (or retropleural retroperitoneal) approach, resecting the rib two vertebral levels above the upper instrumented vertebrae.
2. The sympathetic chain is mobilized laterally with the psoas.
3. The segmental vessels are temporarily occluded and, provided that there are no monitoring changes, ligated.
4. The disks are exposed to the far side to allow a full annulectomy. The bodies, however, are not exposed much beyond the midline.
5. A full 360-degree diskectomy and annulectomy are done, exposing the posterior longitudinal ligament.
6. Screws are then placed within the vertebral body, with the end screws being placed first. Care is taken to place the longitudinal axis of the screw parallel to the end plate and at the apex of the vertebral body.
7. Screw placement is started with an awl and continued with a 5.5 mm tap, continuing until the tip just exits the far side of the cortex. The first one third of the hole is tapped with a 7.0 mm tap, and a 7.0 mm closed top screw with a washer is inserted. The screw must protrude through the opposite cortex by a thread or two. The same process is then repeated at the lower end vertebra.
8. A rod of proper length is cut and contoured to recreate the sagittal-plane angular position of the normal spine. It is then positioned in the end vertebra and used as a guide to locate the entry point for the intermediate screws.
9. Open-ended intermediate screws are inserted in a fashion similar to the end screws, taking care that their travel is parallel to the end screws.
10. The rod is back entered through the upper screw and then the lower screw and seated into the intermediate open screws. The open screws are capped, and the rod

is rotated to place the sagittal-plane contour of the rod in the sagittal plane. An intermediate set screw is tightened to secure the new position of the rod.

11. As the remaining screws are tightened about the rod, it is essential that the disk spaces be opened completely. A Cobb elevator can be used to pry open the disk space.

12. Rib corticocancellous autograft is used to completely fill the disk spaces. This is done using the tenth rib (the usual site of entry), the twelfth rib taken from inside the chest, and the eighth rib taken from outside the chest.

13. The disk spaces are compressed to provide anterior column load sharing. Care should be taken to be sure the set screws are visited at least twice for the end-closed connections and three times for the center-capped connections.

14. Closure is in the standard manner, using chest tubes if the chest has been entered or a retropleural Hemovac if a retropleural retroperitoneal exposure has been done.

15. Aftercare consists in an overnight intensive care stay with the patient sitting out of bed the next morning. A cast or brace is used at the physician's discretion. Activities are restricted for 6 to 12 months, until there is clear indication of graft incorporation.

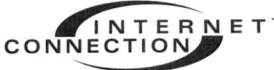

National Association of Orthopedic Nurses (NAON):
http://inurse.com/~naon/

American Academy of Orthopedic Surgeons:
http://www.aaos.org/

Orthopaedic Surgery Case Studies:
http://www.grandrounds.com/3no5.html

Charlotte Orthopedic Specialists: http://www.cosortho.com

Southerna California Orthopedic Institute:
http://www.scoi.com/

Chapter 6: Rheumatology/Orthopedics: http://indy. radiology.uiowa.edu/Providers/ClinRef/FPHandbook/06.html

Center for Arthroscopic Surgery:
http://mmink.cts.com/mmink/dossiers/cas.html

Scoliosis:
http://www.rad.washington.edu/Books/Approach/Scoliosis.html

Wheeless' Textbook of Orthopaedics:
http://www.medmedia.com/

Orthopaedics Today:
http://www.slackinc.com/bone/ortoday/othome.htm

Tissue Engineering: http://www.pittsburgh-tissue.net/

Association of Rehabilitation Nurses (ARN):
http://www.rehabnurse.org/

American Physical Therapy Association: http://www.apta.org

Prosthetics Research Study:
http://weber.u.washington.edu/~prs/

Dr. Pribut's Running Injuries:
http://www.clark.net/pub/pribut/spsport.html

National Osteoporosis Foundation: http://www.nof.org

Orthopedic Surgery News Group: news:sci.med.orthopedics

REFERENCES

1. Ahl, T., Dalen, N., Jorbeck, H., & Hoborn, J. (1995). Air contamination during hip and knee arthroplasties: horizontal laminar flow vs. randomized conventional ventilation. *Acta Orthopaedica Scandinavica, 66*(1), 17-20.

2. American Association of Tissue Banks. (1997). *Technical manual for surgical bone banking.* Arlington, Va.: the Association.

3. American Academy of Orthopadic Surgeons. (1997). Rosemont, Ill: the Academy.

4. An, Y.H., & Friedman, R.J. (1996). Prevention of sepsis in total joint arthroplasty. *Journal of Hospital Infection, 33,* 93-108.

5. Asher, M.A. (1996). *Surgical technique for anterior segmental instrumentation of thoracolumbar and lumbar scoliosis using the Anterior Isola Spinal System.* Cleveland, Ohio: Acromed Corp.

6. *AORN standards, recommended practices and guidelines.* (1998). Denver: Association of Operating Room Nurses.

7. Babbitt, A.M. (1997). Osteoporosis: diagnosis and treatment. *Journal of Bone Joint Surgery, American volume, 79*(4), 634-635.

8. Bridwell, K.H. (1997). Spinal instrumentation in the management of adolescent scoliosis. *Clinical Orthopaedics, 335,* 64-72.

9. Brown, M.D., & Seltzer, D.G. (1991). Perioperative care in lumbar spine surgery. *Orthopedic Clinics of North America, 22*(2), 353-358.

10. Carr, E.C., & Thomas, V.I. (1997). Anticipating and experiencing postoperative pain: the patient's perspective. *Journal of Clinical Nursing, 6*(3), 191-201.

11. Chapman, M.W. (1993). *Operative orthopedics.* Philadelphia: Lippincott.

12. Crenshaw, A.H. (1992). *Campbell's operative orthopaedics.* St. Louis: Mosby.

13. Dienst, M., Wozasek, G.E., & Seligson, D. (1997). Dynamic external fixation for distal radius fractures. *Clinical Orthopaedics, 338,* 160-171.

14. Estebe, J., & Malledant, Y. (1996). Pneumatic tourniquets in orthopedics. *Annales Françaises d' Anesthésie et de Réanimation, 15*(2), 162-178.

15. Frank, S.A. Body temperature and clinical outcome in the perioperative period. Presented at *Consensus Conference on Thermoregulation,* Bethesda, Md., Feb 7, 1998.

16. Gregory, B. (1994). *Mosby's perioperative nursing series: Orthopedic surgery,* St. Louis: Mosby.

17. Gustillo, R., & Templeman, D. (1993). *Fractures and dislocations.* St. Louis: Mosby.

18. Haasblek, J.F. (1997). Adolescent idiopathic scoliosis. *Postgraduate Medicine, 101*(6), 207-209.

19. Haddad, F.S., Cobb, A.G., Bentley, G., & et al. (1996). Hypersensitivity in aseptic loosening of total hip replacements: the role of the constituents of bone cement. *Journal of Bone and Joint Surgery, British volume, 78*(4), 546-549.

20. Hagen, K.S., & Treston-Aurand, J.A. (1995). A comparison of two skin preps used in cardiac surgical procedures. *AORN Journal, 62,* 392-402.

21. Horne, M. (1996). Involving physicians in clinical pathways: an example for perioperative knee arthroplasty. *Joint Commission Journal on Quality Improvement, 22*(2), 115-124.

22. Howmedica. (1995). *Surgical simplex,* P. Rutherford, NJ.: How-medica, Inc.
23. Johnson, L.L. (1993). *Diagnostic and surgical arthroscopy: the knee and other joints.* St. Louis: Mosby.
24. Mathias, J.M. (1998). Build variance tracking into pathway program. *OR Manager, 14*(1), 21-22.
25. Mistain, P., Duijnhouwer, E., Wijkel D., et al. (1997). The problems of elderly people at home one week after discharge from an acute care setting, *Journal of Advanced Nursing, 25,* 1233-1240.
26. McGinley, S., Baus, E., Gyza, K., et al. (1997). Multidisciplinary discharge planning: developing a process. *Nursing Management, 27*(5), 57-60.
27. Mourad, L.A. (1991). *Orthopaedic disorders.* St. Louis: Mosby.
28. Nolan, P. (1998). Competencies drive decision-making. *Nursing Management, 29*(3), 27-29.
29. Oishi, C.S., Carrion, W.V., & Hoaglund, F.T. (1993). Use of parenteral prophylactic antibiotics in clean orthopedic surgery: a review of the literature. *Clinical Orthopaedics and Related Research, 296,* 249-255.
30. Shelbourne, K.D., & Patel, D.V. (1996). Rehabilitation after autogenous bone-patellar tendon-bone ACL reconstruction. *Instructional Course Lectures, 45,* 263-273.
31. Sherk, H.H. (1990). *Lasers in orthopedics.* Philadelphia: Lippincott.
32. Sherk, H.H. (1995). The effects of lasers and electrosurgical devices on human meniscal tissue. *Clinical Orthopaedics and Related Research, 310,* 14-20.
33. Smith, J.E. (1990). Applying the continuous passive motion device. *Orthopedic Nursing, 9*(3), 54.
34. Springfield, D.S. (1997). Allograft reconstructions. *Seminars in Surgical Oncology, 13*(1), 11-17.
35. Thibodeau, G.A., & Patton, K.T. (1994). *Anatomy and physiology,* (ed. 2). St. Louis: Mosby.
36. Trufant, J.E., & Wilson, M.C. Total joint patient family education program. Presented at the AORN Congress, Orlando, Fla., April 2, 1998.
37. Weaver, J.K., & Derkash, R.S. (1994). Don't forget the Bristow-Latarjet procedure. *Clinical Orthopaedics and Related Research, 308,* 102-110.

CHAPTER TWENTY THREE | # Neurosurgery

Ruth E. Vaiden

PERIOPERATIVE NURSES MUST understand the structure and function of the nervous system to provide intelligent, safe, humanistic care for neurosurgical patients. From a range of variables of normal development they must identify those critical for each patient and recognize and respond to a variety of dependency needs, such as the normal response to preoperative sedation, as well as pathologic conditions such as paralysis, aphasia, and coma. Based on an understanding of the many pathologic conditions that result in surgical intervention, perioperative nurses must plan and manage complex patient care. They must be familiar with the use, care, working order, and safety factors of sophisticated instrumentation. They need to appreciate the limitations and stresses facing neurosurgeons. Anticipating and responding to potential complications inherent in specific patients, procedures, and neurosurgical emergencies require great speed but the same care and precision as elective situations. General information to assist perioperative nurses to function effectively in their own clinical settings is presented within this chapter.

SURGICAL ANATOMY

The nervous system, the most complex and least understood of body systems, is divided structurally into the central nervous system (brain and spinal cord) and the peripheral nervous system (cranial and spinal nerves).

Nervous system tissue is composed of neurons and neuroglial cells that support the neurons. The brain and spinal cord are protected by the skull and vertebral columns respectively. The cranial nerves originate within the brain and emerge through openings in the skull to run peripherally. The spinal nerves that emerge from the spinal cord through the vertebral foramina also run peripherally. In this chapter, therefore, peripheral nerves are those outside the cranial cavity and vertebral canal.

The nervous system is divided functionally into voluntary and autonomic (involuntary) systems. The nervous system functions as the communication system for the rest of the body. The functions of all body systems are dependent, in part, on nervous system function. In turn, the nervous system is directly dependent on circulatory system function for life-sustaining glucose and oxygen. Nervous system functions include orientation, coordination, conceptual thought, emotion, memory, and reflex response.

Within the framework of neurosurgical techniques, logical divisions of the nervous system are the head, or cranium; the back, or spine; and the peripheral nerves. These subdivisions lend themselves to meaningful discussion of supporting structures, body positions, instrumentation, and other considerations useful to the nurse providing care for neurosurgical patients during the intraoperative phase of care.

Head

Scalp layers of the head (Fig. 23-1) include skin, subcutaneous tissue, galea, and occipitofrontal musculature. Scalp skin is thick. The subcutaneous tissue, which is exceptionally dense, tough, and vascular, is firmly attached to the galea. Most of the blood vessels lie superficial to the galea. The subgaleal space contains loose areolar tissue that permits mobility of the scalp. It is in this bloodless plane that the standard craniotomy scalp flap is hinged. The pericranium, or outer periosteum of the skull, separates the galea from the cranium.

The arterial supply of the scalp comes from the external carotid artery through the superficial temporal, posterior auricular, occipital, frontal, and supraorbital branches. Most veins roughly follow the course of the arteries, except emissary veins, which drain directly through the skull into the intracranial venous sinuses. Unlike the arteries, the surface veins of the brain have many large anastomoses. The scalp, the extracranial arteries, and portions of the dura mater are the only pain-sensitive structures that cover the brain. The brain itself is insensate.

The skull is formed by 24 bones, joined by serrated bony seams called *sutures*. Eight bones form the walls of the cranial cavity, which houses the brain. There are four single bones—frontal, occipital, ethmoid, and sphenoid—and four paired bones—temporal and parietal (Fig. 23-2). The coronal suture joins the frontal and parietal bones. The squamous sutures border the squamous part of the temporal bones. The lambdoid suture joins the occipital and parietal bones. The sagittal suture lies in the medial plane and joins the two parietal bones (Fig. 23-3).

At the top of the skull in front of and behind the parietal bones are the anterior and posterior fontanelles, which are

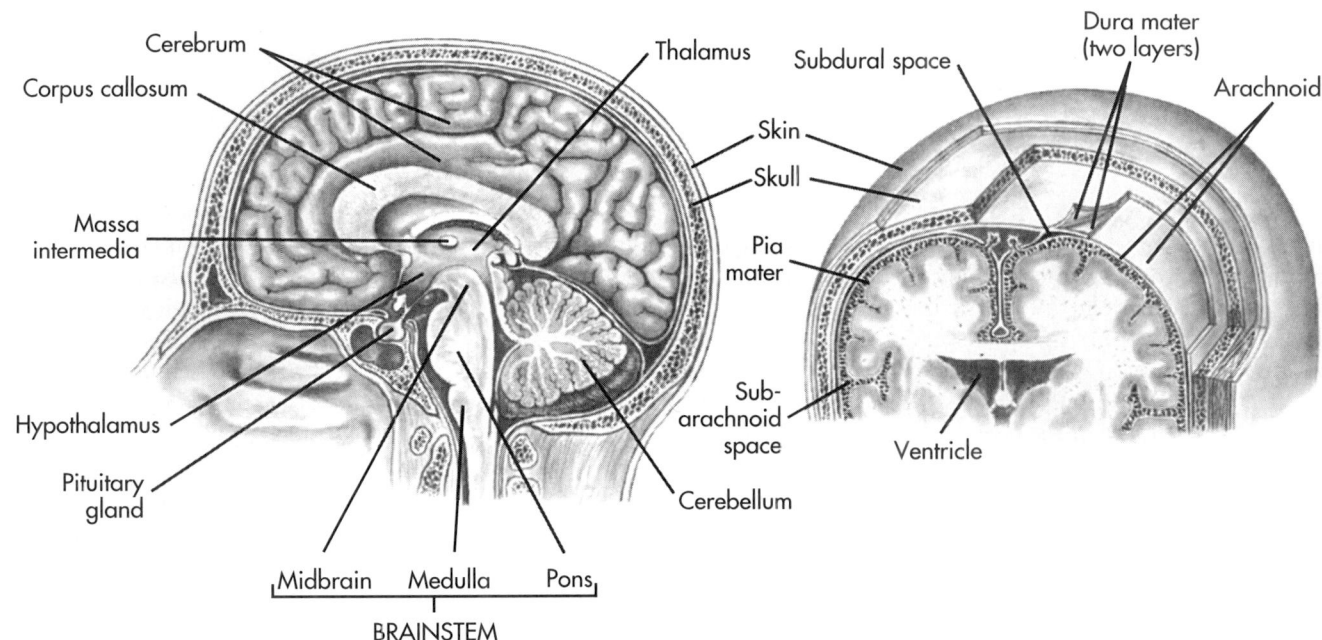

FIGURE 23-1 Scalp is composed of following layers: skin, subcutaneous tissue, galea, and periosteum of skull. Skull bone has three tables: outer, diploë (or spongy layer), and inner. Dura mater lies beneath skull and completely encapsulates brain. Other structures are identified for reference and are described in text.

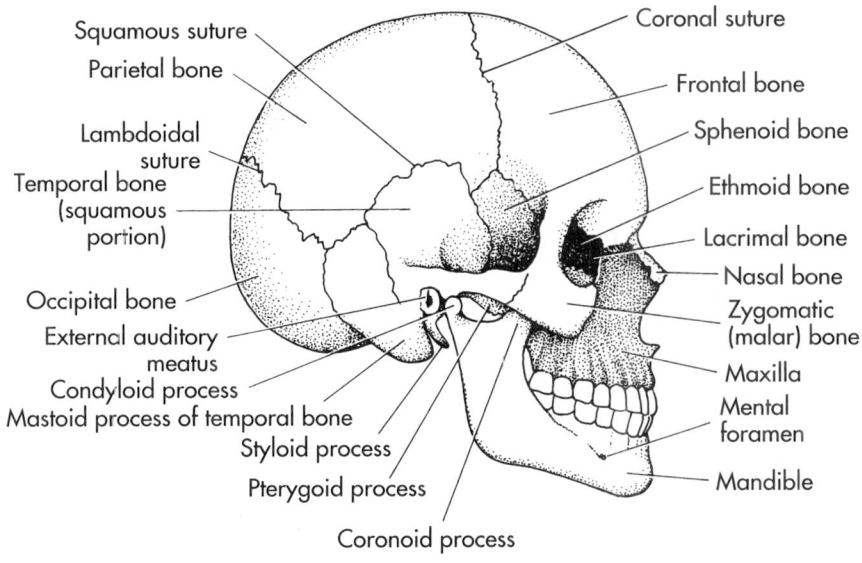

FIGURE 23-2 Skull viewed from right side.

open at birth. The posterior fontanelle is generally closed by 2 months and the anterior by about 18 months after birth. If the suture lines close prematurely, the skull cannot expand as the brain grows. This condition, called *craniosynostosis*, may demand early surgical intervention (see Chapter 29).

The skull is ovoid and is wider in back than in front. The flattened, irregular bones consist of two tables of compact bone that enclose a layer of spongy bone, or diploë (see Fig. 23-1).

The interior of the skull is anatomically divided into three cranial fossae: anterior, middle, and posterior (Fig. 23-4). The anterior fossa is limited posteriorly by the sphenoid ridge, along which pituitary tumors and aneurysms of the circle of Willis are generally approached. The frontal lobes and olfactory bulbs and tracts lie in the anterior fossa. The temporal lobes lie in the middle fossa, which is shaped like a butterfly. The sella turcica, formed by the sphenoid bone, is the most central part of the middle fossa and houses the pituitary gland. The floor and lateral walls of the middle fossa are shaped from the greater wings of the sphenoid bone and parts of the temporal bone, which house the internal and middle ear structures (see Fig. 23-4). The posterior fossa, the largest and deepest fossa, is formed by the occipital, sphenoid, and petrous portions of the temporal bones; the cerebellum and brainstem lie here, as many cranial nerves do. The foramen magnum, the largest opening in the skull, permits the spinal cord to join the brainstem in the posterior fossa. There are numerous other openings in the base of the skull for passage of arteries, veins, and cranial nerves (see Fig. 23-4).

Between the skull and brain are the meninges and three covering membranes: the dura mater, arachnoid, and pia mater (see Fig. 23-1). The dura mater is a tough, shiny, fibrous membrane that is close to the inner surface of the skull and folds to separate the cranial cavity into compartments. The largest fold is the falx cerebri, an arch-shaped, vertically placed, midline structure separating the right and left cerebral hemispheres. A smaller fold of dura mater, the falx cerebelli, separates the cerebellar hemispheres vertically. A transverse fold, the tentorium cerebelli, forms the roof of the posterior fossa. The tentorium supports the temporal lobe and occipital lobes of the cerebral hemispheres. Below the tentorium lie the cerebellum and brainstem. Structures above the tentorium are referred to as *supratentorial*, and those below as

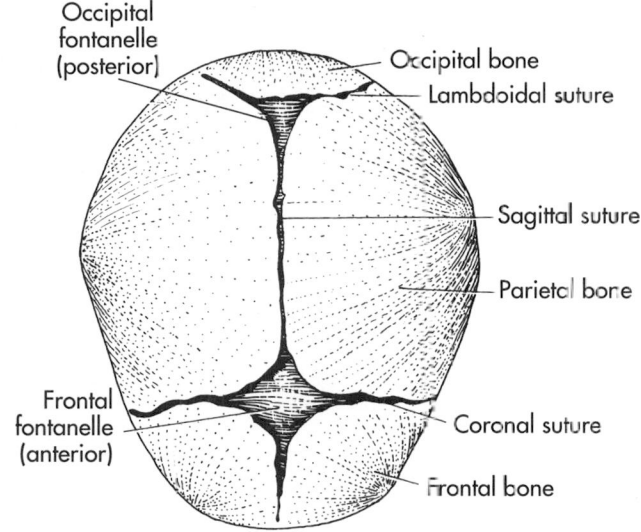

FIGURE 23-3   Skull at birth viewed from above.

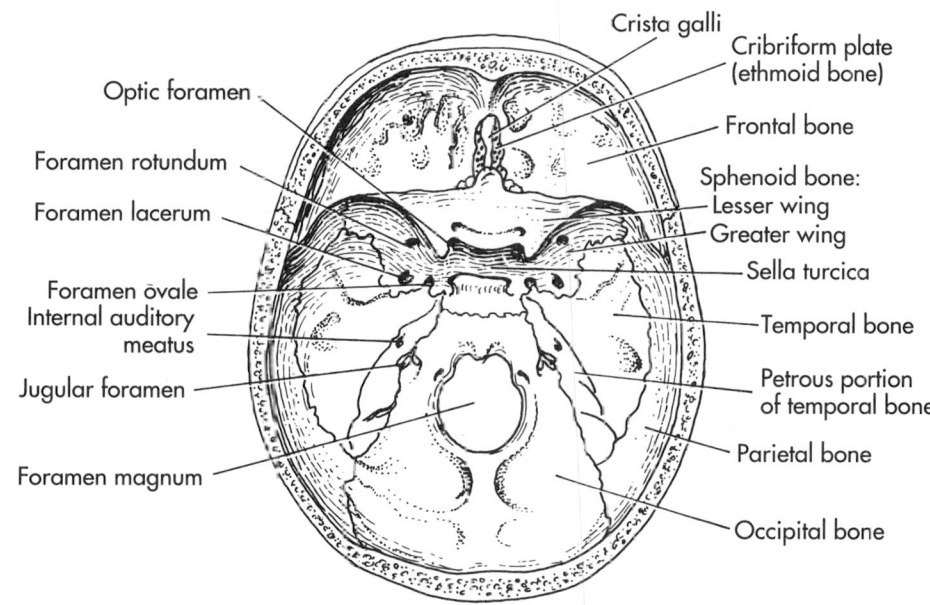

FIGURE 23-4   Floor of cranial cavity.

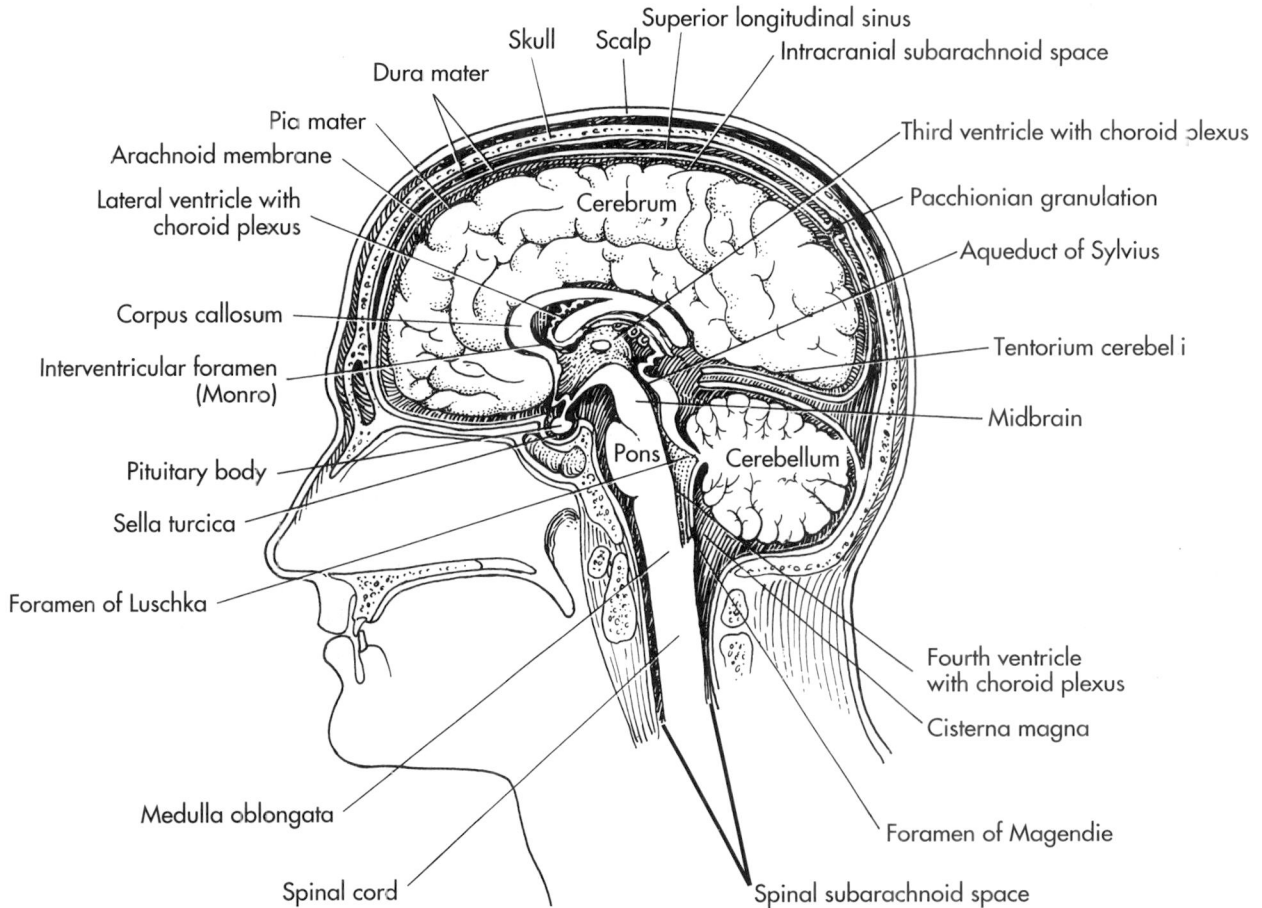

FIGURE 23-5 Sagittal section of head showing cerebrospinal fluid spaces and their relationship to venous circulation and principal subdivision of the brain and its coverings.

infratentorial (Fig. 23-5). At margins of these dural folds lie large venous sinuses that drain blood from the intracranial structures into the jugular veins. Several arteries also lie within the layers of the dura. The largest is the middle meningeal, a source of serious epidural hemorrhage if torn by an overlying skull fracture. The rigid skull makes hemorrhage and swelling in the brain critical. The volume of the intracranial cavity is fixed. Increasing the intracranial contents by a hemorrhage, tumor, or edema may lead to serious intracranial pressure problems. Pressure on brain tissue may cause irreparable damage.

Beneath the dura mater is a fine membrane called the *arachnoid.* The outer layer of arachnoid closely approximates the dura mater. The inner layer forms innumerable weblike filaments that bridge to the surface of the brain (see Fig. 23-1). The outer surface of the arachnoid membrane adheres closely to the dura mater with no space normally between the two membranes. The inner surface is separated from the pia mater beneath it by the subarachnoid space, which is filled with cerebrospinal fluid (CSF) that bathes the brain. Around the base of the brain, particularly, this space becomes enlarged to form cisterns.

The major intracranial nerves and blood vessels pass through these compartments. Intracranial approaches can be charted in terms of the basal cisterns.

The pia mater, the innermost membrane, is like gossamer and attaches to the gray matter, dipping into the sulci and gyri. The pia mater has a rich vascular network that helps form the choroid plexus of the ventricles.

The brain is divided into the cerebral cortex, basal ganglia, hypothalamus, midbrain, brainstem, and cerebellum (see Figs. 23-5 and 23-6).

The right and left cerebral hemispheres are the largest parts of the brain. Each hemisphere is composed of cerebral cortex and is divided into frontal, parietal, occipital, and temporal lobes, insula, rhinencephalon, basal ganglia, and hypothalamus. The two hemispheres are divided by a longitudinal fissure and joined underneath the falx by a large transverse bundle of nerve fibers, the corpus callosum (see Fig. 23-6). Each of the cerebral hemispheres controls sensation and motor activity to and receives sensory stimuli from the opposite half of the body.

The surfaces of the hemispheres form convolutions called *gyri* and intervening furrows called *sulci.* Two sulci of

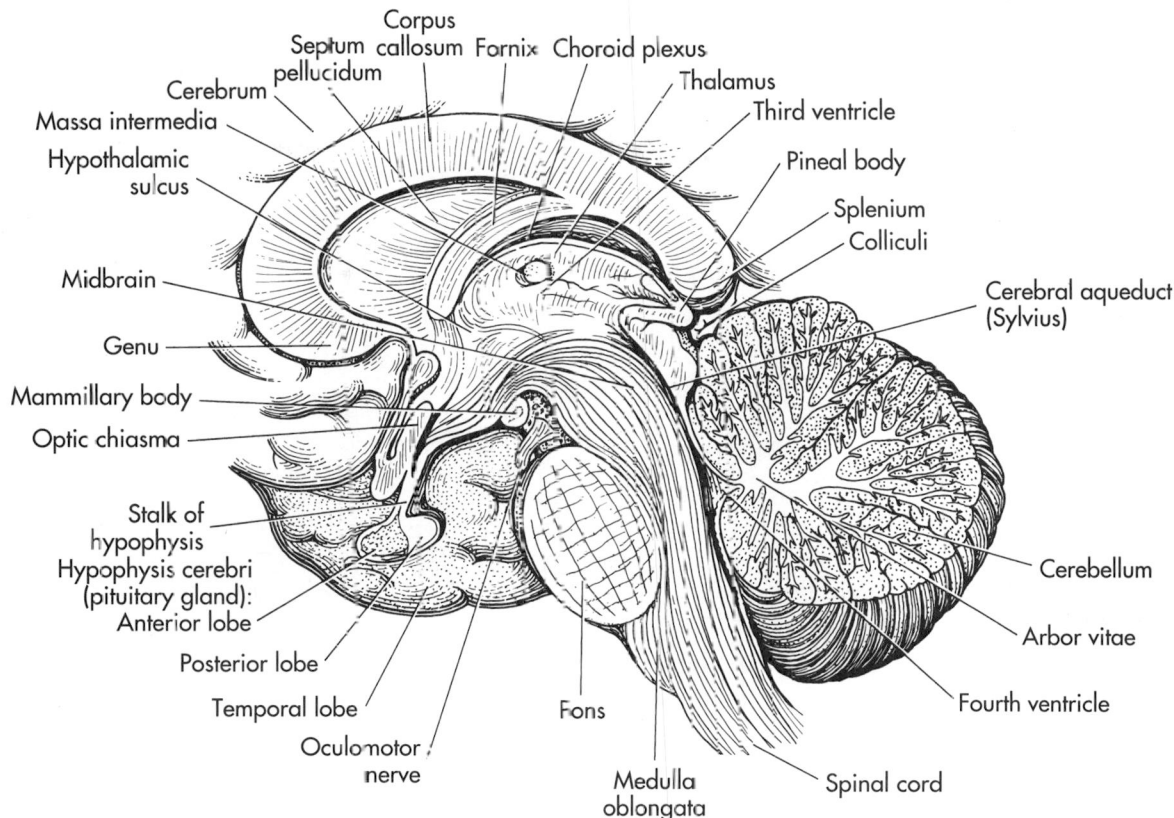

FIGURE 23-6 Sagittal section through midline of brain showing structures around third ventricle including corpus callosum, thalamus, and hypothalamus.

anatomic importance to the surgeon are the central sulcus, or fissure of Rolando, which separates the motor from the sensory cortex, and the lateral sulcus, or fissure of Sylvius, which marks off the temporal lobe (Fig. 23-7). The insula (island of Reil) lies deep within the lateral sulcus and can be exposed when the upper and lower lips of the fissure are separated. The frontal lobe is anterior to the central sulcus and controls the higher functions of intellect and abstract reasoning. The motor cortex lies anterior to the central sulcus. Destruction leads to loss of voluntary motor function on the opposite side of the body (Fig. 23-8).

Posterior to the central sulcus is the parietal lobe, extending back to the parietooccipital fissure. This area contains the final receiving and integrating station for sensory impulses from the contralateral side of the body. The occipital lobe lies posterior to the parietooccipital fissure. It receives and integrates visual impulses and registers them as meaningful images (see Figs. 23-7 and 23-8).

Inferior to the lateral sulcus, in the middle fossa, is the temporal lobe. Lesions of the left temporal lobe in right-handed persons and in many left-handed persons may affect the comprehension and verbalization of words, resulting in aphasia. Rhinencephalic structures, such as the anterior limbic area, may exert an inhibitory effect on brain mechanisms in the expression of emotions, such as

anger. Restlessness and hyperactivity may result from lesions of this area. The rhinencephalon has many connections with the hypothalamus. Malfunctions may affect sexual behavior, emotions, and motivation. Loss of recent memory may indicate a lesion of this area.

The convoluted surface of the cerebrum consists of gray matter, called the *cerebral cortex*, which contains the cell bodies of the many nerve pathways of the brain. The underlying white matter contains millions of myelinated nerve axons and is relatively avascular compared with the cortex. The nerve pathways, or fiber tracts, are of three types: (1) commissural fibers, which pass from one cerebral hemisphere to the other; (2) association fibers, which connect regions of gyri and lobes longitudinally within a cerebral hemisphere; and (3) projection fibers, including the great motor and sensory systems, which run vertically to connect the cortical regions with other portions of the central nervous system.

In prefrontal lobotomy, association fibers in the frontal lobe were divided to effect changes in personality that may be beneficial in certain psychiatric disorders. Cingulotomy, in which the cingulum is interrupted, also may be performed for treatment of these disorders.

Deep in the brain are five basal ganglia, or collections of nuclei, of the extrapyramidal system. Three of them, the caudate nucleus, putamen, and globus pallidus, collectively

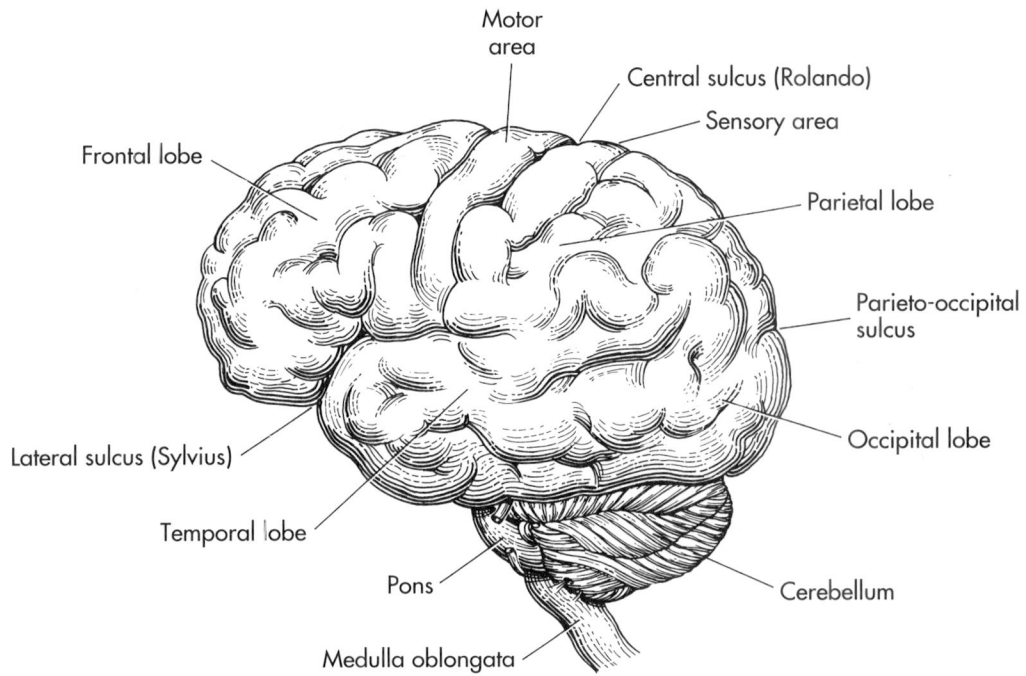

FIGURE 23-7   Lateral view of cerebral hemisphere (showing lobes and principal fissures), cerebellum, pons, and medulla oblongata.

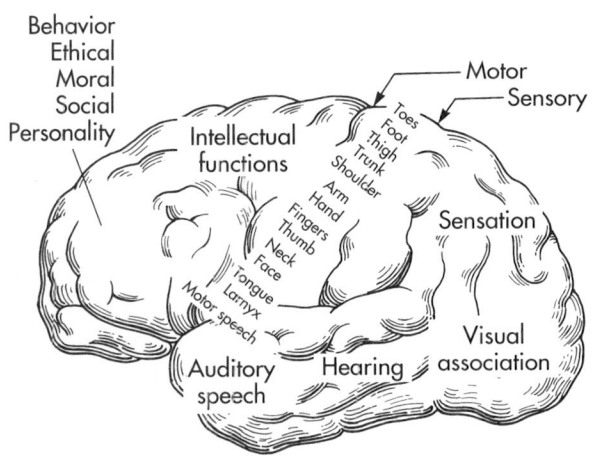

FIGURE 23-8   Principal functional subdivisions of cerebral hemispheres.

referred to as the *corpus striatum*, associate with the thalamus for fine, involuntary motor control (see Fig. 23-6). Lesions here may cause rigidity of the skeletal muscles and various types of spontaneous tremors. Sections of the basal ganglia and thalamus can be selectively destroyed surgically in an effort to relieve the tremors and rigidity associated with multiple sclerosis, Parkinson's disease, various forms of cerebellar degeneration, and late effects of severe brain trauma. In addition to rhythmic processing of brain activity and its influence on affect and higher brain activity, the thalamus is the major relay station for incoming sensory stimuli. Many of these stimuli are subsequently relayed to a final destination in the parietal cortex. Because of its central role in perception of body sensations, surgical lesions can be made in the thalamus in an attempt to alleviate pain.

Along the floor of the third ventricle is the hypothalamus (see Fig. 23-6), which is principally concerned with the autonomic regulation of the body's internal environment and is intimately connected with the pituitary gland.

The short, stocky portion of the brain, between the cerebral hemispheres and pons, is the midbrain (see Fig. 23-5), also referred to as the *mesencephalon*. It is composed of the cerebral peduncles, numerous nerve tracts and nuclei, and association centers that control the majority of eye movements. The hindbrain, or brainstem, immediately below the midbrain, consists of the pons and medulla oblongata (see Fig. 23-7). The midbrain and brainstem form the floor of the fourth ventricle in the posterior fossa of the skull and contain many large efferent and afferent tracts and nuclei of most cranial nerves. The brainstem contains the cardiovascular and respiratory regulatory centers. Surgery directly on the brainstem is extremely dangerous.

The cerebellum, which occupies most of the posterior fossa, forms the roof of the fourth ventricle (see Figs. 23-6 and 23-7). It has two lateral lobes and a medial portion, the vermis. The fissures of the cerebellum are small and run transversely. The cerebellum is principally concerned with balance and coordination of movement. It has many complex connections with higher and lower centers and exerts its influence unilaterally, in contrast to the cerebral hemispheres, which act contralaterally. At least half the brain tumors in children originate in the cerebellum. In

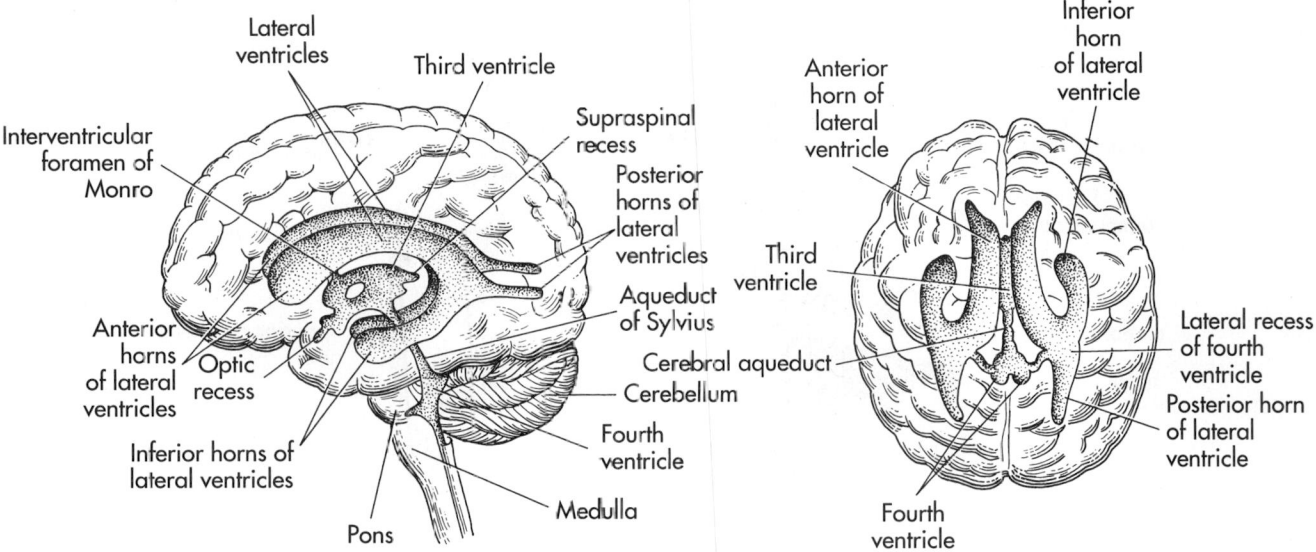

FIGURE 23-9   Ventricular system showing its relationship to various parts of brain.

adults and children the most common surgical lesions in this area are tumors and abscesses. By splitting the vermis in the exact midline, a satisfactory exposure of tumors that lie in the fourth ventricle is obtained without sacrificing the important cerebellar functions.

Cerebrospinal fluid system

Within the brain are four communicating cavities, or ventricles, filled with CSF. In the lower medial portion of each cerebral hemisphere lies a large lateral ventricle, which resembles a wishbone and is separated anteriorly from its counterpart by a thin pellucid septum (Fig. 23-9). Each lateral ventricle has a body and three horns: frontal, occipital, and temporal. Below the bodies of the lateral ventricles is a central cleft, or third ventricle. It communicates anteriorly with the lateral ventricles through the foramen of Monro and posteriorly with the fourth ventricle through the aqueduct of Sylvius, a long narrow channel passing through the midbrain. The fourth ventricle is a rhomboid cavity in the posterior fossa, between the cerebellum and the brainstem. In the roof of the fourth ventricle is the foramen of Magendie, an opening into the cisterna magna; at the lateral margins are the two foramina of Luschka, which open into the cisterna pontis.

Much of the CSF originates in the choroid plexuses of the ventricles. These are tufted, vascular structures that allow certain fluid elements of the blood to pass through their ependymal linings. The choroid plexus is found along the floor in each lateral ventricle, on the roof of the third ventricle, and in the posterior portion of the fourth ventricle. Most of the fluid is formed in the lateral ventricles and flows through the interventricular foramen of Monro to the third ventricle and through the aqueduct of Sylvius to the fourth ventricle, where it escapes into the

subarachnoid space of the basal cisterns through the foramina of Magendie and Luschka. From the basal cisterns the fluid flows around the spinal cord, over the cerebellar lobes, around the medulla and the base of the brain, and over the cerebral hemispheres in the subarachnoid space. The fluid is absorbed into the venous circulation through villi of the arachnoid (pacchionian granulations) into the great dural venous sinuses, particularly the superior sagittal sinus, and by diffusion through perivascular, perineural, and periradicular channels (see Fig. 23-1).

The total amount of circulating CSF averages 125 to 150 ml in the adult. Each lateral ventricle contains 10 to 15 ml, the rest of the ventricular system contains 5 ml, the cranial subarachnoid space averages about 25 to 35 ml, and the spinal subarachnoid space contains about 75 to 90 ml. The ventricular fluid normally has 5 to 15 mg/dl protein content, whereas the spinal fluid has 25 to 45 mg/dl. These values may be considerably elevated in pathologic conditions of the central nervous system.

The characteristics of normal spinal fluid are as follows:

- Appearance: clear and colorless
- Pressure: 70 to 200 mm H_2O
- pH: 7.35 to 7.4
- Specific gravity: 1.005 to 1.009
- Glucose: 50 to 75 mg/dl (⅔ of blood glucose)
- Chlorides: 120 to 130 mEq/L
- Cells: up to 10/ml (lymphocytes only)
- Protein: lumbar, 15 to 45 mg/dl; cisternal, 10 to 25 mg/dl; ventricular, 5 to 15 mg/dl
- Culture: negative
- Gamma globulin: 6% to 13% of total protein

Spinal fluid bathes the brain and spinal cord, helps support the weight of the brain, and acts as a cushion for

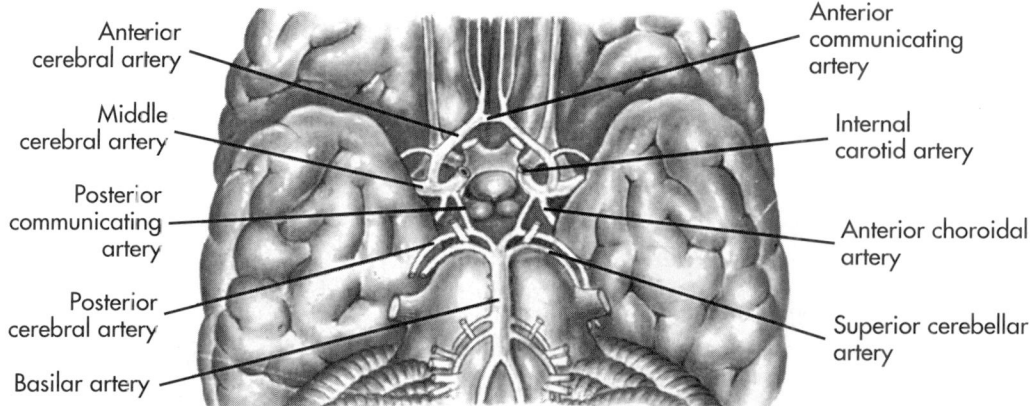

FIGURE 23-10   Principal cerebral arteries and circle of Willis.

the brain and spinal cord by absorbing some of the force of external trauma. By variation in its volume, it aids in keeping intracranial pressure relatively constant. If the brain atrophies, the CSF increases in amount to fill the dead space; if the brain swells, the CSF decreases in amount to compensate for the increase in brain mass. The fluid can carry certain drugs to diseased parts of the brain. It does not, however, play a significant role in supplying nutrition to the structures that it bathes.

The rate of absorption and production of CSF is related to the osmotic and hydrostatic pressure of the blood. When intracranial pressure rises, an intravenous injection of hypertonic mannitol or a nonosmotic diuretic is employed to dehydrate the blood and decrease the volume of CSF.

Elevations in CSF pressure can be caused by an expanding mass within the skull, such as a tumor, hemorrhage, or cerebral edema; an increase in formation of fluid, as in meningitis, encephalitis, and other febrile conditions; an increase in venous pressure within the skull from an obstruction to normal venous drainage; a blockage of absorption by inflammatory conditions of the arachnoid and perivascular spaces; any mechanical obstruction of the ventricular or subarachnoidal fluid pathways; or problems with the absorption of CSF. Increase in CSF production or decrease in CSF absorption can lead to hydrocephalus. Hydrocephalus can be classified as either communicating (normal CSF pathways open) or noncommunicating (obstruction of CSF pathways). The appropriate surgical procedure depends on the precise type of hydrocephalus.

Blood supply

The arterial supply to the brain, which requires 20% more oxygen than any other organ, enters the cranium through the two internal carotid arteries anteriorly and the two vertebral arteries posteriorly. These communicate at the base of the brain through the circle of Willis (Fig. 23-10), which ensures continuity of the circulation if any one of the four main channels is interrupted. However, these connections are extremely variable and do not always have functional anastomoses. The main branches for distribution of blood to each hemisphere of the brain from the internal carotid arteries are the anterior and middle cerebral arteries. Each artery nourishes a specific area of the brain (Fig. 23-11). The anterior cerebral artery supplies the anterior two thirds of the medial surface and adjacent region over the convexity of the hemisphere, thus including about half of the frontal and parietal lobes. The middle cerebral artery supplies most of the lateral surface of the hemisphere, including half of the frontal, parietal, and temporal lobes. The posterior cerebral artery, which originates off the basilar artery, supplies the occipital lobe and the remaining half of the temporal lobe, principally on the inferior and medial surfaces. The brainstem and cerebellum are supplied by branches of the basilar and vertebral arteries.

The circle of Willis is of particular interest surgically because of the development of aneurysms in this area. An aneurysm is a dilatation in the wall of a large artery. Aneurysms usually develop in or near the crotch of a bifurcation of the circle of Willis. It is believed that the weakness develops because of the superimposition of two lesions: a congenital absence of the media and a degeneration of the internal elastic lamina that normally strengthens the arterial wall. Erosion of the lamina results from the wear and tear of pulsatile pressure.

The most common sites of intracranial aneurysms are (1) adjacent to the anterior communicating artery, (2) at the junction of the posterior communicating artery and the internal carotid artery, (3) at the origin of the anterior cerebral arteries, (4) at the first bifurcation of the middle cerebral artery, and (5) on the basilar arteries.

The cerebral veins do not parallel the arteries as the veins do in most other parts of the body. The external cortical veins anastomose freely in the pia mater, forming larger cerebral veins, and as such they pierce the arachnoid membrane, cross the subdural space, and empty into the great dural venous sinuses. A subdural hemorrhage after head trauma may arise from disruption of these bridging vessels; an epidural hemorrhage often results from lacera-

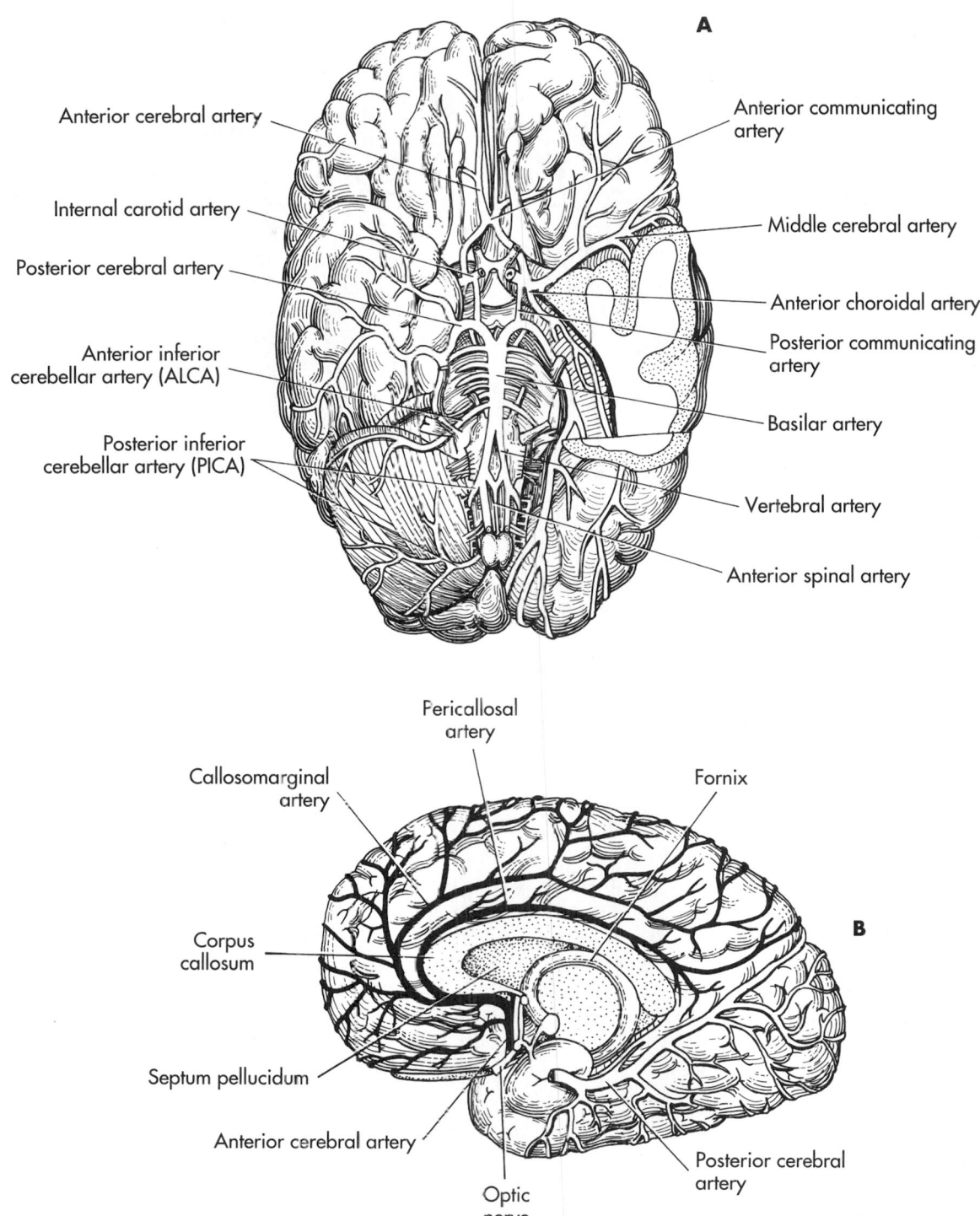

A

Anterior cerebral artery

Internal carotid artery

Posterior cerebral artery

Anterior inferior
cerebellar artery (ALCA)

Posterior inferior
cerebellar artery (PICA)

Anterior communicating
artery

Middle cerebral artery

Anterior choroidal artery

Posterior communicating
artery

Basilar artery

Vertebral artery

Anterior spinal artery

Pericallosal
artery

Callosomarginal
artery

Corpus
callosum

Septum pellucidum

Anterior cerebral artery

Optic
nerve

Fornix

B

Posterior cerebral
artery

FIGURE 23-11   **A**, Arteries of the inferior surface of the brain. Left half of cerebellum and part of left temporal lobe have been removed. **B**, Arteries of medial surface of brain. Anterior cerebral artery and its branches are shown in black; posterior cerebral artery and its branches are shown in white.

Continued

tions of the middle meningeal artery, a branch of the external carotid artery that supplies the dura mater. The deep cerebral veins, which drain the interior of the hemispheres, empty principally into the great vein of Galen and the inferior sagittal sinus (Figs. 23-12 and 23-13).

The blood transports oxygen, nutrients, and other substances necessary for the proper functioning of living tissue. The needs of the brain for oxygen and glucose are critical. The brain can store only small amounts of oxygen and energy-producing nutrients. Constant flow of blood to the brain must be maintained.

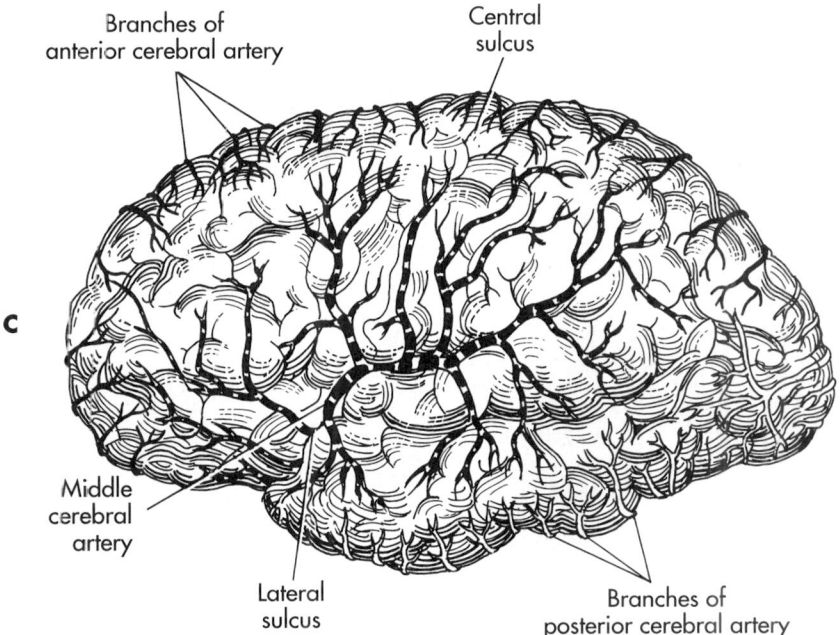

FIGURE 23-11, cont'd   **C,** Arteries of lateral surface of brain. Middle cerebral artery and its branches are shown striped; small branches of anterior cerebral artery reaching around from medial surface are shown in black; those of posterior cerebral artery are shown in white.

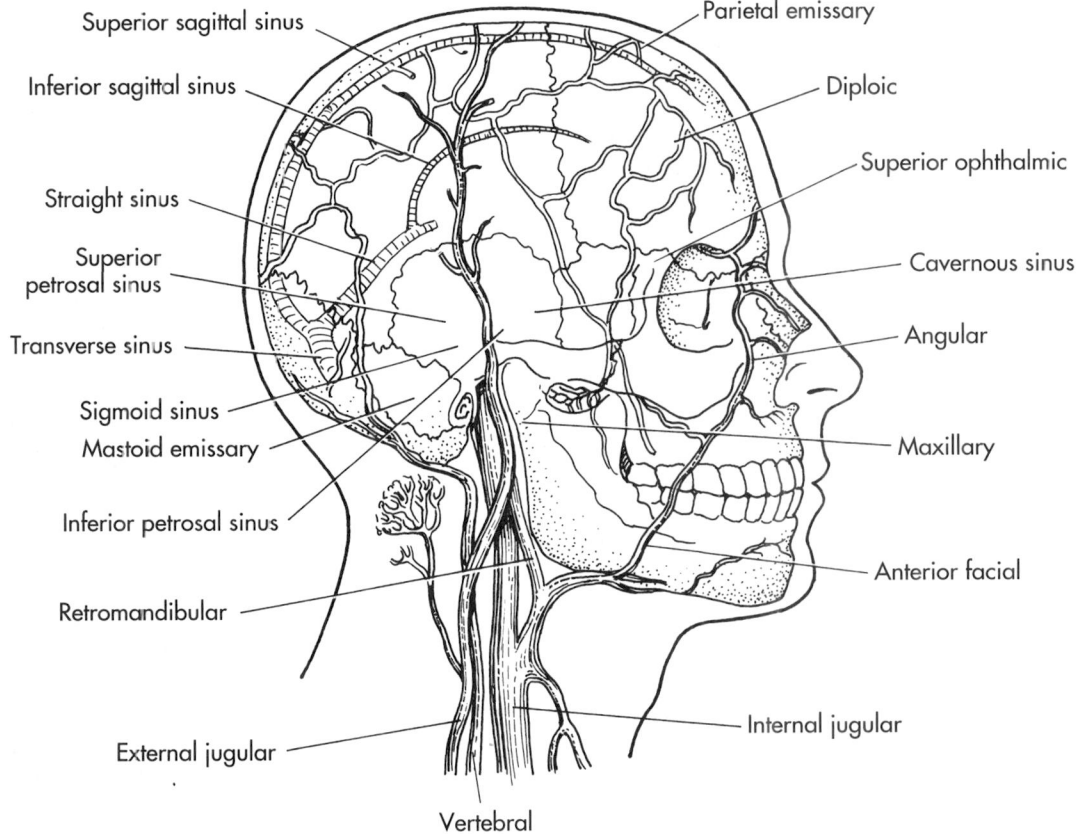

FIGURE 23-12   Semischematic projection of large veins of head. Deep veins and dural sinuses are projected on skull. Notice connection (emissary veins) between superficial and deep veins.

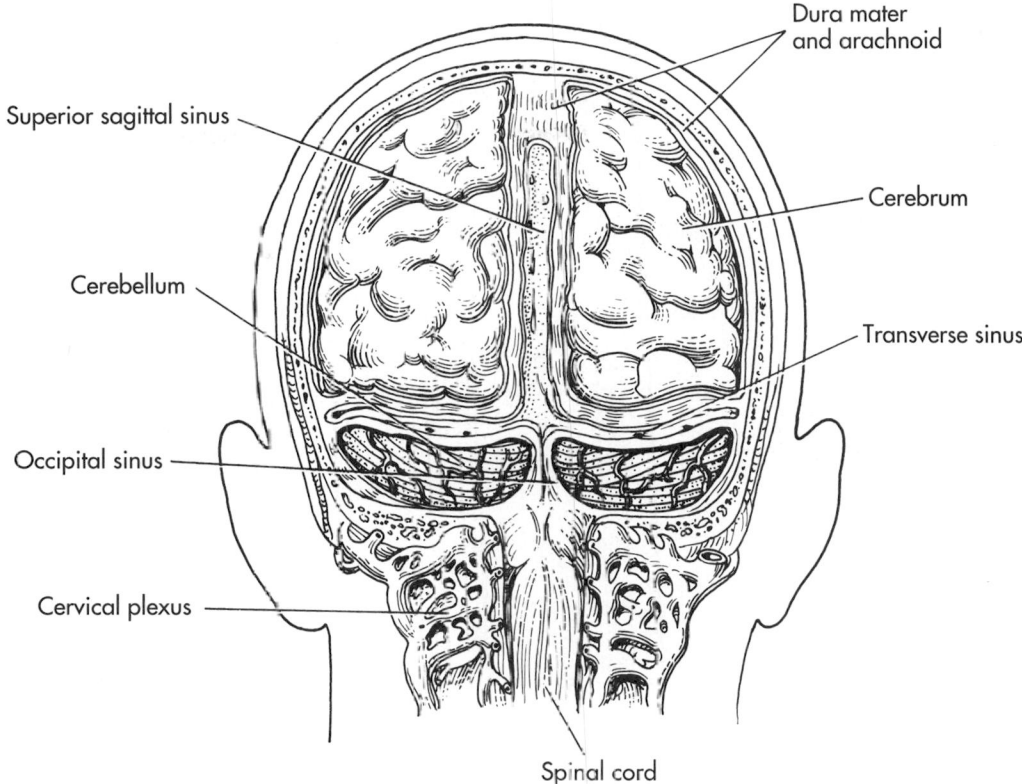

Superior sagittal sinus
Cerebellum
Occipital sinus
Cervical plexus
Dura mater and arachnoid
Cerebrum
Transverse sinus
Spinal cord

FIGURE 23-13   Venous sinuses shown in relation to brain and skull.

The brain uses oxygen in the metabolism of glucose, the chief source of energy. Protein and fat metabolism plays little part in energy production. In the face of an oxygen deficit, the survival time of central nervous system tissue is very short. In the face of low blood glucose, central nervous system function is compromised and unconsciousness results.

Generally, all factors affecting the systemic blood pressure indirectly affect the cerebral circulation. The brain normally receives 20% of the cardiac output. The cerebral blood flow is kept constant by an autoregulation phenomenon such that increases in blood pressure lead to vasoconstriction of cerebral arteries and decreases in blood pressure cause cerebral vasodilatation to maintain a relatively constant cerebral blood flow. When the mean arterial pressure falls below 60 mm Hg, the autoregulation mechanism usually fails. Thus controlled hypotension may be safely used in intracranial surgery.

Cranial nerves

Twelve pairs of cranial nerves arise within the cranial cavity (Fig. 23-14). From a surgical standpoint, they are considered with the head.

First Cranial Nerve

The olfactory nerve, a fiber tract of the brain, is located under the frontal lobe on the cribriform plate of the ethmoid bone. It transmits the sense of smell. Frontal lobe tumors, fractures of the anterior fossa of the skull, and lesions of the nasal cavity may affect the olfactory nerve.

Second Cranial Nerve

The optic nerve is a fiber tract of the brain. Originating in the ganglion cells of the retina, it passes through the optic foramen in the apex of the orbit to reach the optic chiasma, where a partial crossing of the fibers occurs, so the fibers from the nasal half of each retina pass to the opposite side. Posterior to the chiasma, the visual pathway is called the *optic tract*; still farther back, it becomes the optic radiation. Lesions in various parts of this pathway produce characteristic defects in the visual fields. For example, a lesion of the chiasma usually destroys the temporal vision of each eye (bitemporal hemianopia), whereas a lesion of the occipital lobe produces impairment of vision (homonymous hemianopia) affecting the right or left halves of the visual fields of both eyes.

Lesions that affect the optic nerve and are treated by neurosurgery include primary gliomas of the nerve, pituitary tumors that press on the optic chiasma, and occasionally meningiomas in the region of the sella turcica and olfactory groove. The optic nerves and chiasma are best exposed through a frontal craniotomy, along the floor of the anterior fossa, or through a frontotemporal approach along the sphenoid ridge.

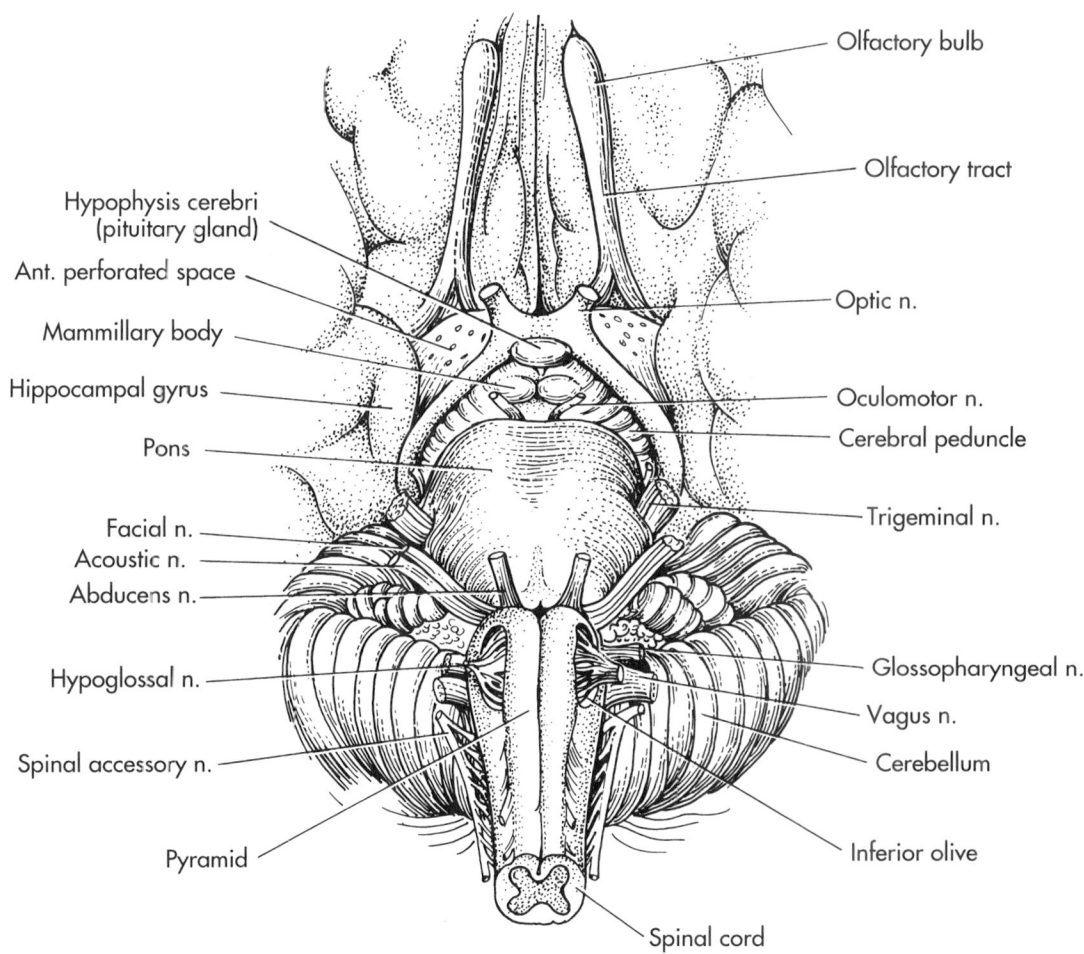

Hypophysis cerebri
(pituitary gland)

Ant. perforated space

Mammillary body

Hippocampal gyrus

Pons

Facial n.
Acoustic n.
Abducens n.

Hypoglossal n.

Spinal accessory n.

Pyramid

Olfactory bulb

Olfactory tract

Optic n.

Oculomotor n.
Cerebral peduncle

Trigeminal n.

Glossopharyngeal n.

Vagus n.

Cerebellum

Inferior olive

Spinal cord

FIGURE 23-14   Ventral surface of brain showing attachment of cranial nerves.

Third, Fourth, and Sixth Cranial Nerves

These three pairs of nerves—the oculomotor, the trochlear, and the abducens respectively—are conveniently considered together because they are the motor nerves to the muscles of the eyes. They are affected by many toxic, inflammatory, vascular, and neoplastic lesions. The third nerve may be affected by aneurysms of the internal carotid artery, and pressure against this nerve accounts for pupillary dilatation when temporal lobe herniation resulting from increased intracranial pressure is present.

Fifth Cranial Nerve

The trigeminal nerve has two functions: (1) sensory supply to the forehead, eyes, meninges, face, jaw, teeth, hard palate, buccal mucosa, tongue, nose, nasal mucosa, and maxillary sinus and (2) motor innervation of the muscles of mastication. The sensory fibers that arise from cells in the gasserian ganglion travel along the medial wall of the middle cranial fossa and then extend peripherally in three divisions: ophthalmic, maxillary, and mandibular. Behind the ganglion the fibers enter the brainstem by way

of the sensory root. The motor root, which originates from cells in the brainstem, follows the course of the larger sensory component (Fig. 23-15).

Trigeminal neuralgia (tic douloureux) is characterized by excruciating, piercing paroxysms of pain, affecting one or more of the major peripheral divisions. The recurrent attacks are usually brought on by stimulation of trigger zones present about the face, nares, lips, and teeth. This affliction, of unknown cause, tends to occur unilaterally and in older persons. Medical treatment is frequently unsuccessful. A great variety of neurosurgical procedures have been proposed for its control. Peripheral neurectomies of the supraorbital or infraorbital nerves may easily be performed with the patient under local anesthesia, but the effect is temporary because the nerves regenerate. Trigeminal neuralgia can also be treated by a posterior fossa approach using the operating microscope. The microscope allows decompression of the trigeminal nerve from normal surrounding blood vessels and selection of its various fibers. Sensations of pain and temperature are eliminated, and the sensation of touch and corneal reflex

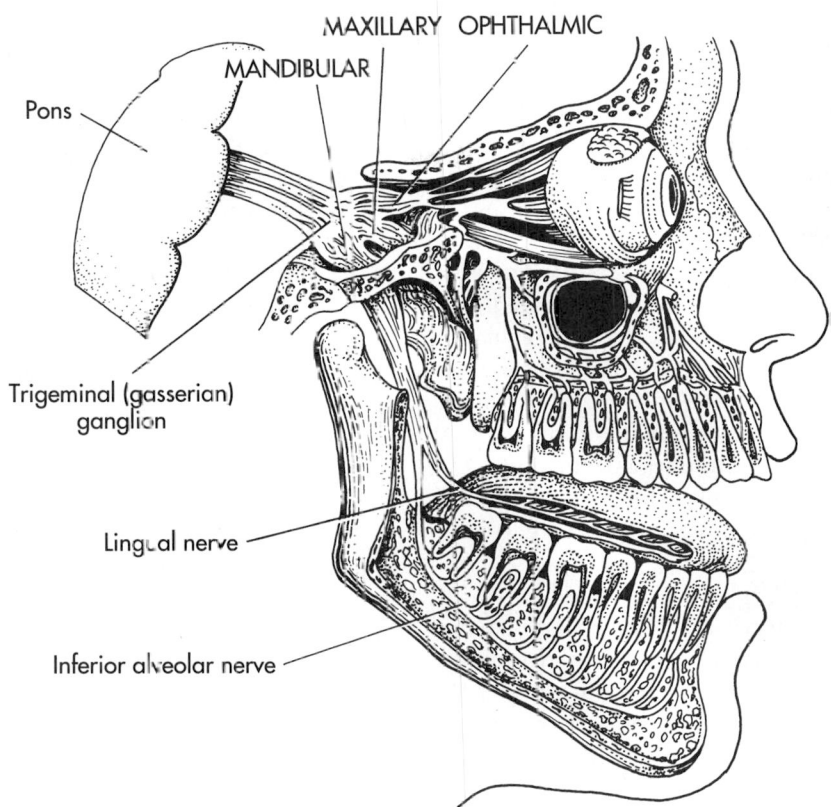

FIGURE 23-15 Trigeminal (fifth cranial) nerve and its three main divisions.

are preserved. Trigeminal neuralgia can also be treated by retrogasserian rhizotomy with radiofrequency current and chemical rhizolysis.

Seventh Cranial Nerve

The facial nerve supplies the musculature of the face and the anterior two thirds of the tongue (for taste). It originates in the brainstem, passes through the skull with the eighth nerve by way of the internal acoustic meatus, continues along the facial canal, and exits just posterior to the parotid gland. The nerve may be damaged by acoustic neurinomas, fractures at the base of the skull, mastoid infections, and surgical procedures in the vicinity of the parotid gland.

Bell's palsy, a facial lower motor neuron paralysis, can affect the seventh nerve. It may last for a few weeks to a few months, but recovery usually takes place. When permanent interruption of the nerve occurs, useful operations for restoration of function include spinal accessory–facial and hypoglossal-facial anastomosis. These operations are performed high in the neck behind the parotid gland by use of the operating microscope.

Eighth Cranial Nerve

The acoustic nerve has two parts, both sensory—the cochlear for hearing and the vestibular for balance. The former receives stimuli from the organ of Corti, the latter

from the semicircular canals. The major surgical lesion of the eighth nerve is acoustic neurinoma, a histologically benign tumor growing from the nerve sheath at its entrance into the internal auditory meatus. This tumors arises deep in the angle between the cerebellum and pons. Symptoms may include unilateral deafness, tinnitus, unilateral impairment of cerebellar function, numbness of the face from involvement of the fifth cranial nerve, and, late in the course, papilledema caused by increased intracranial pressure.

The operative approach is usually through a unilateral suboccipital craniectomy; in some instances a translabyrinth approach may be used. Great care must be taken to prevent injury to the pons, and an attempt is made to preserve the facial nerve. Meniere's disease is an affliction of the eighth nerve characterized by a recurrent and usually progressive group of symptoms including dizziness and a sensation of fullness or pressure in the ears. When medical measures fail to alleviate the problem, section of the eighth nerve may be performed; this procedure has given consistently excellent results.

Ninth Cranial Nerve

The glossopharyngeal nerve supplies the sense of taste to the posterior third of the tongue and sensation to the tonsils and pharyngeal region and partially innervates the pharyngeal muscles. Rarely it is involved in a painful tic similar to trigeminal tic. Its sensory component can be sectioned for this reason, to treat a hypersensitive carotid sinus, or, along with the fifth nerve, to treat painful malignancies of the face, mouth, and pharynx. The ninth nerve lies near the eighth nerve in the posterior fossa and is exposed in a similar way.

Tenth Cranial Nerve

The vagus nerve has many motor and sensory functions, chief among which are innervation of pharyngeal and laryngeal musculature, control of heart rate, and regulation of acid secretion of the stomach. In neck surgery the surgeon carefully avoids the recurrent laryngeal branch; in gastric surgery the surgeon may sever the vagus nerve at the lower end of the esophagus to treat a peptic ulcer. The neurosurgeon is concerned mainly with preventing damage to the vagus nerve during posterior fossa surgery.

Eleventh Cranial Nerve

The spinal accessory nerve is a motor nerve to the sternocleidomastoid and trapezius muscles. To restore mobility to the face, it may be anastomosed to the peripheral end of a damaged facial nerve.

Twelfth Cranial Nerve

The hypoglossal nerve innervates the musculature of the tongue. Its neurosurgical interest is similar to that of the spinal accessory nerve.

The contents of the cranial nerves are demonstrated in Table 23-1.[4]

Pathologic lesions of the brain

Brain tumors are not as rare, nor is their prognosis as poor, as is often believed. Early diagnosis simplifies surgical treatment because increased intracranial pressure and severe neurologic changes are not usually present. Brain tumors are either malignant or benign, depending on the cell type. Primary tumors generally do not resemble the carcinomas and sarcomas found elsewhere in the body and rarely metastasize outside the central nervous system. If both primary and metastatic tumors of the brain and its covering membranes are included in the term *intracranial tumors*, such tumors may be classified pathologically as germ cell, mesodermal, neuroepithelial, metastatic, and miscellaneous as follows:

1. Germ cell tumors
   a. Teratoma is a congenital tumor containing embryonic elements.
   b. Germinoma is a neoplasm arising from germ cells.
   c. Embryonal carcinoma is a tumor arising from premature exoderm.
   d. Choriocarcinoma is an extremely rare, very malignant neoplasm.
   e. Craniopharyngioma occurs in children and adults and arises from the region of the pituitary stalk; it is

usually cystic; calcification above the sella turcica is often seen on x-ray films. In addition to headache, vertigo, vomiting, and papilledema, diabetes insipidus and visual field changes are common.

2. Meningeal lesions. Meningioma is a slow-growing tumor, originating in the arachnoidal tissue; it is very vascular and may adhere to the dural venous sinuses or major arteries, making its complete removal difficult.
3. Neural sheath tumor. Neurinoma usually arises from the neurilemma sheath cells of the vestibular portion of the eighth cranial nerve within the auditory meatus, grows to fill the cerebellopontine angle, and may indent the brainstem.
4. Vascular tumors
   a. Angioma is an often congenital arteriovenous malformation.
   b. Hemangioblastoma may be solid or cystic; it is likely to occur in cerebellar hemispheres; sometimes it is present in association with angiomas of the retina and other organs.
5. Neuroepithelial tumors
   a. Gliomas
      (1) Glioblastoma multiforme is an infiltrative, fast-growing, rapidly recurring cerebral tumor that occurs most frequently in middle age. It may invade both cerebral hemispheres by crossing in the corpus callosum. Areas of necrosis are characteristic. Astrocytomas and oligodendrogliomas may transform into this malignant tumor with time.
      (2) Medulloblastoma is a fast-growing, rapidly recurring tumor of the vermis of the cerebellum and fourth ventricle that usually occurs in young children. It characteristically metastasizes into the subarachnoid spaces, usually spreading to the base of the brain by this route.
      (3) Ependymoma occurs most frequently in children and is likely to arise in or near the ventricular walls. It commonly occurs in the fourth ventricle, where it abuts or involves vital medullary centers. It also frequently metastasizes into the subarachnoid spaces.
      (4) Astrocytoma usually occurs in the cerebellum of children and the cerebrum of adults. It is often cystic and discrete in children, infiltrating and ill defined in adults.
      (5) Oligodendroglioma is usually found in the cerebral hemispheres and is infiltrating but occasionally moderately well defined.
      (6) Others not mentioned include choroid plexus papillomas, pinealomas, and microgliomas.
   b. Pituitary tumors
      (1) Chromophobe tumor is relatively common in the anterior pituitary glands of adults. It causes compression of the pituitary, adjacent optic chiasma, and hypothalamus. The last may lead to diabetes insipidus.

TABLE 23-1 | Contents of the Cranial Nerves

NERVE	FUNCTIONAL COMPONENT	ORIGIN OR TERMINATION WITHIN CNS	PERIPHERAL SENSORY OR MOTOR ENDING
I	SVA	Olfactory bulb	Olfactory epithelium
II	SSA	Lateral geniculate nucleus and superior colliculus	Originates in ganglion cells of retina
III	(G) SE	Oculomotor nucleus	Superior, inferior, and medial recti; inferior oblique; levator palpebrae superioris
	GVE	Edinger-Westphal nucleus (part of oculomotor nucleus)	Sphincter pupillae, ciliary muscle*
IV	(G) SE	Trochlear nucleus	Superior oblique
V	GSA	Spinal and main sensory nuclei	Skin and deep tissues of head; dura mater
		Mesencephalic nucleus	Muscle spindles and other mechanoreceptors
	SVE	Trigeminal motor nucleus	Muscles of mastication, tensor tympani, and a few others
VI	(G) SE	Abducens nucleus	Lateral rectus
VII	GSA	Spinal trigeminal nucleus	Outer ear
	SVA	Solitary nucleus	Taste buds of anterior two thirds of tongue
	GVA	Solitary nucleus	Small portion of nasopharynx
	GVE	Superior salivatory nucleus	Submandibular, sublingual salivary glands; lacrimal gland*
	SVE	Facial motor nucleus	Muscles of facial expression; stapedius
VIII	SSA	Cochlear and vestibular nuclei	Organ of Corti; cristae of semicircular canals; maculae of utricle and saccule
IX	GSA	Spinal trigeminal nucleus	Outer ear
	SVA	Solitary nucleus	Taste buds of posterior third of tongue
	GVA	Solitary and spinal trigeminal nuclei	Carotid body and sinus; mucous membranes of nasal and oral pharynx and middle ear
	GVE	Inferior salivatory nucleus	Parotid gland*
	SVE	Nucleus ambiguus	Pharynx (stylopharyngeus)
X	GSA	Spinal trigeminal nucleus	Outer ear
	SVA	Solitary nucleus	Taste buds of epiglottis
	GVA	Solitary and spinal trigeminal nuclei	Thoracic and abdominal viscera; mucous membranes of larynx and laryngeal pharynx
	GVE	Dorsal motor nucleus	Thoracic and abdominal viscera*
	SVE	Nucleus ambiguus	Larynx and pharynx; heart*
Cranial XI	SVE	Nucleus ambiguus	Larynx and pharynx
Spinal XI	SVE	Accessory nucleus, cervical cord	Sternocleidomastoid; trapezius
XII	(G) SE	Hypoglossal nucleus	Muscles of tongue

From Nolte, J. (1988). *The human brain: an introduction to its functional anatomy* (ed. 2). St. Louis: Mosby.
*Final destination after synapse in a parasympathetic ganglion.
GSA, General somatic afferent; fibers are related to receptors for pain, temperature, and mechanical stimuli in somatic structures such as skin muscles, and joints; *GSE*, general somatic efferent; fibers innervate skeletal muscles; *GVA*, general visceral afferent; fibers are related to receptors in visceral structures such as the walls of the digestive tract; *GVE*, general visceral efferent; fibers are preganglionic autonomic; *SSA*, special somatic afferent; fibers are related to the special senses of sight, hearing and equilibrium; *SVA*, special visceral afferent; fibers are related to the special senses of smell and taste; *SVE*, special visceral efferent; fibers innervate the branchiomeric muscles; muscles of the larynx, pharynx, and face are branchiomeric muscles.

(2) Eosinophilic adenomas are secretory, causing an excessive amount of growth hormone in the serum.

(3) Basophilic adenomas are responsible for the excessive secretion of corticotropic, gonadotropic, and thyrotropic hormones. Acromegaly or, less commonly, Cushing's syndrome may occur and cause the patient to seek help long before the tumor has expanded sufficiently to compromise the optic chiasma.

(4) Prolactinoma or prolactin cell adenoma exhibits considerable differences in clinical presentation depending on the sex of the patient. In women of reproductive age the onset of amenorrhea and galactorrhea with associated infertility is an obvious sign. The diagnosis of a prolactinoma is established early in the course. In men the clinical endocrinal symptoms, which include decreased libido and impotence, are not as conspicuous and initially may be disregarded by the

patient. As a result, male patients frequently do not seek medical attention until the tumors are large and have spread beyond the confines of the sella.

(5) Metastatic tumors usually arise from carcinoma, more rarely from sarcoma, and occasionally from melanomas and retinal tumors. The most common sources are bronchogenic carcinoma and carcinoma of the breast.

Tumors not discussed here are eosinophilic granulomas, tuberculomas, and other granulomas; brain abscesses; colloid cysts; fibrous dysplasia; and lymphomas. A brain lesion is diagnosed by history, neurologic examination, and diagnostic studies. The manifestations of an intracranial tumor fall into two classes: those resulting from irritation or impairment of function in specific areas of the brain directly affected by the tumor and those resulting from diffuse increased intracranial pressure.

Lesions in the left frontotemporal region, where motor speech originates, lead to aphasia; occipital tumors produce hemianoptic visual defects; large frontal lobe tumors may cause striking personality changes.

Cortical tumors frequently produce focal seizures of diagnostic value. The onset of epileptiform seizures in an adult is often associated with an intracranial neoplasm. Pituitary tumors characteristically press on the optic chiasma and impair the temporal vision of each eye. They disturb pituitary glandular function, resulting in hypopituitary states, pituitary dwarfism, or acromegaly. Posterior fossa tumors often manifest their presence by blocking the CSF circulation, but they may also destroy cerebellar function, resulting in incoordination, ataxia, scanning speech, and deafness.

Back

The spinal column consists of 33 vertebrae: seven cervical, twelve thoracic, five lumbar, five sacral (fused as one), and one coccygeal (fused from four small vertebrae) (Fig. 23-16).

The first cervical vertebra, or atlas, supports the skull. The second cervical vertebra, or axis, can be identified by its odontoid process, a vertical projection extending into the foramen of the atlas like a stick in a hoop; it rests against the anterior tubercle. Ligaments hold the two together but allow considerable rotational movement.

The other cervical, thoracic, and lumbar vertebrae are more alike in structure. Each has a body, an oval block of spongy bone situated anteriorly. An intervertebral disk, a fibrocartilaginous elastic cushion, separates one body from another (Figs. 23-17 and 23-18). The spinal cord lies in a canal formed by the vertebral bodies, pedicles, and laminae. Articular surfaces or facets project from the pedicles and form joints with the facets of the vertebrae above and below. Transverse processes extend laterally and serve as hitching posts for muscles and ligaments. Spinous processes extend posteriorly (see Fig. 23-17) and can be palpated in all except obese persons. The vertebrae are held together by multiple ligaments and muscles. Motion of the spine occurs at the articular facets and through the elastic intervertebral disks (see Fig. 23-18).

The spinal cord is protected by this bony framework. The dura mater is separated from its bony surroundings by a layer of epidural fat. Beneath the dura mater is the arachnoid, a continuation of the same structure in the head. The subarachnoid space contains spinal fluid. A thin layer of pia mater adheres to the cord, and CSF also circulates from the fourth ventricle into the central canal of the cord.

The spinal cord is a downward prolongation of the brainstem, starting at the upper border of the atlas and ending at the upper border of the second lumbar vertebra. The cord is oval in cross section. It is slightly flattened in the anteroposterior diameter. A cross section looks like a gray H surrounded by a white mantle split in the midline, anteriorly and posteriorly, by sulci (Fig. 23-19).

The peripheral white matter carries long myelinated motor and sensory tracts; the central gray matter consists of nerve cell bodies and short unmyelinated fibers (see Figs. 23-16 and 23-19). The principal long pathways are the laterally placed pyramidal tracts, carrying impulses down from the cerebral cortex to the motor neurons of the cord; the dorsal ascending columns, mediating sensations of touch and proprioception; and the anterolaterally placed spinothalamic tracts, carrying pain and temperature sensations to the thalamus, the sensory receiving station of the brain (Fig. 23-20).

At each vertebral level are two pairs of spinal nerves (see Fig. 23-19): an anterior or motor root, the cell bodies of which lie in the anterior horn of the spinal gray matter; and a posterior or sensory root, the cell bodies of which lie in the spinal ganglia in the intervertebral foramina, through which the nerves exit from the spinal canal and emerge from the cord. Each pair of roots forms one spinal nerve. The cervical nerves pass out horizontally, but at each lower level they take on an increasingly oblique and downward direction. In the lumbar region the course of the nerves is nearly vertical, forming the cauda equina (see Fig. 23-16). This phenomenon is explained by the fact that the spinal cord, which fills the entire spinal canal in the fetus, grows at a slower rate than the bony spine, thus leaving the lower nerves a progressively longer course to their exit.

The vasculature of the spinal cord and vertebral column is a rich, delicate network. The arterial blood supply to the spinal cord arises from the vertebral arteries as the anterior spinal artery and the posterior spinal arteries. These vessels branch and anastomose on both sides of the cord and within the substance of the cord. They also branch into anterior and posterior radicular arteries that form spinal rami as they accompany the spinal nerve roots through the intervertebral foramina.

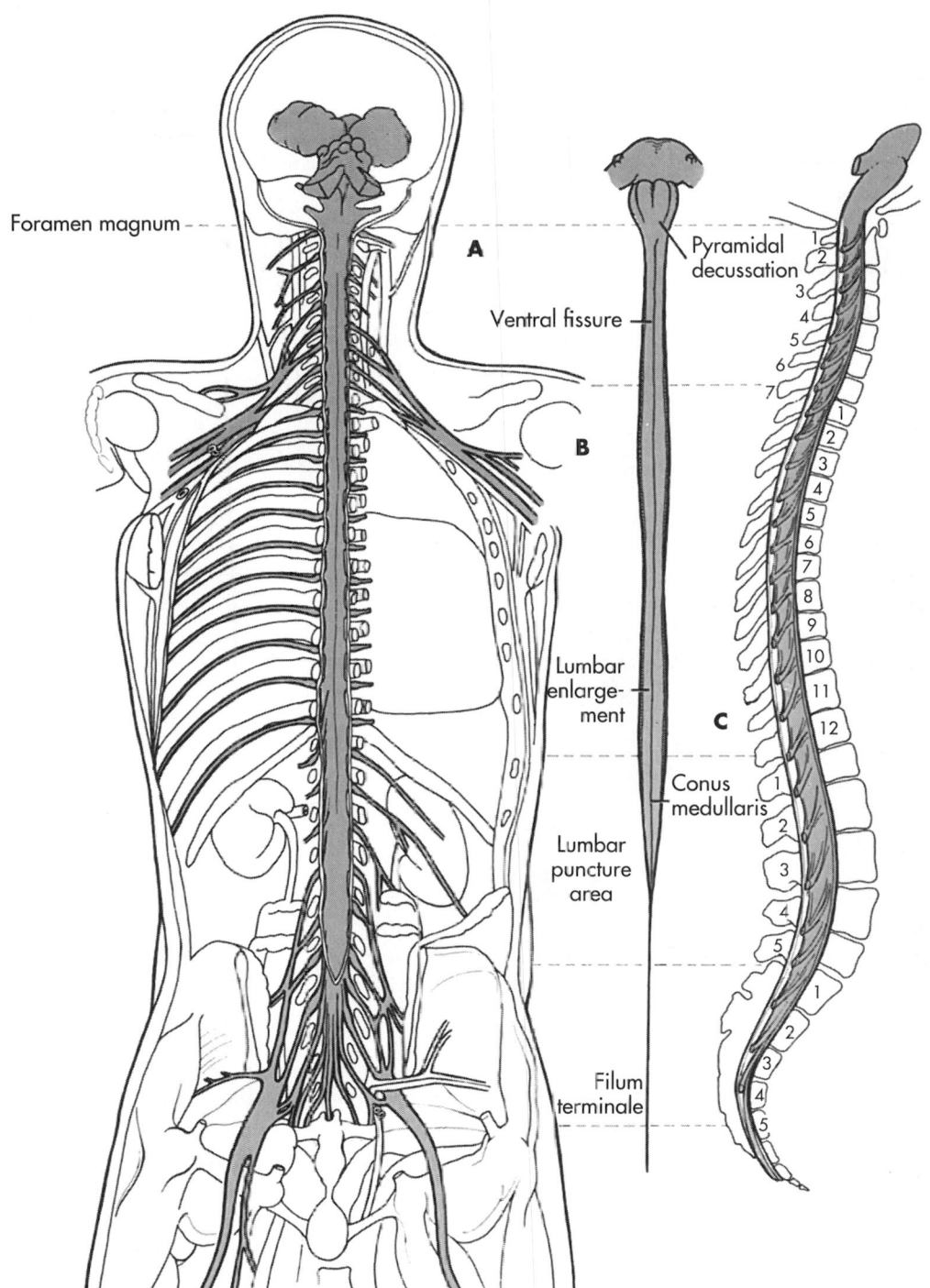

FIGURE 23-16   Posterior view of brainstem and spinal cord. **A,** Torso dissected from back is shown. Dura mater has been opened and cord exposed. Levels concerned can be easily determined by referring to ribs on left side of thorax. Cord proper terminates opposite body of second lumbar vertebra (**B**) as conus medullaris. **B,** Ventral surface of cord stripped of dura mater and arachnoid. It is symmetric in structure, two halves of which are separated by ventral fissure. This fissure stops at foramen magnum. Caudally, pia mater leaves conus medullaris as glistening thread, or filum terminale. **C,** Cord is exposed from lateral side. Dura mater has been opened. Since cord is shorter than canal and spinal nerves leave through intervertebral foramina, one at a time, lowest portion of canal is occupied only by a bundlelike accumulation of nerve roots—cauda equina. Caudal end of dural sac, enclosing spinal cord and cauda equina, lies somewhere between bodies of first and third sacral vertebrae. Size and position of the three views correspond, and elimination of major vertebral levels is indicated by transverse lines for all three figures.

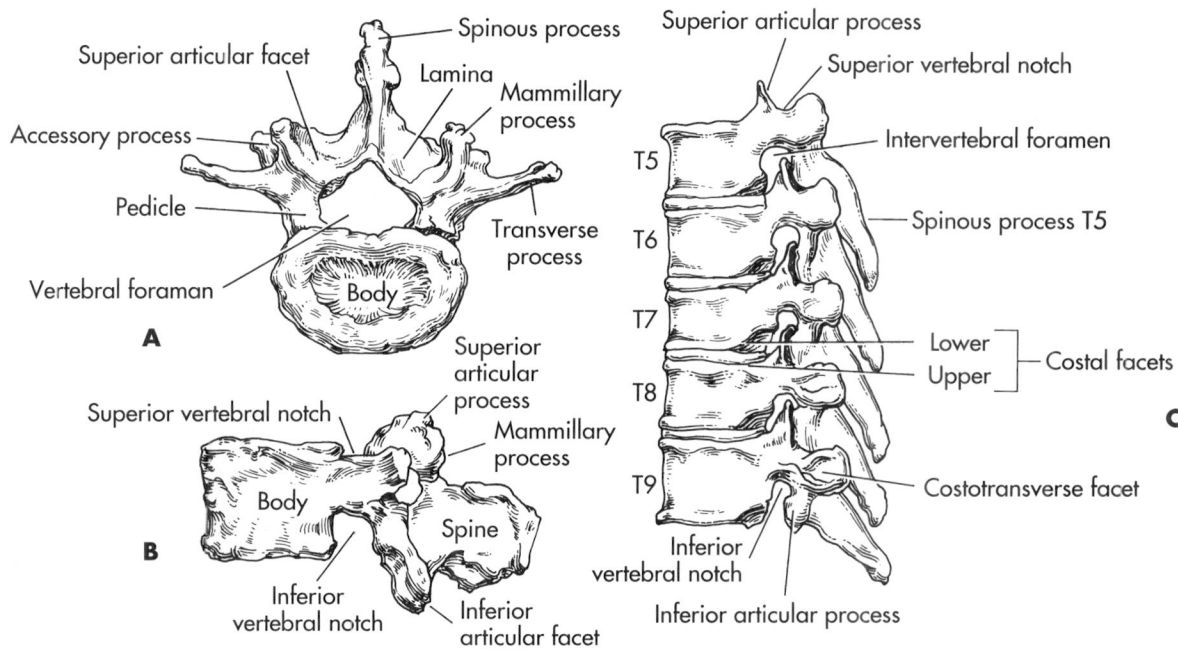

FIGURE 23-17   **A**, Fourth lumbar vertebra from above. **B**, Fourth lumbar vertebra from side. **C**, Fifth to ninth thoracic vertebrae, showing relationships of various parts.

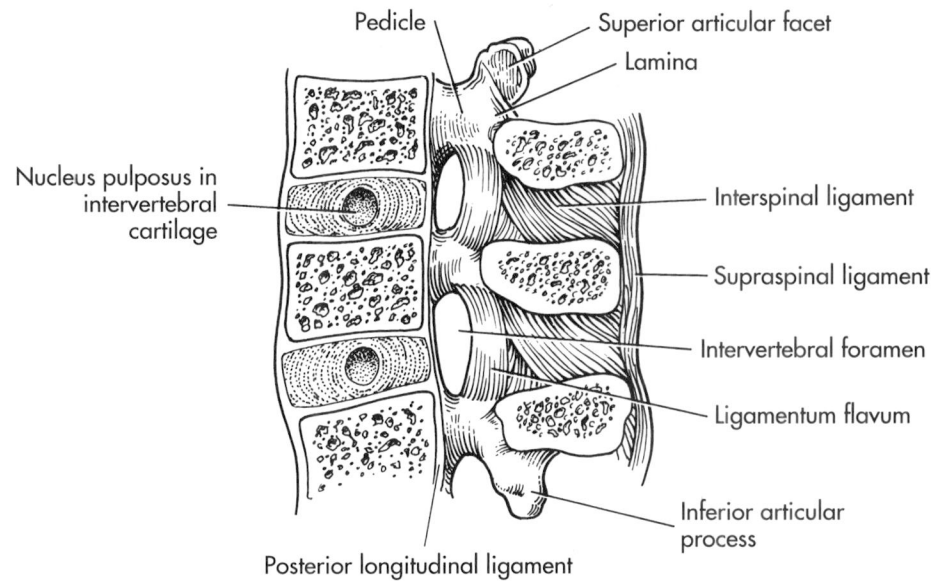

FIGURE 23-18   Median section through three lumbar vertebrae, showing intervertebral disks (nuclei pulposi).

A series of venous plexuses surround and innervate the spinal cord at each level in the vertebral canal. They anastomose with each other and form the intervertebral veins as they leave through the intervertebral foramina with the spinal nerves to join the intercostal, lumbar, and sacral veins. The lateral longitudinal veins near the foramen magnum empty into the inferior petrosal sinus and cerebellar veins. The venous network innervates the bony structures and musculature as well as the spinal cord and nerve roots. Venous bleeding during spinal surgery is a potential problem for which the perioperative nurse must be prepared.

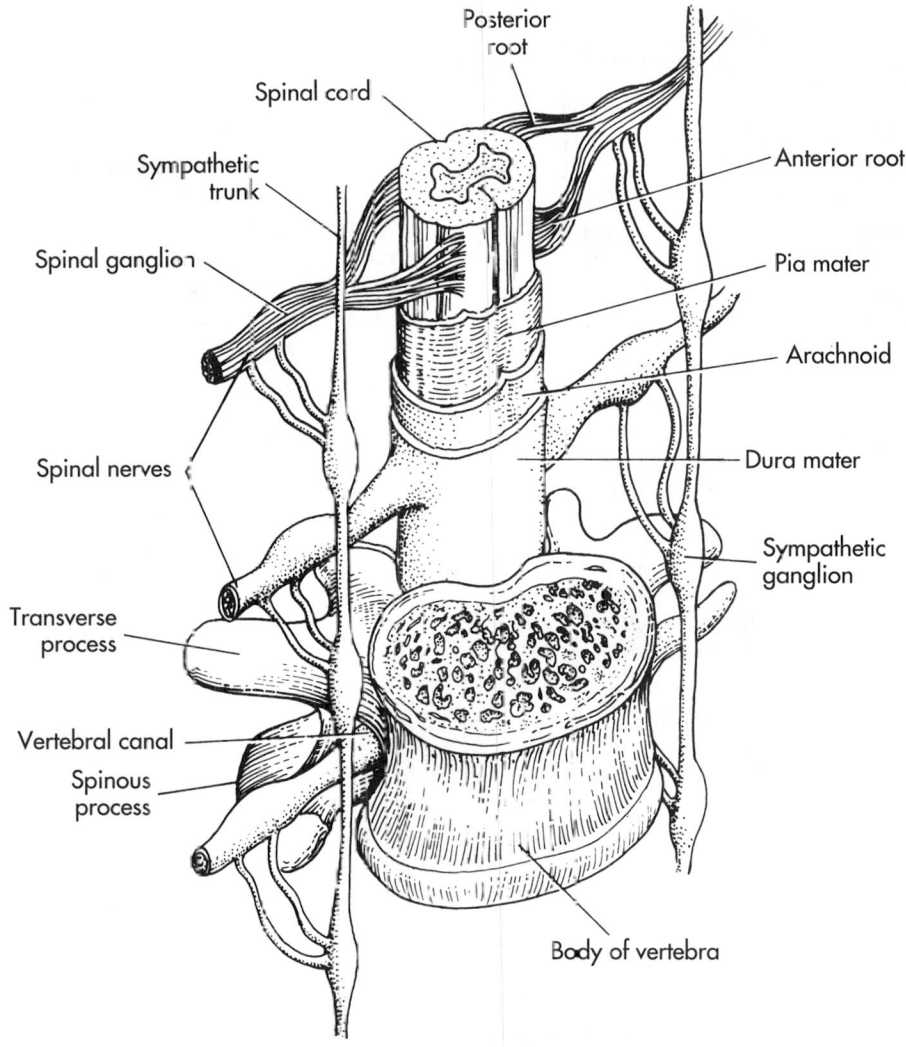

Posterior root

Spinal cord

Sympathetic trunk

Spinal ganglion

Spinal nerves

Transverse process

Vertebral canal

Spinous process

Anterior root

Pia mater

Arachnoid

Dura mater

Sympathetic ganglion

Body of vertebra

FIGURE 23-19 Spinal cord, showing meninges, formation of spinal nerves, and relationships to vertebra and to sympathetic trunk and ganglia.

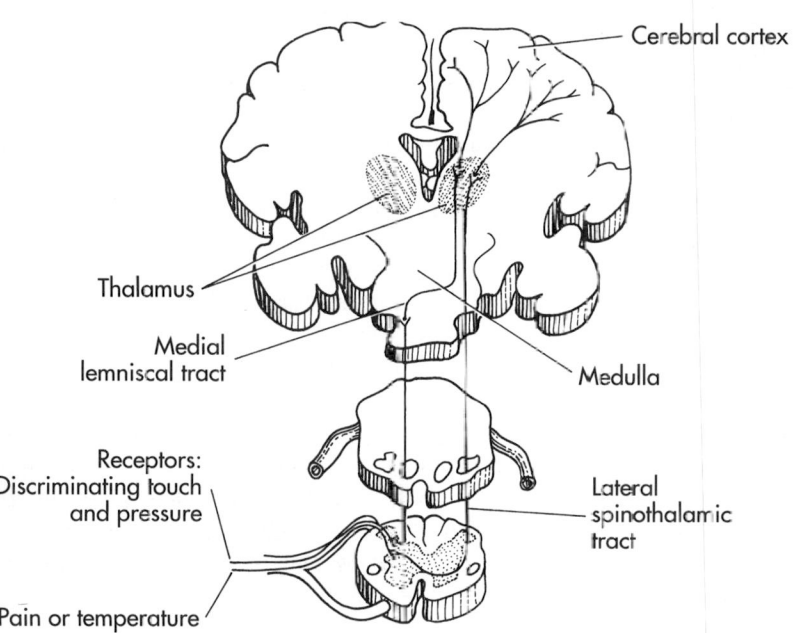

Cerebral cortex

Thalamus

Medial lemniscal tract

Receptors: Discriminating touch and pressure

Pain or temperature

Medulla

Lateral spinothalmic tract

FIGURE 23-20 Lateral spinothalmic and medial lemniscal neural tracts.

23-1 RESEARCH HIGHLIGHT

Researchers from the University of California at San Diego School of Medicine and the Salk Institute for Biological Studies have reported the first successful use of gene therapy to achieve partial recovery from spinal cord injuries. In this study, rats with spinal cord injuries had a sample of normal skin cells removed and cultured and then genetically modified to produce the growth factor neurotrophin-3 (NT-3). When grafted back into the rats, the modified cells secreted NT-3 at the site of the spinal cord injuries, which in turn stimulated axon regrowth, resulting in some recovery of walking ability. In addition, the genetically modified cells were also found to deliver NT-3 continuously for several months, further enhancing the regeneration of injured axons and the partial restoration of function.

Promotion of the regrowth of cut or damaged axons is the goal in spinal injury research. The results of this research indicate that cellular delivery of NT-3 through gene therapy can restore function by promoting the sustained growth of axons. The findings of this study can have important applications for the perioperative nursing care of the patient with a spinal cord injury.

From Grill, R., Murai, K., Blesch, A., et al. (1997, July 15). Cellular delivery of neurotrophin-3 promotes corticospinal axonal growth and partial fractional recovery after spinal cord injury. *Journal of Neuroscience, 17*(4), 5560-5572.

Pathologic lesions of the spinal cord and adjacent structures

Operations are performed to correct congenital malformations, injuries, tumors, herniated and degenerative intervertebral disks, abscesses, and intractable pain.

The most common congenital lesion encountered is a lumbar meningocele, or meningomyelocele, a failure of the union of the vertebral arches during fetal development. The fluid-filled, thin-walled sac often contains neural elements. Surgical correction is necessary when the sac lining is so thin that there is a potential or actual CSF leak. The operation consists of excising the sac wall to preserve adhering nerves, closing the dura mater, and reinforcing the closure with fascial flaps swung from the paraspinal muscles. Skin closure without tension is essential for primary healing. Large skin and subcutaneous flaps must occasionally be fashioned to ensure healing.

Injuries to the spinal cord are serious. No regeneration of destroyed or divided nerve tracts occurs. However, researchers have recently reported the successful use of gene therapy to promote recovery from spinal cord injuries (Research Highlight 23-1). Recovery may take place with lesser degrees of injury, such as contusion or compression. Surgery can be of value in preventing further damage by

debridement of penetrating wounds, removal of foreign bodies, relief of pressure on the cord or roots, open reduction of certain dislocations and fractures, and measures aimed at stabilizing the spine. In cervical injuries skeletal traction by means of tongs applied to the skull is often the preferred treatment.

Spinal cord tumors are classified according to location as extradural (outside the dura mater) or intradural (inside the dura mater). Intradural tumors may be either extramedullary (outside the cord) or intramedullary (within the cord). Extradural tumors include sarcomas and carcinomas, which may be metastatic from adjacent structures in or about the vertebrae. Other extradural lesions include Hodgkin's disease, lipomas, neurofibromas, chondromas, angiomas, abscesses, and granulomas.

Intradural tumors can be extramedullary, in which case they are usually benign and originate from the dura mater and arachnoid surrounding the cord and from the root sheaths of spinal nerves. Neurinomas are especially common in the thoracocervical area and may be part of generalized neurofibromatosis. Meningiomas also commonly occur in intradural extramedullary locations. Less frequently, lipomas or other types of tumors are found. Gliomas are the most common intramedullary tumors and have a less favorable prognosis. These tumors infiltrate the cord tissue and are much more difficult to remove than extramedullary tumors.

The majority of intradural tumors are extramedullary and benign and, if diagnosed early before severe neurologic deficits occur, offer an excellent prognosis. They manifest their presence by pain of a radicular nature and various motor and sensory disabilities below their segmental locations.

Cord tumors frequently produce spinal fluid blockage and can be pinpointed accurately with MRI, which is now the procedure of choice with or without enhancement. Intraspinal injection of contrast material (myelography) is another option. A standard laminectomy is used for exposure and removal.

The rare surgical infections of the spinal cord take the form of extradural abscesses and granulomas. Treatment is by a combination of excision, drainage, chemotherapy, and occasionally spinal fusion.

The most frequently encountered neurosurgical problem is the herniated intervertebral disk. Because of weakness or rupture of the circular ligament (annulus fibrosus), which confines the soft center of the disk (nucleus pulposus), herniation of the latter may occur and give rise to pain from nerve root compression. When pain is severe or nerve damage excessive, surgical excision of the disk offers the most satisfactory relief. The procedure entails interlaminar exposure and piecemeal removal of the displaced nucleus. If the spine is unstable or there are other incontrovertible reasons for operative stabilization of the bony spine, a fusion of one type or another may be combined with the disk surgery (see Chapter 22).

Although infrequently done, another method of treating disk disease is chemonucleolysis, a technique whereby primary lumbar intervertebral disk disease is treated by an intradiskal injection of chymopapain, a proteolytic enzyme in the form of a sterile lyophilized powder. However, the injection of chymopapain into the lumbar nucleus pulposus is not an innocuous procedure. Hypersensitivity to the drug and anaphylactic reactions have been reported. The patient needs to be checked for allergies to meat tenderizer, since this would demonstrate the sensitivity to the drug. Reports of transverse myelitis and subsequent paraplegia associated with chymopapain injection have raised serious questions about its use in young and otherwise healthy patients. A newer concept is that of percutaneous lumbar diskectomy, through a posterolateral approach. The method entails gaining access to the disk space through the use of an introduction system and cannulas. A 2 mm aspiration probe (called a *Nucleotome*) is then placed through the cannula into the disk space, and the nucleus pulposus is aspirated. Patients who have had previous surgery at the same level are not candidates for this approach.

Certain painful spinal lesions, usually of a malignant nature, can be controlled by epidural opiates, by Duragesic patches, temporarily or permanently with a pump, or by dividing the pain fibers supplying the affected area. It may be accomplished by sectioning the sensory roots intraspinally (posterior rhizotomy) or by incising the spinothalamic tracts (anterolateral cordotomy) that carry pain and temperature impulses. A laminectomy is necessary for exposure.

Peripheral Nerves

Within the context of this discussion the peripheral nervous system includes the cranial nerves outside the cranial cavity, the spinal nerves, the autonomic nerves, and the ganglia. This division is artificial and only for the purpose of delineating surgical approaches. The cranial nerves have been described under the section on the head because all arise within the cranial cavity, and most are approached neurosurgically through the head. There are 31 pairs of spinal nerves, each pair numbered for the level of the spinal column at which it emerges: cervical one (C1) to eight (C8), thoracic one (T1) to twelve (T12), lumbar one (L1) to five (L5), sacral one (S1) to five (S5), and coccygeal one. The thoracic region is sometimes referred to as the dorsal region, with D1 being synonymous with T1 and so on. The first pair of cervical spine nerves emerges between C1 and the occipital bone. The eighth cervical nerves emerge from the intervertebral foramina between C7 and T1. The first thoracic nerves emerge between T1 and T2.

In the cervical and lumbosacral regions the spinal nerves regroup in a plexiform manner before they form the peripheral nerves of the upper and lower extremities; those in the thoracic region form cutaneous and intercostal nerves. The principal nerves of the upper plexus include the musculocutaneous, median, ulnar, and radial; those of the lumbosacral plexus include the obturator, femoral, and sciatic.

Each spinal nerve divides into anterior, posterior, and white rami. Anterior and posterior rami contain voluntary fibers; white rami contain autonomic fibers. Posterior rami further branch into nerves going to the muscles, skin, and posterior surfaces of the head, neck, and trunk. Most anterior rami branch to the skeletal muscles and the skin of extremities and anterior and lateral surfaces. In the process they form plexuses, such as the brachial and sacral plexuses. Spinal nerves contain sensory dendrites and motor axons; some have somatic axons, and some have axons of preganglionic autonomic motor neurons.

The autonomic (involuntary) nervous system consists of all the efferent nerves, through which the cardiovascular apparatus, viscera, glands of internal secretion, and peripheral involuntary muscles are innervated (Fig. 23-21). A major anatomic difference between the somatic and autonomic nervous systems is that in the former an impulse from the brainstem or spinal cord reaches the end organ through a single neuron, whereas in the latter an impulse passes through two neurons—the first ending in an autonomic ganglion and the second running from the ganglion to the end organ. Some of the ganglia lie adjacent to the vertebral column to form the sympathetic trunks or chains; others are closely associated with the end organs.

The preganglionic neurons from the brainstem, which go out along the cranial nerves, and those from the second, third, and fourth sacral segments to the pelvic viscera end in ganglia in proximity to their end organs; thus their postganglionic fibers are very short. This is known as the *parasympathetic*, or *craniosacral*, division of the autonomic nervous system. The preganglionic fibers from the thoracic and lumbar spinal cord end in the paravertebral ganglia, making up the sympathetic chain, and their postganglionic fibers are relatively long. This is termed the *sympathetic*, or *thoracolumbar*, division of the autonomic nervous system.

The two divisions are distinct anatomically and physiologically. The chemical substance mediating transmission of impulses at most postganglionic sympathetic nerve endings is norepinephrine, and the one at all parasympathetic and preganglionic sympathetic neurons is acetylcholine.

The majority of organs have dual innervation, part from the craniosacral and part from the thoracolumbar divisions. The functions of these two systems are antagonistic. Together they work to maintain homeostasis. In general, the thoracolumbar division functions as an emergency protection mechanism, always ready to combat physical or psychologic stress. The craniosacral division functions to conserve energy when the body is in a state of relaxation.

Stimuli arising from internal organs or from outside the body traverse visceral and somatic afferent nerve fibers to

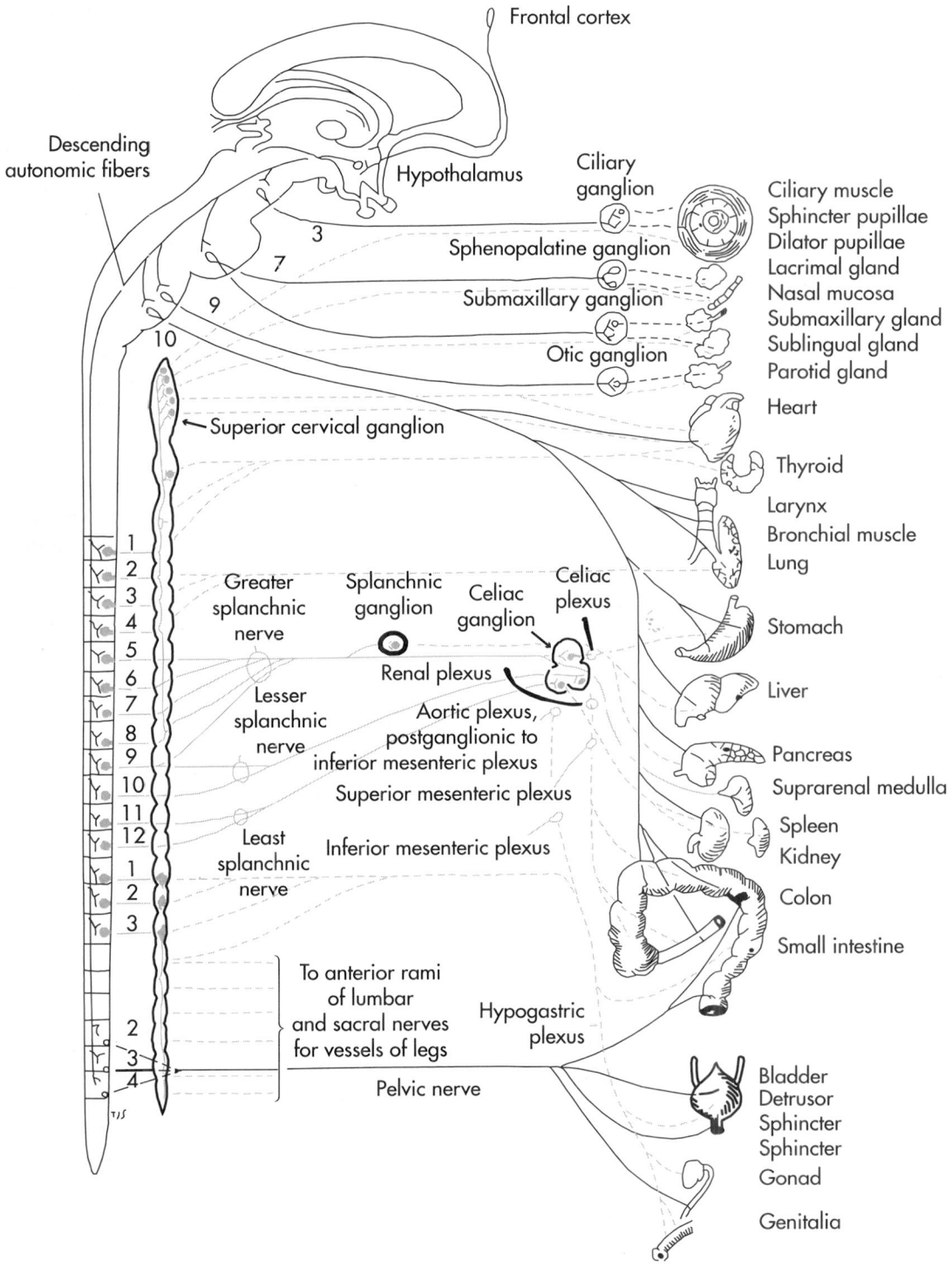

FIGURE 23-21 Sympathetic division of the autonomic nervous system.

make reflex connections with preganglionic autonomic neurons in the brainstem and spinal cord. Such stimuli trigger activity of these involuntary systems automatically. When these automatic mechanisms break down or overact, surgery may be indicated. Thoracolumbar sympa-

thectomy was once performed in hypertension to try to decrease blood vessel tone and lower the blood pressure. Vagotomy is done to decrease acid secretion to the stomach in peptic ulcer patients. Lumbar sympathectomy is used to relieve vasospastic disorders of the legs.

PERIOPERATIVE NURSING CONSIDERATIONS

Assessment

Communication between the perioperative nurse and surgeon, either directly or through a knowledgeable person, such as a clinical nurse specialist, operating room supervisor, privately employed nurse, RNFA, or resident who has direct communication with the surgeon, is essential for intelligently planning care for the neurosurgical patient in the operating room. Information the perioperative nurse needs before the arrival of the patient in the operating room includes the diagnosis; the diagnostic studies done and reports needed at the time of operation; the age, size, level of consciousness, physical disabilities resulting from neuropathologic conditions (as well as those from other causes), and communication barriers of the patient; the specific surgical approach and position to be used; the need for any special equipment, instruments, and supplies not ordinarily used; the amount of blood ordered and available; the method or methods planned to reduce intracranial pressure in the case of cranial surgery; the need for radiologic support during the procedure; and the planned preliminary procedures, such as carotid ligation, lumbar puncture, placement of monitoring lines, and Foley catheter insertion. This information permits the perioperative nurse to plan for needed equipment, instruments, and supplies.

Most diagnostic procedures are performed before the patient arrives in the operating room. Of greatest significance to the perioperative nurse are radiologic studies that produce either positive or negative images the surgeon can use during the operation to locate the pathologic condition. The perioperative nurse is responsible for having these images in the operating room before the procedure begins. The studies include the following:

1. *Myelography.* Injection of contrast medium into the spinal subarachnoid space to demonstrate a defect by radiography.
2. *Angiography (arteriography).* Injection of contrast medium into the brachial, carotid, vertebral, or femoral arteries to study the intracranial blood vessels for size, location, and configuration and to allow diagnosis of space-occupying lesions and vascular abnormalities.
   a. *Digital subtraction angiography (DSA).* A computerized radiologic procedure. An intravenous rather than arterial injection is required; a contrast medium injection to allow examination of selected arterial circulation is used. DSA provides an alternative to cerebral angiography for high-risk patients by using computer technology.
   b. *Magnetic resonance angiography (MRA).* MRA may prove to be a sensitive screening procedure for carotid stenosis. It can detect dissection of cranial

cervical vessels, as well as permit follow-up study in a noninvasive fashion and guide treatment.
   c. *Three-dimensional computerized tomography (CT) angiography.* Contrast-enhanced CT brain scan data are used to generate a three-dimensional image of the intracranial vasculature with minimal risk to the patient.
   d. *Stereoscopic display of MRA.* Recent advances in magnetic resonance imaging (MRI) permit high-resolution imaging of blood flow. Projection angiograms can be produced to overcome the tomographic nature of conventional MR scans. These angiograms are similar to plain x-ray films or digital subtraction angiograms in the demonstration of blood vessels, but the three-dimensional information inherent in them is partially lost in single projections. Stereoscopic image pairs allow the clinician to perceive the relative distance of vessels to one another. MRA permits perception of vascular anatomy in three dimensions.
3. *CT scan.* Use of x-ray studies with or without instilled contrast medium and computer technology to produce a sequential series of positive images of transverse sections of the brain and spinal cord in which differences in tissue density can be detected and deviations from normal identified. This study remains the criterion standard for evaluation of acute head injury.
4. *Isotope brain scan.* Injection of radioactive substance intravenously to demonstrate brain lesions.
5. *Echoencephalography.* Method of recording referred ultrasound from reflecting surfaces; especially helpful in the identification of subdural hematomas.
6. *Echo doppler scanning.* Noninvasive technique used to assess the blood flow in the carotid artery. This procedure can be done in or out of the surgical suite.
7. *MRI.* Use of powerful magnetic waves to reproduce details of the human body with no known risk to patients; uses no radiation. Advances in MRI scanning provide enhancement of the scan with the use of gadolinium. Many patients experience extreme feelings of claustrophobia during MRI.
8. *Pneumonencephalography (PEG).* Injection of air into the subarachnoid space, usually through a lumbar or cisternal puncture, to outline the ventricular system and the cranial subarachnoid space to identify deviations from normal. Because of advances in radiologic techniques, this procedure is very seldom used.
9. *Ventriculography.* Injection of air directly into the lateral ventricles when a block exists between the spinal canal and the lateral ventricles. It is seldom used but remains an excellent tool if CT or MRI cannot be obtained.
10. *Venography.* Dural sinus studies for narrowing sinuses and interference with cranial drainage, which often occur in lesions of the posterior fossa. This study has been essentially replaced with newer MRI software.

Nursing Diagnosis

Five nursing diagnoses to be considered in caring for the neurosurgical patient are as follows:

- Anxiety related to surgery or surgical outcome
- Knowledge deficit related to diagnostic tests and surgical procedures
- Risk for ineffective breathing patterns related to location of tumor, surgical position, or effects of general anesthesia
- Risk for pain related to pathophysiologic alterations
- Risk for infection related to surgical intervention

Outcome Identification

Outcomes identified for the selected nursing diagnoses could be stated as follows:

- The patient's anxiety will be reduced or controlled.
- The patient or family will verbalize knowledge regarding diagnostic and surgical procedures.
- The patient will maintain effective breathing patterns.
- The patient will report a reduction in pain.
- The patient will be free from signs and symptoms of infection.

Planning

Preparation can significantly reduce both anesthesia and intraoperative time for the patient as well as physical and psychologic stress for both the surgeon and the perioperative nurse. Planning for the patient's care in the operating room is based on the results of nursing assessment and the identification of relevant nursing diagnoses. The plan of care then identifies desired outcomes derived from the nursing diagnoses; priorities are set and nursing interventions designed to assist the patient to reach the desired outcomes. Nursing interventions identified for the patient's plan of care may include reassessment, teaching, counseling, referrals, and specific interventions to assist the patient in achieving patient care outcomes. The Sample Care Plan shown on p. 937 could be utilized by the perioperative nurse for the patient who is undergoing a neurosurgical procedure.

Implementation

The perioperative nurse plays a vital role in maintaining blood volume, body temperature, and fluid balance in neurosurgical patients. The role of maintaining blood volume includes planning for minimizing and monitoring blood loss as well as for blood replacement. The surgeon may minimize blood loss by infiltrating the tissues at the site of incision with normal saline solution; minimizing or eliminating periosteal stripping and carefully attending to intracranial emissary veins and sinuses; and using electrosurgery and bipolar coagulation, bone wax, Gelfoam, thrombin, or Surgicel. The surgeon's preferences for instruments and supplies must be prepared and ready for use before needed. Sponges from the operative field must be continuously placed within view of the anesthesia provider or weighed as they are discarded from the field. Blood or blood products must be available in the surgical suite. A blood warmer must be ready to use as careful, accurate fluid replacement therapy is carried out. When the anesthesiologist is unable to see the operative field (which is usually the situation during any cranial surgery), the perioperative nurse must inform the anesthesia provider immediately of active bleeding at the operative site.

Patients come to the operating room fearful and apprehensive about the outcome of the surgical procedure and its effect on them and their lifestyle. Both male and female patients are devastated by having their hair removed. During this procedure the perioperative nurse should provide psychologic support and give realistic reassurance and information to both conscious, responsive patients and patients who may be incoherent or unconscious but still hear what is going on around them and feel what is being done to them. Hair removal from the head, like all other forms of preoperative preparation, should be done as close to the time of skin incision as possible to decrease the possibility of postoperative wound infection. Some surgeons prefer complete hair removal because dressings are easier to apply, hair regrowth is more even, a better wig fit can be obtained, and it is far easier to prepare a sterile field around such an operative site. However, because of the severe disturbances in body image caused by total hair removal, an effort should be made to facilitate a compromise between patient and surgeon. Whenever possible, minimal hair removal is recommended. There may be a relationship between hair removal and postoperative recovery, especially in the areas of orientation, social interaction, and compliance. Also, when the patient's wishes are considered, the patient has a degree of control over what is happening.

An aged person undergoing neurosurgical intervention brings a potential range of problems such a hearing, sight, and mobility deficiencies unrelated to the neuropathologic condition. Responses to stimuli generally are slower in the elderly. The skin is more prone to pressure injury. The ability to heal may be impaired. More time and greater care must be taken with older patients. Communication can be established and reassurance given by touching and by being nearby while the patient is conscious. Vigilant monitoring of blood loss, temperature, and urine output is also required in caring for the older patient in the operating room. Surgery may be performed with the patient under local anesthesia, and the perioperative nurse may be responsible for monitoring vital signs, as well as for providing a personal communication link for the patient. Sitting with the patient and explaining the procedure and the sensations that will be experienced makes the patient more comfortable and cooperative and diminishes fears.

Among neurosurgical patients are those who have little or no apparent loss of function, those who are coping with

SAMPLE CARE PLAN

Nursing Diagnosis: Anxiety related to surgery or surgical outcome

Outcome: The patient's anxiety will be reduced or controlled.

Interventions:

Broadly classify the patient's anxiety (low, moderate, high).

Provide reassurance and explanations; repeat as necessary.

Provide ongoing opportunity for patient (and family) to ask questions and express fears.

Involve other support persons (social worker, case manager, chaplain) as appropriate.

Determine the patient's coping skills.

Assist the patient to utilize personally effective coping skills.

Use touch to communicate caring (as appropriate).

Nursing Diagnosis: Knowledge deficit related to diagnostic tests and surgical procedures

Outcome: The patient or family will verbalize knowledge regarding diagnostic tests and surgical procedure.

Interventions:

Determine patient or family knowledge level (and desire for knowledge).

Correct misinformation; refer to other health care team members as appropriate.

Identify patient or family readiness and motivation to learn.

Provide information about procedures; use understandable terms.

Explain perioperative routine; include both factual information and expected sensations associated with tests, surgical procedure, perioperative environment, and postoperative care.

Base psychoeducational interventions on individual needs.

Nursing Diagnosis: Risk for ineffective breathing patterns related to location of tumor, surgical position, or effects of general anesthesia

Outcome: The patient will maintain effective breathing patterns.

Interventions:

Provide appropriate positioning accessories; assist in their placement.

Monitor arterial blood gases (ABGs); interpret and report variations from expected values.

Review results of pulse oximetry for blood oxygen saturation.

Collaborate with anesthesiologist in monitoring endtidal volume carbon dioxide.

Maintain open suction line.

Observe respiratory rate, depth, and characteristics of breath sounds.

Encourage patient to cough and breathe deeply on emergence from anesthesia.

Communicate with PACU regarding postoperative requirements for ventilatory assistance.

Check airway patency frequently during transport to PACU.

Nursing Diagnosis: Risk for pain related to pathophysiologic alterations

Outcome: The patient will report a reduction in pain.

Interventions:

Determine effectiveness of preoperative medications; communicate ineffectiveness.

Administer additionally prescribed medications to control pain or anxiety; monitor patient response.

Assist patient to utilize personally effective pain control measures.

Provide physical comfort measures (such as warm blankets) and emotional support.

Explain postoperative regimens for control of pain.

Nursing Diagnosis: Risk for infection related to surgical intervention

Outcome: The patient will be free from signs and symptoms of infection.

Interventions:

Adhere to strict aseptic technique.

Implement environmental precautions.

Control traffic patterns.

Document wound classification.

Identify and correct breaks in technique.

Dress wound, intravenous line sites, and drain exit sites aseptically.

Monitor for postoperative indications of infection (elevated temperature; redness, swelling, warmth, or drainage at incision site; persistent incisional pain).

Provide patient or family with specific information regarding wound care and the signs and symptoms that should be reported.

---

chronic pain and are looking forward to the operation for the relief it will bring, and those who are totally or partially dependent for everything because they are unconscious, quadriplegic, or aphasic. If pain is present, the perioperative nurse should know the type and site of the pain and aim to make the patient as comfortable as possible while

conscious. If the patient is acutely and severely traumatized, the perioperative nurse must be aware of injuries other than those for which the patient is being treated neurosurgically so that these injuries can be taken into consideration. A perioperative nurse with prior knowledge of a given situation is better prepared to cope with that situation and can plan individualized care based on that knowledge.

Basic neurosurgical maneuvers

Scientific advances that enable surgeons to control pain, hemorrhage, infection, and other physiologic responses have contributed largely to the neurosurgeon's ability to operate successfully on the nervous system. The extent of a modern neurosurgical operation may be determined not so much by the physiologic hazards involved as by the degree of neurologic disability that may be expected after surgery. Knowing the hazards and having everything ready in advance will enhance the ability of the surgeon to achieve a favorable outcome.

Preliminary Procedures

A number of procedures or therapeutic measures may be performed by the neurosurgeon or other member of the team in a holding or induction room before positioning, prepping, and draping take place. It is important that the perioperative nurse know why these procedures are done in order to anticipate them and be prepared to facilitate them.

A Foley catheter is often inserted into the bladder to monitor urinary output during the procedure. It is essential for prolonged procedures and when mannitol is to be given intravenously, so that the bladder does not become distended. A Foley catheter is also required when hypothermia or hypotension will be induced, when excessive bleeding is anticipated, and in trauma patients for continuous assessment of kidney function.

A right atrial or central venous pressure line is required for management of air embolism. An air embolus can occur in any position, but there is an increased risk when the operative field is above the heart. A left atrial pressure line may also be inserted in the operating room immediately before the surgical procedure is begun.

When excessive intracranial bleeding is a possibility, the neurosurgeon may choose carotid cutdown and temporary ligation or tourniquet placement for occlusion of the carotid arteries during bleeding. Carotid cutdown is a separate surgical procedure and requires a special sterile setup, including drapes and instruments. Procedures that may require such management include intracranial vascular surgery and removal of meningiomas.

In some situations CSF drainage may be required. This can be done by placement of a ventricular cannula, such as the Scott or Seletz, or by placement of a spinal needle in the lower lumbar spinal canal. The stylette of either needle is left in place until drainage is required. The surgeon can remove the ventricular stylette, but the perioperative nurse must be able to remove the spinal needle stylette. When the lumbar puncture method is used, the patient is placed in a semilateral position and stabilized, so that the patient does not roll onto the needle and the perioperative nurse can remove the stylette without contaminating it during

the procedure. An extension tubing and stopcock can be attached to the needle at the time of lumbar puncture. When this is done, the tubing and stopcock are supported so that traction is not put on the needle, and they are placed where they are accessible to the perioperative nurse or anesthesia provider. The stopcock can be opened for drainage. Another alternative to drainage is to place a lumbar drain rather than leave a hard metal needle in the back or a cannula in the brain.

Induced hypotension may be required to manage bleeding. Intracranial vascular surgery and removal of some tumors also may require induced hypotension. Sodium nitroprusside (Nipride) is an effective agent. Very little of the drug is required to produce an immediate and dramatic hypotensive state. Recovery from the effects of the drug is immediate. When mixed in solution for intravenous administration, sodium nitroprusside is unstable in light. The perioperative nurse must have a roll of aluminum foil available to cover the intravenous bottle and tubing completely when the drug is hanging and in use or ready for immediate use; an electronic device to measure and control the amount administered must also be set up.

Some surgeons prefer to use antibiotics in the immediate preoperative period. A second-generation cephalosporin, Ancef, is the most common drug of choice.

Skin Preparation

If head hair must be removed, it is best removed after the patient has arrived in the surgery department but before arrival in an operating room. The hair is first clipped with electric clippers, which are cleaned and disinfected after each use. The hair is placed in a container, labeled with the patient's name, and kept with the patient after surgery. The scalp is then shaved using warm, soapy water and either a straight razor or several disposable safety razors. As soon as the patient experiences any pulling, the razor blade should be changed to prevent any abrasion to the skin and for the patient's comfort. The perioperative nurse should explain to the patient exactly what is being done and what sensations to expect during the procedure.

For surgery on the cervical spine it is possible to secure long hair on top of the head and remove neck hair with clippers to a level even with the top of the ears or just below the occipital protuberance. Postoperatively patients with long hair can comb it down over the shaved area until the hair regrows.

Patients undergoing thoracic or lumbar spine surgery may not need to be shaved. If hair is present, it can be removed by a depilatory or clipping just before surgery. After hair removal the skin should be inspected carefully for any signs of inflammation or infection. If any such signs are noted, they should be reported to the surgeon immediately.

An antiseptic skin prep is done after the patient is positioned and before draping. Skin prepping may be done by the perioperative nurse, surgeon, or resident. General principles and precautions cited in Chapter 4 apply to neurosurgical preps, regardless of who performs them.

Many neurosurgeons mark the incision line with a marking pencil, a marking solution and wooden stick, or a scalpel. If a marking solution is used, indigo carmine, gentian violet, or brilliant green is recommended. Methylene blue should never be found in a neurosurgical operating room because it produces an inflammatory reaction in central nervous system tissue and could be disastrous if accidentally injected into the subarachnoid space, for example.

After marking, the surgeon may inject the incision site and the sites for application of towel clamps with a local anesthetic agent or with normal saline solution. Any solution will apply pressure within the tissues and decrease bleeding at the time of incision. The local anesthetic agent has the additional effect of decreasing the effect of the stimulus of the skin incision.

Positioning

The basic body positions and their modifications are used in neurosurgery. The perioperative nurse must know the position for each procedure; the hazards and precautions of each position; and the equipment, supportive positioning devices, and time necessary to place a patient in a given position (see Chapter 5). General considerations of special importance in positioning for neurosurgery include protecting the eyes from pressure, chemical burns, and corneal abrasions; maintaining joints in functional alignment with no pressure or tension on superficial nerves and vessels; and checking the Foley catheter for tension and kinks to ensure drainage.

The dorsal recumbent, or supine, position or some modification of it is used for supratentorial craniotomy, subtemporal decompression, and anterior cervical fusion. The lateral position is used for thoracic and lumbar laminectomy by some surgeons and for lumbar sympathectomy. Modifications of the prone position can be used for lumbar, thoracic, and cervical laminectomy and for posterior fossa craniectomy. The sitting, or upright, position can be used for cervical laminectomy, posterior fossa craniectomy, temporal craniectomy, and ventriculography. Only specific aspects of the sitting position for neurosurgical procedures and the knee-chest position, a modification of the prone position, are covered in this chapter.

The extreme sitting, or upright, position may be the neurosurgeon's choice for infratentorial cranial surgery and posterior cervical laminectomy when acute trauma is not the cause of cervical cord disease. Advantages of this position include optimum visibility of the operative field and decreased blood loss because of the lowered arterial and venous pressures. However, hypotensive changes also pose potential problems: some patients cannot tolerate the upright position under general anesthesia; thus the patient is slowly placed in this position as the anesthesia provider

monitors the blood pressure. Most patients have a drop in arterial pressure but rapidly adapt to the position; those who do not are placed in the prone position. In the sitting position the venous pressure in the head and neck may be negative, predisposing to air embolism. Other potential problems with this position include neck flexion with airway compromise and difficulty in achieving and maintaining functional alignment.

Preoperatively, elastic bandages, wrapped from the patient's toes to groin, special tensor stockings, such as thromboembolic disease (TED) hose, or sequential compression stockings may be applied. All these help prevent venous stasis in the lower extremities and help maintain the blood pressure. Other precautions during positioning and throughout the procedure include checking the heels, soles, and popliteal areas to prevent pressure; checking male genitals to ensure that pressure will not compromise circulation and cause necrosis and female breasts to prevent any unnecessary pressure; preventing thighs from contacting the metal crossbar table attachment; stabilizing the head in the headrest; and stabilizing the shoulders and torso to prevent neck flexion.

Preparations should be made in collaboration with the anesthesia provider to manage air embolism if this complication should occur. The patient may be placed in a G (gravity) suit before positioning to prevent this complication. The G suit also assists in maintaining the blood pressure. A right atrial line can be placed under direct-vision fluoroscopy in either the cardiac catheterization laboratory or the radiology department; before arrival of the patient in the operating room, or in the operating room, using the image intensifier. After anesthesia induction, the anesthesia care provider may place an esophageal stethoscope or attach the patient to a Doppler unit to hear air entering the right atrium. The air can be withdrawn through the atrial line with a 50 ml syringe and a three-way stopcock connection. If the management of air embolism includes repositioning the patient with the surgical wound open, the repositioning must be accomplished quickly, without endangering the patient in other ways, such as contamination of the surgical wound, displacement of a joint, or dislodgment of the endotracheal tube.

The most common position for lumbar and thoracic laminectomy is prone. Both legs are wrapped with elastic bandages, or tensor hose are used to prevent venous stasis in the extremities.

Anesthesia induction and intubation take place on the transport vehicle. The patient is then placed on the OR bed in the prone position. Special bed attachment supports or a chest roll must be placed under the chest on each side from the shoulder to the iliac crest to permit lung expansion during the procedure. The bottom of the bed is dropped to about a 25-degree angle. The patient's knees are flexed, and the lower legs elevated and supported on two large pillows and the bed mattress, under which the footboard is placed at a right angle to the bed. The knees are padded with foam. The arms are flexed at the elbows and supported by pillows on wide armboards. Care is taken to prevent pressure or tension on the brachial plexus. The Wilson back frame, Kambin, or Andrews spinal frame can be used. The patient is placed prone on the frame with pillows under the legs and pillows or sheets supporting each arm. For surgery on the neck and posterior part of the skull, the foot of the bed is not dropped; the ankles and feet are supported on a large pillow; and the arms are secured at the patient's sides, protecting the ulnar, median, and radial nerves. A horseshoe or Mayfield point headrest may be used.

The major problems encountered with the prone position include an increase in venous pressure and bleeding at the operative site, peripheral venous stasis, and decrease in vital capacity. Precautions include checking female breasts, male genitals, and knees to prevent pressure on these areas; avoiding hyperextension of shoulders and pressure on the brachial plexus when turning the patient to begin positioning and during the procedure; preventing abduction of the arms and occlusion of the subclavian and axillary arteries; and protecting the eyes from pressure, corneal abrasions, and chemical burns.

The knee-chest, or tuck, position is also used for lumbar laminectomy. This is a modification of the prone position, in which the patient's hips and knees are flexed so that the body is supported on the thighs and lower legs, with the abdomen and chest hanging free or supported on chest rolls. The Hicks spinal surgery frame ("butt board") may be used for the knee-chest position, as well as the Andrews spinal frame or table. Advantages of this position include decreased bleeding because of the collapse of epidural veins, better exposure resulting from hyperflexion of the spine, absence of pressure on the vena cava, and increased ease of ventilation. Operating time is usually reduced when this position is used.

Disadvantages of the knee-chest position include the difficulty of maintaining physical stability on the OR bed, hypotension, and pooling of blood in the lower extremities.

Draping

Most neurosurgeons do their own draping. Draping for some procedures is complex and requires the cooperation of surgeon, assistant, and scrub nurse. Four or more towels are placed around the operative site. They may be secured by disposable skin staples, small towel clamps, or silk sutures on a heavy cutting needle. When sutures are used, the surgeon also needs heavy, 6-inch toothed tissue forceps and suture scissors. Forceps, scissors, needle holders, and needles are discarded after towels have been secured in place.

A plastic adhesive drape may be placed either before or after the towels. The skin must be completely dry for the drape to adhere tightly to the skin.

Fluid-impervious barrier drape sheets and towels are essential. If an overhead instrument table is used, it should be covered with a sheet large enough that the front edge can be fanfolded at the front edge of the table until the table is brought forward over the patient toward the operative site. The fanfolded sheet can then be secured at the lower border of the operative site to bridge the gap between the unsterile undersurface of the table and the sterile field. Mayo stands should also be covered with effective barriers. The particulars of draping for neurosurgical procedures vary and are influenced by the patient's position, the surgeon's preferences, and what is available in each hospital. Therefore a detailed description of the draping for each procedure is not provided here. The particulars of draping for each procedure should be clearly described on the neurosurgeon's preference card. Doubts can be clarified by communication with the neurosurgeon before the operation.

As a general rule, neurosurgeons prefer to have all equipment ready before making the incision. Therefore they can be helpful to the perioperative nurse in attaching and hooking up suction tubings, electrosurgical cords, and other equipment that will be needed for the operation.

Hemostasis

Meticulous hemostasis is of particular importance in neurosurgery. The first consideration is control of hemorrhage from the highly vascular scalp. Compression of the edges of the wound with gauze sponges and fingers during the initial incision is followed by application of hemostatic clips and clamps. When clips are used, they are applied so that they include the galea and skin edge, whereas clamps are attached directly to the galea and then everted. Before the incision is made, normal saline solution or a local anesthetic agent may be injected to minimize scalp bleeding.

Bone wax, a hemostatic material described in Chapter 6, is prepared for all cranial and spinal cord operations. The surgeon firmly rubs the wax into the bleeding surface of the bone after all periosteum has been scraped off. When the skull flap has been elevated, bone wax is also rubbed into the diploë to control bleeding from the bone edge. During spinal surgery, bone wax is used on the cut edges of the laminae.

Electrosurgery is routine for neurosurgical procedures. Perioperative nurses must understand the uses and hazards of the electrosurgical unit and be familiar with the safety measures. Electrocoagulation may be used to stop bleeding in the galea, in the periosteum, on the surface of the dura, on the spinal cord, and in the brain. The coagulation current seals the blood vessels. The electrical current is applied to the forceps, a metal suction tip, or other instrument, which acts as a conducting tool. To be effective, the coagulating current must contact the vessel in a dry field. For this reason, suctioning is necessary to remove blood as the contact is made between the instrument carrying the current and the bleeding point.

Bipolar electrosurgical units are frequently used (Fig. 23-22). Bipolar units provide a completely isolated

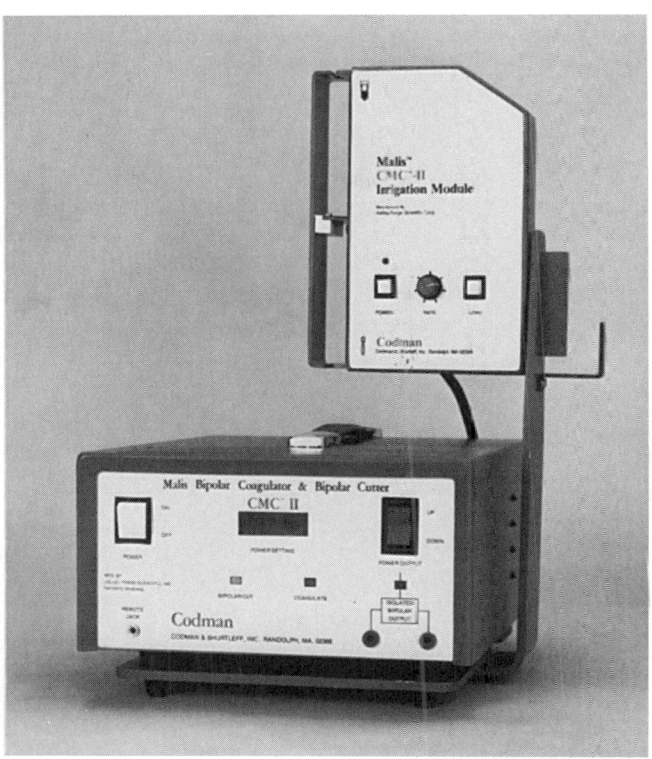

FIGURE 23-22 Malis bipolar coagulator and bipolar cutter, with irrigation module.

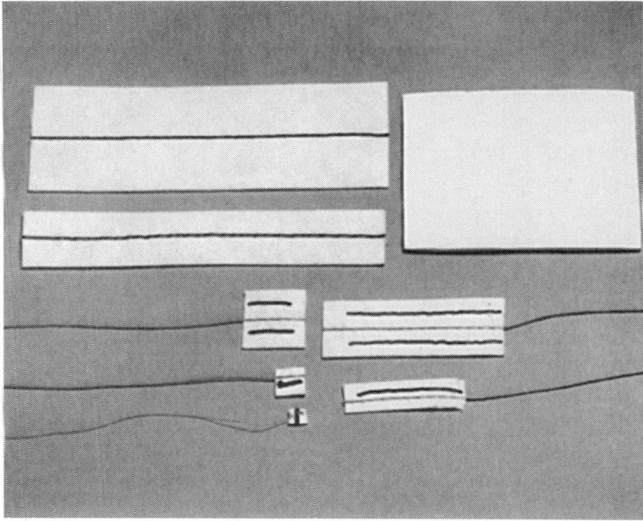

FIGURE 23-23 Cottonoid strips and neuro patties.

output with negligible leakage of current between the tips of the forceps, permitting use of coagulating current in proximity to structures where ordinary unipolar coagulation would be hazardous. Lactated Ringer's or normal saline solution irrigation is used during bipolar coagulation to minimize tissue heating, shrinkage, drying, and adherence to the forceps. Some bipolar units have built-in irrigating systems. Need for a dispersive pad is eliminated. The use of the bipolar coagulation technique allows hemostasis of almost any size vessel encountered. Vessels as large as the superficial temporal artery, as well as those too small for suture or clip ligation, may be coagulated with bipolar units.

Electrosurgery is also used for cutting with a lower power setting. When the surgeon is using a cutting electrode to remove a tumor, the circulating nurse should stand by the machine to adjust the settings as needed. As the surgeon uses the cutting electrode, an assistant holds a suction tip to one side of the area of dissection to remove smoke.

Gauze sponges are used to control bleeding before the skull or spinal canal is entered. Coarse gauze sponges injure fragile tissues such as the brain and spinal cord, so wet compressed rayon cotton (cottonoid) pledgets or strips are used in place of gauze sponges to control bleeding beneath the skull and around the spinal cord. Sterile cottonoid strips and pledgets, or patties, must be available in a variety of sizes (Fig. 23-23). Strips are usually 6 inches long, although some surgeons prefer them 3 inches in length. The standard widths are ¼, ½, ¾, and 1 inch. Strips have

x-ray–detectable markers or strings attached. Pledgets should have both x-ray–detectable markers and strings attached.

Standard sizes for pledgets are ¼ × ¼ inch, ½ × ½ inch, ¾ × ¾ inch, and 1 × 1 inch. All strips and pledgets must be counted. Some surgeons prefer to use Biocal or Telfa strips, which the nurse cuts to size before use. During the procedure the nurse maintains a supply of these special neurosurgical sponges, thoroughly soaked with normal saline or lactated Ringer's solution, within reach of the surgeon's forceps. They may be displayed on a waterproof surface, such as a towel; a sterile inverted metal basin (emesis basin, small bowl); a plastic drape, such as 3M or Vi-Drape; a piece of rubber clipped to a folded towel; or a patty plate, a flat piece of metal that attaches to the Mayo tray with two small towel clamps. The surgeon may prefer that the nurse keep a supply of these moist sponges on the palm or back of one hand and extend them toward the surgeon as needed. The sponges are aligned on the display surface in order of size. As soon as one is used, it is replaced. Loose, wet cotton balls may be used as a temporary pack or tamponade in a bleeding tumor bed after a tumor has been removed. The gentle pressure of the cotton balls along with time and patience on the part of the surgeon may stop bleeding not controllable by other means. The scrub nurse is responsible for counting the number of cotton balls placed in the tumor bed and ensuring that none is left behind at closure.

A variety of hemostatic clips is available and used by neurosurgeons to occlude both superficial and deep vessels. The original clip used by Cushing and later modified by McKenzie is made of silver. Newer clips such as the Samuels hemoclip and the ligaclip are of tantalum or an alloy that is compatible with the MRI scanner. The scrub nurse removes the clips from a special cartridge with the appropriate applicator and passes them to the surgeon for application to a vessel. Such clips enable the surgeon to occlude vessels in areas difficult to reach by other means

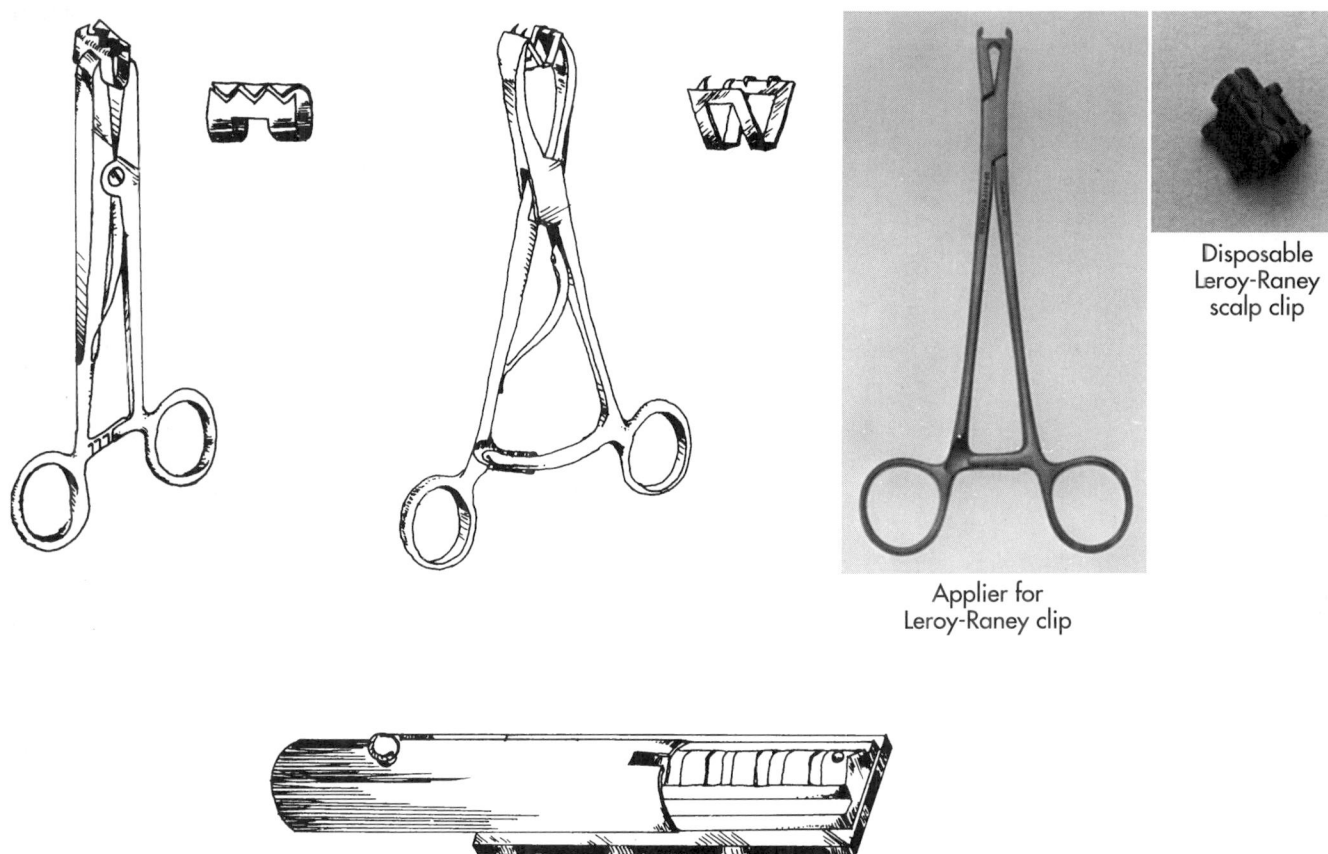

Disposable
Leroy-Raney
scalp clip

Applier for
Leroy-Raney clip

FIGURE 23-24   Scalp clip appliers and clips, disposable Leroy-Raney scalp clip, and applier for Leroy-Raney scalp clip.

and to ligate superficial vessels of the brain before cutting them and without destroying any surrounding tissues. Clips can be obtained in a variety of sizes.

Hemostatic scalp clips include Raney, Adson, and LeRoy clips. Autoclips and Michel clips are still used occasionally (Fig. 23-24). There are also plastic disposable scalp clips of the Raney and Leroy-Raney types. Each type of clip has a specific clip applier by which the clips are placed on the scalp edges. At time of closure clips are removed by a hemostat, a special clip remover, or the applier, which simultaneously serves as a remover. A minimum of two clip appliers is essential; the scrub nurse loads one clip applier while the surgeon is using the other to place the clip on the scalp. The Adson clips are loaded on the appliers from a special rack. After use they must be reshaped before replacement on the clip rack; there is a special instrument for this purpose. The Raney and Michel clips are loaded by hand. If the Raney clips are nondisposable, they are difficult to clean by hand and should be placed in an ultrasonic cleaner or soaked in hydrogen peroxide.

Numerous special clips are used for permanent or temporary occlusion of vessels or an aneurysm neck in the surgical treatment of intracranial aneurysm (see pp. 957-958).

Neurosurgeons almost routinely use certain hemostatic agents in addition to mechanical hemostasis. Gelfoam is one of these agents. It comes in two forms: a powder and a compressed sponge. The sponge is produced in three sizes: #12, #50, and #100. The sponge form can be applied to an oozing surface dry or saturated with saline solution or topical thrombin. The larger pieces of Gelfoam are cut into a variety of sizes of strips and pledgets. The surgeon's preference dictates the exact method of preparation and use. Gelfoam is absorbable and can be left in the body.

Surgicel, a rayonlike cellulose gauze, and Oxycel, an absorbable hemostatic agent that comes in both cotton and gauze forms, are used to control bleeding from oozing surfaces, vessels, and sinuses in the brain and spinal canal. These hemostatic substances are also cut into suitable sizes and shapes and are handed to the surgeon dry, followed by a moist cottonoid strip or patty. The hemostatic material adheres to the bleeding area as gentle pressure is applied to the cottonoid material for several minutes.

Pieces of fresh muscle tissue can be used to tampon and control bleeding where the usual forms of hemostasis are not possible.

Most surgeons use polyglactin 910 synthetic absorbable, black braided nylon, or silk suture material for traction sutures and wound closure.

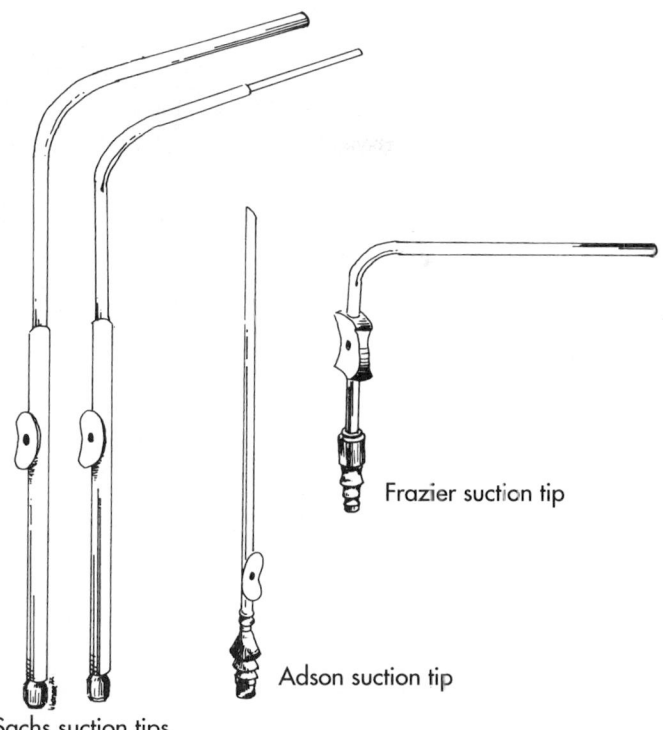

Sachs suction tips

Frazier suction tip

Adson suction tip

FIGURE 23-25   Suction tips.

Irrigating the wound with lactated Ringer's or normal saline solution may facilitate hemostasis. This procedure definitely helps the surgeon identify active bleeding points. Two completely filled bulb or Asepto syringes should always be within reach of the surgeon. Suction is the best means of keeping the wound dry and permitting control of bleeding. Therefore suction and irrigation are used together.

Metal suction tips, such as the Cone, Sachs, Frazier, Bucy, and Adson (Fig. 23-25), are used because they not only keep the wound dry but also can be used to conduct coagulation current from a monopolar unit to the bleeding point. The Bucy-Frazier tip is insulated and attached to both suction and electrosurgical units to become the active coagulating electrode. Use of the suction-coagulation unit is limited to areas in which gross coagulation can be done safely, for example, during the opening phase of a surgical procedure.

Suction can be used to remove necrotic or traumatized brain tissue or soft brain tumors rapidly after a sample has been obtained for pathologic examination. It is also useful in evaluating abscess cavities, removing fluid from a ventricle or the subarachnoid space, holding a solid tumor during its removal, and applying compression to a bleeding vessel.

Many neurosurgeons irrigate surgical wounds with an antibiotic solution before wound closure. The antibiotic must be mixed with irrigation solution according to the surgeon's preference so that it is ready for use when

needed. Gelfoam may be soaked in antibiotic solution before use.

Equipment

An operating room used for neurosurgical procedures should be large enough to accommodate the equipment needed for procedures done by the neurosurgeons on the hospital staff. The emphasis of this discussion is equipment that is necessary for neurosurgery in any setting.

Essential built-in equipment includes a minimum of eight electrical outlets per wall, four overhead spotlights, six single or three double x-ray view boxes, and four wall or ceiling vacuum suction outlets capable of high negative pressure. Other equipment that can be built in if the situation demands includes a two-way telephone communication line, a ceiling-mounted operating microscope with camera, a closed-circuit television unit with monitor, an electrocardiogram-electroencephalogram monitor with readouts, and a wall or ceiling source of nitrogen or compressed air to operate air-powered equipment. Additionally, many operating rooms now have computer consoles for three-dimensional reformation and stereotaxis, EMG, evoked potentials, and spinal cord monitoring. Consideration must be given to enough room for the equipment in the rooms that are designated for neurosurgery.

Some basic mobile equipment is needed for any setting in which neurosurgery is done. An OR bed and complete set of bed attachments and neurosurgical headrests are essential. The best headrest is one that can be adapted for use in any body position, such as the Gardner and the Mayfield skull clamp (Fig. 23-26, *B*). Each of these headrests has a three-pin suspension and skull clamp that attaches to a headrest bed attachment for secure fixation of the skull during the operation. This is especially useful when the patient is placed in a sitting position. Two or three sterile pins are placed in the head after the insertion sites are prepared with an antiseptic, such as an iodophor. The headrest skull clamp is first attached to the pins and then to the bed attachment. Precautions during insertion of the pins include avoiding the frontal sinuses, superficial temporal arteries, and the eyes. In many instances, especially for supratentorial craniotomy, the head can be stabilized by a rubber doughnut. A mobile cart should be used for storage of the neurosurgical headrests and bed parts as well as any other positioning devices and aids used by the neurosurgeon.

One special neurosurgical overhead instrument table, such as the Mayfield table (Fig. 23-27), is preferable, but two large Mayo trays can be used for any neurosurgical procedure. One large instrument back table is a must. It should be at least 6 to 8 inches higher than the standard table because the scrub nurse must frequently work on a high lift to see the operative field and perform effectively. The extra height of the back table enables the perioperative nurse to maintain a sterile field and to work more comfortably.

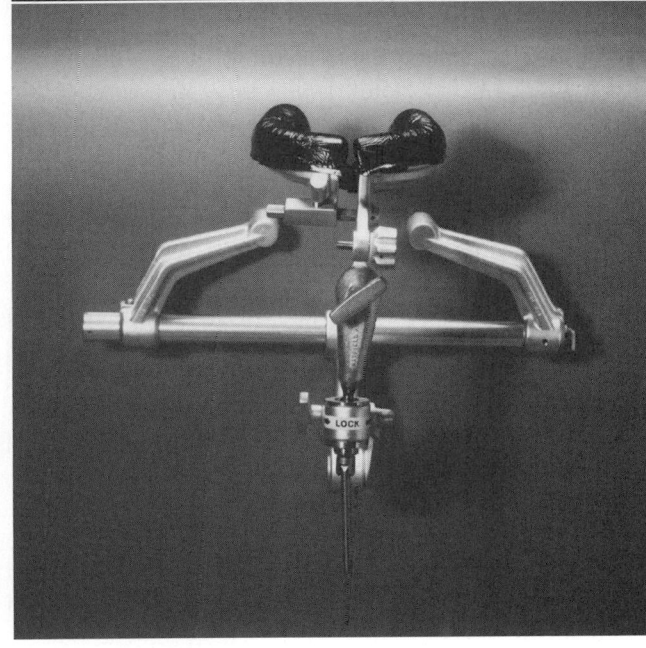

FIGURE 23-26 **A,** Three-pin suspension skull clamps for stabilizing head during neurosurgical procedures. **B,** Mayfield headrest.

Eight to ten footstools are needed. They can be arranged side by side or on top of each other for the safety, efficiency, and comfort of the personnel. Kickbuckets are needed for trash and sponges. Also useful are two small utility tables for preparation and special equipment and supplies.

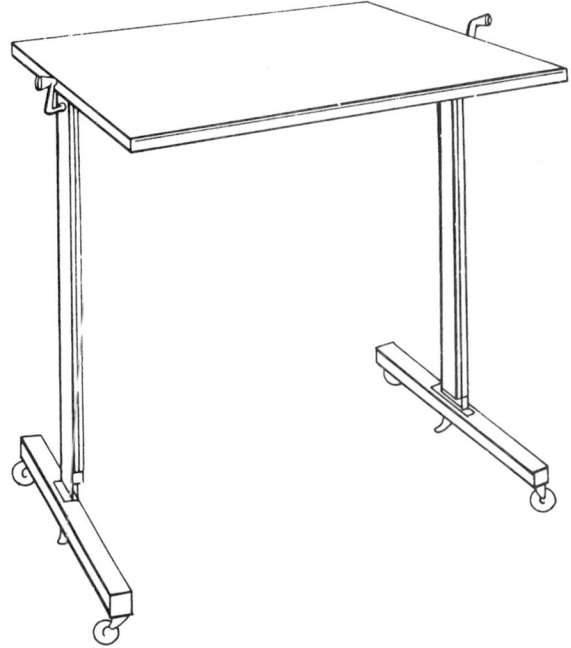

FIGURE 23-27   Mayfield overhead instrument table.

A cooling-heating unit with two blankets, such as the K-thermia unit, should be available for use. An electronic temperature-monitoring device with esophageal, intraaural, and rectal probes is essential.

Other essential equipment includes a monopolar electrosurgical unit, a bipolar electrosurgical unit, at least one fiberoptic headlight, and one fiberoptic light source for lighted retractors and telescopes, if they are used. Also needed is an operating microscope such as the Zeiss, a tank of nitrogen, if not built in, with a special pressure gauge for operating air-powered instruments, four pressure bags and bulb pumps for infusion of blood, two blood-warming units, one or two electronic intravenous rate control units such as I-Vac units, a solution warmer, and a nerve stimulator. A cryosurgical unit, an image intensifier, and a stereotaxic apparatus may be needed if the surgical procedure requires them. A laser, ultrasonic surgical aspirator, and intraoperative ultrasound should be available (Fig. 23-28).

Instrumentation

Scientific developments in other fields have been applied to the health care delivery system in general. Some of the developments with application to neurosurgery in the forms of specialized instrumentation and equipment have been discussed previously. A few items require further discussion.

Air-powered instrumentation has become popular with neurosurgeons over the years since the first Hall air drill was developed. Modifications of the original instrument continue today. These instruments decrease open wound

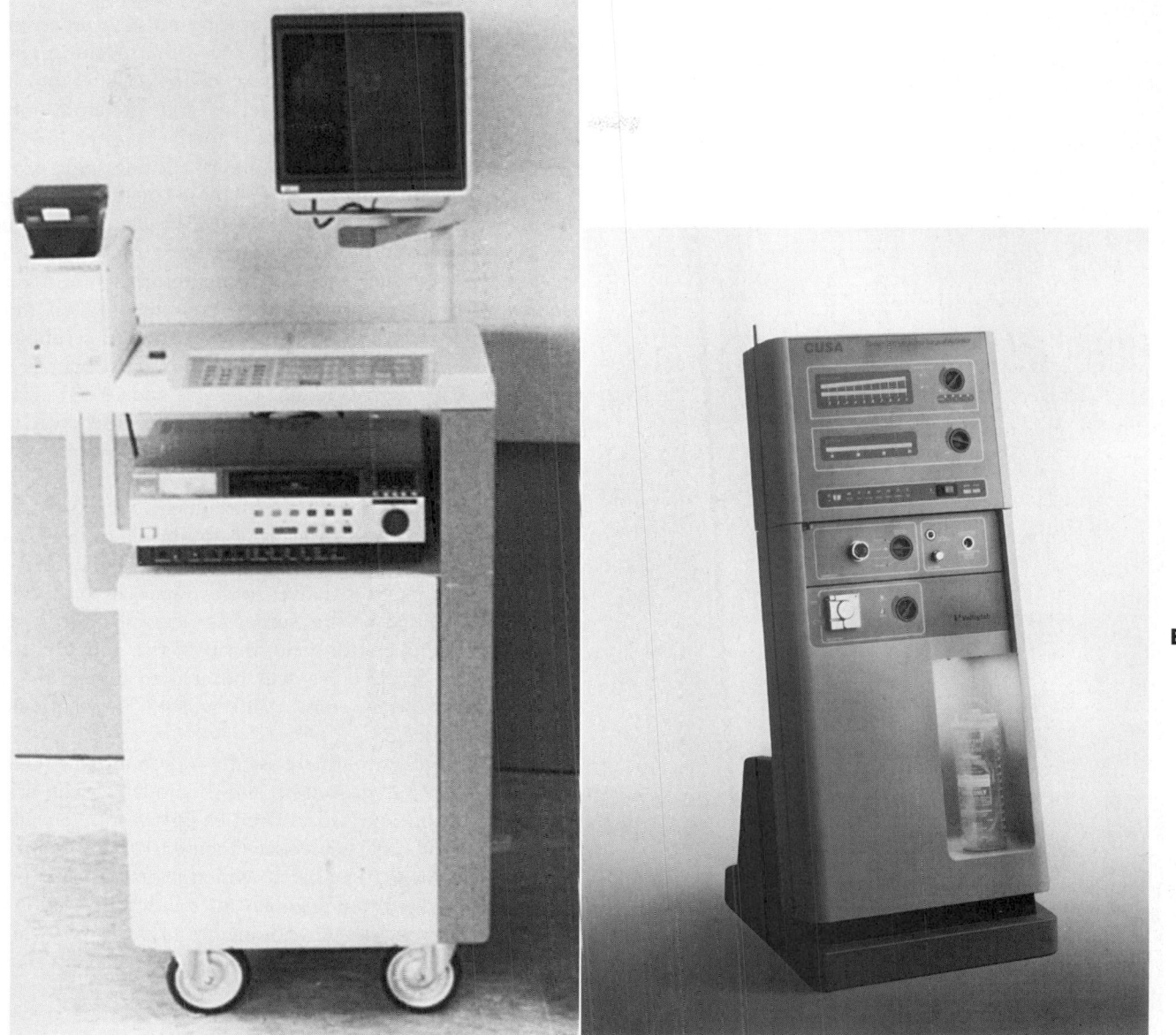

FIGURE 23-28   **A**, Intraoperative ultrasonograph. **B**, CUSA 200 Ultrasonic Surgical Aspirator.

time and anesthesia time for the patient and conserve energy for the surgeon.

The basic air driver has been adapted by means of special attachments for neurosurgery. Because improvements and new developments in air-powered instruments are ongoing, specific instructions for use and care of such equipment should be obtained from the manufacturer at the time of purchase. Basic information is included here.

The Hall Surgairtome 200 (Fig. 23-29) can be used for precision cutting, shaping, and repair of bone. Its use increases the ease of bone work and reduces operating time. Compressed nitrogen is the power source, as with other air-powered equipment. The Hall Surgairtome 200 can be used to widen the graft area in anterior fusions and to unroof the auditory canal in eighth cranial nerve surgery. For use in less accessible areas, such as the sphenoidal sinus, pituitary fossa, and vertebral bodies, 20-degree and 90-degree angle attachments are available. A range of burrs and guards is available.

The Crainotome may still be used by surgeon choice, and it offers perforator drive for drilling burr holes. Both 12 mm and 7 mm perforators are available in disposable and reusable forms. The perforator driver attachment can be removed and a saw blade and dura guard attached to adapt the instrument for cutting a craniotomy bone flap. The saw blade is interchangeable with a wire-pass drill bit for drilling holes and placing wires, when a bone flap is to be wired in place. A cranioplasty burr and skull contour burr as well as guards for each type of burr are available.

Although seldom used now, electrically powered instruments were popular and widely used before the introduction of the air-powered models.

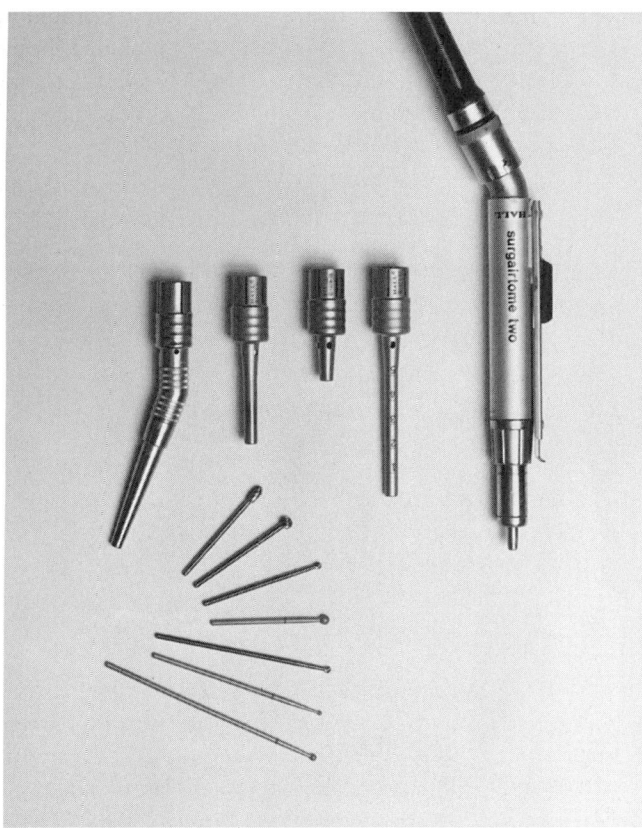

FIGURE 23-29   Hall Surgitome 200 with attachments.

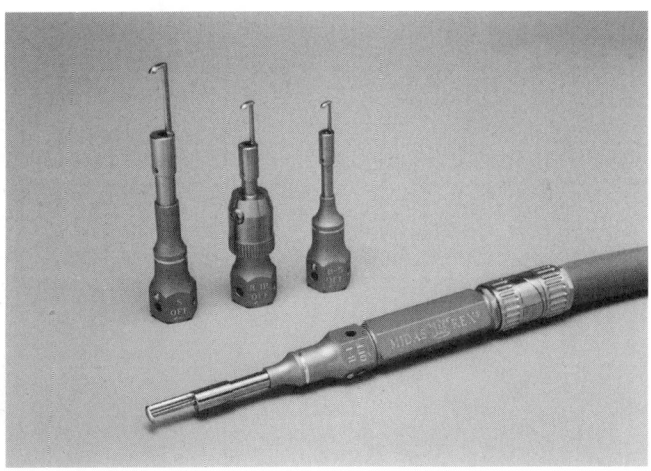

FIGURE 23-30   Midas Rex Drill with attachments.

Another versatile pneumatic tool is the Midas Rex instrument (Fig. 23-30). The variety of disposable cutting tools of this foot–controlled instrument and its attachments provides the neurosurgeon with a wide capability in bone cutting, including small rectangular holes in place of burr holes, bone flaps of any size and shaping, and unroofing areas such as the sphenoid wing. Additionally, large craniotomy flaps can be turned with only a single burr hole. Manufacturer's precautions and instructions must be followed.

The operating microscope (see Chapter 18) has revolutionized neurosurgery, making possible procedures never done before and making other neurosurgical procedures on vessels, such as aneurysm surgery, and surgery on nerves more precise and therefore more successful.

The lens system for neurosurgery and the angle of the microscope are different from those used in otologic surgery. If a microscope is shared by neurologic and otologic services, the perioperative nurse must be able to adapt the microscope for use in neurosurgery by attachment of the appropriate pieces, and the surgeon must check it for focal length and focus before scrubbing. Disposable drapes are available for the microscope, as are assistant and observer lenses. Cameras and closed-circuit television monitors are also available for use with the operating microscope if the situation warrants such sophisticated equipment.

The routine use of video cameras, recorders, and television monitors, if available, is invaluable to teach staff and enhance interest and understanding of the surgical procedure by perioperative nurses who are otherwise unable to visualize the surgeon's actions directly. By viewing the operative field through the monitor, the experienced scrub nurse will be able to anticipate the neurosurgeon's next move and will therefore provide better assistance.

Many surgeons routinely use the carbon dioxide (CO_2) laser for precise dissection and hemostasis. The laser produces a concentrated infrared energy beam, generated by CO_2, that can be precisely focused on any point at which it is aimed. The beam, which is made visible by a superimposed red aiming light, causes flash vaporization of cellular water at 100° C. Advantages of the laser include improved hemostasis and healing with decreased tissue trauma, swelling, and risk of metastasis.

The potassium titanyl phosphate (KTP) laser also has proved to be a valuable tool for the neurosurgeon. Postoperative morbidity is minimal. The laser is especially advantageous in microvascular surgery and is used to occlude vessels less than 0.5 mm in diameter in operations for aneurysms and arteriovenous malformations as well as to remove tumors with minimal or no damage to surrounding structures. Tissue damage depends on amounts of energy generated and exposure duration.

Precautions include the need to wear protective glasses or plastic goggles, specific to the laser being used, to prevent accidental damage to eyes of personnel in the room and the need to keep all cottonoid, sponge, and towel materials thoroughly damp to prevent fire that could result from contact between a dry combustible material and the beam. The CO_2 and other gas sources must be checked before use to ensure adequate supply for the procedure. Nonflammable anesthetic agents must be used. Smoke evacuators should be available to remove the smoke generated.

Direct image intensification is essential for an increasing number of neurosurgical procedures, such as placement of nerve-stimulator electrodes in brain or spinal areas and stereotaxic procedures. If possible, a C-arm and monitor should be available in the operating room. Otherwise these procedures can be done in the radiology department. Procedures requiring use of the CT scan can also be done in the radiology department.

Choice of instrumentation for a given neurosurgical procedure is largely controlled by the surgeon or, in some operating rooms, by the chief of the department. Exactly what the neurosurgeon needs for a specific procedure is highly individual. Factors that influence the choices include training, experience, type of setting in which the surgery is performed, pathologic condition of the patient, surgical approach planned, and equipment available.

Some hospitals provide a full range of highly specialized neurosurgical instrumentation; some supply only instruments that can be used in orthopedic, otologic, and nasal surgery as well as in neurosurgery. Many neurosurgeons in private practice carry some or all of their own special instruments from hospital to hospital.

Usually several instruments can be used to perform one function. The choice depends on what is available and the surgeon's preference. Therefore only instrument types and examples of each type are listed here. The exact instrument list for any neurosurgeon for each procedure must be written by the perioperative nurse in collaboration with that surgeon.

A hospital with an active neurosurgical service has its own basic craniotomy instrument list. The perioperative nurse should use that list and add the special preferences of a given neurosurgeon.

In addition to the basic types of instruments essential for supratentorial craniotomy (Figs. 23-31 to 23-34), suture scissors, wire scissors, and 6-inch Russian forceps should be included. A bone punch (Cone or Ingram), a drill guide and dura protector (Adson or Hamlin), a twist drill that fits the Hudson brace or a Raney brace and perforator, hemostatic clips and applicators, trephines, burr hole covers (Silastic, such as the Todd-Crue buttons, or tantalum). Ray pituitary curettes, a Rayport dura knife, pituitary forceps (Adson or D'Errico), Bonney forceps, Penfield watchmaker's forceps, Hartmann forceps, monopolar electrosurgical bayonet forceps (Davis, Raney, Hoen, Jansen), bulldog clamps, angled dura scissors (Taylor, Frazier, DeBakey, Potts-Smith), and many other instruments that a given neurosurgeon may desire can be included.

Many neurosurgeons prefer Allis forceps, rather than towel clamps or Peers clamps, to attach suction, electrosurgical pencils, and other devices to the drapes. Allis forceps used for this purpose should not be used for any other surgical procedures. They can be marked for neurosurgery and kept with the special neurosurgical instruments. They will not effectively hold tissue, such as the edge of the small bowel, after continued use on drape materials. Two 10 ml

Luer-Lok and two 10 ml plain-tipped syringes should be included in every craniotomy setup. Also included should be six to 12 rubber bands, one or two Penrose drains, two medicine cups, suture material and needles of the surgeon's choice, and dressing headrolls (Kling or Kerlix).

Many neurosurgeons use magnifying loupes. They are made on a custom basis and are usually the personal property of the surgeon.

Posterior fossa or infratentorial craniectomy requires the same instrumentation as supratentorial craniotomy, minus saws, saw handles, and saw guides. A cerebellar extension for the Hudson brace must be included, as well as a larger assortment of double-action and Kerrison rongeurs

Additional instruments required for laminectomy, anterior fusion, surgery of peripheral nerves, microsurgery, and aneurysm surgery are included in the descriptions of these surgical procedures. An example of a back-table setup for craniotomy is shown in Fig. 23-35.

Evaluation

After the surgical procedure is completed, the patient is transported to the ICU or PACU. The patient is evaluated for the previously established outcomes. Bony prominences and pressure points are checked for skin integrity. A report along with documentation is given to the PACU nurse. Included are the outcomes from the identified nursing diagnoses. If the outcomes were met, they may be communicated as follows:

- The patient demonstrated a reduction in anxiety, verbalized feeling of being less anxious, coped with perioperative routines adequately, and verbalized an understanding of the planned procedure or procedures.
- The patient or family verbalized knowledge of diagnostic and surgical procedures and had realistic expectations of tests, routines, and postoperative care.
- The patient maintained effective breathing patterns; ventilation was maintained, arterial blood gases (ABGs) were within normal limits, and breath sounds were bilateral.
- The patient will continue to report a reduction in pain, ask for pain medication, and verbalize relief or absence of pain.
- The patient will exhibit no signs and symptoms of infection; the wound will be clean and well healed.

Patient and Family Education and Discharge Planning

Patient and family education is the key to helping the patient return to as normal a life as possible. Because of the numerous neurosurgical procedures in this chapter, it would be difficult to describe patient and family teaching pertinent to each procedure. Therefore this important aspect in the care of the patient is described in general.

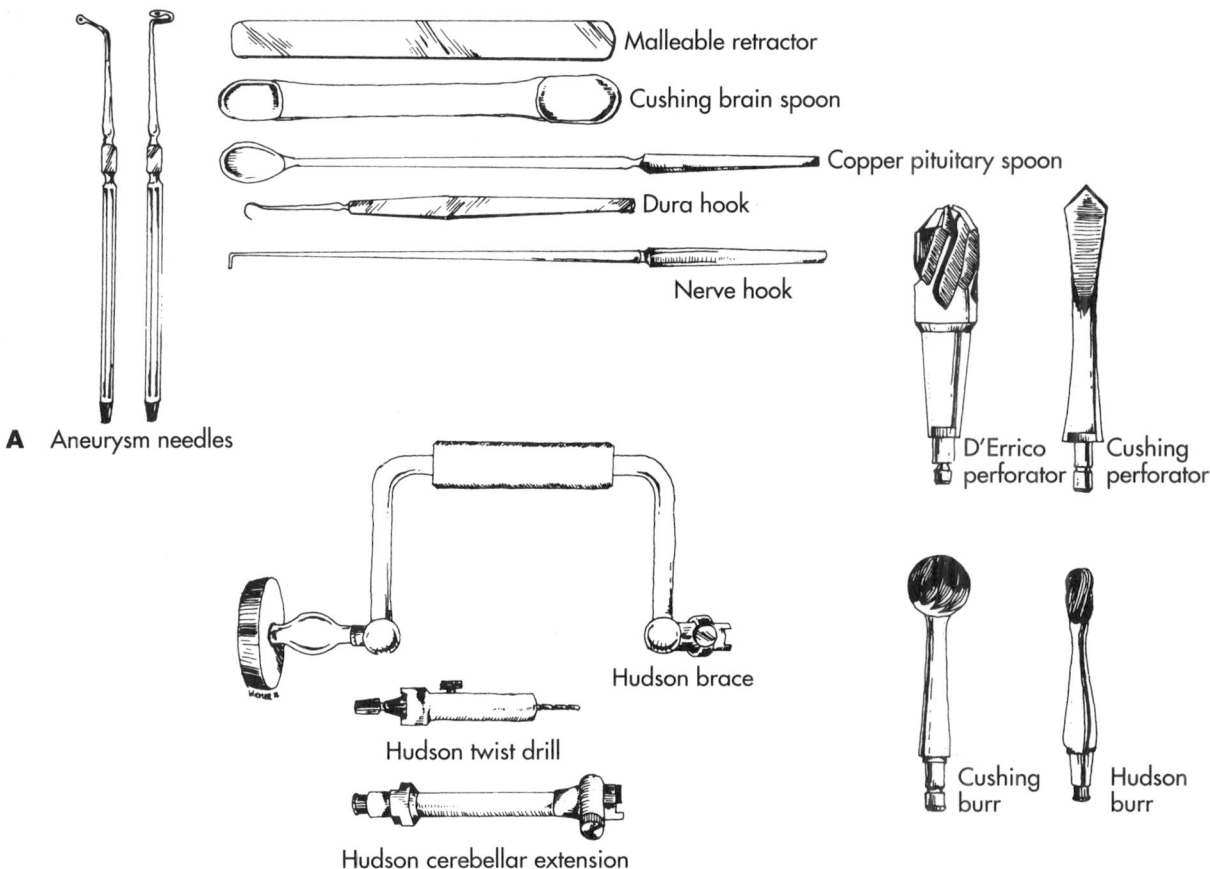

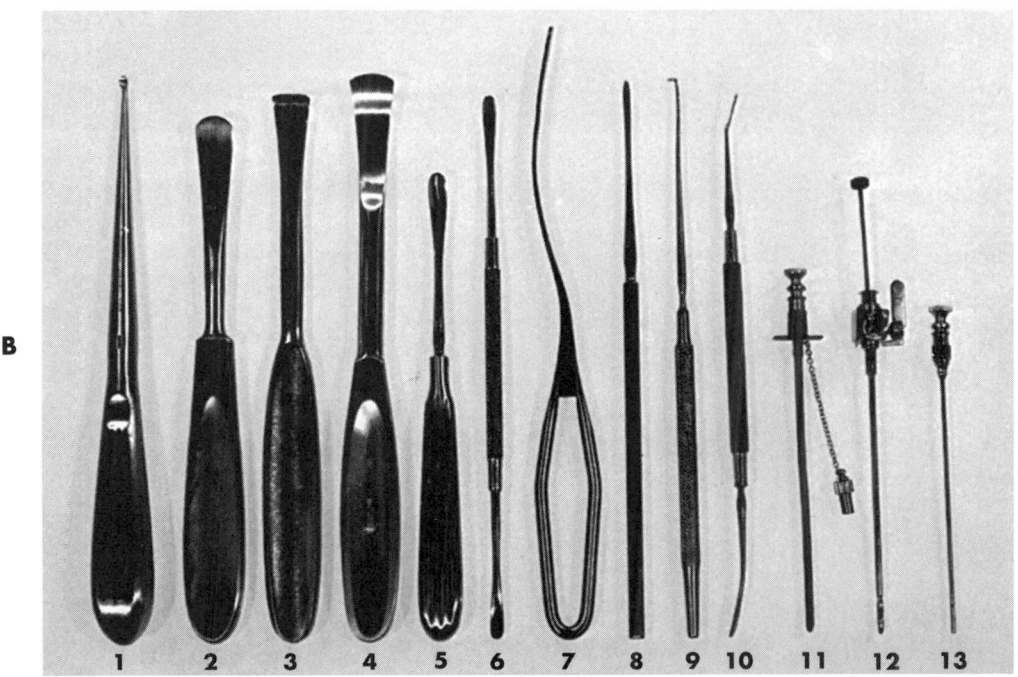

FIGURE 23-31 **A**, Some basic instruments for craniotomy. **B**, *1*, Spinal curette, straight; *2*, Cushing periosteal elevator, blunt; *3*, Cushing periosteal elevator, sharp; *4*, Adson periosteal elevator, wide; *5*, Adson elevator #3 (joker); *6*, Freer elevator; *7*, Sachs dura separator; *8*, Sunday staphylorrhaphy elevator; *9*, nerve hook; *10*, Olivecrona double-ended dissector; *11*, Scott ventricular cannula; *12*, Seletz ventricular cannula; *13*, Cone ventricular needle.

As soon as the need for surgery is identified, a multidimensional education program should begin as soon as possible and must include the patient's family or significant others. Teaching should address the psychosocial and physiologic aspects of the patient's life. The plan should offer opportunities for the patient to develop new skills, coping mechanisms, and behaviors to adapt to aspects of temporary or permanent neurologic deficit. Factors that may influence the patient's ability to learn include the neurologic status, particularly in relation to sensory deficits and pain, and developmental level.

The education program begins with the assessment of the patient and develops into a tool used to identify the patient's and family's needs. The plan should include any areas that could cause conflict with the patient's cultural and personal beliefs.

Discharge options must consider the potential of transfer to a rehabilitation center for continued extensive therapy or discharge to return home with assistance and continuation of patient rehabilitation. Patients with severe alterations in neurologic function may require long-term care.

The patient and family require much support, care, and concern during the process, and all should be encouraged to express their feelings regarding the reality of the situation and their fears and concerns.

SURGICAL INTERVENTIONS

It is not possible in this chapter to provide a detailed approach to each neurosurgical procedure. Specific neurosurgical procedures are numerous, and each has many modifications or variations. The operating surgeon decides exactly which procedure and what variation will be performed. Basic general approaches, however, are limited and can be described in detail. Therefore only a few step-by-step descriptions of basic approaches are presented. The perioperative nurse who is familiar with neurosurgical anatomy and pathologic conditions can learn these basic approaches and adapt them to the specific procedure.

HEAD SURGERY

Burr Holes

Burr holes are placed to remove a localized fluid collection beneath the dura mater. Fluid not composed of clot can be easily evacuated through a burr hole. Burr

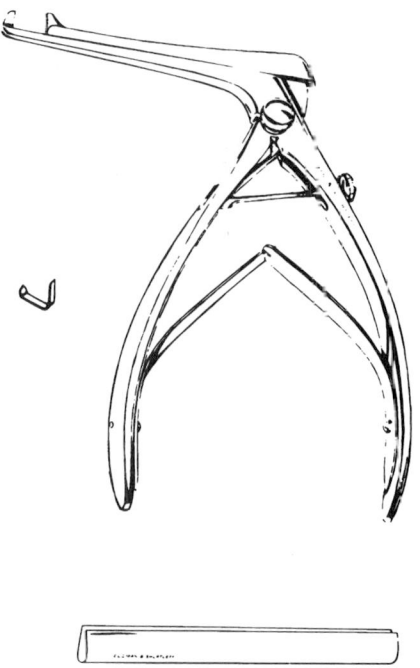

FIGURE 23-32 Setup for craniosynostosis may include Ingraham-Fowler tantalum clips, Ingraham-Fowler guillotine applicators, and preformed silicone strip.

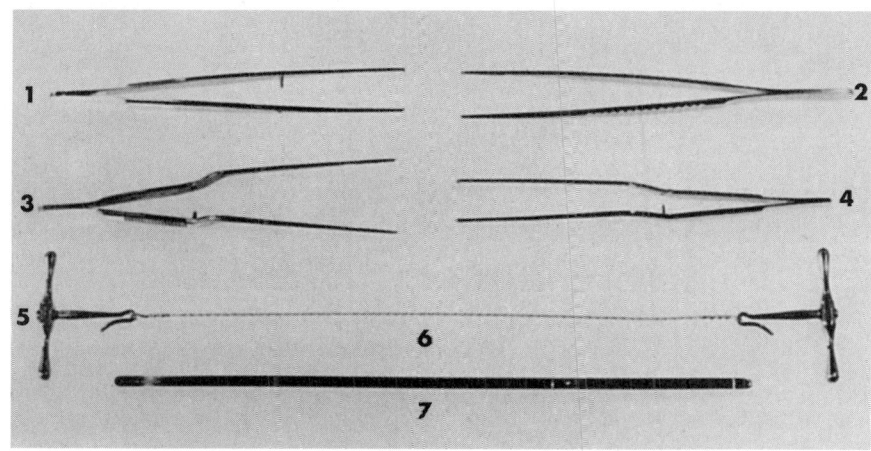

FIGURE 23-33 *1*, Cushing tissue forceps; *2*, Cushing dressing forceps; *3*, Cushing bayonet dressing forceps; *4*, Cushing bayonet tissue forceps; *5*, Gigli saw handle; *6*, Gigli saw wire; *7*, Bailey saw guide.

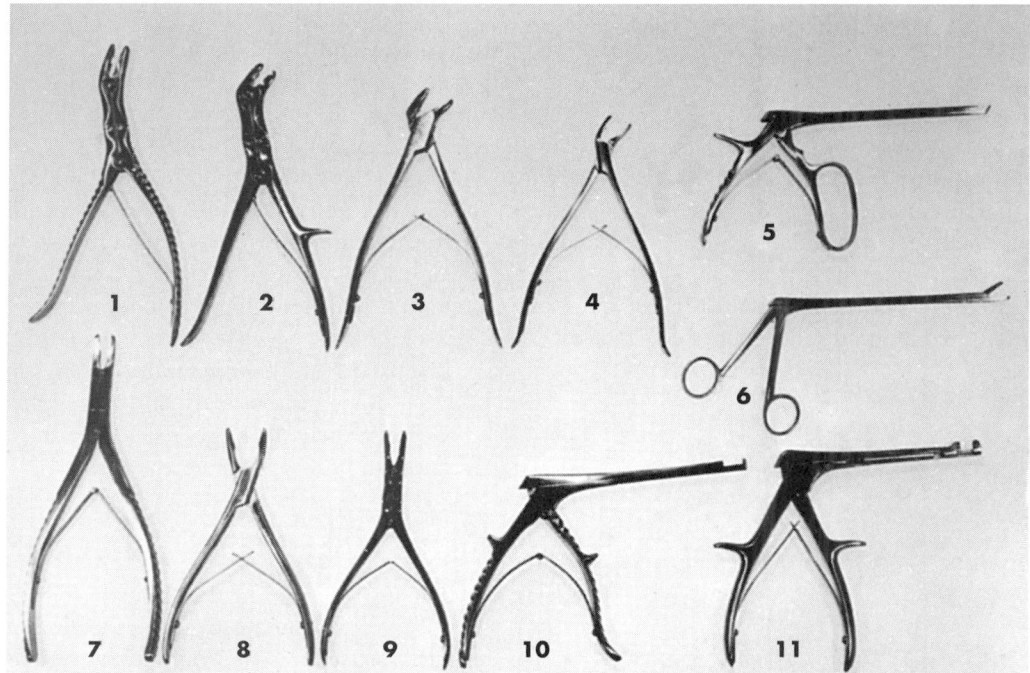

FIGURE 23-34   *1*, Leksell rongeur; *2*, Stille gooseneck rongeur; *3*, Bacon rongeur; *4*, Stookey cranial rongeur; *5*, Cloward 40-degree angle punch rongeur; *6*, pituitary disk rongeur; *7*, Fulton rongeur; *8*, Lempert rongeur; *9*, Zaufal-Jansen rongeur; *10*, Kerrison rongeur; *11*, Raney punch.

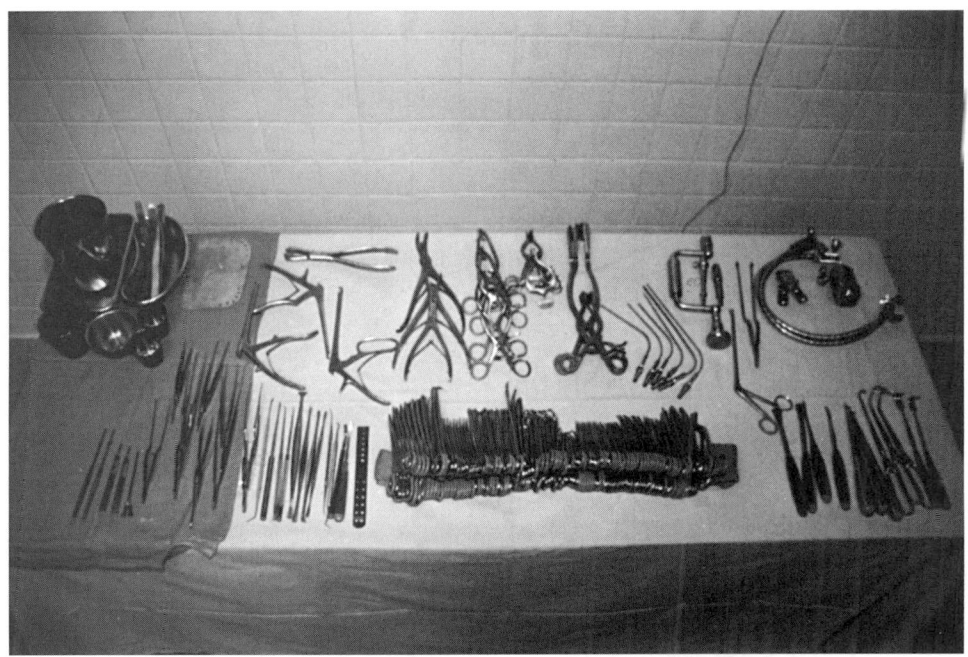

FIGURE 23-35   Back-table instrument setup for craniotomy.

holes are also made to tap a lateral ventricle to relieve pressure. Burr holes are used by many surgeons when treating a brain abscess. The abscess may be aspirated, and antibiotics instilled. Other surgeons prefer to treat abscess by craniotomy. Frequently burr holes are used to locate or drain subdural hematomas. However, a craniectomy is usually necessary to gain adequate exposure in these cases (Fig. 23-36). A burr hole is one of the steps in procedures to shunt ventricular fluid to another body system for absorption or elimination.

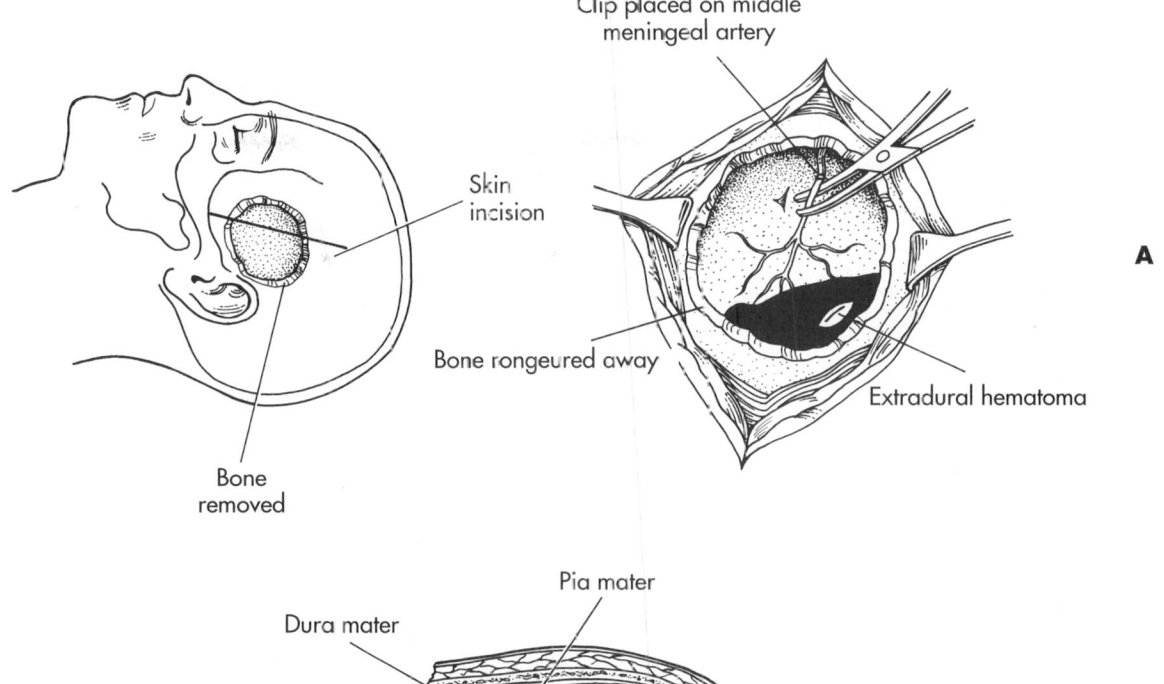

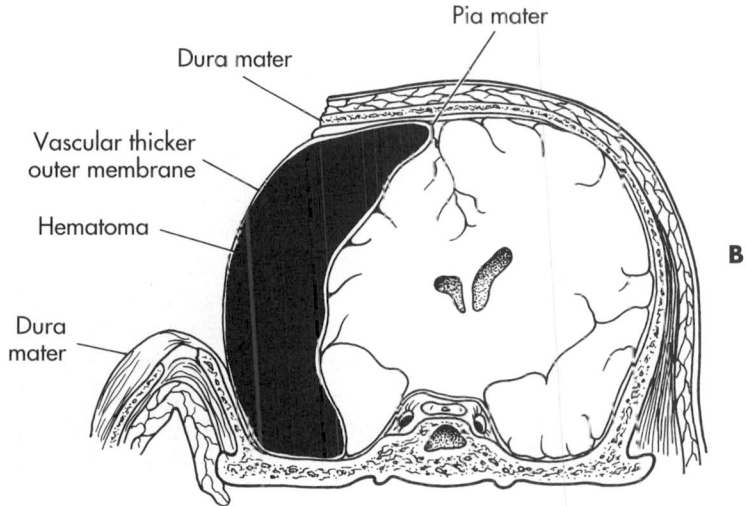

FIGURE 23-36   **A,** Extradural hematoma. **B,** Subdural hematoma.

Burr holes are placed to introduce air into the lateral ventricles for ventriculography (Fig. 23-37). The air or appropriate contrast medium make the ventricles visible in radiographic studies.

Craniectomy

Craniectomy is the formation of an opening into the skull. This term usually applies when the opening is larger than the average burr hole. A piece of bone is cut with a circular saw that attaches to a Hudson brace. Procedures performed by craniectomy include prefrontal lobotomy, topectomy, cingulotomy, leukotomy, and thalamotomy. Today some of these procedures may be a part of stereotaxic neurosurgery.

Craniotomy

Craniotomy is an incision into the skull to expose and surgically treat intracranial disease.

Procedural considerations

Depending on the location of the pathologic condition, a craniotomy may be frontal, parietal, occipital, temporal, or a combination of two or more of these. When turning a scalp flap for a craniotomy, the surgeon may peel the scalp back off the pericranium; the bone flap is then elevated with the overlying muscles still attached (osteoplastic), or the periosteum may be stripped off the skull before the bone flap (free flap) is turned.

The bone plate may be separated from the soft tissues, removed from the skull, and set aside for replacement at the end of the procedure. It may be placed in an antibiotic solution or an iodophor solution or wrapped in a saline-moistened sponge or one that has been saturated with an antibiotic solution or an iodophor solution. The bone plate is not removed from the sterile field. If it is not replaced, it may be frozen in a sterile container or saved and stored in a marked, unsterile container to use as a

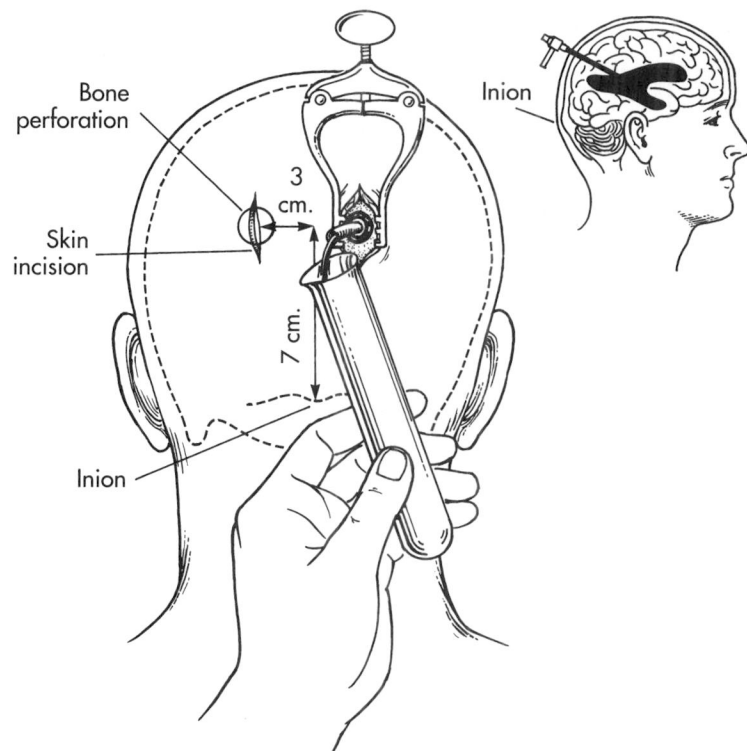

FIGURE 23-37 Occipital burr holes for ventriculography.

template for forming a cranioplastic plate at a later date. The defect can be repaired without use of this template, however. If the bone is not separated from the soft tissues, it is turned back with the temporal muscle and soft tissues.

Operative procedure

After draping and attachment of suction and electrosurgical cords, the procedure is begun.

1. The surgeon and the assistant apply digital pressure over folded 4 × 4 inch radiopaque sponges on both sides of the incision line. The skin and galea are incised in segments, with the length of each segment being equal to that over which the finger pressure is applied. The tissue edges are held with 6-inch toothed forceps as scalp clips are placed on the flap edges. Hemostatic clamps are placed on the outside edge of the incision in adults and are grouped in segments and secured together by rubber bands placed around the handles or by a Penrose drain or open 4 × 4 inch sponge threaded through the handles and tied or clamped together with heavy forceps, such as a Pean (Fig. 23-38). Any remaining active arterial bleeding is controlled by electrocoagulation. If the incision extends into the temporal area, bleeding in the temporal muscle is managed by electrocoagulation, hemostats, tamponade, or suture ligature. Mayo scissors can be used to incise temporal muscle and fascia.
2. The soft tissue is peeled off the periosteum by sharp or blunt dissection or by electrodissection (see Fig.

23-38). The scalp flap is turned back over folded sponges and retracted by use of small towel clamps and rubber bands or muscle hooks on rubber bands. In either case the traction is maintained by securing the rubber band to the drapes with heavy forceps. The flap may be covered with a moist sponge or Telfa strips and a sterile towel. Bleeding is controlled by electrocoagulation.

3. When a free bone flap is planned, the muscle and periosteum are incised. Muscle and periosteum are elevated with the skin-galea flap, turned back, and retracted as a unit, as described previously.
4. The periosteum and muscle are incised with a scalpel or electrosurgical knife except at the inferior margins, which are left intact to preserve the blood supply to the bone flap. The periosteum is stripped from the bone at the incision line with a periosteal elevator. Bone wax is used to control bleeding.
5. The scalp edges and muscle are retracted from the bone incision line by a Sachs or Cushing retractor. Two or more burr holes are made with either a hand or power cranial drill (Figs. 23-39 to 23-41). As each hole is drilled, the assistant must hold the patient's head to diminish the agitation and prevent displacement from the headrest. A great deal of heat is generated by the friction of the perforator or burr against the bone. The scrub nurse or assistant must irrigate the drilling site to counteract the heat and remove bone dust, which collects as the holes are made. Some surgeons prefer that the scrub nurse

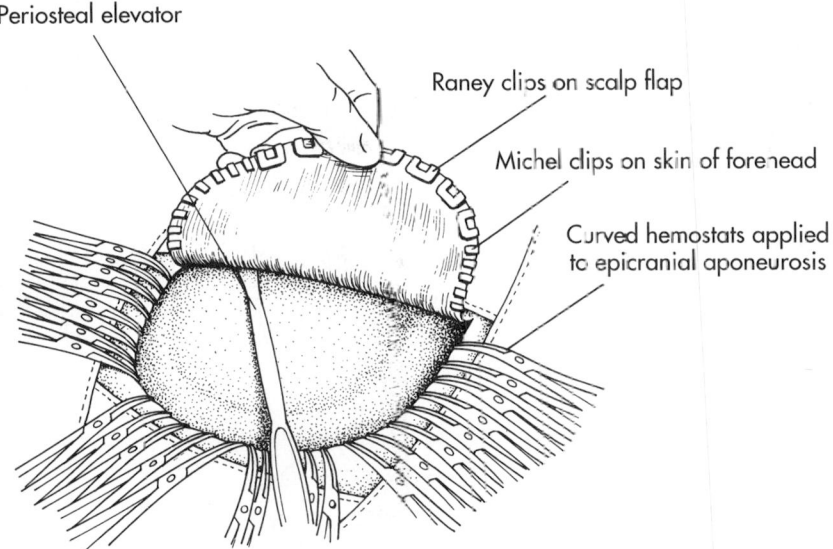

Periosteal elevator

Raney clips on scalp flap

Michel clips on skin of forehead

Curved hemostats applied to epicranial aponeurosis

FIGURE 23-38   Elevation of scalp flap. Hemostats on outer rim of incision and Raney clips and Michel clips on scalp flap.

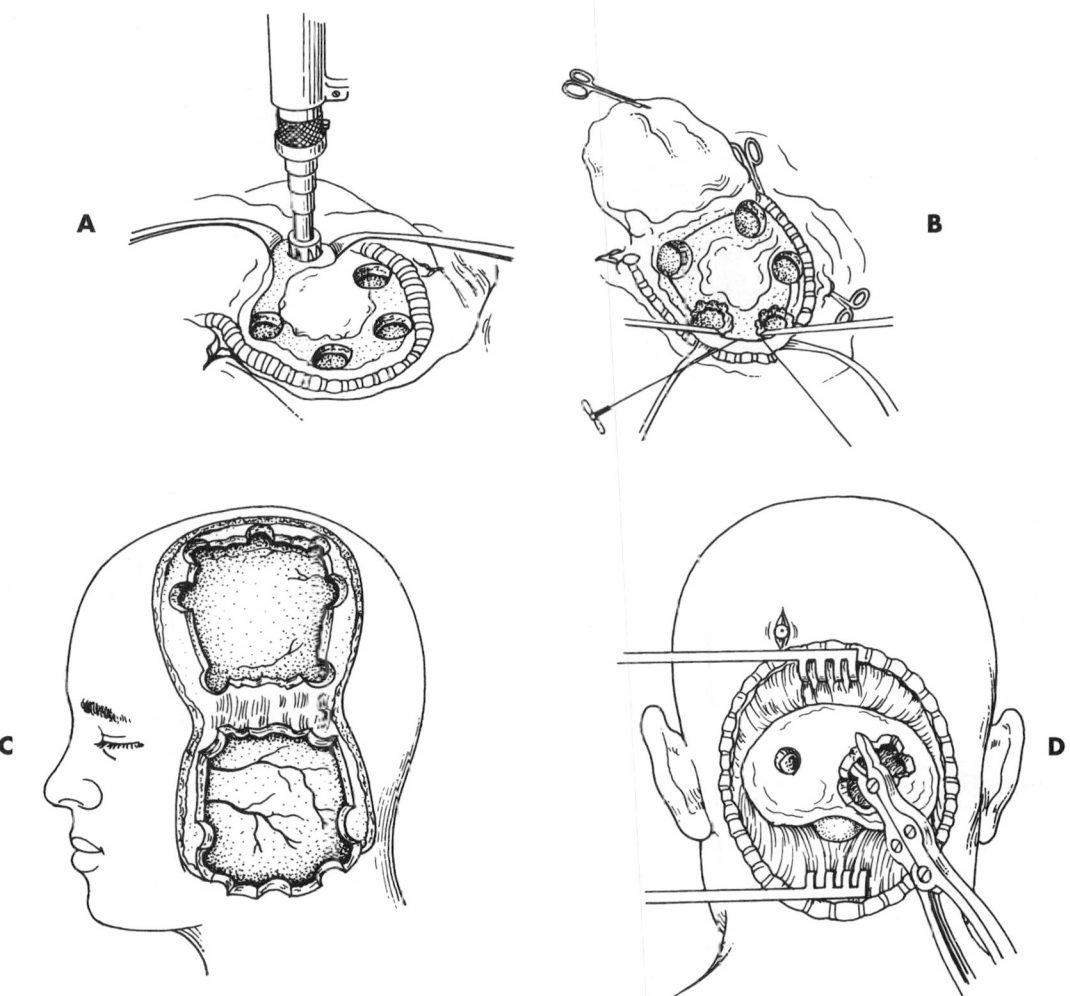

A

B

C

D

FIGURE 23-39   Techniques of cranial surgery. **A**, Drilling burr holes. **B**, Using the Gigli saw. **C**, Bone flap turned down. **D**, Modification for cerebellar craniotomy.

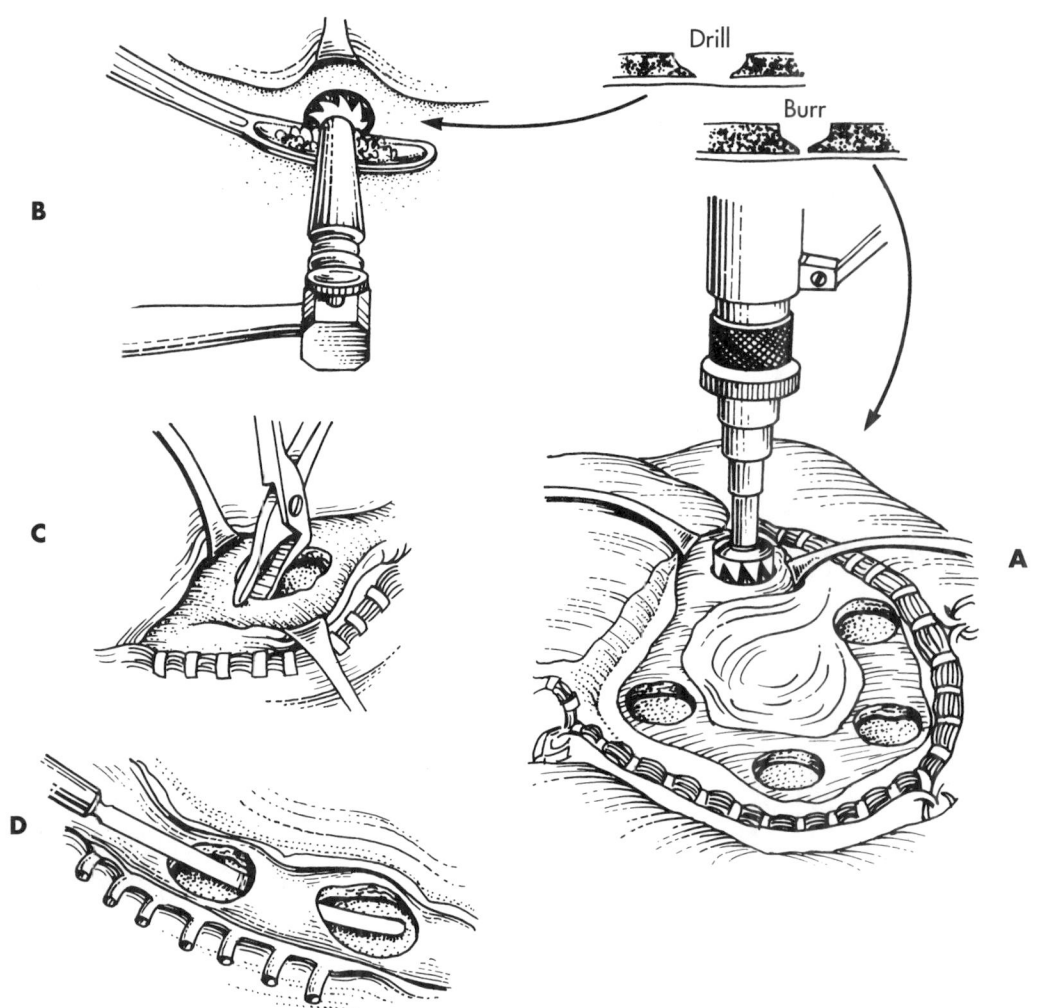

FIGURE 23-40   Methods of making osteoplastic flap (craniotomy). **A**, Using electric drill to make burr hole. **B**, Using hand perforator to make burr hole. **C**, Using rongeur to enlarge burr hole. **D**, Separating dura mater from skull.

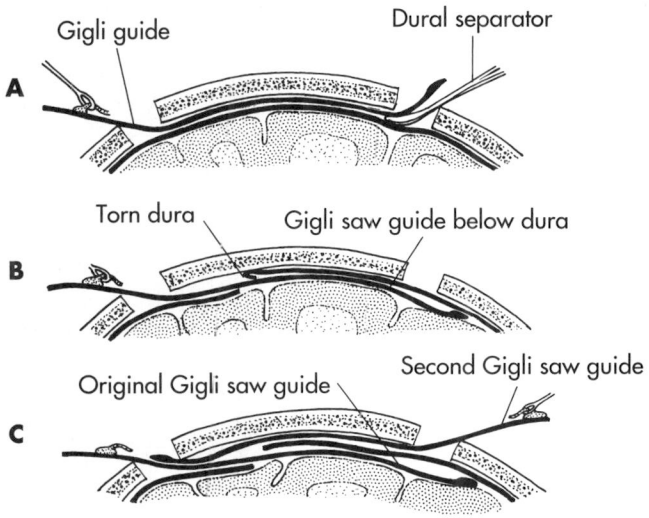

FIGURE 23-41   Gigli saw insertion. **A** to **C**, Steps to be taken if Gigli saw tears dura mater.

collect the bone dust for replacement in the burr holes at closure. The dust is placed in a medicine glass and kept moist with a small amount of normal saline solution. A large-gauge suction tip is used to remove both irrigating solution and debris from the field. As the inner table is perforated and the dura exposed, the burr hole may be temporarily tamponed with bone wax or a cottonoid strip or patty. Each hole is eventually debrided by a #0 or 00 bone curette or small periosteal elevator (joker). The dura mater is freed at the margins with a #3 Adson elevator, #3 Penfield dissector, or right-angle Frazier elevator or similar instrument. The hole is irrigated and suction applied simultaneously. Active bleeding points in the bone are identified, and bone wax is applied.

6. When all burr holes have been made, the bone flap is cut by sawing between holes after the dura mater has been separated from the bone by a dural separator, such as the Sachs, or by a #3 Penfield dissector. Dural

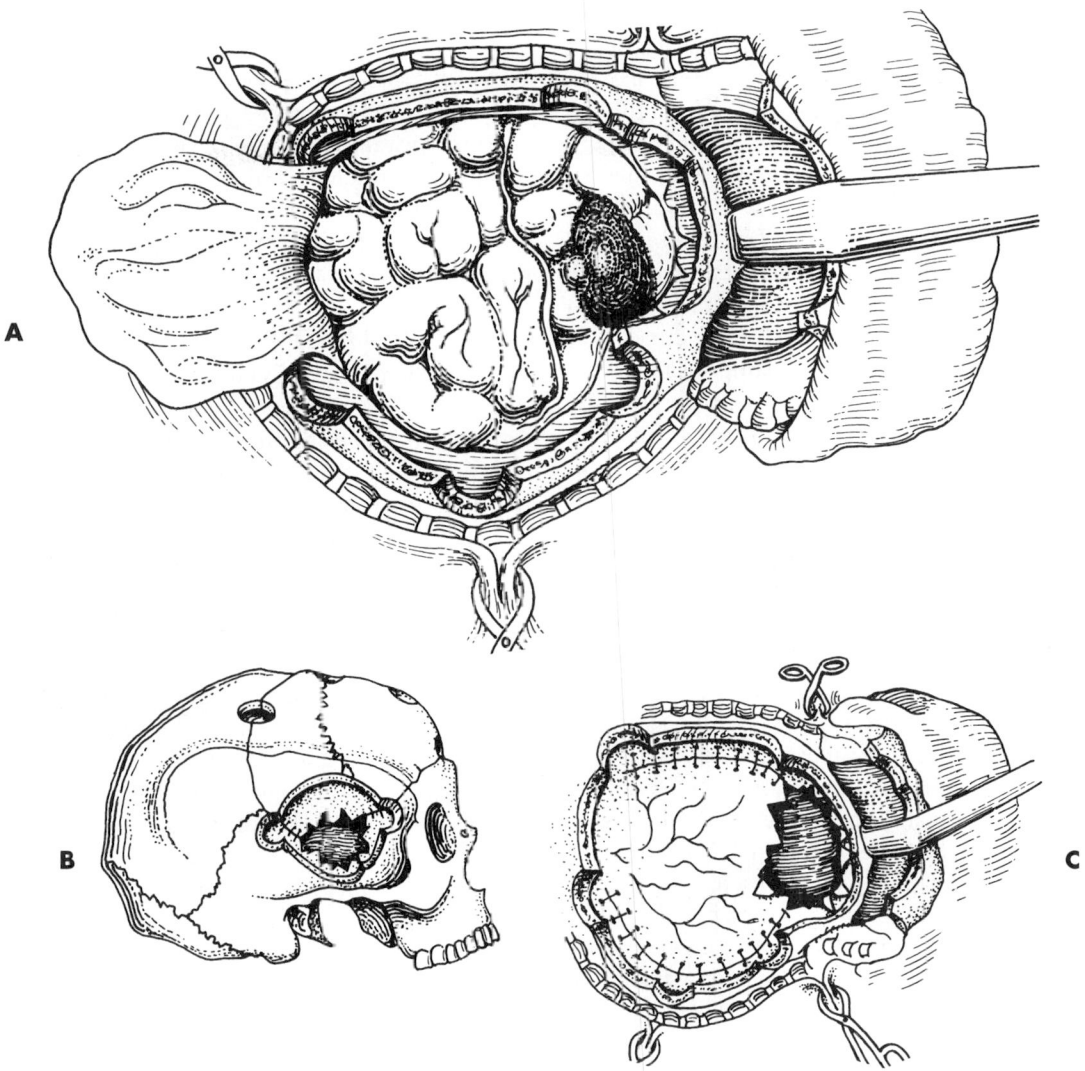

FIGURE 23-42 Craniotomy with subtemporal decompression. **A,** Malignant cerebral tumor exposed. **B,** Bony defect. **C,** Dural defect.

separation is done to prevent tearing of the dura mater, especially over venous sinuses. Using a rongeur, the surgeon may cut channels into the two burr holes at the inferior edge of the planned bone flap under the muscle. When the rest of the bone flap has been sawed, this segment can be easily cracked as the bone is elevated and turned back. If the sawing is done by hand, a dural separator is passed from one hole to the next under the bone. A saw guide-passer with a saw attached is passed from one hole to the next in the same manner. The saw is detached from the guide, saw handles are attached to both ends of the saw, and the bone is incised by sawing in a back-and-forth motion. Friction generates heat, so irrigation and suction must be used during the process. The procedure is repeated until all segments but the one under the muscle have been cut. Usually a new saw is used each time. An air craniotome or Midas Rex drill can also be used for the opening. Irrigation and suction are required as the

bone flap is cut. Soft-tissue edges are retracted with Sachs or Cushing retractors.

7. The bone flap with muscle attached is lifted off the dura mater by two periosteal elevators. As it is forced up and back, the bridge of bone under the muscle cracks. Bleeding from the bone is controlled with bone wax. A double-action rongeur is used to remove sharp, irregular edges where the bone cracked. The bone flap is covered with a moist sponge, cottonoid material, or Telfa pads and then a clean sterile towel and is retracted in the same manner as the scalp flap.

8. The dura mater is irrigated. Moist cottonoid strips or patties or Telfa pads may be inserted between the dura mater and bone and folded back to cover the exposed bone edges. Clean sterile towels may be placed around the operative site.

9. The dura mater is opened (Fig. 23-42). A dura hook may be used to elevate the dura mater from the brain, and a small nick is made in the dura mater with a #15

blade on a #3 or #7 knife handle; or a small opening may be made in the dura mater without elevating it, after which the dural edges are grasped with straight mosquito hemostats or two Adson or Cushing forceps with teeth and are elevated. A narrow, moist cottonoid strip is inserted with smooth forceps (bayonet or Cushing) into the opening to protect the brain as the dura mater is incised and elevated. The dural incision can be made with Metzenbaum scissors, special dura scissors, or a Rayport dura knife. Usually traction sutures are placed at the outer edge of the dura mater and are tagged with small bulldog clamps or mosquito hemostats. Sometimes the tag instruments are attached to the drapes to increase traction and keep tension on them. As the dural veins are approached during dural opening, they are ligated or coagulated before cutting. Ligation is done with hemostatic clips such as Weck Hemoclips, McKenzie clips, or Ligaclips. The brain surface is protected by moist cottonoid strips.

10. The surgeon places cottonoid strips and brain retractors, self-retaining (Fig. 23-43) and manual, appropriately while working toward visualizing the particular pathologic entity.

11. Brain spoons, Cushing pituitary spoons, and Ray curettes as well as pituitary rongeurs or other tumor forceps must be available for tumor removal. Also, a selection of dissectors, Cushing and Gerald forceps, and a bipolar coagulation unit are used. Completely filled irrigating syringes and a full range of moist cottonoid patties and strips must be within easy reach of the surgeon and the assistant. After correction of the pathologic condition and control of bleeding, the brain may be irrigated with an antibiotic solution of the surgeon's choice.

12. The dura mater is usually closed by running or by interrupted sutures of #4-0 silk, 4-0 polyglactin 910 suture, or 4-0 black braided nylon. Under some conditions, dural substitutes may be used. A drain may or may not be used. Epidural tack-up sutures are usually placed around the edge of the craniotomy defect to close the epidural dead space. This is usually done before the opening of the dura.

13. The bone flap may or may not be replaced. If swelling is anticipated, it is usually not replaced. If the flap is free and replaced, holes may be drilled in it, and the skull and suture material are inserted to secure it in place. Titanium plates and screws are also available for fixation of flaps. The craniotome or Midas Rex can be used for this purpose. During drilling a dura protector is used on the skull side. A brain spoon can serve as a dura protector.

14. Periosteum and muscle are approximated with #2-0 or 3-0 polyglactin 910 synthetic absorbable suture or #2-0 or 3-0 silk or Surgilon. The galea is closed with the same sutures as above. Skin closure can be interrupted or continuous and of silk or synthetic suture material, such as nylon, or skin staples.

Craniotomy for cerebrospinal rhinorrhea

Cerebrospinal rhinorrhea occurs when there is a tear of the dura mater, with evagination of the torn arachnoid through the dura mater into a hole or fracture in the skull communicating with one of the nasal sinuses or the nasal cavity. This results in leakage of CSF from the nose, which is frequently seen with a basal skull fracture. Repairing the defect is necessary to prevent air from being trapped under pressure in the brain and to prevent intracranial infection.

Operative Procedure

1. Usually a bifrontal craniotomy is carried out, and the dura mater is opened. The frontal lobes are elevated until the defect can be visualized. The surgeon may elect to use the microscope.
2. The dura mater is dissected from the orbital and cribriform plates.
3. The defect in the bone is defined, and the bony defect is repaired with a split-thickness graft from the skull or may be filled with methyl methacrylate or covered with tantalum mesh.
4. The dural defect may be closed with sutures, but usually some type of patch is placed over it. A piece of muscle, pericranium, fascia, gelatin foam, silicone sheeting, or freeze-dried dura substitute may be used. These may be sutured or glued. Some surgeons do not fasten the patch into place.
5. The dural incision is sutured, and the wound is closed.

A similar procedure is carried out in the temporal or suboccipital region to repair a defect in cerebrospinal otorrhea.

Craniotomy for intracranial aneurysm

An aneurysm is a vascular dilatation usually caused by a local defect in the arterial vascular wall. Within the cranial cavity an aneurysm may impinge on the third nerve or the optic chiasm. Hemorrhage into the subarachnoid space, causing sudden, severe headache, is generally the first evidence of an intracranial aneurysm.

Modern neurosurgical techniques have made operations on intracranial aneurysms more feasible. Fatal hemorrhage is the greatest hazard of the condition and of the operation. To prevent this, control of blood pressure as well as vascular supply to the region beyond the limits of the lesion may be required. Occasionally control of the cerebral circulation at the level of the cervical carotid artery is desired. The artery may be exposed and controlled by means of preplaced ligatures or clamps that can be tightened to occlude the vessel if bleeding occurs at the aneurysm site during the operation. This is a separate preliminary surgical procedure.

Procedural Considerations

Aneurysm clips and appliers of the surgeon's choice must be included with the instrumentation. Figs. 23-44 and 23-45 illustrate a few of the clips and appliers available.

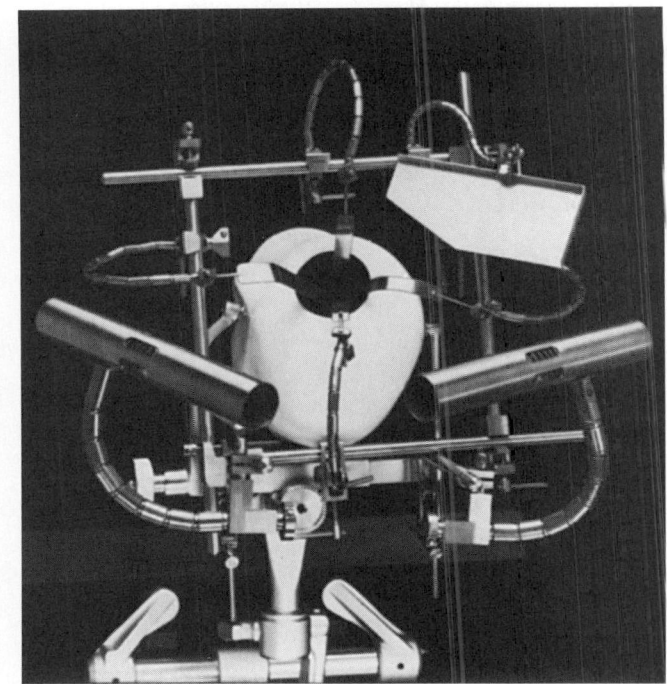

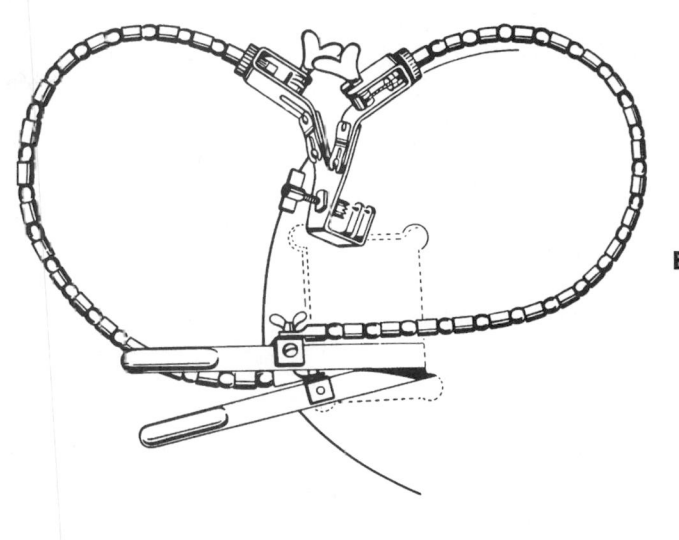

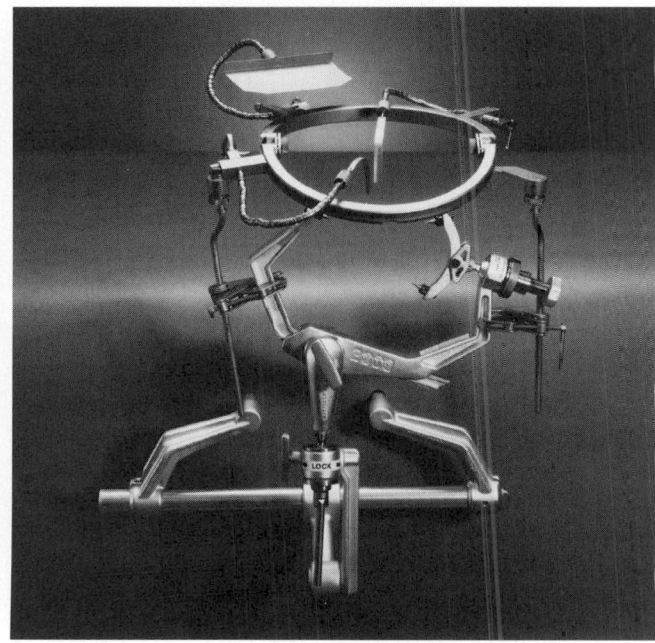

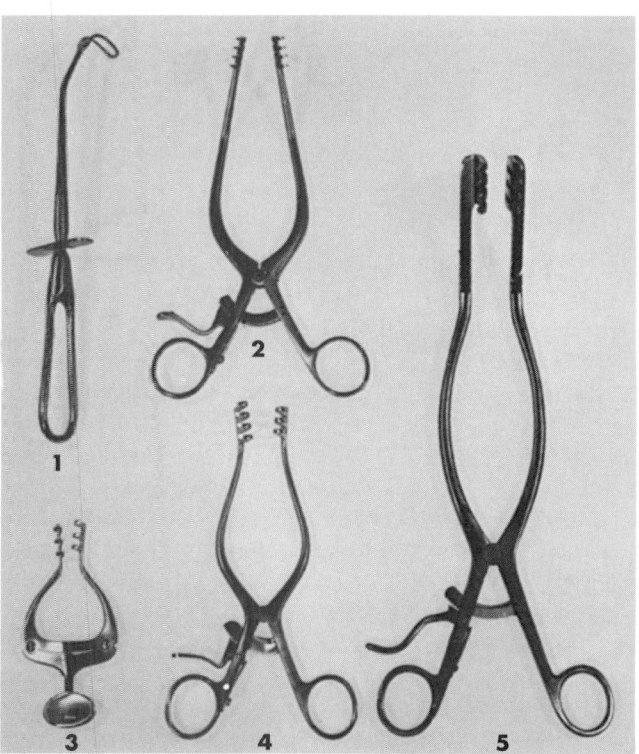

FIGURE 23–43 **A**, Greenberg retractor with blades. **B**, Leyla-Yasargil self-retaining retractor. **C**, Budde halo retractor with attachments. **D**, Retractors: *1*, Cushing subtemporal decompression retractor; *2*, Adson cerebellar retractor; *3*, Jansen mastoid retractor; *4*, Weitlaner retractor; *5*, Beckman laminectomy retractor.

A minimum of two appliers for each type of clip must be included; both temporary and permanent clips must be available. Temporary clips include Mayfield, McFadden, Drake, Yasargil, Sugita, and Schwartz, but Heifetz, Sundt-Kees, Olivecrona, Housepian, Scoville, Yasargil Phynox, and Sugita are types of permanent aneurysm clips. Today most clips have been updated with an alloy that is MRI compatible. Permanent clips can be removed from the vessel if necessary. The clip appliers serve as clip removers.

Aneurysm clips should never be compressed between the fingers. Clips should be compressed only when seated in their appliers. Once a clip has been compressed, it should be discarded. Clips that have been compressed may

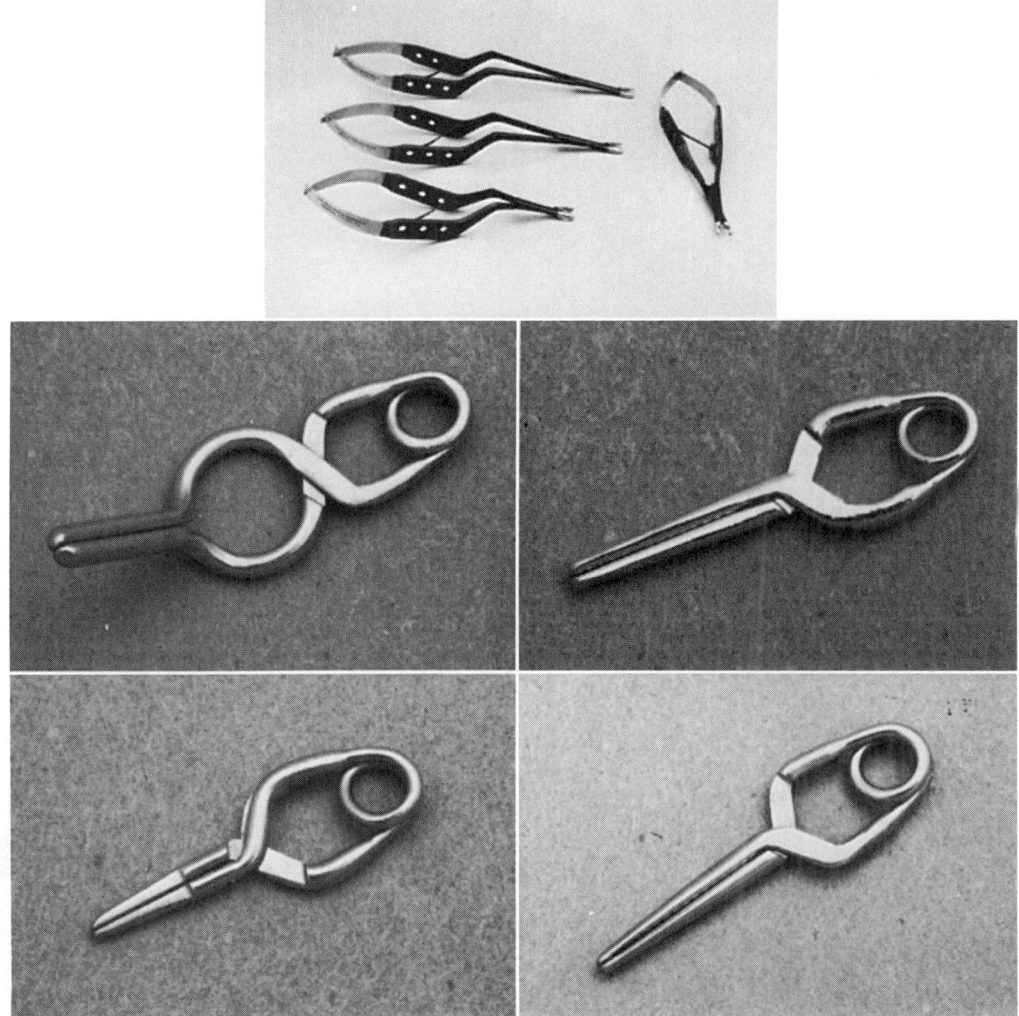

FIGURE 23-44   Yasargil microaneurysm, standard aneurysm clips and appliers.

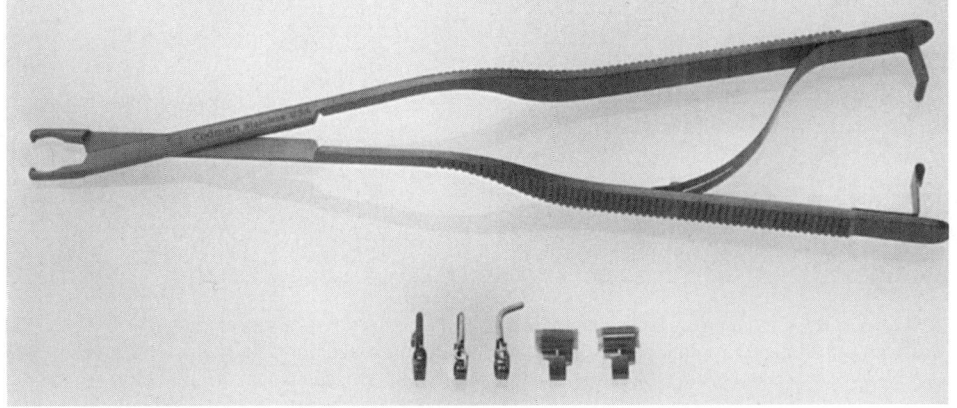

FIGURE 23-45   Sundt aneurysm clips and applier.

be sprung and may slip, causing complications such as bleeding or compression of another vessel or a nerve.

The full armamentarium of aneurysm-occlusion tools should be available for the surgeon. Besides clips, fast-setting aneuroplastic resinous material, a piece of temporal muscle, ligature carriers, or any other material requested by the surgeon should be in the room and ready to use. Fine silk ligatures and hemostatic clips, with or without bipolar coagulation of the neck of the aneurysm, have also been used successfully.

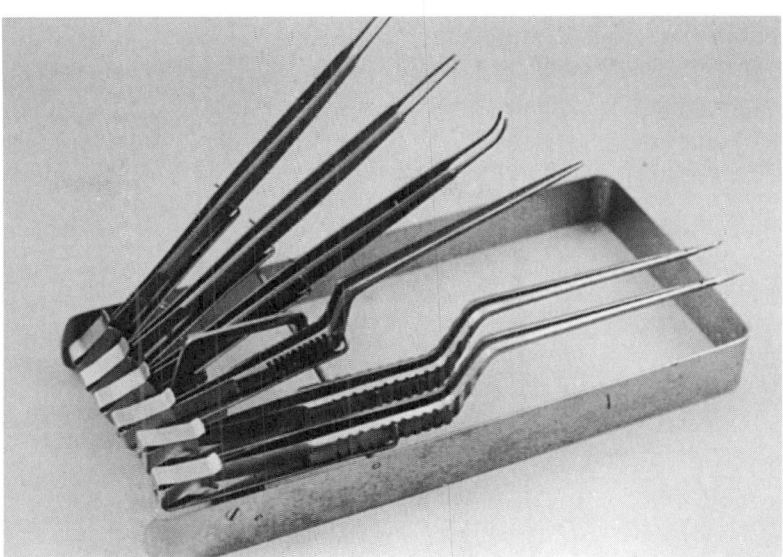

FIGURE 23-46 Microscissors and forceps in rack.

A basic craniotomy setup is required in addition to the special items mentioned. Supplementary suction must be immediately available on the field to prevent hemorrhage from obscuring the surgeon's vision if the aneurysm dome ruptures during operation and for removing smoke resulting from laser dissection. A cell saver unit should be available for reprocessing of blood for replacement when significant blood loss is expected.

Operative Procedure

1. A frontal, frontotemporal, or bifrontal craniotomy may be done to approach an aneurysm in the area of the circle of Willis. The bifrontal approach requires extra scalp clips and hemostatic forceps. All aneurysm instruments preferred by the surgeon must be included.

2. After the dura mater has been opened, a self-retaining brain retractor is placed, and the optic nerve and subarachnoid cisterns are exposed. The olfactory nerve may be coagulated and divided with a long scissors for better exposure.

3. The operating microscope is positioned. Microinstruments, including a micropolar bayonet, are used (Figs. 23-46 to 23-56).

4. Bridging veins are coagulated with bipolar coagulating forceps. Irrigation, which may be a part of the bipolar unit, is necessary during bipolar coagulation.

5. The covering arachnoidal webs are dissected away with microdissectors, hooks, elevators, scissors, knives, forceps, a diamond microknife, and an irrigating bipolar unit.

6. Careful dissection of the arachnoid and clear visualization of the neck of the aneurysm without rupture of the dome are the aims of the surgeon.

7. The parent arteries are identified and freed so that they can be occluded with a temporary clip if neces-

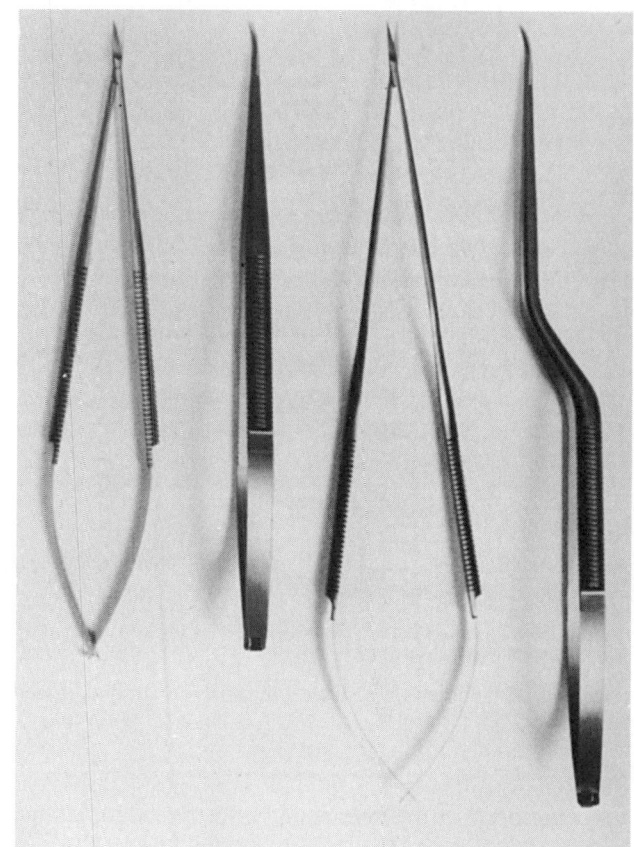

FIGURE 23-47 Rhoton titanium microscissors.

sary. Other structures, such as the optic chiasma and optic nerves, are identified.

8. As the surgeon works slowly toward the dome and neck of the aneurysm, the patient's blood pressure can be lowered for easier control of hemorrhage, should the aneurysm rupture.

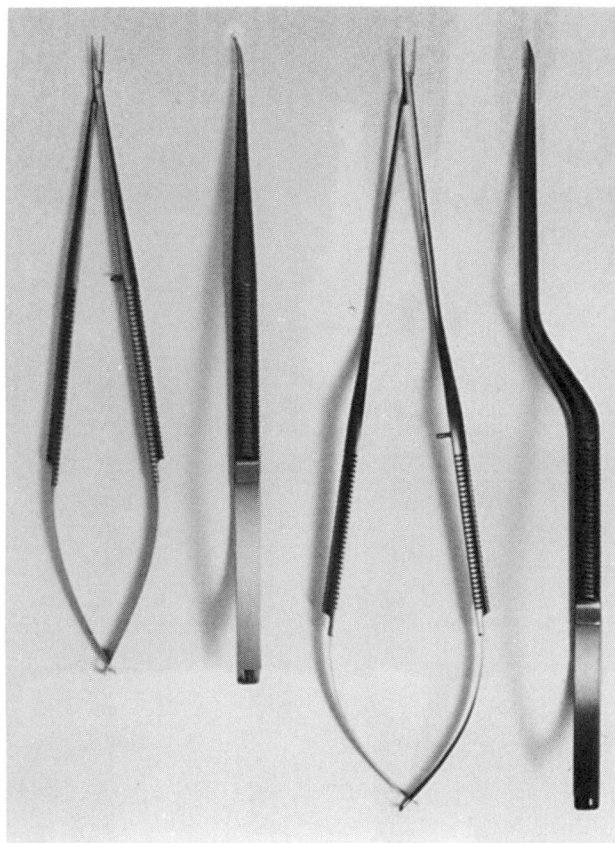

FIGURE 23-48 Rhoton microsurgical needle holders.

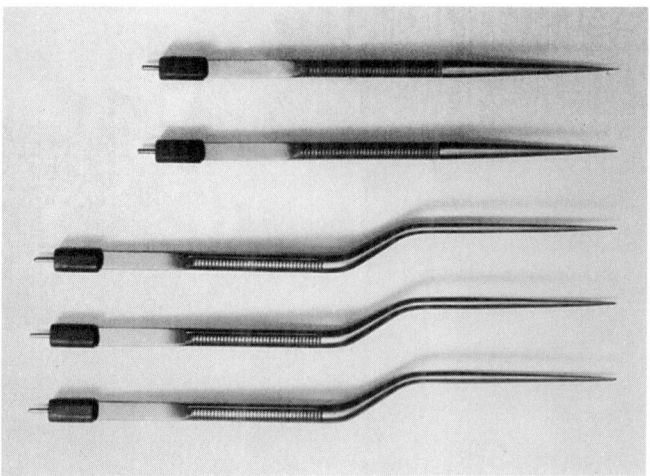

FIGURE 23-50 Rhoton microsurgical bipolar forceps, straight and bayonet.

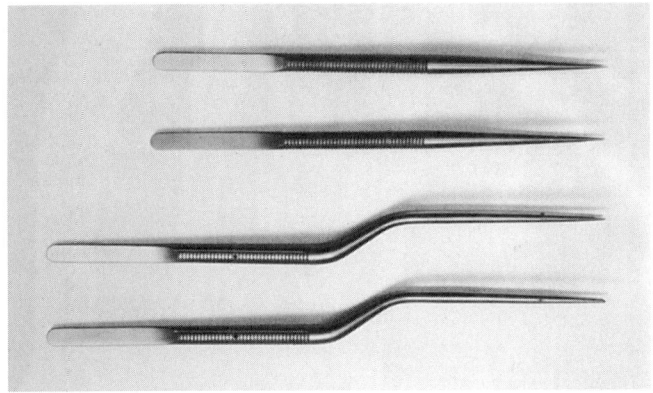

FIGURE 23-49 Rhoton microsurgical forceps, straight and bayonet.

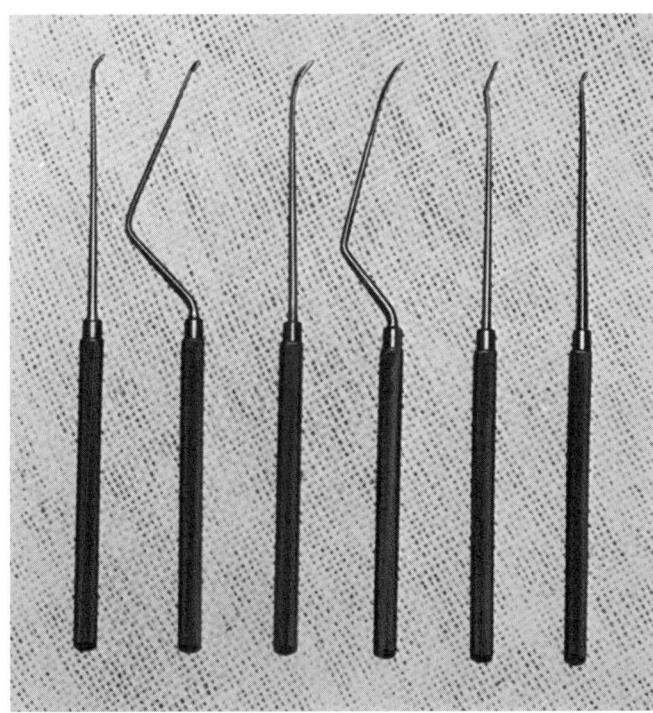

FIGURE 23-51 Malis microsurgical instruments. *Left to right*, Semisharp dissector, curette, two elevators, sharp dissector, round dissector.

9a. If the neck of the aneurysm can be isolated, a clip is placed across it. Clips such as the Sundt-Kees and Heifetz have Teflon linings and can be used to approach the aneurysm from a 180-degree angle to avoid excessive manipulation and traction of the parent vessel, if the neck is on the underside of the vessel. These clips support the vessel and serve as a clip graft.

9b. When clipping is not feasible, wrapping the aneurysm with muslin has good results.

10. As soon as the aneurysm has been occluded, the blood pressure is returned to normal, and the aneurysm site is checked for bleeding. When the surgeon is satisfied that the operative field is dry, wound closure is begun.

Craniotomy for arteriovenous malformation

An arteriovenous malformation consists of thin-walled vascular channels that connect arteries and veins without the usual intervening capillaries. These vascular lesions may be microscopic or massive.

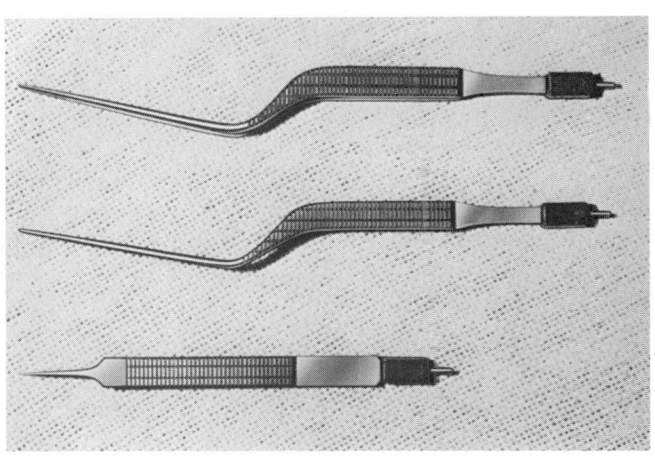

FIGURE 23-52   Malis titanium bipolar forceps.

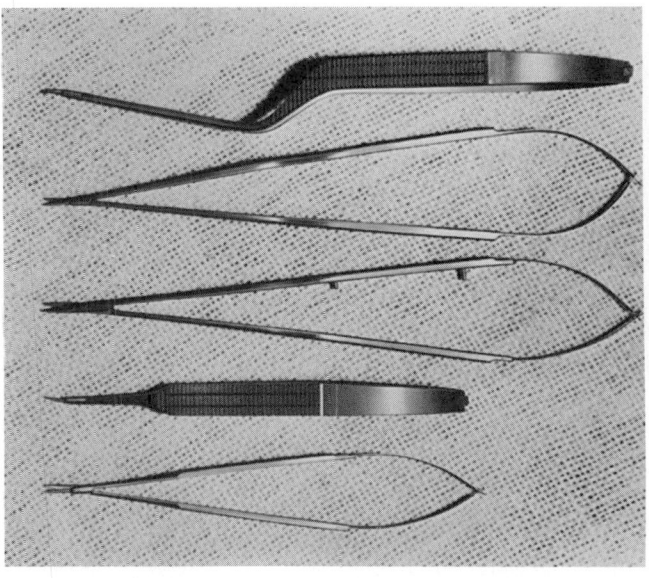

FIGURE 23-54   Malis microsurgical scissors.

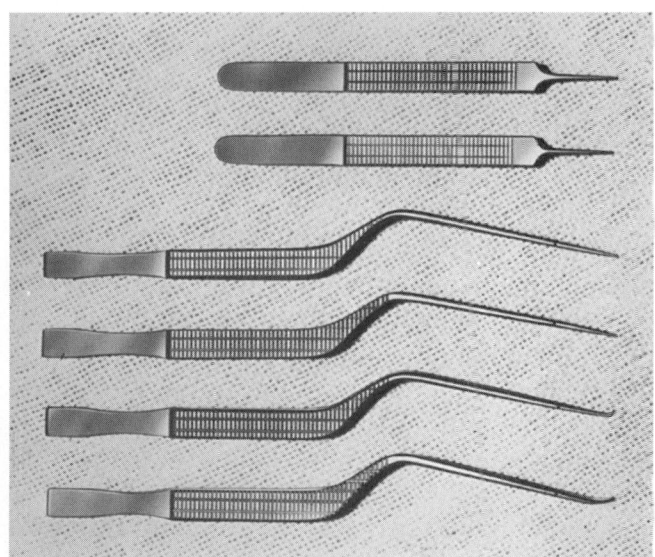

FIGURE 23-53   Malis microforceps (titanium), straight and bayonet.

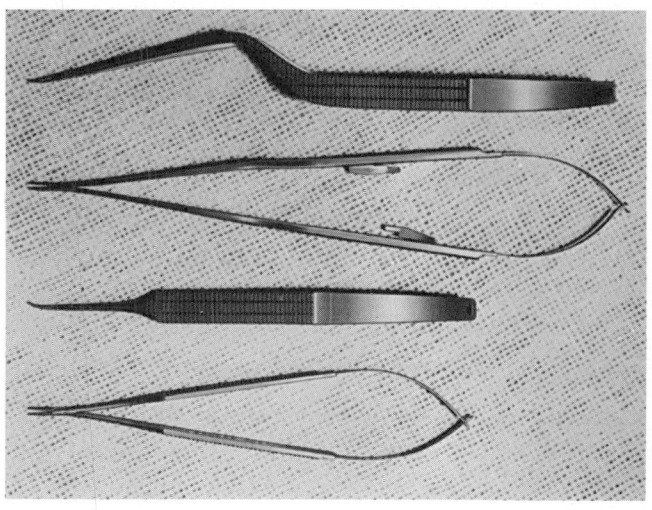

FIGURE 23-55   Malis microsurgical needle holders.

Malformations vary widely in size, area of involvement, and structure. Arteriovenous fistulas may be congenital or may result from trauma or disease. Vascular anomalies may also give rise to subarachnoid or intracerebral hemorrhage or may have extensive irritative effects and cause focal or generalized seizures.

These lesions are difficult to treat successfully. Feeding vessels can be clipped with or without partial removal of the lesion. Total removal, when possible, gives best results. Microsurgical techniques and the laser have made total removal without devastating injury to surrounding brain tissue and vessels possible in many cases.

Other methods of treating these malformations have been tried. One successful method has been with the Gamma knife. Only a few health care facilities offer this procedure; however the technology is becoming more available. Another method is preoperative embolization, which makes dissection much easier.

Operative Procedure

1. A supratentorial or infratentorial craniotomy is done, depending on the location of the lesion.
2. The feeding arteries are exposed a distance from the malformation, traced toward it, and then occluded a short distance before they penetrate its substance. This spares as many of the arteries to the brain as possible. The feeding arteries may be occluded by clipping, electrosurgical coagulation, ligation, or laser beam coagulation.
3. The malformation is dissected out with suction and

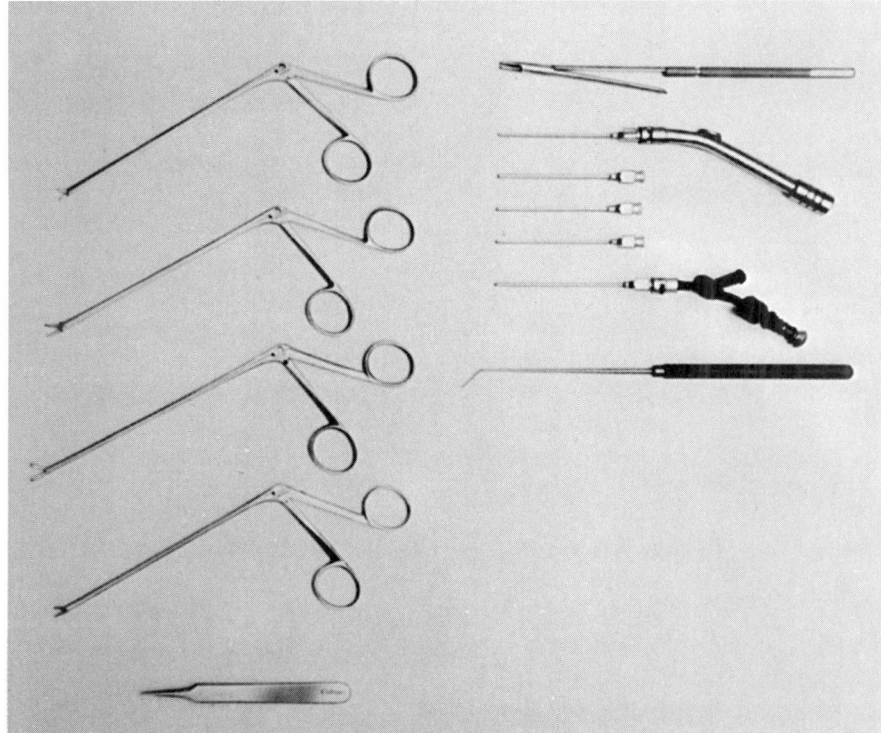

FIGURE 23-56 Microinstruments for neurosurgical procedures. *Bottom to top, left,* Forceps, rongeurs, and scissors; *right,* arachnoid knife, Malis suction-coagulation handle and four tips, Cadac microsuction handle and tip, blade breaker and holder.

bayonet forceps. Additional vessels are clipped or coagulated along the way. Usually one or more draining veins are left to be ligated as the last step in the removal. Closure and dressing are as described for craniotomy.

Craniotomy for intracranial revascularization

Although infrequently performed, the microbypass technique, developed in 1967, is used to shunt blood flow around an occluded portion of the internal carotid artery or the middle cerebral artery by anastomosing the superficial temporal artery to the middle cerebral artery distal to the occlusion. The procedure may also be used for revascularization for giant aneurysm, arteriovenous malformations, and tumor.

Procedural Considerations

Craniotomy for intracranial revascularization, although brief in description, is long and tedious; 7 hours is not unusual. Positioning is crucial to prevent pressure on superficial nerves, vessels, and vulnerable skin areas. Blood gas monitoring and arterial pressure readings are done routinely during the procedure. An arterial line may be placed before the patient's arrival in the surgery department or as a preliminary procedure in the operating room. Sterile and unsterile probes for the Doppler ultrasonic scanners should be available.

Operative Procedure

1. The first stage is reflection of the scalp flap on the operative side to expose the superficial temporal artery for dissection. Care must be taken in placing the hemostatic scalp clips to make sure that they are farther apart than usual to prevent compromise of the scalp circulation after diversion of the flow of the temporal artery. Care also must be taken to prevent injury to the temporal artery as the scalp incision is made and the flap is reflected.

2. After the superficial temporal artery is identified, the microscope is positioned, and the microinstrumentation is put to use.

3. The portion of the temporal artery to be used is freed but not occluded until the time of anastomosis. It may be supported and covered with Gelfoam or cottonoid material soaked in a papaverine solution. Papaverine helps prevent vessel spasm.

4. The temporal muscle is incised and retracted with fishhook retractors to begin the second stage of the procedure.

5. A burr hole is made into the frontotemporal area and enlarged with a rongeur.

6. The dura mater is opened and anchored over the bone edges with silk or black braided nylon sutures. The self-retaining brain retractor is used.

7. The middle cerebral artery is located, and a branch

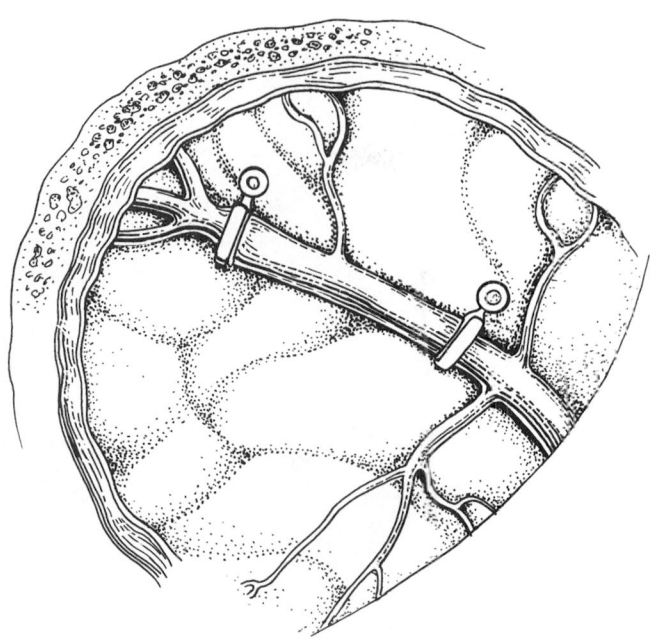

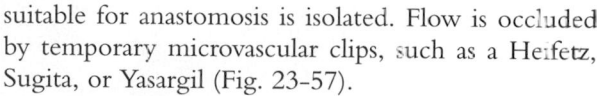

FIGURE 23-57   Exposure of middle cerebral artery with clips.

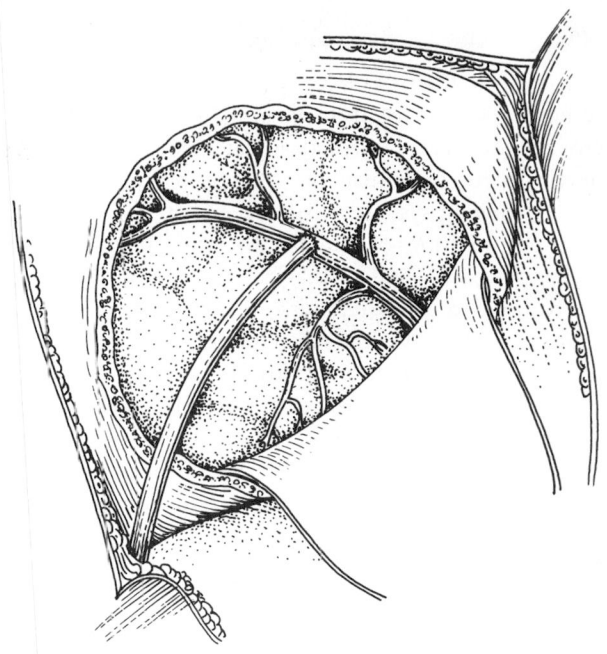

FIGURE 23-58   Final anastomosis of superficial temporal artery to middle cerebral artery.

suitable for anastomosis is isolated. Flow is occluded by temporary microvascular clips, such as a Heifetz, Sugita, or Yasargil (Fig. 23-57).

8. Flow also is occluded in the superficial temporal artery, the artery is cut, and an end-to-side anastomosis is completed with very fine suture material, such as #10-0 monofilament nylon (Fig. 23-58).

9. The temporary microvascular clips are removed. The vessels are observed for patency and flow.

10. The wound is closed, and dressings are applied.

Craniotomy for pituitary tumor (craniopharyngioma, optic glioma, and other suprasellar and parasellar tumors)
Procedural Considerations

The setup is as for craniotomy with these additional pituitary instruments: Ray curettes (ring, sharp); angulated suction tips, right and left; large and small spinal needles, #22 or #24; curettes, small, #0 through #4-0; and a Luer-Lok syringe, 10 ml.

Operative Procedure

1. Either a bifrontal or a unilateral incision is made into the frontal or frontotemporal region. Most unilateral approaches are carried out from the right side.

2. Wet brain retractors over moist cottonoids are inserted for exposure of the optic chiasma and the pituitary gland. The frontal and often the temporal lobes are retracted. The olfactory nerve may be coagulated and divided with scissors.

3. A DeMartel, Edinborough, Yasargil, or Greenberg

self-retaining retractor is placed to maintain exposure. Aneurysm clips and applicators should be available to control unexpected bleeding from major vessels. The microscope may be moved into place.

4. Using a syringe with moistened plunger and a #22 or 24 spinal needle, the surgeon attempts to aspirate the contents of the tumor to guard against inadvertently entering an aneurysm or vessel.

5. The tumor capsule is coagulated for hemostasis and incised with a #11 blade on a long knife handle. With a pituitary rongeur or cup forceps, the tumor is removed.

6. Small stainless steel, copper, or Ray curettes, as well as suction, may be used during tumor removal.

7. A wide clip may be applied to the stalk of the pituitary, which may then be cut distally. A long angulated scissors is especially helpful for this.

8. If the tumor capsule is to be removed, bayonet forceps, cup forceps, nerve hooks, and suction aid in the dissection.

9. Closure and dressing are as described for craniotomy.

For pituitary adenoma with a prefixed chiasma, the surgeon may elect to remove the anterior wall of the sphenoidal sinus and sella turcica with an air drill to gain access to the tumor.

In the case of craniopharyngioma, extreme caution must be used in removing fluid from the capsule because the fluid is extremely irritating and may cause chemical leptomeningitis. Calcified pieces of tumor are dissected and removed in the same manner as the capsule of a pituitary adenoma. This is an extremely difficult procedure because of deposits on the carotid arteries, optic nerves,

23-2 RESEARCH HIGHLIGHT

In more than 90% of primary malignant brain tumors death occurs from local recurrence within a 2 cm margin. A new method of delivery has been developed to maximize the benefit of chemotherapy while reducing systemic toxicity. This is the implantation, at the time of surgery for tumor removal, of biodegradable polymers that release chemotherapy to the tumor site over the course of several weeks. Initial clinical studies have indicated that patients receive the benefit of chemotherapy to the brain tumor without suffering the inconvenience or systemic complications of prolonged chemotherapy. The patient receives two types of therapy—surgery and chemotherapy—at the same time. Additionally, these studies indicate that survival may be increased.

The approach of using biodegradable polymers to deliver prolonged local concentrations of a drug while minimizing systemic exposure has many potential applications. For example, research is underway to develop various forms of biodegradable polymers capable of releasing drugs such as antineoplastics, antibiotics, and steroids over hours, weeks, months, or years. They also will be designed in various forms, (such as microspheres), not only to treat brain tumors but also for use in many types of cancer. They will have the potential to be implanted stereotactically or infused angiographically.

From Barker, E. (1994). *Neuroscience nursing*. St. Louis: Mosby.

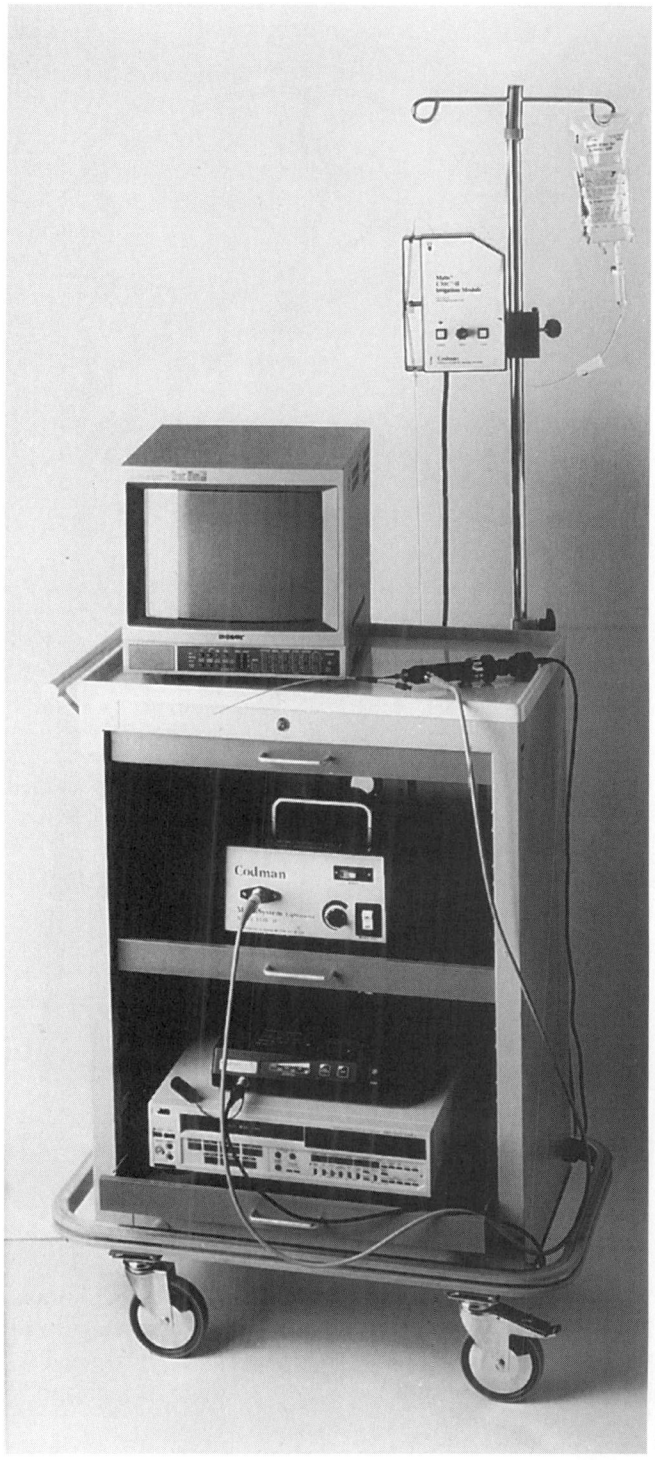

FIGURE 23-59 Neuroendoscopy system.

and optic chiasma. The tumor capsule is often left behind on the hypothalamus to avoid stripping off blood vessels supplying this structure. Many moist cottonoid strips are used to protect the surrounding areas from the cystic contents.

Suprasellar meningiomas usually arise from the tuberculum sellae just anterior to the optic nerves and chiasma. Tumor removal is similar to that of a pituitary adenoma except that the electrosurgical cutting loop may be used to excavate the interior of the tumor. After the tumor has been removed, the site of its attachment to the dura is thoroughly coagulated to prevent recurrence. Other meningiomas arising at the base of the skull are treated by similar techniques.

Biodegradable polymers that release chemotherapeutic agents over several weeks are being implanted in patients with primary brain tumors at the time of surgery for tumor removal. Studies indicate that the survival rate may be increased with this treatment modality (Research Highlight 23-2).

Less invasive approaches to intracranial surgery are being developed and performed. Endoscopic intracranial surgery was first addressed around the turn of the century,

but recently the technique has been enhanced and has gained popularity among neurosurgeons.[2]

Laser-assisted neuroendoscopy has proved to be a valuable tool in both diagnosis and treatment of central nervous system conditions in and also adjacent to the ventricular system. The neuroendoscope has three ports: one for viewing, one for illumination, and one for pulsed irrigation and introduction of a laser fiber (Fig. 23-59).

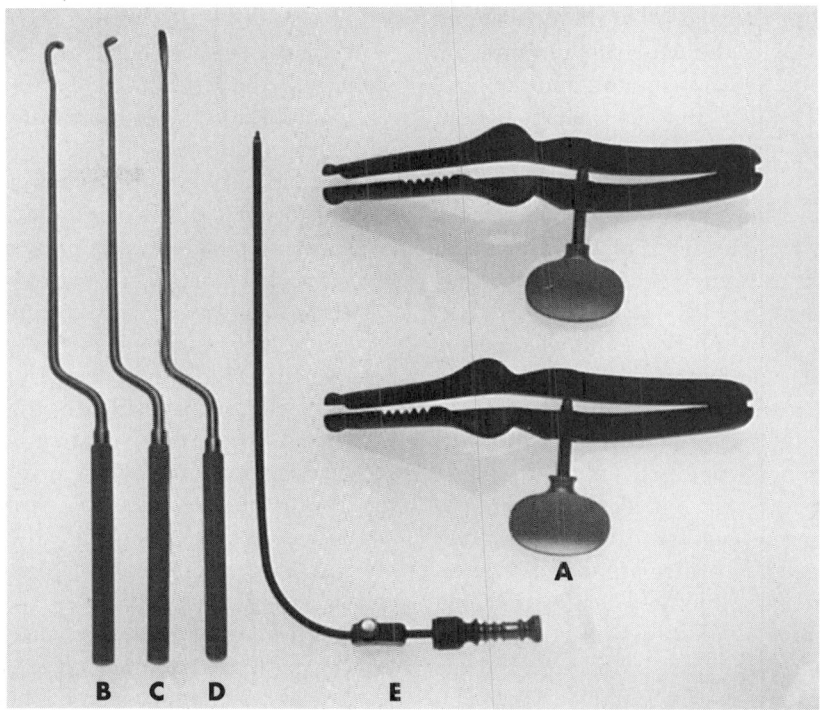

FIGURE 23-60   Special instruments for transsphenoidal hypophysectomy. **A**, Hardy's modified Cushing bivalve speculum. **B**, Hardy's enucleator. **C**, Hardy's enucleator. **D**, Hardy's dissector. **E**, Hardy's suction tubes.

Neuroendoscopy can be used in diagnosing small seeding tumors, cysts, and infectious granulation, which may be seen before detection is made by MRI or CT imaging. Biopsy samples from small tumors can be collected with microforceps introduced through the endoscope. Other applications include the following:

- Placement of new ventricular shunt catheter
- Removal of proximal shunt occluded by choroid plexus
- Choroid coagulation/plexectomy
- Third ventriculostomy
- Transseptal fenestration
- Ventriculocystostomy
- Tumor biopsy and excision

It is of utmost importance that the perioperative nurse have a systematic method to manage the extensive setup and implementation of neuroendoscopy procedures.[3]

Transsphenoidal Hypophysectomy

Endocrine pituitary disorders, such as Cushing's syndrome, acromegaly, malignant exophthalmos, and hypopituitarism resulting from intrasellar tumors as well as nonpituitary disorders such as advanced metastatic carcinoma of the breast and prostate, diabetic retinopathy, and uncontrollable severe diabetes have been successfully treated by transsphenoidal hypophysectomy. Rapid access to the sella turcica is achieved. Complete extracapsular enucleation of the pituitary in cases of hypophysectomy and possible complete removal of small pituitary tumors, with the remaining normal portion of the gland being left

intact, can be obtained. Patients are relatively free from pain after surgery. No visible scar remains.

Procedural considerations

Transsphenoidal hypophysectomy is performed with the patient under light general endotracheal anesthesia, combined with a local anesthetic. The patient is placed in a semisitting position, with head against the headrest. A portable image intensifier is used. The horizontal beam is centered on the sella turcica. A subnasal midline rhinoseptal approach is used.

The face, mouth, and nasal cavity are prepared with an antiseptic solution. Infiltration of the nasal mucosa and the gingiva with a local anesthetic agent containing 1:2000 epinephrine is helpful in initiating submucosal elevation, as well as diminishing oozing from the mucosa. A sterile adhesive plastic drape is applied to the entire face with additional sterile drapes to ensure a relatively sterile operative field. Sterile sponges or cotton is placed in the patient's mouth so that only the upper gum margin is exposed.

A biopsy setup is required as well as special instruments (Fig. 23-60). The operating microscope is used for the cranial portion of the procedure.

Operative procedure

1. Using the biopsy setup on a separate small Mayo table, the surgeon may take a small piece of muscle from the previously prepared thigh to be used later in the procedure. This is kept in a moist sponge.

2. An incision is made in the middle of the upper gum margin. The soft tissues of the upper lip and nose are elevated from the bone with an elevator, and the nasal septum is exposed. The nasal mucosa is elevated from either side of the nasal septum, which is flanked by the blades of a Cushing bivalved speculum. The inferior third of the anterior cartilaginous septum and osseous vomer are resected, as is the floor of the sphenoidal sinus, exposing the sinus cavity. The floor of the sella turcica can be identified.

3. The floor is opened with a sphenoidal punch, and the dura mater is incised. The hypophyseal cavity should be opened only in patients undergoing surgery for pituitary adenoma. In these patients the gland is explored, and the tumor is identified and removed.

4. The extracapsular cleavage plane is identified, and the superior surface of the pituitary is dissected until the stalk and the diaphragmatic orifice are found. Cotton pledgets are applied for exposure, hemostasis, and protection of structures.

5. The stalk is sectioned low with a sickle knife, and the lateral posterior and inferior surfaces of the pituitary are dissected with an enucleator.

6. The gland is removed in toto, and the sellar cavity may be packed with muscle obtained previously from the thigh to prevent CSF leakage. The floor is reconstructed with cartilage from the nasal septum.

7. Antibiotic powder may be used and nasal packing introduced for 2 days. The gingiva incision is closed with suture of the surgeon's preference.

Some surgeons prefer to perform this operation by means of a lateral rhinotomy with a transantral-transsphenoidal approach. An ear, nose, and throat (ENT) surgeon may do the initial opening, depending on surgeon preference. If an ENT surgeon does assist, a separate setup is available.

Craniectomy

Craniectomy is incision into the skull and removal of bone by enlarging one or more burr holes using rongeurs to gain access to the underlying structures.

A craniectomy procedure may be required to remove tumors, hematomas, scars, and infections of the bone. Craniectomy is also indicated as treatment for craniosynostosis in infants and to relieve pressure on the brain from depressed bone or internal hemorrhage resulting from trauma. Today large craniotomies may be performed for acute trauma.

Craniectomy with evacuation of epidural or subdural hematoma

After trauma, decompression of the brain, as well as removal and drainage of blood clots and collections of liquefied blood from outside or beneath the dura mater, is accomplished.

Operative Procedure

1. A linear or small horseshoe incision is made over the site of the lesion. The initial procedure is similar to craniotomy. One or more burr holes are made. A bone flap is not turned.

2. If a blood clot or collection of bloody fluid is found outside or beneath the dura mater, the burr hole is further enlarged, with a Kerrison or double-action rongeur, until adequate exposure is obtained. Bone edges are waxed, and cottonoid strips are put into position along the edges.

3. Clot and fluid are evacuated, and hemostasis is accomplished with coagulation or the use of hemostatic clips.

4. In cases of chronic subdural hematoma the inner and outer membranes are stripped and coagulated.

5. The brain is irrigated using catheters or employing an Asepto or bulb syringe directly. Large amounts of saline irrigating solution are used until the return appears clear.

6. A silver or a hemostatic clip may be placed on the cortex at the site of a small incision. Another clip is placed on the dura mater. These are tag clips that are visible on postoperative x-ray films to check the bleeding site.

7. A small drain or a polyethylene or red rubber catheter may be inserted subdurally for additional drainage, or a closed drainage system, such as the Jackson-Pratt, may be used through a separate stab wound in the skin posterior to the incision. Additional burr holes are made during the course of the procedure to be sure clots in other areas do not remain undetected and untreated.

Suboccipital craniectomy for posterior fossa exploration

Perforation and removal of the posterior occipital bone and exposure of the foramen magnum and arch of the atlas are done to remove a lesion in the posterior fossa (Fig. 23-61).

Procedural Considerations

Depending on the type and size of the lesion, the exposure may be unilateral or bilateral. The operation may include the removal of the arch of the atlas. This approach gives the surgeon access to the fourth ventricle, the cerebellum, the brainstem, and the cranial nerves.

The sitting position may be preferred, but the park bench position is also utilized. An extra-high instrument table or two Mayo stands and standing stool are necessary for the nurse.

Operative Procedure

1. Before the initial surgical incision, an occipital burr hole is done for placement of a ventricular catheter. This can be done as a separate procedure or concurrently with the procedure.

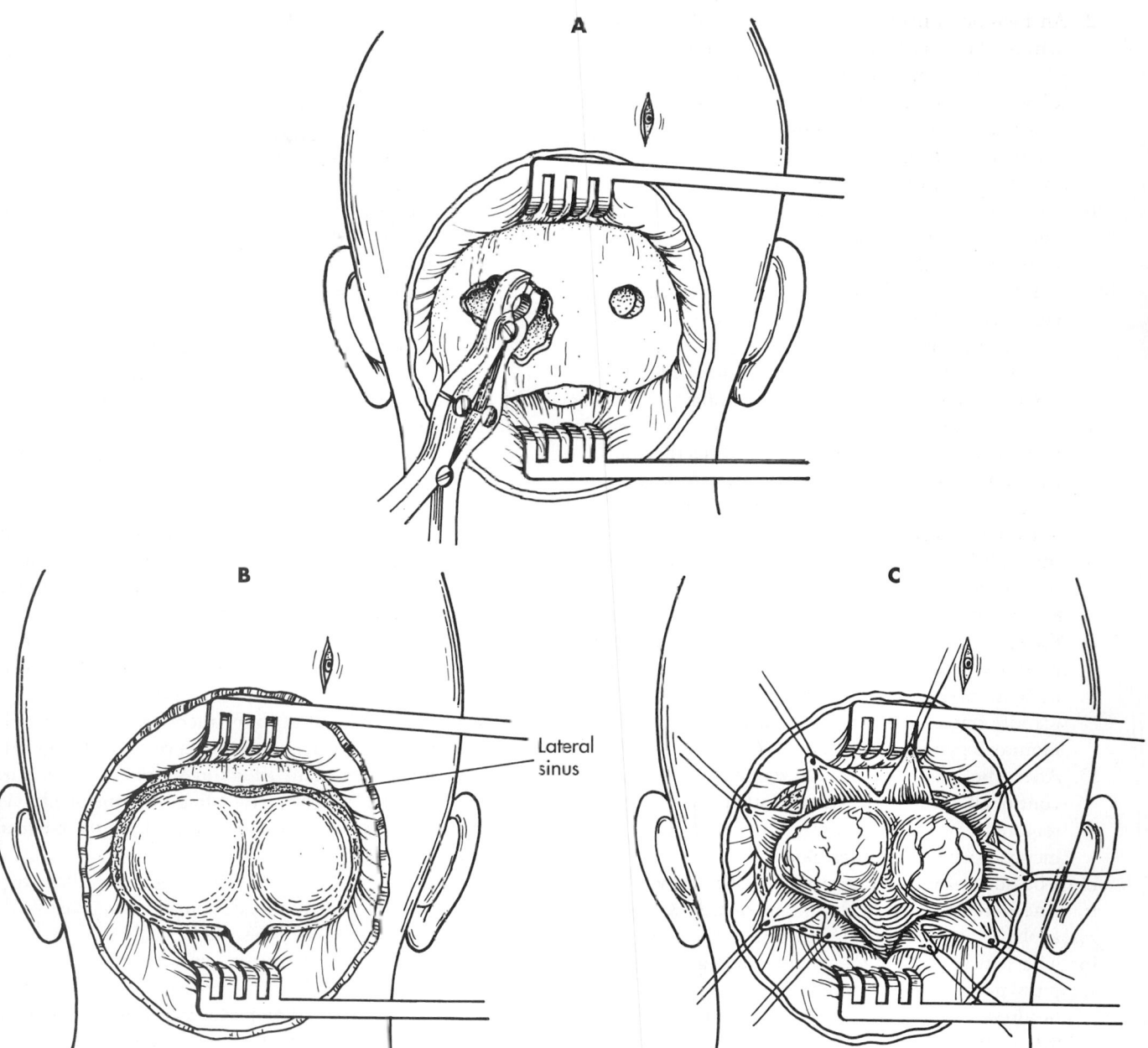

A

B

Lateral
sinus

C

FIGURE 23–61   Suboccipital craniectomy. **A**, Craniectomy being performed. **B**, Dura mater exposed. **C**, Dura mater incised and cerebellum exposed.

2. The incision may be made from mastoid tip to mastoid tip, in an arch curving upward 2 cm above the external occipital protuberance.
3. Scalp bleeding is controlled, and the skin flap is retracted with the Weitlaner retractors.
4. A periosteal elevator is used to free the muscles, which are then divided with an electrosurgical blade using cutting current. The incision is deepened. A self-retaining retractor is used. The laminae of the first two or three cervical vertebrae may be exposed.
5. One or more holes are drilled in the occipital bone. If a Hudson brace is used, the cerebellar extension is

attached. The Midas Rex (see Fig 23-30) or Anspach drill is very beneficial for this approach because it reduces the time needed to make the opening.
6. The dura mater is stripped from the bone. A double-action rongeur, Raney punch, Kerrison punch, or Leksell rongeur is used to enlarge the hole and smooth the edges.
7. Osseous and cerebellar venous bleeding is controlled at each step with bone wax, Gelfoam, and electrocoagulation to prevent air embolism.
8. The dura mater is opened. A small brain spoon or cottonoid strip is used to protect the brain as the initial

nick is extended with scalpel or scissors. The dural incision is continued until the cerebellar hemispheres, the vermis, and the tonsils can be visualized. Hemostatic clips are used on the dura mater as necessary. Dural traction sutures are placed.

9. The cisterna magna is opened, emptied of spinal fluid, and protected with a cottonoid strip.

10. The cerebellar hemispheres are inspected. Bleeding is controlled with the bipolar coagulator. A needle may be introduced through a small coagulated incision into the cerebellar hemisphere in an attempt to palpate or tap a deep lesion.

11. Brain retractors over cottonoid strips are placed for exposure. The handle of the retractor must be kept dry to avoid slippage in the surgeon's hand. However, the inserted edge should be wet to prevent damage or tears in the brain surface. These retractors may be positioned in areas that control respiration or other vital functions, so every effort must be made to avoid jarring these instruments in the operative field. When the pathologic entity is identified, a self-retaining retractor may be placed.

12. Long bayonet forceps, bayonet cup forceps, pituitary forceps, suction, and the electrosurgical loop tips may be used to remove the lesion. Clips may be used to aid in hemostasis. A nerve stimulator may be used to identify cranial nerves; evoked potentials for brainstem monitoring are becoming routine.

13. After the lesion has been removed and bleeding controlled, further checking for adequate hemostasis is required. Venous pressure in the patient's head is increased by the anesthesiologist.

14. The dura mater may be partially or completely closed. The muscle, fascia, and skin are closed. A dressing is applied.

15. The patient must remain anesthetized until the supine position is achieved and the prongs of the headrest are removed. Particular attention must be given to the patient's head when these prongs are removed to prevent tearing the scalp or damaging the eyes.

Subtemporal craniectomy for trigeminal exploration or rhizotomy

Trigeminal neuralgia (tic douloureux, fifth cranial nerve pain) is a condition characterized by brief, repeated attacks of excruciating pain in the face. Temporary relief of trigeminal neuralgia may be obtained by interruption of branches of the nerve divisions (ophthalmic, maxillary, and mandibular) by means of alcohol injection or surgical sectioning. This approach may also be used for exploration for trigeminal neuromas.

Procedural Considerations

The patient may be placed in the supine or sitting position, depending on the surgeon's preference.

Operative Procedure

1. A vertical temporal incision extending from the zygomatic process and through the temporal muscles and periosteum is made.

2. The soft tissue is freed from the bone with a periosteal elevator. The bone exposure is maintained with a self-retaining retractor.

3. A burr hole is made. The dura mater is freed from the underside of the temporal bone.

4. The burr hole is enlarged, with a double-action rongeur, to a diameter of about 2½ inches.

5. With a moist brain retractor, the dura mater overlying the temporal lobe is retracted upward. By means of blunt dissection with cottonoids held in bayonet forceps, the dura mater is elevated from the bony floor of the middle fossa.

6. The brain retractor is replaced by a self-retaining brain retractor placed deeper into the wound to hold up the temporal lobe and dura mater. The microscope provides light as well as magnification.

7. As the dura mater is elevated, the middle meningeal artery is seen as it leaves the foramen spinosum to join the dura mater. It is coagulated with bipolar bayonet forceps and may be clipped before being divided. A cottonoid or wax plug is packed into the foramen spinosum.

8. Additional blunt dissection uncovers the mandibular division of the trigeminal nerve and finally the trigeminal (gasserian) ganglion within its own dural sheath (dura propria). Bleeding is controlled with cottonoids and a hemostatic material such as Gelfoam and thrombin.

9. Some surgeons terminate the procedure after stripping the ganglion and its dura mater from that of the overlying temporal lobe. (The ganglion may be injected with saline solution, and the dura mater may be split.)

10. If a root section is to be performed, a #11 blade on a long knife handle is used to make an incision into the lateral rim of the dura propria. The sensory and motor roots of the nerve are defined with a fine nerve hook. The mandibular and maxillary sections of the root are usually divided. These are elevated with a nerve hook and divided with fine scissors or a fine blade. The ophthalmic portion of the root is spared, as is the motor root.

11. Absolute alcohol may be injected into the affected divisions of the nerve just distal to the ganglion.

12. Saline solution is injected into the dura mater overlying the temporal lobe to distend it.

13. The incision is closed, and dressings are applied.

Suboccipital craniectomy and decompression for trigeminal rhizotomy

Some surgeons prefer to section the posterior root of the trigeminal nerve by the suboccipital route.

Procedural Considerations

The position of the patient for suboccipital craniectomy is sitting, prone, or semilateral. To be prepared, the perioperative nurse must know during the planning phase (usually the day before the procedure is scheduled) which position the surgeon plans to use.

Operative Procedure

1. The incision is made vertically behind the mastoid process. A trephine or burr hole is made and enlarged with a rongeur.
2. The dura mater is opened. The cisterna magna is pierced to empty the CSF and permit backward retraction of the cerebellum. A brain spoon, brain spatula, or lighted retractor over moist strips of cottonoid is used to gently lift the cerebellar hemisphere. The eighth nerve is readily seen. The fifth nerve is approached by opening the arachnoid of the cisterna pontis and suctioning out the fluid. Veins are protected and bleeding is controlled by pressure over cottonoid strips.
3. The nerve and the vessels around it are identified. The nerve is decompressed by coagulating the vessel over the nerve or separating the vessel from the nerve with a Teflon pledget. The microscope facilitates microvascular decompression. The motor root medial and anterior to the sensory root is preserved.
4. The wound is closed.

Suboccipital craniectomy and glossopharyngeal nerve section

Posterior fossa exploration for glossopharyngeal neuralgia is occasionally necessary. The same posterior fossa approach is used as for trigeminal neuralgia. The cerebellar hemisphere of the affected side is gently elevated upward and toward the midline. The ninth, tenth, and eleventh nerves are identified and defined with bayonet forceps, nerve hooks, and fine dissectors. The ninth nerve and a portion of the tenth are consecutively elevated with a nerve hook and divided with a fine-tipped scissors.

Suboccipital craniectomy for acoustic neuroma

Usually the acoustic neuroma arises from the vestibular portion of the eighth cranial nerve within the auditory meatus. It is desirable, although not always possible, to remove the complete tumor without damage to the facial nerve.

Operative Procedure

1. The posterior fossa approach may be used. A unilateral straight paramedian incision is made.
2. The cerebellum is retracted gently upward with brain retractors and is cushioned with moist cottonoids. The lower cranial nerves are defined with a nerve or aneurysm hook. A cottonoid is placed over these nerves to protect them. Veins draining the tumor into the superior petrosal sinus are identified and either clipped or coagulated and cut.
3. The tumor is excavated and resected by methods similar to those employed to remove a pituitary adenoma.
4. A nerve stimulator may be used to identify the facial nerve. Use of the operating microscope is advantageous because of the many nerves and vessels in the area.
5. A high-speed air drill may be used to unroof the auditory canal and expose the remaining tumor. Constant irrigation is mandatory during drilling.

Very small tumors confined to the auditory canal may be approached by drilling directly through the temporal bone to open the auditory canal within the bone and avoid the posterior fossa.

Suboccipital craniectomy for Meniere's disease

Meniere's disease is characterized by recurrent explosive attacks of vertigo associated with nausea, vomiting, tinnitus, and progressive deafness. It is usually unilateral. The cause is obscure, and in intractable cases surgical section or partial section of the eighth nerve (acoustic) may be performed for relief. However, surgery is not often performed for Meniere's disease.

Operative Procedure

1. The cerebellum is approached through a lateral vertical incision behind the ear. The cerebellum on the affected side is retracted.
2. The eighth nerve is exposed with bayonet forceps and gentle manipulation. The nerve is freed from the arachnoid of the lateral cistern. It is separated from the underlying structures with a blunt nerve hook. Care is taken to prevent traction on the nearby seventh nerve (facial).
3. With fine scissors the vestibular fibers in the anterior half of the nerve are divided over a nerve hook. If the patient has useful hearing, the posterior auditory branches are preserved. Tinnitus may be relieved by section of the anterior fibers of the auditory portion of the nerve.
4. The dura mater and wound are closed.

Cranioplasty

Cranioplasty is performed for repair of a skull defect resulting from trauma, malformation, or a surgical procedure. Cranial defects covered by muscular areas need not be repaired. The purposes of cranioplasty are to relieve headache, vertigo, fear of injury, and local tenderness or throbbing; to prevent secondary injury to the underlying brain; and for cosmetic effect.

Procedural considerations

Many materials have been used to repair skull defects, including bone and cartilage, celluloid, metals such as Vitallium and tantalum, and synthetic resins such as methyl methacrylate and silicone rubber. All involve technical problems. The use of commercially prepared cranioplastic synthetics that supply the needed chemicals and mixing containers has simplified the procedures of shaping and molding the prosthesis. Sometimes heavy wire mesh is cut to the shape of the defect, and the methyl methacrylate is molded over the mesh.

Operative procedure

1. A scalp flap is turned, and the bony defect is exposed.
2. The edges of the defect are trimmed, and a ledge is formed to seat the prosthesis.
3. After the bone defect has been prepared so that it is slightly saucerized, the methyl methacrylate is mixed when one volume of liquid monomer is added to one volume of the powdered polymer. When this has formed a doughy mass, it is dropped into a sterile polyethylene bag. The soft plastic is then rolled onto a flat surface into the desired shape, leaving the thickness to the approximate depth of the skull edges. A sterile test tube, syringe barrel, or other round object can be used, although a stainless steel roller is preferred because of its weight and ease of use.
4. The soft cranioplastic material in the bag is placed over the skull defect and, through light pressing with the ends of the fingers, is fitted into the missing skull area. The plastic bag is stretched by assistants as the surgeon molds the plate into the defect and forms an overlapping bevel edge. This overlapping fringe keeps the plate from falling inside the skull, as the skull saucerization does.
5. When the heat of the chemical reactions begins, the plate is lifted out of the bony wound and removed from the polyethylene bag. Cool saline should be used on the flap while the exothermic reaction takes place.
6. When cool enough to handle, the excess material is trimmed away with bone rongeurs or cut with a saw and placed in the cranial defect.
7. A sterile carborundum wheel attached to the electrical bone saw or craniotome is used to smooth the rough spots and bevel the edges so that the plate will blend gradually with the skull.
8. Mixing and fitting the plate take about 7 minutes, as hardening does. Sutures may be used to hold the plate in place, generally at three or more points.

Microneurosurgery

Adaptation of the operating microscope for neurosurgery has resulted in improvement of many neurosurgical procedures and made new procedures possible. For years neurosurgeons have worn magnifying loupes to see small structures. Loupes usually have a magnification of 2 or 2.8. The microscope has a variety of magnifications ranging from 6 to 40, providing flexibility and precision. The coaxial illumination overcomes the difficulties of lighting neurosurgical wounds.

Use of the microscope restricts the surgeon's field of vision and mobility; therefore the scrub nurse must be proficient. The operative field, unless video monitoring is available, cannot be seen. The scrub nurse must understand the surgical procedure, know the anatomy, know the names and uses of all the microinstruments, and be able to place each instrument in the surgeon's hand without delay so that the surgeon will be able to use the instrument without readjusting it. The scrub nurse must make it possible for the surgeon to perform the operation without looking away from the operating field. Instruments must be kept free from blood and tissue during use because the microscope also magnifies debris on the instruments, occluding the structure the surgeon is about to approach. The perioperative nursing team must understand the degree of stress these difficult procedures place on the neurosurgeon.

Microneurosurgical instruments are expensive and delicate. Instructions for handling, cleaning, sterilizing, and storing these instruments should be followed. An instrument that is sprung, bent, dulled, hooked, or in any way damaged must never be handed to a surgeon for use but must be repaired or replaced.

Existing microsurgical instruments have been modified and adapted to the requirements of neurosurgery. These instruments often possess the following characteristics: bayonet shape, so that the surgeon's hand remains outside the line of vision and the beam of the microscope light; finely sprung and fluted grip; long length for access to deep structures; and slender and delicate tips that take up as little space as possible.

Very fine microsutures are available. The neurosurgeon may want to open the suture pack and ready the suture for use. However, the scrub nurse should be able to open and handle a delicate suture without damaging it. Each time the surgeon must look away and then back to the surgical field, open wound time and anesthesia time are increased while the surgeon becomes reoriented to the field. Therefore the assistance the scrub nurse gives the surgeon saves time and directly benefits the patient.

Microsurgical techniques have been applied to cranial, spinal, and peripheral nerve operations. Perhaps microneurovascular surgery is the area in which the most progress has been made. However, patient outcomes after microsurgical procedures on cranial nerves, spinal nerves, and cord tumors and especially for repair of peripheral nerve injuries have been enhanced.

Some procedures in which microsurgery is of value are posterior fossa explorations, especially for tumors of the fourth ventricle or cerebellopontine angle; translabyrinthine and transpetrosal removal of small acoustic neuromas, with resulting preservation of the facial nerve; and transsphenoidal hypophysectomy and transsphenoidal operations for small intracranial tumors, such as pituitary adenomas or even craniopharyngiomas. Transclival operations are also performed. Small vessel endarterectomy, cerebral arterial bypass, cerebral aneurysm surgery, and excision of arteriovenous malformations are done under the microscope. Microsurgery also has advantages in the treatment of tumors and arteriovenous malformations of the spinal cord.

Stereotaxic Procedures

The use of complex mechanisms to locate and destroy target structures in the brain is known as *stereotactics*. Predetermined anatomic landmarks are used as guides. Special head-fixation devices have been developed by surgeons and engineers for use with radiography, fluoroscopy, CT scans, and MRI to permit accurate placement of a probe directed at the target area. Stereotaxic procedures can also be done on the spinal cord. Common target areas for the stereotaxic approach include tumors, the basal ganglia, the thalamus, the hypophysis, aneurysms, and anterolateral spinal tracts. Target areas undergo biopsy or are destroyed by chemical or mechanical means or electrically stimulated to control intractable pain. Stereotaxic procedures are also done to place electrodes in various regions of the brain to determine the site of origin of seizures. Lesions in target areas are made to perform biopsies and remove tumors, alleviate pain, abolish movement disorders, change endocrine balance to reverse such conditions as retinopathy, acromegaly, and endocrine-sensitive cancers, and obliterate aneurysms.[1]

Operative procedure

The patient's head is placed into the stereotaxic frame, and the patient is taken to the MRI or CT room, where the target is located and computer coordinates are determined. The computer then determines target trajectory. The patient is then taken to the operating room, and the stereotaxic procedure with precise coordinates is performed. The probe is checked by the same method after it is believed to rest on target (Fig. 23-62).

Hollow cannulas, coagulating electrodes, cryosurgical probes, wire loops, and other lesion-producing or biopsy instruments have been introduced for the destruction of areas in the brain. Temporary and permanent nerve-stimulator electrodes are also introduced to augment the pain-control function of the central nervous system. These instruments are introduced through a burr hole or twist-drill hole in the skull.

Continuing advancements in technology allow for the use of the laser with stereotaxic equipment and endoscopic equipment. The numerous stereotaxic frames available include the BRW, CRW, Leksell, Patel, Pelorsus, and Reichert Mundinger. Along with stereotactic surgery comes a new era in surgical navigation and information delivery. This technology provides 3-dimensional visualization of anatomic features with real-time localization information (Fig. 23-63).

Surgery of the globus pallidus, basal ganglia, and thalamus

Pallidotomy is incision into the globus pallidus, usually by electrosurgery. Chemopallidectomy is introduction of a sclerosing solution through a rigid catheter or cannula to produce a lesion. Thalamotomy is incision into the thalamus. Chemothalamectomy is creation of a lesion in the region of the ventrolateral nucleus of the thalamus by means of a chemical solution such as alcohol with iophendylate. This approach is still effective but not done as much as in the past. Surgical intervention is intended to interrupt the nerve pathways and alleviate the crippling locomotor symptoms of persistent, intractable tremor or rigidity associated with multiple sclerosis, severe brain trauma, Parkinson's disease, and various types of cerebellar degeneration. Studies are being conducted on fetal pituitary allografts and transcortical intraventricular adrenal medullary grafting in the treatment of Parkinson's disease. Some new treatment frontiers pose difficult ethical questions for neuroscience research; these will be an ongoing dilemma in the development of new treatment protocols. Operations of this type are also performed on the thalamus in an attempt to relieve pain.

Procedural Considerations

The patient must be conscious and cooperative to permit careful examination and observation of response to the procedure and the effects of the symptoms. Local anesthesia is used. The patient may be in a supine or semisitting position.

Operative Procedure

1. The patient's head is positioned and secured in the stereotaxic frame.
2. A skin incision and burr hole are completed as for ventriculography.
3. It may be necessary to take ventriculograms (however, CT and MRI scans have essentially replaced ventriculograms) in addition to viewing the position of the cannulas or needles.
4. When the correct position has been achieved, tests or reversible lesions may be attempted. The patient's response is observed. Finally, the definitive lesion is created at the selected site by means of electrosurgery, chemical solutions, or a cryogenic unit.
5. The dura mater and incision are closed.

Cryosurgery

Cryosurgery is the use of subfreezing temperatures in the treatment of disease to create a lesion. It is used in neurosurgery for transsphenoidal destruction of the pituitary gland in patients with acromegaly, diabetic retinopathy, and metastatic breast carcinoma. It can also be used for the destruction of the posterior portion of the thalamus for the treatment of Parkinson's disease or other involuntary movement disorders.

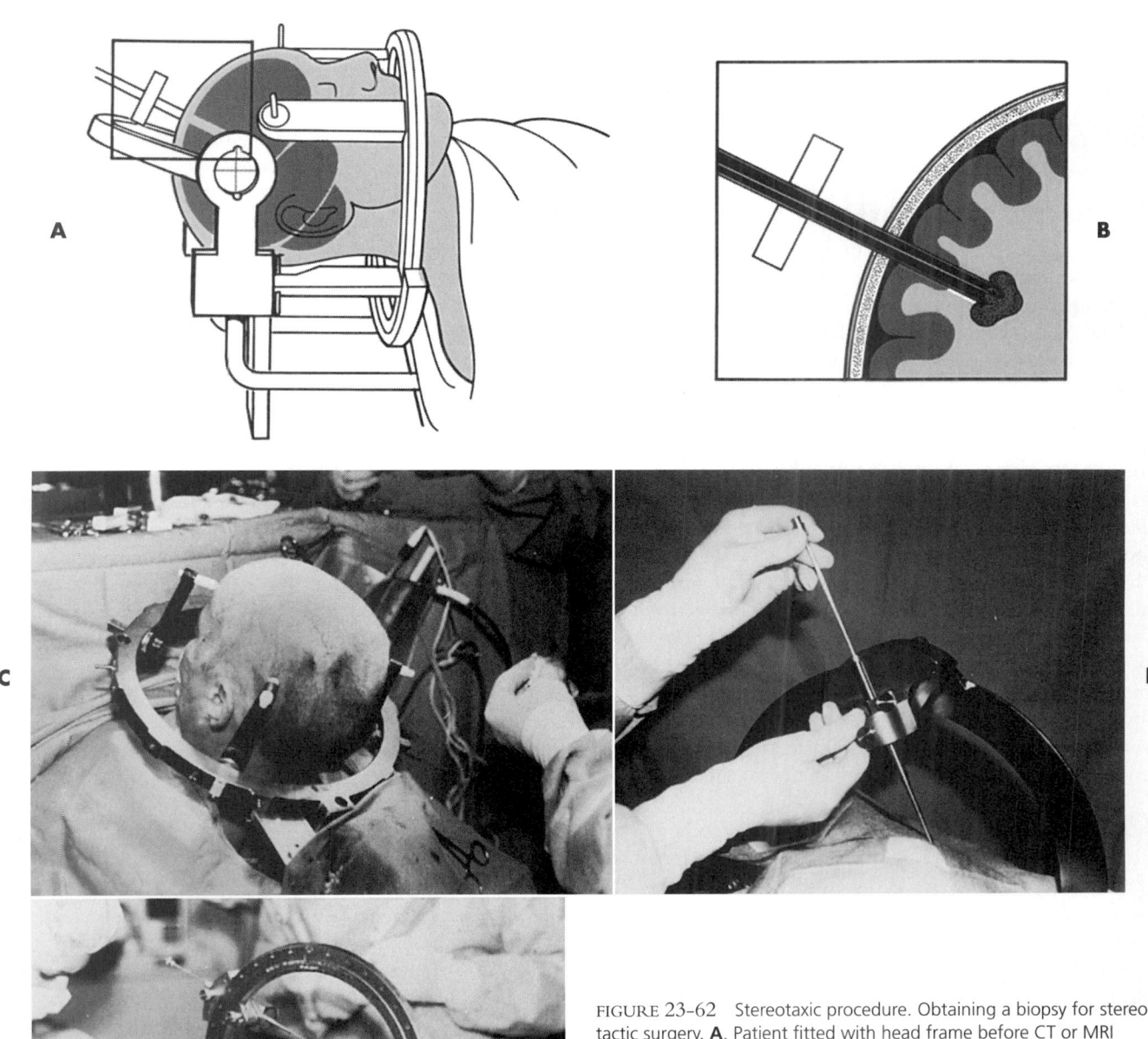

FIGURE 23-62 Stereotaxic procedure. Obtaining a biopsy for stereo-tactic surgery. **A,** Patient fitted with head frame before CT or MRI scanning. **B,** After the imaging procedure establishes landmarks, a stereotactic biopsy is performed. **C,** Awake patient in the sitting position for application of the BRW frame for stereotactic brain biopsy. **D,** Stereotactic surgical procedure with needle insertion for biopsy. **E,** Stereotactic surgical procedure with arc sytem placed on phantom base to demonstrate and check accuracy of biopsy needle with *xyz* coordinates for precise depth and angle.

Transsphenoidal cryosurgery of the pituitary gland

Transsphenoidal cryosurgery is of special benefit to the patient suffering from metastatic carcinoma of the breast. These patients are most likely to respond if they have benefited from previous hormonal therapy or oophorectomy. In the patient with diabetic retinopathy, transsphenoidal cryosurgery is indicated when further laser beam coagulation of retinal lesions is considered useless. With acromegaly, if optic nerve or chiasma compression is present, a craniotomy is usually necessary.

Patients may undergo retrograde jugular venography before surgery to outline the cavernous sinuses and carotid

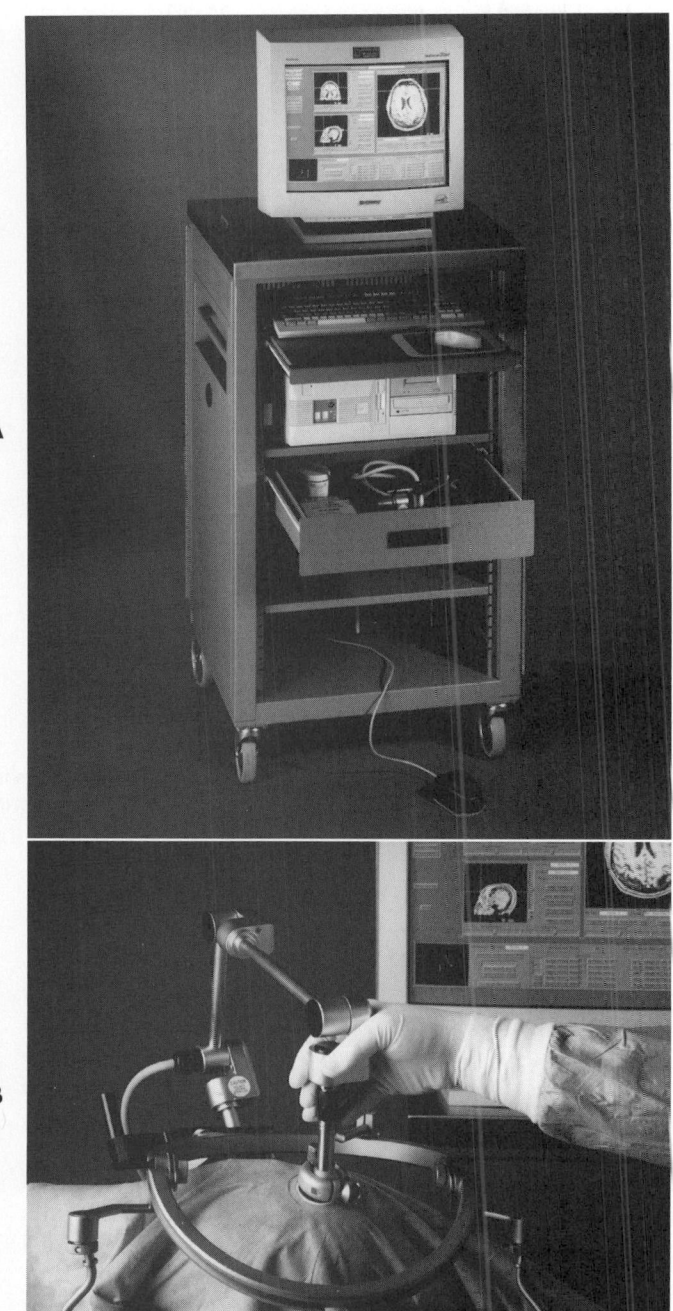

FIGURE 23-63 **A** & **B**, Mayfield ACCISS-Surgical navigator and information delivery system.

arteries. Patients with tumors must also have contrast CT scanning.

The advantages of transsphenoidal cryosurgery follow:

1. Candidates in poor physical condition tolerate this procedure better than a craniotomy because it is less traumatic. Local rather than general anesthesia may be used.
2. Mortality and morbidity are low.
3. Complete destruction can be achieved with fair

certainty in neoplastic glands and good certainty in normal glands.

Procedural Considerations

Surgery is performed with fluoroscopic control. The patient is under local anesthesia supplemented with neuroleptanalgesia. Transtracheal anesthesia is used before insertion of an endotracheal tube for maintenance of a patent airway during the procedure. The patient is instructed to answer questions with hand signals.

Operative Procedure

1. A topical local anesthetic administered with cotton applicators and 1% lidocaine injections through long needles is used to anesthetize the nasal and nasopharyngeal mucosa.
2. The head is placed in the stereotaxic head holder and fixed after injection of local anesthetic in the skin at the points of fixation.
3. Preliminary x-ray films of the skull are taken to be sure that proper positioning has been achieved.
4. A guide is introduced, and a hole is drilled into the sphenoidal sinus and the floor of the sella turcica through the nasal vault. The guide is positioned fluoroscopically.
5. A cryoprobe is introduced through the guide into the pituitary gland, and its position is confirmed with radiographs. The temperature of the probe is lowered to 18° or 19° C for 12 to 15 minutes. The probe can be used to feel the exact location of the dura mater surrounding the pituitary gland laterally and the diaphragm of the sella turcica superiorly.
6. The probe may be introduced to several depths of penetration into the sella turcica, and additional lesions are made. Additional holes may be drilled for further lesions.
7. The probe is withdrawn, and the nasal vault is inspected for bleeding. It can be packed with nasal packing. Antibiotics can be instilled before packing.

Patients are kept supine for 2 to 3 days and prescribed a regimen of prophylactic antibiotics and cortisone replacement. Complications are meningitis secondary to CSF leakage, extraocular palsy, damage to the optic nerve, and injury to cranial vessels such as the carotid and cavernous sinus. These can be prevented by an accurate preoperative evaluation and precise probe placement during surgery.

Shunt Operations

Hydrocephalus is a pathologic condition in which there is an increase in the amount of CSF in the cranial cavity because of excessive production of, inadequate absorption of, or an obstruction that interferes with the flow of the fluid through the ventricular system.

Noncommunicating, or internal, hydrocephalus results from obstruction within the ventricular system.

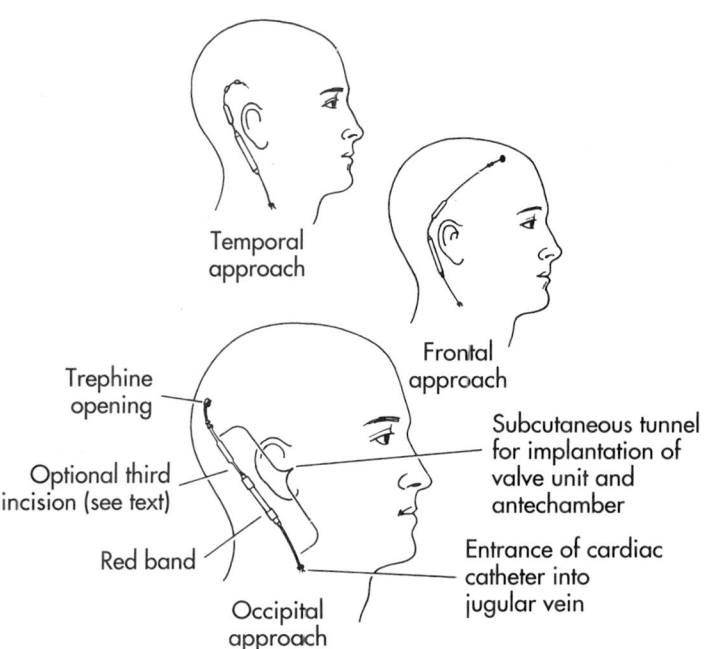

FIGURE 23-64   Placement of ventriculoatrial shunt.

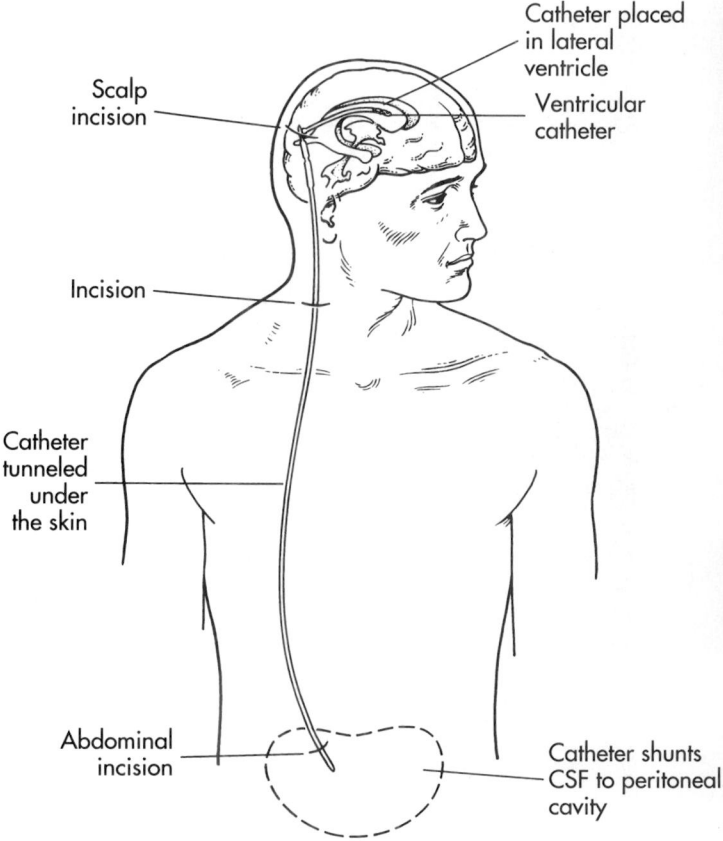

FIGURE 23-65   Patient with ventriculoperitoneal (VP) shunt.

Ventricular fluid does not communicate with subarachnoid fluid.

Communicating, or external, hydrocephalus results from an obstruction outside the ventricular system. All the ventricles are enlarged, and ventricular and subarachnoid fluids freely communicate. Normal pressure hydrocephalus results from malabsorption of CSF.

Currently the two most widely used methods to divert excessive CSF from ventricles to other body cavities from which it can be absorbed are ventriculoatrial (ventriculocardiac) (Fig. 23-64) and ventriculoperitoneal shunts. A catheter is inserted into the ventricular system (usually a lateral ventricle) and connected to a distal catheter that is placed in the right atrium of the heart or the peritoneal cavity (Fig. 23-65). Ventriculoatrial shunts are not used as much as in the past but are still a good alternative for treatment of CSF conditions.

A valve system is used to direct the flow of CSF and regulate the ventricular fluid pressure by opening within a preset range and draining the excess fluid into the atrium or peritoneum. The valve system may be a separate unit, such as the Holter valve, or Hakim or Denver system. The unit may be placed between the ventricular and distal catheters under the scalp just behind the ear (see Fig. 23-64) or may be incorporated into the distal catheter (Fig. 23-66).

Usually a reservoir is inserted into the system between the ventricular catheter and the valve. The reservoir is also placed under the scalp just behind the ear or in a burr hole that was made to tap the lateral ventricle. The reservoir can be punctured through the scalp with a 25- or 26-gauge Huber needle to irrigate and clear an obstruction in the ventricular catheter, to introduce a contrast medium for an

x-ray check of patency, to inject medication into the ventricle, or to serve as a flushing device when digital compression is applied (Fig. 23-67). Currently, the Ommaya reservoir is being utilized for the introduction of chemotherapeutic agents and for drainage of cystic brain tumors.

The valve assembly must be checked for patency and pressure before implantation. Each manufacturer provides specific instructions, which must be followed. As with all implantable devices, the shunt assembly must be kept free from lint, glove powder, and other potential foreign bodies that could cause a reaction in the patient's tissues.

Neurosurgeons and engineers frequently modify and improve shunt assemblies.

Valves are manufactured with pressure ranges of high, medium, low, and extra low. Slit-valve catheters have three pressure ranges: high, medium, and low. All shunt systems and parts can be purchased sterile.

Other procedures that are sometimes done to correct hydrocephalus include cauterization of the choroid plexus of the lateral ventricles by placing a lensed ventriculoscope or laser into the ventricle through a burr hole to visualize and destroy the production site of CSF; lumbar subarachnoid shunt, in which a laminectomy is done and the CSF is diverted into the peritoneal cavity; and ventriculocisternostomy, or Torkildsen procedure, in which a catheter is

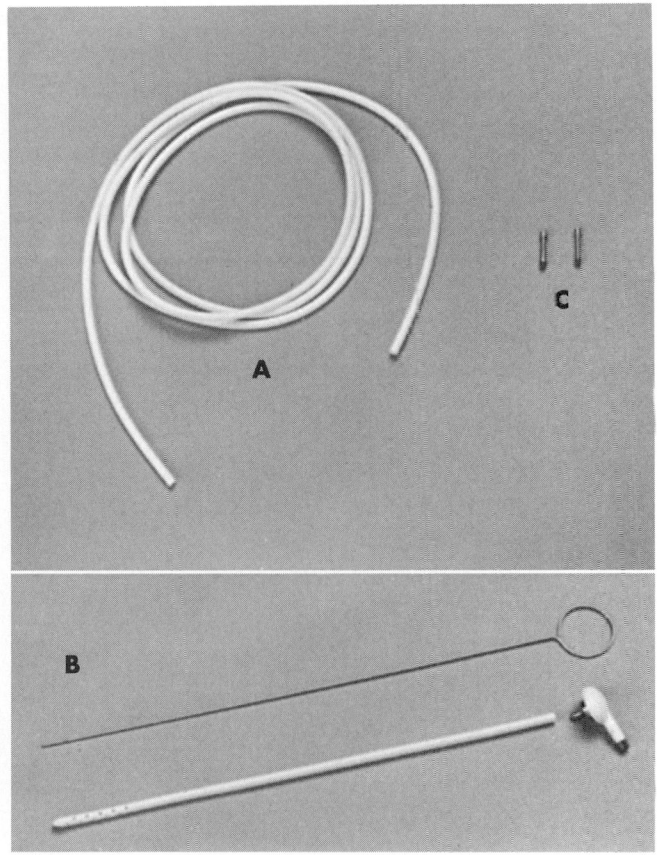

FIGURE 23-66   Shunt is made from silicone tubing of special formula and consists of three parts. **A**, Peritoneal catheter. **B**, Ventricular with side perforations. **C**, Connector. Materials used in shunt can be steam sterilized.

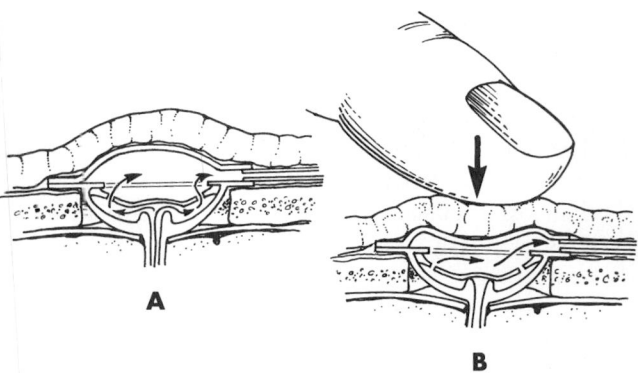

FIGURE 23-67   Pudenz valve flushing device for ventricular shunts. **A**, Flanged silicone capsule and diaphragm valve are shaped to fit into burr hole in skull. **B**, Pressure on capsule closes ventricular inlet and flushes shunt tube.

placed to shunt fluid from a lateral ventricle to the cisterna magna. Endoscopic third ventriculostomy fenestrating the floor of the third ventricle into the cistern space is an excellent procedure for communicating hydrocephalus.

Ventriculoatrial shunt
Procedural Considerations

Insertion of a ventriculoatrial shunt is carried out with the patient in a modified supine position. The head is usually slightly elevated and turned to the left and may be supported on a doughnut. An x-ray film of the chest is taken to validate correct placement of the distal catheter, or the catheter can be placed under direct-vision fluoroscopy with the image intensifier.

Operative Procedure

When the distal slit-valve catheter is used, an incision is made into the neck to isolate the facial or the internal or external jugular vein. The atrial (distal) catheter is filled with normal saline solution, clamped with a bulldog clamp to prevent air from entering the circulatory system, and threaded into the right atrium through the isolated vein. Most catheters have a radiopaque tip for easy identification

of placement during radiography. The catheter should lie at the T6 or T7 level.

Access is gained to the right lateral ventricle through a burr hole or twist-drill hole. The ventricular catheter is placed and connected to a reservoir. A tunnel is made under the skin from the burr hole to the neck incision with uterine packing forceps or a special tunneling device appropriate for the specific assembly being used. The atrial catheter is pulled through the tunnel to the burr hole and connected to the reservoir. When a separate valve, such as the Holter, is used, the ventricular part of the procedure is carried out first. A special valve introducer and tube passer have been designed for use with the Holter assembly.

A single-catheter shunt system without a reservoir is also available. The distal end is a slit valve, and the proximal end is a ventricular catheter.

Ventriculoperitoneal shunts

The ventricular portion of this procedure is the same as for ventriculoatrial shunts. The distal catheter is much longer than that for ventriculoatrial shunts and is threaded from the ventricular puncture site under the scalp and superficial tissues of the neck, chest, and abdomen to the abdominal incision. The tip of the distal catheter may be placed under the liver.

Some precautions that must be taken during the valve-implantation procedures include the following:

1. Trapping of air in the valve assembly unit should be prevented.
2. Storage fluid surrounding the valve should be removed, pumped out of the valve, and replaced with lactated Ringer's solution.
3. Extreme care should be used in handling the unit. It should never be placed on gauze or linen, to avoid lint or other foreign body. The unit is always placed in a basin and should also be kept covered.

4. Lubricants should never be used on the unit. The patient's body fluid adequately lubricates the device.

5. The valve must be properly oriented. It permits only one-way passage of fluid.

6. The valve system must not be pumped excessively immediately after surgery. This can cause too rapid a fluid loss, leading to a rapid decrease in ventricular size. This is poorly tolerated and may lead to subdural hemorrhage.

Frequently, shunts must be revised. Some shunts become obstructed. Others become disconnected or malfunction mechanically in some way. The growth of infants and children may require revision of distal tubings.

BACK SURGERY

Laminectomy

Laminectomy is removal of one or more of the vertebral laminae to expose the spinal canal. Laminectomy, hemi-laminectomy, and the interlaminar approach are performed to reach the spinal cord and its adjacent structures to treat compression fracture, dislocation, herniated nucleus pulposus, and cord tumor, as well as for spinal cord stimulation and insertion of infusion pumps for pain control. Section of the spinal nerves, including cordotomy and rhizotomy, requires similar surgical exposure. Laminectomy is also done to insert subarachnoid shunts for hydrocephalus or pseudotumor cerebri.

Procedural considerations

Laminectomy can be done with the patient in the prone, lateral, knee-chest, or sitting position. It is performed on the cervical, thoracic, or lumbar spine. Laminectomy instruments include the basic neurosurgical set, the back retractor of the surgeon's choice, and an assortment of specialty rongeurs.

Operative procedures

Laminectomy for Herniated Disk (Nucleus Pulposus)

1. A midline vertical or transverse incision is made at the operative site.

2. Hemostatic forceps may be placed on the underside of the skin edge and everted for hemostasis. Deeper vessels are usually electrocoagulated.

3. Two self-retaining retractors (Cone, Weitlaner, or Adson) are inserted for exposure.

4. The fascia is incised in the midline with Mayo scissors, electrosurgical cutting tip, or a scalpel.

5. One side of the spinous processes is exposed by sharp dissection.

6. The paraspinous muscles and periosteum are stripped off the laminae with a knife and sharp periosteal elevators. Cutting current dissection with the electrosurgical unit may be used.

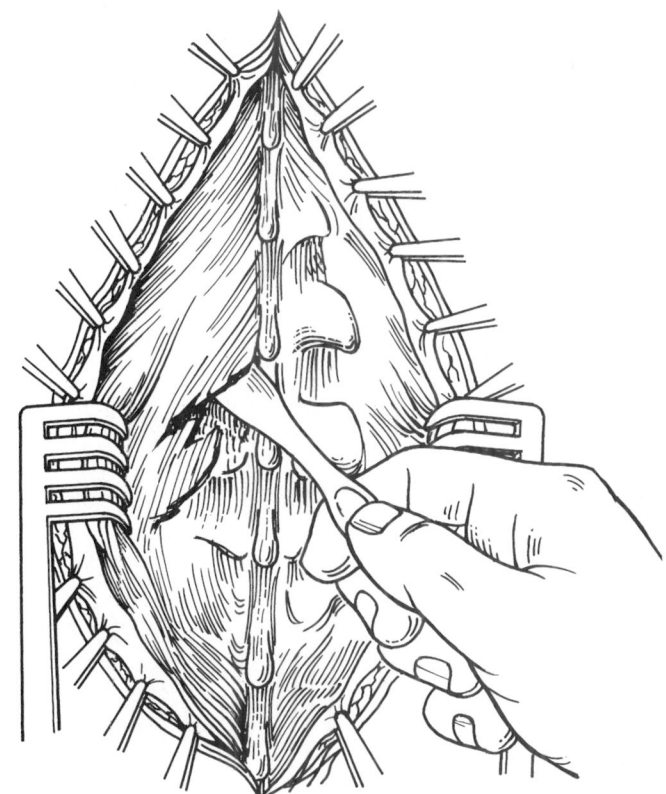

FIGURE 23-68 Laminectomy, exposing vertebrae by dissecting muscle away from spine.

7. As each area is stripped, a gauze sponge is packed around the bony structures with a periosteal elevator to aid in blunt dissection and to tampon bleeding. The paraspinous muscles are dissected from all the laminae (Fig. 23-68). In disk surgery this may be done only on one side, the side of the lesion.

8. A laminectomy retractor is then placed in position. A Scoville (with a blade on the tissue side and a slightly shorter hook on the bone side), Tower, Crank, or Beckman-Adson retractor can be used.

9. Cottonoid strips or patties are placed in the extremes of the field for hemostasis.

10. The edges of the laminae overlying the interspace with the herniated disk are defined with a curette. A partial hemilaminectomy of these laminal edges extending out into the lateral gutter of the spinal canal is performed with a Schwartz-Kerrison rongeur. The bone edges are waxed.

11. The flaval ligament is grasped with vascular bayonet forceps with teeth, and a #15 blade on a #7 knife handle is used to incise it as close to the midline as possible. Cottonoid strips or patties are passed through this incision to protect the underlying dura, and a window is cut into the flaval ligament with a #15 blade on a #7 knife handle (Fig. 23-69).

12. Additional ligaments out in the lateral gutter of the spinal canal may be removed with a large curette or a

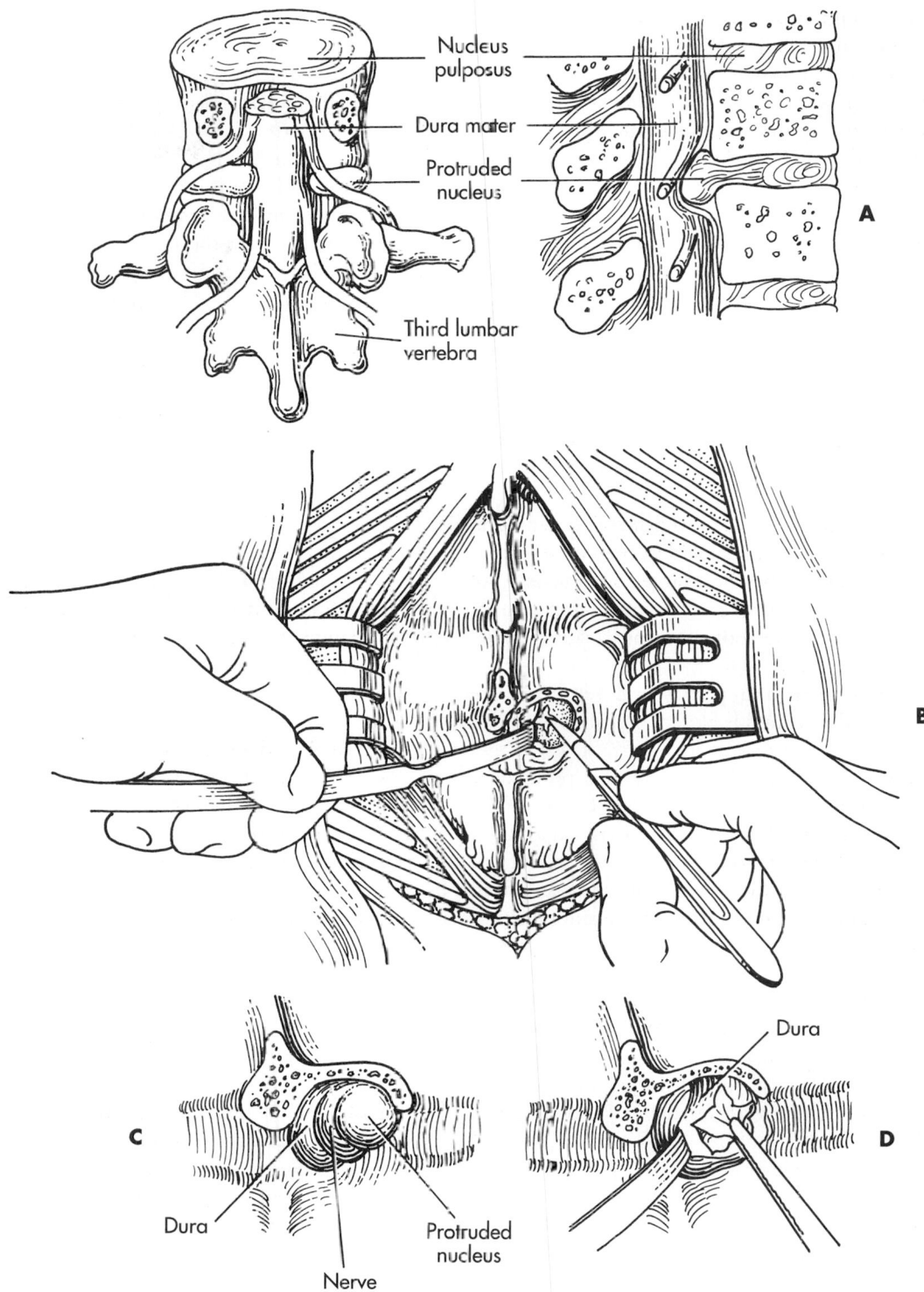

FIGURE 23-69 **A**, Normal and herniated nucleus pulposus (disk). **B**, Window has been made in lamina, and ligament has been incised to expose underlying dura mater and nerve root. **C**, Relationship of dura mater, nerve root, and protruded nucleus pulposus (disk). **D**, Retraction of nerve root over dura mater and removal of disk.

Cloward punch after first protecting the dural sac and nerve root with a cottonoid strip.

13. A dural elevator and a Love or copper nerve root retractor are used to retract the nerve root and dural sac to expose the disk space.

14. Epidural veins are controlled by packing with narrow cottonoid strips and if necessary by careful coagulation with a bipolar bayonet.

15. Any herniated fragment of disk is removed with a pituitary rongeur.

16. After coagulation of its surface, an opening is cut into the posterior aspect of the interspace with a #11 or 15 blade on a #7 knife handle.

17. Pituitary rongeurs, straight and angled, narrow and wide, are used to remove the disk material from the interspace.

18. Straight and angled Scoville and ring curettes help to further clean out the interspace. Disk material so loosened is removed with the pituitary rongeurs.

19. The area is irrigated with lactated Ringer's or normal saline solution, and the interspace is explored with a suction tip.

20. The nerve roots and extradural space are explored with a blunt nerve hook.

21. If no further specimen is obtained, hemostasis is secured with cottonoid strips or patties. If possible, neither gelatin sponge nor gauze nor other hemostatic material is used.

22. The cottonoid strips are removed from the epidural space, the bed is unflexed, and the area is further irrigated. A change of position sometimes causes more disk material to protrude, and the interspace is reexposed with a nerve root retractor to rule out this possibility.

23. All cottonoid strips and patties and retractors are removed, and the wound is closed.

For cervical or thoracic disks, only the protruding fragment is removed and limited if any exploration of the interspace is performed. The reason is that attempts of adequate interspace exploration require retraction of the dural sac, which contains the spinal cord at these levels. Such retraction would result in cord injury and paralysis. For a thoracic disk a costotransversectomy or transthoracic approach is used.

Laminectomy for Spinal Cord Tumors

1. The fascial incision is made in the midline, both sides of the spinous processes are dissected out, and the paraspinous muscles are taken down bilaterally, one side at a time.

2. One or more double-bladed Scoville or Beckman-Adson self-retaining retractors are placed to maintain the bony exposure.

3. A midline laminectomy is performed, with the spinous processes excised with a Horsley bone cutter. Various rongeurs (such as Leksell, double-action, Cloward) are used to remove the laminae after the edges are defined with a curette. The Midas Rex drill may also be used. The bone edges are waxed.

4. The remaining flaval ligament is removed with scissors, scalpel, and Kerrison or Cloward rongeurs. Epidural fat is electrocoagulated and if necessary removed with dissecting scissors, so that the dura mater is exposed fully.

5. A wide moist cottonoid strip is placed over the superficial soft tissues and muscle down to the bone bordering the exposed dura mater. This provides additional hemostasis.

6. The dura mater is elevated with a small hook and nicked with a #15 knife blade. A grooved director is inserted beneath the dura mater, and the dural incision is extended over it using long forceps and fine scissors. Alternatively, the surgeon may lengthen the incision by pulling apart the two edges of the dural incision with bayonet forceps or by pushing at the ends of this incision with the edge of a dural elevator. Traction sutures of #4-0 silk or nylon on dura needles are placed in the dural edges, and the cord is exposed (Fig. 23-70).

7. The cord is explored for the pathologic area. Aspiration through a #22 needle on a plain-tipped syringe may be carried out. The tumor may be encountered extradurally or intradurally. Whenever possible, the tumor mass is dissected free and removed by suction, the dissecting scissors, the cutting electrosurgical forceps, cottonoid, small (pituitary) scoops, curettes, pituitary rongeurs, or an ultrasonic aspirator. Intraoperative ultrasonography may also be used to locate intraaxial tumors or cyst cavities. Bleeding is controlled with a moist cottonoid, hemostatic clips, gelatin gauze, and topical hemostatics. Bipolar coagulation is used around the nerves and spinal cord. The spinal subarachnoid space may be explored with a small rubber catheter to detect blockage.

8. The wound is irrigated with normal saline or lactated Ringer's solution, Asepto syringes, and suction.

9. Hemostasis is obtained; the dura mater is closed with a #4-0 or 5-0 silk, #4-0 black braided nylon, or #4-0 polyglactin 910 synthetic absorbable suture.

10. The incision is checked for further bleeding, and the paraspinous muscles are approximated with #0 polyglactin 910 synthetic absorbable suture or #2-0 silk. The remainder of the wound is closed.

In the case of extradural tumors, intradural exploration may be omitted. The operating microscope may be used, especially on intradural tumors and vascular anomalies. The laser also may be used and should be available, along with intraoperative ultrasonography and ultrasonic aspiration.

Cervical Cordotomy (Schwartz Technique, Thoracic Cordotomy, Rhizotomy)

Cervical cordotomy is division of the spinothalamic tract for the treatment of intractable pain. Pain management techniques, epidural administration of opiates, or percutaneous cordotomy may be initiated for pain management. High cervical cordotomy is an effective surgical procedure. Rhizotomy is interruption of the roots

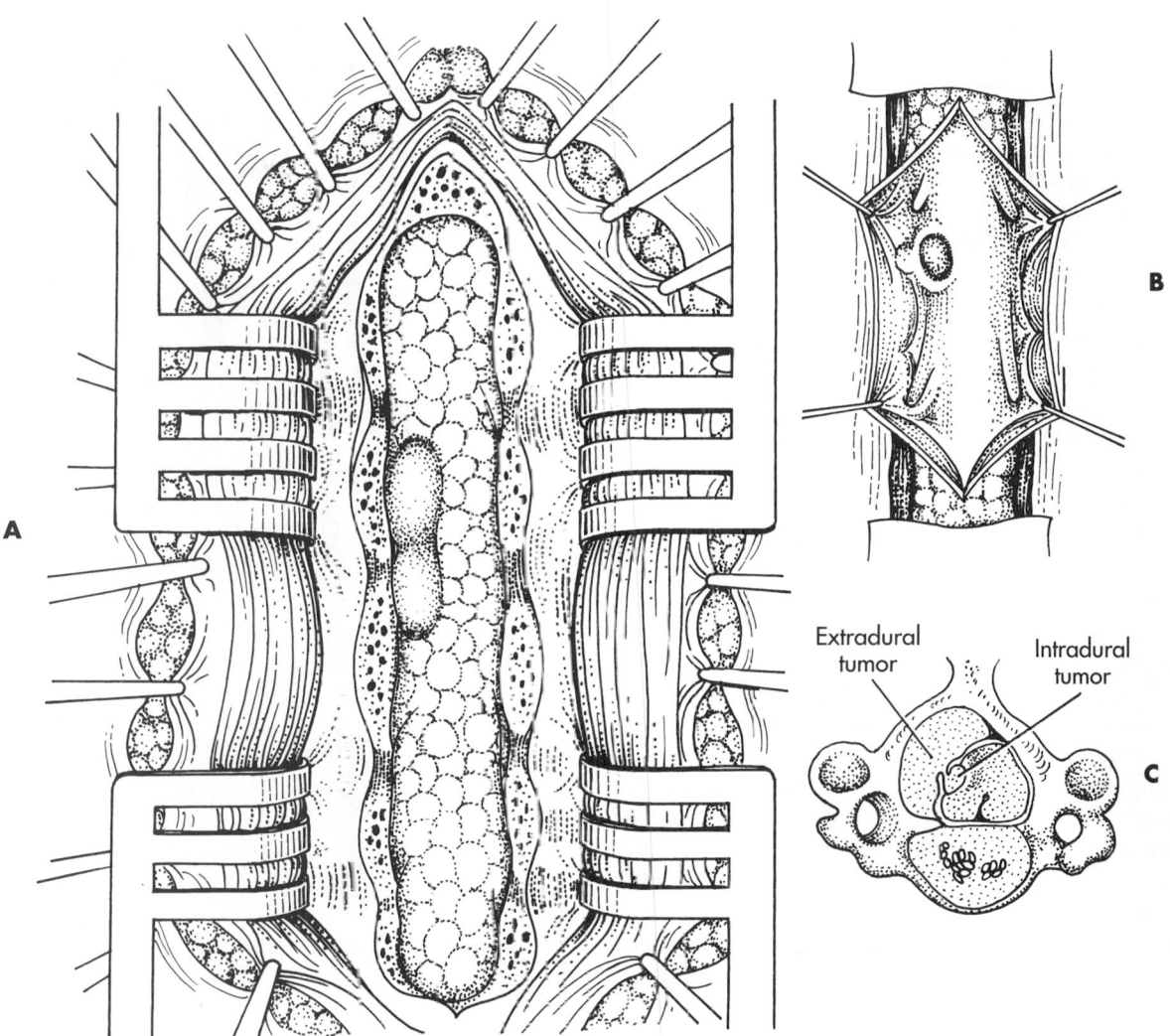

FIGURE 23-70 **A**, Laminectomy completed: dura mater and tumor exposed. **B**, Dura mater incised and retracted, revealing pia arachnoid over spinal cord and part of tumor. **C**, Diagram of cross-section of tumor site and location of extradural and intradural pathologic areas.

of the spinal nerves within the spinal canal. Anterior rhizotomy is division of the anterior or motor spinal nerve roots for the relief of spasm; posterior rhizotomy is division of the posterior or sensory spinal nerve roots for the relief of intractable pain. Other pain management techniques that can be effective are implantable morphine pumps and variable block approaches.

Procedural considerations

Cervical cordotomy may be performed with the patient under general anesthesia, but, to permit intraoperative testing of the level of analgesia achieved, local anesthesia is preferred. The perioperative nurse should keep an accurate account of the amount of local anesthetic agent used. In a very ill or apprehensive patient, a drop in blood pressure or cardiac symptoms may develop if too much local anesthetic is injected.

The patient is placed in a prone position, with head slightly flexed to a level below the horizontal level of the cervical spine. It is essential to keep the patient as comfortable as possible and to offer reassurance frequently.

Operative procedure

1. The skin is infiltrated with a local anesthetic agent, the incision line is marked, and longer needles are used to block the second and third cervical nerves at their points of emergence from the spinal canal.
2. A midline incision is used. Hemostatic forceps are placed to control bleeding, and the Weitlaner retractor is inserted for exposure.
3. Using the electrosurgical unit (cutting current) with the spatula blade, the surgeon separates the muscles from one side of the arches and laminae of the first and second cervical vertebrae. An angled periosteal elevator may be used for further dissection. A gauze

sponge may be packed into the wound to enhance the dissection as well as to aid hemostasis.

4. A Scoville hemilaminectomy retractor with short hooks and longer blade is inserted between the midline structures and the reflected paraspinous muscles. The flexion of the head is increased when the retractor is inserted.

5. The Schwartz self-retaining retractor (modified Gelpi) is placed, with the multitoothed end in the occipital bone and the sharp point penetrating the spinous process of C2 to widen the interlaminar space between C1 and C2 vertebrae. (For additional exposure it may be necessary to remove some of the laminae with a Kerrison rongeur.)

6. Large, moist cottonoid strips are placed over the superficial tissues and muscle down to the bone bordering the exposed dura mater.

7. With the use of a dural hook, the dural incision is made with a #7 knife handle and a #15 blade. Vascular or Metzenbaum scissors are used to lengthen the incision.

8. With #4-0 silk stay sutures on an ophthalmic needle, the dural edges are retracted and secured with curved or straight mosquito hemostats.

9. While suctioning is being performed on cottonoid strips to remove spinal fluid, the dentate ligament is identified at its dural attachment with bayonet forceps and followed to the cord and left attached to prevent distortion of the cord.

10. Fine bayonet forceps (Gerald) are used to elevate the dentate attachment to provide visualization of the anterolateral quadrant of the cord and the anterior nerve rootlets.

11. The cord is incised with a slightly curved cordotomy knife (Fig. 23-71).

12. After the incision is made, the patient is checked for adequacy of the level of analgesia. If the level is not satisfactory, the cord incision is deepened.

13. Hemostasis is obtained, the dural incision is closed, retractors are removed, and the wound is checked for bleeding and is closed.

As technology improves, the laser is being utilized in performing this procedure. This procedure can also be done percutaneously in radiology.

For bilateral cordotomy, the muscles are separated from both sides of the arches and laminae of the vertebrae. A double-bladed Scoville retractor is used, and the Schwartz retractor (modified Gelpi) is placed according to the side of the cord being approached. The cordotomy is performed on one side and then on the other. With bilateral high cervical cordotomy, falls in blood pressure and respiratory difficulty may occur.

High thoracic cordotomy is performed unilaterally or bilaterally in a similar manner, but a hemilaminectomy or total laminectomy at two levels must usually be performed

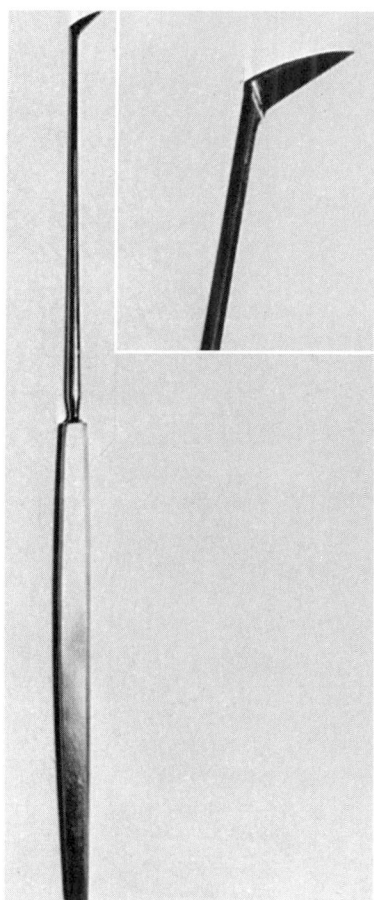

FIGURE 23-71   Schwartz cordotomy knife.

to gain adequate exposure. The lateral or prone position may be used.

Rhizotomy is performed through a similar exposure with the appropriate nerve roots dissected free of any large radicular vessels, held up with a nerve hook, crushed with a hemostatic forceps, and divided with fine-tipped scissors. A silver clip may be placed on the distal ends of the roots before division. This aids in hemostasis and permits subsequent radiologic visualization of the extent and precise level of the root section (Fig. 23-72).

Removal of Anterior Cervical Disk with Fusion (Cloward Technique)

This procedure is done to relieve pain in the neck, shoulder, and arm caused by cervical spondylosis or a herniated disk. It entails removal of the disk and fusion of the vertebral bodies. Bone dowels for the fusion are obtained from the patient's iliac crest or from a bone bank.

Procedural considerations

The patient is placed in the supine position, with the head turned very slightly to the left and with the right hip elevated for exposure of the iliac crest (if the bone dowel is

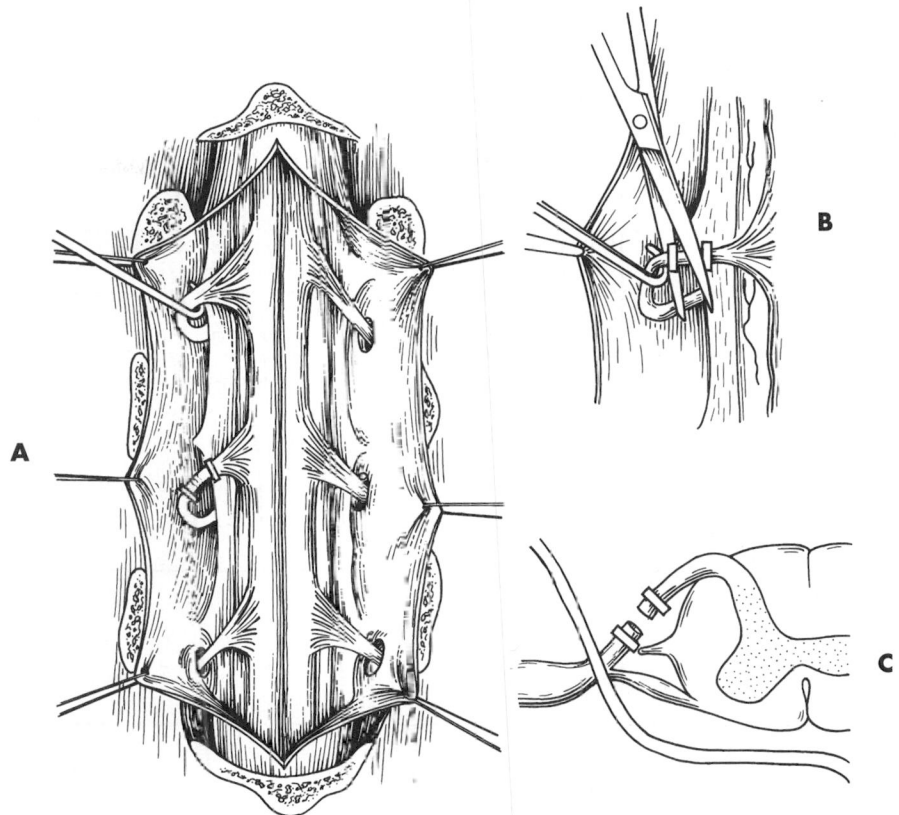

FIGURE 23-72 Posterior rhizotomy after laminectomy. **A,** Spinal cord and roots exposed. **B,** Posterior root identified. **C,** Cross-section of spinal cord and divided posterior root.

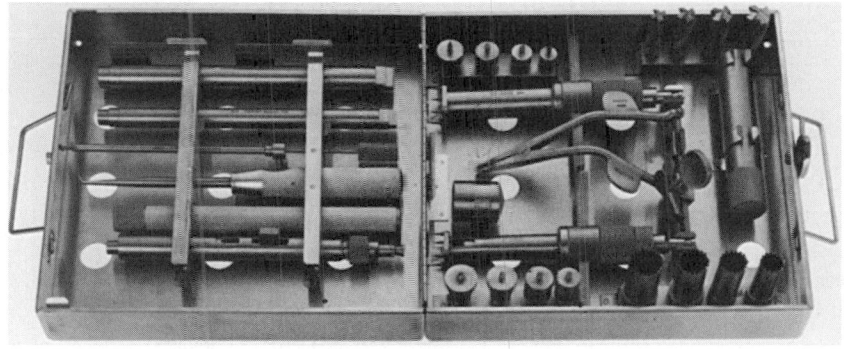

FIGURE 23-73 Instruments for anterior cervical disk removal with fusion. *Left side,* Cloward dowel cutter shaft, dowel ejector, osteophyte elevator, depth gauge, guard guide (large, small). *Right side, bottom to top,* Dowel ejector pins, dowel cutter pins, cervical drill guards (small and large), drill guard cap, drill shaft, cervical drills, crossbar handle, dowel cutter shaft guard, vertebra spreader, and spanner wrench.

to be taken from the iliac crest). The basic minor dissecting set is used, plus the instruments shown in Fig. 23-73. A clinical pathway for patients undergoing anterior cervical diskectomy is shown in Fig. 23-74.

Operative procedure

1. A transverse skin incision is made on one side of the neck (usually the right) directly over the involved disk space; curved mosquito hemostats or Michel clips are placed on the skin edges for hemostasis.

2. A Weitlaner retractor is placed, and the platysma muscle is divided with Metzenbaum scissors and tissue forceps with teeth or with the electrosurgical cutting blade.

3. The medial edge of the sternocleidomastoid muscle is defined with the scissors by blunt and sharp dissection.

4. A vertical plane of dissection between the carotid sheath laterally and the trachea and esophagus medially is created by blunt finger dissection. This

Vanderbilt University Medical Center

ANTERIOR CERVICAL DISKECTOMY

DRG Number: _____

ELOS: _____

	Pre Op (Outpatient)	**Day of Surgery** (OR → RR → 11S)	**Post Op: Day One** (11S → Home)	**Follow Up: 6 Weeks** (Clinic)
Goals:	Complete tests and labs within 30 days of surgery Review data when tests are complete 1-4 days pre op Results WNL Pre op teaching teaching complete	Patient in holding room by 6 a.m.	Lab results available by 5 a.m. rounds Stable neuro, metab, CV, and resp status	Patient able to return to work
Labs:	SMA7 CBC with diff and Plts PT, PTT UA T and S			
Tests	History and Physical CXR and EKG • No CXR for pts <35 unless indicated by history Myleogram/MRI			
Treatments		X-Ray in OR Standard RR care SCD and Ted Hose Volurex q 1° WA (RN/Other)	Standard 11S set-up and care Teds →	
Activity	Ad Lib	Up to chair	Ambulate	
Diet	NPO at 12 MN night of surgery	Advance as tolerated	Regular	
Consults	Anesthesia			
Meds/IV		IV (D/C after antibiotic) Antibiotic - Ancef (until drain out) Stool Softener Pain Med (IV) Anesthesia Meds	Stool Softener (PO) Pain Med (PO)	
Teaching and D/C Planning	Procedure Plan of care Post Op restrictions VUMC orientation Provide D/C instruction sheet Home care needs	11S routines	11S routines Review plan of care Self Care Wound Care and precautions Family teaching - safety Procedure/Disease process D/C needs evaluation and planning	Return to work
Discharge Planning		OR Supplies Laminectomy Tray J Vac Reservoir Cord Bipolar Disp. Pencil Electrode Anesthesia Supplies IMED sgl channel IMED tubing	Respiratory Equipment	
Patient Flow	Complete tests + labs within 30 days of surgery Review data when tests are complete (1-4 days pre op)	Holding Room at 6 a.m. First dose of antibiotics in OR pre op	Criteria for D/C 11S: • Independent with ADL's	

FIGURE 23-74 Clinical pathway for anterior cervical diskectomy.

plane is held open with Cloward hand retractors, Meyerding finger retractors, or U.S. Army retractors.

5. The anterior surface of the spine is identified, and the long muscles of the neck are peeled off the anterior surface of the spine with periosteal elevators. Bleeders are coagulated with a dural elevator or bayonet forceps.

6. A 20-gauge spinal needle is inserted a short distance into the disk space, and a lateral x-ray examination is taken to determine the level of the exposure. At this time a C-arm may be brought in to give instantaneous localization of the desired level.

7. While x-ray films are being developed, the neck incision is covered, an incision is made over the iliac crest, and straight hemostats are applied and retracted.

8. Soft tissue is dissected until the crest is reached using Mayo scissors, tissue forceps, electrosurgical cutting blade, and Richardson retractors for exposure.

9. A Hudson brace with the Cloward dowel cutter is used to remove the bone graft. (Care must be exercised to use dowel cutter, Cloward guide, and cervical drill guards matched for size.) The dowel should have cortex at both ends. The dowel hole is inspected and waxed if needed. The incision is packed with gauze sponges and covered.

10. The Cloward self-retaining retractors (two long and two short blades) are inserted into the neck incision. The right blade should be slightly longer than the left. Care is used to protect the carotid artery and the esophagus. A combination of sharp and dull blades is used to acquire the best retraction. If a toothed blade is used, the teeth are carefully hooked beneath the long muscle of the neck.

11. A #15 or 11 blade on a #7 knife handle is used to cut into the disk space; a fine pituitary rongeur is used to remove the disk material, which is saved and weighed as a specimen. A vertebral spreader is inserted into the vertebral space to widen the area, and further disk material is removed with the rongeur or small curettes (angled or straight, nos. 0 to 4-0) until the entire surface of both vertebrae are clean. A Surgairtome with small burr may also be used.

12. The Cloward bone guide is inserted into the disk space to measure its depth.

13. After the drill guard is adjusted so that the drill can protrude no farther than the measured depth of the interspace, the cervical drill guard is inserted around the disk space, with the aid of a mallet, until the points catch the vertebral bodies above and below the interspace.

14. After the guard is in place, the vertebral spreader is removed or spread to a more limited degree.

15. The Cloward drill on a Hudson brace is inserted into the guard, and the hole is drilled. (The bone dust on the drill point is inspected and saved in a medicine glass.) Cottonoid strips or topical hemostatics are used for active bleeders. Bone wax should not be used on the walls of the disk hole. Thrombin-soaked cottonoid pledgets may help control bleeding.

16. The bottom of the hole is checked for further disk or cartilaginous material, which is removed. The guide may be removed and replaced, and drilling may be done several times until the desired depth is reached. The drill and guide are then removed.

17. Further bone is removed by use of the Cloward cervical punch or curettes until complete anterior decompression of the nerve root or dural sac is obtained. Nerve hooks may be used here for demonstration of adequate dissection. The Surgitome 200 or Midas Rex may also be used.

18. The depth of the hole is measured and compared with the dowel. The dowel may be trimmed with a drill, rongeur, or rasp. The shaped dowel attached to the impactor is inserted into the hole and tapped into place. The double-edged impactor is used to drive the dowel in deeper if necessary. The spreader is removed, and bone dust may be applied.

19. Hemostasis is obtained and the wound irrigated; the vertebral spreader and retractors are removed, and both incisions are closed.

Other instrumentation designs and techniques have been developed for the anterior approach to cervical disk disease. The perioperative nurse needs to be aware of these to accommodate the neurosurgeon's preference.

CAROTID SURGERY OF THE NECK
Carotid Artery Ligation

Carotid artery ligation is performed to occlude the internal carotid artery. It may be done to control anticipated hemorrhage during intracranial surgery for vascular anomalies. A permanent occlusion may be necessary for the control of intracranial hemorrhage or small, repeated strokes from an intracranial lesion.

Procedural considerations

Special clamps are available for gradual occlusion of the artery. Occlusion may protect the patient from debilitating or fatal intracranial hemorrhage from aneurysm and may be used to treat carotid-cavernous fistula. Only a basic minor instrument set is used.

Operative procedure

1. The skin is incised, and a Weitlaner retractor is inserted for exposure.
2. The carotid artery is freed. A small Penrose tubing, umbilical tape, or vessel loop is passed around the vessel for retraction.
3a. For *temporary* control of the carotid artery (during procedures for very large aneurysms or arteriovenous anomalies), an umbilical tape is passed around the vessel

and fixed using the Roper-Rumel tourniquet in such a manner that occlusion can be accomplished immediately if necessary.

3b. For *permanent* occlusion, two heavy silk ligatures are used, and the artery may be divided between ligatures. Transfixing suture ligatures may be used as well if the artery is divided.

4. The incision is closed, and a dressing is applied.

Carotid Surgery for Carotid-Cavernous Fistula

Ligation of the common carotid artery is one mode of surgical treatment for a carotid-cavernous fistula.

Another form of surgical treatment is to embolize the fistula. In either case, internal carotid ligation is usually done after satisfactory placement of the embolus. In some cases a frontotemporal craniotomy is also performed, and the internal carotid artery is clipped intracranially as well. Interventional radiology can also perform superselective anterior balloon occlusions.

Endarterectomy is another procedure involving the cerebral circulation, although not directly involving the brain and cranial nerves (see Chapter 26). Endarterectomy consists in exposing the carotid artery in the neck at the site of occlusion, incising the vessel, and removing the associated sclerotic tissue. Electroencephalographic (EEG) or evoked response monitoring may be used intraoperatively.

PERIPHERAL NERVE SURGERY

Sympathectomy

Sympathectomy is exision of a portion of the sympathetic division of the autonomic nervous system. Most sympathectomies are performed on the paravertebral chain and are named for the region resected, such as cervical, thoracolumbar, and lumbar. The periarterial sympathectomy, vagotomy, and presacral neurectomy are other procedures that are occasionally performed on the autonomic system.

The principal diseases treated by sympathectomy are vascular disorders of the extremities and intractable pain from certain nerve injuries, chronic abdominal conditions, and hyperhidrosis.

Procedural considerations

The position of the patient depends on the region to be resected. Basic dissecting instruments and the microscope are used. For retropleural and transthoracic approaches, rib-resecting instruments are added (Fig. 23-75).

For the thoracic approach, Beckman or Scoville

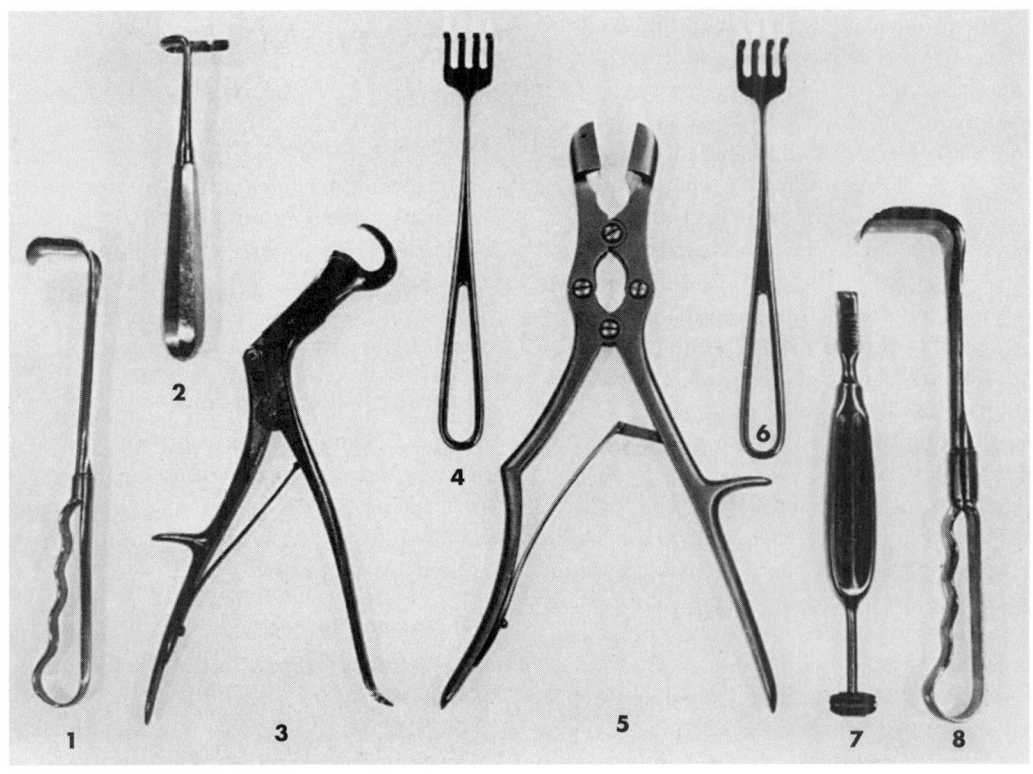

FIGURE 23-75   Instruments for rib resection. *1*, Richardson retractor; *2*, Doyen rib raspatory; *3*, Stille rib shears; *4*, blunt rake retractors; *5*, Sauerbruch rib rongeur; *6*, blunt rake retractor; *7*, Alexander costal periosteotome; *8*, Richardson retractor.

laminectomy retractors and an assortment of hand-held retractors including malleables, Deaver's, and Richardson's are added. For the abdominal approach, Balfour self-retaining retractors are added.

Cervicothoracic Sympathectomy (Dorsal)

Dorsal sympathectomy entails removal of the cervico-thoracic chain, often from the fourth cervical to the third thoracic ganglion. Sympathetic denervation of the upper extremities and heart may be accomplished by cervicotho-racic sympathectomy. The vasospastic phenomenon of Raynaud's disease is relieved by this procedure. It also may be beneficial in relieving intractable angina pectoris.

Procedural considerations

For the anterior approach, both the laminectomy set and rib instruments are used, plus deep retractors and a nerve stimulator. The setup for the posterior approach is as for the anterior approach, plus rib-resecting instruments, periosteal elevators, small rib retractors, a firm rubber pad, and OR bed attachments for the posterolateral position.

Operative procedures

Anterior Approach

1. The patient is placed in a supine position with the head rotated to the opposite side, as in mastoidectomy (see Chapter 19). General endotracheal anesthesia is necessary because there is a possibility of puncturing the pleura.
2. A transverse incision is made one fingerbreadth above the clavicle, the clavicular head of the sternocleidomas-toid muscle is severed, and the deep cervical fascia is divided.
3. The phrenic nerve and the jugular vein are protected, and the anterior scalene muscle is divided to expose and isolate the underlying subclavian artery. The thyroid axis, one of its branches, is ligated and divided.
4. The stellate ganglion, deep against the vertebral body, is brought into view and lifted on a nerve hook. The sympathetic chain is traced upward to the middle cervical ganglion and divided. Deep dissection behind the pleura exposes the upper thoracic ganglia, which are removed to below the third thoracic ganglion. Clips may be placed on the sympathetic nerves before their division.
5. The wound is closed according to the surgeon's preference.

Posterior Approach

1. The patient is placed in the lateral position, and a paravertebral incision is centered over the third rib. The trapezius muscle is divided, and the rhomboid is split in line with its fibers. The third and fourth ribs are isolated extrapleurally, and the posterior 4 to 5 cm is resected.

The transverse processes may be removed to provide better exposure.

2. The sympathetic trunk, which lies on the anterolateral aspect of the vertebral body, is reached by carefully reflecting the pleura. The trunk is picked up on a nerve hook, traced up and down, and removed, usually from the stellate ganglion to the fourth thoracic ganglion. Clips may be applied to the nerve before the fibers are severed.
3. A firm rubber tube may be left in the wound during closure. Suctioning apparatus is applied to this tube as the last deep fascial suture is drawn tight; all air is aspirated, and the tube is quickly withdrawn.
4. The subcutaneous tissue and skin edges are closed.

Nerve Repairs

Peripheral nerve injuries are the most common indication for this surgery. Nerve tumors are rare in comparison. During wartime, injuries of nerves assume particular importance because of their frequency and disabling results.

When the continuity of a nerve is destroyed, function distal to the site of injury is lost. Recovery will occur only if regeneration of nerve axons takes place from the healthy proximal segments. These axons must grow down the axis cylinders of the nerve beyond the injury if they are to reinnervate their end organs and allow function to return.

When a nerve is divided, the cut ends retract, become scarred, and form neuromas. Regenerating axons from the proximal segment cannot bridge such a gap or penetrate the scar tissue. An unobstructed path down the axis cylinder must be made available if nerves are ever again to move muscles or transmit sensation. All procedures are directed toward obtaining the best possible conditions for regeneration.

Procedural Considerations

A basic dissecting instrument set, microinstruments, a microscope, and a nerve stimulator are used.

For lesser procedures such as spinal-accessory-facial anastomosis in the neck, division of the volar carpal ligament for median nerve compression at the wrist, or repair of a small digital nerve, suitable modification may be made.

The positioning, skin prep, and draping of the patient depend on the site of the injury. A large area is prepped.

General anesthesia is usually preferred, with the patient positioned for maximum accessibility to the injured nerve. Exposure must be adequate because considerable mobilization of the nerve is often necessary. A dry field may be achieved using a tourniquet on the involved extremity.

Operative Procedure

The site of injury is explored, with careful attention to hemostasis. Nerve ends are dissected from surrounding scar tissue, and neuromas are excised. Moist umbilical tapes,

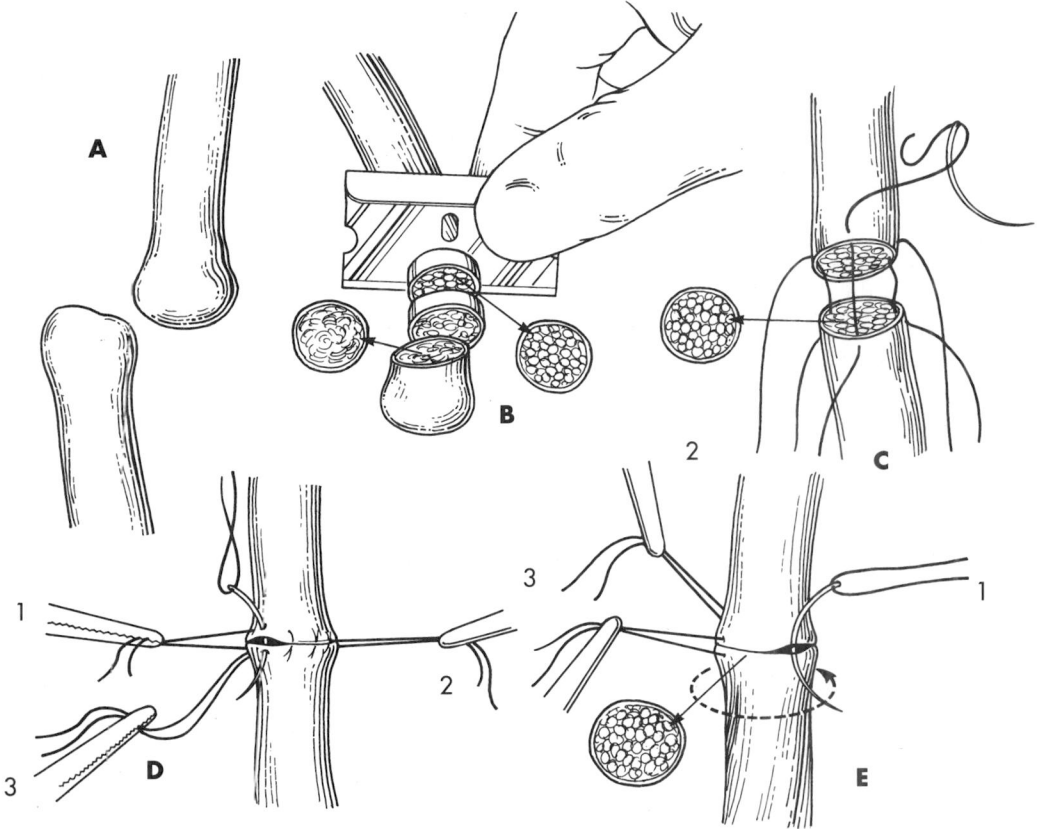

FIGURE 23-76 Nerve repair. **A**, Divided nerve with neuroma. **B**, Serial resection of neuroma to healthy nerve fibers. **C**, Placement of sutures in epineurium. **D** and **E**, Approximation and tying of sutures.

vessel loops, or Penrose tubing may be passed about the nerve to handle it more easily and with less trauma.

The nerve repair (anastomosis) is made with multiple fine sutures placed only through the nerve sheath or epineurium (Fig. 23-76). Tension at the suture line is eliminated by maneuvers such as freeing up a long length of nerve on either side of the point of injury, transposition of the nerve to shorten its course, appropriate positioning of the extremity with plaster splinting during the postoperative period, and, rarely, use of a nerve graft. Some surgeons apply a cuff of inert material such as silicone about the anastomosis.

Hypoglossal facial nerve anastomosis

Hypoglossal facial nerve anastomosis is performed to restore function to an injured facial nerve. With certain lesions in the posterior fossa and during some procedures on the posterior fossa, the facial nerve may be damaged.

Operative Procedure

1. An incision is made over the anterior edge of the sternocleidomastoid muscle, extending from the mastoid process downward for a distance of approximately 11 to 12 cm.
2. The fascia and muscles are divided, and further dissection is carried out until the hypoglossal nerve is exposed and divided distally.

3. The facial nerve is exposed and divided close to its exit from the stylomastoid foramen deep to the front of the mastoid process.
4. The proximal end of the hypoglossal nerve is anastomosed to the distal end of the facial nerve with fine arterial or nerve sutures, and the wound is closed.

Occasionally a surgeon uses the accessory or even the phrenic nerve instead of the hypoglossal nerve. Microsurgical techniques and instruments are used.

Carpal tunnel syndrome

Carpal tunnel syndrome is a condition of the hand in which the median nerve is compressed by the transverse carpal ligament or compressed by displacement of the lunate bone or a volar carpal ganglion. Decompression of the nerve is done by removing part of the roof of the fibrous sheath of the ligament or the offending bone or ganglion. Another excellent option for decompression is the scoping procedure, which is gaining popularity in some areas of the country.

Procedural Considerations

The patient is placed in the supine position with the operative arm extended on a hand table or armboard. Local, regional, or general anesthesia may be used.

Operative Procedure

1. A longitudinal skin incision is made in the thenar palm crease. This runs perpendicular to and stops at the most distal transverse skin crease in the wrist. This incision generally suffices but may be extended into an L or a T.
2. A Weitlaner, mastoid, or self-retaining spring-action retractor is placed.
3. The fibers of the carpal ligament are divided transversely in blunt fashion at the most proximal point of exposure. A hemostat is introduced through this opening in the ligament, pointed distally, and spread. This protects the underlying median nerve. The ligament is divided between the jaws of the hemostat with Mayo or plastic Metzenbaum scissors.
4. The incision is closed with fine sutures, and a bulky dressing is applied, with the fingers visible.

Ulnar nerve transposition at the elbow

Because of traumatic or anatomic problems, the ulnar nerve may be predisposed to irritation resulting in chronic discomfort. In such instances the position of the nerve can be changed to provide protection and comfort.

Procedural Considerations

The patient is placed in the supine position. The arm may be supported in a functional position, with Webril and elastic bandages to attach it to the anesthesia screen, or it may be left free for the surgeon to manipulate during the procedure. The inner, posterior aspect of the upper and lower arm must be exposed for the operation.

Operative Procedure

1. A long incision is made, and the nerve is dissected free from the surrounding soft tissues with Metzenbaum scissors and hemostatic forceps. Moist umbilical tapes, vessel loops, or Penrose tubing is passed around the freed segment of the nerve to aid in handling it for further dissection until a satisfactory length of nerve has been freed from above to below the elbow.
2. The muscle and fascia entered by the nerve at each end of the field may be slit with scissors to prevent tethering and kinking at these points after the nerve has been transposed.
3. A fascial flap overlying the medial epicondyle of the humerus is cut and elevated, and the nerve is transposed beneath it.
4. The fascia is then loosely reapproximated to the fascial edge remaining on the epicondyle with #3-0 silk or #2-0 polyglactin 910 synthetic absorbable suture.
5. The wound is closed in layers.

An alternative procedure, medial epicondylectomy is sometimes performed. In this case the nerve is not dissected out, but the medial epicondyle of the humerus is removed with a rongeur, and the residual bone is waxed. The fascia and muscle tending to tether or kink the nerve, particularly distally, may be slit with scissors, as in the transposition procedure.

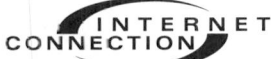

American Association of Neuroscience Nurses: http://www.aann.org

National Spinal Cord Injury Hotline: http://members.aol.com/scihotline

University of Chicago Neuroanatomy Collection: http://http.bsd.uchicago.edu/~pmason/neuro.html

The Whole Brain Atlas: http://www.med.harvard.edu/AANLIB/home.html

Massachusetts General Hospital Department of Neurosurgery: http://neurosurgery.mgh.harvard.edu

Neurosciences on the Internet: http://www.neuroguide.com

Neurosource: http://www.neurosource.com

Neurosurgery://On-Call: http://www.neurosurgery.org

Robert's Neurology Listings: http://mediswww.meds.cwru.edu/dept/neurology/robslist.html

The National Rehabilitation Information Center: http://www.cais.net/naric/

National Headache Foundation: http://www.headaches.org

American Council for Headache Education: http://www.achenet.org

REFERENCES

1. Barker, E. (1994). *Neuroscience nursing*. St. Louis: Mosby.
2. Bradley, W., & Wilkins, R. (1997). *Yearbook of neurology and neurosurgery*. St. Louis: Mosby.
3. Manwaring, K., & Crone, K. (1992). *Neuroendoscopy* (vol. 1). New York: Mary Ann Liebert Co.
4. Nolte, J. (1993). *The human brain: an introduction to its functional anatomy* (ed. 3). St. Louis: Mosby.

CHAPTER TWENTY FOUR

Plastic and Reconstructive Surgery

Katherine J. Donahoe

PATIENTS WHO EXPERIENCE plastic and reconstructive surgery have the dual concern of restoration of a normal appearance and the desire to achieve cosmetic improvement, hence the term *esthetic* surgery. The field of plastic and reconstructive surgery has experienced rapid advancement in recent years. Patients who require emergency surgery as well as those undergoing elective cosmetic procedures have benefited from innovative and unique technologies and techniques. Experimental reconstructive techniques continue to be developed to afford potential new reconstructive options. Perioperative nurses have the opportunity to become partners in this pioneering field of plastic and reconstructive surgery as it continues to expand.

The word *plastic* is derived from the Greek *plastikos*, which means 'pertaining to molded, formed, or contoured'. Plastic surgery deals with the healing, reconstruction, restoration of function, and correction of disfigurement or scarring resulting from trauma or acquired or congenital defects (see Chapter 29 for a discussion of pediatric plastic and reconstructive surgery). Plastic and reconstructive surgery has the goal of restoring normal function and appearance, thus contributing to the patient's body image, self-esteem, and quality of life. Psychosocial integrity is often interwoven with the person's perception of his or her physical appearance. It has been suggested that cosmetic surgery improves body image as well as self-esteem, which is important to physical health. Body image may be defined as the sum of both conscious and unconscious attitudes a person has toward his or her body.[9] These attitudes are central to the concept of self. A person's feelings that one's body, or a part of it, is too big or too small, attractive or unattractive, can influence the person's feelings, anxieties, and values. These influence self-concept and can lead to adaptive or maladaptive responses (Fig. 24-1). Part of perioperative nursing care for the patient undergoing plastic or reconstructive surgery is to assist the patient in obtaining a positive self-concept and realizing his or her potential, despite the sometimes disfigurement from injury. The effects of aging, cosmetically displeasing to some people, may seriously affect their self-image; feelings of unattractiveness may diminish self-esteem and contribute to a negative body image. The perioperative nurse caring for the patient undergoing cosmetic plastic surgery and reconstruction needs to possess creativity, curiosity, insight, and an understanding of the human psyche. Because of its relationship to psychosocial integrity, plastic surgery has been called the *surgery of the psyche*.

Plastic and reconstructive surgery is not limited either to a single anatomic or biologic system or to a single operative technique. Rather, it relies on the basic techniques of surgery and a view of the patient as a whole biopsychosocial being. Only the anatomy of the hand is discussed in detail in this chapter (see the hand surgery section, p. 1030). Other anatomic relationships are described in the chapters relating to surgical intervention for a specific body system.

A wide variety of operations are standard parts of plastic and reconstructive surgery. The advancement of microsurgical techniques has expanded the repertoire of the surgeon to include sophisticated procedures in replantation of limbs and digits, microvascular free flaps, and the like to restore and retain functional use of esthetic configuration. Breast augmentation, reconstruction, and reduction are included in this chapter. Tissue expanders are discussed with breast reconstruction, although they may be used in other areas of reconstruction. The esthetic problems, varieties of acquired defects, diversity of operative techniques, and the psychologic responses of patients offer unique learning experiences and challenges for providing perioperative nursing care.

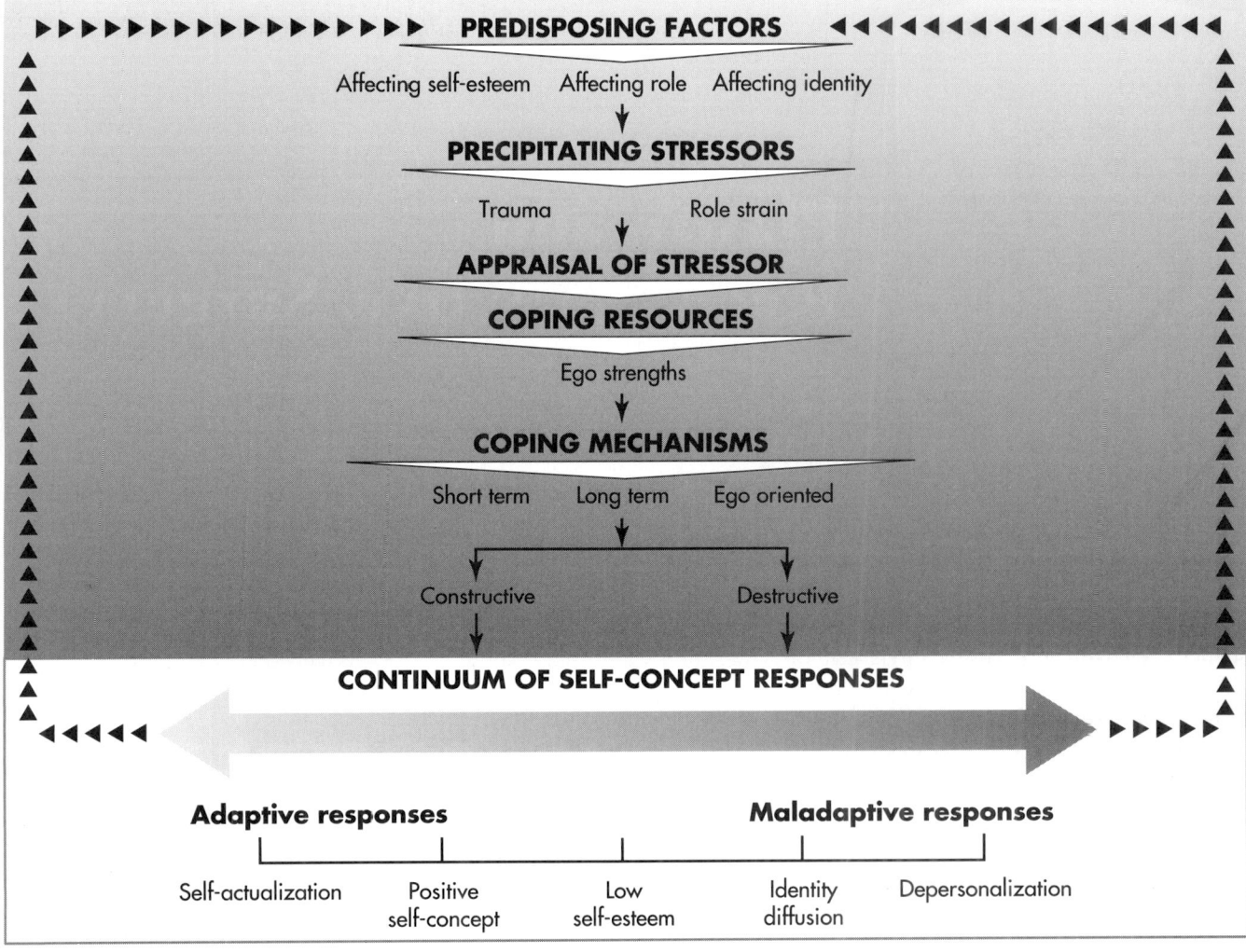

FIGURE 24-1   The Stuart Stress Adaptation Model related to self-concept responses.

PERIOPERATIVE NURSING CONSIDERATIONS

The nursing process is a deliberate, systematic method of individualizing nursing care. Through the nursing process the perioperative nurse is able to focus on unique responses of the patient to the planned surgical intervention. Each step of the nursing process is sequential in that the steps that follow it depend on information gathered and conclusions reached in each successive step. It is an ongoing, dynamic process responsive to both the individual patient and changes within that patient's status.

Assessment

During assessment the perioperative nurse gathers and analyzes data and information that lead to the identification of actual or high-risk health problems or nursing diagnoses. The emphasis of this data collection is on preoperative, intraoperative, and postoperative events. In general, the perioperative nurse is concerned with the patient's ability to communicate, with religious, ethnic, or cultural preferences, and with current health problems, risk factors, knowledge level, mobility limitations, skin integrity, sensory and perceptual status, emotional status, and overall physical condition.[8] Preoperative and postoperative visits by the perioperative nurse provide a sound basis for better understanding the patient, assessing his or her problems, planning care that meets individual needs, and assessing the effectiveness of that care. Preoperative education helps to alleviate much of the fear and anxiety usually associated with a surgical intervention. Patients undergoing reconstructive plastic surgery often are experiencing a disturbance in their body image. The procedure may be elective or urgent as a result of trauma. The perioperative nurse must assess the patient for both physical and psychologic effects from reconstructive and esthetic surgery and incorporate patient findings into a plan of care.

Nursing Diagnosis

Nursing diagnoses that relate to the patient undergoing plastic and reconstructive surgery might include the following:

- Body image disturbance
- Anxiety related to surgical intervention or outcome
- Knowledge deficit related to perioperative events
- Risk for injury related to surgical positioning
- Risk for altered tissue perfusion related to surgical intervention

Outcome Identification

Nursing diagnoses lead to the formulation of desired or expected patient outcomes. These are desirable and measurable patient states, including biologic or physiologic states; psychologic, cultural, and spiritual aspects; and the knowledge or skills related to these states. As such, the patient outcome indicates progress toward or resolution of the nursing diagnosis. When possible, outcomes should be mutually formulated with the patient, family, and other health care providers. Such formulations should be realistic, involve consideration of the patient's present and potential capabilities and resources, and provide direction for continuity of care,[1] as well as determining satisfaction with that care (Research Highlight 24-1). For the selected nursing diagnoses, the outcomes might be stated as follows:

- The patient will acknowledge feelings about altered structure/function.
- The patient's anxiety will be reduced.
- The patient will verbalize an understanding of the sequence of perioperative events.
- The patient will be free from injury related to the surgical position.
- The patient's tissue perfusion will be maintained and/or restored.

Planning

Once nursing diagnoses and desired outcomes are identified, the plan of care is designed for the specific patient. Planning involves setting priorities, identifying nursing interventions, and documenting the nursing care plan. Perioperative nurses often begin the early stages of planning as they are admitting the patient to the surgical suite. While assessing the patient, the nurse may also be planning possible nursing interventions for identified patient problems. A Sample Care Plan for the patient undergoing plastic and reconstructive surgery might be as shown on p. 992.

Critical paths (also referred to as clinical paths or pathways) are structured outlines or plans of care that are usually based on research, consensus, best practice, and outcome achievement. Their use in planning perioperative

24-1 RESEARCH HIGHLIGHT

Nurses employed in surgery units should be aware of factors influencing patients' assessments of their experiences. Once identified, these factors must be incorporated into the delivery of nursing care. Common determinants of patient satisfaction include support and kindness from nurses, perceived competence of nurses, prompt answers to call lights, and straightforward answers to patients' questions. Patients' definitions of quality of care thus appear to be related to their perceptions of factors associated with physical and psychological well-being. Because patient satisfaction with and expectations of care are valid indicators of quality nursing care, a 21-item questionnaire was designed to assess the effectiveness of nursing care in an outpatient surgery center.

The 4 constructs of the instrument for measuring patient satisfaction are caring, defined as an interpersonal interaction or therapeutic process between nurse and patients, family members, or care partners; continuity of care, defined as the care and interventions coordinated throughout the perioperative process; competency of nurses, defined as patients' perceptions of the behavior and manner in which services, information, and care are delivered; and education of patients and family members, defined as the ability of nurses to enable patients and family members to make informed decisions about treatment. Questions in the caring domain revolve around respect, concern, compassion, acceptance, and individualized care that is sensitive to patients' and family members' needs and differences. In the second construct, questions pertain to aspects of care and information related to services, treatments, and outcomes. Questions in the competency domain focus on nursing interactions that decrease patients' physical and emotional anxiety and discomfort. In the fourth construct, questions are related to the quality of preoperative and postoperative information and education, the goal of which is to help patients and family members understand care interventions and comply with treatment.

Content validity and test-retest reliability have been established for this instrument. Use of this tool to assess patients' responses to care can help the perioperative nurse improve care delivery and hence patient satisfaction.

From Forbes, M.L., & Brown, H.N. (1995). Developing an instrument for measuring patient satisfaction, *AORN Journal, 61,* 737-743.

SAMPLE CARE PLAN

Nursing Diagnosis: Body image disturbance
Outcome: The patient will acknowledge feelings about altered structure or function.
Interventions:

Assist patient in identifying and discussing feelings, stressors, and perception of physical deformity.

Provide environment (privacy, supportive listening) conducive to expression of feelings.

Help patient identify significance of culture, religion, sex, and age on perceived changes in body structure or function or image.

Determine patient's body image expectations and whether expectations are realistic; clarify unrealistic expectations or misconceptions.

Convey sense of respect for abilities and strengths in coping with problems or concerns.

Assist patient to separate physical appearance from feelings of personal worth, self-concept and self-esteem (as appropriate).

Refer the patient to other health professionals (clergy, social worker, psychiatric liaison) or support groups as appropriate.

Nursing Diagnosis: Anxiety related to surgical intervention, outcome
Outcome: The patient's anxiety will be reduced.
Interventions:

Broadly classify the patient's anxiety (mild, moderate, severe).

Seek to understand the patient's perception of the stressors or stressful situation or event.

Introduce self and other members of the surgical team.

Explain all perioperative events and any sensations likely to be experienced.

Determine the patient's normal coping patterns.

Communicate with the patient in a calm, unhurried, reassuring manner.

Encourage the patient to ventilate feelings and concerns; listen attentively.

Reduce distracting stimuli in the perioperative environment.

If the patient is awake, provide reassurance and information about the progress of the surgery; implement mechanism for family progress reports also.

Provide comfort measures (such as warm blankets, soft music that the patient prefers).

Use touch as appropriate (such as softly stroking the hand).

Encourage and assist the patient to use personally effective coping strategies (such as meditation, guided imagery, relaxation).

Nursing Diagnosis: Knowledge deficit related to perioperative events
Outcome: The patient will verbalize an understanding of the sequence of perioperative events.
Interventions:

Verify surgical consent with operating room schedule and patient's statement of planned surgery.

Solicit the patient's questions; answer or refer questions as appropriate.

Explain the sequence of perioperative events and their purpose, as appropriate (such as holding area, operating room attire, insertion of lines and attachment of monitoring devices, type of anesthesia, postoperative recovery unit, and protocols).

Provide sensory (what the patient will hear and feel, using lay terms) as well as factual procedure-related information.

Whenever possible, provide printed material to reinforce patient education (preoperative routines, explanations of surgical intervention, postoperative management of pain, discharge instructions).

Nursing Diagnosis: Risk for injury related to surgical positioning
Outcome: The patient will be free from injury related to the surgical position.
Interventions:

Determine whether the patient has any mobility limitations; adapt surgical position accordingly.

When possible, have patient assume surgical position before induction of general anesthesia; observe areas of discomfort and adapt position accordingly.

Secure the patient to the OR bed; reapply restraints after positional change.

Observe the patient's nutritional status, body height and weight, skin integrity, and adequacy of protective tissue at dependent pressure sites.

Apply protective padding to OR bed, dependent pressure sites, and vulnerable neurovascular bundles.

Prevent the compression of body parts against one another (such as crossed legs), the hard surface of the OR bed, positioning accessories.

Maintain the patient in good body alignment; reassess body alignment after positional changes.

Keep sheets under patient dry and wrinkle free.

Provide adequate assistance to safely transfer the patient to and from the OR bed.

Nursing Diagnosis: Risk for altered tissue perfusion related to surgical intervention (microvascular surgery, grafts)

Continued

SAMPLE CARE PLAN—cont'd

Outcome: The patient's tissue perfusion will be maintained or restored.

Interventions:

Notice any sensory or perceptual alterations in the affected body part; document them.

Maintain body temperature with warming device, reflective blankets, and the like.

Warm intravenous fluids, blood and blood products, and irrigating fluids.

Increase the temperature in the operating room as indicated.

Monitor the patient's core temperature.

Provide intraoperative medications as prescribed for local irrigation (such as heparinized saline); label all medications on the sterile field and document their administration.

Monitor tissue perfusion (as by Doppler ultrasound) as prescribed and flap ischemic time; record results.

Notice any swelling, change in color or temperature, or drainage from graft sites before discharge from the operating room.

Provide warm blankets for the patient at the conclusion of the surgical procedure.

Teach the patient or the family how to care for the incision, including signs and symptoms of infection, graft failure (as applicable).

---

patient care contributes to some degree of assurance that consistency will characterize patient treatment and care. A clinical pathway for the patient undergoing a skin graft is presented in Fig. 24-2 as one example of the efforts in which perioperative nurses in plastic and reconstructive surgery are involved to provide efficient and cost-effective patient care.

Implementation

The planning and implementation phases of perioperative patient care are closely interrelated. Implementing a plan of care in the surgical setting involves gathering required patient care items, providing antimicrobial skin antisepsis, creating and maintaining a sterile field, initiating counts of surgical items, properly disposing of surgical specimens, classifying the patient's wound, dispensing medications, monitoring the patient, and collaborating with other members of the health care team to ensure a safe, efficient environment and outcome for the patient.

Preoperative skin preparation

Most surgical interventions require that the operative site and adjacent areas be cleansed before surgery. This treatment may be prescribed by the physician to be carried out before surgery by the patient. Special attention is given to the fingernails for patients undergoing hand surgery; to hair for surgery of the head, face, or neck, and to oral hygiene for surgery in or near the mouth. The perioperative nurse should verify with the patient that the prescribed regimens have been carried out. The operative site should be inspected for any rashes, bruises, or other skin conditions. Shaving is avoided, if possible, because it creates an access for the entry of bacteria into the operative site. The eyebrows and eyelashes, in particular, are left intact to preserve facial appearance and expression. Either a povidone-iodine solution, an iodine-alcohol mixture, chlorhexidine, or another broad-spectrum agent may be selected for antimicrobial skin preparation. The use of chlorhexidine should be avoided around the ears and eyes; it has been reported to cause increased intraocular pressure, resulting in blindness.

Positioning and draping

The OR bed must be positioned so that remaining space in the room can comfortably accommodate anesthetic equipment, members of the surgical team, instrument tables, and any adjunct equipment (hand table, drills, microscope, laser) to be used. The patient is carefully positioned on the OR bed so that all operative sites may be appropriately exposed and the airway easily observable and accessible.

Correct draping procedures depend on the location of the operative site or sites. Disposable drapes (see Chapter 4) are often used because of their barrier qualities, ease of handling and storage, and versatility in adapting to a variety of plastic surgery procedures. However, choosing single-use disposable drapes or reusable drapes must be balanced with environmental concerns about resource use and waste disposal. Analyses tracking cradle-to-grave influence on resource use, energy consumption, and contribution to the waste system should be reviewed by perioperative nurses as they participate in selection and use of single-use or reusable draping systems for the plastic and reconstructive surgery patient.[2]

Two of the most frequently used draping techniques in plastic surgery are the head drape and the hand drape. Both of these draping techniques have the goal of providing maximum mobility of the operative part. The head drape includes a fluid-resistant drape that encircles the head and the addition of a drape to cover the remainder of the body. The following techniques represent methods of obtaining maximum accessibility and sterile coverage for facial surgery.

1. A barrier sheet, folded in half, and two towels are placed beneath the patient's head with the towels

DRG Number: __458__

AMLOS: __19 days__

GMLOS: __14 days__

VANDERBILT UNIVERSITY MEDICAL CENTER

Skin Graft

T < 98.6 > 101.5, SBP < 90 > 180, DBP < 50 > 110, P < 60 > 130, UOP < 30 cc/hr
or change in NV status

Condition: _____   Allergies: _____

Diagnosis: _____   Additional Dx: _____

	Pre-Op	Post-Op to 72 Hours Immediate Post-Op	72 Hours to Removal of Burn Pack	Staple Removal to Discharge
Goals:	Voice pain relief			Adequate pain/itch relief
	VS Stable			
	Wounds w/o infection			
	NPO	SBP 90-160 no active bleed		Ambulate-3x day
	Anesthesia consult complete	UOP> 30 ea/hr		D/C sheet complete
	Labs WNL	Palpable pulses		Home Health finalized
	Operative permit signed	T < 101.5°		Self ADL/self showering
	and witnessed	Labs WNL		Verbalize knowledge re:
	Verbalized understanding	Tolerate p.o. diet		skin care for D/C
	of OR procedure	Donor sites without s/sx		Graft adhered [if not adhered repeat
		infection		this pathway]
		Tolerate ROM exercise		Begin ambulation/mobility
		Home Health evaluation begun	Up to chair	Pt/family performs dsg change
		Begin reviewing D/C instructions	Afebrile	per assistance
			Continue reviewing D/C instructions	
Consults:	Anesthesia	Dietician		
	OT			
	PT			
	Case Manager			
	Social Worker			
Labs/ Test:	Type & Cross			
	Pre-op labs as indicated			
Diet:	NPO after midnight	NPO advance as tolerated toward high calorie, high protein		
Treatments:	Burn care BID	VS q 4° x 24° then q 8°, q 4° T		Burn care BID per pt family
	Remove burn dsgs prior to	Burn care to open areas BID		Staples out
	OR, wrap in dry towels	Burn packs to STSG areas	Burn pack removal	
	VS q 4°	I & O q 8°		
	Hydrotherapy	Heat lamp/air to exposed donor site		Self showering
	Complete OR checklist	CDB q 2° w/a		Measurement for pressure
	Start IV (if applicable)	Splints		garments
		OT		
		PT	Weight QOD	
Meds/IV:	IVF	Change to heplock with po intake		D/C heplock after staple removal
	Topical Abx	Topical Abx		
	Analgesic IV	Analgesic IV	Begin Weaning	D/C
	Analgesic po	Analgesic po		
	Antipyretic	Antipyretic/Antiemetics		D/C
	Antipruritic	Antipruritic		
	LOC	LOC		D/C
	Pre-Op medication	Topical emollient		
		Consider PCA Pump		
		IV Antibiotics		
Activity:	Bedrest	Bedrest x 24°		
	Rom exercises	Position for comfort		
	Complete OR checklist	Expose donor site after		
	No smoking	post-op (if xeroform)		
	Review CP with MD			
		Bedrest (for LE burns)		ROM exercises
		ROM to donor site		
		Up to chair with donor		
		sites ace-wrapped		Ambulate 3x/day
Equipment:		Heat lamp (if xeroform)		Supplies for D/C
	Consider need for therapeutic	PCA pump (for consideration)		
	Bed ( )			
	IV pump/pole	D/C		
	B/P cuff, stethoscope		Scale	
	Ambu - Bag			
Teaching/ D/C Planning:	Pre-op teaching	Reinforce teaching about	Teach pt/family:	
	Teach about C/DB	donor site	Burn/skin care	
	Orient family where to wait	Reinforce pain mgt. teaching	Exercise	
	Infection control		Nutrition	
	Reinforce OR pre-op teaching	Evaluate need for family	Infection Control	
		conference	Importance of pressure garments	
	Answer D/C questions from			Dsg change performed by pt/family
	family/pt.			Home Health Finalized
				Teach about D/C meds when ordered
				Prescriptions given to pt/family
				D/C instruction review
				D/C sheet complete
				F/U clinic appointment

Revised Skin Graft 2/9/96 Burn

© 1996 Vanderbilt University Medical Center. All Rights Reserved.

MC 4877 (7/96)

FIGURE 24–2   Clinical pathway for the patient undergoing skin graft.

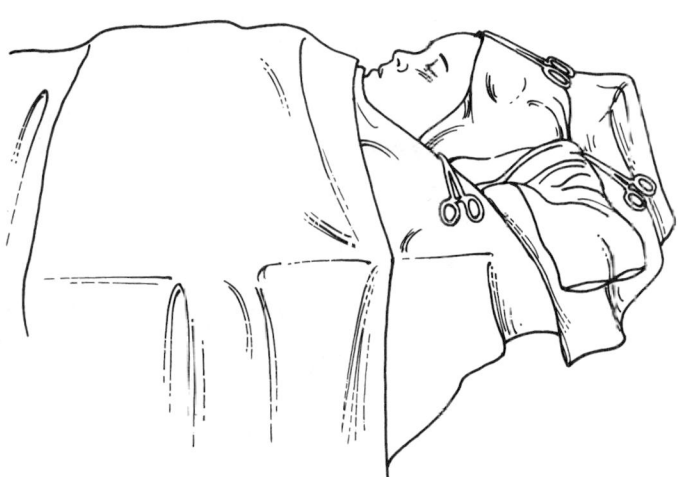

FIGURE 24-3   Head drape.

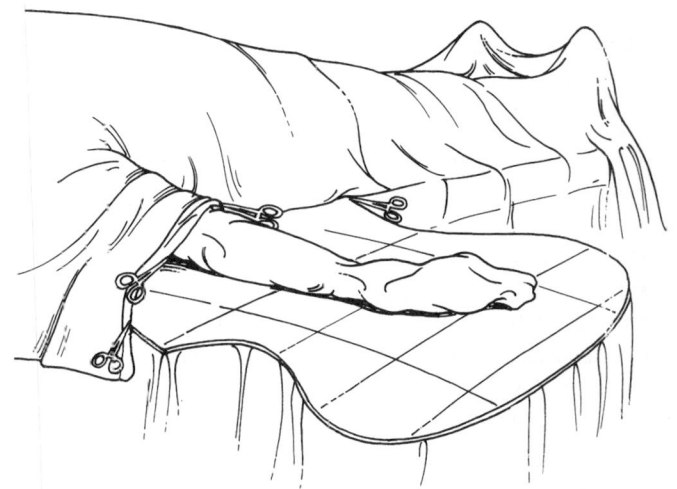

FIGURE 24-4   Hand drape.

uppermost. The folded barrier sheet covers the headrest or head portion of the OR bed. One towel is brought around the patient's head on each side to cover all hair, leaving the entire face (and ears, as necessary) exposed; the towel is then secured with towel clamps. For craniofacial procedures a towel folded lengthwise in quarters may be placed under the head to assist with moving the head from side to side. Two additional towels are then placed diagonally across the neck just under the chin and secured to each other in the middle over the neck on each side to the towel around the head with towel clamps. A full sheet is then added to cover the patient from neck to feet (Fig. 24-3).

2. The head portion of the drape is placed as described above. A split, or U, drape is added to cover the patient from neck to feet.

   a. The hand drape, described below, can be applied to either upper or lower extremities, as required by the surgical procedure. A commercially prepared extremity drape that has an aperture incorporated into the drape may be substituted for the procedure described in steps 3 to 5.

   b. Before a hand drape is begun, a pneumatic tourniquet cuff is often applied to the upper arm over padding. The patient is supine on the OR bed, with the affected arm extended and supported on a hand table. While an assistant holds the patient's arm with both hands around the tourniquet cuff, the skin preparation solution is applied from fingertips to tourniquet cuff. Care is taken to keep the cuff dry and free of solution.

   c. The following comprises the hand drape (Fig. 24-4):

      (1) Two folded barrier sheets are used to cover the hand table. The first sheet is placed with the folded edge nearest the patient (thus forming a cuff) and lies directly beneath the tourniquet.

      (2) Double-thickness, 4-inch stockinette is used to cover the extremity, and the edge is rolled over the tourniquet.

      (3) The upper arm and upper half of the body are covered by a folded sheet, with the folded edge placed across the part of the stockinette that covers the tourniquet cuff.

      (4) A small towel clamp that grasps the edge of the folded top sheet, the stockinette, and the edge of the cuff of the bottom sheet is placed on each side of the arm. This excludes the tourniquet cuff from the sterile field.

      (5) The remainder of the body is covered with one or two additional sheets.

Dressings

Dressings are an essential part of the operative procedure in plastic surgery and may contribute to the ultimate outcome of the surgical intervention. Dressings are usually applied while the patient is still anesthetized. In general, the dressing should accomplish the following five goals: (1) immobilize the part, (2) apply even pressure over the wound, (3) collect drainage, (4) provide comfort for the patient, and (5) protect the wound.

Pressure dressings are essential in the elimination of dead space, the prevention of seroma and hematoma formation, and the prevention of third spacing associated with liposuction and reconstructive procedures involving transfer of large muscle or tissue flaps. In some cases pressure can be achieved by the use of catheters or drains placed within the operative site and connected to closed-wound suction devices, such as a Hemovac or Jackson-Pratt. In smaller wounds a butterfly cannula may be inserted into the operative site, with the needle end placed into a red-topped tube such as a blood collection tube, which has a vacuum (evacuated tube).

The perioperative nurse should be familiar with the

owing common general dressing supplies available in sterile form:

- Nonadherent gauze (such as Betadine gauze, Adaptic, NuGauze, Xeroform, Biobrane, Scarlet Red)
- Petrolatum gauze, ½ inch (or other packing material, such as Merocel sponge for nasal packing)
- Telfa
- Fine mesh gauze
- Interface
- Gauze dressing sponges, 4 × 4 inches, 2 × 2 inches
- Kling, Kerlix fluff, and Kerlix gauze rolls (2, 4, and 6 inches wide)
- Abdominal pads (most commonly used is 5 × 8 inches)
- Skin tapes, flesh colored and regular (⅛, ¼, ½, and 1 inch wide)
- Cotton sheets and balls
- Webril

Also required are the following:

- Tape (adhesive, plain and waterproof, paper, silk, and foam)
- Benzoin spray or swab
- Ace bandages
- Coban
- Casting supplies (as required for postoperative immobilization)
- Abdominal binders and other postoperative garments
- Slings

Anesthesia

Many plastic surgery interventions are performed after the administration of local, topical, or regional anesthesia accompanied by intravenous conscious sedation administered by either an anesthesia staff member or the perioperative nurse. An anesthetic history should be obtained by the anesthesia provider and documented in the patient record. Local anesthetics can cause allergic reaction, or cardiovascular, central nervous system, and respiratory depression, or toxicity. Institutional policy and procedures for monitoring the patient by the perioperative nurse should indicate criteria for patient selection, monitoring responsibilities and documentation requirements, frequency of recording monitored data, medications that can be administered by the perioperative nurse, and perioperative nurse-credentialing requirements (such as Advanced Cardiac Life Support training).

Most patients have an intravenous line in place and appropriate monitors attached, including a blood pressure cuff, cardiac monitor leads, and a pulse oximeter (see Chapter 7). Emergency drugs, oxygen, suction equipment and catheters, and resuscitation equipment should be available before the administration of the anesthetic or sedation. All medications, including those on the sterile field, should be clearly labeled with drug name and strength. Medications administered from the sterile field or by the perioperative nurse should be appropriately

documented (name of medication, dosage, route, time, patient response, ordering physician) in the patient record, as should cardiac rate and rhythm, blood pressure, pulse rate, respiratory rate, oxygen saturation (SaO_2), level of consciousness, type and amount of IV fluid administered, and any significant or untoward reactions and their resolution.[6]

Patients receiving local anesthesia with or without sedation must have baseline data recorded on admission to the operating room and at prescribed intervals thereafter (such as every 5 minutes during intravenous sedation; every 15 minutes during local anesthesia unaccompanied by sedation). The perioperative nurse who is monitoring the patient or administering the intravenous sedation should have no additional responsibilities such as circulating; attention should be focused on monitoring patient response to drug therapy.

Drugs most frequently administered for local anesthesia are lidocaine (Xylocaine) 0.5%, 1%, and 2% and bupivacaine (Marcaine) 0.25%, 0.5%, and 0.75%. These drugs block the generation and conduction of impulses through nerve fibers. The patient's vital signs and state of consciousness should be closely monitored; early signs of central nervous system (CNS) toxicity include restlessness, numbness or tingling of the mouth, and lightheadedness. CNS stimulation may be followed by CNS depression; the patient may become drowsy or unconscious and hypotensive and demonstrate bradycardia and arrhythmias on the ECG monitor. Before administration of these drugs the perioperative nurse should review the patient record and query the patient regarding hepatic impairment, cardiac or endocrine disease, and history of drug allergy.

Local anesthetics may be combined with epinephrine to slow vascular absorption at the site of injection, prolong the duration of anesthesia, and decrease bleeding in the operative field. Because of its vasoconstrictive properties, epinephrine is contraindicated in surgery where it may compromise blood supply in an area with already decreased vascularity; in regional anesthesia, including digital nerve blocks; in patients with hypertension or cardiac arrhythmias; and for patients receiving monoamine oxidase (MAO) inhibitors. The volatile anesthetics halothane and enflurane potentiate myocardial sensitivity to circulating catecholamines. Therefore the anesthesia provider must be alerted before the injection of local anesthetics with epinephrine.

Drugs used for topical anesthesia include cocaine 4% and tetracaine (Pontocaine) 2%. With topical anesthesia the agent is applied or sprayed onto the surface as a solution. It is useful for certain plastic surgery procedures on the ear and nose; it is suitable for use on mucous membranes but not unbroken skin. Tetracaine has a duration of 1 to 3 hours. Cocaine, a vasoconstrictor, is a short-acting local anesthetic with a duration of 1 to 2 hours.

Drugs commonly prescribed for sedation accompanying the administration of local anesthesia include diazepam (Valium), midazolam (Versed), fentanyl (Sublimaze), and meperidine (Demerol). Diazepam is a CNS depressant; it provides sedation, light anesthesia, and anterograde amnesia during the surgical intervention. The CNS side effects are dose related; transient drowsiness, dizziness, ataxia, fatigue, and confusion may be observed. Apnea may occur, especially in the elderly surgical patient. Diazepam is contraindicated in any patient with respiratory depression or hypersensitivity. Intravenous diazepam should be administered slowly to avoid irritation, swelling, venous thrombosis, or phlebitis at the injection site. Midazolam is shorter acting than diazepam and less likely to cause pain or tissue irritation at the injection site. Its primary adverse reaction is respiratory depression; appropriate dosage and careful monitoring are essential with this agent. Elderly patients are particularly sensitive to midazolam-induced respiratory depression, which may be delayed for many hours; in conscious sedation, the total dose of midazolam rarely exceeds 3.5 mg with elderly patients.[5] Fentanyl is a potent synthetic narcotic analgesic, altering the perception of and response to pain. The patient must be closely observed for respiratory depression, depressed cough reflex, and skeletal muscle rigidity. Fentanyl must be administered slowly to avoid intercostal muscle rigidity. Extreme response may require the administration of a muscle relaxant and respiratory resuscitation. Meperidine produces analgesia as well as sedation. The patient should be closely observed for respiratory depression, hypotension, dizziness, and nausea. Narcotics, including meperidine, should not be administered to patients taking tricyclics or MAO inhibitors (within 14 days of MAO inhibitor use). Unpredictable and sometimes fatal complications such as cardiovascular collapse, seizures, and death may occur.

Implant materials

During surgical reconstruction autogenous (autologous) tissue may be taken from one part of the patient's body and replanted in another part. This tissue has always been considered the most desirable implantation material. Homologous tissue is taken from the same species. Alloplastic materials are inert foreign substances that are readily available, leave no donor defect, are biodegradable, and do not undergo resorption. Implant materials should be noncarcinogenic, nontoxic, nonallergenic, nonimmunogenic, mechanically reliable, capable of resisting strain, biocompatible, sterilizable, and capable of being shaped into a desired shape or form.

Silicone-filled implants (for breast, chin, and testicular uses) have been voluntarily removed from the market by the manufacturer as a result of the Food and Drug Administration (FDA) investigations that occurred in 1992. The correlation between silicone and breast cancer detection, connective tissue disorders, and autoimmune disorders has yet to be substantiated. The effect of these investigations with regard to saline-filled silicone shell implants has yet to be determined. Investigations of the use of silicone as an option for implant material are still being conducted.

Other implant materials used in plastic surgery include plastics such as Dacron and Marlex, biologic materials such as collagen, metals such as stainless steel, Vitallium, titanium, and tantalum, and ceramics.

The perioperative nurse must exercise care when handling materials for implantation. Alloplastic implant materials generally are available prepackaged and sterile from the manufacturer. They must be meticulously handled to prevent contamination. Powder must be wiped from surgical gloves and the implant inspected for any defects and placed on a lint-free surface. Breast prostheses and tissue expanders made from silicone should be placed into a container with sterile saline or antibiotic solution on the sterile field. If the expander or implant needs to be sterilized, the manufacturer's directions must be followed. A basic procedure is as follows. The perioperative nurse must put on gloves (oil from the skin may cause an inflammatory response), wash the expander or implant in a pure soap (such as Ivory), and rinse it with distilled water. Then 10 ml of normal saline should be placed in the outer lumen with the fill tube of the expander. This tube should be kept in place during sterilization to allow for the exchange of pressures during the sterilization process, preventing rupture. The expander or implant should then be placed on a lint-free surface and sterilized according to manufacturer's instructions. The expander or implant should be rinsed thoroughly with normal saline before implantation in the patient. Tissue expanders and implants should not be resterilized with ethylene oxide.

Special mechanical devices

Many special mechanical devices are used in plastic surgery. The perioperative nurse must be familiar with the operation and safety requirements of all equipment used. The manufacturer's instructions for proper sterilization methods and for special care after use must be followed. Each piece of equipment must be kept in working order. The following types of mechanical devices are used in plastic surgery.

Dermatomes

Used for removing split-thickness skin grafts from donor sites, dermatomes are of three basic types: knife, drum, and motor driven.

1. Knife dermatomes
   a. Ferris-Smith (Fig. 24-5). Grafts obtained in freehand manner; sterile blades supplied by manufacturer
   b. Humby or Watson. With adjustable roller to control thickness of graft
   c. Weck (Fig. 24-6). Uses straight razor blades with interchangeable guards (0.008, 0.010, and 0.012 inch) to obtain small grafts; also used for debridement of burn wounds
2. Drum type of dermatomes. Operate on the principle of fixing outer surface of skin to half of a metal drum and

...en moving rotating blade back and forth close to surface of the drum to obtain split-thickness skin graft

   a. Reese (Fig. 24-7). Tape containing adhesive is fixed to drum; dermatome cement is applied to skin in thin layer and allowed to dry for 3 minutes; distance between blade and drum (thickness of graft) is adjusted by inserting shim (0.008 to 0.034 inch) adjacent to blade in carrying arm; sterile dermatome tapes, cement, and blades available from manufacturer

3. Motor-driven dermatomes. Graft obtained with knife blade that moves back and forth like the blade of a hair cutter; power supplied by electricity or compressed gas; long sterile cable serves as drive shaft and runs between dermatome and its power source; motor activated by foot pedal or hand control

   a. Zimmer dermatome. Motor located in the handle, sterile blades provided by the manufacturer; consists of four templates (varying in sizes from 1 to 4 inches, determined by the size of graft needed) and one

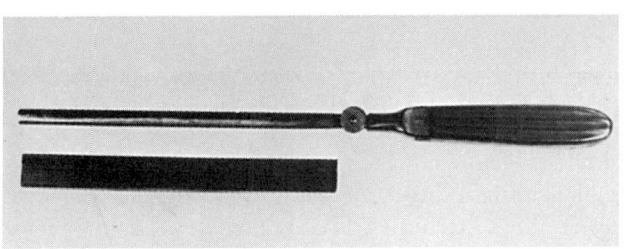

FIGURE 24-5 Ferris-Smith knife dermatome handle and blade (straight razor).

screwdriver that secures template on top of the blade; depth of graft desired can be determined by a calibrated lever on the handle

   b. Brown air dermatome (Fig. 24-8). Usually powered by compressed air; sterile blades provided by the manufacturer; blade is secured in the handle with a specially designed wrench; depth of the graft can be determined by adjusting the calibrating knobs on the handle; can be steam sterilized

   c. Padgett dermatome. Motor is located in the handle; dermatome may be nitrogen powered or electric; if the dermatome is driven by electricity, the manufacturer's recommendations must be followed for sterilization; sterile blades are also available from the company, and different-sized templates are included; calibration is accomplished by adjusting the knob on the head of the dermatome

Insertion of the knife blade and guards of shims with any dermatome is often done by the surgeon. It is also the surgeon's responsibility to make the final blade adjustment and alignment and to remove the knife blade after obtaining a graft and before any instrument cleansing procedures are begun by perioperative personnel. The blade should be disposed of in an appropriate puncture-resistant container.

Skin Meshers

There are several types of skin meshers available (Fig. 24-9), each designed to produce multiple uniform slits in a skin graft, approximately 0.05 inch apart, which allow for the expansion of multiple apertures in the graft,

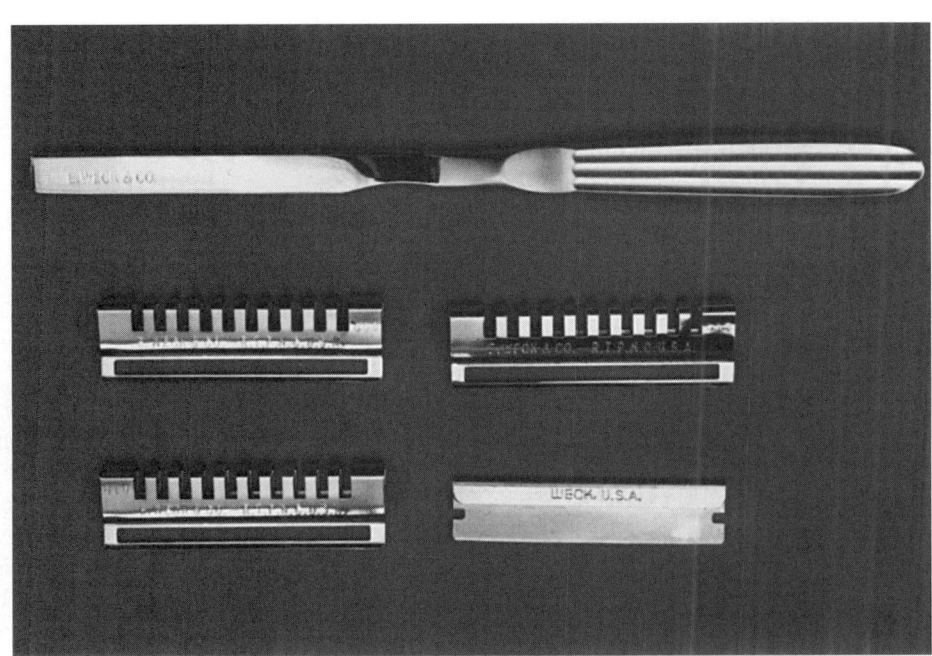

FIGURE 24-6 Weck dermatome handle, guards, and blade (straight razor).

permitting the skin graft to stretch and cover a larger area and facilitating drainage. The graft is placed on the carrier and passed through the mesher. Sterile carriers for meshers are supplied by the manufacturer. They are usually available in several sizes, which determine the expansion ratio of the skin graft (with 3:1 and 1.5:1 ratios being the most commonly used).

Pneumatic-Powered Instruments
(Fig. 24-10, *A* to *D*)

Pneumatic-powered instruments use an inert, nonflammable, and explosion-free compressed gas as their power source. The motor may be activated by a foot pedal or hand control.

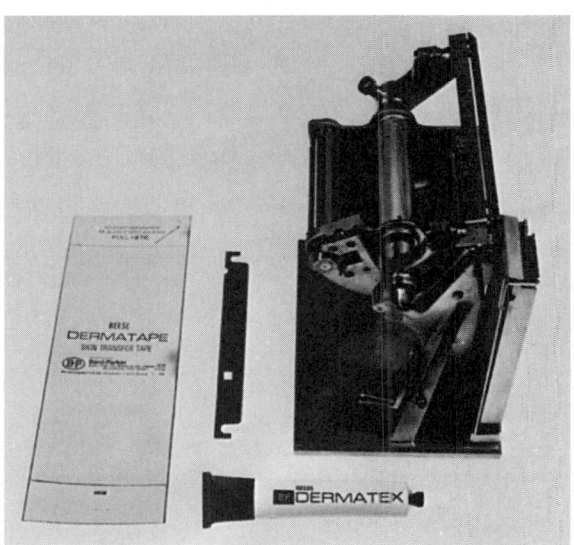

FIGURE 24-7   Reese dermatome on stand, with tape, blade, and glue; shims are stored at lower right of dermatome stand.

The various attachments may be gas or steam sterilized, as recommended by the manufacturer (not immersed in liquid). The following attachments may be used in plastic surgery:

- Wire driver and bone drill
- Oscillating saw
- Derma-Tattoo (used with reciprocating-saw handpiece)
- Reciprocating saw
- Dermabrader
- Sagittal saw

The Hall II air drill (Fig. 24-10, *E*) is pneumatic powered; the motor is activated by a pedal or a handpiece. Burrs and drill points of varied sizes are available for precision cutting and shaping of bone or for drilling holes in bone for wire passing. The drill may be steam or gas sterilized (not immersed in liquid).

A pneumatic tourniquet with an inflatable cuff is used with most hand surgery procedures as well as in other upper and lower extremity surgical interventions. The tourniquet is described on p. 1031 in the hand surgery section (see also Chapter 22).

Bipolar Coagulation Unit

Bipolar electrosurgery is the use of electrical current where the circuit is completed by means of two parallel poles located close to one another. One pole is positive; the other is negative. The flow of current is restricted between these two poles, which are most often the tines of the bipolar forceps. Because the poles are so close, low voltages are used to achieve the tissue effect. Since electrical current does not flow through the patient, a return electrode (dispersive pad) is not necessary. This makes bipolar electrosurgery very safe and permits precise coagulation. The bipolar coagulation unit is further described in Chapter 23.

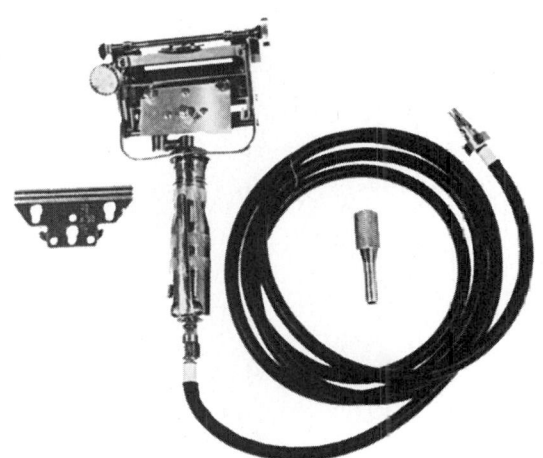

FIGURE 24-8   Brown air dermatome and hose assembly with blade and check for securing blade.

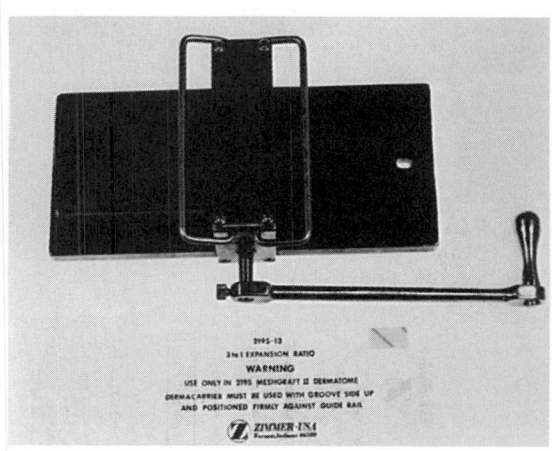

FIGURE 24-9   Zimmer mesh graft II dermatome and dermacarrier with 3:1 skin expansion ratio.

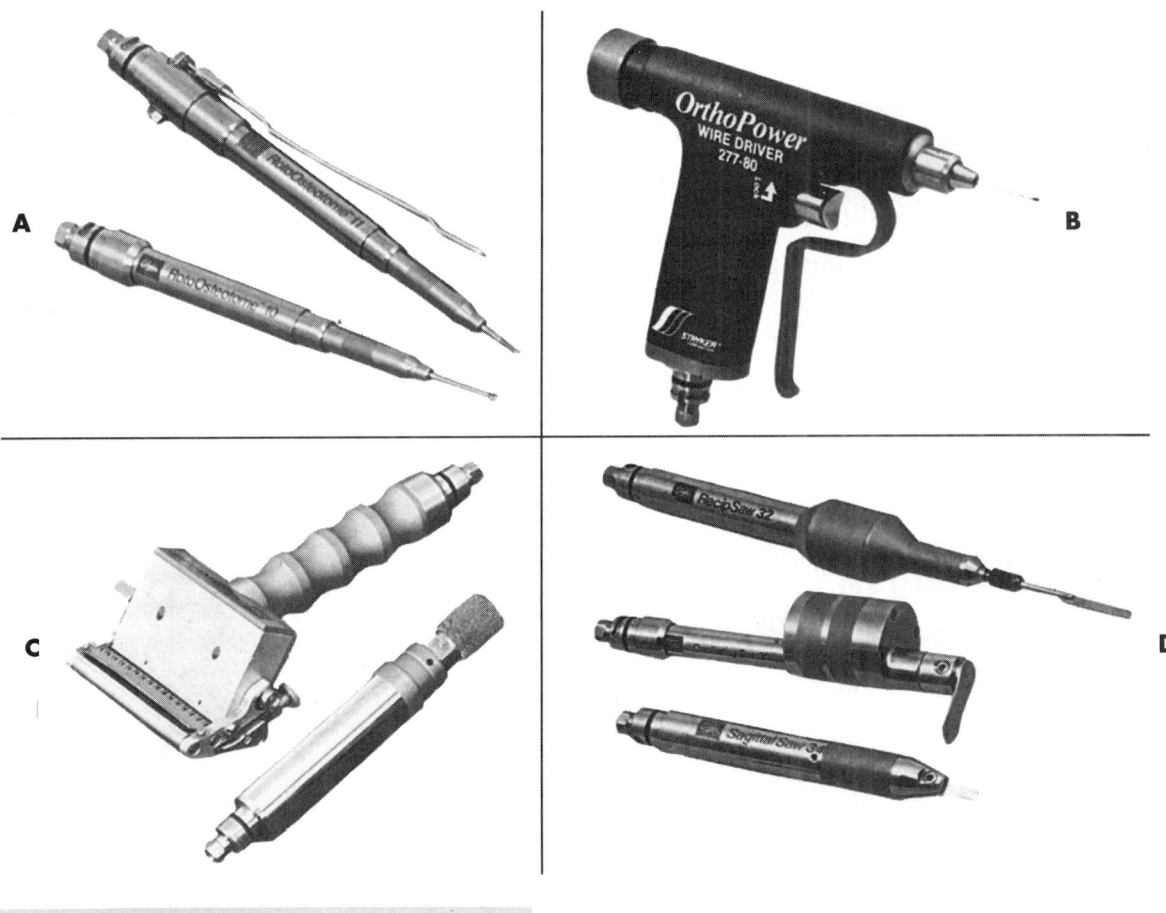

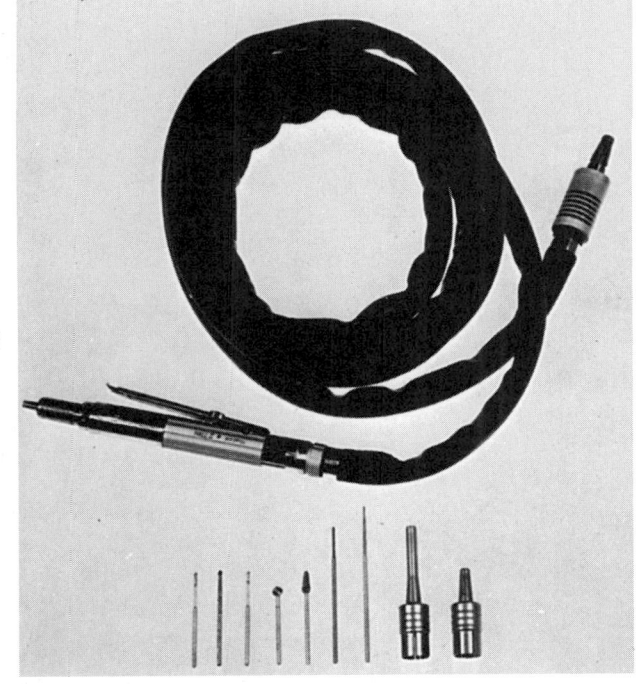

FIGURE 24–10   **A** to **D**, Pneumatic-powered instruments. **E**, Hall II air drill and hose assembly with assorted burrs and long and medium burr guards.

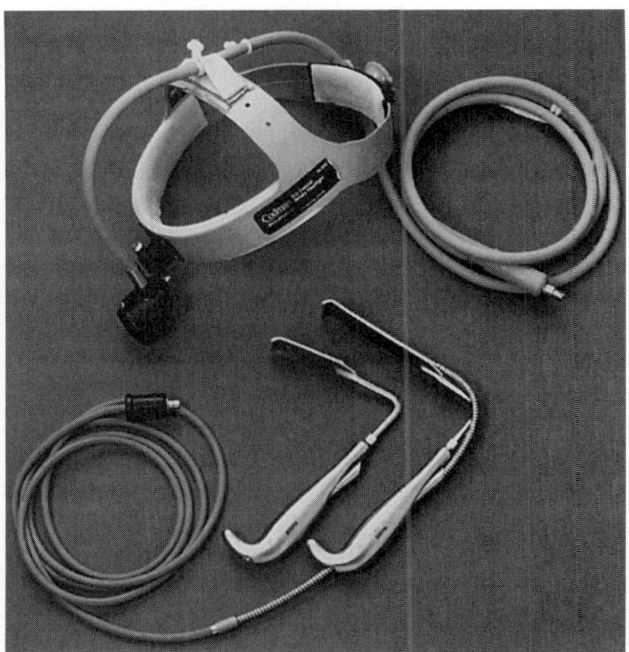

FIGURE 24-11 Fiberoptic equipment. *Top*, Headlight; *bottom*, mammary retractors and cord.

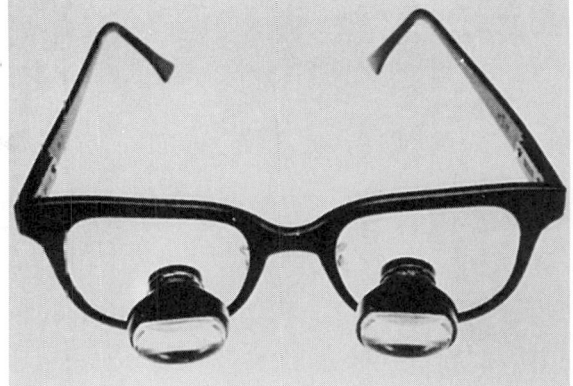

FIGURE 24-12 Loupes, used for magnification.

Fiberoptic Instruments (Fig. 24-11)

The light source is described in Chapter 25. Examples of fiberoptic instrument attachments used in plastic surgery include a headlight for rhinoplasties, augmentation mammoplasties, and other procedures; a mammary retractor for augmentation mammoplasties; a rhytidectomy retractor; abdominoplasty retractors; and endoscopic face and forehead fiberoptic instrumentation.

Loupes (Fig. 24-12)

Loupes are magnifying lenses used by many plastic surgeons for microvascular surgery and nerve repairs and in numerous other instances where cosmetic results are improved by the magnification effect.

Woods Lamp (Fig. 24-13)

The Woods lamp is an ultraviolet lamp used in determining viability of skin flaps in a darkened room. After intravenous injection of 20 ml of 5% sodium fluorescein, the blood vessels appear bright purple (the skin appears yellow). Sodium fluorescein is excreted in the urine, and patients should be informed of this.

Electrosurgical Unit

The electrosurgical unit (ESU) and safety features are described in Chapters 2 and 3.

Microscope

The microscope is frequently used in nerve repairs and microsurgical anastomoses. Chapter 18 provides a full description of operating microscopes.

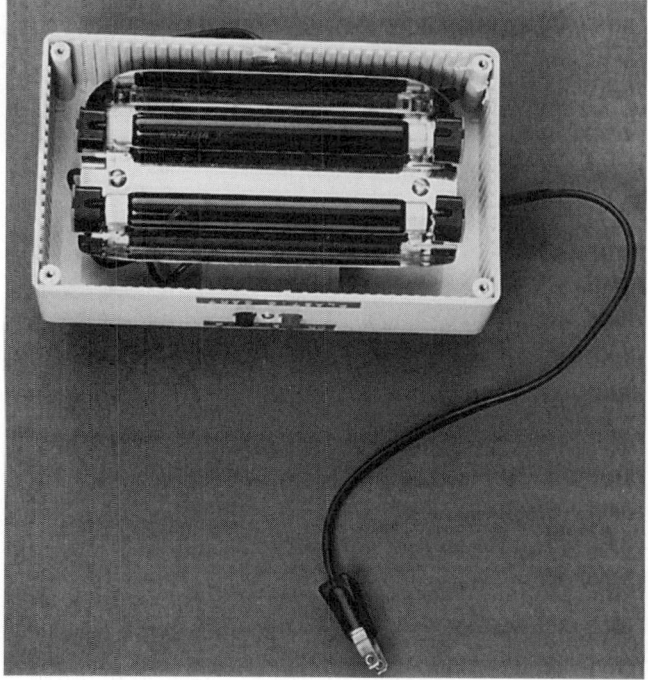

FIGURE 24-13 Wood's lamp and cord assembly.

Instrumentation

Three types of sterile basic instrument trays (Figs. 24-14 to 24-16) are kept available in the plastic surgery operating room. With modification by addition of instruments for specific operations, these trays suffice for all plastic surgery operations.

Special Supplies

Surgeon- and procedure-specific, special supplies are frequently added to instrument setups for plastic and reconstructive procedures. These commonly include the following:

- Marking pen or methylene blue
- X-ray film, unexposed (for pattern making; this can be steam sterilized)

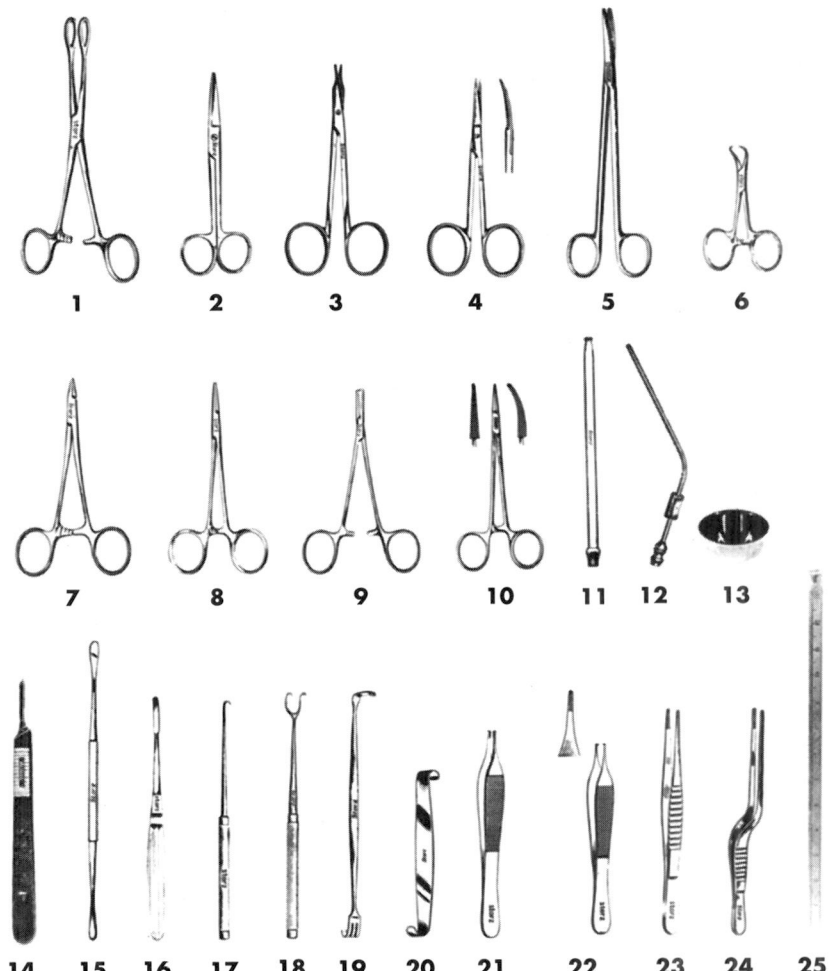

FIGURE 24-14   Plastic local instrument set. *1*, Sponge-holding forceps; *2*, Brown dissecting scissors; *3*, Stevens tenotomy scissors; *4*, straight and curved iris scissors; *5*, Metzenbaum scissors; *6*, towel clamp; *7*, Brown needle holder; *8*, Webster needle holder; *9*, straight mosquito hemostat with teeth; *10*, straight and curved mosquito hemostats; *11*, Anthony suction tip; *12*, Frazier-Ferguson suction tip; *13*, small bowl; *14*, Bard-Parker knife handle no. 3; *15*, Freer septal elevator; *16*, Joseph periosteal elevator; *17*, single skin hook; *18*, double skin hook; *19*, Senn-Kanavel retractor; *20*, S-shaped retractor; *21*, Brown-Adson tissue forceps; *22*, Adson tissue and dressing forceps; *23*, dressing forceps; *24*, bayonet dressing forceps; *25*, ruler.

- Local anesthetic of choice for injection, with syringes and needles
- ESU, with active electrode (pencil) and tip of choice, with tip cleaner

Evaluation

During the surgical intervention, the perioperative nurse is constantly evaluating the patient's response to nursing interventions, anesthesia, and the surgery itself. Progress or lack of progress toward the identified patient outcomes is continuously assessed. The results of this ongoing evaluation enable the perioperative nurse to reassess the patient, reorder priorities of patient care, establish new patient outcomes, and revise the perioperative care plan.

At the conclusion of the surgical intervention the perioperative nurse reviews whether identified patient outcomes have been achieved. The patient's skin integrity is assessed; dressings are applied and their integrity is established before discharge from the operating room. Any drains or tubes incorporated in the dressing should be noted. Infusion sites are inspected, and the type of infusing solution, flow rate, and amount infused are noted in the patient record. Documentation of local anesthetics, sedation, or other medications received by the patient is similarly performed. The patient's response during the perioperative period is noted; any unusual or untoward responses are reported to the nurse in the discharge unit. The transport vehicle is obtained; any special equipment needed for patient transport is also obtained and checked for proper functioning. Warm blankets may be provided, and the patient is gently moved to the transport vehicle.

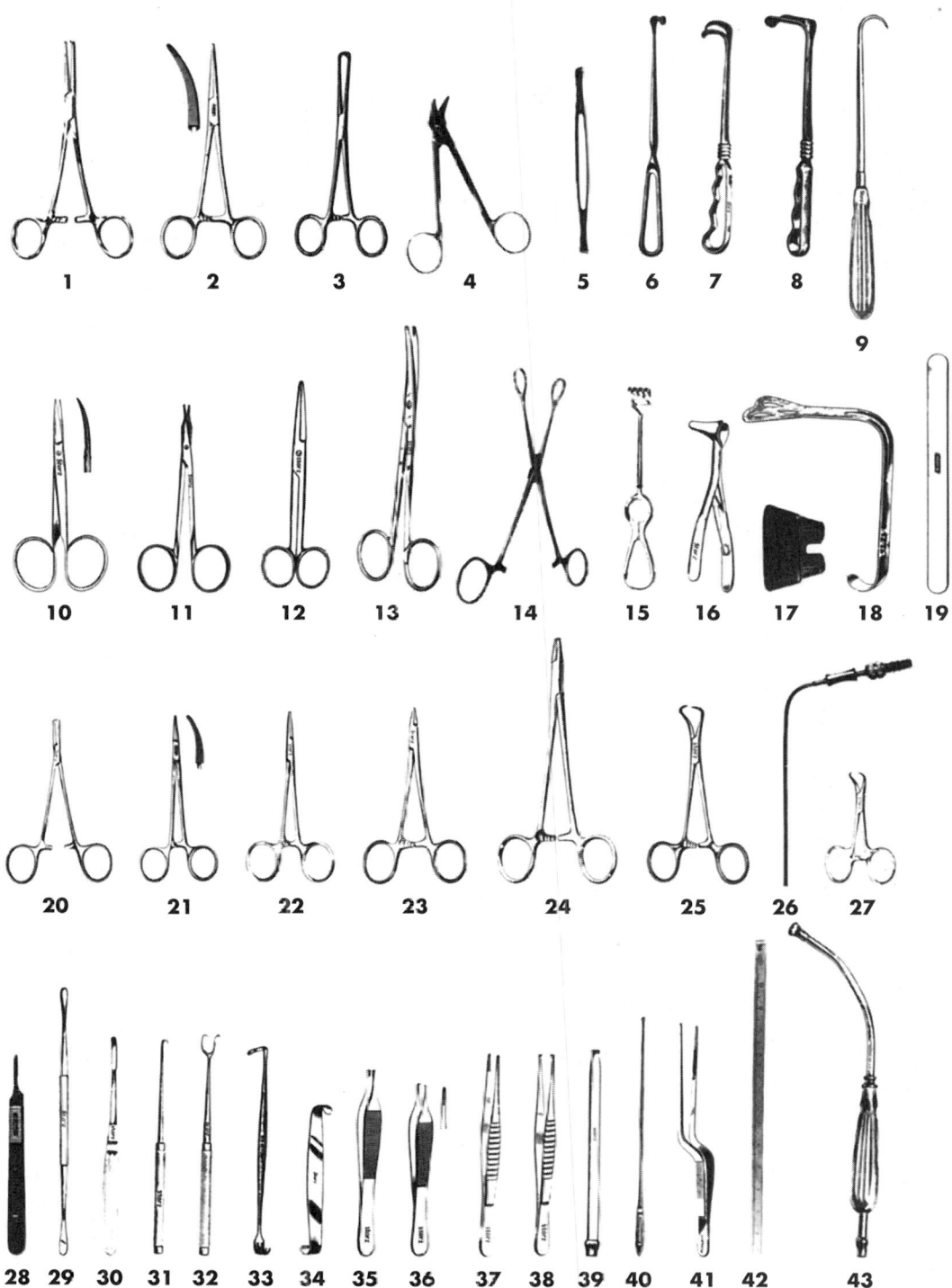

FIGURE 24–15 Basic plastic instrument set. *1,* Ochsner forceps; *2,* straight and curved Kelly hemostats; *3,* Allis forceps; *4,* wire suture scissors; *5,* Army-Navy retractor; *6,* Cushing vein retractor; *7* and *8,* Richardson retractors; *9,* jaw hook; *10,* straight and curved iris scissors; *11,* Stevens tenotomy scissors; *12,* straight Mayo scissors; *13,* curved Metzenbaum scissors; *14,* sponge-holding forceps; *15,* rake retractor with blunt prongs; *16,* nasal speculum; *17,* bite block; *18,* Weider tongue depressor; *19,* ribbon malleable retractor; *20,* Halsted forceps with teeth; *21,* straight and curved mosquito hemostats; *22,* Webster needle holder; *23,* Brown needle holder; *24,* Mayo-Hegar needle holder; *25,* large towel clamp; *26,* Frazier-Ferguson suction tip; *27,* small towel clamp; *28,* Bard-Parker knife handle no. 3; *29,* Freer septal elevator; *30,* Joseph periosteal elevator; *31,* single skin hook; *32,* double skin hook; *33,* Senn-Kanavel retractor; *34,* S-shaped retractor; *35,* Brown-Adson tissue forceps; *36,* Adson tissue and dressing forceps; *37,* dressing forceps; *38,* tissue forceps with teeth; *39,* Anthony suction tip; *40,* silver probe; *41,* bayonet dressing forceps; *42,* ruler; *43,* Yankauer suction tube.

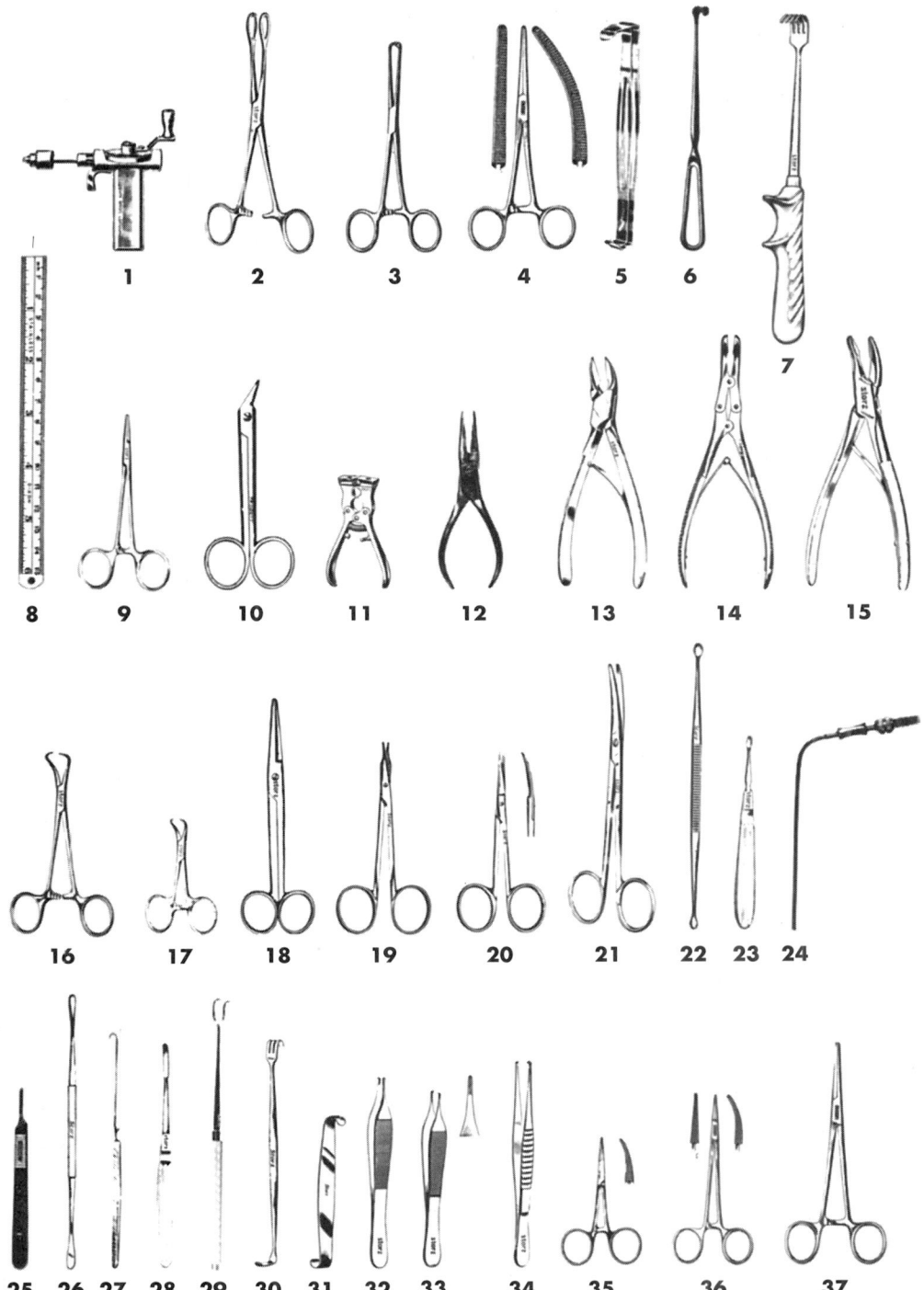

FIGURE 24–16 Plastic hand instrument set. *1,* Bunnell hand drill; *2,* sponge-holding forceps; *3,* Allis forceps; *4,* straight and curved Kelly hemostats; *5,* Army-Navy retractors; *6,* Cushing vein retractor; *7,* rake retractor with blunt prongs; *8,* ruler; *9,* Webster needle holder; *10,* wire suture scissors; *11,* Kirschner wire cutter; *12,* needle-nosed pliers; *13,* bone-cutting forceps; *14,* Ruskin rongeur; *15,* Lempert rongeur; *16,* large towel clamp; *17,* small towel clamp; *18,* straight Mayo scissors; *19,* Stevens tenotomy scissors; *20,* straight and curved iris scissors; *21,* curved Metzenbaum scissors; *22* and *23,* curettes; *24,* Frazier-Ferguson suction tip; *25,* Barc-Parker knife handle no. 3; *26,* Freer septal elevator; *27,* single skin hook; *28,* Joseph periosteal elevator; *29,* double skin hook; *30,* Senn-Kanavel retractor; *31,* S-shaped retractor; *32,* Brown-Adson tissue forceps; *33,* Adson tissue and dressing forceps; *34,* tissue forceps with teeth; *35,* straight and curved Hartmann mosquito hemostats; *36,* straight and curved mosquito hemostats; *37,* Ochsner forceps.

The patient who is recovering from general anesthesia is placed in a safe position on the vehicle; the awake patient should be assisted to a position of comfort.

The perioperative nurse should give the report to the nurse in the discharge unit. Areas requiring ongoing patient observation should be noted in this report; the patient's preoperative, intraoperative, and immediate postoperative status is reported also. Using the Sample Care Plan introduced earlier in this chapter, the perioperative nurse may give part of the report based on patient outcomes. If they were achieved, they may be stated as follows:

- The patient acknowledged feelings about altered body structure or function.
- The patient's anxiety was reduced.
- The patient verbalized an understanding of perioperative events.
- The patient was free from injury related to the surgical position.
- Tissue perfusion at the graft and surgical site was maintained or restored.

Patient and Family Education and Discharge Planning

The importance of patient and family education and planning for discharge (Box 24-1) has become a priority perioperative nursing consideration. As more procedures are performed on an ambulatory basis, preparation for home and self-care need to be accomplished in a time-efficient yet effective manner[10] (Research Highlight 24-2). In general, all patients undergoing a plastic or reconstructive surgical intervention require information regarding the care of the operative site or sites, activity levels and any activity restrictions, symptoms to expect after the surgical intervention and their management, signs and symptoms that must be brought to the attention of the surgeon (or other health care professional), what to look for and anticipate as normal wound drainage and appearance and what might signal an infection, care of drains or drain sites and expected amounts of drainage, any dietary restrictions, and medication instructions. Teaching strategies and content should be individualized for the intervention and for the individual patient (Box 24-2). The time, place, and date of the first follow-up care appointment should be provided along with the phone number of the appropriate person to call in the event of postprocedure problems, concerns, or questions. Plastic surgery encompasses both esthetic and major reconstructive surgery. Sample teaching guides for postoperative wound care at home (Box 24-3) represent one example of the kinds of patient and family education materials perioperative nurses may develop.

BOX 24-1	Discharge Planning

Definition

Preparation for moving a patient from one level of care to another within or outside the current health care agency

Activities

Assist patient/family/significant others to prepare for discharge

Collaborate with the physician, patient/family/significant others, and other health team members in planning for continuity of health care

Coordinate efforts of different health care providers to ensure a timely discharge

Identify patient's and primary caregiver's understanding of knowledge or skills required postdischarge

Identify patient teaching needed for postdischarge care

Monitor readiness for discharge

Communicate patient's discharge plans as appropriate

Document patient's discharge plans on chart

Formulate a maintenance plan for postdischarge follow-up

Assist patient/family/significant others in planning for the supportive environment necessary to provide the patient's posthospital care

Develop a plan that considers the health care, social, and financial needs of patient

Arrange for postdischarge evaluation as appropriate

Encourage self-care as appropriate

Arrange discharge to next level of care

Arrange for caregiver support as appropriate

Discuss financial resources if arrangements for health care are needed after discharge

Coordinate referrals relevant to linkages among health care providers

From McCloskey, J.C., & Bulechek, G.M. (1996). *Iowa intervention project: nursing interventions classification (NIC)* (ed. 2). St. Louis: Mosby.

SURGICAL INTERVENTIONS REPLACEMENT OF LOST TISSUE (SKIN GRAFT)

Free Skin Graft

Skin grafting provides an effective way to cover a wound if vascularity is adequate, infection is absent, and hemostasis is achieved. Skin from the donor site is detached from its blood supply and placed in the recipient site, where it develops a new blood supply from the base of the wound. Color match, contour, and durability of the graft are all considerations in selection of an appropriate donor area.

Skin grafts can be either split-thickness or full-thickness grafts (Fig. 24-17) A split-thickness (or partial-thickness) skin graft contains epidermis and only a portion of the dermis of the donor site; it varies from a thin graft to a

24-2 RESEARCH HIGHLIGHT

Patient education and teaching has long been a cornerstone of perioperative nursing. As early as the 1970s, nursing conducted numerous studies on the best methods of preoperative patient teaching. In the 1990s, the prevalence of ambulatory surgery has altered research priorities. Shortened stays, same-day surgery, and office-based surgery require the need for perioperative patient education that includes home care and what the patient and family need to know to successfully recover and recuperate after discharge. In 1996, an estimated half of the 700,000 cosmetic plastic surgery procedures performed in this country were done in the surgeon's office (How safe is cosmetic surgery in the office? [1998]. *OR Manager, 14*[4], 8). Thus questions of when to teach, what to teach, and how to teach it, and assessing the effectiveness of that teaching become critically important for plastic and reconstructive surgical patients.

This study examined clinical results of patients who were discharged from care within 24 hours. Based on patient responses to the nature of their preparedness for home care and what to expect, the researcher recommended three critical elements for patient education in ambulatory surgery populations: (1) instilling confidence in the patient and family, (2) using and developing preoperative strategies for postoperative care, and (3) focusing on expected limits in activity levels.

From Kleinbeck, S.V.M. Monitoring ambulatory patients after discharge. Presented at AORN Congress, Orlando, Fla., April 1, 1998.

BOX 24-2 | **Teaching: Individual**

Definition

Planning, implementation, and evaluation of a teaching program designed to address a patient's particular needs

Activities

Establish rapport
Establish teacher credibility as appropriate
Determine the patient's learning needs
Appraise the patient's current level of knowledge and understanding of content
Appraise the patient's educational level
Appraise the patient's cognitive, psychomotor, and affective abilities/disabilities
Determine the patient's ability to learn specific information (i.e., developmental level, physiologic status, orientation, pain, fatigue, unfulfilled basic needs, emotional state, adaptation to illness)
Determine the patient's motivation to learn specific information (i.e., health beliefs, past noncompliance, bad experiences with health care/learning, conflicting goals)
Enhance the patient's readiness to learn as appropriate
Set mutual, realistic learning goals with the patient
Identify learning objectives necessary to reach goals
Determine the sequence for presenting the information
Appraise the patient's learning style
Select appropriate teaching methods/strategies
Select appropriate educational materials
Tailor the content to the patient's cognitive, psychomotor, and/or affective abilities/disabilities
Adjust instruction to facilitate learning as appropriate
Provide an environment conducive to learning
Instruct the patient when appropriate
Evaluate the patient's achievement of the stated objectives
Reinforce behavior as appropriate
Correct information misinterpretations as appropriate
Provide time for the patient to ask questions and discuss concerns
Select new teaching methods/strategies if previous ones were ineffective
Refer the patient to other specialists/agencies to meet the learning objectives as appropriate
Document the content presented, the written materials provided, and the patient's understanding of the information or patient behaviors that indicate learning on the permanent medical record
Include the family/significant others as appropriate

From McCloskey, J.C., & Bulechek, G.M. (1996). *Iowa intervention project: nursing interventions classification (NIC)* (ed. 2). St. Louis: Mosby.

thick graft. Although this type of graft becomes vascularized more rapidly and the donor site heals more rapidly than a full-thickness graft, it may exhibit postgraft contraction, be minimally resistant to surface trauma, and look the least like normal skin in texture, suppleness, pore pattern, hair growth, and other characteristics. A split-thickness skin graft (STSG) may be meshed; meshed grafts can expand to many times their normal size. Meshing allows the graft to be placed on an irregular recipient area; however, its appearance may be esthetically undesirable. A full-thickness skin graft (FTSG) contains both epidermis and dermis; any remaining subcutaneous tissue is trimmed before the FTSG is applied to the graft site. The advantages of this type of graft are that it causes minimal contracture, can be used in areas of flexion, has a greater ability to withstand trauma, can add tissue where there has been a loss or padding is required, and is esthetically more acceptable than an STSG. The donor site can be closed primarily, leaving a minimal defect. Other types of grafts

that are available for surgical reconstruction include bone, cartilage, nerve, tendon, and autologous fat grafts. Referred to as composite grafts, these are also free tissue grafts that must reestablish vascularity in the recipient area.

The donor site for an STSG heals by regeneration of epithelium from dermal elements that remain intact.

BOX 24-3 | Postoperative Wound Care at Home

By the time of discharge, you should be educated in all aspects of wound care. Your ability to clean, dress, irrigate, monitor, and pack the wound area depends on the location and size of the wound. Should you be unable to care properly for the wound, a home care manager or nurse can be contacted.

You should pay strict attention to the following home care procedures:

- Medications should be taken as prescribed unless otherwise indicated by your physician.
- The proper dressing and bandages should be applied as explained by your health care provider before you were discharged. Be sure to use the bandages, tape, topical ointments, and irrigation solutions recommended by your physician, all of which can be bought at your local pharmacy or ordered from a home care company.
- When changing the dressing, follow these guidelines:
  - Wash your hands
  - Wear gloves
  - Properly dispose of the old dressing
  - Clean the area as explained by the physician or nurse before discharge
  - Apply the new dressing as specified

It is important that you look for early signs of infection, hemorrhage, or dehiscence (separation or rupture of the surgical incision or wound closure). Be sure to contact your physician or home care provider if you have any questions.

This box may be copied for free distribution to patients and families. All rights reserved.
From Mosby. (1997). *Mosby's patient teaching guides, update II*, St. Louis: Mosby.

Therefore only a dressing is placed over this donor site. Because no dermal elements remain when an FTSG is taken, this donor site does not heal spontaneously. It heals either when the wound edges of the donor site are sutured together (primary closure) or when an STSG is applied over it. A scar remains at the donor site of a skin graft. Therefore donor sites that are covered by clothing are generally chosen.

For a graft to survive, the vascularity of the recipient area must be adequate, contact between the graft and recipient bed must be maintained, and the graft-bed unit must be adequately immobilized.

Color, temperature, signs of infection, blanching of the skin, excessive pain and discomfort, edema, vasoconstriction, and venous congestion should be noted and any change reported to the surgeon.

Documentation of any changes should be made. If the patient is discharged to home after surgery, patient and family education should include reportable signs and symptoms of potential complications.

A stent or tie-over dressing is often placed over a skin graft (Fig. 24-18). This exerts even pressure, ensuring good contact between graft and recipient site. It also eliminates potential shearing forces at the graft and recipient site interface that might disrupt new blood vessels growing into the graft.

Procedural considerations

A plastic local instrument set is required, plus a dermatome of choice, a skin mesher, a marking pen, and sterile unexposed x-ray film.

The patient is positioned so that both donor and recipient sites are well exposed. Both areas are prepped and draped to maintain adequate exposure and mobility, as required.

Operative procedure

1. The recipient site is prepared as necessary. This step may involve excision of a benign or malignant skin tumor, débridement of an open wound, or release of a scar contracture.
2. Careful planning and marking before harvesting the graft from the recipient site are essential. When feasible, a pattern of the recipient site is made with sterile unexposed x-ray film. This pattern is transferred to the donor site and outlined with a marking pen.
3. STSGs are harvested with a Weck knife or dermatome of the surgeon's choice.
4. Moist sponges soaked in normal saline, an antibiotic solution, or 20 mg of phenylephrine HCl (Neo-Synephrine) per 1000 ml of normal saline may be applied to the donor sites to aid hemostasis. A small amount of methylene blue may be placed in the solution of Neo-Synephrine as a marker to identify it from other solutions on the sterile field. Topical thrombin may also be used to aid in hemostasis. It comes prepackaged and ready to attach to a sprayer or sponges may be soaked in thrombin solution. Topical thrombin is for topical use only and not for injection. These sponges are removed, and the donor site is covered with Biobrane or Opsite.
5. If the graft is to be meshed, it is now applied to specifically supplied carriers for use with certain skin meshers.
6. A graft that is not immediately applied to the recipient site dries quickly, particularly a meshed graft. Therefore grafts should be kept in moist gauze sponges contained in a small basin to prevent inadvertent loss of the graft. Meshed skin should not be removed from its carrier until it is applied directly to the recipient site. Whether applied as a sheet or meshed, STSG may be sutured or stapled with a skin stapler. Nonadherent gauze is usually applied as the first layer of dressing over a graft. Moist dressings should be applied to all meshed grafts to prevent desiccation and loss of the graft.
7. Fat adherent to the graft is trimmed. The graft is applied to the recipient site and usually sutured at the

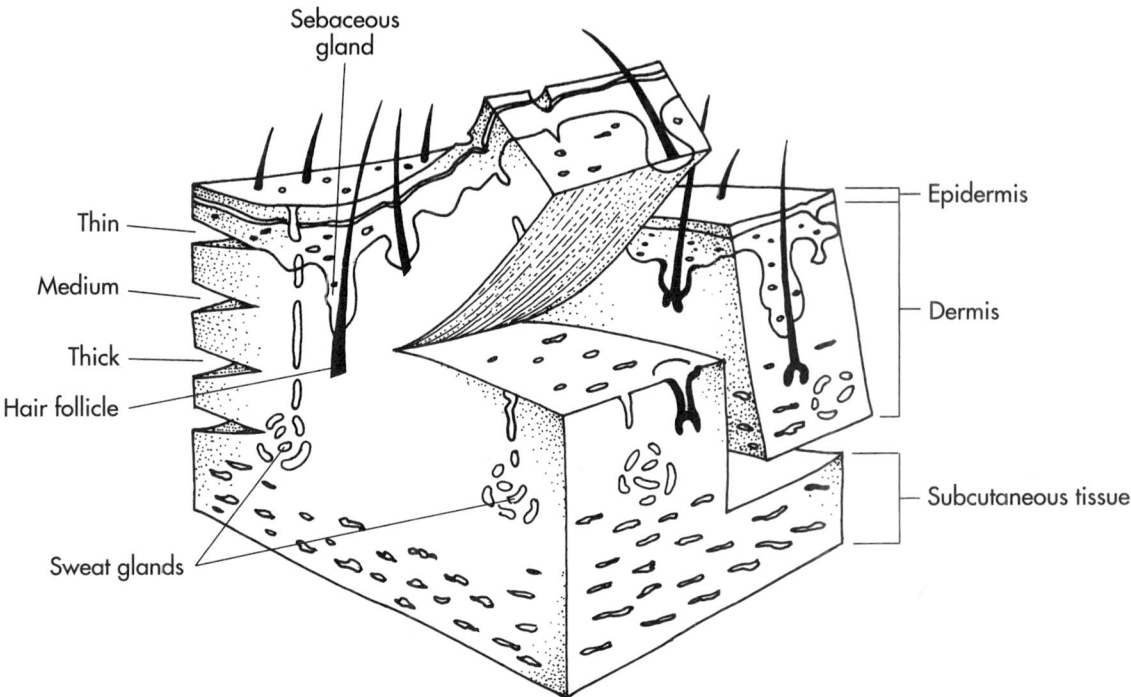

FIGURE 24-17   Split-thickness and full-thickness skin grafts.

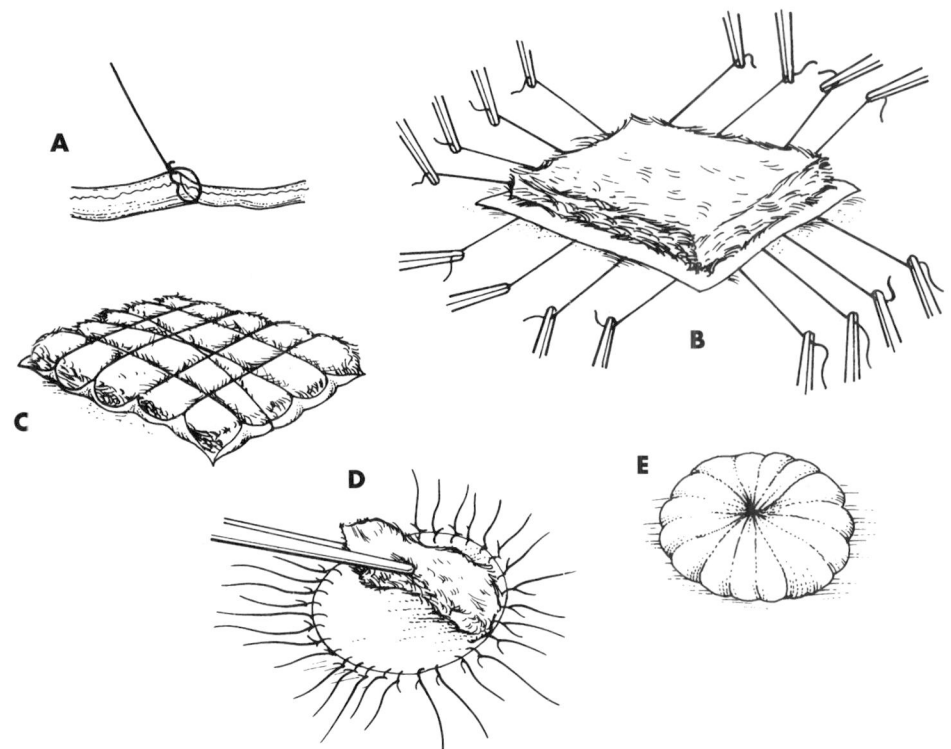

FIGURE 24-18   **A,** Method of fixation of skin graft to edges of wound. **B,** Nonadherent dressing is applied over skin graft, and on this a generous pad of acrylic fiber. **C,** Long ends of suture are tied over fiber to produce area of pressure between graft and base. **D,** Similar dressing is applied to circular graft. **E,** Long suture ends are tied over circular graft (often called "stent" dressing).

edges, and these sutures are left long to tie over a stent dressing. Blood clots beneath the graft are removed by saline irrigation before the dressing is applied.

Preservation of Skin Grafts

A skin graft may be harvested but not used immediately. Skin can be obtained from the patient on whom it is to be grafted (autograft) or from a living or nonliving donor unrelated to the recipient (allograft). Skin that is obtained for future grafting must be preserved and stored in a safe, controlled environment until it is used. Although a general procedure is described below, each facility should establish protocols for preserving, maintaining, and storing tissue. Issues of consent, medical contraindications, and screening criteria should be included in these protocols.[2]

Preservation procedure

The setup should include the skin specimen and the following items:

- Sterile 3-inch rolled gauze
- Adhesive tape for sealing and labeling container
- Basin with isotonic solution
- Sterile container with screw cap
- Storage solution or preservative (as appropriate)

Operative procedure

1. The skin should be kept on the instrument table until it is ready for storage.
2. The skin must be kept moist with an isotonic solution such as balanced salt solution or saline at all times.
3. The skin is gently flattened, smoothed out, and placed on a piece of roller gauze moistened with the isotonic solution, with its external surface facing downward.
4. The scrub person rolls the gauze and skin loosely, places the roll in the sterile container, and secures the cap.
5. The circulating nurse labels the jar with the donor's name and hospital number, location of donor site, date of collection, any preservative used and its concentration, and size of graft.
6. If the surgeon anticipates using the preserved skin within 14 days, it may be stored in a refrigerator at between 1° and 10° C (34° and 50° F) until it is used. An alternative method is to place the skin in a tissue medium such as McCoy's; the tissue may then be stored in a refrigerator at between 1° and 10° C (34° and 50° F) for 30 days until it is used.
7. If the surgeon does not anticipate using the skin within 14 days, it can be maintained by one of several long-term storage methods. One method is to place the skin in a cryoprotectant (such as ethylene glycol) for 1 to 2 hours at 4° C (39° F), gradually cool the skin to -70° C (-94° F), and then store in a liquid nitrogen freezer.

Flaps

The term *flap* refers to tissue that is detached from one area of the body and transferred to the recipient area with either part or all of its original blood supply intact or reestablished (Fig. 24-19); thus they have a self-contained vascular system. The base or pedicle of the flap is that portion through which the blood supply enters or exits. Because flaps carry their own blood supply, they are usually used to cover recipient sites that have poor vascularity and full-thickness tissue loss. Flaps are used for reconstruction or wound closure. They are useful for covering exposed bone, tendon, or nerve. They may be used if operating through the wound may be necessary at a later date to repair underlying structures. Flaps containing skin and subcutaneous tissue retain more properties of normal skin and shrink less than skin grafts. Flaps, however, have some disadvantages, such as bulky appearance, failure to match tissue of the recipient site in texture or color, and the possibility of requiring multiple operations and prolonged hospitalization.

Flaps may be classified according to blood supply. *Random pattern flaps* consist of skin and subcutaneous tissue vascularized by random perforators with limited length-to-width ratio. *Axial pattern flaps* have a well-defined arteriovenous supply along the long axis; they can be comparatively long in relation to width. Flaps may also be classified according to position or how they are rotated after elevation. *Advancement flaps* are cut and advanced to reconstruct a nearby defect. *Transposition flaps* are advanced along an axis that forms an angle to the flap's original position. *Rotation flaps* are similar to transposition flaps but are semicircular and rotate along a greater axis. *Island flaps* of isolated sections of skin and subcutaneous tissue are tunneled beneath the skin to new sites. *Pedicle flaps* were the forerunners of muscle and musculocutaneous flaps. These consist of skin and underlying muscle; they are very mobile and can be rotated into distant defects. *Free flaps* are actually a form of tissue transplantation. Using microvascular techniques, a defined amount of skin, muscle, or bone can be isolated, totally detached, and reattached at the recipient site by microvascular anastomoses between recipient-site blood vessels and the major vessels that supply the flap. The vascular pedicle may contain functional nerves, yielding sensory flaps to provide protective sensation or motor flaps to restore function. Bone and joints may be transplanted as free flaps, as in the case of toe-to-thumb transfers.

Procedural considerations

A basic plastic instrument set is required, plus the following:

- ESU
- Marking pen
- Extra hemostats

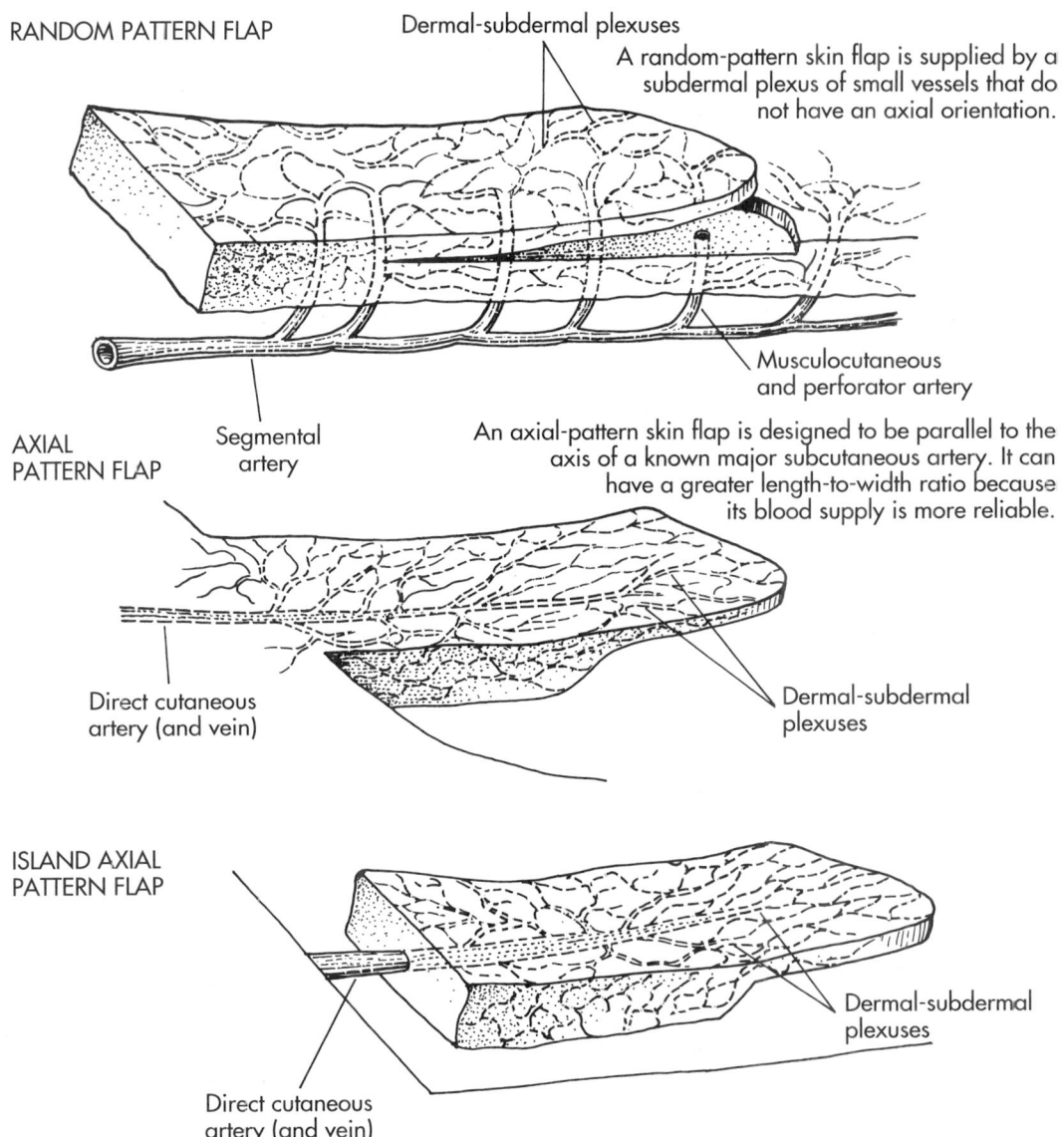

RANDOM PATTERN FLAP

Dermal-subdermal plexuses

A random-pattern skin flap is supplied by a subdermal plexus of small vessels that do not have an axial orientation.

Musculocutaneous and perforator artery

Segmental artery

AXIAL PATTERN FLAP

An axial-pattern skin flap is designed to be parallel to the axis of a known major subcutaneous artery. It can have a greater length-to-width ratio because its blood supply is more reliable.

Direct cutaneous artery (and vein)

Dermal-subdermal plexuses

ISLAND AXIAL PATTERN FLAP

Dermal-subdermal plexuses

Direct cutaneous artery (and vein)

FIGURE 24–19 Types of flaps. *Top,* Random-pattern flap. A random-pattern skin flap is supplied by a subdermal plexus of small vessels that do not have an axial orientation. *Middle,* Axial-pattern flap. An axial-pattern skin flap is designed parallel to the axis of a known major subcutaneous artery. It can have a greater length-to-width ratio because its blood supply is more reliable. *Bottom,* Island axial pattern flap.

- X-ray film, unexposed (sterile)
- Dermatome of choice
- Skin mesher
- Microvascular instruments (as appropriate)

Positioning, prepping, and draping of the patient are carried out to maintain adequate exposure and mobility of both the flap donor and recipient sites.

Operative procedure

1. The recipient site is prepared in the same manner as for a skin graft.
2. When feasible, a pattern of the recipient site is made and transferred to the donor area.
3. The flap is incised, elevated, and transferred to the recipient site. The edges of the flap are sutured to the periphery of the recipient site.
4. The flap donor site is repaired by approximating the skin edges directly or by covering the defect with a skin graft or another flap.
5. Drains are usually placed under flaps.
6. Dressings are applied with particular attention given to immobilization of the flap, which may require stockinette, padding, or plaster of Paris.
7. When a pedicle flap is divided, the surgeon may want to determine the adequacy of circulation within the flap. One can check by placing rubber-shod clamps across the base of the pedicle and injecting 20 ml of

5% sodium fluorescein intravenously. After 10 minutes have elapsed, all lights in the operating room are turned off, and a Woods lamp is held over the flap to determine the presence or absence of fluorescence within the flap. Fluorescein may be injected locally for the same purpose.

Composite Graft

Composite grafts are composed of skin and underlying tissues that are completely separated from the blood supply of the donor site and transplanted to another area of the body. The survival of a composite graft depends on ingrowth of new blood vessels from the recipient site around the periphery of the graft. Therefore, composite grafts are usually small so that no portion of the graft is greater than 1 cm from its periphery. An example of compound tissues used as composite grafts is hair transplants, composed of skin, fat, and hair follicles, which are used to treat male pattern baldness. The term *composite* thus indicates a defect that requires a graft be brought to the area to meet more than one type of tissue deficiency.

Procedural considerations

A plastic local instrument set is required, plus the following:

- Marking pen
- X-ray film, unexposed (sterile)

Positioning, prepping, and draping of the patient are such that adequate exposure of both donor and recipient sites is achieved.

Operative procedure

1. The recipient site is prepared by excising tissue, such as a scar or a benign or malignant skin lesion.
2. When feasible, a pattern of the recipient site is made and transferred to the donor site.
3. The composite graft is excised. The donor site is either closed by approximating its skin edges or left unsutured (as in hair transplant donor sites).
4. Meanwhile, the composite graft is kept in a moist sponge until it is sutured to the edges of the recipient site.
5. Dressings of choice are applied to the composite graft and donor site.

BREAST RECONSTRUCTION

The loss of a breast because of cancer may have a devastating affect on a woman. Breasts are symbolic of a woman's femininity and sexuality. Change in body image resulting from mastectomy is one of the most difficult psychologic aspects of dealing with breast cancer. The patient who selects breast reconstruction must realize that after reconstructive surgery the reconstructed breast will resemble a mound and should be as symmetric as possible to the contralateral side but will not be the same as her preoperative breast. A reduction mammoplasty on the unaffected breast may be done to achieve symmetry.

Breast reconstruction can be performed immediately after mastectomy or can be delayed. The patient's physical condition and preference dictate this decision, just as the need for chemotherapy or radiation therapy does. Contraindications to breast reconstruction may include metastasis to major organs such as liver, bone, or lung. The use of chemotherapy and radiation does not preclude reconstruction but may delay it somewhat as a result of the healing processes.

Reconstruction of the breast can be accomplished in three ways: available tissue and an implant, tissue expanders, or flaps. Use of available tissue is the easiest procedure; however, insufficient tissue remains after mastectomy in numerous patients. When sufficient tissue exists, an implant of the appropriate size may be placed under the remaining skin flap or muscle, with the contralateral side adjusted accordingly by either a reduction mammoplasty or mastopexy to achieve symmetry if the patient so chooses.

Breast Reconstruction using Tissue Expanders

Mastectomy may leave a shortage of skin that prevents creation of a beast mound. For these patients, extra tissue can be created locally with the use of tissue expanders. Tissue expansion is a technique used to stretch normal tissue that is adjacent to a defect, mechanically creating redundancy of normal tissue to correct the defect. For breast reconstruction the expander is basically the same shape as a breast prosthesis. The expander may have a metal-backed, self-sealing silicone valve at its dome or a small, dome-shaped reservoir with a fill tube that is positioned subcutaneously at a distance from the expander but connected to it. In either case, weekly percutaneous injections of normal saline are placed in the expander until the tissue has reached the desired maximum stretch, usually based on a 3:1 ratio. When the desired stretch has been accomplished, the temporary tissue expander is removed, and a permanent implant is placed.

A combination tissue expander and permanent prosthesis is also available. The procedure of expansion is the same as with a temporary tissue expander; however, when the tissue has reached desired maximum expansion, a portion of the saline fill is removed to achieve a size and "settling" of the reconstructed breast at the inframammary fold so that the tissue resembles the contralateral breast. Potential complications associated with the use of tissue expanders include infection, extrusion, deflation, flipped ports, and hematoma formation.[4]

Procedural considerations

A basic plastic instrument set is used. The breast-shape expander is supplied in a sterile package from the

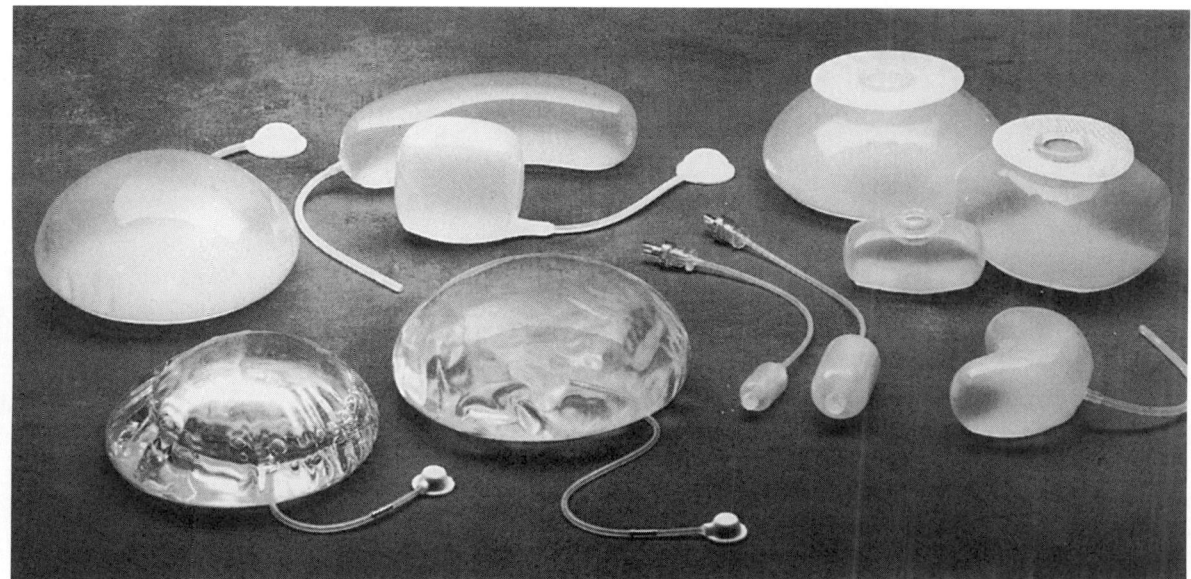

FIGURE 24-20 Tissue expanders are inflatable plastic reservoirs of various shapes and volumes that are implanted under the skin. The skin over the expander is stretched during a period of several weeks as the expander is gradually filled by percutaneous injection of saline into an incorporated part of remote-fill port. Expanders are useful for breast reconstruction.

manufacturer and is available in a variety of sizes (Fig. 24-20). The care of the tissue expander is the same as that for other implantable devices. The patient is positioned supine with the arms extended on armboards. Prepping and draping are carried out in the routine manner to expose both breasts and axilla.

Operative procedure

1. A submuscular pocket is created for the temporary expander. In addition, a tunnel and pocket are created at an adjacent site from the main pocket for the placement of the injection dome and the connecting tube.
2. The tissue expander is tested before insertion for watertight integrity.
3. The expander is then inserted, the reservoir positioned subcutaneously and connected, the wound closed, and the expander filled with sterile saline solution until slight blanching of the skin is achieved. The amount is recorded on the patient record. On occasion, the surgeon may choose to instill 3 to 5 ml of methylene blue into the expander, which can help to identify the proper location of the fill tube postoperatively.
4. Additional inflation of the tissue expander usually begins 2 to 3 weeks after initial placement when healing of the incision line has started and thereafter on an average of every 7 days. The time from implant insertion until complete fill varies according to the desired maximum stretch.
5. After the desired expansion has occurred, the temporary expander is exchanged for a permanent prosthesis.

Breast Reconstruction using Myocutaneous Flaps

Flaps are described by the types of tissue they contain, their blood supply, and the method by which they are moved from the donor to the recipient site. The latissimus dorsi myocutaneous flap is a single-stage reconstruction of the breast after mastectomy. Since the flap consists of skin combined with muscle, it is described as *myocutaneous*. This flap is used when significant tissue deficiency occurs after a mastectomy. The latissimus dorsi muscle is a wide, flat muscle extending over the midthoracic portion of the back and inserting into the humerus; its blood supply comes from the thoracodorsal artery and perforators from the upper lumbar arteries and the intercostal vessels. This rich vascularity allows the surgeon flexibility in orienting and positioning the flap to the pattern of the deficit on the anterior chest wall. Latissimus dorsi flaps for breast reconstruction may be used with an internal breast prosthesis, with or without adjustment in the size of the contralateral breast.

Procedural considerations

The skin island and area of dissection for the latissimus dorsi flap are drawn on the patient's back before prepping and draping. The patient is placed in a lateral position with the arm on the operative side extended and elevated on a sling support. Pressure points are padded and protected by the use of pillows and sheet rolls, and the patient is stabilized on the OR bed. The patient is prepped and draped to expose the affected breast area and muscle and the donor site.

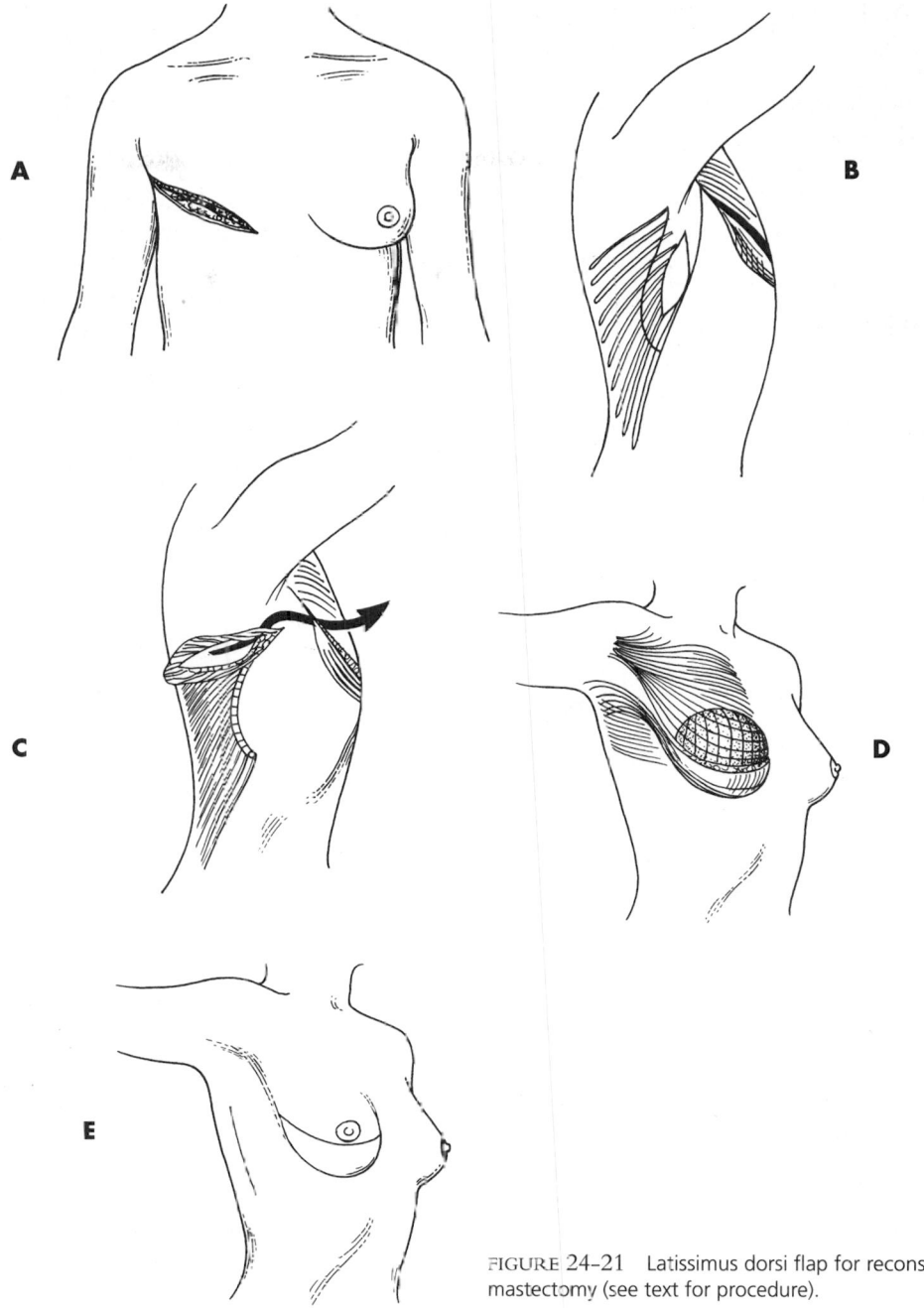

FIGURE 24-21 Latissimus dorsi flap for reconstruction after mastectomy (see text for procedure).

A basic plastic instrument set is used, plus long Metzenbaum scissors, long DeBakey forceps, vascular instruments, Deaver retractors, Freeman areolar markers, lighted breast retractors or a headlight, a Doppler probe, and a second ESU.

Two surgical teams may work simultaneously, one freeing the muscle flap and the other preparing the recipient site.

Operative procedure (Fig. 24-21)

1. Initially the island of skin is incised transversely across the back, with care being taken so that the resulting scar will be covered by a bra or bathing suit.

2. The muscle, subcuticular fat, and fascia are then freed from the overlying skin by undermining so that part or all of the muscle may be mobilized.

3. The skin island and the muscle are then tunneled under the axilla to the chest wall (Fig. 24-21, C). The insertion of the muscle on the humerus and accompanying blood vessels are left undisturbed. The latissimus dorsi muscle fills the space left by the missing pectoralis muscle.

4. The island of skin is oriented to the recipient site, and both are sutured into place (Fig. 24-21, D).

5. A saline-filled implant is placed under the muscle before suturing to reconstruct the breast mound.

6. The wound is drained by closed-wound suction catheters.

7. The nipple-areola complex may also be reconstructed by sharing the nipple on the unaffected side or by using groin or auricular tissue. It can be done at the time of reconstruction or at a later date as a minor procedure under local anesthesia (Fig. 24-21, *E*).

Transverse Rectus Abdominis Myocutaneous Flap

The transverse rectus abdominis myocutaneous (TRAM) flap is a single-stage reconstruction of a postmastectomy breast using the transverse rectus abdomi-

nis muscle. This flap gives the patient and plastic surgeon an alternative to the latissimus dorsi flap by taking excess tissue from the lower abdomen to construct the breast, usually without the need for an implant (Fig. 24-22).

Procedural considerations

Markings on the patient are made preoperatively with the patient in an upright position. A basic plastic instrument set is used as for the latissimus dorsi flap. The patient is positioned supine with arms extended on armboards. Positioning the patient for this procedure is particularly difficult because of the need to promote closure of the abdominal wound, support circulation to the flap, and protect the patient from injury. The OR bed is

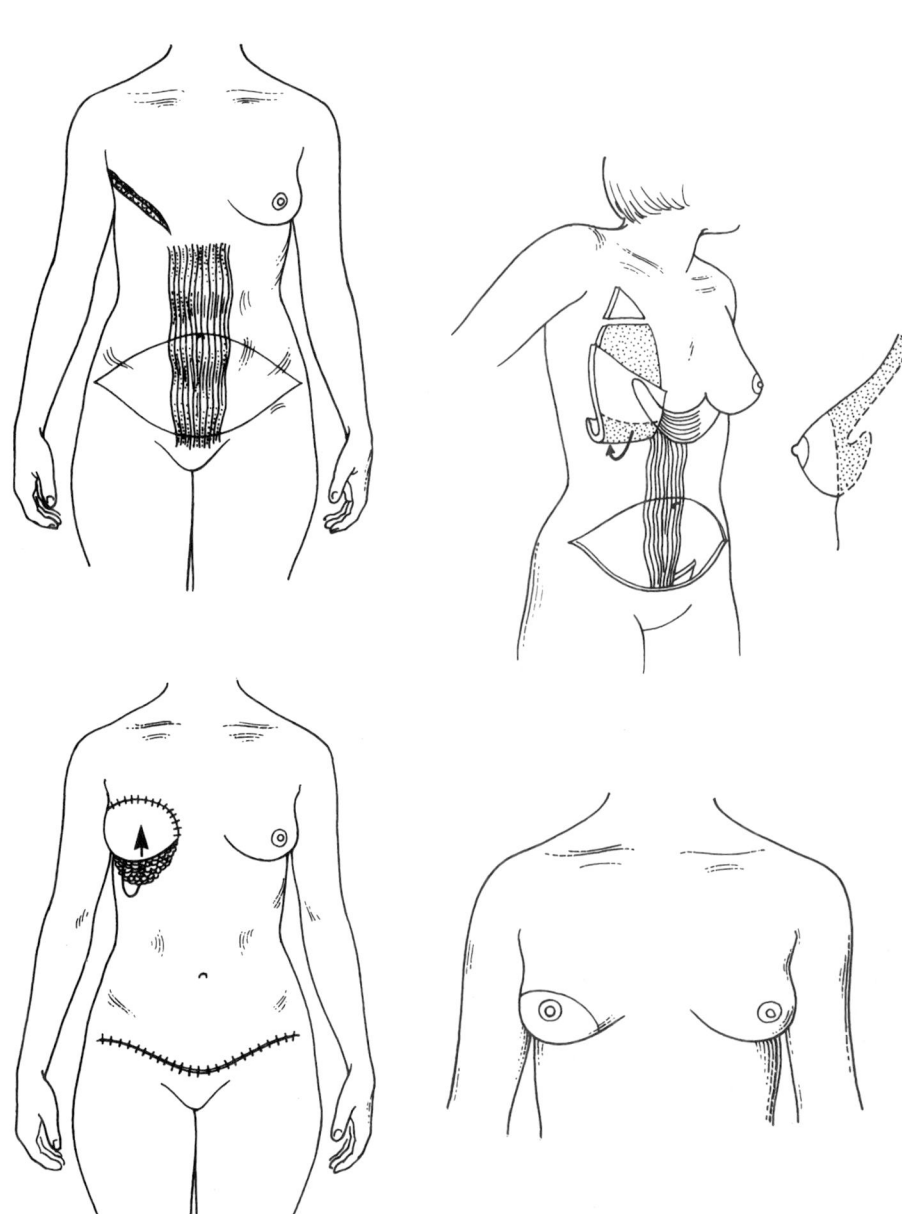

FIGURE 24-22   TRAM flap for postmastectomy breast reconstruction.

often flexed; additional padding of the lower extremities may be required. The chest and abdomen are prepped and draped simultaneously.

Operative procedure

1. The skin from the mastectomy scar is excised.
2. The transverse rectus abdominis muscle is dissected and tunneled subcutaneously to the midline of the abdomen.
3. The flap is brought to the chest wall and sutured medially; the thinnest portion of the flap is superior and medial, and the thickest portion is inferior and lateral.
4. Because of the amount of tissue available, an implant is often unnecessary.

There are alternative approaches to the TRAM flap. With the pedicle approach the TRAM flap is elevated on a vascular pedicle and rotated into place. With the free approach the TRAM flap is separated from the superior epigastric vessels and anastomosed to the vessels of the chest. A supercharged flap involves elevating the TRAM flap on its vascular pedicle, rotating it into position on the chest, and anastomosing vessels to augment blood supply to the flap. With the free or supercharged TRAM flap the microscope, microvascular instruments, Wood's lamp, and loupes need to be available.

Nipple Reconstruction

This procedure may be done at the time of the original reconstruction, but most surgeons believe that they have a better result if it is done as a secondary procedure after the reconstruction has healed and symmetry is achieved. Tissue may be harvested from donor sites such as the groin, auricular area, labia, big toe, or contralateral nipple. Tattooing may complete the reconstruction.

Augmentation Mammoplasty

Breast augmentation is done for hypomastia, to correct breast asymmetry, and to recreate the breast after mastectomy. A saline-filled prosthesis is inserted to enlarge or form the breast mound. Placing the implant under the pectoralis muscle contributes to softness (Fig. 24-23).

Procedural considerations

A basic plastic instrument set is used, plus lighted fiberoptic retractors. The breast implants are packaged in sterile containers from the manufacturer and given to the scrub nurse when breast size is determined. The patient is placed in a supine position. The arms may be extended on armboards to approximately 60 degrees. Alternatively, the hands may be placed over the lower abdomen, the elbows protected with foam padding, and the arms gently secured with adhesive tape to the OR bed. Prepping and draping are carried out in the routine manner to expose the operative site.

Operative procedure

Augmentation mammoplasty is done through circumareolar, inframammary, or axillary incisions. Either the underlying breast tissue or the pectoralis muscle from the chest wall is elevated. A pocket is dissected, and the implant is placed in the pocket. Electrocoagulation is used to achieve hemostasis. The pocket may be irrigated with an antibiotic solution before placement of the implant. The wound is closed in layers, and a light gauze dressing is applied. A bra or an Ace wrap may be used for support.

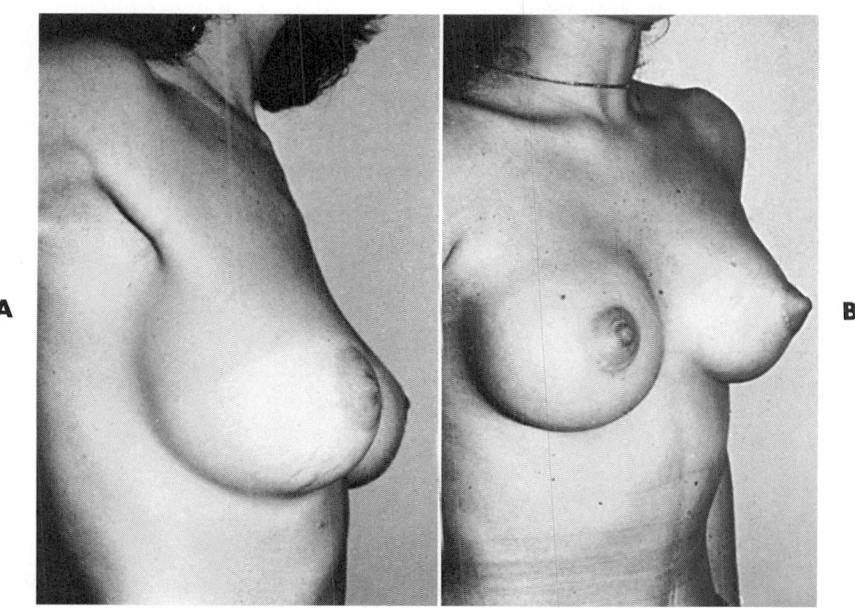

FIGURE 24-23 **A,** Augmentation mammoplasty implant under muscle. **B,** Implant under breast tissue.

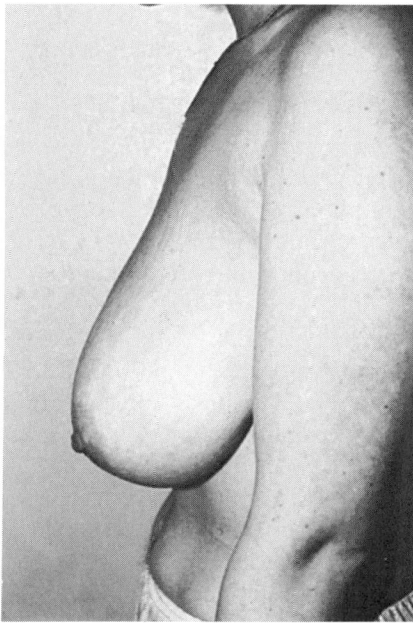

FIGURE 24-24 Patient with pendulous breasts before reduction mammoplasty.

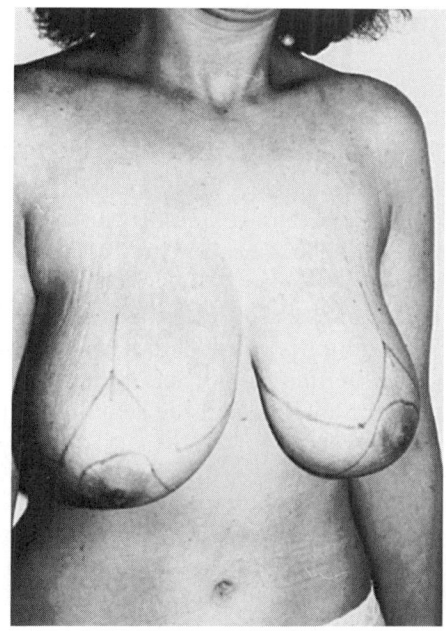

FIGURE 24-25 Area of excision marked before surgery.

Reduction Mammoplasty

Reduction mammoplasty is indicated for the patient with gigantomastia or macromastia resulting with back pain, intertrigo, or deep grooving in the shoulders from the weight of the breasts. The procedure may also be performed to achieve symmetry after a mastectomy on the contralateral side. Excessive breast tissue and its overlying skin is excised, with reconstruction of the breast contour, size, shape, and symmetry (Fig. 24-24). Preoperatively the patient needs to be aware that the scars will be visible and that she may have a slight degree of asymmetry. Autologous blood should be available and the patient typed and crossmatched before undergoing anesthesia.

Procedural considerations

A basic plastic instrument set is used with the addition of a "cookie cutter" areola marker or a "keyhole" pattern marker, a marking pen, skin stapler, tape measure, ESU, and two closed-wound suction systems. A scale for weighing specimens should also be available, and tissue from each side should be carefully weighed and marked appropriately.

The patient is placed in a supine position with arms slightly extended on padded armboards. The hips should be positioned at the break in the OR bed so that the patient may be raised to a sitting position if necessary. Standard prepping and draping are done. Care should be taken not to remove the preoperative markings.

Operative procedure

1. The skin to be excised, as well as the new site for the nipple, is marked (Fig. 24-25).
2. The skin between the new and the old nipple sites is

incised and removed, with the nipple remaining attached to the underlying breast tissue. On patients with very large breasts the nipples are removed and then reapplied as free grafts when the reduction is complete.
3. The redundant segment of breast tissue inferior to the nipple is excised through an inverted-T incision. Tissue from each breast is measured and kept separately.
4. The nipple and adjacent tissue are mobilized and sutured in place.
5. The medial and lateral skin edges are approximated in a vertical suture line inferior to the nipple.
6. The inframammary elliptical incision is trimmed and closed transversely (Fig. 24-26). Closed-wound suction catheters may be placed. The wound is dressed.

Reduction for Gynecomastia

Gynecomastia is a relatively common pathologic condition that consists of bilateral or unilateral enlargement of the male breast. It occurs primarily during puberty or after the age of 40. Although it may be produced by a variety of diseases, it is usually related to excessive hormone production or alterations in hormonal balance. It may also be seen in elderly men and in men after excessive use of marijuana. All subareolar fibroglandular tissue is removed, and the resultant defect is surgically reconstructed. The patient may be positioned in a supine position or semi-Fowler's position, according to the surgeon's preference. Supplies and equipment needed are the same as those for a simple mastectomy, plus a basic plastic instrument set. Because suction-assisted lipectomy (SAL) may be used for contouring, suction cannulas, associated supplies, and an aspirator should also be available.

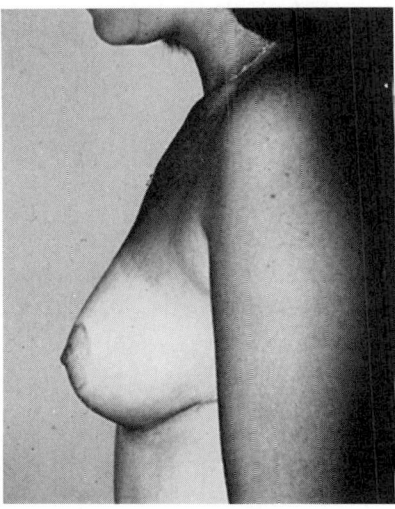
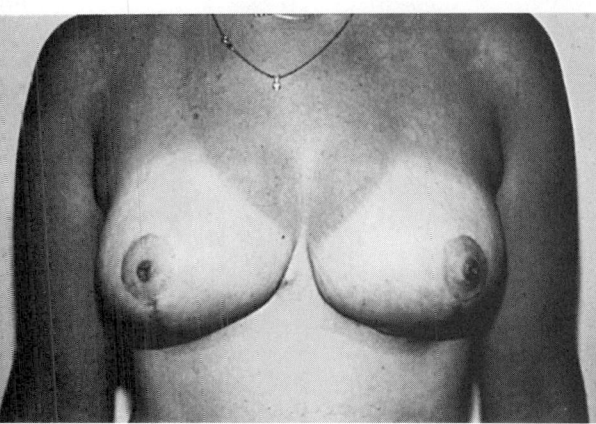

FIGURE 24-26   Postoperative reduction mammoplasty.

Operative procedure

1. A periareolar incision is made. Through this incision the fibrous and ductal attachments of the underlying glandular tissue to the nipple are divided.
2. A cuff of fatty tissue is left attached to the underlying nipple surface to protect the blood supply.
3. The breast tissue mass is then gently dissected. Carrying the dissection to the pectoralis fascia is usually necessary to remove the entire mass.
4. Hemostasis is carefully achieved.
5. When all subcutaneous tissue has been mobilized, a three-layer closure is carried out. A small drain may be inserted to prevent hematoma formation. A firm pressure dressing is applied.

SURGERY FOR MAXILLOFACIAL TRAUMA

Reduction of Nasal Fracture

Usually a closed reduction of the bony nasal fragments is performed by digital and instrumental manipulation Occasionally an open reduction with interosseous wire fixation of nasal bone fragments is necessary. A nasal fracture may involve a fracture of the nasal bones or cartilage (including the septum). Closed reduction of a nasal fracture is most often performed under topical and local anesthesia.

Procedural considerations

A plastic local instrument set is required, plus the following:

- 2 nasal specula, 1 short and 1 long
- 1 Brown nasal splint
- 1 Asch forceps or rubber-shod Kelly hemostat
- Nasal packing or nasal struts of choice

- 4 metal applicator sticks and wisps of cotton (or cotton-tipped applicators)
- Topical and local anesthetic agents of choice

The patient is placed in the supine position. An intravenous infusion is started, and a blood pressure cuff is applied. The head drape is used.

Operative procedure

1. Topical anesthesia for the nasal mucosa and nerve block anesthesia around the nose are administered.
2. Asch forceps are introduced intranasally to elevate the bony fragments while with digital pressure the surgeon's other hand molds the bones into position.
3. The nasal septum is inspected and realigned with the Asch forceps, if necessary.
4. Bilateral anterior nasal packs are placed.
5. Half-inch tape strips are applied over the skin of the nose, followed by application of the nasal splint and a nasal drip pad.

Reduction of Mandibular Fractures

The purpose of treatment for a mandibular fracture is to restore the patient's preinjury dental occlusion. With some types of fractures, a closed reduction with immobilization by means of intermaxillary fixation is sufficient for treatment. With a majority of mandibular fractures, however, an open reduction with wire fixation is necessary, plus supplemental intermaxillary fixation to achieve adequate immobilization for healing.

Intermaxillary fixation is most often accomplished when arch bars are applied to the maxillary and mandibular teeth. Stainless steel wires (#24 or #25) are placed around the necks of the teeth and are ligated around the arch bars to hold the latter in place. Latex bands are attached to the tongs on the maxillary and mandibular arch bars to fix the teeth in occlusion (Fig. 24-27). If the patient is edentulous,

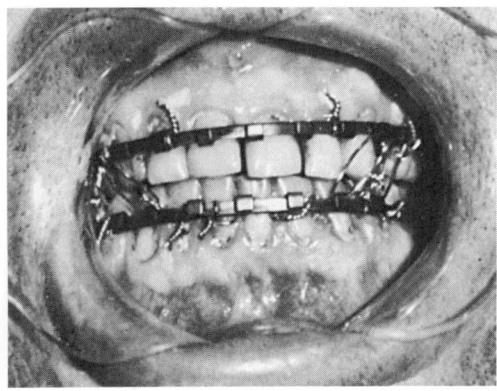

FIGURE 24-27 Teeth in occlusion with arch bars in place. Tongs on arch bars will accept latex bands, which maintain occlusion for several weeks (wires around tongs are shown).

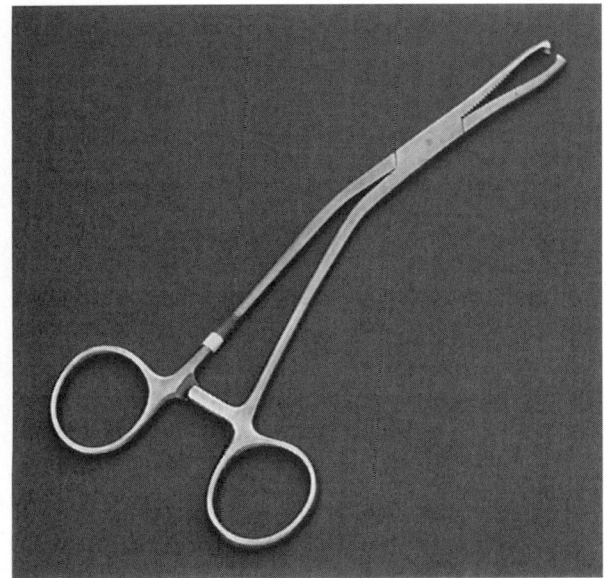

FIGURE 24-28 Dingman bone-holding forceps used in reduction of mandibular fractures.

arch bars are attached to dentures or specially fabricated dental splints. The dentures or splints are held in place by means of wires placed around the mandible (for the mandibular arch bar) and through the nasal spine and around the zygomatic arches (for the maxillary arch bar). Scissors or wire cutters must be sent with the patient to PACU to prevent aspiration, should the patient vomit or choke.

Procedural considerations–open reduction

A basic plastic instrument set, plus the following instruments and supplies, is needed for an open reduction of a fractured mandible: a Hall II air drill; two Dingman bone-holding forceps (Fig. 24-28); a nerve stimulator; a marking pen; stainless steel wires, #24, #26, and #28; the ESU; epinephrine 1:200,000 for injection; and a rigid fixation system.

For the application of arch bars or other types of interdental wiring techniques, a separate Mayo setup with the following instruments and supplies is required: a set of coil arch bars and latex bands; stainless steel wire, #25 or #26; two Mayo-Hegar needle holders, 8 inches; a wire suture scissors, 4¾ inches; a wire twister; a Yankauer suction tube; two Weider tongue depressors, large and small; six mosquito hemostats, curved, 5¼ inches; a Brown fascia needle (if dentures or splints are used); a Freer septal elevator; and a small drain.

If arch bars are applied before the open reduction is performed, this latter setup must be kept completely separate from the instruments used for the open reduction. Because the mouth is a contaminated area, a complete change of gowns, gloves, and drapes is necessary after the intraoral procedure.

The patient is placed in the supine position on the operating room bed. The head drape is used.

Operative procedure

1. Arch bars may be applied before or after the open reduction.
2. A line inferior and parallel to the lower border of the mandible at the fracture site is marked, and the area is infiltrated with epinephrine 1:200,000 for hemostasis.
3. The incision is made so that the inferior border of the mandible is exposed. The nerve stimulator may be used to aid in identification of the marginal mandibular branch of the facial nerve in fractures of the posterior body and angle of the mandible.
4. The fracture is reduced by manipulation. Holes are drilled into the mandible on each side of the fracture line with the Hall II air drill while an assistant holds the reduced fracture with the aid of Dingman bone-holding forceps.
5. Stainless steel wire is inserted through the holes and twisted tightly to secure the fracture fragments in anatomic alignment.
6. In the event that rigid fixation is desired with the use of plates and screws, the appropriate drill bit, tap, and depth gauge are chosen. With these items the proper-sized prosthesis is placed and the fracture is approximated, aligned, and placed in anatomic position.
7. A small drain is sometimes placed into the wound, and the wound is closed in layers (periosteum, platysma muscle, and skin).
8. The latex bands may be applied to the arch bars at this time but more frequently are applied later, after the patient is fully awake and reactive.
9. A moderate compression dressing is applied to cover the submandibular wound and drain.

Reduction of Maxillary Fractures

Maxillary fractures are usually classified as follows: (1) Lefort I, or transverse maxillary fracture; (2) LeFort II, or pyramidal maxillary fracture, and (3) LeFort III, or

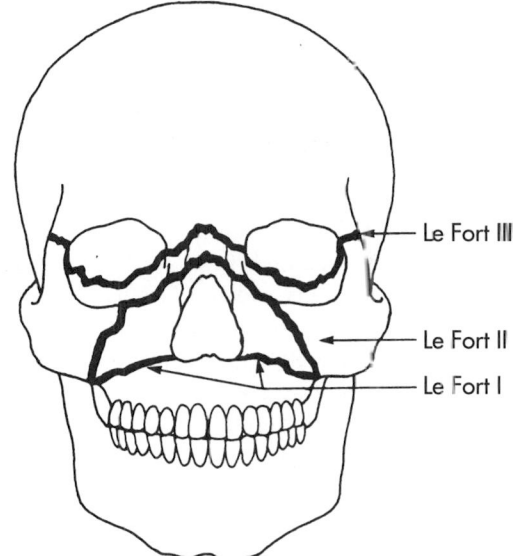

FIGURE 24-29 Le Fort's classification of maxillary fractures.

craniofacial disjunction, which includes fractures of both zygomas and the nose (Fig. 24-29). A maxillary fracture produces malocclusion, just as a mandibular fracture does. In addition, depending on the severity of the fracture, it may produce considerable deformity of the middle of the face, usually perceived as a flattening or smashed-in appearance.

Closed reduction with intermaxillary fixation suffices for treatment of LeFort I and some LeFort II fractures. The more severe LeFort II and all LeFort III fractures require open reduction in addition to intermaxillary fixation.

Procedural considerations

The basic plastic instrument set is required as well as a Hall II air drill or Elane drill; stainless steel wires, #25, #26, and #28; a Rowe maxillary forceps, right and left; a Brown fascia needle; polyethylene buttons; a small foam rubber pad; a marking pen or methylene blue; the ESU; epinephrine 1:200,000 for injection; periosteal elevators; and a rigid fixation system.

A separate Mayo setup for the application of arch bars is required, as described for reduction of mandibular fractures.

The patient is placed in the supine position on the OR bed. The head drape is used.

Operative procedure

Arch bars are applied before or after the open reduction, or they may be the only mode of treatment in closed reduction. In addition to ligating the maxillary arch bar to the teeth, it must also be suspended from stable bones superior to the fractured maxilla (which is unstable). In LeFort I fractures, suspension may be around both zygomatic arches by passage of percutaneous wires. In LeFort II and III fractures, suspension wires are placed

through holes drilled bilaterally into the zygomatic process of the frontal bone. This requires incisions into both lateral eyebrow areas. The following description pertains to open reduction of LeFort II and III fractures.

1. After injection of epinephrine 1:200,000 for hemostasis, bilateral incisions are made to expose the infraorbital rims and frontozygomatic suture lines.
2. The Rowe maxillary forceps are applied intranasally and intraorally to disimpact and reduce the maxilla. Holes are drilled into bone on each side of fracture lines along the infraorbital rim (and frontozygomatic area for LeFort III fractures, after reducing the zygomatic fractures).
3. Stainless steel wires are passed through these holes and twisted down tightly to maintain the reduction.
4. Suspension wires are passed from the eyebrow incisions, behind the zygomatic arches, and into the mouth with the Brown fascia needle. A pullout wire is looped through each suspension wire within the eyebrow incision, brought out through the skin near the hairline, and tied down over a polyethylene button and foam rubber padding. Self-tapping screws, mini-compression plates, and bone grafts may also be used, based on the surgeon's preference. Incisions are closed.
5. When indicated, reduction of a nasal fracture is then performed.

Reduction of Zygomatic Fractures

Fractures of the zygoma (the cheek or malar bone) are corrected by either closed or open reduction. The two most common types of zygomatic fractures are depressed fractures of the arch and separation at or near the zygomaticofrontal, zygomaticomaxillary, and zygomaticotemporal suture lines, which constitutes a trimalar fracture. Although fractures of the zygoma can interfere with the ability to open and close the mouth properly, their chief consequence is a flattening of the cheek on the involved side, which results from a depressed trimalar or zygomatic arch fracture. Treatment is directed toward elevating the depressed fracture and maintaining the reduction. Closed reduction is the procedure used for treatment of zygomatic arch fractures, whereas most trimalar fractures are reduced by means of open reduction with internal fixation.

Procedural considerations

A plastic instrument set, a Suraci zygoma hook-elevator, and a jaw hook are required for a closed reduction. A basic plastic instrument set, along with the following instruments and supplies, is required for an open reduction: a Hall II air drill; stainless steel wires, #26, #28, and #30; the Suraci zygoma hook-elevator; a jaw hook; a Kerrison rongeur; two Blair retractors; the bipolar ESU; a marking pen; epinephrine 1:200,000 for injection; and a mini-plating rigid fixation set.

The patient is placed in the supine position on the operating room bed. The head drape is used.

Operative procedure

Closed reduction is performed by elevating the depressed fracture with a percutaneous bone hook. Stabilization of a trimalar fracture may then be achieved by inserting a transantral Kirschner wire from the fractured side to the normal side.

The technique of open reduction of a trimalar fracture is as follows:

1. Incisions are marked along the lateral area of the eyebrow and lower eyelid over the zygomaticofrontal suture line and zygomaticomaxillary suture line (infraorbital rim) fractures respectively.
2. After injection with epinephrine 1:200,000 for hemostasis, incisions are made down to bone, and suture lines are identified and exposed.
3. The depressed zygoma is elevated with a Kelly hemostat or periosteal elevator placed behind the body of the zygoma through the lateral eyebrow incision. Bone hooks placed percutaneously or at the fracture sites may be used instead.
4. Holes are drilled into bone on each side of the fracture lines. Stainless steel wires are passed through the hole and twisted down tightly to maintain the reduction. (Reduction and stabilization of two of the three fractures are sufficient.) An alternative method of stabilization of the fractures is interosseous wiring of the zygomaticofrontal fracture and placement of a transmural Kirschner wire.
5. Incisions are closed.
6. An eye-patch dressing may be applied.

Reduction of Orbital Floor Fractures

The orbital floor is the eggshell-thin bone on which the eye and periorbital tissues rest. It separates the orbit from the maxillary antrum. Orbital floor fractures usually occur in combination with fractures of the infraorbital rim (maxillary and zygomatic fractures). An isolated depressed orbital floor fracture with an intact infraorbital rim is called a *blowout fracture*.

Symptoms of orbital floor fractures are diplopia and enophthalmos. Diplopia is caused by entrapment of periorbital fat and extraocular muscles in the fracture line, which restricts movement of the eyeball. Enophthalmos usually results from a fracture extensive enough to allow herniation of periorbital fat into the maxillary antrum, which gives the eye a sunken appearance. Treatment is directed toward relief of these symptoms.

Because the orbital floor is so thin, comminuted fractures occur frequently and segments of bone may be irretrievably lost into the maxillary antrum. If the floor cannot be reconstructed by elevating the bony fragments,

its integrity must be restored with an implant (cartilage graft, bone graft, or alloplastic material).

Procedural considerations

A basic plastic instrument set is required, as well as two Blair retractors, the Hall II air drill, alloplastic material of choice (Teflon or Silastic sheet), a marking pen or methylene blue, a bipolar ESU, epinephrine 1:200,000 for injection, and a rigid fixation system.

In addition, instruments and supplies listed for reduction of maxillary and zygomatic fractures may also be needed because orbital floor fractures often occur in combination with these fractures.

The patient is placed in the supine position on the OR bed. The head drape is used.

Operative procedure

1. A lower eyelid incision is marked, and the eyelid is injected with epinephrine 1:200,000 for hemostasis and incised down to the infraorbital rim.
2. Periosteum is elevated from the infraorbital rim and orbital floor.
3. The fracture is identified, and any entrapped periorbital tissues are reduced by gentle traction.
4. Continuity of the orbital floor is reestablished by reducing the fracture, replacing any bone chips if possible, or inserting an autogenous graft or alloplastic implant.
5. The orbital floor implant is secured anteriorly to the infraorbital rim with a suture after a hole has been drilled into the bone.
6. The incision is closed in one layer (skin).
7. An eye-patch dressing may be applied.

ELECTIVE ORTHOGNATHIC SURGERY

A large number of patients are afflicted with either acquired or congenital facial defects that affect the maxilla or the mandible, or both. The condition of many of these patients can be improved dramatically with orthodontic care; however, many also require surgical rearrangement of the maxilla or mandible.

Psychosocial and functional deficits are related to abnormalities of the maxilla and mandible. Surgical correction of these defects can improve the quality of life for these patients. Surgery is usually delayed until an adequate number of permanent teeth are in place for postoperative immobilization. Proper preoperative planning is of great importance to these patients.

Operative procedure

1. Arch bars are applied for postoperative immobilization.
2. Intraoral incisions provide exposure.
3. The maxilla or mandible is cut as indicated by the preoperative workup.

4. Bone is advanced or set back to a predetermined position.
5. Bones are wired in place with grafts in defects as needed.

SURGERY FOR ACUTE BURNS

A majority of burns result from exposure to high temperatures, which injures the skin. Thermal skin injury may be caused by flame, scalding, or direct contact with a hot object. Similar destruction of skin can result from contact with chemicals such as acid or alkali or contact with an electrical current. The latter, however, often involves extensive destruction of the underlying tissue and physiologic systems in addition to the skin.

Intact skin provides protection against the environment for all underlying tissues and organs. It aids in heat regulation, prevents water loss, and is the major barrier against bacterial invasion. Burn patients are therefore some of the most acutely ill patients brought to the operating room. The greater the degree of injury to the skin,

expressed in percentage of total body surface area (TBSA) and depth of burn, the more severe the injury. The most common method of measuring TBSA is by use of the rule of nines (Fig. 24-30).

Partial-thickness (first- and second-degree) burns heal by regeneration of skin from dermal elements that remain intact. Full-thickness (third-degree) burns require skin grafting to heal because no dermal elements remain intact. Both partial- and full-thickness burns may require débridement of necrotic tissue (eschar) before healing can occur by skin regeneration or grafting. Allograft may be used to cover the burned area during the initial healing process. However, the allograft must be carefully tested for immunodeficiency diseases. Xenograft (such as pig skin) may also be used for covering the burned area.

Procedural considerations

The essentials of skin grafting are discussed in the section on free skin grafts. This section therefore deals only with the procedure for débridement of burn wounds.

A basic plastic instrument set is required, plus a knife

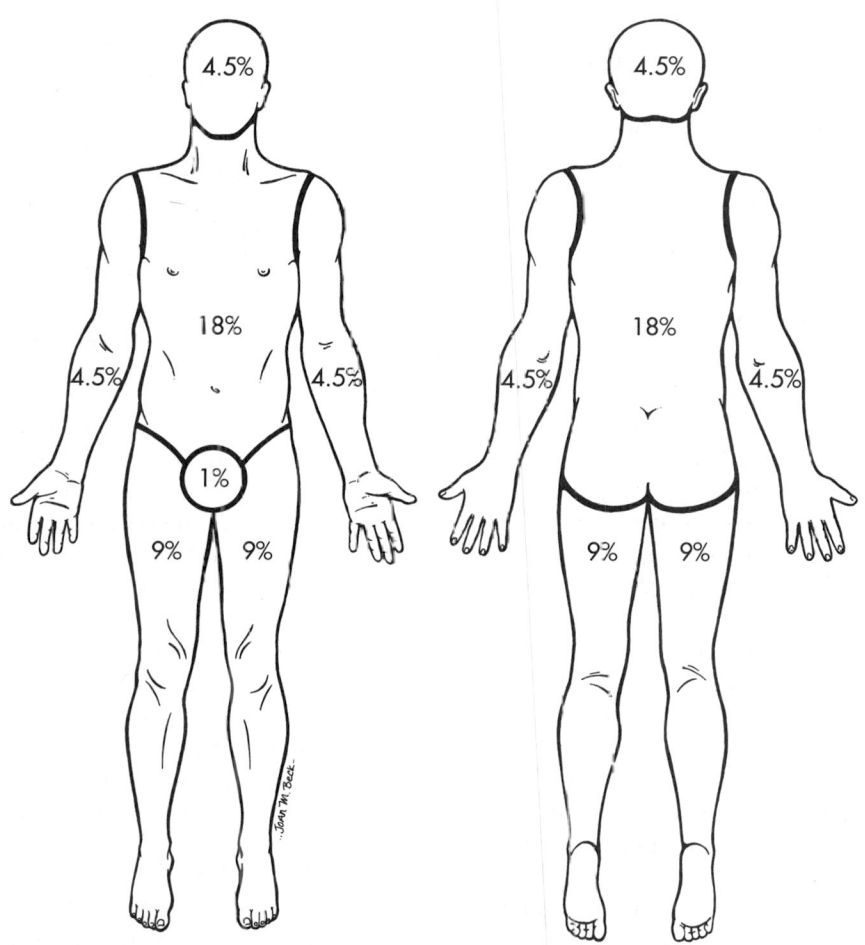

FIGURE 24-30   The "rule of nines." Dividing the body into 11 areas of 9% each helps one to estimate the amount of skin surface burned in an adult.

dermatome, an ESU, topical thrombin solution, a pneumatic tourniquet for isolated extremity burns, and a topical antimicrobial agent of choice.

Because most burn wounds become infected within a few days, burns are contaminated, and appropriate operating room procedures are followed.

Most burn patients arrive in the operating room with dressings covering their wounds. These are removed after the patient has been anesthetized to minimize pain and loss of body heat through the open burn wounds. The temperature in the operating room should be constantly monitored so that the patient's normal body temperature is maintained. The loss of heat from the body is increased by the lack of intact skin caused by a burn.

Operative procedure

1a. Nonviable tissue is excised down to underlying muscle fascia.

1b. An alternative method is tangential excision of the burn wound, which is performed with a knife dermatome. This type of excision is usually carried down only to subcutaneous fat, rather than to fascia.

2. Hemostasis is obtained with electrocoagulation or use of topical thrombin solution.

3. Dressings saturated with the topical antimicrobial agent of choice are applied.

Although skin grafting may be done at the time of wound débridement, it is usually performed several days later, particularly in burns that are extensive.

Cultured Epithelial Autografting (CEA)

In the event that the patient has been massively burned (greater than 90% of the body surface) or has a wound that would be open 21 days after injury, the need for coverage is critical. A skin biopsy (about the size of a postage stamp) is taken from the axilla, groin, postauricular area, and the sole of the foot. These areas, even in the situations of massive burn injuries, are sometimes available. The biopsy is then sent to a specific technologic laboratory where the full-thickness biopsy is placed in a specially developed culture medium, maintained nutritionally, and allowed to grow. Through the course of 21 days and fastidious care of the cultured skin by the technology lab, the patient's wounds can be expected to be covered.

Procedural considerations

The previously described considerations for acute burn surgery can be followed. The cultured skin, when ready to be placed on the patient, is transported to the institution in a box that maintains a controlled atmosphere. The cultured skin, placed in individual plastic containers in the atmosphere-controlled box, is positioned on the patient's wound and stapled in place with nylon netting, and the dressings are applied. Documentation of the

number of cultured skin pieces as well as their location is done by use of photography and notation on the patient's record.

Operative procedure

1. The dressings, Biobrane, or pig skin (if applicable) is removed to expose the burn wound.

2. The cultured skin is applied.

3. The cultured skin is secured with nylon netting, which is stapled in place.

4. Hemostasis is achieved with electrocoagulation and topical hemostatic solutions.

5. The wound is dressed using large pieces of flat gauze, Webril, and Kling wrap.

ESTHETIC SURGERY

Esthetic surgery is usually performed with the patient under local anesthesia with conscious sedation. The perioperative nurse must be prepared to monitor the patient during the procedure. Baseline vital signs should be recorded on the operating room record. A blood pressure cuff, pulse oximeter, and cardiac monitor electrodes should be placed. Intravenous fluids should be started. The operating room should be kept quiet and patient privacy protected. Care should be taken to avoid conversation that could be misinterpreted by the patient.

Rhinoplasty

Deformities of the external nose and nasal septum may be congenital or secondary to previous trauma (Fig. 24-31). The goal of rhinoplasty is to improve the appearance of the external nose. This is accomplished by reshaping the underlying framework of the nose, which allows the overlying skin and subcutaneous tissue to redrape over the new framework. Reshaping the nasal skeleton usually includes rasping down of a dorsal hump, partial excision of lateral and alar cartilages, shortening of the septum, and osteotomy of nasal bones. A procedure to alter the nasal septum, septoplasty, or submucous resection (SMR), often accompanies rhinoplasty.

The goal of SMR is to improve the nasal airway by resecting a segment of septal cartilage. Septoplasty reshapes the existing septal cartilage; it may aid in altering the appearance of the nose or in improving the airway.

Rhinoplasty is performed through incisions made inside the nose or outside the nose (open rhinoplasty). Small external incisions at the alar bases and near the nasal bridge are also used to narrow the nose.

Procedural considerations

A plastic local instrument set is required, along with special rhinoplasty instruments (Fig. 24-32). A nasal splint, nasal packing, and fiberoptic headlight are also needed.

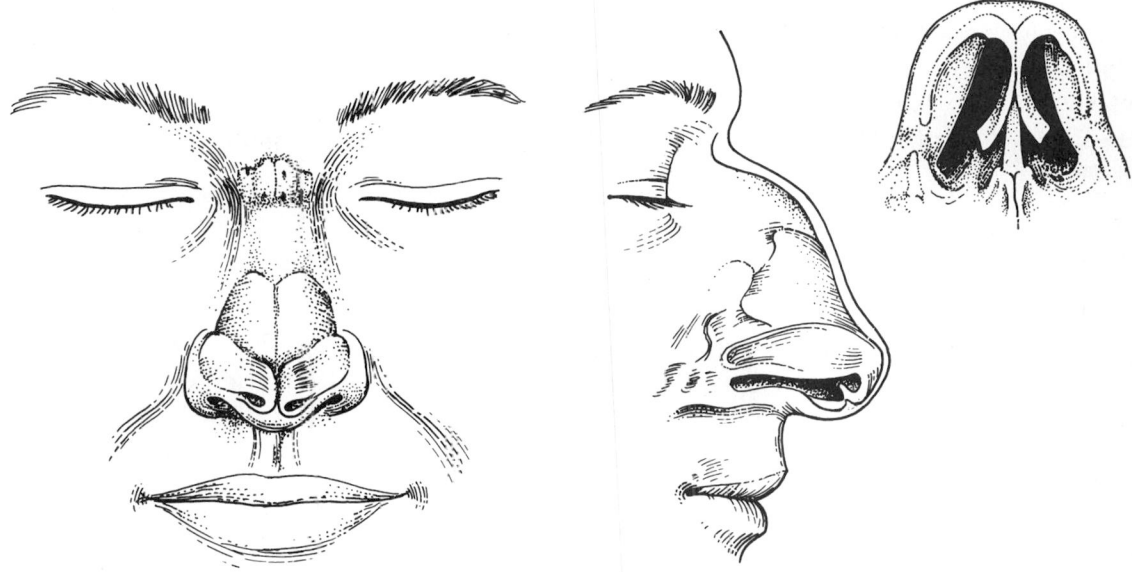

FIGURE 24-31   Skeleton of abnormal nose with soft tissues superimposed.

Rhinoplasty may be performed with the patient under local anesthesia. A separate local anesthetic setup should contain a bayonet forceps; sponges; the local anesthetic of choice, topical and local; needles, 30 gauge and 25 gauge (1½ inches); petrolatum gauze for nasal packing; an atomizer (optional); and a 10 ml syringe.

Intravenous fluids are started, and a blood pressure cuff, pulse oximeter, and cardiac monitor electrodes are placed. Allergies are screened for and baseline vital signs obtained before initiation of local anesthesia.

From this setup (before scrubbing), the surgeon can do the preliminary nasal preparation, inject the local anesthetic, and pack the nose with gauze or cotton soaked in 4% cocaine solution. With this procedure the local anesthesia can take effect while the surgeon is scrubbing.

The patient is placed in the supine position on the OR bed. The face is prepped, and an ophthalmic ointment may be placed in the eyes to diminish the potential for irritation. The head drape is used. The surgeon may use a headlight while performing the operation.

Operative procedure
Intranasal

1. Topical and local anesthetics are administered by the surgeon. The topical anesthetic is applied with applicator sticks or an atomizer.
2. Intranasal incisions are made, and the skin and soft tissues of the nose are elevated from the underlying nasal bones and cartilage.
3. The tip of the nose is reshaped by excising portions of the alar and lateral cartilages on each side.
4. The nasal dorsum (hump) is reduced by removing portions of the bone and septum.

5. The nasal bridge is narrowed by means of medial and lateral osteotomies of the nasal bones.
6. The intranasal incisions are sutured.
7. Bilateral anterior nasal packs are inserted, and a nasal splint and drip pad (moustache dressing) applied. Cool compresses may be immediately applied to decrease swelling and bruising.

If an SMR is performed at the time of rhinoplasty, it usually immediately precedes step 2. Septoplasty may be performed at any time during the operative procedure.

Blepharoplasty

The aging process causes a sagging or relaxation of eyelid skin and the orbital septum. As the latter becomes weaker, it allows periorbital fat to bulge. These changes are perceived as baggy eyelids, which give the patient a chronically tired appearance. The goal of blepharoplasty is to improve the patient's appearance by removing loose skin and protruding periorbital fat in the upper and lower eyelids. The upper eyelid skin can be so redundant that it encroaches on the patient's field of vision. Blepharoplasty is often performed with rhytidectomy.

Procedural considerations

A plastic local instrument set is required, as well as two Blair retractors, a bipolar or monopolar ESU, a marking pen, and a local anesthetic. Blepharoplasty is usually performed with the patient under local anesthesia with conscious sedation. Intravenous fluids are started, and a blood pressure cuff, pulse oximeter, and cardiac monitor electrodes are applied. Allergies are screened for and baseline vital signs recorded. The patient is placed in the

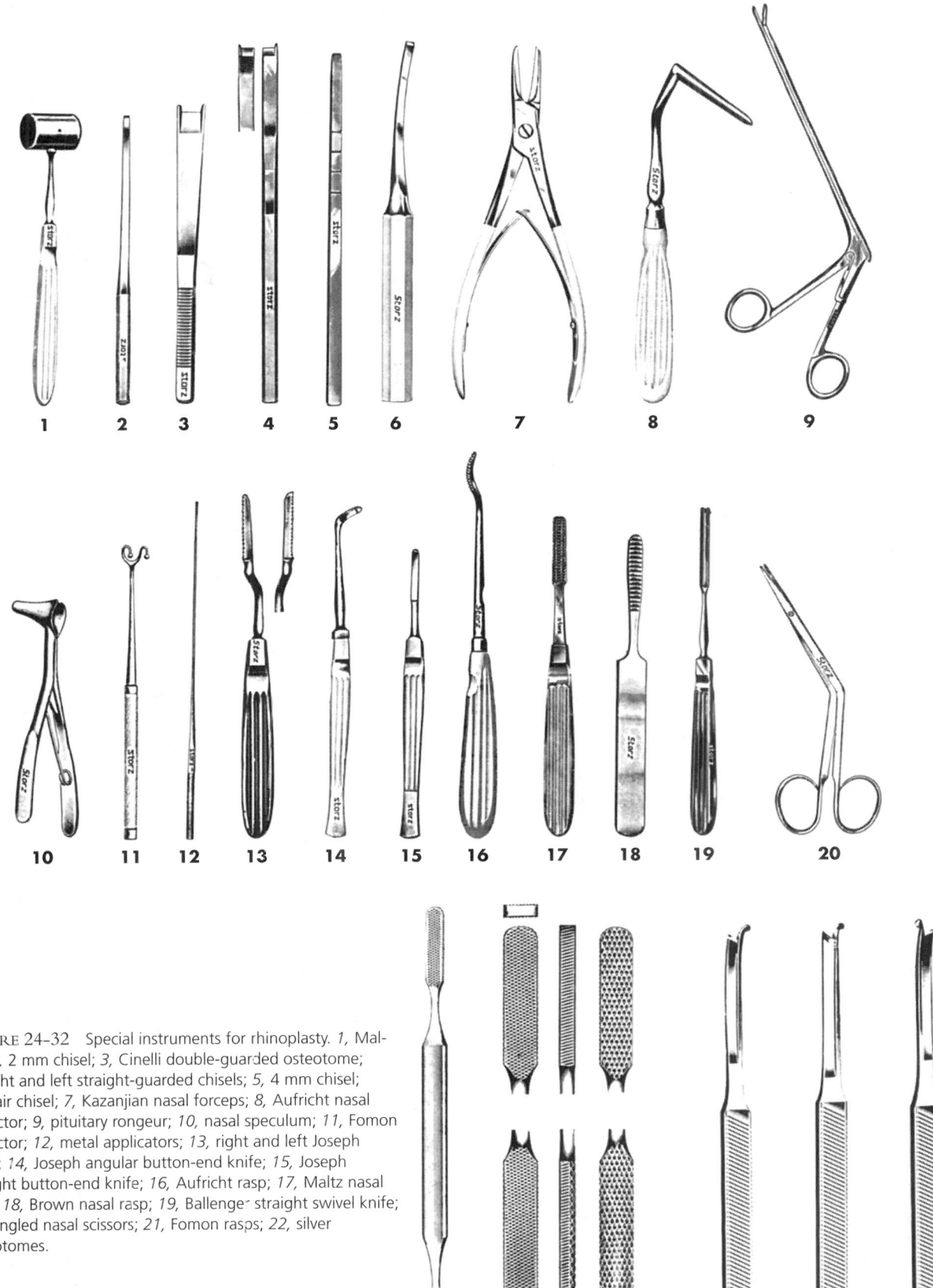

FIGURE 24–32   Special instruments for rhinoplasty. *1*, Mallet; *2*, 2 mm chisel; *3*, Cinelli double-guarded osteotome; *4*, right and left straight-guarded chisels; *5*, 4 mm chisel; *6*, Blair chisel; *7*, Kazanjian nasal forceps; *8*, Aufricht nasal retractor; *9*, pituitary rongeur; *10*, nasal speculum; *11*, Fomon retractor; *12*, metal applicators; *13*, right and left Joseph saws; *14*, Joseph angular button-end knife; *15*, Joseph straight button-end knife; *16*, Aufricht rasp; *17*, Maltz nasal rasp; *18*, Brown nasal rasp; *19*, Ballenger straight swivel knife; *20*, angled nasal scissors; *21*, Fomon rasps; *22*, silver osteotomes.

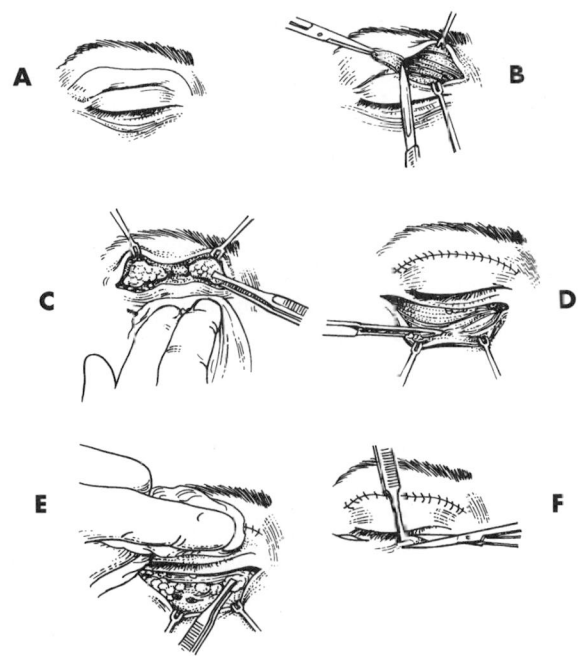

FIGURE 24-33 Blepharoplasty for baggy eyelids. **A,** Areas of proposed skin excision marked with methylene blue or marking pen. **B,** Strip of skin excised from upper lid; fat pad shining through orbital fascia and orbicular muscle of eye. **C,** Orbital fascia opened in two places (medially and laterally). Pressure on eyeball causes fat pads to bulge. They are eased out meticulously. **D,** Upper lid incision sutured with continuous no. 6-0 silk. Orbicular muscle fibers are separated from skin. **E,** Orbital fascia opened; fat pads bulge because of digital pressure and are teased out meticulously. **F,** Skin tailored to fit and sutured.

supine position on the OR bed. The face is prepped, and the head drape is used.

Operative procedure (Fig. 24-33)

1. The local anesthetic is injected after the incision lines have been marked bilaterally.
2. An ellipse of excess skin is excised from the upper eyelids.
3. After a strip of the orbicularis oculi muscle and orbital septum is incised or removed, protruding periorbital fat is excised and coagulated.
4. The upper eyelid incisions are sutured in one layer.
5. The lower eyelid incisions are made close to the ciliary margin or through a transconjunctival approach when only fat is to be excised.
6. A skin flap or skin-muscle flap is elevated away from the orbicularis oculi muscle.
7. Protruding periorbital fat is excised from beneath the orbicularis muscle.
8. The skin flaps are draped over the lower eyelids, and any excess skin is excised. Removal of too much skin from the lower eyelid can cause an ectropion.
9. The lower eyelid incisions are sutured in one layer.
10. Finely crushed ice on moist gauze 4 × 4 pads may be

applied to the eyes; other means of reducing swelling, such as cold compresses or a mechanical cold mask, may be similarly applied.

Rhytidectomy (Facelift)

As the aging process progresses, the skin of the face and neck becomes loose and redundant. This is particularly noticeable in the "jowl" areas and just beneath the chin. A rhytidectomy is designed to improve the patient's appearance by removing some of the excess skin and sometimes the excess fat of the neck. Rather than excising the redundant skin directly, incisions adjacent to or within hairlines are used so that the scars are virtually indiscernible.

Procedural considerations

A basic plastic instrument set is required, along with Gorney or Kaye facelift scissors, two Deaver retractors (1 inch), two Army-Navy retractors, two Cushing tissue forceps (7 inches), two Brown-Adson forceps, two Cushing dressing forceps (7 inches), six Burlisher clamps (curved), a rhytidectomy retractor (optional), long Metzenbaum scissors, a marking pen, the bipolar ESU, a fiberoptic light source, local anesthetic agent of choice, and a skin stapler.

A rhytidectomy may be performed with local anesthesia with conscious sedation or use of general anesthesia. Intravenous fluids are started, and a blood pressure cuff, a pulse oximeter, and cardiac monitor leads are applied. The patient is placed in the supine position on the OR bed. The hair and face are prepped, and the head drape is used. Minimal or no hair is shaved.

Operative procedure (Figs. 24-34 and 24-35)

1. Bilateral incision lines are marked from the temporal scalp, in front of the ear in a natural skin-wrinkle line, around the earlobe, onto the posterior surface of the ear, and into the occipital scalp.
2. The incision lines, both temples, cheeks, upper neck, and the submental area are injected with the local anesthetic agent.
3. After the incisions are made, large flaps of skin and subcutaneous tissue are elevated from the face and upper third of the neck, meeting in the midline in the submental area and exposing the SMAS (superficial muscular aponeurotic system) and platysma. The SMAS and platysma are often tightened, trimmed, and sutured behind and above the ears.
4. The edges of the flap are grasped with Allis forceps, and superior and posterior traction is placed on the flaps. The excess fat is removed, the platysma is plicated in the midline, and the neck is contoured. Suction may be used for the contouring.
5. Excess skin at the flap edges is excised, which pulls tight the tissue in the previously redundant areas.
6. Drains, if used, are inserted.

7. Incisions are closed in one or two layers.
8. A moderate pressure dressing is applied.

Dermabrasion

Sanding or planing of the skin is done primarily to smooth scars and surface irregularities of the skin. Dermabrasion is most commonly performed to improve

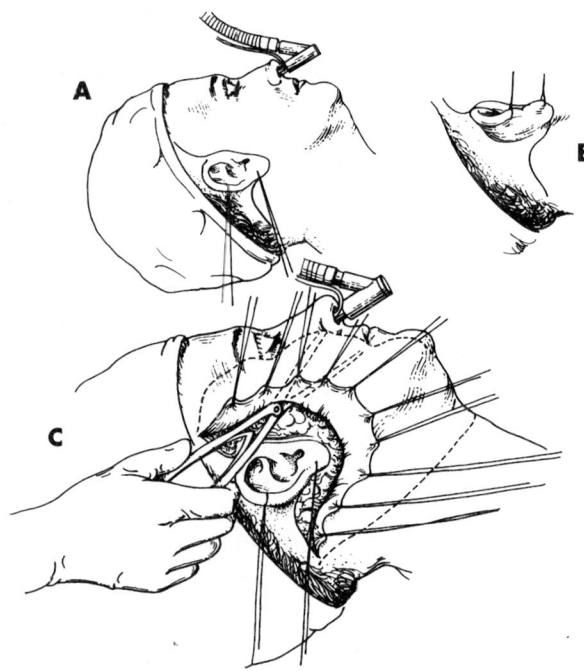

FIGURE 24-34 Rhytidectomy: line of incision and undermining. **A,** Traction sutures of no. 4-0 silk placed into auricle; temporal incision curved posteriorly for better support of upward pull. **B,** Incision carried under earlobe and then curved posteriorly upward and then caudad toward midline. **C,** Skin undermined almost to nasolabial fold, to area of mental foramen, and to midline of neck as far down as thyroid cartilage. Care is taken to avoid injury to submandibular branches of facial nerve and facial artery.

the appearance of facial scars, especially the irregular scars resulting from acne vulgaris. It may also be used for the removal of foreign-body tattoos. It is less successfully used for removal of professional body tattoos and to smooth fine wrinkle lines of the face. In these instances, laser resurfacing may be selected.

The goal in treating irregular surfaces with dermabrasion is to sand or plane down the high points of elevations so that the low ones appear less deep. Dermabrasion removes epidermis and a portion of the dermis of the skin. Healing occurs from residual dermal elements, as in partial-thickness burns or split-thickness skin-graft donor sites.

Procedural considerations

Instrumentation includes a plastic local instrument set, dermabrader, marking pen, and protective goggles. The procedure may be performed with the patient under general or local anesthesia. The patient is positioned and draped so that the area to be dermabraded is well exposed.

Operative procedure

1. The bases of pitted scars and depressions are marked.
2. The skin is planed with the dermabrader.
3. A single layer of the dressing of choice is applied to the dermabraded area.

Scar Revision

Scar revision involves the rearranging or reshaping of an existing scar by means of a scar revision procedure so that the scar is not as noticeable. The simplest form of scar revision is excision of an existing scar and simple resuturing of the wound. This may improve scars that are wide.

The Z-plasty is the most widely used method of scar revision (Fig. 24-36). It breaks up linear scars, rearranging

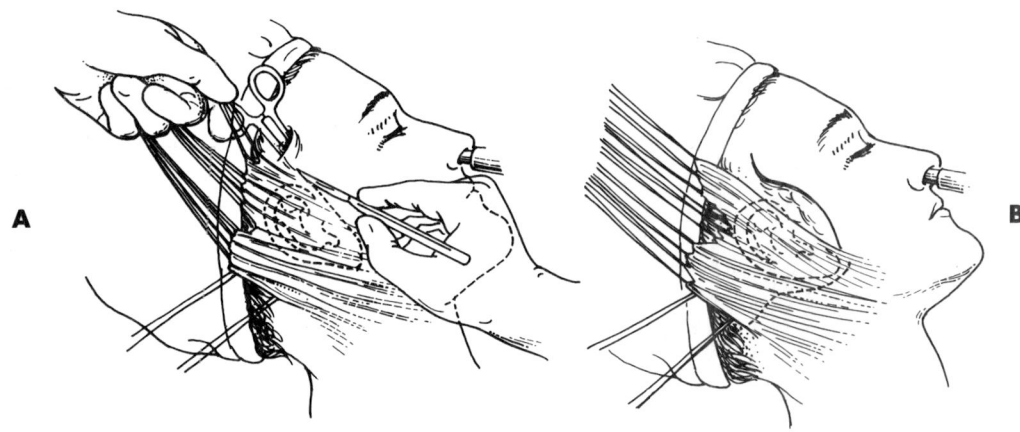

FIGURE 24-35 Rhytidectomy: removal of superfluous skin. **A,** Skin drawn upward to proper degree of tension and incision made along posterior margin of clamp. **B,** Incision continued upward around posterior margin of auricle and then backward to excise skin specimen.

them so that the central limb of the Z lies in the same direction as a natural skin line. Scars that are parallel to skin lines are less noticeable than scars that are perpendicular to skin lines. A contracted scar line can also be lengthened with a Z-plasty.

Procedural considerations

A plastic local instrument set and a marking pen are required. The procedure may be performed under local or general anesthesia. The patient is positioned, prepped, and draped so that the scar that is to be revised is well exposed.

Operative procedure

1. The pattern for the planned revision is marked.
2. The scar is excised.
3. The surrounding tissue is undermined, and the wound

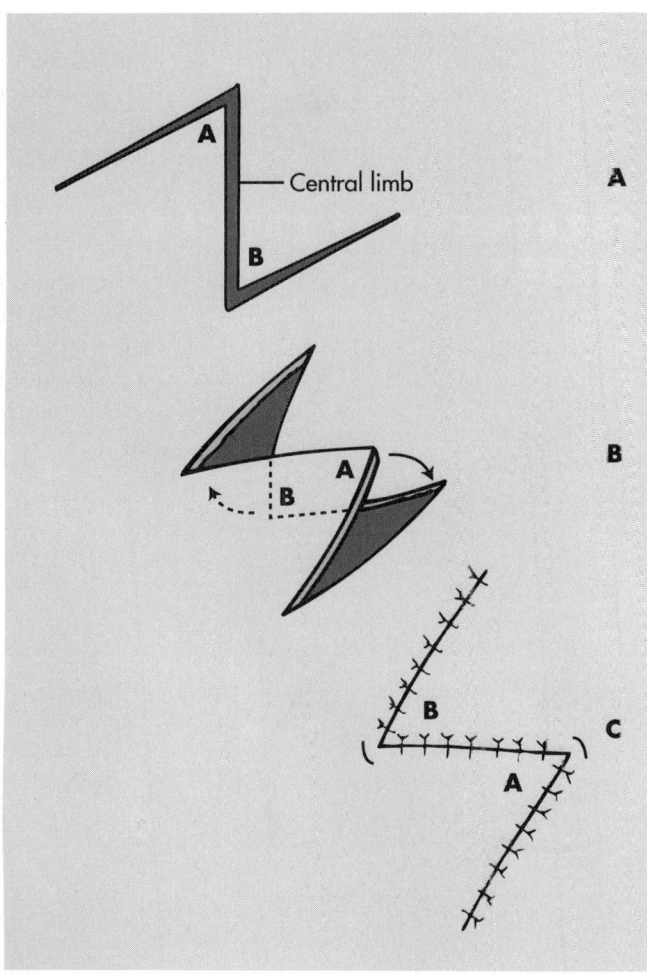

FIGURE 24-36 Z-plasty for scar revision. **A,** The central limb of the Z-plasty is over the scar that needs to be revised. **B,** Two other limbs are incised, each equal in length to the central limb and diverging from it at an equal angle. The flaps are then transposed. **C,** Flaps transposed, and original Z rotated 90 degrees and reversed.

edges are approximated according to the surgeon's markings.

4. Dressings may or may not be applied.

Abdominoplasty

Abdominoplasty is particularly useful in improving the appearance (and to a certain extent, function) of persons who have lost a great deal of weight. Obesity produces distention and stretching of the skin of the abdomen. Although weight loss reduces the volume of the underlying fat, it does not produce concomitant reduction in the excess surface area of the overlying skin, resulting from destruction or insufficiency of elastic fibers in the skin. The stretched skin remains as an apron that hangs from the lower abdomen, sometimes as far as the knees. The rectus abdominis fascia is also stretched in obese patients, and weight loss does not restore its integrity.

Abdominoplasty is usually performed to remove redundant skin and fat of the lower abdomen; it also repairs any laxity of the rectus muscle. The open procedure is described below; endoscopic abdominoplasty is performed for patients with smaller protrusions who do not have a large pannulus or require pannulectomy.

Procedural considerations

A basic plastic instrument set is required, as well as extra retractors and clamping instruments, an ESU, and a marking pen. Sequential compression devices or antiembolism hose are usually in place or applied in the operating room. The patient is placed in the supine position with slight flexion at the hips. Draping is such that the entire abdomen, lower costal margins, upper thighs, and both anterior iliac spines are exposed.

Operative procedure

1. A low, transverse abdominal incision across both inguinal areas laterally and the superior border of the mons pubis in the midline is marked and incised down to fascia.
2. A large flap of skin and subcutaneous tissue is elevated away from the fascia of the anterior abdominal wall.
3. The umbilicus is left in its normal position.
4. The abdominal flap is elevated further until the xiphoid process of the sternum and the lower costal margins are reached.
5. If diastasis of the rectus abdominis fascia is present, plication is performed from the xiphoid process to the mons pubis.
6. The flap of abdominal skin and subcutaneous tissue is pulled inferiorly, and excess tissue is excised.
7. A small incision is made in the midline of the flap to accommodate the umbilicus, which is then sutured peripherally to the flap.
8. Drains may or may not be used, followed by closure of the lower abdominal incision in two layers.

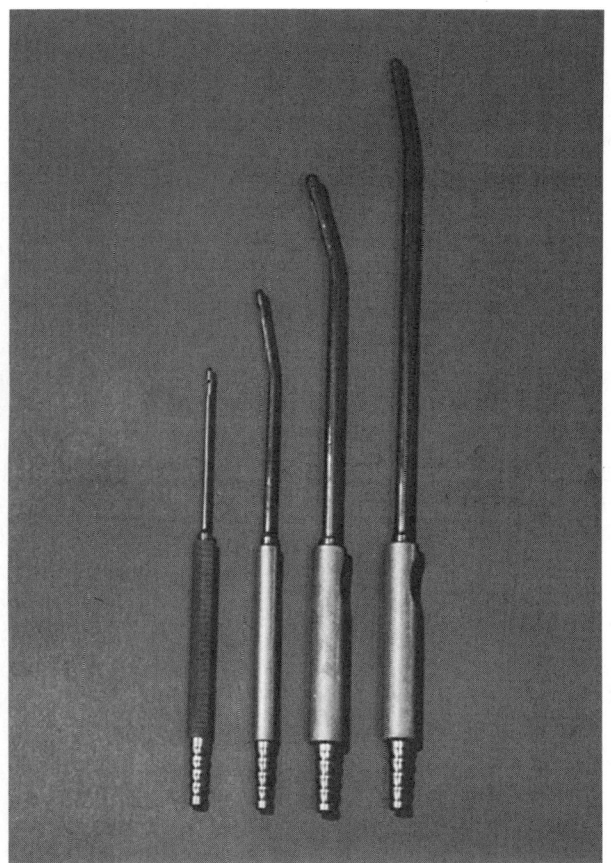

FIGURE 24-37   Suction lipectomy cannulas.

9. Postoperatively the patient is placed in the hospital bed in high Fowler's position.

Suction Lipectomy

In this body-contouring technique, a slender cannula is inserted into the subcutaneous layer, and fat is aspirated by vacuum. Suction lipectomy may be used for body contouring on the buttocks, flanks, abdomen, thighs, upper arms, knees, ankles, breasts (after reduction mammoplasty), and chin. Suction lipectomy is not a substitute for weight loss, and it is not a cure for obesity. Plastic surgeons prefer to do this procedure on relatively young patients, those under 40 years of age, because the skin of younger patients is more elastic and shapes itself easily to the newly contoured frame. The procedure may be done in an acute care, ambulatory surgery facility or the surgeon's office-based surgical suite.

Immediate preoperative preparation includes asking the patient to stand while the area of deformity is outlined. Two lines are usually drawn on the skin surface, one delineating the major area of defect, the other placed a short distance outside the first area. These lines make it easier for the plastic surgeon to make a smooth transition toward the normal tissue by adjusting the amount of fat removed from the center to the periphery of the deformity. The patient may remain standing and be prepped circumferentially with a spray bottle of warm iodophor solution. Care should be taken to protect the patient's privacy.

Procedural considerations

A plastic local instrument set is used. A general anesthetic is administered.

Operative procedure

1. A small incision from ½ to 1 inch long is made in the area closest to the deformity that can best be concealed.
2. A suction curette or blunt cannula (Fig. 24-37) is inserted through the incision.
3. The curette is attached to a firm suction tubing and connected to the aspirating (suction) unit (Fig. 24-38).
4. The high vacuum pressure created by the unit causes the fat cells to emulsify so that they can be suctioned through the vacuum opening near the rounded tip of the curette.
5. The incision is closed by one or two sutures, and a bulky pressure dressing is applied to the area.
6. Compression garments may be applied to maintain even pressure. Taping may also be used, based on the surgeon's preference. The compression garment or dressing usually remains on for 2 to 4 weeks.

TREATMENT OF PRESSURE ULCERS

Pressure ulcers result from prolonged compression of soft tissues overlying bony prominences (Fig. 24-39). However, whether excessive pressure is sufficient to create an ulcer depends on the intensity and duration of the pressure as well as tissue tolerance. Other factors that contribute to pressure ulcer development are shearing force, friction, and nutritional debilitation.[3] The most common sites of pressure ulcers are the sacrum, the ischium, the trochanter, the malleolus, and the heel. Surgical interventions for pressure ulcers are usually based on ulcer staging (also referred to as grading). In stage I the ulcer involves the epidermis and has soft-tissue swelling that is irregular and ill defined; heat and erythema at the ulcer site are characteristic. A stage II ulcer involves the epidermis and dermis but not the subcutaneous fat. Stage III ulcers show full-thickness skin loss with injury to underlying tissue layers and may contain necrotic material. Thorough debridement is performed, and intravenous antibiotic therapy is instituted. Although debrided stage III ulcers often heal on their own, surgical excision and closure may be done to prevent a lengthy spontaneous closure, which may result in a weak, unstable scar, with resultant recurrence. Stage IV ulcers are the deepest, requiring more radical débridement. Adequate soft-tissue cover may be obtained by either split-thickness or full-thickness skin grafting or tissue flaps. Tissue expansion

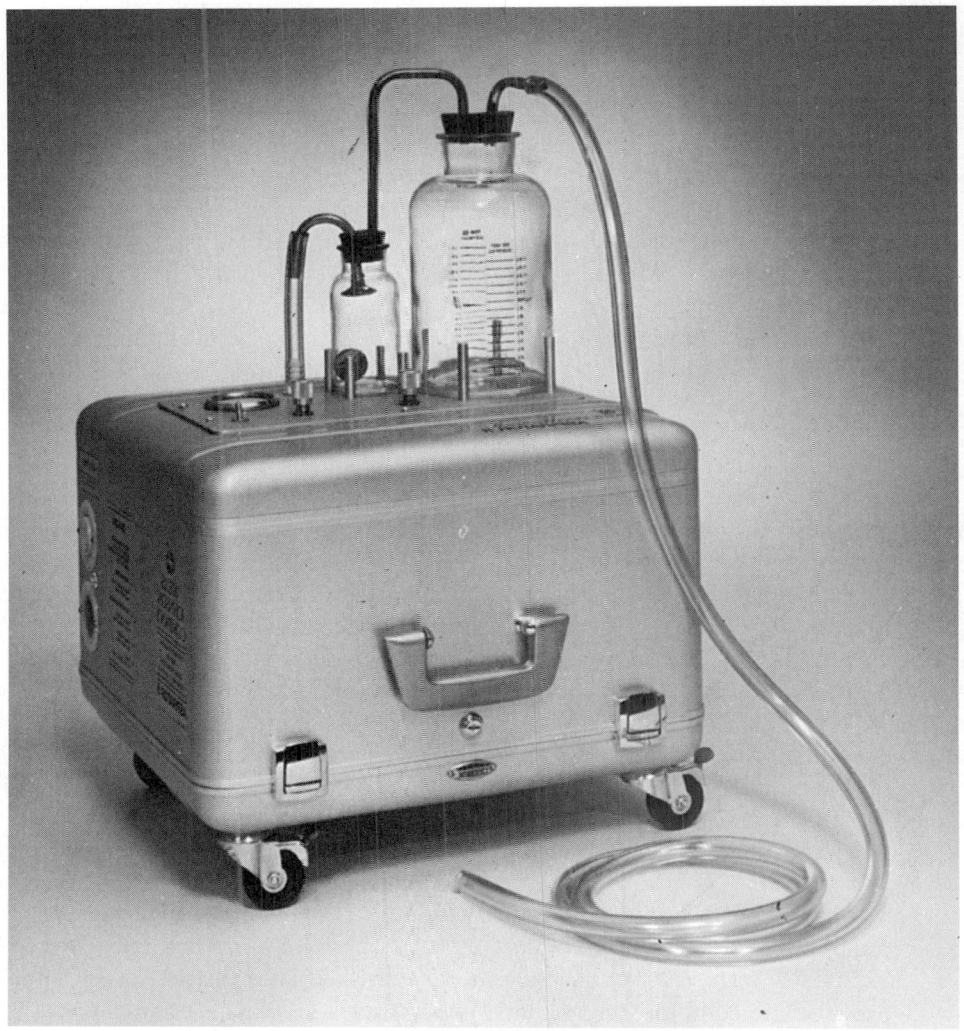

FIGURE 24-38 Suction lipectomy vacuum machine and tubing.

may be utilized where there is not enough tissue adjacent to the ulcer site to provide flap coverage.

An alternative to the standard surgical approach is the use of the carbon dioxide laser. The laser offers the advantage of minimizing blood loss and possibly reducing infection rates in the presence of gross contamination.

Although many techniques and flaps are surgical options, basic principles apply to all pressure ulcer closure procedures. The following procedure is for an adjacent flap.

Procedural considerations

A basic plastic instrument set is required, as well as assorted sizes of osteotomes (straight and curved), a mallet, the gigli saw and handle, assorted curettes, a key periosteal elevator, duckbill rongeur, bone wax, the dermatome of choice, the ESU, a marking pen, and a closed-wound drainage system. The patient is positioned and draped so that the pressure ulcer, adjacent flap donor site, and a skin-graft donor site are well exposed.

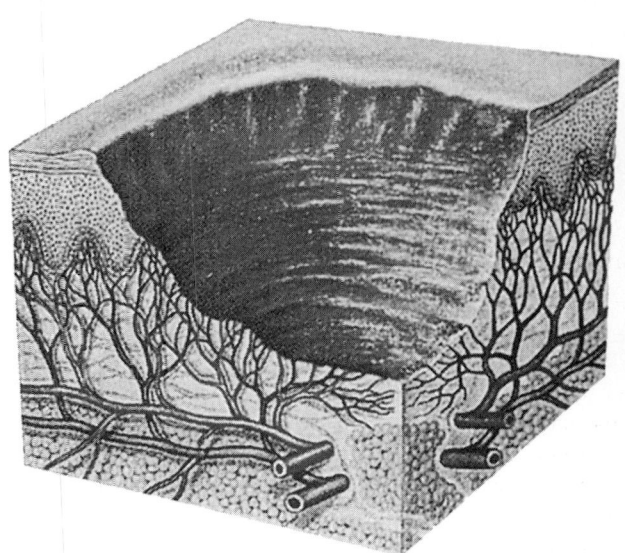

FIGURE 24-39 Pressure ulcers often appear after blood flow to an area slows or is obstructed because of pressure on bony prominences. Infections often follow, as lack of blood flow causes tissue damage or death.

Operative procedure

1. The area to be excised and the local flap are outlined.
2. The ulcer is excised along with the underlying bony prominence.
3. Large suction catheters are placed into the defect left by excision of the ulcer and beneath the flap.
4. The flap is sutured in place.
5. An STSG is usually used to resurface the flap donor site.
6. A stent dressing is placed over the skin graft, and gauze dressings or a plastic spray dressing are applied over the suture lines of the flap.

SEX REASSIGNMENT

Transsexualism defines the condition in which an individual with chromosomes and internal and external organs normal to one sex identifies psychologically and socially with attributes of the opposite sex. Reassignment of sex by means of surgery is the last step to be taken in treatment of transsexuals. It is performed only after the patient has been treated with hormones of the opposite sex, has experienced a period of cross-sex living, and has had intensive psychiatric evaluation. Most institutions performing this type of surgery have sex-identity teams who evaluate and treat transsexuals. These teams usually include a variety of professionals: psychiatrist, psychologist, endocrinologist, plastic surgeon, urologist, gynecologist, and social worker.

The surgical techniques for assignment of male to female are technically easier. A breast augmentation may be performed if hormone therapy has not sufficiently changed breast size. Construction of the neovagina includes radical penectomy, bilateral orchiectomy, urethroplasty, perineal dissection, creation of a neovaginal vault, vaginoplasty, and vulvoplasty.

The surgical technique for female to male is technically more difficult and requires multiple surgical procedures. Considerations that must be addressed are twofold: a neophallus that will allow the patient to stand to void must be constructed and a phallus that will permit stimulation of a sexual partner during intercourse. This may require a radial artery forearm free flap with a later-stage surgical insertion of a penile prosthesis for attaining an erection.

HAND SURGERY

Plastic surgery of the hand is directed toward restoration of function. It deals with the treatment of acute injuries and reconstruction in established deformities. A systematic surgical approach for the restoration of hand function includes (1) replacement of lost tissue covering; (2) restoration of bony architecture; (3) repair of severed nerves; (4) restoration of the motor unit, either by tendon repair, tendon graft, or tendon transfer; and (5) replantation of severed digits.

Surgical Anatomy

The functional unit in hand surgery consists of the hand, digits, wrist, and forearm. Each of these structures has a radial and an ulnar side, as determined by its position in relation to the radius and ulna of the forearm, rather than a lateral and medial side. Each also has a dorsal and volar, or palmar, surface. To avoid confusion, the digits of the hand are referred to as the thumb and the index, long, ring, and little fingers.

The skeletal framework of the hand and wrist consists of three distinct parts: (1) the metacarpals, or bones of the hand; (2) the phalanges, or bones of the digits; and (3) the carpals, or bones of the wrist (Fig. 24-40). The five metacarpals articulate distally with the proximal phalanges of each digit at the metacarpophalangeal (MP) joints. The two bones of the thumb are the proximal phalanx and the distal phalanx, which articulate at the interphalangeal (IP) joint. Each of the four fingers contains three bones: a proximal phalanx, a middle phalanx, and a distal phalanx. Each finger therefore has three joints: (1) the metacarpophalangeal joint, (2) the proximal interphalangeal (PIP) joint between the proximal and middle phalanges, and (3) the distal interphalangeal (DIP) joint between the middle and distal phalanges.

The carpus (wrist) consists of eight bones arranged in two rows. The proximal row includes the scaphoid (navicular), lunate, triquetrum, and pisiform. The distal row includes the trapezium (greater multiangular), trapezoid (lesser multiangular), capitate, and hamate. The metacarpals articulate proximally with the distal row of carpal bones. The proximal row of carpal bones articulates with the radius and ulna of the forearm.

Motion of the thumb and fingers is achieved through the action of muscles intrinsic and extrinsic to the hand. The intrinsic muscles are those with muscle bellies that lie within the hand: (1) the interosseous and lumbrical muscles of the hand, which flex the MP joints while extending the PIP and DIP joints and permit spreading and approximation of the fingers; (2) the muscles of the thenar eminence, which aid in adduction, abduction, flexion, and opposition of the thumb; and (3) the muscles of the hypothenar eminence, which aid in abduction, flexion, and opposition of the little finger.

The extrinsic muscles are so called because the muscle bellies are located in the forearm, whereas the tendons pass into the hand, dorsally beneath the extensor retinaculum (Fig. 24-41), and volarly beneath the flexor retinaculum (Fig. 24-42) at the wrist, to insert on the phalanges of the thumb and fingers. The dorsal group consists of the extensor tendons, which extend the finger MP joints and the thumb MP and IP joints. The volar group consists of the flexor tendons, one for the thumb and two to each finger. The paired finger flexors are the superficial (sublimis) flexor tendons, which flex the PIP joints, and the deep (profundus) flexor tendons, which flex the DIP

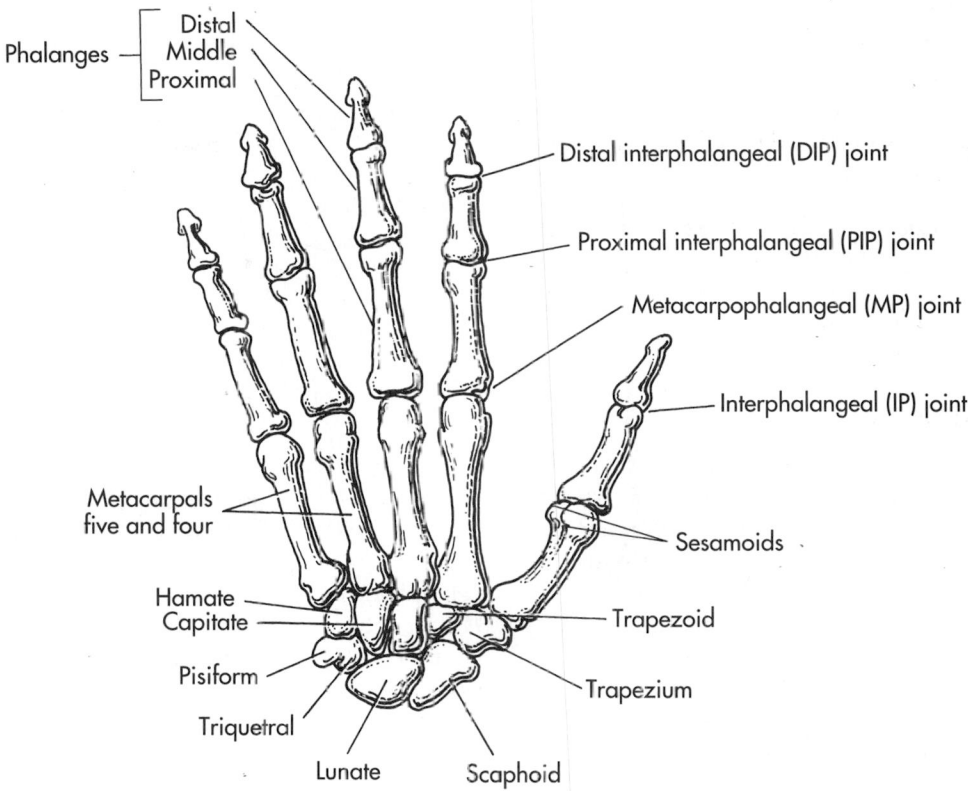

FIGURE 24–40   Skeleton of wrist and hand, palmar view.

joints. In addition to the finger and thumb flexors and extensors, other muscles of the forearm have tendinous insertions that work to abduct the thumb and flex and extend the wrist.

Although hand movements are achieved by the action of various muscles and their tendons, muscle function depends on adequate innervation of the muscle belly. The motor nerves of the hand are (1) the radial nerve to the extensors, (2) the median nerve to a majority of the flexor tendons and a few intrinsic muscles, and (3) the ulnar nerve to a majority of the intrinsic muscles and remaining flexors.

Sensation in the hand is provided by the same three nerves: (1) the radial nerve supplies the dorsal radial hand and fingers; (2) the median nerve, the volar (palmar) radial hand and digits (thumb, index, long, and radial side of the ring finger); and (3) the ulnar nerve, the remaining dorsal and volar ulnar hand and fingers. As the terminal sensory branches of the median and ulnar nerves enter the thumb and fingers, they are called *digital nerves* (see Fig. 24-42).

The principal blood supply for the hand is from the radial and ulnar arteries that form a superficial and deep palmar arch in the hand, giving off terminal branches to both sides of each digit, called *digital arteries* after they enter the fingers and thumb. A rich network of dorsal veins serves to return blood from the hand.

A minimum of skin and subcutaneous tissue covers the dorsum of the hand and digits. The skin covering the volar (palmar) surface is anchored to underlying fascia in areas of skin folds. Because of these fascial attachments, the skin and subcutaneous fat pads of the volar (palmar) surface do not move about during flexion and grasping of an object. The palmar fascia is a thick fibrous structure overlying the blood vessels, tendons, and nerves in the palm of the hand, to which skin is anchored, principally at the palmar skin creases. The palmar fascia sends extensions into each digit.

Special Equipment
Tourniquet

Because it renders the operative field relatively bloodless, a tourniquet is almost essential in dealing with the complex, delicate, and vital structures within the hand. The tourniquet may be of the pneumatic type, inflated with compressed gas, the pressure of which can be determined with an accurate gauge. Each tourniquet must be checked at regular intervals against a tourniquet test gauge or a mercury manometer to maintain the accuracy of its gauge. Electrically powered tourniquets are also available; these units have self-testing mechanisms and continuous readouts of tourniquet time and pressure. The tourniquet can be a dangerous device when not in good working order and when improperly used.

The arm cuff of the tourniquet should be smooth and broad so that pressure is distributed evenly over a wide

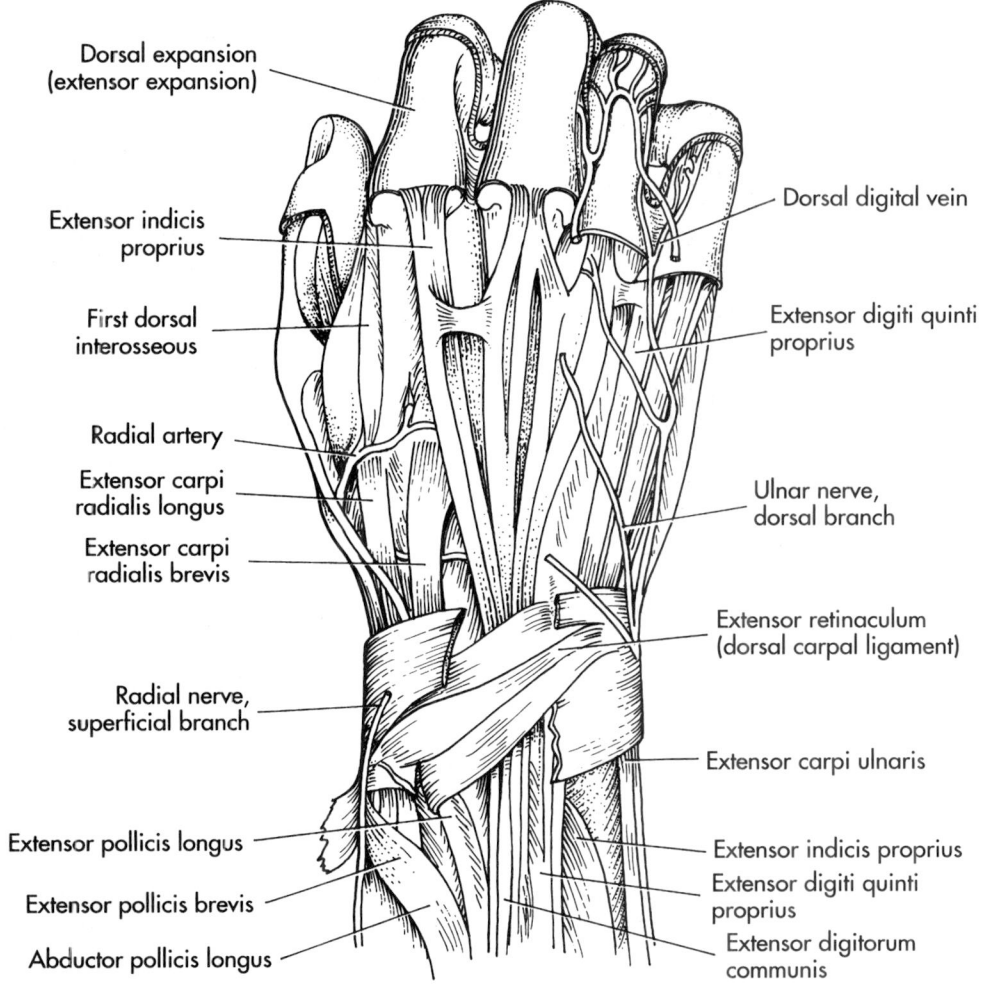

FIGURE 24-41 Dorsum of hand and wrist; finger and long thumb extensor tendons pass under extensor retinaculum at wrist.

area. Sheet cotton (Webril) or a tourniquet cover may be wrapped smoothly around the limb where the tourniquet will be applied. It should be placed as far proximally on the arm as possible, where a greater amount of soft tissue provides padding for underlying nerves and blood vessels as they are compressed against bone when the tourniquet cuff is inflated. There should be no kinking of the tubing between the cuff and gas-regulating mechanism. To prevent a chemical burn, antimicrobial solutions used for skin preparation should not be allowed to run beneath the tourniquet cuff.

The arm is exsanguinated by progressively wrapping the arm from fingertips to tourniquet cuff (distal to proximal) with a 3-inch Esmarch rubber bandage. The tourniquet is quickly inflated to prevent filling of superficial veins before occlusion of the arterial blood flow. The Esmarch bandage is removed after inflation of the tourniquet cuff. The amount of pressure used to inflate the tourniquet depends on the size of the extremity and the patient's age and systolic blood pressure.

Tourniquet time should be kept to a minimum. Times

of inflation and deflation should be recorded. After completion of the surgical maneuver that required use of the tourniquet, deflation of the cuff should be accompanied by total removal of the tourniquet cuff from the arm. If the cuff is left on the arm after being deflated, it may cause some obstruction to the return of venous blood, which is perceived as increased bleeding at the operative site.

Hand operating table

The hand table is used for most hand operations. This may be designed to clamp onto the frame of the OR bed (legless) or have adjustable legs that allow fitting to any standard operating room bed level (Fig. 24-43). The surgeon and assistants sit during the operation. A stainless steel pan with drain and plug may be placed in the hand table to facilitate irrigation of wounds.

Pulsatile irrigation

When the situation arises that a wound must be copiously irrigated, an electrically powered pulsatile

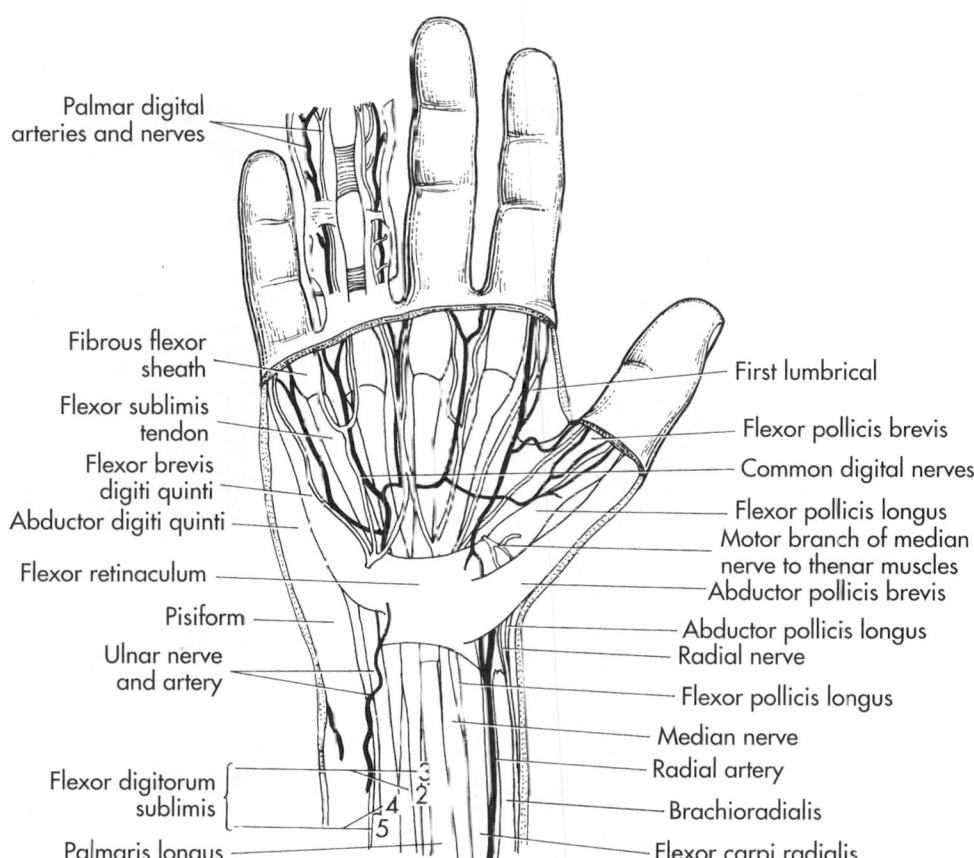

Palmar digital arteries and nerves

Fibrous flexor sheath

Flexor sublimis tendon

Flexor brevis digiti quinti

Abductor digiti quinti

Flexor retinaculum

Pisiform

Ulnar nerve and artery

Flexor digitorum sublimis

Palmaris longus

First lumbrical

Flexor pollicis brevis

Common digital nerves

Flexor pollicis longus

Motor branch of median nerve to thenar muscles

Abductor pollicis brevis

Abductor pollicis longus

Radial nerve

Flexor pollicis longus

Median nerve

Radial artery

Brachioradialis

Flexor carpi radialis

FIGURE 24-42   Volar (palmar) surface of hand and wrist. Median nerve, finger, and long thumb flexor tendons pass beneath flexor retinaculum (transverse carpal ligament) at wrist.

irrigation system can be employed. These systems are packaged in sterile, disposable kits, including pistol grip handles, assorted-size irrigation tips, splash shields, spiked tubing for the solutions, and suction tubings. Antibiotics can be added to the irrigation solutions according to physician preference. Protective barriers should be used by the perioperative team to prevent splash exposure as recommended in Standard Precautions (see Chapter 4).

Intravenous Regional Anesthesia

Intravenous regional anesthesia (see Chapter 7) is often used for hand operations and may be administered by the surgeon or an anesthesiologist. A pneumatic tourniquet with a double cuff and dual control valves and tubing is used. A butterfly needle is inserted into a vein of the affected extremity and secured with tape. The position of the needle within the vein is verified by irrigating with sterile saline solution in a 10 ml syringe, which is left attached to the tubing of the butterfly needle. An Esmarch bandage is used to exsanguinate the extremity, and the proximal cuff of the tourniquet is inflated. After removal of the Esmarch bandage, 0.5% lidocaine is injected intravenously through the butterfly needle (usual dosage is

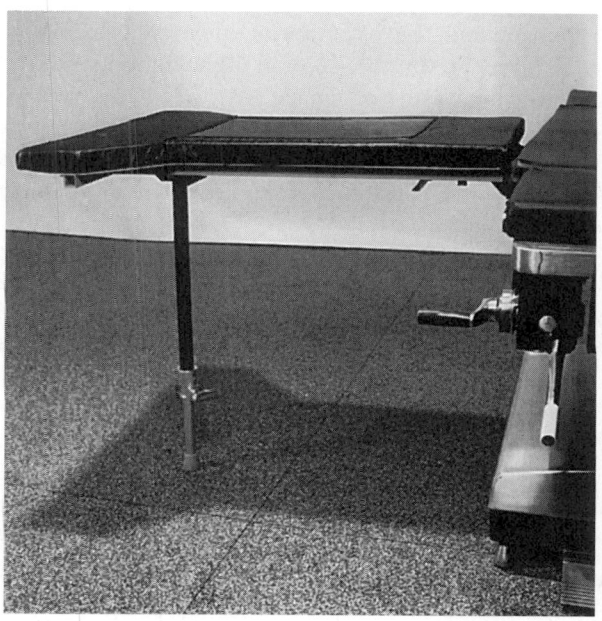

FIGURE 24-43   Boyes-Parker hand operating table. Central segment slides out so that stainless steel pan can be inserted during wound irrigation.

3 mg/kg of body weight, not exceeding a total dose of 250 mg). The butterfly needle is removed, and pressure is applied at the venipuncture site for several minutes. Prepping and draping of the patient usually follow.

The advantage of a tourniquet with a double cuff is as follows: When the patient experiences moderate discomfort from the proximal cuff pressure (approximately 30 minutes after inflation of the cuff), the distal cuff may be inflated. The distal cuff lies over an anesthetized area on the arm, and the patient's discomfort should be reduced. After inflation of the distal cuff, the proximal cuff is deflated.

Dressings and Immobilization

Basic conditions for good wound healing after hand surgery are immobilization and elevation. Adequate immobilization achieves support and splinting to protect against both active and passive motion. With most hand operations, because of many closely related movements, immobilizing the entire hand, fingers, wrist, and distal two thirds of the forearm is usually necessary. This immobilization is often maintained for 3 or 4 weeks after surgery. Application of the means of immobilization must therefore be performed with care while the patient is still anesthetized. Although plaster of Paris may be used to achieve immobilization, many surgeons prefer a soft, bulky hand dressing. Steps in the application of a hand dressing are as follows:

1. An assistant supports the hand and elevates it by flexing the elbow and resting it on the hand table.
2. Nonadherent gauze is applied over incisions.
3. Gauze dressing sponges in thin layers are placed between the fingers to prevent maceration. These sponges must be of uniform thickness proximally to distally to prevent pressure on digital blood vessels.
4. A thicker layer of gauze is placed between the thumb and index finger to prevent an adduction contracture of the thumb. In addition to abduction, the thumb is also rotated into opposition as the dressing is applied.
5. A bulky dressing is placed in the palm of the hand to support the PIP and DIP joints of the fingers in extension. It may also be added to the thumb-index finger web space to maintain thumb abduction. Folded abdominal pads are placed vertically across the dorsal and volar surfaces of the wrist for support.
6. Two Kling gauze rolls are wrapped around the hand and forearm so that the MP joints are in approximately 90 degrees flexion, the PIP and DIP joints are extended, the thumb is in abduction and opposition, and the wrist is in a neutral position. All fingertips must be exposed to permit inspection for determining viability.
7. Inch-wide strips of adhesive tape are applied vertically over the dressing (to avoid constricting the bands).

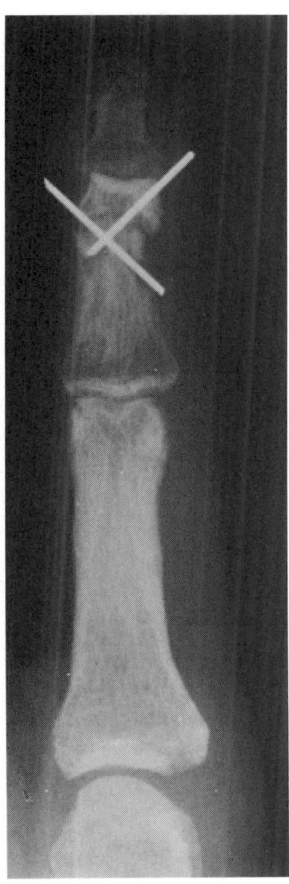

FIGURE 24-44 Radiograph shows fracture of middle phalanx of index finger after open reduction, with internal fixation by means of crossed Kirschner wires across fracture site.

Surgical Interventions
Treatment of fractures

Fractures within the scope of hand surgery may involve the phalanges in the fingers, the metacarpals in the hand, and the carpals in the wrist. The basis for treatment of any fracture is reduction of the fracture and immobilization until healing occurs.

Reduction of a fracture may be closed or open. Closed reduction is performed by manipulating the fracture fragments beneath intact skin and subcutaneous tissue. X-ray studies verify the reduction. One performs open reduction by making an incision, visualizing the fracture site, and then manipulating the fragments under direct vision. Radiographs are usually also obtained after open reduction.

Immobilization of a fracture may be external or internal. External methods include splinting and casting. Internal immobilization in hand fractures is usually accomplished by inserting Kirschner wires (Fig. 24-44). This may be the best method by which a reduction can be stabilized. It has the additional advantage of allowing motion in a maximum number of hand joints while

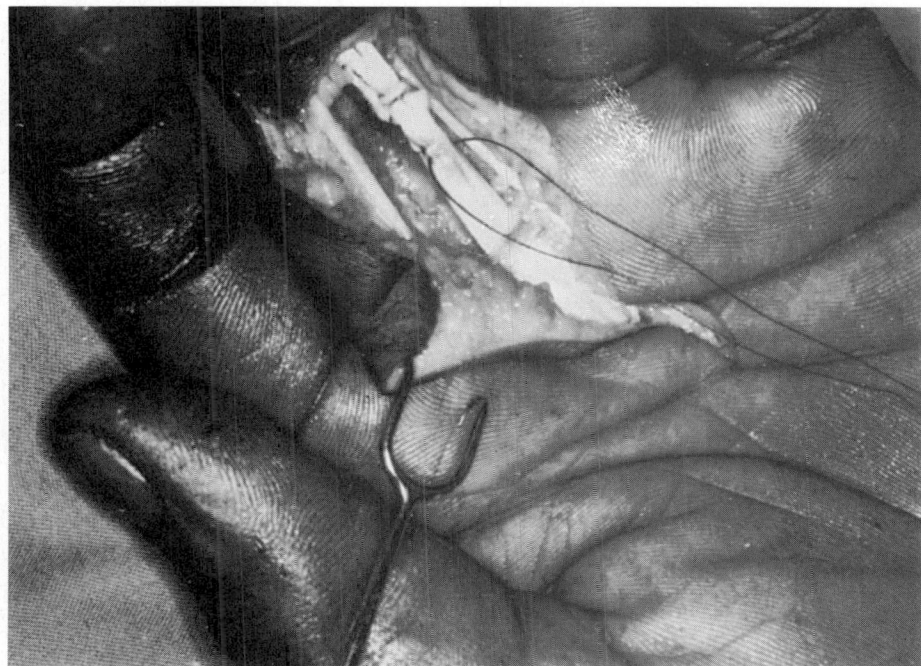

FIGURE 24-45   Primary repair of flexor profundus tendon of long finger in distal area of palm.

immobilizing only the injured part, thus preventing unnecessary joint stiffness.

Procedural Considerations

A plastic hand instrument set, a Kirschner wire driver and wires, an Esmarch bandage, and a marking pen are required. The patient is placed in the supine position on the OR bed, with the arm extended on a hand table. The hand drape is used.

Operative Procedure (open reduction, internal fixation)

1. The incision is marked.
2. The pneumatic tourniquet is inflated after exsanguination.
3. The incision is made, and the fracture is exposed.
4. The fracture is reduced by manipulating the fragments digitally or instrumentally under direct vision.
5. While an assistant holds the reduced fracture, Kirschner wires are driven into bone, usually across the fracture site. (Miniscrews and plates may also be used as internal fixation.)
6. After radiographs are obtained to verify the fracture reduction and immobilization, the Kirschner wires are cut off so that the ends are buried beneath skin or with a short segment protruding through skin. This segment is twisted down with needle-nosed pliers. (Fluoroscopy is also a frequently used option for these procedures.)
7. The incision is sutured in one layer (skin).
8. A hand dressing is applied.

Tendon repair

When continuity of a tendon is interrupted by avulsion or laceration, a specific active movement of one or more joints of the hand is lost. The treatment is tendon repair. Primary flexor or extensor tendon repair is usually performed at the time of injury or within several hours of the acute injury. When adequate tendon length is present on each side of the laceration, repair is performed by suturing the tendon ends together (Fig. 24-45). When the laceration is near the bony insertion of the tendon, the distal tendon segment is too short to permit adequate purchase for a suture. In this case tendon repair is performed by reinserting the proximal end of the tendon into bone.

Procedural Considerations

A plastic hand instrument set, an Esmarch bandage, a marking pen, and #3-0 or #4-0, double-armed, nonabsorbable suture on Keith needles are required. The patient is placed in the supine position on the OR bed, with the arm extended on a hand table. The hand drape is used.

Operative Procedure

1. The skin laceration is usually enlarged to permit adequate exposure of the tendon laceration, after the skin extensions for the laceration are marked and the tourniquet is inflated.
2. An additional incision in the hand or wrist or both may be necessary to identify the retracted proximal tendon end.

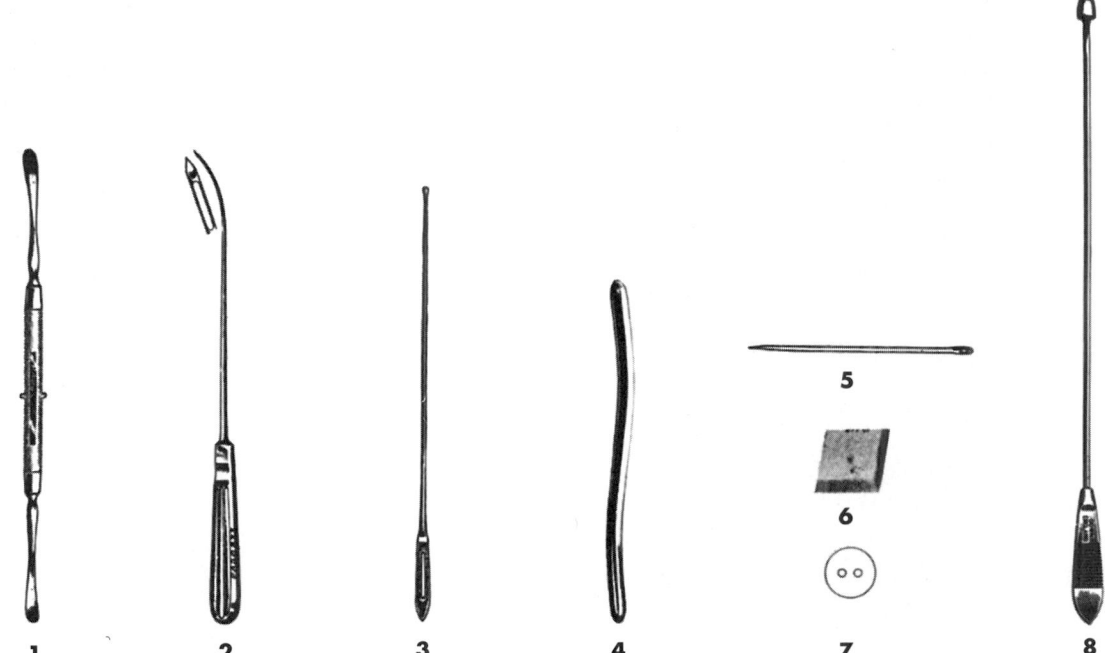

FIGURE 24-46   Special instruments for flexor tendon graft. *1,* Freer septal elevator (with hole); *2,* Sanders-Brown fascia needle; *3,* silver probe; *4,* no. 6 Hegar dilator (with hole); *5,* Keith needle; *6,* foam rubber; *7,* polyethylene button; *8,* Brand tendon stripper.

3. The tendon is repaired by placing a #3-0 or #4-0, double-armed, nonabsorbable suture through the tendon ends and approximating the ends. A pullout suture may or may not be placed through the tendon suture.
4. Incisions are closed in one layer.
5. A hand dressing is applied.

Flexor tendon graft

A graft is used to restore function when the original tendon is incapable of so doing because of a large gap between ends of a lacerated tendon or because of a failed primary tendon repair. Although extensor tendon grafts are possible, most free tendon grafts are flexor profundus and flexor pollicis longus tendon grafts. A gap large enough to preclude approximation by direct suturing of the tendon ends results from loss of a segment of tendon at the time of injury or from shortening of the proximal tendon end if too much time has elapsed since the original injury. A failed primary tendon repair is usually caused by scar tissue that inhibits adequate tendon gliding. Tendon gliding must be sufficient to produce appropriate joint movement when the muscle belly of the tendon contracts. If a great deal of scar tissue is present in the tendon bed, a free tendon graft also may fail to glide sufficiently to produce adequate joint movement. In this case a rod may be inserted into the tendon bed. The scar tissue that forms around the rod creates a pseudosheath through which a tendon graft is placed 6 to 8 weeks later. The pseudosheath often permits better tendon gliding.

The most commonly used donor tendon for a free graft is the palmaris longus tendon in the wrist and forearm. The plantaris tendon in the leg is also frequently used. Toe extensor tendons are used less commonly.

Procedural Considerations

A plastic hand instrument set is required, along with special instruments for flexor tendon graft (Fig. 24-46). The patient is placed in the supine position on the OR bed, with the arm extended on a hand table. The hand drape is used. If the plantaris tendon or a toe extensor tendon is to be used as the donor tendon, the lower extremity also must be prepped and draped. Use of a pneumatic tourniquet on the leg is optional.

Operative Procedure

1. After marking incisions and inflating the pneumatic tourniquet, the surgeon makes a distal incision to expose the insertion of the flexor profundus tendon into the distal phalanx, and a proximal incision is made in the hand or wrist or both.
2. Scar tissue in the tendon bed is excised.
3. If the flexor tendon bed is not deemed suitable for a tendon graft, a rod is inserted and sutured distally to the profundus tendon remnant attached to the distal phalanx (Fig. 24-47).
4. If the tendon bed is suitable or a rod has previously been inserted, a free tendon graft is obtained with a tendon stripper.
5. Approximation of the proximal tendon end and graft is performed in the palm or wrist.

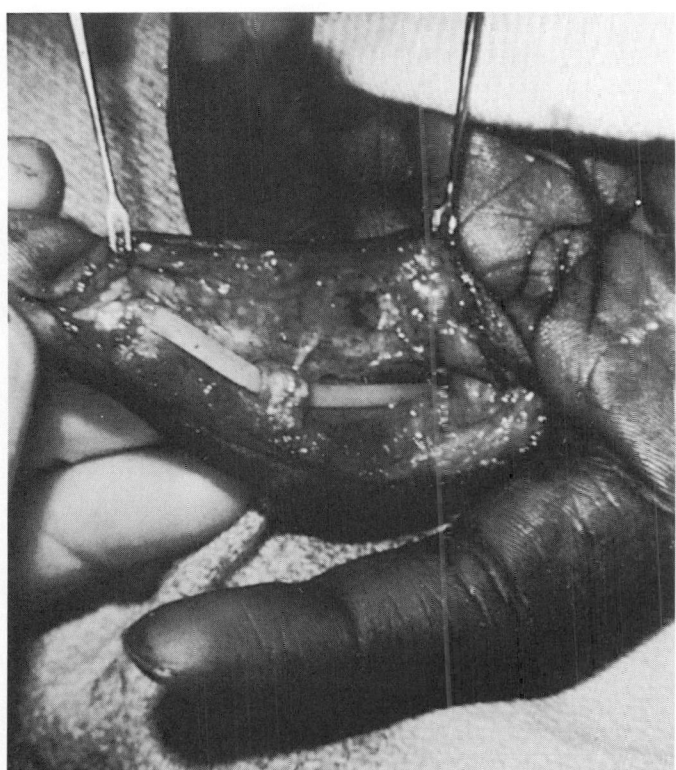

FIGURE 24-47 Silicone rod placed into profundus tendon bed of long finger in preparation for flexor tendon grafting.

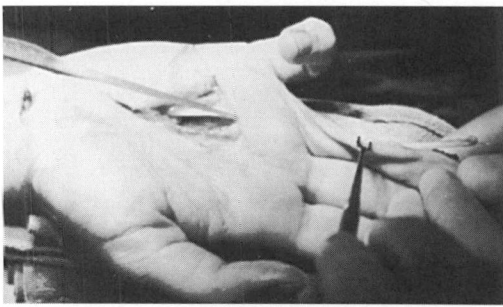

FIGURE 24-48 Flexor tendon graft being threaded through profundus tendon bed of ring finger from palm to distal phalanx. Palmaris longus tendon has been obtained with Brand tendon stripper through small wrist incision.

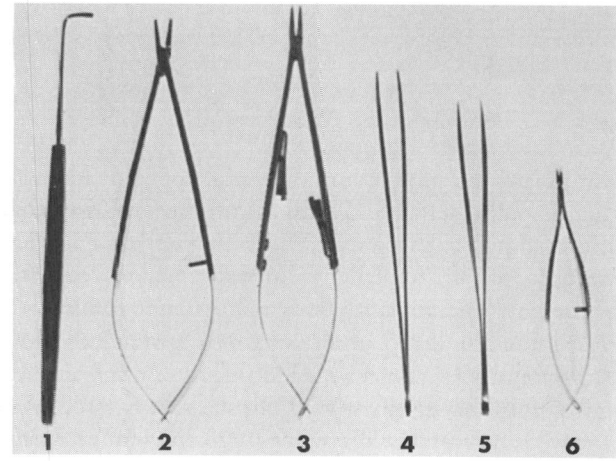

FIGURE 24-49 Special instruments for nerve repair and grafting. *1,* Von Graefe muscle hook; *2,* Castroviejo needle holder without lock; *3,* Castroviejo needle holder with lock; *4* and *5,* jeweler's forceps; *6,* Castroviejo-Vannas scissors.

6. The graft is threaded through the tendon bed to the distal phalanx (Fig. 24-48), where it is inserted after the tension of the graft has been carefully adjusted.
7. The incisions are closed in one layer.
8. A hand dressing is applied.

Peripheral nerve repair and grafting

Nerve repair is done by direct approximation of nerve or severed nerve ends or by means of a nerve graft to attempt to restore continuity of a nerve in the hand, wrist, or forearm and regain sensation or motor function.

Procedural Considerations

A plastic hand instrument set is required, along with the special instruments shown in Fig. 24-49 A sterile razor blade, marking pen, nerve stimulator, Esmarch bandage, and loupes or operating microscope also will be needed. The patient is placed in the supine position on the OR bed, with the arm extended on a hand table. The hand drape is used. If a nerve graft is to be used, a lower extremity is also prepped and draped. Use of a pneumatic tourniquet on the leg is optional.

Operative Procedure

1. After incisions are marked and the tourniquet is inflated, the proximal and distal nerve ends are exposed.
2. Devitalized nerve tissue or scar at the severed nerve ends is resected sharply with a sterile razor blade, back to normal nerve tissue, where individual nerve bundles can be visualized.
3. With the aid of loupes or the operating microscope, individual nerve bundles are approximated (Fig. 24-50) with a fine, nonabsorbable suture (usually #7-0 to #10-0 nylon).
4. If a nerve graft is used, it is obtained through a series of short transverse incisions or one long vertical incision along the posterolateral aspect of the leg. Approximation of the nerve bundles between the graft and proximal and distal nerve ends is performed as in step 3.
5. The incisions are sutured, and dressings are applied. The hand dressing is applied so that tension at the site of repair is prevented.

Implant arthroplasty

Destruction of the cartilage that forms the articular surface of a joint results in stiffness and pain during movement of the joint. Traumatic arthritis and rheumatoid

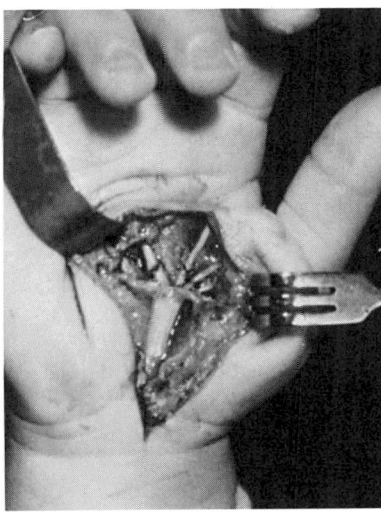

FIGURE 24-50 Severed branches of median nerve have been reapproximated with fine sutures.

arthritis are the most common causes of destruction of articular joint surfaces. Excision of the diseased joint surface affords relief of pain and improves joint motion. Insertion of an implant is an adjunct to resection arthroplasty. The implant serves as a dynamic joint spacer, not a joint prosthesis. In severe cases custom total joint prostheses may be used.

The most commonly used implants in hand surgery are flexible implants made of Silastic. Flexible implants available for arthroplasty within the scope of hand surgery are finger joints (for MP and PIP joints), wrist joint, carpal trapezium, lunate, and navicular (scaphoid).

Procedural Considerations

A plastic hand instrument set is required, along with alloplastic rasps, an oscillating bone saw, the Hall II drill with Swanson burrs, alloplastic implant of choice with sizer, an Esmarch bandage, and a marking pen. The patient is placed in the supine position on the OR bed, with the arm extended on a hand table. The hand drape is used.

Operative Procedure

1. After the incision line is marked and the pneumatic tourniquet is inflated, the involved joint is exposed through an appropriate incision.
2. In finger joint resection arthroplasty, the joint surfaces are excised together with comprehensive soft tissue release of the joint capsule. In resection arthroplasty of a carpal bone, the involved bone is completely excised.
3. In finger joint arthroplasty, the medullary canals of the two adjacent bones are reamed with the Hall II drill with Swanson burrs. In carpal bone implant resection arthroplasty, holes are reamed in one appropriate adjacent bone.

4. The two stems of a finger or wrist joint implant or the single stem of a carpal bone implant is seated in adjacent bones.
5. Soft tissues of the joint capsule (ligaments, tendons) are repaired.
6. The skin incisions are closed.
7. A hand dressing is applied.

Palmar fasciectomy

Dupuytren's contracture is a progressive disease involving the palmar fascia and the digital extensions of the palmar fascia. It usually begins with a small nodular thickening in the palm, most frequently in line with the ring finger. With progression of the disease, additional nodules appear, usually with skin adherent to them. Subsequent contracted longitudinal bands of palmar fascia may appear beneath the skin. When the digital extensions of the palmar fascia become involved in the disease process, flexion contractures of the finger MP and PIP joints result.

The cause of Dupuytren's contracture is unknown. One or both hands may be involved. The disease may also be present in the foot in the form of nodules and cords involving the plantar fascia. It does not result in contracture of the toes, however, because the plantar fascia has no digital (toe) extensions.

Surgery is the preferred treatment for Dupuytren's contracture, preferably at an early stage in the disease before irreparable joint damage occurs as the result of prolonged fixed flexion contracture. Surgical procedures include fasciotomy (simple division of contracted bands) or partial or total excision of the palmar fascia. In long-standing disease with irreversible joint changes, amputation of the finger may be the only treatment possible.

Procedural Considerations

A plastic hand instrument set is required, plus an Esmarch bandage and a marking pen. The patient is placed in the supine position on the OR bed, with the arm extended on a hand table. The hand drape is used.

Operative Procedure (Fig. 24-51)

1. Incision lines are marked, often with several Z-plasties to lengthen the involved skin of the finger and palm (as for scar revision).
2. The tourniquet is inflated.
3. After incisions are made, flaps of skin and subcutaneous tissue are carefully elevated to preserve their blood supply, with exposure of the fibrotic palmar fascia and its digital extensions.
4. Part or all of the palmar fascia and digital extensions is excised.
5. The tourniquet is usually released before skin closure so that hemostasis can be obtained. Incisions are sutured. A shortage of skin is sometimes noted at this point, in which case coverage by means of an FTSG is required.

A   **B**   **C**

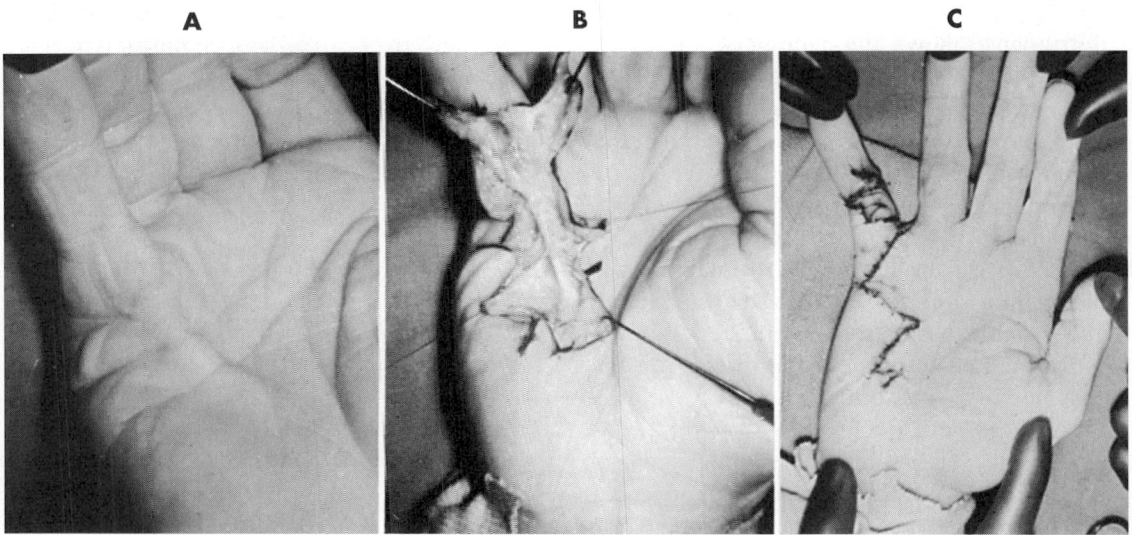

FIGURE 24-51 Dupuytren's contracture involving palmar fascia and its digital extensions into little finger. **A,** Cord and nodules in palm with mild flexion contracture of little finger. **B,** Contracted band of palmar fascia exposed. **C,** Wound closure with multiple Z-plasties to lengthen contracted skin.

6. If skin grafts are used, they are stented, and then a hand dressing is applied.

Carpal tunnel release

The transverse carpal ligament is incised or excised, with or without synovectomy, to relieve the symptom complex produced by compression of the median nerve within the carpal canal at the wrist. The carpal tunnel is located along the volar surface of the wrist.

Its rigid boundaries consist of carpal bones along three sides and the transverse carpal ligament along the fourth (volar) side. The median nerve, superficial and deep finger flexors, and the long thumb flexor tendon pass through the carpal tunnel before entering the hand. Any condition that decreases the size of the canal, such as fracture of a carpal bone, or increases its volume, such as the hypertrophic synovitis of rheumatoid arthritis, may cause pressure on the median nerve with resultant symptoms of carpal tunnel syndrome.

The symptoms of median nerve compression at the wrist are usually pain and paresthesia in the thumb, the index finger, the long finger, and the radial half of the ring finger. Night pain is common, interrupting the patient's normal sleep patterns. Long-standing median nerve compression may result in hand weakness, paresthesia on raising the hands, and thenar muscle atrophy. The condition may be unilateral or bilateral.

The procedure to release carpal ligament structures may include the use of endoscopic equipment. The necessary equipment includes video camera, monitor, telescopic lenses, probes, fiberoptic light cords, fiberoptic light source, and small sheaths or obturators. The same considerations with regard to use of the tourniquet as well as draping and prepping routines remain.

Procedural Considerations

A plastic hand instrument set is required, plus an Esmarch bandage and a marking pen. The patient is placed in the supine position on the OR bed, with the arm extended on a hand table. The hand and forearm are prepped to the elbow. The hand drape is used. The procedure is commonly performed as an ambulatory one with the patient receiving an axillary block or intravenous regional anesthesia, along with conscious sedation.

Operative Procedures

1. After appropriate skin marking and inflation of the pneumatic tourniquet, an incision is made across the volar wrist surface and base of the palm for adequate exposure of the transverse carpal ligament.
2. The transverse carpal ligament is incised along its entire length. A segment of it may be excised.
3. Synovectomy of structures within the carpal canal may or may not be performed.
4. The incision is closed in one layer.
5. A hand dressing is applied.

Endoscopic Carpal Tunnel Release

After appropriate skin marking and inflation of the pneumatic tourniquet, an incision is made in the wrist flexion crease. Blunt dissection of subcutaneous tissue is performed and a Ragnell retractor or self-retaining retractor is employed for visualization. Incision through the fascia is then completed, and the deeper end of the

Ragnell retractor is placed into the wound. Insertion of dissecting instruments allows the tenosynovium to be bluntly dissected off the transverse carpal ligament and the distal forearm fascia from the proximal incision to the distal extent of the transverse carpal ligament. At this time the slotted cannula is introduced into the carpal tunnel. The hand and cannula assembly are moved as a unit, and the hand is hyperflexed. Utilization of a hand-holding device can be helpful in maintaining this position. The distal incision is determined by palpation of the tip of the cannula assembly. This incision is made into the dermis using an instrument that presses on the palmar arch. Removal of the obturator leaves behind a slotted cannula whose design protects vulnerable structures but allows entry of endoscopes, probes, and endoscopic knives. Placement of the lens is done by attaching the light cord to the telescope and handing off to the circulator the other end of the cord to be placed in the light source. The camera is placed on the eyepiece of the lens, and the appropriate end of the camera cord is placed into the outlet on the video system. If moisture collects on the distal end of the endoscope, cotton-tipped applicators are inserted as needed. With the assistance of the video monitor, appropriate endoscopic knives are used to accomplish the release. After the carpal tunnel release is completed, the obturator is reinserted into the cannula, both are removed, and the incisions are closed. The procedure is completed with steps 4 and 5 as described above.

MICROSURGICAL REPLANTATION

Reconstructive microsurgery involves the use of an operating microscope and special microvascular instruments to reconstruct or replant tissue lost through injury or disease. Today's skilled microsurgeons can successfully anastomose the ends of a vessel measuring less than 1 mm in diameter. The success of microsurgery depends on several factors: (1) the individual and collective experiences of the surgical team and the members' ability to work together, relieving each other as necessary during long operations; (2) the surgeon's knowledge of the physiology of the microcirculation; (3) many hours of practice in the laboratory by the surgical team; and (4) the availability of proper microscopes, microvascular instruments (Fig. 24-52), and microvascular suture.

Replantation of Amputated Body Part

Replantation is an attempt to reattach a completely amputated digit or body part. Revascularization is the procedure performed on incomplete amputations, when the part remains attached to the body by skin, artery, vein, or nerve. Good candidates for replantation are those with the following amputations: (1) thumb, (2) multiple digits (Fig. 24-53), (3) a cut through the palm, (4) wrist or

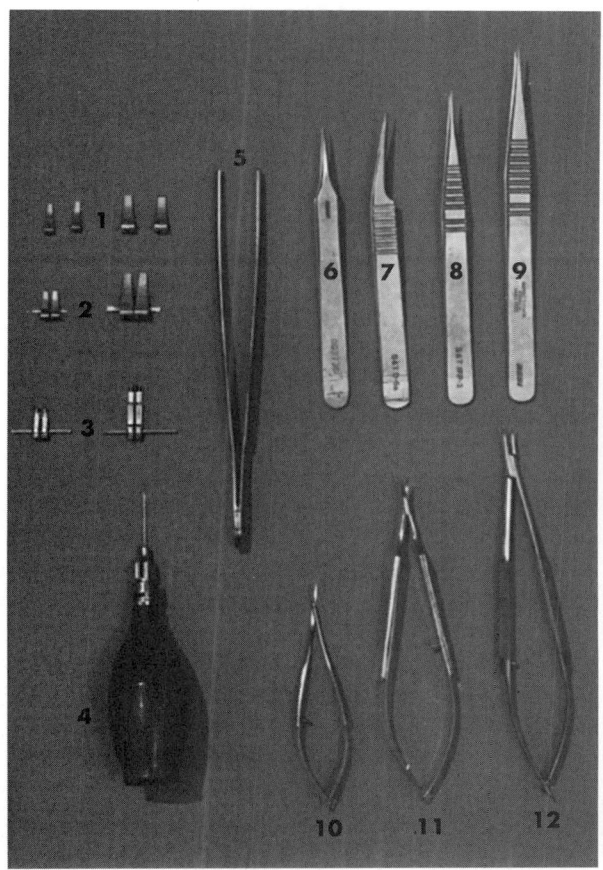

FIGURE 24-52 Microvascular instruments. *1,* Single vessel clamps; *2,* approximator clamps; *3,* nerve approximator clamps; *4,* Bishop-Harmon irrigating bulb and cannula tip; *5,* clamp-applying forceps; *6,* jeweler's forceps; *7,* Acland vessel dilator; *8* and *9,* Pierce tissue forceps; *10,* Vannas scissors; *11,* Castroviejo-Vannas scissors; *12,* Barraquet needle holder.

forearm, (5) elbow and above the elbow, and (6) almost any body part of a child.

The success of digital replantation depends primarily on the microsurgical repair of one digital artery and two digital veins. Replantation of an amputated part is ideally performed within 4 to 6 hours after injury, but success has been reported up to 24 hours after injury if the amputated part has been cooled. Proper care of the amputated body part or parts before surgery is vital to successful replantation (Fig. 24-54). The ultimate aim of replantation is the restitution of function beyond that provided by a prosthesis.

Procedural considerations

A regional anesthesia is usually given to replantation patients if the anticipated length of surgery so permits. Because of the length of these surgeries (12 to 16 hours), positioning is important. The OR bed and armboards should be carefully padded with egg-crate foam or a gel-filled mattress to support the supine patient. The surgeon may request the room temperature to be between

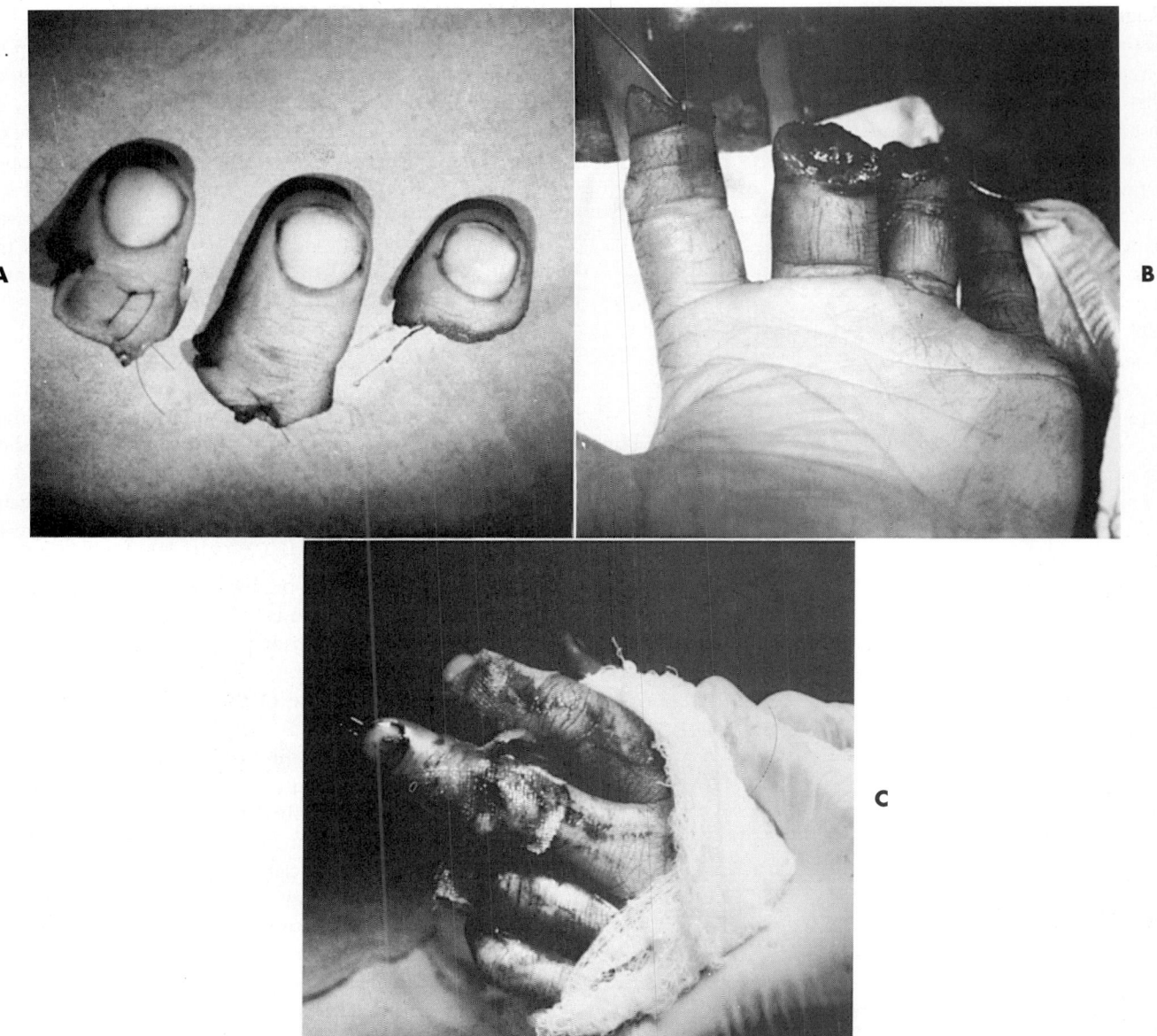

FIGURE 24-53 **A,** Complete amputation of three digits from hand. **B,** Hand after amputation. **C,** Reattachment of three completely amputated digits to the hand.

75° and 80° F before the patient arrives because the warm room will reduce vasoconstriction in the extremities. A warming device, such as warm forced air, is usually applied to keep the patient's body temperature between 98.6° and 101° F. The surgeon usually brings the amputated part to the operating room before the patient arrives to ensure ample time for preparation of the amputated part for replantation.

Instrumentation includes a plastic hand instrument set, microvascular instruments, a Kirschner wire driver, Kirschner wires, an operating microscope, and a bipolar ESU.

A pneumatic tourniquet cuff is placed on the patient's upper arm, and a hand drape is used.

Operative procedure

1. Bone ends are shortened to eliminate tension on vascular anastomoses to be done later; the bone is stabilized by means of internal fixation with Kirschner wires.
2. Flexor and extensor tendon repairs are usually performed next.
3. The digital nerves are repaired with the aid of loupes or the operating microscope.
4. With microsurgical instruments and techniques, two digital veins are repaired, followed by repair of one digital artery. If ischemic time has been prolonged, digital vessel repair may precede repair of tendons and nerves.

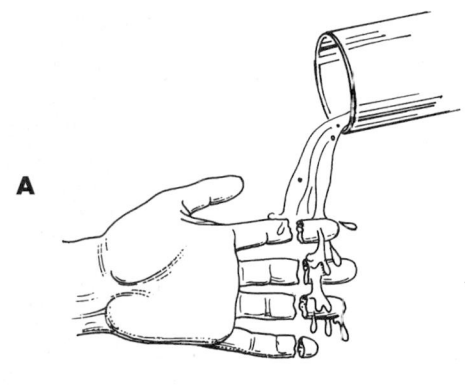

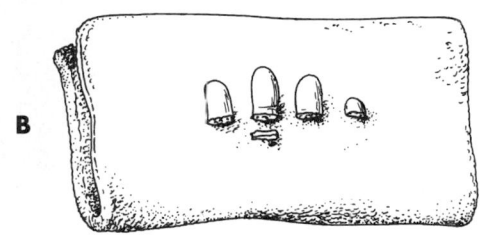

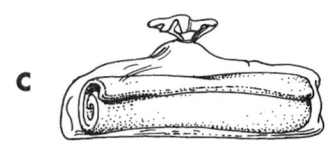

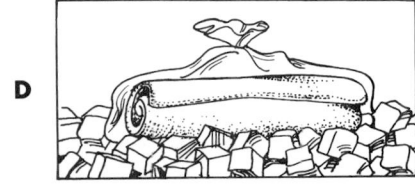

FIGURE 24-54 All severed body parts should be sought, including small pieces of mangled tissue. The following steps should be performed: **A,** rinse; **B,** wrap in moist towel; **C,** place in towel in clean plastic bag and seal; **D,** cool on ice. The iced bag should be sent to the replantation center with the patient.

5. The skin is sutured.
6. A bulky supportive hand dressing is applied.

Toe-to-Hand Transfer

The reconstructive procedure of toe-to-hand transfer involves surgical removal of a single toe or multiple toes and anastomosing of the vessels of the toes to those on the hand to restore finger and thumb functions. It is lengthy surgery (12 to 16 hours), entailing a two-team approach, one at the foot for toe removal and one at the recipient site, the hand.

Procedural considerations

The patient is placed in the supine position on the OR bed. The patient is placed on an anticoagulation regimen during the anastomosis procedure. Two tourniquets are needed, one on the thigh of the operative foot and one on the operative arm. Both extremities are separately prepped and draped. Instrumentation includes a plastic hand set, microvascular instruments, power Kirschner wire driver, and Kirschner wires. Additional equipment includes the operating microscope, two tourniquet power sources, two bipolar ESUs, marking pen, and Esmarch bandage.

Operative procedure

1. The surgeon preparing the hand determines adequate blood flow and vessel location on the thumb or finger site (Fig. 24-55, *A*). This may prevent a needless amputation of the toe.
2. Appropriate skin flaps are incised to expose the veins on the dorsum of the hand and clamped with vessel microclips.
3. The radial artery or branches are dissected out and prepared for anastomosis.
4. The flexor and extensor pollicis longus tendons are located and transfixed.
5. The bone at the base of the thumb is prepared for the toe.
6. The nerves to the thumb are dissected out with adequate length for suturing without tension.
7. The toe is circumscribed with a racket-shaped incision (Fig. 24-55, *B*), and the veins are isolated through the dorsal aspect and clamped with micro-vessel clips.
8. The extensor tendon is dissected proximally and transsected over the base of the metatarsal.
9. The dorsalis pedis artery is dissected to the digital vessels with ligation of all branches of that vessel to prepare for the anastomosis.
10. On the plantar surface the digital nerves and flexor tendons are transsected at levels of adequate length for anastomosis (Fig. 24-55, *C*).
11. The toe is transsected at the level previously determined for adequate length of the thumb.
12. The toe vessels are anastomosed microsurgically to the thumb vessels. The toe is attached to the thumb area by Kirschner wires (Fig. 24-55, *D*).

An esthetic and functionally effective hand can be achieved through this procedure (Fig. 24-55, *E*).

Free Jejunal Tissue Transfer

Reconstructive problems in patients undergoing laryngectomy and upper cervical esophagectomy can be adequately solved by free jejunal transfer. Modern microsurgical techniques greatly improve the success rate. Free jejunal transfers have proved beneficial in the following:

- Patients with massive resection of the laryngopharynx when resection may extend into the oropharynx or even

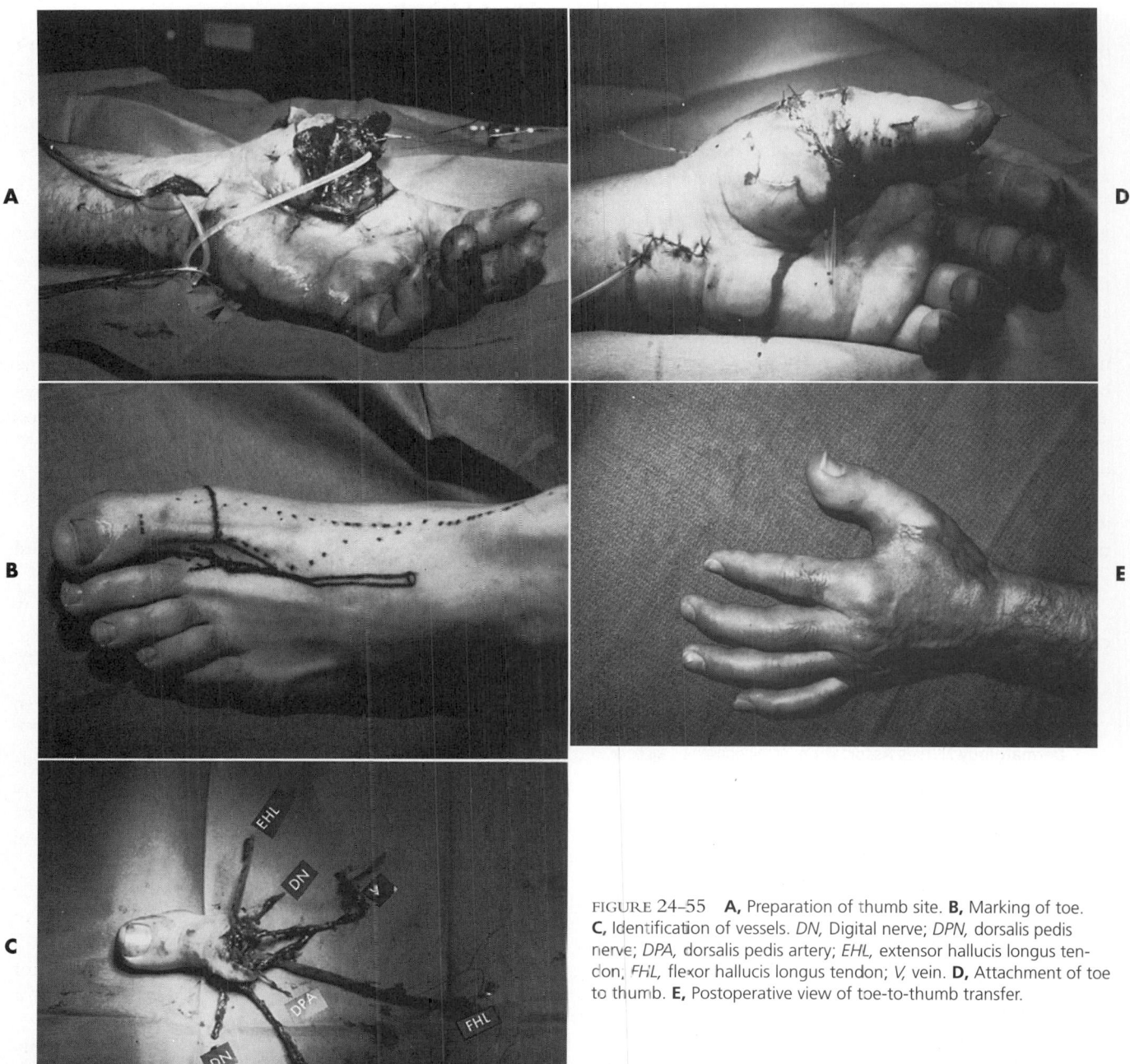

FIGURE 24–55   **A,** Preparation of thumb site. **B,** Marking of toe. **C,** Identification of vessels. *DN,* Digital nerve; *DPN,* dorsalis pedis nerve; *DPA,* dorsalis pedis artery; *EHL,* extensor hallucis longus tendon; *FHL,* flexor hallucis longus tendon; *V,* vein. **D,** Attachment of toe to thumb. **E,** Postoperative view of toe-to-thumb transfer.

the lower nasopharynx and encompass a large portion of the cervical esophagus
- Patients with radiation failure in whom laryngopharyngoesophagectomy is required
- Patients with secondary reconstruction of the hypopharynx or cervical esophagus in whom other methods have failed because of flap necrosis or radiation
- Patients in whom primary pharyngoesophageal radiation has resulted in hypopharyngeal stricture unresponsive to dilatation
- Isolated cases in which a large area of oral lining is lost

Procedural considerations

The patient is positioned, prepped, and draped for laryngectomy with the abdomen exposed. The abdomen is covered with sterile towels during laryngectomy. When laryngectomy is completed (see Chapter 21), all instruments and drapes are discarded after the wound has been covered with sterile towels. The patient is again prepped and draped for the free tissue graft.

The basic plastic instrument set is used, plus abdominal instruments for the graft and microsurgical and vascular instruments for the graft anastomosis. The operating

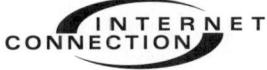

microscope or loupes may be used for preparation of the graft and graft placement.

Operative procedure

A two-team approach is used whenever possible. Neck dissection is carried out, at which time donor vessels are identified and preserved. The abdomen is opened, and the ligament of Treitz is located. A suitable segment is identified in the first 2 feet of jejunum with a single dominant vascular pedicle. The segment with its pedicle is resected, and bowel continuity is reestablished. The abdomen is closed as the microsurgeon prepares the bowel vessel for anastomosis. The donor-recipient vessels in the neck are prepared using the microscope. The proximal bowel anastomosis is made, followed by the vascular anastomosis. When the microvascular clamps are removed, pulsation of the mesenteric vessels and peristalsis should begin. The distal bowel anastomosis is then done. The neck is closed, leaving a small Silastic window over the jejunal segment to allow for close, postoperative observation of the transplant.

INTERNET CONNECTION

American Society of Plastic and Reconstructive Surgical Nurses: http://inurse.com/~asprsn

Dermatology Nurses Association: email dna@mail.ajj.com

FDA Breast Implant Information: http://www.fda.gov/oca/breastimplants/bitac.html

The Mole Hill: http://www.health.ufl.edu/hs/molehill.htm

The Plastic Surgery Link: http://www.nvpc.nl/plink

Plastic Surgery Info Service: http://www.plasticsurgery.org/

American Society of Plastic and Reconstructive Surgeons: http://www.plasticsurgery.org

American Society for Aesthetic Plastic Surgery Home Page: http://surgery.org/

Tissue Engineering: http://www.pittsburgh-tissue.net/

American Cancer Society: http://www.cancer.org

REFERENCES

1. American Nurses Association. (1998). *Standards of clinical nursing practice.* Washington, D.C.: the Association.
2. *AORN standards, recommended practices, and guidelines.* (1998). Denver: the Association.
3. Clyne BD: Updating pressure ulcer care, letter to the Editor. *AJN 98*(1), 1998, 16C.
4. Hidalgo, D.A., & Disa, J.J. Plastic surgical reconstruction. In Wilmore, D., et al. (Ed.). (1998). *American College of Surgeons Care of the Surgical Patient,* vol. 2. New York: Scientific American Medicine.
5. Hodgson, B.B., Kizior, R.J., & Kingdon, R.T. (1997). *Nurse's drug handbook,* Philadelphia, Saunders.
6. Janikowski, D.L., & Rockefeller, C.A. (1998). Awake and talking: ambulatory surgery and conscious sedation, *Nursing Economic$, 16*(1), 37-42.
7. Kleinbeck, S.V.M., & Eelle, K.R. (1997). Monitoring postdischarge ambulatory surgical recovery: costs and outcomes. *Surgical Services Management, 3*(3), 33-35.
8. Smyth, S. Plastic and reconstructive surgery. In Rothrock, J.C. (Ed). (1996). *Perioperative nursing care planning,* (ed. 2). St. Louis: Mosby.
9. Stuart, G.W., & Laraia, M.T. (1998). *Stuart and Sundeen's principles and practices of psychiatric nursing* (ed. 6). St. Louis: Mosby.
10. Surgery in transition. (1998). *Surgical Services Management, 4*(1), 56.

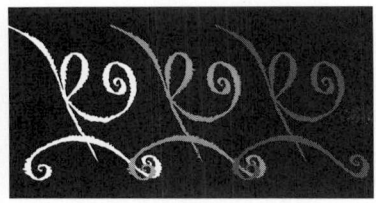

CHAPTER TWENTY FIVE

Thoracic Surgery

Brenda Gregory Dawes

THORACIC SURGERY, LIKE other specialties, has evolved with the development of surgical techniques and treatments, such as blood transfusion, anesthetic delivery, and screening procedures. The first thoracic procedure, recorded in 1499, was an unsuccessful excision of a herniation of the lung. From that time, the physiologic effect on the lungs and perceived difficulty entering the chest resulted in hesitancy to perform thoracic procedures. Until the 1880s, the only thoracic procedures performed were for drainage of empyema and of lung abscess or treatment of traumatic chest injury. In 1823, the first purposeful resection of a part of the lung for accidental injury was reported by Milton Antony, and in 1861, the French surgeon Péan removed part of a lung for tumor.

Treatment of tuberculosis (TB), which has been attempted for centuries, also provided reasons for developments in thoracic procedures. Thoracoplasty became widely used as a means of collapsing the lungs for treatment of TB followed by other forms of treatment. In 1907 an article was published describing surgical techniques for access to the thoracic cavity. In 1913, Jacobeus is credited with dividing adhesions with a cautery passed through one cannula while through another he passed a cystoscope-like instrument he called a *thoracoscope*. Student textbooks in the 1920s contained only a short paragraph on cancer of the lung. From that time until the first successful pneumonectomy in 1933 there were many attempts to remove carcinomas with limited success.[11]

During the past 50 years the understanding of pathophysiology and improved techniques has expanded the field of thoracic surgery. The thoracic specialty extends beyond the surgical arena into infectious disease, trauma, and oncology. Improved technology, such as use of lasers in the 1970s, the advent of video-assisted thoracoscopic procedures, and the determination to treat diseases previously considered untreatable with surgery continues to improve the recovery rate for patients experiencing thoracic diseases. As the ability to treat lung diseases has improved, the responsibilities of the perioperative nurse have expanded, resulting in accomplishments throughout the years that have provided an extensive knowledge base and specialized perioperative practitioners.

SURGICAL ANATOMY

The skeletal framework of the thorax is formed anteriorly by the sternum and costal cartilages, laterally by the 12 pairs of ribs, and posteriorly by the 12 thoracic vertebrae (Figs. 25-1 and 25-2). This airtight compartment is enclosed in the root of the neck by Sibson's fascia and is separated from the abdomen by the diaphragm.

The sternum forms the anterior thoracic wall in the midline. It consists of three parts: (1) the upper part, or manubrium; (2) the body, or gladiolus; and (3) the lower cartilage, or xiphoid process. The manubrium articulates with the clavicles and the first two ribs on each side; the gladiolus articulates with the remaining true

ribs by separate costal cartilages; and the xiphoid fuses with the gladiolus in early development and is attached to the diaphragm by the substernal ligament (Figs. 25-1 and 25-3).

Normally the lateral walls of the thorax are formed by the 12 pairs of ribs. Posteriorly each pair of ribs articulates with its corresponding thoracic vertebrae (see Fig. 25-2). Anteriorly the first seven ribs articulate with the sternum. The eighth, ninth, and tenth ribs articulate with the costal cartilages of the rib above; however, the eleventh and twelfth are not fixed to the costal arch (see Fig. 25-1).

The muscles of each hemithorax (Figs. 25-3 and 25-4) include the 11 external and 11 internal intercostal muscles,

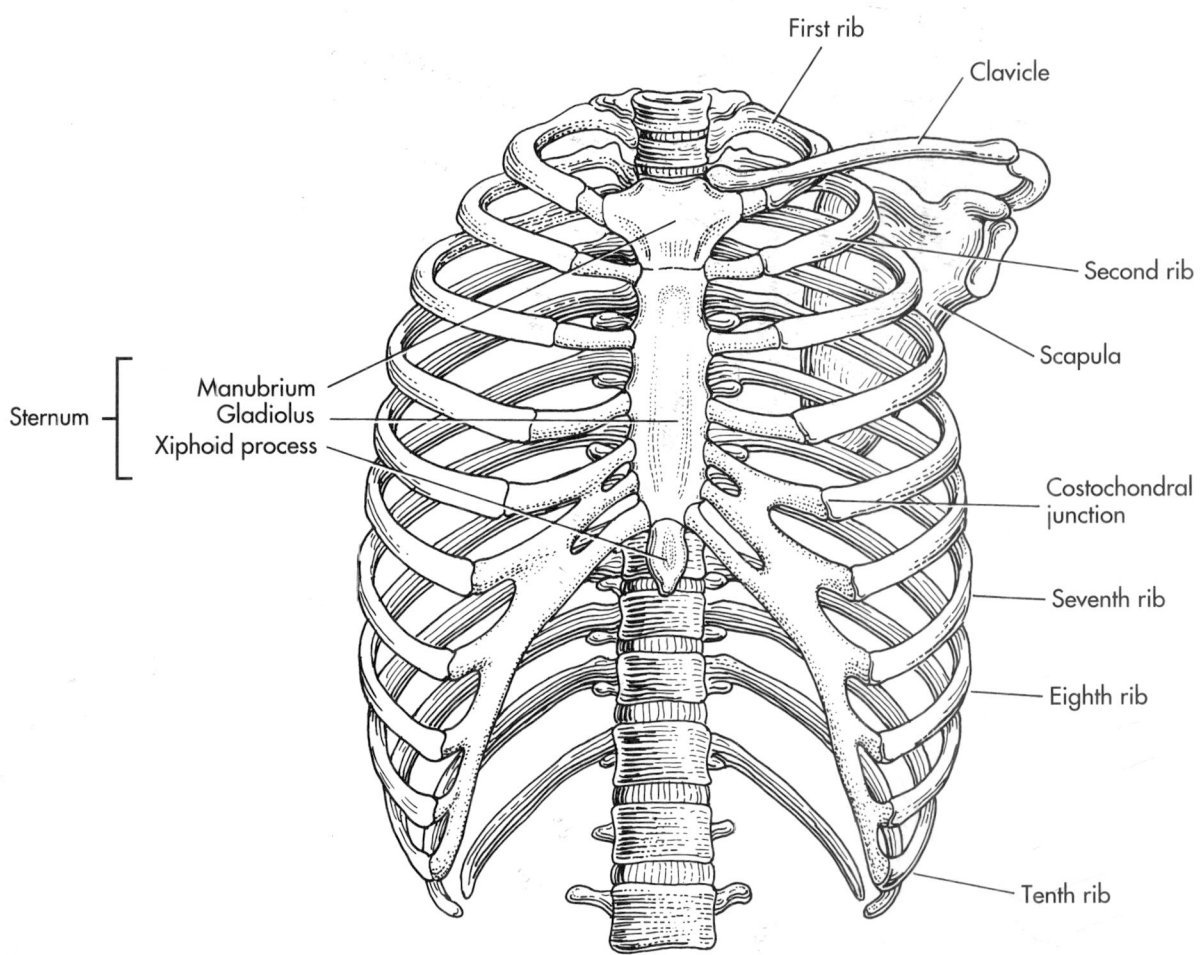

First rib

Clavicle

Second rib

Scapula

Costochondral junction

Seventh rib

Eighth rib

Tenth rib

Manubrium
Gladiolus
Xiphoid process

Sternum

FIGURE 25-1   Bony thorax.

which fill the spaces between the ribs. An intercostal artery, vein, and nerve accompany each intercostal muscle. The arteries communicate with the internal thoracic artery anteriorly and arise from the aorta posteriorly. The intercostal veins follow the course of the arteries and communicate with the mammary veins anteriorly and with the azygos and hemiazygos veins posteriorly.

During surgery great care is taken to prevent injury to the intercostal nerve, which passes forward and alongside the posterior intercostal artery and shares with the superior branch of the artery the intercostal groove on the inferior edge of the corresponding rib. When the nerve must be disturbed, an anesthetic agent may be injected to prevent postoperative pain.

The thoracic outlet is a junction bound by the manubrium anteriorly and by the first ribs anterolaterally and posteriorly by the first thoracic vertebrae and posterior angles of the first ribs of the space. The great vessels of the head, neck, and arm pass through this space. Compression of these structures causes thoracic outlet syndrome.

The chest cavity is subdivided into the right and left pleural cavities, which contain the lungs, separated by the mediastinum, which lies medially between the two pleural

membranes. The parietal pleura, the membrane that lines the inner surface of each hemithorax, is adjacent to the inner surfaces of the ribs posteriorly and the mediastinum medially and covers the surface of the diaphragm except at the central portion. Part of the parietal membrane is reflected back at the root of each lung to form a sac around it. This reflection is called the *visceral pleura*. A serous secretion, pleural fluid provides lubrication between these two membranes to minimize friction. Approximately 0.1 to 0.2 ml/kg of body weight of fluid exists in the pleural space.

The lungs are the essential organs of respiration. The base of each lung rests on the diaphragm, whereas its apex (upper end) projects into the base of the neck at a level above the first rib. The bronchus, the nerves, the lymphatics, and the pulmonary and bronchial vessels enter and leave the lung on the mediastinal surface in a structure known as the *hilum*, or root, of the lung. Deep fissures divide the spongy, porous lung into lobes. The primary bronchi divide and then subdivide into each lobe and eventually become bronchioles. The right lung has an upper, middle, and lower lobe; the left lung has only an upper and lower lobe (Fig. 25-5). However, the lungs are

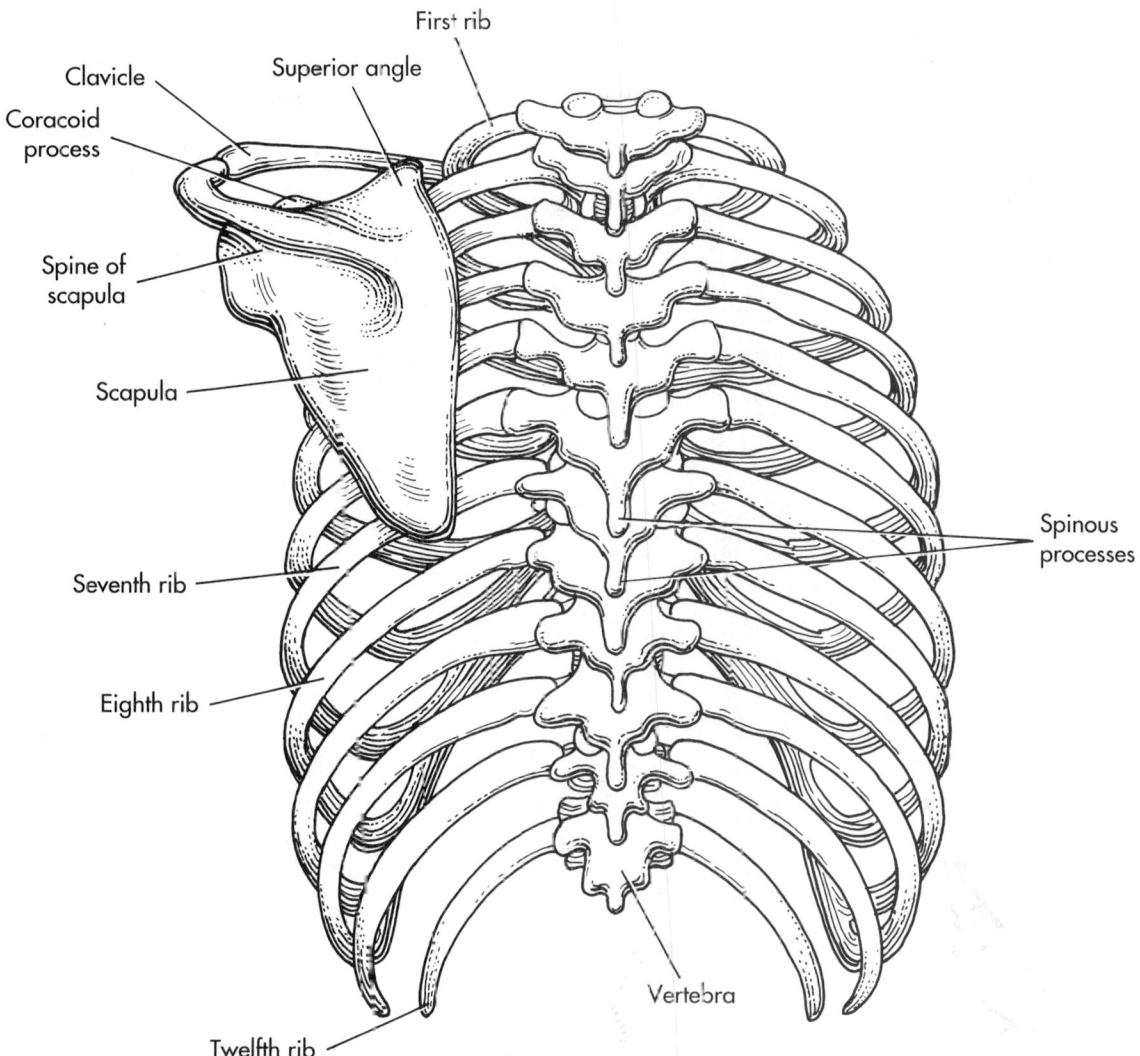

FIGURE 25-2 Posterior view of bony thorax.

similar in that each is composed of 10 major segments. Each segment extends to the pleural surface, expanding in volume from its center to its peripheral edges. Each segment also has its own bronchus and branches of the pulmonary artery and vein.

The bronchial arteries, arising from the aorta, supply nourishment to the lungs. They vary in their number and course. The arrangement may include two branches to the left lung and one branch to the right lung, which later branches into two, or there may be one or two branches for each lung. The pulmonary arteries carry the blood to the pulmonary parenchyma, and the pulmonary veins transport the oxygenated blood to the left atrium.

The nerves of the lungs are a part of the autonomic nervous system (see Chapter 23). They regulate constriction and relaxation of the bronchi and of the blood vessels within the lungs.

Although the thoracic cavity is an airtight space, the lungs inspire outside air through the nasal passages, trachea,

and bronchi. The main function of the lungs is to exchange carbon dioxide for oxygen. Normally, as the thorax expands, the lungs also expand as air is drawn in; during expiration the thorax relaxes, and the lungs passively contract as air is forced out. Inspiration normally takes place when the intrathoracic pressure is slightly below atmospheric pressure (76 cm Hg, or 760 mm Hg) and when a partial vacuum exists between the parietal and visceral pleural (intrathoracic) surfaces. As the muscles of inspiration contract to enlarge the chest cage, the lungs passively follow the diaphragm and chest wall because of decreased intrathoracic pressure. The acts of inspiration and expiration are the result of air moving in and out of the lung, causing pressure to equalize with that of the atmosphere at the end of expiration (Fig. 25-6).

The normal intrapleural pressure varies from −9 to −12 cm H_2O during inspiration and from about −3 to −6 cm H_2O during expiration. The greatest amount of air that can be expired after a maximum inspiration is termed

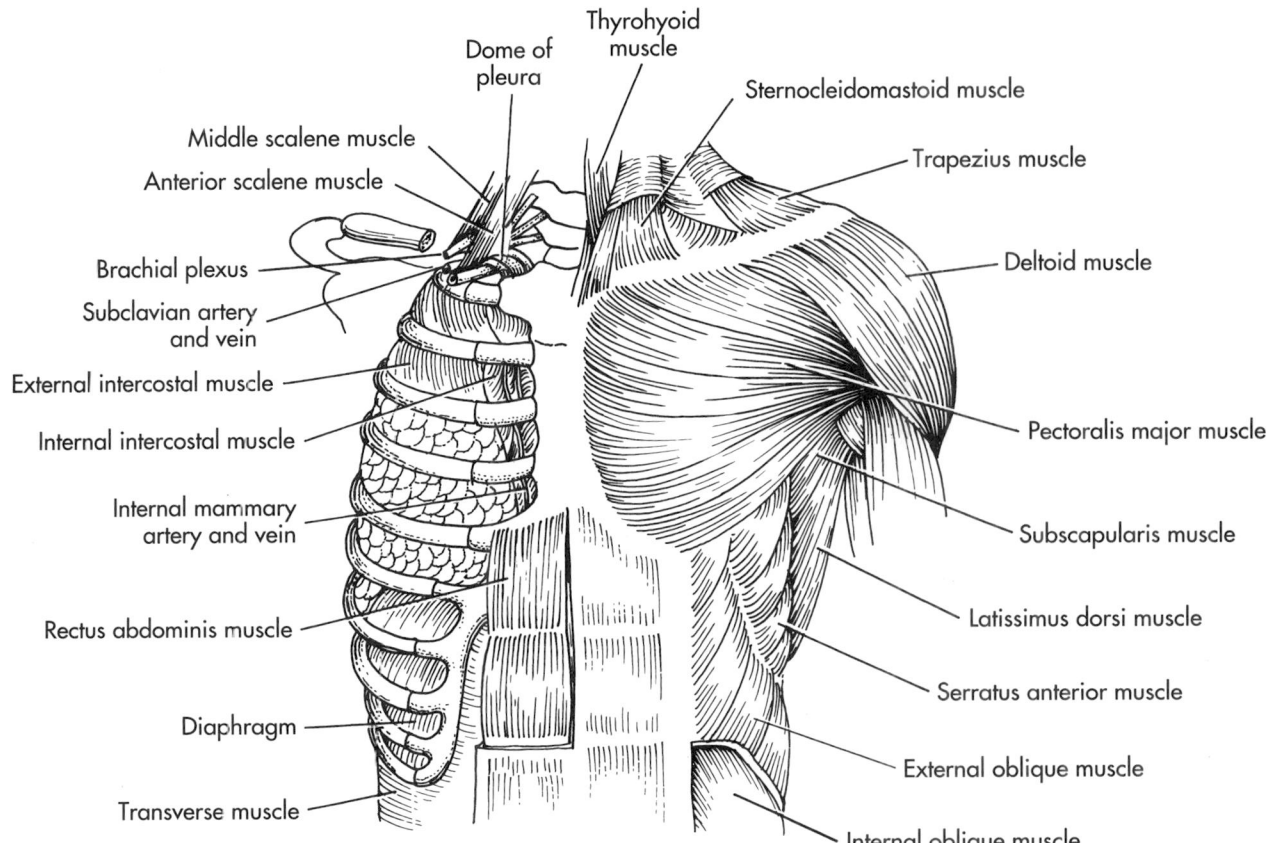

FIGURE 25-3   Anterior view of thorax and contiguous portions of base of neck and anterior abdominal wall. *Right half,* Superficial layer of muscles and fascia; *left half,* relations of deep muscles of neck and abdomen to rib cage, intercostal muscles, diaphragm, and internal mammary vessels; relations of muscles, nerves, and vessels with first rib; and anterior relations of lung.

the *vital capacity* and the volume of gas remaining in the lungs after maximal expiration is *residual volume.* Size, age, sex, and pulmonary disease of the patient influence vital capacity. Any condition that interferes with the normally negative intrapleural pressure affects respiratory function.

PERIOPERATIVE NURSING CONSIDERATIONS

Assessment

During assessment the perioperative nurse gathers information (patient data) that is important to planning patient care. Signs and symptoms demonstrated by the patient are confirmed by the perioperative nurse during the admission assessment. The perioperative nurse may begin data collection through a review of the patient's medical record, including results of the history, physical examination, laboratory tests, other diagnostic workups, and the nursing history and assessment. It is valuable to assess the patient's understanding of the disease process and of the anticipated procedure. It is also important to assess emotional status, since patients may be asymptomatic, which creates an atmosphere for denial. A focused

assessment of the respiratory system should be included during the physical assessment. The nurse questions the patient or otherwise confirms the presence of an increased frequency of cough, increase in sputum production, recurrent hemoptysis, malaise, shortness of breath, substernal chest discomfort, weight loss, poor appetite, adequacy of nutrition, and hypoxia. The results of the physical examination of the chest should be reviewed; the perioperative nurse may auscultate the chest and confirm the presence of crackles or wheezes on inspiration or expiration.

The review of diagnostic and laboratory tests may include the chest x-ray films, sputum analysis confirmed during bronchoscopy, cytology reports, and pulmonary function studies.[10] The chest x-ray film remains an indispensable diagnostic tool and will be needed in the operating room. This film outlines the lesion, if any is present, and defines its shape and space-occupying nature (tracheal shift). The presence of air in the hilar region, pleural effusion, or atelectasis may also be confirmed by radiologic evidence. Sputum analysis for culture and sensitivity may alert the perioperative nurse to an infectious process; cytologic examination may confirm a malignancy. The patient may have already undergone

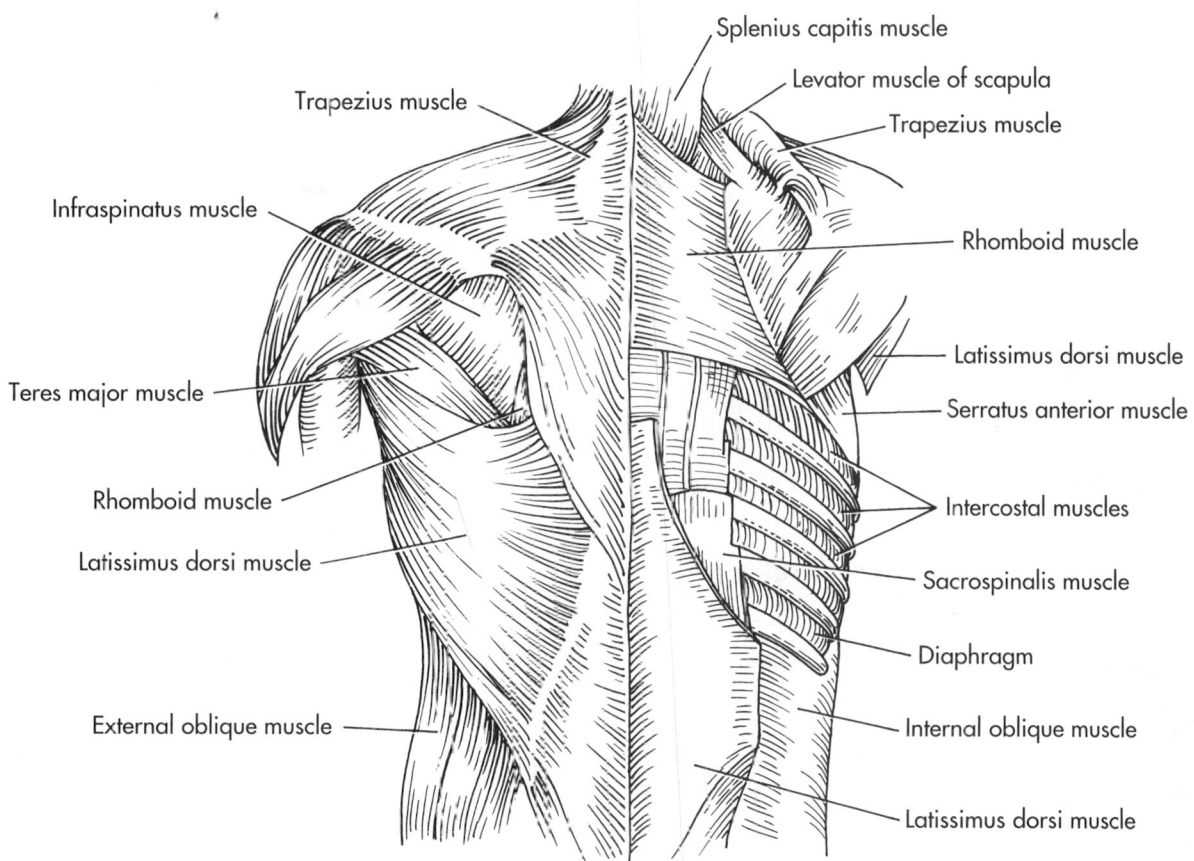

Splenius capitis muscle

Levator muscle of scapula

Trapezius muscle

Trapezius muscle

Rhomboid muscle

Infraspinatus muscle

Latissimus dorsi muscle

Serratus anterior muscle

Teres major muscle

Intercostal muscles

Rhomboid muscle

Sacrospinalis muscle

Latissimus dorsi muscle

Diaphragm

External oblique muscle

Internal oblique muscle

Latissimus dorsi muscle

FIGURE 25-4   Posterior view of thorax and contiguous portions of neck and abdominal wall. *Left half*, Superficial muscles; *right half*, deeper muscles.

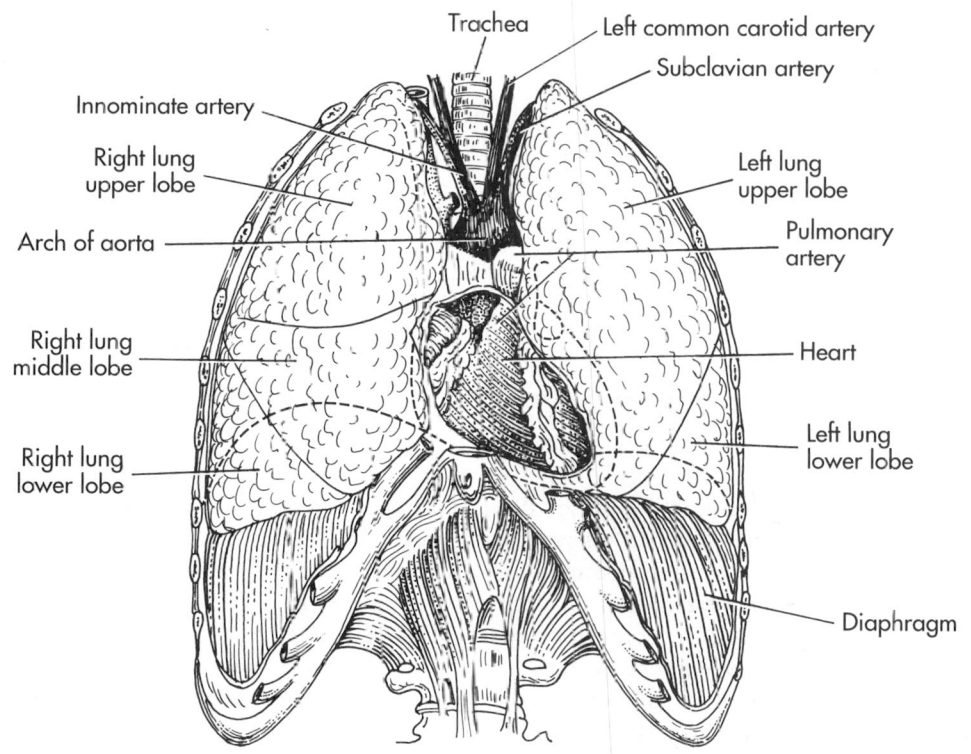

Trachea

Left common carotid artery

Subclavian artery

Innominate artery

Right lung upper lobe

Left lung upper lobe

Arch of aorta

Pulmonary artery

Right lung middle lobe

Heart

Right lung lower lobe

Left lung lower lobe

Diaphragm

FIGURE 25-5   Organs of thoracic cavity. Part of pericardium has been removed to expose heart.

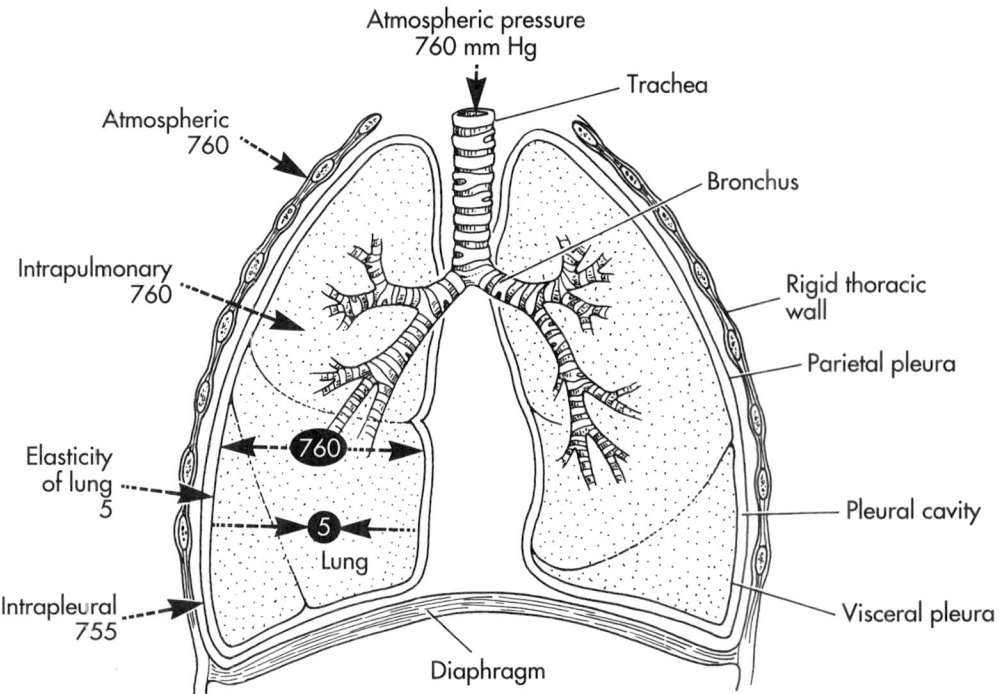

Atmospheric pressure
760 mm Hg

Trachea

Atmospheric
760

Bronchus

Intrapulmonary
760

Rigid thoracic
wall

Parietal pleura

Elasticity
of lung
5

760

Pleural cavity

5

Lung

Intrapleural
755

Visceral pleura

Diaphragm

FIGURE 25–6   Thoracic cavity structures showing intrapulmonary and intrapleural pressures with chest wall in resting position.

TABLE 25–1	Normal Results of Laboratory Studies for Assessment of Patients Undergoing Thoracic Procedures	
TEST	**NORMAL RESULTS**	**PURPOSE**
Pulmonary Function Tests		
Vital capacity (VC)	>4 L	Detect abnormalities in respiratory function
Maximum voluntary ventilation (MVV)	>80 L/min	Determine extent of pulmonary abnormality
Maximum midexpiratory flow (MMF)	>2 L/sec	
Forced expiratory flow	>32 L	
Forced expiratory flow, 1 sec (FEV$_1$)	>71 L	
Perfusion Studies—Arterial Blood Gases		
pH	7.35-7.45	Indicate respiratory and metabolic disturbances
Pco_2	35-45	
HCO_3	21-28	
Po_2	80-100	
O_2 saturation	95%-100%	

diagnostic bronchoscopy or mediastinoscopy; if so, the results should be reviewed for acid-fast bacillus smear, culture, bronchial washing, and biopsy results. Computerized tomographic (CT) scans of the chest, as well as of the brain, liver, and abdomen, may reveal the presence or absence of metastasis, pleural calcification, thickening, or plaque; radioisotope scans may have been done for similar reasons. Magnetic resonance imaging (MRI) detects vascular relationships to masses or vascular lesions. The results of pulmonary function tests and arterial blood gases should be reviewed[13] (Table 25-1). Ventilation and perfusion studies show the distribution of each function in the lung. These results assist the perioperative nurse in collaborating with the surgical team to maintain effective gas exchange during the surgical intervention. The results are also valuable in predicting postoperative respiratory function and metabolic responses. Patients hospitalized for surgery related to carcinoma may have received

25-1 RESEARCH HIGHLIGHT

It is believed that smoking cessation is valuable in decreasing pulmonary complications, stabilizing pulmonary function, decreasing risk of myocardial infarction, and potentially improving response to oncologic therapy. A study conducted by Dresler et al. assessed patients for smoking habits and followed them during the postoperative course to determine the effects of presurgery cessation. Of the 345 patients with a smoking history, 86% remained nonsmoking after surgery. Of the 44 patients who had remained or started smoking postoperatively, 61% did not stop before surgery. In the 17.5-month follow-up study, 85% of the patients who quit between 2 weeks to 3 months preoperatively remained nonsmoking postoperatively. The researchers concluded that patients who did not quit smoking preoperatively are at significant risk of continuing to smoke postoperatively. The longer that patients are nonsmoking preoperatively, the more likely they will continue not smoking postoperatively.

From Dresler, C.M., Bailey, M., & Roper, C.R. (1996). Smoking cessation and lung cancer resection, *Chest, 110*(5), 1199-1202.

chemotherapy or radiation therapy before surgery. Assessment of the skin and the patient's general condition is important in preventing perioperative complications.

The patient's and family's knowledge and understanding of the surgical procedure and expected outcomes should be determined. Their willingness to participate in the patient's care and to assist with accomplishing the desired outcomes should be determined. Smoking habits (Research Highlight 25-1) and pain tolerance are two areas that should be assessed to determine necessary teaching or tools that will assist in achieving positive postoperative outcomes.

After a general and focused review of the patient's medical record and patient interview, the perioperative nurse formulates nursing diagnoses. These statements reflect problems that will require perioperative nursing intervention, either independently or collaboratively with other members of the surgical team. Nursing diagnoses should be individualized and prioritized for each patient.

Nursing Diagnosis

Nursing diagnoses related to the care of patients undergoing thoracic surgery might include the following:

- Risk for impaired gas exchange related to the surgical intervention
- Risk for impaired skin integrity related to surgical positioning, length of surgical intervention, or use of chemical antimicrobial agents on the skin

- Fluid-volume excess related to decreased surface area of the lung for perfusion and administration of IV fluids during surgery
- Risk for infection related to inadequate secondary defenses (presence of existing disease process) and surgical disruption of tissues

Outcome Identification

Outcomes identified for the selected nursing diagnosis could be stated as follows:

- The patient will experience adequate gas exchange during the surgical procedure.
- The patient's skin integrity will be maintained.
- The patient will maintain appropriate fluid balance.
- The patient will be free from infection.

Planning

A Sample Care Plan for a patient undergoing thoracic surgery is included on p. 1052.

Implementation

During implementation of the care plan the perioperative nurse is concerned with both preparatory patient considerations (such as procedure, explanation and teaching for the patient, positioning, presurgical diagnostic interventions, and draping) and the requirements of the surgical intervention (medication delivery; instrument, equipment, and supply availability). These patient care needs are coordinated with the other nursing interventions identified in the specific patient care plan.

Endoscopy

Endoscopy is use of a scope for visualization. Thoracic endoscopy includes use of the bronchoscope, mediastinoscope, or thoracoscope.

Medications

The procedure may be completed using topical, local, monitored anesthesia care (MAC) or general anesthesia. The topical (or local) anesthetic setup should include a headlight for visualization, laryngeal mirrors of various sizes, a lingual spatula, sprays with straight and curved cannulas, and anesthetic drugs, as ordered. Other items include the laryngeal syringe with straight and curved cannulas, Jackson cross-action forceps, and the Schindler pharyngeal anesthetizer, if desired. A small basin with warm water can be used to prevent fogging of the scope. Luer-Lok syringes, 10 ml, and needles, 20 and 22 gauge, are needed for transtracheal injection.

The anesthetic drugs frequently used are lidocaine (Xylocaine), procaine (Novocain), and tetracaine (Pontocaine, Cetacaine) with or without epinephrine[14] (Table 25-2). Pauses of 3 to 4 minutes are taken between applications of the anesthetic agent to the tongue, palate, and pharynx and then to the larynx and to the trachea.

S A M P L E   C A R E   P L A N

Nursing Diagnosis: Risk for impaired gas exchange related to surgical intervention

Outcome: The patient will experience adequate gas exchange during the surgical procedure.

Interventions:

Determine the preoperative status of gas exchange by reviewing laboratory results and assessing the patient; report deviations of studies.

Obtain chest x-ray films for the intraoperative period.

Obtain a double-lumen endotracheal tube with a soft, inflatable cuff.

Obtain humidifier for ventilator gases.

Obtain equipment for and monitor arterial blood gases (ABGs).

Obtain equipment for and assist with patient preparation for hemodynamic monitoring: ECG, CO_2 analyzer, pulse oximeter, arterial pressure, central venous pressure; evaluate results provided by these monitoring devices during the procedure.

Obtain equipment for temperature monitoring; monitor temperature during procedure.

Obtain thermal unit; check equipment before procedure; monitor during procedure.

Place ECG monitoring pads; monitor for arrhythmias.

Position the patient to provide access to the endotracheal tube, enable efficient ventilatory function, and prevent injury.

Obtain and label specimens (ABG, blood count) to be sent to laboratory; evaluate results of tests and report abnormal values.

Nursing Diagnosis: Risk for impaired skin integrity related to surgical positioning, length of surgical intervention, and use of chemical antimicrobial agents on the skin.

Outcome: The patient's skin integrity will be maintained.

Interventions:

Observe skin integrity and condition preoperatively.

Determine presence of preexisting conditions that could compromise skin integrity (age, obesity, diabetes, allergies, radiation therapy).

Apply principles of positioning for efficient circulatory function for lateral or supine position during the procedure; protect vulnerable neurovascular bundles.

Identify and pad the pressure sites:

1. *Lateral position:* ear, acromion process, iliac crest, greater trochanter, medial and lateral condyles, malleolus
2. *Supine position:* occiput, scapula, olecranon, sacrum, ischial tuberosity, calcaneus.

Stabilize the patient in lateral position on the OR bed; check for tape sensitivity if adhesive tape is used.

Position the patient in the best possible body alignment to allow visualization of the operative field

1. Assess for preexisting conditions (joint implants, arthritis, restricted movement).
2. Stabilize the patient in lateral position (beanbag, sandbag, soft shoulder roll, pillows between knees).
3. Flex the upper arm slightly (not exceeding 90-degree extension) above the head on a raised padded armboard or supported on padding.
4. Use adequate number of individuals to position the patient for the lateral position.

Consider principles of placement when placing the electrosurgical dispersive pad; shave the area if necessary.

If hair must be removed from the operative site, use clippers or a depilatory (check patient sensitivity); shave the patient with wet shave if a razor must be used.

Prevent pooling of skin prep solutions at the bedline, site of ECG electrodes, or electrosurgical dispersive pad.

Decrease surgical time by anticipating needs of the patient and surgical team.

Observe skin integrity and condition postoperatively; compare to preoperative status.

Nursing Diagnosis: Fluid-volume excess related to decreased surface area of the lung for perfusion and administration of IV fluids during surgery

Outcome: The patient will maintain appropriate fluid balance.

Interventions:

Insert indwelling urinary catheter; use aseptic technique.

Position drainage bag off floor, where it is readily observable.

Monitor urinary output hourly during the procedure; report output less than 30 ml/hour.

Provide access for administration of IV fluids; assist with administration and insertion of lines.

Monitor results of hemodynamic parameters; report appropriately.

Monitor blood loss during the procedure; report appropriately.

Provide blood (including autologous) or blood products for fluid replacement; assist in replacement therapy and patient monitoring.

Observe for symptoms of shock (hypotension, abnormal ECG); report symptoms and initiate corrective nursing actions.

Observe for symptoms of excess blood loss (rapid, weak pulse; rapid respirations; cool, moist skin; and early, slight rise in blood pressure); report symptoms and initiate corrective nursing actions.

Continued

S A M P L E   C A R E   P L A N — c o n t ' d

Observe for symptoms of fluid excess (tachycardia, increased blood pressure); report symptoms and initiate corrective nursing actions.

Have available and administer furosemide (Lasix) and other diuretic agents as prescribed; monitor for therapeutic results.

Nursing Diagnosis: Risk for infection related to inadequate secondary defenses (presence of existing disease process) and surgical disruption of tissues

Outcome: The patient will be free from infection.

Interventions:

Create and maintain a sterile field.

Wear proper operating room attire.

Practice aseptic technique when opening supplies, moving about the sterile field, completing skin preparation, catheterizing the patient, and inserting intravenous lines.

Complete skin preparation at the incision site and point of insertion of monitoring lines to decrease microbial contamination.

Monitor traffic patterns; limit the number of persons entering and leaving the operating room.

Administer antibiotic of choice for irrigation and intravenous administration; check for patient allergies; record all medications administered by the perioperative nurse or from the sterile field.

Decrease surgical time by anticipating patient needs.

Monitor sterile technique of team members; initiate corrective action for breaks in technique.

Obtain appropriate suture; consider whether patient is obese, malnourished, or presenting with symptoms of a secondary disease process when selecting suture.

TABLE 25-2 | **Medications Used as Anesthetic for Bronchoscopy**

MEDICATION	PURPOSE	SIDE EFFECTS	DOSAGE
Lidocaine HCl (Xylocaine)	Topical anesthetic	Swelling, burning, irritation, rash, edema	Varies (1-2 oz)
Procaine (Novocain)	Local anesthetic	Anxiety, restlessness, loss of consciousness, drowsiness, rash, blurred vision, status asthmaticus, respiratory arrest	Varies (10 ml)
Tetracaine/tetracaine HCl (Cetacaine, Pontocaine)	Control of gagging	Rash, irritation, sensitization	Varies (1 oz)

The anesthetic agent is applied by means of a spray or laryngeal syringe with a straight or curved cannula.

Some physicians prefer to have the patient sit upright and gargle with the topical anesthetic mixture, rinse it around in the mouth, and then expectorate it, thereby producing a partial anesthesia of the buccal mucosa and pharynx.

For direct bronchoscopy a long metal cannula attached to a syringe is generally used to apply the anesthetic agent to the surface of the vocal cords; then the agent is injected through the anesthetized glottis into the trachea. This act causes the patient to produce a sharp, sudden cough.

For intrabronchial anesthesia a portion of the anesthetic agent is introduced through the bronchoscope.

Refer to Chapter 7 for perioperative nursing considerations when monitoring the patient receiving local or monitored anesthesia care.

Draping

Aseptic technique is used during an endoscopy. The principles of draping for other procedures are followed (see Chapter 4).

Instrumentation

Instruments are designed for direct inspection and observation of the larynx, trachea, bronchi, or mediastinum; to remove secretions; to obtain washings or tissue for bacterial and cytologic studies; or to remove tissue. They are also designed to remove foreign bodies.

Bronchoscope

The standard bronchoscope is a rigid speculum used for visualizing the tracheobronchial tree. The rigid bronchoscope might be selected for biopsy of a large central mass, removal of a foreign object, or provision a mechanism for hemorrhage control during biopsy of a vascular mass. The rigid bronchoscope remains the instrument of choice for removal of foreign bodies in infants and children. A fiberoptic light carrier is inserted into the bronchoscope to illuminate the distal opening. A side channel has been incorporated into the bronchoscope to permit aeration of the lungs with oxygen or anesthetic gases (Fig. 25-7). An additional device, the Sanders Venturi system, which is available to the anesthesia provider, provides adequate patient observation and ventilation during bronchoscopies

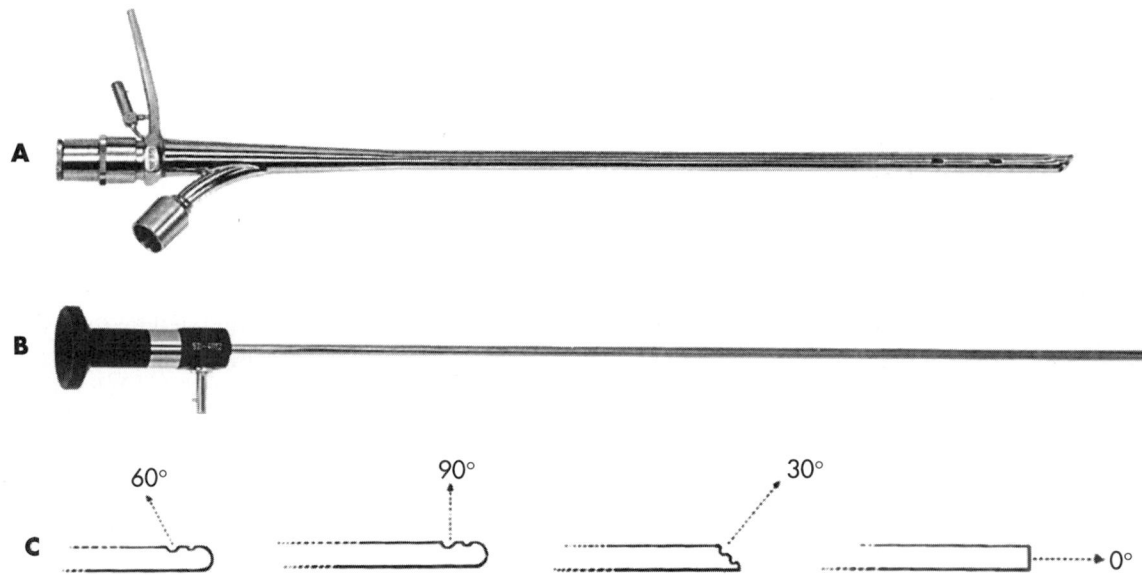

FIGURE 25-7   Instruments for bronchoscopy. **A**, Holinger ventilating fiberoptic bronchoscope. **B**, Fiberoptic light carrier. **C**, Fiberoptic bronchoscopic telescopes: forward oblique 60 degree, lateral 90 degree, right-angle 30 degree, and forward 0 degree.

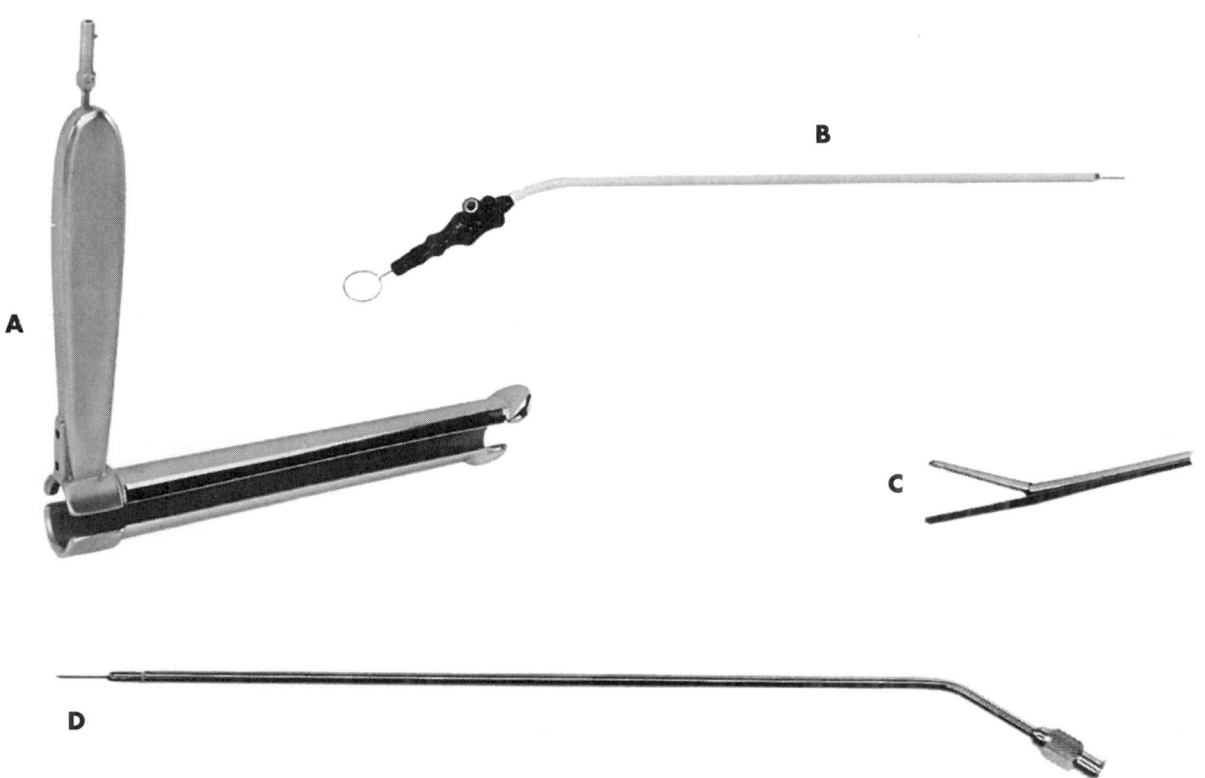

FIGURE 25-8   Instruments for mediastinoscopy. **A**, Carlens mediastinoscope. **B**, Insulated suction tube. **C**, Jackson laryngeal forceps. **D**, Aspirating needle.

and laryngoscopies. Fiberoptic telescopes permit visualization of the upper, middle, and lower lobe bronchi. They can be passed in patients with jaw deformity or cervical bone rigidity with less difficulty than the rigid scope can. Flexible fiberoptic bronchoscopes are being used with increased frequency, as is video endoscopy.

Mediastinoscope

The mediastinoscope is used to view lymph nodes or masses in the superior mediastinum. The instrument is a hollow tube with a fiberoptic light carrier (Fig. 25-8). A fiberoptic light source with a light-intensity dial provides power and control of illumination (Fig. 25-9).

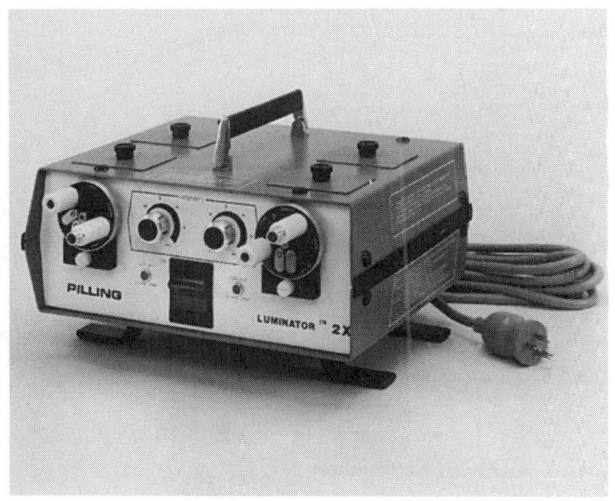

FIGURE 25-9 Fiberoptic light source with multipurpose adapter that accepts several types of fiberoptic light cords.

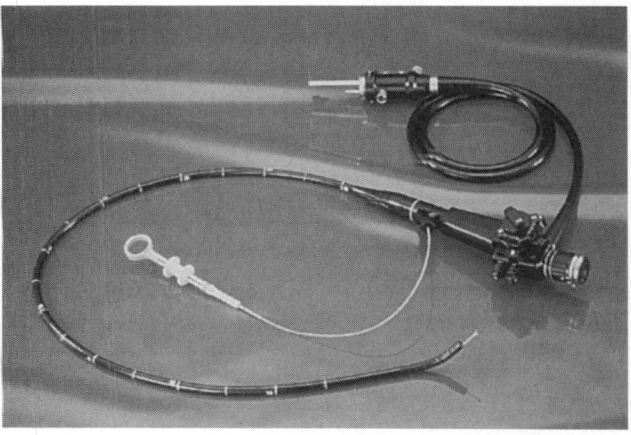

FIGURE 25-10 Flexible endoscope with cold light source cord.

Thoracoscope

The thoracoscope facilitates an endoscopic approach to visualization of the thoracic cavity for diagnosis of pleural disease or treatment of conditions. The need for a thoracotomy incision is eliminated. The thoracoscope is used with video equipment, including a monitor and light source.

Lasers

The Nd:YAG or CO_2 laser can be used for treating tracheobronchial lesions with use of a bronchoscope. Obstruction of the mainstem bronchus and trachea caused by benign and malignant lesions can effectively be treated. Use of laser equipment requires a thorough understanding of the equipment, safety issues, responsibilities, and the procedure (see Chapter 3).

Fiberoptic light carriers, cord, and light source

Each standard scope requires a fiberoptic light carrier, cord, and light source. Duplicates of each, along with the appropriate replacement light bulbs for the light source, should be available for immediate use. The light source (Figs. 25-9 and 25-10) should be tested periodically and immediately before use.

Sponge carriers and sponges

The metal sponge carrier (Fig. 25-11) consists of two parts: an inner rod, which has two jaws protruding from its distal end, and an outer band, which is screwed down on the inner rod so that a sponge can be held securely within the jaws. Small gauze sponges are used to keep the field dry, remove secretions, and apply a topical anesthetic agent.

Specimen collectors

Cytologic specimen collectors, such as the Clerf (see Fig. 25-11) or Lukens, are used to hold secretions as they are obtained.

Aspirators

Aspirating tubes of different lengths and designs (see Fig. 25-11) are used to remove secretions and collect material for microscopic examination and cultures. The straight aspirating tube with one or two openings at the distal end is used to remove material from the pharynx, larynx, and esophagus. The curved aspirating tube with a flexible tip is used to remove secretions from the upper and dorsal orifices of the bronchi.

Forceps

Various types of forceps are designed to remove foreign bodies or tissues for histologic study. Biting tip forceps may be used to secure tissue for pathologic study. Forceps with jaws that veer laterally at about a 45-degree angle from the instrument's axis permit visualization during the biopsy maneuver. Bronchoesophageal forceps (Fig. 25-12) consist of a stylette, a cannula with a handle, a screw, a locknut, and a set screw. Forceps for laryngeal and bronchial regions are designed to remove tissue specimens.

Handling, Terminal Disinfection, and Care
Handling of instruments

To ensure long life of the optical system of endoscopes, one should keep each instrument straight at all times when not in use. Flexible endoscopes should never be severely bent.

When a telescope is sent for repair, it must be properly packed in a padded instrument case and placed within a padded carton to ensure protection of the lens system during transportation. A direct blow can break the objective window or lenses of telescopic endoscopes. The junction of the flexible and rigid portions of the scope is the most vulnerable point.

During use the patient might bite down while the flexible portion of the scope is being passed. A specially designed mouthpiece may be used to prevent damage to the scope. The sheath covering the flexible part

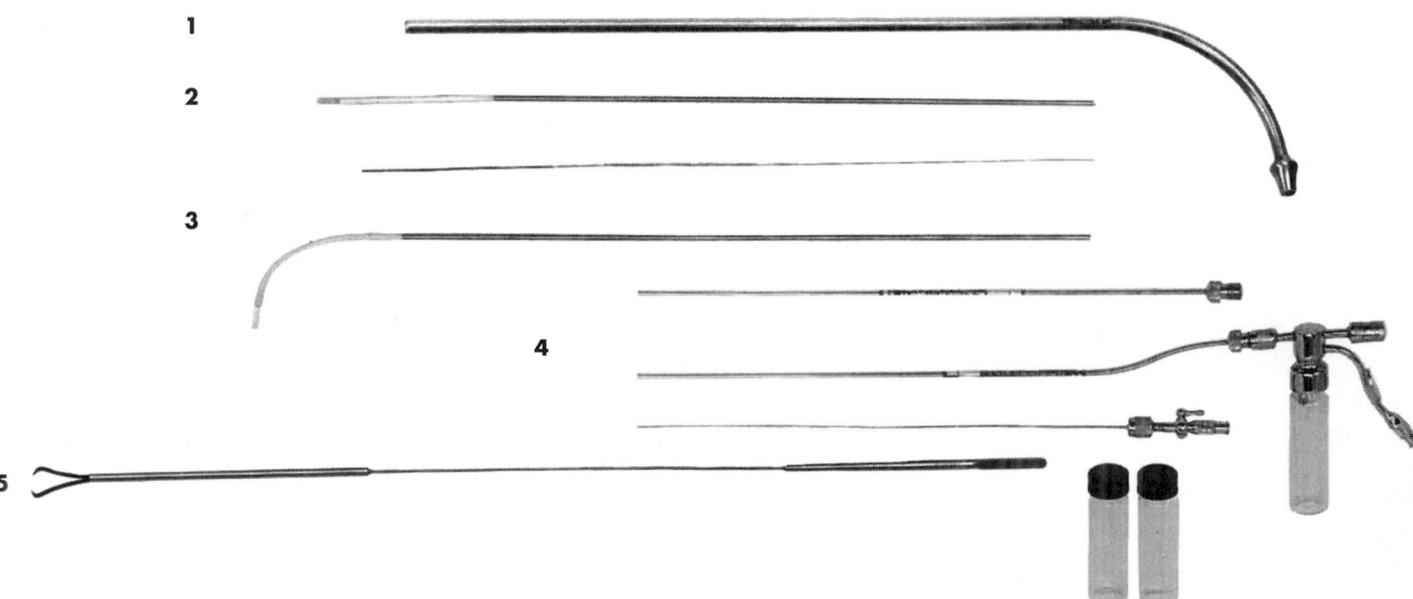

FIGURE 25–11 Aspirating tubes for bronchoscopy. *1*, Jackson open-end; *2*, straight flexible tip; *3*, curved flexible tip; *4*, cancer cell specimen collector, *5*, Jackson sponge carrier.

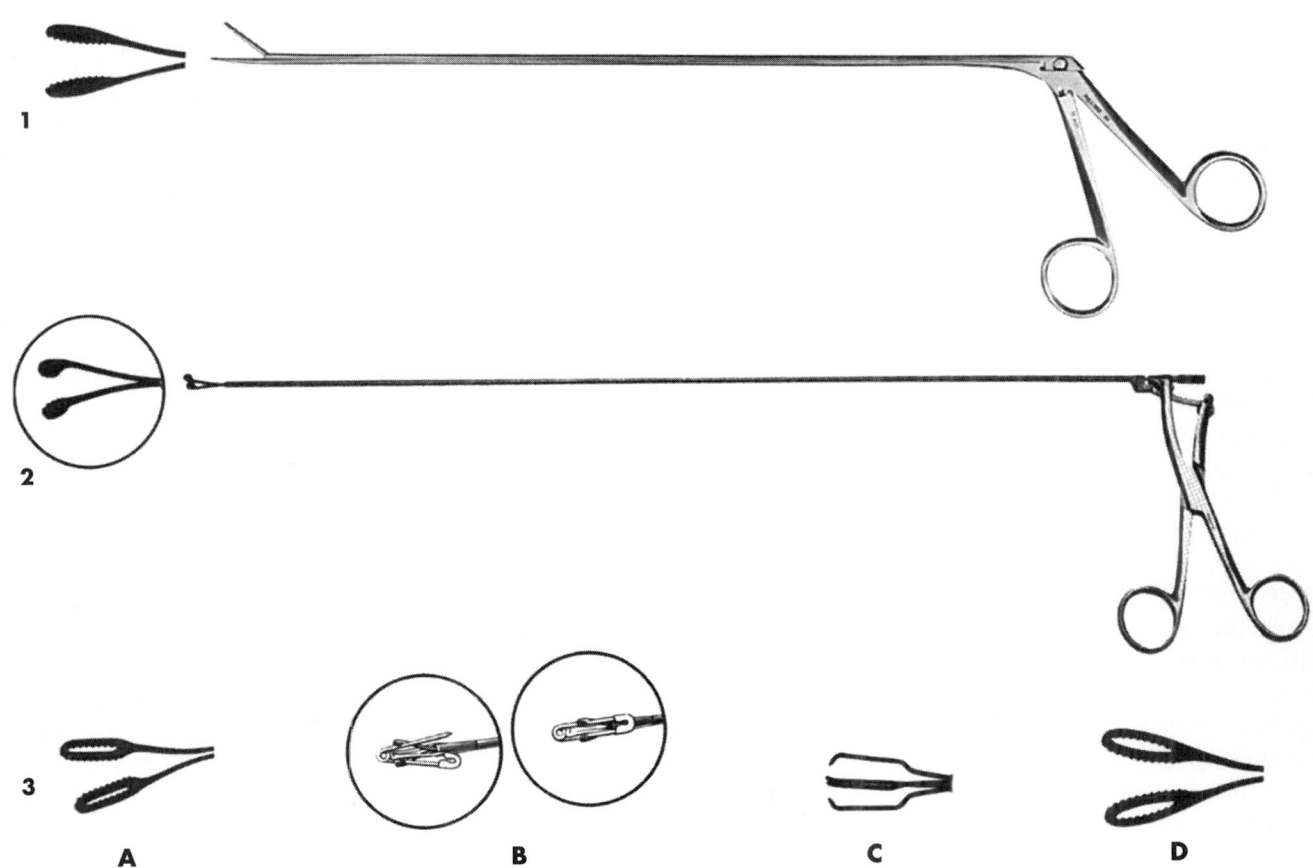

FIGURE 25–12 Forceps for bronchoscopy. **1**, Jackson forward grasping forceps with serrated, cupped jaws; **2**, Jackson side-curved grasping forceps; **3**, forceps for foreign-body removal: **A**, Jackson fenestrated peanut-grasping forceps; **B**, Clerf-Arrowsmith safety pin closer; **C**, Gordon bead grasping forceps; **D**, Jackson fenestrated meat-grasping forceps.

may become perforated after contact. When a new covering is needed, the instrument should be sent to the manufacturer.

Preparing endoscopes for terminal storage

The manufacturer's procedures for cleaning, terminally disinfecting, and terminally sterilizing flexible or rigid endoscopes should be followed. Usually, both the flexible and rigid scopes can be cleaned with soap and water. A soft brush designed to clean the lumen is used for rigid scopes. Both types can be terminally cleaned by using a glutaraldehyde solution in a designated endoscope washer or peracetic acid in that type of sterilization system. Thorough rinsing and drying is required before storage.

Cleaning a telescopic endoscope

The scope is held vertically by its ocular end and is wiped repeatedly with downward strokes using gauze sponges or a soft brush saturated with surgical soap and water. Special attention is given to surface joints and crevices that may retain mucus. The scope is then dried thoroughly with clean gauze sponges.

Optical telescopes should never undergo steam sterilization. Only those sterilizing agents that are recommended by the manufacturer should be used. Sterilization can be achieved by use of a chemical such as ethylene oxide or peracetic acid.

Cleaning aspirating tubes and sponge carriers

These instruments are cleaned and flushed with soap and water and are sterilized by steam or gas. Special care must be given to spiral-tipped aspirators. All bent or broken-tipped aspirators should be sent to the manufacturer for repair.

The sponge carrier collar must be unscrewed before it is cleaned. After sterilization the threads of the carrier are oiled. The carrier is reassembled and stored lying straight.

Cleaning forceps

The forceps may be placed in an ultrasonic cleaner. After cleaning, each forceps is taken apart, one at a time, by unscrewing the nut and removing the stylette. All parts are examined carefully, and noncorrosive solvent oil is applied to the joint of the forceps. Each forceps is reassembled and the action tested; then it is stored lying straight with jaws open. Forceps in good condition should have (1) jaws closing together in parallel position; (2) handles touching slightly when the jaws are closed; (3) jaws merging into the cannula when the forcep is closed and protruding widely without expanding the spring when it is open; (4) the end nut, located in the stylette, in place; (5) the side screw tight; and (6) the distal end and jaws' edges smooth on finger examination.

Setting and testing the illumination

To test the fiberoptic light carrier and telescope, the instrument should be held vertically by the ocular end.

The endoscope should always be tested immediately before passage into the patient. The light-intensity dial should be set at the proper level, as specified by the manufacturer. The light source should be switched on and off to test its function. During a procedure, the light source should be in standby mode whenever it is not in active use.

Postprocedure Concerns

Patient safety during and after endoscopy under topical, local anesthesia or monitored anesthesia care is a concern attributable to medications administered. The gag reflex may not return for 2 to 3 hours. The patient may be positioned on the side or with the head of the bed elevated to promote drainage of secretions. The patient should be restricted from any oral intake until the gag reflex has returned. During bronchoscopy, particularly with a rigid bronchoscope, teeth could be loosened or oral structures damaged. The lips, teeth, and oral mucosa should be examined to ensure undisturbed integrity. Patients are also anxious to know the results of the procedure and benefit from the nurse's openness and willingness to discuss a patient's feelings and perceptions.

Thoracotomy

Positioning

Thoracotomies can be performed with the patient in one of three common positions. The type of position is determined by the operative procedure planned. The three basic approaches are (1) posterolateral thoracotomy, (2) anterolateral thoracotomy (Fig. 25-13), and (3) median sternotomy. The prone position can also provide access in some procedures.

Draping

The drapes may be a fenestrated sheet or single sheets surrounding the incision site. A magnetic pad may be placed on the drapes below the incision site when the patient is placed in lateral position to prevent instruments from falling from the field.

Instrumentation

Instrumentation for thoracic surgery includes the laparotomy instrument set (see Chapter 11), and specialty items (Figs. 25-14 and 25-15). Instruments used for a thoracotomy or chest procedure include a combination of delicate and heavy instruments. The delicate instruments are used to cut tissue and vessels or to clamp tissue in a traumatic or nontraumatic manner. The heavier instruments are used for bone cutting, dissecting or retracting. Instrumentation must also be available for hemostasis and suturing of all types of tissue.

Perioperative nursing staff should determine the thoracic surgery arrangement of items on the instrument table and Mayo stand; this arrangement should be an effective standard method that applies principles of work simplification and thorough knowledge of procedures.

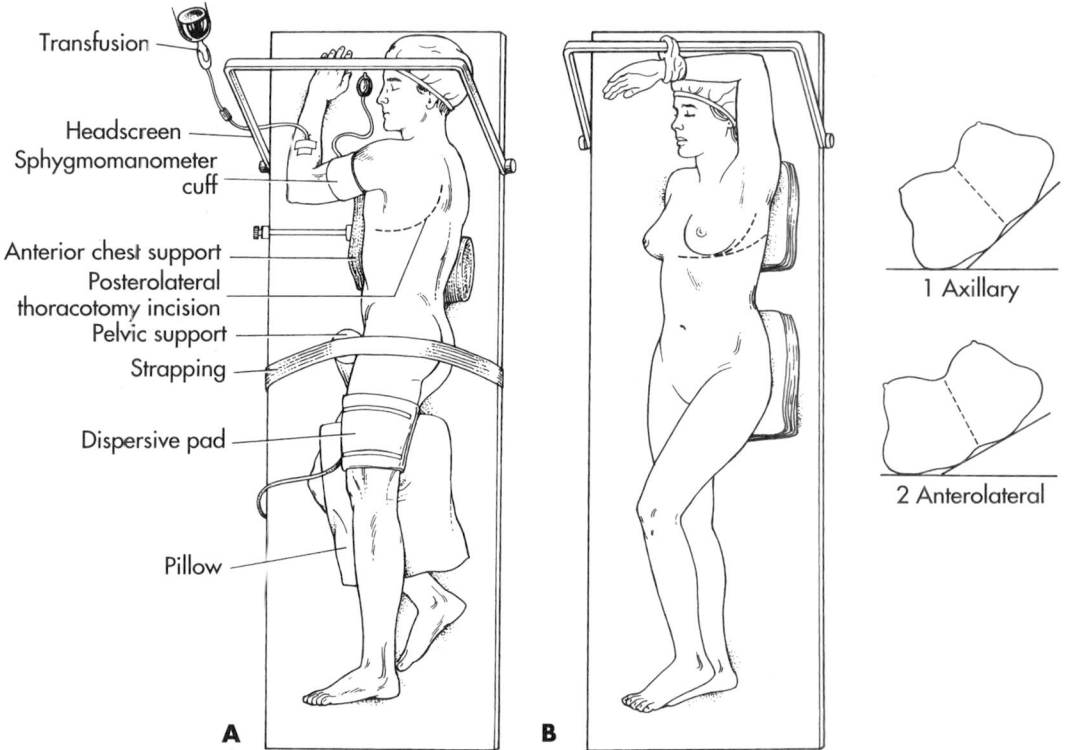

FIGURE 25-13   Positions for thoracotomy incisions. **A,** Lateral position for posterolateral incision. **B,** Semilateral position for axillary or anterolateral position.

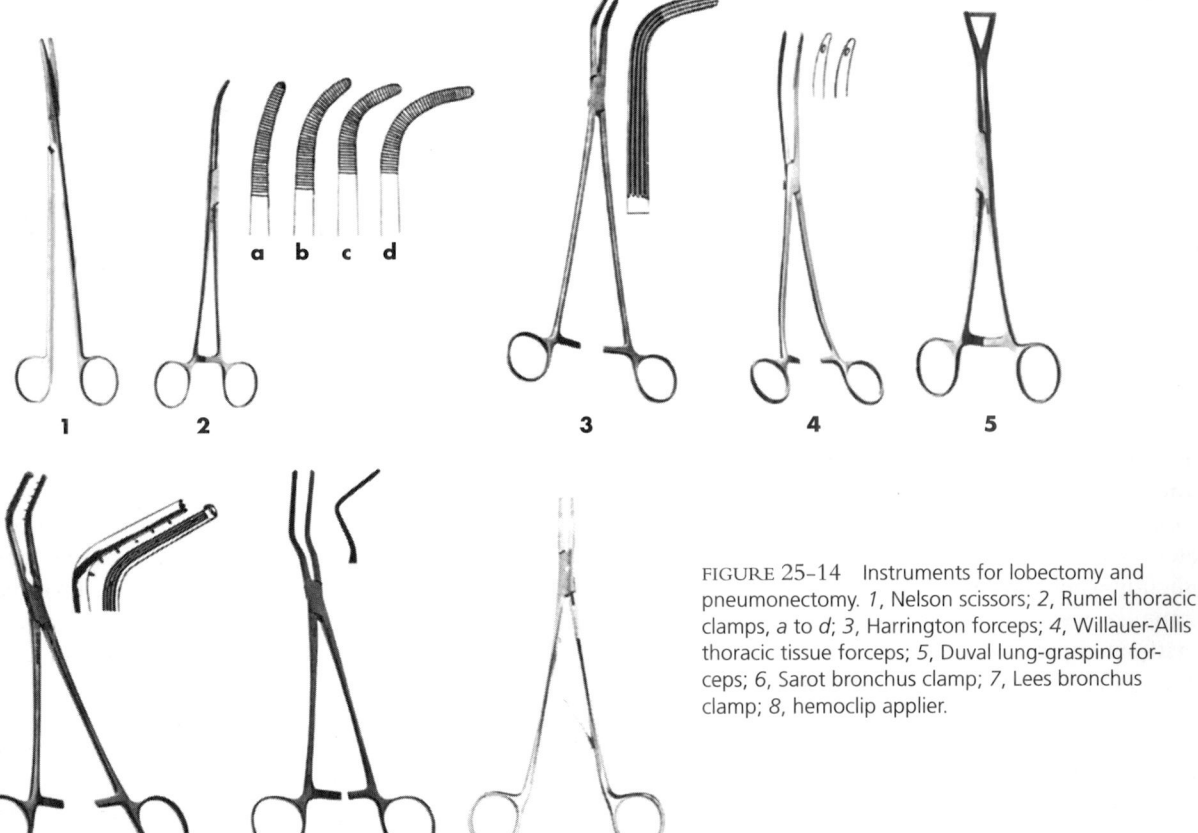

FIGURE 25-14   Instruments for lobectomy and pneumonectomy. *1,* Nelson scissors; *2,* Rumel thoracic clamps, *a* to *d*; *3,* Harrington forceps; *4,* Willauer-Allis thoracic tissue forceps; *5,* Duval lung-grasping forceps; *6,* Sarot bronchus clamp; *7,* Lees bronchus clamp; *8,* hemoclip applier.

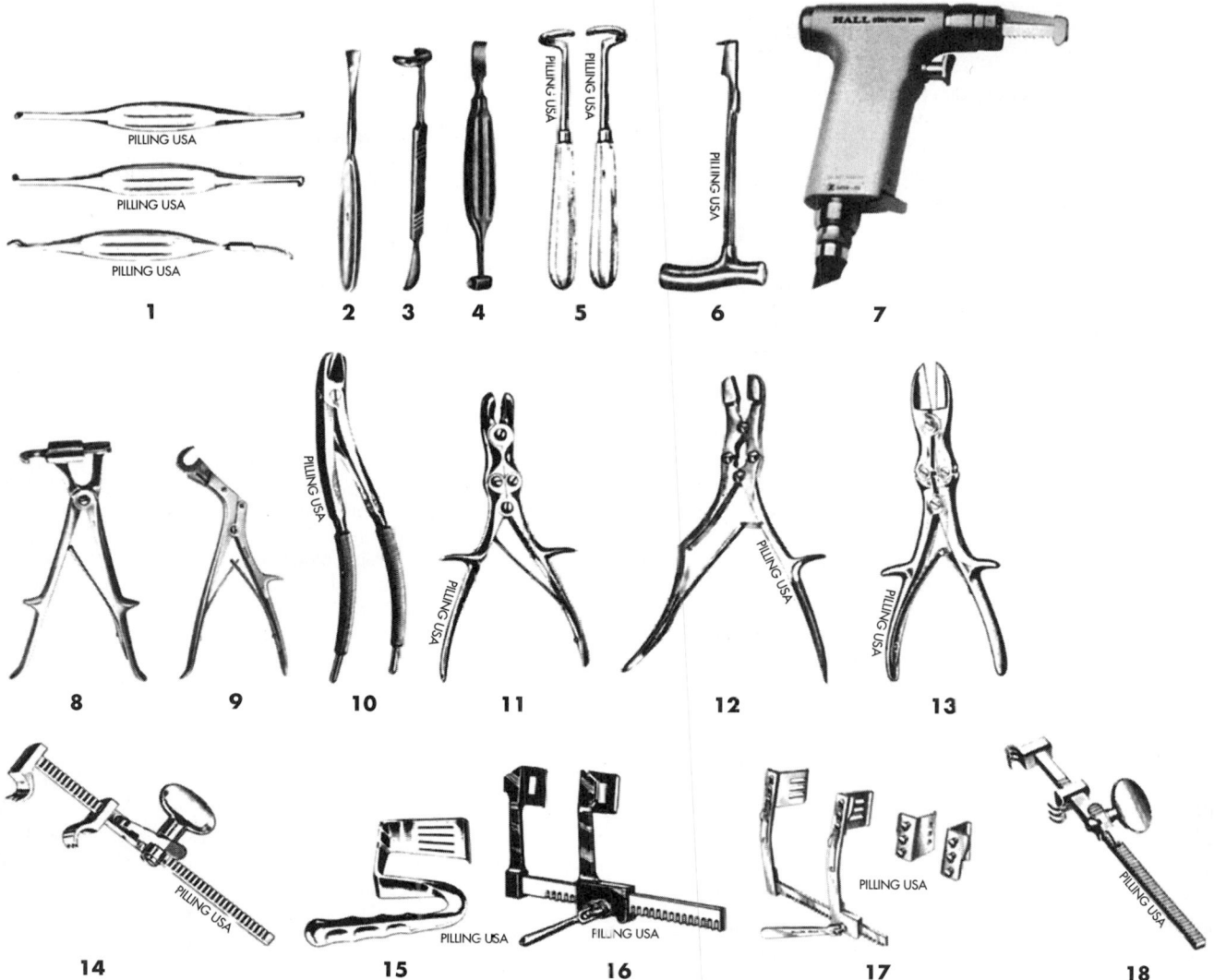

FIGURE 25-15   Instruments for thoracotomy. *1*, Overholt elevators, #1, #2, and #3; *2*, Langenbeck periosteal elevator; *3*, Matson rib elevator and stripper; *4*, Alexander costal periosteotome; *5*, Doyen rib raspatories, right and left; *6*, Lebsche sternal knife; *7*, sternal saw; *8*, Sauerbruch rib shear; *9*, Giertz (first rib) rib guillotine; *10*, Bethune rib shears; *11*, Stille-Luer bone rongeur; *12*, Sauerbruch rib rongeur; *13*, Stille-Liston bone-cutting forceps, straight; *14*, Bailey rib spreader; *15*, Davidson scapula retractor; *16*, Finochietto rib retractor; *17*, Burford rib retractor with two sets detachable blades; *18*, Bailey rib retractor.

Chest Drainage Systems

In the presence of restrictive and obstructive pulmonary disease, the lung may not fully expand or contract, causing a reduction in alveolar ventilation with resultant hypoxia. Other conditions that interfere with respiratory function are mucus, a foreign body in a bronchus, closed pneumothorax (simple and tension types), open pneumothorax, hemothorax, and multiple rib injuries that produce paradoxic motion of the thoracic cage, or flail chest (Fig. 25-16).

The normal function of the lungs is supported by elasticity and negative intrapleural pressure. Collapse of the normal lung follows any condition that reduces or eliminates the negative intrapleural pressure if the lung is not adherent to the chest wall. When the pleural space is filled with air, reducing the negative pressure, the lung collapses. This action may cause complete collapse if the pressure within the intrathoracic (pleural) space becomes positive.

A diminished negative pressure or occurrence of actual positive pressure in one pleural space may cause the mediastinum or trachea to shift toward the opposite side. When this happens, not only does the affected lung collapse because of a positive pressure in the pleural space, but the function of the lung on the opposite side may also be impaired as a result of compression by the shifted mediastinum. Tension pneumothorax can produce serious effects as air continues to escape from the lung into the intrapleural space. The air is unable to return to the bronchi to be exhaled, thereby increasing the intrapleural

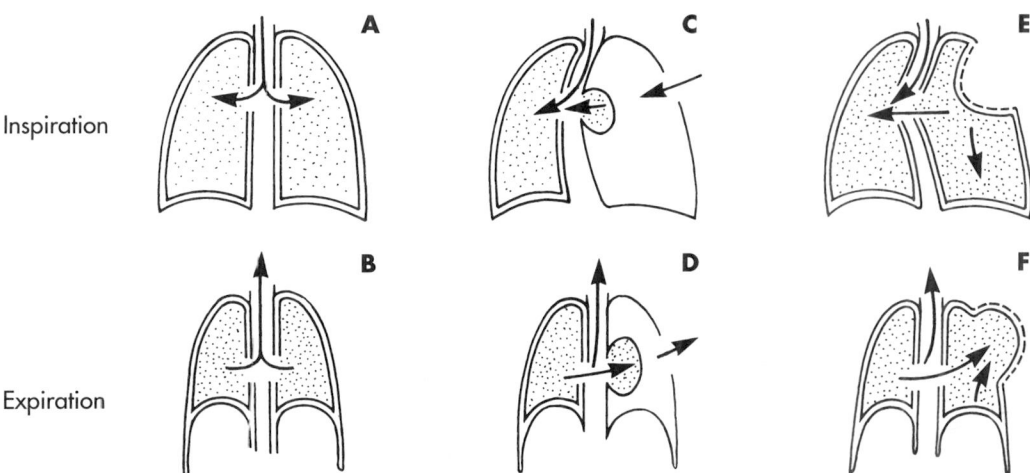

FIGURE 25-16   Pathophysiology of severe chest injuries. **A** and **B**, Normal physiology of inspiration and expiration. **C** and **D**, Open (sucking) wound of thorax. On inspiration, air at atmospheric pressure rushes in through defect (**C**), collapsing lung. Next, positive pressure causes mediastinum to shift, compressing opposite lung. On expiration (**D**) air from lung on uninjured side reenters collapsed lung and is rebreathed in next inspiration. Impaired cardiopulmonary function in presence of sucking wound of chest is caused by (1) collapse of lung on injured side, (2) partial collapse of opposite lung, (3) increased functional dead space caused by rebreathing of unoxygenated air from collapsed lung, and (4) diminished venous return to right side of heart. **E** and **F**, Primary effect of paradoxical motion resulting from flail or stove-in chest is diminution of pulmonary ventilation and extensive rebreathing from one lung to the other. Venous return to right side of heart is impaired. Appropriate treatment requires intubation of trachea and use of volume-limited ventilator.

pressure. When a large opening in the chest wall allows direct communication of the pleural space with atmospheric pressure, it may cause death if the mediastinum becomes mobile. The exposure of the pleural space to atmospheric pressure collapses the affected lung. The positive pressure is also transmitted to the mediastinum, which in turn shifts toward the opposite side and may cause the opposite lung to collapse.

Paradoxic motion of the chest results from severe instability of the chest wall because of multiple and often bilateral rib fractures; with inspiration, partial collapse of the thoracic space occurs. The blunt injury that caused the multiple rib fractures also causes severe contusion of the lung itself. This contusion contributes to impairment of lung function by affecting gas exchange, which may result in severe, life-threatening hypoxia.

One or more chest catheters (tubes) may be inserted for postoperative closed chest drainage.[12] The chest tubes provide a conduit for drainage of air, blood, and other fluid from the intrapleural or mediastinal space and reestablishment of negative pressure in the intrapleural space.[8] Drainage systems use three mechanisms to drain fluid and air from the pleural cavity: positive expiratory pressure, gravity, and suction. The chest tubes are connected to a sterile water-seal or gravity-drainage system. Water-seal suction may be necessary when a persistent air leak cannot be controlled by drainage alone. Historically a two- or three-bottle system was used to accomplish this. Several compact, disposable units are available that function like the three-bottle system; these units are preferable because

they are easier and safer to use. The principles of operation remain the same and can be described more easily using the bottle-system model (Fig. 25-17, *A*). The first bottle collects the drainage from the intrapleural space, the second bottle provides the water seal, and the third provides the suction control determined by the level of water. The disposable units have three or four compartments for drainage, water seal, and suction (see Fig. 25-17, *B*).

If two chest tubes are inserted, they may be attached by a Y connector to a single drainage unit or attached individually to two separate units. All connections should be banded or otherwise secured to ensure an intact system (Fig. 25-18). The drainage system must be sterile and maintained in a position lower than the patient's body to prevent air and fluid from reentering the chest cavity. Chest tubes are generally removed within 5 to 7 days.

Monitoring

During a thoracotomy the patient requires constant monitoring of laboratory results (ABGs), temperature, blood loss, and urine output. The results are communicated with other team members for continuity of care.

Blood Replacement

Blood replacement therapy during or after the procedure may be required because of extensive tissue dissection and removal in a highly vascular area. A patient may have autologous blood ordered; however, the diagnosis may prohibit patient donation of his or her own blood. The

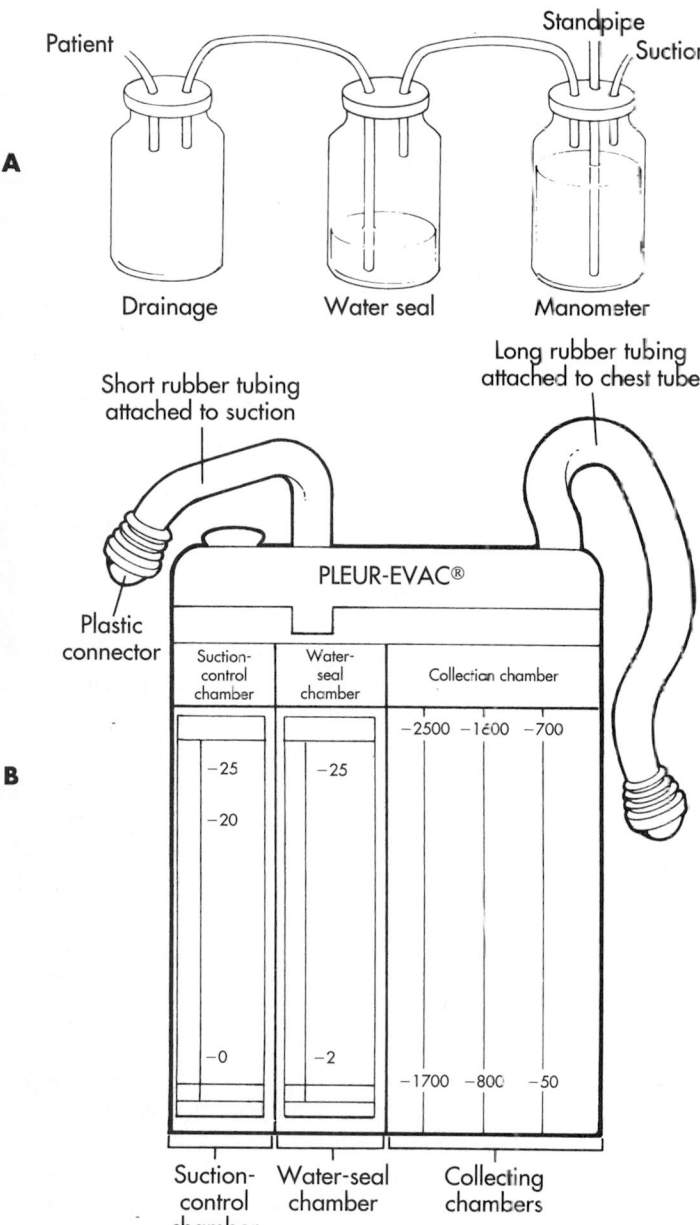

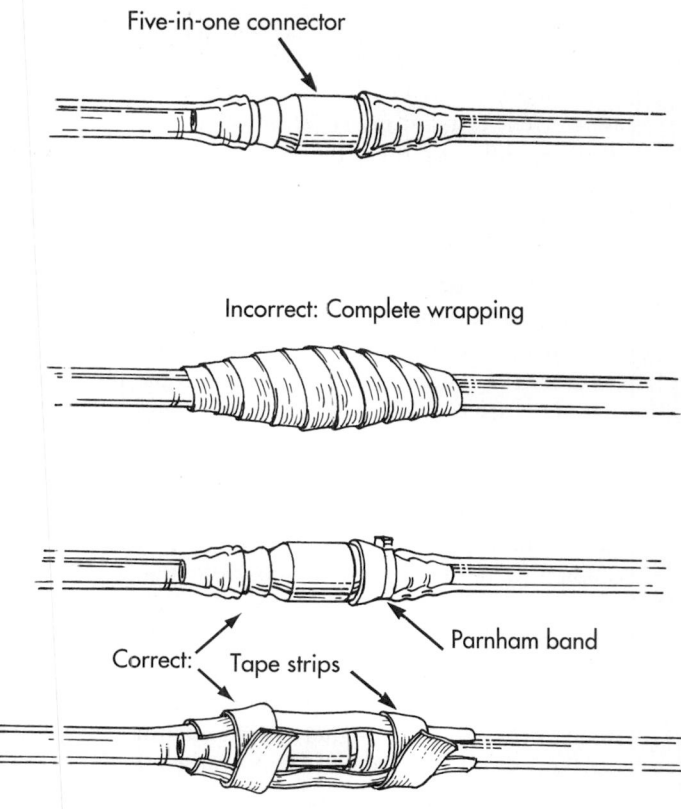

FIGURE 25-18 Method of securing chest tubes after connection to water-seal drainage system.

FIGURE 25-17 **A**, Method of draining pleural space, using triple-bottle system as model. **B**, Commercial chest drainage system.

blood type and amount of blood ordered before the procedure should be noted and its availability confirmed. During the procedure, every effort should be made to control and monitor bleeding. If blood collection or reinfusion systems are used, the manufacturer's instructions and institutional protocols should be followed.

Postprocedure Concerns

Patients are transferred to the PACU using care not to dislodge the chest tube, urinary catheter, or monitoring equipment. The endotracheal tube may remain in place to maintain an adequate air exchange. Air exchange and effective ventilation are two immediate needs of the

patient after thoracotomy. The thoracotomy is considered a painful procedure and, when coupled with muscle injury, affects functional capacity (Research Highlight 25-2). A postprocedure epidural catheter with monitoring or injection of a local anesthetic at the completion of wound closure for pain management should improve the comfort level of the patient as postoperative activities are encouraged.

Patients are often anxious about their limitations, the environment, and the results of the procedure. Patients and families will benefit from preoperative teaching about pain management techniques and use of the pain assessment tool, as well as being allowed to discuss their feelings and needs. Family members should be informed of the patient's status as soon as possible after the procedure.

Documentation

Documentation of perioperative care includes assessment of the patient upon admission to the operating room, nursing interventions, and postoperative evaluation. Documentation for a patient undergoing a thoracotomy specifically addresses positioning aids used, position of the patient, medications administered, results of laboratory tests completed, special equipment used, urine output, blood replacement, insertion of chest tubes and drainage systems, and postoperative evaluation of patient care outcomes.

25-2 RESEARCH HIGHLIGHT

Pain is associated with a thoracotomy and considered a deterrent to rapid return of function postoperatively. Patients differ in their descriptions of intensity and responses to pain therapy. Two different studies described the findings after thoracotomy with posterolateral approach. One study measured the superficial abdominal reflexes and assessed postoperative pain intensity according to a numeric rating scale and the postoperative opioid dose. The abdominal reflexes were measured to assess intercostal nerve impairment, believed to have an effect on postoperative pain. The second study compared pain after a thoracotomy procedure with a posterolateral approach with pain after other procedures by means of a median laparotomy approach. The subjective and objective perception was studied by use of the patient-controlled analgesia data and a visual analog scale (VAS). It was found that patients with complete disappearance of the superficial abdominal reflexes experienced more severe postoperative pain than those in whom reflexes were maintained. It is believed that higher pain intensity may be attributable to intercostal nerve impairment. The patients with a posterolateral approach did not experience more pain than those with a median laparotomy incision; thus increased pain medication should not be necessary.

From Salzer, G.M., Klingler, P., Klinger, A., et al. (1997). Pain treatment after thoracotomy: Is it a special problem? *Annals of Thoracic Surgery, 63*(12), 1411-1414; Benedetti, F., Amanzio, M., & Casadio, C. (1997). Postoperative pain and superficial abdominal reflexes after posterolateral thoracotomy. *Annals of Thoracic Surgery, 64*(1), 207-210.

Transfer Report

The patient is transferred from the operating room to the PACU after thoracotomy. The report to the PACU nurse is often a collaborative effort of the nurse and anesthesia provider. The perioperative nurse reports the patient's preoperative status, including anxiety level and understanding of the procedure, to assist the PACU nurse in meeting the emotional needs of the patient. A description of the position of the patient during the procedure provides criteria for assessment and evaluation of mobility. Results of immediate postoperative assessment including skin integrity, location and type of dressing applied, location and type of drains, blood loss, fluid replacement, medications administered, and laboratory results obtained during the procedure are reported as a baseline control for assessment in the PACU. The PACU nurse must be informed of the procedure performed, particularly if it varies from the anticipated or scheduled

procedure. The perioperative care plan should be reviewed and patient outcomes reported.

Evaluation

At the completion of the surgical procedure, the perioperative nursing goals are evaluated. They may be restated as brief outcomes. For the goals identified for the patient undergoing thoracic surgery, outcomes could be as follows:

- The patient's gas exchange was unimpaired; ventilation-to-perfusion ratios were adequate as evidenced by laboratory results and vital signs within normal limits; skin, nailbeds, and mucosa were pink; lung fields were clear bilaterally; and chest excursion was normal.
- The patient's skin integrity was maintained; reddened or discolored skin and other signs of altered tissue perfusion were not present.
- Fluid balance was maintained; there were no fluid excesses or deficits; mental orientation was consistent with preoperative level; serum electrolytes and arterial blood gases were within normal limits and urinary output was stable.
- A postoperative wound infection will not be experienced; the incision site will remain approximated and dry, without redness, drainage, or undue tenderness. (This is a long-term goal, and its evaluation will require the collaboration of the nurse in the patient care unit.)

Patient and Family Education and Discharge Planning

Discharge status will be determined by the type of procedure being performed. Patient concerns include mobility, pain management, and outpatient care. After a bronchoscopy, patients will be discharged within hours of the procedure. Their main concerns might be the results of biopsy and diagnosis. The patient and family should be aware of the length of time until results will be available and the method used to obtain those results. Patients should also be reminded of the need to rest for 2 to 3 days after the procedure. Side effects might result from medications used for conscious sedation or untoward intraoperative outcomes (for example, the patient may experience bloody sputum, difficulty in breathing). In addition, patients should be reminded that their throats might feel numb 2 to 3 hours after the procedure and difficult swallowing will subside.

After a surgical procedure (such as thoracoscopy or thoracotomy), patients will ambulate within 4 to 6 hours after the procedure; length of time until discharge might be a few days to a few weeks. Patients who progress without difficulty after a thoracoscopy or thoracotomy will be monitored for drainage from the chest tubes, and for pain management or complications that are a result of surgery. Postoperative air leaks or pulmonary infections will delay discharge from the healthcare setting. In-home nursing care is initiated to monitor oxygen levels, wound care needs, and pain management. The patient may have been discharged with supplemental oxygen. This would require that the patient be weaned and demonstrate satisfactory ambulatory SaO_2 rates of 88% to 90%. An informal ambulation program might be supervised by homecare nurses.

SURGICAL INTERVENTIONS

ENDOSCOPY (DIAGNOSTIC OR THERAPEUTIC)

Endoscopy refers to examination of hollow body organs or cavities with instruments that permit visual inspection of their contents and walls. The endoscopic procedures pertinent to thoracic surgery are bronchoscopy, mediastinoscopy, and thoracoscopy. Each endoscopist has preferences regarding the type of endoscope, positioning of the patient, type of anesthetic, and equipment. Invasive diagnostic or therapeutic measures enhance the decision to pursue surgical intervention by providing information related to the disease process, including histologic characteristics, location of the lesion, and lesion extent. Therapeutic endoscopy provides treatment by removal of the lesion or foreign body.

Standard Bronchoscopy using Rigid Bronchoscope

Standard bronchoscopy is the direct visualization of the mucosa of the trachea, the main bronchi and their openings, and most of the segmental bronchi and includes removal of material for microscopic study if necessary.

Bronchoscopy is an integral part of the examination of patients with pulmonary symptoms such as persistent cough or wheezing, hemoptysis, obstruction, and abnormal roentgenographic changes. Common causes of bleeding (hemoptysis) are bronchiectasis, carcinoma, and tuberculosis. Congenital anomalies and suspected presence of a foreign body, especially in infants and children, are responsible for emergency examination of the respiratory tract.

Bronchoscopy is done to determine the presence of a lesion in the tracheobronchial passages, to identify and localize that lesion accurately, and to observe periodically the effects of therapy. In suspected carcinoma the aspirated secretions obtained by bronchoscopy may contain malignant cells.

Procedural considerations

Bronchoscopy on an adult patient may be completed with the patient under local anesthesia or monitored anesthesia care; a child usually receives general anesthesia. The adult patient receiving local anesthesia may experience discomfort and anxiety. To reduce anxiety, personnel

should be introduced, intraoperative activities explained, and reassurance provided to the patient. The oral structures, including the teeth and lips, should be assessed for integrity. Loose teeth may require removal before or during the procedure.

Intravenous sedatives or analgesics may be administered during the procedure. See Chapter 7 for perioperative nursing considerations when the patient is receiving local or monitored anesthesia care.

The patient may be positioned either in supine position, with the shoulders elevated on a small roll or a sandbag to gently extend the head and neck, or in the sitting position.

The setup includes the bronchoscope (see Fig. 25-7), telescopes of desired types, fiberoptic light cords, and the fiberoptic light source. Other supplies that will be needed are suction tubing, aspirating tubes (see Fig. 25-11), specimen collectors (see Fig. 25-11), sponge carriers (see Fig. 25-11), and the desired type of forceps (see Fig. 25-12).

The bronchoscopist risks contamination in the presence of communicable diseases. For this reason, the endoscopist and assistants should wear face masks and eyeglasses, goggles, or a transparent shield attached to a headband. With increasing numbers of patients with tuberculosis, particulate respirators are recommended as protective devices. Aseptic technique is used to prevent cross-contamination.

Operative procedure (Fig. 25-19)

1. The head is placed in position for visualization of the bronchus, to the left when the right main bronchi are inspected and to the right when the left bronchi are inspected. The head is lowered for inspection of the middle lobe.
2. The bronchoscope is inserted over the surface of the tongue, usually through the right corner of the mouth. The patient's lip is retracted from the upper teeth with a finger of the endoscopist's left hand. The epiglottis is identified and elevated with the tip of the bronchoscope.
3. The distal end of the scope is passed through the true vocal cords of the larynx, and the upper tracheal rings are viewed. A small amount of anesthetic solution may be sprayed through the tube on the carina of the trachea and into the bronchus with the bronchial atomizer or spray. The patient's head is moved to the left to obtain a view of the right bronchi. The right-angle telescope is inserted with the light adjusted into the bronchoscope. The optical system should be kept free from precipitated moisture.
4. The segmental bronchial orifices of the upper right lobe bronchi are viewed, and the telescope is removed. Suction and aspirating tubes are introduced to clear the field of vision.
5. The middle lobe branches are inspected by inserting an oblique 45-degree angle telescope or right-angle

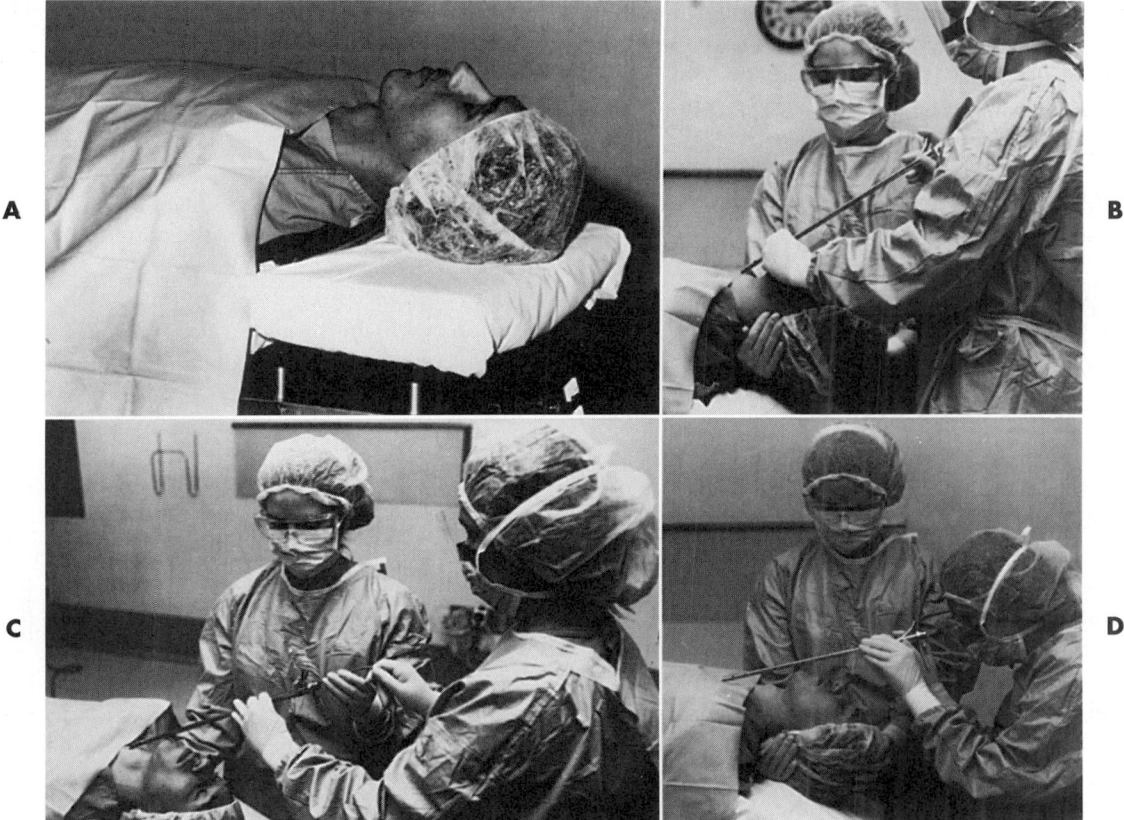

FIGURE 25-19   **A**, Patient positioned with shoulder at table break for bronchoscopy. A shoulder roll or sandbag can be placed beneath the patient's shoulders. **B**, Initial position with head held high and supported. **C**, Assistance is provided as the forceps or suction is guided while the head is supported. **D**, Position assumed as the endoscope is inserted; the head will be raised or lowered as the anatomy is viewed.

telescope and advancing it. The patient's head is lowered to view the right middle lobe or turned to the right to view the left main bronchus.

6. Secretions are aspirated for study. Biopsy forceps are used if indicated; foreign bodies are removed with forceps.

7. The bronchoscope is removed. The patient's face is cleansed. If able, the patient is encouraged to sit on the edge of the OR bed before transfer to the stretcher. An emesis basin and sponges should be provided for the patient's use. Assistance and support should be provided to the patient to prevent a fall.

Bronchoscopy using Flexible Bronchoscope

Flexible bronchoscopy is done to view structures that cannot be observed with a rigid scope. Flexible bronchoscopy may be performed in addition to a standard rigid bronchoscopy or as an independent procedure. If performed separately, the patient may remain on the transporting stretcher during the procedure. The bron-

choscopy is completed for the same reasons as a rigid bronchoscopy.

Procedural considerations

Patient considerations are as described for rigid bronchoscopy. Instruments and equipment used include the flexible bronchoscope, fiberoptic light source, flexible biopsy forceps, flexible brush (optional; if used, slides and alcohol are necessary to collect specimen), specimen collectors, syringe for wash, and suction tubing with collection tube attached to collect the wash specimen.

Operative procedure

1. The lubricated bronchoscope is passed through the adapter on the endotracheal tube, which is held secure by the anesthesia provider.

2. The suction tube is positioned with the specimen collector attached for collection of bronchial washings. When indicated, the suction tubing is connected to the bronchoscope; the container for collection is held securely in an upright position to prevent loss of the specimen through the suction.

3. Approximately 5 ml of saline solution is injected into the channel. Suction is quickly reapplied. This procedure may be repeated.
4. After completion of the procedure, specimen containers are labeled and sent to the laboratory.

Mediastinoscopy

Mediastinoscopy is the direct visualization and possible biopsy of lymph nodes or tumors at the tracheobronchial junction, under the carina of the trachea, or on the upper lobe bronchi or subdivisions. Mediastinoscopy may precede an exploratory thoracotomy in known cases of lung carcinoma. Patients with positive findings may be treated with radiation or chemotherapy, as indicated.

Procedural considerations

The setup for mediastinoscopy includes a set of instruments for making an incision, cutting, retracting, and suturing similar to those needed for a minor procedure. In addition, the desired type of mediastinoscope, fiberoptic light cords, fiberoptic light source, suction tubing, aspirating tubes, biopsy forceps, electrosurgical unit, and an endocardiac needle, 20 gauge, 8 inches, are required.

The patient is placed under endotracheal anesthesia and positioned as for a tracheostomy (see Chapter 21).

Operative procedure

1. A short (approximately 2 cm) transverse incision is made above the suprasternal notch, and the pretracheal fascia is exposed.
2. The pretracheal fascia is incised.
3. Tunneling is accomplished alongside the trachea by blunt (digital) dissection into the mediastinum.
4. The mediastinoscope is introduced under direct vision deep to the fascial plane and advanced along the side of the trachea toward the mediastinum.
5. The scope is manipulated to visualize the tracheal bifurcation, bronchi, aortic arch, and associated lymph nodes.
6. Lymph nodal tissue is located for biopsy and aspirated with a small-gauge needle and syringe for positive identification of a nonvascular structure.
7. A biopsy forceps is inserted through the scope, and a tissue specimen is excised. Pressure can be applied to the excision site with a bronchus sponge on a holder. The mediastinum is reinspected for bleeding.
8. The mediastinoscope is withdrawn.
9. Subcutaneous tissue is sutured with absorbable sutures. The skin is approximated and sutured with ligature on a cutting needle.
10. A small dressing is applied.

Thoracoscopy

Video-assisted thoracic surgery (VATS) has been recognized for many benefits including decreased pain,

25-3 RESEARCH HIGHLIGHT

A questionnaire was mailed to members of the General Thoracic Surgery Club in November 1995 to determine their perception of the use of video-assisted thoracic surgery (VATS). The respondents were also asked to rate their preference for use of VATS. Of the 200 respondents, 54.1% are seeing the same use of video-assisted thoracic surgery as it was 1 year previously; and 33.5% are seeing an increase in usage. Video-assisted thoracic surgery was rated as highest as the preferable approach for diagnosis of indeterminate pleural masses, lung biopsy for diffuse disease in non–ventilator dependent patients, treatment of spontaneous pneumothorax, sympathectomy, and therapeutic management of malignant pleural effusion. The study also rated those procedures for which the surgeons identified the use of VATS as acceptable or investigatory. It is believed that there are many indications for use of VATS, yet there continues to be a limitation of usage.

From Mack, M.J., Scruggs, G.R., Kelly, K.M., et al. (1997). Video assisted thoracic surgery: Has technology found its place? *Annals of Thoracic Surgery, 64*(1), 211-215.

shortened hospital stay, and reduced morbidity. Its use has been significantly expanded since 1990 (Research Highlight 25-3). Thoracoscopy is indicated for diagnosis of pleural disease or treatment of pleural conditions such as cysts, blebs and effusions. Pleurodesis with instillation of talc,[16-18] tetracycline, or other sclerosing treatment can be accomplished through the thoracoscope. VATS is also used for biopsy of mediastinal masses, to perform wedge resections, pericardectomy, and cervical sympathectomy, to obtain hemostasis, and to evacuate blood clots or divide adhesions.[3,15]

Procedural considerations

Endoscopic instrumentation and equipment used for a thoracoscopy include the 5 and 10 mm lenses, light cord, camera, graspers, dissectors, scissors, ligators, and endoscopic soft-tissue instruments (scissors, hemostats, suction tips, retractors). Accessory equipment for video (television monitors, videocassette recorder, printer, light source for camera and lens, slave television monitor) and insufflation are also used. The patient is positioned supine, semilaterally, or laterally, depending on the anatomic structures involved.

Operative procedure

1. A 2 to 3 cm incision is made between the fifth and seventh intercostal spaces for insertion of the 10 or

12 mm trocar. The 0–degree lens is inserted to view the site to determine the approach.

2. If the procedure can be completed by thoracoscopy, puncture sites are made for insertion of additional trocars to allow instrument manipulation. The size of trocars and types of instruments depend on the diagnosis.

3. A chest tube is inserted through one of the surgical puncture sites and secured to the skin.

LUNG SURGERY

Thoracotomy

Thoracotomy involves an incision in the chest wall through a median sternotomy and a lateral or posterolateral incision for the purpose of operating on the lungs. Intraoperative patient care is similar for various thoracotomy procedures, with consideration of the patient's history and disease process, planned procedure, and individualized patient needs. Basic thoracic instrumentation is used and may include a sternal saw and stapling devices. Preparation by the anesthesia care provider with careful monitoring of the patient is a priority. Insertions of a double-lumen endotracheal tube, an arterial line for monitoring arterial blood gas samples, and a central venous line to ensure patent access for fluids are procedures performed by the anesthesia care provider. An epidural catheter may be inserted for intraoperative and postoperative pain management. Patient preparation by the surgical team includes positioning, placement of devices for prevention of complications (such as sequential compression stockings, a thermal blanket, and a dispersive pad), insertion of a urinary catheter, and on-going evaluation of patient care.

Pneumonectomy

Pneumonectomy is removal of an entire lung, usually to treat malignant neoplasms. Other reasons for removal include an extensive unilateral bronchiectasis involving the greater part of one lung, drainage of an extensive chronic pulmonary abscess involving portions of one or more lobes, selected benign tumors, and treatment of any extensive unilateral lesion. Other resections are often combined with pneumonectomy, such as resection of mediastinal lymph nodes, resections of portions of the chest wall or diaphragm, and removal of parietal pleura. A clinical pathway for pneumonectomy is shown in Fig. 25-20.

Procedural Considerations

The basic thoracic instrumentation is used. The patient is placed in the lateral position for a posterolateral incision.

Operative Procedure

1. The skin, subcutaneous tissue, and muscle are incised by scalpel, suction, and electrodissection. Hemostasis

is attained. If a rib is to be excised, the procedure discussed later is implemented.

2. The ribs and tissue are protected with moist sponges; the rib retractor is placed (Fig. 25-21) and opened slowly.

3. The lung is mobilized when peripheral adhesions are freed and the pulmonary ligament is divided. Dissection to the hilum of the involved lobe is carried out.

4. The superior pulmonary vein is gently retracted, and the pulmonary artery is dissected.

5. The branches of the pulmonary artery and vein of the involved lobe are clamped, doubly ligated, and divided with fine right-angled vascular clamps, scissors, and nonabsorbable suture.

6. The inferior pulmonary vein is exposed by incising the hilar pleura and retracting the lung anteriorly. The inferior pulmonary vein is clamped, doubly ligated, and divided.

7. The bronchus clamp is applied, and the bronchus near the tracheal bifurcation is divided. The stump is closed with atraumatic nonabsorbable mattress sutures or bronchus staples. If staples are applied, the scalpel is used to complete division of the bronchus. The lung is removed from the chest.

8. The pleural space is irrigated with normal saline to check for hemostasis and air leaks during positive pressure inspiration.

9. A pleural flap is created and sutured over the bronchial stump. Other methods of securing the bronchus might be used.

10. Hemostasis is ensured in the pleural space.

11. Chest tubes (28 to 30 Fr) are inserted into the pleural space and brought through a stab wound at the eighth or ninth interspace near the anterior axillary line (Fig. 25-22). An upper tube is inserted through a second stab wound if indicated to evaluate leaking air. The tubes are secured with heavy sutures and connected to water-seal drainage after closure of the pleural space.

12. The rib approximator (Fig. 25-23) is placed, and closure is begun with interrupted sutures.

13. The muscle, subcutaneous tissue, and skin are closed. Drains are anchored to the chest wall with suture.

14. The dressing is applied.

15. Chest tube connections are secured with Parnham bands or tape (see Fig. 25-18) and labeled (anterior or posterior).

Lobectomy (left upper)

Lobectomy is excision of one or more lobes of the lung. It is performed to remove metastatic involvement when the tumor is peripherally located and hilar nodes are not involved. Other conditions affecting the lung and resulting in lobectomy might be bronchiectasis, giant emphysematous blebs or bullae, large centrally located benign tumor,

Vanderbilt University Medical Center

Lobectomy/Pneumonectomy

DRG Number: _____

ELOS: _____

	Preop (Outpatient)	Day of operation (OR)	Day of operation (PACU/9N)	Postop day 1 (9N)	Postop day 2 (9N)	Postop day 3-7 (9N → Home)	Follow-up: 1 month (CV Clinic)
Goals:	Preop testing completed within 30 days of operation Recheck labs within 2-4 days preop if abnormal Results available (in one folder) for review 2-4 days preop Preop test results WNL Patient contacted by case manager 2-3 days preop Patient/family talk with surgeon preop Consent form signed Patient/family teaching is completed	EMA: Pt in admitting 3 hrs preop/holding room 2 hrs preop Complete in holding room: Shave, IV Art line, anesthesia meds, sub ! heparin, SCD hose Family aware of where to wait and approx. time of operation Pt tolerates operation without complications	Hemodynamically stable No arrhythmias Temp WNL Pain controlled Good oxygenation and ventilation Extubate per anesthesia protocol	Transfer to 9N by 12 noon	Air/fluid leak resolved Remove chest tubes No pneumothorax Oxygen off	Criteria for D/C: Afebrile No arrhythmias ADL's with minimal assist Patient/family competent with meds D/C from 9N by 9 a.m. when Complete D/C planning and teaching Schedule F/U appointment	
Labs:	SMA 6, 12 CBC, diff, plts PT, PTT UA T+C 2 units PRBC	After intubation with DL ET tube, ABG on one lung, Q 30 min PCV if EBL > 300 ml	30 minutes postop then Q 6° × 4 (if intub) Q12 if extub: ABG PCV	Chem 7 CBC ABG		Night before D/C: SMA 7 CBC	
Tests	CXR, CT Scan, PET Scan? PFT's, Bronchoscopy History and physical	Pathology	Immediately postop: portable CXR	AP portable ──────────→ CXR		Day before D/C: CXR—PA/lat	
Diet	NPO after 12 MN night before operation	NPO	NPO If intubated, clear liqs. if awake & extubated	Regular diet			
Activity	Ad Lib		OOB in chair if extubated	OOB in chair tid	Ambulate tid		
Treatments	Hibiclens soap scrubs (two), night before operation	Skin shave prep Ventilator SaO$_2$ monitor CT/Pleuravac Cardiac monitor NG tube Foley Central line Incision care	Do not remove dressing × 48 hr				
Consultations	Surgeon Anesthesiologist Case manager Occ. cardiologist						
Meds/IV	Premed for sleep night before operation per anesthesiologist	Holding room: IV (started in holding room) Preop anesthesia Sub Q heparin Ancef in OR before incision	IV fl ──────────────────────→ Ancef 1 gram IV Q8h × 9 doses postop MgSO$_4$ PCA or IV Epidural Sub Q heparin, 5000u, Q12h		DC/IV after antibiotics Percocet PO D/C telemetry Stool softener		

FIGURE 25–20 Clinical pathway for lobectomy or pneumonectomy. *Continued*

	Preop (Outpatient)	Day of operation (OR)	Day of operation (PACU/9N)	Postop day 1 (9N)	Postop day 2 (9N)	Postop day 3-7 (9N → Home)	Follow-up: 1 month (CV Clinic)
Equipment and Supplies	Soap scrub Incentive spirometer	Shave/prep kit IV start/IV tubing Ventilator Invasive monitoring Kit-2 Pleuravac Foley/urine bag OR supplies Anesthesia supplies Double-lumen ET tube Epidural catheter SCD hose & device	Pulse oximeter Face mask (O₂) IMED PCA pump/tubing	Nasal O₂ ⟶ ⟶ D/C ⟶ D/C	D/C D/C	**HOME CARE INSTRUCTION** Incision care Antiembolus precautions Progressive exercise per Pt Hygiene When/how to notify physician Medications Diet per dietary Follow-up visit schedule	
Teaching/ D/C Plan	Procedure Plan of care Recovery after D/C VUMC orientation ACS lung cancer booklet Incentive spirometery teaching		Incentive spirometery Orient family to 9N		Begin home care instruction		

FIGURE 25-20, cont'd   Clinical pathway for lobectomy or pneumonectomy.

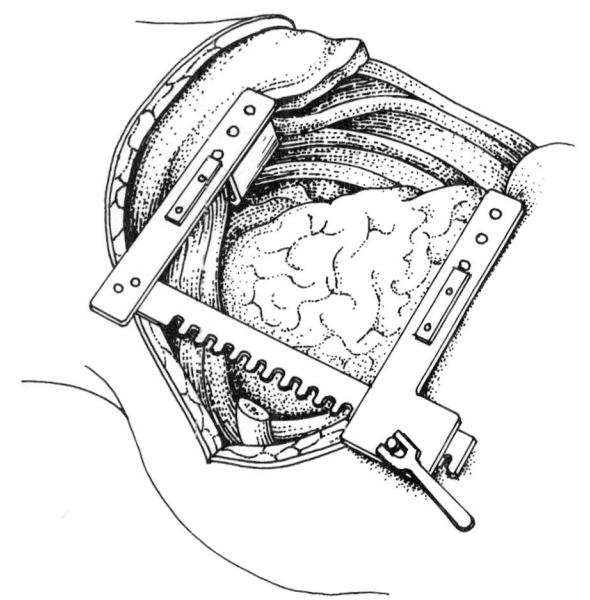

FIGURE 25-21   Rib retractor placed for thoracotomy.

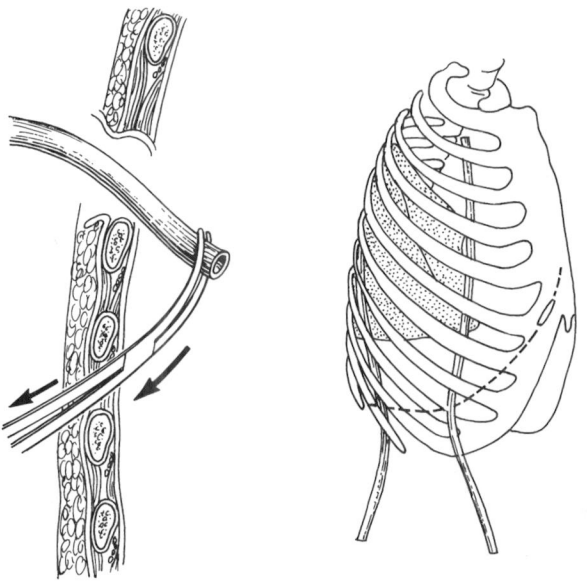

FIGURE 25-22   Introduction of chest drainage tube through a stab wound; placement of apical and basal drainage tubes after upper and middle lobectomy.

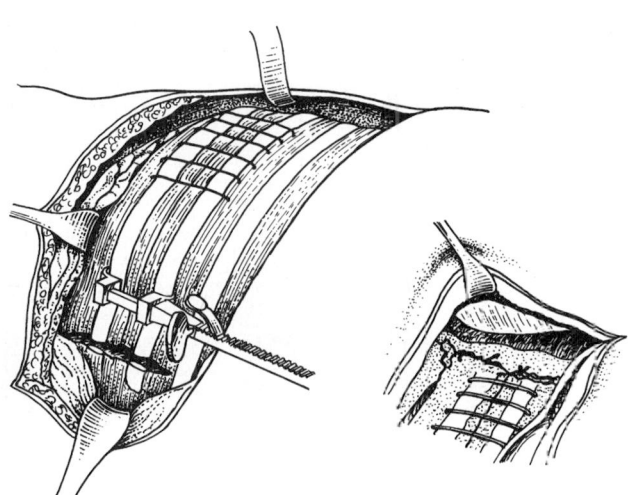

FIGURE 25-23 Rib approximator placed for closure of incision. Heavy-gauge suture used for closure of ribs.

fungal infections, and congenital anomalies. Lesser consideration is given for lobectomy of the middle lobe because of bronchial division involvement.

Procedural Considerations

Basic thoracic instrumentation is used. The patient is placed in a lateral position for a posterolateral incision; the supine position may be used for upper and middle lobe resections. The procedure varies with the specific lobe to be removed depending on the anatomic structure.

Operative Procedure

1. The skin, subcutaneous tissue, and muscle are incised using scalpel, suction, and electrodissection. Hemostasis is attained. If a rib is to be excised, the procedure already discussed is implemented.
2. The ribs and tissue are protected with sponges. The rib retractor is placed and opened slowly.
3. The pleura is entered, and peripheral adhesions are freed with scissors, blunt dissection, or a sponge on a sponge-holding forceps.
4. The hilar pleura is incised and separated.
5. The branches of the pulmonary arteries and veins are isolated, clamped, double ligated, and divided with fine, right-angled vascular clamps, scissors, and nonabsorbable suture.
6. The main trunk of the pulmonary artery is identified as is the fissure between the lobes.
7. The bronchus clamp is applied. The remaining lung is inflated to identify the line of demarcation. The bronchus is divided with a scalpel or heavy scissors.
8. Bronchial secretions are suctioned.
9. The bronchus is closed with atraumatic, nonabsorbable mattress sutures or bronchus staples. If staples are applied, the scalpel is used to complete division of the bronchus.

10. Incomplete fissures are divided between hemostats with fine Metzenbaum scissors. Edges may be sutured closed.
11. A pleural flap is created and sutured over the bronchial stump. Other methods of securing the bronchus might be used.
12. The pleural cavity is thoroughly irrigated with normal saline, and hemostasis is ensured. The remaining lobes are inflated to check for air leaks, and the degree of expansion of the remaining lobes is assessed.
13. The pleural space is irrigated, and the procedure is completed as for a pneumonectomy.

Segmental resection

Segmental resection is removal of one or more anatomic subdivisions of the pulmonary lobe. It conserves healthy, functioning pulmonary tissue by sparing remaining segments. Segmental resection is indicated for any benign lesion with segmental distribution or diseased tissue affecting only one segment of the lung with compromised cardiorespiratory reserve. The most common cause for removal is bronchiectasis. Other conditions requiring removal include chronic, localized inflammation and congenital cysts or blebs.

Procedural Considerations

Basic thoracotomy instrumentation is used. The patient is placed in lateral position for an incision appropriate for the area of tissue to be removed.

Operative Procedure

1. The skin, subcutaneous tissue, and muscle are incised with scalpel, suction, and electrodissection.
2. The parietal pleura is incised with a scalpel and scissors. Adhesions are divided with sharp or blunt dissection.
3. The segmental artery is identified to provide accurate identification of the bronchus of the diseased segment.
4. The segmental pulmonary vein and branches are ligated.
5. The bronchus is clamped with the bronchus clamp, and the remaining lung is inflated. The intersegmental boundary is confirmed, and proper placement of the clamp is ensured.
6. The visceral pleura is incised around the diseased segment, beginning anterior to the hilum and progressing toward the periphery. Exposure is facilitated with malleable or other type of retractors. The intersegmental vessels are clamped with thoracic hemostats and ligated.
7. The segmental bronchus is transsected. The stump is closed with atraumatic, nonabsorbable mattress sutures or bronchus staples (Fig. 25-24).
8. Dissection is continued to separate segmental surfaces, and vessels are ligated as needed. The segment of the lung is removed.

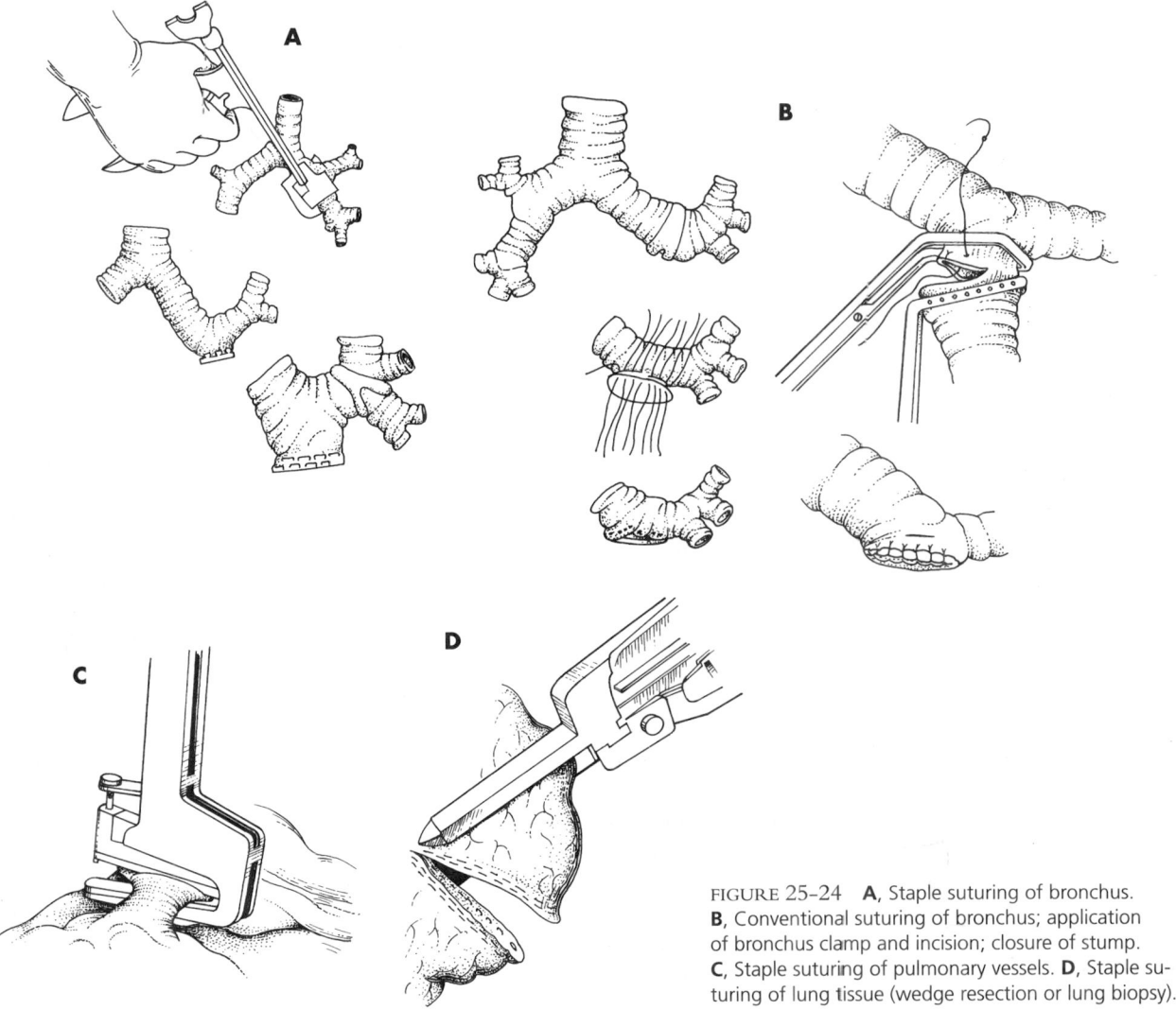

FIGURE 25-24 **A**, Staple suturing of bronchus. **B**, Conventional suturing of bronchus; application of bronchus clamp and incision; closure of stump. **C**, Staple suturing of pulmonary vessels. **D**, Staple suturing of lung tissue (wedge resection or lung biopsy).

9. A pleural flap is created and sutured over the bronchial stump. Other methods of securing the bronchus may be used.
10. The lung is reinflated and irrigated with normal saline. Bleeding is controlled with ligatures or hemoclips.
11. The procedure is completed as for pneumonectomy.

Wedge resection

Wedge resection is removal of a wedge-shaped section of parenchyma that includes the identified lesion, without regard for intersegmental planes. The resection is used for removal of small, peripherally located benign primary tumors, peripherally located inflammatory disease, and biopsy in chronic diffuse lung disease.

Procedural Considerations

Thoracic instrumentation is used. The patient is positioned to allow access to the operative site with consideration of the area of lung to be removed.

Operative Procedure

1. The skin, subcutaneous tissue, and muscle are incised using a scalpel, suction, and electrodissection.
2. The rib retractor is placed.
3. Bleeding is controlled, and small bronchi are secured with clamps and ligature. Large bronchi are ligated or sutured to prevent persistent air leak.
4a. The wedge is outlined for excision, with a margin of normal tissue left, using one of the following techniques.
4b. Long hemostatic clamps are applied in three rows to outline the wedge. Excision is accomplished with a scalpel. The tissue is sutured with a running absorbable suture behind the clamps before removal. The edges of the tissue are oversewn with a continuous or interrupted suture (Fig. 25-25).
4c. The lobe is grasped with a lung clamp, and the thoracic stapling instrument is applied to the parenchymal portion of the lung. Staples are applied, and the wedge is excised with the scalpel. Staples are

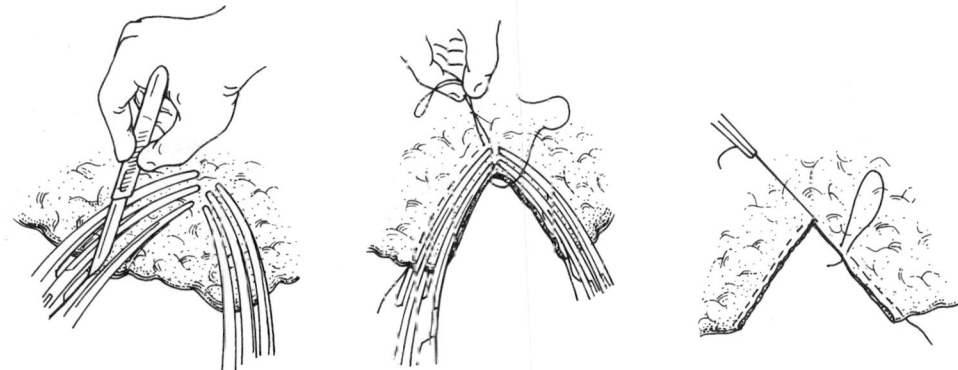

FIGURE 25-25 Wedge resection. Clamps applied to edge of lung tissue to be excised with scalpel and sutured with a running suture and oversewn.

reapplied to the opposite side of the lesion adjoining the staple lines.

5. The specimen is removed. Air leaks are checked by irrigation and inspection. Bleeding is controlled with ligation or hemoclips. The procedure is completed as for pneumonectomy.

Lung Volume Reduction Surgery

Lung volume reduction surgery (LVRS) is an alternative surgical treatment for patients with chronic pulmonary emphysema.[4,5] The procedure may also be referred to as *lung volume reduction pneumoplasty or pneumonectomy*. Candidates for the procedure have progressive severe dyspnea, secondary to pulmonary dysfunction; medical management is ineffective; and disease distribution is limited to target areas of severity. The procedure can be performed through a median sternotomy, lateral thoracotomy or transverse anterior thoracotomy incision. The patient's compromised status attributable to malnourishment requires particular attention to padding and protection of skin and bony prominences and the use of appropriate devices to prevent injury.

Procedural considerations

The basic thoracotomy setup and instrumentation are used. In addition, bovine pericardium strips are prepared (Research Highlight 25-4).

Operative procedure

1. The lungs are exposed through a transverse anterior thoracotomy incision using the sternal saw to separate the sternum. Adhesiotomies are performed, and the inferior pulmonary ligaments incised.
2. The lungs are deflated to visualize the portions of the lung where air is trapped in emphysematous lung tissue.
3. A lung-grasping forceps is used to hold the portion of the lung to be excised. A surgical stapling device is lined with bovine pericardium and positioned on either side of the lung. The stapling of emphysema-

25-4 RESEARCH HIGHLIGHT

Postoperative air leak is a prevalent problem in patients after lung volume reduction surgery or other procedures for emphysema. There have been attempts to decrease the duration of postoperative air leaks by using several techniques. The most recent method is the use of strips of bovine pericardium on the staple lines. This study was a prospective randomization of 123 patients undergoing stapled thoracoscopic unilateral lung volume reduction procedures. Preoperative characteristics of the patient's disease and respiratory function were similar. The length of time before chest tube removal was evaluated and compared to the improvement in air leaks at the staple lines. The length of stay was compared to determine cost of this technique. The researchers concluded that the bovine pericardial sleeves used to buttress staple lines in thoracoscopic unilateral lung volume reduction procedures resulted in shorter duration of postoperative leaks.

From Hazelrigg, S.R., Boley, T.M., Naunheim, K.S., et al. (1997). Effect of bovine pericardial strips on air leak after stapled pulmonary resection. *Annals of Thoracic Surgery, 63*(6), 1573-1575.

tous lung tissue continues, and staple lines are overlapped to prevent air leaks.
4. The lung is reinflated to identify air leaks. If air leaks are found, the lung is deflated, and the stapling procedure continues.
5. One or two chest tubes are placed into each pleural space. The chest tubes are connected to water-seal drainage systems without suction.
6. The ribs and sternum are reapproximated using stainless steel surgical wire. The muscle layer, subcutaneous tissue, and skin layer are closed.[1]

Lung Biopsy

Lung biopsy is resection of a small portion of the lung for diagnosis. The biopsy allows removal of relatively large

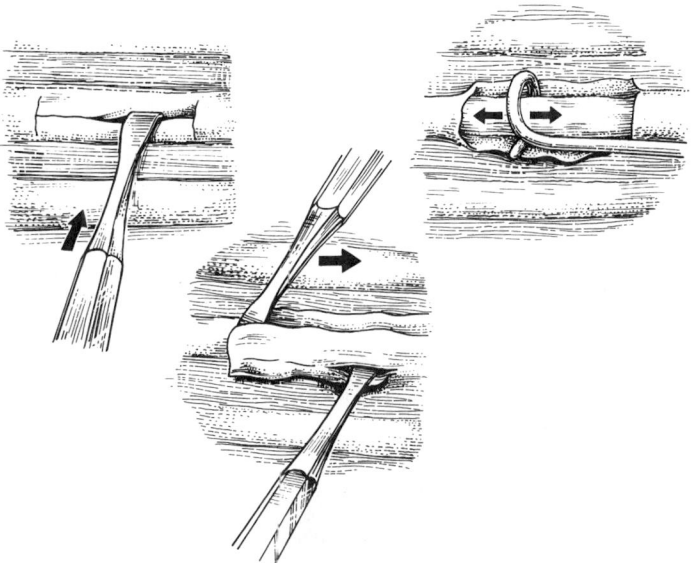

FIGURE 25-26 Separation of muscles of rib with a periosteal elevator and rib stripper.

specimens for microscopic examination of the lung tissue. Indications include failure of closed methods (needle biopsy) for diagnosis, and the presence of small localized lesions that can be removed by biopsy.

Procedural considerations

In addition to the basic instrument setup, a rib retractor, lung-grasping forceps, and dissecting scissors are used. The patient is positioned in a semilateral position for anterolateral incision.

Operative procedure

1. A short incision (approximately 5 cm) is made at the fifth intercostal space. The pleura is incised; the ribs are retracted.
2. The lung is secured and pulled out the opening with the Duval lung clamp.
3. Samples from one or more segments of the lung are taken for biopsy with application of a Satinsky clamp or application of staples with a stapling device. The tissue to be removed is excised with a scalpel. After application of the clamp, tissue edges are approximated with absorbable suture.
4. Bleeding is controlled by the application of a moist sponge at the incision site. The area is irrigated and inspected for air leaks.
5. The chest tube (28 to 30 Fr) is inserted and connected to suction.
6. The incision is closed, the chest tube is anchored to the chest wall, and a dressing is applied.

Decortication

Decortication of the lung is removal of any fibrinous deposit or restrictive membrane on the visceral and parietal

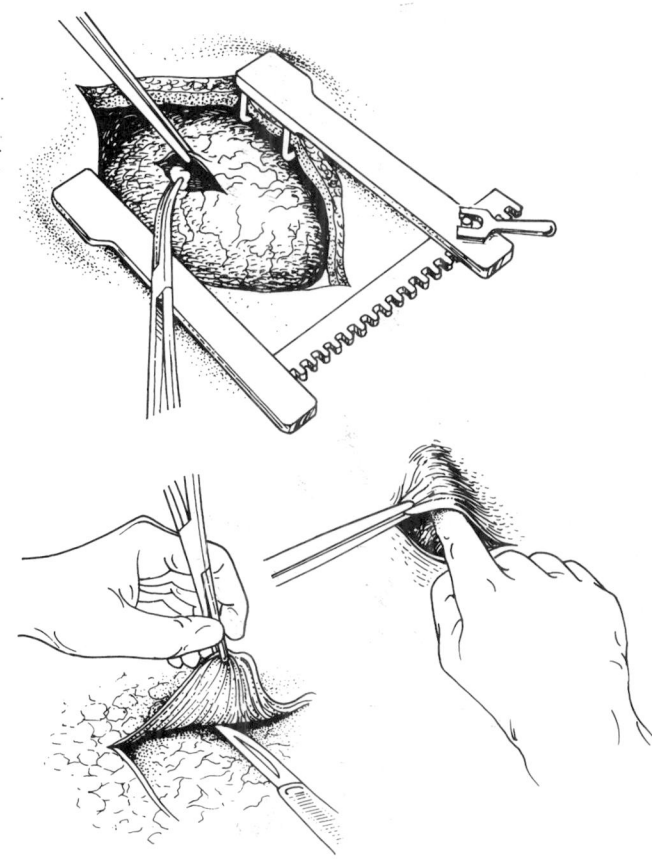

FIGURE 25-27 Decortication. Methods of separating fibrous membrane from visceral pleura.

pleura that interferes with pulmonary ventilatory function. The procedure results in blood loss and trauma and should be used only if the underlying lung is healthy. The objective is to return the lung to near-normal function.

Procedural considerations

The basic thoracic instrumentation is used. The patient is placed in a lateral position for a posterolateral incision.

Operative procedure

1. The skin, subcutaneous tissue, and muscle are incised with the scalpel, suction, and electrodissection.
2. A rib, usually the fifth or sixth, is stripped (Fig. 25-26) and resected.
3. The ribs and tissue are protected with moist sponges. The rib retractor is placed and slowly opened.
4. Parietal adhesions are divided to the margins of the lung, mediastinal surface, and pericardium with thoracic scissors, forceps, and a moist sponge on sponge-holding forceps.
5. The fibrous membrane is incised and separated from the visceral pleura using blunt and sharp dissection and handling the tissues gently (Fig. 25-27). The procedure is completed as for pneumonectomy.

TABLE 25-3 | Antineoplastic Medications Administered for Sclerosing Therapy

MEDICATION	DOSAGE	SIDE EFFECTS
Bleomycin sulfate (Blenoxane)	60-90 mg	Nausea, vomiting, anorexia, weight loss, rash, alopecia, fibrosis, pneumonitis, pulmonary toxicity, fever, chills
Uracil mustard (nitrogen mustard)	None recommended topically	Thrombocytopenia, leukopenia, anemia, nausea, amenorrhea, azoospermia, vomiting, diarrhea, alopecia, pruritus, rash
Thiotepa	10-15 mg	Dizziness, nausea, vomiting, anorexia, hematuria, amenorrhea, azoospermia
Fluorouracil (5-FU)	None recommended	Thrombocytopenia, leukopenia, anemia, myelosuppression, amenorrhea, hemorrhage, renal failure, rash, fever, lethargy, malaise

Drainage of Empyema

Drainage of empyema is treatment for purulent effusion associated with acute or chronic infection. Empyema (other than a pure tuberculous type) must be drained to prevent fibrothorax and further treatment with decortication. Acute empyema could be the result of lung abscess, pneumonia, or infection after thoracotomy. The procedure can be accomplished with the patient receiving local anesthesia when the infection is not extensive. Prolonged intrapleural infection results in chronic empyema, which can create additional complications such as mediastinal shift, difficulty in swallowing, respiratory limitations, erosion into the bronchus, and deformity of the chest. Sclerosing therapy may be instilled to promote mesothelial inflammation and fibrosis. The agent used must have the least toxicity and best patient tolerance. Medications used might include bleomycin, thiotepa, cytarabine and cisplatin, doxycycline, or doxorubicin (Table 25-3). Talc poudrage may be the treatment of choice for patients able to tolerate additional procedures and who experience relief of pleural effusion by thoracentesis.[16]

Procedural considerations

If the patient is anesthetized, the basic thoracic instrumentation is used. The patient is placed in a lateral position for an anterolateral incision. The chest cavity is irrigated profusely during and upon completion of the procedure.

Operative procedure

1. The skin and tissues are incised with a scalpel to expose the affected area of the lung. Suction is used to prevent spillage of drainage from the chest.
2. The pleural space is obliterated, and an inflammatory response is created by stripping the parietal pleura from the visceral pleura by sharp or blunt dissection and by inserting a catheter and instilling a sclerosing substance.
3. The incision site is closed as for other thoracotomy procedures.
4. A dressing is applied.

Open Thoracostomy (Partial Rib Resection)

Partial rib resection is removal of a portion of selected rib or ribs through an open thoracostomy incision to allow healing and reinflation of an infected lung. The procedure is performed for treatment of chronic empyemic lesions to establish a mechanism for continuous drainage.

Procedural considerations

The basic thoracic instrument set and bone-cutting instruments are used. The patient is placed in a lateral position for a posterolateral incision. The surgical procedure can be completed with the patient under local anesthesia.

Operative procedure

1. The skin, subcutaneous tissue, and muscle are incised by scalpel, suction, and electrodissection.
2. The rib is resected, and the pleura is incised. Suction is used to control anticipated drainage.
3. Aerobic and anaerobic swabs for culture and sensitivity are obtained. The chest cavity is irrigated.
4. A large chest tube is inserted through the pleural opening. The incision is closed or packed open (depending on the extent of disease process).
5. The chest tube is secured with a suture of heavy-gauge material on a cutting needle when it is passed through the incision and tied around the tube.
6. The chest tube is connected to a water-seal drainage system, and connections are secured.
7. A dressing is applied. An increased number of layers of dressing to absorb drainage may be necessary.

Closed Thoracostomy (Intercostal Drainage)

Closed thoracostomy is insertion of a chest catheter through an intercostal space for establishment of closed drainage. The procedure provides continuous aspiration of air, blood, or infectious fluid from the pleural cavity.

Indications are treatment of spontaneous pneumothorax, traumatic hemothorax, pleural effusion, and acute empyema. If the pleural effusion is malignant, an appropriate sclerosing agent (doxycycline, bleomycin) is required.

Procedural considerations

The thoracostomy may not take place in an operating room setting. A local anesthesia set including syringes, needles, and an anesthetic agent of choice for local injection will be needed. The basic instrument set is used, in addition to disposable chest catheters, water-seal drainage system, two aspirating needles, and culture tubes. The patient is placed in a lateral or sitting position (see Chapter 5).

Operative procedure

1. The correct depth of insertion is gauged; the catheter is marked. The operative site is anesthetized.
2. An aspirating needle attached to a syringe is introduced into the chest cavity to verify the presence of purulent drainage, air, or blood.
3. The skin is incised, and a clamp is introduced through the incision into the intercostal space and pleural cavity.
4. A catheter that fits the incision site without space around the circumference is inserted. The catheter is clamped to prevent egress of air as it is inserted into the cavity.
5. The incision site is sutured, and the catheter is secured.
6. The catheter is attached to water-seal drainage and the tubing secured. The clamp is removed and a dressing is applied.

Decompression for Thoracic Outlet Syndrome

Thoracic outlet syndrome is a compression of subclavian vessels and brachial plexus at the superior aperture of the thorax. The cause of compression is usually the first rib, either caused by a congenital deformity or a traumatic injury resulting in anatomic changes. Symptoms depend on whether nerves, blood vessels, or both are compressed at the thoracic outlet. Decompression is accomplished through partial or entire removal of the rib.

Procedural considerations

Soft-tissue and bone instrumentation is used. The patient is positioned in a lateral decubitus position.

Operative procedure

1. The skin and subcutaneous tissue are incised with the scalpel using suction and electrodissection. Soft-tissue dissection continues to identify the neurovascular bundle.
2. The first rib is meticulously dissected subperiosteally using the periosteal elevator with or without the rib elevator and stripper with or without rib raspatories, avoiding undue traction in the brachial plexus and damage to the subclavian artery or vein.
3. A wedge is taken from the midportion, or the rib is removed in its entirety using the rib shears.
4. A drain is placed, and the incision is closed. A dressing is applied.

Excision of Mediastinal Lesion

Excision of a mediastinal lesion is the removal of a lesion from the mediastinum, which is divided into superior, anterior, middle, and posterior sections. A mediastinoscopy could determine the diagnosis of an anterior mediastinal lesion. Indications for excision of a mediastinal lesion include cystic hygroma, thymoma, lymphoma, and neurogenic tumor.

Procedural considerations

The thoracic instrumentation is used. A procedure on the superior mediastinum might require use of thyroid instruments (see Chapter 16). The patient is placed in a supine position for a median sternotomy incision (lateral position alternatively may be used).

Operative procedure
Thymoma

1. The skin and subcutaneous tissue are incised with the scalpel along with suction and electrodissection.
2. The sternum is transsected with a power saw or sternal knife (Fig. 25-28). Bleeding is controlled at the bone edges with bone wax.
3. The thymus gland is dissected; vessels are clamped, ligated, and divided. The gland is removed.
4. The incision is closed. The sternum is reapproximated and closed with heavy wire. The skin is sutured closed. A dressing is applied.

Lung Transplantation

Since the mid-1980s there has been expanded experience with both single-lung transplantation (SLT) and double-lung transplantation (DLT). Indications for SLT include restrictive lung disease, emphysema, pulmonary hypertension and other nonseptic end-stage pulmonary diseases.[7] Bilateral lung transplantation is indicated for cystic fibrosis or patients with a chronic infection in end-stage pulmonary failure. The procedure involves the allografting of one or both lungs from a cadaver or brain-dead donor. Success has been recognized with donor contribution from living relatives for persons who are experiencing chronic disease and who have a high risk on the donor transplantation list.[7] Contraindications for a transplantation include multisystem disease other than the lung, history of carcinoma or sarcoma, current infection, significant renal or hepatic dysfunction, cigarette smoking within 3 or 4 months, drug or alcohol abuse, psychologic instability or poor medication compliance. One-year survival rates for SLT have increased to about 90%.[6] Early

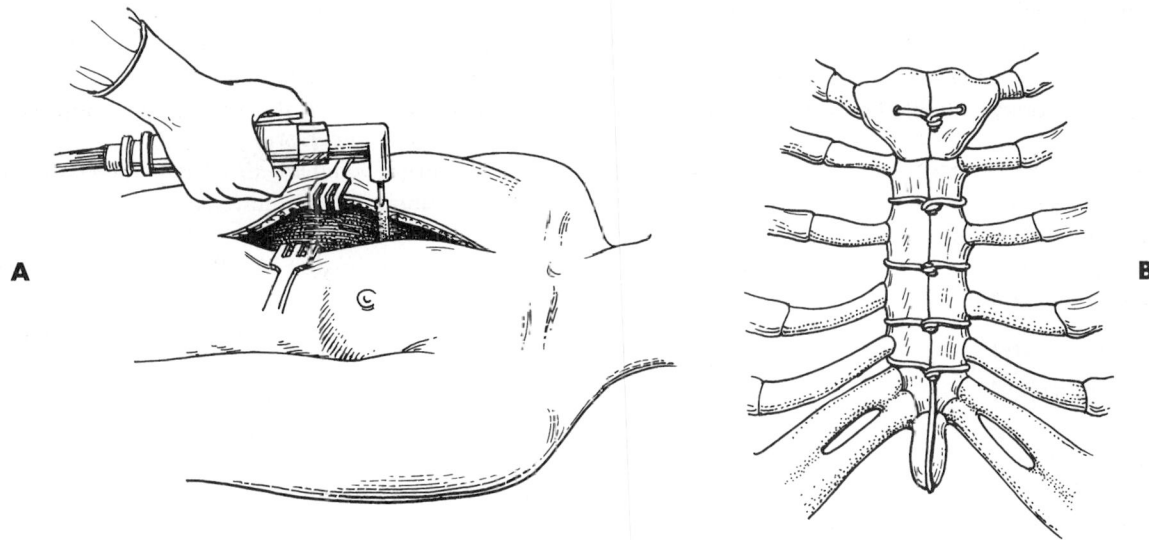

FIGURE 25-28   Median sternotomy. **A,** Incision with power saw. **B,** Closure with heavy-gauge wire.

and late airway anastomosis complications can slow the patient's progress (Research Highlight 25-5). Although there is increasing success with the surgical technique, it is anticipated that future application of lung transplantation techniques will be limited by donor supply. As the field of lung transplantation continues to evolve, questions will need to be answered regarding quality of life after transplantation and whether the single or double procedure is best in the long run for patients with chronic obstructive lung disease and primary pulmonary hypertension. Major issues include the shortage of suitable donors, improved methods for early detection of chronic rejection, and improved immunosuppressive agents and regimens.

The success of lung transplantation depends on the multidisciplinary efforts of surgeons, anesthesiologists, harvest and donor teams, nursing personnel, social workers, and many others.[2] The United Network for Organ Sharing has recommended the following institutional resources for a lung transplant program:

- A lung-transplantation team with expertise in complex thoracic surgical problems; individuals having prior experience with clinical LT are desirable.
- A pulmonary medicine section with individuals who have expertise in managing chronic lung disease and in pulmonary rehabilitation; an institutional program in pulmonary rehabilitation and in prevention of chronic lung disease is desirable.
- Institutional experience with solid-organ transplantation in general is essential; this implies the presence and active participation of experts in infectious disease, clinical immunology, and psychiatry as well as nursing personnel with experience in the care of lung-transplantation recipients.
- Staff with experience in complex cardiac surgery; the presence of staff with experience in cardiac transplantation or cardiopulmonary transplantation is desirable.

25-5 RESEARCH HIGHLIGHT

Airway complications after lung transplantation have decreased with changes in surgical technique and experience with lung transplantation. Despite these changes, airway complications remain a significant source of morbidity and occasional mortality. The pathophysiology leading to airway complications is not understood; therefore multiple methods have been implemented to prevent the complications, without full understanding of the correlation of benefits. A retrospective review of 119 consecutive patients undergoing pulmonary transplantation was conducted. These patients had undergone single-lung or bilateral sequential lung transplantation. The researchers identified treatments being used to include stenting, bronchodilatation, laser debridement, rigid bronchoscopic debridement, operative revision, and growth factor application. It is determined that airway complications can be managed with a good outcome if recognized early. An algorithm summarizing treatment interventions for airway anastomotic complications was developed.

From Kshettry, V.R., Kroshus, T.J., Hertz, M.I., et al. (1997). Early and late airway complications after lung transplantation: incidence and management. *Annals of Thoracic Surgery, 63*(6), 1567-1583.

- An intensive care unit with expertise in managing postoperative general thoracic surgical patients, including immunosuppressed patients and their pulmonary problems; the capability for extracorporeal membrane oxygenation treatments is desirable.
- At least two clinically experienced thoracic anesthesiologists assigned to the lung transplantation program.

Procedural considerations

Selection of the donor, recipients, lung preservation, and administration of anesthetic are considerations in this procedure. The nursing care plan is modified considerably for each patient, since nursing personnel are caring for two patients with different needs. Recipient patients will have been started preoperatively on immunosuppressive therapy and infection prophylaxis. The patient's positioning will vary for the techniques being employed. The instrumentation is like that used for a thoracotomy.[9]

Operative procedures (single-lung transplantation)
Donor Harvesting

1. The patient is prepped from chin to knees and laterally to the midaxillary line. A median sternotomy incision or thoracotomy incision may be used.
2. The pleura are opened longitudinally posterior to the sternum, and the pericardium is divided back to the hilum on both sides. The inferior pulmonary ligament is taken down, pleural adhesions are incised, and the proximal pulmonary arteries are dissected at their origin.
3. After heparinization and hypotensive anesthesia, the superior vena cava is ligated and divided, and heavy silk ties are placed around each vessel.
4. The aortic arch is dissected free, and the ligamentum arteriosum is divided. The anterior and inferior margins of the pulmonary artery are separated from the main artery and ascending aorta. Umbilical tapes are placed around the pulmonary artery and aorta. A pursestring suture is placed for infusion of the cardioplegia solution in the heart.
5. Once the cardioplegia and pulmonoplegia delivery is complete, the heart is prepared for removal; veins and arteries are separated, and the heart is removed and placed in cold Collins solution.
6. The pulmonary arteries are dissected free from the mediastinum to the hilum anteriorly and then posteriorly to the anterior aorta and hilum. The trachea is dissected free. The lungs are inflated before stapling and dissection. The lungs are removed and immersed in cold Collins solution.

Recipient Preparation and Transplantation

1. The patient is positioned laterally, and the area is prepped for exposure of the chest and abdomen (nipple line to knees).
2. An incision is made for a thoracotomy. The procedure depends on which lung is to be removed. If the right lung is being removed, the pulmonary vein is isolated extrapericardially; the pulmonary artery is isolated as close to the lung as possible. The azygos vein is ligated and divided, and the pulmonary artery is dissected.
3. If the left lung is being removed, the ligamentum arteriosum is divided.

4. The lung to be removed is collapsed, and the proximal pulmonary artery is occluded. If instability occurs after occlusion, partial femoral arteriovenous bypass is initiated. If the patient remains stable, the pneumonectomy is performed.
5. Pulmonary veins are divided extrapericardially. The first branch of the pulmonary artery and descending branch are separated. One preserves the blood supply to the bronchus by not dissecting tissue around the bronchus.
6. The bronchus is divided and the lung removed. The pericardium is opened around the pulmonary veins to allow room for the atrial clamp.
7. Inferior and superior pulmonary veins are incised and joined.
8. Three anastomoses are completed for a single lung transplant: bronchus to bronchus, pulmonary artery to pulmonary artery, and recipient pulmonary veins to donor atrial cuff. Techniques used to minimize bronchial anastomotic complications include shortening the donor bronchial stump, reinforcing the anastomosis with a vascularized tissue pedicle such as omentum or intercostal muscle pedicle flap, or using an intussuscepting bronchial anastomosis technique.
9. After anastomoses and restoration of circulation, the lung is fully inflated and observed.
10. After closure of the chest, the patient is examined with a bronchoscope to remove secretions and to ensure that the anastomosis is intact.

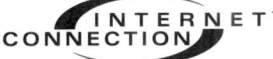

Respiratory Nursing Society: email rnsatpns@aol.com

Society of Thoracic Surgeons: http://www.sts.org

Respiratory Care Web:
http://www.hsc.missouri.edu/shrp/rtwww/rcweb/docs/rcweb.html

International Lung Sounds Association:
http://www.umanitoba.ca/medicine/pediatrics/ILSA

Medical Matrix Pulmonology:
http://www.slackinc.com/matrix/SPECIAL/PULMONAR.html

American College of Chest Physicians:
http://www.chestnet.org

Virtual World Congress Chest Diseases CME Program:
http:www.accp-vwc.org/

American Cancer Society: http://www.cancer.org

Medicine Online: http://www.meds.com/

REFERENCES

1. Allen, G.M. (1996). Surgical treatment of emphysema using bovine pericardium strips. *AORN Journal, 63*(2), 373-388.

2. Cooper, J.D. (1993). Commentary on DATTA lung transplantation assessment. *Abstracts of Clinical Care Guidelines, 5*(4), 11-12.

3. de Campos, J.M., Laert, F., Werebe, E., et al. (1997). Thoracoscopy in children and adolescents. *Chest, 111*(2), 494-497.

4. Dickey, D.M. (1996). Bilateral lung volume reduction surgery for treatment of emphysema. *AORN Journal, 63*(2), 355-372.

5. Graling, P.R., Hetrick, V.L., & Kiernan, P.D. (1996). Bilateral lung volume reduction surgery. *AORN Journal, 63*(2), 389-404.

6. Grover, F.L., Fullerton, D.A., Zamora, M.R., et al. (1997). The past, present and future of lung transplantation. *American Journal of Surgery, 173*(6), 523-533.

7. Kirchner, S.A. (1991). Living related lung transplantation: a new dimension in single lung transplantation. *AORN Journal, 54*(4), 704-714.

8. Lewis, R.J. (1993). Perspectives in the evolution of video assisted thoracic surgery. *Chest Surgery Clinics of North America, 3*(2), 207-213.

9. Lloyd-Jones, H., Wheeldon, D.R., Smith, J.A., et al. (1996). An approach to the retrieval of thoracic organs for transplantation. *AORN Journal, 63*(2), 416-426.

10. LoCicero, J., et al. (Eds.). (1992). Diagnostic procedures for thoracic disease. *Chest Surgery Clinics of North America, 2*(3), 443-699.

11. Meade, R.H. (1961). *History of thoracic surgery*. Springfield, Ill.: Charles C Thomas.

12. Munnell, E.R. (1997). Thoracic drainage. *Annals of Thoracic Surgery, 63*(5), 1497-1502.

13. Pagana, K.D., & Pagana, T.J. (1997). *Mosby's diagnostic and laboratory test references*. St. Louis: Mosby.

14. Skidmore-Roth, L. (1994). *Mosby's nursing drug reference*. St. Louis: Mosby.

15. Tampinco-Golos, I. (1992). Endoscopic thoracotomy: a new approach to thoracic surgery. *AORN Journal, 55*(5), 1167-1180.

16. Tampinco-Golos, I. (1995). Talc poudrage for treatment of pleural effusion in selected patients. *AORN Journal, 62*(1), 83-91.

17. Viallat, J.R., Rey, F., Astoul, P., et al. (1996). Thoracoscopic talc poudrage pleurodesis for malignant effusions. *Chest, 110*(6), 1387-1393.

18. West, M.A., Sharma, S., Aohn, J., et al. (1997). A randomized trial of empyema therapy. *Chest, 111*(6), 1548-1551.

CHAPTER TWENTY SIX

Vascular Surgery

Beth Ann MacVittie

THE HISTORY OF vascular surgery can be traced as far back as 600 to 800 B.C. During this time, an Indian surgeon, Sushruta, not only wrote the first surgical text, but also was the first to control hemorrhage with hemp fiber ties and use boiling oil to cauterize bleeding. Through the years, many attempts were made to repair arteries and veins but these efforts failed because of sepsis and thrombosis. Consider the following examples of important discoveries in an attempt to place our current practices in perspective: Lister's principles of asepsis were not reported until 1867, and McLean did not discover Heparin until 1916. and even then it was too toxic for clinical use until 1940. Thromboendarterectomy, first performed by Dos Santos in 1946, was not adequately refined for widespread use until Fogarty developed the Fogarty embolectomy catheter in 1963. Carotid endarterectomy, a common peripheral vascular procedure in the United States today, was first reported by DeBakey in 1953.[18] Peripheral vascular surgery has developed rapidly since these early discoveries.

Improved patient outcomes are enhanced by the current strides in angiography, great improvements in surgical and anesthesia techniques, and the growth of monitoring and intensive care medicine. Preoperative cardiac assessments and intraoperative cardiac monitoring (such as pulmonary artery catheters, echocardiography) have increased the safety of invasive procedures. Limb-salvage is more aggressive and often delays or prevents limb amputations. Great strides have been made in saving limb function by the combining of bypass with free-flap coverage of large nonhealing foot or leg ulcers. Free flaps are done by the plastic surgeon either simultaneously or soon after arterial reconstruction (see Chapter 24). Advances in prosthetic technology and rehabilitation are improving the outlook for patients undergoing lower extremity amputation.[26] Blood salvage techniques have expanded with the advent of cell-saving and autotransfusion devices. Reinfusion of a patient's own blood was first utilized in 1818 in London by James Blundell. Refined techniques and increased concern about the safety of banked blood have stimulated widespread utilization of blood salvage. Shed blood is collected, washed of clotting factors and debris, and returned to the patient as packed red blood cells (RBCs).[1]

Peripheral vascular surgery includes interventions to both the arterial and venous systems of the vasculature, excluding the heart itself (see Chapter 27). Vascular disease takes many forms and can best be organized into acute and chronic venous insufficiency and acute and chronic arterial insufficiency. Peripheral vascular disease (PVD) usually refers to arterial insufficiency attributed to atherosclerosis, which can affect any artery. Although all facets of the etiology of PVD have yet to be elucidated, risk factors include diabetes mellitus, tobacco use in any form or amount, hypertension (HTN), genetics or family history, diet, and elevated cholesterol.[33]

In the last decade, many new technologies have been introduced. Laser-assisted balloon angioplasty (LABA), to open arterial occlusions, was widely used until clinical results indicated that there were short-lived patency and often deleterious effects in the small vessels of the leg.[58] This technique has essentially been abandoned with the exception of iliac artery angioplasty, which seems to be beneficial for patients with isolated lesions up to 5 cm long or at risk for a more invasive procedure. Early results show that percutaneous balloon angioplasty is as successful without the laser.[50] Subsequent studies vary in the lesion location, lesion size, and other patient-selection criteria. The current literature suggests that balloon angioplasty is appropriate in iliac artery and carefully selected femoropopliteal lesions.[49]

Other endovascular procedures recently introduced include angioscopy, mechanical atherectomy, and the placement of intravascular stents and stent grafts (Box 26-1). Angioscopy, the endoscopic visualization of vessels, began in the mid-1980s and has developed as catheters and micro-optics have advanced. Angioscopes that are 0.8 to 3.3 mm in diameter have been developed to permit visualization of small vessels with high-resolution images. Not a treatment mode in itself, it may be useful to predict the prognosis of vascular bypass procedures and detect technical problems that lend themselves to correction intraoperatively.[58] Peripheral mechanical atherectomy may be performed percutaneously or by arteriotomy to remove plaque by pulverizing and debulking of an atheromatous lesion. Four devices are currently approved by the FDA (TracWright System, Auth Rotabator, Simpson Atherocath, and Transluminal Extraction Catheter). Although touted initially as an alternative to balloon angioplasty, atherectomy devices tend to be traumatic resulting in neointimal hyperplasia and restenosis.[49]

The placement of intravascular stents is increasing in popularity. A variety of stents or intravascular supports have been developing since the 1960s in an attempt to alleviate the drawbacks of angioplasty: elastic recoil and intimal dissection. Three types are currently being utilized: spring-loaded stainless steel stents, thermally expanded metal stents, and balloon-expandable stents. Successful placement of stents has been performed in the iliac arteries and veins and superior vena cava. Large, high-flow vessels seem to benefit most. Stents are being used to treat failed angioplasties and to repair intimal flaps, dissections, and recoil.[58]

The field of vascular surgery is expanding and responding to the demands for less invasive procedures (Research Highlight 26-1). One of the areas of critical importance to advancement is that of imaging. Duplex scanners, intravascular ultrasonography (IVUS), and improved computerized tomography (CT) and magnetic resonance imaging (MRI) will someday provide painless and more accurate information for the diagnosis, treatment planning, and evaluation of vascular disease. In addition, the less invasive interventions need improved guidance techniques to assist the surgeon and interventional radiologists.[58]

SURGICAL ANATOMY

Basic knowledge of anatomy is essential for all phases of the care of the vascular patient. See Fig. 26-1 to review the principal arteries and veins. Arteries and veins have three layers:

- Tunica intima (innermost layer)
- Tunica media (muscular middle layer)
- Tunica adventitia (fibrous outer layer)

Arteries differ from veins in function and slightly in structure (Fig. 26-2). Structurally, arteries have a thicker muscle layer and more elastic fibers than veins have and therefore are thicker walled than veins are. The properties of elasticity and distensibility enable the vessels to compensate for changes in blood pressure and volume. Because of the thicker muscle layer, severed arteries are capable of contracting and constricting enough to stop hemorrhage. In contrast, veins are more fragile than arteries and whether traumatic or iatrogenic, venous bleeding can be difficult to control. Another difference is the presence of semilunar intimal folds, or valves, in veins that prevent backflow. Veins and arteries are nourished by a

tiny network of vessels, the vasa vasorum, as well as from the intraluminal blood flow. Both are regulated by the autonomic nervous system with veins having fewer nerve fibers than arteries have. The two systems are connected (except for the pulmonary artery): arteries, carrying oxygenated blood, branch into smaller arteries and then

---

BOX 26-1	**Endovascular Procedures**

Embolectomy
Endarterectomy
Balloon angioplasty
Atherectomy
Stent placement
Bypass graft insertion

26-1 RESEARCH HIGHLIGHT

ENDOVASCULAR STENT GRAFTS AS TREATMENT FOR ABDOMINAL AORTIC ANEURYSMS

154 patients were involved in a prospective clinical trial to define the value of treating abdominal aortic aneurysms by placement of an endovascular stent-graft rather than by the standard abdominal surgical approach. The graft was made of nitinol metal covered with polyester fabric. The grafts were placed via the femoral arteries under fluoroscopic guidance. Successful placement was defined as complete exclusion of the aortic aneurysm. Twenty one patients had straight grafts placed, and 133 had bifurcated grafts. Three procedures had to be converted to open abdominal surgery. There were 13 minor complications and 3 major complications including one death. The conclusion was that this is a technically feasible intervention and may be especially recommended for patients in a high surgical risk group.

From Blum, U., Voshage, G., Lammer, J., et al. (1997). Endoluminal stent-grafts for infrarenal abdominal aortic aneurysms. *New England Journal of Medicine, 336*(1), 13-20.

arterioles, and then capillaries to venules to veins. The work of exchanging nutrients and metabolic wastes is done at the capillary level.[55]

Blood flow is a complex process dependent on many factors. Blood flow that travels parallel to the vessel wall, relatively undisturbed, is referred to as *laminar*. When flow is disrupted by an obstruction, stenosis, curve, or bifurcation, the particle motion is referred to as *turbulent*. Turbulence may be evidenced by the presence of a bruit,

by auscultation, or by a characteristic Doppler signal. Flow is dependent on blood viscosity, vessel wall resistance, and the peripheral resistance of the arterioles. There must be a difference in pressures or a pressure gradient to allow blood to flow. The contraction of the left ventricle provides this gradient. The negative pressure created by the relaxed right ventricle assists in venous return by creating a suctioning effect, and the skeletal and visceral muscles help propel venous return toward the heart.

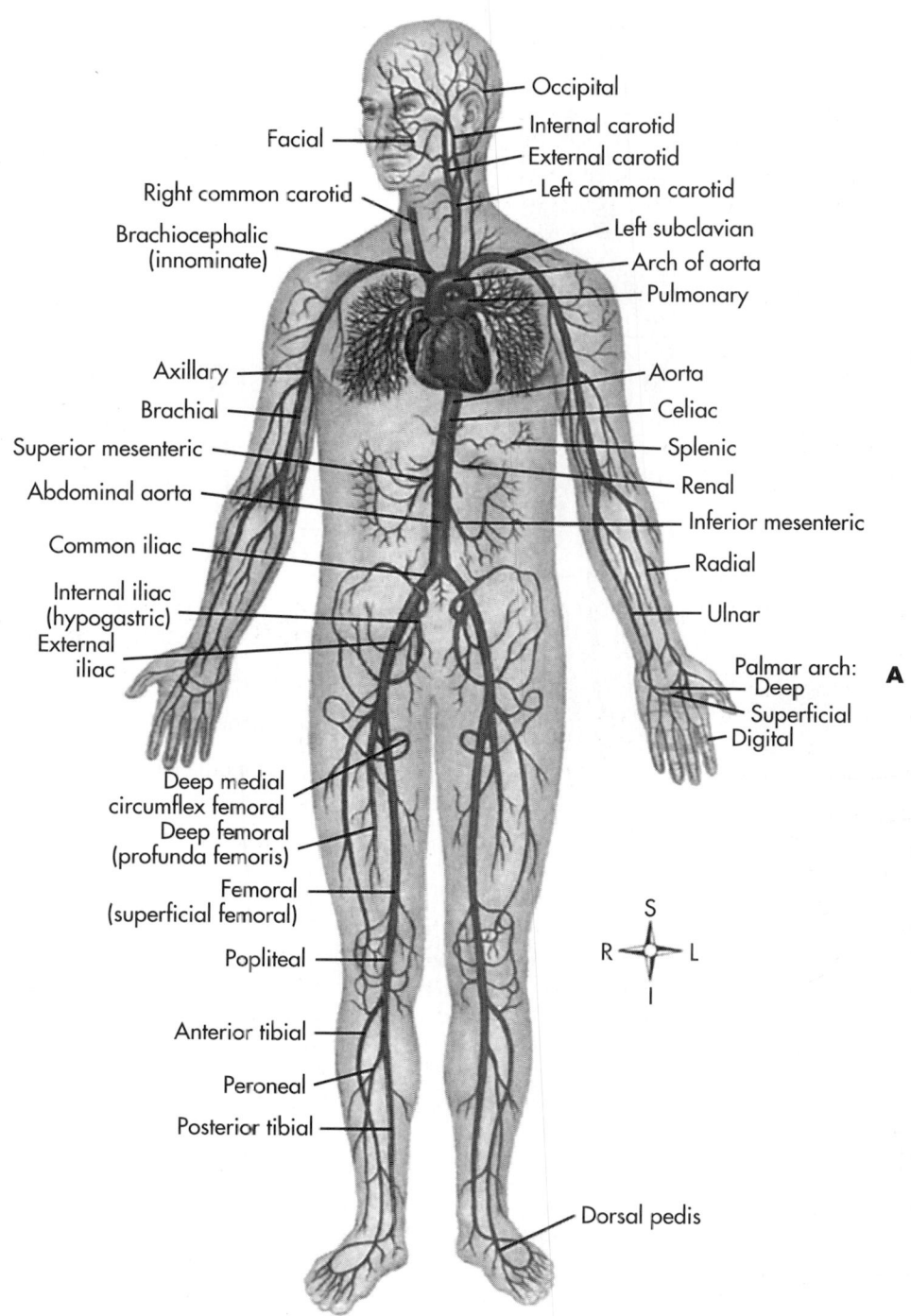

FIGURE 26-1   **A,** Principal arteries of the body.   *Continued*

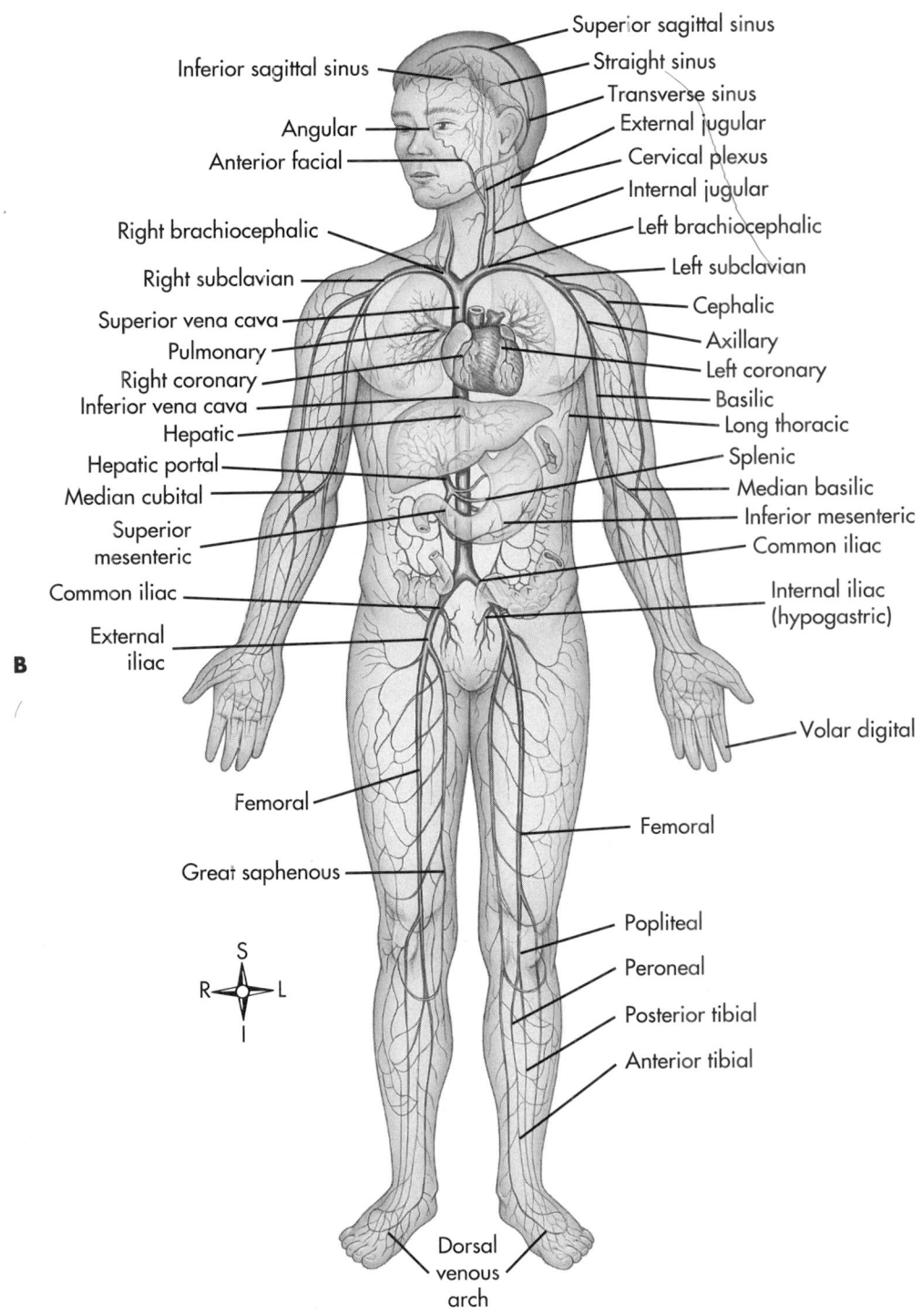

Superior sagittal sinus

Inferior sagittal sinus

Straight sinus

Transverse sinus

External jugular

Angular

Anterior facial

Cervical plexus

Internal jugular

Right brachiocephalic

Left brachiocephalic

Right subclavian

Left subclavian

Superior vena cava

Cephalic

Pulmonary

Axillary

Right coronary

Left coronary

Inferior vena cava

Basilic

Hepatic

Long thoracic

Hepatic portal

Splenic

Median cubital

Median basilic

Superior mesenteric

Inferior mesenteric

Common iliac

Common iliac

Internal iliac (hypogastric)

External iliac

Volar digital

Femoral

Femoral

Great saphenous

Popliteal

Peroneal

Posterior tibial

Anterior tibial

Dorsal venous arch

FIGURE 26-1, cont'd   **B**, Principal veins of the body.

Arterial Disease

Acute

Arterial insufficiency may be acute as in embolic disease or chronic as in atherosclerosis. Emboli may arise from the heart, as in atrial fibrillation, but occasionally result from a myocardial infarction (MI). Atherosclerotic plaque can also break loose from other areas and result in an acute arterial blockage. Patients with acute arterial occlusion usually present with the onset of the five *P*s: sudden severe pain, pulselessness, paresthesia, paralysis, and pallor of an extremity.[48] Heparin is the mainstay to prevent the enlargement of emboli to allow time for collateral blood flow to develop. However, in the threatened limb, there are basically two options: surgical removal of the clot

ARTERY

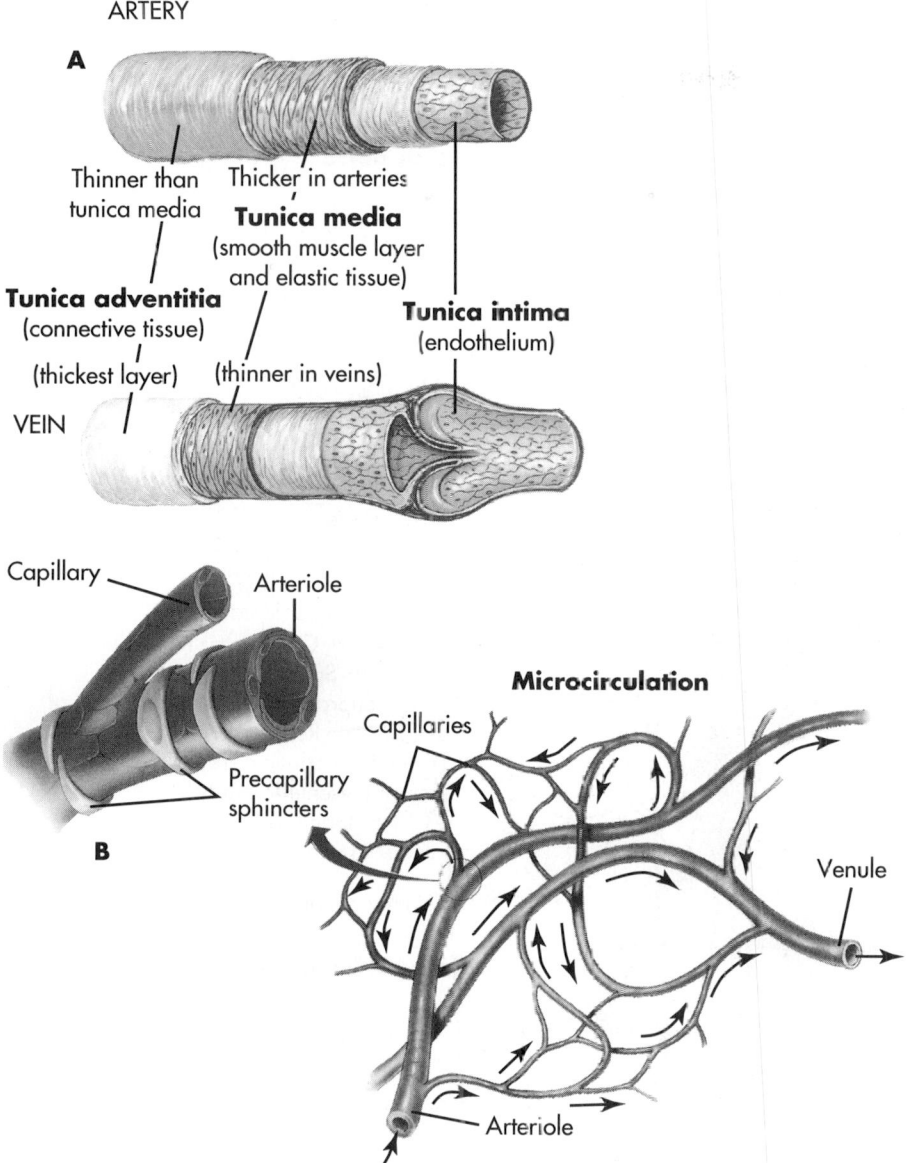

A

Thinner than tunica media

Thicker in arteries

Tunica media
(smooth muscle layer and elastic tissue)

Tunica adventitia
(connective tissue)

Tunica intima
(endothelium)

(thickest layer)

(thinner in veins)

VEIN

Capillary

Arteriole

Microcirculation

Capillaries

Precapillary sphincters

B

Venule

Arteriole

FIGURE 26-2   **A**, Layers of artery and vein. Drawings of a sectioned artery and vein show the three layers of large vessel walls. **B**, Microcirculation. The smaller blood vessels—arterioles, capillaries, and venules—cannot be observed without magnification. Notice that the control of bloodflow through any particular region of a capillary network can be regulated by the relative contraction of precapillary sphincters in the walls of the arterioles (*inset*). Notice also that capillaries have a wall composed of only a single layer of flattened cells, whereas the walls of the larger vessels also have a smooth layer.

(embolectomy), or chemical removal of the clot with the use of a thrombolytic drug. If the limb reaches the point where the muscle is rigid, the limb is not salvageable, and amputation is a lifesaving procedure.[9]

Chronic

Chronic arterial insufficiency (ischemia) occurs because of the deposition of calcium and cholesterol within the wall of the artery. *Arteriosclerosis* is a natural part of the aging process whereby the arteries lose their full elasticity. This should not be confused with *atherosclerosis obliterans*, which is a pathologic process that affects the intimal layer of the artery with the buildup of a fibrous plaque of lipids that can calcify and necrose. *Atherosclerosis* is the most common cause of occlusive disease; the probable mechanism may be initial damage to the intima and subsequent activation and aggregation of the body's platelets. Inflam-

mation follows with the deposition of lipoproteins forming an atheroma. Calcification of this lesion leads to the development of an atherosclerotic plaque. The process is a gradual one, and a localized lesion is usually indicative of systemic disease. The body develops a network of collateral vessels as an adaptive mechanism to supply the tissues with oxygenated blood. Many theories have been postulated to explain the process of atherogenesis. The inflammatory process of intimal injury, as described above, seems to be the current and most widely accepted hypothesis. Smoking has a definite link to atherogenesis, but whether this is attributable to an immunologic response or a direct toxic reaction has yet to be proved. Some research implicates hypertension as a cause, whereas others identify it as a result. Besides the smoker, the diabetic patient is also prone to PVD. Many mechanisms contribute to atherogenesis in the diabetic: hyperglycemia

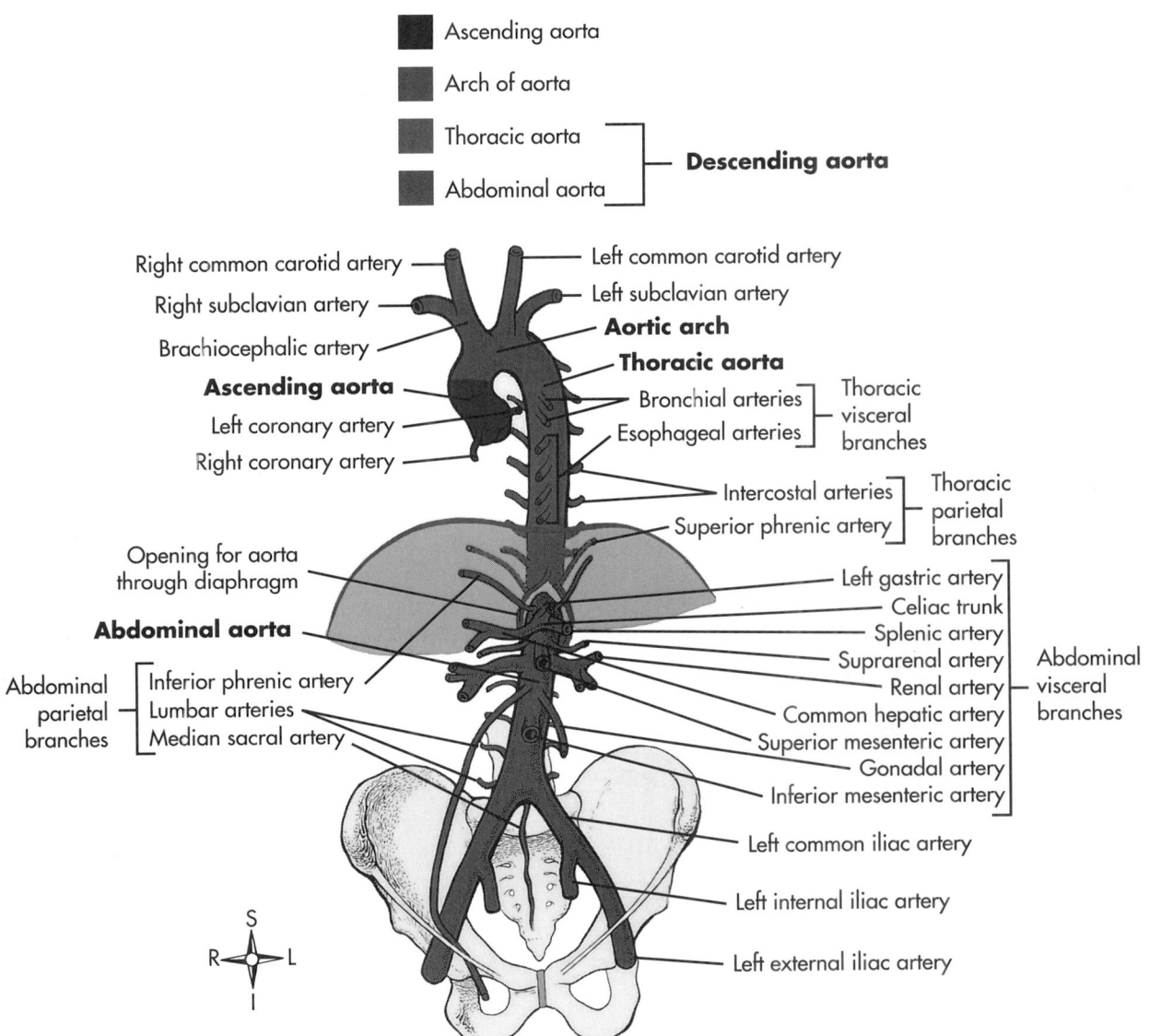

Ascending aorta

Arch of aorta

Thoracic aorta

Abdominal aorta

Descending aorta

Right common carotid artery —
Right subclavian artery —
Brachiocephalic artery —

Ascending aorta
Left coronary artery
Right coronary artery

— Left common carotid artery
— Left subclavian artery
Aortic arch
Thoracic aorta
Bronchial arteries
Esophageal arteries

Thoracic visceral branches

Intercostal arteries
Superior phrenic artery

Thoracic parietal branches

Opening for aorta through diaphragm

Abdominal aorta

Abdominal parietal branches
Inferior phrenic artery
Lumbar arteries
Median sacral artery

Left gastric artery
Celiac trunk
Splenic artery
Suprarenal artery
Renal artery
Common hepatic artery
Superior mesenteric artery
Gonadal artery
Inferior mesenteric artery

Abdominal visceral branches

Left common iliac artery

Left internal iliac artery

Left external iliac artery

S
R — L
I

FIGURE 26-3 The aorta. The aorta is the main systemic artery, serving as a trunk from which other arteries branch. Blood is conducted from the heart first through the ascending aorta and then through the thoracic and abdominal segments of the descending aorta.

alters the platelet function and could increase thrombosis, and insulin triggers increased smooth muscle cholesterol synthesis.[11] Most of the vascular surgeon's practice revolves around the results of this type of chronic arterial insufficiency and aneurysmal disease.

Aneurysmal disease

The cause of aneurysmal disease was previously attributed to a progression of atherosclerosis. More current evidence proposes that atherosclerosis is a concurrent finding with aneurysmal disease and not the causative factor. Genetic factors and alterations in the actual structure of the aorta are important findings.[2] Aneurysms are dilatations of artery walls and may be dissecting (a tear allows blood to seep between vessel layers) or false, that is,

pseudoaneurysms (a tear goes through all layers). They occur most frequently in the abdominal aorta but are also found in the thoracic aorta, iliac, femoral, and popliteal arteries.[37] More men than women are affected, and aneurysmal disease tends to be a disease of older patients. In 1977, Clifton noted a familial tendency that subsequent research has verified. As many as 18% of patients with abdominal aortic aneurysms have a first-degree relative similarly diagnosed.[57]

Abdominal aortic aneurysms occur primarily below the renal arteries (Fig. 26-3). An aneurysm involves intimal damage of the aorta and weakening of the media or elastic portion (collagen and elastin defects) of the arterial wall.[37] Gradually the vessel wall in the damaged area expands, and atheroma develops within the aneurysm sac. An abdominal aortic aneurysm has minimal symptoms and is generally discovered on routine history and physical examination. Mortality is low with elective resection of the aneurysm. Dissection and rupture of the aneurysm dramatically increase operative mortality.

Arterial insufficiency

The initial and most important symptom of vascular disease in the aortoiliac vessels and distal arteries is *intermittent claudication*. The term *claudication* is derived from the Latin word *claudicare*, which means 'to limp'. This is the most common symptom of lower extremity PVD and occurs with exercise distal to the arterial obstruction. The pain is located in the working muscle, occurs with the same amount of exercise each time, and is relieved with rest. This is referred to as functional ischemia; blood flow is adequate at rest but inadequate to sustain exercise. The increased muscle demand for oxygen with exercise cannot be met distally to the arterial obstruction. Anaerobic metabolism occurs, and muscle cramping develops. Surgery is not usually performed for claudication unless it is unusually disabling. The second symptom, *rest pain*, which is located in the foot, develops as the vascular disease progresses. At this stage the ischemia is termed critical.[33] Rest pain occurs without exercise and is a constant discomfort, often aggravated at night. The body is now unable to meet the oxygen needs of distal tissues even at rest. Rest pain may be somewhat relieved by analgesics or by lowering the legs off the bed. Gravity assists in increasing the tissue perfusion and oxygen supply to decrease the pain. Unless the vascular disease is corrected, nonhealing ulcers and gangrene can develop. Gangrene occurs when the arterial vessels are unable to meet the oxygen needs of distal tissues even at complete rest.

Stroke

Stroke is the third leading cause of death in the United States. Cerebrovascular disease may manifest itself as a transient ischemic attack (TIA) or as a major or minor stroke. A TIA is an episode of neurologic dysfunction that resolves in 24 hours. It may be caused by atheromatous debris or a thromboembolism from a carotid artery or vertebral basilar system. Vascular lesions in the carotid artery occur primarily at the bifurcation of the common carotid artery into the internal and external carotid artery. The internal carotid artery supplies the brain with its oxygen needs. Obstruction in this arterial vessel leads to cerebrovascular insufficiency. The anatomy of the blood supply to the brain is shown in Fig. 26-4. The right and left carotid and vertebral arteries supply the brain. This supply is protected by the existence of the circle of Willis. The first major branch of the internal carotid artery is the ophthalmic artery. Thromboembolic events that affect this artery may result in visual disturbances or ocular TIAs, or "amaurosis fugax." Clinical conditions that generally indicate the need for a carotid endarterectomy are transient cerebral ischemia, asymptomatic severe stenoses, and stable strokes (Research Highlight 26-2).

Venous Disease
Acute

Acute venous insufficiency is caused by a clot in the deep venous system or deep venous thrombosis (DVT). This can be a diagnosis of DVT, phlebitis, thrombophlebitis, or phlebothrombosis, which merely indicates that there is a clot, usually in the lower extremity. Virchow, a pathologist, identified three conditions that give rise to vein clots. These conditions or risk factors are endothelial injury, stasis, hypercoagulability, or a combination. The cause of hypercoagulability is sometimes unknown but seen in patients with tissue trauma (such as surgery, burns, stroke), malignancy, sepsis, pregnancy or estrogen usage, and diabetes mellitus.[27] The patient may be asymptomatic or present with limb swelling, pain, and a skin color change. The danger lies in the potential emboli migrating to the right ventricle and proceeding to the lungs. Pulmonary emboli (PE) can be fatal. PE has been reported to be responsible for approximately 50,000 to 200,000 deaths and 300,000 hospitalizations per year.[24,52] The majority of these originate in the lower extremities. The usual treatment is medical: the use of heparin and bedrest. In cases that preclude the use of systemic heparin or in which heparin is ineffective, the surgical insertion of a vena cava filter may be indicated.

Chronic venous insufficiency

Patients with chronic venous insufficiency (CVI) have not been treated surgically as often as patients with arterial disease for several reasons. CVI is not life or limb threatening. Only recently have improved imaging techniques (such as duplex ultrasonography) allowed better diagnoses of the precise problem. There was a misconception that venous surgery contributed to thromboembolism.[35] The treatment of the majority of venous disorders is nonsurgical and aimed at increasing venous return and decreasing edema.[31] Chronic venous insufficiency, which presents with stasis ulcers from postphlebitic syndrome, usually occurs in one leg. The leg is usually very swollen with a cyclic edema, unlike lymphedema, which does not change visibly by morning from leg elevation. Stasis ulcers and hyperpigmentation usually are found in the "gaiter" area and above the medial malleolus on the leg. The condition is caused by incompetent perforator valves. The perforating veins connect the superficial and deep venous systems. The usual management is to apply 20 to 30 mm Hg of external pressure by means of special pressure stockings. Surgical intervention, valvuloplasty (direct repair of the valve) or valve transposition or transplantation (moving a valve from the arm to the leg), or perforator interruptions are occasionally performed but have had limited success. Patient selection is critical, and long-term results are mixed.[35]

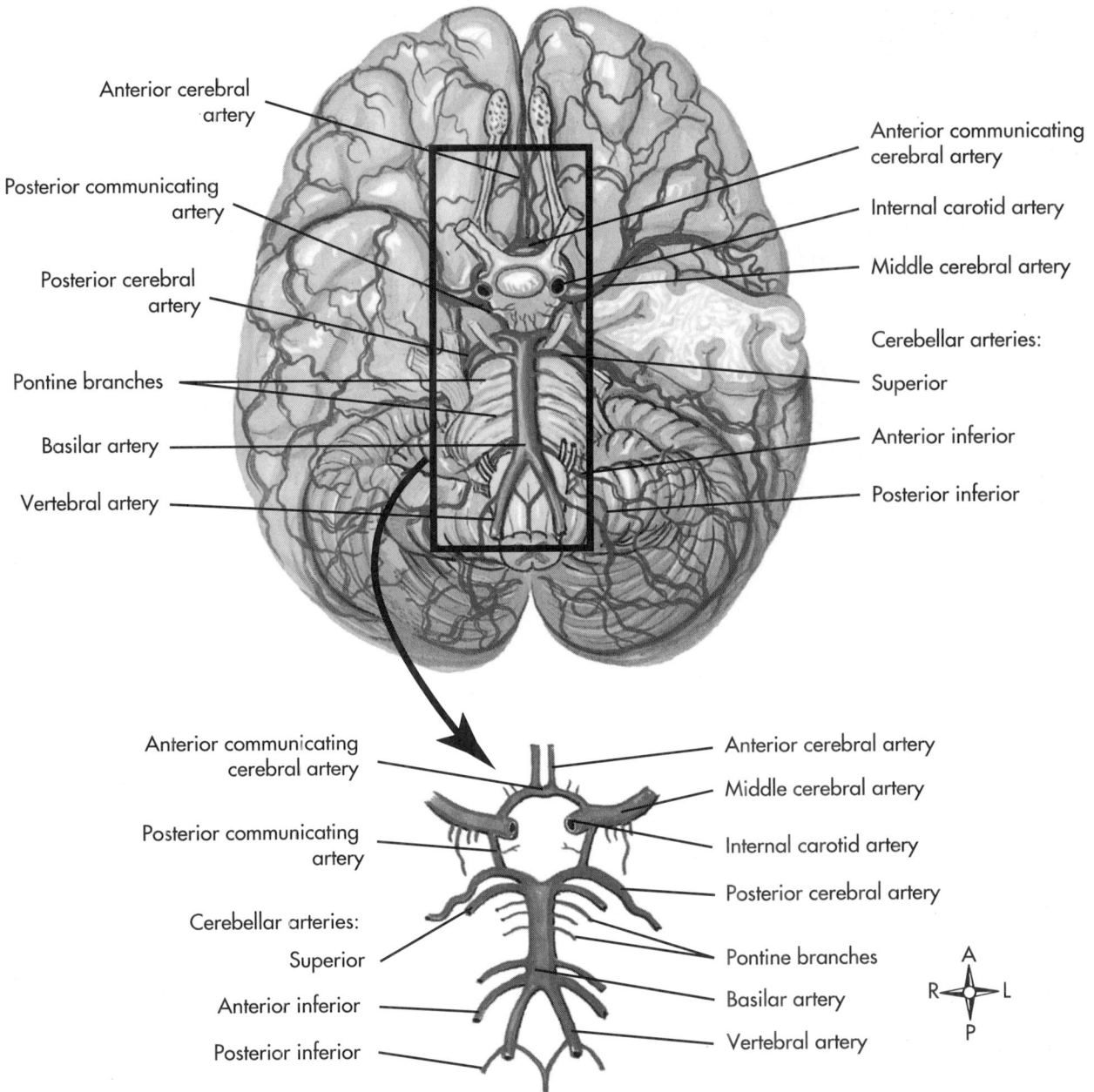

FIGURE 26-4   Arteries at the base of the brain. The arteries that compose the circle of Willis are the two anterior cerebral arteries joined to each other by the anterior communicating cerebral artery and to the posterior cerebral arteries by the posterior communicating arteries.

PERIOPERATIVE NURSING CONSIDERATIONS

Assessment

Nursing responsibilities

A preoperative assessment is necessary for an adequate understanding of the patient's disease, the patient's response, and the proposed surgical procedure. Knowledge of vascular disease and its progression assists the perioperative nurse in performing a comprehensive assessment and

developing a plan of care for patients undergoing surgical procedures.

The perioperative nurse should assess the patient for the development and extent of vascular symptoms. Medical conditions including cardiac, renal, pulmonary, coagulation status, and allergies must be assessed to ensure that the patient can tolerate a possible angiogram, since the contrast medium is toxic, and increased fluid volumes are needed if angioscopy is planned. This is a shared responsibility of the nursing, surgical, and anesthesia team members. The

26-2 RESEARCH HIGHLIGHT

ASYMPTOMATIC CAROTID ATHEROSCLEROSIS STUDY

The Asymptomatic Carotid Atherosclerosis Study (ACAS) was conducted between 1987 and 1993. Thirty-nine clinical sites in the United States and Canada were part of a prospective, randomized trial. Of patients with asymptomatic carotid artery stenoses of 60% or more, 1662 were randomized to either medical or surgical treatment. The medical treatment was administration of daily aspirin and management of risk factors. The surgical group received the medical management interventions and underwent carotid endarterectomy. The surgical group had a 5% risk of stroke, and the medical group had an 11% risk. Surgical intervention is clearly indicated for patients with a 60% or greater carotid artery stenosis if the patient's general health status is not a contraindication. These patients will have a significantly decreased risk of stroke if surgery is performed under conditions of less than 3% morbidity and mortality and the risk factors are aggressively managed.

From Executive Committee for Asymptomatic Carotid Atherosclerosis Study. (1995). Endarterectomy for asymptomatic carotid artery stenosis, *JAMA, 273*(18), 1421-1428.

BOX 26-2 | Chart Review

The nurse will review the surgical patient's chart for the following items:

- Correct and current chart
- Surgical consent
- History and physical examination
- Baseline vital signs (include height and weight)
- Mental status
- Medications
- Allergies or adverse reactions to drugs, topical agents, or other substances
- Skin tone and integrity
- Physical limitations
- Laboratory data (blood work, ECG report, urinalysis, ultrasound or x-ray studies, or other pertinent tests)
- Religious preferences
- Nursing plan of care or other notations from transferring nurse
- Presence or disposition of prosthetic devices (hearing aids, dentures, glasses, etc.)

patient's nutritional status, use of alcohol and cigarettes, and the existence of any skin lesions should also be identified. Preoperative location, grading, and marking of distal peripheral pulses can assist the nurse with intraoperative assessment of tissue perfusion. The perioperative nurse must be able to efficiently assess the patient and his or her specific needs. This includes time to perform an adequate chart review (Box 26-2). The first sight of the patient may give much information but must be confirmed by thorough assessment to avoid mistaken assumptions. The patient must be greeted by name, and such identification must be confirmed by the patient, when possible, and by a name band and the medical record. Comfort should be the next most important assessment before any interview is continued. This is caring and will promote the establishment of a nurse-patient rapport and facilitate obtaining accurate and complete information. Patient acuity will also affect the prioritizing of the assessments and interactions. Safety is always the first priority. The surgical procedure must be confirmed and the patient's understanding assessed. Informed consent is not a piece of paper with a signature. Written requirements for informed consent vary by region and institution. The nurse must follow the policies of the institution, but his or her role as advocate mandates that he or she determine that the patient comprehend the pending intervention to the best of his or her ability. Inaccuracies or misconceptions must be clarified before proceeding with surgery. The Patient's Bill

of Rights specifies that the patient has the right to receive information about treatment that is pertinent, up to date, and clear to him or her.[3] The surgeon is responsible for providing this information. Written documentation may be in the form of a narrative description by the physician or a preprinted form that the patient or legal alternate signs. A consent is designed to protect the patient by allowing clarification in writing of the proposed procedure. It is not legal proof that the patient is truly informed; however, it does lend support that the patient gave permission. Consents that are valid and obtained freely and from a competent person remain in effect for as long as the person still agrees to the surgery or procedure. This may vary by institutional modification.[3] Complex decision making and the availability of new technologies may make informed consent difficult.

After reviewing the results of the patient's physical examination, the perioperative nurse should verify signs and symptoms of vascular disease that need to be considered during intraoperative care. Muscle and skin atrophy, the presence of tissue ulceration or necrosis, pain, neurovascular status, skin color and temperature, and other integumentary changes should be noted. Elderly, cachectic, and obese patients are at increased risk for pressure injuries.

The nurse should assess the patient's mental status and determine the level of understanding and emotional response to the surgery. Vascular patients usually have

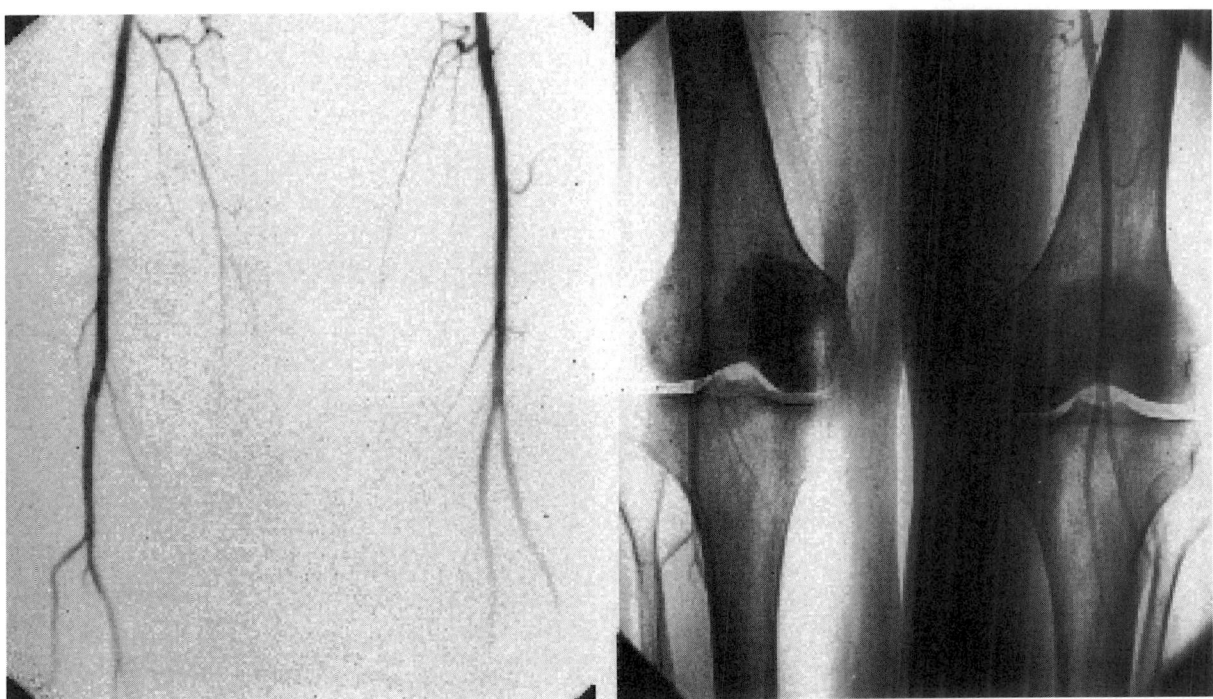

FIGURE 26-5 Digital subtraction angiography.

systemic disease, and the fear of a stroke (carotid endarterectomy), amputation (ischemic limb), or other complications may be a realistic concern. A skin assessment should include notation of color, integrity, pain, and pulses. Any musculoskeletal problems that could preclude patients moving themselves to the OR bed and any weaknesses that may have resulted from a stroke or that would modify the positioning for surgery should be noted. Reinforcement or correction of misunderstandings is possible only if the nurse identifies the patient's current level of knowledge. Identification of the patient's fears and concerns helps the nurse with planning appropriate nursing interventions.

Vascular surgery can be lengthy. Attention to the maintenance of the patient's tissue and skin integrity as well as body temperature is important. The patient's extremities should be assessed for color, temperature, and strength of pedal pulses before the surgical procedure. This assessment evaluates tissue perfusion distal to the arterial obstruction. When the perioperative nurse knows such assessment will be required, it should be performed during the initial preparation of the patient to provide for baseline comparisons.

Preoperative tests

A variety of tests may be required to plan for surgical interventions. Segmental pressure measurements give partial anatomic information in that they assist in locating lesions. Hemodynamic tests provide information on the flow of blood, such as that to the brain or an extremity and the effects on flow caused by a vascular lesion.

Invasive diagnostic tests may be performed preopera-

tively to identify the extent and location of the patient's peripheral vascular disease. The introduction of contrast media through a catheter into the arterial or venous system of the patient facilitates this visualization. Angiography also involves the injection of contrast media into the patient's arterial system and the taking of serial radiographics of the movement of the dye through the arteries (Fig. 26-5). Digital subtraction angiography is one such technique that uses a computer to make the image along with contrast injection. Usually the left side of the film shows the bone for orientation and the right side subtracts the density of the bone and soft tissue to allow a clearer view of the vessels. Arteriography provides information on arterial anatomy and the location of stenotic or occluded vessels and assists the surgeon in planning bypass procedures. It may also be valuable to document a surgical outcome. A venogram (contrast venography) is performed to show venous abnormalities in extremities, the vena cava, and the hepatic or renal systems. Ascending venography can differentiate between acute and chronic thrombosis, and define anatomy. Descending venography assesses valve competence of lower extremities.

Ultrasonography is done to obtain information about structures through the emission of high-frequency sound waves. These sound waves are reflected or bounced back to the probe or transducer that emits them and are electronically transformed into an image.

Doppler scanning

The Doppler effect, initially described by Christian Johann Doppler (1903-1953), is the *change in the frequency* of echo signals that occurs whenever there is a *change in the distance* between the source of a sound and the receiving object.[41] The probe, or transducer, is aimed toward the blood vessel at an angle of 45 to 60 degrees. This directs an ultrasound beam that is reflected back to the probe by moving RBCs. The velocity of the flow of cells is converted into an audible signal heard through a speaker. The signal is described as a swishing sound.[43] The sound is called a signal, not a pulse. The tip of the probe is made of an element called a ceramic piezoelectric crystal. This can send, receive, and convert signals when an electric current is applied. The element becomes thicker and thinner, thus resulting in a pressure wave converted to an audible signal.[41] The simplest form is the continuous wave (CW) Doppler probe. It has two elements; one sends a high frequency wave and the other receives it. In a pulsed Doppler probe, the same element sends and receives signals. The pulsed Doppler probe has the advantage of being able to differentiate between vessels of different depths. A normal arterial Doppler signal is either biphasic or triphasic. The first sound corresponds to systolic flow and is forward moving and of high velocity. The second sound is related to early diastole and has a lesser reversal of flow. The third is later diastole and is a smaller, forward flowing and of a lower velocity. The pitch is described as rising quickly in systole and dropping quickly in early diastole. An abnormal signal, indicating stenosis or occlusion, is heard as low pitched and monophasic. These abnormal arterial signals may sound like venous signals.[61] The Doppler probe can provide information in three forms: the audible signal, a visible graph printout similar to an ECG tracing, and a spectral analysis that appears on a screen and may be recorded on paper as well.[5] The Doppler transducer is the most widely used instrument for vascular study. It has the advantages of being readily available, inexpensive, and easy to use. A small portable, battery unit is durable and can be transported and stored easily. When used on intact skin, a water-soluble gel is needed to conduct a signal. Probes can be used directly on a vessel intraoperatively. The probes are heat sensitive and must be sterilized accordingly to be used intraoperatively on the sterile field, or they may be inserted into a sterile sleeve or probe cover. If they are handled gently, the probes have a reasonable life span. Care must be taken to protect the sensitive tip from being dropped or crushed. The biggest drawback of the Doppler probe is a negative finding in the presence of a stenotic lesion pronounced enough to produce a flow disturbance that results in an altered signal. A bruit is a sound disturbance that is sometimes described as a low-pitched blowing sound. It can be heard through a stethoscope over an area of blood flow turbulence that occurs at points of vessel stenoses. Bruits do not provide information on the extent of a lesion, only that an abnormal flow may exist. They occur at points of significant stenosis and are not heard when severe flow restriction or total flow occlusion occurs.[61] The Doppler probe is noninvasive and painless for patients. For venous assessment, CW Doppler probe can identify the presence and location of venous obstruction and allow one to assess the severity. It is a good screening tool because it is fast, easy, and inexpensive. It cannot differentiate between veins of different depths.

B-mode ultrasonography

B-mode is brightness modulation, a technique in ultrasound imaging that projects a two-dimensional image on an oscilloscope screen. The image appears as dots from the echoes of the signal. The strength of the echo is shown by the intensity and brightness of the dots on the screen.[5]

Duplex ultrasonography

A duplex ultrasound machine is a combination of the pulsed Doppler image and the so-called real-time B-mode image ultrasonogram. Real time simply refers to the image projecting the current, undelayed information. B-mode image is best when the probe is perpendicular to the vessel, but the Doppler probe does not pick up signals at a perpendicular angle. Some manipulation of the probe angle is required to obtain the best results.[41] Color duplex imaging converts the detected signals caused by blood flow into a color depending on the direction of flow. Flow toward the probe may be displayed as red, away from the probe as blue, and turbulence as multiple colors. This imaging provides both hemodynamic and anatomic information.[5] This technology is also used in transesophageal echocardiography.

Pulse volume recording (PVR), or sequential volume plethysmography

A plethysmograph measures and records the changes in the sizes and volumes in extremities by measuring the blood volumes at blood pressure cuffs placed at intervals along the extremity. The methods include electrical impedance, mercury in Silastic strain gauges, air or fluid displacement, and others. It is used to determine the location of an arterial lesion and estimate the severity of the disease.[5] This test requires careful limb positioning and a cooperative patient. Impedance or air plethysmography is used to quantify venous outflow from the extremity. Venous outflow is decreased in the presence of venous thrombosis. It also tests for valve function. A negative study is a good predictor of low risk for PE.

This test is inexpensive, has good predictive value, and is accurate in detecting thrombosis. It has the disadvantage of a high rate of false-positive results in the presence of old deep venous thrombosis (DVT), congestive heart failure (CHF), and external compression.

Magnetic resonance imaging

MRI measures the behavior of atoms in a strong magnetic field. This test provides detailed and three-dimensional images of anatomy for evaluation of carotid, aortic, and lower extremity disease. An MRI provides more detail than ultrasonography or CT scan and avoids the complications of contrast injection and exposure to x rays. It is superior to CT scan for cerebral and spinal disease. One of the disadvantages is that it is contraindicated for patients with pacemakers or metal cerebral aneurysm clips, and vena cava filters may cause large image artifacts.

Nursing Diagnosis

Nursing diagnoses related to the care of patients undergoing vascular surgery might include the following:

- Anxiety related to the surgical intervention and its outcomes.
- Risk for altered body temperature (hypothermia) related to surgical exposure and anesthesia.
- Risk for fluid volume deficit related to loss of body fluids.
- Risk for impaired skin integrity and altered tissue perfusion related to surgical positioning, diagnosis, and vascular clamping.

Based on the perioperative nurse's assessment, the identification and prioritization of nursing diagnoses aid in the development of an individualized plan of care.

Outcome Identification

Outcomes identified for the selected nursing diagnoses could be stated as follows:

- The patient will have all questions answered. The patient will verbalize decreased anxiety and understanding of surgical procedure and perioperative routines. The patient will exhibit increased relaxation as shown by facial expression or other body language.
- The patient's body temperature will remain within normal limits as evidenced by postoperative temperature equitable to preoperative level and absence of postoperative shivering.
- Fluid balance will be maintained as evidenced by postoperative pulses equitable to preoperative level, hourly urine output of at least 30 ml, and good skin turgor.
- Skin integrity will be maintained. Skin temperature and color will be within normal limits. No pressure lesions will be in evidence, and electrosurgical return-electrode site will be intact.

Planning

Some of the outcomes will have been achieved at the end of the intraoperative phase. Others require ongoing evaluation during the postoperative phase. Because perioperative nursing practice is collaborative, the perioperative nurse develops a plan of care that extends from the admission to the surgical suite through safe recovery from surgery. Some patient goals are measured immediately upon discharge from the operating room; others require the collaboration of the postanesthesia care unit (PACU)

or unit nurse for final evaluation. The perioperative nurse thus develops and contributes to a comprehensive, holistic plan of patient care. Such care planning provides evidence of quality patient care and provides a mechanism of communication and continuity of care with other healthcare professionals. Before the patient is brought into the operating room, the perioperative nurse should procure the necessary medical and surgical supplies and equipment for the intended surgical intervention. Because the need for an arteriogram or fluoroscopy for endovascular procedures is a possibility, the vascular patient should be on an appropriate operating room bed with x-ray capabilities. The perioperative nurse needs to coordinate the availability of x-ray personnel. Appropriate contrast media, catheters, and impermeable sterile x-ray covers must be available. Radiation-protection devices, such as lead aprons and shields, should also be used for the patient, when possible, and for the surgical team members. A Sample Care Plan for the patient undergoing vascular surgery, utilizing the suggested nursing diagnoses, is shown on p. 1091.

Arterial procedures, especially those that involve the aorta, may place the patient at risk for significant blood loss. The nurse should consider the availability of blood-replacement products. It may be prudent to have blood products in the OR before the surgical procedure. The use of rapid infusion systems or blood salvage equipment should be determined and planned.

Implementation
Intraoperative monitoring

Intraoperative monitoring for vascular patients consists in the use of the basic ECG, pulse oximeter, and blood pressure cuff. For patients undergoing saphenous vein stripping or amputation, these are usually adequate. For lengthy procedures, as in arterial bypass or reconstruction, an arterial line is usually placed percutaneously into the radial artery. This is kept open by a heparin drip line attached to a transducer, and a waveform monitor reads out the systolic and diastolic pressures. The monitor also calculates the mean arterial pressure (MAP), which aids in the evaluation of the perfusion of systemic and cardiac circulation. This arterial line also allows easy access for collecting specimens for arterial blood gas analysis. The electrocardiogram and direct arterial lines are used for monitoring and assessment. Continuous assessment of the patient's arterial pressure is a critical part of the surgical procedure. Pulmonary capillary wedge pressure as an index of left atrial pressure (LAP) may be monitored depending on the patient's physiologic status. A general anesthetic may be administered, and the patient intubated; local or regional anesthesia may also be used, depending on the surgical intervention. Epidural catheters are placed to provide intraoperative anesthesia that can be augmented to accommodate increased surgical time as opposed to a spinal that provides a finite period of anesthesia. Epidural

SAMPLE CARE PLAN

Nursing Diagnosis: Anxiety related to the surgical intervention and its outcomes

Outcome: Patient will verbalize decreased anxiety.

Interventions:

Include the family, significant other, or both, in explanations of perioperative routines.

Allow time for patient's questions; provide explanations or make appropriate referral.

Observe verbal and nonverbal indications of anxiety; assist the patient with anxiety-reducing techniques such as rhythmic breathing and relaxation.

Encourage ventilation of concerns and fears.

Provide emotional support and supportive nursing measures (such as touch).

Demonstrate warmth, calmness, and acceptance of the patient's anxiety.

Maintain a quiet environment.

Document patient's reactions.

Nursing Diagnosis: Risk for altered body temperature (hypothermia) related to surgical exposure and anesthesia

Outcome: The patient's body temperature will remain within normal limits during the intraoperative phase.

Interventions:

Limit the patient's physical exposure; expose only those body surfaces required for skin preparation.

Cover the patient's head with a blanket or cap.

Use warmed skin preparation solutions (as applicable to agent being used).

Place a warming device (such as a padded hyperthermia blanket) on the OR bed.

Provide the anesthesiologist with a fluid warmer.

Monitor the patient's temperature.

Use warm saline for irrigation.

Provide warm blankets at the end of the surgical procedure.

Nursing Diagnosis: Risk for fluid volume deficit related to loss of body fluids

Outcome: The patient will maintain fluid balance.

Interventions:

Determine the availability of replacement blood or blood products.

Assist with the insertion of intravenous lines and fluid replacement therapy. Keep IV lines patent.

Estimate blood loss on sponges and drapes.

Initiate autotransfusion or utilization of cell-saver as required.

Record the amount of irrigation used.

Document the contents of the suction canisters.

Monitor and document hourly urine output; communicate results of all outcome measurements.

Monitor vital signs and oxygen saturation; assist with the collection and interpretation of intraoperative blood analyses.

Nursing Diagnosis: Risk for impaired skin integrity and altered tissue perfusion related to surgical positioning, diagnosis, and vascular clamping

Outcome: The patient will maintain skin integrity and tissue perfusion.

Interventions:

Document the patient's preoperative skin condition and tissue perfusion.

Position the patient on a cushioning device (gel-filled or eggcrate mattress) on the operating room bed.

Keep OR bed sheets dry and wrinkle free.

Pad all bony prominences.

Maintain body alignment.

Place restraining straps snugly but not tightly.

Protect vulnerable neurovascular bundles from compression.

Check and record tissue perfusion (color, temperature, pulses) as required.

Elevate drapes off the patient's toes; use appropriate positioning accessories.

Reassess and document the patient's postoperative skin condition and tissue perfusion.

---

catheters may be left in place postoperatively for pain management as well. Because many patients undergoing vascular surgery have generalized atherosclerotic disease, the nurse should be constantly alert for cardiac arrhythmias and blood pressure changes. Acid-base balance and pulmonary gas exchange may be assessed from the arterial blood gas analysis (ABG). This may be especially important in the patients on ventilators.[3]

A central venous pressure catheter (CVP) or various types of pulmonary artery (PA) catheters may be inserted, usually via the right internal jugular vein. The CVP line allows assessment of blood volume and vascular tone. The more sophisticated PA catheters (that is, the Swan-Ganz)

can monitor cardiac output, fluid balance, and the cardiac response to drugs. These would be used for aortic surgery or patients with cardiac disease.

The carotid endarterectomy patient can be monitored with electroencephalography (EEG). This allows immediate observation of slowing of the brain waves caused by cerebral ischemia or reduced perfusion. The surgeon may elect to place a temporary shunt in the artery if this occurs during clamping. This could reduce the chances of perioperative stroke.

Transesophageal echocardiography may be used to monitor the heart noninvasively during aortic surgery. The device looks similar to a bronchoscope and can be passed down the esophagus to provide an ultrasonic image. The cardiac structures, blood flow, wall motion, and great vessels can be observed. The equipment is very expensive and requires highly skilled personnel and thus may not be available in many settings. Its use intraoperatively to detect myocardial ischemia is in question and in need of further study.[44]

A urinary catheter should be inserted, especially if the proposed procedure involves the renal arteries or clamping of the aorta above the renal arteries, if considerable blood loss is anticipated, or if the planned procedure time is lengthy or whenever spinal or epidural anesthesia is used because they delay the patient's ability to void voluntarily. Urinary catheterization facilitates accurate hourly measurements of urine during and after the surgical procedure and assists in the assessment of renal perfusion and fluid status.

Positioning

Positioning of the patient undergoing vascular surgery is of particular importance because of restricted circulation distal to the area of arterial obstruction and a generalized state of poor circulation. Particular care must be exercised in positioning elderly patients (see Chapter 30). Awareness of joint range-of-motion limitations attributable to immobility or joint surgery is critical even for a procedure as routine as Foley catheter insertion. Again, preoperative assessment can prevent injury and decrease OR time. Whenever possible, the nurse should have the patient demonstrate the ability to assume the position for the proposed procedure while the patient is awake and able to provide feedback. A footboard may be applied to the operating room bed to prevent the weight of drapes resting on the patient's lower extremities. For a carotid endarterectomy, the patient's head may be supported on a head support. A roll may be placed between the scapulae. For surgical procedures involving a lower extremity, the patient's thigh may be externally rotated and abducted with the knee flexed. A small bolster may be used under the knee to support the patient's leg. Proper skeletal alignment during surgery prevents injury to the neuromuscular system. Attention to the skin overlying bony prominences, especially the heels, sacrum and elbows, and the use of proper supports and pads prevent injury to the patient. Because of the lengthy nature of these procedures, an eggcrate mattress or gel-filled pad can be placed on the operating room bed to help prevent patient injury. For the same reasons, members of the scrubbed team should also be cognizant of heavy instruments and drapes resting on the patient's body and take measures to avoid pressure injuries (see Chapter 5).

Skin preparation and draping

Skin preparation for vascular surgery may be extensive. For abdominal aortic surgery, the patient's skin is prepared from the nipple line to the midthigh area. For peripheral vascular surgery on the lower extremities, the patient is prepped from the umbilicus to the feet. The patient's legs are prepared circumferentially. For carotid surgery, the patient is prepped from the ear and chin on the affected side to below the clavicle. Draping should permit the surgeon free access to involved areas. For example, abdominal surgery may also require exposure of the groin region for possible exploration of the femoral arteries. A femoral-popliteal bypass on one leg may require access to the other leg for harvesting of the saphenous vein. Impervious drapes should be used to prevent contamination of the surgical field from blood and irrigation fluids.

Medications and solutions

Medications and solutions on the sterile field should always be labeled. Heparin is the most common drug used in vascular surgery. It may be given as an IV bolus to systemically anticoagulate the patient. When administered parenterally, it has an immediate onset of action and peaks in minutes. It has a 2- to 6-hour duration. Because it is metabolized in the liver and excreted by the kidneys, the effects of heparin may be prolonged in patients with liver and renal disease. The anticoagulant effects may be monitored by measurement of the activated partial thromboplastin time (APTT) or partial thromboplastin time (PTT).[43] Patients are anticoagulated just before the placement of a vascular clamp to prevent a thromboembolic event. Systemic heparin may or may not need to be reversed at the end of the surgical procedure. Monitoring the activated clotting time (ACT) intraoperatively provides useful data for judging the need for reversal or additional heparin. Heparin is reversed by protamine sulfate.

Since protamine sulfate is derived from fish sperm and testes, caution is advised when administering protamine to patients who are allergic to fish or have received protamine-containing insulin. One milligram of protamine neutralizes 100 mg of heparin. The dose should be calculated to offset half of the last dose of heparin. Protamine must be given slowly, at a maximum of 50 mg in 10 minutes, or it may cause dyspnea, flushing, bradycardia, and severe hypotension. Another reason for monitoring heparin is that protamine, given in the absence of circulating heparin, acts as an anticoagulant and could delay hemostasis intraoperatively.[43]

Heparinized saline solution is used as an irrigation. It may be used to irrigate a blood vessel lumen during surgery, usually after the patient has been systemically heparinized. It is also commonly utilized to flush the lumen of tubes used to shunt blood. The probable mechanism is twofold by creating a negative charge on the tubing wall and by interfering with platelet adherence.[10] The strength of the heparin solution will vary according to the manufacturers' recommendations for certain implant devices or by surgeon preference. A reasonable range is 250 to 1000 units in 250 ml of normal saline.

There are differing ideas on solutions with which to

distend, irrigate, or store vein grafts. Some surgeons prefer a cold solution to decrease the metabolic demands of the vessel, whereas others believe this may lead to spasm. Spasm may be of particular concern when working with the small vessels of the distal leg or foot. Papaverine HCl may be added to a heparinized saline for its direct antispasmodic effect on the smooth muscle of the vessel wall and its vasodilating properties.[51] A reasonable dose is 120 mg in 250 ml saline. The pressure of a hand-held syringe to distend vein grafts has been viewed as a potential cause of graft failure or graft stenosis because this causes endothelial damage. Papaverine HCl, as a smooth muscle relaxant, allows distention at a lower pressure and may decrease the risk of injury.[13] Concentrations for infiltration range from 0.05 to 0.6 mg/ml or 12.5 to 150 mg per 250 ml of solution. The literature suggests that more studies are needed to determine whether cold (4° C) or warm storage solutions are better and exactly what the ideal vein storage solution is.[53]

Blood coagulation is controlled by intravascular and extravascular (intrinsic and extrinsic) mechanisms. Injury to the endothelium, such as trauma or atherosclerosis, can trigger this mechanism (intrinsic). The extrinsic coagulation mechanism is triggered by the insult of surgery to tissue and vessels, which precipitates exposure of tissue thromboplastin, which results in a clot forming.[55]

Topical hemostatic agents may be needed. Absorbable hemostatics are effective by creating an environment that promotes the adhesion of platelets. An absorbable gelatin sponge, such as Gelfoam, may be applied to a bleeding surface to provide a matrix into which clots form. It may be applied dry, moistened with saline, or soaked in a topical thrombin-saline solution. One hundred to 2000 NIH units of thrombin per milliliter of saline or blood may be applied to control bleeding.[51]

Infections of prosthetic vascular grafts are rare but are extremely serious. Infection may be life threatening for patients with aortic grafts or limb threatening in lower extremity procedures. Protecting the prosthetic graft from contact with the skin is essential to prevent bacterial contamination.[29] Prophylactic IV antibiotic administration within 1 hour of the surgical incision has been shown to be effective.[8]

Vascular prostheses

Vascular grafting materials and techniques are of major importance to the field of vascular surgery for bypass procedures and reconstruction. The understanding, study and comparison of new prosthetic grafts, utilization and preparation of autogenous grafts, and knowledge of long-term patency rates cannot be overly emphasized. Grafts are made in varying sizes and configurations; they may be conduits that are straight, tapered, or in the shape of a Y called *bifurcated*, or they may be pieces of material cut for use as a patch. The arteriotomy of a carotid endarterectomy may be closed primarily or with a patch of either vein or synthetic fabric. In aortic surgery, a straight tube or a bifurcated synthetic graft is used. Dacron (polyester) grafts are the usual choice and have been used successfully for over 35 years. The large vessels have high flow rates and thus have a low incidence of thrombus formation and excellent graft-patency rate. The search for the ideal vascular graft continues. Some desired characteristics are that they are reasonably priced, readily available in a variety of sizes and suitable for use anywhere in the body. They need to be biocompatible and hypoallergenic and survive repeated sterilizations. The surgeon's preference would also include ease of handling, that is, elastic, easy to sew, and nonfraying. An implanted graft should last a lifetime and permit blood passage without clotting or infection.[32]

Prosthetic grafts are nonantigenic; tissue incorporates well, which helps prevent infection, and such grafts generally resist thrombosis. For years, knitted polyester grafts were preferred over woven polyester because they were easier to handle, although they had to be preclotted because of their high porosity. Woven grafts are somewhat stronger and bleed less through the fabric interstices but can be more inflexible. Newer grafts have been developed to incorporate the best of both by utilizing a velour polyester. They are also being impregnated with albumin, collagen, or gelatin to provide ease in handling without the need to preclot. Preclotting is usually accomplished by submerging of the graft into a basin of blood collected before systemic heparinization. This makes the graft impervious by allowing fibrin to fill in the fabric spaces.[3]

The other popular prosthetic material is polytetrafluoroethylene (PTFE), which is available in straight, tapered, and bifurcated styles of varying lengths and may have external support rings to prevent compression.[3] These grafts do not stretch, and needle-hole bleeding may be troublesome.

Human allografts were tried in the 1950s for aortic replacement but ultimately failed because of thrombosis, calcification, or aneurysm development.[60] Human umbilical cord vein grafts are commercially available for patients who have no veins available because of previous bypass procedures, saphenous vein stripping, or poor quality or size of available veins. Manufacturers' instructions must be followed to rid the umbilical grafts of preservative by being rinsed.[3]

Volumes have been written on vascular grafts, and the reader should consider this chapter an introduction only. The American National Standards Institute, the Food and Drug Administration, and Association for the Advancement of Medical Instrumentation are a few of the organizations active in setting standards and regulating usage and development of grafts. Randomized trials to determine the best grafting choices and techniques require many years of patient follow-up study.[60]

Autogenous vein grafting for infrainguinal bypass is considered the criterion standard. Undamaged endothelial

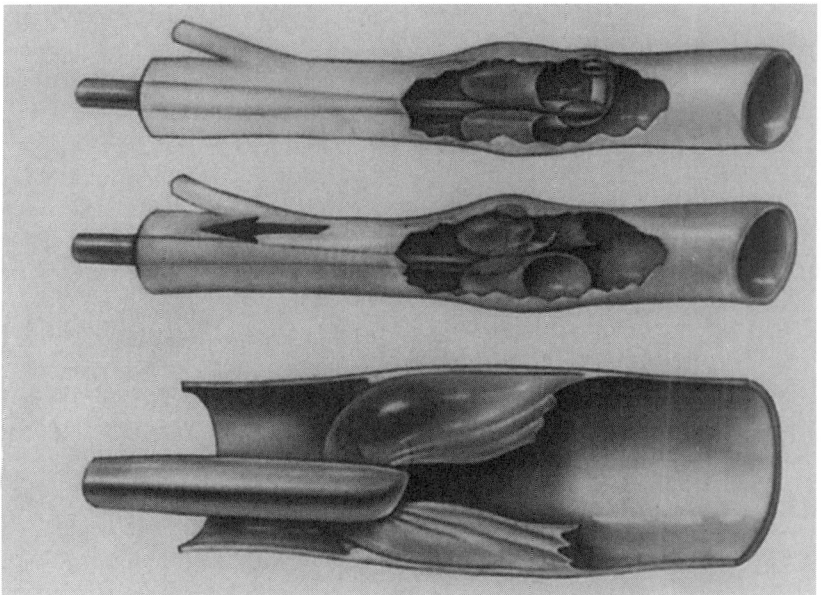

FIGURE 26-6   Valve incision with valvulotome.

cells inhibit the clotting mechanism by the natural release of fibrinolytic substances and plasminogen factors.[3] Two methods of grafting veins have been extensively studied, and the results are not totally conclusive that one method is better than the other. These are the in situ graft and the reversed vein graft. The in situ method leaves the vein in its place, side branches are ligated to prevent arteriovenous fistulas, and the valves that would impede arterial flow are disrupted with instruments specifically designed to cut valves, called *valvulotomes* (Fig. 26-6). Reoperation is more frequent with the in situ method because of missed valves and residual arteriovenous fistulas.[28] Reversal of a vein graft is performed per surgeon preference or when it must be harvested from the contralateral limb. Vein grafts are clearly mandated in the below-knee (BK) bypass procedures.[6] Above-knee (AK) bypasses may use PTFE or other synthetic graft for vein sparing or in high-risk patients who may not tolerate the longer vein harvesting or have a life expectancy of less than 3 years.[60] According to Stanley et al.,[54] damage that contributes to graft failure may be caused by the so-called atraumatic clamps used. Rubber, plastic, or hydrostatic jaw clamps are best for protecting vein grafts from injury. Distal bypasses, particularly those in diabetics, are more successful today as a result of improved tissue handling. The use of the pneumatic tourniquet as an alternative to clamping the vessels may improve results. Although there is an increased awareness of this among vascular surgeons, no randomized study has been undertaken to verify this.[23]

Sutures

Most vascular sutures are made of synthetic, nonabsorbable materials such as Dacron, polyester, polytetrafluoroethylene (PTFE), and polypropylene. Vascular sutures have swaged-on needles of various sizes and are available in sizes 0 to 8-0. The suture may be single armed or double armed (that is, a needle on one or both ends). The size and curve of the needle depend on the vessel and its location. Teflon felt or leftover pieces of graft material (synthetic or vein) may be used as pledgets or buttresses under a suture.[3] They are used when tissue is friable to keep the suture from tearing through or when an anastomosis leaks and needs a better seal. The pledget may be loaded onto the vascular suture or added by the surgeon to a suture already in use. The pledget remains on the suture line[39] (Fig. 26-7).

Vascular monitoring equipment

Assessing blood flow through diseased vessels by palpation is often difficult. Physical assessment of the patient's hemodynamic status during surgery can be further complicated by spasm of the vessel walls, the cool environment of the operating room, and alterations in blood pressure caused by hemorrhage. Vascular monitoring equipment can be used by the surgeon in the operating room to evaluate tissue perfusion and flow. The Doppler device is critical when pulses cannot be palpated. Using a coupling gel, the unsterile Doppler probe can be placed on the patient's skin distal to the surgical site. Some probes can be sterilized and used directly in the surgical wound to assess the flow in an arterial graft or determine whether the blood supply to the intestines or other structures is intact after aortic surgery. Besides providing an audible signal, the Doppler probe can provide a permanent record of the sound if a recorder is attached. The unit is inexpensive and easily transported. Surgical personnel can use the Doppler probe after minimal training.

An EEG accurately determines reduced cerebral perfusion during a carotid endarterectomy. This enables the

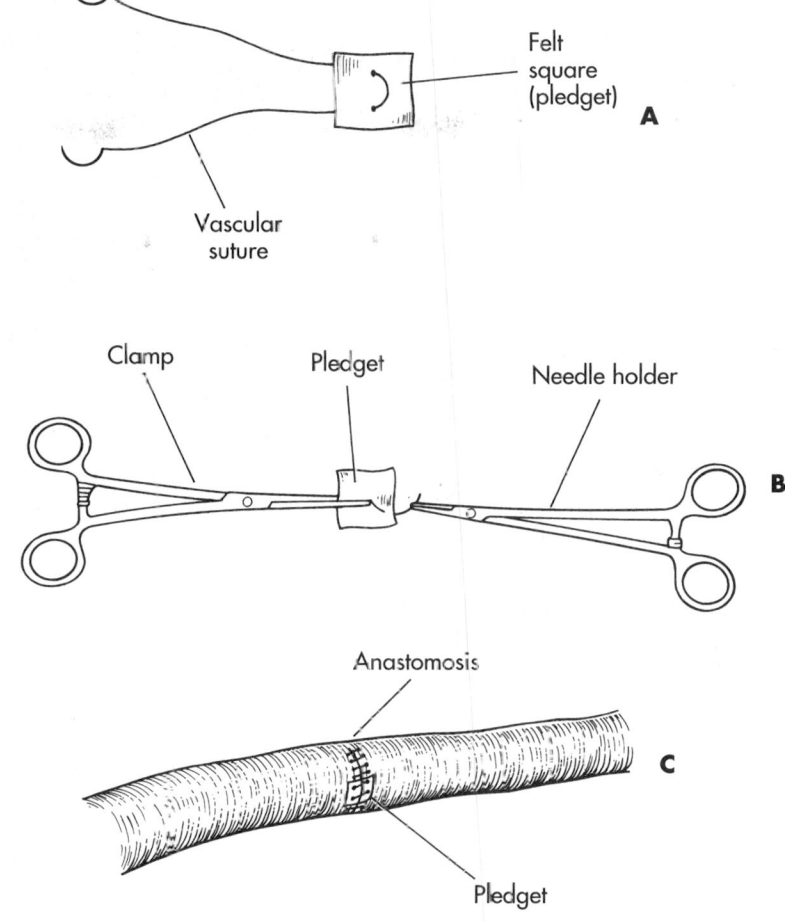

FIGURE 26-7 Pledgeted suture. **A,** Double-armed vascular suture prepared with pledget. **B,** Technique for surgeon to add pledget to suture already in use. **C,** Appearance of suture line with pledget in place.

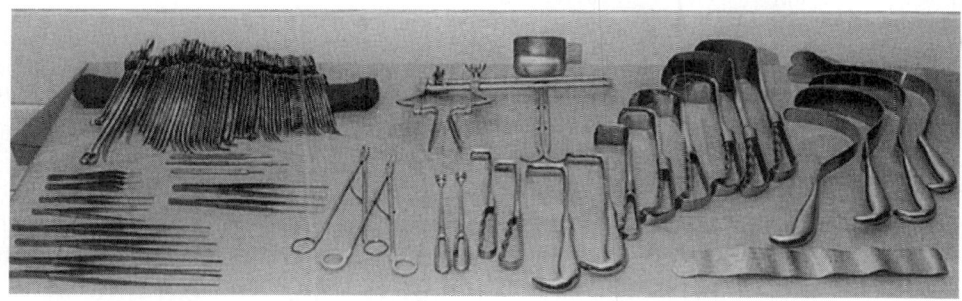

FIGURE 26-8 Basic laparotomy instrument set.

surgeon to decide whether to use a temporary shunt in the carotid artery or if the patient can tolerate clamping. Trained personnel are necessary to operate this equipment.

Instrumentation

The most efficient setup to have is a basic laparotomy set (Fig. 26-8) for scissors, clamps, and retractors (see Chapter 6) and a vascular set (Fig. 26-9) as the foundation for all vascular procedures. The items specific to each surgical procedure are then added. For abdominal surgery, a large self-retaining retractor (that is, an Omni-tract or Bookwalter) should be added. Additional individually wrapped, sterile aortic clamps wrapped individually and sterile and some long clamps (cystic duct and right angle) and long forceps for larger patients should be available in the OR. For peripheral procedures, a variety of Weitlaner self-retaining retractors should be available. Carotid surgery requires carotid shunt clamps and microforceps for

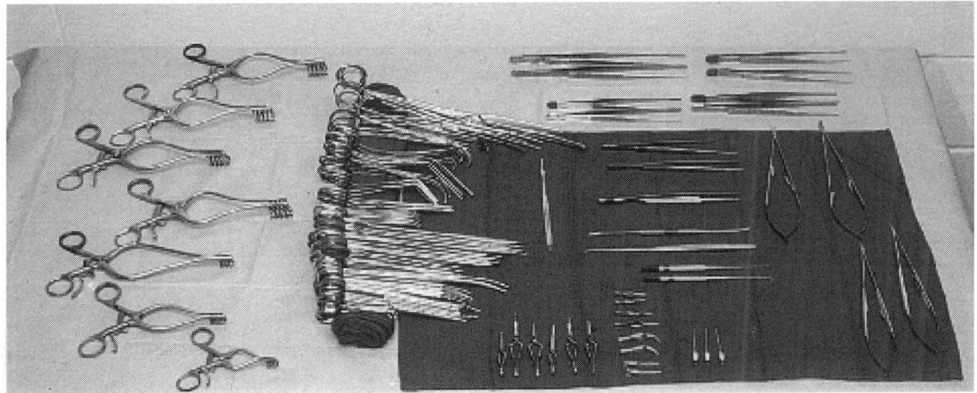

FIGURE 26-9   Basic vascular instrument set.

peeling plaque from the artery. One may use the saphenous vein as a graft conduit by removing and reversing it or by using it in situ. A variety of instruments is available for disrupting the valves to permit arterial flow in the in situ procedure. Amputations do not require vascular instrumentation. A minor basic set and appropriately sized bone instruments are needed.

Documentation

During the implementation of perioperative nursing care, documentation of patient problems and nursing actions addressing these identified problems is important. Every nursing assessment and intervention should be recorded.

Every patient is identified and assessed for allergies; the surgical procedure is verified; and any other interventions performed by the nurse for patient safety and mandated by institution policy are documented. A brief mental status exam is especially important for vascular patients who are at risk for stroke. For a patient undergoing vascular surgery, possible areas to document include the preoperative and postoperative assessment of the integrity of the patient's skin, the presence or absence of peripheral pulses, the surgical position and positioning devices used, fluid intake and output, and the achievement of patient goals. During surgery, various local anesthetic drugs and irrigating solutions, such as thrombin, antibiotic, and heparin solutions, may be used. The scrub nurse should label each container with the solution type and strength. The circulating nurse maintains an accurate record of the solutions used and the amounts administered. The type, size, and serial and lot numbers of vascular implants should be documented according to institutional policy and procedure.

The care provided in the operating room should complement the patient's care preoperatively and postoperatively.

Evaluation

Evaluation is an ongoing process during which the perioperative nurse determines the extent to which the patient goals are met. This phase is continuous throughout implementation of the nursing process. Assessing, observing, and appraising are actions of the perioperative nurse for this phase.

The conclusion of the intraoperative phase is the transfer of the care of the peripheral vascular patient to colleagues in the PACU or the intensive care unit. A nursing report should be given when the perioperative nurse transfers the care of the patient to other individuals. The report should include identification of the patient, the surgical procedure performed, any allergies or special needs, and the achievement of patient outcomes. The outcomes identified for the stated nursing diagnoses could be documented as follows:

- The patient verbalized understanding of the surgical procedure and routines. All questions were answered to the patient's satisfaction. The patient appeared more calm as evidenced by facial expression and other body language.
- Temperature remained within normal limits.
- Fluid balance was maintained. Intake and output were documented.
- Skin intact, no lesions or reddened areas; skin color, temperature, and turgor were adequate.

Patient and Family Education and Discharge Planning
Overview

All postoperative patients need basic instruction on care of surgical wounds, identification of the signs and symptoms of infection, review of medications, follow-up appointments, and a means to contact healthcare providers. Proper hand washing should be reviewed and emphasized to prevent wound infection. Patients who have undergone a lower-extremity arterial bypass are most interested in information that will assist them in recognizing, preventing, and managing complications. They need instruction on incisional care and bathing to optimize incisional healing. Many have had experience with slow healing of wounds because of their arterial disease. Pain, sleep disturbances, and fatigue have been identified as important areas for instruction. One study to determine discharge teaching needs in this population showed that patients are capable of identifying their discharge learning needs in the preoperative period.[19] Patients should be taught to manage the discomfort of incisions and leg swelling to prevent sleep disturbances. The need to balance activity and rest should be emphasized. Patients in the immediate postoperative period are often receptive to counseling on risk-factor modification. Cessation of smoking is an important step to improved wound healing and slowing the progression of the occlusive disease process. The nurse should assess the patient for learning needs about control of hypertension and diabetes and stress and support lifestyle modifications that are attainable and individualized for each patient. Patients may be fearful of limb loss. Providing realistic goals without overwhelming demands will be most productive. Patients must *believe* that their efforts will make a difference in improving their quality of life for lifestyle changes to be sustained.[15]

Patient and family education related to postoperative activities and discharge planning for specific vascular procedures follow.

Varicose vein surgery

- Provide instruction on the proper way to wrap an Ace bandage, the timing of rest and leg elevation, and how to apply manual pressure if bleeding occurs.

Carotid endarterectomy

- Teach patient about possibility of reperfusion headaches (patients may fear that they are having recurrent symptoms unless they know about this possibility).
- Explain that activity may return to normal as tolerated, driving may be resumed when neck discomfort no longer restricts range of motion, and the surgeon has examined patient 2 weeks postoperatively.
- Explain that fatigue for 4 to 6 weeks after surgery is normal.
- Explain incision care: keep incision clean and dry, may shower with transparent dressing in place. Remove transparent dressing in 3 to 4 days. Wash incision with soap and water; pat gently to dry. Avoid the use of powder and lotion. Do not shave over incision until it is well healed.
- Explain that the numbness around the incision and extending to the ear is normal.
- Teach the patient about any cranial nerve deficits that he or she may experience: as a result of manipulation of nerves during surgery. Assist the patient in understanding the difference between an intraoperative stroke and cranial nerve deficits; that is, nerve injury or trauma from surgical manipulation occurs on the same side as surgery except for eye symptoms. Use diagrams and pictures to review pertinent anatomy.

- Encourage relevant lifestyle changes as indicated, that is low-cholesterol diet, review of diabetic diet, smoking cessation.
- Teach the patient and family to observe for and report any new symptoms, TIAs, mental-status changes, personality changes, or speech difficulties.
- If a synthetic patch is in place, explain that the patient will need antibiotics before dental procedures or scope procedures. Instruct the patient to notify dentists and other healthcare providers of this need.

Abdominal aortic aneurysm resection

1. Explain postoperative care procedures:
   a. Intubated and ventilated for 12 hours (varies with setting and surgeon preference).
   b. Monitor cardiac, respiratory, and renal function.
   c. NPO and nasogastric tube until bowel signs and flatus; advance as tolerated.
   d. Assess lower-extremity perfusion hourly.
   e. Assess pain and provide relief; provide periods of rest.
   f. Bedrest, out of bed on postoperative day 2; ambulate on postoperative day 3.
2. Discharge planning:
   a. Reassure patient that feelings of fatigue are normal and take weeks to resolve.
   b. Incision care. Showering is permitted. Use soap and water only and pat dry. Protect incision from oils, lotions, and powder. If Steri-Strips are in place, showering is permitted. The strips will peel away in about 5 days.
   c. Activity with specific restrictions per surgeon.
      (1) Avoid lifting over 5 to 10 pounds for 6 weeks to allow abdominal healing.
      (2) Walk to increase strength and improve circulation; progress gradually.
      (3) Climb stairs and walk out of doors as desired.
      (4) Avoid sitting for more than 1 or 2 hours.
      (5) Avoid crossing legs.
      (6) Driving requires permission from surgeon, usually after first office visit and when patient is no longer taking pain medication.
   d. Smokers should be counseled about the profound effect of smoking on vascular disease and wound healing.
   e. Review all medications and any dietary recommendations.
   f. Antibiotics may be prescribed before any endoscopy procedures, surgery, or dental procedures.
   g. Instruct patient in foot care.
   h. Notify surgeon of the following:
      (1) Changes in wounds (such as redness, swelling, increased tenderness, bleeding, and drainage).
      (2) Fever.
      (3) Change in bowel habits.

*Arterial reconstructive procedures
of the lower extremity*

1. Explain importance of control of diabetes and hypertension.
2. Stress importance of smoking cessation.
3. Teach signs and symptoms of graft failure; teach patient and family to assess pulses.
4. Teach foot care and protection:
   a. Inspect daily (use mirror-assistive methods or have family member help)
   b. Observe for cracks, ulcers, blisters, rashes, or discoloration
   c. Trim nails properly for prevention of ingrown toenails.
   d. Shoes must fit properly (avoid walking barefoot).
   e. Avoid tight socks or hose.
5. Explain incisional care.
6. Teach proper use and application of Ace wraps for leg swelling (normal after surgery).
7. Discuss pain management, sleep disruption, fatigue.
8. Driving with surgeon's approval, after follow-up office visit (approximately 2 weeks postoperatively).
9. No heavy lifting, vigorous exercise, or prolonged upright sitting; walking, stair climbing, and going out of doors is permissible as able.
10. Encourage gentle range-of-motion exercise of leg to prevent flexion contractures
11. Showering is permitted.
12. Diet: resume previous diet, review special diets with patient (diabetic, low salt, low fat); reinforce role of adequate nutrition in wound healing.
13. Notify surgeon of the following:
    a. Return of preoperative symptoms.
    b. Wound changes (redness, swelling, drainage).
    c. Fever.
    d. Change in color, temperature, sensation or use of leg, foot, or toes.
14. Antibiotics may be recommended before any dental or endoscopic procedures if a synthetic graft was implanted.

SURGICAL INTERVENTIONS
ABDOMINAL AORTIC ANEURYSM RESECTION

Abdominal aortic aneurysmectomy is surgical obliteration of the aneurysm, which may or may not include the iliac arteries, with insertion of a synthetic prosthesis to reestablish functional continuity. The majority of abdominal aortic aneurysms begin below the renal arteries, and many extend to involve the bifurcation and common iliac arteries. Severe back pain, along with symptoms of hypotension, shock, and distal vascular insufficiency, usually indicates rupture and represents a true emergency condition. The prime surgical consideration when a

rupture occurs is the control of hemorrhage by occlusion of the aorta proximal to the point of rupture. Abdominal aortic aneurysms (AAAs) are usually asymptomatic and found on routine physical examination. They occur more frequently in men than in women. Aneurysmal disease is caused by a disruption of the media, which structurally weakens the aortic wall. Aneurysmal aortas are found to have a significantly decreased amount of collagen and elastin in the vessel wall.[25] Aneurysms occur most often in the abdominal aorta, thoracic aorta, and the popliteal arteries.[3] An aneurysm with a diameter of 6 cm or more (2 cm is considered normal) has a 42% chance to rupture in 5 years.[16] Rupture carries a 50% mortality. Risks from AAA surgery include massive hemorrhage, injury to the ureters, renal failure, spinal cord ischemia, and death. Since PVD is systemic, it is not surprising that patients with aneurysms often have concomitant coronary artery disease. Patients are at risk of myocardial ischemia, myocardial infarction, hypotension, and hypertension.[25] Myocardial infarction is the leading cause of death after AAA repair; therefore it is imperative that a patient with cardiac symptoms or ECG abnormalities have a thorough preoperative cardiac assessment.[42]

The nurse must be alert to the fact that at the time the aortic clamp is released to permit distal flow "declamping shock" or severe hypotension may occur. This may be attributable to inadequate volume replacement, the sudden reestablishment of flow to vasodilated distal vessels, potassium, or the release of acidic metabolites. This and hemorrhage have been proposed as a the causes of renal failure from acute tubular necrosis.[42]

Procedural considerations

The patient is placed in the supine position. The skin is prepped for a midline abdominal incision, and draping is completed to permit access to the groin region for possible exploration of femoral arteries. The pedal pulses should be marked before the beginning of the procedure so that they may be located immediately if the surgeon requests a check of the pulses. This assessment of pulses can be done manually or with an ultrasonic instrument (Doppler probe).

Operative procedure

1. The abdomen is opened through a midline incision (Fig. 26-10, *A*) from the xiphoid process to the symphysis pubis. Hemostasis is accomplished, and exploration is completed as described for laparotomy (see Chapter 11).
2. An abdominal self-retaining retractor is inserted into the wound. If necessary for exposure, a portion of the small bowel can be placed outside the abdomen and covered with moist laparotomy packs.
3. The parietal peritoneum is incised over the aorta and extended superiorly to expose the aneurysm and also inferiorly over the bifurcation and beyond the iliac

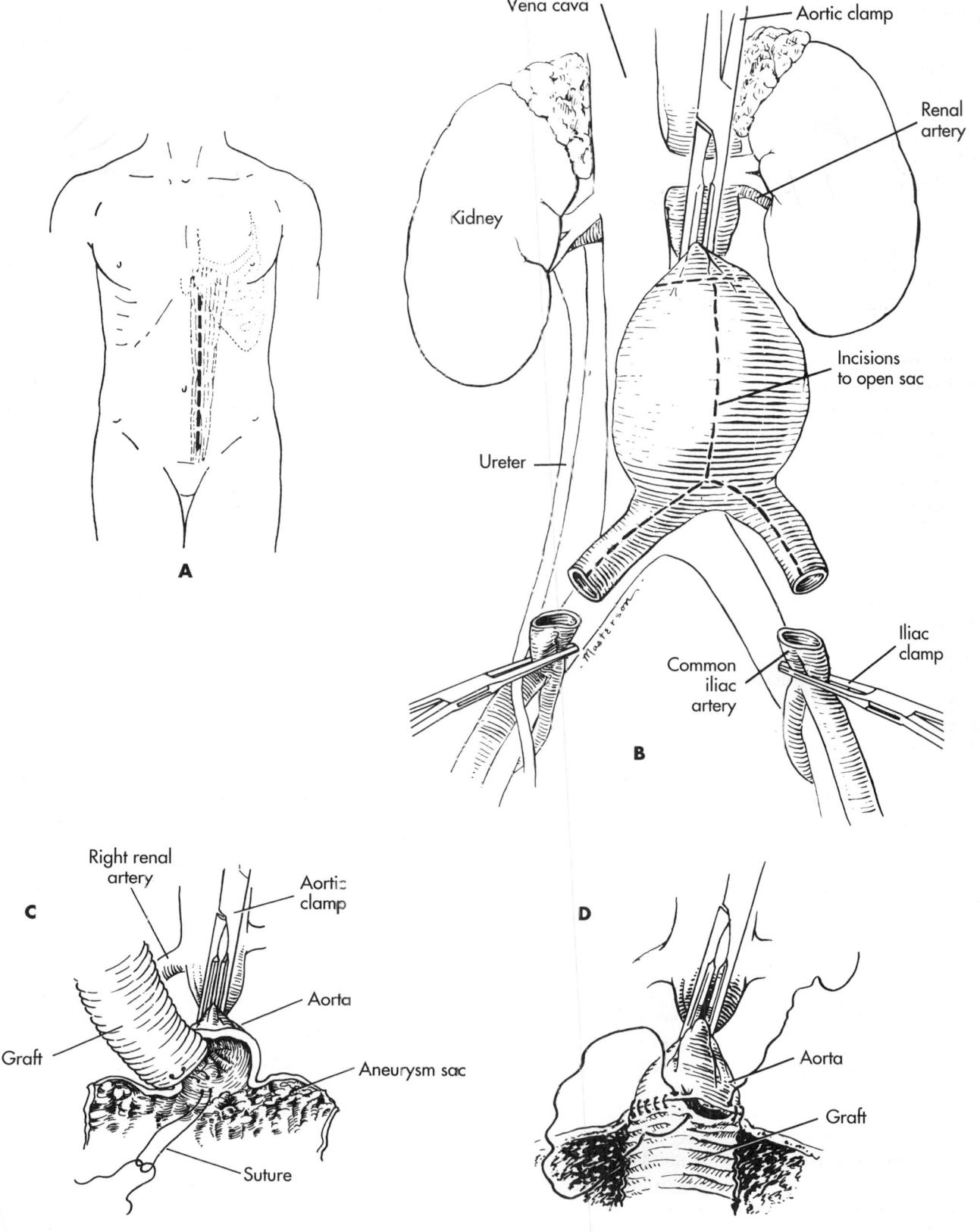

FIGURE 26-10   Resection of abdominal aortic aneurysm. **A**, Midline abdominal incision. **B**, Aneurysm sac is opened. **C**, Prosthetic graft is sewn to back wall of aorta, creating a cuff. **D**, Completion of aortic graft anastomosis.

Continued

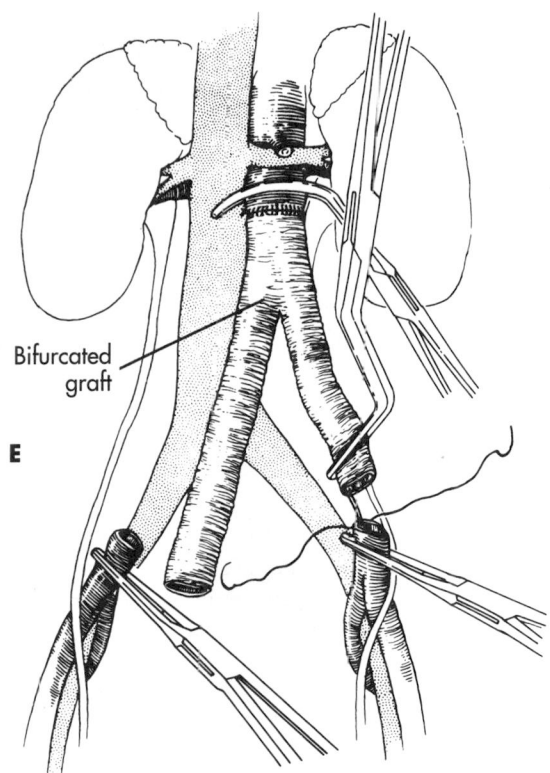

FIGURE 26-10, cont'd Resection of abdominal aortic aneurysm. **E**, Iliac artery anastomosis.

arteries. Metzenbaum scissors, smooth forceps, and hemostats are used.

4. Careful blunt and sharp dissection is continued to expose the aorta above the aneurysm to permit placement of an aortic clamp. The renal artery and ureters are avoided. The iliac vessels and bifurcation are inspected for evidence of small aneurysms, thrombosis, and calcification.

5. An aortic clamp such as a DeBakey, Fogarty, or Satinsky is applied and closed. Opening of the aneurysm is undertaken with a scalpel or electrosurgical blade and heavy scissors (Fig. 26-10, B).

6. The aneurysm is completely opened, and all atheromatous and thrombotic material is removed. The aneurysm walls may be excised but usually are left in place for eventual coverage of the prosthesis. In either case the posterior aspect of the aorta is left intact (Fig. 26-10, C). Bleeding is controlled, especially from the lumbar vessels, which enter posteriorly.

7. A prosthetic graft of appropriate size is prepared for insertion. If the aneurysm does not involve the aortic bifurcation, a straight tubular graft is used; otherwise a bifurcated or Y-shaped graft is necessary. Preclotting of a knitted graft may be accomplished by immersing the graft into a small quantity of the patient's own blood before systemic heparinization.

8. The aortic cuff is prepared for anastomosis by irrigating it with heparinized saline solution and by removing all fibrotic plaques. One or two vascular

sutures (double armed) are used to accomplish the anastomosis by a through-and-through continuous suture (Fig. 26-10, D). Additional interrupted sutures may be needed if the anastomosis leaks on completion.

9. The distal vessels are opened and inspected for backbleeding, and heparinized saline solution may be injected to prevent clotting.

10. Each limb of the graft is anastomosed to the iliac artery, using a smaller vascular suture and similar technique. After the first side of the anastomosis has been completed, blood is permitted to circulate, and the remaining limb of the graft is clamped to prevent leaking during the last part of the anastomosis (Fig. 26-10, E).

11. The aneurysm is closed over the graft.

12. The abdominal wound is closed.

FEMORAL-POPLITEAL AND FEMORAL-TIBIAL BYPASS

Femoral-popliteal bypass is the restoration of blood flow to the leg with a graft bypassing the occluded section of the femoral artery. The bypass may be a saphenous vein or straight synthetic graft. The patency of an outflow artery must be demonstrated for a successful bypass procedure. If popliteal patency is doubtful, artery exploration is necessary as the first procedure. Involvement of the popliteal artery may necessitate the exposure and use of the tibial vessels for the lower anastomosis. If this occurs, the procedure could require the use of microvascular instruments and technique.

Procedural considerations

The patient is placed in a supine position. The hip is externally rotated and abducted with the knee flexed. Prepping and draping include the entire groin and leg. The instrument setup includes the basic minor and vascular sets, plus the following: Gelpi retractors, Garrett or Weitlaner retractors, a tunneler, and supplies and equipment for operative arteriograms.

Operative procedures
Exploration of Common Femoral Artery

1. A vertical incision, extending downward about 3 to 5 inches along the medial aspect of the thigh, is made over the femoral artery below the inguinal area, and a self-retaining retractor is inserted (Fig. 26-11).

2. The common femoral artery is located, and the artery is dissected in both directions for complete exposure.

3. Moist umbilical tapes or vessel loops are passed around the common femoral, the superficial femoral, and the deep femoral arteries.

Exploration of Above-Knee Popliteal Artery

1. A vertical incision is made along the medial aspect of the lower area of the thigh. If the popliteal artery is

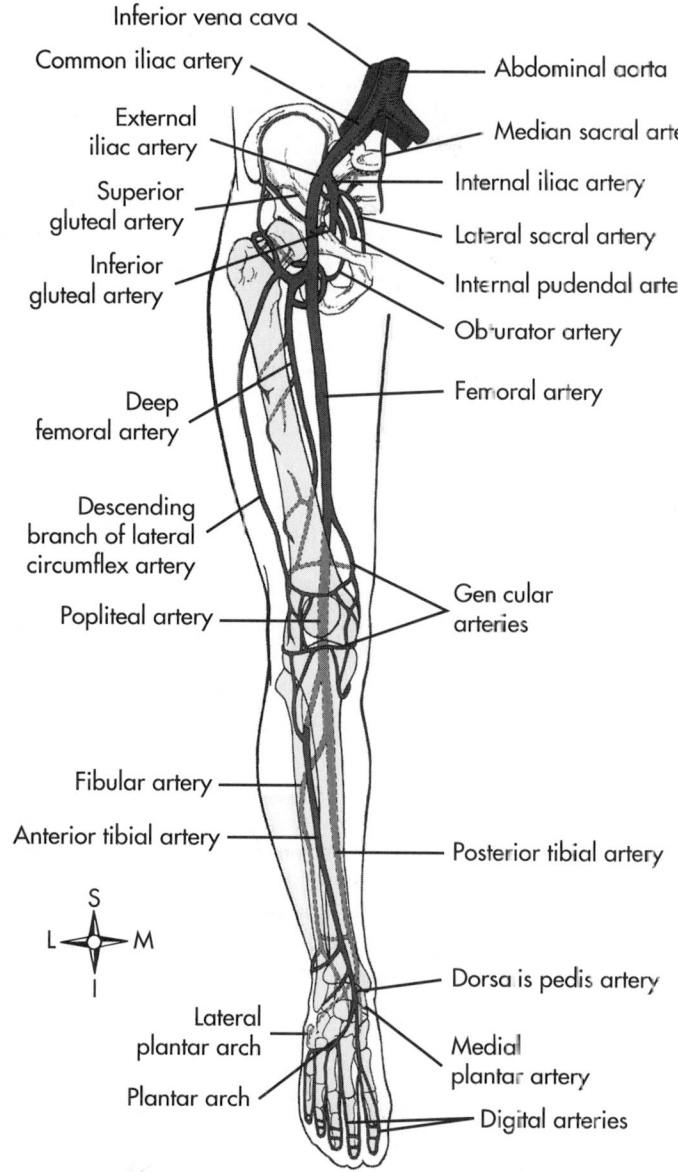

Inferior vena cava
Common iliac artery
External iliac artery
Superior gluteal artery
Inferior gluteal artery
Deep femoral artery
Descending branch of lateral circumflex artery
Popliteal artery
Fibular artery
Anterior tibial artery
Lateral plantar arch
Plantar arch

Abdominal aorta
Median sacral artery
Internal iliac artery
Lateral sacral artery
Internal pudendal artery
Obturator artery
Femoral artery
Genicular arteries
Posterior tibial artery
Dorsalis pedis artery
Medial plantar artery
Digital arteries

S
L — M
I

FIGURE 26-11   Major arteries of the lower extremity.

diseased, an incision below the knee is necessary to expose the distal popliteal artery.

2. A Weitlaner retractor is used to retract the muscles and expose the artery.

3. The knee is flexed, the popliteal artery is dissected free, and a moist umbilical tape is passed around the popliteal artery. It may be desirable at this time to perform arteriograms if doubt exists about the patency of the popliteal artery or distal arterial tree.

4. The saphenous vein is exposed when the femoral and popliteal incisions the length of the thigh are joined or through multiple short incisions along the medial area of the thigh. If the vein is suitable, the necessary length is resected or prepared for in situ grafting. If a prosthesis is used, the length and size are determined, and the graft may be preclotted as previously described.

5. The saphenous vein is prepared for use by carefully ligating side branches with fine silk. Finally, because of venous valves, the vein is reversed so that the end originally in the groin is anastomosed to the popliteal artery.

6. For a synthetic graft, the tunneler is passed beneath the sartorius muscle from the popliteal fossa to the groin.

7. The graft is carefully pulled through the tunnel and positioned to prevent kinks or twists.

8. An incision is made into the femoral artery with a #11 knife blade and extended with a Potts angulated scissors.

9. The graft is anastomosed to the artery with fine vascular sutures.

10. The knee is flexed, and vascular clamps are placed on the popliteal artery at the site of the distal anastomosis.

11. An incision is made into the popliteal artery as explained for the femoral arteriotomy.

12. The graft is sutured to the popliteal (or tibial) artery, and before completion the femoral occluding clamp is momentarily opened to eliminate air and debris.

13. All occluding clamps are removed, and the graft is assessed for anastomotic leaks.

14. The incision is closed as described previously.

Femoral-Popliteal Bypass In Situ

In situ femoral-popliteal bypass is the restoration of blood flow to the leg, bypassing an occluded portion of the femoral artery with a patient's saphenous vein, which remains in place. The procedure includes incising the venous valves and interrupting the venous tributaries. The adequacy of the patient's saphenous vein can be validated before the surgical procedure by an ultrasound duplex scan. Varicose veins or a previous saphenous vein ligation and stripping are contraindications to the procedure. The advantages of a vein-bypass procedure include increased graft availability and improved patency. A disadvantage is the time-consuming aspect of this technique. Valves can be incised with microvascular scissors, a Mills valvulotome, or a leather in situ valve cutter kit. An angioscope may be used to monitor the lysis of valve leaflets.

Operative procedure

1. The procedure is like that for a femoral-popliteal bypass. The groin incision is extended downward over the course of the saphenous vein. A skin bridge may be left between the groin and the popliteal incisions.

2. The saphenous vein is exposed and divided at its proximal and distal ends. Venous tributaries are occluded with vessel clips, such as hemoclips, or fine nonabsorbable sutures.

3. The valvulotome is passed from below to the top, usually through side branches. The valvulotome is used to incise the internal valve (see Fig. 26-6). In angioscopically assisted bypass, valve lysis is done under direct vision.

4. The saphenous vein is distended with heparinized

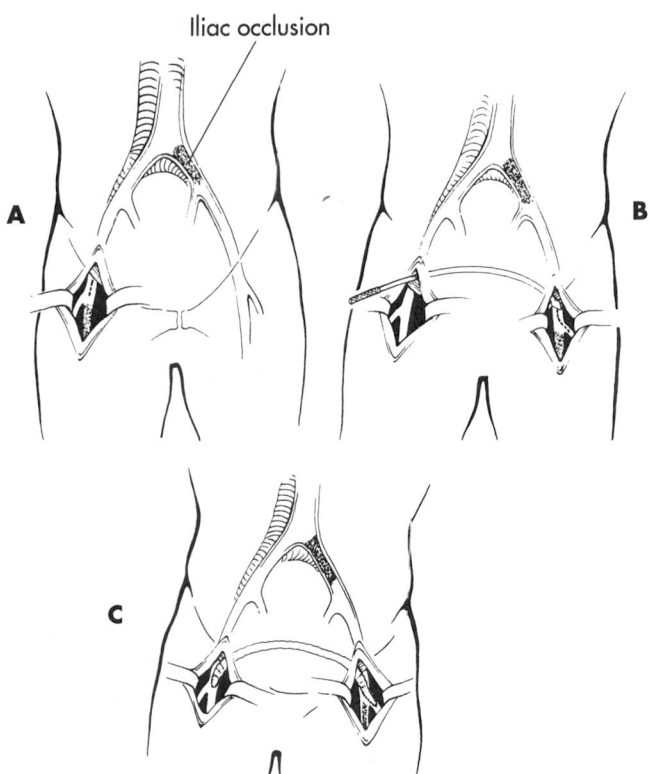

FIGURE 26-12   Femorofemoral bypass to restore blood flow to left leg. **A,** Left iliac artery occlusion and right femoral artery exposure. **B,** Exposure of the right and left femoral arteries: tunneling device creating a path for the graft in the subcutaneous tissue. **C,** Femoro-femoral bypass graft in place.

saline, papaverine, or heparinized blood to identify any valvular obstruction or open venous tributary. Another pass of the valve cutter alleviates the obstruction. Open branches of the saphenous vein can also be ligated with vessel clips or fine nonabsorbable sutures.

5. The incompetent saphenous vein is used to bypass the occluded segment of the femoral artery (see steps 11 to 14 of the femoral-popliteal bypass procedure).

FEMOROFEMORAL BYPASS

Femorofemoral bypass is an extraanatomic (a route that is outside the normal path) bypass that is performed to restore blood flow to one leg when an inflow procedure is necessary but a major aortic procedure is not desired or surgical risks for the patient are high because of a complicated medical condition or technical problems with the procedure (Fig. 26-12). Severe cardiac or pulmonary disease may prevent the patient from undergoing a more extensive procedure. Subcutaneous vascular grafting is an option in these conditions because the procedure bypasses normal vascular anatomy and can be done under local anesthesia with adjunct sedation. The patient must have one good iliac artery for inflow for a femorofemoral bypass

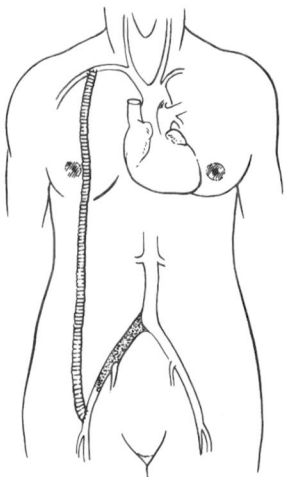

FIGURE 26-13   Axillofemoral bypass graft for right iliac artery occlusion.

to be considered. Another extraanatomic procedure that can be done in these instances is an axillofemoral bypass involving the subcutaneous placement of a prosthesis from the axillary artery to the femoral artery on the same side (Fig. 26-13).

Procedural considerations

The patient is positioned on the operating room bed in a supine position. For a femorofemoral bypass, a small pad is placed under each knee. The area prepared for surgery extends from the umbilicus to midthigh area. The genitalia are covered with a sterile towel.

Operative procedure

1. A longitudinal incision is made over each femoral artery from the inguinal ligament to just below the femoral bifurcation.
2. Each common femoral, superficial femoral, and deep femoral artery is dissected free, mobilized, and secured with umbilical tapes or vessel loops.
3. The graft tunnel between the two femoral arteries is created across the symphysis pubis in the subcutaneous tissue. This tunnel is created with digital dissection, scissors dissection, or the passage of a clamp or tunneler across the preperitoneal space.
4. A Dacron or PTFE vascular graft is passed through the subcutaneous tunnel with care to prevent kinking of the graft.
5. Vascular clamps are placed on the common femoral, superficial femoral, and deep femoral arteries. A longitudinal arteriotomy is made in the common femoral artery.
6. An end-to-side anastomosis using nonabsorbable vascular sutures is performed to join the graft with the common femoral artery. A similar anastomosis is done on the other side.
7. After the clamps are released and flow is restored, the

patient's pulses are checked; the circulating nurse may be asked to inspect the patient's feet.

8. The femoral incisions are closed.

ARTERIAL EMBOLECTOMY

Arterial embolectomy entails an incision made in the affected artery to remove thromboembolic material (Fig. 26-14) and restore blood flow. Emboli may be clot particles, a foreign body, air, fat, or a tumor that circulates through the bloodstream and becomes lodged as the vessel decreases in size. More often the direct source is a cardiac mural thrombus, associated with cardiac or vascular disease. Pain or numbness distal to the obstruction is the initial symptom, accompanied by other signs of vascular occlusion, such as pallor and absence of pulses.

Procedural considerations

The patient is placed in the supine position, the skin area is prepped, and draping is completed to permit access to the affected area. The instrument setup includes the basic instrument and vascular sets, including Fogarty embolectomy catheters.

Operative procedure

1. The initial incision is completed, and the artery is carefully exposed to permit the application of vascular clamps (Fig. 26-14, *A* and *B*).
2. An incision is made into the artery with a #11 blade and a Potts scissors. A Fogarty catheter is carefully inserted beyond the point of clot proximally and distally. The balloon is inflated, and the catheter is withdrawn along with the detached clot (Fig. 26-14, *C* and *D*).
3. As backflow is obtained, a vascular clamp is applied below the arteriotomy (Fig. 26-14, *E*).
4. The artery may be flushed by injection of heparinized saline solution through a small irrigating catheter. Angioscopy or an arteriogram may or may not be requested at this time.
5. The arterial closure is completed with vascular sutures (Fig. 26-14, *F*). The wound closure is accomplished in the usual manner, and dressings are applied.

AMPUTATION

Amputations involving the lower extremity are performed to eliminate ischemic, gangrenous, necrotic, or infected tissue, relieve pain, and promote maximum independence. Amputations may be necessary because of trauma or malignancy. It is critical to verify the correct limb for this procedure. Since these are often performed under regional anesthesia, the nurse must be sure that the patient does not witness the wrapping or transport of the amputated limb. Toes or partial foot amputations may be done in certain instances, but often a BK or AK

amputation is indicated. The Syme amputation, through the ankle, is seldom performed because of improved prosthetics and rehabilitation that favor midcalf amputation.[36] The level is based on the patient's health, the level of vascularity, and potential for healing and rehabilitation. Severe infection or toxemia may require amputation as a life-saving procedure. Operative risks for amputation are higher than for reconstruction possibly because of more extensive vascular disease.[45] BK amputations are best done at the junction of the upper and middle third of the lower leg. This allows an immediate postoperative prosthesis, aids in better healing, and may reduce phantom limb pain. AK amputations may be at the middle or lower third of the thigh. Flaps are tailored to provide fascial and skin coverage to cushion the smoothed end of the bone. Meticulous hemostasis and drainage are needed to decrease hematoma formation, since healing is both problematic and critical in these patients. Diabetics are at highest risk for amputation because of their neuropathy, altered response to infection, and vascular insufficiency. Diabetics are 20 times more likely to have vascular disease than the general population. Minor trauma to the feet is the most common cause of diabetic foot ulcers.[21]

Operative procedure

1. The level of amputation is determined, and the incision line is marked to create a long posterior flap for a BK amputation. For an AK amputation, the anterior and posterior flaps are fairly equal (Fig. 26-15).
2. The incision is made. Muscle and soft tissue are divided. Periosteum is raised with an elevator.
3. Bones are cut, with beveling of their anterior aspect and smoothing with a rongeur and rasp.
4. The wound is irrigated, and hemostasis is achieved.
5. A drain may be inserted.
6. Fascia is closed with interrupted sutures.
7. Skin is approximated and closed with interrupted suture or staples.
8. An immediate postoperative stump dressing may be applied.

CAROTID ENDARTERECTOMY

Carotid endarterectomy is the removal of an atheroma at the carotid artery bifurcation to increase cerebral perfusion and decrease the risk of embolization. A clinical pathway for carotid endarterectomy is shown in Fig. 26-16. Lessening the likelihood of any transient or permanent neurologic deficit is a major concern during a carotid endarterectomy. The use of a temporary carotid artery shunt, such as an Argyle (Fig. 26-17) or Javid shunt, allows for a continuous blood flow through the carotid artery and to the brain. Some disadvantages in using this temporary device are the additional dissection necessary for its placement and the possibility of dislodging debris when the shunt is inserted as well as a difficult view of the

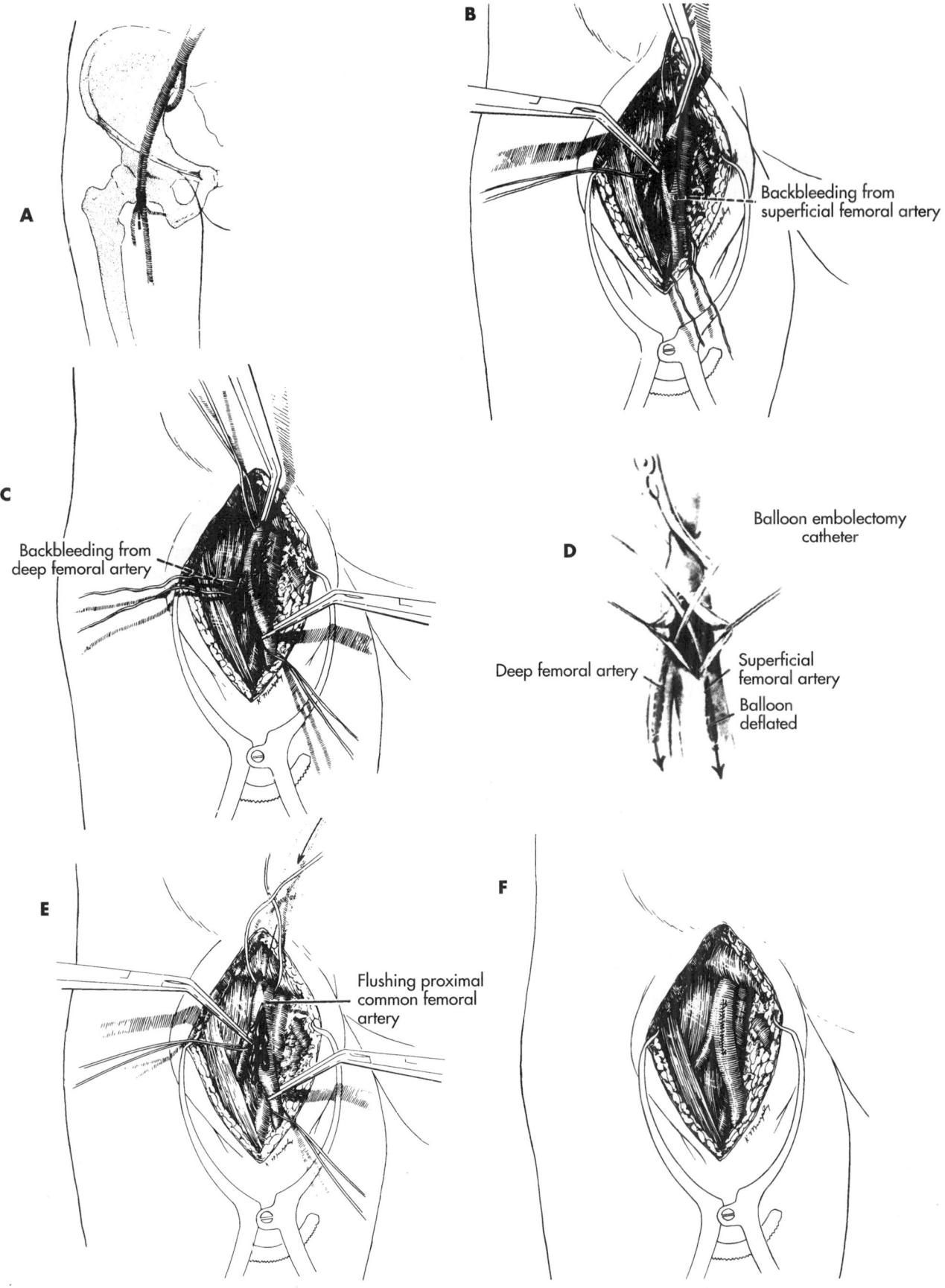

FIGURE 26-14 Femoral embolectomy. **A,** Femoral arteriotomy. **B,** Clamp on common femoral and deep femoral (profunda femoris) arteries. Backflow of blood from superficial femoral artery (SFA) is checked. **C,** Clamp on common femoral artery and SFA. Backflow of blood from deep femoral artery is checked. **D,** Balloon embolectomy catheters are passed into SFA and profunda. **E,** Proximal (common femoral artery) is unclamped and flushed. **F,** Arteriotomy is closed.

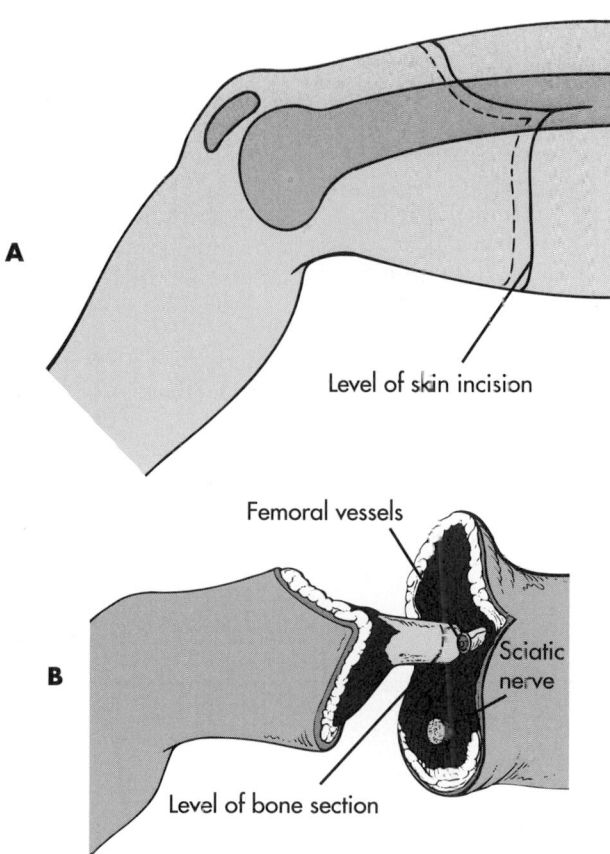

A

Level of skin incision

Femoral vessels

B

Sciatic nerve

Level of bone section

FIGURE 26-15 Leg amputation, above knee, through the middle third of the thigh. **A**, Level of skin incision. **B**, Level of bone resection.

endarterectomy end point and increased difficulty in suturing a patch.

Two techniques that facilitate continual assessment of cerebral perfusion are the use of cervical block anesthesia or electroencephalography. A conscious patient under cervical block anesthesia can be observed for neurologic deficits encountered during the procedure. In addition, the patient under general anesthesia can be monitored with an EEG. If either method demonstrates reduced cerebral perfusion, the surgeon may decide to use a temporary carotid artery shunt. The shunting device should always be available and sterile at the beginning of the procedure.

Procedural considerations

The patient is placed on the operating room bed in a supine position with the head supported on a head support. The head is turned away from the operative side, and the neck may be slightly hyperextended. A roll may be placed between the scapulae.

Operative procedure

1. A longitudinal incision is made over the area of the carotid bifurcation (Fig. 26-18, *A*). The Weitlaner self-retaining retractor may be placed for exposure.

2. With Metzenbaum scissors, the soft tissue is dissected for exposure of the carotid artery and its bifurcation (Fig. 26-18, *B*).

3. A moistened umbilical tape or vessel loop is passed around the vessel for ease of handling. The patient is systemically heparinized.

4. The external, common, and internal carotid arteries are clamped.

5. With a #11 scalpel blade, an arteriotomy is made over the stenotic area. The incision is lengthened with a Potts angulated scissors to expose the full extent of the occluding plaque.

6. With a blunt dissector, the plaque or plaques are dissected free from the arterial wall. Heparin solution is used as an irrigant to clean the intima.

7. The arteriotomy is closed with fine vascular sutures. A synthetic (polyester or polytetrafluoroethylene) or autogenous (vein) patch graft may be used to restore the arterial lumen if it is small (Fig. 26-19). Before complete closure, blood flow is temporarily restored through the arteries to wash away any free plaques, air, or thrombi. For this to be done, the occluding clamps are opened and closed individually, with flushing of any debris away from the internal carotid artery. The closure of the arteriotomy is completed (Fig. 26-20).

8. The occluding clamps are removed from the external and common carotid arteries; *the internal carotid artery clamp is removed last.* This sequence ensures that any minor debris missed will be flushed harmlessly into the external rather than the internal carotid artery.

9. Additional interrupted sutures may be needed to control leakage.

10. A drain is inserted via a separate stab incision.

11. The wound closure is accomplished in the usual manner, and dressings are applied.

CAROTID ENDARTERECTOMY WITH SHUNT

Operative procedure

1-5. The first five steps as described for carotid endarterectomy are followed.

6. A piece of tubing (polyethylene or Silastic) with a suture tied around its center or a commercially prepared shunt device is inserted into the common carotid artery and the internal carotid artery to maintain cerebral blood flow and is held with vessel loops or shunt clamps (Fig. 26-21).

7. The plaque is removed as described for carotid endarterectomy.

8. The arteriotomy is closed with or without a patch.

9. Before the arteriotomy closure is completed, the shunt clamp or vessel loop on the internal carotid artery is released, and the shunt is removed. The external carotid occluding clamp is removed, followed

1. Focus of clinical path: Carotid endarterectomy

2. Timeline:		Preoperative: 60-90 minutes	Intraoperative: 90-120 minutes	Postoperative: 60-90 minutes
3. Patient Care Problems		Preoperative:	Intraoperative:	Postoperative:
A. Carotid stenosis List existing neurodeficit _____ _____ _____

B. Risk for altered cerebral perfusion

C. Risk for fluid - volume excess

D. Risk for injury | 4. I N T E R V E N T I O N S | • Identify patient

• Reinforce patient and family teaching

• Confirm operative site

• Secure results of diagnostic tests: arteriogram, labs, ECG

• Document baseline neuroassessment

• Assess skin integrity | • Utilize safety measures
• Safe transport/transfer
• Head/neck/arm positioning with appropriate aids
• Electrosurgical dispersive pad
• Containment of surgical prep solutions

• Assist anesthesia provider
  — With induction
  — With hemodynamic monitoring

• Prepare skin at surgical incision site

• Appropriate use of intraoperative medication/fluids/devices
  — Heparin
  — Surgicel
  — Lidocaine
  — IV fluids
  — Shunts

• Create and maintain sterile field

• Perform counts

• Communicate with family | • VS q15min

• Neurocheck q30min

• Assess wound drainage q30min

• Observe for signs of tracheal edema q30min

• Assess skin integrity |
| 5. E X P E C T E D   O U T C O M E S | | Immediate:
• Free from physical, chemical, or electrical injury

• Normothermic

• Maintain preoperative level of neurofunction

• Free of hematoma at incision site | Discharge from PACU:
• Maintain VS within acceptable baseline limits

• Free of hematoma at incision site

• Freedom from or slight tracheal edema | |
| 6. V A R I A N C E S | | For concurrent intervention:
• Preoperative and postoperative neurofunction

• Impaired skin integrity

• Return to OR for hemostasis | For retrospective analysis:
• New postoperative onset of neurodeficit

• Impaired skin integrity

• Return to OR for hemostasis | |

VS, Vital signs.

FIGURE 26–16   Clinical pathway for carotid endarterectomy.

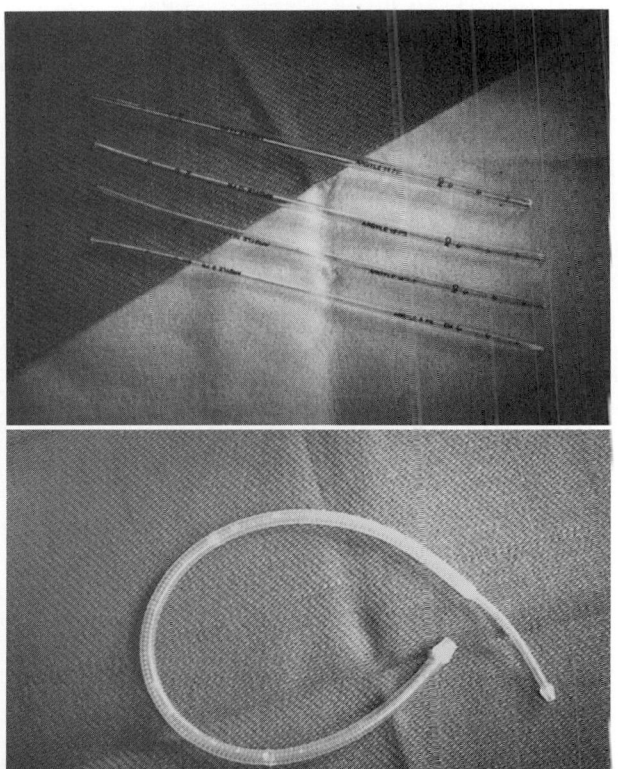

FIGURE 26-17   Example of temporary carotid artery shunts that are used to permit blood flow during carotid endarterectomy procedures.

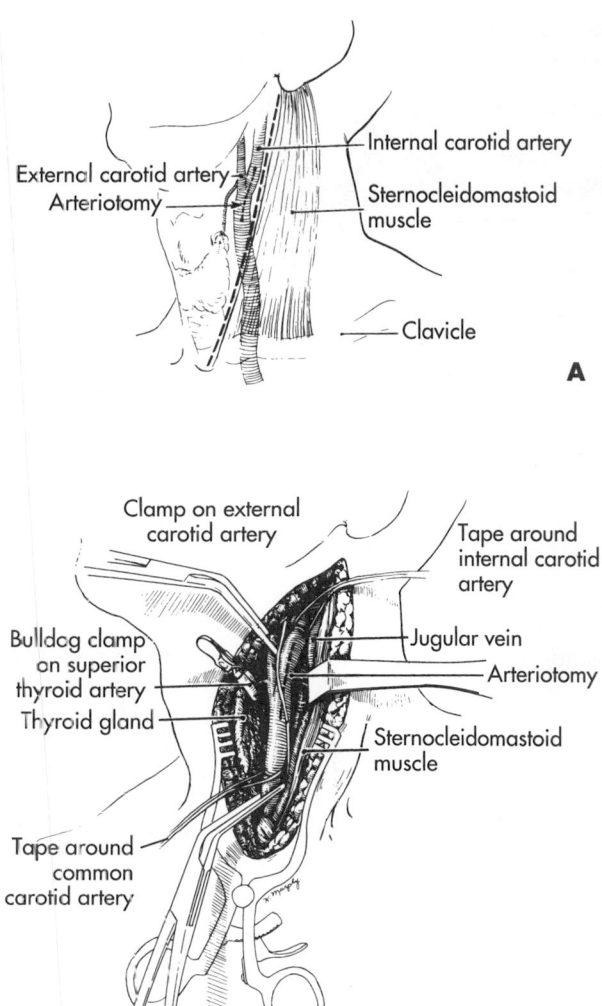

FIGURE 26-18   Left carotid endarterectomy. **A,** Incision and anatomy. **B,** Exposure of carotid bifurcation.

by the common carotid artery clamp, and last, the internal carotid artery occluding clamp.

10. The wound is closed in the usual manner.

ARTERIOVENOUS FISTULA

Arteriovenous fistulas, direct connections between an artery and a vein, are the standard means of vascular access for long-term renal dialysis. The dilated vein would then be used for direct cannulation with large-bore needles for hemodialysis. This method is preferable to an external shunt, which carries a high risk of thrombosis and infection. An alternative is created by a conduit between an artery and a vein, referred to as an *arteriovenous shunt*, or *bridge fistula.*[22] The best access is achieved using the patient's own vessels and creating a subcutaneous connection between the artery and vein. Other choices include using a bovine carotid artery, human umbilical vein graft, or a synthetic vascular graft, usually PTFE (polytetrafluoroethylene).[4] Approximately 80% of all fistulas placed (including revisions) use PTFE.[38] Four anastomoses that can be created between the artery and vein include side of artery to side of vein, end of artery to side of vein, end of vein to side of artery, and end of vein to end of artery (spatulated)[17] (Fig. 26-22). The Brescia-Cimino fistula is a connection between the radial artery and cephalic vein at

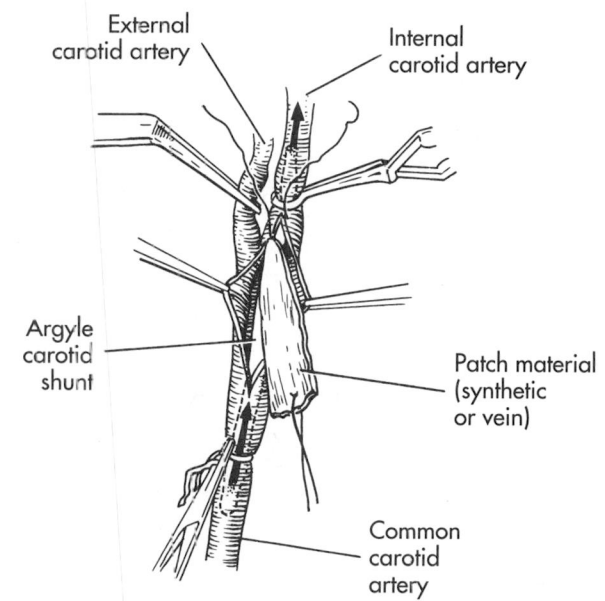

FIGURE 26-19   Left carotid endarterectomy illustrating initial placement and suturing of a patch (a shunt is in place).

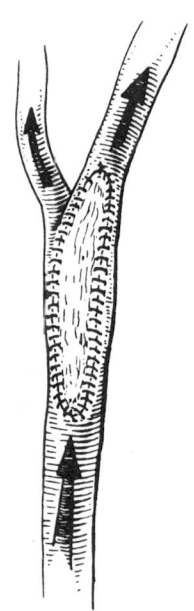

FIGURE 26-20 Left carotid endarterectomy (patch angioplasty) with patch sewn in place.

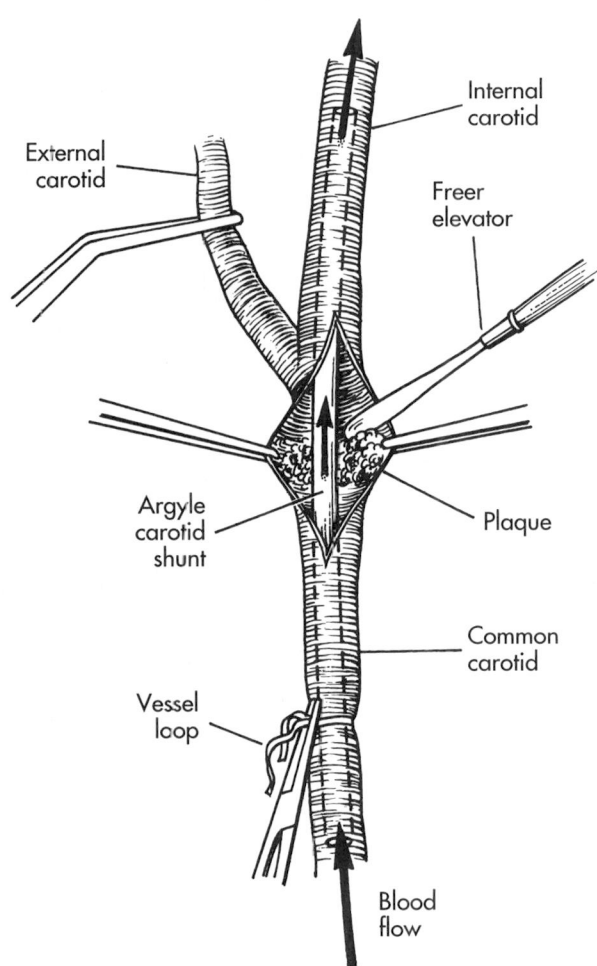

FIGURE 26-21 Left carotid endarterectomy. Argyle carotid shunt in place to allow blood flow to the brain. Stenotic plaque being removed with Freer elevator.

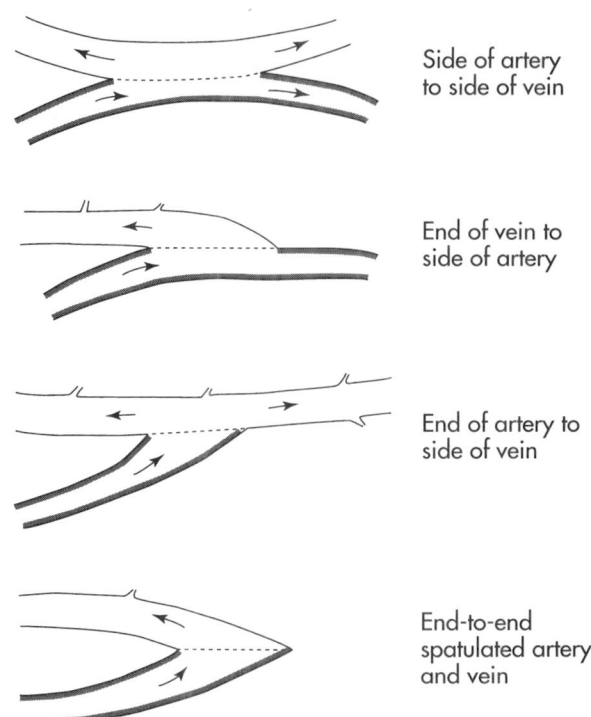

Side of artery to side of vein

End of vein to side of artery

End of artery to side of vein

End-to-end spatulated artery and vein

FIGURE 26-22 Four types of anastomoses between radial artery and cephalic vein.

Arteriovenous anastomosis

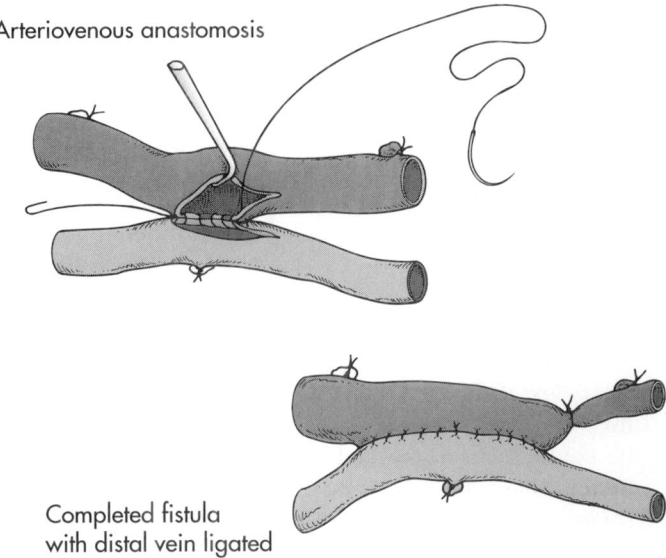

Completed fistula with distal vein ligated

FIGURE 26-23 Arteriovenous anastomosis. The artery is anastomosed to the vein.

the wrist (Fig. 26–23). A basic principle of creating a fistula is to start in the distal arm and move proximally with subsequent fistulas. These include ulnar artery to basilic vein and brachial artery to brachial or cephalic vein[14] (Fig. 26–24).

Arteriovenous fistulas are indicated for long-term renal dialysis access. Patients with end-stage renal disease have their creatinine clearance levels followed. When the

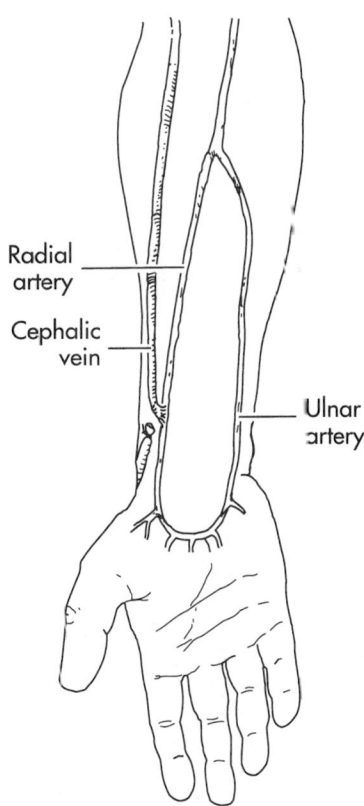

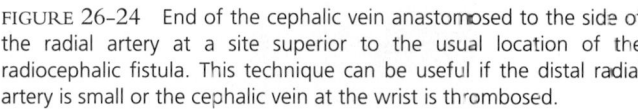

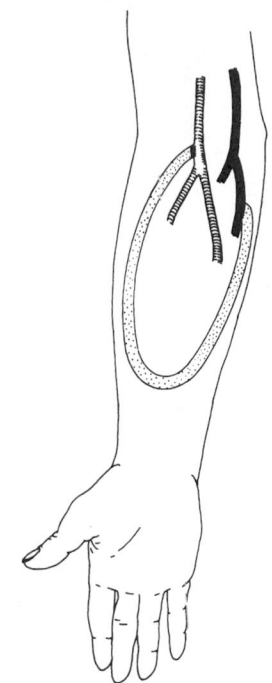

FIGURE 26-24 End of the cephalic vein anastomosed to the side of the radial artery at a site superior to the usual location of the radiocephalic fistula. This technique can be useful if the distal radial artery is small or the cephalic vein at the wrist is thrombosed.

FIGURE 26-25 An example of a loop fistula. A synthetic graft has been used to create a loop brachiocephalic fistula.

creatinine clearance falls to 10 ml/min, a Cimino fistula may be created in anticipation of the need for dialysis. A Cimino (or Brescia-Cimino) type of fistula has proved to have the longest patency and lowest infection rate. It is created to connect the patient's artery to a vein that will "arterialize" or dilate and become thick walled (its muscle layer hypertrophies). This occurs from the high rate of blood flow delivered by the connection to the artery. The arterialization, or maturation process, necessary to allow the fistula to withstand the repeated needle punctures of dialysis takes about 3 weeks.[17]

Bridge fistulas do not need to mature and therefore are available for immediate dialysis use. For connections between an artery and a vein that are in proximity, a U-shaped graft is placed. Grafts that are far apart require a straight or slightly curved graft. Patency rates for bridge grafts using PTFE grafts are reported to be 70% to 80% at 1 year, which is comparable with the Cimino fistula in comparable patients. Although saphenous vein, umbilical vein graft, and bovine carotid artery are used, the PTFE grafts work the best and are most commonly used for bridge fistulas.[4] Some surgeons prefer to use a specially designed PTFE step-graft, or tapered graft. These have a short segment of 4 mm in diameter at one end and the majority of the graft with a 7 mm diameter. This graft may

avoid steal or an output or flow rate that is so high it causes cardiac overload.[59] Primary sites for bridge fistulas include the upper arm between the brachial artery and axillary vein and the forearm between the brachial artery and antecubital vein or brachial artery and basilic vein (Fig. 26-25). The axillofemoral graft for dialysis is reserved for those patients who have exhausted other fistula sites. A regular-walled (versus a thin-walled) graft is placed from the axillary artery to the common femoral vein. PTFE grafts may be used immediately, but it may be better to wait 2 weeks for anastomotic healing to occur.

The side-to-side fistula was the original subcutaneous method introduced by Brescia in 1966. The side-to-side fistula is technically the easiest to perform and creates the highest flow rate. The arterial end–to–vein side fistula decreases the incidence of distal arterial "steal" but has a lower flow rate. The arterial side–to–vein end fistula is technically more difficult to create but has a lower incidence of venous hypertension. The end-to-end construction has the lowest rate of either venous hypertension or steal but also has the lowest flow rate.[4] There is a trend toward performing fewer side-to-side fistulas and more artery side-to-vein end fistulas.[40]

Because the patency of fistulas is limited, dialysis patients return for revision or embolectomy in attempts to

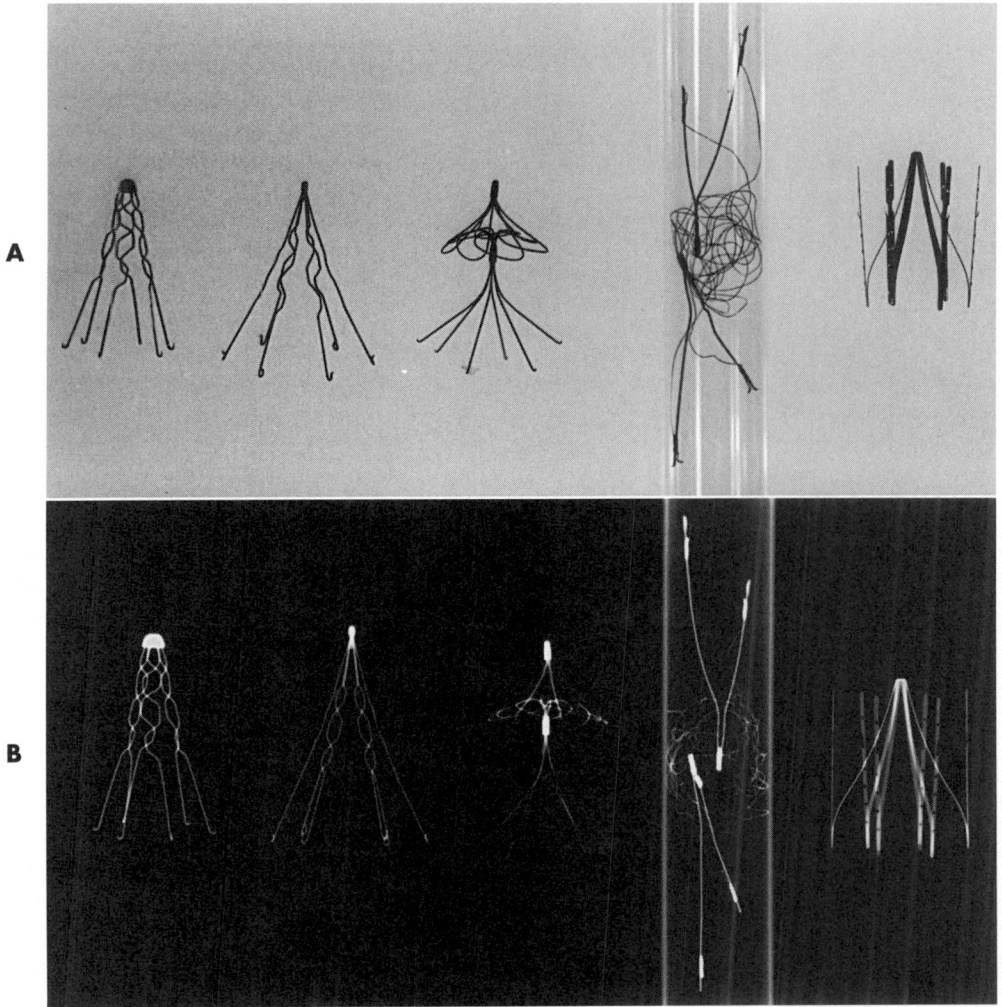

FIGURE 26-26 Vena cava filters. **A**, Actual filters. **B**, Radiographic images. *Left to right*, Kimray-Greenfield, Titanium Greenfield, Simon nitinol, Gianturco-Bird's Nest, and Vena Tech.

salvage their function. Unfortunately the success rate for salvage is low and access may be better managed by the creation of another site or a bridge fistula.[4] Risk factors for complications include being female, black, over 65 years, and diabetic.[38,46] Treatment for the most common complication, stenosis, is surgery. Stenosis usually results in thrombosis, and these are considered a single problem. Stenosis most often involves the venous anastomosis, and a patch angioplasty is usually performed to revise a thrombosed fistula. Other complications include aneurysm and pseudoaneurysm formation, infection, steal syndrome, and high–output CHF.[34]

VENA CAVA FILTER INSERTION

Vena cava filter insertion entails the partial occlusion of the inferior vena cava with an intravascular filter, such as a Greenfield filter, inserted under fluoroscopy with local or monitored anesthesia care. The Greenfield device offers the option of jugular or femoral vein insertion, and the correct kit must be selected. In patients for whom heparin therapy is either contraindicated or not effective, the vena cava filter is the treatment of choice to capture emboli that arise from the pelvis and lower extremities to prevent pulmonary emboli. Several types of filters have been used during the past 20 years. Currently five types have FDA approval for insertion (Fig. 26-26). The Greenfield filter is the most successful and widely used device, and the mortality and morbidity have been extremely low. The device has progressed from the earlier design that required an incision and venotomy to the current percutaneous titanium vena cava filter. The filter maintains a patent vena cava but prevents PE by trapping the emboli at the apex of the device.

Patient and family education regarding postoperative care and functions is essential (Box 26-3).

Procedural considerations

The patient is placed in the supine position on a radiopaque OR bed to permit fluoroscopic visualization at the level of the renal veins. This procedure may be performed in the OR, radiology suite, or the ICU for

| BOX 26-3 | Postoperative Patient Teaching for Vena Cava Filter Insertion |

For a femoral vein insertion site, do not bend leg for about 8 hours.

Avoid strenuous activity or lifting more than 5 pounds.

Expect that bruising of the insertion site may occur because this is common in patients who are or have been receiving anticoagulant therapy.

Apply pressure using appropriate method if bleeding at insertion site occurs.

Report signs of local infection or significant bleeding.

Elevate affected leg and wear elastic stockings to relieve lower extremity swelling, which may be temporary side effect of the underlying DVT.

Understand the purpose and proper way to wear support stockings.

Report sudden or severe leg swelling.

From MacVittie, B.A. (1998). *Vascular surgery.* St. Louis: Mosby.

critical patients. The head is turned to the left for jugular vein insertion or the groin is exposed for femoral vein insertion. The right femoral is preferred over the left because the anatomy of the left vein often makes threading the filter more difficult. Local anesthesia, heparinized saline to flush device lumens, and contrast medium should be available. Since this is a percutaneous insertion, no instruments are needed.

Operative procedure

1. The right groin area is prepped and draped and infiltrated with local anesthesia.
2. An 18-gauge entry needle is used for right femoral venotomy.
3. The guidewire is inserted and advanced to a level above the renal veins under fluoroscopic guidance.
4. The sheath or dilator is inserted over guidewire after all lumens have been flushed with heparin solution.
5. The sheath is removed, and the introducer catheter is inserted and advanced to the implantation site.
6. This catheter carries the preloaded, radiopaque carrier capsule. The sheath is retracted, the filter discharged, and sheath removed.
7. Pressure is applied to the puncture site for approximately 5 minutes or until hemostasis is achieved.

VARICOSE VEIN EXCISION AND STRIPPING

The saphenous trunk may be ligated and divided with subsequent stripping and excision. A series of cup-shaped valves maintains the venous blood flow in a direction toward the heart. Varicose veins are described as primary or secondary. Primary varicose veins are more prevalent and are not associated with a pathologic condition of the deeper venous system, that is, postthrombotic syndrome or

a history of deep venous thrombosis (DVT). Secondary varicose veins are believed to be a result of insufficiency of the deep venous system. Disease may prevent the normal functioning of these valves, resulting in distention. The veins gradually become dilated. Those in the lower extremities are most frequently affected, particularly the long saphenous vein. The incidence is estimated at 2% in Western populations, with women being affected two and one half times as often as men are. Callam,[7] in an extensive review of the literature, reports the following as risk factors: female sex, increased age, pregnancy, geographic location, and race (more prevalent in whites). Obesity and family history are *not* risk factors. Conclusions are difficult to reach because of the varied criteria used to study the disease. However, it appears that lifestyle may play an important role. Criado and Johnson[12] found that "chair sitting" with its resultant increase in ankle venous pressure may be worse than "ground sitting." This may imply that industrial versus nonindustrialized societies are at greater risk. Family history has not been substantiated in well-controlled studies, but this impression has existed because patients with varicose veins are more likely to be asked about relatives with similar symptoms. Climate has been ruled out as a cause. Different populations, when moved to an industrial lifestyle, develop associated health problems. Affluence, diet, exercise, and environmental variables seem to be contributing factors.[20] Dilatation of the saphenous vein produces venous stasis, which may be followed by secondary complications, such as stasis ulcers. Venous obstruction causes an increase in venous pressure, which leads to an increase in capillary pressure. This causes fluid to leak from the capillaries and produce edema.[47] The objective of surgical intervention is to remove the diseased veins, thus preventing ulceration, secondary edema, pain, and fatigue in the extremity.

Procedural considerations

Before sedation or entrance into the operating room, the patient should stand, and the varicose veins should be marked with an indelible marker. This ensures adequate visualization for complete removal of the varicosities,[30] since the patient is often placed in Trendelenburg's position intraoperatively to decrease venous congestion, which could interfere with visualization of the varicosities. The patient is placed on the operating room bed in a supine position with the legs slightly abducted. Ligation or stripping of the lesser saphenous veins and branches may require placing the patient in the prone position. Multiple small incisions are made over the identified varicosities, and the affected vein segments are removed. This is becoming the procedure of choice. Stripping indicates removal of a long segment of vein by means of a special device. Drapes are placed to enable flexing and lifting at the knee. Instruments include the basic minor instrument setup, plus the following: Weitlaner self-retaining retractors, #11 blades, skin hooks, mosquito hemostats, vein strippers with various tips available, and elastic bandages.

Operative procedure

1. The incision is made in the upper area of the thigh, parallel to the crease in the groin. Bleeding vessels are clamped and ligated.

2. The saphenous vein is identified and isolated. Margins of the wound are separated with a Weitlaner self-retaining retractor.

3. The saphenous vein branches are doubly ligated with black silk ties or transfixed, clamped, and divided. The proximal stump is dissected upward to the point at which it enters the femoral vein, where it is carefully ligated.

4. If the saphenous vein is to be excised, an incision is made at its distal portion at the ankle, and the vein is identified, ligated, and divided.

5. A vein stripper is inserted and advanced to the proximal end of the vein in the groin, where it is secured with a heavy suture, and the tip is attached.

6. As the stripper is pulled up the leg, external compression is applied.

7. Tributaries may be excised through numerous small incisions along the course of the vein.

8. The groin wound is closed in layers and other small incisions are closed with skin sutures or staples. Dressings and circular compression bandages are applied.

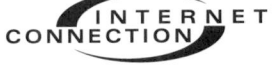

Society of Vascular Nursing: email svnatpns@aol.com

The University of Kansas Vascular Surgery Program:
http://www.kumc.edu/vsurg/

USC Center for Vascular Disease:
http://www.surgery.usc.edu/divisions/vas/VASCULAR.HTM

Vascular Surgical Society of Great Britain & Ireland:
http://www.vssgbi.co.uk/

The Merck Manual (Chapter on vascular disease):
http://www.merck.com

Stroke:
http://netsrv.casi.sti.nasa.gov/thesaurus/S/word15061.html
http://www.nutrimed.com/STROKE.HTM

Peripheral Vascular Disease:
http://www.fhcrc.org/~cvdeab/chpt06.html

REFERENCES

1. Almgren, C.C., & Borgini, L. (1994). Intraoperative nursing care of the vascular patient. In Fahey, V.A. (Ed.). *Vascular nursing* (ed. 2). Philadelphia: W.B. Saunders.

2. Anderson, L.A. (1994). An update on the cause of abdominal aortic aneurysms, *Journal of Vascular Nursing, 12*(4), 95-100.

3. Atkinson, L. J., & Fortunato, N. (1996). *Berry & Kohn's operating room technique* (ed. 8). St. Louis: Mosby.

4. Bennion, R.S., Williams, R.A., & Wilson, S.E. (1994). Principles of vascular access surgery. In Veith, F.J., Hobson, R.W., Williams, R.A., & Wilson, S.E. (Eds.). *Vascular surgery principles and practice* (ed. 2). New York: McGraw-Hill.

5. Blackburn, D.R., & Peterson-Kennedy, L. (1994). Noninvasive vascular testing. In Fahey, V.A., (Ed.). *Vascular nursing* (ed. 2). Philadelphia: W.B. Saunders.

6. Brewster, D.C. (1995). Prosthetic grafts. In Rutherford, R.B. (Ed.). *Vascular surgery* (ed. 4). Philadelphia: W.B. Saunders.

7. Callam, M.J. (1994). Epidemiology of varicose veins. *British Journal of Surgery, 81*, 167-173.

8. Calligaro, K.D., DeLaurentis, D.A., & Veith, F.J. (1995). Infected infrainguinal grafts. In Ouriel, K. (Ed.). *Lower extremity vascular disease.* Philadelphia: W.B. Saunders.

9. Cambria, R.P. (1989). Acute lower extremity ischemia. In Brewster, D.C. (Ed). *Common problems in vascular surgery.* St. Louis: Mosby.

10. Clark, J.B., Queener, S.F., & Karb, V.B. (1994). *Pharmacological basis of nursing practice* (ed. 4). Philadelphia: Mosby.

11. Clements, D.L., & Verhaeghe, R. (1993). Atherosclerosis and other occlusive diseases. In Clements, D.L., & Shepherd, J.T. (Eds.). (1993). *Vascular diseases in the limbs: mechanisms and principles of treatment.* St. Louis: Mosby.

12. Criado, E., & Johnson, G. Jr. (1991). Venous disease. *Current Problems in Surgery, 28*(5), 335-400.

13. Cunningham, J.N., Catinella, F.P., Nathan, I.M., & Spencer, F.C. (1981). Proposed mechanism for early vein graft thrombosis. *Surgical Forum, 32,* 239-241.

14. Doyle, J.E. (1994). Vascular access surgery. In Fahey, V.A. (Ed.). *Vascular nursing* (ed. 2). Philadelphia: W.B. Saunders.

15. Emma, L.A. (1992). Chronic arterial occlusive disease. *Journal of Cardiovascular Nursing, 7*(1), 14-24.

16. Fellows, E. (1995). Abdominal aortic aneurysms: warning flags to watch for, *American Journal of Nursing, 95*(5), 26-33.

17. Fernando, H.C., & Fernando, O.N. (1996). Arteriovenous fistulas by direct anastomosis for hemodialysis access. In Wilson, S.E. (Ed.). *Vascular access: principles and practice* (ed. 3). St. Louis: Mosby.

18. Friedman, S.G. (1989). *A history of vascular surgery.* New York: Futura.

19. Galloway, S., Bubela, N., McKibbon, A., et al. (1995). Symptom distress, anxiety, depression, and discharge information needs after peripheral arterial bypass. *Journal of Vascular Nursing, 13*(2), 35-40.

20. Geelhoed, G.W., & Burkitt, D.P. (1991). Varicose veins: a reappraisal from a global perspective. *Southern Medical Journal, 84*(9), 1131-1134.

21. Gibbons, G.W., Marcaccio, E.J., & Habershaw, G.M. (1995). Management of the diabetic foot. In Callow, A.D., & Ernst, C.B. (Eds.). *Vascular surgery: theory and practice.* Stamford, Conn.: Appleton & Lange.

22. Gordon, I.L. (1996). Physiology of the arteriovenous fistula. In Wilson, S.E. (Ed.). *Vascular access: principles and practice* (ed. 3). St. Louis: Mosby.

23. Green, R.M. (1993). Personal communication, April 29, 1993, Rochester, N.Y.

24. Greenfield, L.J., & Proctor, M.C. (1996). Venous interruption. In Haimovici, H. (Ed) *Haimovici's vascular surgery: principles and techniques* (ed. 4). Cambridge, Mass.: Blackwell Science.

25. Hatswell, E.M. (1994). Abdominal aortic aneurysm surgery. Part 1. An overview and discussion of immediate and postoperative complications. *Heart and Lung, 23*(3): 228-239.

26. Helt, J. (1994). Amputation in the vascular patient. In Fahey, V.A. (Ed.). *Vascular nursing* (ed. 2). Philadelphia: W.B. Saunders.

27. Humphrey, P.W., & Silver, D. (1995). Antithrombotic therapy. In Rutherford, R.B. (Ed.). *Vascular surgery* (ed. 4). Philadelphia: W.B. Saunders.

28. Jacobs, D.L., & Towne, J.B. (1995). Femoropopliteal bypass. In Ouriel, K. (Ed.). *Lower extremity vascular disease.* Philadelphia: W.B. Saunders.

29. Jicha, D.L., & Stoney, R.J. (1995). Infected aortic grafts. In Ouriel, K. (Ed.). *Lower extremity vascular disease.* Philadelphia: W.B. Saunders.

30. Johnson, G., Jr., & Rutherford, R.B. (1995). Varicose veins: patient selection and treatment. In Rutherford, R.B. (Ed.). *Vascular surgery* (ed. 4). Philadelphia: W.B. Saunders.

31. Karp, D.L., & Fahey, V.A. (1994). Chronic venous disease. In Fahey, V.A. (Ed.). *Vascular nursing* (ed. 2). Philadelphia: W.B. Saunders.

32. Kempczinski, R.F. (1995). Vascular grafts. In Rutherford, R.B. (Ed.). *Vascular surgery* (ed. 4). Philadelphia: W.B. Saunders.

33. Kempczinski, R.F., & Bernhard, V.M. (1995). Management of chronic ischemia of the lower extremities: introduction and general considerations. In Rutherford, R.B. (Ed.). *Vascular surgery* (ed. 4). Philadelphia: W.B. Saunders.

34. Kempe, D.A., Durham, J.D., & Mann, D.J (1996). Thrombolysis and percutaneous transluminal angioplasty. In Wilson, S.E. (Ed.). *Vascular access: principles and practice* (ed. 3). St. Louis: Mosby.

35. Kistner, R.L., & Eklof, B. (1995). Operative procedures and their results in managing chronic venous insufficiency. In Callow, A.D., & Ernst, C.B. (Eds). *Vascular surgery: theory and practice*. Stamford, Conn.: Appleton & Lange.

36. Krajewski, L.P., & Olin, J.W. (1996). Atherosclerosis of the aorta and lower-extremity arteries. In Young, J.R., Olin, J.W., & Bartholomew, J.R. (Eds.). *Peripheral vascular diseases* (ed. 2). St. Louis, Mosby.

37. Krupski, W.C. (1995). Arterial aneurysms. In Rutherford, R.B. (Ed.). *Vascular surgery* (ed. 4). Philadelphia: W.B. Saunders.

38. Lazarus, J.M., Denker, B.M., & Owen, W.F. (1996). Hemodialysis. In Brenner, B.M. (Ed.). *The kidney* (ed. 5). Philadelphia: W.B. Saunders.

39. MacVittie, B.A. (1998). *Mosby's perioperative nursing series: vascular surgery*. St. Louis: Mosby.

40. McEwen, D.R. (1994). Arteriovenous fistula: vascular access for long-term hemodialysis. *AORN Journal, 59*(1), 225-237.

41. McGraw, D.J., & Rubin, B.G. (1995). The Doppler principle and sonographic imaging: applications in the noninvasive vascular laboratory. In Callow, A.D., & Ernst, C.B. (Eds.). *Vascular surgery: theory and practice*. Stamford, Conn.: Appleton & Lange.

42. Mitchell, M.B., Rutherford, R.B., & Krupski, W.C. (1995). Infrarenal abdominal aortic aneurysms. In Rutherford, R.B. (Ed.). *Vascular surgery* (ed. 4). Philadelphia: W.B. Saunders.

43. Pagana, K.D., & Pagana, T. J. (1997). *Mosby's diagnostic and laboratory test reference* (ed. 3). St. Louis: Mosby.

44. Paul, S.D., & Eagle, K.A. (1995). Modalities for assessment of cardiac risk in vascular surgery. In Callow, A.D., & Ernst, C.B. (Eds). *Vascular surgery: theory and practice*. Stamford, Conn.: Appleton & Lange.

45. Pevec, W.C. (1995). Morbidity associated with vascular surgery. In Callow, A..D., & Ernst, C.B. (Eds). *Vascular surgery: theory and practice*. Stamford, Conn.: Appleton & Lange.

46. Rocco, M.V., Bleyer, A.J., & Burkart, J.M. (1996). Utilization of inpatient and outpatient resources for the management of hemodialysis access complications. *American Journal of Kidney Diseases, 28*(2), 250-256.

47. Rohrer, M.J. (1994). The systemic venous system: basic considerations. In Fahey, V.A. (Ed.). *Vascular nursing* (ed. 2). Philadelphia: W.B. Saunders.

48. Rutherford, R.B. (1995). The vascular consultation. In Rutherford, R.B. (Ed.). *Vascular surgery* (ed. 4). Philadelphia: W.B. Saunders.

49. Rutherford, R.B., Durham, J.D., & Kumpe, D.A. (1995). Endovascular interventions for lower extremity ischemia. In Rutherford, R.B. (Ed.). *Vascular surgery* (ed. 4). Philadelphia: W.B. Saunders.

50. Self, S.B., & Seeger, J.M. (1992). Laser angioplasty. *Surgical Clinics of North America, 2*(4), 851-868.

51. Shannon, M.T., Wilson, B.A., & Stang, C.L. (1995). *Govani & Hayes: drugs and nursing implications* (ed. 8). Norwalk, Conn: Appleton-Century-Crofts.

52. Shortell, C.K. (1995). Pulmonary embolism and vena caval interruption. In Ouriel, K. (Ed.). *Lower extremity vascular disease*. Philadelphia: W.B. Saunders.

53. Stanley, J.C., Sottiurai, V., Fry, R.E., & Fry, W.J. (1975). Comparative evolution of vein graft preparation media: electron and microscopic studies. *Journal of Surgical Research, 18*(3), 235-246.

54. Stanley, J.C., Lindenauer, S.M., Graham, L.M., et al. (1991). Biologic and synthetic vascular grafts. In Moore, W.S. (Ed.). *Vascular surgery: a comprehensive review*. Philadelphia: W.B. Saunders.

55. Thibodeau, G.A., & Patton, K.T. (1996). *Anatomy and physiology* (ed. 3). St. Louis: Mosby.

56. Verhaeghe, R., Verstraete, M. (1993). Hemostasis, thrombosis, and anti-thrombotic and thrombolytic therapy. In Clement, D.L., & Shepherd, J.T. (Eds). *Vascular diseases in the limbs: mechanisms and principles of treatment*. St. Louis: Mosby.

57. Webster, M.W., St. Jean, P.L., Steed, D.L., et al. (1991). Abdominal aortic aneurysm: results of a family study, *Journal of Vascular Surgery, 13* 366.

58. White, R.A. (1995). Endovascular visualization and therapy. In Callow, A.D., & Ernst, C.B. (Eds). *Vascular surgery: theory and practice*. Stamford, Conn.: Appleton & Lange.

59. Wilson, S.E. (1996). Vascular interposition (bridge fistulas) for hemodialysis. In Wilson, S.E. (Ed.). *Vascular access: principles and practice* (ed. 3). St. Louis: Mosby.

60. Wright, C.B., Dunn, E.J., Ketterhagen, J.P., et al. (1987). The regulatory environment for vascular grafts. In Sawyer, P.N. (Ed.). *Modern vascular grafts*. New York: McGraw-Hill.

61. Zierer, R.E., & Sumner, D.S. (1995). Physiologic assessment of peripheral occlusive disease. In Rutherford, R.B. (Ed.). *Vascular surgery* (ed. 4). Philadelphia: W.B. Saunders.

CHAPTER TWENTY SEVEN

Cardiac Surgery

Patricia C. Seifert

CARDIAC SURGERY HAS been affected by cost-driven changes in health care, endoscopic and video technology, societal demands for less traumatic interventions, and the rapid growth of minimally invasive techniques for the treatment of acquired heart disease.[53,79] This growing trend has not replaced the need for traditional "open" techniques; rather it has expanded the treatment options for coronary artery disease, valvular dysfunction, thoracic aneurysms, conduction disturbances, congenital abnormalities, and end-stage cardiac disease. Newer technologies employing lasers, genetic engineering, and heterograft replacement organs have increased the available therapeutic interventions.

SURGICAL ANATOMY

The heart (Fig. 27-1) is a four-chambered muscular organ that acts as a power pump for the circulatory system. It is enclosed in a pericardial sac within the mediastinum, which lies between the lungs, posterior to the sternum, and anterior to the vertebrae, esophagus, and descending portion of the aorta. The diaphragm is positioned below the heart (Fig. 27-2). The cardiac wall is composed of three layers: the epicardium, the outer lining; the myocardium, or muscular layer, which is the important functional layer; and the endocardium, the inner lining (Fig. 27-3). Two thirds of the heart is located to the left of the midline, and the remaining third to the right. Although functionally divided into right and left halves, the heart is rotated to the left, with the right side located anteriorly and the left side relatively posterior.

Each half of the heart contains an upper and lower communicating chamber: the atrium and the ventricle. The right atrium receives desaturated blood from the inferior and superior venae cavae and from the coronary circulation via the coronary sinus. The left atrium receives oxygenated blood from the lungs via the pulmonary veins. From the atria, blood flows through the atrioventricular valves into the ventricles.

The left ventricle pumps blood into the major vessels of the *systemic circulatory system*: the aorta and its main branches to the head, upper extremities, abdominal organs, and lower extremities. The right and left internal (thoracic) mammary arteries, used as grafts during coronary bypass surgery, branch off the subclavian arteries and course behind and parallel to the edges of the sternum. The arteries of the circulatory system subdivide into arterioles and eventually into capillaries, where internal respiration and metabolic exchange occur. From the capillary beds, desaturated blood flows into the venules and veins and finally returns to the right atrium.

In the *pulmonary circulatory system*, blood is pumped from the right ventricle through the pulmonary valve into the main pulmonary artery. It divides into the right and left pulmonary arteries, which further subdivide into arterioles and the capillaries of the lungs. External respiration occurs in the capillary beds, where carbon dioxide is exchanged for oxygen. Freshly oxygenated blood from the lungs flows through the pulmonary veins into the left atrium.

The *coronary circulation* (Fig. 27-4) supplies oxygen and nutrients to the myocardium. The heart receives its blood supply from the left and right coronary arteries, which originate in the sinuses of Valsalva behind the cusps of the aortic valve in the ascending aorta. The left main coronary artery divides into the left anterior descending coronary artery and the circumflex coronary artery; along with the right coronary artery, these arteries represent the three main vessels of the coronary arterial system. Depending on the severity of the lesion, atherosclerotic plaques within

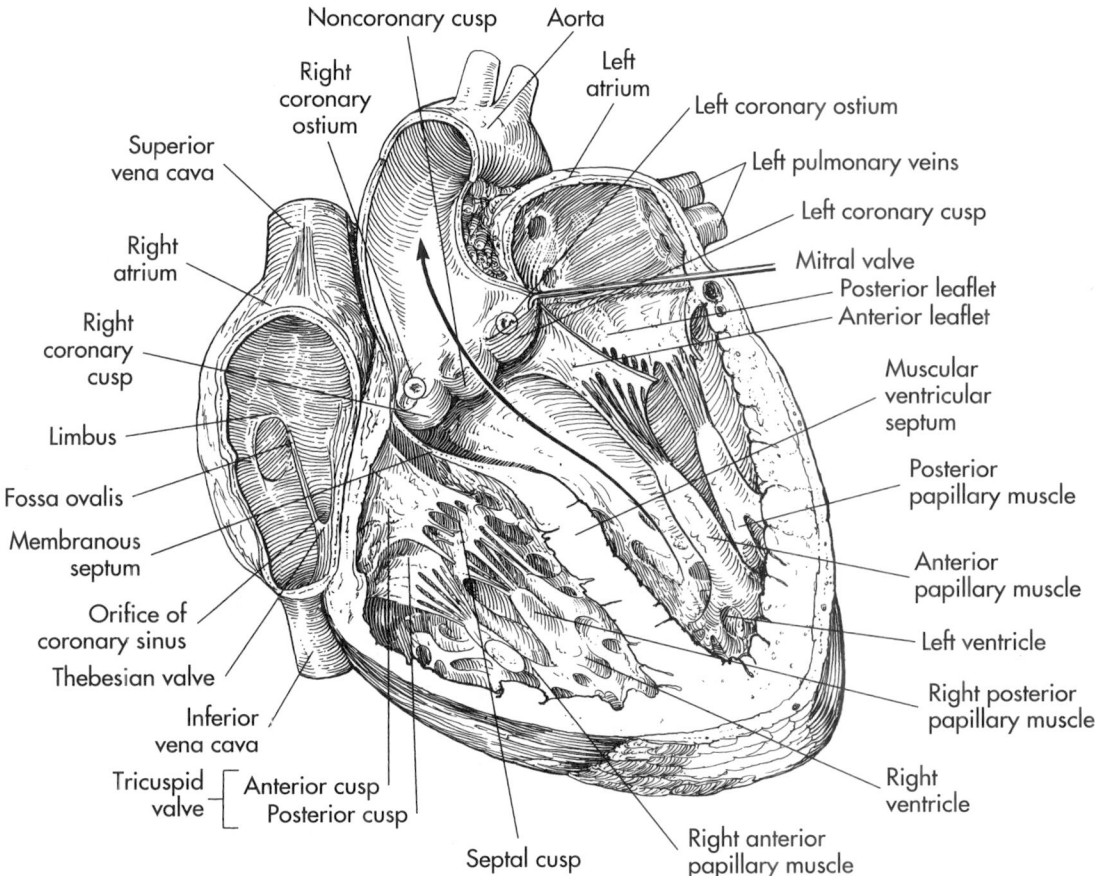

FIGURE 27-1   Frontal view of the heart. Systemic venous blood returns to the heart via the inferior and superior venae cavae. It enters the right atrium, flows through the tricuspid valve into the right ventricle, and is ejected through the pulmonic valve (not shown) into the pulmonary circulation. The blood is oxygenated in the lungs and returns to the left atrium through the pulmonary veins. From the left atrium, it flows through the mitral valve into the left ventricle, where it is ejected through the aortic valve into the aorta and the systemic circulation.

these arteries jeopardize myocardial blood flow and oxygenation, producing ischemic pain (in many cases) and irreversible damage if untreated.

The main coronary arteries are situated in the epicardium, which facilitates their accessibility during coronary bypass procedures. From these arteries arise the septal perforators and other branches that penetrate the entire myocardium. The cardiac veins empty into the right atrium via the coronary sinus; the thebesian veins, prominent in the walls of the right atrium and the right ventricle, open directly into these chambers.

Nerve impulses to the heart travel from the medulla oblongata (see Chapter 23) along the middle cervical nerve, which is composed of sympathetic fibers, and the vagus nerve, composed of parasympathetic fibers. The sympathetic nerves promote an increase in the force and rate of contraction, and the parasympathetic fibers control the heart rate. Running vertically along the right and left sides of the pericardium are major branches of the phrenic nerve, which innervate the diaphragm and stimulate it to contract. Identifying this nerve is important for protecting

the diaphragm in procedures in which the lateral pericardium is incised or excised. Within the myocardium itself, certain areas of tissue are modified to form a *conduction system* (Fig. 27-5). The process of excitation and contraction originates in the sinoatrial (SA) node, located in the area where the superior vena cava meets the right atrium. The impulse spreads to the atria through the internodal pathways and travels to the atrioventricular (AV) junction (which contains the AV node) located medially to the entrance of the coronary sinus in the right atrium, close to the tricuspid valve. From the AV junction, the impulse spreads to the bundle of His, which extends down the right side of the interventricular septum. The bundle divides into the right and left bundle branches, which terminate in a network of fibers called the *Purkinje system*. The Purkinje fibers are spread throughout the inner surface of both ventricles and the papillary muscles, which when stimulated produce contraction of the heart muscle. The location of conduction tissue is clinically significant during surgical repair of atrial or ventricular septal defects.

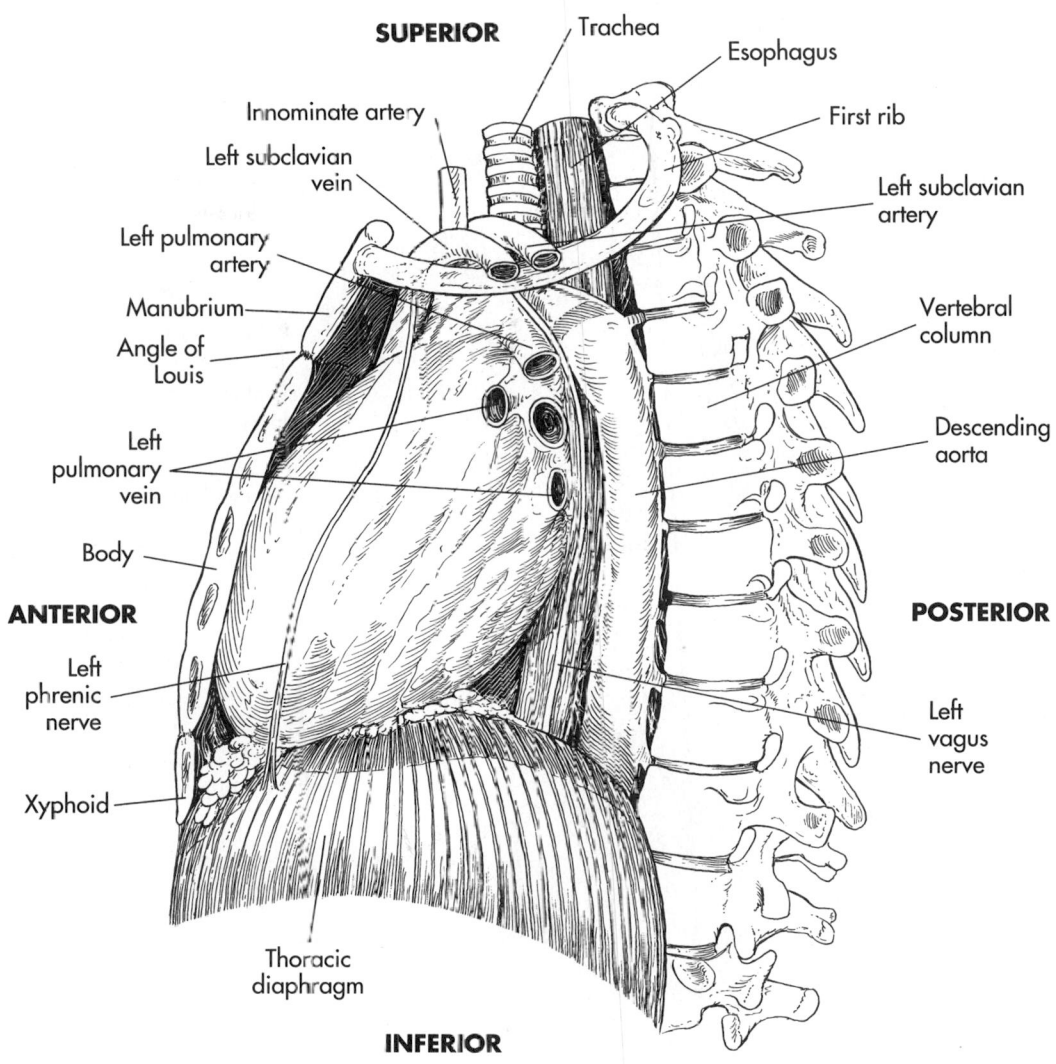

SUPERIOR

Trachea

Esophagus

Innominate artery

First rib

Left subclavian vein

Left subclavian artery

Left pulmonary artery

Manubrium

Vertebral column

Angle of Louis

Left pulmonary vein

Descending aorta

Body

ANTERIOR

POSTERIOR

Left phrenic nerve

Left vagus nerve

Xyphoid

Thoracic diaphragm

INFERIOR

FIGURE 27-2   Regions of the mediastinum.

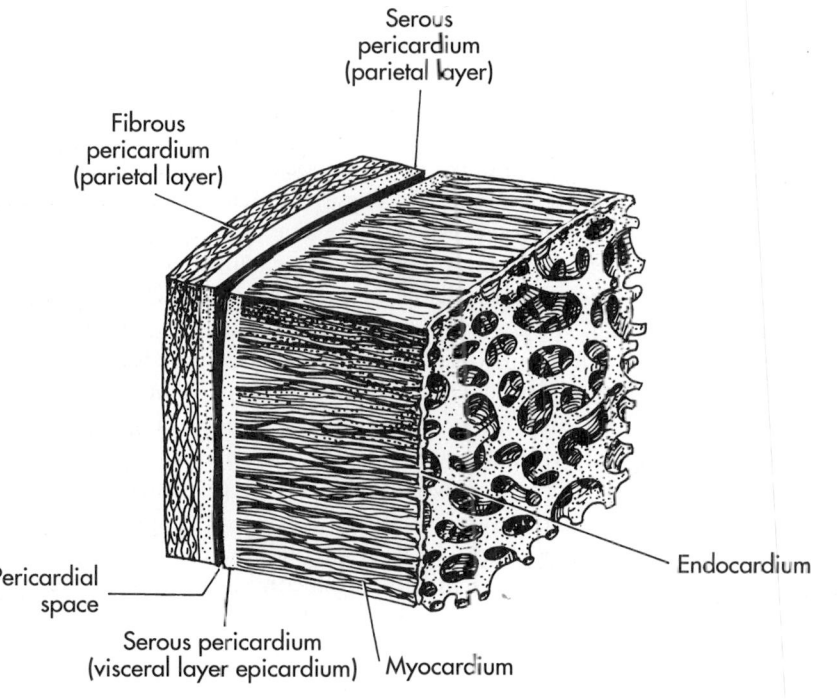

Serous pericardium (parietal layer)

Fibrous pericardium (parietal layer)

FIGURE 27-3   Cross section of cardiac muscle showing its three layers (endocardium, myocardium, and epicardium) and pericardium.

Pericardial space

Endocardium

Serous pericardium (visceral layer epicardium)

Myocardium

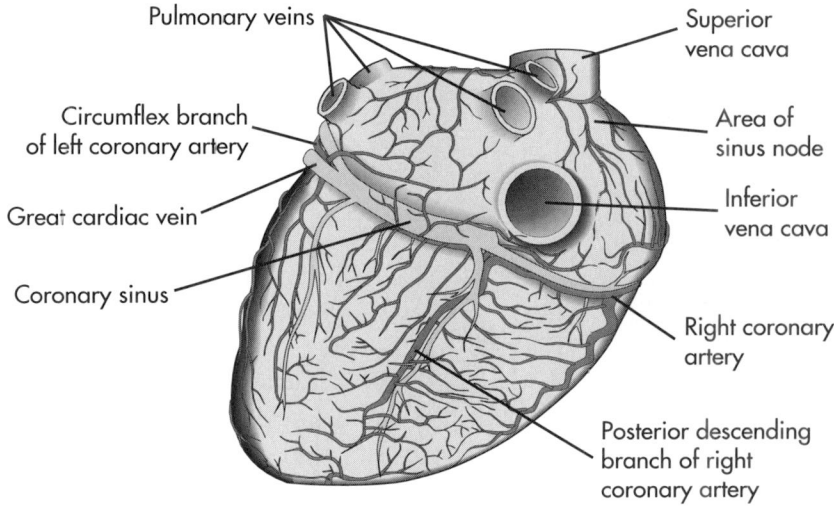

POSTERIOR VIEW

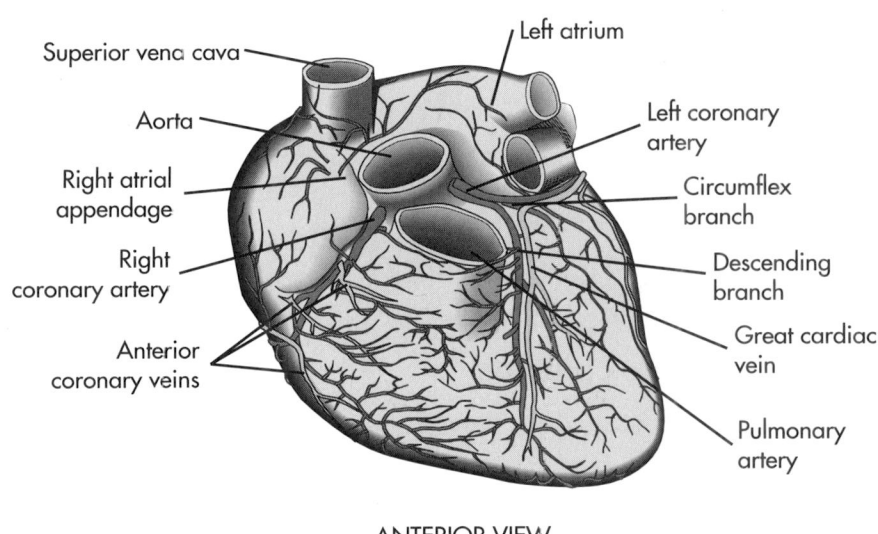

ANTERIOR VIEW

FIGURE 27-4 Anterior and posterior surfaces of the heart, illustrating the location and distribution of the principle coronary arteries.

During myocardial contraction and relaxation, unidirectional blood flow is maintained by the four cardiac valves (Figs. 27-6 and 27-7). The atrioventricular valves are located between the atria and the ventricles. The right atrioventricular valve is called the *tricuspid valve* and contains three leaflets. The left atrioventricular valve, called the *mitral valve*, consists of two leaflets (see Fig. 27-6). Each of these valves is a complex system consisting of a fibrous annulus surrounding the valve orifice, the valve cusps or leaflets, the chordae tendineae, and the papillary muscles, which anchor the valve to the inner ventricular wall (see Fig. 27-1). When the ventricle contracts, these muscles and the chordae tendineae, connected to the valve leaflets, prevent the leaflets from everting into the atrium. All parts of the system must be functioning for the valve to work properly.

The semilunar valves are located at the outlets of the left and right ventricles. These valves are known as the aortic and pulmonic valves respectively. They are less complex than the atrioventricular valves, and they open and close passively with the cyclic fluctuations in the blood pressure and volume that occur during systole and diastole.

Abnormalities such as stenosis, insufficiency, or a combination of both impair the mechanical function of the valves. Stenosed valves have leaflets that are fibrous and stiff, with uneven and adherent margins. Insufficient or incompetent valves, such as those with leaflet degeneration or perforations, dilated annuli, or ruptured chordae tendineae, produce regurgitation of blood into the originating chamber. These conditions, or a combination of stenosis and insufficiency, strain the myocardium by increasing intracardiac pressure, volume, and workload.

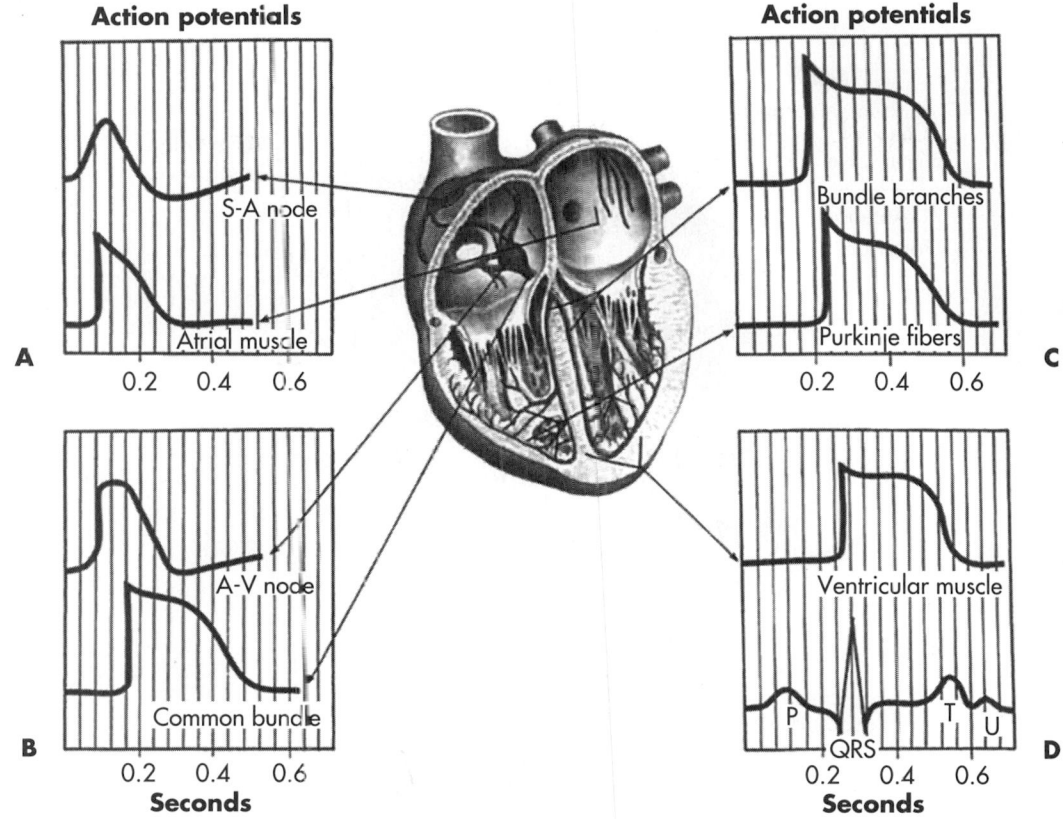

FIGURE 27-5 Heart with normal conduction pathways and transmembrane action potential of sinoatrial (SA) node (**A**), atrioventricular (AV) node (AV junction) (**B**), bundle branches (**C**), and ventricular muscle (**D**).

Any of the four valves may be congenitally deformed. Acquired valvular heart disease most commonly affects the mitral and aortic valves and is believed to be caused by the increased stress associated with the higher pressures within the left chambers of the heart.

PERIOPERATIVE NURSING CONSIDERATIONS

Specialized nursing considerations that are indicated for thoracic operations (see Chapter 25) also apply to cardiac surgery.

Assessment

Because the severity of pathologic changes varies among patients throughout the life span, knowledge of physical derangements, psychosocial concerns, and functional health patterns enables the nurse to plan care and manage the patient perioperatively. The perioperative nursing database should include the patient's biopsychosocial history, the physical examination, and results from laboratory tests.

History

The history includes information about the patient's health status as well as the response to the disease and the recommended intervention. Patients with cardiac disease may display symptoms including ischemic chest pain (angina pectoris), fatigue, dyspnea, and syncope. Depending on their severity, these symptoms affect the patient's functional status and ability to engage in activities of daily living (Box 27-1). Atypical chest pain is more likely in women than in men[33] and may be attributable to vasospastic angina or mitral valve prolapse. Coronary artery disease is unusual in premenopausal women, but after cessation of menses the risk is similar to that of men.[43]

A cardiovascular disease risk factor profile (Table 27-1) is helpful in planning care for hospitalization and discharge by focusing on areas that might require further patient education. A history of rheumatic fever or frequent tonsillitis as a child is significant because the sequelae of rheumatic fever and streptococcal infections can lead to damage of the cardiac valves. The presence of diabetes is notable because this disease affects the vascular system and may retard healing and predispose the patient to infection. Hypertension and obesity increase the workload of the heart; obesity may also increase the risk for postoperative infection because adipose tissue is poorly vascularized. Mental stress has been increasingly implicated in the development of myocardial ischemia.[49]

Risk factors associated with postoperative infection include previous cardiac surgery, duration of surgery and cardiopulmonary bypass, blood transfusion, postoperative blood loss, and length of preoperative hospitalization.[38,66]

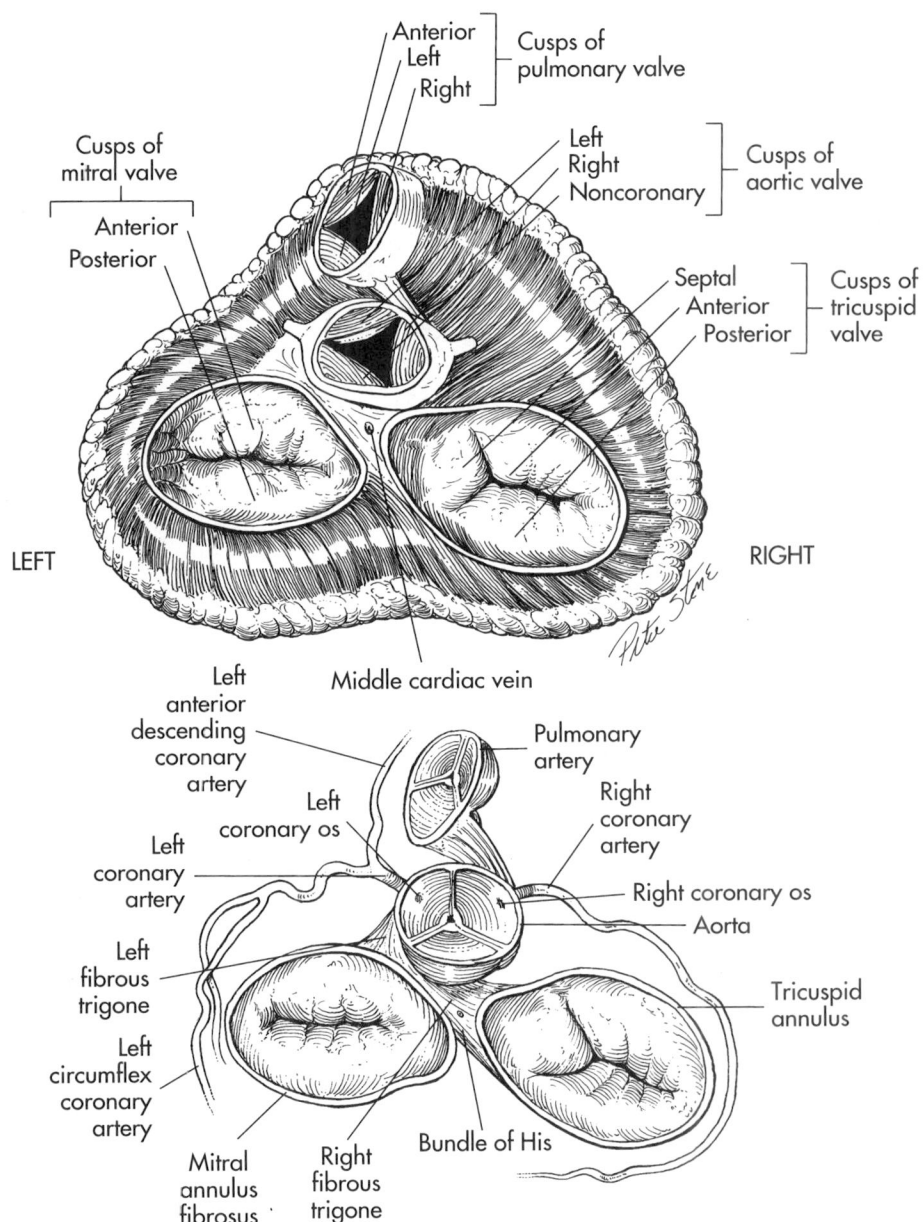

FIGURE 27-6 Superior view of cardiac valves. Pulmonary (*top*), aortic (*middle*), mitral (*bottom left*), and tricuspid (*bottom right*).

Female sex, obesity, diabetes mellitus, and arterial occlusive disease of the legs are significant risk factors for impaired wound healing at the saphenous venectomy site after coronary bypass surgery.[29] Another study included bilateral internal mammary artery (IMA) grafts, obesity, and postoperative inotropic support as risk factors for impaired wound healing.[61]

The patient's knowledge and understanding of the disease process and its effect on his or her functional, physiologic, and psychologic status should also be part of perioperative nursing assessment. The patient's personal strengths, external resources, and coping strategies should be determined. The perioperative nurse should note any cultural, ethnic, spiritual, or religious beliefs that are relevant to perioperative patient care.

Physical examination

The physical assessment provides the perioperative nurse with baseline data and information about potential problems that might require intervention. Table 27-2 lists some normal, age-specific changes in the very young or the elderly that should be differentiated from pathologic conditions.[3-6] Chapter 29 describes pediatric cardiac surgery.

The appearance of the skin offers clues to cardiovascular status. Dryness, coolness, diaphoresis, paleness, edema,

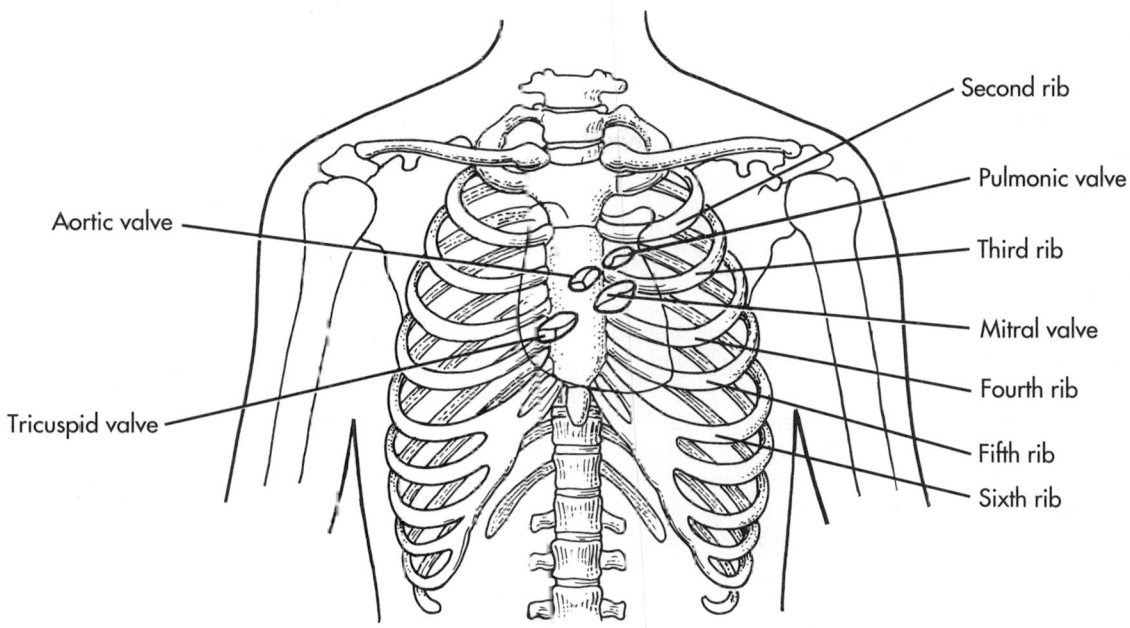

FIGURE 27-7 Anatomic position of cardiac valves. Notice relationship of left ventricular apex to fourth and fifth ribs, a frequent site for minimally invasive incisions.

BOX 27-1 | **New York Heart Association Functional Classification System (NYHA Class)**

Class I

Patients with cardiac disease do not display symptoms of syncope, undue fatigue, dyspnea, or anginal pain with ordinary physical activity.

Class II

Patients with cardiac disease are comfortable at rest but display the above symptoms during ordinary physical activity.

Class III

Patients with cardiac disease, although comfortable at rest, are considerably limited functionally and display symptoms with less than ordinary exercise.

Class IV

Patients with cardiac disease are unable to engage in any physical activity without discomfort and may have symptoms of cardiac insufficiency even at rest.

Adapted from the New York Heart Association (1964). *Diseases of the heart and blood vessels: nomenclature and criteria for diagnosis* (ed. 6). Boston: Little, Brown & Co.

TABLE 27-1 | **Risk Factors for Coronary Artery Disease**

NONMODIFIABLE	MODIFIABLE
Age	Elevated serum cholesterol
Sex*	Hypertension
Family history	Cigarette smoking
Race	Obesity
	Elevated serum lipids
	Diabetes mellitus
	Psychologic stress
	Personality type

Adapted from Kinney, M.R., Packa, D.R. (Eds.). (1996). *Comprehensive cardiac care,* (ed. 8). St. Louis: Mosby.
*Postmenopausal women have risk similar to that of men.

---

poor capillary refill, bruising, and petechiae can reflect impaired cardiovascular function. Visual problems and headaches may be related to inadequate cardiac output, atherosclerotic disease, or medications such as digitalis. The presence of chronic or local infection should be identified; if untreated, these may become potential sources of postoperative infection.

Nutritional status is assessed to determine increased risk for infection, skin breakdown, or other complications.

The patient's level of consciousness, memory, comprehension, and emotional status should be assessed. Confusion, restlessness, slurred speech, numbness, and paralysis can signal impaired perfusion. Their presence preoperatively should be noted by the perioperative nurse.

During respiratory assessment the perioperative nurse should note the use of accessory muscles or nostril flaring and auscultate breath sounds. Adventitious sounds such as crackles and wheezes may point to pulmonary edema. Orthopnea, shortness of breath, or dyspnea may require elevation of the head of the stretcher and assistance during transfer onto the OR bed. If the patient is receiving

TABLE 27-2 | **Physiologic Features of the Very Young and the Very Old (compared with the adult)**

VERY YOUNG	VERY OLD	VERY YOUNG	VERY OLD
Cardiovascular System		**Respiratory System—cont'd**	
Myocardium		Higher oxygen consumption	Reduced vital capacity, maximum ventilation volume
Less contractile tissue	Increased subendocardial fat		
Less compliant	Increased heart weight		
Cardiac output increased by faster heart rate	Reduced resting cardiac output	Short, narrow airway obstructed easily	
Valves		**Renal System**	
Less tension created by papillary muscle	Fibrous thickening, calcification of leaflets and annulus	Glomeruli small and immature	Fewer functional glomeruli
Coronary arteries		Tubular concentration of fluids and electrolytes diminished	Reduced renal blood flow and glomerular filtration rate
Rarely, anomalies of coronary arteries	Coronary arteriosclerosis, atherosclerosis; tortuous epicardial arteries	Unable to excrete increased electrolytes and hydrogen ions (acids)	Impaired ability to excrete increased amount of water and electrolytes; reduced ability to secrete hydrogen ions
Conduction system			
Impulse conduction faster	Impulse conduction slower		
Blood volume		**Other**	
Total circulating small amount, volume per kilogram of body weight relatively greater	Reduced plasma volume Reduced blood water content	*Temperature control*	
		Immature regulating system: rapid heat loss	Decreased control
Respiratory System		*Metabolic rate*	
Inadequate cough reflex	Decreased ability to eliminate secretions	Higher	Lower
		Stress response	
Increased chest wall compliance, decreased pulmonary compliance	Increased chest wall rigidity, decreased lung compliance	Decreased phagocytic capability of leukocytes	Limited capability to retain homeostasis
		Immature immunoglobulin synthesis	Decreased adrenal activity

Source: Association of Operating Room Nurses, Inc. (1997). *The geriatric patient; The neonate, infant, and toddler patients; The premature infant patient,* Denver, Colo.: AORN, Inc., 1997.

oxygen, the flow rate and method of administration should be observed. Alleviating pain is a prime consideration in the care of the cardiovascular patient because pain is a myocardial stressor. A patient with angina may come to the operating room with nitroglycerin tablets or transdermal patches. Cold also increases the work load of the heart because the shivering that accompanies chilling elevates the metabolic rate; the patient should be kept warm.

Heart sounds, murmurs, and friction rubs provide clues to congenital, ischemic, or valvular heart disease or pericarditis. The patient may complain of palpitations. Apical, radial, or femoral pulses also reflect cardiac function; their rate, rhythm, and quality should be determined. The presence of cyanosis or peripheral edema should be noted.

The blood pressure may be high, normal, or low. The hypertensive patient may have left ventricular hypertrophy, and the hypotensive patient may display changes in neurologic, gastrointestinal, and renal function. Blood pressures should be checked bilaterally. Unequal pressures in the arms may be a contraindication for the use of the internal mammary artery as a bypass graft on the side of the

lower blood pressure, where perfusion may not be optimal. Patients with dissections or aneurysms may have unequal carotid, femoral, brachial, or radial artery blood pressures when the lesion occludes one or more of these vascular branches.

Because cardiac function affects all the body's organ systems, assessment of the patient should be comprehensive whenever possible. A thorough assessment also alerts the physician and perioperative nurse to the need for special diagnostic tests and laboratory procedures.

Diagnostic studies

Most patients referred for surgery have had clinical evaluations including both invasive and noninvasive studies (Table 27-3). After the history and physical assessment, a resting electrocardiogram (ECG) is ordered. An exercise ECG (stress test) is often performed because ST-segment changes indicating myocardial ischemia may be apparent only during or after exercise. In patients with intractable arrhythmias, electrophysiology (EP) studies may be performed to locate the site of irritable atrial or ventricular foci that can be surgically ablated or excised or controlled

TABLE 27-3 | **Diagnostic Tests Commonly Performed for Cardiovascular Disorders***

	CORONARY ARTERY DISEASE	VALVULAR HEART DISEASE	CONDUCTION DISTURBANCE	THORACIC ANEURYSM	CONGENITAL HEART DISEASE (CHILD AND ADULT)
Resting ECG	X	X	X	X	X
Exercise ECG (stress test)	X		X		X
Chest radiography	X	X	X	X	X
Aortography	X			X	X
Echocardiogram	X	X	X	X	X
Resting MUGA	X				
Exercise thallium	X				X
Exercise MUGA	X				
CAT scan				X	
PET scan with stress	X				
MRI					X
Electrophysiology			X		
Cardiac catheterization	X	X	X	X	X

Adapted from Kinney, M.R., & Packa, D.R. (Eds.). (1996). *Comprehensive cardiac care*, (ed. 8). St. Louis: Mosby.

*Tests may not be limited to only those disorders designated.

CAT, Computerized axial tomography; *ECG*, electrocardiogram; *MRI*, magnetic resonance imaging; *MUGA*, multiple uptake gated acquisition; *PET*, positron emission tomography.

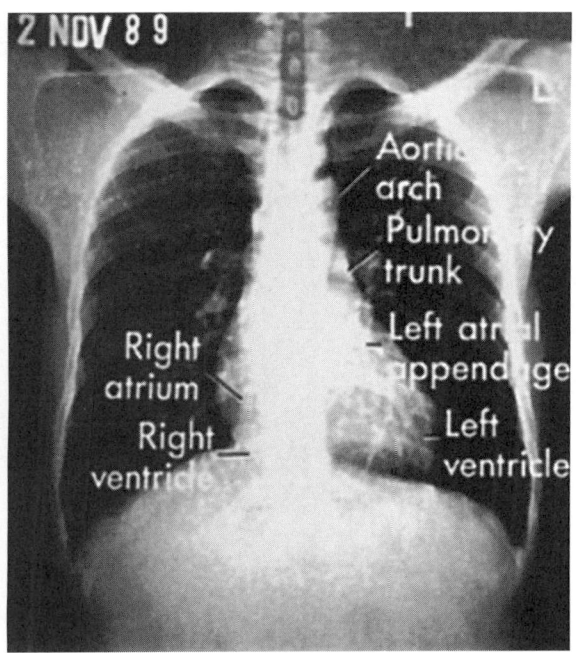

FIGURE 27-8   Anteroposterior chest radiograph (normal).

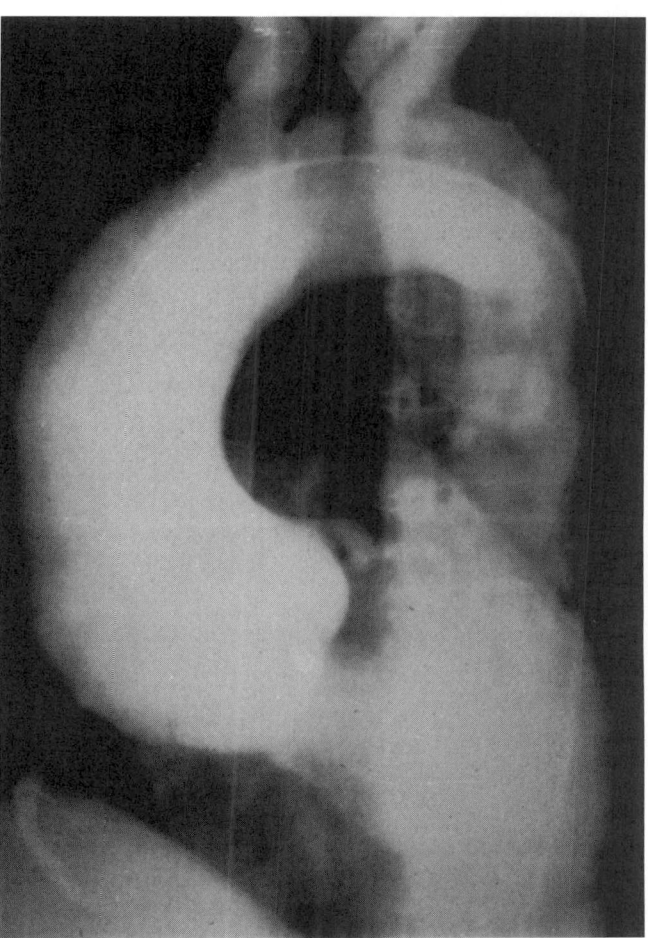

FIGURE 27-10   Aortogram of ascending aortic dissection, with aortic valve insufficiency. Notice regurgitation of dye into left ventricle.

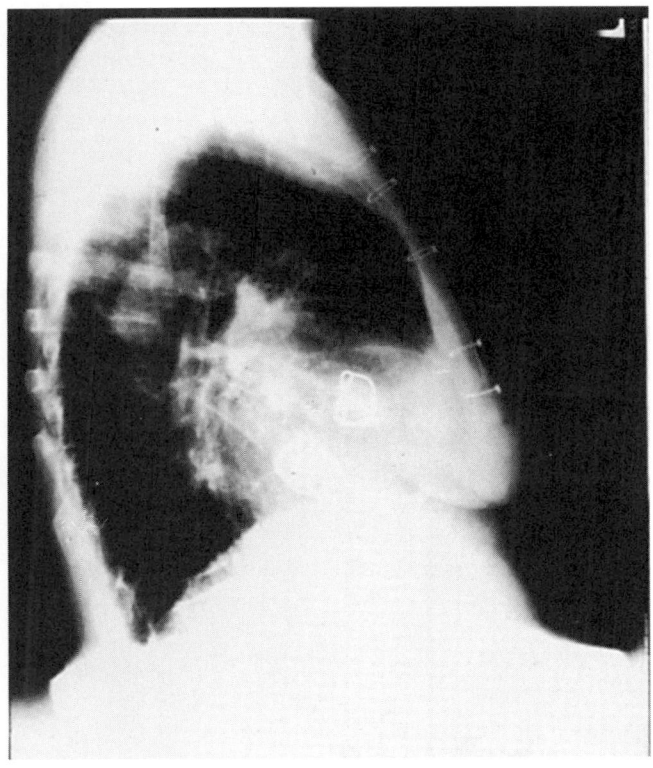

FIGURE 27-9   Anteroposterior chest radiograph. Notice chest wires and pericardial adhesions from previous median sternotomy.

with pharmacologic therapy. EP studies are also performed to determine the need for internal defibrillators or antitachycardia devices.

Chest roentgenography provides information about the size of the cardiac chambers, thoracic aorta, and pulmonary vasculature as well as the presence of calcium in valves, pericardium, coronary arteries, and aorta (Fig. 27-8). Lateral chest radiographs of patients with prior sternal operations demonstrate the chest wires and extent of pericardial adhesions (Fig. 27-9). In patients with suspected aortic or other vascular abnormalities, a computerized tomography (CT) scan of the chest with intravenous contrast is used to create x-ray serial "slices" of the body area under study. CT scan is contraindicated in very unstable patients because the patient's position in the CT tubelike machine makes access to the patient difficult.

Arteriography with radiographic contrast material (dye) may also be performed to determine the size and location of the lesion and the site of the intimal tear in aortic dissections (Fig. 27-10); digital subtraction angiography (DSA) can provide exceptionally clear images and requires less contrast material. Magnetic resonance imaging (MRI) can also be employed to image vascular structures.[60]

Echocardiography is a noninvasive test that evaluates both the structure and function of the heart by transmitting sound waves to the heart and measuring those sound waves reflected back to the transducer (Fig. 27-11). They

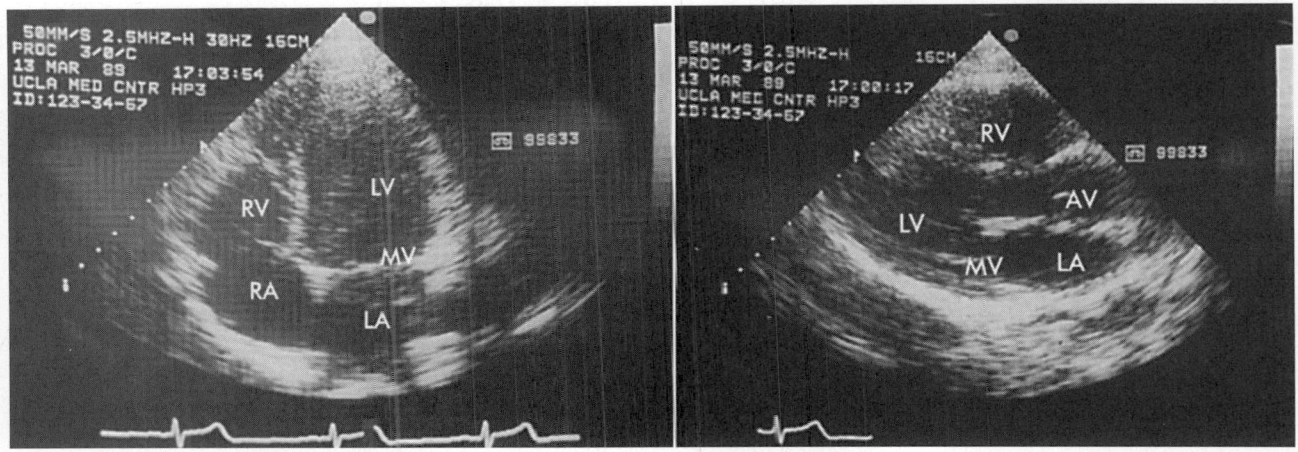

FIGURE 27-11   Two-dimensional echocardiography showing two views of the cardiac chambers. *LA*, Left atrium; *LV*, left ventricle; *MV*, mitral valve; *RA*, right atrium; *RV*, right ventricle

are processed by the transducer, which creates visual images of the structure's movements. This test is commonly used to assess ventricular and valvular function before, during, and after surgery and to determine the degree of valvular stenosis or regurgitation. It can also demonstrate a tumor, thrombus, or air in the ventricular or atrial cavities. Color-flow Doppler techniques have greatly enhanced the functional assessment of valvular performance. Transesophageal echocardiography (TEE) is commonly used to evaluate the effectiveness of valve repairs and to diagnose valvular disorders. Echocardiography is becoming the gold standard for diagnosing valvular disorders.

Radionuclide imaging is employed to illustrate wall motion and blood flow through the heart and to quantify cardiac function. These noninvasive techniques are generally well tolerated by patients, especially when they may be too unstable to withstand a cardiac catheterization. They may also be used as a complement to catheterization. Tests include the multiple uptake gated acquisition (MUGA) scan (also known as *blood pool imaging*) and exercise thallium perfusion scintigraphy. In the MUGA, multiple images are viewed to evaluate regional and global wall motion of the heart and to determine the ejection fraction.[60] Exercise thallium perfusion scintigraphy provides additional information about the function of the heart in patients with coronary artery disease (CAD) by reflecting deficits in myocardial perfusion at rest and after exercise. The procedure is similar to a MUGA except that there is an exercise portion of the study. Patients unable to exercise may be stressed pharmacologically.

Cardiac catheterization provides definitive information about the extent and location of ischemic and congenital heart disease and is often an adjunct to echocardiography for diagnosing valvular heart disease. A radiopaque plastic catheter is inserted retrogradely through the aortic valve into the left side of the heart by a percutaneous puncture or

a cutdown to the vessels of the brachial artery (Sones's technique) or the femoral artery (Judkins's technique). The right side of the heart is approached by a venous route. To perform coronary angiography that demonstrates coronary anatomy, a contrast medium is injected into the coronary ostia. Obstructions (Fig. 27-12), flow, and distal perfusion can be assessed. Ventriculography illustrates contractile weaknesses of the ventricles as well as shunting and regurgitation of blood. These studies are used to assess the degree of myocardial dysfunction and to plan interventions such as coronary artery bypass grafting, valve repair or replacement, repair of congenital anomalies, and cardiac transplantation. The cardiologist can compute the orifice of a stenosed valve, or determine the degree of regurgitation of an incompetent valve.

Ventricular, atrial, and pulmonary pressures are recorded, and cardiac output and ejection fraction are estimated (Box 27-2 and Table 27-4). Oxygen saturation of cardiac chambers and the ratio of pulmonary to systemic blood flow (Q_p/Q_s) are calculated in patients with shunts and congenital or acquired defects. Cinearteriograms record the movement of the heart, and cut films from these cines may be displayed in the operating room during surgery.

The cardiac catheterization laboratory has also become the site for more aggressive interventional therapies related to evolving and acute myocardial infarctions. Coronary thrombolysis with streptokinase and tissue plasminogen activator can dissolve fresh blood clots and reopen, or recanalize, the artery. Percutaneous transluminal coronary angioplasty (PTCA) with or without insertion of intracoronary stents may be performed to dilate the artery. Laser angioplasty and atherectomy to excise intraluminal plaque may also be employed. In many instances these interventions may obviate the need for surgical bypass grafting, although restenosis after PTCA is not uncommon; eventually the patient may require surgical revascularization.

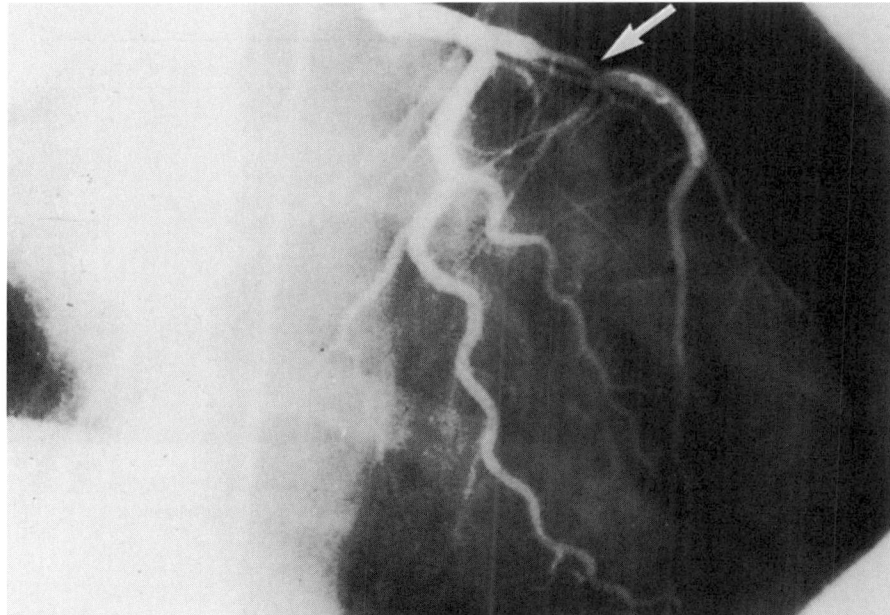

FIGURE 27-12   Right anterior oblique (RAO) view of left coronary artery injection demonstrating high-grade stenosis of the left anterior descending coronary artery (arrow) at the lead of the first septal perforator.

| BOX 27-2 | Hemodynamic Concepts |

Cardiac Output

The amount of blood (in liters) ejected by the left ventricle per minute; product of heart rate times the stroke volume.

Cardiac Index

The cardiac output corrected for differences in body size.

Preload

The volume of blood in the ventricle at the end of diastole; the pressure of blood in the ventricle at the end of the diastole. Central venous pressure (CVP) measures right-sided heart preload; pulmonary artery wedge pressure (PAWP) indirectly measures left-sided heart preload.

Afterload

The impedance, or resistance, the heart must overcome to pump blood into the systemic circulation; the left ventricular wall tension during systole; systemic vascular resistance.

Contractility

The inotropic state of the heart; the ability of the ventricle to pump.

Ejection Fraction

The percentage of end-diastolic volume ejected into the systemic circulation; indicator of ventricular function.

Operating room availability is often recommended for PTCA, stent insertion, and atherectomy.

EP studies are performed to diagnose conduction disturbances and to provide therapeutic interventions (such as radiofrequency ablation of accessory pathways seen in Wolff-Parkinson-White syndrome).

Laboratory tests

Preoperative laboratory tests are used to assess physiologic function (Table 27-5). Hematologic tests include a detailed coagulation profile to uncover hemorrhagic disorders. In patients who have been taking aspirin or dipyridamole, platelet activity has been decreased; this alerts the perioperative nurse to anticipate prolonged bleeding necessitating infusion of this blood product. The patient's blood type is also determined, and the appropriate order is placed with the blood bank. Precautions are taken to test the blood for viral contamination and for cold antibodies that could produce agglutination of the patient's blood during surgery when the patient is cooled to hypothermic temperatures.

Liver and kidney function test results may be abnormal in patients with chronic heart failure, possibly because of congestion related to right heart failure in the former and reduced blood flow in the latter. Progressive improvement in hepatic and renal function is anticipated with successful operative intervention. Blood glucose levels are tested and monitored closely, especially in patients with diabetes mellitus.

Additional perioperative laboratory examinations may include arterial blood gases and enzyme markers of myocardial damage (such as the creatine kinase MB isoenzyme, known as *MB bands*), especially in the presence of persistent angina.[46] Pulmonary function tests are performed to determine baseline data and to plan postoperative care. Postoperative respiratory function may be impaired as a result of the use of extracorporeal circulation and stasis of lung secretions that accompany prolonged surgery.

Nursing Diagnosis

After a comprehensive review of individual patient data, the perioperative nurse identifies relevant nursing diag-

TABLE 27-4 | Cardiac Catheterization Data

HEMODYNAMIC DATA	NORMAL VALUES		
Flow			
Cardiac output (CO)	4.0-8.0 L/min		
Cardiac index (CI)	2.5-4.0 L/min/m^2		
Ejection fraction (EF)	60%-70%		
Left ventricular end-diastolic volume (LVEDV)	90-180 ml		
Stroke volume (SV)	60-130 ml/beat		
Stroke volume index (SVI)	35-70 ml/beat/m^2		
	SYSTOLIC	**DIASTOLIC**	**MEAN**
Resistances			
Systemic vascular resistance (SVR)	<20 Wood units		
Total pulmonary resistance	<3.5 Wood units		
Pulmonary vascular resistance (PVR)	<2.0 Wood units		
Shunts (Q_P/Q_S)			
Pulmonary flow/systemic flow		1:1	
Oxygen Saturations			
Venae cavae		70%	
Right atrium		70%	
Right ventricle		70%	
Pulmonary artery		70%	
Pulmonary veins		97%	
Left atrium		97%	
Left ventricle		97%	
Aorta		97%	
Valve Orifices (Adult)			
Aortic	2-4 cm^2		
Mitral	4-6 cm^2		
Tricuspid	10 cm^2		
Pressures (mm Hg)			
Venae cavae			0-5
Right atrium (RA)			2-6
Right ventricle (RV)	20-30	0-5	
Pulmonary artery (PA)	20-30	10-20	10-15
Pulmonary artery wedge pressure (PAWP)			4-12
Left atrium (LA)			4-12
Left ventricle (LV)	120	0-5	
Left ventricular end-diastolic pressure (LVEDP)			5-12
Aorta	120-140	60-80	70-90
Brachial artery	120	70	
Femoral artery	125	75	

Angiographic Data	Findings
Coronary arteries	Anatomy/function coronary vascular bed: distal coronary flow; AV fistula; atherosclerosis; anomalous origin of coronary arteries
Ventriculography	Anatomy/function of ventricles and associated structures; LV aneurysm; congenital abnormalities; valvular stenosis/regurgitation; shunts
Valvular angiography	Intact mitral/triscuspid complex; valvular incompetence/stenosis/regurgitation
Pulmonary angiography	Pulmonary embolism, congenital abnormalities
Aortography	Patency of aortic branches; normal mobility, competence, and anatomy of aortic valve; aneurysms: saccular, fusiform; origin of aortic dissection; shunts or anomalous connections; congenital defect or obstructions

Adapted from Pagana, K.D., & Pagana, T.J. (1997). *Mosby's diagnostic and laboratory test reference*, (ed. 3). St. Louis: Mosby.

TABLE 27-5 | **Laboratory Data**

TEST	NORMAL VALUES	TEST	NORMAL VALUES
Arterial blood gases (ABGs)		Creatinine (urine, 24 hour)	
pH	7.38-7.44	Male	20-26 mg/kg/24 hr
P_{O_2}	95-100 mm Hg	Female	14-22 mg/kg/24 hr
P_{CO_2}	35-40 mm Hg	Electrolytes	
Blood chemistry		Potassium (K)	3.8-5.0 mEq/L
Glucose (fasting)	70-110 mg/dl	Sodium (Na)	136-142 mEq/L
Protein (total)	6.8-8.5 g/dl	Chloride (Cl)	95-103 mEq/L
Blood urea nitrogen (BUN)	8.0-25 mg/dl	Magnesium (Mg)	1.5-2.0 mEq/L
Uric acid	3.0-7.0 mg/dl	Lipids	
Cardiac enzymes		Cholesterol	<200 mg/dl
Creatine phosphokinase	<70 IU/L	Triglycerides	10-190 mg/dl
(CPK)		Phospholipids	150-380 mg/dl
CPK-MB (isoenzyme)	0-7 IU/L	Free fatty acids	9.0-15.0 mM/L
Coagulation profile		Liver function	
Platelet count	150,000-400,000/μL	Albumin (serum)	3.5-5.0 g/dl
Prothrombin time (PT)	Depends on thromboplastin reagent used; typically 9.5-12.0 sec	Alkaline phosphatase	20-90 IU/L
		Globulin (serum)	2.3-3.5 g/dl
		Serum bilirubin (total)	0.2-1.4 mg/dl
Thrombin time	Depends on concentration of thrombin reagent used; typically 20-29 sec		
Partial thromboplastin time (PTT)	Depends on phospholipid reagent used; typically 60-85 sec	Pulmonary function (Normal values vary depending on the patient's age, sex, weight, and race. The following are generally calculated.)	
		Residual volume (RV)	
Activated PTT	Depends on activator and phospholipid reagents used; typically 20-35 sec	Tidal volume (TV)	
		Expiratory reserve volume (ERV)	
		Inspiratory reserve volume (IRV)	
Complete blood count (CBC)		Total lung capacity (TLC)	
Hemoglobin (Hgb)		Vital capacity (VC)	
Male	13.5-18.0 g/dl	Urinalysis	
Female	12.0-16.0 g/dl	Color	Amber, yellow
Hemotocrit (Hct)		Clarity	Clear
Male	42%-52%	pH	4.6-8.0
Female	35%-47%	Specific gravity (SG)	1.002-1.035
Red blood cells (RBC)		Protein	0.0-8.0 mg/dl
Male	4.6-6.2×10^6/μL	Sugar, ketones, RBC, WBC,	Negative
Female	4.2-5.4×10^6/μL	casts	
White blood cells (WBC)	4.5-11.0×10^3/μL		

Adapted from Pagana, K.D., & Pagana, T.J. (1997). *Mosby's diagnostic and laboratory test reference,* (ed. 3). St. Louis: Mosby.

noses, from which the perioperative plan for patient care is derived (see Sample Care Plan on p. 1129).

For the patient undergoing cardiac surgery, the nursing diagnoses might be as follows:

- Decreased cardiac output related to mechanical factors (altered preload, afterload, contractility, heart rate)
- Risk for infection (wound) related to surgical disruption of tissues
- Risk for injury related to perioperative positioning
- Knowledge deficit related to perioperative events
- Risk for impaired tissue integrity related to cardiopulmonary bypass and hypothermia

Outcome Identification

Outcomes for the selected nursing diagnoses might be stated as follows:

- Patient will demonstrate an adequate cardiac output.
- Patient will be free from wound infection.
- Patient will be free from injury from surgical position.
- Patient will describe perioperative events.
- Patient's tissue integrity will be maintained.

Each additional nursing diagnosis should have a corresponding outcome statement. The outcome should be measurable, with criteria by which to evaluate its achievement. For example, for the outcome "The patient

SAMPLE CARE PLAN

Nursing Diagnosis: Decreased cardiac output related to mechanical factors (altered preload, afterload, contractility, heart rate)

Expected Outcome: Patient will demonstrate an adequate cardiac output.

Interventions:

Check clotting function, coagulation profile, and electrolyte values.

Monitor blood pressures (arterial, CVP, PAWP) and ECG.

Measure and report blood loss (such as suction and sponges).

Maintain adequate supply and assist with administration of replacement blood or blood products.

Follow institutional protocol for allergic blood reaction.

Have topical hemostatic agents available.

Have inotropic and antidysrhythmic medications available; assist with administration.

Use autotransfusion system per protocol.

Monitor, report, and record urine output and chest tube drainage; keep tubes and catheters patent.

Have available defibrillator (with appropriate internal and external paddles and settings), fibrillator, external pacemaker, temporary epicardial pacemakers leads, and appropriate ECG cables for cardioversion and intraaortic balloon pump.

Nursing Diagnosis: Risk for wound infection related to surgical disruption of tissues

Expected Outcome: Patient will be free from wound infection.

Interventions:

Verify that prescribed preoperative prophylactic antibiotic has been administered.

Dress all invasive arterial and venous lines.

Use depilatories or electric clippers to remove hair at the surgical site; avoid razors if possible.

Routinely, prepare anatomic area to knees (or lower if leg vein needed) with antimicrobial antiseptic agent.

Monitor aseptic technique; correct breaks.

Have available prescribed topical antibiotics.

If the OR bed is raised, lowered, or turned from side to side, take measures to maintain sterility of field.

Confine and contain instruments used in groin or leg; change gown and gloves when moving from lower extremities to chest.

Protect sterility of closed urinary drainage system.

Maintain sterility of instrument setup until patient discharged from operating room.

Maintain documentation of all implants.

During patient rewarming, avoid excessive heat loss: cover exposed areas, irrigate with warm solutions, increase room temperature.

Nursing Diagnosis: Risk for injury related to perioperative positioning.

Expected Outcome: Patient will be free from injury caused by perioperative positioning.

Interventions:

Obtain and prepare appropriate positioning accessories.

Maintain proper body alignment.

Pad and protect vulnerable neurovascular bundles and dependent pressure areas.

Prevent pooling of skin preparation agents at bedlines.

Pad thermia blanket.

Keep all surfaces dry and wrinkle free.

Ensure patency and security of peripheral and central lines, catheters, and electrosurgical dispersive pad on positional changes.

Have adequate personnel to assist with positional changes; lift (do not pull) patient during all positioning maneuvers.

Safely secure patient to OR bed; ensure patient stability.

Nursing Diagnosis: Knowledge deficit related to perioperative events

Expected Outcome: Patient will describe perioperative events.

Interventions:

Explain or describe the following events:

NPO status

Administration and effects of preoperative medication

Transport to operating room

Holding area

Insertion of peripheral, arterial, and venous lines

Operating room environment (temperature, staff, attire, equipment)

Induction of anesthesia

Skin preparation

Anticipated length of surgery

Minimally invasive versus standard cardiac procedures

Surgical intensive care unit and patient status (for example, unable to talk while intubated and plans for alternative methods of communication)

Determine patient's desire for additional knowledge (respect denial).

Answer questions; clarify misperceptions.

Know where family or significant other will be waiting during surgery, provide communication per institutional protocol.

SAMPLE CARE PLAN—CONT'D

Nursing Diagnosis: Risk for impaired tissue integrity related to cardiopulmonary bypass or hypothermia

Expected Outcome: Patient's tissue integrity will be maintained.

Interventions:

Place thermia blanket on OR bed.

Preoperatively, provide warm blankets as required.

Expose only those body areas required for surgical intervention.

Monitor patient's temperature (esophageal, pulmonary, rectal, bladder, or ventricular septal).

Adjust room temperature as needed.

Inspect cardiopulmonary bypass lines for patency and presence of particulate matter; alert surgeon as indicated.

Avoid large ice particles on heart.

Use solutions of appropiate temperature when irrigating the heart (cold during hypothermia arrest; warm before and after arrest); warm throughout for "warm heart" surgery.

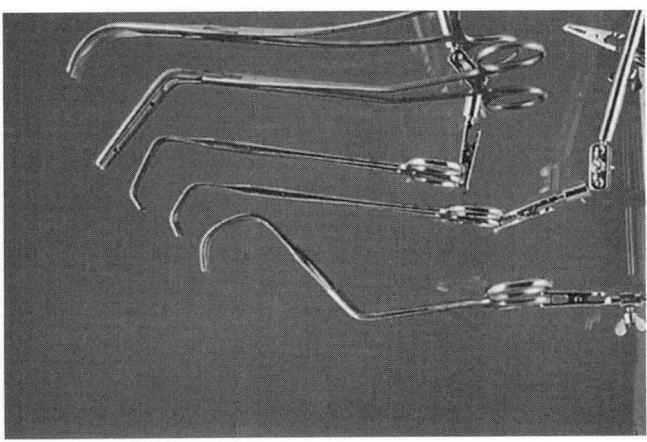

FIGURE 27-13 Cardiovascular clamps (*top to bottom*): Semb suture passer, Fogarty cross-clamp (angled), Beck partial occlusion clamp (medium and small), Lambert-Kay partial occlusion clamp.

will demonstrate adequate cardiac output," the perioperative nurse might identify criteria such as vital signs and hemodynamic status consistent with or better than preoperative parameters; fluid and electrolyte balance consistent with preoperative levels; absence of rate, rhythm, or conduction defects; absence of iatrogenic injury to the heart; and normal clotting parameters. Each of these criteria becomes evidence that the outcome was achieved. When outcomes are evaluated, they should be documented in the perioperative record. Some outcomes will have been achieved at the conclusion of the surgical procedure; others require ongoing evaluation in the postoperative period to be adequately measured. The evaluation section on p. 1149 indicates the requirement for ongoing goal measurement by the use of "will" rather than stating the outcome as having been achieved.

Planning

Once the diagnoses and outcomes have been established, a plan of care is devised that will enable the perioperative nurse to achieve the goals that have been set.[69] Patient and family needs, elicited from interviews when possible, should be integrated into the planning. The perioperative nurse will need to identify criteria specific to the patient for each of the stated outcomes in the Sample Care Plan.

Implementation

Some considerations, other than those previously mentioned, can be useful in implementing the perioperative plan of care for patients undergoing cardiac surgery.

Special facilities

The operating room must be large enough to accommodate bulky, highly specialized equipment while maintaining aseptic technique. Multiple electrical outlets, auxiliary lighting, and additional suction outlets should be available.

Instrumentation and equipment

The basic setup described for thoracic procedures (see Chapter 25) is used, along with some specialized cardiovascular instruments and equipment.

Vascular clamps, which are designed to occlude blood flow partially or completely, must be maintained in good condition if they are to prevent fracture of the delicate intima of the blood vessels and still retain their specific holding qualities. There are many variations in construction of vascular instruments. The jaws may consist of single or double rows of fine, sharp, or blunt teeth or special cross-hatching or longitudinal serrations. The working angles of the clamps also vary. All clamps are designed to hold the vessels securely and without trauma (Fig. 27-13).

Minimally invasive procedures require special instrumentation to access the heart via smaller incisions (Fig. 27-14). Retractors, dissecting instruments, suturing devices, and vascular clamps are available.

There are sternal and rib retractors to meet specific needs. Internal mammary artery (IMA) retractors expose the retrosternal artery bed by elevating the sternal border (Fig. 27-15). Some sternal retractors have attachments that

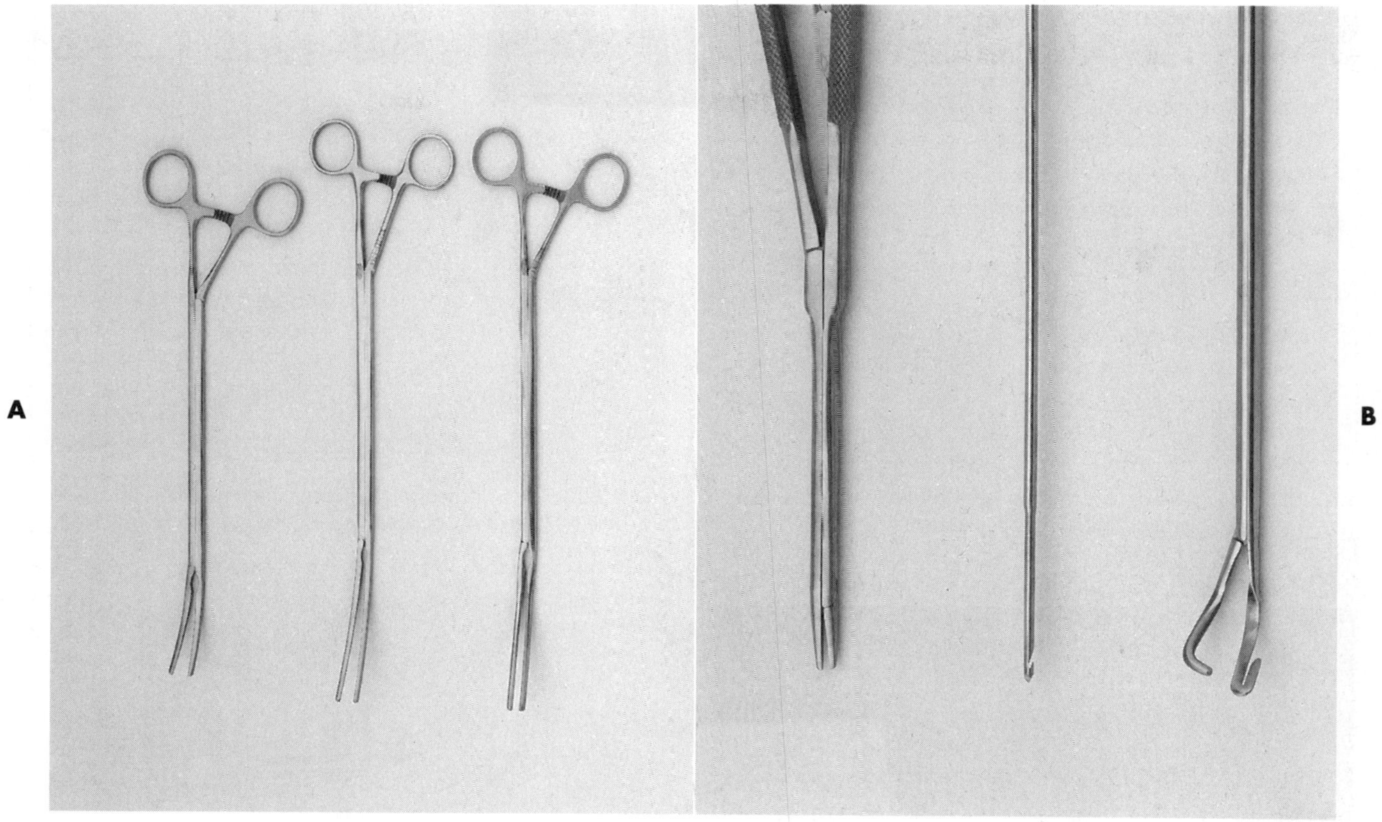

FIGURE 27-14 **A**, Transthoracic DeBakey vascular clamps are designed to pass through the chest wall via smaller incisions for minimally invasive procedures. **B**, Close-up view of minimally invasive needle holder, trocar/suture puller, and knot slider.

provide improved exposure of the left atrium during mitral valve replacement (MVR) (Fig. 27-16). Exposure of the left or right atrium, or the aortic root, may also be accomplished with hand-held retractors. Special rib spreaders provide exposure for minithoracotomy procedures (Fig. 27-17).

Other equipment commonly used (or available) for cardiac surgery includes the following:

- Sternal saw and motor
- Slush machine
- Autotransfusion system
- Electrical fibrillator
- DC defibrillator and internal paddles (Fig. 27-18)
- Thermia unit
- External and internal pulse pacemaker generator (single and dual chamber)
- Pump oxygenator
- Epicardial pacemaker leads (temporary and permanent)
- Fiberoptic headlight and light source
- Intraaortic balloon pump
- Mechanical assist pumps
- Transesophageal echocardiography (TEE)
- Intraoperative mapping, testing equipment for dysrhythmia surgery

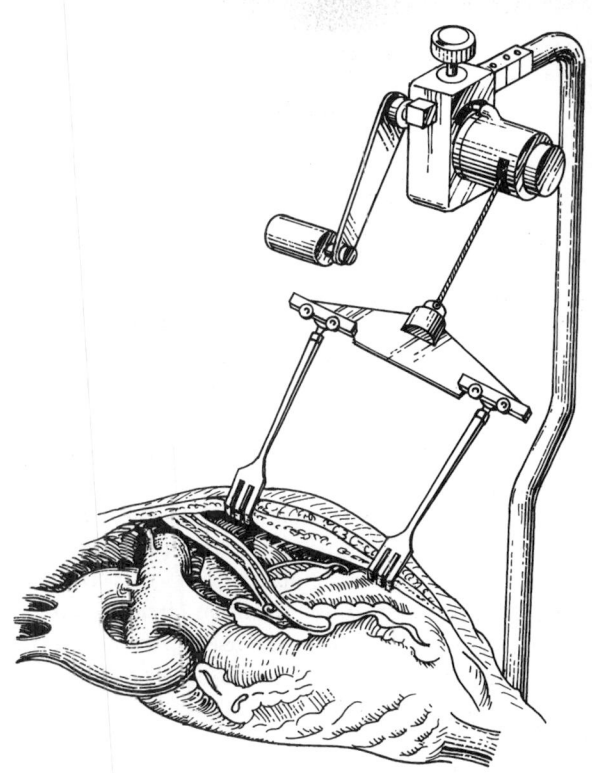

FIGURE 27-15 Retractor used to elevate sternal border for exposure of the internal mammary artery.

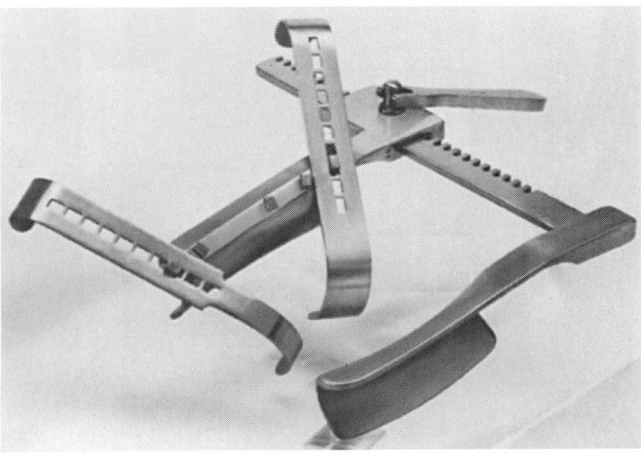

FIGURE 27-16 Sternal self-retaining retractor with attachments for left atrial retraction during mitral valve replacement.

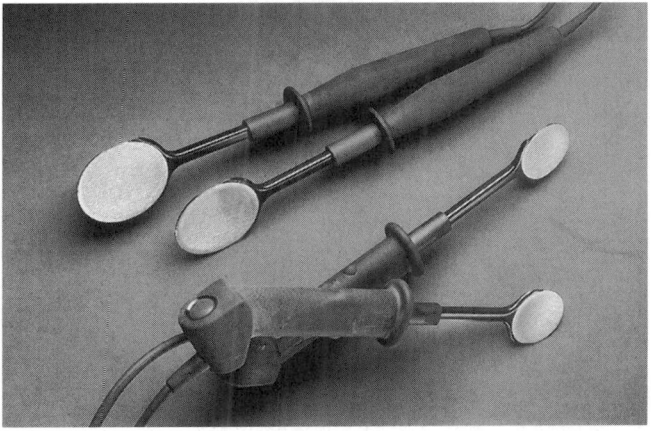

FIGURE 27-18 Switched and switchless internal defibrillator paddles are available in an array of sizes. Smaller internal paddles are used for infants and children.

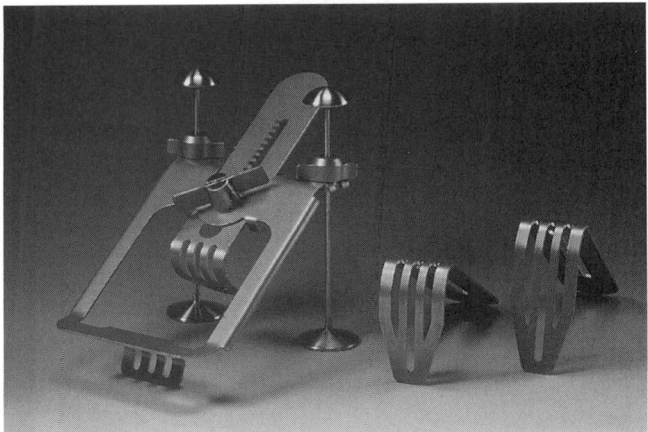

FIGURE 27-17 Minimally invasive rib retractor provides access to the internal mammary artery.

- Thoracoscopes equipment
- Video equipment

Suture materials

A variety of nonabsorbable cardiovascular sutures with atraumatic needles are available from most suture manufacturers. Synthetic sutures of Teflon, Dacron, polyester, or polypropylene are usually selected for insertion of prostheses and for vascular anastomoses. Most sutures are double armed with a needle on each end. Because of the number of stitches required for prosthetic valve placement, alternately colored suture may be helpful to avoid confusion. Vessel loops and umbilical tapes are commonly used to identify and to retract blood vessels and other structures. Wire is used to approximate the sternum (Fig. 27-19), with plastic or nylon bands occasionally added to reinforce fragile bone. Skin staplers may be used to close skin incisions; a staple remover must accompany the patient to the recovery area if staples have been used to close the chest.

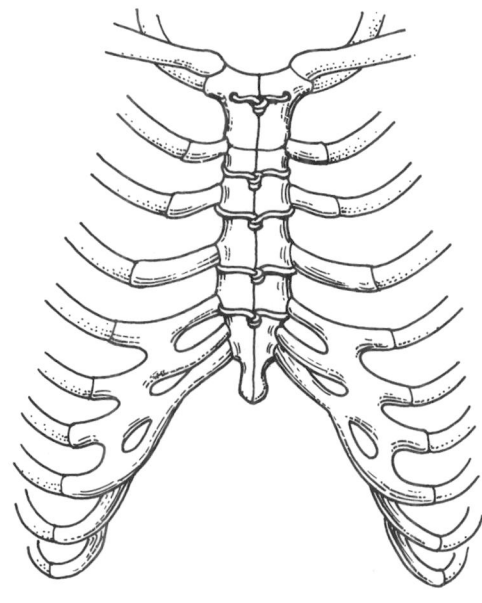

FIGURE 27-19 Technique for wire closure of the sternum. In selected patients in whom disruption may be anticipated, such as elderly, obese, malnourished persons, two or more heavy bands of nylon may be passed around the sternum and secured by a twisted stainless steel wire, in addition to the wire sutures. A figure-of-eight technique may also be employed.

Supplies

The following supplies are generally used in most cardiac procedures. Depending on surgeon preference, other items may be added or substituted.

- Rubbershods
- Pill sponges
- Various-sized Silastic or polyvinyl chloride tubing
- Tourniquet catheters
- Disposable drapes
- Foot control and hand control electrosurgical pencils
- Adapters, connectors, stopcocks

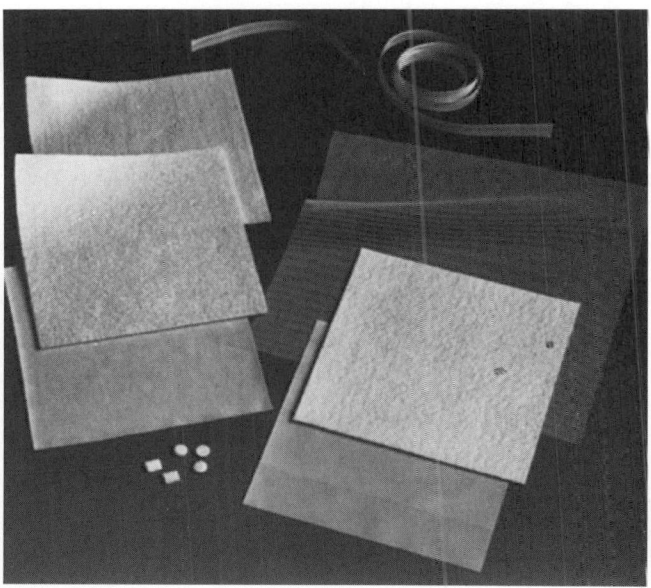

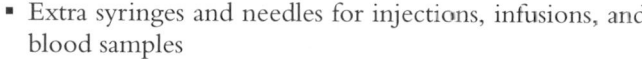

FIGURE 27-20 Assorted prosthetic materials to repair intracardiac and extracardiac defects: tapes, Teflon and Dacron patches, and pledgets.

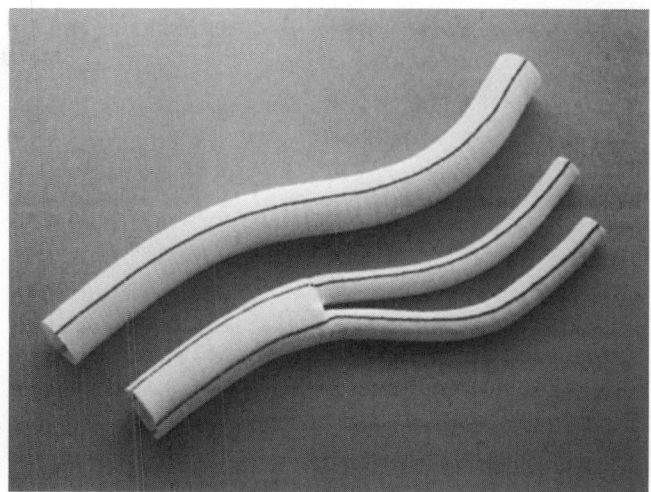

FIGURE 27-21 Straight and bifurcated arterial tube grafts.

- Extra syringes and needles for injections, infusions, and blood samples
- Marking pen to identify anastomotic sites and mark grafts
- Irrigation cannulas
- Disposable vascular (bulldog) clamps
- Coronary occluders and stabilizers
- Autotransfusion supplies
- Chest tubes, chest drainage system
- Topical hemostatic agents

Prosthetic material

In addition to these general supplies, special supplies are needed for repair or replacement of cardiovascular structures. Intracardiac patches, heart valves, and synthetic grafts should be handled with care to prevent damage or the introduction of foreign materials. Teflon, a fluorocarbon fiber, and Dacron, a polyester fiber, are available in a variety of meshes, fabrics, felts, tapes, and sutures and are also combined with other materials in prosthetic heart valves (Fig. 27-20).

Teflon patches are made in a variety of forms for intracardiac and outflow tract use. Varying degrees of firmness, thickness, and porosity are available for specific uses. Low reactivity, strength retention, and tissue acceptance are important properties to be considered in the selection of such patches.

Dacron arterial grafts are commonly used in cardiac surgery, although reinforced expanded polytetrafluorethylene (PTFE) grafts are also available. There are two types of Dacron grafts: knitted and woven. Woven prosthetic grafts are usually employed when the patient has been fully heparinized because the interstices of woven grafts are tighter than those in knitted grafts, and bleeding is usually

reduced. The advantages of knitted grafts are that they do not fray as readily as woven grafts when cut, they are easier to handle, and they reendothelialize more quickly than woven grafts do. Grafts are available in a variety of sizes and may be straight or bifurcated (Fig. 27-21). Knitted and woven grafts impregnated with collagen to reduce interstitial bleeding are useful in the thoracic aorta and do not have to be preclotted, even when the patient is fully heparinized for cardiopulmonary bypass. Graft sizers are available for determining the correct size.

Tube grafts reinforced at one or both ends with metal rings have been used in surgery for thoracic and abdominal aneurysms; the intraaortic device is anchored in place with nylon tapes tied around the rings. Some surgeons may elect to insert a few interrupted stitches to further secure the prosthesis. If one end of the graft has no ring or the ring has been cut, routine anastomotic techniques are used (Fig. 27-22).

Valve prostheses

Valve prostheses are selected according to their hemodynamics, thromboresistance, ease of insertion, anatomic suitability, and patient acceptability.[73] Most mechanical prostheses employ a tilting disk or ball-and-cage design. Prosthetic valves allow complete closure with slight regurgitation to prevent stasis of blood (Figs. 27-23 to 27-26). Porcine and bovine prostheses (Figs. 27-27 to 27-29) are also available. Porcine valves (see Fig. 27-27) consist of an aortic valve from a pig, which is sutured to a Dacron-covered stent; bovine pericardial valves (see Fig. 27-28) are created by cutting leaflet-shaped pieces from bovine pericardium and sewing them onto a stent (stentless allografts and bioprostheses are also available). The advantage of these biologic valves is that long-term

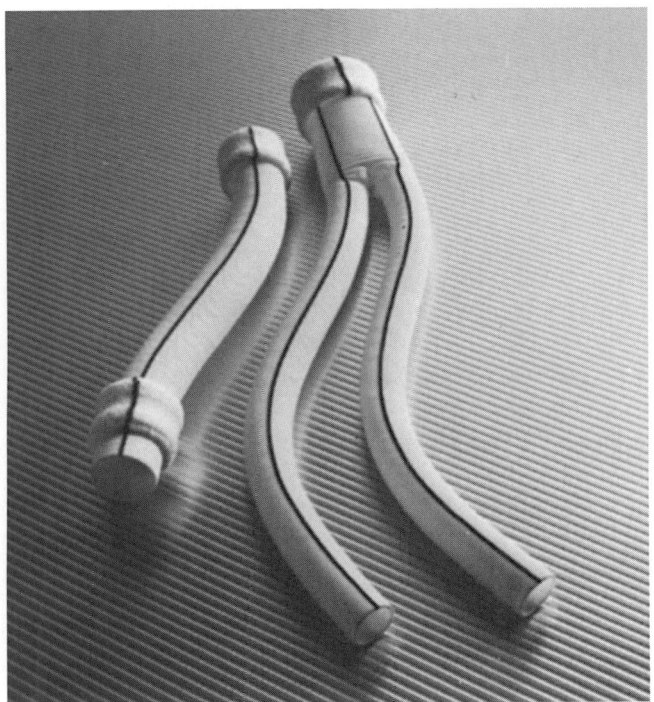

FIGURE 27-22   Ringed intraaortic prostheses, straight and bifurcated, for emergency repair of aortic aneurysms.

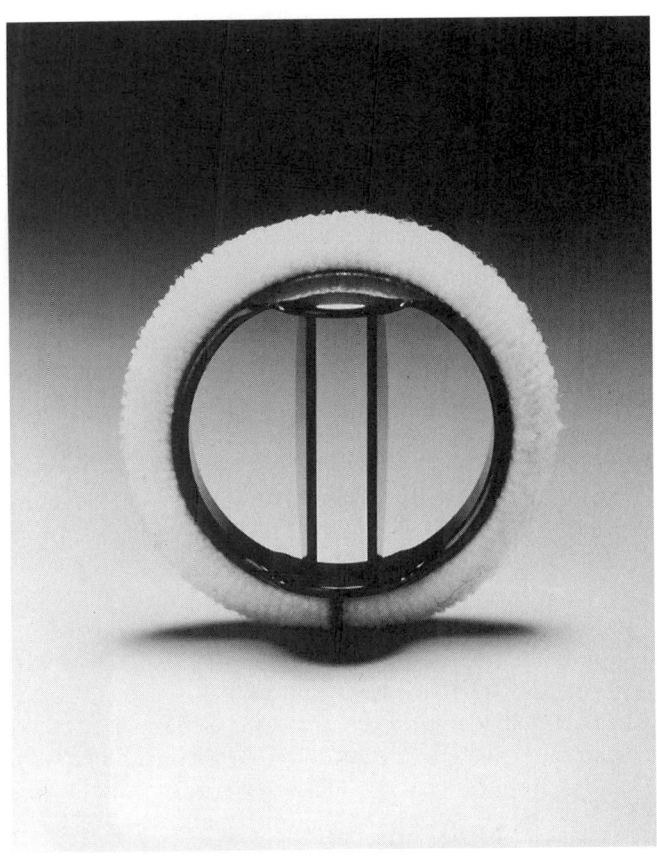

FIGURE 27-23   St. Jude Medical bileaflet tilting disc valve prosthesis.

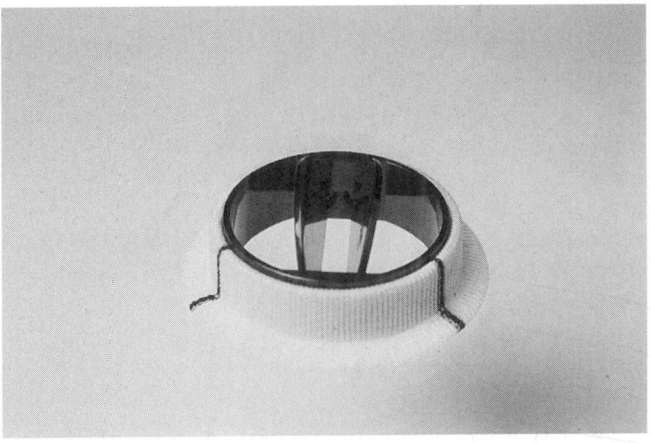

FIGURE 27-24   Carbomedics supra-annular aortic prosthesis designed for the small aortic root.

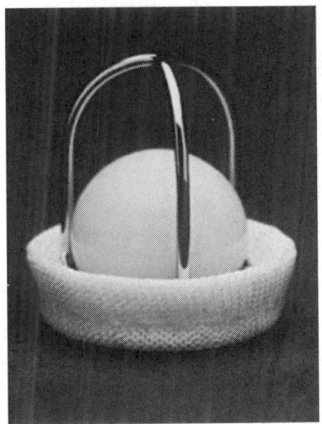

FIGURE 27-25   Starr-Edwards ball-cage aortic valve prosthesis.

anticoagulants are not necessary in most patients.[58] Obturators for sizing prosthetic valves as well as valve holders are specific to the prostheses (see Figs. 27-26, B and 27-29). Table 27-6 compares biologic and mechanical prosthetic heart valves.

Aortic valve allografts (homografts) are used with increasing frequency because of their advantages: little or no risk of thromboembolism, optimal hemodynamic function, no need for anticoagulation drugs, and no risk of sudden catastrophic failure. Moreover, they demonstrate a lower incidence of infective endocarditis than mechanical or biologic valves do, and their long-term durability is superior to that of bioprostheses.[59] Allograft root replacement is also a valuable technique in the setting of prosthetic valve endocarditis.[31] The entire ascending aorta and valve (Fig. 27-30) or the valve alone (Fig. 27-31) may be inserted. Allografts are cryopreserved and must be thawed in saline according to the vendor's protocol before implantation.

Conduits consisting of mechanical or biologic aortic valves attached to a tube graft (Fig. 27-32) are used in

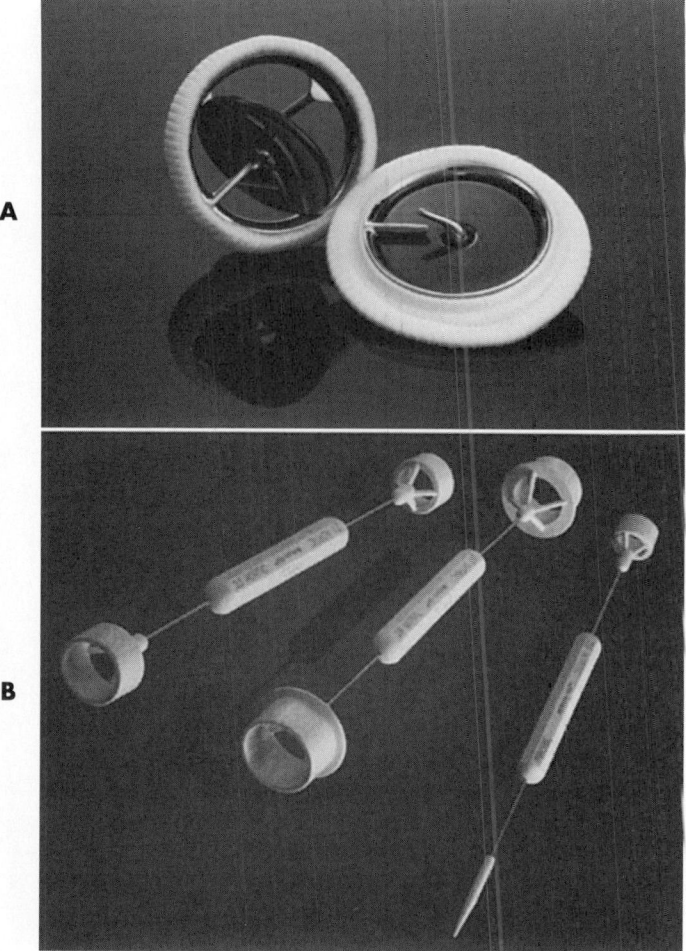

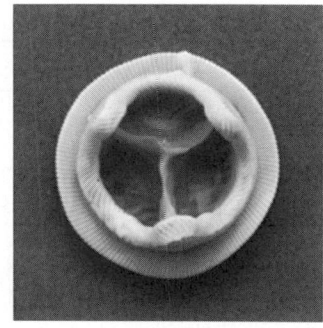

FIGURE 27-27   Hancock porcine bioprosthesis.

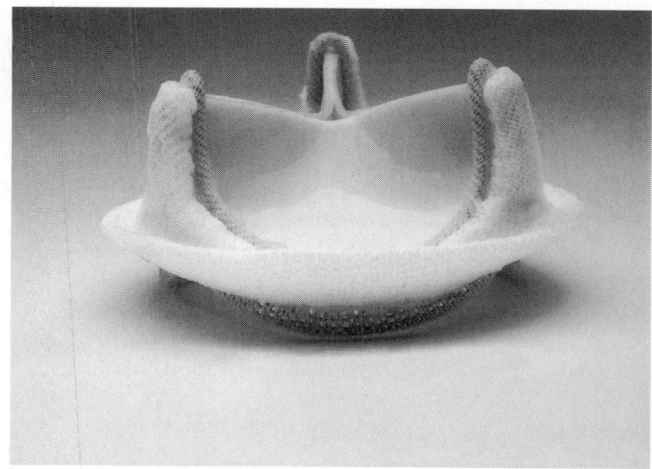

FIGURE 27-28   Carpentier-Edwards bovine pericardial aortic bioprosthesis.

FIGURE 27-26 **A**, Medtronic-Hall tilting disk valve prosthesis. **B**, Double-ended sizing obturators for the Medtronic-Hall prosthesis (*left, center*) and probe (*right*) to test leaflet movement. All valve prostheses have sizing obturators specific to the prosthesis itself.

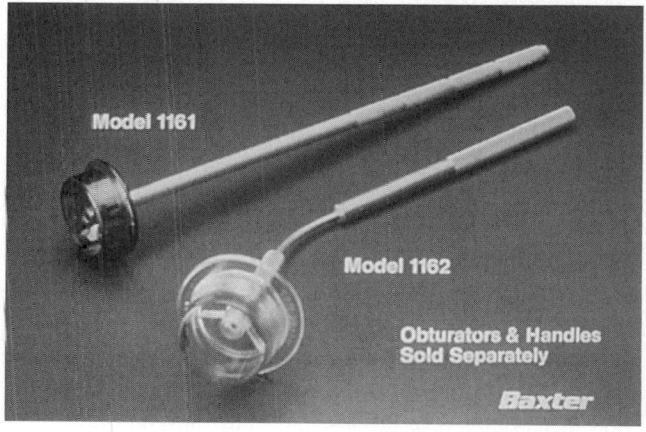

FIGURE 27-29   Obturators for Carpentier-Edwards porcine bioprosthesis.

procedures such as repair of aortic dissections requiring replacement of the aortic valve and ascending aorta. If vein grafts must be inserted into the conduit or if a direct coronary ostial anastomosis is required, an eye cautery is used to make the opening into the graft and at the same time heat-seal the cut edges of the prosthesis. Conduits with biologic valves interposed between tube graft material may be used when patients are at increased risk for bleeding complications from chronic anticoagulation. Allograft conduits may be used for these procedures as well.

In addition to the use of allografts to avoid the complications associated with prosthetic valve replacement, valve repair rather than replacement is preferred when possible, resulting in greater use of mitral and tricuspid annuloplasty rings (Fig. 27-33) to restore valvular competence. Obturators specific to each kind of annuloplasty ring are used to size the annulus.

Safety considerations include storing prosthetic materials in a clean, protected environment and utilizing them according to manufacturers' instructions. Before implantation, biologic valves must be rinsed in three saline baths to remove the glutaraldehyde storage solution. During insertion they should be kept moist with saline. Mechanical valves should be protected from scratching and other injury.

TABLE 27-6 | Commonly Used Mechanical and Biologic Valve Prostheses

| | BALL AND CAGE | TILTING DISK | |
	STARR-EDWARDS	MEDTRONIC-HALL, OMNISCIENCE	CARBOMEDICS ST. JUDE MEDICAL
Mechanical			
Model/description	6120 mitral; 1260 aortic	Spherical tilting disk	Bileaflet tilting disk
Advantages	Long-term durability	Long-term durability	Long-term durability
	Good hemodynamics	Good hemodynamics in all sizes	Good hemodynamics in all sizes
	Inaudible	Low profile	Low TE rate for a mechanical valve
	Least risk of sudden thrombosis		Low profile
Disadvantages	Anticoagulation required	Anticoagulation required	Anticoagulation strongly recommended
	Higher incidence of TE than disk valves	Sudden thrombosis	Sudden thrombosis
		Noisy	Some noise
	Suboptimal hemodynamics in small aortic sizes (less than 23 mm)	Higher risk of TE in mitral position	Higher risk of TE in mitral position
	High profile not optimal in small LV or aortic root	If Coumadin (warfarin sodium) must be discontinued, there is increased risk of catastrophic thrombosis	If Coumadin must be discontinued, there is increased risk of catastrophic thrombosis
	Higher risk of TE in mitral position		
Special considerations	Sizers and handles specific to prosthesis; must be sterilized	Sizers and handles specific to prosthesis; must be sterilized	Sizers and handles specific to prosthesis; must be sterilized
	Poppet of aortic valve removable to facilitate tying sutures; replaced before aorta closed; mitral poppet not removable		
	Aortic model has 3 struts; mitral has 4		
Resterilization	See manufacturer's instructions	See manufacturer's instructions	See manufacturer's instructions

Adapted from Vongpatanasin, W., Hillis, L.D., & Lange, R.A. (1996). Prosthetic heart valves. *New England Journal of Medicine, 335*(6), 407–416.
LV, Left ventricle; *TE,* thromboembolism.

Preinduction care

The patient is brought to the operating room suite, where a preoperative assessment is performed, and the perioperative nurse reviews the chart for completion and documentation of informed consent, advance directives, laboratory results, diagnostic data, and other pertinent information. Preoperatively, cardiac surgical patients may exhibit more stress and anxiety than other types of patients. Perioperative nurses should anticipate and prepare for this reaction because anxiety increases myocardial oxygen consumption.[7] Efforts to reduce the family's anxiety level are also important and result in less emotional stress being transmitted to the patient.

A peripheral arterial pressure line and venous infusion lines are inserted. A local anesthetic may be used at the insertion sites, and a sedative may be injected intravenously.

Admission to the operating room

Depending on the amount of sedation received preoperatively, the patient may require assistance onto the OR bed. Warm blankets should be provided for comfort and to reduce shivering. After application of the ECG leads and the pulse oximeter finger cot, the hands, elbows, and feet can be padded. The perioperative nurse confirms that the peripheral arterial pressure line and the pulse oximeter are performing properly; repositioning the arms is performed as necessary and proper position confirmed with the anesthesia care provider.

Anesthesia induction

The choice of anesthetic agent or agents depends on the cardiovascular effects of the anesthetic and the patient's hemodynamics and general health. Because the period of induction is one of the most critical during the procedure, close monitoring of the patient is required, especially for patients with ventricular ischemia from congenital or acquired disease. Anesthetic management focuses on keeping myocardial oxygen demand low and the oxygen supply high.[45] (See Chapter 7 for additional considerations related to anesthesia care monitoring.)

Monitoring

Maximal monitoring of hemodynamic and other variables is indicated during cardiac surgery (Table 27-7). After intubation (or before, depending on anesthesia preference), additional pressure lines may be inserted to measure central venous pressure and pulmonary artery

TABLE 27-6 | Commonly Used Mechanical and Biologic Valve Prostheses—cont'd

	HETEROGRAFT		ALLOGRAFT (HOMOGRAFT)
	CARPENTIER-EDWARDS; HANCOCK	CARPENTIER-EDWARDS PERICARDIAL VALVE	
Biologic			
Model description	Porcine heterograft (from excised pig aortic valves, mounted on stent)	2700 aortic bovine pericardium (cut and shaped into a trileaflet valve, mounted on stent)	Aortic valve allograft (cadaver, organ donor, excised cardiomyopathic heart from transplant recipient)
Advantages	Incidence of TE very low; anti-coagulation rare after AVR No hemolysis Good hemodynamics Central flow Gradual failure allows elective reoperation	Incidence of TE very low; anti-coagulation rare after AVR No hemolysis Good hemodynamics in all sizes Central flow Gradual failure allows elective reoperation Residual gradient minimal	Incidence of TE very low; anticoagulation rare (used mainly for AVR) No hemolysis Excellent hemodynamics (especially with stentless technique) Central flow Gradual failure allows elective reoperation No residual gradient
Disadvantages	Durability less than 15 years Accelerated fibrocalcific degeneration in children and patients with hypertension or on chronic renal dialysis Suboptimal hemodynamics and residual gradient in smaller sizes (less than 23 mm aorta or 29 mm mitral) May be contraindicated in small, hypertrophied LV	Durability not yet established Available only for AVR Accelerated calcification may be a problem in children, renal patients, or those with hypertension	Limited durability Limited availability
Special considerations	Sizers and handles specific to prosthesis; must be sterilized Before insertion, must be rinsed in saline to remove glutar-aldehyde storage solution Frequent irrigation recommended to prevent drying Diets low in calcium recommended for children, renal patients	Approved for aortic position only Sizers and handles specific to prosthesis; must be sterilized Before insertion, must be rinsed in saline to remove glutaralde-hyde storage solution Frequent irrigation recommended to prevent drying Diets low in calcium recommended for children, renal patients	No specific sizers; may use sizers for heterografts Cryopreserved allograft must be thawed per protocol Used for aortic valve replacement; stent attached for use in the mitral and tricuspid position
Resterilization	Not recommended	Not recommended	Not recommended

AVR, Aortic valve replacement.

pressures. Peripheral and central arterial and venous pressures are usually monitored directly by means of a transducer and oscilloscope. Perioperative nurses may be required to assist with the preparation and placement of central lines; they should observe the ECG monitors for signs of ventricular irritability, such as ectopy or tachycardia, and be prepared to assist with defibrillation of the patient if necessary. If the patient cannot be resuscitated, the chest is opened rapidly and internal cardiac massage is performed. A urinary drainage catheter is inserted for monitoring renal function, especially during and after cardiopulmonary bypass. It may contain a thermistor

temperature probe. Other temperature probes may be placed, usually in the esophagus, nasopharynx, or rectum. Temperatures can also be recorded from the pulmonary artery catheters and the arterial infusion line of the bypass circuit. Ventricular septal temperatures may be recorded while the patient's heart is arrested.

The skin is carefully inspected before ECG and electrosurgical (ESU) dispersive pads are placed. Bony prominences, such as the coccyx and the back of the head, are padded to prevent pressure necrosis resulting from hypoperfusion and hypothermia during bypass. Because elderly patients are especially vulnerable to skin

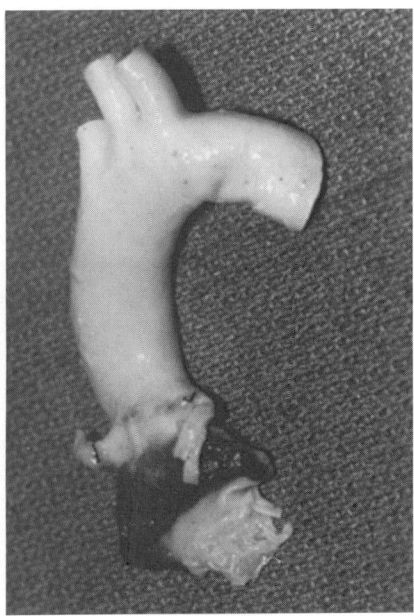

FIGURE 27–30 Aortic allograft (homograft) with aortic valve and arch vessels attached.

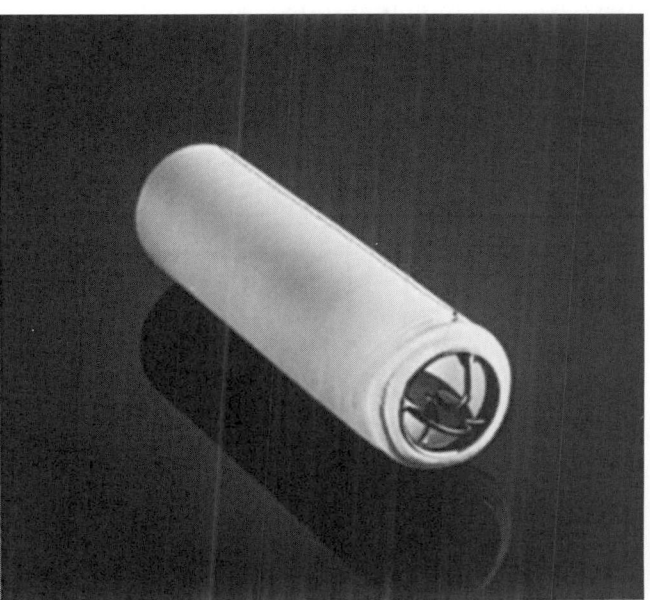

FIGURE 27–32 Valved conduit with Medtronic-Hall tilting disk valve prosthesis.

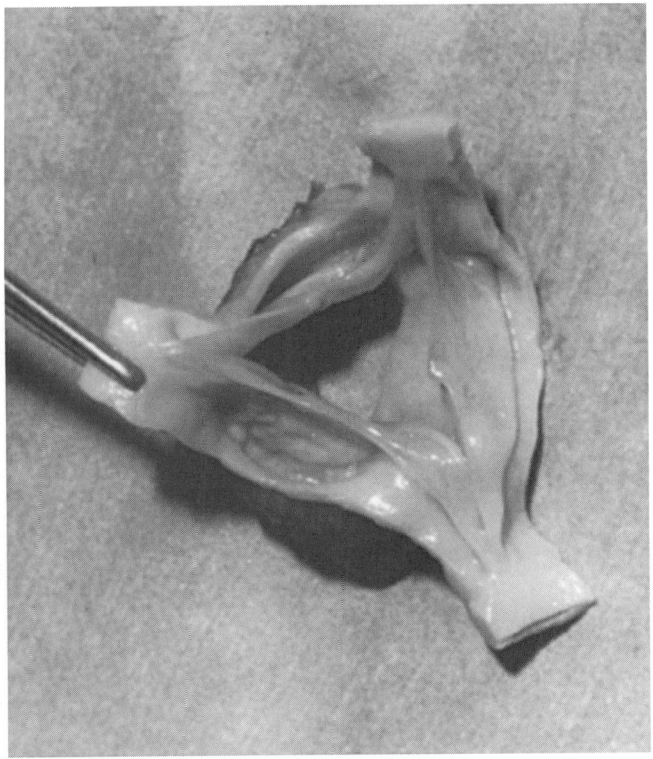

FIGURE 27–31 Aortic valve allograft (homograft).

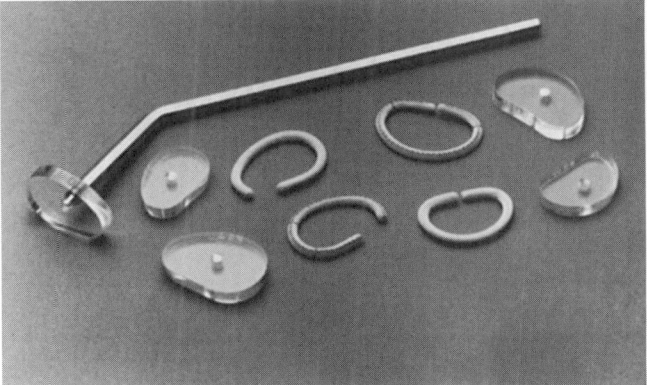

FIGURE 27–33 Carpentier-Edwards "classic" tricuspid and mitral annuloplasty rings, sizers, and sizer handle. The tricuspid rings are notched in the area corresponding to conduction tissue in the tricuspid annulus to avoid suture injury.

breakdown, additional precautions to avoid pressure injuries are recommended.[3]

Positioning

The supine position provides optimum exposure for the institution of cardiopulmonary bypass and the surgical repair of the heart and great vessels. In addition, there is less respiratory impairment and discomfort with this approach. When the supine position is used, the hands and arms are tucked along either side of the body. The legs may be slightly "frog-legged" to provide access to the femoral arteries for insertion of pressure lines, or intraaortic balloon pump lines or to excise the saphenous vein. Measures to avoid venous stasis ulcers (especially in the elderly, debilitated, or obese patient) include padding of the coccyx and application of heel protectors. Measures to protect the occipital area from pressure ulcers include placing pillows under the head and readjusting the head during surgery (Research Highlight 27-1). Significant factors associated with the development of pressure ulcers include diabetes mellitus; lower preoperative hemoglobin, hematocrit, and serum albumin levels; and the presence of intraaortic balloon pumps.[50]

TABLE 27-7 | Perioperative Patient Monitoring

MONITORING DEVICE	LOCATION	MEASURES
Electrocardiogram (ECG)	Lateral, posterior electrode placement	Electrical activity of heart
Arterial line	Peripheral	Arterial blood pressure (direct)
	Radial artery	
	Central	
	Femoral artery	
	Aorta (with needle attached to pressure tubing, or with sensor in bypass circuit)	
Blood pressure (BP) cuff	Upper arm	Arterial BP (indirect)
Central venous pressure (CVP) line	Right atrium (RA)	RA pressure (e.g., CVP)
Pulmonary artery (PA) catheter	RA (proximal port)	RA pressure (e.g., CVP)
(Swan-Ganz)	Right ventricle (RV) (midline port)	RV pressure
	Distal PA (distal port)	PA and pulmonary artery wedge pressure (PAWP)
		Indirect measure of left atrial and left ventricular (LV) pressure
		Cardiac output
Left atrial (LA) line	Left atrium	LA, LV pressure
Pulse oximeter	Finger, ear lobe	Oxygen saturation of arterial hemoglobin
Urinary drainage catheter	Urinary bladder	Urine output, renal perfusion/function
Temperature probes	Esophagus	Temperature (core and peripheral)
	Urinary bladder	
	Rectum	
	Ventricular septum	
	Bypass circuit	
	Pulmonary artery catheter	
Electroencephalogram (EEG)	Head	Electrical activity of brain

27-1 RESEARCH HIGHLIGHT

Steinmetz and Langemo designed a descriptive study to evaluate occipital capillary tissue interface pressures (TIPs) in patients undergoing coronary artery bypass grafting (CABG). A convenience sample of 25 adults scheduled for nonemergent CABG consented to participate in the study. Preoperative American Society of Anesthesiologists (ASA) physical status classification was P3 and P4; approximately 50% of subjects had a history of hypertension, and 20% had diabetes mellitus. The number of bypass grafts ranged from one to six per subject.

Each subject was placed in the supine position on the operating room (OR) bed. An electropneumatic sensor was placed on the bony prominence of the subject's occiput. The subject's head was then placed on a standard synthetic pillow, and one pillowcase was placed between the sensor and the subject's occiput. Occipital capillary TIP and mean arterial pressure was measured (1) before anesthesia induction (AI), (2) within 10 minutes after AI, (3) after the subject was placed on cardiopulmonary bypass (CPB), (4) every 30 minutes while on CPB, (5) immediately after termination of CPB, and (6) before closure of the chest incision.

The researchers found significant changes in TIP, which was highest during the anesthesia-induction period and lowest during CPB and immediately after termination of CPB. The results of this study indicate that CABG patients may be at risk for pressure ulcers and alopecia related to prolonged immobility, underlying circulatory impairment, and unresponsiveness to somatic stimuli signaling inadequate tissue oxygenation. Recommendations include repositioning patients' heads every 30 minutes and replication of the study in patients who are not cooled and placed on CPB (as may occur in some forms of minimally invasive CABG procedures performed on a "beating" heart).

From Steinmetz, J.A., & Langemo, D.K. (1996). Changes in occipital capillary perfusion pressure during coronary artery bypass graft surgery. *Advances in Wound Care, 9,* 28-32.

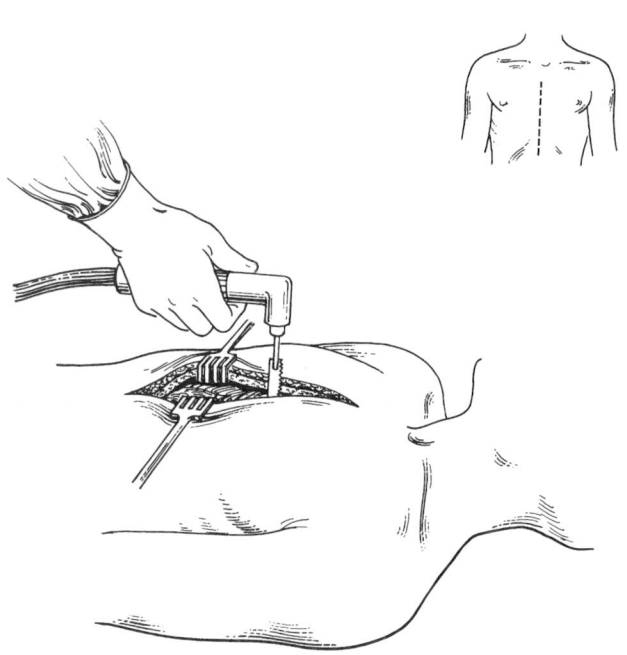

FIGURE 27-34   Median sternotomy with sternal saw.

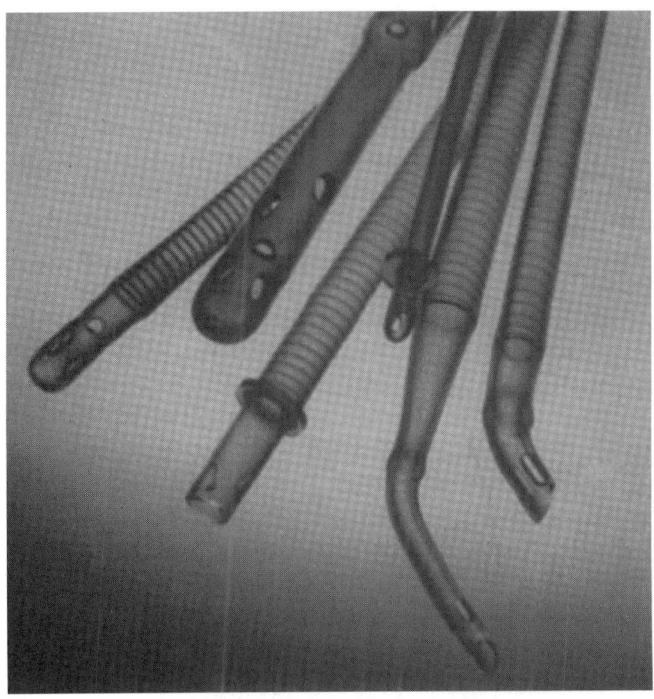

FIGURE 27-35   Arterial and venous perfusion cannulas.

The thoracotomy position is used for some minimally invasive procedures and surgery on the descending thoracic aorta. The presence of severe mediastinal adhesions may also necessitate this approach in some repeat valve operations.[35] Thoracotomy positioning aids should be available to position arms and legs per surgeon protocol (see Chapter 25).

Prepping and draping

For procedures requiring excision of the saphenous vein, the prep extends from the jaw to the toes and includes the anterior (or lateral) area of the chest, abdomen, groin, and legs. The legs and feet are prepped circumferentially and the chest and abdomen from bedline to bedline.

In procedures not requiring saphenous vein excision, the prep extends to the knees to give the surgeon access to the femoral artery or saphenous vein in the thigh area. Femoral artery access may be required for arterial pressure monitoring or insertion of an intraaortic balloon. Saphenous vein exposure facilitates access should a bypass conduit be required. In the lateral position, the patient is prepped bedline to bedline anteriorly and posteriorly to the knees.

After the prep, the patient is draped so that the anterior area of the chest, abdomen, and inguinal area are accessible. The perineum is covered, and a towel may be placed across the umbilicus to connect the side drapes. When the saphenous vein is to be excised, both legs remain exposed, with only the feet covered. When draping, the perioperative nurse should consider the

placement of bypass lines so that they remain securely attached and do not become contaminated. A small drape or towel may be placed over the groin area when access to it is not immediately necessary. If, later, the femoral artery needs to be accessed, the drape can be discarded.

Incisions

Both standard median sternotomy and mini- or full thoracotomy incisions may be used, depending on surgeon preference and type of procedure.

Median Sternotomy

The skin incision extends from the sternal notch to the linea alba below the xiphoid process (Fig. 27-34). The sternum is divided with a saw, and a sternal retractor is inserted. If the internal mammary artery or the saphenous vein will be used, they are made available at this time. The pericardium is incised and retracted with sutures.

In repeat sternotomies, adhesions from a previous cardiac operation must be dissected. The sternum may be split with a vibrating saw and the retrosternal tissue cut free. Increased risk of fibrillation from manipulation of the heart and bleeding and laceration of the ventricle should alert the perioperative nurse to the possibility of instituting femoral vein–femoral artery bypass (discussed later). If the patient fibrillates during dissection, sterile external paddles or internal-external paddles may be needed if two internal paddles cannot be inserted into the scarred, adherent pericardium. In the latter case, an external paddle is placed behind the patient before the prep, one internal paddle is placed on the anterior surface of the heart, and the patient

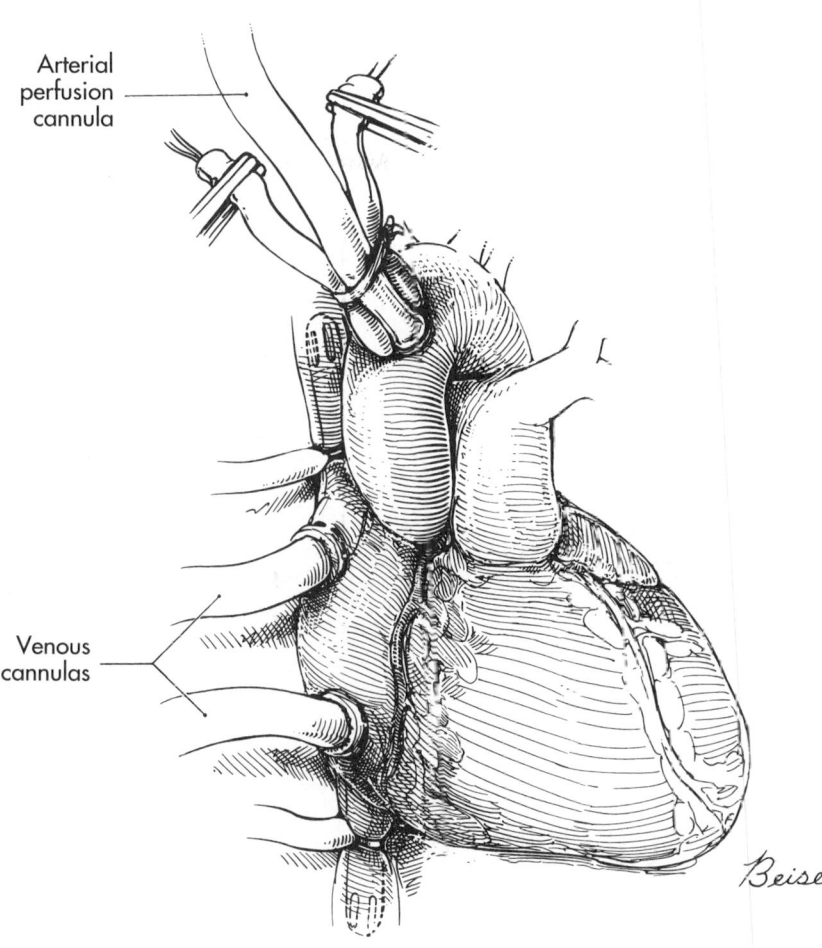

Arterial
perfusion
cannula

Venous
cannulas

Beisel

FIGURE 27-36   Bicaval cannulation of the superior and inferior venae cavae; aortic cannulation.

is defibrillated. Occasionally, two internal paddles can be used if the pleura is opened; one paddle tip is inserted through the pleural opening and placed against the heart, and the second is positioned on top of the heart.

Anteroposterior and lateral chest radiographs are useful to determine the extent of retrosternal adhesions and to count the number of chest wires for removal (see Fig. 27-9). On occasion a patient presents for repeat mitral valve surgery. If the initial operation was performed through a thoracotomy incision, sternal adhesions may be minimal or nonexistent, and the special precautions associated with repeat sternotomy may not be necessary.

Minithoracotomy

For minimally invasive cardiac procedures, a variety of smaller (up to approximately 8 cm) incisions can be used. These include anterolateral chest incisions small enough for the insertion of specially designed retractors and instruments (see Fig. 27-14). At this stage of development of minimally invasive technology, cardiac procedures are commonly performed through smaller incisions but still under direct visualization by the surgeon using special instruments. Video-assisted techniques are being rapidly developed and tested but are not commonly employed in the clinical setting.

Cardiopulmonary bypass

The temporary substitution of a pump oxygenator for the heart and lungs allows the surgeon to stop the heart to perform cardiac procedures under direct vision in a relatively dry, motionless field. It also allows the surgeon to manipulate the heart (which can result in inefficient contraction and reduce cardiac output) without jeopardizing perfusion to the rest of the body.[72]

Under some circumstances, access to the anteroapical portion of the heart can be achieved without manipulation of the heart and the attendant risk of inducing ventricular fibrillation. These situations can allow the surgeon to create coronary artery bypass grafts to the anterolateral coronary arteries without the use of cardiopulmonary bypass (CPB) and induced cardiac arrest and forms the basis for minimally invasive procedures performed on a beating heart (discussed later).

In traditional CPB circuits, systemic venous return to the heart flows by gravity drainage through cannulas (Fig. 27-35) placed in the superior and inferior venae cavae (Fig. 27-36) or through a single two-stage cannula in the right atrium (Fig. 27-37) into tubing connected to the bypass machine. Blood is oxygenated, filtered, warmed or cooled, and pumped back into the systemic circulation through a cannula placed in the ascending aorta or

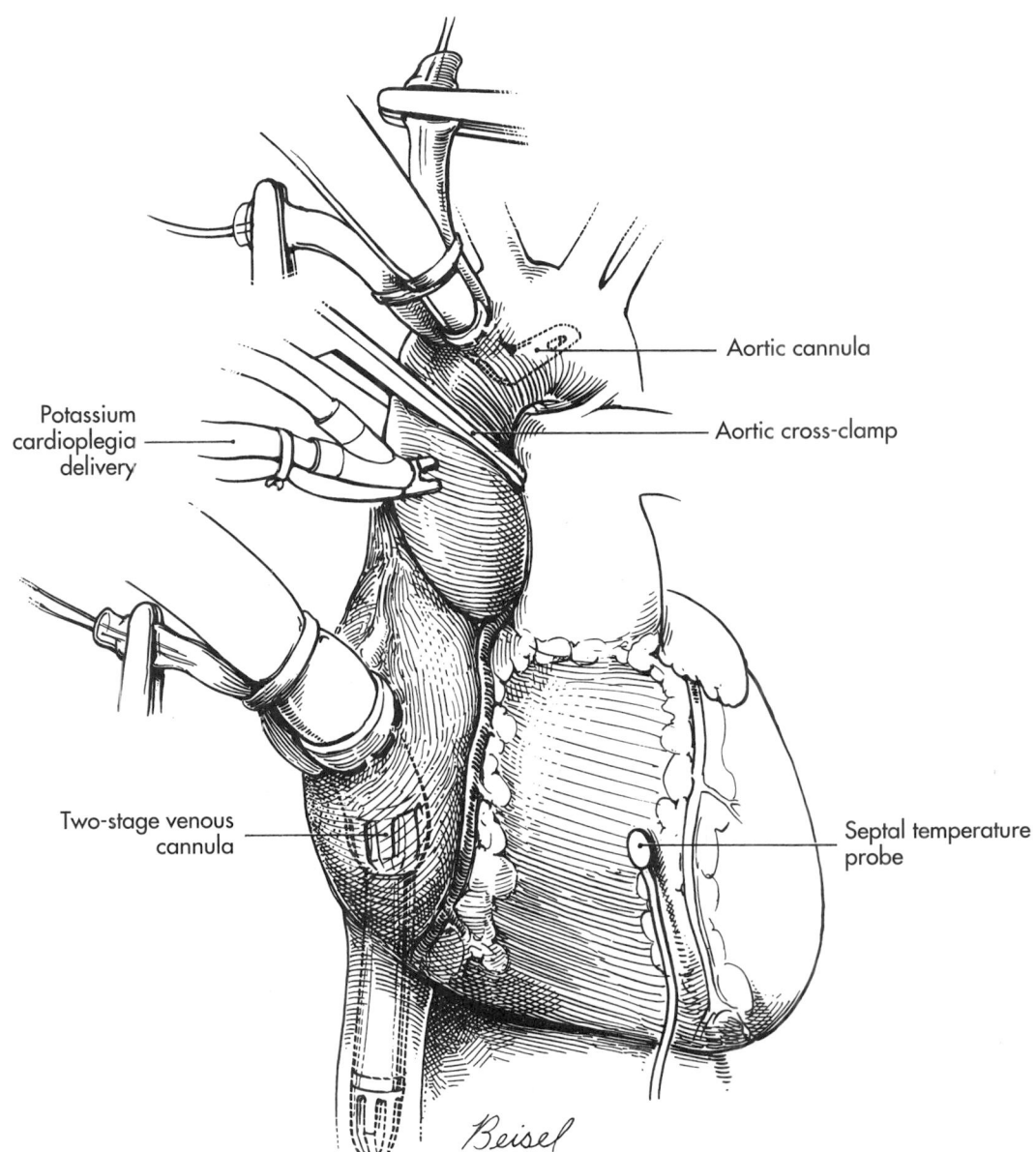

Potassium cardioplegia delivery

Aortic cannula

Aortic cross-clamp

Two-stage venous cannula

Septal temperature probe

Beisel

FIGURE 27-37 Diagram showing aortic and venous cannulas during aortic cross-clamping. Also shown is antegrade cardioplegic solution delivery catheter in the aorta proximal to the cross-clamp and a temperature probe. The single (two-stage) venous cannula has openings in the distal end of the cannula to drain the inferior vena cava; the openings in the midportion (right atrial area) of the cannula drain the superior vena cava and the coronary sinus venous return.

occasionally in the femoral artery (Fig. 27-38). Because blood is oxygenated by the CPB machine, the lungs do not need to function and can be deflated to provide better exposure of the mediastinal structures.

A percutaneous method of instituting femoral vein–femoral artery CPB can be used for minimally invasive procedures (Fig. 27-39) and in emergency situations where the environment is not conducive to traditional CPB methods (as in the cardiac catheterization laboratory, the intensive care unit, and the emergency department). The system employs thin-walled, wire-reinforced catheters inserted into the femoral vein and artery. Gravity drainage

is impeded by the resistance of the small-bore cannula used in the femoral vein; to overcome this, a centrifugal pump may be used to actively siphon blood to the pump oxygenator.

By diverting blood away from the heart, CPB also decompresses the ventricles, thereby reducing myocardial wall tension, which is a significant determinant of myocardial oxygen demand. This principle is evident when cardiopulmonary bypass or other means of ventricular support are employed to "rest" the heart. Further decompression is achieved by venting of the left ventricle to remove air and accumulated thebesian and bronchial

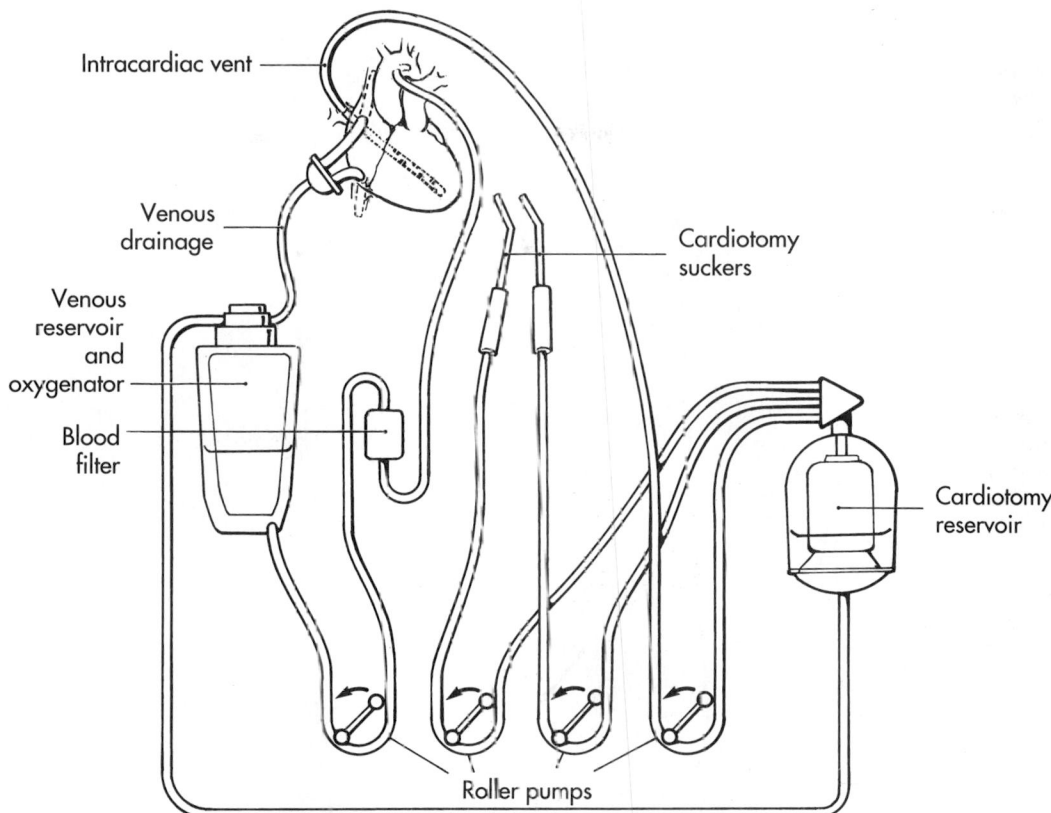

Intracardiac vent

Venous drainage

Venous reservoir and oxygenator

Blood filter

Cardiotomy suckers

Cardiotomy reservoir

Roller pumps

FIGURE 27-38   Cardiopulmonary bypass circuit. Venous blood is drained by gravity from the right atrium or venae cavae into an oxygenator that incorporates a blood reservoir and a heat exchanger, which warms or cools the blood as needed. The ventilating gas flowing into the oxygenator removes carbon dioxide and adds oxygen to the blood. Saturated blood leaves the oxygenator and is pumped from the reservoir into the arterial system by the use of a roller pump. Filters and monitors are incorporated into the circuit. Additional roller pumps are used to suction shed blood from the pericardial well and the intracardiac chambers (cardiotomy suckers); the blood is returned to the cardiotomy reservoir. Another roller pump is used to vent air and blood through a right superior pulmonary venous catheter that is inserted into the left ventricle.

venous return as well as systemic return flowing around the venous cannulas (Fig. 27-40). The venting catheter is inserted into the left ventricle via the right superior pulmonary vein or, less commonly, through the left ventricular apex. The venting line is connected to the suction lines of the bypass machine. A small venting catheter may also be inserted into the ascending aorta to remove air. Occasionally a vent is inserted into the pulmonary artery. Venting can reduce the incidence of gaseous emboli.

Membrane oxygenators (Fig. 27-41) are used for gas exchange that removes carbon dioxide and adds oxygen to the blood. Gases diffuse through a semipermeable membrane that separates the oxygenating gas and the venous blood. Although membrane oxygenators preserve platelet and red blood cell function better than the older "bubble" oxygenators, there is considerable morbidity associated with the use of CPB. Extracorporeal circulation causes fluid retention and intercompartmental fluid shifts, multiple organ dysfunction, showers of microemboli, inflam-

matory responses, and unique bleeding complications. The mechanism of injury is believed to be related to the exposure of the blood to the abnormal surfaces of the bypass circuit, hypothermia, and altered blood flow. These can initiate a systemic inflammatory response (complement activation), which releases vasoactive substances. Attempts to minimize the inflammatory reaction have focused on modifying the activation of platelets and blood factors that play a major role in initiating the response.[34] These complications have stimulated the development of "beating heart" techniques for myocardial revascularization that do not employ CPB.

Two types of pumps are available: roller pumps and centrifugal pumps. Roller pumps have roller heads that propel blood forward by compressing blood-filled tubing against a smooth, metal housing. Centrifugal pumps use cones or blades that rotate at high speed to produce forward flow. All pumps produce some hemolysis from turbulence and shear forces, but careful calibration and minimal use of connectors can provide relatively

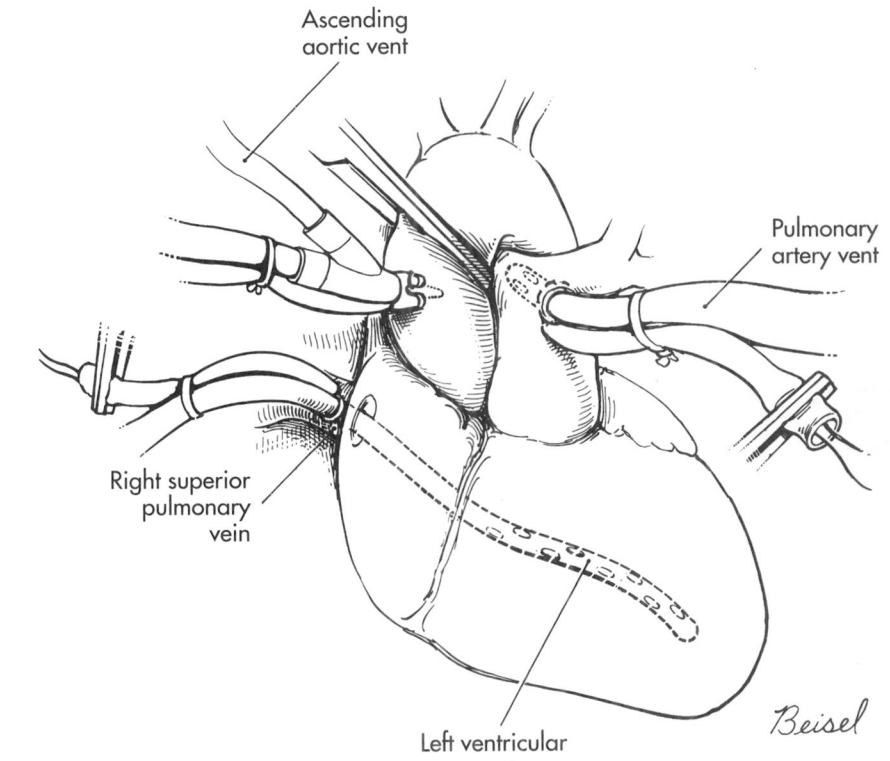

FIGURE 27-39 **A**, Endovascular cardiopulmonary bypass and myocardial protection system (see text). **B**, Intracardiac placement of catheters.

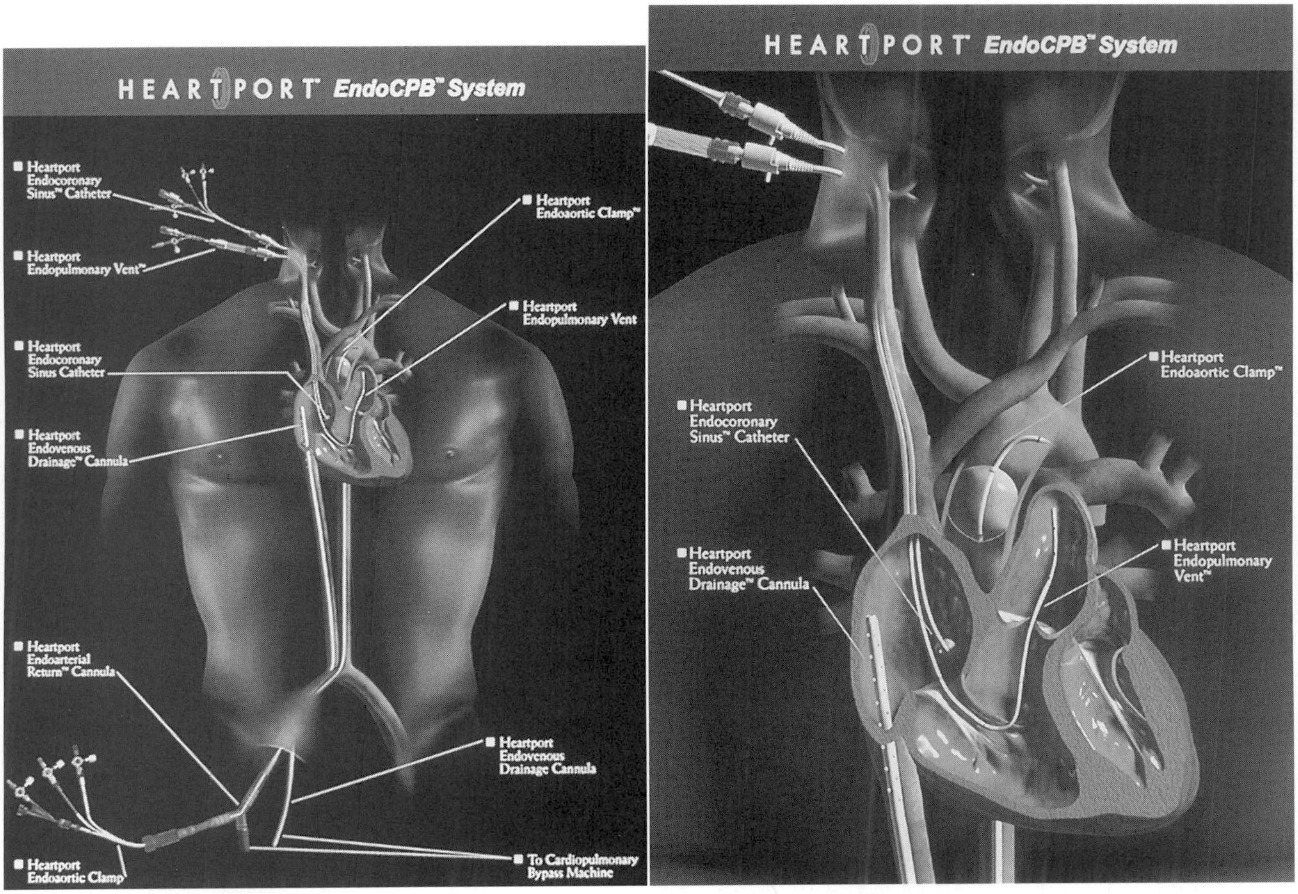

FIGURE 27-40 Types of venting catheters.

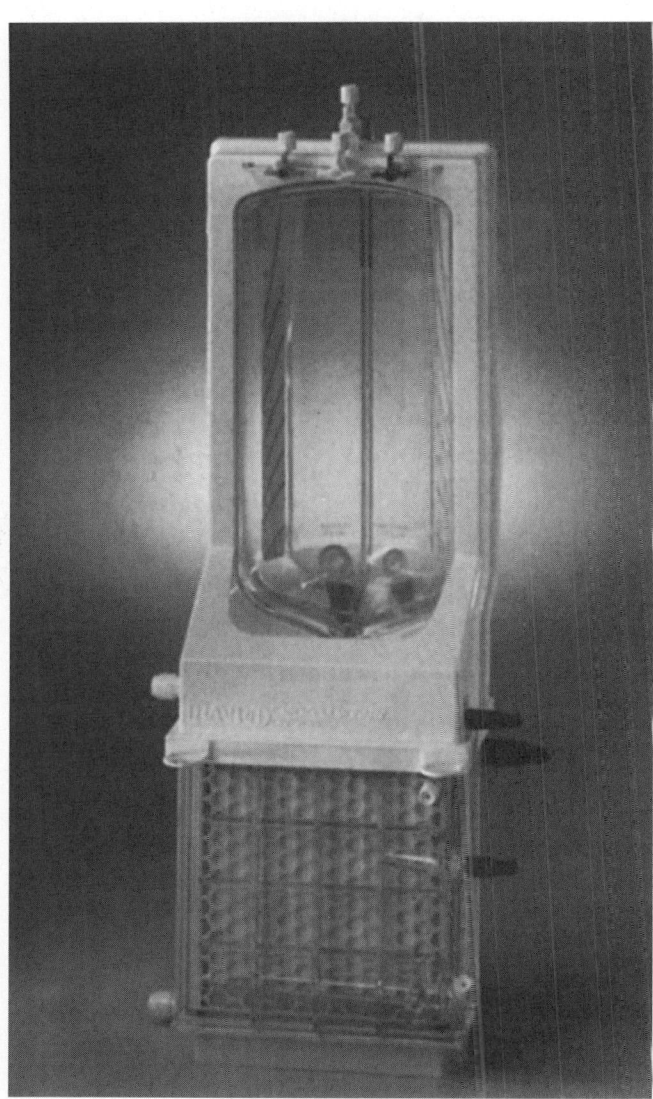

FIGURE 27-41   Membrane oxygenator.

atraumatic flow for short periods of time (such as less than 6 hours). Arterial blood flow on bypass is nonpulsatile (there are no systolic and diastolic intervals) and will be manifested by a mean arterial wave form on the oscilloscope during CPB. Modifications to the bypass circuit can be made to imitate pulsatile flow, but improved outcomes have been difficult to demonstrate.[72]

Suction lines are ordinarily used during CPB to return lost blood to the venous reservoir and the oxygenator (see Fig. 27-38). These lines usually combine conventional hand-held suction tubes and ventricular decompression lines or sumps (see Fig. 27-40). Before the initiation of CPB, the entire extracorporeal circuit must be primed, or rendered free of air, to prevent air emboli. The priming solution is usually a combination of colloid and crystalloid fluids with a balanced electrolyte component. This produces hemodilution, which reduces the amount of bank blood being used. Other advantages include reducing the number of homologous serum reactions and the incidence of hepatitis and human immunodeficiency virus

(HIV) as well as providing better perfusion of the capillary beds because of reduced blood viscosity. Hematocrits as low as 20% may be adequate during CPB, but once CPB is terminated, transfusion of red blood cells may be required to enhance the blood's oxygen-carrying capacity.[72]

The amount and kind of drugs used in the priming solution vary among institutions, but heparin is routinely added to block clot formation in the bypass circuit. Heparin-coated circuits are also available. Anticoagulation is routinely monitored during bypass, and more heparin is given as needed to maintain an activated clotting time (ACT) exceeding 600 seconds. Other ingredients are added to maintain normal pH and electrolytes.

Arterial blood flow rates are estimated according to the patient's height, weight, and body surface area. Depending on the arterial and venous pressure values and the results of blood gas determinations, the flow is adjusted.

Myocardial protection

Improvement in the results of cardiac surgery are attributable in great part to progress made in the protection of the myocardium. Coronary circulatory interruptions, ischemia, and hypoperfusion accompanying induced cardiac arrest are often necessary to permit the surgeon sufficient time to repair cardiac lesions under direct vision. Unless measures are taken to protect the myocardium during these periods, irreversible damage can result. The two main protective strategies are cooling the heart (and the rest of the body) to reduce metabolic demand, and rapidly arresting the heart so that myocardial energy resources are preserved.[14]

Hypothermia

Hypothermia in cardiac surgery is the deliberate reduction of body temperature for therapeutic purposes. A moderate degree of hypothermia, to 28° C (82.4° F), permits reduction of oxygen consumption by 50%. At 20° C (68° F) there is a further reduction of about 25%. Systemic circulatory cooling is achieved with the heat exchanger of the heart-lung machine. When very cold temperatures (less than 20° C) are desired for myocardial protection in prolonged complex cases, additional surface cooling of the heart with topical application of cold saline/slush or continuous irrigation of the pericardial wall can be used. Large ice chips in pericardial irrigants should be avoided to prevent injury to the phrenic nerve and cardiac tissue.

Insulation pads placed behind the heart can reduce heat conduction from relatively warmer organs. Transmural cooling of the heart is achieved with cardioplegia (discussed later).

Ventricular fibrillation can occur during the cooling process although it is less likely at temperatures above 32° C (89.6° F). Other complications are related to the adverse effects that hypothermia has on coagulation and wound healing; this may delay hemostasis after heparin reversal and impact recuperation.[57]

Cardioplegic Arrest

Rapidly arresting the heart during diastole is beneficial because an arrested heart uses less energy than a fibrillating or beating heart. Cardioplegia with hypothermia can reduce energy requirements even further, according to Buckberg.[14] A few authors have supported the use of normothermic cardioplegic arrest without the concomitant use of hypothermia.[40,54] Both "warm" and "cold" heart-surgery proponents concur that infusing a warm initial bolus of cardioplegia acts as a form of active resuscitation in energy-depleted hearts. There is also concurrence that providing a warm terminal bolus of cardioplegia helps to avoid reperfusion injury (caused by oxygen-free radicals and lactic acid buildup) by providing oxygen and other nutrients to the heart. The controversy lies in the use of normothermic cardioplegia during the period of arrest when the actual surgical repair or bypass construction occurs.[14,54] Proponents of warm arrest techniques seek to avoid the complications associated with hypothermia; warm cardioplegia is delivered continuously while the surgical repair is performed. Opponents of continuous warm cardioplegia cite the technical difficulty associated with a constant flow of cardioplegia obscuring the surgical site. It is suggested that if cardioplegia infusions are even momentarily interrupted to enhance visualization myocardial protection is jeopardized. These authors favor intermittent cold cardioplegia infusions.

Cardioplegia Delivery

Cardioplegic arrest is accomplished by infusing the coronary arteries with a 4° C to 10° C (39.2° F to 50° F) solution containing potassium (2 to 50 mEq/L) and buffering agents to counteract ischemic acidosis. Potassium acts by depolarizing the myocardial cell membrane and arresting the heart in diastole.

Delivery of the solution may be by the antegrade or the retrograde route (Fig. 27-42). With antegrade delivery, a needle is inserted into the aortic root proximal to the aortic cross-clamp; the cardioplegic solution is infused under pressure that closes the aortic valve leaflets. The only remaining route for the solution is into the right and left coronary arteries and the coronary circulation (see Fig. 27-37). If the aortic valve does not close properly, the cardioplegic solution will flow preferentially into the left ventricular chamber causing distention; in these cases direct cannulation of the coronary ostia is performed. Direct infusion into vein grafts protects the myocardium distal to coronary lesions and enhances transmural cooling. Retrograde infusion is achieved with a catheter placed transatrially into the coronary sinus; the perfusate enters the coronary venous sytem and flows through the myocardial circulation, leaving through the coronary ostia. The retrograde route is especially useful in the presence of coronary artery obstructions and left ventricular hypertrophy.

When the heart is sufficiently arrested, the ECG reflects

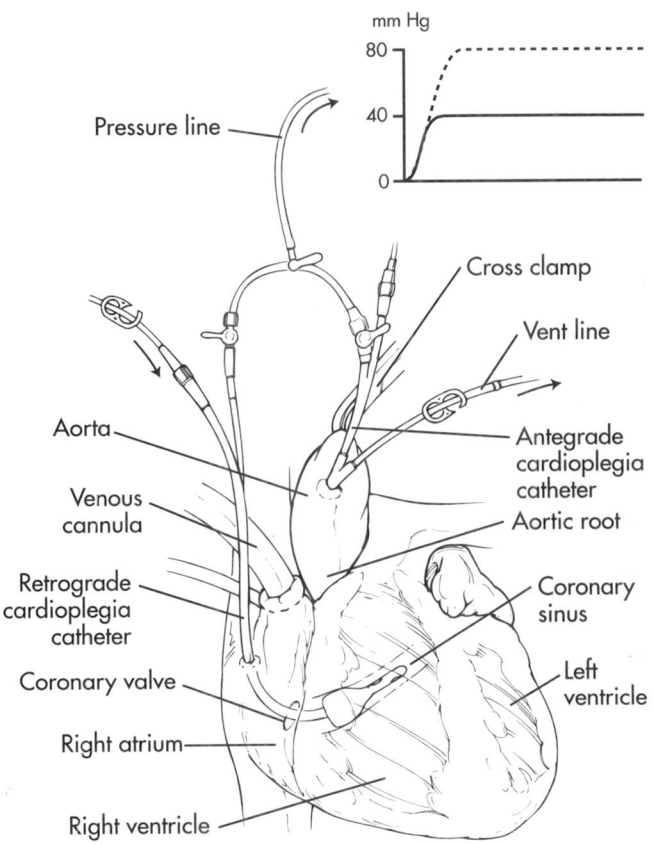

FIGURE 27-42   Antegrade-retrograde cardioplegia system. The antegrade cardioplegia catheter is inserted into the aorta proximally to the cross-clamp; the catheter is Y-ed into a vent line and into the retrograde cardioplegia catheter, which is inserted transatrially into the coronary sinus. The coronary sinus pressure is monitored; it should remain at pressure under 50 mm Hg.

a straight line; when electrical activity is noticed on the monitor (fine fibrillation), the cardioplegic solution is reinfused when continued cooling is desired (approximately every 15 to 20 minutes).

Minimally invasive techniques for myocardial protection have also been developed (see Fig. 27-39, A and B). Percutaneously inserted catheters can infuse antegrade cardioplegic solution through a catheter threaded into the aortic root; retrograde cardioplegic solution is infused through a catheter threaded from the internal jugular vein into the superior vena cava, right atrium, and the coronary sinus.

Circulatory Arrest

In some highly complex procedures lasting more than 45 minutes, such as those involving the aortic arch, it may be impossible to place an occluding clamp across the aorta. In these cases, circulatory arrest may be used to maintain a dry operative site. Because all blood flow will be interrupted, additional protection is required to protect myocardial, cerebral, and other tissue from ischemia.

The patient is cooled with the heat exchanger to approximately 18° C (65° F), at which point the bypass pump is turned off. The incision is made, and the repair is performed. The small amount of collateral drainage entering the field can be removed with a suction catheter. When the repair is completed, air is removed, and CPB is slowly reinstituted. Rewarming is performed at a rate of approximately 1 celsius degree every 3 minutes.

Cerebroplegia

Circulatory arrest poses additional risk to the brain. Cerebral protection, cerebroplegia, is provided by the infusion of oxygenated blood retrogradely to the brain via the superior vena cava cannula. Because CPB is temporarily halted, the vena cava cannula is not needed to drain venous blood and can be connected to the source of oxygenated blood for cerebral infusion. After the repair is completed, the venous cannula can be used again to drain venous return when CPB is reestablished.[67]

Termination of CPB

Near the end of the repair, the heart is allowed to rewarm while the perfusionist rewarms the patient systemically with the oxygenator's heat exchanger. Air is evacuated from the left ventricle and the proximal portion of the aorta. The cross-clamp is removed. The heart often converts spontaneously to sinus rhythm, but internal defibrillation may be necessary. Temporary epicardial pacing wires may be sutured to the right atrial appendage or the right ventricle; these are used postoperatively if the patient has transient dysrhythmias.

When the heart is contracting, the patient is gradually weaned from CPB. Ventilation of the lungs is restarted. Venous flow is gradually reduced by clamping the venous line or lines, and a commensurate reduction in arterial flow is made by the perfusionist. When heart action is sufficient and systemic and pulmonary blood pressures are stabilized, the bypass is terminated, and the cannulas are removed.

Measures to actively promote body heat retention are implemented to enhance clotting mechanisms, immune function, and oxygenation (Research Highlight 27-2). Maintenance of normothermia has also been recommended to reduce the risk of postoperative infection.[48,57]

Closing

After hemostasis is achieved, catheters are inserted into the pericardium for mediastinal drainage of shed blood. If either or both pleura have been entered, chest tubes are inserted to drain shed blood entering from the pericardium and to create negative intrapleural pressure to faciliate lung expansion. The tubes are connected to straight or Y connectors to a water-seal drainage system (see Chapter 25) or an autotransfusion drainage system.

Chest closure in median sternotomy is achieved with wire sutures (see Fig. 27-19). The wire sutures are twisted, excess wire is cut, and the wire ends are buried into the sternal periosteum. Some surgeons use small metal

---

27-2 RESEARCH HIGHLIGHT

This double-blind study on 200 patients 18 to 80 years of age undergoing elective colorectal surgery has profound implications for cardiac surgery. Cardiac patients are often cooled to reduce oxygen consumption and to protect tissue from ischemia.

The authors randomly assigned patients to the (1) hypothermia group, in which the core temperature was allowed to decrease to approximately 34.5° C, and (2) normothermia group in which the core temperature was actively maintained near 36.5° C with the use of fluid warmers and forced air covers. Postoperatively the patients' wounds were evaluated daily until discharge from the hospital and in the clinic after 2 weeks. Surgical wound infections (defined as wounds containing culture-positive pus) were found in 18 of 96 patients (19%) assigned to the hypothermia group but only in 6 of 104 patients (5.7%) assigned to the normothermia group ($p = 0.009$). The duration of hospitalization was prolonged by 2.6 days (approximately 20%) in the hypothermia group ($p = 0.01$).

Mild perioperative hypothermia may increase the risk of surgical wound infection by triggering thermoregulatory vasoconstriction, which decreases subcutaneous oxygenation and impairs oxidative killing of microbes by neutrophils. Hypothermia also directly impairs immune function and the production of antibodies. Hypothermia can also increase blood loss and the need for transfusion during surgery by impairing the function of platelets and the activity of clotting factors.

Implications for perioperative cardiac nurses include implemeting heat-retention strategies such as intravenrous fluid warmers and warmed topical irrigating solutions, covering exposed body areas outside the immediate surgical site, applying head coverings, increasing room temperature during rewarming from cardiopulmonary bypass, and employing warming blankets.

From Kurz, A., Sessler, D.I., & Lenhardt, R., for the Study of Wound Infection and Temperature Group (1996). Perioperative normothermia to reduce the incidence of surgical-wound infection and shorten hospitalization. *New England Journal of Medicine, 334*(19), 1209-1215.

---

crimpers to approximate and hold the wires (rather than twisting and burying the wire ends).

The linea alba is closed with suture. A layer of sutures is placed to approximate the fascia over the sternum; the subcutaneous tissue and skin are closed. If metal staples are used on the skin, a staple remover should accompany the patient to the recovery area. Thoracotomy incisions are closed in standard fashion (Chapter 25).

BOX 27-3 | **Patient Transfer Report**

PROCEDURE (include source of autogenous grafts) _____

MONITORING DEVICES (LOCATION)

CVP _____ ARTERIAL LINE _____ SWAN _____ PERIPHERAL _____

HEMODYNAMICS

BP _____ PAP _____ PAD _____ PAWP _____ CO _____ CI _____ CVP _____ Svo_2 _____

INTRAOPERATIVE OCCURRENCES

BLOOD LOSS _____ URINE _____ DYSRHYTHMIAS _____ BYPASS

PROBLEMS _____ DEFIB X's _____ LO TEMP _____ HI TEMP _____

CROSS-CLAMP TIME _____ PUMP TIME _____

BLOOD: GIVEN _____ AVAILABLE _____ AUTOTRANSFUSION

TOTALS: _____ ml _____ Units

COMPONENTS: FFP _____ PLATELETS _____ CRYO _____

ADDITIONAL ORDERED (TYPE) _____

MEDICATIONS

NEO _____ DOPAMINE _____ DOBUTAMINE _____ LIDOCAINE _____ NITRO _____

LEVOPHED _____ EPINEPHRINE _____ NITROPRUSSIDE _____ INOCOR _____

DDAVP _____ OTHER _____

TUBES/DRAINS: MEDIASTINAL _____ PLEURAL (Rt/Lt) _____

EPICARDIAL LEADS: ATRIAL _____ VENTRICULAR _____

PACING: YES/NO   RATE _____

LABS:

K^+ _____ Na^+ _____ Glu _____ Hgb _____ Hct _____

PATIENT CONCERNS _____

_____

ADDITIONAL INFORMATION _____

ICU BED # _____ ETA _____

REPORTED BY _____

To _____ TIME _____

BP, Blood pressure; CI, cardiac index; CO, cardiac output; CRYO, cryoprecipitate; CVP, central venous pressure; DDAVP, l-deamino-8-D-arginine vasopressin (e.g., Desmopressin); ETA, estimated time of arrival; FFP, fresh frozen plasma; Glu, glucose; Hct, hemotocrit; Hgb, hemoglobin; K^+, potassium; ml, milliliters; Na^+, sodium; NEO, Neo-Synephrine; Nitro, nitroglycerine; PAD, pulmonary artery diastolic pressure; PAP, pulmonary artery pressure; PAWP, pulmonary artery wedge pressure; Svo_2, percent saturation of mixed venous blood; SWAN, Swan-Ganz (pulmonary artery) catheter.

Before transferring the patient, the perioperative nurse telephones a report to the recovery area, usually the cardiovascular intensive care unit (CVICU). Box 27-3 lists information commonly supplied. The patient's special concerns and fears as well as significant physiologic alterations should be communicated.

Perioperative documentation follows the standard protocol and includes a description of the procedure performed and identification of medications and all implanted material (with lot and serial numbers). Hospital policy should be followed to ensure compliance with the Safe Medical Devices Act.

Evaluation

Evaluation of perioperative care includes the determination of whether the patient met the outcomes identified in the care plan. Such evaluation assists perioperative nurses in determining if the nursing interventions designed for a specific patient were successful. This type of data collection becomes the basis of the development of future plans of care for similar patients. Evaluation should be documented in the perioperative record. For the nursing diagnoses and the subsequent plan of care presented in this chapter for the cardiac surgery patient, those outcome statements might be as follows:

- The patient demonstrated adequate cardiac output.
- The patient will be free from wound infection.
- The patient was free from injury related to the surgical position.
- The patient described perioperative events.
- The patient's skin integrity was maintained.

Patient and Family Education and Discharge Planning

With hospital length of stay shortened from 1 week or more to 4 or 5 days, patient education and preparation for home care maintenance has become even more critical for enhancing positive patient outcomes. Many patients are admitted to the cardiac service on the day of surgery; teaching sessions can be scheduled before admission along with preoperative laboratory testing (Research Highlight 27-3).

The perioperative nurse acts to reinforce, review, clarify, and add to important information and instructions the patient and family or significant other needs in planning for surgery, recovery, and discharge. Research by Kuperberg and Grubbs[47] suggested that patients may be hesitant to complain of pain and request pain medication; perioperative nurses can anticipate patients' concerns about pain and encourage them to ask for pain medications.[24,39] Although patients undergoing repeat operation have had previous experience with cardiac surgery, they also have significant learning needs.[12] Information about newer techniques such as minimally invasive cardiac

27-3 RESEARCH HIGHLIGHT

Moore reviewed 18 published articles and one published dissertation describing interventions to promote recovery after coronary artery bypass grafting (CABG). The author performed a computerized search of MEDLINE Express from 1980 to 1996, the *Cumulative Index of Nursing and Allied Health Literature-CD* from 1980 to 1996, and psychologic literature journal articles from 1980 to 1996. Only experimental studies of CABG patients with control or comparison groups were included; all the studies used convenience samples. Studies related to cardiac rehabilitation programs were not included.

The author found that preparatory information was the intervention most frequently tested. There was clear evidence that information interventions designed to increase an individual's knowledge about managing recovery experiences during the first postoperative month at home and about coronary artery disease risk-factor modification were effective. Findings also supported the greater effectiveness of structured versus unstructured instruction in increasing knowledge. However, information alone did not change behavior, and the effect of preparatory information on mood states during recovery were unclear. In addition, the studies included few women, elders, and minority races.

As hospital length of stay (LOS) becomes shorter and the use of minimally invasive technology increases, perioperative nurses can play a pivotal role in helping patients to recover more quickly and to promote cardiovascular disease prevention and health promotion through structured educational experiences. The effectiveness of these educational sessions may be enhanced by collaboration between perioperative and critical care nurses and strategies that focus on behavior modification in men and women, elders, and minority races.

From Moore, S.M. (1997). Effects of interventions to promote recovery in coronary artery bypass surgical patients. *Journal of Cardiovascular Nursing, 12*(1), 59-70.

surgery, with or without the use of cardiopulmonary bypass, should be provided (Box 27-4).

Patients undergoing prosthetic valve replacement may require long-term anticoagulation. Important information includes drug dosage, reportable signs and symptoms of complications and side effects (such as bleeding, poor healing), and follow-up protocols for monitoring bleeding times.[68]

The patient's ability to cough and breathe deeply should be determined; the patient should be taught to use a cough pillow or splinting techniques. Required lifestyle changes should be reviewed, and the patient's feelings about these modifications elicited. The perioperative nurse should

BOX 27-4	Patient Teaching Considerations for Minimally Invasive Surgery	
	Beating Heart	**Arrested Heart**
Definition	CABG without CPB or induced cardiac arrest; HR and contractile force may be pharmacologically reduced to enhance technical precision	CABG with CPB and endovascular technique for CPB and induced cardiac arrest
Indications	Single-, double-vessel disease, angioplasty contraindicated, medical problems, poor anatomy, accessible target arteries (LAD), previous CABG with blocked grafts	Single-, double-vessel disease, angioplasty contraindicated, need to stop the heart to enhance technical precision, accessible target arteries, mitral valve
Contraindications	Complex lesions, posterior targets*	Highly complex lesions, posterior targets*
Incisions	1 to 3 small right or left rib or submammary incisions ministernotomy (cephalad or caudad)	1 to 3 small rib incisions, 1 to 2 groin incisions
CPB	No; available on standby	Yes
Cardioplegia	No	Yes
Procedure time	2 to 3 hours or more	2 to 3 hours or more
Hospital LOS	3 to 5 days (versus 5 to 10 for sternotomy)	3 to 5 days (versus 5 to 10 for sternotomy)
Advantages	Avoids CPB, ischemic arrest, and hypothermia	Allows repair of more complex lesions without the technical challenge of a moving heart
Potential complications and disadvantages	Learning curve, technically more challenging, may cause VF, may have to revert to standard sternotomy with CPB and induced arrest	Learning curve, technically more challenging, may have to revert to standard sternotomy, potential for dissection of cannulated arteries
Discharge planning	Anticipated faster recovery of 1 to 2 weeks (versus 4 to 12 weeks for sternotomy) earlier ambulation, need to identify reportable signs and symptoms (angina, difficulty breathing)	Anticipated faster recovery of 1 to 2 weeks (versus 4 to 12 weeks for sternotomy), earlier ambulation, need to identify reportable signs and symptoms (angina, difficulty breathing)

Data from product literature from CardioThoracic Systems, Cupertino, Calif.; Heartport, Redwood City, Calif.; Johnson & Johnson, Ethicon Endo-Surgery, Inc, Somerville, N.J.; Snowden Pencer, DSP, Tucker, Ga.; United States Surgical Corporation, Norwalk, Conn.
*In some patients with double- or triple-vessel disease, the LAD and diagonal are revascularized with minimally invasive surgical techniques; the posterior coronary arteries may be stented in the cardiac catheterization laboratory postoperatively.
CABG, Coronary artery bypass grafting; *CPB,* cardiopulmonary bypass; *HR,* heart rate; *LAD,* left anterior descending (coronary artery); *LOS,* length of stay; *VF,* ventricular fibrillation

verify that the patient knows reportable signs and symptoms associated with the specific procedure and understands prescribed medications, dosages and times, potential side effects, and signs and symptoms of complications. Any misconceptions should be clarified or referred to an appropriate source. The family or significant other's ability and willingness to assist the patient in home care maintenance should be queried; referrals to an agency for assistance at home may be required.

SURGICAL INTERVENTIONS

The following section describes operations for acquired forms of heart disease. Both traditional "open" procedures and minimally invasive techniques are described. Traditional procedures are performed through a median sternotomy incision using aorto-caval CPB (see Fig. 27-37) and antegrade-retrograde cardioplegia (see Fig. 27-42) with routine chest drainage and closure. Minimally invasive procedures are described for CPB, saphenous vein harvesting, coronary artery bypass grafting, and MVR. These procedures may be performed through an anterior left or right thoracotomy; some lesions may be approached through a cephalad or caudal ministernotomy.

EXTRACORPOREAL CIRCULATION PROCEDURES

Operative procedures
Aorto-Cava Cannulation via Sternotomy

1. A longitudinal pericardial incision is made, and the pericardial edges are retracted by suture to the chest wall.
2. The aorta, if it is to be cannulated for arterial blood return to the patient, is partially dissected from the pulmonary artery. If there are atrial adhesions, these are dissected.
3. Purse-string sutures are placed in the aorta (twice) and right atrium (or both venae cavae) for the eventual placement of the perfusion cannulas. Tourniquets are placed over the suture ends and held with a hemostat.
4. The ascending aorta is cannulated for the arterial blood return. If the aorta is not calcified, a partial occlusion

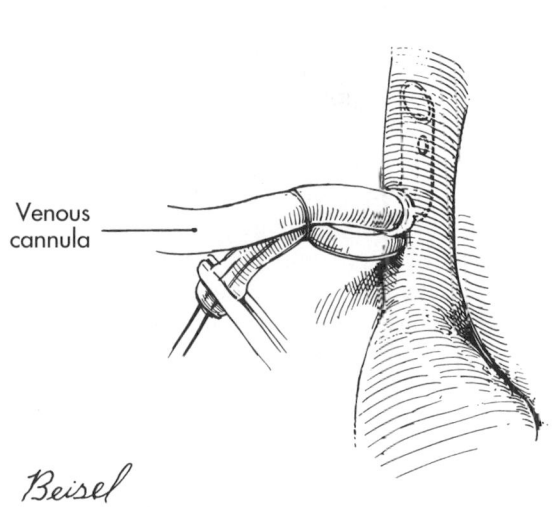

Venous cannula

Beisel

FIGURE 27-43   Right-angle cannula in superior vena cava.

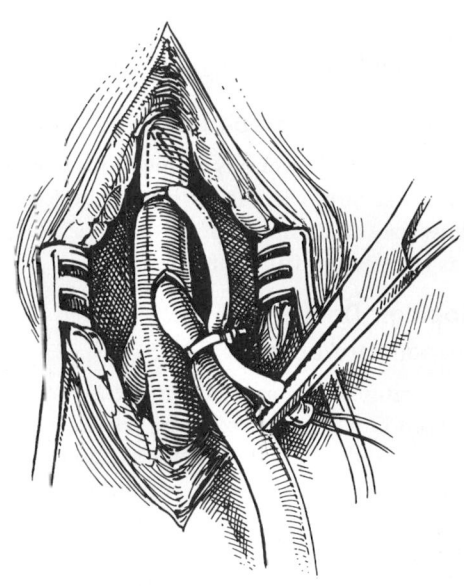

FIGURE 27-44   Cannulation of femoral artery.

clamp may be used to isolate a segment of the aortic wall. (Calcium may be seen on a radiograph and is palpable at operation.) The wall is incised, the cannula is inserted, and the purse-string suture is firmly secured with the tourniquet. It is important to have the distal end of the cannula clamped before it is inserted into the aorta to prevent backbleeding from the aorta. To prevent air emboli, the arterial connection is made under a saline drip, or by having the perfusionist slowly pump priming solution out of the arterial line.

Arterial cannulation is generally performed before the cava cannulation so that direct access for blood replacement is available if needed.

5. Venous cannulation: for the venous return to the pump–oxygenator, an incision is made into the right atrial appendage, and the two-stage cannula (see Fig. 27-37) is inserted into the atrium. The distal end of the cannula is placed into the inferior vena cava. The purse-string suture is secured with a tourniquet, and the catheter is permitted to fill partially with blood before being connected to the venous line.

When double cannulation is used, a second incision is made into the atrial wall within the purse-string suture, and the cannulas are placed in the inferior and superior venae cavae (see Fig. 27-36). To force all venous return into the cannulas, umbilical tapes with tourniquets may be placed around each cava and then tightened. This forces all systemic venous return to enter the cannulas, producing total CPB. Coronary sinus venous return from the heart is vented with an intracardiac vent (see Fig. 27-40).

6. In procedures where greater exposure of the right atrium is required (such as tricuspid valve surgery, closure of atrial septal defects in adults), a right-angled

cannula may be inserted into the superior vena cava (Fig. 27-43).

Femoral Vein–Femoral Artery Cannulation

1. A vertical or oblique incision is made into the femoral triangle, and the femoral vein and artery are exposed. Umbilical compression tapes are passed around the vessels above and below the proposed venotomy and arteriotomy. Vascular clamps may be applied above and below the incision into each vessel.

2. An incision is made into the femoral artery, and the perfusion catheter (occluded distally with a tubing clamp) is inserted retrogradely into the artery as the proximal clamp or tourniquet is released. The proximal tourniquet is tightened (Fig. 27-44). The cannula is connected to the arterial line.

3. An incision is made into the femoral vein, and the venous catheter is inserted into the vein as the proximal clamp or tourniquet is released. After the cannula is in place, the proximal tourniquet is tightened to prevent bleeding from the venotomy. The cannula is occluded at the distal end with a tubing clamp to prevent bleeding from the cannula. The cannula is connected to the venous line, and the tubing clamp is removed.

Minimally invasive cannulation

Femoral cannulation techniques are employed. Femoral arterial cannulation is as described above. Venous drainage is achieved with an extended catheter inserted into the exposed femoral vein, and the distal tip is advanced to the superior vena cava (SVC) (see Fig. 27-39). Side ports along the distal portion of the cannula allow drainage of blood from the SVC, the right atrium, and the inferior vena cava (IVC). Because of the higher resistance to drainage flow compared to right atrial cannulation, a centrifugal pump is used to augment venous drainage.[62]

Pump-oxygenator preparation

After the arterial and venous connections are completed and the lines secured, bypass is slowly begun, and the desired flow rate is gradually achieved. Perfusion flow is adjusted as necessary during the operation.

Cardioplegic Delivery
Antegrade cardioplegia

A purse-string suture and tourniquet is placed into the anterior ascending aorta proximally to the aortic cross-clamp, and a needle-tipped catheter is inserted (see Fig. 27-42). Both the catheter and the cardioplegic tubing are flushed to remove residual air. The catheter tubing is Y-ed into a vent line so that alternatively the needle can be used to infuse the cardioplegic solution into the aortic root or vent air and blood from the left ventricle. Hand-held cardioplegic cannulas may be used to infuse cardioplegic solution directly into the coronary ostia. Because of the risk of injuring ostial tissue with this technique, it is rarely used; retrograde delivery is the preferred alternative.

Retrograde cardioplegia

A purse-string suture is placed into the lateral wall of the right atrium, and a tourniquet is applied to the suture. A stab wound is made into the atrium, and the retrograde catheter is inserted and palpated into the coronary sinus. Blood is aspirated from the catheter, and the catheter is connected to the flushed retrograde infusion line and to a pressure line. Infusion pressure should be less than 50 mm Hg.[14] Because a full right atrium facilitates insertion of the catheter, insertion is performed before the initiation of CPB when possible. If the patient is already on CPB, the surgeon can fill the atrium by clamping the venous drainage line momentarily, thereby diverting blood into the heart.

Minimally invasive endovascular antegrade-retrograde cardioplegia

Peters et al.[62] describe a system of endovascular multi-lumen catheters designed to infuse solutions, vent air and blood, measure intravascular pressures, and occlude the aorta (see Fig. 27-39). Fluoroscopy is employed to confirm proper catheter placement.

The intravascular aortic catheter has three lumens. The first lumen has an inflatable balloon at the tip that, when inflated inside the vessel, occludes the aorta and serves as an internal "cross-clamp." The second lumen can be used either to infuse antegrade cardioplegic solution or to vent the ventricle. The third lumen is used to measure aortic root pressure. The catheter is introduced into the femoral artery and advanced into the ascending aorta. Either the femoral artery used for arterial inflow may be accessed, or the contralateral femoral artery is used.

The triple-lumen coronary sinus retrograde cardiople-gic catheter is inserted percutaneously through the jugular vein into the SVC. The catheter is guided into the coronary sinus under fluoroscopy. One lumen allows manual catheter balloon inflation; another lumen is used to infuse retroplegic solution; and the third lumen measures coronary sinus pressure.

A third, pulmonary artery, catheter is used as a venting-and-decompression device. It is inserted into the jugular vein (through a separate sheath from the retrograde catheter) and advanced into the main pulmonary artery.

These catheter systems allow surgeons to use minimally invasive techniques to treat lesions, such as mitral valve disease, that cannot be performed safely with a beating heart.

Termination of CPB

1. After the intracardiac procedure has been completed, all air is evacuated from the left ventricle. A warm dose of cardioplegic solution may be given, after which the cross-clamp is removed.
2. Defibrillation is often spontaneous with removal of the aortic cross-clamp and the entry of warm blood into the coronary circulation. If not, internal defibrillation is necessary. Endovascular, minimally invasive procedures will require external defibrillation with sterile external paddles. Temporary epicardial pacing wires are attached to the atrium and to the ventricle.
3. Venous flow to the pump is reduced. Arterial flow is also reduced to equal the venous return. When heart action is sufficient and systemic arterial blood pressure is stabilized, venous return is further reduced, and the patient is taken off bypass by clamping all lines and stopping the pump.
4. As the cannulation catheters are removed, the purse-string sutures are tightened and tied. Additional sutures may be required for hemostasis.
5. Chest tubes are inserted into the pericardium (and the pleural cavity if the pleura has been opened).
6. Protamine sulfate, a heparin antagonist, is administered.
7. The pericardium is usually left open so that accumulating drainage does not produce cardiac tamponade.

Closure of Femoral Incisions

1. The femoral catheters are removed, and the arteriotomies are closed with nonabsorbable cardiovascular suture. Compression tapes and bulldog clamps, if used, are removed.
2. The incision is closed with absorbable sutures, and the skin is closed with interrupted or continuous sutures.
3. Dressings are applied to all incisions.

PERICARDIECTOMY

Pericardiectomy is the partial excision of the adhered, thickened fibrotic pericardium to relieve constriction of compressed heart and large blood vessels.

Myocardial contractility is restricted by the adhered

portions of the scarred, thickened pericardium. As the pericardial space is obliterated and calcification of the pericardium occurs, the heart is further compressed. Ascites, elevated venous pressure, decreased arterial pressure, edema, and hepatic enlargement result. This condition is usually caused by chronic pericarditis, which may be of tubercular, rheumatic, viral, or neoplastic origin.

Procedural considerations

Occasionally bypass may be requested on a standby basis, but usually the supplies and instruments for bypass are not needed.

Operative procedure

1. The lungs are displaced laterally, and the right and left phrenic nerves are identified and carefully protected. The pericardium is incised.
2. The outer thickened pericardium is removed as indicated. Cartilage scissors may be required. The fibrous portions adhering to the atria and ventricles are carefully dissected with dry dissectors and scissors. Caution is exercised to prevent perforation of the atria and right ventricle; thus small areas of adherent pericardium may be retained.
3. Dissection is continued, and the large blood vessels are exposed and freed as indicated.
4. Drainage catheters are placed near the heart or through the pleural spaces. Connections to the water-seal drainage system are established as described in Chapter 25.

SURGERY FOR CORONARY ARTERY DISEASE

The growth of minimally invasive surgical techniques, increasingly accompanied by interventional cardiologic procedures, is most evident in the treatment of coronary artery disease (CAD). Revascularization of the ischemic myocardium can be achieved in new ways, thereby expanding treatment options for those patients in whom standard revascularization techniques are contraindicated. These techniques include transmyocardial laser revascularization[21] and balloon angioplasty, atherectomy, and stent insertion.[9] Port-access, endoscopic, and video-assisted technology can be used with smaller thoracic or sternal incisions and has been adapted to saphenous vein excision.[1] Newer treatments also include the choice of performing surgery on beating hearts (without the use of CPB) or on arrested hearts with CPB and myocardial protection provided by minimally invasive systems (see Fig. 27-39). Advantages of the minimally invasive techniques include more cosmetic incisions, less perioperative bleeding, fewer surgical wound infections, and earlier postoperative ambulation; disadvantages are that these procedures are more technically challenging and may prolong operative time.[20] Thus not all surgeons will use these newer techniques,[70] but there is a growing demand for a choice of interventions from consumers and payers.

Standard surgical treatment of coronary artery disease includes myocardial revascularization with coronary artery bypass grafting (CABG) by use of the autogenous saphenous vein, the internal (thoracic) mammary artery (IMA), the radial artery, and other autogenous arterial and venous conduits. CABG often alleviates angina pectoris and can prolong life in certain subsets of patients such as those with disease of the left main and left anterior descending coronary arteries.[15,42] The IMA demonstrates excellent long-term patency,[17,52] and this has promoted the use of arterial conduits such as the radial artery, the gastroepiploic artery,[13] and the inferior epigastric artery,[41] but the saphenous vein remains an effective conduit when multiple grafts are needed. The increasing number of reoperations for coronary artery disease has also stimulated the use of alternative conduits[37,64] (Box 27-5). Coronary artery instruments are added to the basic setup for cardiac surgery.

Other ischemia-related disorders requiring surgery include mitral valve regurgitation (MR), dysrhythmias, left ventricular aneurysms, and ventricular septal defects (VSDs).

CABG with Arterial and Venous Conduits

A clinical pathway (Fig. 27-45) can be used to guide the perioperative nurse caring for patients undergoing CABG.[13,75,80]

Operative procedure

1. A median sternotomy is performed as described.
2. Conduit preparation
   a. *IMA.* The IMA is dissected free from its retrosternal bed (Fig. 27-46). A special retractor, such as the one shown in Fig. 27-15, can be used to expose the IMA until the necessary length is obtained. Occasionally, both right and left IMAs are used. Heparin is given before arterial grafts are clamped and cut to prevent intraluminal thrombosis.

   Minimally invasive IMA dissection is performed with a special retractor (see Fig. 27-17) inserted into

---

BOX 27-5	Alternative Conduits for Use as Coronary Bypass Grafts

Splenic artery
Lesser saphenous vein
Cephalic vein
Basilic vein
Greater saphenous vein allografts (homografts)
Synthetic grafts (e.g., Dacron, PTFE)

Adapted from Bryan, A.J., Angelini, G.D. (1996). Vascular biology of coronary artery bypass conduits: new solutions to old problems? *Advances in Cardiac Surgery, 8,* 47-80.

Coronary Artery Bypass Graft (CABG) Clinical Path

FOCUS	PREOPERATIVE (before incision)	INTRAOPERATIVE	POSTOPERATIVE
Assessment	History & physical Review diagnostic & lab reports Preop check list	Physiologic assessment continuous	Assess skin and pressure points, ESU pad site & temperature
Tests	Chest x-ray film Cardiac catheterization report Electrocardiogram (ECG) Laboratory tests: complete blood count (CBC), chemistry/electrolytes, urinalysis, arterial blood gases (ABG's), hematology, prothrombin times (PT, APPT), other tests as ordered History & physical examination Height & weight 4 units packed red blood cells typed & cross matched, tested for cold antibodies	ABG's, CBC, activated clotting time (ACT) electrolytes, PT, APPT ECG, monitoring lines Maintain blood/blood product availability as requested	ACT, PT, APPT, chest x-ray film, coagulation profile as needed ECG, monitoring lines
Medications	Induction anesthetic agents Cardiac drugs, induction antibiotics Cardioplegia ordered & available Heparin, protamine sulfate Papaverine Topical antibiotic	Topical hemostatic agents available Perfusion drugs per protocol Additional heparin, papaverine, & other drugs as needed Antibiotic irrigation	Medications requested for CVICU
Treatments	Arterial pressure line (A-line), central venous pressure (CVP) line, pulmonary artery (PA) line per protocol Hair clipped along incision sites Hypo/hyperthermia blanket Skin prep chin to toes Draping per protocol Perfusion set-up per protocol Urinary drainage catheter inserted Nasogastric tube in OR	Femoral pressure line supplies available Intra-aortic balloon supplies available ESU to desired setting Cool patient as requested; rewarm before end of bypass Chest tube insertion Monitor urine output	Dress all lines Activate chest drain
Safety	Dependent areas & elbows/hands padded Supine position with maintenance of musculoskeletal functional status Intra-aortic balloon pump (IABP) and pacer available in OR Autotransfusion device set-up ESU pads to bilateral buttocks Defibrillator turned on Verify equipment function (eg, saw, headlight, ESU) All medications labeled	Avoid leaning on patient or placing heavy objects on body Salvage heparinized blood for autotransfusion Defibrillator settings confirmed	Maintain sterility of back table until patient leaves room Cover naked pacer wires Dress & secure all tubes, lines & incisions Measure chest drainage

FIGURE 27–45   Clinical pathway for CABG.

Continued

FOCUS	PREOPERATIVE (before incision)	INTRAOPERATIVE	POSTOPERATIVE
Teaching/Discharge Plan	Orient to surgery Assess knowledge of CABG Patient/family teaching; Orientation to waiting area; Preparation for post-op condition of patient	Update family on surgical progress	Notify CVICU of estimated time of arrival Prepare post-op bed (monitor, oxygen, drugs) Reinforce teaching; solicit tips for improvement
Expected Outcomes*	Maintain hemodynamic stability on induction Anxiety reduced Necessary resources available	Hemodynamically stable Desired temperature maintained Aseptic technique maintained Patient injury-free Absence of foreign bodies	Hemodynamically stable Temperature maintained Skin integrity maintained Injury-free

*Variances to be documented on perioperative record and may specify if related to patient, care giver(s), or system (see Fujihara & Fahndrick, 1998).

FIGURE 27-45, cont'd   Clinical pathway for CABG.

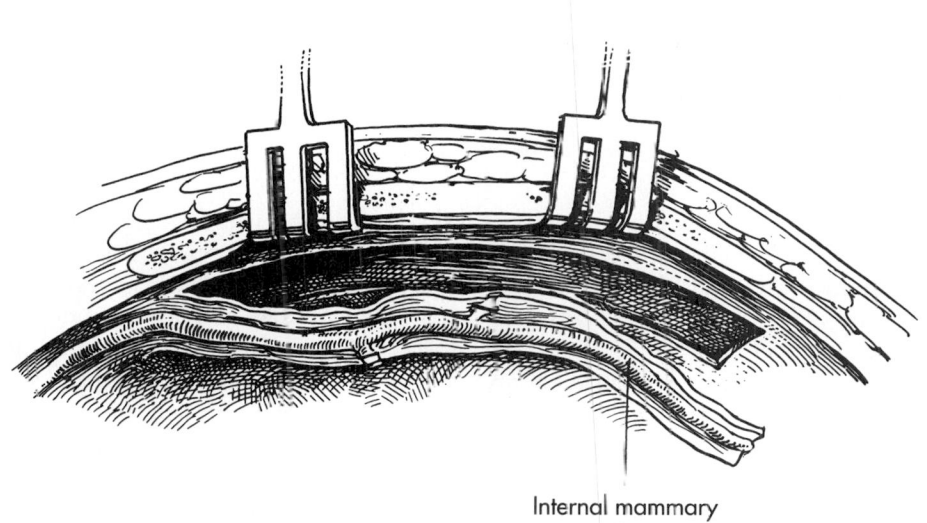

Internal mammary
artery

FIGURE 27-46   Dissection of internal mammary artery (IMA). Bleeding from side branches is controlled by vascular clips on the IMA side and cautery on the sternal side. Dilute solution of papaverine is sprayed onto or into lumen of IMA to dilate the artery and reduce muscular spasm. The IMA pedicle is placed in the pleural cavity until needed for anastomosis.

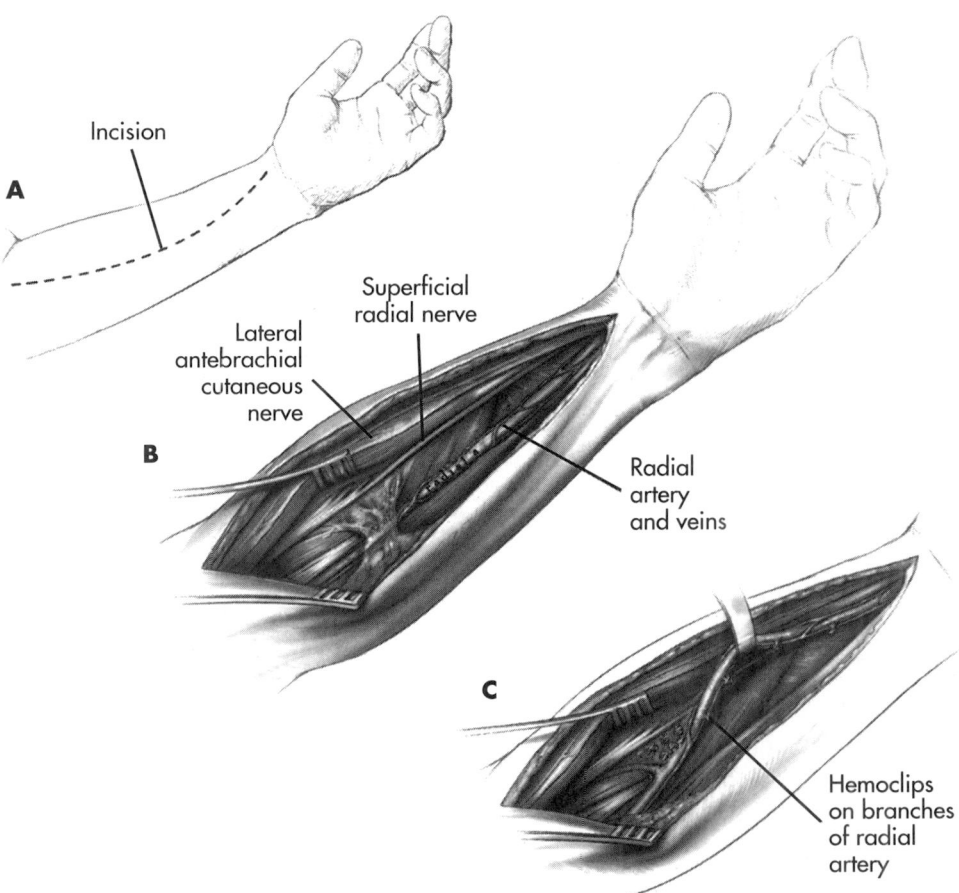

FIGURE 27-47 Dissection of radial artery. Before removal of the radial artery, an Allen's test is performed to ensure that the ulnar artery will provide sufficient blood flow to the hand if the radial artery is excised: the radial and ulnar arteries are compressed to produce blanching of the hand. The ulnar artery is released while compression is maintained on the radial artery. The skin on the palm of the hand should immediately become red as blood flow is restored through the ulnar artery to the hand. **A,** Incision line. **B,** Deep forearm dissection exposes the radial artery and vein pedicle. **C,** Radial artery pedicle is mobilized, and the multiple side branches are clipped on the arm and artery side. The artery is removed and may be irrigated with a vasodilator. A continuous intravenous infusion of diltiazem helps to prevent vasoconstriction of the artery.

the left anterior thoracic incision at the level of the fourth intercostal space. A light source is usually required to visualize the proximal IMA. Ligation of arterial branches and venous tributaries is performed with hemostatic clips and electrocoagulation.

b. *Radial artery.* A longitudinal incision is made 3 cm distally to the elbow crease lateral to the biceps tendon, ending 1 cm before the wrist crease (Fig. 27-47). The artery is exposed and mobilized with a vessel loop and harvested as a pedicle with adjacent veins and fatty tissue. The artery is ligated proximally and distally after systemic heparinization. Papaverine may be injected into the lumen to reduce spasm. The arm is closed over a small suction drain.[32,37]

c. *Gastroepiploic artery.* When an additional arterial conduit is required, the gastroepiploic artery may be used (Fig. 27-48).

d. *Saphenous vein.* The necessary length of saphenous vein is harvested from one or both legs (Fig. 27-49),

and tributaries are ligated. The distal end of the vein is identified to place the vein in a reversed position so that the semilunar valves do not interfere with the flow of blood. The vein is flushed with heparinized blood or saline and kept moist until needed.

Minimally invasive saphenous vein harvesting is performed through one to three incisions over the vein at the knee and at the ankle and the groin if necessary (Fig. 27-50). The vein is located under direct vision; the remaining length of vein is excised by means of video-assisted endoscopy and endoscopic scissors. An endoscopic clip applier is used to clip tributaries on the leg side; tributaries on the vein side may be clipped or ligated with suture after removal from the leg. To reduce postoperative tunnel dead space and minimize fluid accumulation, the leg is wrapped with a pressure bandage.[1]

3. Cardiopulmonary bypass with mild hypothermia is instituted. If CABG is performed without CPB, the

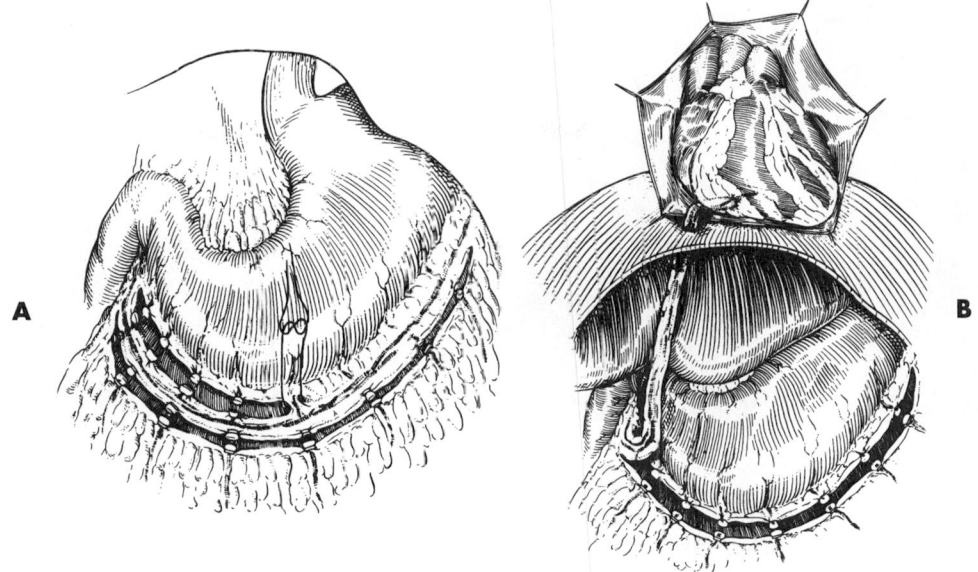

FIGURE 27-48   Right gastroepiploic artery mobilization. **A,** Branches to the stomach are divided with clamps and ties; omental branches may be divided with a staple gun. The gastroepiploic pedicle is isolated proximally to its origin from the gastroduodenal artery. **B,** The pedicle is brought up into the pericardium and anastomosed to the right coronary artery (shown here). The artery can also be grafted to the distal right and the left anterior descending coronary arteries.

patient is not cooled. CPB standby is usually available. Antegrade-retrograde cardioplegic solution is infused after the aorta is cross-clamped.

4. Coronary anastomoses. Anastomoses using saphenous vein, free arterial grafts, and in situ arterial grafts (such as IMA and gastroepiploic artery) are performed.
   a. The affected coronary artery is identified, and a small incision is made into the artery. The graft conduit is beveled to approximate the incision (side-to-side jump grafts may be performed as well).
   b. The anastomosis is made with fine cardiovascular sutures (Fig. 27-51). Before the anastomosis is completed, the distal coronary artery may be probed to ensure patency.
   c. Steps a and b are repeated for each subsequent anastomosis.
5. The distal anastomosis of the IMA to the coronary artery is done as described for the anastomosis of the saphenous vein graft to the coronary artery. No aortic (proximal) anastomosis is required because the IMA remains intact at its takeoff from the subclavian artery.
6. Aortic anastomoses
   a. Aortic anastomoses may be performed while the aorta is cross clamped; or the aortic clamp is removed, the heart is defibrillated, and the anastomoses are completed after each distal (coronary) anastomosis. When the proximal (aortic) anastomoses are performed on a beating heart, the aorta is partially occluded with an angled vascular clamp, and a small segment is resected, approximately the diameter of the vein graft. An aortic punch may be used for this (Fig. 27-52).

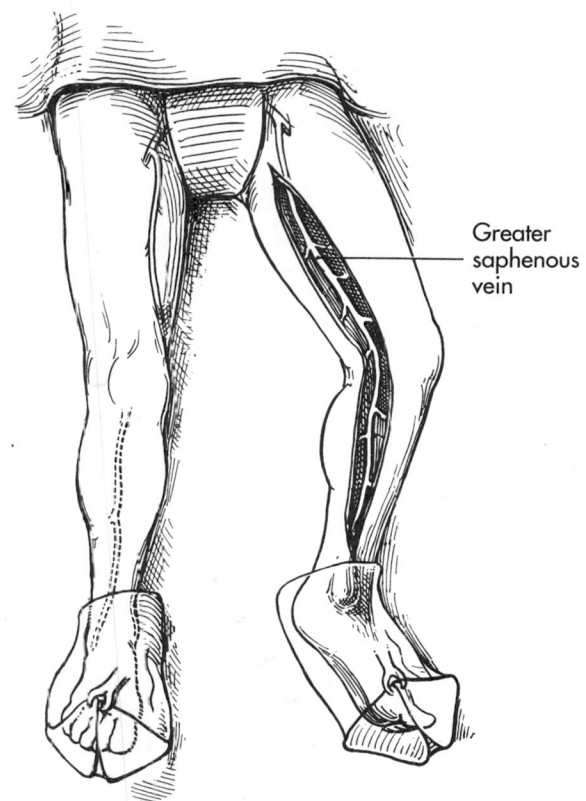

Greater saphenous vein

FIGURE 27-49   Excision of the greater saphenous vein.

   b. The conduit is anastomosed, end to side, to the aorta with fine vascular sutures. The partial occlusion clamp is removed, so that the proximal portion of the vein can fill with blood. Needle aspiration of the vein graft is performed to

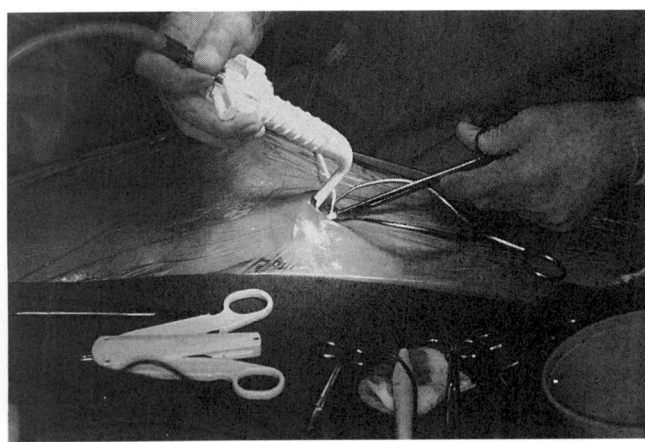

FIGURE 27-50 Minimally invasive saphenous vein harvesting. An incision is made medially to the knee over the saphenous vein. A lighted retractor is inserted to illuminate the vein, which is excised under direct vision. An endoscope with video monitoring capability can also be used. Vein tributaries are ligated with clips.

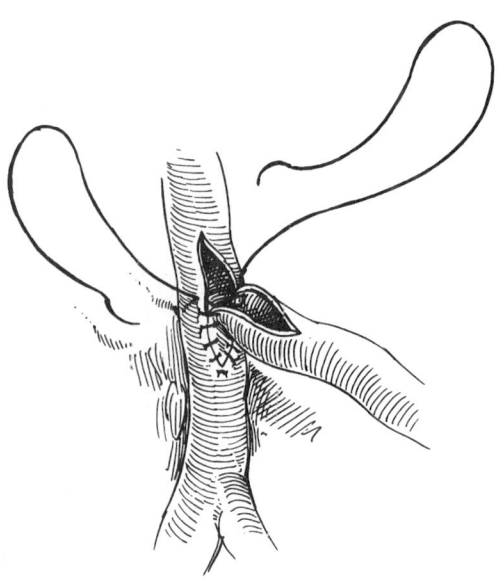

FIGURE 27-51 End-to-side coronary anastomosis with bypass graft conduit.

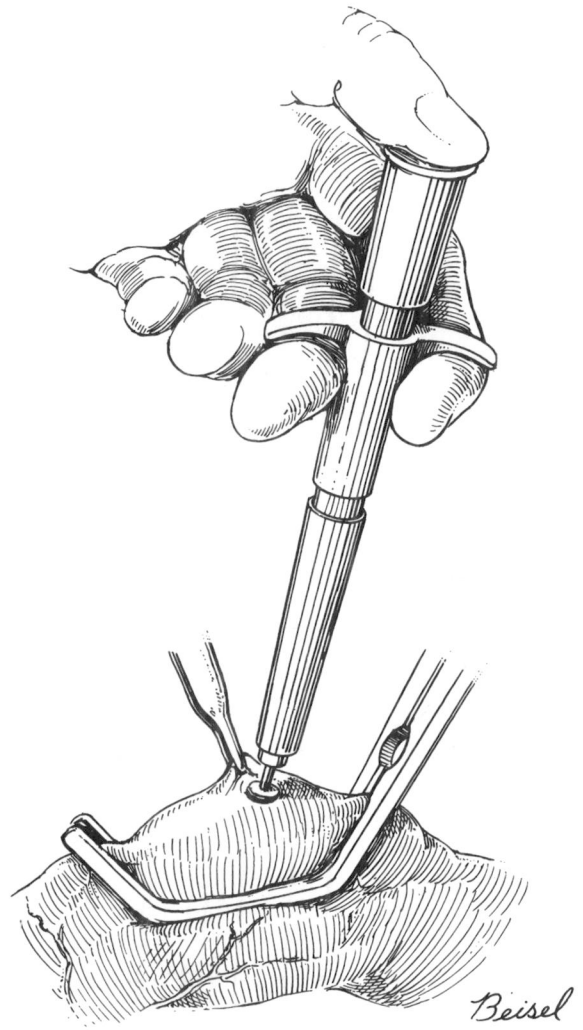

FIGURE 27-52 Proximal anastomosis of bypass graft. A partial occlusion clamp isolates the portion of the ascending aorta where the aortotomy is to be made with the punch.

prevent air from entering the coronary circulation (Fig. 27-53).
c. When proximal anastomoses are performed during a single period of cross-clamping, air is aspirated from the grafts before the cross-clamp is removed.
7. The aortic anastomoses of the vein grafts are usually marked with clips or rings for future identification.
8. Cardiopulmonary bypass is discontinued, and the sternum is closed.
9. Minimally invasive procedures
a. These are indicated in patients with lesions easily accessible through an anterior thoracotomy, such as narrowings in the left anterior descending (LAD) and diagonal coronary arteries. When endovascular CPB and cardioplegic solution is used, more lateral and posterior arteries (obtuse marginal and right coronary arteries) may be grafted because ventricular fibrillation secondary to stimulation of the heart is obviated with induced cardioplegic arrest. A double-lumen endotracheal tube may be inserted so that the left lung can be hypoventilated to enhance visualization of the LAD (and the IMA).[16]
b. In a beating heart CABG,[23,77,78] cardiac contraction poses a technical difficulty for the surgeon in creating a precise anastomosis. Various coronary stabilizers are available to reduce the motion of the heart in the vicinity of the anastomosis (Fig. 27-54). These are often attached to the retractor, thereby freeing the hands of the surgeon to sew.[10] Pharmacologic cardiac motion reduction may be employed; beta-blocker drugs and adenosine have been used by some surgeons.[11] The anastomosis of the IMA to the LAD is performed under direct, albeit limited, vision.

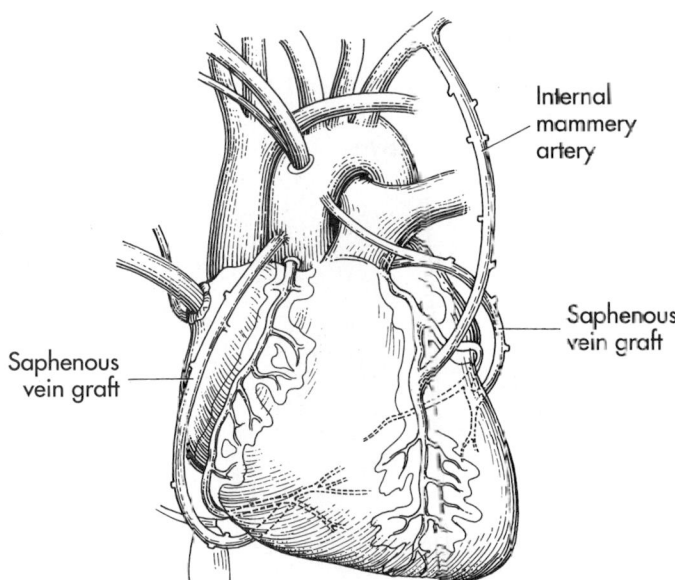

FIGURE 27-53 Coronary artery bypass grafts with reversed saphenous vein and the left internal mammary artery.

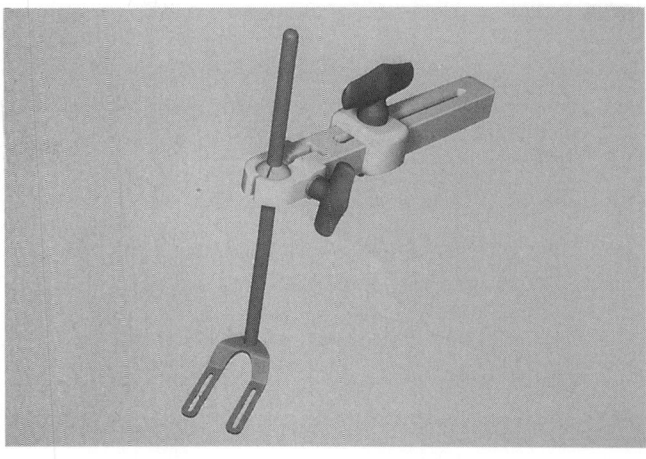

FIGURE 27-54 Coronary anastomotic site stabilizer. Used during beating-heart bypass surgery. The horseshoe-shaped foot has a nonsmooth surface to provide an atraumatic grip on the epicardium, reduce the movement of the beating heart, and isolate the target coronary artery site for anastomosis.

c. In arrested heart procedures, the IMA-to-LAD anastomosis is constructed on a quiet heart. Access to the graft site is through one or more left anterior thoracic ports.[62] Fig. 27-55 illustrates this technique compared with traditional open-chest techniques.

Ventricular Aneurysmectomy

Ventricular aneurysmectomy is the excision of an aneurysmic portion of the left ventricle and reinforcement with synthetic patch material (Fig. 27-56). An aneurysm of the left ventricle occasionally develops after a severe myocardial infarction in which part of the myocardium is replaced by thin scar tissue. The scar may stretch as a result of the left ventricular pressure, thus forming an aneurysm. The aneurysm is usually adherent to the pericardium, and it may not be possible to dissect it free until cardiopulmonary bypass has been established.

Procedural considerations

The patient is placed in the supine position. The setup is as described for open-heart surgery, plus Teflon felt strips to bolster the suture line, pledgets, and #0 cardiovascular sutures on a large needle. Occasionally, patch closure of the ventriculotomy is performed (endoaneurysmorrhaphy); synthetic patch material and 3-0 or 4-0 polypropylene sutures are used.

Operative procedure

1. A median sternotomy is performed, and CPB is begun as described.
2. The scar tissue of the ventricle is excised, and any clot is removed carefully (Fig. 27-56, A and B).
3. A cuff of scar tissue is left, through which heavy cardiovascular sutures reinforced with Teflon felt pledgets are passed (Fig. 27-55, C).
4. The left ventricle may be vented with an apical catheter; after the ventricle is de-aired, the catheter is removed, and closure of the incision completed.

Postinfarction ventricular septal defect (VSD)

Ventricular septal (or free-wall) rupture is a catastrophic complication of myocardial infarction, creating an acute left-to-right shunt and cardiac failure requiring emergency surgery. The defect is closed with a prosthetic patch.[27]

SURGERY FOR THE MITRAL VALVE

Mitral stenosis, the most common acquired valvular lesion, is a narrowing of the valve orifice such that it causes impedance to forward blood flow. It is often caused by rheumatic fever. The normal opening in the valve is about 5 cm^2. As the disease progresses, the mitral valve becomes a narrow slit in a fibrotic plaque, severely limiting blood flow into the left ventricle. Mitral stenosis causes a rise in pressure and dilatation of the left atrium. This pressure is transmitted throughout the pulmonary vascular bed, with subsequent pulmonary hypertension, right ventricular hypertrophy, and possibly tricuspid valve regurgitation.

The major symptoms are dyspnea, fatigue, and orthopnea. Late findings are severe pulmonary congestion and right ventricular failure. A characteristic diastolic murmur is heard, and atrial fibrillation is not unusual. Thromboembolism may result from stasis of blood in the left atrial appendage. Later findings are severe pulmonary congestion and right ventricular failure.[46]

Mitral regurgitation occurs when the valve leaflets do not close properly or when the leaflets are perforated and

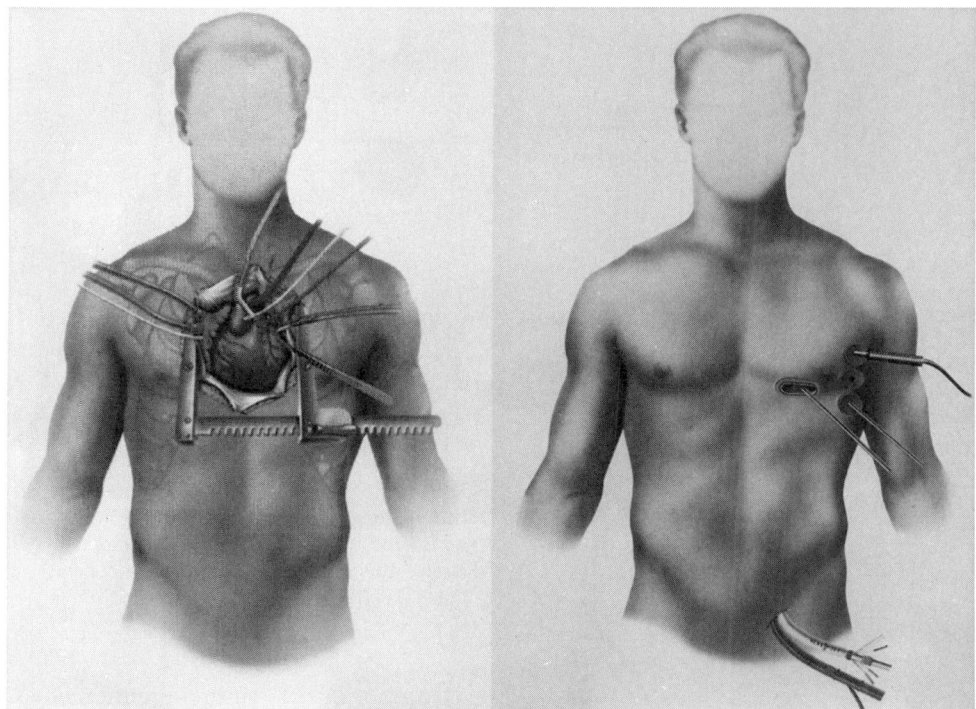

FIGURE 27-55 Traditional sternotomy (*left*) compared with minimally invasive incisions (*right*) that provide access to the heart and to the femoral artery and vein.

blood escapes back into the left atrium during ventricular systole. During ventricular diastole, blood volume entering the left ventricle is augmented by the blood regurgitated into the left atrium. Mitral regurgitation may accompany mitral stenosis or be attributable to leaflet tears, annular dilatation, or elongated or ruptured chordae. Ischemic heart disease may produce papillary muscle dysfunction, which prevents sufficient anchoring of the leaflets in the closed position. Symptoms include those seen with stenosis and with left ventricular dilatation from the increased volume load on the left ventricle.

The surgeon's selection of the procedure (repair or replacement) is determined by the stage of disease, presence or absence of calcification, history of thromboembolism and dysrhythmia, ability to tolerate chronic anticoagulation, and any associated pathologic defects.

Reparative procedures that preserve the native valve are widely employed because the complications associated with prosthetic replacement and anticoagulation can be avoided. The technique selected must be tailored to the unique pathophysiologic findings; therefore the surgeon carefully evaluates the leaflets and related structures at the time of surgery before deciding on which procedure to perform. Because there is always a possibility that the valve may have to be replaced, instruments (and prostheses) for replacement as well as repairs should be available. Also included are atrial hand-held or self-retaining retractors, obturators for sizing prosthetic rings and valves, sizer or prosthesis handles, and special sutures if requested. Bicaval cannulation is used to enhance exposure of the operative field and to decompress the heart (see Fig. 27-36). TEE

can be used to confirm efficacy of the repair after the cross-clamp is removed and the heart resumes beating and again after bypass is discontinued. TEE can also be used to detect the presence of air (seen as white specks) within the cardiac chambers.

Mitral Valve Repairs

Open commissurotomy of the mitral valve for mitral stenosis

Open commissurotomy is the separation of fused, adherent leaflets of the mitral valve under direct vision.

Procedural Considerations

The patient is placed in a supine position for a median sternotomy. The setup is as described for open-heart procedures, with mitral valve instruments.

Operative Procedure

1. A median sternotomy is performed, and bicaval cannulation is performed for cardiopulmonary bypass.
2. The left atrium is incised, and the valve is inspected; in some cases, a transseptal approach (right atrium to left atrium) may be used.
3. Fused leaflets are separated with vascular forceps and scissors or a knife (Fig. 27-57). A dilator may be used to enlarge the mitral valve orifice.
4. The valve is again inspected for any resultant insufficiency.
5. The left atrium is closed with a continuous cardiovascular suture.

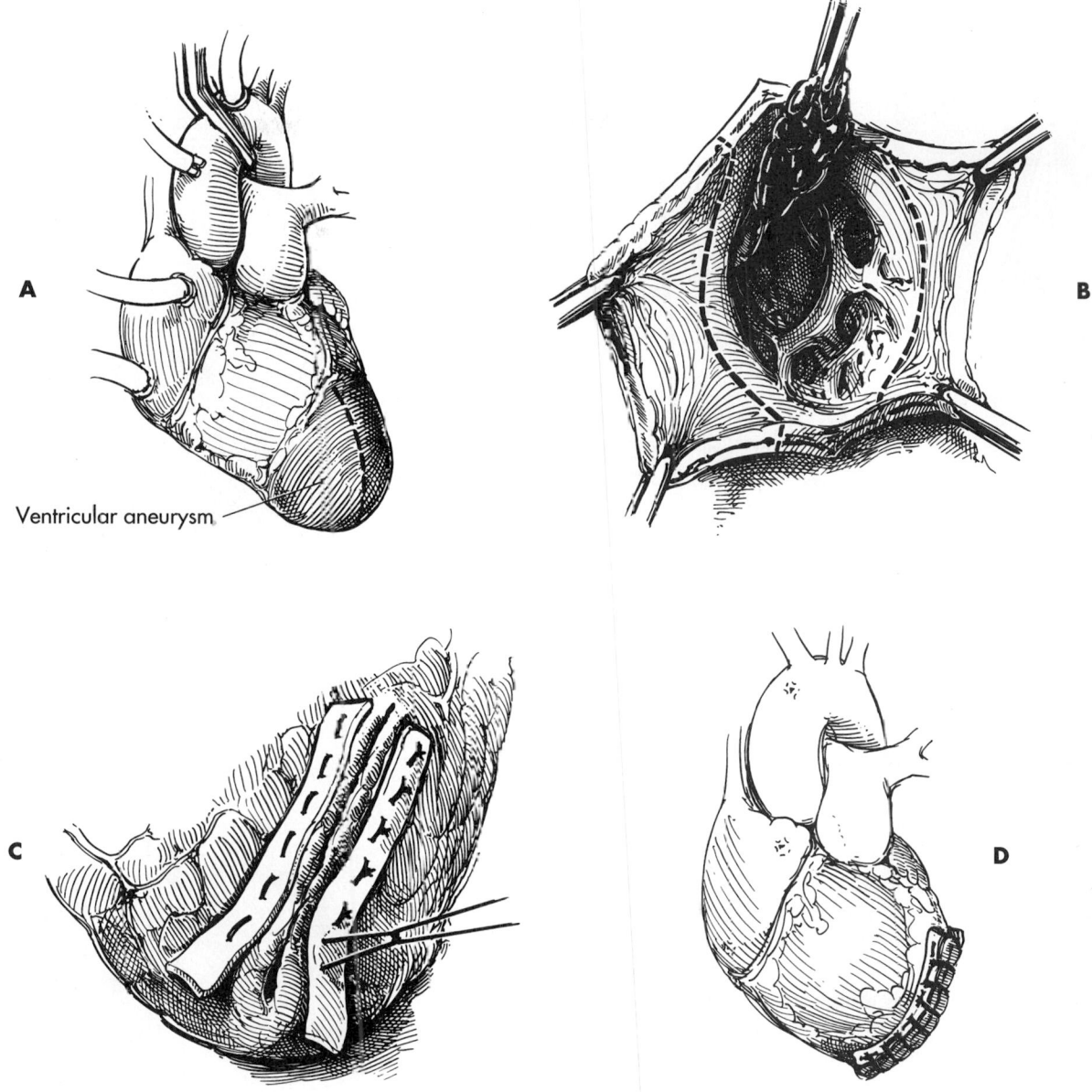

Ventricular aneurysm

FIGURE 27-56   Repair of left ventricular aneurysm (see text).

Mitral annuloplasty for mitral regurgitation

Mitral annuloplasty is the reduction of a dilated annulus (commonly involving the posterior leaflet) by inserting a prosthetic ring (see Fig. 27-33). Techniques created by Carpentier[19] continue to be widely used, just as more current techniques are.[28]

Operative Procedure

1. The left atrium is incised, and sump suctions are inserted into the atrial cavity to remove blood.
2. The annulus, leaflets, chordae, and the rest of the mitral complex are inspected.
3. If there is generalized annular dilatation, an annuloplasty ring is inserted. An obturator is used to determine the appropriate-sized ring (Fig. 27-58, *A*).

Interrupted sutures are placed around the circumference of the annulus and then into the ring (Fig. 27-58, *B*). When the stitches are tied, the excess annular tissue of the posterior leaflet is evenly drawn up against the prosthesis (Fig. 27-58, *C*).

4. The valve is inspected for competency with a bulb syringe filled with saline to distend the ventricle. The left atrium is closed.

Mitral valvuloplasty repairs for mitral regurgitation

Mitral valvuloplasty is the repair of the valve leaflets or related structures. Selection of the appropriate repair for perforated or redundant valve leaflets or for shortened or

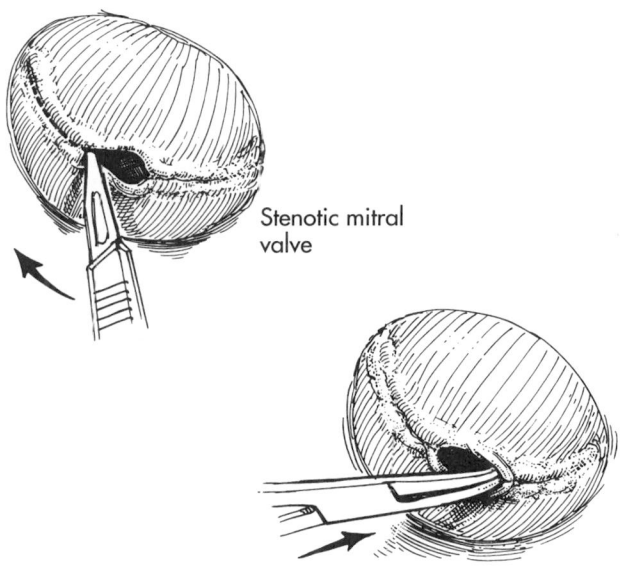

FIGURE 27-57   Mitral commissurotomy (see text).

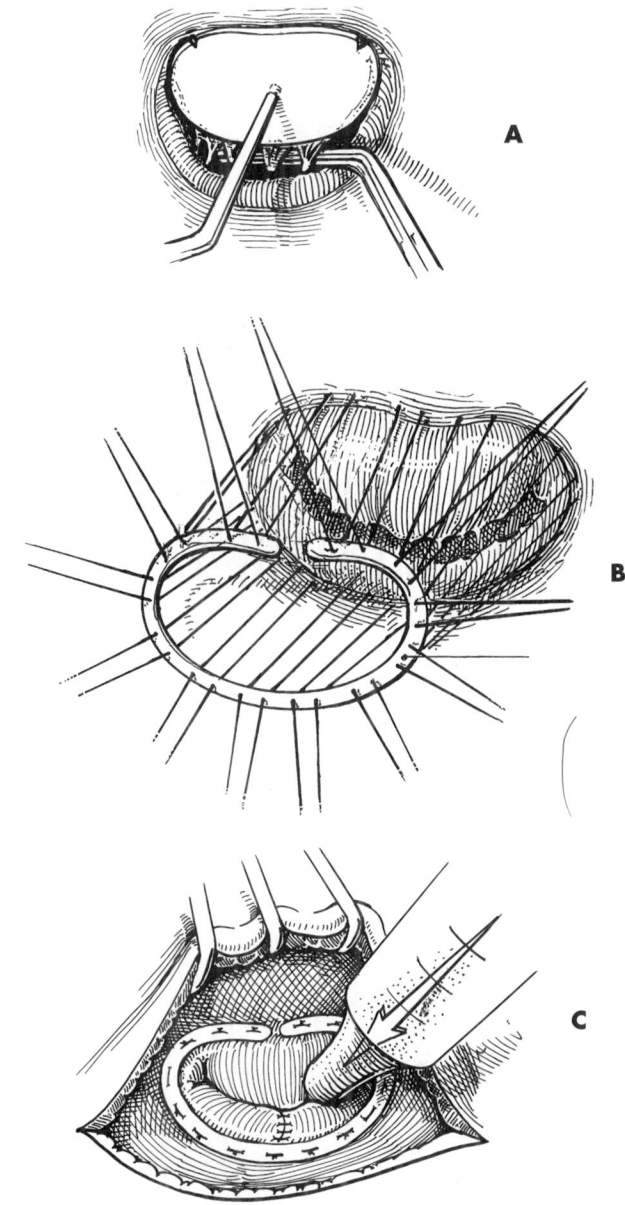

FIGURE 27-58   Mitral valve annuloplasty (see text).

elongated chordae tendineae requires careful assessment and evaluation of the abnormalities present.

Operative Procedure

1. Perforated leaflets can be patched with pericardium.
2. Redundant leaflet tissue can be resected (Fig. 27-59). The cut edges are sewn together, and the corresponding annular segment is plicated. An annuloplasty ring is inserted to reinforce the leaflet repair and reduce annular dilatation (see Fig. 27-58).
3. Shortened, fused chordae tendineae can be lengthened and mobilized by their division into secondary chordae or by incising the tip of the papillary muscles.
4. Redundant tissue of elongated chordae may be implanted into the papillary muscle head or folded over itself and secured with a suture (Fig. 27-60).
5. A chordal flip procedure (Fig. 27-61) can be used to reestablish chordal attachment to the anterior leaflet. A section of the posterior leaflet with attached chordae is cut, swung over to the anterior leaflet, and sewn onto the anterior leaflet. The remaining posterior leaflet defect is closed with suture (as in step #2 above).

Mitral Valve Replacement

Mitral valve replacement (MVR) is the excision of the mitral valve leaflets and replacement with a mechanical or biologic prosthesis. Generally the mural (posterior) leaflet and associated chordae and papillary muscles are retained to maintain ventricular configuration, thereby enhancing postoperative ventricular function. If possible, the anterior leaflet is also retained if it is not too heavily calcified.

Median sternotomy is performed in most cases, but right thoracotomy incisions are useful in selected cases.[23]

Minimally invasive procedures on the mitral valve can also utilize right thoracotomy incisions or ports.

Procedural considerations

Although the surgeon may intend to implant a specific type of prosthesis, patient-related factors (Box 27-6) or prosthetic valve complications (Box 27-7) may modify the plan.[58] A complete range of valves should be available as well as saline to rinse the glutaraldehyde storage solution from biologic prostheses, should they be used. Pledgeted sutures of alternating colors are used. Venting catheters and aspirating needles are used to remove air from the heart and ascending aorta. A small dental mirror may be used after a

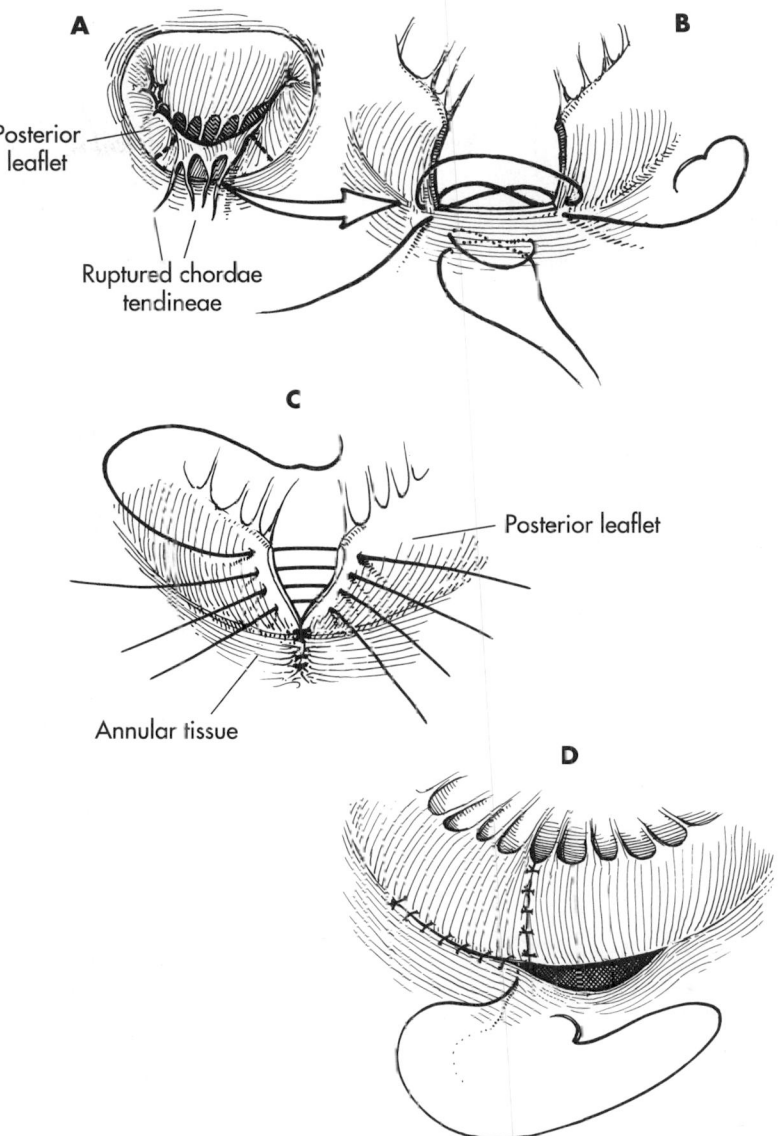

FIGURE 27-59   Quadrangular resection of nonsupported posterior leaflet tissue caused by ruptured chordae tendineae (see text). A similar technique can be used to resect *redundant* tissue causing mitral regurgitation.

bioprosthesis has been implanted to ensure that sutures are not caught in the subvalvular structures.

Operative procedure

Double venous cannulation (Fig. 27-62, *A*) is used.

1. The aorta is cross clamped, and cardioplegic solution is infused through the aortic root or, more commonly, retrograde through the coronary sinus.
2. The left atrium is incised along the interatrial groove to expose the mitral valve (Fig. 27-62, *A*).
3. The valve is assesseed, and the anterior leaflet is excised. The posterior leaflet is often retained to enhance the ventricular configuration and postoperative function.

Occasionally the anterior leaflet is retained. Rongeurs may be used to debride heavy calcification; loose debris is removed. A margin of the valve annulus is retained to insert fixation sutures to the prosthesis (Fig. 27-62, *B*).

4. A valve sizer is used to determine the correct size of the prosthesis, which is delivered to the field.
5. Nonabsorbable cardiovascular sutures (15 to 20) are placed in the retained margin of the valve and then placed into the sewing ring of the prosthesis.
6. The sutures are held taut (and moistened) as the prosthesis is guided into position and secured, and the sutures are tied and cut (Fig. 27-62, *C*).
7. Continuous nonabsorbable sutures are used to partially close the atriotomy. The patient is placed in reverse Trendelenburg's position, and the lungs are inflated to

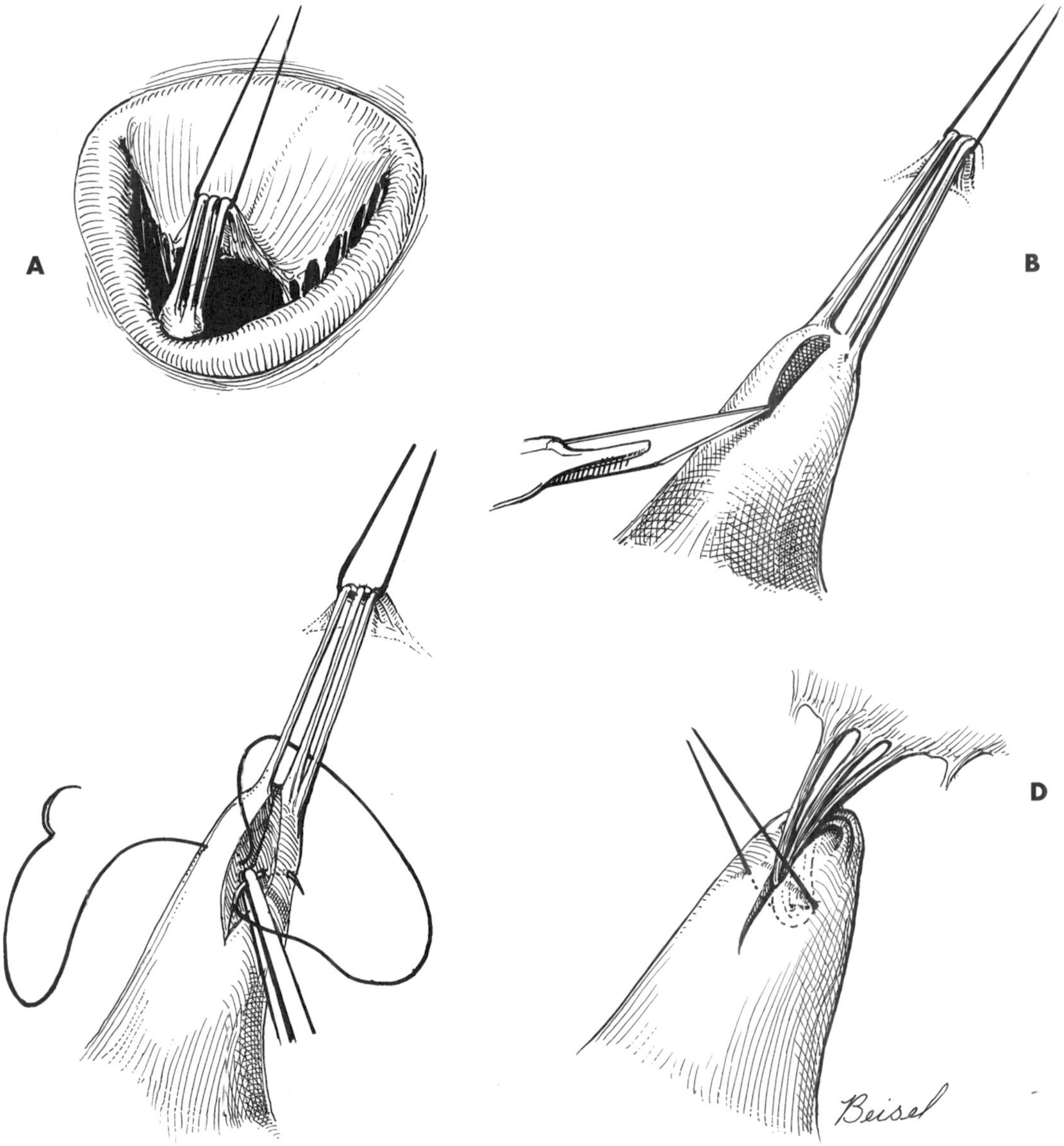

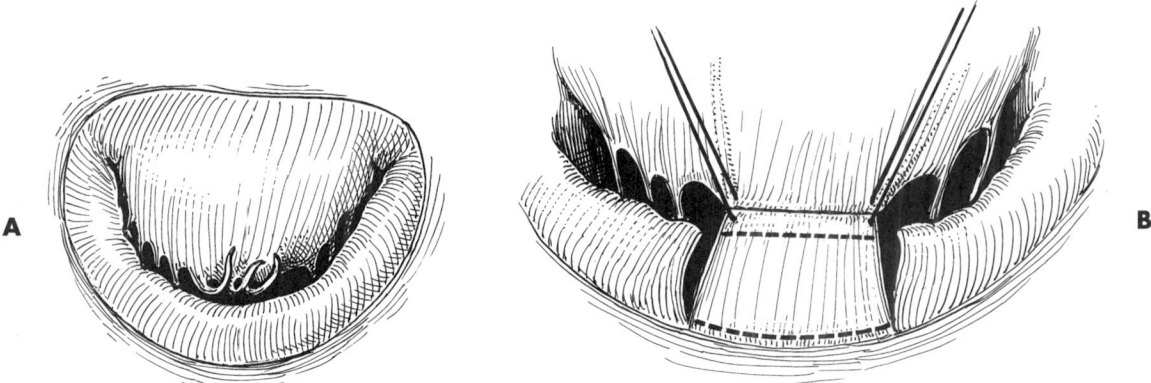

FIGURE 27-60   Chordal shortening technique (see text).

FIGURE 27-61   Chordal flip procedure. Although portions of the posterior leaflet can be resected with success, the same is not true of the anterior leaflet because the shape of the valve and the coaptation margin are altered. **A**, When there are ruptured chordae of the *anterior* leaflet of the mitral valve, the flip procedure can be used to reestablish chordal support for the anterior leaflet. **B**, A portion of normal posterior leaflet tissue with attached chordae is cut, swung over, and sewn onto the flail segment of the anterior leaflet. The posterior leaflet defect is repaired as previously illustrated in Fig. 27-59.

BOX 27-6	Patient-Related Factors and Risks

Age

Sex

Residence

History of atrial fibrillation

Endocarditis (preoperative)

Connective tissue disorders (e.g., myxomatous changes)

Congenital anomalies (e.g., bicuspid aortic valve)

Enlarged left atrium

Left atrial thrombus

Left ventricular function (e.g., functional class, myocardial infarction, congestive heart failure)

Syncope

Anticoagulation compliance

Preexisting medical problems (e.g., diabetes mellitus, hypertension, hepatic or renal disease)

Valve lesion

Previous cardiac surgery

Adapted from Rao, V., Christakis, G.T., Weisel, R.D., et al. (1996). Changing pattern of valve surgery. *Circulation, 94*(suppl. II), II113- II120.

BOX 27-7	Valve-Related Risks and Complications

Thromboembolism

Anticoagulation-related hemorrhage

Prosthetic valve endocarditis

Periprosthetic leak

Prosthetic failure

Adapted from Vongpatanasin, W., Hillis, L.D., & Lange, R.A. (1996). Prosthetic heart valves. *New England Journal of Medicine, 335*(6), 407-416.

remove air from the pulmonary veins and atrium. Air is aspirated from the left ventricle through a hypodermic needle or vent catheter, and the atrial closure is completed.

SURGERY FOR THE TRICUSPID VALVE

Tricuspid Valve Annuloplasty

Tricuspid valve annuloplasty is the reduction of a dilated annulus with a suture technique or a prosthetic ring. Tricuspid valve regurgitation may be caused by bacterial or viral endocarditis. It may be the functional result of mitral valve disease; after mitral valve correction, tricuspid valve function may return to normal. If the tricuspid valve does not regain competence after mitral valve surgery or if

tricuspid annular dilatation occurs, repairs similar to mitral annuloplasty may be performed. Caution is taken to avoid injury to the conduction tissue in the area of the atrioventricular (AV) node.

Operative procedure

1. Double venous cannulas are inserted so that they do not cross one another in the right atrium, and occluding tapes are tightened around the cavae and cannulas to prevent venous return from entering the right atrium and obscuring the surgical site. A right-angled venous cannula (see Fig. 27-43) may be placed into the superior vena cava to enhance exposure.
2. The right atrium is opened longitudinally to expose the tricuspid valve. Sump suctions are inserted to remove coronary sinus drainage.
3a. In the DeVega technique[65] (Fig. 27-63) a double-armed, felt-pledgeted suture is placed in the valve annulus, beginning at the anteroseptal commissure and continued around to the level of the coronary sinus orifice. The remaining arm of suture is similarly placed. The suture is tied over a pledget with sufficient tension to reduce the annular area to the size desired.
3b. In the Carpentier[19] or Cosgrove[55] technique a prosthetic ring is inserted in a manner similar to mitral valve annuloplasty (see Fig. 27-58).
4. Saline may be injected into the ventricle to test the competence of the repair, and TEE is also employed.
5. The right atrium is closed with nonabsorbable suture.

SURGERY FOR THE AORTIC VALVE

Aortic stenosis produces obstruction of the left ventricular outflow. Whether caused by rheumatic fever, a congenital bicuspid valve, or calcific degeneration, the fused valve leaflets present an increasing pressure load on the ventricle. To compensate, the ventricle hypertrophies so that it can generate sufficient pressure to eject blood through the narrowed opening. When disease is severe, large pressure gradients are often measured during cardiac catheterization, with differences in systolic pressures between the ventricle and the aorta reaching 50 mm Hg or greater. In the early stages of the disease, a systolic aortic murmur may be heard, but patients are rarely symptomatic; eventually fatigue, exertional dyspnea, angina pectoris, syncope, and congestive heart failure may develop, presenting a grave prognosis. Sudden death is not uncommon.[63]

Repair of the aortic valve is difficult because of the precise closing mechanism of the aortic valve leaflets. Total valve excision and replacement with a prosthesis or an allograft is commonly performed. Patch enlargement of the small aortic root enhances long-term survival.[71]

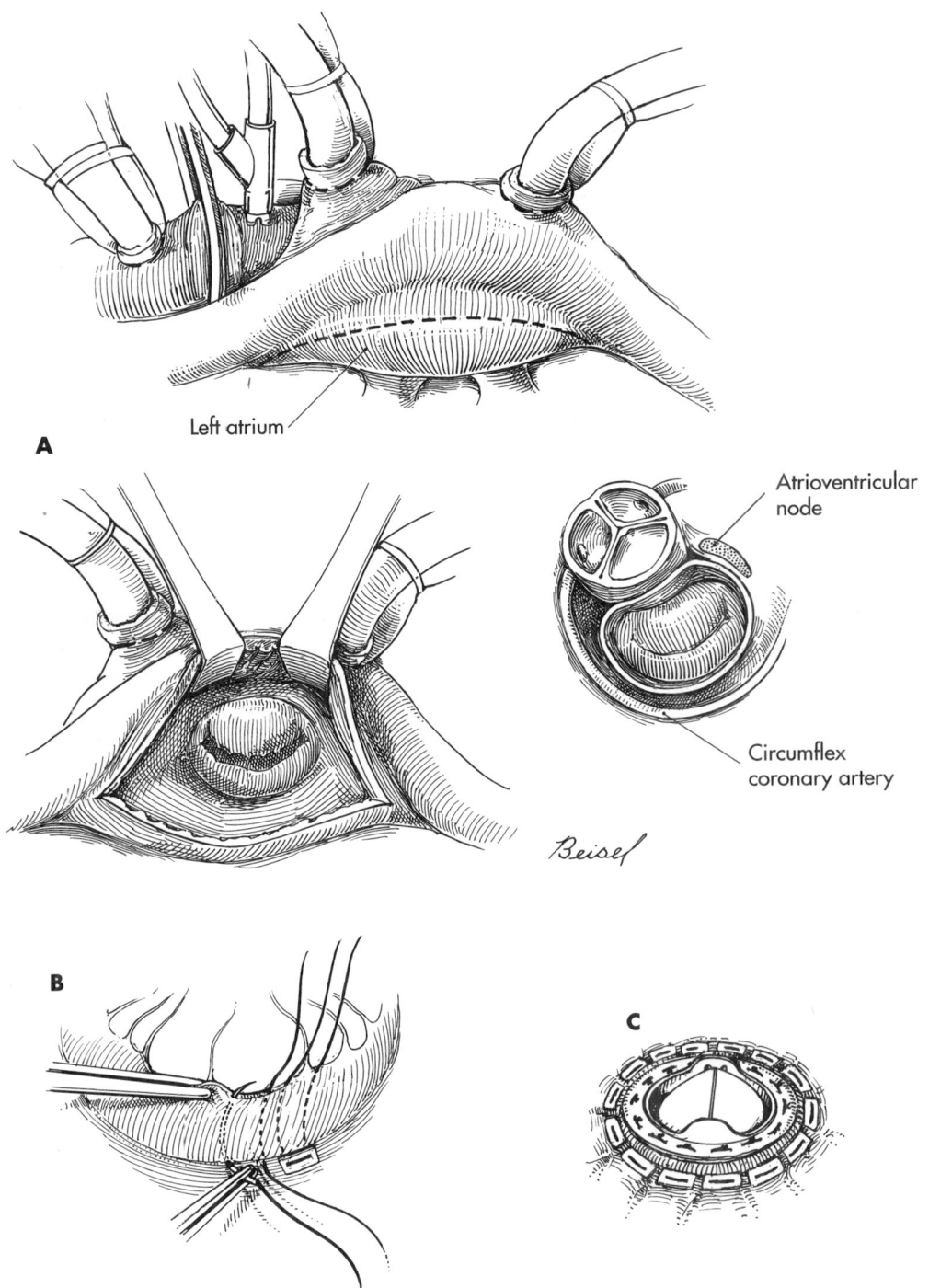

FIGURE 27-62 Mitral valve replacement. **A,** Line of incision and cannulation for bypass, anatomic relationship between mitral and aortic valve with location of conduction node, and exposure of valve. **B,** Placement of pledgeted double-armed sutures in native valve annulus. **C,** Completed valve replacement.

Occasionally, the patient's own pulmonary valve is used as an autograft replacement of the aortic valve; the pulmonary valve is then replaced with an allograft.

Aortic Valve Replacement

The aortic valve is excised and replaced with a mechanical or biologic prosthesis or an aortic valve allograft or autograft.

Procedural considerations

To the basic setup are added the following:

- Aortic valve instruments
- Aortic valves, sizers, and holders
- Coronary artery retrograde-infusion cannula and venting catheters
- Saline to rinse biologic prostheses or allografts

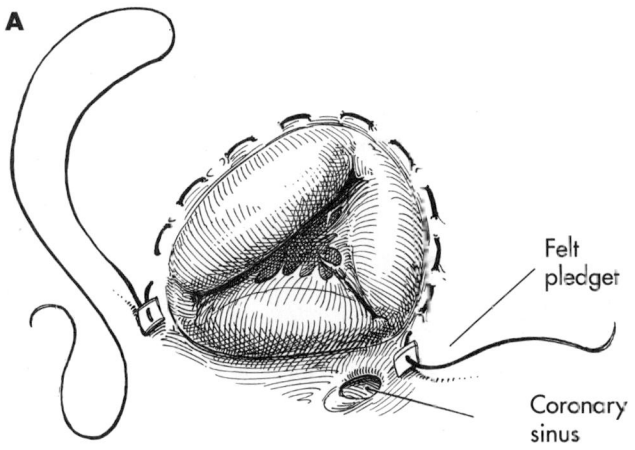

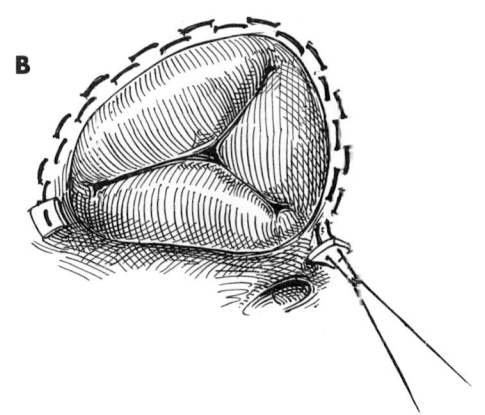

FIGURE 27-63   De Vega tricuspid valve suture annuloplasty.

Operative procedure

1. After the institution of CPB, a left ventricular vent is inserted through a stab wound into the right pulmonary vein, and the tip is advanced into the left ventricle. A retroplegia catheter is inserted into the coronary sinus (Fig. 27-64, *A*).

2. The aorta is cross clamped. If aortic insufficiency is present, the initial bolus of cardioplegic solution is infused retrogradely; subsequent cardioplegic infusions are also given retrogradely. Occasionally, direct coronary perfusion (Fig. 27-64, *B*) is given if a retrograde catheter cannot be inserted.

   If aortic stenosis is present, the initial bolus of cardioplegic solution may be infused by needle through the aorta into the aortic root. Once the heart is arrested, the aorta is opened.

3. The native valve is inspected. Calcium is debrided with scissors or rongeurs. The valve is carefully excised to avoid injury to the annulus and underlying structures (Fig. 27-64, *C*). Narrow packing may be used in the left ventricle to confine small, loose, calcified fragments

that could subsequently embolize. Instruments should be wiped clean frequently.

4. The annulus is sized, the proper prosthesis selected, and a prosthesis holder attached.

5a. If a biologic valve is selected, it is delivered to the field and rinsed in three saline baths of at least 2 minutes each. Biologic valves should be kept moist with frequent saline irrigation.

5b. If an allograft is used, it is delivered to the field and thawed in saline baths according to protocol.[59]

5c. If a mechanical valve is chosen, it may be placed in an antibiotic solution until inserted (antibiotic solutions are not recommended for biologic valves).

6a. The new valve is implanted (Fig. 27-64, *D* and *E*) by use of a technique similar to that previously described for mitral valve replacement.

6b. If the aortic annulus is too small to accept a prosthesis of adequate size, the annulus and proximal portion of the ascending aorta can be enlarged.[32,74] A patch of bovine pericardium or Dacron graft is placed longitudinally in the proximal anterior ascending aorta where the aortic annulus has been cut (Fig. 27-65, *A* and *B*). The valve prosthesis is sutured to the natural annulus and then to the patch (Fig. 27-65, *C*). The patch is sutured to the remaining edges of the aortotomy (Fig. 27-65, *D*).

7. The aorta is closed with nonabsorbable sutures, and the cross-clamp is removed (Fig. 27-64, *F*).

8. The left side of the heart is deaired (by vent, by moving the OR bed side to side, or by other maneuvers chosen by the surgeon). The patient is placed in Trendelenburg's position, and the lungs are inflated. The heart is not allowed to eject blood until the surgeon is satisfied that no air remains within the left ventricle. The heart is defibrillated if it does not resume beating spontaneously.

9. Rewarming of the heart continues, the venting catheter or catheters are removed, and the chest is closed in the routine manner.

Combined Surgery

When CABG is to be performed with AVR, the procedure is done in the following order:

1. The diseased valve is excised, the annulus sized, and the prosthesis selected.
2. Distal coronary anastomoses are performed.
3. The prosthetic valve is inserted.
4. The aorta (or left atrium in MVR) is closed.
5. The proximal coronary anastomoses are inserted into the aorta, after which the aortic cross-clamp is removed.

Double Valve Replacement

When the *aortic and mitral valves are both replaced,* the valves are first excised and the annuli sized. Then the mitral valve is implanted, followed by the aortic valve. The aorta

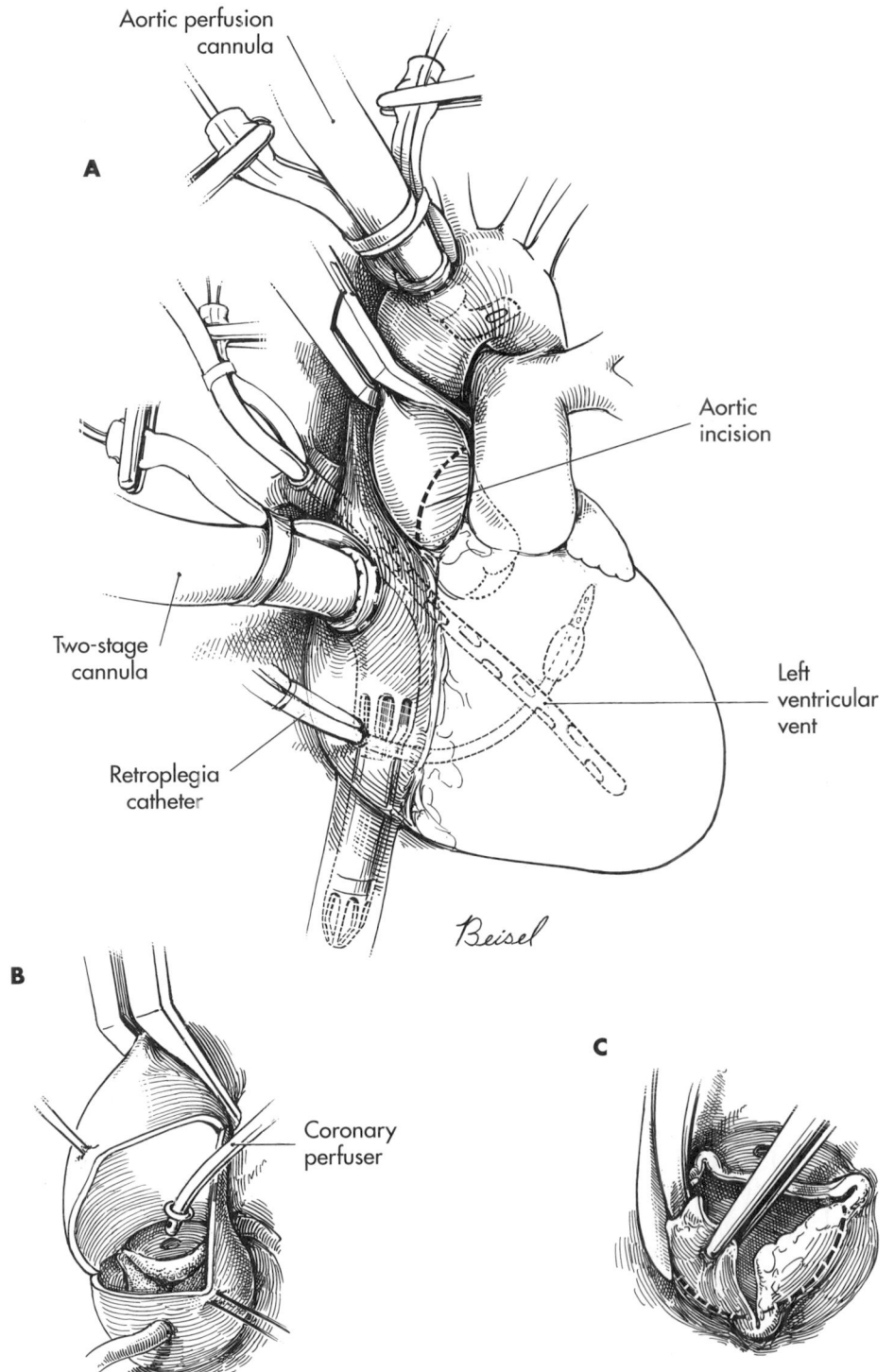

Aortic perfusion
cannula

A

Aortic
incision

Two-stage
cannula

Left
ventricular
vent

Retroplegia
catheter

Beisel

B

Coronary
perfuser

C

FIGURE 27–64 **A**, Cannulation, retrograde cardioplegia, and vent sites for aortic valve procedures. Notice incision line. **B**, If retrograde cardioplegia is not used, hand-held coronary ostial catheters can deliver antegrade cardioplegic solution. **C**, Diseased valve is completely excised.   *Continued*

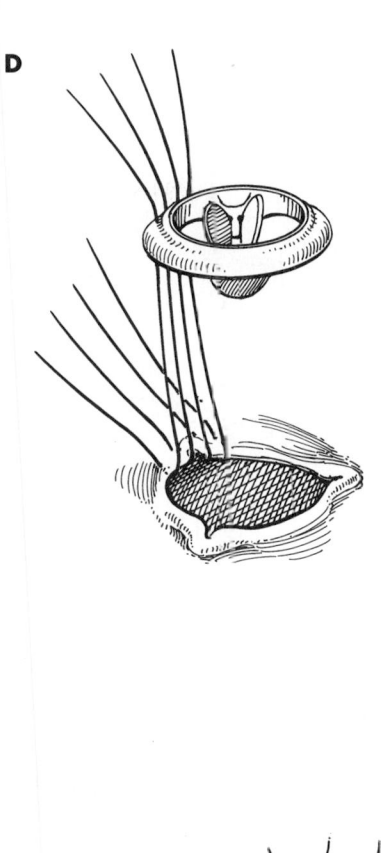

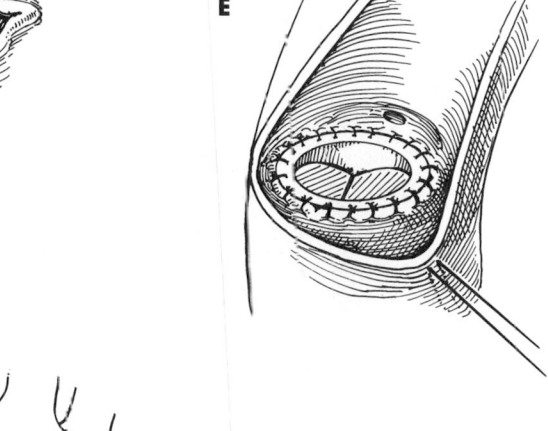

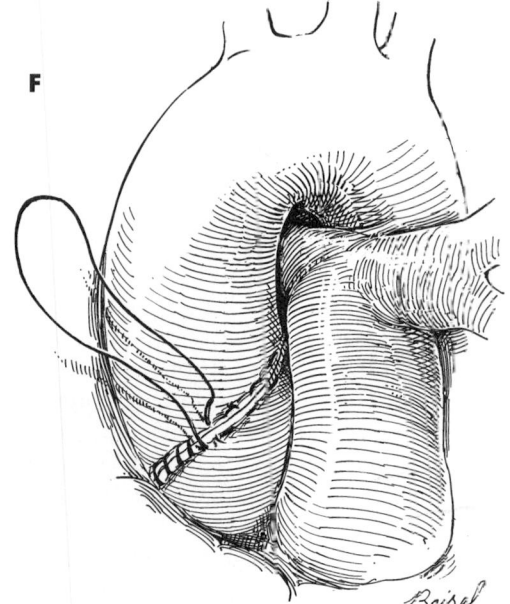

FIGURE 27-64, cont'd   **D**, Sutures are placed in the valve annulus and the prosthetic sewing ring. **E**, Stitches are tied and cut. **F**, Closure of the aortic suture line.

is closed, and after sufficient de-airing of the left ventricle the left atrium is closed.

SURGERY FOR THE THORACIC AORTA

Thoracic aortic aneurysmectomy is excision of an aneurysmal portion of the ascending, arch, or descending thoracic aorta and replacement with a prosthetic graft, valve-graft conduit, or intraaortic prosthesis. Collagen-impregnated grafts have significantly reduced interstitial bleeding and obviated the need for preclotting techniques.

Aneurysms may be caused by atherosclerosis, arteriosclerosis, trauma, infection, or medial degeneration.[32] *Atherosclerosis* affects large and medium arteries with intimal deposits of plaques containing cholesterol, lipoid material, and lipophages. *Arteriosclerosis* is a condition characterized by loss of elasticity and by thickening and hardening of the arteries. Both conditions may lead to aneurysm formation within any artery.

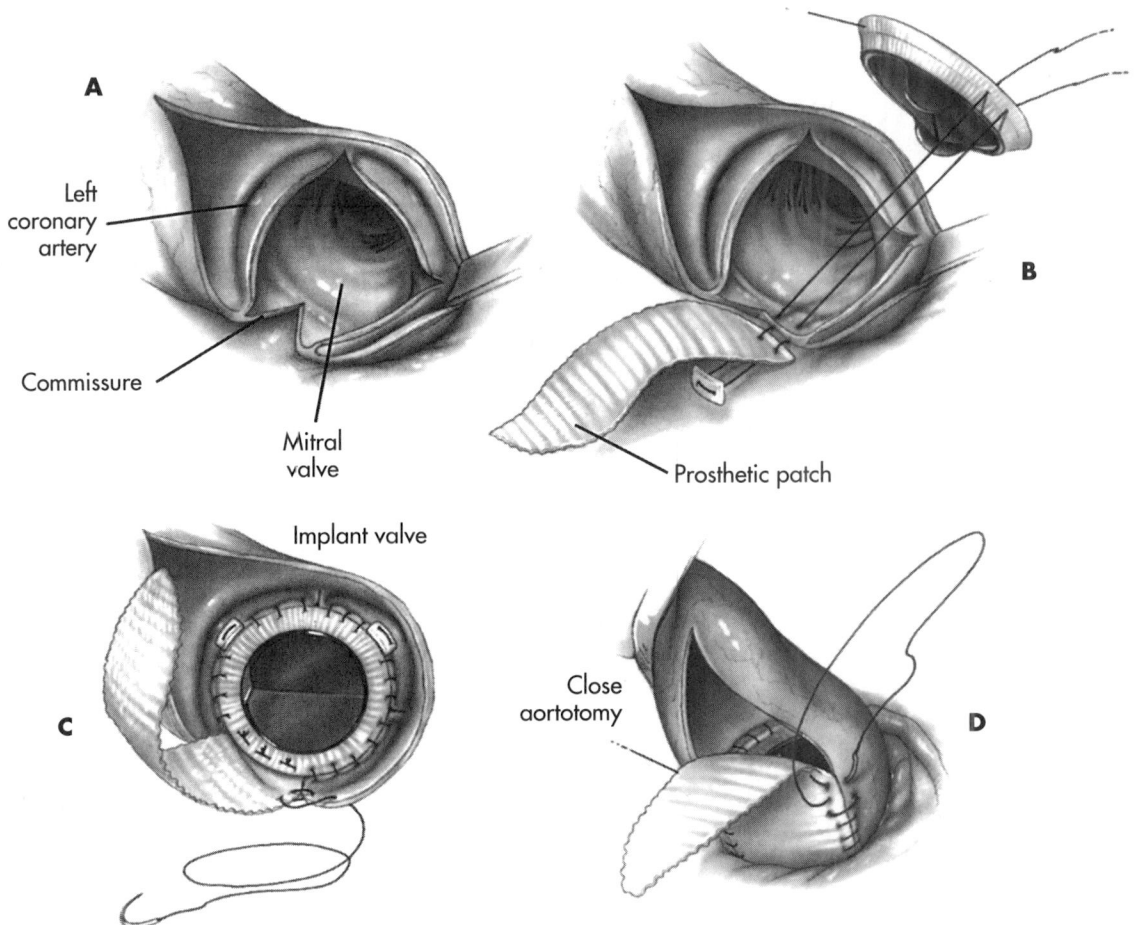

FIGURE 27-65 Technique for aortic enlargement (Nicks-Nuñez operation). **A,** The aortotomy is extended through the commissure separating the left and noncoronary cusps. **B,** A prosthetic patch is sewn into the cut portion of the aorta and into the prosthetic valve. **C,** The prosthetic valve is seated, and the stitches are tied and cut. **D,** The patch is incorporated into the aortotomy closure.

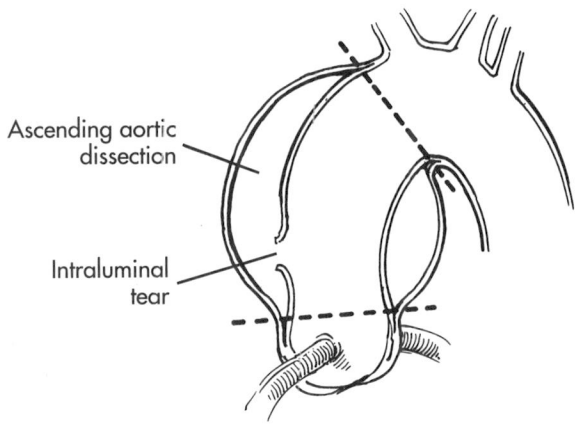

FIGURE 27-66 Aortic dissection.

Aortic *dissection* is a unique entity and is related to degenerative changes in the medial layer of the artery. These changes predispose the artery to tearing of the intimal layer with subsequent dissection of the vessel wall by blood entering it through the tear.[76]

Surgical intervention becomes necessary when presenting symptoms indicate a compromised circulation or danger of rupture; generally, medical management with hypotensive agents to reduce stress on the vessel is the preferred initial treatment until surgical repair can be performed.

Aneurysms can be characterized morphologically as follows: (1) saccular—a sac type of formation with a narrowed neck projecting from the side of the artery and (2) fusiform—a spindleshaped formation with complete circumferential involvement of the artery. Aortic dissections involve a splitting of the intima of the aorta, permitting blood to pass between the layers of the wall to form a false channel; as the channel extends and enlarges, the blood flow is obstructed (see Figs. 27-10 and 27-66).

Procedural considerations

Several methods of surgical treatment are described in Crawford's classic study.[26] In situations where ascending aortic aneurysm or aortic dissection produces annular dilatation with subsequent aortic valve insufficiency, a

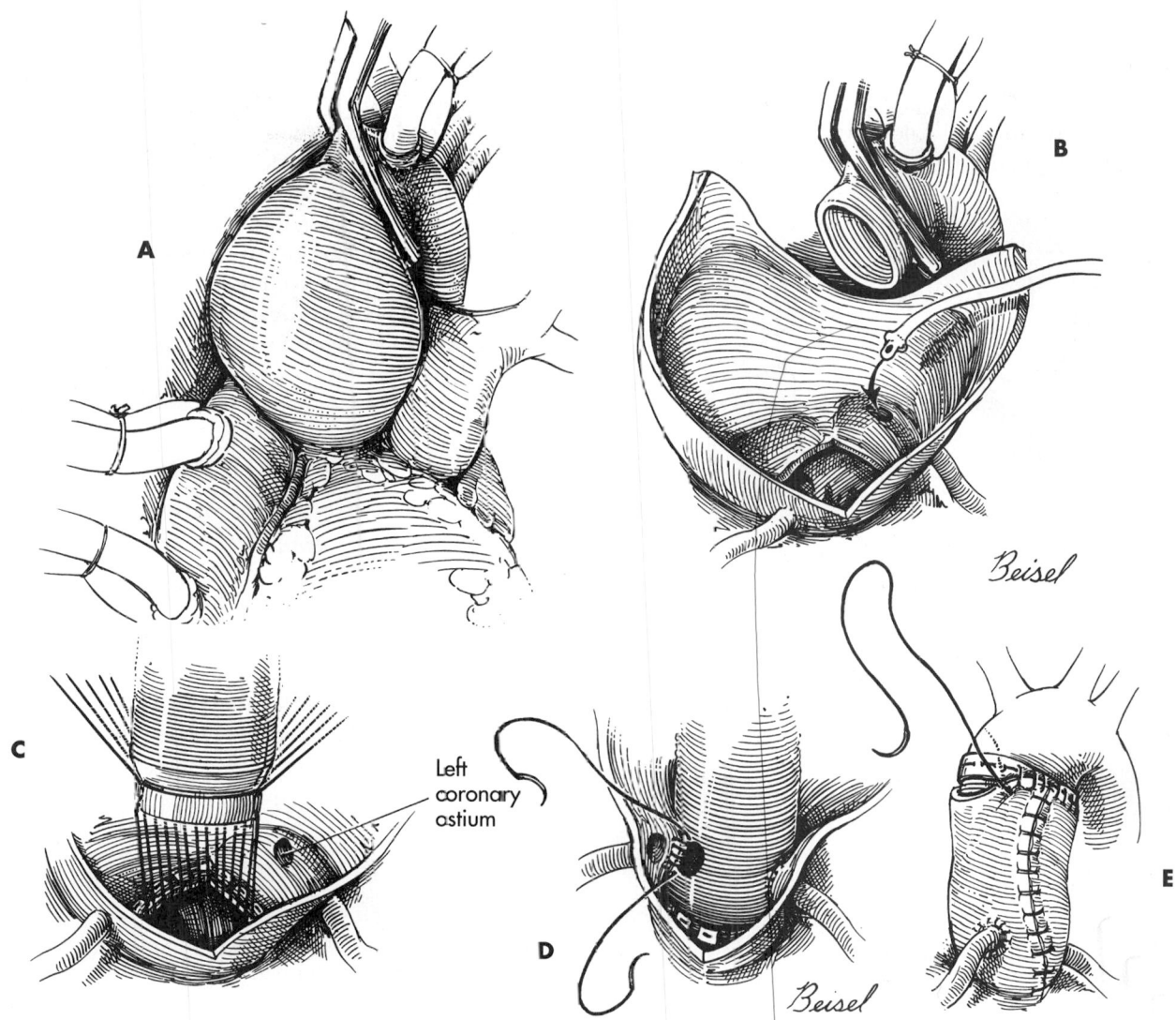

FIGURE 27-67   Bentall-Bono procedure (see text).

Bentall-Bono procedure with a valved conduit (see Fig. 27-32) may be performed to replace the aortic valve and the aneurysmal aorta (Fig. 27-67). Retrograde cardioplegia is usually employed; if necessary, selective coronary infusion may be used. This procedure necessitates reimplanting the right and left coronary ostia into the prosthetic graft. In patients with coronary artery disease, vein grafts may be inserted and anastomosed proximally to the prosthesis.

The type of CPB depends on the location of the aneurysm. Generally the atrium is cannulated for venous return, and the femoral artery is used for arterial inflow (because the weakened ascending aorta cannot be safely cannulated). Deep hypothermia with circulatory arrest and cerebroplegia may be needed to protect heart and brain in particularly complex lesions of the aortic arch. In aneurysms involving the aortic arch, placement of a cross-clamp is difficult.

In descending thoracic aortic aneurysms, the heart is not arrested; it continues beating to perfuse the upper body. Femoral bypass may be instituted to perfuse the kidneys and lower extremities; normothermia is maintained. In some patients, a transluminally placed endovascular stent is a feasible alternative to open procedures.[51]

Repair of Ascending Thoracic Aortic Aneurysm or Dissection
Procedural considerations

To the basic setup are added aneurysm instruments. Valve instruments, coronary instruments, and an array of tube grafts, valves, or valved conduits should be available. Bicaval cannulation for venous drainage is preferred, but if the cavae cannot be safely accessed, the femoral vein is used initially for venous drainage. Once the aneurysm is controlled, the femoral venous line can be Y-ed to a vena cava catheter.

Operative procedure

1. The patient is positioned for a median sternotomy.
2. Cannulation for CPB is performed.
3. The sternum is opened, and the aneurysm is inspected.
4a. If the aortic annulus is not involved, the aneurysm is incised longitudinally, and a woven graft is anasto-

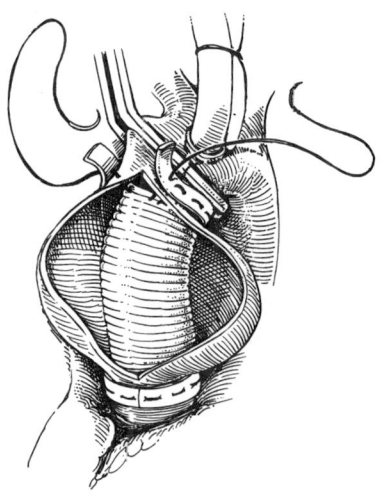

FIGURE 27-68 Resection and graft repair of ascending aortic aneurysm.

mosed proximally and distally to the healthy aorta (Fig. 27-68). Felt strips incorporated into the anastomosis may be used to bolster friable tissue.

4b. If the aortic annulus is involved, the ascending aorta is incised to the annulus. The leaflets are excised, and the annulus is measured. The proximal end of a valved conduit is inserted (see Fig. 27-67, *C*). An eye cautery is used to create openings in the graft at the location of the right and left coronary ostia, which are anastomosed to the graft (see Fig. 27-67, *D*). (If the patient has concomitant coronary artery disease, saphenous vein grafts are inserted.) The distal end of the conduit is sutured to healthy aorta, and the aneurysmal remnant may be wrapped around the conduit (see Fig. 27-67, *E*).

5. Bypass is discontinued, and all incisions are closed.

Repair of Aortic Arch Aneurysm
Procedural considerations

Aneurysm instruments and woven grafts are available. If deep hypothermia is to be used, the patient's face and head may be covered with bags of ice at the beginning of the procedure. Precautions (such as padding) to prevent frostbite are instituted. The location of the aneurysm will determine the positioning. Aneurysms of the proximal

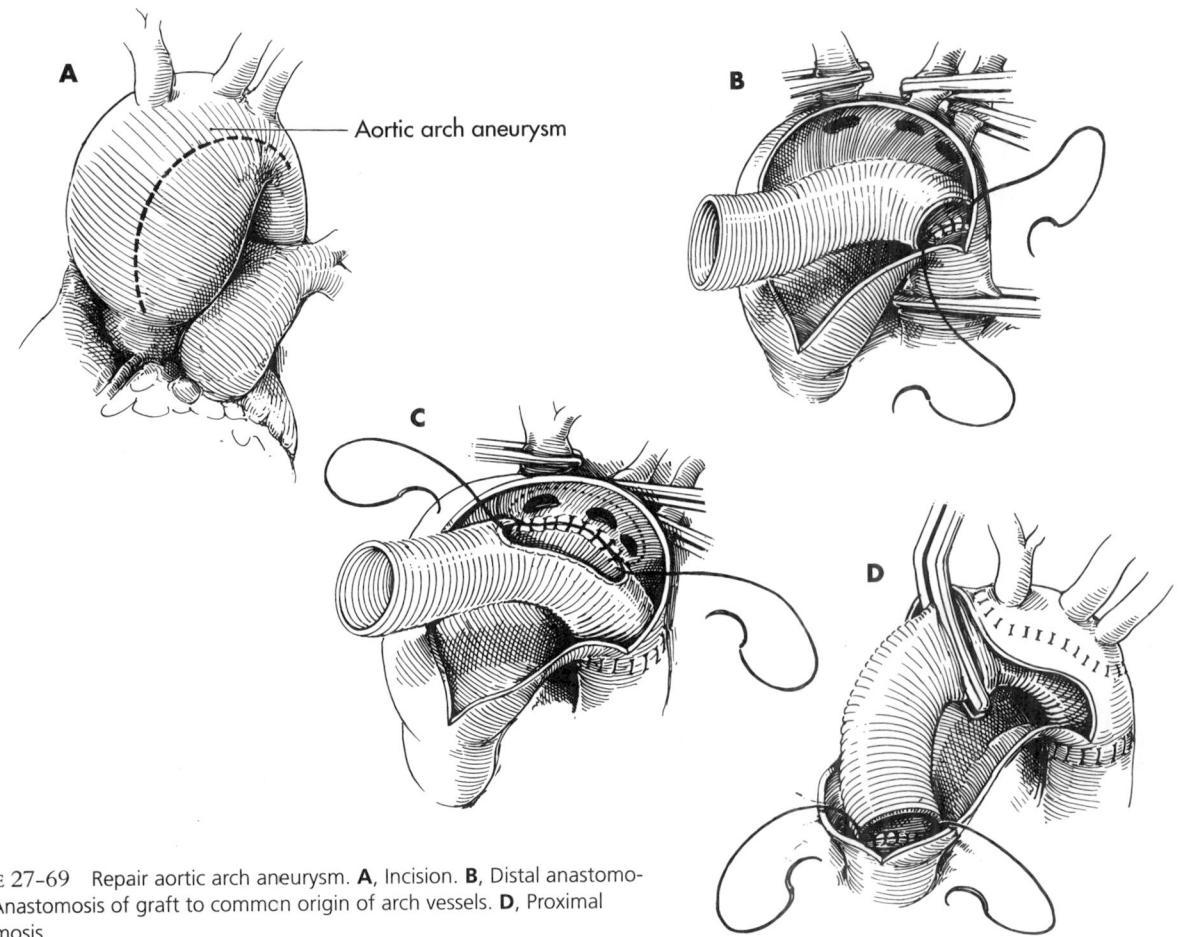

FIGURE 27-69 Repair aortic arch aneurysm. **A**, Incision. **B**, Distal anastomosis. **C**, Anastomosis of graft to common origin of arch vessels. **D**, Proximal anastomosis.

arch can be accessed through a median sternotomy; distal arch aneurysms may require a modified thoracotomy position to optimize exposure.

Operative procedure

1. Cannulation of the right atrium and femoral artery is performed.
2. Once the patient is cooled to the desired temperature, the arch vessels are individually cross-clamped (Fig. 27-69, *A* and *B*). (If circulatory arrest is indicated, cross clamps are not used.) The aneurysm is incised, a tube graft is selected, and the anastomosis to the descending aorta is performed.
3. An opening is made into the side of the graft, and the graft is anastomosed to the common origin of the brachiocephalic, left carotid, and left subclavian vessels. The graft is cross clamped proximally to the arch and de-aired (Fig. 27-69, *C*).
4. The proximal aorta is anastomosed to the graft while the patient is rewarming. The graft is de-aired, and the patient is weaned from bypass (Fig. 27-69, *D*).
5. All incisions are closed.

Repair of Descending Thoracic Aortic Aneurysm
Procedural considerations

Thoracotomy instruments and supplies are added to the basic setup; additional long aortic cross clamps may be needed. Prosthetic grafts are available. The patient is positioned for a left posterolateral thoracotomy. Femoral vein–femoral artery bypass is performed to perfuse the lower body. The heart perfuses the upper body proximal to the aneurysm. Normothermia is maintained.

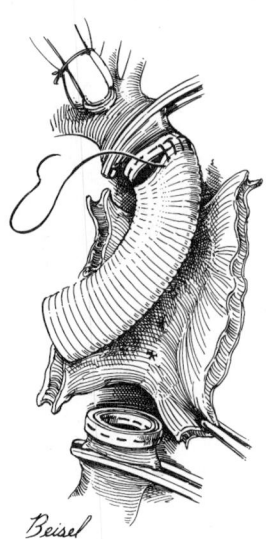

FIGURE 27-70 Resection and graft replacement for descending thoracic aortic aneurysm.

Operative procedure

1. Cannulation for femoral vein–femoral artery bypass is performed.
2. A thoracotomy incision is made, the aneurysm is exposed, and the surrounding structures are inspected. (Occasionally the surgeon makes two thoracotomies for better access to and control of the aorta.) Renal involvement is assessed; if indicated, measures to protect the kidneys are instituted (such as local cooling).
3. Normothermic femoral bypass is initiated.
4. The aneurysm is incised longitudinally, and the aorta is sized.
5a. A woven graft (Fig. 27-70) is inserted, and the aneurysmal remnants are wrapped around the graft.
5b. If an intraaortic prosthesis (see Fig. 27-22) is used, it is inserted into the true aortic lumen, and the aorta is wrapped around the prosthesis. Dacron tapes are used to encircle the aorta and the proximal and distal rings. The tapes are tied, securing the prosthesis. Stay sutures may be inserted to further secure the prosthesis.

MECHANICAL AND BIOLOGIC CIRCULATORY ASSISTANCE

A small percentage of patients cannot be weaned from CPB after open-heart operations, even with the use of inotropic and vasodilator drugs. Other patients have end-stage cardiomyopathy. Various mechanical devices are available to support the circulation while the heart recovers or while the patient awaits cardiac transplantation. Biologic assistance in the form of an autogenous muscle wrap is valuable in some patients who may not be candidates for transplantation. Heart reduction surgery, developed by Batista,[2] is another technique that has been used to treat dilated cardiomyopathy; ongoing research is attempting to provide a fuller understanding of the effect of this procedure on cardiac configuration and function.[30]

Intraaortic Balloon Pump

The most widely used short-term device is the intraaortic balloon pump (IABP). The IABP (Fig. 27-71) employs the principle of counterpulsation to increase coronary blood flow and decrease afterload (such as the resistance the ventricle must overcome to open the aortic valve).

Operative procedure

1. A flexible guidewire is passed through a percutaneous needle into the femoral artery. The needle is removed, and graduated dilators are inserted over the guidewire to dilate the overlying tissue and the artery wall.
2. The IABP catheter (with the furled balloon) is inserted into the artery and advanced to a position just distal to the left subclavian artery. The catheter can be marked at

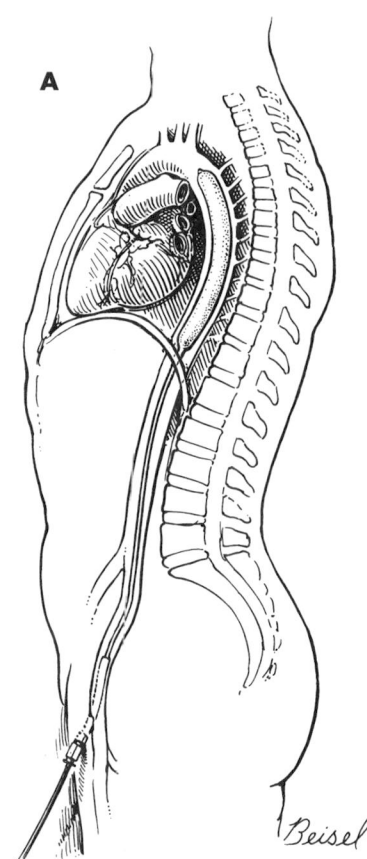

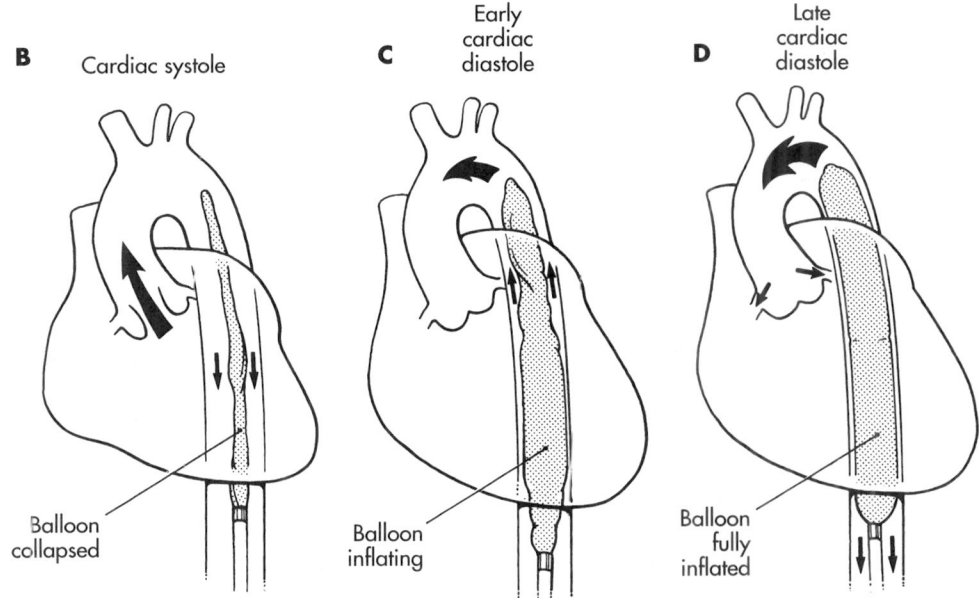

FIGURE 27–71 Phases of balloon pumping. **A,** Balloon inflation occurs from closure of aortic valve to end of diastole. Inflation causes retrograde flow of blood in aorta, increasing coronary perfusion pressure without increasing myocardial work or oxygen demand. Inflation also causes antegrade flow, increasing mean arterial pressure, renal flow, and cerebral flow. **B,** Balloon deflation occurs from just before opening of aortic valve to closure of aortic valve. Deflation encourages antegrade flow, decreasing afterload or resistance to left ventricular ejection. Deflation also decreases oxygen required by left ventricle, shortens systolic ejection, and increases stroke volume. **C** and **D,** When the balloon reinflates, the cycle is repeated.

the proximal end with a silk tie to measure how far the catheter should be inserted.

3. The balloon is unfurled and activated.

Ventricular Assist Device

Ventricular assist devices (VADs) are designed to augment cardiac output and decrease the work load of the heart by diverting blood from the ventricle to an artificial pump that maintains systemic perfusion. One multicenter study[36] demonstrated that patients with selected left VADs (LVAD) can become better transplant candidates because the VADs can enhance anabolism, ambulation, and improved organ function.

Procedural considerations

If patients cannot be weaned from CPB with IAPB, an assist system may be indicated. Cardiac support devices include external centrifugal pumps, and internal pneumatic (Fig. 27-72) or electric-power assist devices. Right or left VADs are available. The device described below is approved for support of the left ventricle when right ventricular function is normal.[32] Prosthetic valves are incorporated into the circuit to maintain unidirectional blood flow.

Operative procedure
Thermo Cardiosystems, Inc., "HeartMate" LVAD

1. A median sternotomy incision is made and extended to the umbilicus (Fig. 27-72, *A*).
2. A preperitoneal pouch is made for placement of the assist device.
3. CPB is established, and the aorta is cross clamped. The atrial septum is inspected for defects, which if found are closed.
4. A Dacron graft is anastomosed to the aorta (Fig. 27-72, *B*).
5. The left ventricular apex is mobilized, and an opening is created in the apex (Fig. 27-72, *C*).
6. A connector is inserted into the apex, and the flange is sewn to the surrounding left ventricular myocardium with pledgeted sutures. The inflow conduit is attached to the apical connector (Fig. 27-72, *D* to *G*).
7. An opening is made into the diaphragm near the location of the apical connector and inflow conduit. The conduit is passed through the diaphragm and attached to the assist device.
8. The aortic graft is attached to the outflow conduit which is connected to the assist device (Fig. 27-72, *H* and *I*).
9. The drive line is tunneled to the left lower quadrant where it exits through the skin. The drive line can be connected to the drive console or to a battery pack. Blood flows from the left ventricular apex, to the device, and back into the body through the aortic conduit (Fig. 27-72, *J*).
10. CPB is discontinued, and incisions are closed.

To remove the pump, the patient is returned to the operating room, the sternotomy is reopened, and the cannulas are removed.

Total Artificial Heart

The total artificial heart (TAH) has not demonstrated great success as a permanent cardiac replacement because of thromboembolism and infection. Long-term right or left VADs have been increasingly employed as a bridge to cardiac transplantation by supporting the circulation while a suitable donor heart can be found.

Biologic Ventricular Support

Among the newer trends in providing ventricular support is the use of latissimus dorsi muscle for cardiomyoplasty (Fig. 27-73). This technique uses electrostimulated skeletal muscle to reinforce or partially replace the heart muscle.[56]

HEART AND HEART-LUNG TRANSPLANTATION
Heart Transplantation (Fig. 27-74)

Orthotopic transplantation (replacing one heart with another) is most commonly performed, but heterotopic (piggyback) and combined heart-lung procedures are done as well. Important considerations continue to be recipient and donor selection, the immune response, and control of infection. Older recipients and donors (over 60 years of age) have demonstrated acceptable morbidity and survival.[3]

Procedural considerations

Individual instrument setups are necessary for the donor and the recipient.

Operative procedures
Donor Heart

The donor heart is exposed through a median sternotomy. The aorta, pulmonary artery, and venae cavae are dissected. The venae cavae are occluded, the left atrium is opened to decompress the ventricle, and the heart is rapidly cooled and arrested.

The heart is excised by incision of the left atrium circumferentially at the level of the pulmonary veins and by severing the aorta and pulmonary artery. The donor heart is immediately placed into cold saline and transported to the site where it will be inserted into the recipient.

Recipient Heart

The recipient is placed on bypass with cannulation of the inferior vena cava and the superior vena cava; cava tapes are placed around the cavae. The patient is cooled to approximately 25° C, and the cava tapes are tightened. The

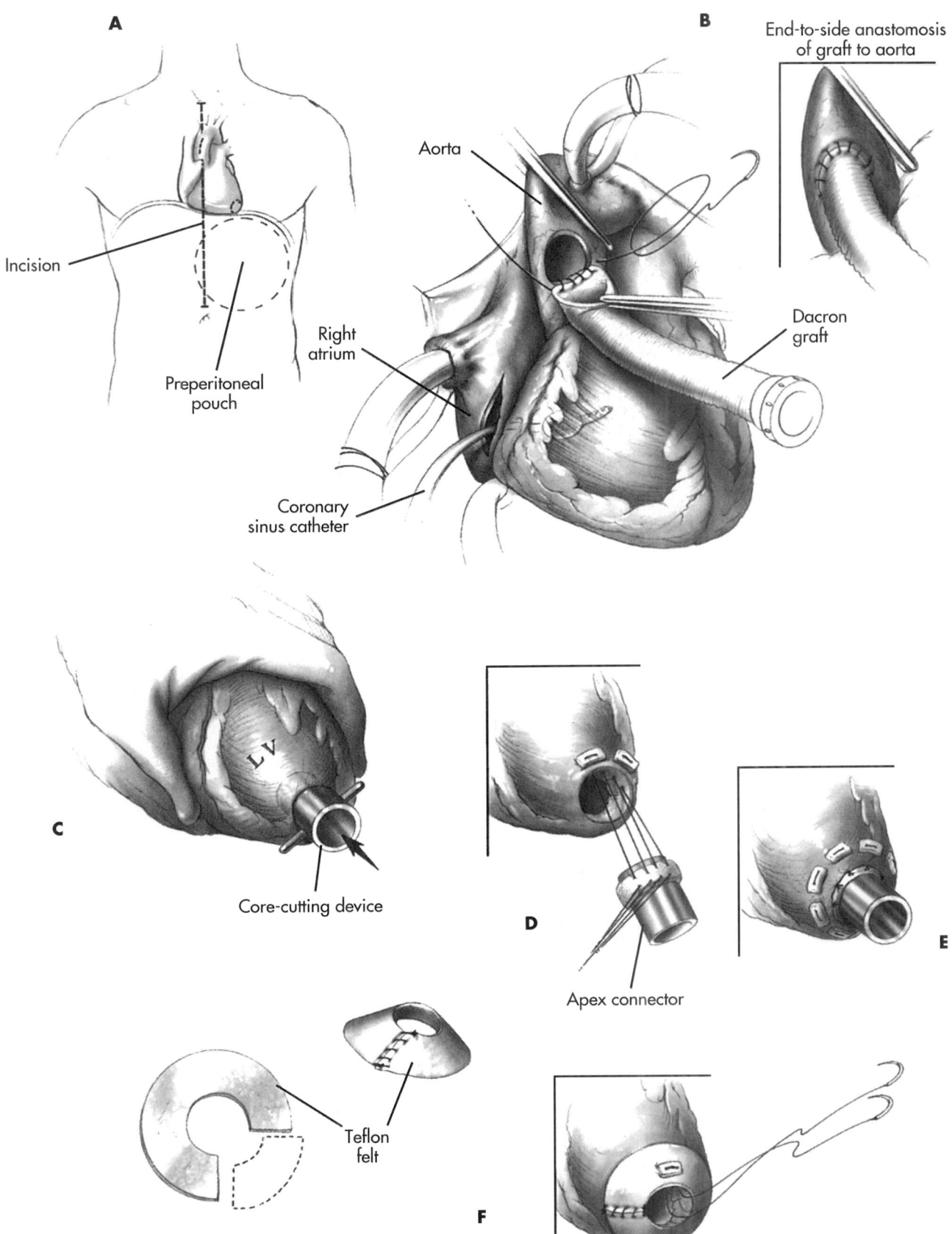

FIGURE 27–72 Left ventricular assist device (see text).

Continued

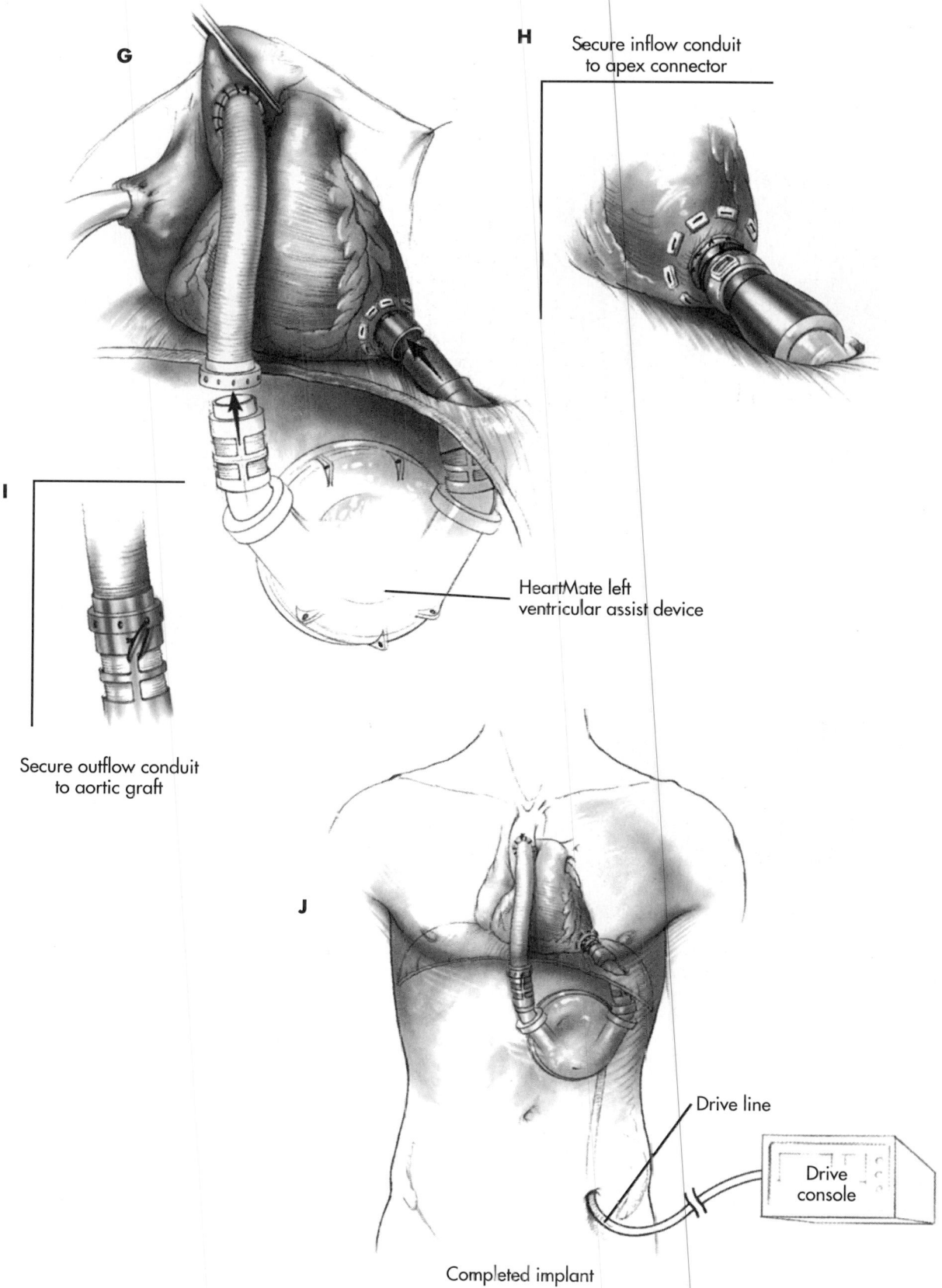

G

H   Secure inflow conduit
to apex connector

I

Secure outflow conduit
to aortic graft

HeartMate left
ventricular assist device

J

Drive line

Drive
console

Completed implant

FIGURE 27-72, cont'd   Left ventricular assist device (see text).

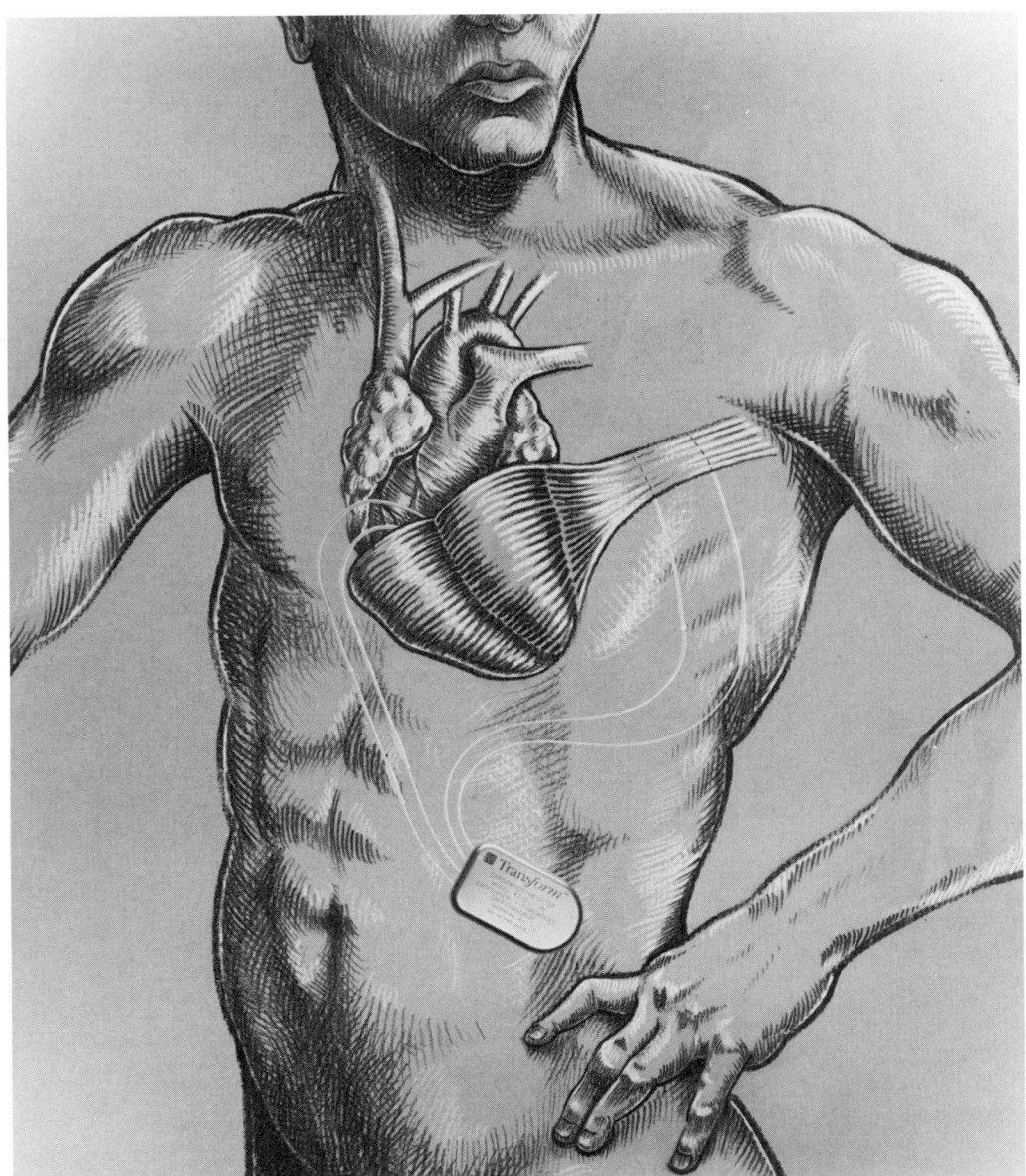

FIGURE 27-73   Cardiomyoplasty. The left latissimus dorsi muscle is dissected from the back and swung around to the heart where it is sewn around the ventricle. This (skeletal) muscle is then transformed into a continuously beating muscle by a cardiomyostimulator that paces the muscle with increasing frequency, allowing the muscle to become fatigue resistant. The muscle wrap squeezes the heart in synchronization with natural electrical impulses moving through the heart muscle.

pulmonary trunk and aorta are dissected immediately above their respective semilunar valves; the atria are incised to leave intact portions of the right and left atrial walls and the atrial septum of the recipient. The recipient heart is then removed.

The donor heart is placed in the pericardial well. The interatrial septum and the left and then the right atrial walls are approximated with running cardiovascular sutures (Fig. 27-74, *A* and *B*). The donor and recipient aortas are similarly joined (Fig. 27-74, *C*). Air is removed from the left side of the heart.

The aortic clamp is removed, and a clamp is placed across the donor pulmonary artery. The cava tape is removed, and vigorous ventricular fibrillation of the donor heart commences. Local cooling of the heart is discontinued at this point, and, before the pulmonary artery is sutured, all atrial suture lines are carefully inspected for significant bleeding areas. The pulmonary arteries are united (Fig. 27-74, *D*), and the clamp is removed. Defibrillation of the ventricles is usually effected with a single DC shock. A needle vent in the ascending aorta allows residual air to escape. The patient is then gradually

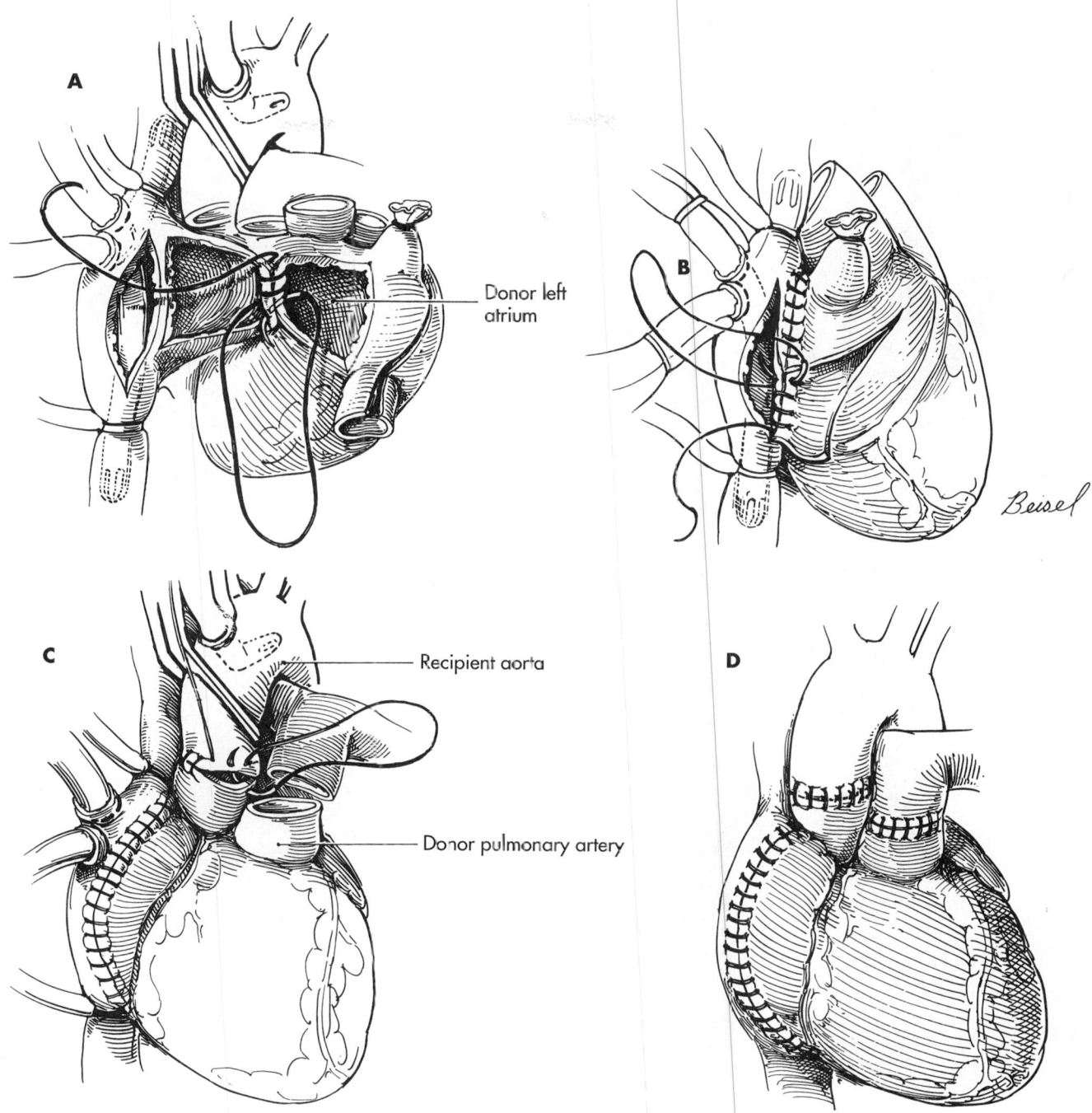

FIGURE 27-74   Heart transplantation. **A**, The recipient and donor left atria are anastomosed. **B**, Anastomosis at the right atria. **C**, Aortic anastomosis **D**, Pulmonary artery anastomosis.

weaned from the bypass. Cannulas are removed from the venae cavae and the aorta. The incisions are closed as described previously.

Heart–Lung Transplantation (Fig. 27-75)

A three-anastomosis technique for combined heart–lung transplantation ensures preservation of the *donor's* sinus node and the *recipient's* recurrent laryngeal, vagus, and phrenic nerves.[32]

Operative procedure

The recipient's diseased heart and lungs are excised separately or en bloc, with care taken not to injure the major nerves listed previously. The recipient's right atrium is saved to create a large atrial cuff for attachment to the donor heart. The bronchi are transsected, and the stumps are clamped to prevent contamination. The trachea is transsected just above the carina. The donor heart and lungs are brought onto the field. The right lung is placed

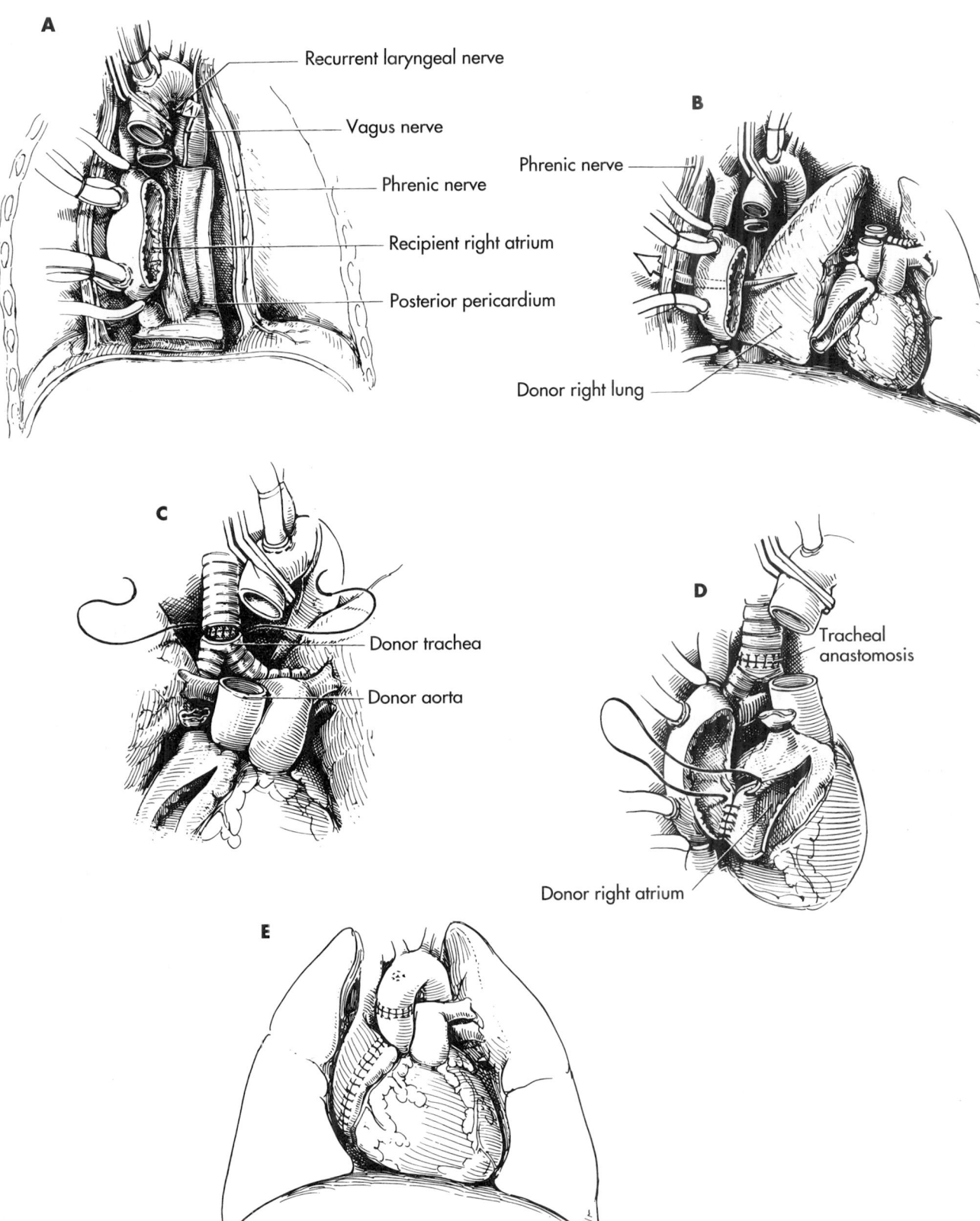

FIGURE 27-75 Heart-lung transplantation. **A**, Recipient's heart and lungs are removed. **B**, Donor organs are placed in the field. **C**, Tracheal anastomosis. **D**, Right atrial anastomosis. **E**, Completed procedures.

in the right pleural space, and the left lung is positioned in the left pleural space. The tracheal and the right atrial anastomoses are performed, and rewarming is begun. The aortic anastomosis is performed, the aorta is de-aired, and the cross-clamp is removed.

SURGERY FOR CONDUCTION DISTURBANCES

Disturbances of the conduction system can affect the rate and rhythm of the contracting heart. Surgical techniques have been developed to treat a variety of supraventricular dysrhythmias (such as atrial fibrillation [AF] and Wolff-Parkinson-White reentry tachycardia), and both ischemic and nonischemic ventricular tachydysrhythmias (such as ventricular tachycardia or fibrillation).[32] Surgical intervention includes the Maze procedure for AF,[44] subendocardial resection of the myocardial dysrhythmogenic focus, ablation of abnormal conduction pathways with radiofrequency or cryotherapy, and the insertion of pacing and antitachycardia-fibrillation devices.

Before surgery the patient's conduction pathways are mapped in the electrophysiology laboratory. These tests can identify aberrant pathways, tachydysrhythmias, the existence of additional pathways, and the effects of medications on the dysrhythmia. At operation the surgeon initiates cardiopulmonary bypass and attaches electrodes to each atrium and ventricle. Intraoperative mapping is performed to verify the suspected dysrhythmia. During surgery for accessory conduction pathways, for example, the pathway is located and dissected, and the surgeon ablates the tissue. After termination of bypass and the achievement of hemostasis, the chest is closed in the routine fashion.

Surgical treatment for AF involves multiple incisions in the atria so that the electrical impulses (which are unable to cross suture lines) are routed from the sinoatrial node to the atrioventricular node. The incisions are then closed with suture, creating a maze that directs the impulses in the desired direction.[25]

Many procedures formerly performed in the operating room are now frequently performed in the cardiac catheterization suite, in particular, insertion of pacemakers and internal cardiovertor defibrillators (ICDs).

Insertion of Permanent Pacemaker

A permanent pacemaker (pulse generator and electrodes) initiates atrial or ventricular contraction, or both types. Complete heart block and bradydysrhythmias (such as slow heart rates) are the most common indications for pacemaker implantation. The development of multiprogramable and physiologic pacemakers has made possible the treatment of many forms of dysrhythmias and neuroconductive disturbances as well as tachydysrhythmias.[46] A temporary pacemaker may also be used for acute forms of heart block and dysrhythmias that occasionally occur during and after cardiac surgery.

Two methods of placing electrodes for permanent cardiac pacing include transvenous and epicardial approaches. The transvenous route is most commonly used because it does not require a major thoracotomy or a general anesthetic and is therefore safer for high-risk patients. Permanent epicardial electrodes may be placed during cardiac operations when the chest is opened and the heart is exposed; a subxiphoid approach may be used to place epicardial leads without having to open the sternum.

Pulse generators (Fig. 27-76) are typically powered by lithium, which lasts 5 to 10 years. Life expectancy depends on the amount of power used and the frequency of demand. The generators are classified into three groups: fixed rate (or asynchronous), ventricular demand, and physiologic. The asynchronous was the first type implanted and fires at a fixed rate, independent of the electrical activity of the heart. A major disadvantage of this type of pacing is competition between the heart's intrinsic beat and the paced beat, possibly resulting in ventricular fibrillation if the paced beat occurs during the T-wave period of the ECG. Ventricular demand pacemakers were developed in response to this problem and fire at a fixed rate only if spontaneous ventricular activity fails. Adding a sensing mechanism to the existing stimulating mechanism makes this type of pacing possible. "Physiologic" pacemakers can stimulate both the atria and the ventricles, maintain atrioventricular synchrony, and can enhance cardiac output by as much as 20%. Pacemakers are also capable of adjusting the rate of stimulation in response to increased metabolic activity (rate-responsive pacers).

There are two types of electrodes: *myocardial (epicardial)*, which are attached to the heart muscle under direct vision, and *endocardial*, which are inserted transvenously. The stimulating and sensing electrodes are located at the tip of the lead, which attaches to the pulse generator.

Pacing systems are also available as *unipolar* or *bipolar*. A pacemaker with one stimulating electrode at the tip of the lead is unipolar. The electrical current flows between the electrode and the pulse generator. A bipolar pacemaker has two stimulating electrodes at the tip of the lead. Electrical current flows between the two electrodes.

Insertion of Transvenous (Endocardial) Pacing Electrodes
Procedural considerations

The patient is placed in the supine position. Continuous ECG monitoring is essential. A defibrillator and emergency drugs should be available because dysrhythmias can occur during catheter insertion. The patient should be made as comfortable as possible because this procedure can sometimes be lengthy and is frequently performed using local or local standby anesthesia (monitored anesthesia care).

Fluoroscopy is required; thus either a portable image intensifier is needed or the procedure is done in the special

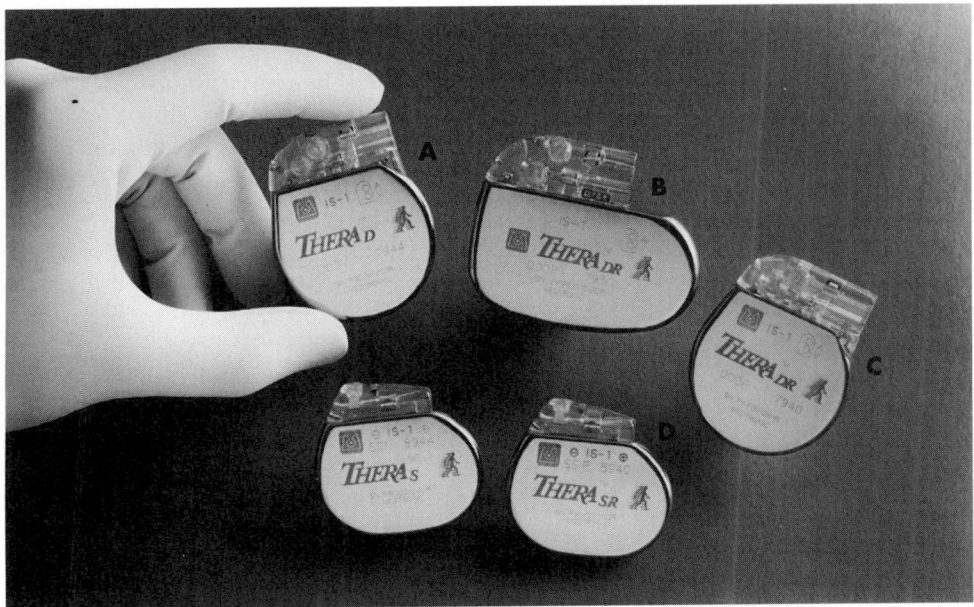

FIGURE 27-76   Pacemaker generators come in a variety of sensing and pacing modes. **A,** The generator (in hand at left) is designed to pace and to maintain synchrony between both chambers of the heart. It can also provide rate-responsive ventricular pacing. **B,** Paces and maintains synchrony between both chambers of the heart; designed to automatically adjust to the body's circulatory needs while automatically switching modes when necessary to prevent an inappropriate heart rate if the atrial rate accelerates dangerously. **C,** A generator smaller than that shown in B. **D,** Single-chamber rate-responsive pacemaker. **E,** Single-chamber generator.

studies section of the radiology or cardiac catheterization department. A minor set of instruments is used, plus the following:

- Vascular dissecting instruments
- Tunneling instrument
- Sterile pacemaker and electrodes
- Introducer set
- External pacemaker (for testing) or a pacing system analyzer (PSA)
- Alligator test cables
- Screwdriver and other accessory items as needed

Operative procedure (Fig. 27-77)

1. The skin and subcutaneous tissue are infiltrated with a local anesthetic, and the patient is placed in Trendelenburg's position (to engorge the vein for easier access and to avoid air emboli).
2. A skin pocket is made close to the subclavian vein (Fig. 27-77, *A*). The vessel may be encircled with a heavy suture.
3. A venotomy is performed with an introducer needle (Fig. 27-77, *B*). A guidewire is threaded to the desired cardiac chamber, and the needle is removed. The pacing electrode is inserted through a peel-away dilator sheath, which is withdrawn after the lead insertion (Fig. 27-77, *C*). The guidewire is withdrawn. A stylette is then inserted to help position the electrode.

4. The electrode is advanced under direct fluoroscopic vision into the right atrium, through the tricuspid valve, and into the right ventricle (Fig. 27-77, *D*).
5. The surgeon attempts to entrap the tip of the electrode in the trabeculae carneae cordis of the right ventricular apex to stabilize it. Once the electrode is positioned and tested with alligator test cables and the pacing analyzer to confirm proper placement and function, the stylette is removed.

   If a dual chamber pacemaker is inserted, the second lead is entrapped in the right atrial appendage (Fig. 27-77, *D*).
6. The electrode or electrodes are brought down and attached to the pulse generator.
7. The pulse generator is placed into the pocket, and the incision may be irrigated with an antibiotic solution. If the pocket must be made farther away from the vein, a tunneling device may be used to thread the electrode to the pocket.
8. The incision is closed in layers with absorbable sutures.

Insertion of Myocardial (Epicardial) Pacing Electrodes

A subxiphoid, left anterior thoracotomy, or sternotomy approach can be used; the setup is as described for placement of endocardial electrodes. The subxiphoid process and left upper quadrant area are infiltrated with the

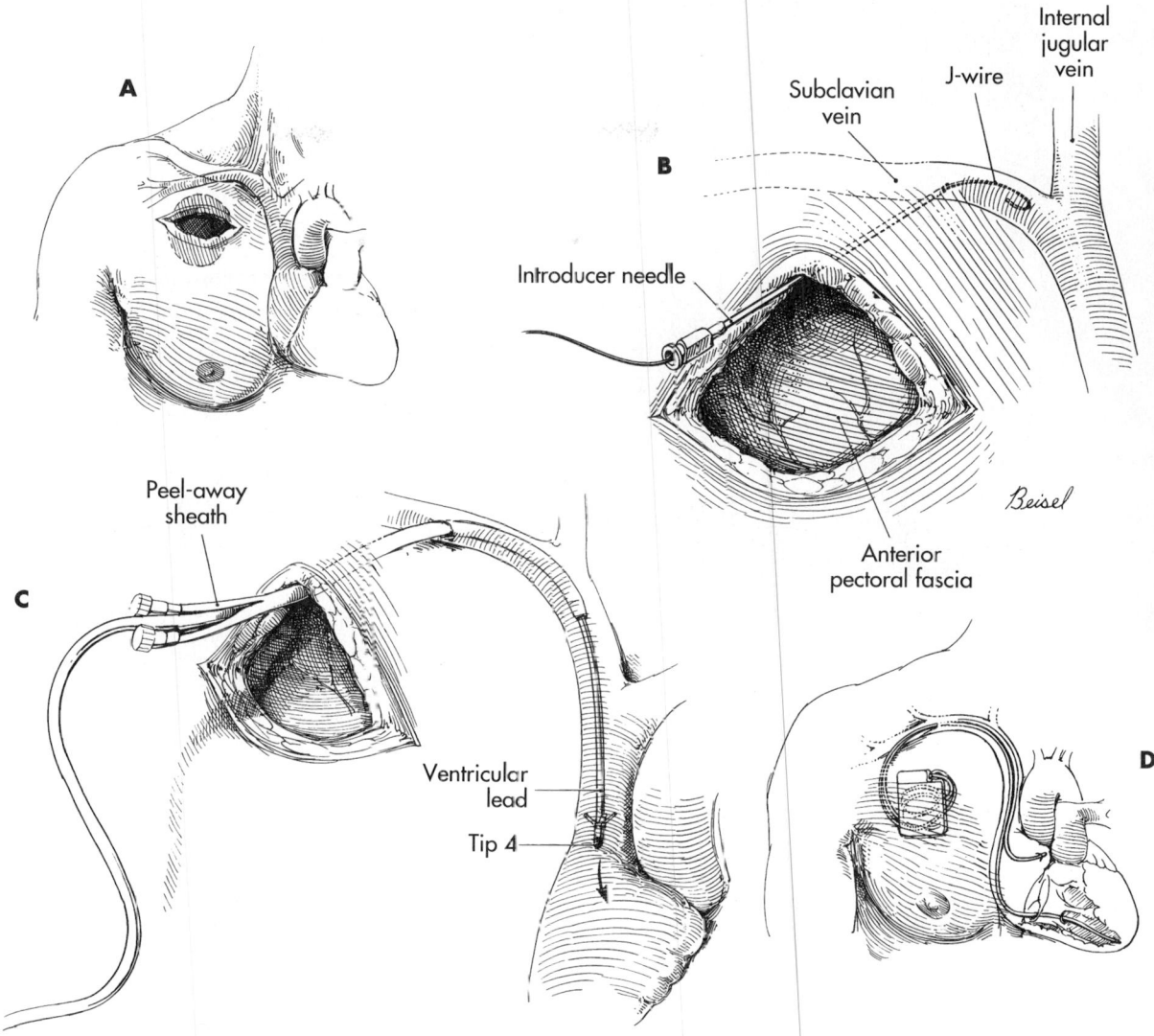

FIGURE 27-77   Insertion of transvenous pacemaker (see text).

anesthetic. A small, transverse incision is made below the xiphoid process and is carried down to the linea alba. A tunnel is created under the xiphoid process to the pericardium, which is incised to expose the heart. The pacing electrode, mounted on its carrier, is screwed into the ventricular myocardium, and the carrier is removed. The remainder of the procedure is as described for insertion of the endocardial electrode.

For the sternotomy approach the mediastinum is opened for a concomitant cardiac procedure, and an area of myocardium is chosen for placement of the pacing electrodes. The electrode tips are screwed into or are sutured to the myocardium and are attached by an appropriate cable to an external pulse generator or pacing analyzer for testing. The pocket and subcutaneous tunnel are created, as described for insertion of the endocardial electrode.

Insertion of Implantable Cardioverter Defibrillator

Many persons who survive sudden cardiac death from malignant ventricular dysrhythmias (ventricular fibrillation and ventricular tachycardia) cannot be helped by surgery or pharmacologic intervention. The implantable cardioverter defibrillator (ICD) is an electronic device designed to monitor cardiac electrical activity and deliver prompt defibrillatory shocks (Fig. 27-78). The ICD differs from a pacemaker in that the former senses ventricular tachycardia or fibrillation and the latter senses asystole.[46] Newer models are capable of tiered therapy, whereby increasingly stronger impulses are delivered depending on the underlying dysrhythmias. These devices are capable of pacing as well as defibrillating (pacing cardioverter defibrillators [PCDs]). The ICD device consists of a generator and sensing and defibrillator electrodes (Fig. 27-79, *A*). Many

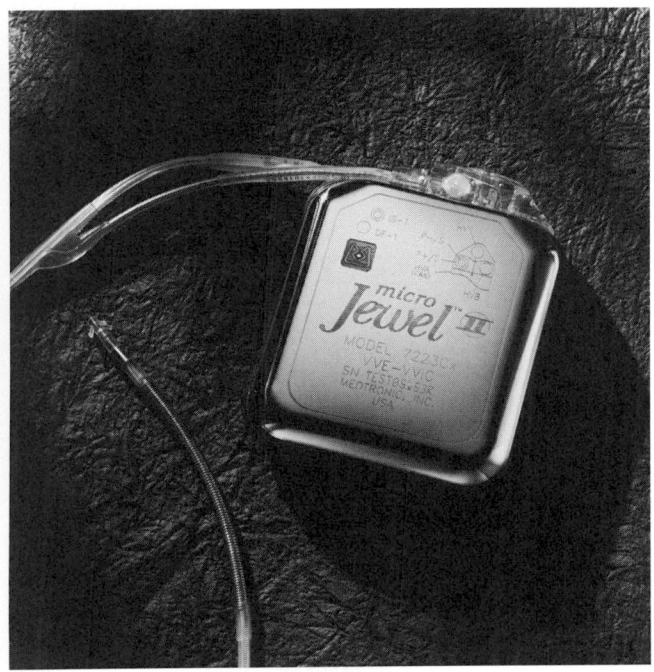

FIGURE 27-78   Internal cardioverter-defibrillator (ICD) is implanted under the skin of the chest to monitor heart action and deliver electrical impulses to correct potentially lethal dysrhythmias such as ventricular tachycardia and ventricular fibrillation. The model shown is about the size of a small pager, weighs 97 grams (about 3½ ounces) and can deliver output of up to 30 joules.

ICD electrodes currently employed consist of transvenous electrodes inserted into the generator much like a transvenous pacemaker system. Myocardial or subcutaneous patches may be added if the transvenous catheters alone do not adequately defibrillate the heart. EP studies are performed before and after insertion to diagnose the dysrhythmia and to evaluate device function respectively.

Operative procedure

The transvenous route with fluoroscopy is the one most commonly employed. Insertion is similar to transvenous pacemaker insertion (Fig. 27-79, *B*). Myocardial sensing and defibrillation electrodes may be used if the patient is undergoing median sternotomy for a cardiac procedure. The thoracotomy approach may be used for patients who have mediastinal adhesions from previous sternal surgery. The subxiphoid approach may also be used. Ventricular shocking patches are sewn to the epicardium anteriorly and posteriorly; the sensing electrodes are often a screw-in design. The generator is housed in a subcutaneous pocket near the umbilicus. The free ends of the lead system are tunneled to the generator and inserted. The device is tested, and the incisions are closed.

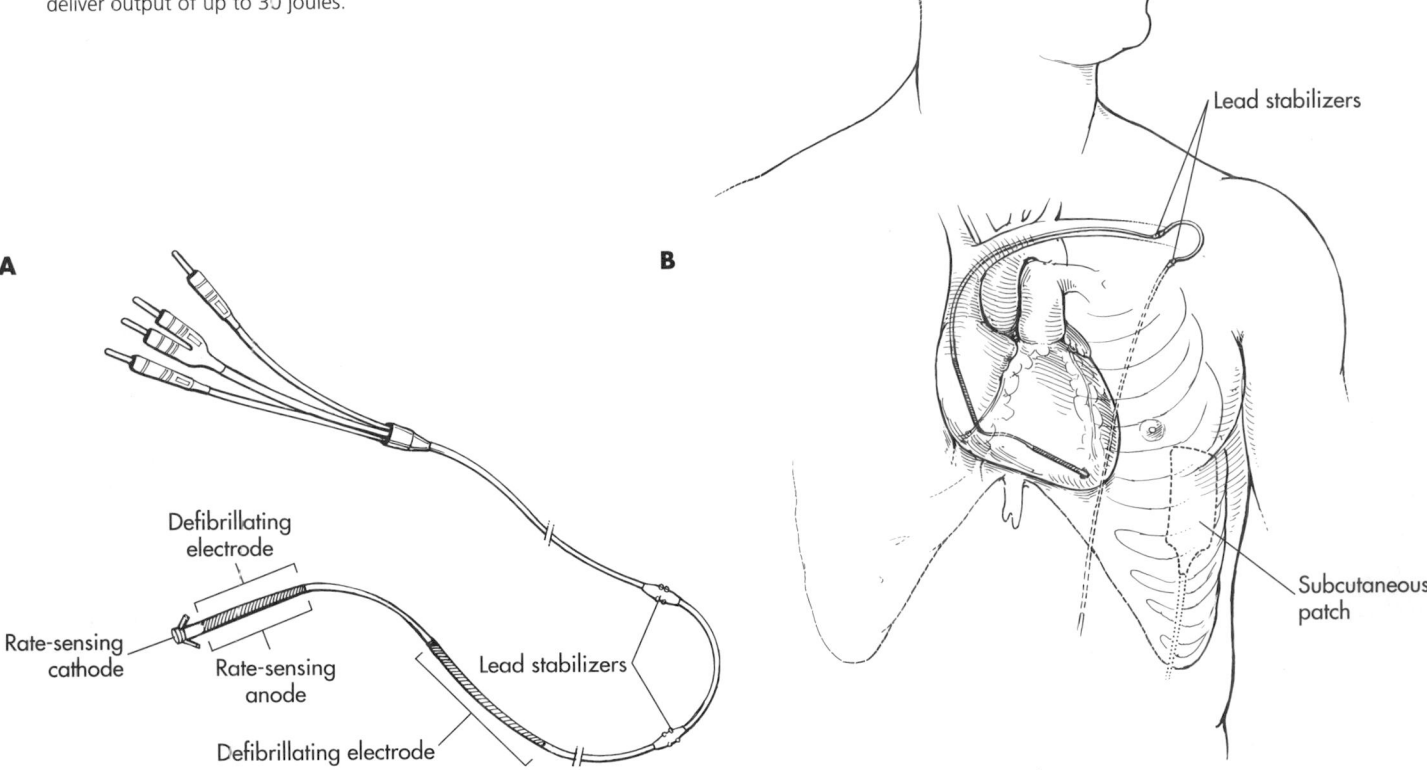

FIGURE 27-79   Nonthoracotomy ICD insertion. **A,** The lead system is composed of sensing and defibrillating electrodes in 1 unit and is inserted transvenously. **B,** The proximal end of the electrodes is tunneled to the abdomen (or the chest) and attached to the generator (not shown). The rate-sensing cathode at the tip relays information to the generator, which initiates an electrical shock by means of the defibrillating electrodes. A second (patch) electrode, placed subcutaneously on the left chest wall, may be necessary if the transvenous electrode alone cannot successfully defibrillate the patient during testing of the unit. If the nonthoracotomy system does not result in suitable defibrillation thresholds, a left thoracotomy or subxiphoid approach may be used to place sensing leads and defibrillation patches directly on the heart.

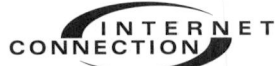

American Heart Association: http://www.amhrt.org

Congenital Heart Disease Information and Resources: http://www.tchin.org

Heart Information Network: http://www.heartinfo.org

Cardiology Compass: http://www.cardiologycompass.com

Heartweb: http://www.heartweb.org

Annals of Thoracic Surgery: http://www.sts.org/annals

Heart Surgery Forum: www.hsforum.com

National Marfan Foundation: http://www.marfan.org

Cardiothoracic Surgery Network: www.ctsnet.org

REFERENCES

1. Allen, K.B., & Shaar, C.J. (1997). Endoscopic saphenous vein harvesting. *Annals of Thoracic Surgery, 64,* 265-266.
2. Altman, L. (1996, June 14). Brazil surgeon develops a bold, promising operation for patients with heart failure. *New York Times,* A16.
3. Association of Operating Room Nurses, Inc. (1997). *The geriatric patient: AORN's age specific competencies series,* Denver, Colo.: AORN, Inc.
4. Association of Operating Room Nurses, Inc. (1997). *The neonate, infant, and toddler patient: AORN's age-specific competencies series,* Denver, Colo.: AORN, Inc.
5. Association of Operating Room Nurses, Inc. (1997). *The premature infant patient: AORN's age-specific competencies series,* Denver, Colo.: AORN, Inc.
6. Association of Operating Room Nurses, Inc. (1997). *The preschool, school-age, and adolescent patient: AORN's age-specific competencies series,* Denver, Colo.: AORN, Inc.
7. Baas, L. (1996). Care of the cardiac patient. In Kinney, M.R., & Packa, D.R. (Eds.). *Comprehensive cardiac care* (ed. 8). St. Louis: Mosby.
8. Bergin, P., Rabinov, M., & Esmore, D. (1995). Cardiac transplantation in patients over 60 years. *Transplantation Proceedings, 27,* 2150-2151.
9. Bittl, J.A. (1996). Advances in coronary angioplasty. *The New England Journal of Medicine, 335*(17), 1290-1302.
10. Borst, C., Jansen, E.W.L., Tulleken, C.A.F., et al. (1996). Coronary artery bypass grafting without cardiopulmonary bypass and without interruption of native coronary flow using a novel anastomosis site restraining device ("Octopus"). *Journal of the American College of Cardiology, 27,* 1356-1364.
11. Borst, C., Santamore, W.P., Smedira, N.G., & Bredee, J.J. (1997). Minimally invasive coronary artery bypass grafting: on the beating heart and via limited access. *Annals of Thoracic Surgery, 63,* S1-S5.
12. Brenner, A.R. (1993). Patient's learning priorities for reoperative coronary artery bypass surgery, *Journal of Cardiovascular Nursing, 7*(2), 1.
13. Bryan, A.J., & Angelini, G.D. (1996). Vascular biology of coronary artery bypass conduits: New solutions to old problems? *Advances in Cardiac Surgery, 8,* 47-80.
14. Buckberg, G.D. (1995). Update on current techniques of myocardial protection. *Annals of Thoracic Surgery, 60,* 805-814.
15. CABRI Trial Participants. (1985). First-year results of CABRI (coronary angioplasty versus bypass revascularization investigation). *Lancet, 346,* 1179-1184.
16. Calafiore, A.M., Di Giammarco, G., Teodori, G., et al. (1996). Left anterior descending coronary artery grafting via left anterior small thoracotomy without cardiopulmonary bypass. *Annals of Thoracic Surgery, 61,* 1658-1665.
17. Cameron, A., Davis, K.B., Green, G., & Schaff, H.V. (1996). Coronary bypass surgery with internal-thoracic-artery grafts—effects on survival over a 15-year period. *New England Journal of Medicine, 334*(4), 216-219.
18. CareMaps used in perioperative patient care. (1997). *OR Manager, 13*(2), 18-20.
19. Carpentier, A. (1983). Cardiac valve surgery: the French correction, *Journal of Thoracic and Cardiovascular Surgery, 86,* 323.
20. Chapek, P.E. (1997). A review of minimally invasive cardiac surgery. *Seminars in Perioperative Nursing, 6*(3), 165-169.
21. Cooley, D.A., Frazier, O.H., Kadipasaoglu, K.A., et al. (1996). Transmyocardial laser revascularization: clinical experience with twelve-month follow-up. *Journal of Thoracic and Cardiovascular Surgery, 111*(4), 791-799.
22. Coulson, A.S., Bakhshay, S., Quarnstrom, J., et al. (1997). Minimally invasive direct coronary artery bypass surgery. *AORN Journal, 66*(6), 1012-1037.
23. Coulson, A.S., Quarnstrom, J.A., Holmes, K., & Henry, J. (1997). Right thoracotomy approach to mitral valve surgical procedures. *AORN Journal, 65*(2), 347-364.
24. Coyne, H.L., Smith, J.F.H., Stein, D., et al. (1998). Describing pain management documentation. *MEDSURG Nursing, 7*(1), 45-51.
25. Cox, J.L., Boineau, J.P., Schuessler, R.B., et al. (1991). Successful surgical treatment of atrial fibrillation: review and clinical update. *Journal of the American Medical Association, 266,* 1976-1980.
26. Crawford, E.S. (1990). The diagnosis and management of aortic dissection. *Journal of the American Medical Association, 264*(9), 2537.
27. David, T.E., Dale, L., & Sun, Z. (1995). Postinfarction ventricular septal rupture: repair by endocardial patch with infarct exclusion. *Journal of Thoracic and Cardiovascular Surgery, 110,* 1315-1322.
28. David, T.E., Feindel, C.M., Armstrong, S., et al. (1995). Reconstruction of the mitral anulus: a ten-year experience. *Journal of Thoracic and Cardiovascular Surgery, 110,* 1323-1332.
29. DeSisto, M.G., Sexton, D.L. (1996). Risk factors for impaired wound healing at the saphenous venectomy site after coronary artery bypass graft surgery. *Cardiovascular Nursing, 32*(6), 37-41.
30. Dickstein, M.L., Spotnitz, H.M., Rose, E.A., & Burkhoff, D. (1997). Heart reduction surgery: An analysis of the impact on cardiac function. *Journal of Thoracic and Cardiovascular Surgery, 113,* 1032-1040.
31. Dossche, K.M., Defauw, J.J., Ernst, S.M., et al. (1997). Allograft root replacement in prosthetic aortic valve endocarditis: a review of 32 patients *Annals of Thoracic Surgery, 63,* 1644-1649.
32. Doty, D.B. (1997). *Cardiac surgery: operative technique.* St Louis: Mosby.
33. Douglas, P.S., & Ginsburg, G.S. (1996). The evaluation of chest pain in women, *New England Journal of Medicine, 334*(20), 1311-1315.
34. Edmunds, L.H. (1995). Why cardiopulmonary bypass makes patients sick: strategies to control the blood-synthetic surface interface. *Advances in Cardiac Surgery, 6,* 131-167.
35. Espersen, C. (1998). The R.N. first assistant in cardiac surgery. In Rothrock, J.C. (Ed.). *The R.N. first assistant: an expanded perioperative role* (ed. 3). Philadelphia: J.B. Lippincott.
36. Frazier, O.H., Rose, E.A., McCarthy, P., et al. (1995). *Annals of Surgery, 222,* 327-338.
37. Fremes, S.E., Christakis, G.T., Del Rizzo, D.F., et al. (1995). The technique of radial artery bypass grafting and early clinical results. *Journal of Cardiac Surgery, 10,* 537-544.
38. Gottlieb, L.J., Beahm, E.K., Krizek, T.J., & Karp, R.B. (1996). Approaches to sternal wound infections. In Karp, R.B., Laks, H., & Wechsler, A.S. *Advances in cardiac surgery,* vol. 7. St. Louis: Mosby.
39. Graling, P.R. (1997). Research review: "Coronary artery bypass patients' perceptions of acute postoperative pain." *AORN Journal, 66*(2), 337-338.
40. Guyton, R.A., Gott, J.P., Brown, W.M., Craver, J.M. (1996). Cold and warm myocardial protection techniques. *Advances in Cardiac Surgery, 7,* 1-29.
41. Hlozek, C.C., & Zacharias, W.M. (1997). The RN first assistant's role during inferior epigastric artery harvesting. *AORN Journal, 65*(1), 26-29.
42. Hueb, W.A., Bellotti, G., de Oliveira, S.A., et al. (1995). The medicine, angioplasty or surgery study (MASS): a prospective, randomized trial of medical therapy, balloon angioplasty or bypass surgery for single proximal left anterior descending artery stenoses. *Journal of the American College of Cardiology, 26,* 1600-1605.

43. Julian, D.G., & Wenger, N.K. (1997). *Women and heart disease*. St. Louis: Mosby.

44. Kawaguchi, A.T., Kosakai, Y., Isobe, F., et al. (1996). Factors affecting rhythm after the Maze procedure for atrial fibrillation. *Circulation, 94*(suppl. II), II139-II142.

45. Kaplan, J.A. (1993). *Cardiac anesthesia* (ed. 3). Philadelphia: W.B. Saunders.

46. Kinney, M.R., Packa, D.R. (Eds.). (1996). *Comprehensive cardiac care* (ed. 8). St. Louis: Mosby.

47. Kuperberg, K.G., & Grubbs, L. (1997). Coronary artery bypass patients' perceptions of acute postoperative pain. *Clinical Nurse Specialist, 11*(3), 116-122.

48. Kurz, A., Sessler, D.I., Lenhardt, R., for the Study of Wound Infection and Temperature Group. (1996). Perioperative normothermia to reduce the incidence of surgical wound infection and shorten hospitalization. *New England Journal of Medicine, 334*(19), 1209-1215.

49. Leor, J., Poole, W.K., & Kloner, R.A. (1996). Sudden cardiac death triggered by an earthquake. *New England Journal of Medicine, 334*(7), 413-419.

50. Lewicki, L.J., Mion, L., Splane, K.G., et al. (1997). Patient risk factors for pressure ulcers during cardiac surgery. *AORN Journal, 65*(5), 933-942.

51. Liston, S.M. (1997). Stent-graft placement procedures for descending thoracic aortic aneurysms. *AORN Journal, 66*(3), 433-444.

52. Loop, F.D., Lytle, B.W., Cosgrove, D.M., et al. (1986). Influence of the internal-mammary-artery graft on 10-year survival and other cardiac events. *New England Journal of Medicine, 314*, 1.

53. Mark, D.B. (1996). Implications of cost in treatment selection for patients with coronary heart disease. *Annals of Thoracic Surgery, 61*, S12-S15.

54. Mauney, M.C., & Kron, I.L. (1995). The physiologic basis of warm cardioplegia. *Annals of Thoracic Surgery, 60*, 819-823.

55. McCarthy, J.F., & Cosgrove, D.M. (1997). Tricuspid valve repair with the Cosgrove-Edwards annuloplasty system. *Annals of Thoracic Surgery, 64*, 267-268.

56. Moreira, L.F.P., & Stolf, N.A.G. (1996). Dynamic cardiomyoplasty. *Advances in Cardiac Surgery, 8*, 147-173.

57. Mortensen, N., & Garrard, C.S. (1996). Colorectal surgery comes in from the cold. *New England Journal of Medicine, 334*(19), 1263-1264.

58. Myken, P.S.U., Larsson, C.K., et al. (1995). Mechanical versus biological valve prostheses: a ten-year comparison regarding function and quality of life. *Annals of Thoracic Surgery, 60*, 447S-452S.

59. O'Brien, M.F. (1995). Allograft aortic root replacement: Standardization and simplification of technique. *Annals of Thoracic Surgery, 60*, 92S-94S.

60. Pagana, K.D., & Pagana, T.J. (1997). *Mosby's diagnostic and laboratory test reference* (ed. 3). St Louis: Mosby.

61. The Parisian Mediastinitis Study Group. (1996). Risk factors for deep sternal wound infection after sternotomy: a prospective, multicenter study. *Journal of Thoracic and Cardiovascular Surgery, 111*, 1200-1207.

62. Peters, W.S., Siegel, L.C., Stevens, J.H., et al. (1997). Closed-chest cardiopulmonary bypass and cardioplegia: basis for less invasive cardiac surgery. *Annals of Thoracic Surgery, 63*, 1748-1754.

63. Piwnica, A., & Westaby, S. (Eds.). (1997). *Surgery for acquired aortic valve disease*. Oxford: Isis Medical Media, Ltd.

64. Pym, J., Brown, P., Pearson, M., et al. (1995). Right gastroepiploic–to–coronary artery bypass: the first decade of use. *Circulation, 92*(suppl. II), II45-II49.

65. Rabago, G., De Vega, N.G., Castillon, L., et al. (1980). The new De Vega technique in tricuspid annuloplasty. *Journal of Thoracic and Cardiovascular Surgery, 21*, 231.

66. Rebollo, M.H., Bernal, J.M., Llorca, J., et al. (1996). Nosocomial infections in patients having cardiovascular operations: a multivariate analysis of risk factors. *Journal of Thoracic and Cardiovascular Surgery, 112*, 908-913.

67. Safi, H.J., Letsou, G.V., Iliopoulos, D.C., et al. (1994). Impact of retrograde cerebral perfusion on ascending aortic and arch aneurysm repair. *Annals of Thoracic Surgery, 63*, 1601-1607.

68. Seifert, P.C. (1994). *Cardiac surgery*. St. Louis: Mosby.

69. Seifert, P.C. (1996). Cardiac surgery. In Rothrock, J.C. *Perioperative nursing care planning*, (ed. 2). St. Louis: Mosby.

70. Shennib, H., Mack, M.J., & Lee, A.G.L. (1997). A survey on minimally invasive coronary artery bypass grafting. *Annals of Thoracic Surgery, 64*, 110-115.

71. Sommers, K.E., & David, T.E. (1997). Aortic valve replacement with patch enlargement of the aortic annulus. *Annals of Thoracic Surgery, 63*, 1608-1612.

72. Utley, J.R., & Gravlee, G.P. (1996). Special considerations in cardiopulmonary bypass, *Advances in Cardiac Surgery, 7*, 87-100.

73. Vongpatanasin, W., Hillis, L.D., & Lange, R.A. (1996). Prosthetic heart valves. *New England Journal of Medicine, 335*(6), 407-416.

74. Waldhausen, J.A., Pierce, W.S., & Campbell, D.B. (1996). *Johnson's surgery of the chest* (ed. 6). St. Louis: Mosby.

75. Wieczorek, P. (1995). Developing critical pathways for the operating room. *AORN Journal, 62*(6), 925-927.

76. Wieczorek, P., Riegel, M.B., Quattro, L., & DeMaio, K. (1997). Marfan's syndrome and surgical repair of ascending aortic aneurysms. *AORN Journal, 64*(6), 895-913.

77. Wisniowski, C. & Stephen, L. (1997). Minimally invasive treatment for coronary artery disease. *AORN Journal, 66*(6), 1002-1009.

78. Woerth, S.T., Cranfill, J.D., & Neal, J.M. (1997). A collaborative approach to minimally invasive direct coronary artery bypass. *AORN Journal, 66*(6), 994-1001.

79. Zenati, M., Domit, T.M., Saul, M., et al. (1997). Resource utilization for minimally invasive direct and standard coronary artery bypass grafting. *Annals of Thoracic Surgery, 63*, S84-S87.

80. Zevola, D.R., Raffia, M., Brown, K., et al. (1997). Clinical pathways and coronary artery bypass surgery. *Critical Care Nurse, 17*(6), 20-33.

UNIT III

SPECIAL CONSIDERATIONS

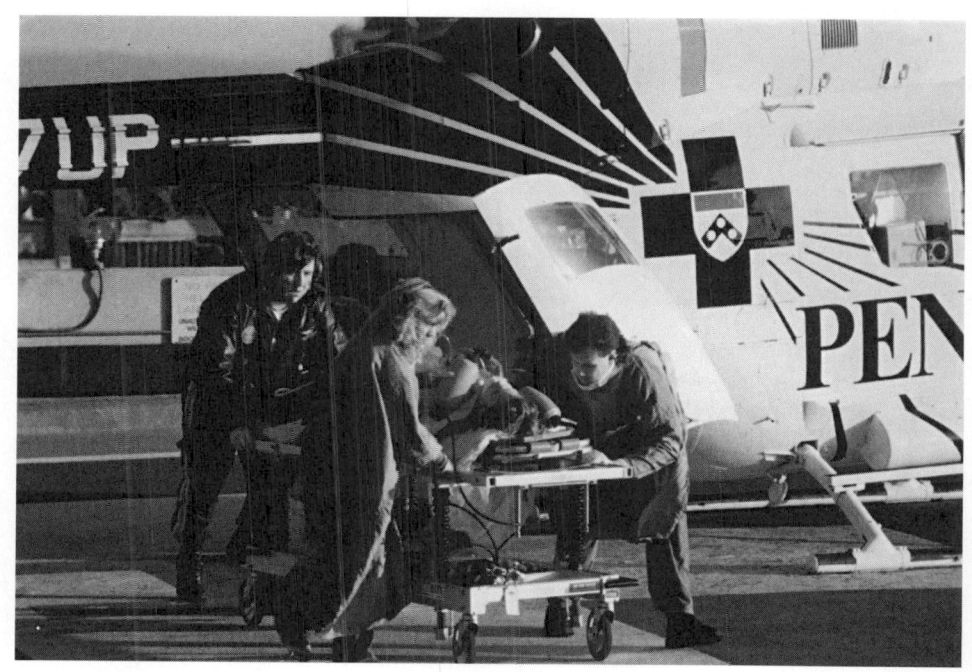

CHAPTER TWENTY EIGHT

Ambulatory Surgery

Denise L. Geuder

THE CONCEPT OF ambulatory surgery has revolutionized the delivery of surgical care, becoming a standard for patient-centered perioperative care delivery models. Although phenomenal growth in ambulatory surgery has occurred since the early 1980s, the concept is referred to as early as 3000 B.C. in writings from Egyptian scrolls. Ambulatory surgery is interwoven within medical and nursing history and is referred to in the Bible and early Indian and Hindu literature. In the United States the initial concept of ambulatory surgery began in 1818 when Massachusetts General Hospital established the first outpatient department. It was not until the 1960s, however, that interest in ambulatory surgery became widespread.

The first freestanding surgical center that was independently owned and operated was the Phoenix Surgicenter (in Phoenix, Arizona), founded by Drs. Wallace Reed and John Ford in 1970. Dr. Reed identified patient selection, types of procedures, anesthesia, careful surgery, well-defined discharge criteria, and appropriate patient follow-up examinations as key concepts in delivering safe care in ambulatory settings.[18] The Phoenix Surgicenter quickly became a prototype for other centers across the country.

Since the advent of the Phoenix Surgicenter, market-driven forces have significantly influenced the resurgence of ambulatory surgery. Continued pressures to reform the health care system, at both federal and state levels, pressures of managed care, the increased presence of capitated payment systems, advances in technology, and public awareness and support of the concept have all been driving factors. In 1982 the federal government enacted the Tax Equity and Fiscal Responsibility Act (TEFRA), which included prospective payment for inpatient care with diagnosis-related groups (DRG's). As a result, Medicare reimbursement for outpatient procedures was higher than that for those performed on an inpatient basis. Third-party payers quickly followed suit, and financial incentives clearly favored surgical care delivery on an outpatient basis.

Concurrently, an explosion of technology such as minimally invasive techniques and new, shorter-acting anesthetic agents contributed to the ability to meet criteria for outpatient procedures. Public acceptance quickly followed as patients were drawn to the user-friendly environment created by successful ambulatory surgery centers. Highly effective marketing fostered public acceptance of the benefits of recuperation at home because the hospital had become the place for the acutely ill.[10] Many procedures that were once considered appropriate only for inpatient treatment are now being performed with great success as ambulatory surgery.

The Association of Operating Room Nurses (AORN) statement on perioperative nursing practice in ambulatory surgery (Box 28-1) outlines the significance and importance of a skilled perioperative nurse who is clinically and professionally competent to provide care to the ambulatory surgery patient in a short time. The care provided should be cost effective, convenient, and efficient, should be consistent with established standards of perioperative nursing practice, and must include the patient and family or significant others throughout the surgical experience. The AORN recognizes the move from "the highest quality care at any price" toward "the best care at the lowest price" that offers safe, efficient care throughout the patient's surgical experience.[2]

In 1966, Ferguson and Kaplan[7] described the ambulatory patient as follows:

One who does not require hospital in-patient care. This presupposes that the patient is able to walk and travel to his home after his treatment, safely, often without aid from other persons. It should be understood from the first that ambulation should not interfere with or retard the required treatment. Ambulatory care does not necessarily mean care in a private office. It may mean treatment given in an adequately equipped and staffed emergency room, outpatient department, or private office, or even in an operating room, to a patient who can return to his home after his treatment.

Today, this definition is still appropriate and adequately describes the ambulatory patient who is discharged with the intention of having postoperative care provided by the patient and family or significant others.

FACILITIES

The acceptance of ambulatory surgery as a strategy for the future has resulted in a proliferation of various models for ambulatory surgery. Paryani et al.[20] refer to a revolution in outpatient care, predicting a continued shift of patient care to outpatient centers. Successful ambulatory surgery models include various types of facilities including hospital integrated, hospital separated, freestanding, office based, and recovery center. Regardless of the ownership or physical location of the facility, several key issues must be considered to ensure success of the facility.[14]

1. Identification of unique clinical niche based on an assessment of community need
2. Active participation by a multidisciplinary surgical advisory committee with representation by all high-volume specialties targeted by the facility
3. Strong anesthesia leadership and participation in daily operations
4. Effective, experienced manager with strong team-building skills
5. Recruitment and retention of qualified, dedicated staff
6. Participative governance structure allowing key-user input to decision making
7. Sound financial management
8. Efficient design
9. Facility and equipment adequate to meet the demand, allowing for growth
10. Design and decor that reflect a patient-oriented, user-friendly alternative to the traditional hospital environment.

Patient condition and type of procedure assist the healthcare team (surgeon, anesthesia provider, perioperative staff) in determining the most appropriate facility. Questions often asked to determine appropriateness of patient selection and facility include the following:[22]

1. Is the facility equipped to deal with emergency situations related to the surgical procedure, patient's condition, and anticipated treatments?
2. Can the procedure be performed without hospitalization?
3. Is the risk to the patient minimal if the procedure is performed at the facility?
4. Will extended recovery be necessary?
5. Are quality standards adhered to at the facility?
6. Does the patient need any special care (such as special equipment) that may not be available at the facility?
7. Do the patient and family or significant others understand and accept the concept of ambulatory surgery?

The intent of ambulatory surgery is for safe, convenient, and cost-effective surgery to be provided at a facility with the patient discharged to a short-term recovery center or home. Patients are carefully screened to be healthy, with no unusual problems that cannot be taken care of in the facility, and the family/significant others need to be willing to monitor, provide treatment as necessary, and care for the patient once discharged.

| BOX 28-1 | **AORN Statement on Perioperative Nursing Practice in Ambulatory Surgery** |

A combination of legislative trends, changes in technology, a more knowledgeable society, and greater professional sophistication has created a climate for change in health care in which the focus is moving from "the highest quality care at any price" toward "the best care at the lowest price." Ambulatory surgery, as an established component of surgical patient care, is one outcome of these changes. As AORN assumes a leadership role in the care of all surgical patients, dynamic, creative, proactive strategies are essential. Perioperative nursing must be practiced in all surgical settings.

Perioperative nursing, of a distinctive nature, is practiced in ambulatory surgery settings. Because of a wellness orientation, teaching, self-care, and responsibility and inclusion of family and support people are emphasized. Our belief is that professional nursing competencies are essential during all three phases of the ambulatory surgery patient's experience. Because of the compressed nursing time frame, technical proficiencies, assessment, judgment, and organizational skills must be highly refined and sophisticated. Ambulatory surgery nurses must also be flexible, accepting of change, and willing to become functional in all patient care areas. Mechanisms to achieve desired patient outcomes may be different from those in the inpatient setting but are equally important. The ambulatory surgery setting serves as a model for perioperative nursing practice and as an ideal clinical laboratory for visualizing the total nursing process in a few hours.

We recognize that today's patient population expects to participate in their own care and that their rights must be respected regardless of practice settings. We believe that ambulatory surgery patients, as well as all surgical patients, should expect to receive:
1. Cost-effective, convenient, efficient care
2. Care consistent with accepted standards of practice, recognizing the patients' rights to be active participants in their plans of care
3. Succinct perioperative education involving family/significant others

From *AORN standards, recommended practices and guidelines* (1998).

Hospital-Integrated Facility

The hospital-integrated facility is the most common system across the country. This setting uses the main operating room suites for ambulatory as well as inpatient surgery. However, many hospitals have different preoperative and postoperative areas that are designated specifically for ambulatory surgery patients. Ambulatory procedures may either be interspersed with inpatient procedures on any given day or done on a day or in an operating room reserved solely for ambulatory patients. The admitting process for these patients may be handled by the hospital's admitting department or by the ambulatory unit itself. In this type of setting family members of both inpatient and ambulatory surgery patients usually share a common waiting area. In addition to admitting ambulatory surgery patients, hospital-integrated facilities may handle the processing of day of surgery (DOS) patients or morning admission patients, who are to be admitted to the hospital after surgery. Preoperative laboratory and diagnostic tests are usually done on an outpatient basis before surgery, and these patients are admitted to the hospital after surgery.

The advantages of a hospital-integrated facility include shared personnel among the different areas, available equipment and supplies, rapid admission to the hospital if necessary, and sharing of cost related to capital budget. However, there is less control of patient scheduling and the potential for delays caused by scheduling ambulatory surgical patients after an inpatient procedure or being canceled in the event of an inpatient surgical emergency.

Hospital-Separated Facility

The hospital-separated facility is affiliated with the hospital but is a separate ambulatory surgery department with designated preoperative, intraoperative, and postoperative areas. The facility may be located within the hospital complex, adjacent to the hospital, or at a satellite location some distance from the hospital. In contrast to the hospital-integrated facility, the hospital-separated facility has a dedicated staff, equipment, policies and procedures, and postanesthesia recovery care area for the ambulatory surgery patient. The facility is physically and organizationally separate from the hospital's main operating room suites and is exclusive for the ambulatory surgery patient population. Advantages of this type of facility include convenient scheduling, availability of hospital services, easy admission of the patient to the hospital if necessary, less likelihood of delay or cancellation as a result of scheduling complications, sharing of certain equipment and services with the main operating room suite, and use for more complicated procedures and high-risk patients.

Freestanding Facility

A freestanding facility is independently owned and operated and is not hospital affiliated. These facilities are operated on a for-profit basis and may be owned by entrepreneurs, physicians, and nurses. The types of ownership vary and generally include corporate, joint venture, or independent. A growing trend has been for healthcare corporation chains to own and operate such facilities. These facilities compose a growing segment of the industry, are conveniently located, and cater to the desires and needs of the patient, while providing safe, quality care that is cost effective.

Office-Based Facility

An office-based facility is much like a freestanding facility but is operated on a smaller scale. These facilities allow for ambulatory surgery to be provided safely and effectively in a surgeon's office. These for-profit facilities often have elaborate equipment, specially trained personnel, and an appropriate inventory of supplies and instrumentation. This type of arrangement may be very advantageous to the physician as a managed care strategy because it allows the physician to capture revenue from facility charges and supplies traditionally charged by the hospital or surgery center.[6] A mobile surgical services program can enhance office-based surgery by providing equipment, disposable supplies, staffing, and sterilization services to nontraditional surgical settings such as offices.[9] This allows the surgeon to provide services such as laser interventions to patients without the capital investment of equipment and the ongoing cost of specialized staff.

Advantages include more schedule flexibility for the surgeon and patient, cost effectiveness of the procedure, and staff with training specific to the procedures being performed. Limitations include strict patient selection criteria and the lack of a regulating agency to assess and determine that standards of quality are being implemented. The American College of Surgeons (ACS) has developed a set of guidelines for office-based surgical facilities that include administration, facility design, ancillary services, surgical care, and quality assurance,[12] which are intended to ensure and maintain superior quality of care for surgical patients undergoing procedures in office-based surgical facilities.

Recovery Center

The concept of a freestanding facility with an adjacent recovery center has become popular in many areas of the country. The recovery center offers an alternative to the patient and family or significant others when skilled nursing care is desired but acute care is unnecessary. The center generally is equipped with private rooms designed with a decor similar to that of a hotel. A family member or significant other is allowed to stay with the patient if desired. The needs of the patient and visitors are catered to (such as meals, telephone, television, stereo, minibar).

Hospital programs have also incorporated the concept of the recovery center into hospital-sponsored ambulatory surgery programs. The amenities are usually the same as those mentioned above, but the facility itself may be part of the hospital building. The patient is usually charged a reduced rate similar to a freestanding recovery center, but the appeal of the hospital program is the proximity to the

---

BOX 28-2 | **Procedures Frequently Performed in Ambulatory Surgery**

General Surgery

Breast biopsy
Hemorrhoidectomy
Laparoscopic procedures
Excisions of lesions

Hernia
Vein stripping
Mastectomy
Temporal artery biopsy

Gynecology

Tubal ligation
Vaginal hysterectomy
Dilatation and curettage
Laparoscopy

Laser conization
Laser vaporization
Laser laparoscopy procedures
Hysteroscopes

Ophthalmology

Cataract extraction
Keratotomy
Photorefractive keratectomy,
   phototherapeutic
   keratectomy
Muscle surgery

Vitrectomies
Entropion or ectropion
Nasal lacrimal duct probe,
   irrigation, stents

Orthopedics

Arthroscopy
Tendon release
Removal of plates, screws
Nerve repair
Ganglion cysts

Hand surgery (carpal tunnel,
   open reduction with
   internal fixation [ORIF])
Ulnar nerve transpositions

Otolaryngology

Tonsillectomy
Adenoidectomy
Nasal polypectomy
Myringotomy
Vocal cord biopsy
Otoplasty
Sinus surgery
Nasal fractures

Tympanomastoidectomy
Excision submandibular
   masses
Diagnostic bronchoscopy
   and laryngoscopy

Plastic Surgery

Nasal fracture reduction
Skin graft
Mammoplasty
Liposuction
Blepharoplasty
Facelift
Miniabdominoplasty

Rhinoplasty and septoplasty
Endoscopic browlift
Endoscopic transaxillary augmenta-
   tion
Laser skin resurfacing

Urology

Cystoscopy
Ureteroscopy
Vasectomy
Biopsy
Circumcision

Dental Surgery

Dental implant
Extractions

Cardiovascular Surgery

Arteriography
Cardiac catheterization

Gastroenterology

Colonoscopy
Bronchoscopy
Esophagoscopy

---

hospital if these services are needed. Another advantage is that hospital-based recovery centers can be used for other procedural areas such as cardiac catheterization and invasive radiology procedures, providing a more consistent patient volume. Consistent patient volume allows for cost-effective staffing and helps justify the overhead costs of the unit.

PATIENT SELECTION

Criteria for appropriate patient selection are essential for safe ambulatory surgery. Because surgical intervention in an ambulatory facility does not decrease the risk for potential complications, each patient should be carefully screened. In the past, patients considered appropriate for ambulatory surgery were young and healthy, having no underlying illness. However, procedures being performed today are more complex and the patients are older and less healthy (Box 28-2).

Those responsible for determining appropriate patient selection include the surgeon, anesthesia provider, and perioperative nurse. The surgeon is responsible for assessing underlying problems that may lead to unexpected complications during the procedure. A patient with complex medical conditions unrelated to the procedure may be scheduled at a hospital-affiliated facility versus a freestanding facility because of the potential for specific complications. Patients with complex medical conditions and underlying disease processes may be determined inappropriate for ambulatory surgery and scheduled in the main operating room. Anesthesia providers are responsible for assessing any known or unknown problems related to the chosen anesthetic course. The perioperative nurse is responsible for assessing and evaluating the patient for factors that could lead to complications throughout the perioperative period.

A commonly used classification system is that of the American Society of Anesthesiologists (ASA) (see Chapter 7). The surgeon, anesthesia provider, or perioperative nurse assigns the patient an ASA physical-status classification. Patients classified as physical status 1 or 2 are perfect candidates for ambulatory surgery. These patients generally pose no great risk for procedures performed with general or local anesthesia or IV conscious sedation. Patients classified as physical status 3 must be carefully evaluated and determined that no untoward event is likely to occur during the intraoperative and postoperative phases. Any concomitant disease must be well managed before the patient is acceptable for ambulatory surgery. Specific risk factors for ambulatory surgery include preoperative drug therapy, hypertension, heart disease and congestive heart failure, bronchopulmonary disease, diabetes, obesity, adrenocortical steroid therapy, alcohol or drug abuse, psychotropic drug therapy, psychiatric illness, family or personal history of either malignant hyperthermia or pseudocholinesterase deficiency. Although the presence of one or more of these risk factors doesn't necessarily preclude a patient from ambulatory surgery, these factors indicate that careful preoperative assessment and home care planning must be performed to minimize complications.[11]

ANESTHESIA

Ambulatory surgery is in part attributable to advances in anesthesia, with the availability of evermore potent and fast-acting agents.[27] Although the ideal anesthetic agent has yet to be discovered, desirable characteristics of anesthesia for the ambulatory patient include a rapid recovery period and few side effects. The anesthesia provider must understand the needs of the ambulatory patient population to facilitate anesthesia delivery that supports rapid recovery with adequate postoperative pain control.

Premedication

Preoperative medication may be prescribed to decrease the patient's anxiety and fear regarding the surgery, separation from family and significant others, pain, the unknown, diagnostic results, and perceived loss of control.[8] Additional advantages include analgesia, amnesia effect (depending on drug and dosage), and often a decreased incidence of postoperative nausea and vomiting. Before the administration of a premedication, the patient should be offered the opportunity to void, since the patient will be limited to a bed, a stretcher, or a recliner after administration of the medication. Because the effects of premedication may generate a longer postoperative recovery period for the patient, use of premedication is

---

BOX 28-3	Anesthetic Agents

Induction Agents

 Thiopental sodium
 Methohexital sodium
 Etomidate
 Ketamine
 Midazolam
 Propofol

Neuromuscular Blocking Agents

 Succinylcholine
 Mivacurium
 Atracurium
 Vecuronium
 Pancuronium
 Nocuronium bromide

Inhalation Agents

 Halothane
 Nitrous oxide
 Enflurane
 Methoxyflurane
 Isoflurane
 Sevoflurane
 Desflurane

---

often avoided. However, a patient experiencing anxiety and apprehension should never be denied premedication if necessary. Other preoperative medications may include antibiotics, anticholinergics, or pitocin for gynecological procedures.

General Anesthesia

General anesthesia renders patients unconscious, relaxed, and unable to perceive pain. For the ambulatory surgery patient receiving general anesthesia, consideration of the anesthetic agent is based, in part, on readiness for timely discharge of the patient. Recently approved agents allow for quick induction, short duration of action, and few effects on the patient's vital signs and are relatively safe to administer (Box 28-3).

Local Anesthesia

Local anesthesia is commonly used for the ambulatory surgery patient. The medication is administered by the surgeon, and the perioperative nurse is responsible for monitoring the patient throughout the procedure. Local anesthetics are classified as either amino esters or amino amides (Box 28-4). Local anesthetics are chosen by the surgeon based on their potency, desired duration of action, and surgery site. Local anesthetic agents are also available with epinephrine for vasoconstriction in the area injected, slowing the rate of absorption of the local anesthetic agent, prolonging its duration of action, and lowering the

BOX 28-4	Local Anesthetic Agents

Amide

Prilocaine
Mepivacaine
Lidocaine
Bupivacaine
Etidocaine
Ropivacaine

Amino Ester

Procaine
Chloroprocaine
Cocaine
Tetracaine

BOX 28-5	Commonly Administered Agents for IV Conscious Sedation

Sedative Hypnotics

Diazepam
Midazolam
Methohexital sodium
Ketamine
Propofol
Florazepam

Narcotics

Fentanyl
Alfentanil
Sufentanil
Nalbuphine
Meperidine

Reversal Agents

Romazicon
Naloxone

incidence of toxicity.[23] The perioperative nurse should monitor the patient for presence of side effects such as central nervous system disturbances, cardiovascular problems, hypersensitivity to the medication, and toxic reaction resulting from high levels of the local anesthetic agent.

Conscious Sedation

The perioperative nurse is responsible for monitoring and often administering medications to achieve intravenous (IV) conscious sedation (Box 28-5). *Conscious sedation* is defined as "a condition where the patient exhibits a depressed level of consciousness, but retains the ability to independently respond appropriately to verbal commands or physical stimulation."[2] For optimal care of the patient receiving IV conscious sedation the following parameters should be monitored: respiratory rate, oxygen saturation, blood pressure, cardiac rate and rhythm, mental status, level of consciousness, pain, and skin condition. Continuous uninterrupted monitoring should be provided by the perioperative nurse responsible for the management of the patient receiving IV conscious sedation. The nurse may be requested to divert attention away from the patient, leaving the potential for subtle symptoms of an impending problem to go unobserved. Therefore a second circulator should be assigned to assume the circulating responsibilities during the procedure so that the perioperative nurse administering conscious sedation is not required to leave the patient or interrupt monitoring.[28]

APPEAL OF AMBULATORY SURGERY

It is estimated that by the year 2000 as many as 70% to 80% of surgical procedures will be performed in ambulatory surgery settings in hospitals, freestanding centers, or surgeon's offices. With safety, efficiency, and cost effectiveness well established, third-party payers not only support, but also encourage (and in many procedures may require) the use of ambulatory surgery facilities by their subscribers. As an incentive for use, higher reimbursement for procedures performed at an ambulatory surgery facility have been provided. However, government agencies, especially those associated with Medicare and Medicaid, are actively involved in discussion and legislation relating to the balance between acceptable care and decreased cost. Current economic incentives clearly favor surgery done on an ambulatory, outpatient basis, but those incentives are expected to change. The Health Care Financing Administration (HCFA) has been investigating the concept of prospective payment for ambulatory patient groups (APGs). Although a definitive date has not been scheduled for implementation of APG prospective payment, the initial plan will include routine surgery, radiology, and other diagnostic services.[5]

Ambulatory surgery is appealing to the patient and family or significant others because there are fewer disruptions of normal daily activities, less separation, less time away from the workplace, and less worry about financial outlays because costly hospital stays are avoided. The ambulatory surgery patient and family or significant others are active participants in the patient's plan of care. Some ambulatory centers routinely schedule weekend surgery, further appealing to patients and their families or significant others who are unable to or desire not to interfere with their work schedules. Convenience and patient satisfaction are hallmarks of ambulatory surgery, making it a model for the healthcare industry's focus on customer-oriented service.

For healthcare professionals, the advantages of ambulatory surgery are multiple. There is convenience and less time away from the office for the surgeon. There is opportunity for anesthesia providers to enter into and specialize in a different arena in which anesthetic agents and techniques are continuously being improved to enhance rapid patient recovery and return to ambulation. There are opportunities for the perioperative nurse to condense and refine nursing skills and to develop nursing practice models that focus on wellness, safety, comfort, patient education, and continuity of care. The emphasis on cross-training, productivity, versatility, and independence is appealing to the motivated perioperative nurse practicing in ambulatory surgery. The patient scheduled for ambulatory surgery has fewer preoperative tests and fewer medications and may be active, awake, and involved in the nurse-patient interaction throughout the entire perioperative period. The opportunities for an expanded role are numerous for the nurse specializing in the care of the ambulatory surgery patient. The recent advent of the acute care nurse practitioner (ACNP), with clinical, education, research, consultation, and referral functions, is one example of a perioperative nursing role that will contribute to reduced costs, improved patient and family or significant other satisfaction, and coordination of care across the continuum in ambulatory surgery settings.[16]

NURSING CARE FOR THE AMBULATORY PATIENT

Perioperative nursing in the ambulatory surgery setting incorporates all elements of the AORN standards of perioperative nursing (Box 28-6). However, the paradigm from which the perioperative nurse manages care of the ambulatory patient is very different from that of the hospitalized patient. The ambulatory patient is essentially healthy and the time spent in the ambulatory setting is relatively short, ranging from a few hours to 1 day (23-hour stay); therefore the plan of care for the ambulatory surgical patient must be organized and efficient. To achieve this condition, many healthcare facilities are incorporating concepts of case management into the planning and implementation of care for patients, both inpatient and outpatient. Care delivered in ambulatory surgery lends itself well to the use of the principles of case management, which provides a framework for care that overlays traditional utilization review, resource management, care management, and outcomes management.[24]

Perhaps the most well-known tool of case management is the clinical pathway. Clinical pathways lend themselves well to care of the perioperative patient. Perioperative patient care has long involved teamwork, standing orders, preference cards, and guidelines for care in the daily work of the surgery suite. Clinical pathways extend these familiar tools into interdisciplinary maps that choreograph the role of each team member, including the patient and family (Fig. 28-1). Expected outcomes are included to help define the expectations of everyone involved. Measurable targets are set for variables such as time, resource consumption, length of stay, and pain management.

Responsibility for most of the preoperative and postoperative care is assumed by the patient and family or significant other. Therefore their education and preparation is an integral part of ambulatory surgery. The education process is continuous, begins preoperatively, and proceeds after the patient is discharged. This allows for both the patient and the caregiver to be prepared for discharge requirements and recovery at home. The ultimate goal of providing education to the patient and family or significant other is to ensure adequate preparation for meeting postoperative care needs and establishing plans for seeking additional assistance, if necessary.

> **BOX 28-6** | **AORN Standards of Perioperative Nursing**
>
> **Standards of Perioperative Clinical Practice**
> Assessment
> Diagnosis
> Outcome identification
> Planning
> Implementation
> Evaluation
>
> **Standards of Perioperative Professional Performance**
> Quality of care
> Performance appraisal
> Education
> Collegiality
> Ethics
> Collaboration
> Research
> Resource use

Preoperative Phase

The surgeon, anesthesia provider, perioperative nurse, and patient should jointly determine the appropriateness of surgical intervention at an ambulatory facility. The patient's or family's fears and concerns regarding ambulatory surgery should be discussed before the decision to perform the procedure; patients should not feel that they are receiving a lesser standard of care because the procedure is scheduled at an ambulatory surgery facility. Once the determination is made to have the procedure at the ambulatory surgery facility, contact with the patient occurs to ensure proper preoperative preparation (Research Highlight 28-1).

Patient and family or significant other education is carried out in a variety of ways at various facilities. Important characteristics of an ideal preoperative preparation program include an accessible physical setting, a standardized process, multidisciplinary involvement, and a program for patient education that enhances involvement in self-care.[15] The following information is presented to the patient by the perioperative nurse, physician, or physician office staff; it is usually reinforced with printed teaching material:

1. Time and nature of surgery
2. Location, parking, and suggested time of arrival at the ambulatory surgery center
3. Food and liquid restrictions
4. Suggested clothing for discharge
5. Necessary items to bring (such as glasses, hearing aids)
6. Instructions regarding valuables
7. Identification of responsible adult escort for discharge
8. Who to call for any questions before the procedure

Care Path: Ambulatory Surgery Center	Date:_____ Phase 1 ≅ 15-30 min Pre-admission	Date:_____ Phase 2 ≅ 30 min DOS-Admit	Phase 3 ≅ 30 >min Intra-operative	Phase 4 ≅ 30 >min Recovery to Discharge
ASSESSMENT	Anesthesia protocol Initiate H&A	Complete H&A Complete Surgical Procedure Care Record Attach previous medical records (if present)	Verify patient ID Check medical record Monitor VS per anesthesia/conscious sedation protocol	Report communicated Check medical record Assess VS and pain rating using 0-5 scale
TEST	EKG Chem 7 H&H			Per anesthesia
DIET	NPO after midnight except for medications	→	→	Ice chips or dependent upon anesthesia type
ACTIVITY	As tolerated	Chair rest or up ad lib unless medicated then assist with activity	Position per procedure	Bed or chair rest W/C upon discharge
TREATMENT	Complete consent form and Terms of Care Verify insurance and physician orders Verify operative site	Verify consents Continue with physician's orders	Monitor per anesthesia or conscious sedation protocol Complete prep Maintain patient safety	Continue assessment Implement physician orders
MED/IV	Meds with sip of water on AM of surgery	Insert IID Pre op medications as ordered	Per anesthesia orders and/or physician	As ordered
CONSULTS	Anesthesia Cardiologist as indicated	Anesthesia visit		Per anesthesia needs or physician
EDUCATION	Physician office Provide AM instruction sheet Review ASC process Answer questions	Reinforce instructions for family/care giver Provide instruction sheet to care giver	→ Explain steps in procedure	Instruct family and/or significant other in post-operative care of the patient
DISCHARGE PLANS	Discharge plans reviewed with patient and care giver as needed Instruct patient to bring driver DOS	Reinforce instructions for family/care giver Reinforce ASC process Assess telephone availability for those living alone	Reinforce prior plans for discharge	Provide appropriate documentation for home care with access information to ER, treatment, and follow-up care
PSYCHOSOCIAL	Provide opportunities for discussion	Satisfy patient/family concerns	Inform family and/or significant other of patient status	Satisfy patient/family concerns
OUTCOME *Signature indicates outcome status*	**Outcome: Patient states understanding of procedure.** ___met ___not met **Lab & EKG completed prior to DOS.** ___met ___not met Signature_____	**Outcome: Responsible person with patient.** ___met ___not met Signature_____	**Outcome: Correct procedure performed.** ___met ___not met Signature_____	**Outcome: Pain rating 0-2 following intervention.** ___met ___not met **Family/caregiver verbalize understanding of home care instructions.** ___met ___not met Signature_____

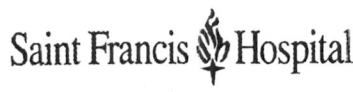

ASC-Gen-D1-9/97
Page 1 of 1

Patient Label

FIGURE 28-1   Clinical pathway for an ambulatory surgery center.

28-1 RESEARCH HIGHLIGHT

The purpose of this study was to identify teaching-content areas that ambulatory surgery patients and their nurses deemed important to the patients' postoperative outcomes and to discover any differences in the patients' and nurses' perceptions. The research objectives were to identify the teaching content that patients perceive as important to receive from nurses in the ambulatory surgery setting, to identify what the nurses perceive as important to teach preoperatively, and to detect differences and commonalities between the two perceptions. The results indicated that patients ranked situational information such as explaining activities and events as the most important teaching-content areas. Nurses ranked psychosocial support, such as dealing with worries and concerns as the most important. Patients preferred to have the teaching conducted before they were admitted for surgery, and the nurses believed that some teaching could take place after admission. This study suggests that initiating teaching earlier in the perioperative process is crucial to the ambulatory surgery patient's perceived satisfaction with postoperative outcomes. Additionally, the perioperative nurse determines what is important to the patient and family or significant other and devises education content to meet these informational needs. Patients in this study preferred situational information, which is concrete and factual, representing what is going to occur during the sequence of patient care events.

From Brumfield, V.C., Kee, C.C., & Johnson, J.Y. (1996). Preoperative patient teaching in ambulatory surgery settings, *AORN Journal, 64*(6), 941-952.

9. Necessary insurance papers to bring
10. Resources available in the home

To assist in data collection and plan individualized care, the patient is asked health-related questions pertaining to pertinent physical disabilities, existing health conditions, previous surgeries and anesthetics with associated responses, and vital information such as height, weight, allergies (foods, medications, latex), and current medications. This preoperative assessment may be completed in various ways, including interviews conducted by telephone, in the preadmission clinic, at the time of admission to the facility, and through completion of written questionnaires. When such preadmission information is obtained before the day of surgery, the admitting process is shortened. Regardless of how the data are collected, they should be documented on the record that will be used the day of surgery to prevent duplication of information (Fig. 28-2).

After admission to the facility and correct identification of the patient, the patient and family or significant other should be given an orientation to the facility and be provided with an explanation of the expected sequence of events. The patient then changes into the appropriate surgical attire (if appropriate), and provisions are made for the safekeeping of clothing and any valuables the patient may have brought. The following assessment parameters are then obtained and documented by the perioperative nurse.

- Observation and assessment of general physical and psychosocial behavior, sensory-perceptual alterations, emotional status, interaction with family, and compliance with preoperative instructions
- Baseline vital signs
- Verification of required laboratory values, radiographs, history, and physical examination
- Administration of preoperative medications as ordered
- Assessment of anxiety and apprehension related to impending surgical procedure
- Assessment of patient knowledge regarding impending surgical procedure, recovery, and postoperative care
- Assessment of patient expectations regarding postoperative pain management
- Development of appropriate plan of care (Fig. 28-3)

An intravenous line or lock may be inserted as ordered. The family or significant other should be permitted to stay with the patient in the preoperative area, and provisions should be made for their comfort. These persons are an integral part of the patient's well-being and should always be included as part of the patient's surgical experience. Colorful surroundings and the promotion of relaxation through means such as music, television, or videos should be provided.

The patient may walk to the surgical suite or be transported by wheelchair or stretcher. The mode of transportation depends on the patient's abilities, the effects of medications if administered, and the policies of the facility. The family or significant others are directed to the waiting area, informed of the approximate time for the procedure, and made comfortable with refreshments, reading material, music, or television.

Intraoperative Phase

Intraoperative nursing care for the ambulatory surgery patient is consistent with the AORN standards and recommended practices for any patient undergoing an operative or other invasive procedure. Perioperative nursing care responsibilities include the following:

- Identify the patient, introduce self, and review chart.
- Report to the physician any relative or absolute contraindications to intraoperative medications that may be used.
- Safely transfer the patient to the OR bed.

**Shaded Areas to be Filled In by
Nurse Assistant / Nurse Technician**

Saint Francis ✤ Hospital · OPAD / ASC
NURSING HISTORY / ASSESSMENT
9264-5862C / 09-96

PATIENT - NAME in FULL	ADMIT - DATE	TIME	PAGE
			1 OF 4
DIAGNOSIS	HEIGHT	WEIGHT	
		cm	kg

SURGERY / PROCEDURE

NPO STATUS   ☐ MIDNIGHT   ☐ MEDICATION TAKEN   OTHER - SPECIFY ☐

HEALTH HISTORY / PERCEPTION / MANAGEMENT   REACTION - DESCRIBE

ALLERGY/ (DRUGS, FOODS, SOAP, LATEX)
SENSITIVITY   ☐ NO   ☐ YES –

☐ SEIZURES   ☐ HEART PROBLEMS   ☐ HIGH BLOOD PRESSURE   ☐ KIDNEY DISEASE   ☐ PSYCHO/SOCIAL NEEDS   DESCRIBE   ☐ OTHER
☐ DIABETES   ☐ BREATHING PROBLEMS   ☐ LIVER DISEASE   ☐ TOBACCO USE   ☐ NONE

COMMENT: PAIN RATING 0 - 5   LOCATION

CURRENT MEDICATION   ☐ See reverse side for additional medication

DRUG - NAME	PURPOSE	FREQUENCY	LAST DOSE	DRUG - NAME	PURPOSE	FREQUENCY	LAST DOSE

COGNITIVE / PERCEPTUAL

VISUAL DEFICIT   HEARING DEFICIT   COMMUNICATION DEFICIT
☐ NA   ☐ NA   ☐ YES   ☐ NO
☐ GLASSES   ☐ HEARING LOSS ☐ R ☐ L   DESCRIBE _____
☐ CONTACTS   ☐ HEARING AIDS ☐ R ☐ L   TRANSLATOR ☐ YES ☐ NO

LEVEL of CONSCIOUSNESS   ☐ PERL   OTHER - SPECIFY
☐ ALERT   ☐ ORIENTED × 4   ☐ DEFERRED ☐

PEDIATRIC PATIENTS   OTHER - SPECIFY

BEHAVIOR   ☐ PLAYFUL   ☐ WITHDRAWN   ☐

COMMUNICABLE DISEASE	HAS HAD NO|YES	EXPOSED TO NO|YES	DATE EXPOSED	IMMUNIZATION UP TO DATE
☐ CHICKEN POX				☐ YES
☐ MUMPS				☐ NO
☐ MEASLES				

TRANSCULTURAL /RELIGIOUS NEEDS   EDUCATIONAL ASSESSMENT
☐ YES ☐ NO DESCRIBE –   COMPLETED ☐ YES ☐ NO

ACTIVITY / EXERCISE   DESCRIBE
STRENGTH / MOBILITY DEFICIT
☐ NO   ☐ YES –

EDEMA ☐ YES ☐ NO
LOCATION

PEDAL PULSES   ☐ DEFERRED   CHARACTER of RESPIRATIONS   DESCRIBE
☐ YES ☐ NO –   ☐ NORMAL ☐

NUTRITION / SKIN

SPECIAL DIET ☐ YES ☐ NO   DESCRIBE

☐ REFERRAL ☐ NA ☐ YES   DESCRIBE

APPEARANCE   OTHER - DESCRIBE
☐ WELL NOURISHED ☐

DENTURES / APPLIANCE ☐ NO ☐ YES

SKIN BREAKDOWN   DESCRIBE
☐ NONE ☐ PRESENT –   ☐ HIGH RISK for SKIN BREAKDOWN

☐ BRUISES –   ☐ RASHES –   ☐ OTHER - SPECIFY

SEXUALITY / REPRODUCTIVE PATTERN   ☐ No Need Identified

FEMALE - PREGNANT   LAST MEN-STRUAL PERIOD if applicable   OTHER - SPECIFY
☐ NO ☐ YES ☐ NA

SELF PERCEPTION / COPING / STRESS

VERBALIZES ANXIETY ABOUT HOSPITAL EXPERIENCE - - - - - - - - ☐ NO   ☐ YES
SOMEONE WILL BE AVAILABLE TO HELP AFTER DISCHARGE - - - ☐ NO   ☐ YES

ASSESSMENT COMPLETED BY RN –   SIGNATURE

CHART PREPARATION CHECKLIST

	OP	OR	NA
ADMISSION -			
SIGNED CONSENT OPERATION - - - - - - - - - - - - - - - - - -			
BLOOD TRANSFUSION - - - - - - - - - - -			
OTHER - SPECIFY _____			
HISTORY and PHYSICAL - - - - - - - - - - - - - - - -			
HEMOGRAM - - - - - - Hgb _____ Hct _____			
SERUM K⁺ _____ Notification if abnormal - - - - - - - -			
OTHER LAB _____			
CHEST X-RAY / MAMMOGRAM - - - - - - - - - - - - - -			
EKG -			
OLD CHARTS - - - - - - - - - - - - - - - - - -			

FAMILY / SIGNIFICANT OTHER / RELATIONSHIP

LOCATION   OTHER - SPECIFY   PHONE NO.
☐ WAITING ROOM ☐

CHECKLIST SUMMARY ☐ ASSESSMENT ☐ PARENT ARMS   ☐ WHEELCHAIR – GURNEY
☐ IV / LOCK ☐ PREOP MED ☐ SKIN PREPARATION ☐ OTHER - SPECIFY

CHECKLIST COMPLETE   TIME ____   RN - SIGNATURE
TO SURGERY / PROCEDURE   TIME ____   RN - SIGNATURE

ADMISSION PREPARATION CHECKLIST

	OP	OR	NA
VITAL SIGNS TIME___ TEMP___ PULSE___ RESP___ BLOOD PRESSURE___/___			
LEGIBLE IDENTIFICATION - - - - - - - -			
BRACELET on WRIST ALLERGY - - - - - - - - - - - - -			
BLOOD - - - - - - - - - - - - -			
JEWELRY REMOVED - If rings, tape securely - - - - - - - - - -			
DENTURES / APPLIANCE OUT - - - - - - - - - - - - - - -			
DISPOSITION –			
HAIRPINS / HAIRPIECE / FALSE EYELASHES REMOVED - - -			
EYEGLASSES / CONTACTS / HEARING AID(s) REMOVED - - -			
DISPOSITION –			
UNDERWEAR REMOVED - HOSPITAL GOWN ON - - - - - - - -			

TIME ___
☐ VOIDED –   ☐ SIDERAILS ELEVATED
                    ☐ FOLEY

CLOTHING   VALUABLES – List   ☐ None   ☐ OPS / RM
☐ OPS / RM ☐ PURSE   ☐ FAMILY
☐ FAMILY   ☐ WALLET   ☐ SECURITY
☐ OFFICE

☐ ORIENTED TO UNIT   ☐ CALL LIGHT WITHIN REACH   ADMITTED BY - SIGNATURE

PATIENT LABEL

FIGURE 28-2 Nursing history and assessment.

ADMITTING SURGERY SERVICES
AMBULATORY SURGERY CENTER

Goals of Preoperative Preparation

The goals of preanesthesia and preoperative preparations focus on a variety of issues such as:

1. Collection of data through assessment and interview as appropriate for age and development.
2. Provision of accurate information to patient and family.
3. Assurance of appropriate preoperative compliance.
4. Promotion of the wellness concept.
5. Improving lines of communication.
6. Provision of emotional support.
7. Reduction of patient anxiety.
8. Decreasing potential for complications.
9. Provision of smooth flow of the surgery schedule.

Outcome Guidelines

Patient or family should identify or describe the planned procedure before transportation to the procedure.

Assessment and Interventions

Admit patient to the room. Orient patient or family to surroundings. If patient is a child, ensure that parent or guardian is present in the room.

Verify patient's identification by checking name bracelet with the chart.

If family or responsible adult is not present, obtain the name and phone number of the person who will be picking up the patient postoperatively.

Assess the patient and complete the Surgical Patient Care Record/Perioperative Record.
  Ascertain compliance to NPO and medication instructions.
  Assessment of patients with existing pulmonary disease should include pulse oximetry as a baseline value for comparison.

For DOS patients, utilize the Admission History and Assessment Record to record the physical assessment and interview with patient or family.

Verify the operative consent with the patient or family and the physician's order.

Assess patient or family understanding of the procedure. Provide information and clarification as needed. Review preoperative teaching and document patient or family understanding.

Start an IV instillation on adults (per standing or individual physician's order). No IV instillation is necessary for local anesthesia unless the conscious sedation technique is used.

Review and analyze assessment data. Notify physician or anesthesia provider of unusual or unexpected conditions.

Communicate with other care providers regarding special needs of the patient or family.

When all preoperative concerns have been addressed, administer preoperative medications.

For patient safety, place bed rails up and instruct patient or family in use of the call light.

Ensure that the physician's preoperative orders have been completed.

When the patient leaves for surgery or procedure, direct the family to the Surgical Family Waiting Room.

Patients receiving conscious sedation should have pulse oximetry monitoring. If patient is over 65 years of age or has cardiac disease, monitor ECG.

PEDIATRIC patients:
  For DOS patients, utilize the Pediatric Admission History and Assessment Record.
  Incorporate parents into all aspects of the patient's care.
  Discuss with parents possible behavior reactions to the surgical experience, including medications and anesthesia.

ELDERLY patients:
  Assess skin condition, nutrition, and hydration.
  Monitor cardiovascular and respiratory status after the preoperative medication has been given.
  Encourage family participation in care to provide emotional support through the surgical experience.
  Observe limitations in mobility.

ORTHOPEDIC patients:
  Implement appropriate care path.
  Complete the shave prep per standing order.
  Bivalve cast if needed.
  Hibiclens/Betadine prep, if ordered.
  Assess skin integrity.
  Assess neurovascular status of involved extremity.
  Orthopedic devices should be labeled and sent to Surgery with the patient if applicable.

GYNECOLOGICAL/GENERAL SURGERY patients:
  Complete the shave prep per standing orders.
  Assess and document pedal pulses and neurovascular status.

ENT patients:
  Assess patient or family history of bleeding tendencies.

A

FIGURE 28–3 **A,** Guidelines for nursing care (GNC).   Continued

NURSING DIAGNOSIS / PROGRESS NOTE | **PROB CODE** — **1** = ANXIETY   **2** = FEAR   **3** = NONCOMPLIANCE   **4** = KNOWLEDGE DEFICIT   **5** =   OTHER - *SPECIFY*   PAGE 2 OF 4

PROB NO.	TIME	ASSESSMENT / PROBLEM IDENTIFICATION	PLAN / IMPLEMENTATION	TIME	OUTCOME / EVALUATION
		Implement GNC— *SPECIFY*			☐ GNC outcome met

B

PREOP MEDICATION   ☐ NONE

TIME	DRUG - NAME	SIGNATURE	TIME	DRUG - NAME	SIGNATURE

LOCK – ☐ IV   ☐ SALINE   CATHETER SIZE _____ gauge   LOCATION

☐ PLA-1000   ☐ ADDITIVE   ☐ NA   *SPECIFY*
☐ D$_5$LR-1000   ☐ *See IV FLOW RECORD*
☐ PIGGYBACK   ☐ OTHER –

START
IV –

SIGNATURE
NURSE –

☐ **PREOPERATIVE TEACHING COMPLETED**

SIGNATURE
NURSE –

COMMENT
....
....
....
....
....
....
....
....
....
....
....
....

PATIENT LABEL

FIGURE 28–3, cont'd   **B,** Nursing diagnosis and progress note.

- Properly position patient and maintain correct body alignment.
- Assist anesthesia personnel as appropriate.
- Administer medications for IV conscious sedation under the direction of a physician.
- Monitor the patient receiving IV conscious sedation and report any changes such as restlessness, cyanosis, pallor, flushing, diaphoresis, nausea, low oxygen saturation, dysrhythmias, and allergic or toxic reaction.
- Monitor for safety precautions, aseptic technique, skin integrity, and fluid and electrolyte balance.
- Document patient care according to facility policy and procedure (Fig. 28-4).
- Maintain AORN standards and recommended practices for the perioperative patient.

It is common practice in ambulatory surgery for the patient to receive IV conscious sedation administered or monitored by the perioperative nurse. In addition to the preoperative assessment parameters previously described, the nurse responsible for managing the care of the patient receiving IV conscious sedation during the intraoperative phase should conduct a thorough nursing assessment (Box 28-7). The goal of this assessment is to determine any contraindications to the administration of IV conscious sedation medications and patient appropriateness for nurse management.

The AORN has developed recommended practices that specifically address monitoring parameters applicable to the ambulatory patient in the intraoperative phase. These include "Recommended practices for managing the patient receiving conscious sedation/analgesia" and "Recommended practices for monitoring the patient receiving local anesthesia."[2] These recommended practices are intended for optimal patient care and should be applied by the perioperative nurse in the ambulatory setting.

Many institutions require specific credentialing for both nurses and physicians involved in the administration of conscious sedation. Credentialing may include specific competency-based education. Janikowski and Rockefeller[17] recommend that key components in conscious sedation and education programs include either a basic or advanced cardiac life-support course that includes airway management, pharmacology, and cardiac dysrhythmia interpretation, anatomy and physiology, preprocedural assessment, review of patient selection criteria and ASA physical status classifications, medications along with dosages, administration rates, onset and duration, adverse effects and contraindications, competency in operating and trouble-shooting essential equipment, medicolegal issues, and management of emergency care. Policy and procedures should be developed and in place based on guidelines and recommendations set forth by external agencies such as the state board of nursing and standards of national nursing associations.

The nurse monitoring the patient receiving conscious sedation should "have no other responsibilities that would require the nurse to leave the patient unattended or compromise continuous patient monitoring during the procedure."[2] The patient's vital signs are monitored by use of electrocardiogram (ECG), pulse oximetry, noninvasive blood pressure monitor, and general observation. The nurse must be familiar with the various types of monitoring equipment and have a basic understanding of ECG interpretation, and oxygen and suction lines should be readily available. A second nurse should be assigned to circulating responsibilities during the procedure.

Postoperative Phase

After completion of the surgical procedure, the patient is transferred to the appropriate recovery area. A complete report on the status of the patient, procedure performed, medications administered, dressings, and allergies is communicated to the receiving nurse by the perioperative nurse or anesthesia provider. Ambulatory surgery is followed by a rapid recovery period, which includes two distinct phases. The first phase is emergence from anesthesia (Fig. 28-5). The second phase allows for readaptation to the environment where the patient is encouraged to sit up, stand, void, and ambulate. Although not always possible, many ambulatory surgery facilities have separate phase 1 and phase 2 recovery areas. The area to which the patient is transferred after surgery is determined by the type of anesthesia administered.

Assessment during phase 1 should be determined and established as a policy and procedure. This will assist staff in utilizing a uniform method of assessing all patients in phase 1. The most common assessment parameters include respiration, circulation, level of consciousness, skin color, and level of voluntary activity. A variety of scoring systems that are simple to use allow for standardized reporting, such as the Aldrete Score (see Chapter 8).

Patients who have received local anesthesia, conscious sedation, or a regional anesthetic may be taken directly to the phase 2 recovery area. The patient is monitored for light-headedness, dizziness, hemorrhage, nausea, vomiting, significant changes in baseline vital signs, pain management, and psychomotor and cognitive function. Methods that may be used to assess psychomotor and cognitive function include paper and pencil test, single reaction time, coordination and attention tests, ability to walk in a straight line, Maddox wing test, flicker fusion test, and psychomotor test. Postoperative nursing care and responsibilities applicable to both phase 1 and phase 2 include the following:

- Assess for inadequate ventilation related to anesthesia or airway obstruction.
- Monitor potential for fluid-volume deficit related to anesthesia or hypovolemia.
- Monitor for injury related to emergence delirium.
- Monitor for alteration in comfort related to pain.

Saint Francis ✚ Hospital *AMBULATORY SURGERY*

OPERATIVE / PERIOP NURSING CARE
363-001

ORSOS NO.	DATE	O.R. NO.	STAFF in O.R. - TIME	PATIENT in O.R. - TIME	SURGERY - START END	PATIENT OUT O.R. - TIME

SPECIALTY ☐ ANESTHESIA ☐ CV ☐ DENTAL ☐ ENT ☐ EYE ☐ GENERAL ☐ GYN ☐ ORTHO ☐ PLASTIC ☐ THOR ☐ URO OTHER - *SPECIFY* ☐

ANESTHESIA ☐ GENERAL ☐ LOCAL ☐ MAC ☐ REGIONAL BLOCK ☐ SPINAL ☐ TOPICAL ☐ NONE **CASE** TYPE ☐ ELECTIVE ☐ URGENT ☐ STAT CLASS / ASA

OPERATION _____

DIAGNOSIS PREOPERATIVE _____
POSTOPERATIVE ☐ SAME

SURGEON	CIRCULATING NURSE	CIRCULATOR-INITIAL COUNT BY - SIGNATURE	FINAL COUNT BY - SIGNATURE
ASSISTING SURGEON	SCRUB NURSE	SCRUB-INITIAL COUNT BY - SIGNATURE	FINAL COUNT BY - SIGNATURE
ANESTHESIA	CIRCULATING / SCRUB RELIEF	SPONGES ☐ CORRECT ☐ INCORRECT ☐ NA	
		NEEDLES ☐ CORRECT ☐ INCORRECT ☐ NA	

IMPLANT

DESCRIPTION	QTY	CATALOG NO.	SERIAL NO.	LOT / LOAD NO.
☐ SEE REVERSE SIDE				

MEDICATION _____

IV CATHETER – SIZE _____ gauge LOCATION _____ ☐ PLA-1000 ☐ LR 500 ☐ NA ☐ OTHER – SPECIFY

TOURNIQUET UP _____ DOWN _____ LOCATION _____ mmHg _____ | **LAB SPECIMEN** TISSUE _____ FROZEN _____ CULTURE _____ CYTOLOGY _____

ASSESSMENT
PATIENT

IDENTIFICATION
☐ CHART
☐ LABEL
☐ VERBAL
☐ ID BRACELET ON

ALLERGY
☐ NKDA
☐ LISTED on CHART
☐ ALLERGY BRACELET ON

MENTAL / EMOTIONAL STATUS
☐ ORIENTED ☐ UNRESPONSIVE
☐ DISORIENTED ☐ AGITATED
☐ SEDATED ☐ ANXIOUS
☐ OTHER - SPECIFY

SKIN INTEGRITY
☐ DRY ☐ CLAMMY
☐ WARM ☐ DUSKY
☐ COOL ☐ NO BREAKDOWN
☐ OTHER - SPECIFY

SKIN INTACT at SURGERY SITE – YES _____ NO - DESCRIBE

PROBLEM IDENTIFICATION
GNC ☐ PERIOPERATIVE OTHER - SPECIFY ☐ PROBLEM - DESCRIBE

SURGERY POSITION
☐ SUPINE ☐ PRONE ☐ LITHOTOMY ☐ LATERAL ☐ JACKNIFE ☐ KNEE-CHEST ☐ FOWLERS ☐ SEMI-FOWLER'S OTHER - SPECIFY ☐

INTERVENTION

PADDING / SUPPORT / RESTRAINT
☐ SAFETY STRAP APPLIED -- _____
☐ FOAM PAD --------
☐ HEADREST ---- _____
☐ PILLOW ------ _____
☐ STIRRUP ------
☐ LEG HOLDER ------- _____
☐ SANDBAG SPECIFY TYPE --- _____
☐ AXILLARY ROLL ----
☐ SHOULDER ROLL
☐ CHEST ROLL - _____
☐ OTHER - SPECIFY

ARM SECURED
☐ ON ARM-BOARD - ☐L ☐R
☐ AT SIDE - ☐L ☐R
☐ ACROSS CHEST - ☐L ☐R
ESU ☐ BIPOLAR – NO. _____ ☐ NA ☐ MONOPOLAR – NO. _____ ☐ PAD - SITE(s) _____ APPLIED BY – NAME

SHAVE ☐ NA SITE _____ SHAVED BY - NAME _____ **PREP AGENT** ☐ NONE ☐ HIBICLENS PHISOHEX ☐ POVIDONE – IODINE ☐ SOAP ☐ SOLUTION ☐ SPRAY ☐ GEL OTHER - SPECIFY ☐

URINARY CATHETER ☐ NA ☐ PRESENT upon ARRIVAL to O.R. ☐ INDWELLING INSERTED – FR _____ ml ☐ STRAIGHT CATHETERIZATION INSERTED BY - NAME _____ TOTAL EMPTIED _____ ml

DRESSING – _____
DRAIN / PACKING –

BODY TEMPERATURE ☐ THERMAL – ☐ BLANKET ☐ LEGGING ☐ CAP WARM BLANKET APPLIED - SITE ☐ ON ARRIVAL to O.R. – ☐ PRIOR to TRANSFER –

EVALUATION
OUTCOME – PATIENT VERIFIES HIS/HER IDENTITY and PROCEDURE ☐ NA ☐ YES – PATIENT EXHIBITS DECREASED ANXIETY by VERBAL or NONVERBAL COMMUNICATION ☐ NA ☐ YES ☐ NO –

COMMENT _____ CIRCULATING NURSE - SIGNATURE

PATIENT TRANSFERRED TO ☐ PACU ☐ DISCHARGE AREA OTHER - SPECIFY ☐

REPORT GIVEN TO – NAME _____

COMMENT – _____

FIGURE 28-4 Operative and perioperative nursing care.

| BOX 28-7 | Nursing Assessment for the Patient Receiving IV Conscious Sedation |

1. Does the patient have any history of:
   Seizure disorder?
   Substance abuse?
   Posttraumatic stress syndrome?
   Cardiovascular problems?
   Liver or kidney problems?
   Respiratory problems?
   Thyroid problems?
   Allergies to medications, food, or latex?
2. Has the patient ever had a bad experience in surgery or an outpatient office such as the dental office?
3. What medications is the patient currently taking?
4. NPO status?
5. Height and weight?
6. Any known medical condition unrelated to the procedure? Is the condition well controlled?
7. What is the patient's perception of their pain tolerance?

- Monitor for nausea and vomiting related to anesthesia or surgical procedure.
- Protect areas sensitized by the administration of a local anesthetic agent.
- Monitor for alteration in circulation related to surgical procedure or dressing or cast.
- Encourage early ambulation and progressive fluid ingestion as appropriate.
- Document plan of care according to facility policy and procedure.
- Supply and review appropriate written discharge instructions.

The perioperative nurse documents the care given and progress of the patient throughout the postoperative phase (see Fig. 28-5). The patient and family or significant other review the discharge instructions with the perioperative nurse, receive clarification, and have the opportunity to ask questions. The patient is discharged when home readiness is determined.

Discharge

Each ambulatory surgery facility must have written guidelines that have been approved by the anesthesia and medical staff to outline criteria for patient discharge (Fig. 28-6). Regulatory agencies such as the Joint Commission on Accreditation of Healthcare Organizations (JCAHO) allow authorized personnel to discharge patients when the criteria are identified. It is unlikely that a physician is available to discharge every ambulatory surgery patient; therefore the authorized person most likely responsible for determining appropriateness of meeting the specified criteria and home readiness is the perioperative nurse.[19] The criteria may be predetermined

as a set of standing discharge orders or written separately as an order by the surgeon. Criteria to determine home readiness are intended to meet the needs of the patient, nursing staff, and facility. The following is a common list of discharge criteria that may be applied to the ambulatory surgery patient:

- Order from the physician
- Stable vital signs
- No evidence of respiratory depression
- Oriented to person, place, and time
- Ability to void, as appropriate
- Ability to take fluids orally, as appropriate
- Ability to dress
- Ability to ambulate without assistance
- Minimal nausea and vomiting
- No excessive pain
- No bleeding or excessive drainage
- Written discharge instructions that include possible complications, activity restrictions, diet, medications, wound care and hygiene, precautions, and plan for follow-up care
- Responsible adult escort

The ambulatory surgery patient should understand that recovery and convalescence are not complete upon discharge. The patient is instructed not to plan to resume usual activities until at least a day after surgery and often longer. Discharge instructions related to possible complications, activity restrictions, diet, medications, wound care, and plan for follow-up care are reviewed and reinforced with the patient and family or significant other. At the time of discharge, written instructions forms are signed and a copy is given to the patient, family member, or significant other. Any additional questions regarding postoperative care are answered.

Although it is anticipated that most patients will return home in the care of family or friends, some patients may require additional assistance from home healthcare agencies. Many ambulatory surgery facilities contract with specific home care agencies to provide various types of assisted care. Possible indications for home healthcare follow-up referral after ambulatory surgery include a lack of support system, the need for complex postoperative care such as dressing change or IV medications, assistance with activities of daily living, or pain management.[21] Home healthcare personnel can assist in meeting the needs of the patient, thus avoiding a hospital stay.

Upon discharge from the facility, patients may be given a questionnaire to be completed at their convenience. The questionnaire provides the facility feedback about its services, any postoperative complications the patient may experience, and any additional comments or suggestions from the patient. It is one way to measure the quality of services provided by the facility. In most ambulatory surgery programs, the perioperative nurse contacts the patient with a follow-up phone call 24 hours after surgery

Saint Francis Hospital *ASC / PACU*
FLOW RECORD   363-002

ACCOMPANIED BY - NAME	SURGEON - NAME	DATE	TIME

PROCEDURE _____

PREOP STATUS / INFORMATION

TIME - ON OFF	VIA □ NASAL CANNULA □ FACE TENT	□ MASK □ FLOW-BY	OTHER - SPECIFY □	L / min — %	ALLERGIES □ NKDA	BRACELET □ ID □ ALLERGY

O_2 –

AIRWAY MANAGEMENT □ NON REQUIRED □ ENDOTRACHEAL □ NASOPHARYNGEAL □ ORAL □ HEADLIFT □ GRASP □ REFLEXES | EXTUBATION at - TIME   BY - NAME | PREOP VITAL SIGNS –   BLOOD PRESSURE /   PULSE

VENTILATOR – □ NA   TIME - ON   OFF   TV O_2 RATE

BREATH SOUNDS	□ RHONCHI	□ STRIDOR	□ WHEEZE	OTHER - DESCRIBE
	□ RALES	□ NORMAL BILAT	□ DIMIINISHED	

POSITION □ SUPINE □ PRONE □ RIGHT SIDE □ LEFT SIDE   OTHER - DESCRIBE

DRESSING □ NA □ See Assessment Notes □ DRY □ INTACT | **WARM BLANKETS** □ | **RESTRAINT** □ LAP BELTS □ WRISTS □   OTHER - SPECIFY | T I M E   ON   OFF

PRESCRIPTION(s) on CHART *list* □ NO □ YES —

HEAD OF BED ↑   TIME   DEGREE | FOOT OF BED ↑   TIME

LEVEL of CONSCIOUSNESS □ RESPONSIVE □ UNRESPONSIVE | **MONITOR** □ ECG □ OTHER - SPECIFY | □ BP CUFF – LOC □ PULSE OXIMETER

CODE —   **A** = ADEQUATE   **S** = SHALLOW   **V** = VENTILATOR

TIME ▶

210
200
190
180
170
160
150
140
130
120
110
100
90
80
70
60
50
40
30
20
10
0
RESP
DEPTH
SaO$_2$
O$_2$
TEMP

C = **C**onsciousness   **A** = **A**irway   **R** = **R**espiration   **C** = **C**irculation   **O** = **O**ral Color

CARCO Criteria Met   □ YES   □ NO

TRANSFER TO –   □ DISCHARGE AREA □   OTHER - SPECIFY   TIME   VIA □ WHEELCHAIR □ WAGON □ CARRIED □   OTHER - SPECIFY

□ DISCHARGE from PACU   PHYSICIAN - SIGNATURE

PRIMARY NURSE - SIGNATURE | RELIEF NURSE - SIGNATURE

INTRAVENOUS FLUIDS

No.	TIME	AMOUNT HOOKED ON	SOLUTION	AMOUNT INFUSED
SITE			TOTAL	

OUTPUT AMOUNT

TIME	VOID	J-P	HEMOVAC	EMESIS	
TOTALS					
		AGGREGATE TOTAL			

PACU
FLOW RECORD
104

FIGURE 28–5   Flow record.   *Continued*

PROBLEM IDENTIFICATION		DESCRIPTION	TIME		DESCRIPTION				
	1 –	INEFFECTIVE AIRWAY CLEARANCE		2 –	PAIN		3 –	FLUID VOLUME DEFICIT / EXCESS	
	4 –	HYPOTHERMIA / HYPERTHERMIA		5 –	ANXIETY		6 –	OTHER - *SPECIFY*	

PLAN	IMPLEMENT GNC ☐ GENERAL ANESTHESIA	☐ SPINAL / EPIDURAL ANESTHESIA	OTHER - *SPECIFY* ☐	☐	☐

TIME	PROB No.	ASSESSMENT / IMPLEMENTATION / OUTCOME	MEDICATION

363-002

FIGURE 28-5, cont'd   Flow record.

to evaluate recovery and general condition and to answer any questions regarding care. The patient is advised to consult the surgeon for any complications related to the surgical procedure. In addition, the perioperative nurse may notify the surgeon regarding the complication. Postoperative calls are an important tool for the ambulatory facility to determine patient satisfaction and effectiveness of care.

PERSONNEL

The recruitment and retention of dedicated staff for the ambulatory surgery setting is of key importance to the success of the facility. Staff working in these settings must be flexible, personable, clinically expert, and able to develop and form relationships with patients and their families or significant others in an abbreviated amount of time. Haas and Hackbarth[13] describe core dimensions of the future staff nurse in clinical practice in ambulatory care as:

1. Enabling daily operations of the facility
2. Performance of technical procedures
3. Implementation of the nursing process
4. Telephone communication skills
5. Advocacy
6. Patient teaching
7. Care coordination

Perioperative nurses in many ambulatory surgery centers are cross-trained to function in all areas of the

NURSING HISTORY / ASSESSMENT – POSTPROCEDURE STATUS

ALLERGIES - *LIST*
☐ No Known Allergies ......

ROOM NO.   ARRIVAL - TIME   VIA
☐ WHEEL CHAIR   ☐ STRETCHER / WAGON   PROCEDURE
☐ CARRIED

COGNITIVE / PERCEPTION   ☐ ORIENTED   ☐ DROWSY   ☐ AWAKE
☐ OTHER – *SPECIFY*

EXTREMITY ELEVATED –   ☐ NA

INTEGRITY
SKIN   ☐ DRY   ☐ CLAMMY   COLOR
☐ WARM   ☐ COOL   ☐ WITHIN NORMAL LIMITS
☐ OTHER –   ☐ DUSKY   ☐ PALE

DRESSING   ☐ DRY   ☐ SLING
☐ NA   ☐ INTACT   ☐ BAND-AID   ☐ ICE BAG
☐ OTHER –   ☐ STERI-STRIP   ☐ PERIPAD

RESPIRA-TIONS   ☐ NORMAL   ☐ SHALLOW   ABDOMEN   ☐ SOFT   ☐ NONTENDER
☐ LABORED   ☐ NA   ☐ FIRM   ☐ DISTENDED

DRAIN   ☐ FOLEY   ☐ NASOGASTRIC   ☐ NA   OTHER - *SPECIFY*
☐ HEMOVAC   ☐ JACKSON-PRATT   ☐

☐ NAUSEA   ☐ VOMITING   ☐ NA

IV   ☐ PLA-1000   ☐ SALINE LOCK   SITE   DISCON-TINUED –   BY
☐ LR-500   ☐ OTHER –   TIME

CAPILLARY REFILL   ☐ BRISK   ☐ SLOW   ☐ NA

☐ ID BRACELET   ☐ GURNEY   ☐ RECLINER
☐ ALLERGY BRACELET   ☐ SIDE RAILS UP   ☐ CALL LIGHT

☐ FAMILY / SIGNIFICANT OTHER PRESENT –   *DESCRIBE*

☐ GNC IMPLEMENTATION   ☐ GNC OUTCOME MET   ☐ *See Page 4*

COMMENT – ......

VITAL SIGNS

TIME	TEMPERATURE	PULSE	RESPIRATION	BLOOD PRESSURE
				/
				/
				/
				/
				/
				/
				/
				/
				/
				/
				/
				/
				/

RATING *0–5*   LOCATION

PAIN –

DRUG NAME	DOSE	ROUTE	TIME	INITIAL

PATIENT / FAMILY EDUCATION

SPECIAL LEARNING NEEDS
☐ PHYSICAL
☐ COGNITIVE
☐ LANGUAGE
☐ NONE

READINESS TO LEARN
☐ MOTIVATED TO LEARN
☐ PARTICIPATIVE
☐ NON-PARTICIPATIVE
☐ EMOTIONAL BARRIER

CONSULT   ☐ NA
☐ DIETARY   ☐ PHYSICAL MEDICINE
☐ SOCIAL SERVICE   ☐ OTHER

☐ Discharge Criteria NOT met – *SPECIFY*

Physician notified – ......

Action taken – *SPECIFY* ......   Admitted to Room No. ......

	TIME	BY - RN INITIAL	☐ WHEELCHAIR	☐ PARENT ARMS
Discharged –			☐ AMBULATORY	☐ STRETCHER

INITIAL	SIGNATURE	TITLE

PATIENT LABEL

DISCHARGE CRITERIA

	YES	NO	NA
Vital signs meet criteria - - - - - - - - - - - - - - -			
Alert and oriented to time, place, person - - - - - - - - - -			
Controlled nausea or vomiting - - - - - - - - - - - - - -			
Pain rating – _____			
Able to void if ordered - - - - - - - - - - - - - - -			
Ambulates appropriately - - - - - - - - - - - - - -			
Dressing dry - - - - - - - - - - - - - - - - - -			
Prescriptions given - - - - - - - - - - - - - - -			
Physician Standard Discharge form given - - - - - - - - -			
Home Care / Discharge Instructions given - - - - - - - - -			
Understanding verbalized by patient / responsible person (person taught) _____			
Responsible person present for escort _____			

FIGURE 28-6   Nursing history and assessment for postprocedure status.   *Continued*

NURSING DIAGNOSIS / PROGRESS NOTE

PROBLEM IDENTIFICATION –   1 = PAIN *SPECIFY*   2 = KNOWLEDGE DEFICIT   3 = NON-COMPLIANCE *SPECIFY*   4 = ALTERED HEALTH MAINTENANCE

5 =   6 =

PROB NO.	√	TIME	ASSESSMENT / PROBLEM IDENTIFICATION	PLAN / IMPLEMENTATION	TIME	OUTCOME / EVALUATION
						☐ GNC outcome met

INITIAL	SIGNATURE	TITLE	INITIAL	SIGNATURE	TITLE	PATIENT LABEL

OPAD/ASC NURSING HISTORY/ASSESSMENT 9264-5862C / 09-96 / PAGE 4

FIGURE 28-6, cont'd   Nursing history and assessment for postprocedure status.

facility. This unique feature of perioperative nursing in ambulatory surgery centers requires exceptional clinical and interpersonal skills.

CONTINUING EDUCATION AND CONTINUOUS QUALITY IMPROVEMENT

Continuing education and staff development for all staff members must be relevant, ongoing, and documented. Staff should annually attend educational programs on CPR, fire and safety, and infection control practices. Other educational opportunities may include staff development programs related to technologic advances, new procedures, IV conscious sedation, updated AORN standards and recommended practices, and continuous quality improvement activities. Ongoing education should also be provided that addresses age-specific and cultural and ethnic aspects of the populations served. Observation and assessment skills are essential in ambulatory surgery nursing and should be updated periodically. Yearly assessment and verification of skills and competencies must be documented.

Performance assessment and improvement, along with

BOX 28-8 | **Quality Assessment and Improvement for the Ambulatory Surgery Patient**

Important Aspect of Care

Preoperative assessment and patient education

Indicators

A preoperative nursing assessment is made for each ambulatory surgical patient.

The patient, family, or significant other learning needs are identified and recorded.

Discharge instructions are written and reviewed with the patient, family, significant other; demonstration of understanding is documented on the nursing care plan.

Important Aspect of Care

Patient safety

Indicators

Patient is free from injury related to positioning, extraneous objects, chemical, physical, and electrical hazards.

Important Aspect of Care

Discharge planning

Indicator

A responsible escort who will accompany the patient when discharged and will be present before the start of surgery.

Important Aspect of Care

Skin integrity and infection management

Indicators

Skin is assessed preoperatively and postoperatively.

Skin assessment is documented on nursing care plan.

Important Aspect of Care

Management of physiologic functions for the patient receiving IV conscious sedation

Indicators

Nasal cannula is in place for all patients.

Vital signs are stable throughout the surgical procedure.

Nausea and vomiting are evaluated.

Level of consciousness is continually assessed.

Management of pain is assessed and documented.

Important Aspect of Care

Customer satisfaction

Indicators

All returned patient questionnaire complaints are recorded, and suggested improvements are noted.

Quarterly patient surveys with comment cards are sent.

Important Aspect of Care

Documentation

Indicators

Nursing record is completed according to established policy and procedures.

Patient response to IV conscious sedation medications is documented.

Consent form is correctly completed.

Physician orders are documented and signed by the nurse.

---

continuing education, promotes high-quality patient care. Standards utilized in quality-improvement activities include structure standards (management of the facility), process standards (what the nurse does for the patient), and outcome standards (what the patient can expect from the nursing care). The facility's performance assessment and improvement program must identify the scope of services provided and important aspects of care (Box 28-8). For effective monitoring and evaluation of care given, quality-improvement activities must identify indicators that will monitor the important aspects of care. Continuous performance assessment and improvement activities are an important part of the care delivered in the ambulatory surgery setting and should look at the service aspect of the facility from the patient's perspective (Research Highlight 28-2). Ambulatory surgery has led perioperative services in the delivery of efficient, cost-effective service. Patient satisfaction tools often lead to opportunities for operational improvement that promote efficiency and customer satisfaction.

The rapid shift and acceptance of ambulatory surgery as an alternative to inpatient care has increased the pressure on ambulatory surgery facilities to demonstrate the best value to payers and patients alike. Value as defined in the healthcare market is a function of cost and quality.[1] Excellence can be defined as using the least-costly combination of human and physical resources[26] that results in optimal outcomes. Outcomes measurement extends beyond traditional measures of quality of surgical programs such as patient satisfaction, morbidity and mortality, and infection rates to examination of quality and costs across the continuum of care for each patient.

DOCUMENTATION

Medicolegal and risk management principles of documentation guide the manager and staff of an ambulatory surgery facility in the development and revision of existing patient records. Using the AORN recommended practices for documentation of perioperative nursing care as a

28-2 RESEARCH HIGHLIGHT

This study describes the development of a 21-item questionnaire to evaluate the effectiveness of nursing care provided in an outpatient surgery center. Four constructs of the instrument for measuring patient satisfaction were caring, continuity of care, competence of nurses, and education of patients and family members. The study findings indicated that patients with previous hospitalization experience had higher expectations of nursing care than first-time patients did. In the application of patient feedback to practice, it was found that patients in their forties perceived education as the domain that best met their needs and expectations. All age groups had equal expectations of caring, competency, and continuity of care. The study suggests that the questionnaires measure patients' opinions of the quality of care they receive, provide nurses with feedback to monitor performance trends as perceived by patients, and help nurses identify areas of practice that need refinement.

From Forbes, M.L., & Brown, H.N. (1995). Developing an instrument for measuring patient satisfaction, *AORN Journal, 61*(4), 737-743.

guide, the following should be included in patient record forms:

- Face sheet (such as demographics)
- Consent for surgical procedure and anesthesia and advance directives
- History and physical examination reports
- Health history
- Applicable laboratory test results
- Preoperative and postoperative instruction sheets
- Preoperative nursing assessment sheet
- Physician order sheet
- Anesthesia record
- Local anesthesia and conscious sedation records
- Intraoperative record
- Postoperative record
- Report of operation
- Pathology report, when applicable

It is very important to streamline forms and documentation, allowing the attention of the team to be focused on the patient, not on documentation. Many ambulatory surgery facilities have become leaders in the development and use of multidisciplinary records that prevent redundancy and duplication of information among the caregivers.[4] The same record often follows the patient through initial contact, preoperative preparation, intraoperative and postanesthesia care, and discharge planning.

Interdisciplinary input into form development and

revision is very important to usability of the form and staff acceptance. All forms should be reviewed periodically and revised as needed.

POLICIES AND PROCEDURES

The purpose of a policy and procedure manual is to provide a framework for daily operation of a facility. The manual should provide information that describes the expected course of action to be followed; as such, it becomes part of the institutional standard of care. A comprehensive policy and procedure manual is an effective tool for communication, education, and prevention of legal issues if correctly followed. Policies and procedures for the ambulatory surgery facility may differ in form and content from institutional hospital regulations because of governing body, ownership, medical staff, accrediting and licensing bodies, and management.

FUTURE TRENDS

Ambulatory surgery will continue to be a driving force in the growth of ambulatory care into the next millennium. As the American health care system undergoes change, the ambulatory surgery arena will feel the effect. Key issues in health care reform include access to service, quality of care, and cost containment. Each affects ambulatory surgery facilities, and strategic plans to maintain continuity and success in the marketplace will need to be developed with foci on consumer need, improving outcomes, and decreasing cost without compromising safety or quality of care. With the continued expansion of technology, particularly in minimally invasive surgery, patients are provided with an alternative modality of treatment, and surgery will continue to be performed outside the operating room in areas such as ancillary departments, mobile units, and physician offices. This will lead to a reshaping of the scope of ambulatory surgery services. Customer-focused care will remain an important component of patient satisfaction for the continued success of ambulatory surgery, as will the mandate to document outcomes of care both from a patient satisfaction and cost perspective.[3] Ambulatory surgery is well positioned for the future because its successes are congruent with the goals of managed care—low-cost, quality care in the appropriate setting.[25]

SUMMARY

Ambulatory surgery will continue to grow and flourish. Perioperative nursing care is the most constant and pervasive part of ambulatory surgical services. Care that was formerly spread over a period of several days is now completed in a few hours. Perioperative nurses practicing in ambulatory surgical care settings will find themselves continuing to adapt to new technology, cross-training, working in an atmosphere of flexible professional roles and teamwork, and managing care across the surgical patient's continuum.

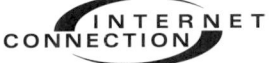

American Academy of Ambulatory Care Nursing: http://www.inurse.com/~AAACN

Case Management Society of America: http://www.cmsa.org

Home Healthcare Nurses Association: e-mail hhna@aol.com

Health World Online: http://www.healthy.net

American Society of Perianesthesia Nurses: http://www.aspan.org

American Hospital Association: http://www.aha.org

REFERENCES

1. Arford, P.H., & Allred, C.A. (1995). Value = quality + cost, *Journal of Nursing Administration, 25*(9), 64-69.

2. *AORN standards, recommended practices, and guidelines.* (1998). Denver, Colo.: Association of Operating Room Nurses.

3. Balicki, B., Kelly, W.P., & Miller, H. (1995, Sept.). Establishing benchmarks for ambulatory surgery costs, *Healthcare Financial Management*, pp. 40-48.

4. Boike, L., Canala, L., Kozminski, K., & Wynd, C.A. (1995). Development of an outpatient perioperative care record, *Journal of Post Anesthesia Nursing, 10*(3), 140-150.

5. Duncan, D.G., & Servais, C.S. (1996, Feb.). Preparing for the new outpatient reimbursement system, *Healthcare Financial Management*, pp. 42-50.

6. Evers, M.L. (1997). In-office surgery—a winning strategy in a managed care environment, *Surgical Services Management, 3*(5), 10-13.

7. Ferguson, L.K., & Kaplan, L. (1966). *Surgery of the ambulatory patient.* Philadelphia: J.B. Lippincott.

8. Fortner, P.A. (1998). Preoperative patient preparation: psychological and educational aspects, *Seminars in Perioperative Nursing, 7*(1), 3-9.

9. Gentner, J. (1995). Mobile surgical service opens the door to new opportunities, *Surgical Services Management, 1*(3), 23-29.

10. Geuder, D.L. (1995). Using resources effectively in ambulatory surgery settings, *Surgical Services Management, 1*(7), 48-52.

11. Goldberg-Alberts, A.L., & Solomon, R.P. (1997). Primer on risk management for ambulatory surgery, *Journal of Ambulatory Care Management, 20*(3), 72-86.

12. *Guidelines for optimal office-based surgery.* (1996). Chicago: American College of Surgeons.

13. Haas, S.A., & Hackbarth, D.P. (1995). Dimensions of the staff nurse role in ambulatory care. Part III. Using research data to design new models of nursing care delivery, *Nursing Economics, 13*(4), 230-241.

14. Hecht, A.D. (1995). Creating greater efficiency in ambulatory surgery, *Journal of Clinical Anesthesia, 7*, 581-584.

15. Hoeksema, J., & Munski, J. (1997). Development of a patient-centered preprocedure program, *AORN Journal, 65*(2), 388-395.

16. Hollinger-Smith, L., & Murphy, M.P. (1998). Implementing a residency program for the acute care nurse practitioner, *MEDSURG Nursing 7*(1), 28-36.

17. Janikowski, D.L., & Rockefeller, C.A. (1998). Awake and talking: ambulatory surgery and conscious sedation, *Nursing Economics, 16*(1), 37-42.

18. Mathias, J.M. (1987). Ambulatory surgery meeting stresses quality of care, *AORN Journal, 45*(5), 1191-1200.

19. Marley, R.A., & Moline, B.M. (1996). Patient discharge from the ambulatory setting, *Journal of Post Anesthesia Nursing, 11*(1), 39-49.

20. Paryani, S. (1995). The revolution in outpatient care, *Journal of Ambulatory Care Management, 18*(6), 58-67.

21. Redmond, M.C. (1995). Using home health agencies to meet patient needs in phase III recovery, *Journal of Post Anesthesia Nursing, 10*(1), 21-26.

22. Reiling, R. (1990). Day surgery and outpatient care. In *American College of Surgeons Care of the Surgical Patient.* New York: Scientific American, Inc.

23. Rivellini, D. (1993). Local and regional anesthesia, *Nursing Clinics of North America, 28*(3), 547-572.

24. Rosenstein, A.H., & Propotnik, T. (1997). Case management, *Journal of Healthcare Resource Management, 15*(2), 11-16.

25. Stout, G. (1996). Ambulatory surgery centers: harbinger of managed care shift, *Journal of Healthcare Resource Management, 14*(1), 9-14.

26. Swan, B.A. (1996). Classifying quality nursing care initiatives: framework for ambulatory surgery nursing practice, *Nursing Economics, 14*(6), 368-372.

27. Van Decar, M.T. (1998). Anesthetic drugs. *Seminars in Perioperative Nursing, 7*(1), 29-38.

28. Waegerle, J.D. (1998). Practical considerations of intravenous sedation for the perioperative nurse. *Seminars in Perioperative Nursing, 7*(1), 21-28.

CHAPTER TWENTY NINE

Pediatric Surgery

Susie S. Maldonado and Cheryl Nygren

THE HIGHLY SPECIALIZED field of pediatric surgery began its dramatic development in the first half of this century. Before this, little distinction was made between the surgical treatment of children and that of adults. Pediatric surgery is now recognized as a separate subspecialty of surgery with board certification status.

The successful and rapid advancements in pediatric surgery can be attributed to improved diagnostic procedures and techniques; better understanding of physiologic, psychologic, and sociologic problems affecting infants, small children, preteens, and adolescents; improvements in newborn intensive care management; increased knowledge about fluid and electrolyte balance, pharmacology, and nutrition, and their effects on various pediatric age groups and the causes and physiology of congenital malformations; improved anesthetic agents and techniques, along with better understanding of their effects on pediatric patients; and improved surgical techniques with more appropriate instrumentation and support equipment and implementation of more effective medical and perioperative nursing care.

The development of high-risk pregnancy centers for mothers with problem pregnancies has resulted in earlier detection of malformations in fetuses as well as of other problems. Earlier detection has led to development of lifesaving operative procedures that can be performed in utero or immediately after delivery.

Current priority research areas in pediatrics include the development of guidelines for management of specific pediatric conditions and development of functional health outcome measures for specific conditions.[2]

PERIOPERATIVE NURSING CONSIDERATIONS

Assessment

The nursing process is the basis for perioperative nursing care of pediatric patients, and the perioperative assessment is the first phase of the nursing process. The goal of a comprehensive nursing assessment is to gather sufficient data to formulate nursing diagnoses from which desired outcomes are identified and care is planned, implemented, and evaluated. The unique aspects of care of the pediatric surgical patient center on the fact that the child is a growing organism. Normally infants and children have higher metabolic rates and different physiologic makeup than those of adults. Their oxygen, fluid, and caloric requirements are greater; add to these the stress of illness or surgery, and these requirements climb even higher. Maintenance of body temperature is of special concern because the temperature control mechanism is

immature in infants and small children. Every effort should be made to limit exposure of the body surface during all surgical procedures. The perioperative nurse must have a good understanding of the normal physical and psychologic parameters for pediatric patients and be able to recognize deviations from these parameters. In addition, the perioperative nurse must be familiar with normal growth and development factors for each age group. During any given day the perioperative nurse may care for all age groups of children—neonates through adolescents.

It is important to remember that the pediatric patient is not a small adult. When caring for them, all members of the surgical team should speak to them on their level of understanding and provide the special emotional support these young patients require.

The preoperative visit is the first step in assessment. For children undergoing an ambulatory surgical procedure, the child and family visit the surgical suite and ambulatory surgical area 1 to 2 weeks before surgery, depending on the developmental level of the child. For children who are inpatients, the perioperative nurse may visit the child and family in the unit. First the patient's chart is reviewed with particular attention given to the patient's age and developmental level, the seriousness of the physical condition, size including height and weight, and a review of the current nursing diagnoses and care plan. A discussion with the primary nurse facilitates data collection, assists in providing continuity of care, and provides the perioperative nurse with information regarding preoperative education done thus far.

The perioperative nurse then interviews the child and family. The purpose of the interview is to gather data, educate, and provide emotional support to both patient and family. The focus of this visit is a discussion of the perioperative process, not necessarily to provide preoperative education regarding the surgical procedure. In pediatric centers preoperative education is often the responsibility of the primary nurse, child life therapists, or clinical nurse specialists. During the preoperative visit the perioperative nurse discusses how the child progresses through the immediate preoperative, intraoperative, and postoperative phases of care. If any questions do arise concerning the surgical procedure, the family is referred to the surgeon, primary nurse, or anesthesia provider for further clarification or reinforcement of previous teaching. The perioperative nurse may briefly describe the roles of staff members, alleviating anxiety to a certain extent by allowing the parents and child to identify a real person behind the mask, gloves, and gown. The family is informed that the child may bring a favorite security object to the operating room and at what point after the operation the child can see the parents. Teaching is always done within a developmental framework, taking into account the cognitive and psychosocial abilities of the child. Medical play items, audiovisual aids, puppets, and photographs are all used in the education process.

Assessment continues when the child arrives in the surgical suite. Because the focus of operative preparation is psychologic rather than pharmacologic, the child usually arrives awake and alert. The perioperative nurse performs an abbreviated physical assessment, focusing on vital signs, cardiopulmonary status, integumentary system, nutritional and metabolic status, and psychologic state. The preoperative checklist is completed, which includes positive patient identification, verification of NPO status, a check of any patient allergies and preoperative laboratory data, communication of deviations from normal, noting of the presence of an informed consent on the chart, and labeling of the child's personal belongings. Throughout this process, the perioperative nurse provides emotional support to the child and family and helps to alleviate fear by administering care with a gentle, calm, trusting approach.

Nursing Diagnosis

At the completion of the assessment phase, the perioperative nurse identifies appropriate nursing diag-

noses based on the patient assessment. Five nursing diagnoses that apply to pediatric patients might be as follows:

- Knowledge deficit related to perioperative events
- Ineffective thermoregulation
- Risk for impaired skin integrity
- Risk for fluid volume deficit
- Risk for injury related to use of electrosurgical unit

Outcome Identification

Perioperative nursing care is predicated on relevant nursing diagnoses. For each nursing diagnosis a desired outcome is identified. Outcomes should be measurable with criteria by which to judge their attainment. Thus for the desired outcome "The patient and family will demonstrate knowledge of perioperative events and the role of various perioperative team members," measurable criteria such as the child and family's ability to describe preoperative preparation and the perioperative routine on the day of surgery, the child's ability to locate the planned site of the surgical incision on a doll, and the child's ability to draw a picture of what he or she expects the surgical site to look like postoperatively might be identified.

Outcomes identified for the selected nursing diagnoses for the pediatric patient could be stated as follows:

- The child and family will demonstrate knowledge of perioperative events and the role of various perioperative team members.
- The child's body temperature will be maintained at an appropriate level during the surgical intervention.
- The child's skin integrity will be maintained.
- The child will remain normovolemic.
- The child will be free from injury related to use of the electrosurgical unit.

Planning

Assessment data, combined with knowledge of the planned surgical procedure, allow the perioperative nurse to anticipate requirements for surgical positioning, instrumentation, equipment and supplies, medications, and activities necessary to prevent injury to the pediatric patient. Along with information about developmental levels and additional information specific to the individual child's physical and psychosocial status, the perioperative nurse develops a plan for patient care during surgery. For the five nursing diagnoses identified a Sample Care Plan has been developed. For each of the desired outcomes the perioperative nurse needs to identify criteria appropriate to the child and surgical setting. A Sample Care Plan for the pediatric patient might be as shown on p. 1213.

Implementation

Age-appropriate communication is important in implementing the pediatric nursing care plan. Implementation begins during the perioperative nursing assessment and continues through discharge to the PACU or other area.

Nursing Diagnosis: Knowledge deficit related to perioperative events

Outcome: The child and family will demonstrate knowledge of perioperative events and the role of various perioperative team members.

Interventions:

Perform preoperative visit and interview; educate the child and family, and provide emotional support.

Utilize audiovisual aids such as photographs, drawings, items for medical play, or a tour of the surgical suite.

Provide explanations on the child's level and at the parent's level of understanding.

Refer to nursing and other interdisciplinary team members to review, reinforce, or supplement preoperative education.

Nursing Diagnosis: Ineffective thermoregulation

Outcome: The child's body temperature will be maintained at an appropriate level during the surgical intervention.

Interventions:

Adjust room temperature approximately an hour before arrival of the child: 26° to 27° C (78.8° to 80.6° F) for infants and newborns; 23° to 24° C (73.4° to 75.2° F) for older children.

Consider wrapping lower extremities in Webril or stockinette and encasing in plastic bag for newborns and infants.

Place hyperthermia blanket on OR bed; adjust blanket temperature to 38° to 40° C (100.4° to 104° F).

Provide radiant heat lamp for use during placement of monitoring lines, induction of anesthesia, positioning, skin preparation, and draping.

Warm blankets, skin preparation solutions, irrigation, and other solutions to body temperature before use.

Use warmers during administration of intravenous fluids and blood products; temperature settings should not exceed 38° C (100.4° F).

Monitor body temperature by rectal, esophageal, tympanic membrane, or other automatic temperature-monitoring device.

Document temperature at prescribed intervals; take appropriate action for temperature extremes.

Nursing Diagnosis: Risk for impaired skin integrity

Outcome: The child's skin integrity will be maintained.

Interventions:

Check for allergies before choosing skin preparation solution.

Prevent skin preparation solutions from pooling at bedline or under child.

Utilize body supports that conform to the size of the child (rolled diapers, towels, sheets, flexible sandbags, foam rolls); use inflatable bag or rolled sheet in place of

kidney rest; use rolled towel for neck or shoulder elevation or support. Maintain all bed sheets and positioning supports dry and wrinkle free.

Provide infant armboards or use padded tongue depressors to stabilize limbs containing intravenous lines.

Position Mayo stand over child's legs and lower part of OR bed to support weight of drapes off child's body.

Use nonwoven, lightweight drapes (when possible) to reduce drape weight.

Determine any skin sensitivity to adhesive before application of self-adhering drapes or adhesive tape.

Have available and use nonallergenic or paper tape as indicated.

Nursing Diagnosis: Risk for fluid volume deficit

Outcome: The child will remain normovolemic.

Interventions:

Maintain and protect patency of intravenous lines.

Review laboratory analyses for results of total blood volume.

Calculate estimated total blood volume using formula of 85 to 90 ml/kg of body weight if total blood volume has not been determined by laboratory tests.

Provide gram scales for weighing sponges discarded from operative field; weigh sponges and report estimated loss.

Provide suction units with reservoirs that measure in 5 to 10 ml increments.

Measure and record quantity of irrigating fluid used.

Provide appropriate amounts of intravenous fluid replacement (such as 250 ml containers).

Measure and record urinary output and output from other drainage tubes.

Send laboratory specimens for analysis as indicated; review results indicating fluid status.

Nursing Diagnosis: Risk for injury related to use of electrosurgical unit

Outcome: The child will be free from injury.

Interventions:

Select appropriate size of adhesive electrosurgery dispersive pad; pad should be able to be molded or contoured to fit application surface yet provide sufficient body mass coverage.

Select pad application site with good tissue mass, as close to operative site as possible; shoulder, buttocks, thigh, or lengthwise on extremity may be selected.

Observe condition of skin at dispersive pad placement site before placement and on pad removal.

Apply dispersive pad with firm but gentle pressure.

Verify that child is not lying on cord or pad connection.

Protect dispersive pad site from pooling of solutions.

Check dispersive pad contact after any positional changes.

The toddler often fears parental separation and abandonment; separation or the surgical intervention may be perceived as a form of punishment. Toddlers fear, among other things, strangers, the dark, and machines. They attribute lifelike qualities to inanimate objects, believing that they, like the toddler, have feelings. Thus a blood pressure cuff that squeezes the child's arm may be perceived to be doing so because it is angry with the toddler. Toddlers may also believe that their body is held together by their skin; anything that violates the skin integrity is feared. For this reason plastic bandages are very important.

Toddlers react with the environment using their senses. The perioperative nurse should allow the toddler to touch and play with objects, such as putting a mask on a teddy bear, as appropriate. Sensory information should be provided in a soft, gentle voice: what things will look like and feel like and what the toddler will touch and hear. A security object is extremely comforting. The operating room should be quiet; background noise should be controlled. Instruments, which are frightening to the toddler, should be kept from view. The toddler should be brought into the room when everything is ready to allow quick induction of anesthesia.

The preschool and school-aged child may still perceive hospitalization or surgery as a punishment; there may be feelings of guilt associated with something the child thinks he or she said or did. Fear of bodily injury and mutilation, loss of control, and the unknown and being left alone characterize these developmental stages. The preschooler benefits from simple and concrete explanations. However, verbal explanations are not enough, and pictures, models, actual equipment, or play are important. Events should be reexplained as they occur; the perioperative nurse cannot assume the preschooler remembers previous explanations.

The school-aged child still fears painful procedures; death may also be a fear at this age. Simple explanations in familiar terms are helpful at this developmental stage; a book or other teaching aid is useful during explanations. This child should be given as many choices as possible (such as letting the child decide into which hand the intravenous line will be inserted or choose desired flavoring for the induction mask).

Adolescents may fear peer rejection, disability, loss of a body part, loss of control and status, altered body image, and perhaps death. They need as much privacy as possible, and their attempts to be independent should be respected. The adolescent may not wish to show any fear. Questions might not be asked while the parents are present. The perioperative nurse should provide explanations and answer questions as reasonably and truthfully as possible. If appropriate, some choices should be allowed, such as wearing underwear to the operating room. The presence of parents during as much of the preoperative period as possible may be very helpful for both young children and parents. Patient care procedures that violate privacy, such as hair removal, skin preparation, and insertion of an indwelling urinary catheter, should be conducted after anesthesia is induced.

Key points in providing perioperative care to pediatric patients include never leaving the child unattended, keeping the room quiet during induction, allowing the child to express fear and fearful behaviors (such as crying), using simple words without double meanings, allowing security objects to remain with the child until induction has been completed, and not being dishonest. If the child asks if something will hurt, explain that it will hurt like something they are familiar with (a bee sting, mosquito bite, and so on). The way children fall asleep during induction is likely to be the way they will wake up; thus all attempts should be made to calm and reassure the child. Parents should be alerted to delays in the surgery schedule; in some instances, the child may be sent back to the pediatric unit if surgery is delayed (Research Highlight 29-1).

Implementing the nursing care plan includes continual assessment and reassessment as well as the initiation of activities that facilitate the surgical intervention and anticipate patient needs. In addition to positioning, surgical skin preparation, creating and maintaining a sterile field, collecting, dispensing, and recording specimens, administering medications, and providing a safe environment, special instruments and sutures must be provided for the pediatric patient.

29-1 RESEARCH HIGHLIGHT

In the past decade ambulatory surgery has increased dramatically. In pediatrics this change brings economic as well as psychologic benefits. However, despite the fact that the child is separated from the family for a minimal amount of time, any type of surgery is a stressful event. The purpose of this study was to explore parents' perceptions of the stressors they and their children experienced as a result of the day surgery experience. A descriptive study was used with the interview conducted in the child's home. The sample was six parents of children ranging from 15 months to 18 years of age undergoing adenoidectomy. The interviews were conducted 1 to 3 days before the child's surgery and 3 to 5 days postoperatively. The interviews consisted of six open-ended questions. In the results of the study parental stressors were identified. Recommendations to decrease these stressors are to provide the family with current and timely information, lessen the period of separation of the child from the parents, and provide privacy and respect of the family's needs and support to the family.

From Maligalig, R.M.L. (1994). Parents' perceptions of the stressors of pediatric ambulatory surgery. *Journal of Post Anesthesia Nursing, 9*(5), 278-282.

Instrumentation

The same types of instruments used in adult surgery are used in pediatric surgery. However, pediatric instruments are usually shorter, have more delicate or less pronounced curves, and are lighter. A complete range of instrument sizes is necessary to make the appropriate size available for each child. Fewer instruments are normally required because incisions in children are shorter and more shallow than those in adults. Use of basic instrument sets, grouped according to types of surgery performed (such as minor or major), facilitates instrument counts. These sets are easily adapted to the patient's needs, as well as the surgeon's needs, and eliminate unnecessary instruments from the sterile field.

The following sets are examples of instrumentation used in surgery. The minor set is used for procedures such as inguinal hernia repair, or pyloromyotomy. The major set is used for major chest and abdominal cases such as tracheoesophageal fistula (TEF) and diaphragmatic hernia repair, omphalocele repair, and resection and pullthrough for Hirschsprung's disease. Smaller and larger instruments should be packaged separately and dispensed to the surgical field as required.

In addition to basic instruments, the minor pediatric instrument set should include a fine, short needle holder; straight and curved strabismus scissors; straight and curved mosquito hemostats; thymus/Lukens, phrenic, and Cushing vein retractors (two of each); and 6-inch Debakey forceps. The major pediatric instrument set should include the components of the minor set, plus additional regular straight and curved mosquito hemostats; Péan forceps; fine and regular Schnidt forceps; right-angled clamp; Lahey gall duct forceps; army-navy, small Deaver, and Richardson retractors (2 of each size); Debakey forceps, 6 inch and 7½ inches; Tuttle forceps; knife handles, #7 and #3; grooved director; tonsil and small Poole suction tubes; and Frazier suction tip, #11.

Sutures

Small sizes of absorbable and nonabsorbable sutures are appropriate for the delicate and fragile tissues of infants and children. Sutures should have attached needles (atraumatic) to reduce tissue damage. The most common sizes are #000 to #5-0 with ½- and ⅜-circle needles. Staples, both pediatric and regular sizes, are often used. Many skin incisions are closed with subcutaneous suture using subcuticular techniques; paper adhesive dressing strips or collodion is then applied. If collodion is used, care must be taken to ensure that the electrosurgical unit has been turned off before collodian is dispensed and applied to the incision line because of its high flammability.

Evaluation

The perioperative nurse evaluates care provided throughout the perioperative period. At the conclusion of the surgical intervention, the skin is inspected, especially at dependent pressure points and at the site of the electrosur-gical dispersive pad. Inspection is carried out to detect any reddened, irritated areas or evidence of compression injury. The temperature of the skin is noted, as is the core temperature. The cardiopulmonary status is closely monitored as the child emerges from anesthesia; the perioperative nurse assists anesthesia personnel during emergence and protects the child from injury. Dry, warm blankets are provided. Hydration status is determined, replacement fluids are administered, and fluid output is noted. The child is transferred to and positioned on the PACU stretcher. The airway is protected, as are tubes, drains, and drainage devices. Supplemental oxygen may be given during transport from OR to PACU (Research Highlight 29-2).

The perioperative nurse provides an oral report to the PACU nurse, focusing on the condition of the child, the response to surgery and anesthesia, presence of catheters and drains, the quality and amount of wound drainage, a description of the dressings applied, and any special needs.

29-2 RESEARCH HIGHLIGHT

An immediate concern for any patient after surgery is airway compromise. This is especially true for pediatric patients who have more acute airway changes than adults. Children are physically smaller than adults, and their airway anatomy is different. The purpose of this study was to identify pediatric patients immediately after surgery who would desaturate to less than 90% when transported from the OR to the PACU and to describe oxygen saturation levels of these patients during the perioperative period. A descriptive correlations design was used. The sample consisted of 45 children between 2 months and 13 years of age who had elective surgery using general anesthesia for more than 1 hour. Oxygen saturations were measured at five different intervals: (1) in the preoperative holding area, (2) in the OR, (3) during transport to the PACU, (4) on arrival, and (5) during the stay in the PACU. The patients were transported without oxygen, except for those intubated or with tracheostomy. Oxygen was administered within 1 minute after arrival to the PACU. Results showed that before administration of oxygen in the PACU 68% of the patients had oxygen saturations at or lower than 95% with 12% of the patients having saturations lower than 90%. As transport time increased, the number of patients with oxygen saturation levels below 95% also increased. Patients under 2 years showed the greatest risk for desaturation. The investigation of the study recommended the use of supplemental oxygen when one is transporting pediatric patients from the OR to the PACU.

From Fossum, S.R., & Knowles, R. (1995). Perioperative oxygen saturation levels of pediatrics patients. *Journal of Post Anesthesia Nursing, 10*(6), 313-319.

Part of this report should focus on the outcomes established in the perioperative care plan. For the care plan presented in this chapter, they might be as follows:

- The child and family demonstrated knowledge of perioperative events and the roles of perioperative team members.
- The child's body temperature was maintained at an appropriate level during the surgical intervention.
- Skin integrity was maintained.
- The child remained normovolemic.
- There was no evidence of injury related to use of the electrosurgical unit.

A summary of this transfer report should be documented.

The perioperative nurse may receive further feedback on the child's progress after the child is discharged from the PACU; this information may be relayed by the surgeon, unit nurse, or clinical nurse specialist. This type of informal feedback helps close the loop of information. It allows the perioperative nurse to informally collect additional data regarding effectiveness of the care plan and provides information about the outcomes of the perioperative care provided.

Patient and Family Education and Discharge Planning

Patient and family teaching varies significantly based on the type of surgery performed. Many hospitals provide special preoperative teaching and orientation sessions for pediatric patients and their parents that help to reduce their stress during the perioperative period. Basics of postoperative care are reviewed with the parents at this time. Parents should be advised to be alert for certain signs and symptoms during the postoperative recovery period that could indicate an infectious process, such as fever, pain, nausea, redness around the incisional area, drainage ("pus") from the wound, or difficulty breathing. These signs and symptoms may develop days or even weeks after surgery. It is important that parents understand the necessity of not ignoring any of these signs and to report them to the surgeon or nurse promptly so that an early diagnosis can be made and treatment prescribed.

Discharge orders are of great variety depending on the type of surgery done and should be followed closely to benefit the patient. Typical discharge orders might include the following:

- No strenuous activity (such as no physical exertion, swimming, contact sports, or bike riding) until released by the doctor. Parents are encouraged to ask during the follow-up visit when the child can resume these activities.
- No school or day care until after the follow-up visit or as instructed by the doctor.

- Wound should be kept clean and dry. (Bandages are sometimes not necessary.)
- Child may take a sponge bath or shower but not a tub bath (to avoid soaking the wound).
- Written discharge instructions are given to parents to reaffirm understanding of discharge orders.
- The phone number of the doctor or nurse will be given to the parents for potential use postoperatively in case a problem should arise.
- An appointment for the child's follow-up visit may be made before discharge or the parents are directed to call the doctor's office to schedule the appointment.

SURGICAL INTERVENTIONS

Pediatric surgery encompasses all specialties but, in general, can be divided into three major areas: congenital malformations or defects, acquired diseases of infancy and childhood, and trauma. Several surgical procedures that may be designated pediatric have been presented in previous chapters of this text under particular specialty headings. Surgical interventions presented here include procedures that are commonly and uniquely performed in the area of pediatric general and cardiac surgery.

CORRECTION OF GASTROINTESTINAL DISORDERS

Central Venous Catheter Placement

The exposure and cannulation of a major vessel for the purpose of inserting and positioning a catheter in the vena cava just above the atrium are indicated for infants and children who require total parenteral nutrition (TPN) because feeding through the gastrointestinal (GI) tract is impossible, inadequate, or hazardous. Common conditions necessitating TPN are bowel fistulas, inadequate intestinal length, chronic diarrhea, extensive burns, and multiple trauma. The TPN fluids are delivered through a central venous catheter to avoid peripheral inflammation and thrombosis. Occasionally a central venous catheter is indicated for infants or children who require chemotherapy, antibiotic therapy, or other long-term IV medical treatment.

The preferred site of placement is the external jugular vein. The internal jugular may be chosen if the external jugular has been used or is too small. From the cannulation site the catheter is tunneled under the skin about 5 to 10 cm. This is done to inhibit contamination of the bloodstream from frequent dressing changes. In cases where the internal or external vein sites are unavailable, the catheter may be placed into the external iliac vein by way of a cutdown in the greater saphenous vein. In these cases the catheter is tunneled out into the abdominal wall.

Procedural considerations

The manufacturer's instructions for handling, preparing, and sterilizing the catheter must be followed. The catheter must not contact linty materials, glove powder, or other foreign matter. Before insertion the catheter is flushed and filled with the infusion solution, special formula, or dextrose 10% in water to prevent air bubbles from entering the circulatory system and to eliminate blood clots in the catheter lumen. The catheter is connected to the pump, and infusion should begin as soon as the catheter is secured. In some instances the catheter is flushed with a dose-dependent (according to the child's size) heparin solution and pump infusion begun in the PACU.

The child is appropriately positioned as dictated by the site chosen for cannulation. The area is prepped and draped.

Operative procedure

1. A transverse incision is made over the lower portion of the medial border of the sternocleidomastoid muscle.
2. The external jugular vein is exposed and prepared for cannulation.
3. Using a long, hollow needle with an obturator (a tendon passer or neurotunneler may be used on a larger child) a subcutaneous tunnel is created, extending from the neck incision to the chest wall medial to the nipple.
4. The obturator is withdrawn, and the catheter is passed through the needle. The needle is removed, and the catheter then lies in the subcutaneous tunnel.
5. The external jugular vein is ligated distally and incised; the catheter is passed into the vein and advanced so that it lies at the point where the superior vena cava enters the atrium.
6. The position of the catheter is then confirmed by radiography in the operating room.
7. The catheter is secured at the exit site on the chest wall with nonabsorbable sutures.
8. Antimicrobial ointment is applied to the exit site, and an occlusive, transparent dressing is placed over this. The catheter is coiled under this dressing to avoid tension on the line and accidental displacement.
9. The infusion pump is connected to the infusing solution before the child is moved from the OR bed or when the child arrives in the PACU.

Repair of Atresia of the Esophagus

Atresia of the esophagus is repaired through a right retropleural thoracotomy, with closure of the TEF and anastomosis of the segments of the esophagus.

This congenital anomaly may arise between the third and sixth weeks of fetal life. Several types are recognized, the most common being an upper segment of esophagus ending in a blind pouch and a lower segment of esophagus communicating by a fistula with the trachea (esophageal atresia with TEF). Ideally this defect is recognized in the first hours of life, but more often the diagnosis is made in the first 36 to 48 hours of life. Drooling, the need for frequent suctioning, and coughing or cyanosis during oral feeding are the most common presentations.[4] Prompt surgical intervention allows the child to breathe and eat without the danger of aspirating mucus, saliva, feedings, or stomach contents.

Procedural considerations

A gastrostomy may be done first to decompress the air-distended stomach, thus facilitating chest movement and ventilation and preventing reflux of stomach contents into the trachea. The patient is then positioned for a right thoracotomy (sometimes rather posteriorly), prepped, and draped. The major instrument set is required, with the addition of baby chest retractors; baby T, regular, and infant malleables; Senn retractors; Gemini mixters; neuromastoid retractors; dilators; vessel loops; ligating clips; cotton-tipped applicators; umbilical tape; appropriate size of chest tube; infant chest drainage system; appropriate size of Malecot catheter; Fogarty catheters; and mineral oil.

Operative procedure

1. The chest is entered through the fourth intercostal space. Removal of the rib is not necessary (Fig. 29-1, A).
2. The pleura is gently dissected off the chest wall (Fig. 29-1, B).
3. As the dissection proceeds posteriorly, the azygos vein is encountered, which is reflected inferiorly after its highest intercostal branches are divided to expose the fistula beneath (Fig. 29-1, C).
4. Tape or silk is passed under the fistula to apply traction gently (Fig. 29-1, D). Dissection of the mediastinum begins with the TEF and distal end of the esophagus. The vagus nerve is an important landmark for the distal end of the esophagus.
5. The fistula is clamped and transsected, leaving a thin cuff of esophageal tissue on the tracheal side to allow closure of the trachea without narrowing it and compromising the lumen of the airway (Fig. 29-1, E).
6. To close the fistula, three or four interrupted atraumatic sutures of 5-0 nonabsorbable suture are used.
7. The upper esophageal pouch is dissected; passage of a nasogastric or Replogle tube by the anesthesia provider aids in its identification.
8. The proximal pouch is then identified and dissected as needed to allow it to reach the distal esophageal segment with minimal tension for anastomoses. At this point the surgeon makes the decision to attempt primary anastomosis. If primary anastomosis is impossible, the distal esophagus is closed and tacked high on the prevertebral fascia. Infrequently the gap between the proximal and distal portions of esophagus is so

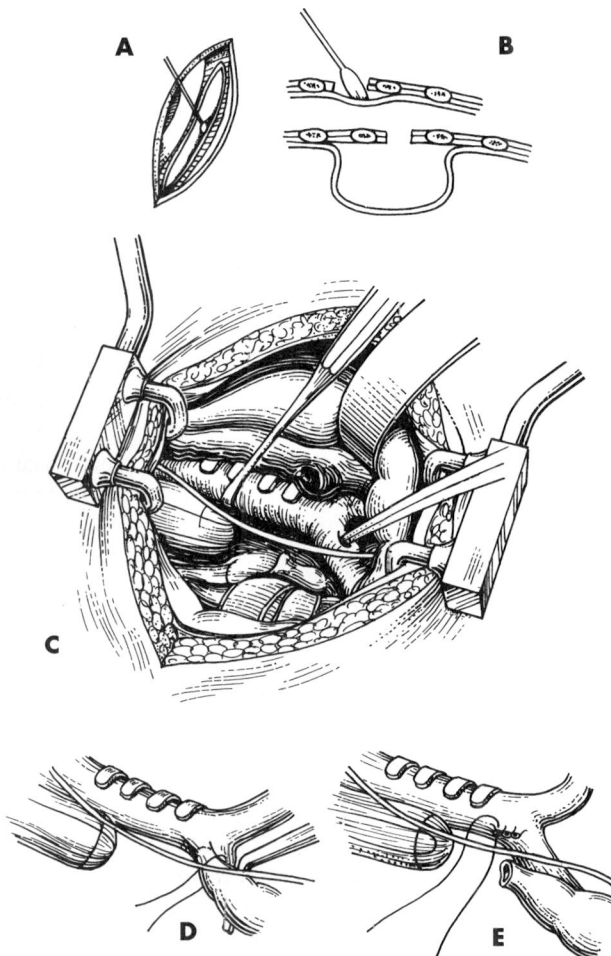

FIGURE 29-1 Repair of atresia of the esophagus. **A,** Incision at fourth intercostal space. **B,** Dissection of pleura off chest wall. **C,** Identification and division of azygos vein to expose fistula beneath. **D,** Traction applied to fistula. **E,** Transsection of fistula leaving 3 mm cuff on trachea.

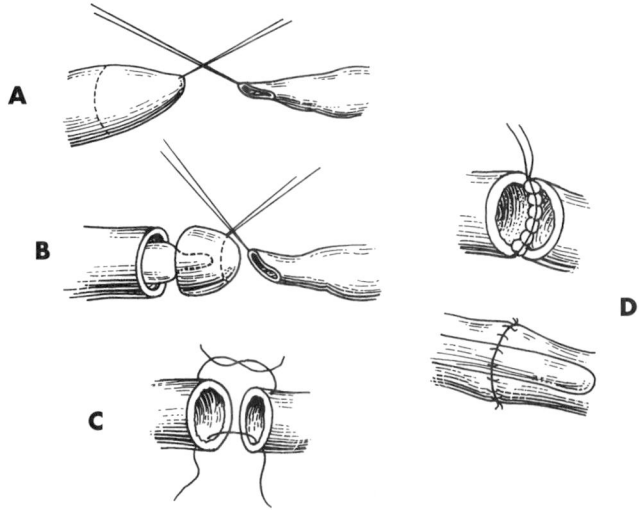

FIGURE 29-2 Primary repair of atresia of the esophagus: single-layer repair. **A,** Traction applied to proximal and distal portions of esophagus. **B,** Blind proximal pouch transsected. **C,** Full-thickness bites of anterior and posterior borders. **D,** Repair completed with Replogle tube in place to allow adequate lumen of esophagus.

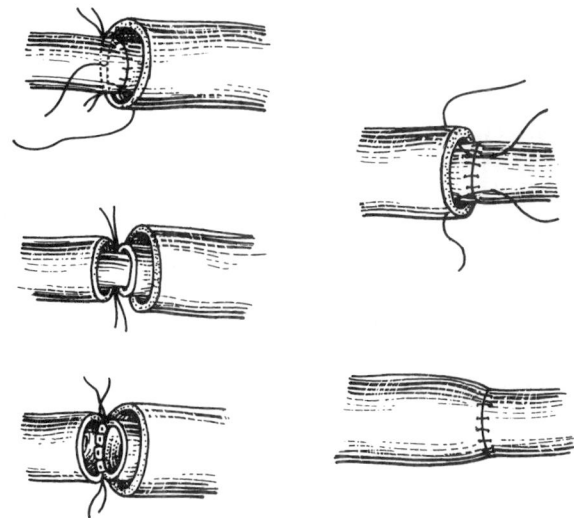

FIGURE 29-3 Haight anastomosis. Mucosal layer of proximal pouch sutured to full thickness of distal esophagus. Muscular sleeve of upper pouch pulled down over inner anastomosis and sutured to muscle of distal esophagus.

long that esophageal replacement is required. In these cases the upper pouch is brought out to the neck in the form of a cervical esophagostomy. When the child reaches 1 year of age, esophageal replacement is attempted through colon interposition or construction of a reverse gastric tube.

9. Primary anastomosis is performed with 5-0 or 6-0 nonabsorbable suture, taking full-thickness bites along anterior and posterior borders (Fig. 29-2). Some surgeons prefer the Haight, or two-layer, anastomosis (Fig. 29-3). The inner layer is composed of the upper pouch mucosa sutured to the full thickness of the distal esophagus. The muscular sleeve of the upper esophagus is then pulled down over the inner anastomosis and sutured to the muscular layer of the inferior esophagus. The incision is irrigated with saline.

10. Some surgeons place a 14 or 16 Fr extrapleural chest tube near the anastomosis through a posterior stab wound. It is secured with sutures to prevent it from putting direct pressure on the anastomosis.

11. Muscle layers are closed with interrupted 5-0 or 6-0 nonabsorbable sutures or continuous 3-0 absorbable suture.

12. Skin is closed with a continuous 5-0 suture, and a collodion dressing or dressing of gauze and tape is applied.

13. The extrapleural chest tube is water sealed after assurance that the number of centimeters of water and the suction-control chamber are appropriate for the size of the infant. A chest x-ray exam is performed.

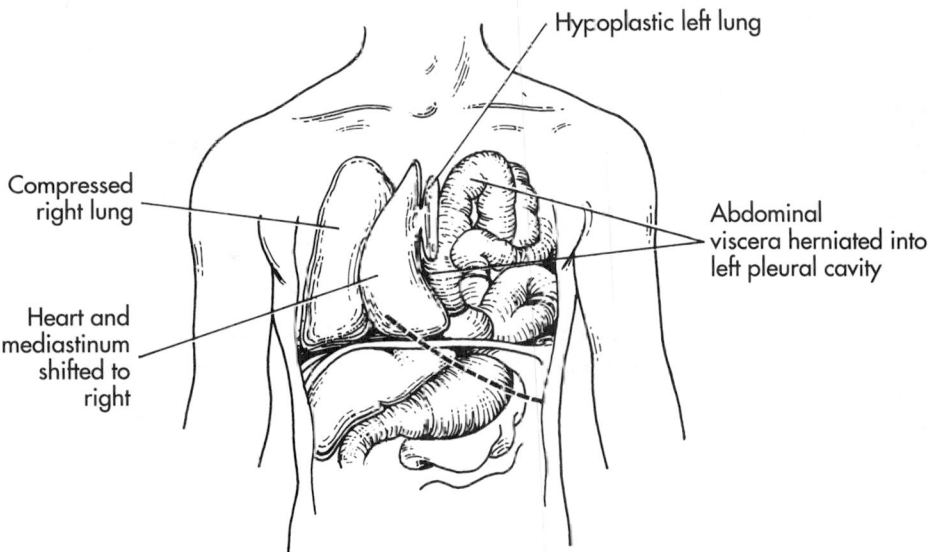

FIGURE 29-4   Diaphragmatic hernia.

Repair of Congenital Diaphragmatic Hernia

A congenital diaphragmatic hernia is repaired by replacement of the displaced viscera into the abdominal cavity with surgical correction of the defect (Fig. 29-4). The conventional surgical repair is through the abdomen. The concurrence of intraabdominal abnormalities is somewhat high in babies with diaphragmatic hernia; therefore treatment is facilitated with an abdominal approach. It is technically easier to extract the viscera from below than to push them out of the thorax. The abnormal intrathoracic intrusion of the abdominal viscera usually causes severe compromise of intrathoracic pulmonary and vascular activities. Therefore urgent restoration of more normal intrathoracic and intraabdominal relationships is the rule in these newborns. The lung may be hypoplastic because of prolonged compression in utero by the displaced abdominal viscera. A residual intrapleural space usually remains for a few days after surgery.

Procedural considerations

A chest tube can be inserted and connected to water-seal drainage. Insertion of a gastrostomy tube minimizes postoperative distention and facilitates feeding. Direct suturing of the margins of the defect is usually possible. Insertion of a prosthetic Silastic sheeting is occasionally required, and the sheeting should be available.

The major instrument set is required, plus the following: medium ligating clips; baby malleables; baby Deavers; appropriate size of chest tube; umbilical tape; infant chest drainage system (may fill to either 3.5 or 5 cm of water based on surgeon's preference); red rubber catheter; and mineral oil. Neuromastoid retractors, chest retractors, bone wax, and Marlex mesh or Silastic sheeting

should be available. The infant is positioned supine on a hyperthermia blanket.

Operative procedure

1. A contralateral chest tube may be placed in the anterior axillary line of the second intercostal space to prevent tension pneumothorax during surgery.
2. A subcostal incision going through all muscle layers is made on the side of the defect.
3. The abdominal viscera are withdrawn from the chest and held downward through the abdominal wound. Because abnormalities of abdominal viscera such as malrotation are associated with diaphragmatic hernia, the surgeon performs careful inspection of the organs at this time. If a malrotation is found, some surgeons prefer to repair it if the clinical condition of the infant allows it.
4. The defect is then carefully inspected, including a search for a hernia sac, which is present in less than 5% of cases. If a sac is identified, it is excised. An ipsilateral chest tube is placed before the diaphragm is closed.
5. The posterior and anterior rims of the diaphragm are identified, and primary closure is performed with mattress sutures of 2-0 nonabsorbable material. If the rim of tissue is too small for mattress sutures, ample sutures of 2-0 or 3-0 nonabsorbable are used. Occasionally, reinforced Silastic sheeting may be needed if sufficient diaphragm is not available for primary closure.
6. Gastrostomy is then performed in most cases.
7. The abdominal wall is then closed. If the musculature cannot accommodate the abdominal viscera, it is left open, and the skin is closed to leave a ventral hernia. In severe cases, the patient may be given extracorporeal membrane oxygenation (ECMO) for several days

before repair of the defect. The infant is returned to the operating room within 7 days for repair of the ventral hernia.

Nissen Fundoplication

Nissen fundoplication is the wrapping of the fundus of the stomach around the esophagus at the gastroesophageal junction. Nissen fundoplication is indicated for infants and children who suffer from severe gastroesophageal reflux disease (GERD). The cause of GERD in these patients is believed to be an inadequate antireflux barrier. The antireflux barrier consists in a combination of anatomic and physiologic factors, including sufficient amount and strength of muscle fibers located in the lower esophageal sphincter, adequate length of the abdominal esophagus, and a high-pressure zone in the lower esophagus. The combination of these factors forms the antireflux barrier and thus prevents GERD. An incompetent antireflux barrier can result in life-threatening complications of GERD, including obstructive apnea, aspiration pneumonia, esophagitis, and failure to thrive. The goal of the Nissen fundoplication is to recreate a competent antireflux barrier.

Procedural considerations

The major instrument set is required, plus the following: medium ligating clips, drain (¼ to ⅜ inch); sterile specimen cup, and appropriate-sized Malecot

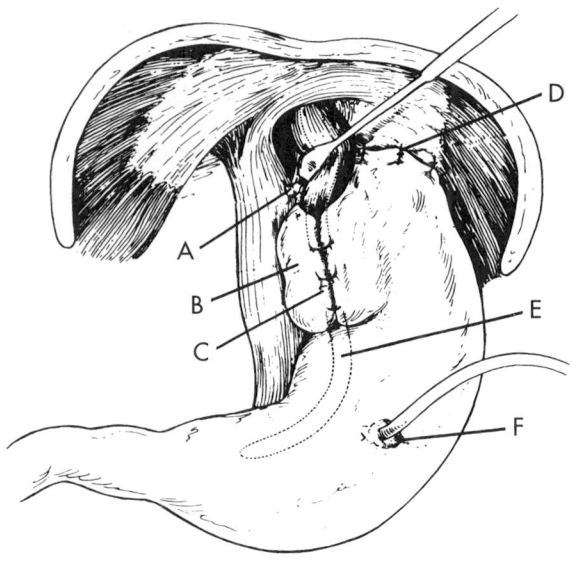

FIGURE 29-5 Salient features of Nissen fundoplication in infants. **A,** Crural sutures to reduce hiatus. **B,** Generous loose, adequate tissue in wrap. **C,** Sutures placed through seromuscular depth of both gastric and esophageal walls. **D,** Sutures to fix fundus to diaphragm. **E,** Appropriate-sized mercury-filled dilator to ensure adequate lumen. **F,** Gastrostomy in all infants and whenever there is any question of gastric outlet problems.

catheter. Have available the following: Deaver retractors, long instruments; self-retaining abdominal retractor systems; and Maloney dilators.

The patient is positioned supine. The surgeon (before scrubbing) or the anesthesia provider (during the procedure) passes the appropriate size of dilator into the esophagus to prevent the wrap from impinging on the lumen of the esophagus (Fig. 29-5).

Operative procedure

1. A left subcostal incision is performed to allow exposure of the lower esophagus to create adequate intraabdominal length.
2. The esophagus is mobilized to create adequate intraabdominal length.
3. The stomach is mobilized to allow loose wrap of the fundus around the esophageal junction; it is used as the lower edge of the wrap.
4. Sutures of 3-0 or 4-0 nonabsorbable are placed through the seromuscular layers of both stomach and esophagus to fix the wrap.
5. Sutures are then placed to tack the fundus to the diaphragm (fundoplication); the posterior fundus is wrapped behind the esophagus and the anterior fundus in front. Two layers of sutures may be used. The first layer passes from the anterior fundus, through the right margin to the posterior fundus. The second layer may be added between the anterior and posterior fundus for additional security.[6]
6. Some surgeons place clips at the level of the gastroesophageal junction and the wrap to aid in follow-up radiographic studies. A gastrostomy is done in most cases. The incision is closed in layers, and a collodion dressing is applied.

Ramstedt-Fredet Pyloromyotomy for Pyloric Stenosis

The Ramstedt-Fredet pyloromyotomy for pyloric stenosis is the incision of the muscles of the pylorus to treat congenital hypertrophy of the pyloric sphincter that is obstructing the stomach. Signs and symptoms of high GI obstruction appear at 2 to 6 weeks of age. The first sign is projectile vomiting that is free of bile. There may be a severe loss of body fluids and electrolyte imbalance, evidenced as hypochloremic, hypokalemic metabolic alkalosis. Once the diagnosis of hypertrophic pyloric stenosis is made, either through physical examination or imaging techniques, surgical correction is planned.

Procedural considerations

The stomach is emptied just before induction of anesthesia, and the nasogastric tube is removed to guard against reflux of gastric contents around the tube during induction. A minor instrument set and a pyloric spreader are used. The patient is prepped in the usual manner.

Operative procedure

1. The abdomen is opened through a right subcostal transverse skin incision. The rectus muscle is retracted or split longitudinally in the middle with spreading clamps, and the peritoneum is opened.
2. After the hypertrophied pylorus is delivered into the wound with a small vein retractor, the prepyloric area is grasped and rotated to expose the anterior superior border of the mass.
3. An incision is made in the serosa on the anterior wall of the pyloric mass from the duodenal junction proximally to a point proximal to the area of hypertrophied muscle (Fig. 29-6, *A*). The circular muscle is spread with the pyloric spreader on the submucosal base, so that all muscle fibers are completely divided (Fig. 29-6, *B*).
4. After completion of the separation the pyloric end of the stomach is returned to the abdomen, and the peritoneum and posterior rectus sheath are closed with a continuous, 3-0 absorbable suture. The anterior rectus sheath is closed with a 4-0 absorbable suture.
5. The skin is closed with fine subcuticular sutures. Small adhesive strips or collodion is applied as dressing.

EMERGENCY GASTROINTESTINAL PROCEDURES

Gastrostomy

Gastrostomy is establishment of a temporary or permanent channel from the gastric lumen to the skin to permit gastric emptying, liquid feeding, or retrograde dilatation of an esophageal stricture. The procedure may be emergent in nature or performed with other surgical procedures to facilitate care of the infant or child after surgery. Placement of the gastrostomy tube may be through an abdominal incision (described below) or percutaneously by means of an endoscope and local anesthesia (PEG). For children receiving long-term gastrostomy feedings a skin-level device (such as Button, Gastroport) may be inserted after the gastrostomy is well established. These devices, which protrude slightly from the abdomen, are more cosmetically acceptable and allow more mobility for the child.

Procedural considerations

A minor instrument set is required, plus a mushroom or Malecot catheter (#14 or #16 for infants and #18, #20, or #22 for older children) and a #11 knife blade on a knife handle. Routine prepping is done.

Operative procedure

1. A short incision is made over the outer border of the left rectus muscle (Fig. 29-7, *A*).
2. The subcutaneous tissues and rectus fascia are exposed with two small retractors (Fig. 29-7, *B*).
3. The anterior rectus fascia is opened, and the rectus muscle is split with clamps for exposure of the posterior rectus sheath (Fig. 29-7, *C*).
4. The peritoneum is opened for exposure of the liver edge and the greater curvature of the stomach (Fig. 29-7, *D*).
5. The stomach is pulled out through the wound with Babcock forceps. A circular purse-string suture of 4-0 nonabsorbable suture is placed; in the center of this a stab wound is made through the gastric wall (Fig. 29-7, *E*).

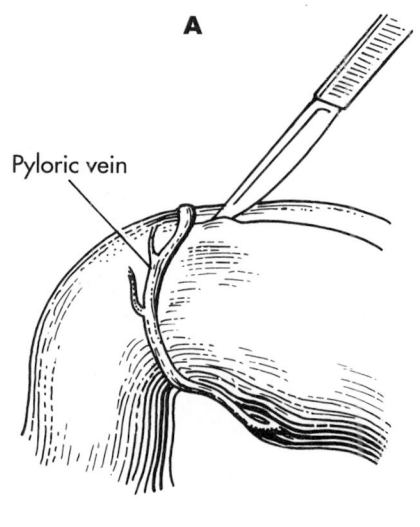

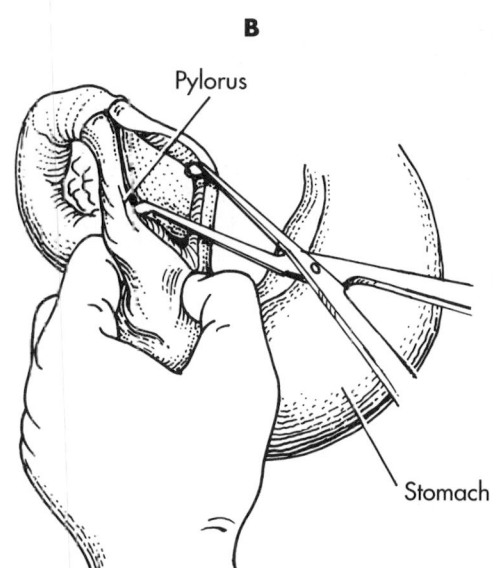

FIGURE 29-6 Operative technique for pyloric stenosis.

6. A mushroom catheter, often with the tip cut off, is inserted into the stomach, and the purse-string suture is tied (Fig. 29-7, *F*).

7. A second purse-string suture is placed outside the previous one, and the same needle is then taken through the peritoneum and the posterior rectus fascia to place the stomach against the peritoneum and thus prevent leaks (Fig. 29-7, *G* and *H*).

8. The catheter is brought out through a left lateral stab wound (see Fig. 29-7, *A*).

9. The stomach wall adjacent to the gastrostomy site is tacked to the undersurface of the peritoneum with interrupted 4-0 nonabsorbable sutures.

10. Routine abdominal closure is performed.

Before the gastrostomy tube is used for feedings, an upper GI study is usually performed to exclude the possibility of distal intestinal atresia.[15]

Omphalocele Repair

Omphalocele is the protrusion of abdominal viscera outside the abdomen into a sac of amniotic membrane and peritoneum at the base of the umbilical cord. There is no skin covering.

Omphalocele occurs during the eleventh week of fetal life when the viscera fail to withdraw from the exocelomic position and occupy the peritoneal cavity. The resulting abdominal wall defect can vary in size from 2 to 15 cm. The sac may contain only a few loops of bowel to nearly all the intestines and the liver and spleen. Associated anomalies include malrotation and abnormal fixation of the bowel.

Since the infant is at risk for hypothermia, hypoglycemia, shock, sepsis, and vascular injury to the bowel, immediate management after birth is necessary.[13] Treatment consists in applying warm saline packs on the sac surface, inserting a nasogastric tube to prevent distention

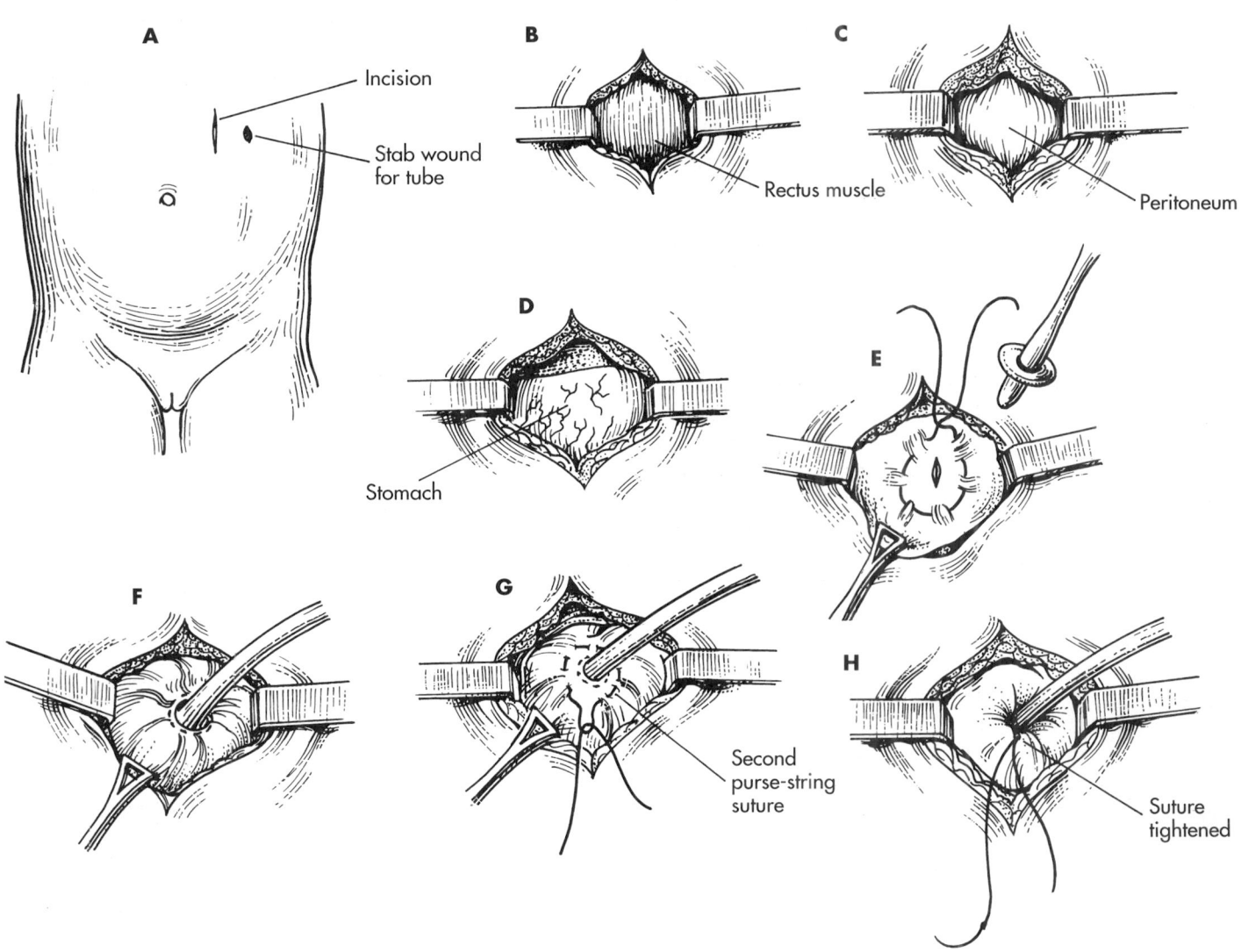

FIGURE 29-7 Gastrostomy. **A,** Incision. **B,** Rectus muscle exposed. **C,** Posterior rectus sheath exposed. **D,** Peritoneum opened. **E,** Purse-string suture placed. **F,** Mushroom catheter inserted. **G,** Second purse-string suture placed. **H,** Suture tightened.

and aspiration, and beginning intravenous access with fluid resuscitation and antibiotic therapy. Surgical intervention is necessary to prevent rupture of the sac, infection, or both. If intrauterine rupture of the sac has occurred, the newborn is kept warm, the bowel is inspected for perforation and torsion, and moist, warm dressings are applied.

An omphalocele is repaired by replacement of the viscera in the abdominal cavity, with reconstruction of the abdominal wall.

Procedural considerations

Particular attention to maintaining body temperature is essential because of the massive exposed surface area from which body heat can be lost. The use of nitrous oxide as an anesthetic agent is avoided during this procedure because it causes increased gas in the intestine, which in turn makes the reduction of abdominal contents into the peritoneal cavity more difficult. Repeated rectal irrigation with warm saline to evacuate meconium from the bowel may be carried out before the abdominal prep.

The major instrument set is required with the addition of the following: baby malleables; ligating clips; and a red rubber catheter. Silastic sheeting, Foley catheter with urimeter, Replogle tube, and a Malecot catheter should be available for potential use.

The infant is positioned supine, and the abdomen, umbilical cord, and sac are gently prepped with a povidone-iodine solution; if the prep solution is warmed, the manufacturer's directions should be followed.

Operative procedure

1. In the presence of small defects, primary closure is attempted. The skin edges are freed, and the sac is excised. Abdominal contents are gently relocated into the peritoneal cavity. The abdominal cavity is closed in layers using 3-0 nonabsorbable suture.
2. In certain cases where the defect is of medium to large size, a primary closure may not be accomplished. In these situations a staged procedure is done using prosthetic reduction. In the first stage the infant is brought to the operating room and positioned and prepped as previously described.
   a. The sac is excised, and the umbilical vein and arteries are ligated.
   b. Gastrostomy may be performed at this time.
   c. A silo is then created with Silastic mesh (Fig. 29-8). The mesh is secured through all layers of the edge of the defect using a continuous locking suture of 2-0 nonabsorbable (Fig. 29-8, *A*). The open end of the silo is closed in the same manner; thus a cylinder of mesh is created extending upward from the abdomen (Fig. 29-8, *B*).
   d. The open end of the cylinder is tied closed with umbilical tape (Fig. 29-8, *C*) or alternatively, attached to a specifically designed roller clamp.
   e. The mesh silo suture line and edge of the defect are wrapped with Kling dipped in an iodophor solution to prevent infection. The infant is transferred to an open Isolette, and the silo is suspended from the top of the Isolette. Plastic wrap is applied to the silo to prevent heat loss.
   f. The infant is then transported to the neonatal intensive care unit, where daily reduction of abdominal contents is performed by adding of a lower tie of umbilical tape or adjustment of the roller clamp. The abdominal viscera are completely reduced within 5 to 10 days, at which time the infant is returned to the operating room for the second stage of repair (Fig. 29-8, *D*).
   g. To avoid an appendectomy in the future on a child with a malrotated colon, an appendectomy may be performed at this time.
   h. The silo is removed, and the fascia is closed with interrupted 2-0 or 3-0 nonabsorbable sutures. The skin is closed with interrupted 4-0 nonabsorbable suture. In an attempt to create an umbilicus, a purse-string suture is utilized in closing the inferior 2 cm of incision.
3. Another technique for treating large omphaloceles is painting the sac and surrounding skin with a 2% solution of merbromin (Mercurochrome) until an

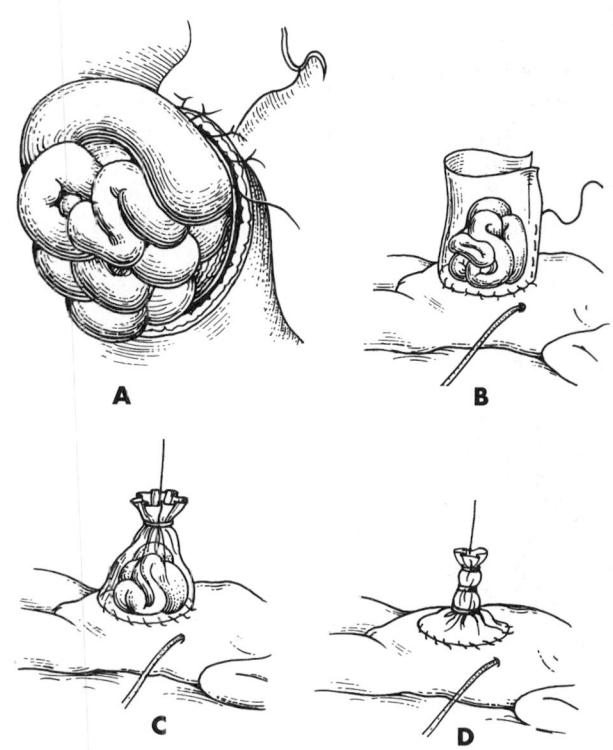

FIGURE 29-8 Staged repair of omphalocele. **A,** Silastic mesh secured to all layers of edge of defect. **B,** Silo closed, creating cylinder of mesh. **C,** Open end of silo tied with umbilical tape. **D,** Lower ties of umbilical tape applied to silo to gradually reduce viscera.

eschar forms to add strength to the sac and resist infection, or the sac may be treated with moist 0.5% silver nitrate dressings. The sac membrane gradually contracts, and skin closes the abdominal wall defect. Later surgery then repairs the abdominal musculature.

REPAIR OF HERNIAS

Umbilical hernia repair

An umbilical hernia, a condition commonly seen in pediatric populations and particularly in African-American children, is corrected by repair of the part of the intestine protruding at the umbilicus. An umbilical hernia is always covered by skin. Small umbilical hernias may be left untreated. They usually close within a few months to a year. If surgical repair is required in a large fascial defect, it may be delayed until the child is at least 2 years of age with some surgeons delaying repair until 4 years of age.

Procedural considerations

Surgical correction of umbilical hernia may be an ambulatory surgical procedure. General anesthesia is used. A minor instrument set is required. The child is prepped as discussed previously. Several variations in technique have been used; an infraumbilical approach is most common and is described below.

Operative procedure

1. An incision is made below the umbilicus through the skin and subcutaneous tissue.
2. Flaps of skin and subcutaneous tissue are mobilized and held back with small retractors to expose the rectus fascia and hernial protrusion.
3. The hernia sac, which is between the rectus muscle sheaths in the midline, is completely freed from all surrounding structures.
4. The hernia sac may be invaginated, dissected free and ligated, or excised.
5. The peritoneum is closed with a continuous suture.
6. The two edges of the rectus fascia are brought together using interrupted 3-0 nonabsorbable sutures.
7. Subcuticular closure of the skin with a continuous, fine, absorbable suture is performed, and a pressure dressing is applied.

Inguinal Hernia Repair

An inguinal hernia is corrected by repair of a protrusion of a hernia sac, containing the intestine, in the inguinal canal. The testis develops high on the posterior wall of the abdomen. It gradually descends into the scrotum. Before the testis enters the inguinal canal, the processus vaginalis projects downward but retains a communication with the peritoneal cavity. The upper part of the processus does not; the remaining sac constitutes an indirect inguinal hernia. In a girl, a similar hernial sac is contiguous with the round ligament.

Procedural consideration

A minor instrument set is used, and routine prepping is done.

Operative procedure

1. An incision is made over the inguinal area in the direction of the skin crease.
2. The subcutaneous tissue is opened, and hemostats are placed on bleeding vessels, which are then ligated or electrocoagulated.
3. Right-angle retractors are placed inferiorly and medially.
4. The external ring is identified, and the external oblique fascia is cleaned and freed with small Metzenbaum scissors.
5. The external oblique fascia is opened with a #15 knife blade on a knife handle, and the upper flap is freed. The lower flap is freed to expose the inguinal ligament.
6. Cord structures are opened at the upper end of the cord. Two forceps are used to grasp tissues at the same level and to separate them.
7. The hernia sac is grasped with a hemostat, and structures of the cord are peeled downward and away from the sac with forceps until the sac is freed. Care is taken to protect the spermatic cord and major vessels as the sac is freed.
8. After the sac is opened and the surgeon's index finger is inserted, the sac is pulled upward. The upward traction is maintained with two or three hemostats.
9. The sac is ligated with 3-0 nonabsorbable suture, and excess sac is removed. Repair of the inguinal canal may be done with nonabsorbable sutures.
10. The subcutaneous tissue is closed with interrupted, fine sutures; closure of the skin is with fine, nonabsorbable subcuticular sutures. Collodion or paper adhesive dressing strips are applied.

REPAIR OF OBSTRUCTIVE DISORDERS

Repair of Intestinal Obstruction

Repair of intestinal obstruction includes (1) untwisting of a volvulus, (2) division of a congenital band, (3) release of an internal hernia, (4) resection of bowel with an anastomosis, and (5) creation of an intestinal stoma.

Intestinal obstruction is the most frequent GI emergency requiring surgery in the newborn. Early recognition is essential. Surgical intervention is usually within the first few hours after birth; delay may increase the risk. Intestinal obstruction can occur in the infant for a variety of reasons: atresia, stenosis, congenital aganglionosis, meconium ileus, or malrotation. Lesions characterized by complete obliteration of intestinal lumen are classified as atresia. Those that produce a narrowing or partial obliteration of the lumen are classified as stenosis.

Procedural considerations

The major instrument set and pediatric intestinal instruments are required, plus culture tubes, syringes, and a 25-gauge needle. Routine prepping is done.

Operative procedure

1. The abdomen is opened through an incision appropriate to the exposure of the particular form of obstruction.
2. Exploration and displacement of the intestines to the abdominal wall help determine the obstructive lesion. With atresia or stenosis, the entire bowel must be examined to rule out multiple areas of involvement.
3. Detorsion or reduction of bowel decompression or resection is performed when indicated.

Reduction of Intussusception

Intussusception is the telescopic invagination of a portion of intestine into an adjacent part with mechanical and vascular impairment. It is relieved by reduction of invaginated bowel by the hydrostatic pressure of a barium enema or by laparotomy and manual manipulation.

Intussusception is the most common cause of intestinal obstruction in the 2-month to 3-year-old age group, and therefore one of the most common surgical emergencies in this age group. A frequent site for intussusception is the ileocecal junction. Intussusception in children is most often idiopathic; other causes may include Meckel's diverticulum, polyps, or hematoma of the bowel. Early diagnosis and reduction are essential to bowel viability.

Procedural considerations

The child is prepped for surgery as described previously. Reduction by barium enema should be attempted only with the full cognizance of the radiologist, surgeon, and pediatrician, with the operating room team on standby. Should reduction not be accomplished, a laparotomy must be done. The major instrument set is used with the addition of pediatric intestinal instruments.

Operative procedure

1. A right lower quadrant transverse or right paramedian incision is made, and the peritoneum is entered (Fig. 29-9, A).

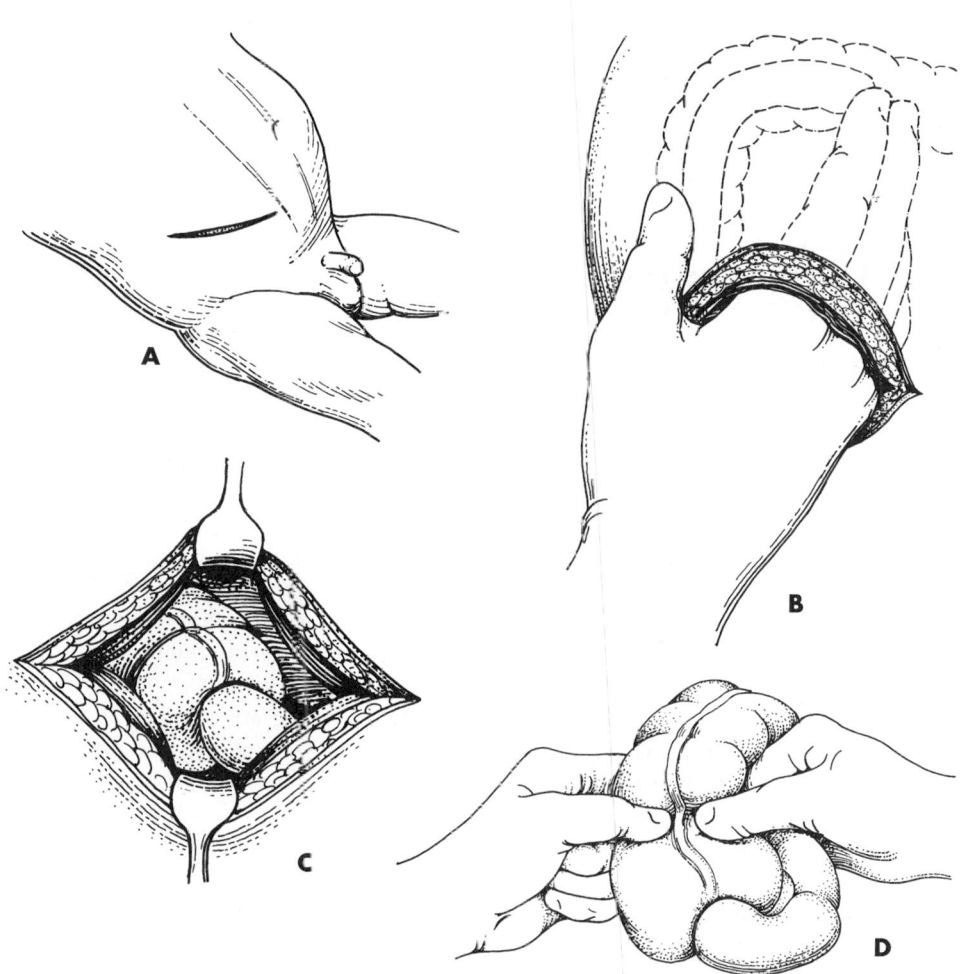

FIGURE 29-9 Reduction of intussusception. **A,** Transverse abdominal incision. **B,** Location of intussusception. **C,** Mass delivered into incision. **D,** Milking reduction.

2. The cecum and ileum are identified; the intussusception is located and elevated with fingers (Fig. 29-9, *B* and *C*).

3. If there is no evidence of bowel compromise, the bowel immediately distal to the intussusception is occluded with one hand and stripped proximally with the other in an attempt to achieve manual reduction (Fig. 29-9, *D*). If the serosa splits during attempted reduction, or if the mass cannot be reduced, bowel resection is done; this may be required in 35% to 41% of children.[14]

4. The abdomen is closed in layers, and the wound is dressed.

Colostomy

Colostomy is the surgical construction of an artificial excretory opening from the colon. Most congenital anomalies that result in colonic obstruction require a temporary colostomy. These include imperforate anus and Hirschsprung's disease. Both conditions ultimately require further pelvic operative procedures, and proper construction of a colostomy is important. In Hirschsprung's disease the colostomy must be placed in a section of bowel containing ganglia.

Procedural considerations

A major instrument set and pediatric intestinal clamps are used. The child is prepped as described previously.

Operative procedure

1. A transverse incision usually is preferred, and the abdomen is entered in the right upper quadrant for a transverse colostomy or the left lower quadrant for a sigmoid colostomy.

2. The loop of colon is freed of peritoneal attachments until it can be brought easily through the abdominal wall without tension.

3. The edges of the mesentery are then sutured to the parietal peritoneum, and the serosa of the colonic loop is sutured with fine absorbable suture materials to the peritoneum and fascia as well as the skin.

4. The colostomy may be sutured immediately. Some surgeons prefer to close the skin under a colostomy loop; others prefer to suture mucosa directly to skin edges. This decision may depend on the location of the colostomy. An important point is that each layer must be securely attached to the serosa of the colon to prevent evisceration and prolapse. The posterior wall of a loop colostomy may be divided by electrosurgery several days after surgery.

Procedures Requiring Colostomy

The following procedures require emergent colostomy at the time of presentation. Definitive repair of the anomaly usually occurs at about 1 year of age.

Resection and pullthrough for Hirschsprung's disease

Resection and pullthrough for Hirschsprung's disease, the definitive surgical procedure, consists in the removal of the aganglionic portion of the bowel and anastomosis of the normal colon to the anus. Hirschsprung's disease is characterized by the absence of ganglion cells in a distal portion of the bowel. The distal colon is more frequently involved, but the disease may encompass the entire colon, with a less favorable prognosis. The absence of ganglion cells results in a lack of peristalsis. The normal proximal colon becomes dilated, and intestinal contents do not pass through the involved segment. The child presents with an abnormally distended abdomen. On barium enema proximal distention of the colon is seen and then a transition zone where the bowel appears funnel shaped, followed by the distal aganglionic segment, which is narrowed. The child is taken to the operating room for a leveling colostomy. Multiple frozen-section biopsy specimens from the muscularis of the proximal portion of the colon are taken to determine the presence of ganglion cells. The colostomy is performed at the most distal portion of the colon that contains ganglion cells. Some surgeons prefer a routine right transverse colostomy at this time and delay frozen-section biopsy specimens until the time of the definitive procedure. The child is returned to the operating room for definitive repair at 1 year of age, if clinical and nutritional status permits.

Several surgical techniques have been devised. Soave's procedure of endorectal pullthrough employs internal bypass of the involved segment. The internal sphincter muscle of the anus is kept intact for continence.

Procedural Considerations

The patient is prepped and draped from the nipples down to and including the buttocks, genitals, perineal area, and upper thighs to permit positioning for the perineal stage without redraping. (Before preparation, the rectum may be irrigated with warm saline solution.)

A folded towel is placed under the buttocks. The patient is placed in the supine position with knees bent and legs in a modified ski position (hips and knees flexed) to facilitate abdominal and perineal approaches without redraping. An indwelling catheter is inserted to keep the bladder empty during the operation.

The *major instrument set*, extra towels and gloves, as well as the following are required: Foley catheter appropriate for size and age of patient; urimeter; Kitner dissectors; small and medium Kocher forceps; 3 ml and 5 ml syringes; 25 g needle; injectable saline; Penrose drain, ¼ inch; sterile safety pins; large dull rakes; small tonsil suction tubes; Hegar dilators. On *second Mayo stand*: a basic minor set; extra curved mosquito hemostats; small needle pad; tonsil hemostats; Penrose drain, ¼ inch; sterile safety pins; hand controlled electrosurgical pencil; suction; muscle stimulator; and nerve stimulator. *Have available*: Deaver retractors;

long instruments; gastrointestinal stapling device (GIA); ligating clips; extra #15 blades; Salem sump; K-Y jelly; rubber catheter (22 to 24 Fr); and mineral oil.

Operative Procedure

1. A left paramedian incision that includes the sigmoid colonic stoma, if present, is made.
2. The stoma is freed from the abdominal wall, and the left portion of the colon is mobilized. (If there is no sigmoid colonic stoma, the extent of aganglionic intestine is established by biopsy and frozen section, and all involved colon is excised. If a stoma is present and the area has already been established as normal, the colon above it constitutes the proximal end of the resection.)
3. The mesocolon and the vessels of the intestine to be resected are divided close to the intestine, with care taken to preserve the blood supply to the rectum (Fig. 29-10, *A*).
4. 4. The mucosal tube is freed from the outer muscular layers by sharp and blunt dissection with Metzenbaum scissors and a gauze-tipped instrument (Fig. 29-10, *B*).
5. A muscular sleeve is transsected, and traction sutures of 4-0 nonabsorbable are placed on the distal edge (Fig. 29-10, *C*). The mucosa is stripped down to the anus. The depth of the dissection may be checked by inserting a finger into the anus (Fig. 29-10, *D*).
6. When the mucosa is adequately freed, the perineal phase is started, and the perineal instrument table is used.
7. The anus is dilated and retracted with Allis forceps. A circumferential incision is made, and the mucosal stripping is completed (Fig. 29-10, *E*).
8. The proximal portion of the intestine is pulled

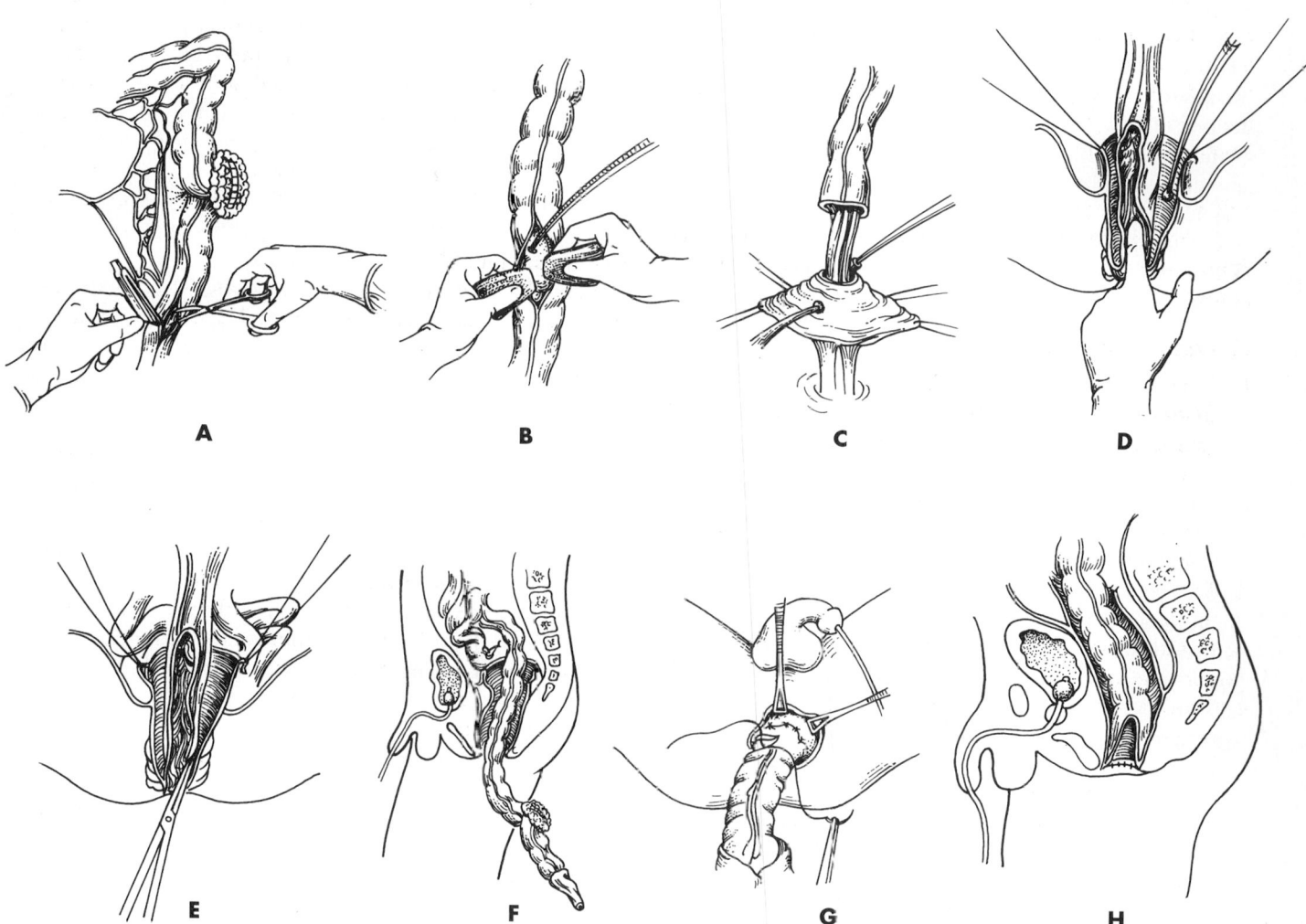

FIGURE 29-10 Pullthrough for Hirschsprung's disease. **A,** Dissection of mucosal tube begun through longitudinal incision. **B,** Gauze-tipped dissecting instrument used to dissect entire circumference of tube. **C,** Muscular sleeve transsected. **D,** Depth of dissection determined by insertion of finger into anus. **E,** Circumferential incision made. **F,** Mucosal tube and proximal portion of colon and stoma pulled through rectal muscular cuff. **G,** Anastomosis performed between all layers of colon and anal mucosa. **H,** Anastomosis completed.

through the rectal muscular sleeve and out the anus (Fig. 29-10, *F*). If the portion of colon to be resected is large, it is excised abdominally before the proximal portion of the intestine is pulled through the anus.

9. Absorbable sutures are used to secure the seromuscular layers of the intussuscepted colon to the rectal muscular cuff. The colon is divided into axial or longitudinal quadrants, and an anastomosis is performed with 3-0 absorbable sutures (Fig. 29-10, *G*).

10. Gowns and gloves are changed, and abdominal instruments are used. The abdominal phase of the operation is completed by approximating the proximal edge of the muscular cuff to the seromuscular layer of the colon with 4-0 nonabsorbable sutures (Fig. 29-10, *H*). The abdomen is closed in the routine manner, without the use of drains.

Repair of imperforate anus

An imperforate anus is repaired by establishing colorectoanal continuity through the external anal sphincter and closure of fistulas, if present. Imperforate anus presents in a variety of forms classified as low, intermediate, and high lesions. Girls commonly have low lesions, and boys primarily exhibit high lesions. A covered anus and anovulvar fistula is an example of a low lesion. A high lesion consists of a blind rectal pouch, a "flat bottom," and a posterior urethral fistula or fistula to the bladder. This type is the most prevalent and the most difficult to repair.

Repair of Low Imperforate Anus in a Girl: Anal Transposition
Procedural considerations

The infant is placed in the lithotomy position with the legs extended on skis. A Foley catheter is inserted, and the perineum is prepped and draped.

The major instrument set is required, with the addition of the following: extra towels; needle-point electrosurgical tip; suction; nasal speculums; small tonsil suction tube; Senn retractors; Foley catheter (check size) and urimeter; Kitner dissectors; Penrose drain, ½ inch; sterile rubber bands with small brass safety pins; K-Y jelly; Hegar dilators; Vaseline gauze; nerve stimulator; and muscle stimulator.

Operative procedure

1. An electrical stimulator is applied to define the center of the true anus.
2. Stay sutures are placed in the fistula, and it is excised using an oval incision (Fig. 29-11, *A*).
3. The bowel is dissected free from surrounding structures, with care taken not to damage the vagina (Fig. 29-11, *B*).
4. When the dissection is complete, a vertical midline incision is performed at the opening of the true anus, and the fibers of the external sphincter are identified (Fig. 29-11, *C*).

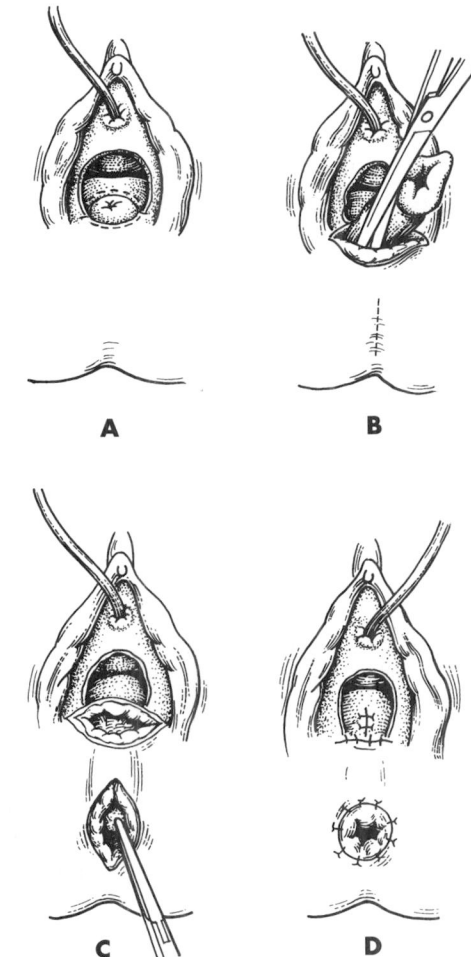

FIGURE 29-11   Anal transposition. **A,** Fistula excised by means of oval incision. **B,** Dissection of bowel from surrounding structures. **C,** Vertical midline incision at site of true anus; identification of external sphincter fibers; mobilized rectum pulled down through subcutaneous tissue to new location. **D,** External sphincter sutured to rectal mucosa; new anus constructed with interrupted sutures through all layers.

5. The mobilized rectum is pulled down through the subcutaneous tissue to its new location.
6. The end of the fistula is amputated. With interrupted sutures of 4-0 nonabsorbable, the external sphincter is sutured to the rectal serosa.
7. Using 4-0 absorbable suture, a new anus is constructed with interrupted sutures through all layers (Fig. 29-11, *D*).
8. A drain may or may not be placed in the anterior incision before it is closed in layers with interrupted 4-0 absorbable sutures.
9. A Hegar dilator is used to calibrate the size of the new anus after closure.

Repair of High Imperforate Anus: Posterior Sagittal Anorectoplasty

When a high imperforate anal anomaly presents, surgical intervention is indicated within 24 to 48 hours of life. A transverse or sigmoid colostomy is performed to irrigate the hiatal lumen and to remove meconium plugs while allowing proximal colon function. After the colostomy, further diagnostic studies, such as cystogram and vaginograms are done. The posterior sagittal anorectoplasty (PSARP) is the definitive surgical procedure and is performed when the condition and size of the child permits, usually around 1 year of age.

The PSARP is a highly technical procedure that utilizes electrostimulation throughout and may require position changes.

Procedural considerations

The child is placed in a prone jackknife position with the hips flexed. Adequate padding must be placed under the hips to avoid compression injury to the femoral nerves.

The major instrument set is required with the addition of the following: Foley catheter (check size) and urimeter; catheter tray; muscle stimulator and probe; needle-point electrosurgical tip; feeding tubes, 5 Fr and 8 Fr; mastoid retractors; Senn retractors; Stevens tenotomy scissors; orthopedic saw; marking pen; Hegar dilators; and K-Y jelly.

Operative procedure (Fig. 29-12)

1. The electrostimulator is used to locate the true anus, and a midsagittal incision is made through the skin from the midsacrum to the anterior border of the anal site.
2. Dissection continues through subcutaneous tissue until the external sphincter muscle layers are identified.
3. With electrostimulation, these fibers are dissected midsagittally, exactly in the midline.
4. A midsagittal split of the coccyx is performed, and the striated muscle complex found beneath the coccyx is incised sagittally along with the visceral endopelvic fascia. Electrostimulation is used to aid in identifying muscle complexes.
5. Next the rectal pouch and urethra are identified, and the bowel is incised vertically to expose the fistulae.
6. The fistula is closed in layers, first the mucosa with interrupted absorbable sutures and then the muscle layer with 5-0 nonabsorbable sutures.
7. The rectum is then mobilized and tapered to allow its placement within the muscle complexes. Tapering consists in excising a wedge of bowel from either the ventral or dorsal surface. The edges are approximated, and the mucosal layer is closed with 5-0 absorbable interrupted sutures. The muscularis layer is closed with interrupted 5-0 nonabsorbable sutures.
8. Again using electrostimulation, the tapered rectum is placed deep within the muscle complex. Then 5-0 nonabsorbable sutures are used to reconstruct the muscles. The seromuscular layer of the bowel is incorporated into these sutures to keep it securely positioned within the muscle complex.
9. The external sphincter muscles and coccyx are reapproximated.
10. Excess bowel is trimmed before it is secured to the skin edges of the anus.
11. Running absorbable subcuticular sutures are used to close the skin.

In cases of very high rectal pouches and fistulas, an abdominal approach may be required. At this point, after the midsagittal incisions and dissections are completed, a rubber tube is placed through the pelvis with one end in the peritoneal cavity and the other through the center of the anus to the skin, where it is temporarily sutured. The child is turned supine, and an abdominal incision is performed. The rectal pouch is mobilized, and the fistula is closed. The bowel is tapered as described previously, and the terminal portion is attached to the rubber tube, which then is used to pull the rectum through the anal orifice. The bowel is sutured to the muscle complex, and reapproximation of the coccyx and external sphincter muscle is done as described earlier.

CORRECTION OF BILIARY ATRESIA

Hepatic Portoenterostomy (Kasai Procedure)

The Kasai procedure is the construction of a bile drainage system by use of an intestinal conduit. Biliary atresia is a disease that results from nonpatent extrahepatic bile ducts that prevent the drainage of bile from the liver and lead to eventual cirrhosis. The Kasai procedure recreates a drainage system using a limb of intestine. This procedure is indicated in patients with extrahepatic biliary atresia who are under 3 months of age. All atretic segments of the existing bile ducts are removed. An operative cholangiogram and frozen-section biopsy of the hepatic duct remnant are prerequisites to the actual procedure.

Procedural considerations

The infant is positioned supine over a radiographic plate. Both a major instrument set and intestinal instruments are required, with the addition of the following: 3-way stopcock; 3, 6, 12 ml and 6 TB syringes; injectable saline; Hypaque dye (mix half dye, half saline); Foley catheter and urimeter; petri dishes; ligating clips; umbilical tape; mineral oil; Jelco catheters, 18 and 20 gauge; sterile light handles or light handle covers; sterile specimen cup; and Taut cholangiogram catheter. Have available the following: Deaver retractors, Kitner or Cherry dissectors, Carmalt hemostats, Kocher forceps, bowel clamps, headlight, drain, Malecot catheter, and Tru-cut biopsy needle.

Operative procedure

1. A right upper quadrant incision is made, and the gallbladder is identified.

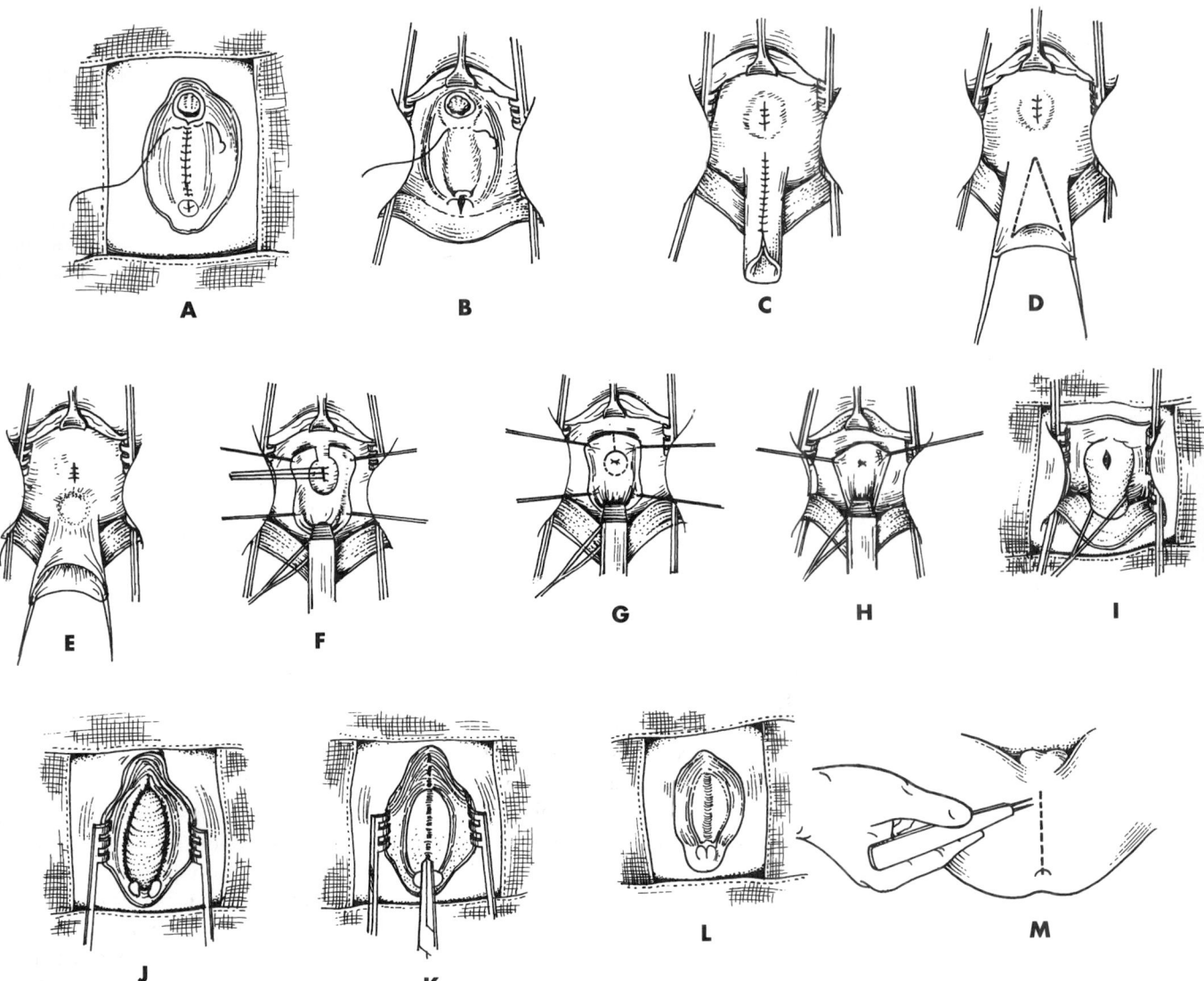

FIGURE 29-12 Posterior sagittal anorectoplasty. **A,** Line of incision and electrical stimulation to determine appropriate anal site. **B,** Midsagittal incision through coccyx and external sphincter fibers of anus, showing striated muscle complex deep to anal site; subcutaneous external sphincter extending about halfway to coccyx; superficial external sphincter inserting on coccyx; levator deeper in midline. **C,** Right-angled forceps beneath levator ani. **D,** All layers of striated muscle partially retracted laterally to expose visceral endopelvic fascia. **E,** Sagittal incision in terminal bowel after proximal dissection around rectum and placement of tape around rectum proximally. **F,** Retracted rectotomy showing fistula site. **G,** Semicircumferential incision through mucosa-submucosa for placement of first sutures to close fistula. **H,** Completed closure of fistula orifice. **I,** *Stippled area* where muscular bowel wall is left in place and *clear area* above where peritoneum may be encountered. **J,** Extent of anterior wedge resection for tapered repair of rectum *(dotted line).* **K,** Approximation of tapered edges of rectum. **L,** First and deepest suture for approximation of levators to establish beginning of canal. **M,** After reapproximation of levator ani to coccyx, interrupted sutures are placed in edges of superficial external sphincter muscle.

2. A small catheter is placed into the gallbladder and secured with a purse-string suture. Radiopaque dye is instilled into the gallbladder, and an x-ray film is taken. The surgeon notes free flow of bile through the ducts and the duodenum. Occasionally free flow of bile will be seen. These patients are then categorized as having correctable biliary atresia. In such situations a liver biopsy is performed, and the incision is closed. The majority of patients with correctable biliary atresia demonstrate progressive improvement. More commonly, though, there is a very small amount of flow or none at all. In these cases of noncorrectable biliary atresia the Kasai procedure is performed.

3. Because of the high incidence of associated anomalies, a thorough inspection of the intraabdominal organs is then performed.

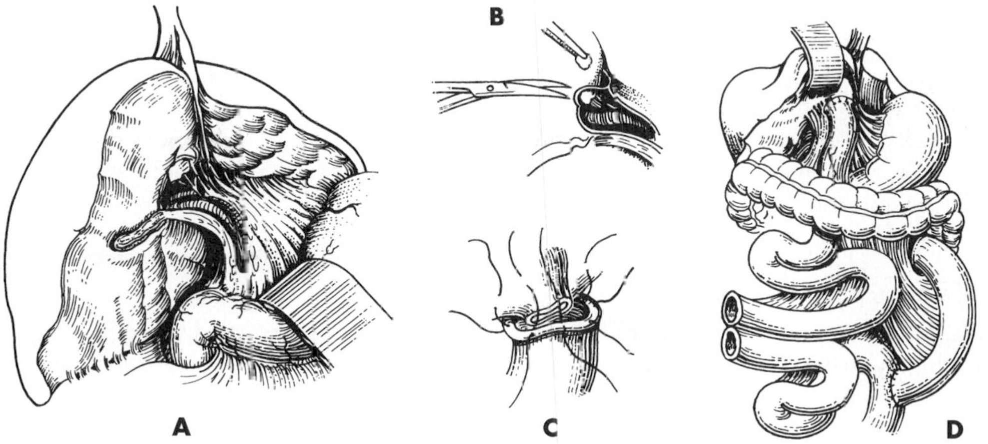

FIGURE 29-13 Kasai procedure. **A,** Exploration of hepaticoduodenal ligament and ligation of drainage structures. **B,** Transsection of hepatic duct remnant using frozen-section biopsy specimens as a guide. **C,** Anastomosis of jejunal conduit at porta hepatis. **D,** Exteriorization of conduit using double-barreled Roux-en-Y approach.

4. The hepatoduodenal ligament is explored, and all drainage structures are ligated (Fig. 29-13, *A*).
5. The hepatic duct remnant is identified and traced to the liver hilum. The remnant is transsected as high as possible using frozen-section biopsy specimens as a guide. Frozen-section biopsy specimens are also obtained at the portahepatis to denote the presence of ductules. Precise identification of this location is essential (Fig. 29-13, *B*).
6. The proximal portion of the jejunum is generally used as the intestinal conduit. A meticulous anastomosis is performed at the portahepatis as previously identified using a single running layer of absorbable sutures (Fig. 29-13, *C*).
7. The conduit is exteriorized with a double-barreled Roux-en-Y approach (Fig. 29-13, *D*).
8. A liver biopsy is then performed.
9. A drain is placed, and the incision is closed in layers.

The procedure described above is one approach of many. Others include exteriorization of the jejunal conduit as a cutaneous jejunostomy and use of double Roux-en-Y loops, avoiding any need for an enterostomy. If none of these procedures is successful, the patient may be a candidate for liver transplantation.

RESECTION OF TUMORS

Nearly two thirds of childhood cancer occurs as solid malignancies. As is always the case, the therapy administered depends on the type of tumor. Examination and judicious investigation of all unusual masses are imperative. Thorough diagnostic workup and prompt definitive treatment may result in cure, even if the tumor is proved malignant. Chemotherapy and radiation therapy are adjuncts to surgical excision of tumors.

Wilms' Tumor

Wilms' tumor, also known as nephroblastoma, is the most common intraabdominal childhood tumor. It presents as a painless mass whose enlargement may laterally distend the abdomen.

Procedural considerations

The child is positioned supine with a roll under the affected side. Both chest and abdomen are prepped. Infrequently the tumor extends into the inferior vena cava as well as the atrium, and in such cases cardiopulmonary bypass should be readily available. Because of the possible need to clamp the inferior vena cava, lines are placed into the arms and neck. Clean gloves and instruments should be available for inspection of the contralateral kidney. Careful attention should be given when handling tumor and lymph nodes to avoid tumor spillage.

Operative procedure

If the tumor is operable, the following aspects are important:

1. The transabdominal approach, which may be extended to a combined transabdominal-transthoracic approach, is used to inspect abdominal contents and clamp the vessels of the renal pedicle before tumor dissection.
2. All suspicious lymph nodes are removed, placed into separate containers, and labeled. If no suspicious nodes are present, biopsy specimens are obtained of those in adjacent areas.
3. The opposite kidney is explored before dissection of the tumor.
4. The extent of the tumor can be marked with hemostatic clips to facilitate radiation therapy.
5. The entire primary tumor is removed if doing so does not place the patient in jeopardy.

6. Any residual tumor is marked with clips.
7. Because of its proximity to the kidney, the adrenal gland is usually removed.
8. The abdominal cavity and viscera are thoroughly inspected for evidence of tumor extension or metastases. Extensive surgery may include partial colectomy or partial resection of the diaphragm.

Neuroblastoma

Neuroblastoma, one of the most common solid tumors of childhood, is a highly malignant tumor. It arises from neural crest tissue and can develop along any sympathetic

ganglion chain, with the most common sites the retroperitoneum and adrenal medulla. The mass is usually firm, irregular, and nontender. It is a silent tumor in its early stages and metastasizes rapidly. Treatment includes an operation to ligate the tumor's blood supply and remove as much of the tumor as possible, as well as chemotherapy and radiation.

Sacrococcygeal Teratoma

A sacrococcygeal teratoma is a tumor that originates early in embryonic cell division. The sacrococcygeal area is the most common extragonadal site of teratoma. The tumor presents as a large protuberance rising from the

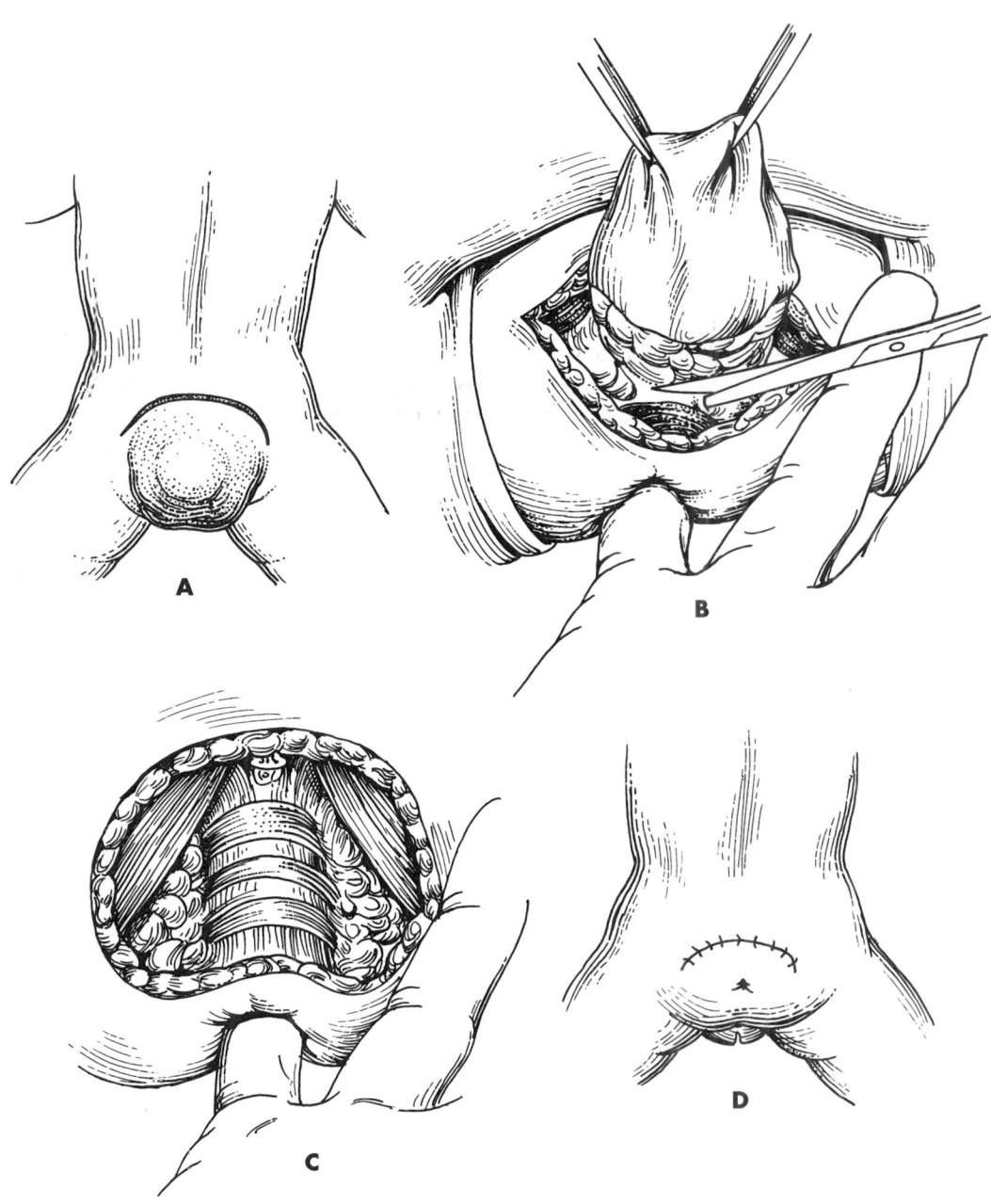

FIGURE 29-14 Excision of sacrococcygeal teratoma. **A,** U-shaped incision. **B,** Dissection of teratoma. **C,** Tumor excised while rectum remains intact. **D,** Closed incisional line.

sacrococcygeal area. It may be irregular or symmetric, varies in size, and may be pedunculated.

A sacrococcygeal teratoma is usually resectable in the newborn but may undergo malignant changes if not removed early in life. Tumors resected in the newborn period show microscopic evidence of malignant cells, but surgical cures have been achieved. Early surgical resection is important because these tumors are not sensitive to irradiation and are only temporarily responsive to chemotherapy.

The tumor is in the area of the sacrum and coccyx but may extend into the pelvis or abdomen. Resection is usually feasible by placing the patient in the Kraske (jackknife) position and excising the tumor mass and coccyx en bloc (Fig. 29-14). Infrequently, in cases where the tumor extends high into the pelvis, an abdominal incision may also be required.

GENITOURINARY SURGERY

Pediatric Cystoscopy

Pediatric cystoscopy is the endoscopic examination of the lower urinary tract of the pediatric patients. The major difference between adult and pediatric cystoscopy is the size of the instruments used and consideration of the small, delicate orifices of the pediatric patients. Indications for pediatric cystoscopy include urinary tract infections, enuresis, urethral valves, vesicoureteral reflux, diverticula,

bladder neck contractures, bladder tumors, and urinary tract obstructions.

Procedural considerations

The cystoscopy setup will have the same type of components as that for the adult cystoscopy patient, except that the size of the cystourethroscope system will be specific to the pediatric patient's needs (Fig. 29-15).

Each pediatric cystourethroscope is designed to fit specific component parts and is very delicate. Therefore the perioperative nurse must be familiar with the proper use of the system and handle the components carefully. The resectoscope loop is commonly used to resect urethral valves and occasionally bladder tumors. The cold knife may be used with the resectoscope to cut urethral strictures and occasionally to resect a urethral valve.

The most common anesthesia used for the pediatric patient is general anesthesia. After induction of anesthesia, the child is placed in a lithotomy or frog-leg position and prepped and draped according to established procedure.

Operative procedure

The pediatric cystourethroscope is lubricated and inserted through the urethra into the bladder. The light cord and irrigation tubing are attached to the telescope and cystoscope and the examination is performed. Most commonly the interior of the bladder is viewed on a

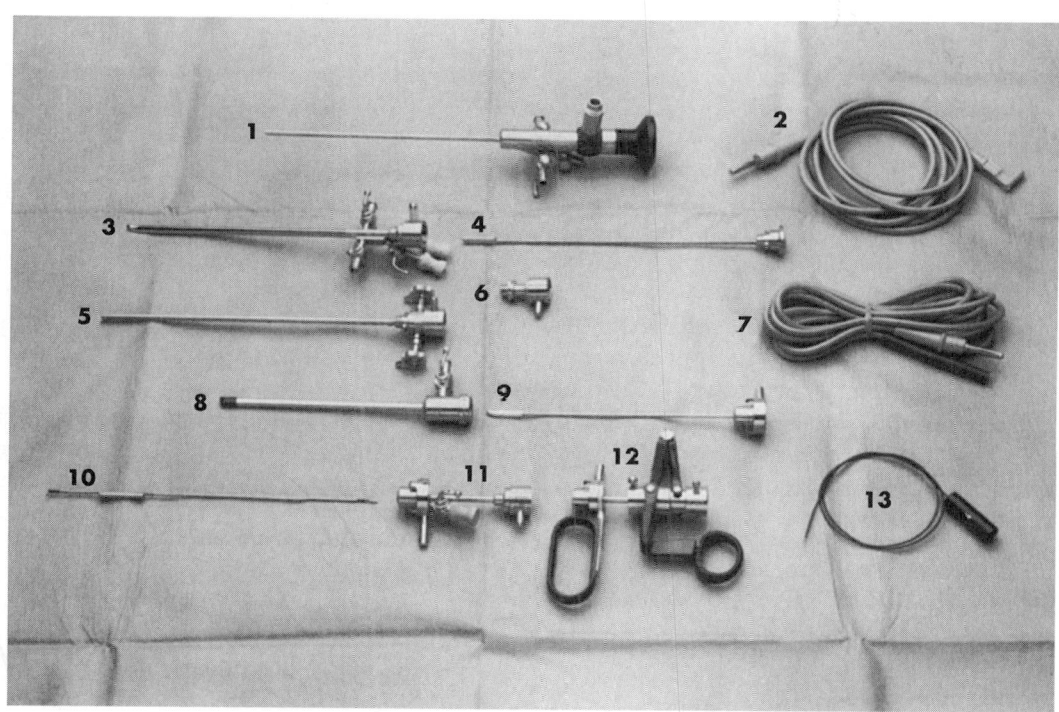

FIGURE 29-15 Pediatric cystoscopy instrumentation. *1*, 8 Fr cystoscope; *2*, fiberoptic light cord; *3* and *4*, 13 Fr cystoscope sheath and obturator; *5*, deflector; *6*, bridge; *7*, high-frequency cable; *8* and *9*, 13 Fr resectoscope sheath and obturator; *10*, resectoscope loop; *11*, bridge; *12*, working element; and *13*, ball-tipped electode.

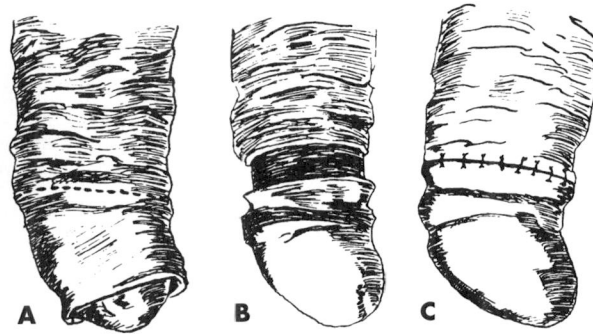

FIGURE 29-16 Circumcision.

video monitor by means of a camera attached to the cystoscope.

Circumcision

Circumcision is the excision of the foreskin (prepuce) of the glans penis. Circumcision may be done prophylactically in infancy. The surgery may be performed for religious reasons, as is required in specific faiths. Provision should be made to observe the religious needs and preferences of the parents.

Circumcision is also performed for the relief of phimosis, a condition in which the orifice of the prepuce is stenosed or too narrow to permit easy retraction behind the glans. Another condition, balanoposthitis, results in an inflamed glans and mucous membrane with purulent discharge and may require circumcision. In addition, circumcision may be done to prevent recurrent paraphimosis, a condition in which the prepuce cannot be reduced easily from a retracted position.

Procedural considerations

Newborns are generally positioned on a specially constructed board that facilitates restraint by immobilizing the limbs and exposing the genitals. Generally, only minimal anesthesia is necessary in this age group. Older children require general anesthesia.

For infants the setup includes fine plastic instruments. A Gomco clamp of the appropriate size, a Plastibell or the Hollister disposable circumcision device may be employed. The Hollister device includes sutures that are sealed in a sterile packet ready for use. For older patients there is no need for the circumcision clamp, and only a plastic instrument set is used. Petrolatum gauze for dressing should be available.

Operative procedure

1. If the prepuce is adherent, a probe or hemostat may be used to break up adhesions. The prepuce is clamped in the dorsal midline and incised toward the coronal mucosa margin (Fig. 29-16, *A*), leaving about 5 cm of coronal mucosa intact. A similar procedure is performed ventrally. The two incisions are then joined

circumferentially. Alternatively a superficial, circumferential incision is made in the skin with a scalpel at the level of the coronal sulcus and mucosa at the base of the glans. The redundant skin is undermined between the circumferential incisions and removed as a compete cuff (Fig. 29-16, *B*).

2. Bleeding vessels are coagulated or clamped with mosquito hemostats and tied with fine absorbable ligatures. Before closure, the area may be cleansed with an appropriate antiseptic solution.

3. The raw edges of the skin incision are approximated to a coronal cuff of mucosal prepuce, generally with 4-0 or 5-0 absorbable sutures on atraumatic plastic cutting or fine GI needles (Fig. 29-16, *C*). The wound is usually dressed with petrolatum gauze or an antibiotic ointment. A penile block with Marcaine is often done for immediate postoperative pain, thus providing a more comfortable "wake-up."

Hypospadias Repair

Hypospadias is a urethral meatus that is proximal to its normal glandular position at the tip of the penis. There are varying degrees of hypospadias. The meatus may be on the ventral surface of the glans, on the corona, anywhere along the shaft, in the scrotum, or even in the perineum. The more proximal the opening, the greater the degree of chordee (downward curvature of the penis). Chordee is caused by fibrous bands that extend from the hypospadiac urethral meatus to the tip of the glans and represent the abnormally developed urethra and its investing layer of Buck's fascia, dartos, and skin. In some cases of clinical curvature, however, these fibrous bands may not be present. Although these curvatures are still termed *chordee*, they are not true fibrous chordee.

The principal methods of hypospadias repair are meatoplasty and glanuloplasty, orthoplasty (release of chordee, thereby straightening the penis), urethroplasty (reconstruction of the urethra), skin cover, and scrotoplasty. These may be done in one- or two-stage repairs depending on the extent of the condition. Recently there has been an increase in efforts to relocate the meatus to the apex of the glans, especially in the more extensive one-stage repair.

One complication of hypospadias repair is urethral fistula formation, which can be repaired without much difficulty. Correction of strictures is more troublesome.

Procedural Considerations

The patient (the majority are infants and young children) is placed in the supine position with legs apart. The urine is diverted with a urethral catheter intraoperatively. The instrument setup varies according to the surgeon's preference. However, a minor set with fine plastic instruments is generally required, and sutures, polyethylene infant feeding tubes, silicone tubing or silicone Foley catheters, and drains may be desired. Owens

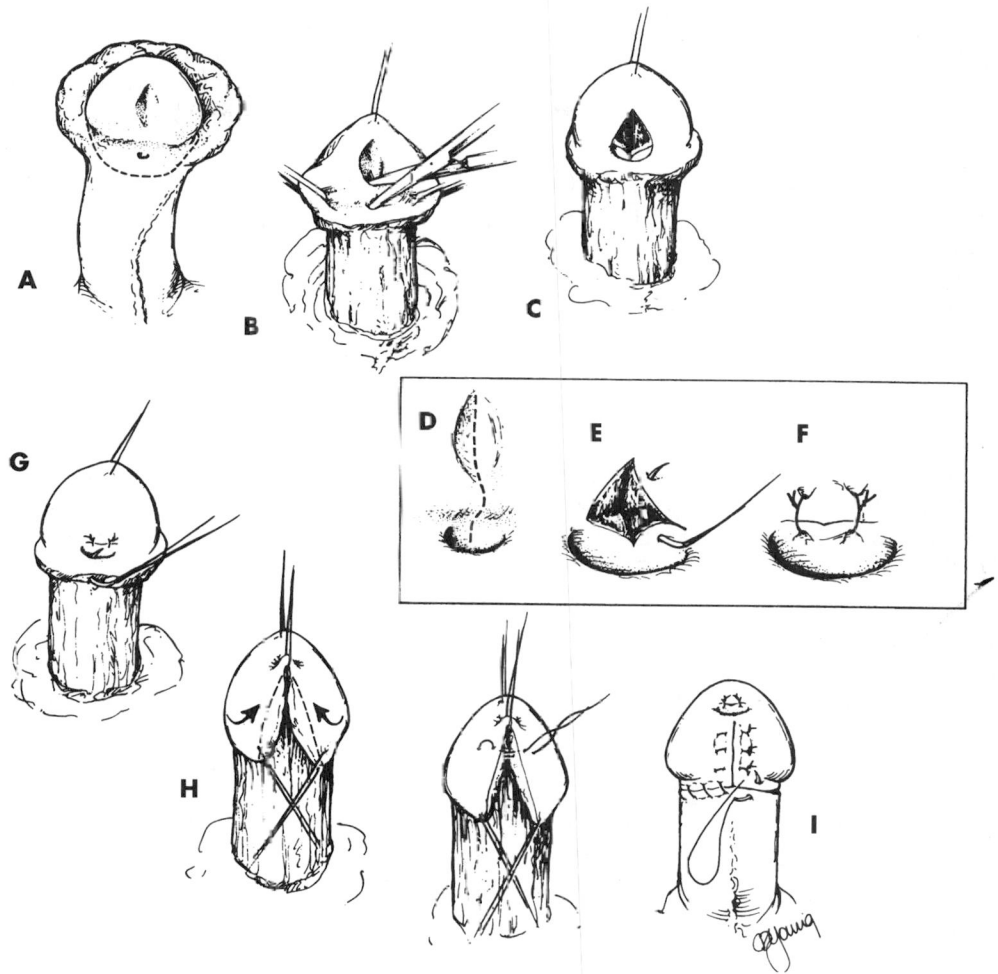

FIGURE 29-17   MAGPI chordee procedure in hypospadias repair.

gauze, Elastomull, Coban, and Elastoplast, as well as adhesive tape, are generally required for the dressing, which is an important part of the hypospadias repair.

Meatoplasty and glanuoplasty (MAGPI procedure)
Operative Procedure

1. A subcoronal, circumferential incision is made about 8 mm proximally to the meatus and corona. The skin is stripped back from the phallus by subcutaneous dissection (Fig. 29-17, *A* to *C*).
2. A bridge of tissue between the meatus and granular groove is made with a transverse closure of the dorsal (upper) meatal edge to the distal granular groove (Fig. 29-17, *D* to *F*).
3. Three traction sutures are placed where the foreskin stops, at the apex of the ventral meatus (on the lower side) and lateral areas of the glans (Fig. 29-17, *G*).
4. The edges of the glans are sutured together ventrally in a V configuration, and the redundant edges are excised (Fig. 29-17, *H*). Vertical mattress sutures are used to approximate the glans beneath the meatus.
5. If foreskin is excessive at the extremities, it may be trimmed, followed by a sleeve style of reapproximation

of the penile skin (Fig. 29-17, *I*). If a ventral skin defect is present, a rotational skin flap closure is used.
6. An indwelling catheter is placed, and the wound is dressed.

Orthoplasty

Orthoplasty is the proper designation for the plastic procedure performed to straighten the penis. Chordee repair is the more common term employed. In true fibrous chordee the penis is curved downward with the meatus and glans in proximity to one another.

Artifical erection is achieved by injecting 0.9% saline solution into the corpus cavernosum. Both corporal bodies fill, making it possible to determine the degree of curvation before and after the resection of the fibrous bands.

Operative Procedure

1. An incision is made circumferentially around the corona and carried distally to the urethral meatus and well below the glans cap (Fig. 29-18, *A*). Dissection continues to the level of the tunica albuginea of the corpora cavernosa.

2. With proximal dissection the adherent fibrous plaque is freed, working in a side-to-side fashion. The urethra is elevated from the corpora during this process (Fig. 29-18, B).

3. The chordee generally surrounds the urethral meatus and often extends for some distance. It is important to free it completely along the entire penile shaft to the penoscrotal junction, or in severe cases into the scrotum or perineum.

4. After release of the chordee the glans penis is closed with 4-0 absorbable sutures in a circular manner (Fig. 29-18, C).

5. If urethroplasty is either delayed or unnecessary, excess dorsal skin is excised (Fig. 29-18, D), and the incision is closed along the dorsal midline with interrupted, absorbable mattress sutures (Fig. 29-18, E). The wound is dressed according to established protocol.

Urethroplasty

Many procedures are described for reconstruction of a urethra. They may be divided into three general groups: adjacent skin flaps, free skin grafts, and mobilized vascular flaps. There are also many combinations of these procedures. In all the procedures some type of temporary urinary diversion, such as a perineal urethrostomy, may be used.

The procedural considerations are the same as those for chordee repair.

Adjacent Skin Flap

It is possible to tubularize skin adjacent to the meatus to create a neourethra in a one-stage repair. Transfer of dorsal skin to the ventrum will also provide graft material close to the meatus. However, this is generally done in two stages, and the vascularity of this thin rotational flap

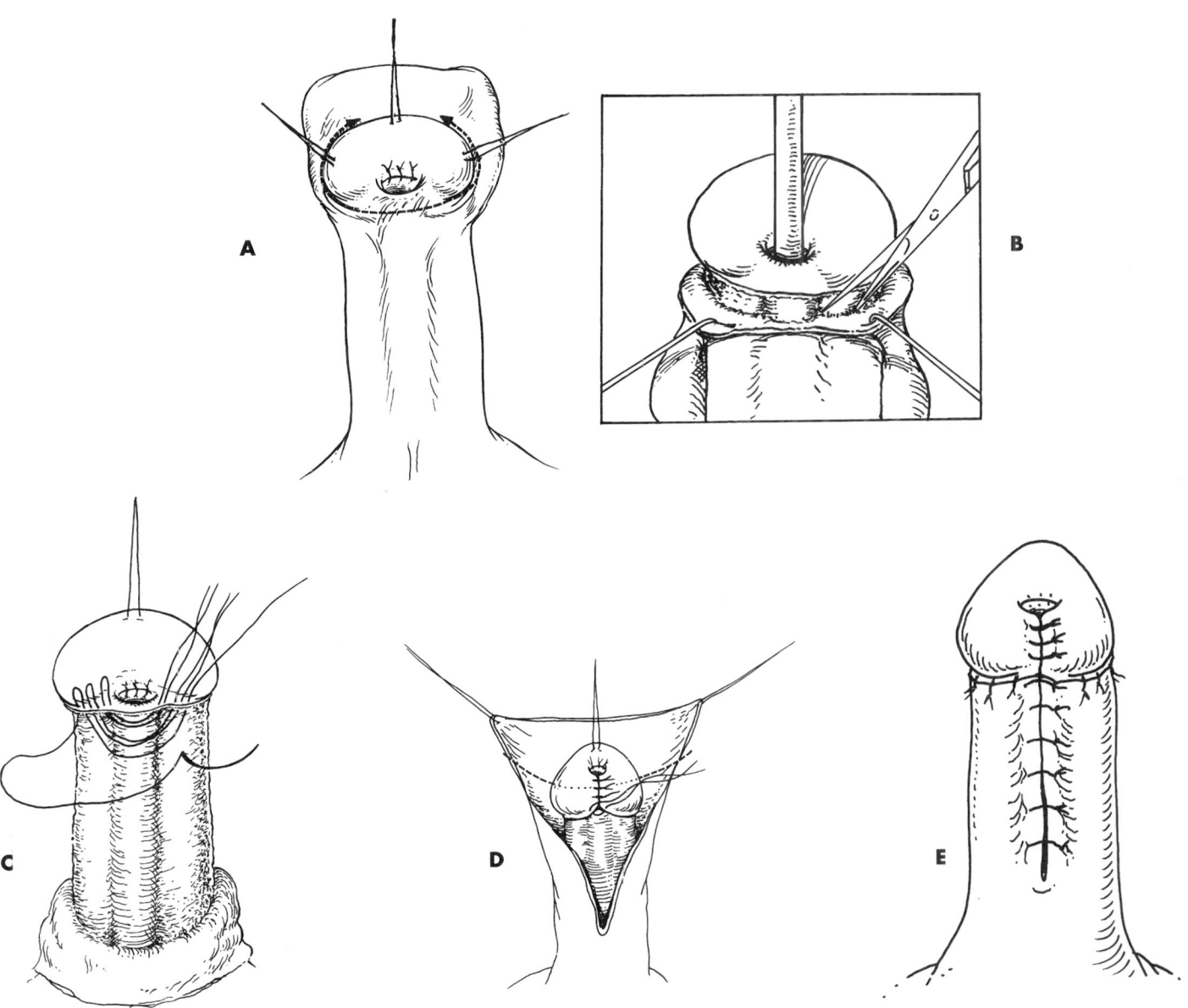

FIGURE 29-18 Orthoplasty.

is less than optimum with results that are prone to complication.

Operative procedure

1. Traction sutures are placed in the tip of the penis and in the glans wings for stabilization and exposure.
2. The distance between the glans tip and the lower edge of the meatus is measured. An outline of the proposed incision is drawn on the penile shaft (Fig. 29-19, *A*). In a one-stage approach the distal length must be increased to compensate for the added penile length after chordee release.
3. An incision is made around the outlined flap and carried proximally to a point on the shaft that corresponds to the distance required to reach the glans tip (Fig. 29-19, *B*). A flap width of 14 to 16 mm is usually sufficient to ensure good circumference of the neourethra.
4. Once incised, the tube is rolled over an 8 or 10 Fr catheter (Fig. 29-19, *B*) with an inverted running stitch of 4-0 or 5-0 absorbable suture.
5. The glans penis is incised, and the glans wings are undermined and freed. The neourethra is carried to the distal portion of the glans and sutured in place (Fig. 29-19, *C*).
6. The glans wings are sutured around the neourethra with absorbable, interrupted mattress sutures. The redundant foreskin is spit down the midline, and the flaps are brought around in a Z-plasty manner (Fig. 29-19, *D*).

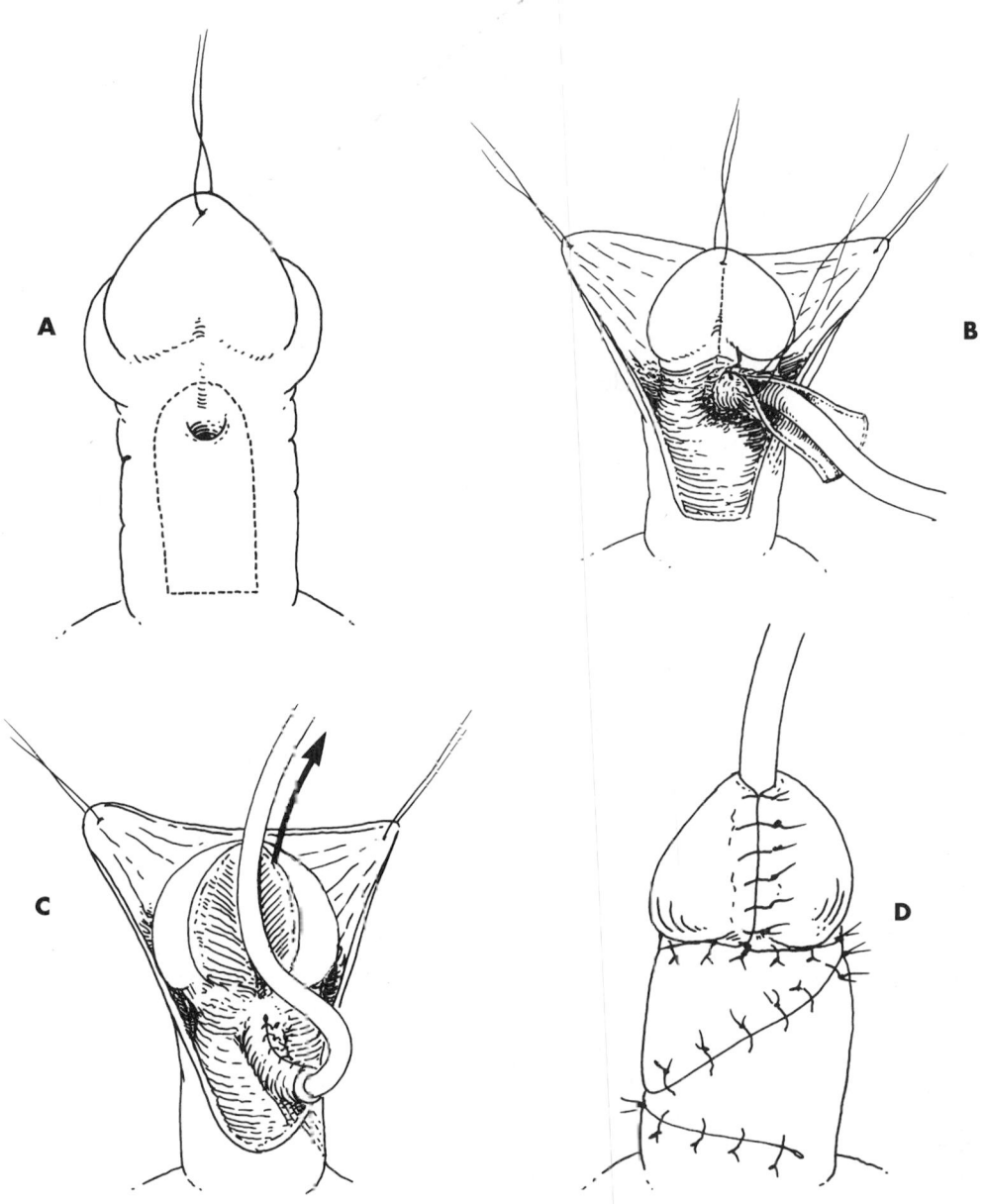

FIGURE 29-19   Urethroplasty with adjacent skin flap.

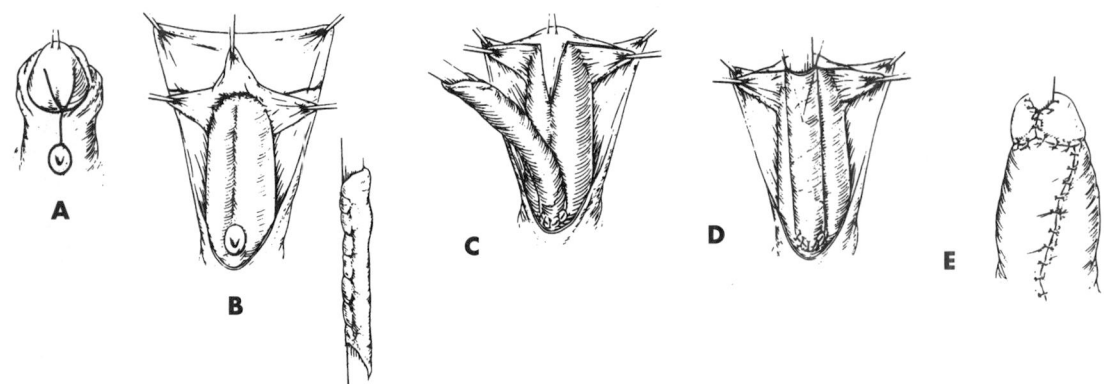

FIGURE 29-20   Urethroplasty with free graft.

7. A dry sterile pressure dressing is applied. The patient can often be discharged on the same day, without the need for an indwelling catheter.

Free Skin Graft

Free skin grafts should be of full thickness. Since the free graft must be revascularized, it is important that it have a perfect skin cover of dorsal, preputial, penile skin that is well vascularized. This type of graft is generally used with a one-stage hypospadias repair.

Operative procedure

1. A V-shaped incision is made on the glans, and the penile skin is mobilized after the chordee release (Fig. 29-20, *A*).
2. Glans wings are developed in a triangular fashion, and ventral preputial skin is used for the full-thickness free graft (Fig. 29-20, *B*).
3. The graft is formed into a neourethra over a stenting catheter (Fig. 29-20, *C*).
4. The graft is anastomosed proximally to the urethra with the suture line of the graft next to the corpora. The middle glans dart is fixed to the corpora (Fig. 29-20, *D*).
5. A meatoplasty with the dorsal glans dart is accomplished.
6. Fine, absorbable, interrupted sutures are placed around the meatus and glans and along the dorsal penile shaft (Fig. 29-20, *E*).
7. The wound is dressed according to established protocol.

Mobilized Vascularized Flaps

Vascularized flaps of preputial or penile skin may be mobilized to the ventrum by leaving them attached to the outer surface of the prepuce or as an island flap. One modification is the transverse preputial island flap neourethra with glans-channel positioning for the meatus. Preputial skin seems to be preferred because of its rich reliable blood supply.

Operative procedure

1. The chordee is released (Fig. 29-21, *A*).
2. Ventral preputial skin is dissected free and fanned out (Fig. 29-21, *B*).
3. The rectangle of skin is rolled into the neourethra and measured (Fig. 29-21, *C*).
4. The island flap is developed by dissection of the subcutaneous tissue from the dorsal penile skin (Fig. 29-21, *D* and *E*).
5. A glans channel is created with plastic scissors in a plane just above the corpora. The glans tissue is removed with the 14 Fr channel, and the island flap urethra is spiraled to the ventrum (Fig. 29-21, *F*).
6. The neourethra is anastomosed proximally to the urethra (Fig. 29-21, *G*).
7. The neourethra is carried to the tip of the glans (Fig. 29-21, *H*).
8. The dorsal penile flaps are transposed laterally to the midline and excess skin is excised. Closure is with fine, absorbable, interrupted mattress sutures around the glans and down the penile shaft (Fig. 29-21, *I*).
9. Dressings are applied according to established protocol.

Skin cover

After orthoplasty and urethroplasty, the penis must be resurfaced with skin. Abundant, excess dorsal foreskin is usually adequate to achieve the desired results.

Operative Procedure

1. Preputial tissue is transposed through a small buttonhole opening in the midline (Fig. 29-22, *A*).
2. The vasculature is spread laterally, and the glans penis is delivered through the hole (Fig. 29-22, *B*).
3. The skin flap is then sutured with fine, absorbable, interrupted mattress sutures (Fig. 29-22, *C*).

Epispadias Repair

An epispadias is the correction of the absence of the dorsal wall of the urethra and the position of the corpora cavernosa, ventral to the urethra. The surgical procedures

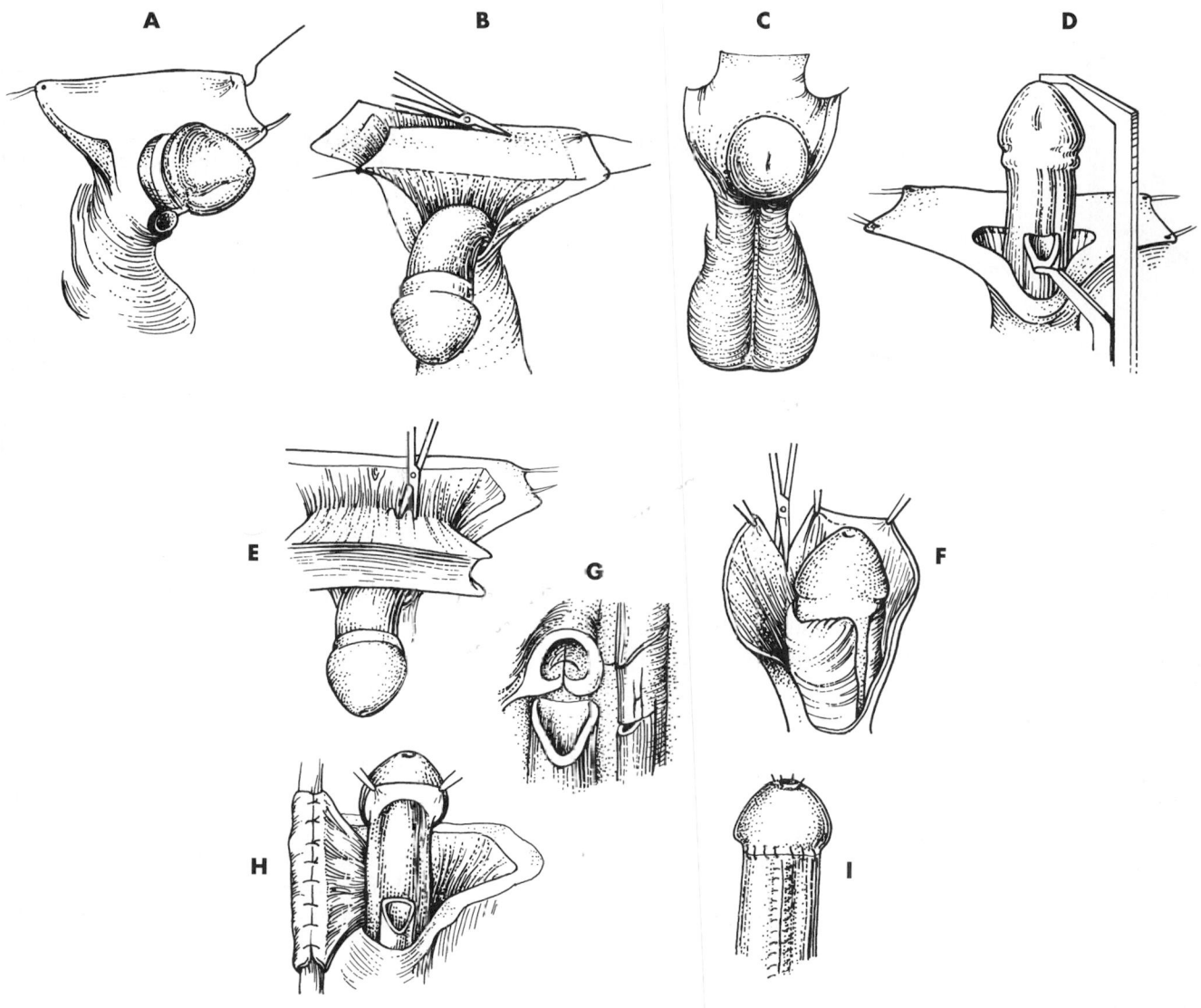

FIGURE 29-21   Urethroplasty, island flap.

employed in the correction of epispadias depend on the extent of the deformity. In mild incomplete defects the repair is the same as a simple hypospadias repair. Complete deformity is always associated with urinary incontinence because of little or no development of the bladder neck; thus the operation is much more involved. The least severe form of the exstrophy-epispadias complex is balanic epispadias, in which the urethra opens on the dorsum of the glans, or penile epispadias, in which the urethra opens on the shaft of the penis. The more severe variety, which occurs when the urethra opens on the proximal end of the shaft or in the penopubic position, is generally associated with severe dorsal chordee and urinary incontinence.

Procedural considerations

The setup for an epispadias repair is as described for hypospadias repair.

Operative procedures
First-Stage Epispadias Repair

1. A vertical incision is made distally to the epispadial meatus and carried circumferentially to the dorsal coronal margin.
2. The foreshortened dorsal urethral strip is lifted off the corpora cavernosa, and the ventral prepuce (foreskin) is rotated dorsally to cover the dorsal skin defect created by penile straightening.

Second-Stage Epispadias Repair

1. A vertical suprapubic incision is made to expose the anterior bladder wall and widened vesical neck. A wedge section of the anterolateral prostatic urethra is removed on either side, so that when it is reconstructed a more normal-caliber prostatic urethra is formed.
2. The roof of the membranous urethra is removed.

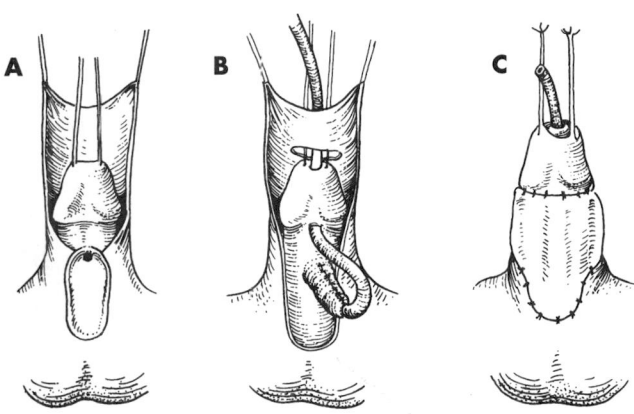

FIGURE 29-22   Skin cover procedure.

3. The prostatic urethra is closed, including muscle that is sutured together in the midline, with absorbable sutures. The bladder is closed so that an indwelling suprapubic catheter is left. The abdomen is closed in layers.
4. The anterior urethra is closed after an appropriate size of octagonal strip of dorsal penile skin is outlined.
5. The remainder of the repair—the creation of the urethra and its coverage with lateral penile skin—is the reverse procedure of a second-stage hypospadias repair.

Bladder Exstrophy Repair

Bladder exstrophy repair corrects a more severe form of epispadias, in which the anterior bladder wall as well as the roof of the urethra are absent. Bladder exstrophy is always accompanied by wide separation of the rectus muscles of the lower abdominal wall and by diastasis of the pubic bone with anterior displacement of the anus. Repair of bladder exstrophy requires an adequate size of bladder for ultimate continence to be achieved. It is preferable to perform this procedure in the neonatal period.

Procedural considerations

The infant is placed in a supine position, and the abdomen and thighs are prepped and draped. Instruments are as required for hypospadias repair.

Operative procedure

1. An incision is made around the exposed bladder medial to the paravesical neck mucosa. The incision is carried distally across the epispadial urethra distal to the verumontanum. The paravesical muscosa is preserved for urethral lengthening. The bladder is then freed from the rectus fascia and the peritoneum. The dorsal chordea is released, and the mobilized paravesical mucosa is apposed in the midline and sutured to the proximal end of the urethra just distal to the verumontanum.
2. The bladder wall is closed vertically in two layers with 3-0 absorbable sutures; a suprapubic tube is inserted for drainage.

3. The bladder neck is loosely reconstructed by approximating the interpubic ligament, which extends between the proximal end of the phallus and the pubic bone.
4. The symphysis pubis is approximated with a heavy #2 nonabsorbable suture. During this step the assistant rotates the iliac bones anteriorly.

Hydrocelectomy

A hydrocele is an abnormal accumulation of fluid within the scrotum. The fluid is contained within the tunica vaginalis. Excessive secretion or accumulation of hydrocele fluid may be the result of infection or trauma. A hydrocelectomy is the excision of the tunica vaginalis of the testis to remove the enlarged, fluid-filled sac. In older patients, the procedure is performed through a scrotal incision.

Procedural considerations

The patient is placed in the supine position. Preparation and draping of the patient include routine cleansing of the external genitals and draping of the patient with a fenestrated sheet. A minor instrument set is required, plus a small drain, a 30 ml syringe with a 20-gauge, 2-inch aspirating needle, and a suspensory dressing.

Operative procedure

1. An anterolateral incision is made in the skin of the scrotum over the hydrocele mass by a scalpel with a #10 or #15 blade (Fig. 29-23, A). Bleeding is controlled with fine-tipped hemostats, and vessels are ligated with 3-0 absorbable ligatures.
2. Small retractors may be placed, after which the fascial layers are incised to expose the tunica vaginalis (Fig. 29-23, B). With fine scissors, forceps, and blunt dissection the hydrocele is dissected free and delivered (Fig. 29-23, C). The sac is opened, and the fluid contents are aspirated.
3. The sac is inverted so that it surrounds the testis, epididymis, and distal cord. Excess tunica vaginalis is excised, and the edges of the tunica are sutured with a continuous 4-0 absorbable suture behind the testicle (Fig. 29-23, D). The testicle is "bottled" by the inverted tunica vaginalis, and this may then be returned to the sac.
4. A drain is placed within the scrotum and brought out through a stab wound in the most dependent portion of the scrotum. The scrotal incision is closed in layers with 3-0 and 4-0 absorbable sutures. A fluff compression dressing contained in a scrotal support (suspensory) aids in reducing postoperative scrotal edema.

Orchiopexy

An orchiopexy (orchidopexy) is the surgical placement and fixation of the testicle in a normal anatomic position in the scrotal sac. If the testis fails to descend into the scrotum during gestation, it is considered undescended. An

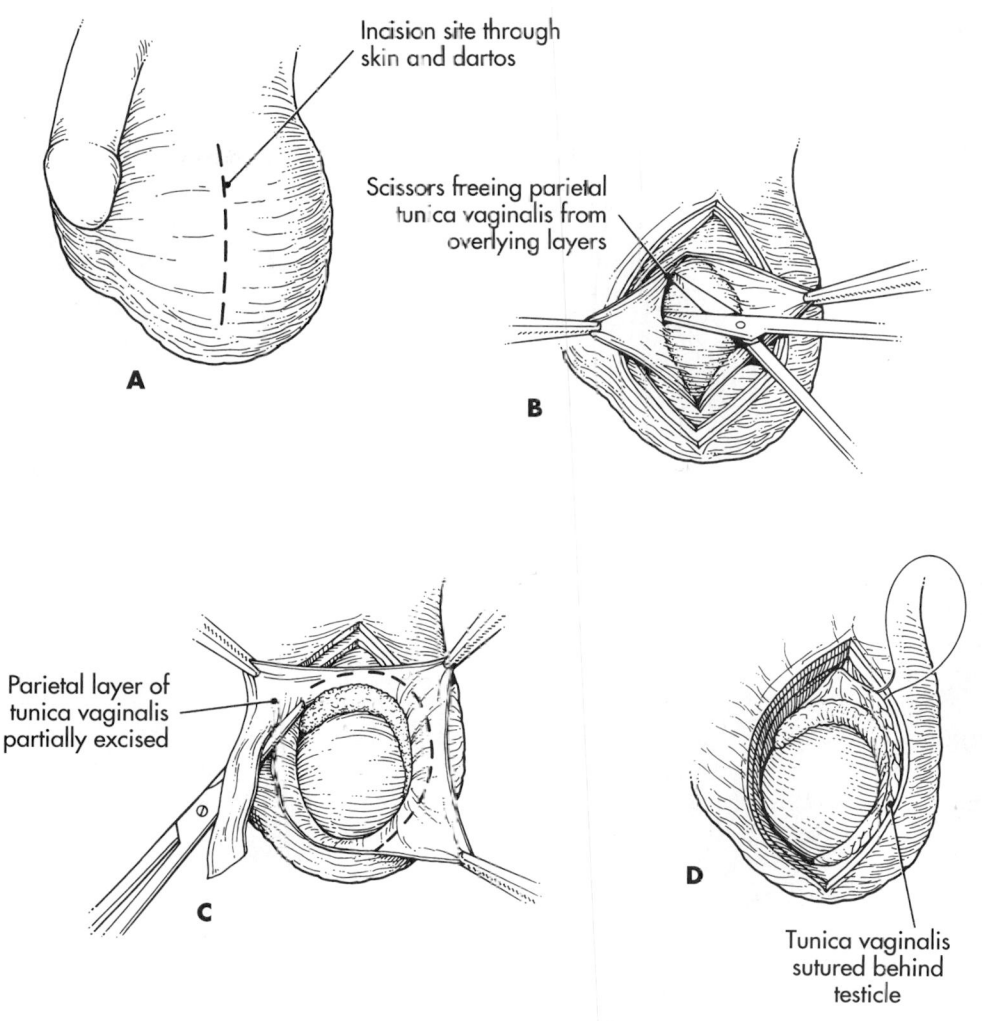

FIGURE 29-23 Hydrocelectomy.

undescended testis becomes arrested somewhere along its normal path of descent. If it is palpable in a position other than its normal path of descent, its position is considered to be ectopic.

A retractile testis has fully descended into the scrotum but retracts out of the scrotum as a result of contraction of the cremaster muscle. Gentle manipulation allows replacement of the testis in the most dependent portion of the scrotum. Retractile testes require no surgical or hormonal treatment.

All testes that are undescended after 1 year, including those that are unresponsive to hormone injections, require surgical placement in the scrotum for optimum maturation. A new technique for determining the position, existence, or size of a "hidden" testes is through laparoscopic examination.

Procedural considerations

The setup is as described for hydrocelectomy. General anesthesia is required. Preparation and draping include the lower abdomen, genitals, and thighs. Because this operation is usually performed on children, a setup containing small, delicate instruments and sutures is required.

Operative procedure

1. An inguinal incision is generally employed for exploration of undescended testes (Fig. 29-24, *A*). Most undescended testes are located in the superficial inguinal pouch or inguinal canal.
2. The external oblique aponeurosis is opened through the external inguinal ring to expose the inguinal canal: the gubernacular attachments of the undescended testis are dissected free as high as the internal inguinal ring or into the abdominal cavity (Fig. 29-24, *B* and *C*).
3. All adhesions and the associated inguinal hernial sac are freed to lengthen the cord, so that the testis is allowed to reach the scrotal cavity. The hernia sac is transsected, twisted, and ligated with sutures (Fig. 29-24, *D* and *E*).
4. To draw vessels into the inguinal canal, more proximally to the scrotum, the floor of the inguinal canal may have to be divided at the internal ring (Fig. 29-24, *F* and *G*).

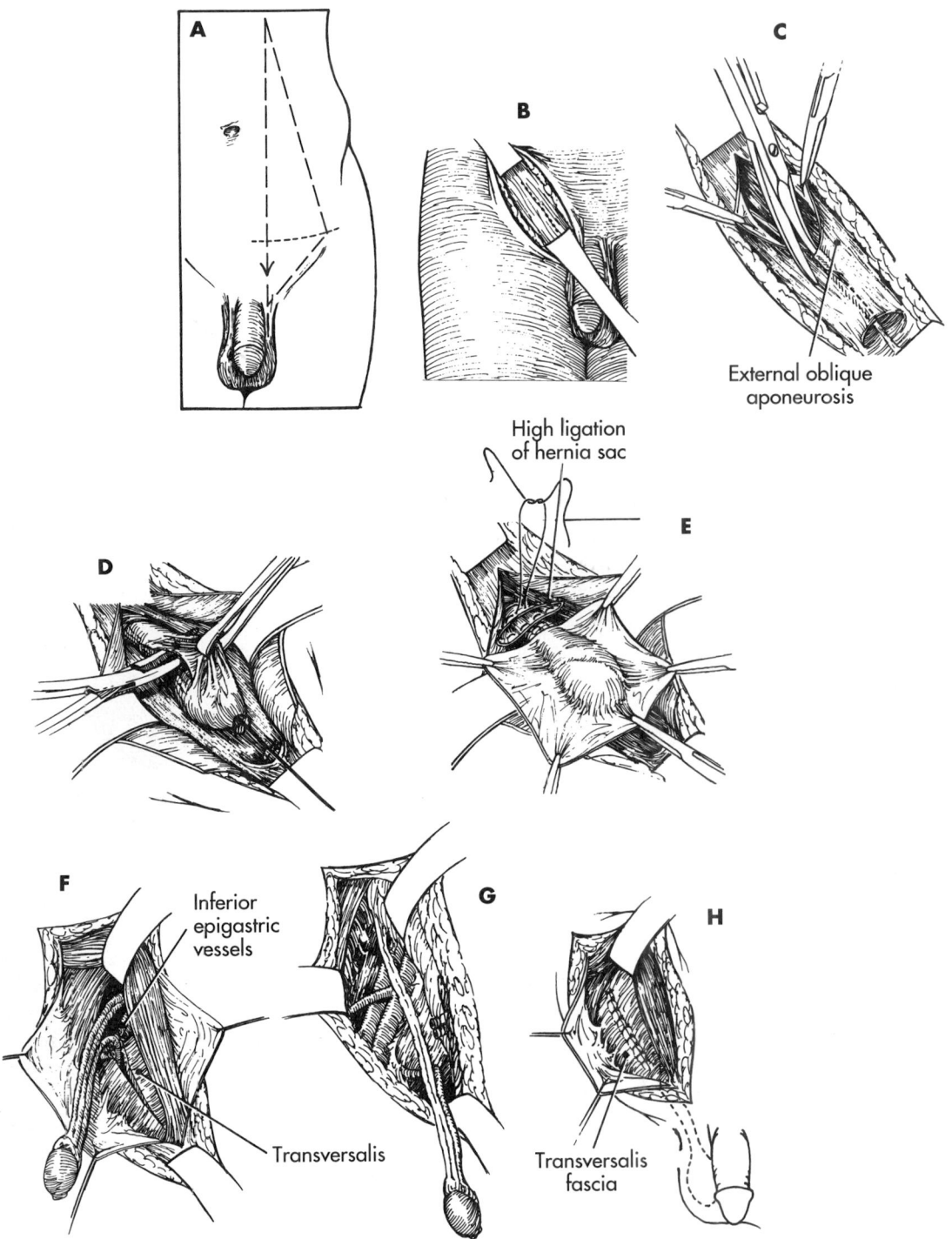

FIGURE 29-24   Orchiopexy.

5. The lateral portion of the internal ring is closed to prevent herniation. A scrotal pocket is created, and the testis is anchored in a normal anatomic position within the scrotum with absorbable sutures (Fig. 29-24, *H*).

NOTE: Orchiopexy may be accomplished by several surgical methods. The dependent portion of the undescended testis may be sutured to the base of the scrotum with absorbable or nonabsorbable sutures brought out through the scrotal wall and tied over a peanut dissector or pledget. The most popular method is to anchor the testis into a dissected subdartos pouch. In this procedure a small midtransverse scrotal incision is made, and space between the skin and dartos muscle is dissected. The testis is then brought through a small hole in the dartos into the subdartos pouch and anchored in position by the traction suture. The overlying skin of the subdartos pouch is closed with fine absorbable suture material. The inguinal incision is repaired in layers with 3-0 absorbable sutures. The skin is closed with a subcuticular suture: Steri-Strips are used for dressing.

EAR, NOSE, AND THROAT PROCEDURES

Myringotomy

Myringotomy is the incision of the tympanic membrane. It is performed to treat otitis media in the presence of an exudate. Serous otitis media can be very difficult to diagnose because it is asymptomatic in pediatric patients. The only symptom may be conductive hearing loss.

Serous otitis media is very common in children between the 6 months and 2 years of age. About 50% to 60% of children in this age group have effusion in the middle ear in the first 2 years of life. The incidence may again peak between 4 and 6 years of age; 30% of children in this age group have fluid in the middle ear with hearing loss at some time.

About 95% of children with serous otitis media have spontaneous resolution. Hearing loss is the main concern when fluid is present in the middle ear. This hearing loss could affect language development and IQ level if fluid persists for a long time. The accepted practice is removal of the fluid and placement of ventilating tubes in the eardrum if the fluid persists more than 8 to 12 weeks and is accompanied by hearing loss.

Otitis media is primarily a pediatric problem, but adult cases are seen. It may respond to one treatment only to return and require another type to therapy. Tympanic fibrosis is common in adults and is a result of repeated infections that have occurred in childhood. Acute otitis media is a collection of infected pus in the middle ear. The patient may have severe pain and bulging of the tympanic membrane (Fig. 29-25). Failure to respond to oral antibiotics and analgesics or other complications such as facial nerve paralysis or labyrinthitis may require a myringotomy. By release of the pus or fluid, hearing is restored, and the infection can be controlled. The procedure may be performed for chronic serous otitis media in which the presence of fluid in the middle ear produces a hearing loss. Frequently, tubes are inserted into the tympanic membrane (Fig. 29-26) to allow ventilation of the middle ear. Care must be taken to avoid getting water in the ears while the tubes are in place. Myringotomy is usually performed on an ambulatory surgery basis.

Procedural considerations

Myringotomy is considered a clean procedure. The patient is usually not prepped or draped. The surgeon may wear gown and gloves or gloves only, depending on the

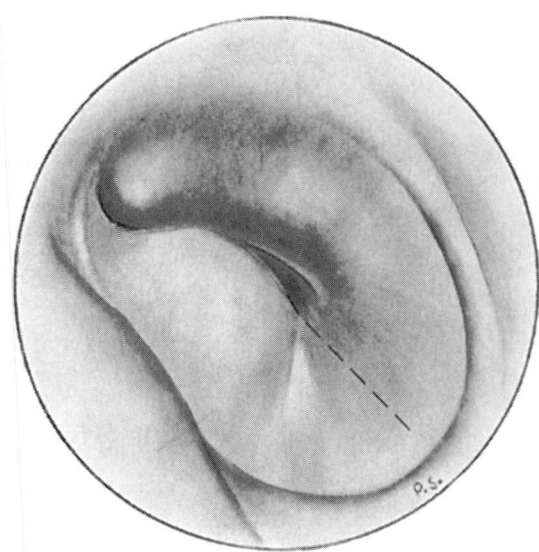

FIGURE 29-25   In purulent otitis media, pus under pressure pushes eardrum outward, resulting in bulging tympanic membrane. *Dotted line,* Radial myringotomy incision.

policy related to Universal Precautions at the institution in which the procedure is performed.

The instrument setup includes the following: myringotomy knife; metal aural applicators; Hartmann aural forceps, delicate type; Buck ear curettes; assorted sizes of aural speculums; Rosen needles; suction tip and tubing; culture tube; and absorbent cotton. Several disposable myringotomy sets are available commercially, are relatively inexpensive, and afford an expedient procedure.

Operative procedure

1. With microscopic visualization, the aural speculum is inserted into the ear canal. The excess cerumen is removed with a wire-loop curette or Toby forceps. With a sharp myringotomy knife a small, curved or radial incision is made in the anterior quadrant of the pars tensa (see Fig. 29-25).
2. A culture may be taken to determine the type of organism present.
3. Pus and fluid are suctioned from the middle ear.
4. A tube may be inserted into the incision with alligator forceps or a tube inserter.
5. Antibiotic drops may be instilled after the positioning of the tube. Several types of disposable myringotomy tubes are available for implantation, depending on the length of time the surgeon wishes the tube to remain in place (see Fig. 29-26). Once the tube falls out, the tympanic membrane incision usually heals.

Tonsillectomy and Adenoidectomy

The palatine tonsils and adenoids are removed by sharp or blunt dissection. Enlarged tonsils and adenoids are usually associated with difficulty in breathing and hearing, chronic colds, enlarged glands of the neck, otitis media, and pressure on the eustachian tubes caused by adenoiditis.

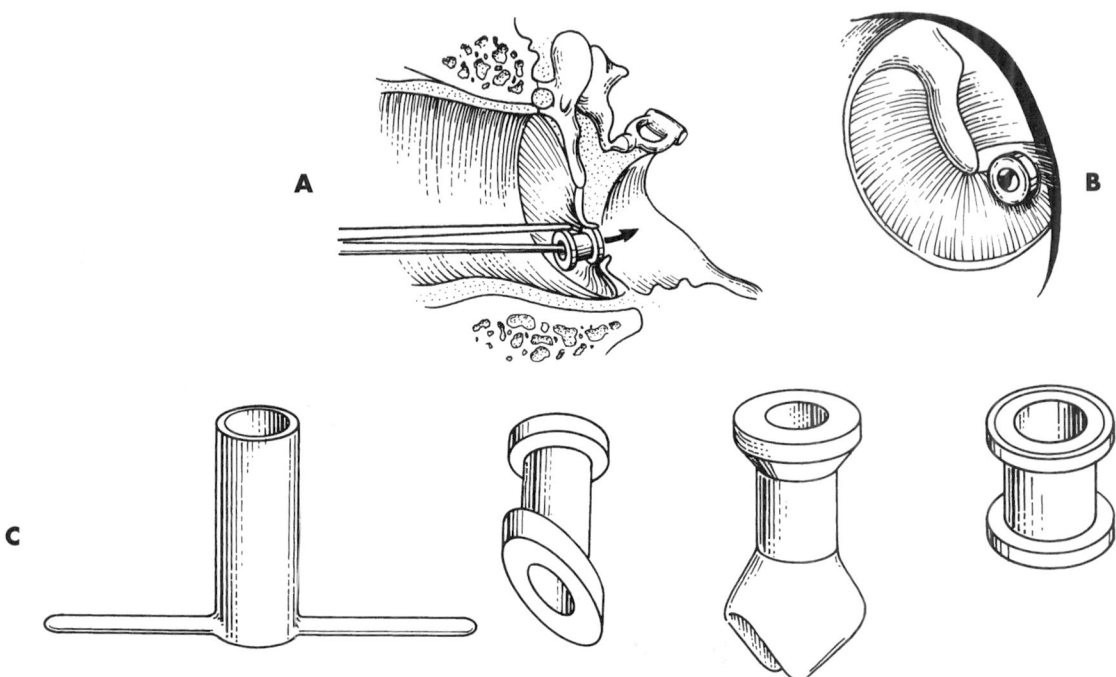

FIGURE 29-26   **A,** Tube (placed on end of alligator forceps) being inserted into tympanic membrane. **B,** Tube in place. **C,** Several types of plastic tubes that may be inserted into tympanic membrane. Purpose of tubes is to aerate middle ear and reduce middle ear infections.

Rheumatism, bronchitis, and hearing loss may be associated with diseased tonsils.

Special preoperative teaching and orientation sessions for pediatric patients have decreased the stress of the perioperative period for children undergoing this surgery. During these sessions parents are instructed in the essentials of postoperative care.

Procedural considerations

The patient is anesthetized and may be placed in slight Trendelenburg's position. The neck is hyperextended when a roll is placed under the shoulders. A small headrest may be necessary if the patient's head is unstable. Typical draping includes application of head drape and an impervious sheet over the patient. The instruments and supplies required include the following (Fig. 29-27): knife handle, #7 with #12 blade; tonsil knife; tonsil snare with additional wires; LaForce or Sluder tonsil guillotines, if desired; Metzenbaum scissors, curved, 7½ inches, or Boettcher scissors; Mayo scissors; adenoid curettes, assorted sizes; Hurd dissector and pillar retractor; sponge-holding forceps; towel clamp; tonsil-grasping forceps, straight and curved; Dean hemostatic forceps; Jennings mouth gag; self-retaining mouth gag with tongue blades, if desired; uvula or palate retractor; tongue depressor; needle holder, 7 inches; Yankauer suction tube with suction tubing; tonsil sponges; gauze sponges; basin set; cold sterile saline solution; electrosurgical handpiece with suction attached; electrosurgical unit; and headlight of surgeon's preference.

Operative procedure (Fig. 29-28)

1. A general anesthetic is used, an endotracheal tube is inserted, the mouth is retracted open with a self-retaining retractor, and the tongue is depressed with a blade retractor. Efficient suction is most important. The metal suction tube is introduced gently and passed along the floor of the mouth, over the base of the tongue, and into the pharynx. During the procedure the suctioning ensures adequate exposure of the operative site and prevents blood from reaching the lungs or stomach.

2. The tonsil is grasped with a pair of tonsil-grasping forceps, and the mucous membrane of the anterior pillar is incised with a knife; the tonsil lobe is freed from its attachments to the pillars with a tonsil dissector, curved scissors, and gauze sponges on a holder. The tonsil is withdrawn with forceps.

3. The posterior pillar is cut with scissors and the tonsil is removed with a snare. In some cases a tonsil guillotine clamp may be used.

4. A tonsil sponge is placed into the fossa with sponge-holding forceps.

5. The vessels are electrocoagulated or bleeding vessels are clamped with tonsil forceps and tied with slipknot absorbable 0 ligatures, and the free ligature ends are cut.

6. The adenoids are removed with an adenotome or curette. Bleeding is controlled by pressure with tonsil sponges, sometimes soaked in a hemostatic solution. (The adenoidectomy may be performed before the tonsillectomy, depending on the surgeon's preference.)

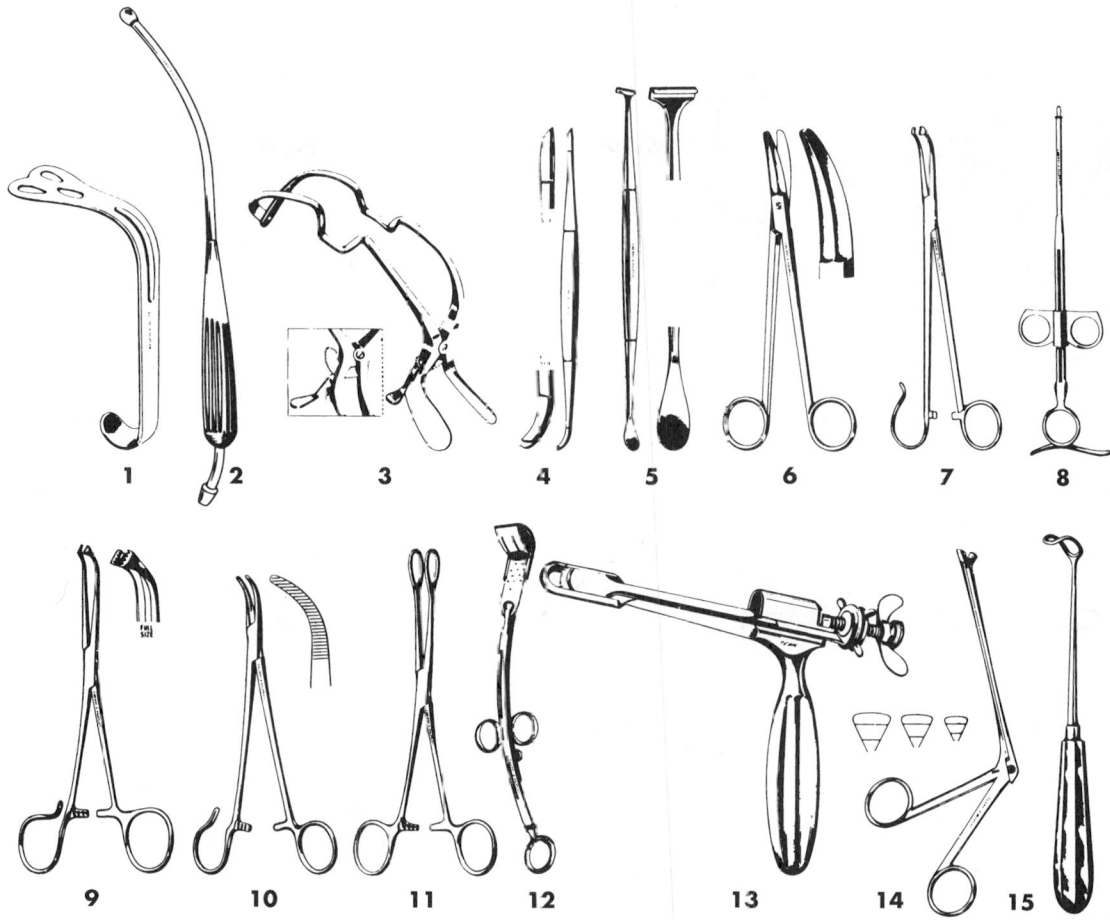

FIGURE 29-27   Instruments for tonsillectomy and adenoidectomy. *1,* Tongue depressor; *2,* Yankauer suction tube; *3,* Jennings mouth gag; *4,* tonsil knife; *5,* Hurd dissector and pillar retractor; *6,* Boettcher tonsil scissors; *7,* White tonsil-grasping forceps; *8,* Eves tonsil snare; *9,* Allis-Coakley forceps, curved; *10,* Dean hemostatic forceps; *11,* Ballenger sponge-holding forceps, serrated jaw; *12,* LaForce adenotome; *13,* Daniel tonsillectome; *14,* adenoid punch; *15,* Barnhill adenoid curette.

7. The fossa is carefully inspected, and any bleeding vessels are cauterized or clamped and tied. Retractors and endotracheal tube are removed, the patient's face is cleaned, and the head is turned to one side. The patient is placed in the semirecumbent (Fowler's) position or on one side, horizontally, to prevent aspiration of blood and venous engorgement postoperatively.

NEUROSURGICAL PROCEDURES

Neuropathologic conditions requiring surgical intervention can be found in any age group. The most common problems requiring neurosurgical procedures in infants and children include meningocele, myelomeningocele, encephalocele, craniosynostosis, hydrocephalus, brain tumors, and trauma. The surgical approach, instruments and equipment required, and steps of the respective operative procedures for pediatric neurosurgery are similar in nature to those required for adult procedures performed for these problems, except for the size of instruments. Consequently

the majority of these procedures are described in Chapter 23.

Perioperative nursing considerations that apply to most neurosurgical procedures are somewhat different for the pediatric patient. The perioperative nurse plays a vital role in maintaining blood volume, body temperature, and fluid balance in pediatric patients. Maintenance of blood volume includes planning and coordinating activities to minimize and monitor blood loss and to facilitate availability of blood for replacement. Sponges from the operative field must be continuously placed within view of the anesthesia provider or weighed as they are discarded from the field. Blood and blood products must be available in the surgical suite. A blood warmer must be ready to use as careful, accurate fluid replacement therapy is carried out.

The perioperative nurse must place a warming blanket on the OR bed before the pediatric patient arrives. If the room temperature can be individually regulated, the thermostat should be set to a temperature about 22° C (72° F) after consultation with the anesthesia provider. The

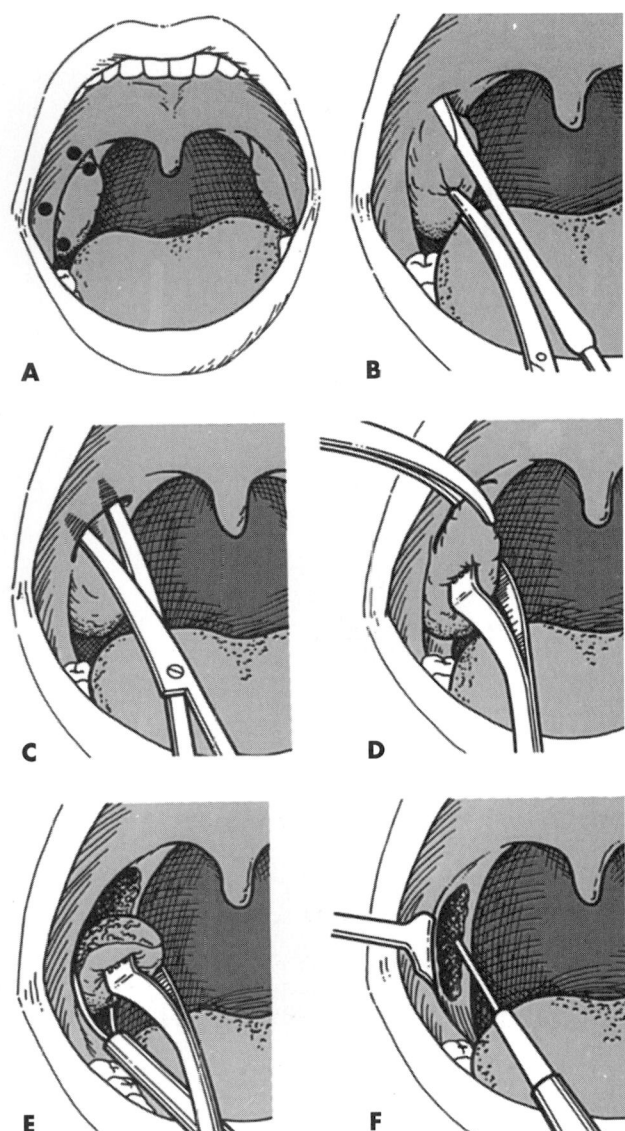

FIGURE 29-28 Surgical method of tonsillectomy. **A,** Local anesthesia infiltration points. **B,** Tonsil knife is used to make an incision at the tonsil anterior pillar superiorly. **C** and **D,** Scissors are used to dissect the superior pole of the tonsil. **E,** A snare is used to separate the tonsil from the lower pole. **F,** Hemostasis is achieved by electrocoagulation or tying of bleeding vessels.

child's body and extremities can be wrapped in plastic materials. Body temperature is monitored with a rectal, intraaural, or esophageal thermistor probe. The thermistor unit must be calibrated and placed within the view of the anesthesia provider before surgery.

Some means to control and monitor fluid intake and output must be planned with the anesthesia provider and neurosurgeon: microdrip intravenous tubing or an electronic drip regulator such as an I-Vac unit may be used for regulating intravenous intake; a Foley catheter may be inserted into the bladder and attached to a urinometer and closed drainage system if the child is to undergo a prolonged procedure; output should be recorded at timed intervals decided on by the perioperative nurse and anesthesia provider and based on the child's general

condition. Irrigation fluid and suction bottle contents are measured and recorded.

Parents of infants and children are usually extremely anxious, just as the families of most surgical patients are. Arrangements by which families can have contact with the patient through a perioperative nurse who has direct access to the operating room during the operation and the postanesthesia recovery relieve anxiety and diminish perceived waiting time for them.

Laminectomy for Meningocele

Malformations such as meningoceles are usually congenital. They are a threat to the life of a newborn infant because the defect may predispose to infection or spinal cord damage. Defects of the cord and spinal nerves are often associated with the condition. There also may be spina bifida, a congenital defect resulting from incomplete closure of the vertebral canal.

Surgery for repair of meningocele is directed at preserving intact the neural elements involved and at closing the cutaneous, muscular, and dural defects. As for other pediatric procedures, small hemostats, retractors, and other instruments are provided. Large bone-cutting instruments may be omitted. The nerve stimulator may be needed.

Craniectomy for Craniosynostosis

Craniectomy for craniosynostosis is performed on infants whose suture lines have closed prematurely. If diagnosis is made shortly after birth, the condition can be corrected by surgical separation of the two involved bones and treatment of the area to prevent resealing until most of the growth of the brain has occurred. The surgeon merely restores the patency of the suture and allows growth of the brain to correct the cosmetic deformity.

Operative procedure

1. After the scalp incision is made over the appropriate skull suture, the dura mater is stripped off the underside of the skull.
2. A generous strip of the bone edges joining to form the fused suture is then removed with heavy scissors, a craniotome, a rongeur, or a Kerrison punch.
3. The bone edges are waxed.
4. Preformed Silastic sheeting can be inserted over the bone edges bordering the craniectomy and sutured or stapled in place.
5. When sutures are used, holes must be placed in the bone edges bordering the craniectomy before the sheeting is placed.

Ventriculoatrial and Ventriculoperitoneal Shunts

The two most widely used pediatric surgical procedures to divert excessive cerebrospinal fluid (CSF) from ventricles to other body cavities from which it can be absorbed are ventriculoatrial (Fig. 29-29) (ventriculocardiac) and ventriculoperitoneal shunts. See Chapter 23 for complete information related to these two procedures.

ORTHOPEDIC PROCEDURES

Congenital Dislocation of the Hip

A congenital dislocation (dysplasia) of the hip (CDH) is an abnormal development present at birth. It is a lateral or upward dislocation of the femoral head from the acetabulum. When alignment is disrupted, soft tissue and bony changes result in contractures of the hip muscles, a shallow acetabulum, and possibly a deformed femoral head. Treatment of congenital dislocation of the hip varies depending on the age of the patient and the stability of the hip. Treatment modalities include application of a Pavlik harness, closed reduction and spica cast application, and surgical correction. Surgery involves soft-tissue release or acetabular and femoral procedures. Many of the total hip systems have congenital dysplastic hip (CDH) implants, which allow joint reconstruction.

Procedural considerations

The patient is usually in the lateral position for these procedures. An anterior incision is usually made for open reduction, whereas a lateral incision is made for the subtrochanteric osteotomy. The surgeon's preference dictates the incision for an innominate osteotomy.

A soft-tissue set and bone set (appropriate for age) are required as well as a total hip set, power reamer and saw, Steinman pins, and CDH implants and instrumentation.

Operative procedures

CDH Total Joint Replacement

Total joint replacement is carried out in similar fashion to the procedure described in Chapter 22.

Open Reduction (Fig. 29-30)

1. The hip joint is opened, and the soft tissue in the acetabulum is excised.
2. The femoral head can then be reduced into the acetabulum and held by suturing of the capsule.

Derotational Osteotomy

A derotational osteotomy is performed when the head is improperly seated in the acetabulum.

1. The femur is placed in internal rotation and divided.
2. The distal fragment is rotated externally to place the knee and foot straight ahead.
3. If the patient is a young child, the osteotomy is frequently performed in the supracondylar region, and the patient is immobilized in a plaster spica cast.
4. For an older child, the osteotomy is frequently done in the subtrochanteric region, and the osteotomized fragments are held with an osteotomy blade plate or an intermediate compression screw. Immobilization may not be necessary.

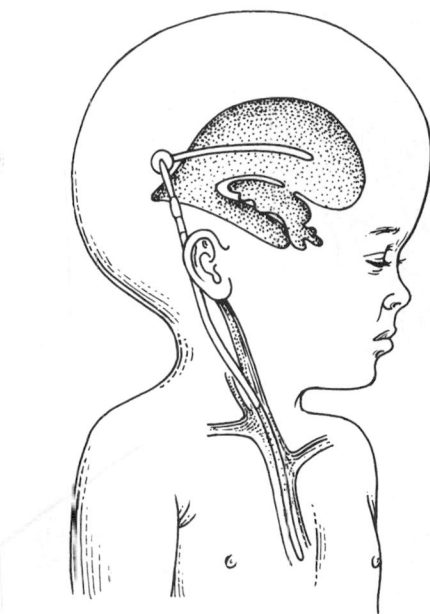

FIGURE 29-29   Placement of ventriculoatrial shunt.

Innominate Osteotomy

1. A complete division of the wing of the ilium is made by an osteotomy from the sciatic notch to the anterior margin of the ilium, superior to the acetabulum.
2. The ilium is then wedged down to increase the depth of the acetabulum when the osteotomy site is opened and a bone graft is inserted.
3. The bone graft is held in place with two heavy wires.
4. Heavy suture is used to close the capsule, and a spica cast is applied for postoperative immobilization.

PLASTIC AND RECONSTRUCTIVE SURGERY

Cleft Lip Repair

The normal upper lip is composed of skin, underlying orbicularis oris muscle, and mucosa. Two skin ridges are sited near the midline outlying the central philtrum of the lip. The vermilion (red portion of the lip) peaks at the philtral ridge on each side and gently curves downward as it reaches the midline to form the Cupid's bow. A deficiency in tissue (skin, muscle, and mucosa) along one or both sides of the upper lip, or rarely in the midline, results in a cleft at the site of this deficiency. The deficiency of tissue present with a cleft lip results in distortion of the Cupid's bow, absence of one or both philtral ridges, and distortion of the lower portion of the nose. Cleft lip is usually associated with a notch or cleft of the underlying alveolus and a cleft of the palate.

Cleft-lip repair is most often performed when the infant is about 3 months of age. Timing of the repair follows the "rule of 10": the infant is 10 weeks of age, weighs 10 pounds, and has a hemoglobin of 10. Early surgical correction aids in feeding and infant-parent bonding. Lip

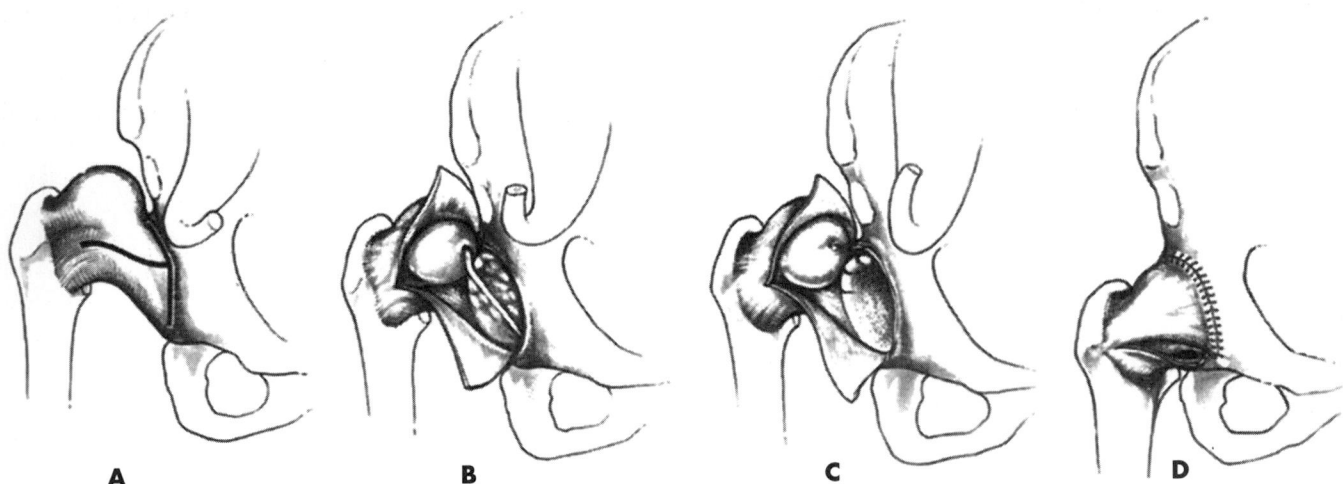

FIGURE 29-30   Repair of congenital hip disorder using open reduction. **A,** T-shaped incision of capsule. **B,** Capsulotomy of the hip and locating the true acetabulum. **C,** Removal of tissue from the depth of the acetabulum. **D,** Capsulorrhaphy.

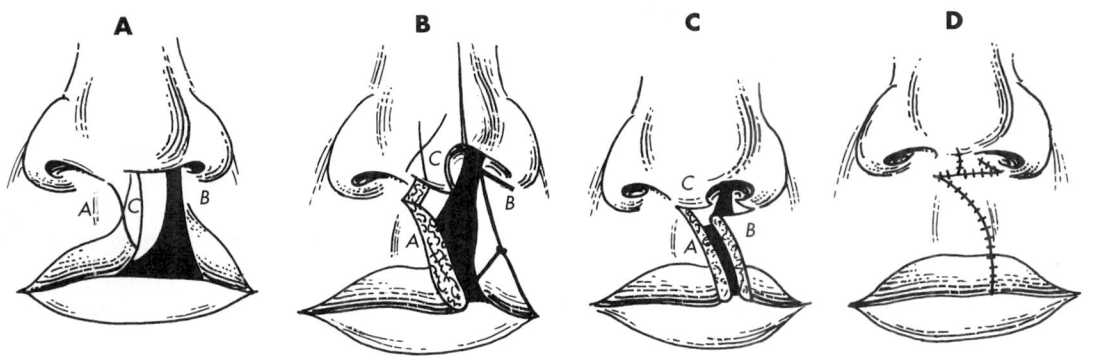

FIGURE 29-31   Rotation-advancement method to correct complete unilateral cleft of lip. **A,** Rotation incision marked so that Cupid's bow-dimple component *A* will rotate down into normal position; flap *C* will advance into columella and then form nostril sill. **B,** Flap *A* has dropped down, flap *C* has advanced into columella, and flap *B* has been marked. **C,** Flap *B* is being advanced into rotation gap, while skin-roll flap is interdigitated at mucocutaneous junction line. **D,** Scar is maneuvered into strategic position where it is hidden at nasal base and floor and philtrum column and interdigitated at mucocutaneous junction.

repair is directed toward rearrangement of existing tissues to approximate the normal lip as closely as possible. Some considerations may also be given to correcting the nasal deformity at the time of the cleft lip repair.

Procedural considerations

A plastic local instrument set is required, plus the following special instruments: Brown lip clamps; calipers; Fomon retractor; skin hooks, double; 5 mm Beaver scalpel handles and blades, #64 and #65; Logan's bow; knife blades, #11; 25 g needle on straight hemostat; marking pen; cotton-tipped application; disposable tongue depressor; methylene blue; and epinephrine 1:200,000 (for injection). The OR bed is usually reversed to create more knee room if the surgeon performs surgery from a sitting position. The patient is placed in the supine position, with the head at the edge of the OR bed. The face is prepped,

and the head drape is used. The surgeon may stand or sit at the patient's side or just above the patient's head during the operation.

Operative procedure

Many types of cleft lip repair are in common use, one of which is illustrated in Fig. 29-31. The following steps are applicable to all lip repairs:

1. Normal landmarks are identified and marked or tattooed. Precise measurements, taken with calipers and a ruler, are made so that corresponding points can be marked along the cleft.
2. The lip may be infiltrated with epinephrine 1:200,000, or lip clamps may be used to aid hemostasis.
3. Incisions are made along the markings for the repair.
4. The abnormal musculature is dissected.

5. Additional dissection along the maxilla and nose may be performed.
6. Closure is done in three layers: muscle, skin, and mucosa. Steri-Strips may be used.
7. A Logan's bow is applied to the cheeks with tape strips. Elbow restraints are placed.

Cleft Palate Repair

The palate is made up of the bony or hard palate anteriorly and the soft palate posteriorly. The alveolus borders the hard palate. A separation or cleft of the palate occurs in the midline and may involve only the soft palate or both hard and soft palates. The alveolus may be cleft on one or both sides.

The major function of the soft palate is to aid in the production of normal speech sounds. An intact hard palate is necessary to prevent escape of air through the nose during speech and to prevent the egress of liquid and food from the nose.

Cleft palate repair is usually performed when the child is 6 months of age and should be achieved before the beginning of speech. Variable factors, including the child's weight and the possibility of other disease processes, can affect the timing of the surgery. The various operations used to achieve surgical closure of the palate all employ tissue adjacent to the cleft (in the form of flaps) and shift it centrally to close the defect.

Procedural considerations

A basic plastic instrument set is required, plus the following special instruments: Dingman mouth gag with assorted blades; Blair palate hook; palate knives; Blair palate elevators, L-shaped, dull and sharp; Burlisher clamps, curved; Crile-Wood needle holders, 6 inches; Stratte needle holder, delicate; Fomon lower lateral scissors, short and long; Cushing tissue forceps; Cushing dressing forceps; Brown forceps; Cottonoids, 1 × 1 inch, with strings; epinephrine 1:200,000 (for injection); marking pen; bipolar electrosurgical unit; and volumetric suction bottle

The patient is placed in the supine position, with the head at the edge of the OR bed. The head drape is used. Many surgeons sit just above the patient's head and cradle the head on their lap (with the patient's neck hyperextended).

Operative procedure

One of the most frequently used cleft palate repairs is illustrated in Fig. 29-32. The following steps are common to all palate repairs:

1. Dingman mouth gag is inserted. Maintenance of the position of the endotracheal tube is crucial at this point. A throat pack may be inserted to absorb blood that may drain into the throat.
2. The outlines of the palatal flaps are marked.

3. The palate is injected with epinephrine 1:200,000 for hemostasis.
4. The flaps are incised and elevated.
5. Closure is in three layers: nasal mucosa, muscle, and palatal mucosa.
6. A large horizontal mattress traction suture is placed through the body of the tongue. If the patient experiences upper airway obstruction after extubation, traction is placed on this suture to pull the tongue forward, rather than insert an airway that might harm the palate repair. The throat pack is removed.

Pharyngeal Flap

When abnormal speech (velopharyngeal insufficiency) results despite a cleft palate repair, a secondary surgical procedure may be necessary to improve speech. Typical "cleft palate speech" is characterized primarily by an excess of air escaping through the nose during speech. This hypernasality often results from insufficient bulk or movement of the muscles of the soft palate. To decrease or eliminate this problem, tissue from the pharynx, in the form of a pharyngeal flap, is added to the soft palate. This flap also reduces the size of the opening between the oropharynx and nasopharynx, thus decreasing or eliminating the nasal escape of air during speech.

A pharyngeal flap repair may be done at any age, but most are done before the patient is 14 years old. A pharyngeal flap also may be part of primary cleft palate repair.

Procedural considerations

The same instruments are needed as for cleft palate repair, plus two 14 Fr red rubber catheters.

Positioning and draping of the patient are as described for cleft palate repair.

Operative procedure

1. The Dingman mouth gag is inserted. A throat pack may be inserted.
2. The palate and posterior wall of the pharynx are injected with epinephrine 1:200,000 for hemostasis.
3. The palate is incised, and the pharyngeal flap is incised and elevated.
4. The pharyngeal wall donor site may be sutured or left open.
5. The pharyngeal flap is sutured to the palate, and the palate is closed.
6. A traction suture is placed through the body of the tongue. The throat pack is removed.

Total Ear Reconstruction

An absent external ear, with either a congenital or a traumatic origin poses to the reconstruction surgical team the dual challenge of being both surgically adept and artistically driven. The patient presents the team with the objective of developing or restoring a part of the

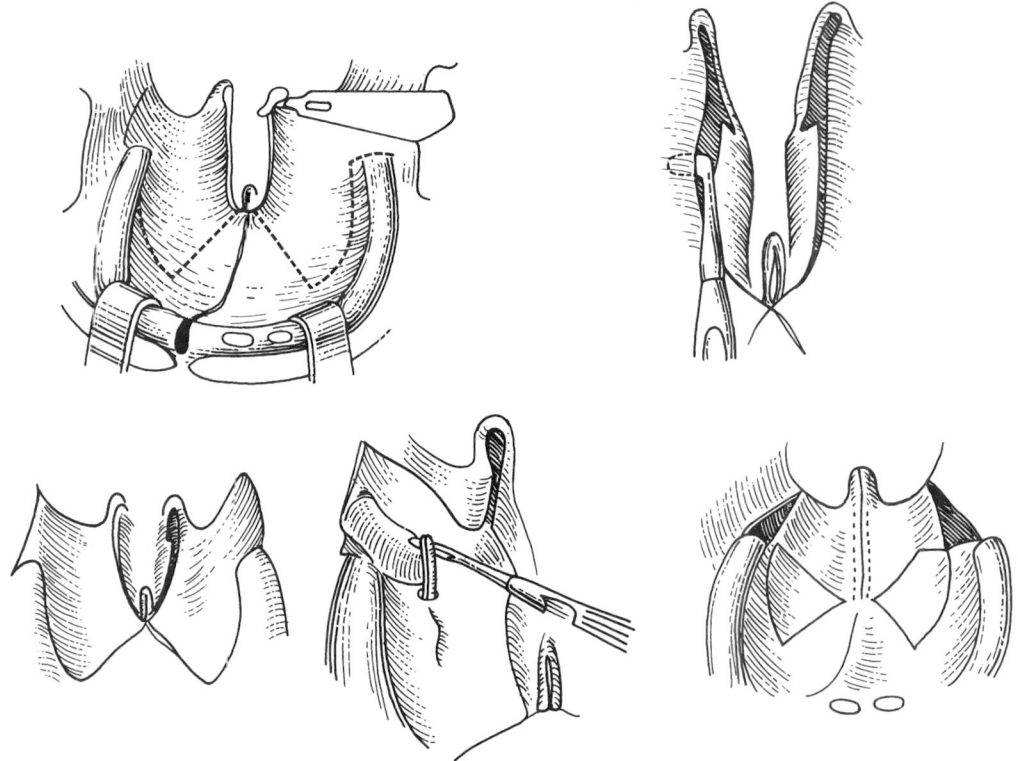

FIGURE 29–32   Closure of cleft of soft palate by V-Y (Wardill-Kilner) palatoplasty. A V-shaped incision is made on oral side of palate; mucoperiosteal flaps are elevated on oral and nasal sides, with preservation of blood vessels; Y-shaped closure (in three layers) closes cleft and lengthens palate.

appearance that will help with self-esteem and confidence in daily interactions as well as enhance hearing, since the external ear funnels sound waves from the environment into the inner ear. Emotional support is a key aspect of the plan of care for these patients.

The external ear comprises skin, subcutaneous tissue, and cartilage. The surgical procedure to create an external ear involves the retrieval of rib cartilage, carving of the cartilage, placement of the newly fashioned ear on the side of the patient's head, and skin grafting and dressing of the operative sites, with continual assessment and reassessment of the preoperative sketches made of the patient's ear with relation to facial structure. This can be accomplished as a one-stage procedure or as a sequence of surgeries. For congenital defects the ideal time for initiating the procedure is between 6 and 10 years of age. In the case of traumatic loss of the external ear (as from burns), the time is individually determined. The option for the use of tissue expanders has been considered in some cases to stretch the skin surface required to cover the ear.

Procedural considerations

The following instruments are required: plastic instrument set (basic), calipers, marking pen, and local anesthesia with epinephrine 1:200,00. Total ear reconstruction with autologous rib cartilage retrieval requires the following additional items: Freer and Key periosteal elevators, rake retractors, Oschner clamps, mallet, osteotomes, chisels, dermatome of choice, wire scissors, unipolar and bipolar electrosurgical unit, Doppler probe with sterile conduction gel for intraoperative use, clear x-ray film, sequential compression boots or antiembolism stockings, Foley catheter, and available blood for transfusion. A gel mattress and a warming blanket should be placed on the OR bed. Preoperative intravenous antibiotics may be prescribed. The patient is supine with the arms tucked securely at the sides. Appropriate padding and protection of vulnerable neurovascular bundles and pressure sites are critical. Use of a sequential compression device and a Bair Hugger or second heating blanket over the lower half of the patient's body should be considered because of the anticipated length of the procedure. Use of a standard head drape and split drape (or U drape) for the patient's torso allows the team access to the auricular area and chest respectively. Usually two instrument tables are used with one being designated for the carving of the rib cartilage. Since the procedure is lengthy (6 to 8 hours on the average), comfortable chairs should be provided for the team. Periodic progress of the procedure should be relayed to the patient's family members in the waiting room.

Operative procedure

1. Preoperative sketches of the ear are done with the use of clear x-ray films. Symmetric and anatomic landmarks are vital considerations in the patterns developed for the reconstruction.
2. Assessment of the vascular integrity of the temporoparietal flap is done preoperatively with an unsterile Doppler pencil and conduction gel.
3. The donor skin graft site is identified and prepped with an antimicrobial scrub.
4. When the sketches are complete, the films are sterilized with care not to remove the markings made by the surgeon.
5. The operative site of the head and chest area are prepped and draped in the usual manner.
6. The temporoparietal fascia flap is lifted, and a sterile Doppler pencil and sterile conduction gel are used to assess the vascular integrity of the flap.
7. Infiltration of the operative sites with local anesthesia with epinephrine 1:200,00 can be used for hemostasis. Epinephrine in greater dosages (such as 1:100,000) is not recommended for use in the area of the flap because of the possible obliteration of the vascular complexes present.
8. Costocartilage retrieval requires preoperative marking of the patient's chest wall (the area of the sixth, seventh, and eighth ribs). The chest wall is incised, and the rib segments are removed with care to preserve the perichondrium. This will encourage bone growth and help to prevent a chest wall defect. The assessment of an intact pleura is critical before closure of the chest. Instillation of saline into the wound is done; if bubbles appear, a chest tube is inserted and attached to a chest drainage system. If still in question, an intraoperative chest x-ray film may be taken to check for a collapsed lung. If bubbles are absent, closure of the wound with the optional injection of local anesthesia to the intercostal areas is performed.
9. While one team closes the chest, another team begins the carving process, using sterile wood-carving tools to accomplish this part of the procedure. The previously marked radiographs are crucial aids for the artistic abilities of the surgeon. The films are the blueprint for the sculpting phase of the procedure. Surgical wire is used to connect the carved pieces of rib cartilage and shaped to resemble the external ear.
10. A skin graft is taken, and the donor site is covered with a dressing of choice.
11. Hemostasis is maintained with the use of electrocoagulation, topical thrombin, and infiltration of local anesthesia with epinephrine.
12. The flap covers the sculpted ear and the skin graft is used to cover any exposed areas (this is a technique used especially with burn patients who have less available skin for coverage).

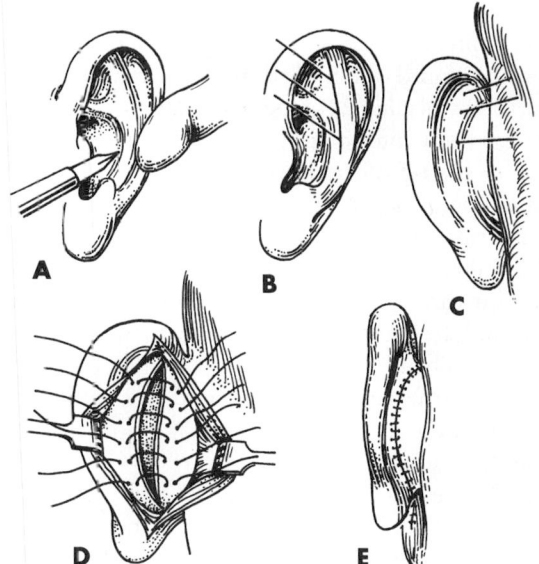

FIGURE 29-33 Otoplasty for correction of protruding ears. **A,** Antihelix defined by application of pressure to ear. **B,** Position of antihelical fold marked by the passage of straight needles through ear. **C,** Needle points visible along posterior surface of ear with ellipse of skin to be excised marked. **D,** Section of ear cartilage incised and scored or excised with sutures placed to hold cartilage back. **E,** Posterior ear incision sutured.

13. Drainage tubes are placed and attached to closed wound suction, or gauze stents wrapped with nonadherent gauze are sutured in place behind the ear. Soft, bulky dressings are applied to the ear and secured with a head wrap of rolled gauze (such as Kerlix); standard dressings are applied to the chest wall.

Otoplasty

A congenital deformity in which the ear protrudes abnormally from the side of the head is generally the result of an absent or insufficiently pronounced antihelical fold of the external ear. The various methods of otoplasty are an attempt at correction by creating an antihelical fold that "pins" the ear back against the side of the head (Fig. 29-33). Protruding ears may be unilateral or bilateral. Otoplasty is usually performed on children just before they start school. It is also performed on adults, in which case either general or local anesthesia may be used.

Procedural considerations

A plastic local instrument set is needed, plus the following: calipers; 22-gauge needle or straight needles, cotton-tipped applicators, methylene blue, marking pen, epinephrine 1:200,00 for injection, and mineral oil.

The patient is placed in the supine position on the OR bed, and a head drape is used, leaving both ears well exposed. The patient's head is turned with the affected ear up and with the lower ear well padded to avoid pressure injury.

Operative procedure

1. The antihelical fold is created when the external ear is bent backward. The position of the antihelical fold is marked by placing 22-gauge or straight needles through the ear from anterior to posterior, applying methylene blue to the tip of the needles, and withdrawing them.
2. An ellipse of skin is excised from the posterior surface of the ear after it has been infiltrated with epinephrine 1:200,000 for hemostasis.
3. The ear cartilage is usually incised near the antihelical fold, and the anterior surface of the cartilage is scored to allow it to bend backward.
4. Sutures are usually placed to hold the cartilage in its new position.
5. The skin incision is closed.
6. A bulky dressing exerting moderate compression on the ears is applied. A nonadherent dressing and fluffs are usually placed behind the ear to avoid pressing the posterior ear surface against the side of the head.
7. A red-topped tube with a butterfly cannula makes a convenient drain for the ear reconstruction and allows the subcutaneous pocket to adhere to the framework beneath.

Repair of Syndactyly

Syndactyly refers to webbing of the digits of the hand or feet. The most common form of syndactyly is symmetric webbing in two otherwise normal hands. It may, however, be associated with other abnormalities in the hand, such as extra fingers (polydactyly) or bony abnormalities. In syndactyly with normal digits a web of skin joins adjacent fingers (Fig. 29-34, *A*); each finger, however, has its own tendons, vessels, nerves, and bony phalanges. Although the skin web may appear loose, a deficiency in skin is always present when surgical separation is undertaken. Plans for taking a skin graft (usually full thickness) should always be made. Surgical separation of syndactyly is performed at any time after approximately 12 months of age.

Toe syndactyly is less often treated surgically than finger syndactyly because proper function of the foot does not require fine movements of individual toes. Although the setup and description that follow are for the repair of finger syndactyly, they can also be applied to the repair of toe syndactyly.

Procedural considerations

A plastic local instrument set is required, plus a marking pen, unexposed x-ray film, a pediatric pneumatic tourniquet, and an Esmarch bandage.

The patient is placed in the supine position on the OR bed with the affected arm extended on a hand table. A pediatric pneumatic tourniquet is used. A hand drape is used, and both inguinal areas are prepped and draped (donor sites for full-thickness skin grafts). Some surgeons prefer to use the wrist or forearm as donor sites.

Operative procedure

1. Skin incisions are marked, and the tourniquet is inflated.
2. The skin in incised, and small flaps at the sides of fingers and in the web are elevated.
3. After these flaps have been sutured into position, patterns of areas of absent skin on the sides of fingers are made and transferred to the skin-graft donor site.
4. The skin graft is taken, and the donor site wound is dealt with appropriately. If a full-thickness skin graft is used, it must be defatted before the graft is sutured in place.
5. Skin grafts are sutured to fingers (Fig. 29-34, *B*).
6. Stent dressings are placed over the skin grafts. The entire hand is immobilized in a bulky dressing (see Chapter 24) or in a long arm plaster cast.

Orbital–Craniofacial Surgery

Some congenital anomalies involve the orbital-craniofacial skeleton. These include (1) hypertelorism

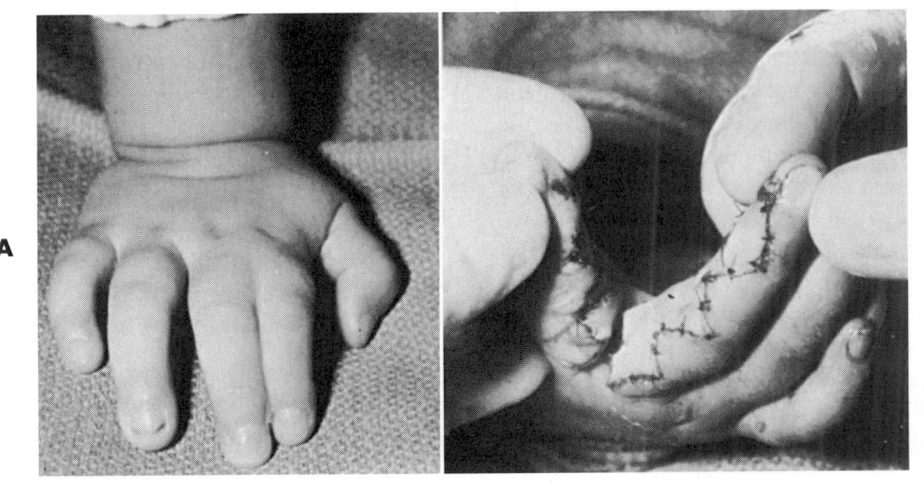

FIGURE 29-34   **A,** Syndactyly involving index and long fingers. **B,** Skin web separated; triangular flaps and skin grafts visible along sides of both fingers.

(Fig. 29-35), in which the distance between the orbits is increased; (2) Crouzon's disease (Fig 29-36), which includes premature closure of the cranial sutures, resulting in an abnormally shaped skull, exophthalmos and hypertelorism, parrot's beak nose, and maxillary hypoplasia; and (3) Apert's syndrome, which includes the same craniofacial deformities as Crouzon's disease with syndactyly or other hand anomalies. Recent advances in plastic surgery make surgical correction of some of these deformities possible.

Binocular vision is normal in humans. It involves the coordinated use of both eyes to obtain a single mental impression of objects. Binocular vision is usually absent in the craniofacial anomalies because of the increased distance between the orbits. The purpose of orbital-craniofacial surgery is to provide the patient with binocular vision, by moving the orbits closer together, and to provide the patient with a more acceptable appearance, by moving the bones of the orbital-craniofacial skeleton into a more normal position. Correction of the deformity seen in Crouzon's disease and Apert's syndrome involves a surgically created Le Fort III maxillary fracture.

Although an extracranial approach may be used, an intracranial approach is used in most cases; therefore a neurosurgeon and a plastic surgeon perform these operations through a bifrontal (coronal) craniotomy approach. A tracheostomy may be done before the start of the procedure. Bone grafts from hips or ribs are necessary to augment areas of bone deficit, which result from movement of the craniofacial skeleton.

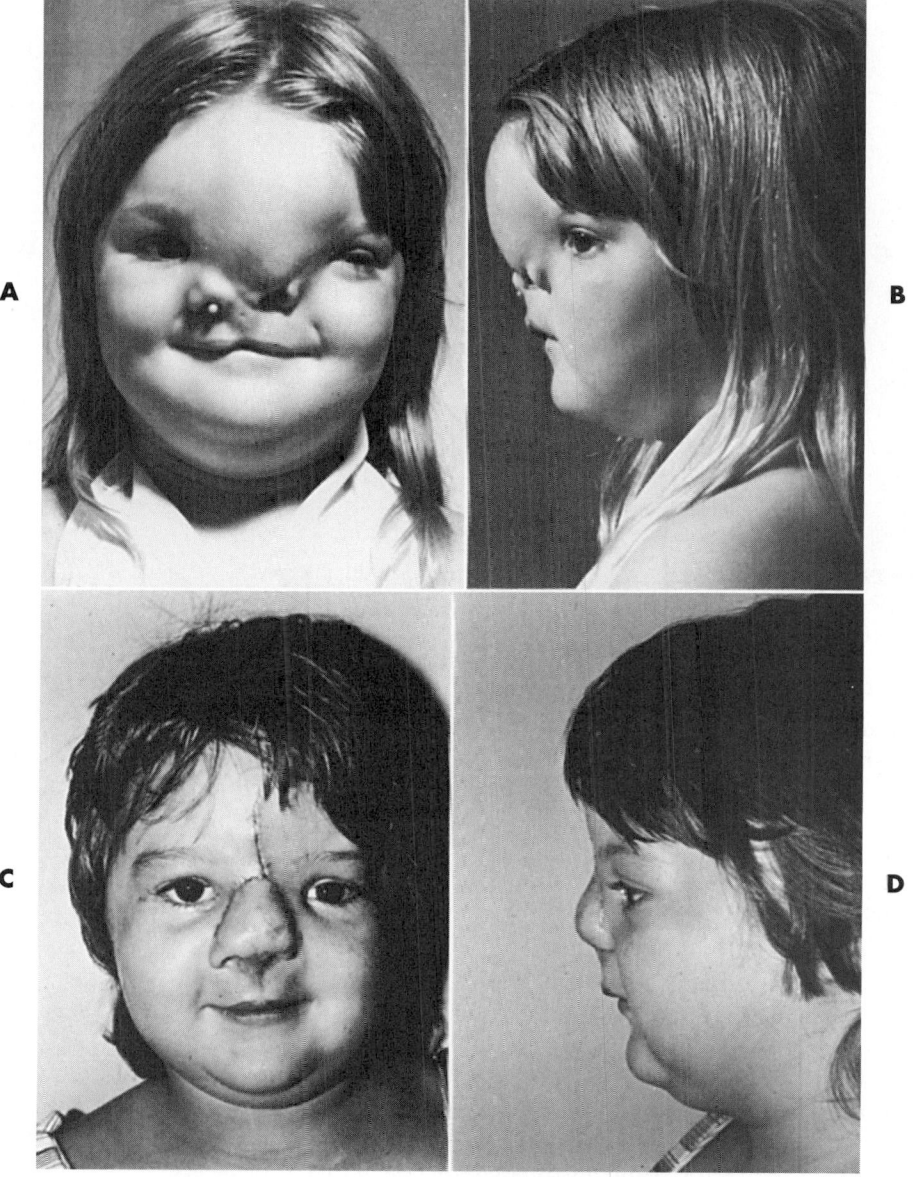

FIGURE 29-35   Hypertelorism. **A** and **B,** Before surgery, front and side views. **C** and **D,** After surgery, front and side views.

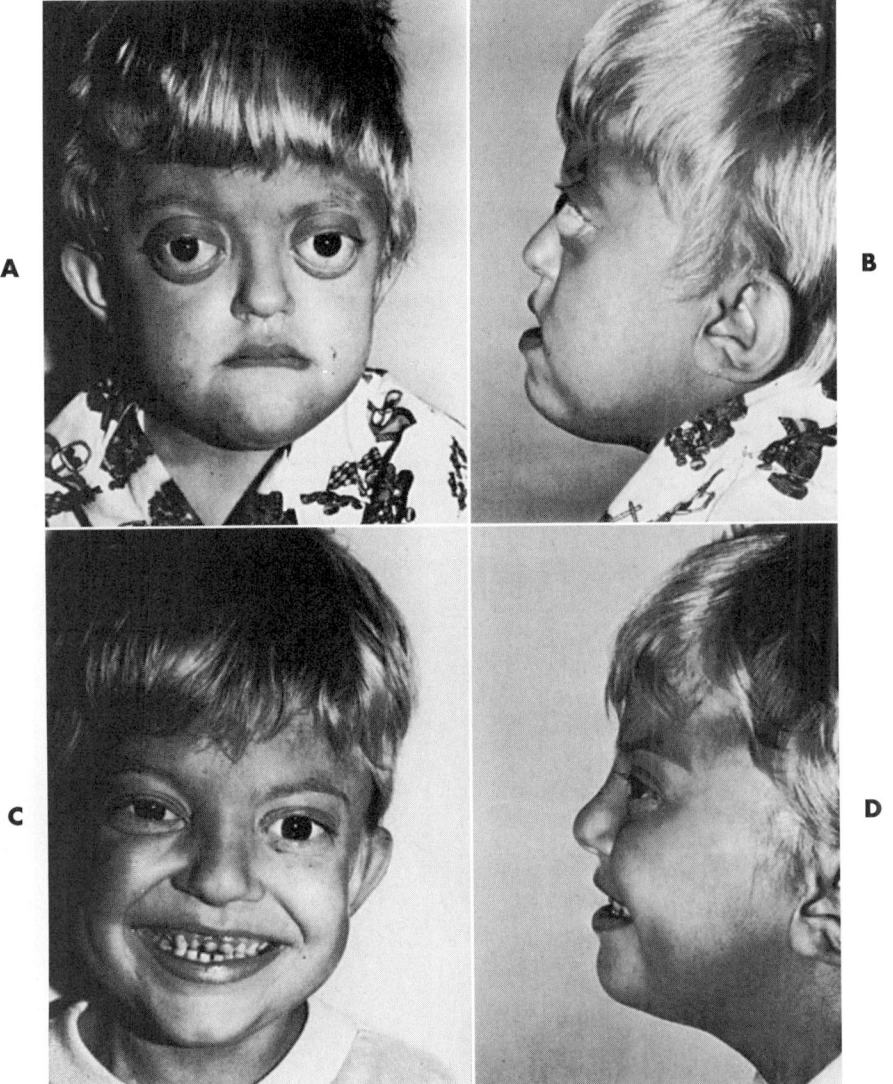

FIGURE 29-36 Crouzon's disease. **A** and **B,** Before surgery, front and side views. **C** and **D,** After surgery, front and side views.

Procedural considerations

These operations are usually performed on children. They are very extensive procedures, often lasting 12 to 14 hours. Blood loss is considerable. Postoperative complications, such as cerebral edema or meningitis can be formidable. The perioperative nurse must pay particular attention to the following important details: (1) insertion of a Foley catheter into the patient's bladder before the operation is started, (2) positioning of the patient on the OR bed so that all bony prominences are well padded, and (3) availability of accurate means for measuring blood loss (usually a volumetric suction bottle and scales for weighing sponges). Use of a sequential compression device and thermia blankets should also be considered.

A basic plastic instrument set, craniectomy instruments and supplies (see Chapter 23) and tracheostomy instruments and supplies (see Chapter 21) are required, plus the following: Hall II air drill; Elane or Midas Rex drill; oscillating and reciprocating saws; osteotomes, assorted sizes, straight and curved; mallet; curettes, assorted; rongeurs, assorted; calipers; Brown fascia needle; set coil arch bars; Rowe maxillary forceps; polyethylene buttons; foam rubber pads, small; volumetric suction bottle; scales for weighing sponges; and a marking pen.

A separate setup is necessary for obtaining the bone graft. It includes a plastic hand instrument set, plus a Weitlaner retractor; curettes, assorted; osteotomes, assorted; mallet; and a Hall II air drill.

The patient is positioned, prepped, and draped as described for bifrontal craniotomy (see Chapter 23). The entire face is left exposed, however, and may temporarily be covered with a plastic drape until the portion of the operation requiring access to the face is reached. The bone graft donor site is also prepped and draped so that both iliac crests and the lower ribs are exposed.

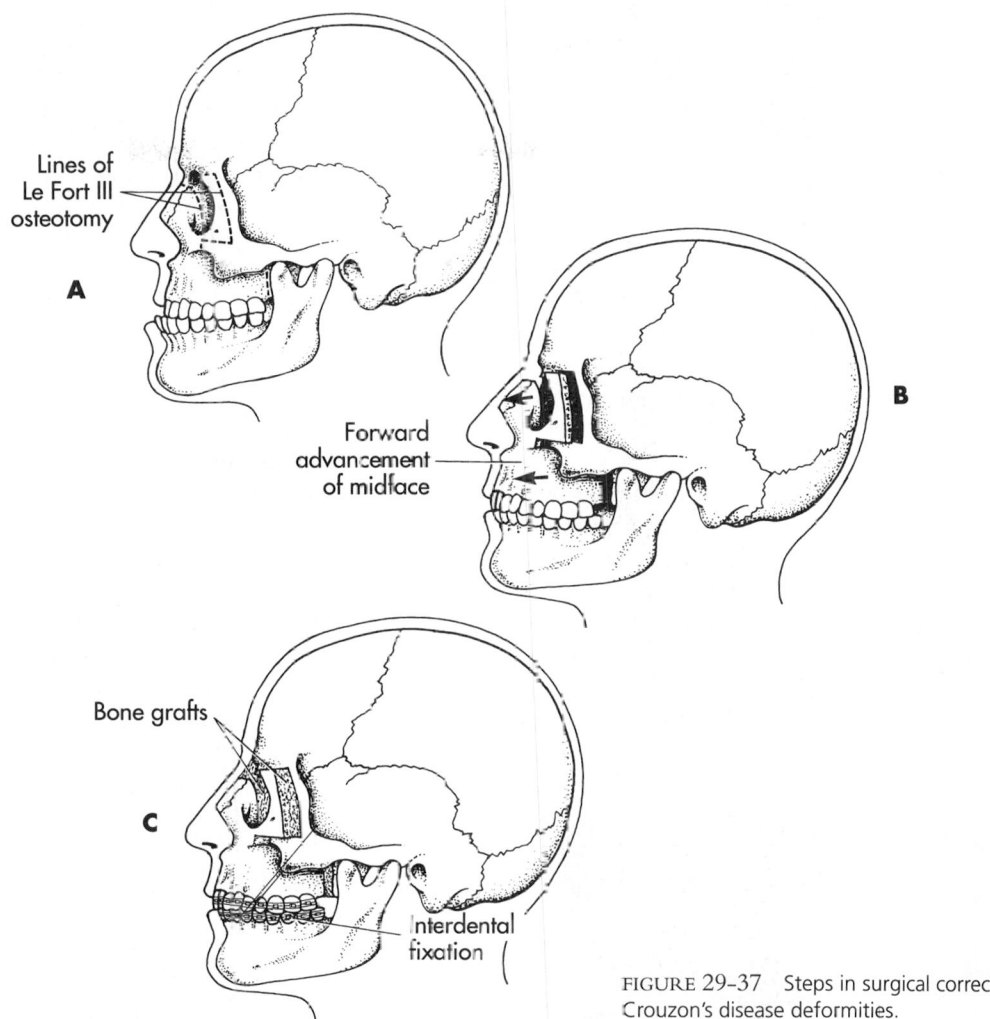

Lines of
Le Fort III
osteotomy

A

B

Forward
advancement
of midface

Bone grafts

C

Interdental
fixation

FIGURE 29-37   Steps in surgical correction of
Crouzon's disease deformities.

Operative procedure

1. Tracheostomy, if required, is performed first, followed by application of arch bars (when indicated as in Crouzon's disease and Apert's syndrome).
2. The bifrontal craniotomy with craniectomy is performed.
3. Orbital osteotomies (Fig. 29-37, *A*) into the anterior cranial fossa are performed bilaterally.
4. Bilateral conjunctival (lower eyelid) and labiogingival sulcus incisions (for Crouzon's disease and Apert's syndrome) are made for other orbital and maxillary osteotomies.
5. The bones of the orbital-craniofacial region are now moved (Fig. 29-37, *B*), based on measurement of the intercanthal distance (in hypertelorism) or occlusion of the teeth (in Crouzon's disease and Apert's syndrome).
6. Bone grafts may be taken from the calvarium, ribs, or hips to augment areas of bone deficit, which result from movement of the craniofacial skeleton.
7. Bone grafts are fixed in place with interosseous wires and by means of intermaxillary fixation applied to arch bars (for Crouzon's disease and Apert's syndrome) (Fig.

29-37, *C*). Rigid plate and screw fixation is another option.
8. The craniotomy, conjunctival, intraoral, and bone-graft donor site incisions are closed.

THORACIC PROCEDURES

Correction of Pectus Excavatum

Pectus excavatum (funnel chest) is a visually obvious defect of the sternum, seen as a deep depression on the chest as a result of posterior displacement of the sternum (Fig. 29-38). It is usually associated with kyphosis. The defect may be asymmetric, most often deeper on the right side, with sternal angulation. In a majority of cases surgical treatment is cosmetic; impaired cardiorespiratory function has been demonstrated in a few cases. The procedure is most commonly performed in patients between 10 and 16 years of age, when children become embarrassed to undress in front of peers. Rigid fixation has become a choice for correction of the defect wherein a metal retaining strut is added to gain chest wall stability and prevent recurrence. This strut must be removed 1 or

2 years later.[3] Other treatments may cosmetically correct the situation over the short term but result in progessive retraction of the sternum.

Procedural considerations

The thoracic instrument set is used. Instruments for lung resection and long instruments are not necessary. The following are added: Gigli saws and handles, osteotomes or chisels, bone hooks, bone-holding forceps, various periosteal elevators, and a fixation rod.

The patient is positioned supine with a portion of the upper chest elevated on a soft roll or sheets. The incision is a median sternotomy or a bilateral inframammary incision.

Operative procedure

1. A vertical midline incision is made from the level of the manubrium to the point below the xiphisternum.
2. A pectoral muscle flap is raised, and origins of the pectoral muscles are detached from the sternum and costal cartilages. The origins of the rectus abdominis muscles are dissected off the lower end of the sternum and costal margins.
3. The deformed costal cartilages are removed completely, but the perichondrium is preserved.

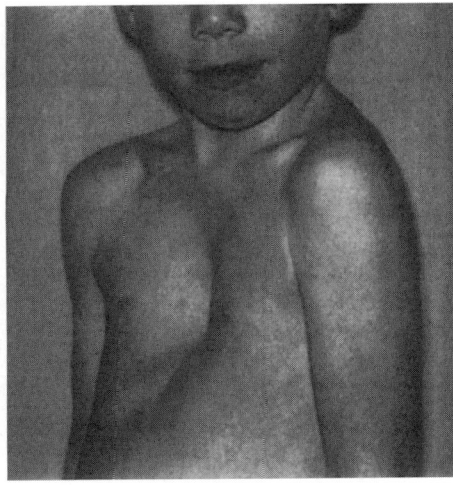

FIGURE 29-38   Patient with pectus excavatum.

4. The lower end of the sternum is elevated, and mediastinal structures and pleura are dissected free.
5. A transverse osteotomy is made through the anterior cortex of the sternum. The sternum is elevated, and the fixation rod is placed behind the sternum at the level of the anterior end of the fourth rib. Sutures are used to fixate the bar and adjacent rib.
6. A vacuum drain is passed into the anterior mediastinal space. The rectus muscles are sutured back to the perichondrium and to the lower end of the sternum.

TRAUMA

Blunt injuries and falls are the most common mechanisms of injury in the child, including pedestrian–motor vehicle accidents.[1] Because of the pliable nature of the skeletal system, if broken bones are present, a severe force of injury must be assumed. Neurologic injuries are the most common in children, but a high index of suspicion is maintained for other severe injuries. Because children have a much smaller reserve than adults have, once a decline in vital functions is noted, demise is rapid (Tables 29-1 and 29-2; Boxes 29-1 and 29-2).

A cuffless endotracheal tube is used in infants and children. One can approximate the size by noting the width of the fifth digit of the hand. IV access is often difficult in the pediatric patient, and an intraosseous line may be started in the emergency department. These lines

TABLE 29-2	Normal Respiration and Heart Rates for the Pediatric Patient	
AGE	RESPIRATION (BREATHS/MINUTE)	HEART RATE (BEATS/MINUTE)
Infant (birth–12 months)	30-60	120-160
Toddler (1-3 years)	25-40	90-140
Preschool-aged child (4-6 years)	22-34	80-110
School-aged child (6-12 years)	18-30	75-100
Adolescent (13-18 years)	12-20	60-100

TABLE 29-1	Sizes for Pediatric Airway Equipment		
AGE	LARYNGOSCOPE	ENDOTRACHEAL TUBE SIZE	SUCTION CATHETER (FRENCH)
Infant (birth–12 months)	Miller 0-1	2.5-4.5 (uncuffed)	5-8
		4.5 (uncuffed)	8
Toddler (1-3 years)	Miller 2		
	Flagg 2		
Preschool-aged child (4-5 years)	Miller 2	5.0 (uncuffed)	10
	Flagg 2		
School-aged child (6-12 years)	Miller 2	5.5-7.0 (uncuffed to 8 years of age)	10-12
	MacIntosh 2		
Adolescent (13-20 years)	MacIntosh 3	7.0-8.0 (cuffed)	12
	Miller 3		

are inserted by use of an intraosseous needle or bone marrow aspirate needle and are placed slightly below the knee on the anterior aspect of the tibia at a 90-degree angle (Fig. 29-39). Stabilization of the line may be difficult, but the line can remain for up to 24 hours and provides rapid access when other routes are too time consuming or difficult to access.

Fluid resuscitation of the pediatric patient as well as types and dosages of medications are based upon body weight. Body size of the patient determines the instrumentation sets required. Pediatric trauma instruments, including vascular clamps and retractors, and suture supplies should be available. Creative problem solving may be required of the perioperative nurse in adaptation of feeding tubes, drains, and other equipment. Maintenance of body temperature is of utmost concern in the pediatric population, and undue skin exposure should be avoided. Fluids for irrigation and IV infusion are warmed. Whenever possible, room temperature is elevated and a head covering of stockinette or other suitable material is used to prevent heat loss.

See Chapter 31 for additional information on care of the trauma patient.

SURGERY FOR CONGENITAL HEART DISEASE

Congenital cardiac abnormalities occur in 1% to 2% of live-born infants and are differentiated on the basis of whether they are cyanotic or acyanotic lesions (Box 29-3).

BOX 29-1 | **Specific Differences Between the Adult and Pediatric Trauma Patient**

- Growth, development and psychologic skills vary with age.
- Children have smaller airways with more soft tissue and a narrowing of the cricoid cartilage. The openings of the trachea and esophagus are closer together, which can make intubation more difficult.
- Children have faster respiratory rates and become hypoxic more quickly.
- The temperature control mechanism is immature in infants and small children.
- Children are easily dehydrated.
- Children have faster heart rates.
- Young children's extremities are likely to appear mottled. This may be a response to cold. Capillary refill may be a better indicator of circulatory status in the child.

BOX 29-2 | **Estimating Blood Pressure for the Pediatric Patient**

Systolic BP (mm Hg) = (2 × Age in years) + 80
Diastolic BP (mm Hg) = ⅔ systolic BP

The cyanosis-producing abnormalities carry a graver prognosis. Cyanosis is present because of a failure of delivery of pulmonary venous return to the systemic circulation (such as transposition of the great vessels) or reduction in the volume of pulmonary blood flow (such as tetralogy of Fallot and tricuspid atresia). The degree of cyanosis is affected by the amount of pulmonary blood flow or the extent of intracardiac mixing of blood through a shunt.

Among the acyanotic group are the obstructive lesions (such as aortic or pulmonary stenosis and coarctation of the aorta) that place an extra burden on the associated ventricle and can lead to heart failure. (Cyanosis may be apparent if the lesion is severe.) Shunt lesions (such as patent ductus arteriosus [PDA], ventricular septal defect [VSD], and atrial septal defect [ASD]) increase pulmonary blood flow. If a large shunt is present, congestive heart failure (CHF) can ensue.

Palliative procedures (described later) attempt to increase or decrease pulmonary blood flow or to increase intracardiac mixing of blood.

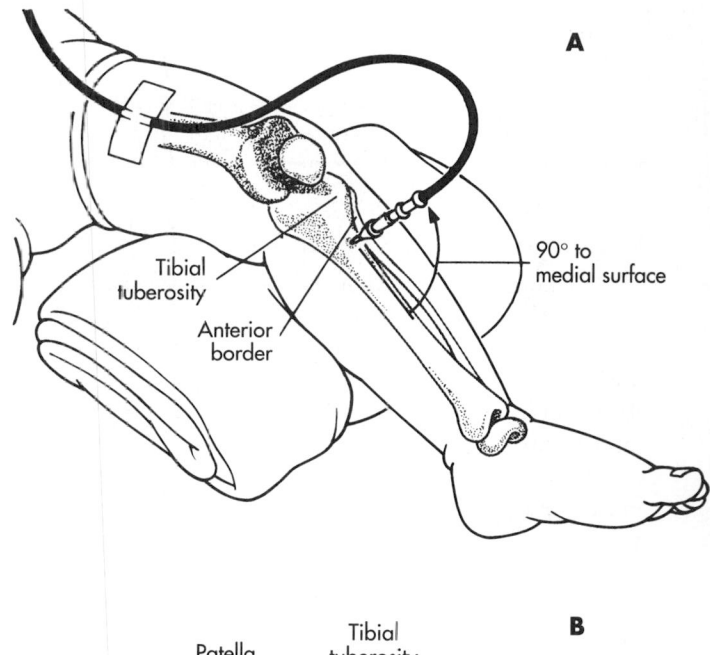

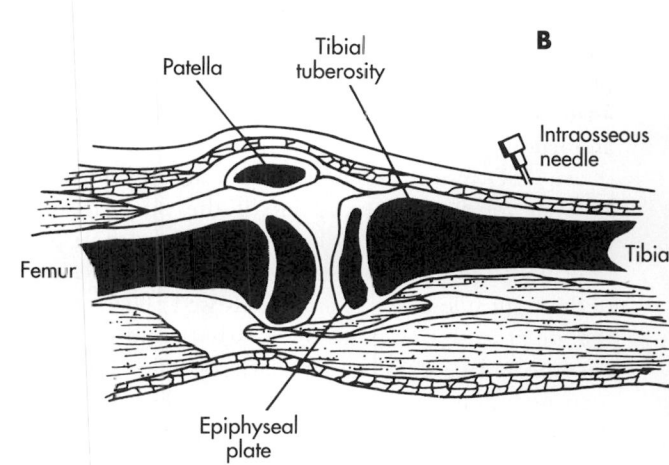

FIGURE 29-39 **A,** Intraosseous infusion technique. **B,** Insertion.

BOX 29-3 | **Congenital Heart Disease Classifications***

Acyanotic Defects

Atrial septal defect (ASD)
Ventricular septal defect (VSD)
Patent ductus arteriosus (PDA)
Atrioventricular canal (AV canal)
Aortic stenosis (AS)
Pulmonary stenosis (PS)
Coarctation of the aorta
Mitral stenosis (MS)

Cyanotic Defects

Tetralogy of Fallot (TOF)
Pulmonary atresia with intact ventricular septum (PA with IVS)
Tricuspid atresia
Interrupted aortic arch (IAA)
Truncus arteriosus
Total anomalous pulmonary venous return (TAPVR)
Hypoplastic left-sided heart syndrome (HLHS)
Transposition of the great arteries (TGA)
Double-outlet right ventricle (DORV)

---

*Congenital heart disease is often classified according to acyanotic or cyanotic hemodynamics. In general, acyanotic lesions involve increased pulmonary blood flow or obstruction to blood flow from the ventricles. The cyanotic lesions involve decreased pulmonary blood flow or mixed blood flow.

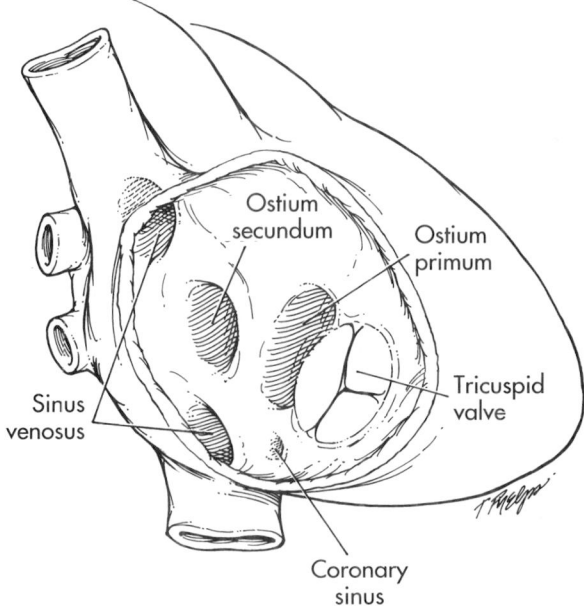

FIGURE 29-40 Various types of atrial septal defects (*ASD*) viewed through the right atrium (ostium secundum, ostium primum, sinus venosus). An unroofed coronary sinus may also act as an ASD.

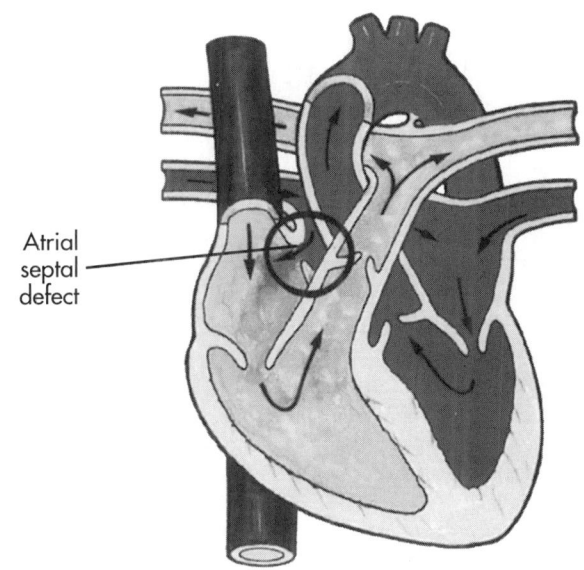

FIGURE 29-41 Atrial septal defect.

Repair of Atrial Septal Defect

Congenital defects in the atrial septum are closed, under direct vision, by a simple suture technique or by insertion of a synthetic prosthetic patch or pericardial patch. An ASD is a common congenital abnormality, and its classification is based on anatomic location and associated abnormalities (Fig. 29-40).

The ostium secundum defect is located in the superior and central portion of the septum. The ostium primum defect is in the lower portion of the atrial septum and is associated with other defects in the atrioventricular canal, usually with a cleft of the mitral valve or occasionally of the tricuspid valve. An accompanying VSD may also be present. The sinus venosus defect is located at the atrium–vena cava junction and is associated with partial anomalous pulmonary venous return.

An ASD results in a left-to-right atrial shunt that may be well tolerated in early life if the opening is small. However, if the defect is large or of the ostium primum type, with a pronounced shunting of blood, the work load of the right side of the heart is increased. The right side of the heart and the pulmonary artery and its branches become enlarged. The vascularity of the lung field is increased, with resulting pulmonary hypertension and subsequent failure of the right side of the heart. At this point the shunt may reverse (Fig. 29-41). In early life the patient may be asymptomatic. The initial symptoms may include fatigue, retardation of normal weight gain, and increased susceptibility to respiratory infections. Later symptoms include those of failure of the right side of the heart and cyanosis with a reverse shunt. A systolic murmur is heard with greatest intensity over the base of the heart. The defect is common in children with trisomy 21, or Down syndrome.

A clinical pathway for pediatric patients undergoing surgical repair of an ASD is shown in Fig. 29-42.

Vanderbilt University Medical Center

Surgical Repair Atrial Septal Defect

DRG Number: _____

ELOS: _____

	Preop (CV Clinic)	Day of Operation (Holding Room) 1-2 Hours	Day of Operation (OR) 4-5 Hours	Day of Operation (CRR)	Postop day 1 (CRR → 6N)	Postop day 2-3 (6N)	Postop day 4 (6N → Home)
Goals	All preop labs/tests completed → results WNL for surgery Pt/family teaching completed Consent form signed	Pt/family to HR by: 1) 6 a.m. if first case or 2) 2 hrs preop Pt ID/allergies verified Preop checklist and orders processed Support to pt/family	Pt safety maintained No injury R/T positioning noted Counts correct Pt tolerates operation without complications	Hemodynamically stable Pain controlled No arrhythmias Stable neuro, metab and resp. status Temp WNL	Extubate in early a.m. and/or when awake/ stable Transfer to 6N in p.m.		Afebrile Eating well Active CXR clear Family support
Treatments			IV Access A-line, CVP placement Foley catheter inserted Bovie pad—skin inspected after removal Warm blanket before transport Incision care—do not remove drsg 24° ———→	Ventilator ———— Oximeter ———— Cardiac Monitor ——— A-line, CVP ———— Foley ———— NG tube ———— CT/Pleur-Evac ——— Peripheral IV ————	Extubate when awake/stable D/C D/C D/C D/C D/C D/C D/C	Room air	
Activity	Ad lib	Bedrest ————————————————————→					
Diet	NPO at MN before surgery	NPO (status verified) ——————————————→			Advance slowly as tolerated ———		———→
Labs	(use clinic lab) Hemogram w/plts PT, PTT SMA-7 UA T+C (4 units PC)	} In pt's chart	Asleep & intubated ABG, PCV Pump primed ABG, PCV, K⁺ Off pump ABG, PCV	1/2 hr postop ABG, PCV, K⁺ Dextrostik Q6h × 4 ABG } × 1 PCV } additional K⁺ } set	Hemogram Chem 7 ABG		Hemogram
Tests	(use clinic radiology) CXR-PA/lat ECG (use ECG done during evaluation) History & Physical	X-ray folder to HR to OR with pt) } In pt's chart		PCXR (immediately postop)	PCXR (after mediastinal CT removed)		CXR (PA and lat)
Consultations	Anesthesiologist CNS/CM Surgeon		CRR—call report when sternal wires placed				Assess by CM before discharge from vicinity
Meds/IV		Preop per anesthesia Cardioplegia—order for use in OR Ancef IV (vancomycin if allergic to Ancef) × 2 doses—to OR with pt ———→	IV fluids ———— Anesthesia drugs Calcium chloride (10%) × 1 amp Heparin (1,000u/ml) × 1 amp Epinephrine (1:1000) × 1 amp Mineral oil × 1 Give after induction and repeat after bypass	——→ D5 W ¼ NS ——→ D5 W ——→ Tylenol (PR) Lasix (IV) Pain med (IV) Ancef × 3 total doses or vancomycin × 2 more doses ——→	——→ ——→ D/C		

FIGURE 29–42 Clinical pathway for repair of atrial septal defect.

Continued

	Preop (CV Clinic)	Day of Operation (Holding Room) 1-2 Hours	Day of Operation (OR) 4-5 Hours	Day of Operation (CRR)	Postop day 1 (CRR → 6N)	Postop day 2-3 (6N)	Postop day 4 (6N → Home)
Teaching/ D/C Plan	Preop instructions Procedure Plan of care Home care evaluation VUMC orientation Pt/family to hotel in vicinity for early a.m. admit (if home not local)	Family instructed of waiting area and anticipated time of surgery		Orient pt/family to CRR	Notify 6N to hold bed for afternoon transfer		Inst to return to clinic in 1 month Discharge to vicinity (or Ronald McDonald House)
Equipment & Supplies		Equipment Anesthesia supplies Ventilator ————— Oximeter ————— IV supplies A-line, CVP supplies Bovie pad & hand control Foley cath with urine meter Pleur-Evac Blood warming coil Fall blood filter Pump oxygenator Paddles—external and internal (age/size appropriate)	Sternal saw—electric Chest tubes Slush basin & supplies Per preference card: • Instrumentation • Sterile supplies • Suture For transport to CRR: • Bed/crib • transport monitor • O₂ tank with Ambu-Bag	Digital thermometer Manual resuscitator IMED II & tubing ——► Head hood ————► Nebulizer ————►	D/C D/C D/C D/C D/C		

FIGURE 29-42, cont'd   Clinical pathway for repair of atrial septal defect.

Procedural considerations

The child is placed in the supine position for a median sternotomy or in a right anterior oblique position for an anterolateral thoracotomy. The instrument setup is as described for basic open-heart surgery (see Chapter 27), with consideration given to the age and size of the child, plus intracardiac patch material, 2 × 2 inches or larger.

Operative procedure (Fig. 29-43)

1. A median sternotomy incision is made, and cardiopulmonary bypass is begun as described. (Infrequently, a right anterolateral incision is performed.) There are many bypass strategies that can be employed. With bicaval cannulation the child remains on bypass during the repair and blood is directed away from the right atrium through cannulas in the superior and inferior venae cavae. However, in this method the cannulas may obstruct the view of the ASD. With single venous cannulation a cannula is placed into the right atrium, and the child remains on bypass during the repair. With this technique the venous line is clamped immediately before the right atrium is incised, and pump suctions are placed into the inferior and superior venae cavae during ASD closure. Deep hypothermic circulatory arrest is usually used in more complicated repairs, such as osteum primum ASD or sinus venosum defects associated with anomalous pulmonary venous return.

2. The right atrium is incised, and the pathologic defect is determined.

3. The defect is closed with a continuous suture, or a patch of pericardium or prosthetic material may be used. By filling the atrium with blood before the atriotomy is completely closed, the surgeon can express air from the atrium. For the ostium primum defect with a cleft mitral valve, repair of the cleft is accomplished by approximation, with use of interrupted sutures.

Repair of Ventricular Septal Defect

Under direct vision a congenital defect in the ventricular septum (Fig. 29-44) is closed by a simple suture technique or, in most instances, by insertion of a synthetic prosthetic or pericardial patch. One of the most common congenital cardiac anomalies, a VSD is of little physiologic importance if small. A murmur is evident, but the patient is otherwise asymptomatic, and the heart size is normal. Larger defects with a significant left-to-right shunt, high right-sided ventricular pressure, increased pulmonary blood flow, and enlarged heart are repaired by surgery (Fig. 29-45). If left uncorrected, pulmonary volume overload results in pulmonary hypertension with subsequent reversal of the shunt to a right-to-left direction and in cyanosis.

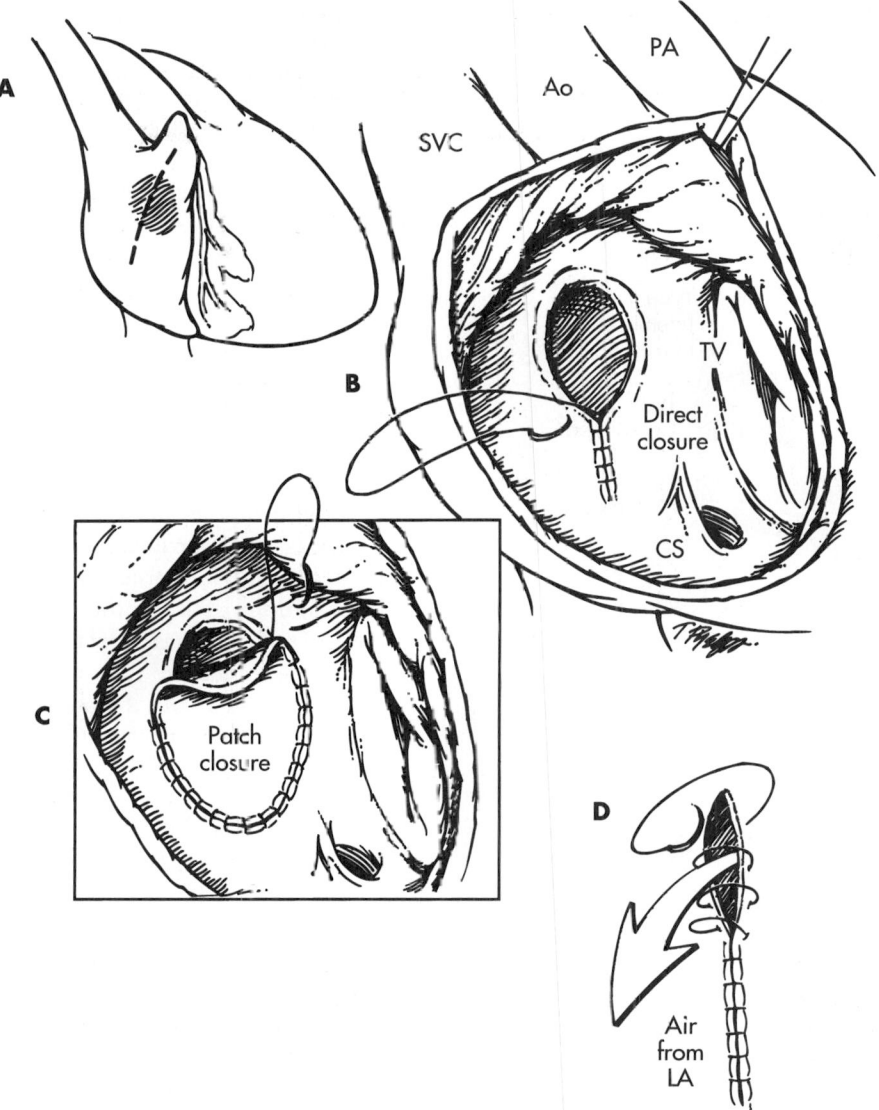

FIGURE 29-43   Surgical procedure for atrial septal defect (ASD) closure. **A,** Incision through right atriotomy. Direct suture closure, **B,** and patch closure, **C,** of secundum ASD. **D,** Deairing of the left atrium. *Ao,* Aorta; *CS,* conduction system; *LA,* left atrium; *PA,* pulmonary artery; *SVC,* superior vena cava; *TV,* tricuspid valve.

Operative procedure (Fig. 29-46)

1. A median sternotomy is performed, and cardiopulmonary bypass is begun as described.
2. The location of the defect determines the location of the incision. For membranous and canal defects, an incision is usually made in the right atrium, the atrium is retracted, and the VSD is identified by use of a pump suction through the tricuspid valve into the right ventricle. For supracrystal VSDs an incision is usually made in the pulmonary artery and may be extended into the right ventricle. A muscular VSD may require an incision in the apex of the heart.
3. A patch is used to close the defect. A continuous 6-0 or 5-0 nonabsorbable suture on a small needle may be

used, or an interrupted suture with or without pledgets, to place the patch. Rarely is the defect closed primarily.
4. Cardiopulmonary bypass is discontinued, and the sternum is closed.

Repair of Complete Atrioventricular (AV) Septal Defects

A-V septal defects (Fig. 29-47) account for 4% of congenital cardiac malformations and represent 30% to 40% of cardiac defects seen in children with Down syndrome. Complete A-V septal defects involve a large atrial septal defect, a large ventricular septal defect, and a common AV valve that straddles both ventricles.[8] The

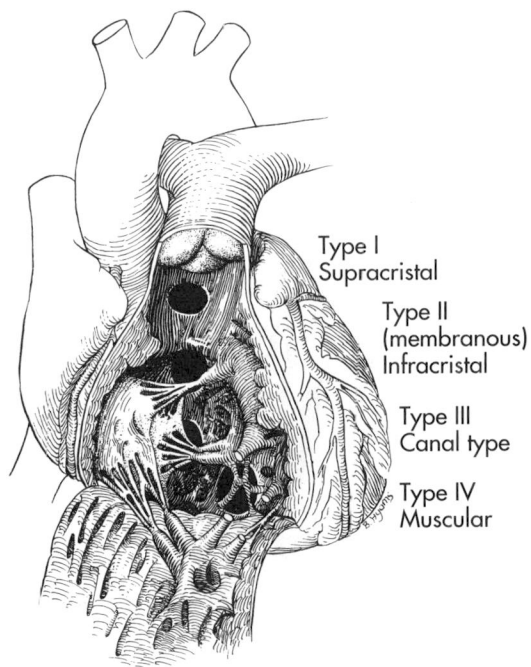

Type I
Supracristal

Type II
(membranous)
Infracristal

Type III
Canal type

Type IV
Muscular

FIGURE 29-44   Ventricular septal defects: anatomic classification.

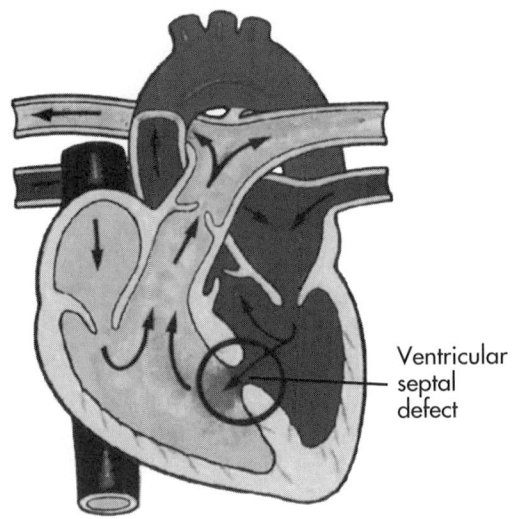

Ventricular
septal
defect

FIGURE 29-45   Ventricular septal defect.

operative procedure depends on the type of common atrioventricular valve and surgeon preference.

Operative procedure

1. A median sternotomy is performed, and cardiopulmonary bypass is begun as described.
2. The right atrium is incised, and the cardiac anatomy is inspected. The AV valve leaflets may be tested at this time by injection of cold saline into the ventricular chambers to float the AV leaflets into a closed position. Suture may be used to approximate the anterior and posterior bridging leaflets.

3. The superior and inferior bridging leaflets may be incised.
4a. If a single-patch repair of a complete AV septal defect is used, a piece of synthetic patch material or the patient's own pericardium is cut to appropriate size and shape. Continuous or interrupted sutures are used to place the patch in the ventricular septum. The bridging AV valve tissues may be secured to the patch with interrupted pledgeted suture or running suture secured with a few interrupted pledgeted stitches. The right side of the AV valve may also be secured to the patch. The left AV valve is tested for competence by use of saline solution, and adjustments are made. The atrial septal defect is then closed by suturing of the superior rim of the patch to the lower rim of the atrial septum.
4b. If a two-patch repair of the complete AV canal defect is used, the ventricular patch may be of synthetic material and the atrial patch may be of autologous pericardium. The synthetic material patch is often placed without division of the common AV valve leaflets. The leaflets are then attached to the crest of the synthetic patch, and the atrial septal defect is closed.
5. The atriotomy is closed using a running suture technique.

Correction of Tetralogy of Fallot

Tetralogy of Fallot is the most common congenital cardiac anomaly in the cyanotic group. Cyanosis, as seen in the superficial vessels of the skin, is the result of shunting unoxygenated blood into the systemic circulation. The essential features of this condition are pulmonary stenosis, high VSD, and overriding of the septal defect by the aorta, with resulting hypertrophy of the right ventricle—all of which may be subdivided into more complex variations (Fig. 29-48). The infundibular form of pulmonary stenosis is a long, localized constricture in the pulmonary outflow tract of the right ventricle. It is the most common type of this anomaly. Valvular stenosis and infundibular stenosis, however, may occur independently.

In tetralogy of Fallot blood flow into the lungs decreases as a result of pulmonary obstruction, and a right-to-left shunt of venous blood from the right ventricle to the left ventricle and aorta occurs. Symptoms of tetralogy are cyanosis, dyspnea, episodes of acute dyspnea with cyanosis, retarded growth, clubbing of extremities, and reduced exercise tolerance. A systolic murmur and secondary polycythemia are usually present. Cardiac catheterization and angiocardiography aid in determining the diagnosis and plan of surgical treatment.

The selection of a palliative or corrective procedure is based on the age and general condition of the patient and the severity of the pulmonary stenosis. The treatment of choice is primary repair; contraindications for primary repair include anomalous origin of the anterior descending coronary artery and presence of pulmonary atresia.

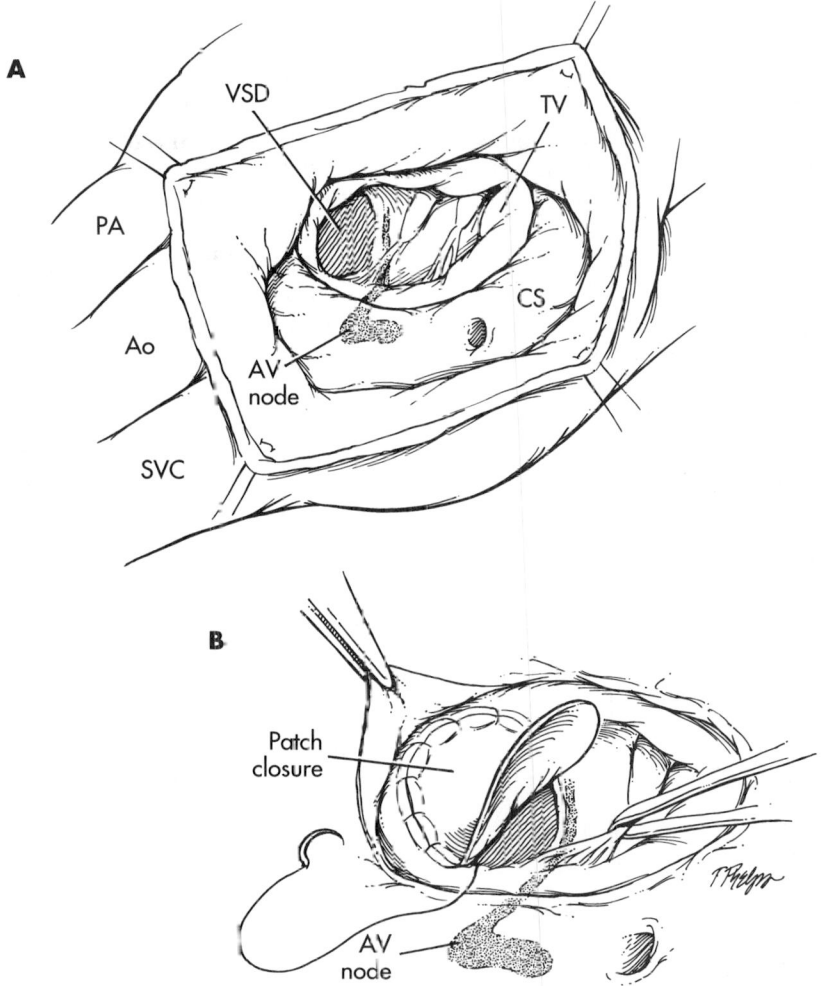

FIGURE 29-46   Ventricular septal defect *(VSD)* closure through the tricuspid valve *(TV)*. **A,** Open site. **B,** Partial closure. *Ao,* aorta; *AV node,* atrioventricular node; *CS,* conduction system; *PA,* pulmonary artery; *SVC,* superior vena cava.

Open corrective repair

The open corrective repair is done under direct vision and is the complete repair of the infundibular stenosis or pulmonary valve stenosis and closure of the VSD.

Procedural Considerations

The child is placed on the OR bed in a supine position. The setup is as described for open-heart surgery, with consideration given to the child's age and size. Additional items to be added to the basic open-heart setup include the following: intracardiac patch, 2 × 2 inches; outflow cardiac patch, 2 × 2 inches; and a felt or Gortex patch, 4 × 4 inches.

Operative Procedure

1. A median sternotomy is performed, and cardiopulmonary bypass with hypothermia is begun as described.
2. A vertical ventriculotomy over the infundibular area is performed (Fig. 29-49, *A*).

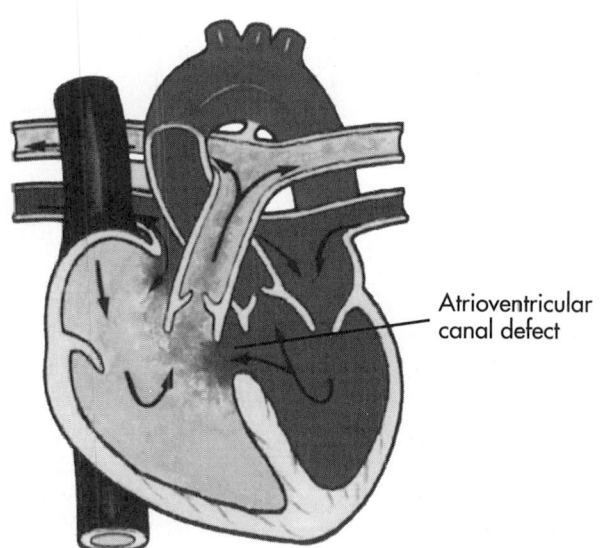

FIGURE 29-47   Atrioventricular canal defect.

3. The VSD is identified. Closure requires an intracardiac patch in almost all instances. This can be of a synthetic material or a piece of pericardium.

4. Interrupted or continuous cardiovascular sutures are placed in the septum with caution because of the danger of suturing a branch of the neuroconductive system.

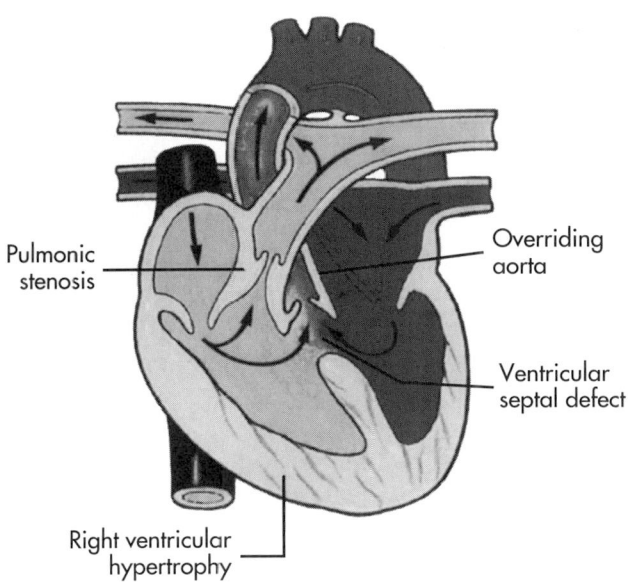

FIGURE 29-48   Tetralogy of Fallot.

5. The hypertrophied infundibular muscle is excised, as completely as possible, from the right ventricular outflow tract. If the pulmonic valve is stenosed, the fused commissures are incised.

6. An estimate is made about whether the right ventricle can be closed primarily or a patch is necessary. If the pulmonic stenosis cannot be relieved adequately by valvulotomy and infundibulectomy, an outflow patch of synthetic material or pulmonary homograft tissue may be needed to enlarge the outflow tract (Fig. 29-49, B). If the pulmonary artery or valve annulus is quite small, it may be necessary to extend the patch across the valve ring to the proximal portion of the pulmonary artery (Fig. 29-49, C).

7. Cardiopulmonary bypass is discontinued, and the sternum is closed.

Operation for Tricuspid Atresia

Failure of the tricuspid valve to develop results in an absence of communication between the right atrium and the right ventricle. Blood flows from the right atrium through an ASD, or a patent foramen ovale, into the left atrium. Some of the left ventrivular blood flows through a VSD to a small right ventricle and then to the lungs (Fig. 29-50). The infant displays cyanosis, periods of dyspnea, easy fatigability, and growth retardation. CHF progresses rapidly.

Palliative operations consist in the use of the Blalock–

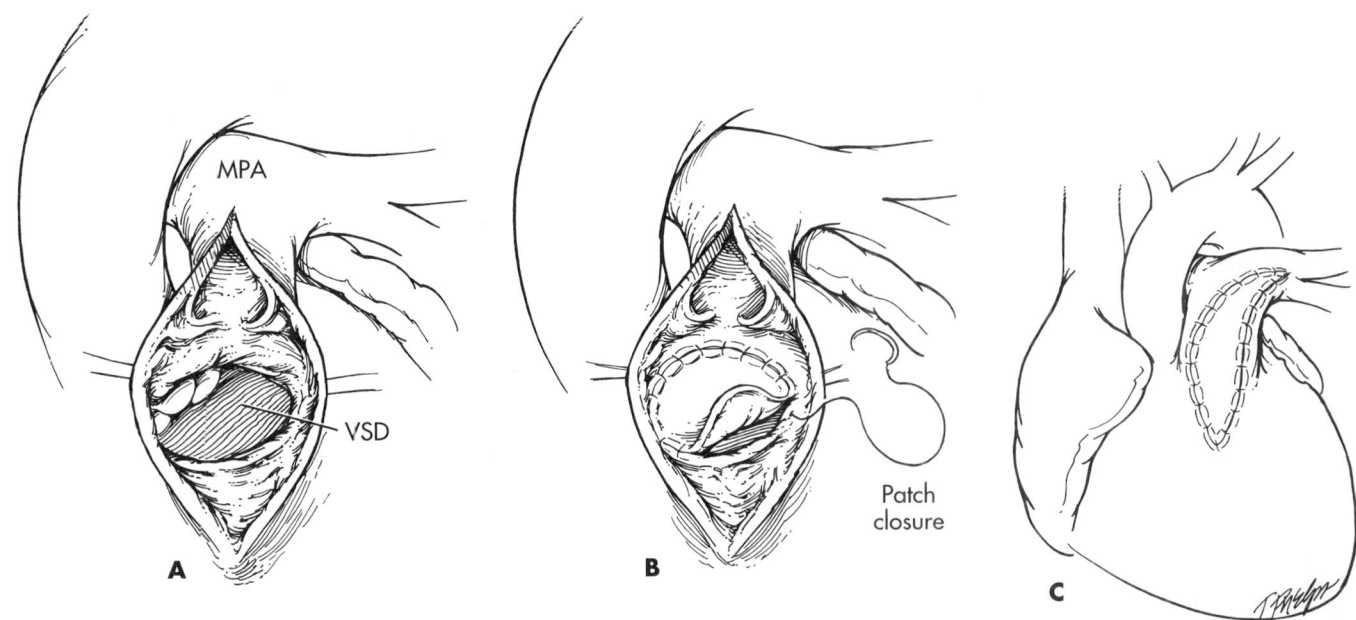

FIGURE 29-49   **A,** The most common ventricular incision used for repair of tetralogy of Fallot is vertical so that it can be extended as shown from the right ventricle across the pulmonary valve annulus and on to the main pulmonary artery *(MPA)*. It is possible to gain adequate exposure to the ventricular septal defect *(VSD)* by extending the incision a short distance beyond the infundibular septum. This "limited ventriculotomy" may help to preserve late right ventricular function yet enable adequate enlargement of the hypoplastic area in the right ventricular outflow tract. **B,** The VSD is closed with a prosthetic patch. Right ventricular outflow obstruction is relieved when the outflow tract is enlarged with a patch as shown. **C,** In some cases, it may be necessary to extend the incision onto the left pulmonary artery and for the patch to be tapered at its most distal extent.

Hanlon procedure (see Fig. 29-68, *C*), which enlarges the ASD or systemic–to–pulmonary artery shunts to relieve the cyanosis. A Fontan procedure, described later in this chapter, will then be performed after the newborn period.

Operations for Transposition of the Great Arteries (TGA)

In the anomaly in which the aorta arises from the right ventricle and the pulmonary artery from the left ventricle, circulation is reversed (Fig. 29-51). However, to sustain life, there must be a communication between the two sides of the heart or major vessels: a patent foramen ovale, PDA, ASD, VSD, or partial transposition of the pulmonary veins, which permits oxygenated blood to enter the systemic circulation.

The newborn with this condition is cyanotic at birth and becomes severely incapacitated, with an enlarged heart that rapidly increases in size and progresses to CHF.

Corrective procedures include the arterial switch, the Senning atrial switch, and the Mustard and the Rastelli procedures. The arterial switch procedure is the most common surgery performed for the TGA during the first week of life.

Palliative procedures that tend to improve intracardiac mixing, thereby increasing the oxygen content of the systemic blood, may be necessary if the surgeon chooses to do the Mustard or Senning procedure in the first few months of life. Palliative procedures include the Blalock-Hanlon procedure and the Rashkind atrial septostomy (see Fig. 29-68, *C*).

For each corrective procedure described, the child is placed on the OR bed in a supine position. The setup is as described for open-heart surgery, with consideration given to the age and size of the patient.

Arterial switch procedure

The surgeon performs anatomic repair of the transposition by switching the pulmonary artery to the right ventricle and the aorta to the left ventricle. The left ventricle must have developed sufficient contractile force to maintain systemic pressure once the procedure is completed. It occurs in patients with VSD and reversible hypertension or in patients in which the procedure is performed during the newborn period. In patients in which the procedure is performed after the newborn period, pulmonary artery banding (see Fig. 29-68, *B*) may first be performed to strengthen the left ventricle. Transfer of the coronary arteries must be accomplished without kinking, torsion, or tension.

Operative Procedure (Fig. 29-52)

1. Median sternotomy and CPB are performed as described.
2. The aorta is dissected away from the main and branch pulmonary arteries.
3. The coronary arteries are inspected, and the site for their transfer into the pulmonary artery is marked.
4. The aorta is cross-clamped and transsected above the sinuses and aortic valve; the pulmonary artery is transsected above the pulmonic valve.
5. The orifices of the coronary arteries with a rim of adjacent aortic wall are excised.
6. The corresponding sinuses of the pulmonary arteries are incised where previously marked. The cuff and coronary artery are then sutured into place. Care is taken not to kink the coronary arteries.
7. The distal aorta is brought behind the pulmonary artery (LeCompte maneuver). The distal aorta is anastomosed to the proximal pulmonary artery (neoaorta).
8. Pericardium or pulmonary homograft tissue is used to

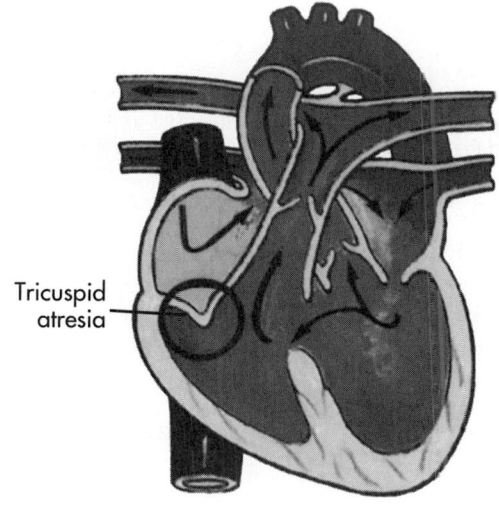

FIGURE 29-50 Tricuspid atresia.

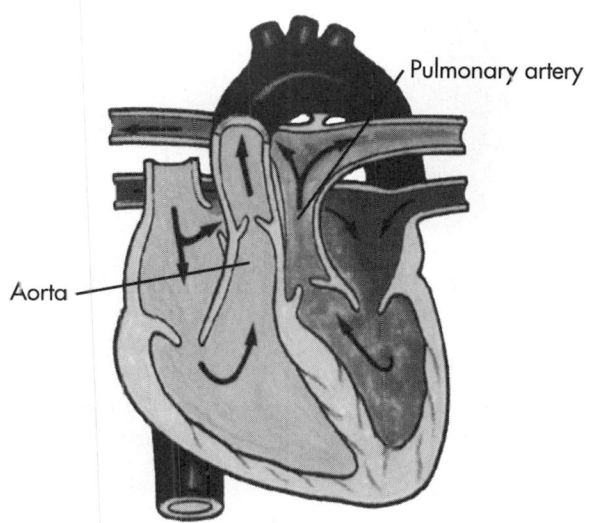

FIGURE 29-51 Transposition of the great arteries.

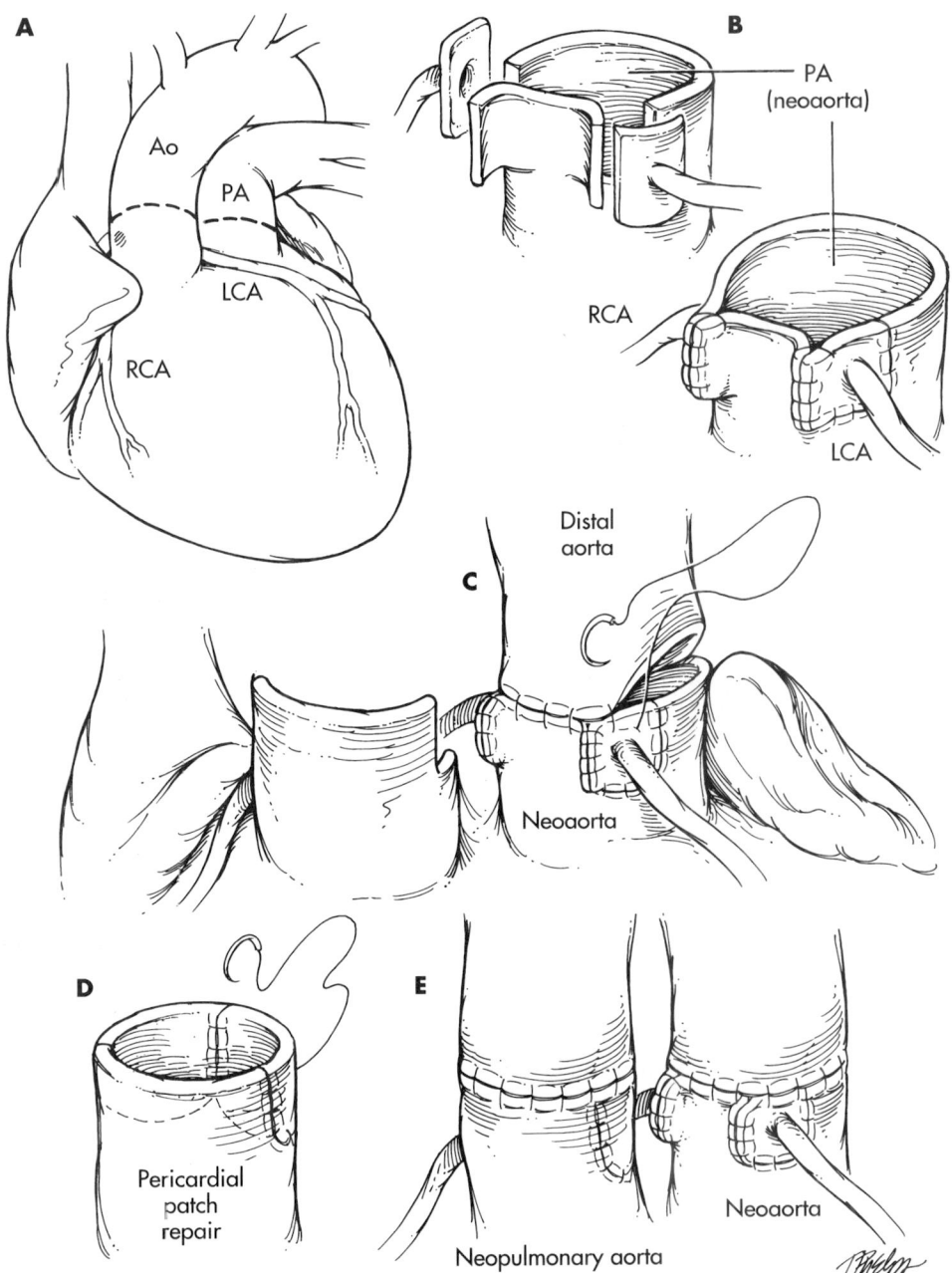

FIGURE 29-52 Technique of the arterial switch operation. **A,** The great arteries are transsected above the sinuses of Valsalva. **B,** The coronaries are excised from the aorta *(Ao)*, transposed posteriorly, and anastomosed to the pulmonary artery *(PA)* (neoaorta). **C,** The distal aorta is brought behind the pulmonary artery (LeCompte maneuver) and anastomosed to the neoaorta. **D,** Separate pericardial patches are sutured to fill in the defects in the aorta created by excision of the coronary arteries. **E,** Completed repair. *RCA,* Right coronary artery; *LCA,* left coronary artery.

enlarge the aorta and patch the defects created by the excision of the coronary ostia.

9. The repair is completed by anastomosing the proximal pulmonary artery to the distal pulmonary artery.

Senning procedure

The Senning alternative inflow procedure redirects venous flow. The Senning operation is sometimes preferred to the Mustard procedure (described on p. 1267)

because it is technically easier to perform and does not require the use of a patch that can eventually cause venous obstruction.

Operative Procedure (Fig. 29-53)

1. A median sternotomy is made, and CPB is instituted.
2. A right atrial incision is made longitudinally, extending to the insertion of the eustachian valve at the orifice of the inferior vena cava.

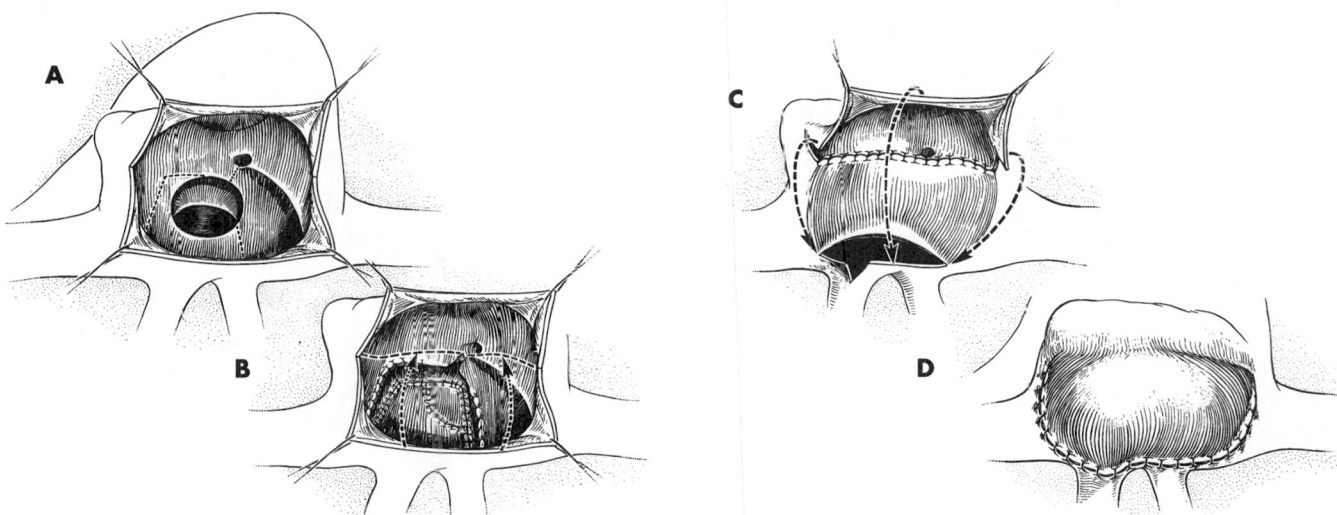

FIGURE 29-53   The Senning procedure. **A,** The atrial septum is cut near the tricuspid valve, so that a flap attached posteriorly between the venae cavae is created. **B,** The flap of atrial septum is sutured to the anterior lip of the orifices of the left pulmonary veins, effectively separating the pulmonary and systemic venous channels. **C,** The posterior edge of the right atrial incision is sutured to the remnant of atrial septum, diverting the systemic venous channel to the mitral valve. **D,** The anterior edge of the right atrial incision (lengthened by short incisions at each corner) is sutured around the vena cava above and below and to the lateral edge of the left atrial incision, completing the pulmonary channel and diversion of pulmonary venous blood to the tricuspid valve area.

3. A lateral atrial septal flap is made and sutured above the left pulmonary veins.

4. The new systemic venous atrium is completed by suturing the edge of the original right atrial incision to the remnant of atrial septum between the mitral and tricuspid valves. This step creates a tube of right atrium containing the venae cavae at each end.

5. Pulmonary venous blood flows around this tube from an opening in front of the right pulmonary veins to the tricuspid valve.

Mustard procedure

Under direct vision the Mustard procedure allows one to excise the remaining segments of the atrial septum; a pericardial or synthetic patch is sutured in place in the atrial cavities creating a baffle so that the venous inflow is reversed. This permits the pulmonary venous return to be redirected into the right ventricle and the systemic venous return to be redirected into the left ventricle (Fig. 29-54). Previous creation of an ASD may serve as a first stage for this procedure. Pericardium or synthetic patch is used as a baffle. Patients with an intact ventricular septum are candidates for an atrial switch type of operation.

Operative Procedure

1. A median sternotomy incision is completed as described.

2. A section of pericardium 2 × 3 inches is harvested.

3. Extracorporeal circulation is established as previously described.

4. A curved incision is made in the wall of the right atrium (Fig. 29-54, *A*).

5. The entire atrial septum is excised. The orifice of the coronary sinus is enlarged (Fig. 29-54, *B* and *C*).

6. Starting at the edge of the left pulmonary vein orifices, the surgeon sutures the baffle between the pulmonary veins and mitral valve, diverting the vena cava blood to the mitral valve and the pulmonary venous return to the tricuspid valve (Fig. 29-54, *D*).

7. An additional section of pericardium or synthetic patch may be placed in the wall of the right atrium that enlarges the new left atrium.

8. Extracorporeal circulation is discontinued, and closures are completed.

Rastelli procedure

In patients with VSD and subpulmonary stenosis the atrial switch operations have not demonstrated favorable results. The Rastelli procedure is an anatomic correction that has the advantage of converting the left ventricle to the systemic pumping chamber. Either a valved conduit or an aortic valve homograft may be used to connect the right ventricle and the pulmonary artery.

Operative Procedure

1. Median sternotomy and CPB are instituted.

2. The pulmonary artery is divided, and the proximal stump is oversewn.

3. The right ventricle is incised high in the outflow tract.

4. A tunnel is created by use of Dacron prosthetic material to direct blood through the VSD into the aorta.

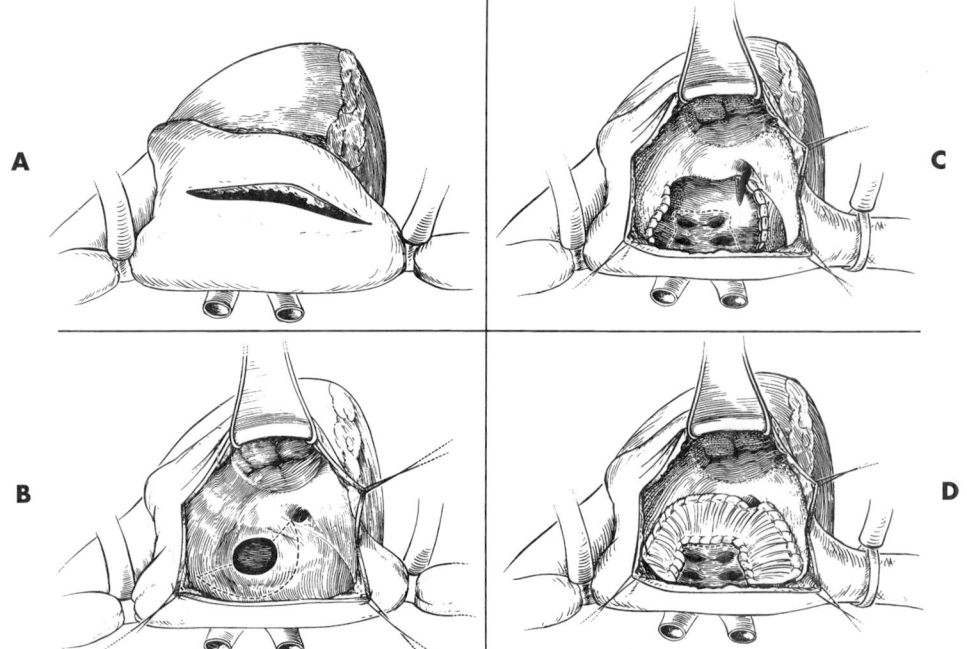

FIGURE 29-54 The Mustard procedure. **A,** The right atrium is opened with a longitudinal incision well away from the sinoatrial node. **B,** The atrial septum is incised from the midpoint on the superior border of the atrial septal defect to the middle of the superior vena cava orifice. All the septum lateral to this incision is excised, with avoidance of the orifices of the right pulmonary veins. The ridge of septum medially is preserved. **C,** The coronary sinus is cut back into the left atrium, and all raw margins of atrial septum are oversewn. The *dotted line* indicates where the baffle will be sutured. **D,** Starting at the anterior lip of the left pulmonary vein orifices, the surgeon sutures the baffle in place, thus diverting the vena cava return to the mitral valve and the pulmonary venous return to the tricuspid valve.

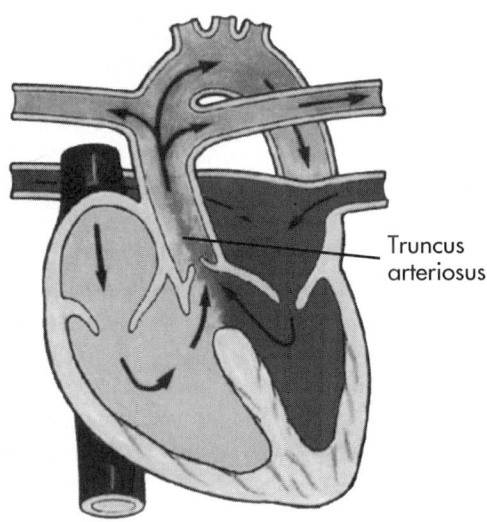

FIGURE 29-55 Truncus arteriosus.

5. An outflow conduit is placed between the right ventricle and the distal portion of the pulmonary artery.

Repair of Truncus Arteriosus

Truncus arteriosus is a retention of the embryologic bulbar trunk. It results from failure of normal septation of this trunk into an aorta and pulmonary artery. In this anomaly a single great vessel leaves the base of the heart through a single semilunar valve. This vessel is situated just above the VSD and receives blood from both ventricles. It gives rise to the coronary arteries and supplies the entire pulmonary and systemic circulations (Fig. 29-55).

Correction is quite successful with a nonvalved conduit of polytetrafluoroethylene (PTFE). The left atrial appendage is opened and used as the floor of the conduit with a patch of pulmonary homograft tissue as a roof over the conduit. With this technique there is no circumferential conduit to replace, and no further surgery is required as the child grows. Small (12 or 14 mm) extracardiac valved conduits may also be used to create a main pulmonary artery; in this instance replacement of the conduit will be required as the child grows.

Infants who do not undergo repair show severe CHF with cyanosis and failure to thrive.

Procedural considerations

The child is placed in the supine position. The basic setup for a sternotomy is used, with consideration given to the child's age and size. Depending on the corrective approach selected, a valved conduit; intracardiac patch material, 2 × 2 inches; and a ½ × 4 inch strip of Teflon felt may be required.

Operative procedure

1. A median sternotomy is performed, and cardiopulmonary bypass is begun as previously described.

2. A cross-clamp is placed on the aorta, the pulmonary artery is excised from the aorta (Fig. 29-56, *A*), and the aortic defect is closed with a double layer of continuous cardiovascular suture. The cross-clamp is removed.
3. A right ventriculotomy is made, and the VSD is repaired (Fig. 29-56, *B*).
4a. If a valved conduit is used, the distal end is anastomosed to the pulmonary artery.
4b. The proximal end of the valved conduit is anastomosed to the right ventriculotomy by use of a Teflon felt buttress, which prevents sutures from cutting through the ventricular wall and enhances hemostasis (Fig. 29-56, *C*).
5. CPB is discontinued, and chest closure is completed.

Open Valvulotomy and Infundibular Resection for Pulmonary Stenosis

Open valvulotomy is the separation of the stenosed leaflets under direct vision; infundibular resection for pulmonary stenosis is excision of the hypertrophied infundibulum.

Procedural considerations

The child is placed in the supine position. The basic setup for a sternotomy is used, with consideration given to the child's age and size.

Operative procedure

1. A median sternotomy is performed, and the cannulations are made for CPB as previously described.
2a. For open valvulotomy the pulmonary artery is opened longitudinally, and the stenotic valve is incised with a scalpel or scissors (Fig. 29-57, *A*).
2b. For infundibular resection, the outflow tract of the right ventricle is opened, and the resection is performed, as described for tetralogy of Fallot (Fig. 29-57, *C*).
2c. A patch of pericardium homograft tissue or synthetic patch material may be used to enlarge the pulmonary outflow tract (Fig. 29-57, *B*).

Other procedures

Some surgeons use a valved conduit for the more severe forms of pulmonary stenosis and atresia. The Rastelli procedure (described previously) may be used to suture the conduit to the right ventricle and to the pulmonary artery, thus bypassing the atretic valve.

Closure of Patent Ductus Arteriosus

Closure of the PDA, an abnormal communication between the aorta and pulmonary artery, is achieved by suture ligation or by division of the ductus. The PDA is an important fetal vascular communication whereby blood is shunted from the pulmonary artery into the aorta during intrauterine life. During fetal life the lungs are inactive, and the blood is oxygenated in the placenta. Normally the

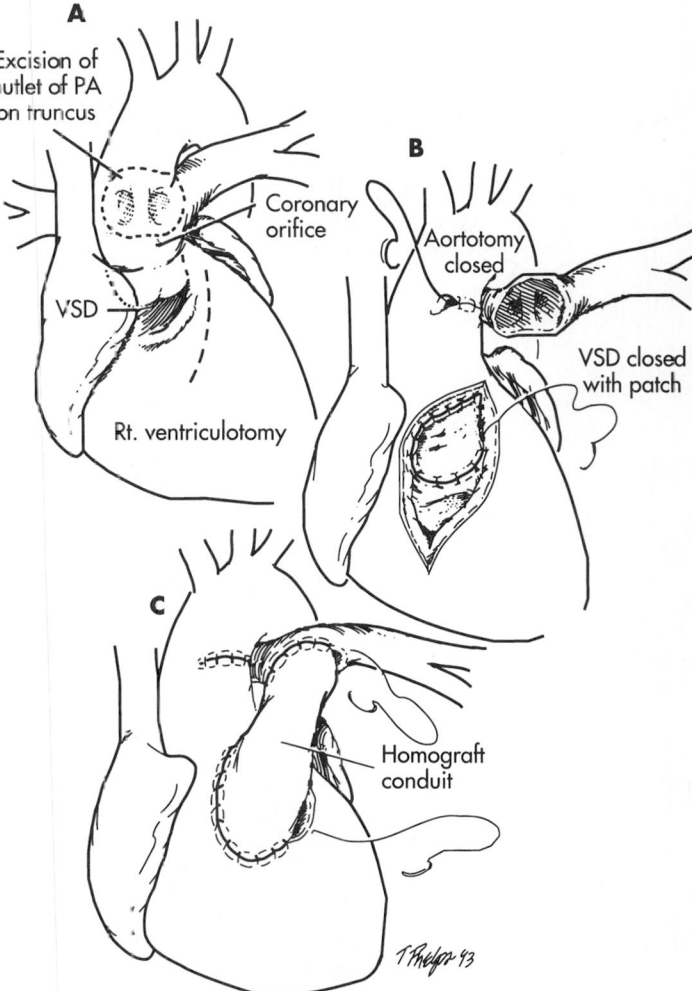

FIGURE 29-56   Complete surgical correction of truncus arteriosus. **A,** The pulmonary artery *(PA)* bifurcation is excised from the truncus. The ventricular septal defect *(VSD)* is exposed through a ventriculotomy. **B,** Aortotomy and VSD closed. **C,** A cryopreserved aortic homograft is anastomosed to the pulmonary artery and ventriculotomy.

muscular coats of the ductus begin to contract soon after birth; the lumen is subsequently obliterated, and blood flow through the shunt ceases.

When the ductus remains patent after birth (Fig. 29-58), it creates a shunt from the aorta through the ductus into the pulmonary circulation. This increases the work of the heart and causes subsequent enlargement and hypertrophy of the left atrium and ventricle. However, when persistent patency of the ductus is associated with other malformations such as tetralogy of Fallot and extreme stenosis of the pulmonary orifice, it is a means of maintaining life. Surgery is not performed if the PDA is serving in a compensatory capacity.

Many children have few symptoms because of the small size of the shunt. A frequent clinical sign associated with this condition is a harsh, continuous murmur. Because the blood is oxygenated passing through the shunt, there is no cyanosis, clubbing, or reduction in peripheral arterial oxygen saturation. However, growth is retarded in children

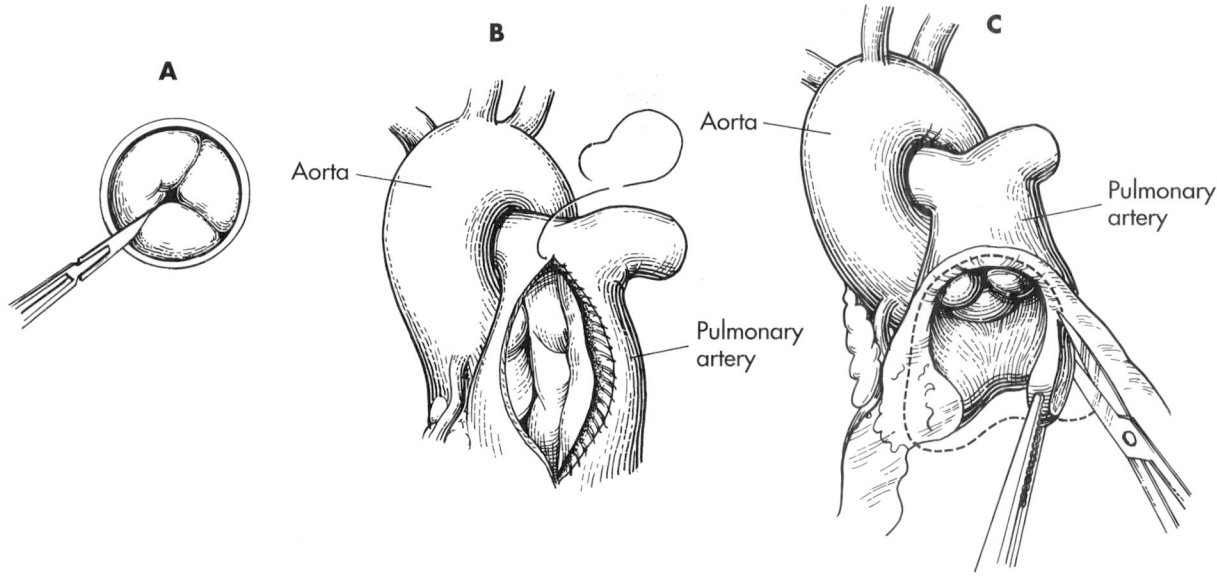

FIGURE 29-57   **A,** Commissurotomy of stenotic valve. Knife is used, and care is taken to incise exactly on commissures. **B,** Diamond-shaped patch being used to enlarge pulmonary outflow tract and pulmonary valve annulus. If vertical pulmonary artery incision is made directly through anterior commissure of valve, three valve cusps remain intact, and some valve competence is retained. **C,** Excision of obstructing infundibular tissue.

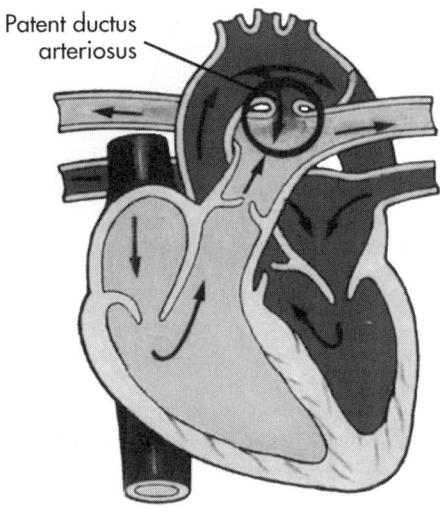

FIGURE 29-58   Patent ductus arteriosus.

who have a large ductus. Other symptoms may include dyspnea, frequent upper respiratory tract infections, palpitation, limited exercise tolerance, and cardiac failure.

Procedural considerations

For newborn infants the surgeon and anesthesia provider may elect to perform this procedure in the intensive care nursery bed because the operation is a short one. However, after the newborn period the surgery is done in the operating room. The child is placed in a right lateral position. The setup is as described, without items for CPB but with special patent ductus clamps. Generally a left posterolateral approach is used; in some cases, however, a left anterolateral approach is used.

Operative procedure

1. The incision is carried through the muscles over the fourth interspace. The chest wall is entered through the third or fourth intercostal space, with use of items as described for thoracotomy (see Chapter 25). The wound edges are protected and retracted with a Finochietto rib spreader.

2. The pleura is incised with Metzenbaum scissors, and the left lung is protected and retracted with a moist pack and a malleable retractor.

3. The mediastinal pleura is opened between the phrenic and vagus nerves over the region of the ductus. The pleura is retracted by insertion of stay sutures. The recurrent laryngeal nerve is identified and protected. The aortic arch and pulmonary artery are dissected with fine scissors and dry dissectors. Fine arterial branches are divided and ligated with curved Crile or mosquito hemostats and nonabsorbable ligatures and cardiac suture ligatures.

4. The parietal pleura overlying the ductus is dissected with fine vascular forceps and scissors. Stay sutures are inserted to facilitate retraction.

5. The adventitial layer of the ductus is dissected free. A small portion of the obscure posterior ductus is carefully freed to admit a right-angle clamp.

6a. For the suture-ligation method (Fig. 29-59, *A*) two ligatures are placed around the ductus, one near the aorta and the other near the pulmonary artery side,

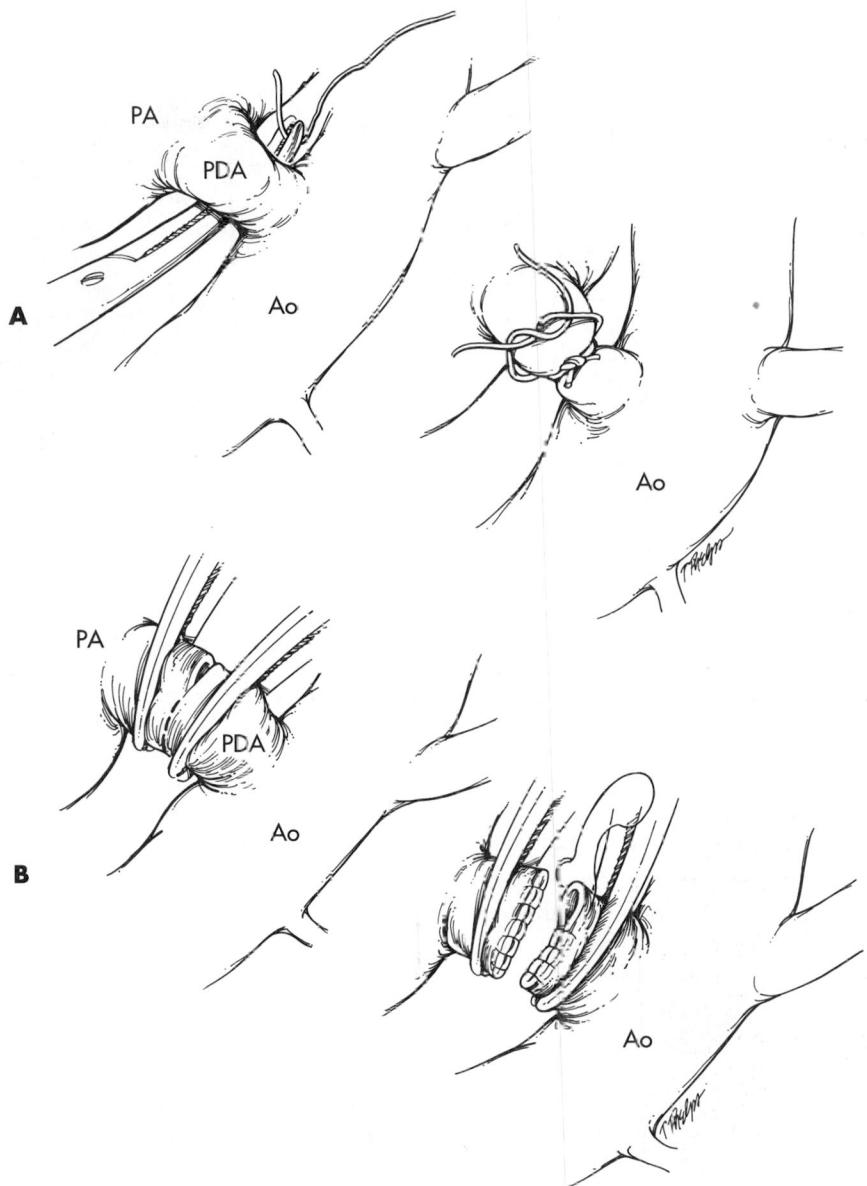

FIGURE 29-59   Surgical correction of patent ductus arteriosus *(PDA)* **A,** Ligation of ductus arteriosus. **B,** Division
of ductus arteriosus. *Ao,* Aorta; *PA,* pulmonary artery.

both of which are tied in place. Between these two
ligatures two transfixion sutures may be inserted.

6b. For the division of the ductus method the patent
ductus clamps are applied as close to the aorta and
pulmonary artery as possible. The ductus is divided
halfway through and partially sutured with mattress
cardiovascular sutures and continued back over the
free edge with an over-and-over whip suture (Fig.
29-59, *B*). After both openings are sutured, a sponge is
held on the area for compression while the patent
ductus clamps are removed.

6c. In premature infants, only a hemoclip may be applied
to the ductus because of the friable nature of the ductal
tissue. The mediastinal pleura is closed with interrupted sutures. The lung is reexpanded, and a chest

catheter is inserted to establish closed drainage. In
newborns reexpansion of the lung may be accomplished by gradual withdrawal of a catheter during
closure; no chest drainage tube is required unless there
is oozing. The chest wall is closed in layers, and
dressings are applied.

Video-Assisted Thoracoscopic Surgery for Patent Ductus Arteriosus

Although thoracoscopy was first described in 1910,[7] the
application of video-assisted thoracoscopic surgery (VATS)
to the pediatric population for cardiovascular repairs did
not occur before this decade. Because of its recent
application in pediatrics, a limited number of cardiac

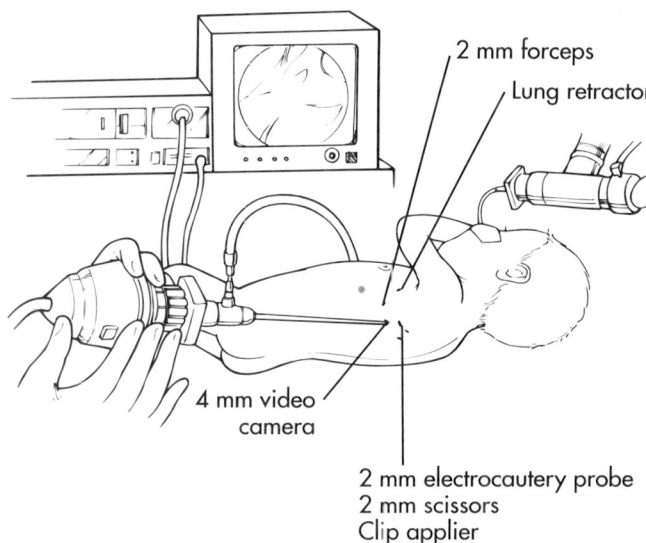

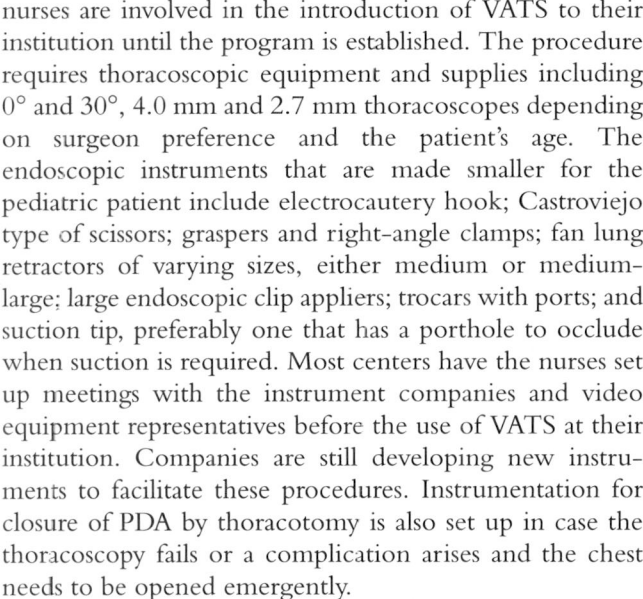

FIGURE 29-60 Video-assisted thoracoscopic approach for PDA ligation.

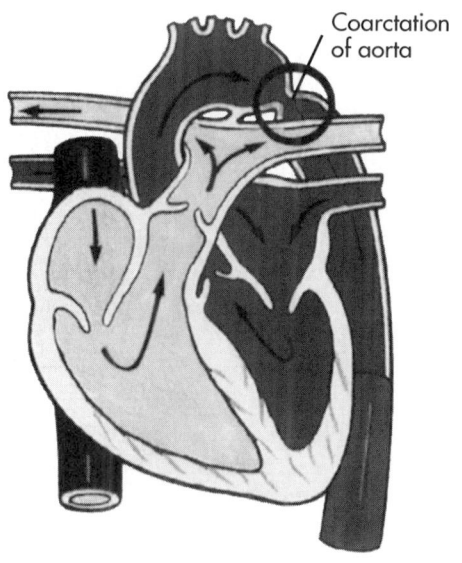

FIGURE 29-61 Coarctation of aorta.

nurses are involved in the introduction of VATS to their institution until the program is established. The procedure requires thoracoscopic equipment and supplies including 0° and 30°, 4.0 mm and 2.7 mm thoracoscopes depending on surgeon preference and the patient's age. The endoscopic instruments that are made smaller for the pediatric patient include electrocautery hook; Castroviejo type of scissors; graspers and right-angle clamps; fan lung retractors of varying sizes, either medium or medium-large; large endoscopic clip appliers; trocars with ports; and suction tip, preferably one that has a porthole to occlude when suction is required. Most centers have the nurses set up meetings with the instrument companies and video equipment representatives before the use of VATS at their institution. Companies are still developing new instruments to facilitate these procedures. Instrumentation for closure of PDA by thoracotomy is also set up in case the thoracoscopy fails or a complication arises and the chest needs to be opened emergently.

Operative procedure (Fig. 29-60)

1. Before the procedure, the television cameras are set up on either side of the OR bed. The patient is placed in a right lateral position. Usually four small incisions are made along the line of the posterolateral thoracotomy incision. Ports are then introduced, and various instrumentation is advanced.
2. The thoracoscope is the first instrument to be advanced so that other instruments can be visualized.
3. The first assistant holds the lung retractor.
4. The second assistant holds the camera. Some institutions use a mechanical articulating arm.
5. The surgeon uses a grasper to elevate the pleura overlying the aorta near the insertion of the PDA and

pulmonary artery, dissects with the electrocautery hook, and also suctions when needed.

6. When the ductus has been clearly identified, the clip applier is inserted, and a clip is applied. A right-angle clamp may first be introduced, and a tie is applied to the duct. More than one clip may be applied.
7. Transesophageal or transthoracic echocardiography is usually performed by a cardiologist before closure of the porthole incisions to assure closure of the ductus. Also, a chest tube will be inserted into the pleural space, the lungs inflated, the chest tube removed or a chest tube may be left in place before porthole incision closures.

Repair of Coarctation of the Aorta

Coarctation of the aorta (Fig. 29-61) may be repaired by excision of a constricted segment of the aorta, plus an end-to-end anastomosis—with or without a graft—to reestablish continuity. In some instances a woven Dacron or PTFE patch may be used to enlarge the aortic diameter at the site of the coarctation, or a subclavian flap is used.

The lesion that narrows or constricts the lumen of the aorta may be classified as infantile or adult. In the infantile type the constriction is long and usually located in the aortic arch proximal to the junction of the aorta and ductus arteriosus. The ductus usually remains patent and may be associated with other cardiac defects. In the adult type the coarctation consists of a constricted area at or just distal to the junction of the aorta and left subclavian artery and the ductus, which is generally closed. This type is compatible with life for a considerable period.

Coarctation of the aorta is a fairly common congenital malformation, and the adult patient suffers from hypertension and complains of dyspnea, palpitation, vertigo,

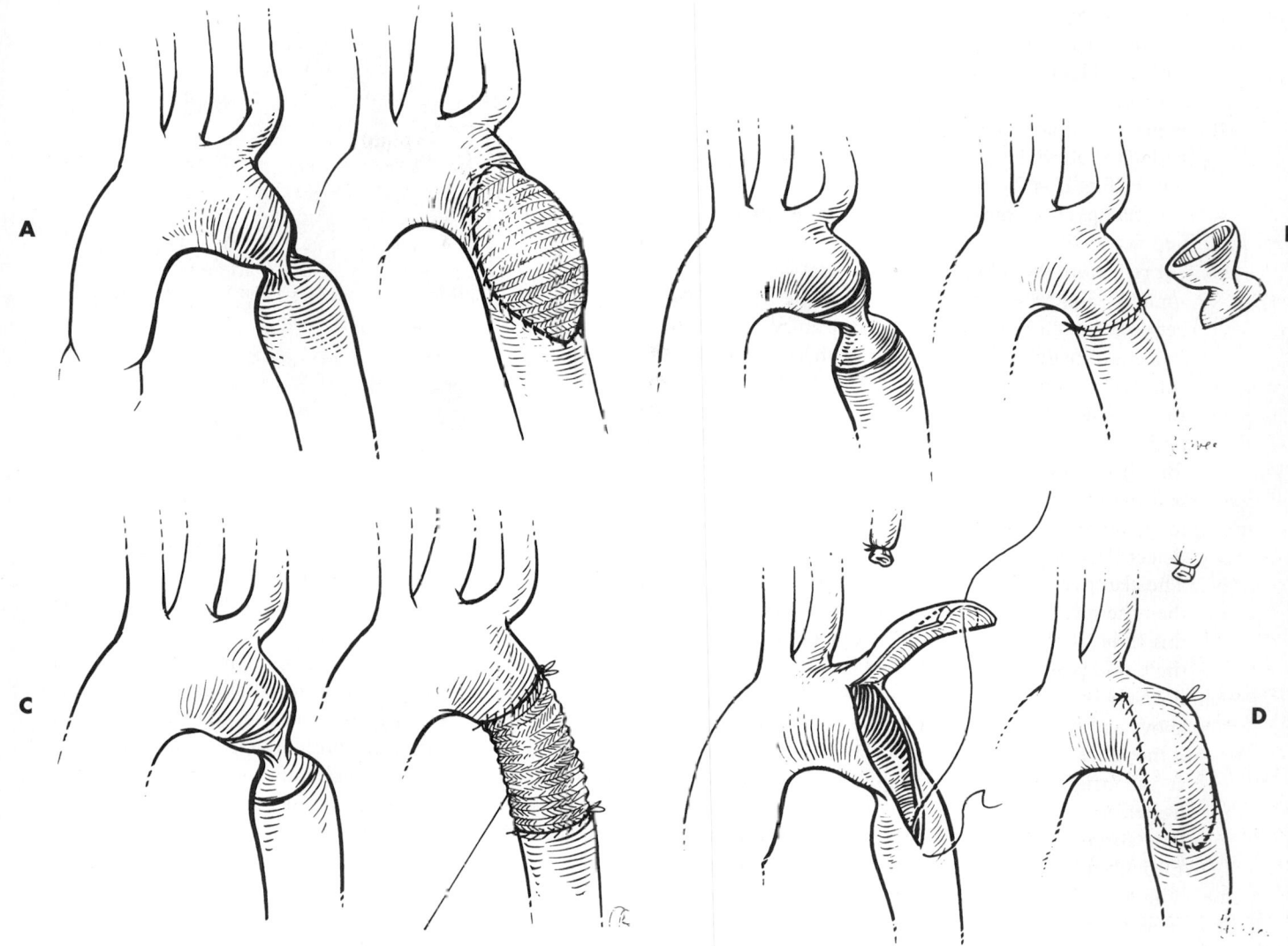

FIGURE 29-62 **A,** Prosthetic patch aortoplasty. **B,** Resection with primary end-to-end anastomosis. **C,** Prosthetic interposition graft. **D,** Subclavian flap aortoplasty.

headache, epistaxis, and weakness. However, when the aorta is almost obstructed, hypertension is manifested in the upper part of the body with hypotension in the lower extremities. With hypertension above the constriction the collateral blood supply, which unites the blood vessels of the shoulder, the upper extremities, and the lower extremities, increases greatly. In so doing the intercostal vessels dilate, allowing their branches to carry blood from the subclavian arteries downward. Occasionally the vessels erode the lower margins of the ribs.

Procedural considerations

The child is placed in the right lateral position. Instrumentation is as described for basic cardiac surgery, plus Teflon or Dacron woven or knitted vascular prostheses in assorted sizes, to be used as necessary when primary anastomosis is not possible. Items for CPB are not needed.

Operative procedure (Fig. 29-62)

1. A left posterolateral incision is carried through the chest wall, as described for thoracotomy. As previously stated, the collateral blood vessels are somewhat enlarged, and bleeding may be profuse. Sponges may be weighed to determine accurate blood replacement, depending on the preference of the anesthesia provider. A Burford or Finochietto retractor is used.

2. The pleura is incised and the lung is retracted. The mediastinal pleura is incised over the constricted portion of the aorta, and the edges are sutured to the chest wall.

3. Careful dissection with fine vascular forceps and dry dissectors is continued to mobilize the aorta and the surrounding intercostal vessels. The laryngeal nerve is identified and protected. The ductus arteriosus is ligated and divided between ductus clamps.

4a. For patch repair the curved or angled vascular clamps are applied, and a longitudinal aortotomy is performed with a #11 knife blade, a Potts scissors, and vascular forceps.

4b. A piece of graft material is inserted, large enough to widen the aorta, by use of a continuous cardiovascular suture (Fig. 29-62, *A*).

4c. The clamps are removed, one at a time, as described in step 5c.

5a. For resection, the curved or angled vascular clamps are applied, and the constricted segment is divided between them. A second set of clamps may be applied above and below, as a safety factor, in fashioning the cuffs for reapproximation.

5b. End-to-end anastomosis (Fig. 29-62, *B*) is accomplished with a continuous, everting mattress technique for the posterior wall and interrupted, everting mattress sutures for the anterior row. If the stricture is long, a synthetic aortic prosthesis is used to bridge the defect (Fig. 29-62, *C*).

5c. The clamps are released slowly, the distal one first and then the proximal one. The blood pressure is noted at this time. Removal of clamps is not completed until the blood pressure is stabilized.

6a. For subclavian flap repairs (Fig. 29-62, *D*) the aorta above and below the patent ductus is dissected out, as is the subclavian artery. The subclavian artery is ligated at the origin of the vertebral artery, which is also ligated.

6b. The aorta is incised distally to the area of narrowing, through the coarctation to the subclavian artery.

6c. The aorta is opened, and the coarctation is excised.

6d. The tip of the subclavian flap is brought down into the aorta and sutured with absorbable or nonabsorbable sutures. The parietal pleura is closed, with a small opening being left at the lower point. Closed drainage is established, and the chest wall is closed in layers. A dressing is applied.

Repair of Hypoplastic Left Heart Syndrome (Fig. 29-63)

Hypoplastic left heart syndrome (HLHS) is the fourth most common congenital heart defect presenting in infancy. HLHS describes a range of congenital cardiac malformations that have in common underdevelopment of the left-sided heart structures, which include aortic valve atresia and stenosis with associated hypoplasia or absence of the left ventricle. The ascending aorta and arch are usually only a few millimeters in diameter and are functionally a branch of the ductus arteriosus–thoracic aorta continuum with blood flowing retrograde through the aortic arch and into the small ascending aorta to the coronary arteries. There is also mitral valve atresia or stenosis present.[5]

Since patency of the ductus arteriosus is needed for systemic circulation, children are maintained on an

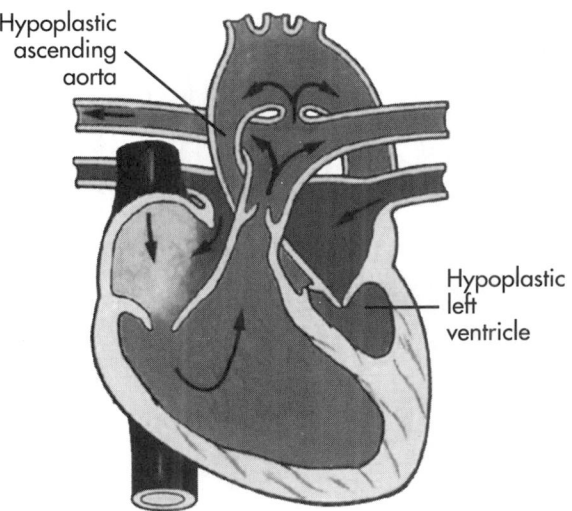

FIGURE 29-63   Hypoplastic left-sided heart syndrome.

infusion of prostaglandin before surgical intervention. If left untreated, a majority of these neonates will die within the first month of life; without surgical intervention the disease is fatal.

It was not until the development of the Fontan procedure, a surgical correction for another form of single ventricle—tricuspid atresia—that long-term survival in patients with HLHS was considered possible. However, because of the neonate's high pulmonary vascular resistance, the Fontan procedure is not a surgical option in the newborn period. A palliative repair (stage I) was developed in the late 1970s by Norwood to prepare the heart for the Fontan procedure.

Two surgical options for patients with HLHS exist: a series of reconstructive procedures or a heart transplant. The series of reconstructive procedures usually involves three stages. Stage I is performed during the newborn period. The goals of stage I are to (1) maintain systemic perfusion, (2) preserve the function of the only ventricle, and (3) allow normal maturation of the pulmonary ventricle. The first goal is met by creating an unobstructed communication between the right ventricle and the systemic circulation. This is accomplished by transsecting the main pulmonary artery and creating a neoaorta from the main pulmonary artery, native aorta, and pulmonary homograft tissue. The other two goals are met by creating a right modified Blalock-Taussig (BT) shunt and a nonrestrictive interatrial communication. These measures allow for adequate pulmonary blood flow and for the pulmonary vascular resistance to decrease as the child grows while they limit the volume interposed on the single ventricle.

The modified Fontan procedure was initially performed on a child at approximately 18 months of age. However, since 1989 a staged approach to the Fontan procedure has been undertaken to minimize the effect of rapid changes in ventricular configuration and diastolic function that can be

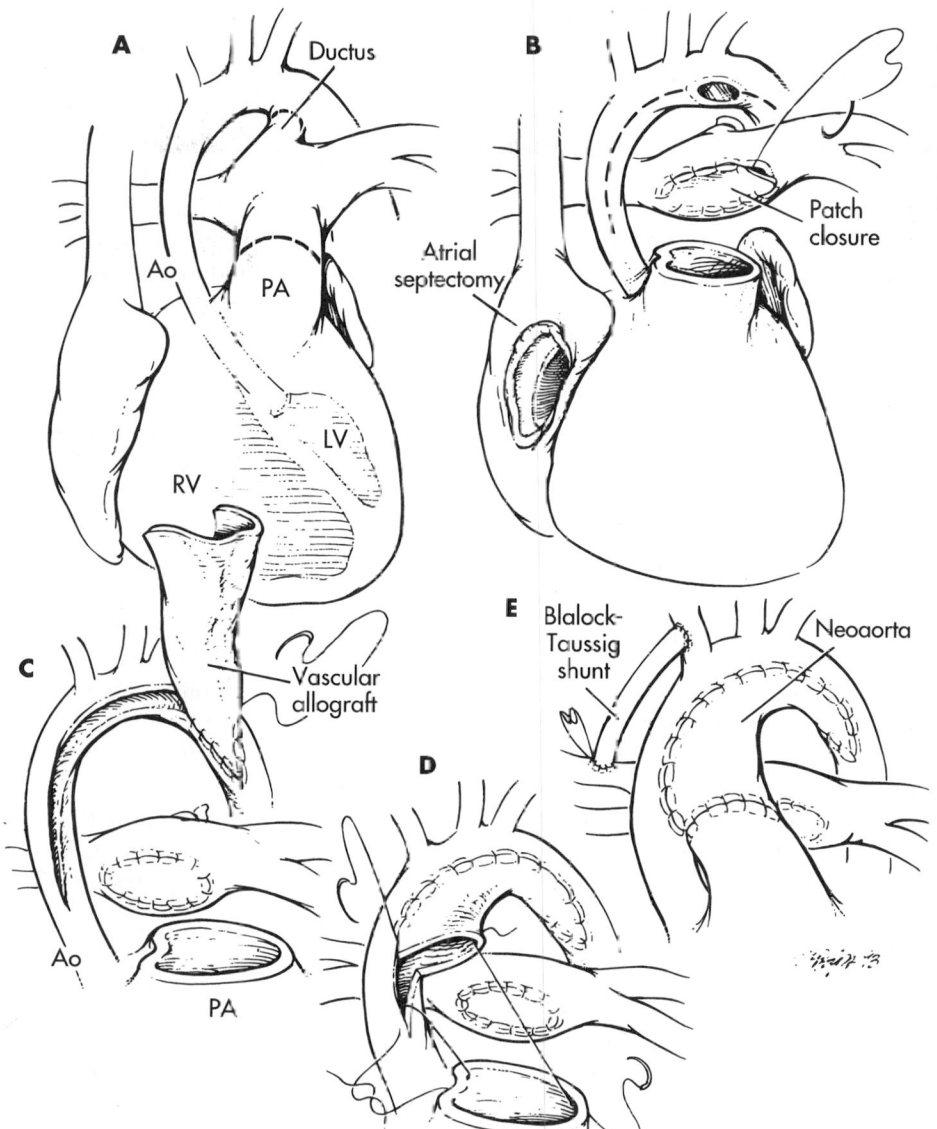

FIGURE 29-64   Stage I Norwood procedure. **A,** Transsection points of the main pulmonary artery *(PA)* and ductus arteriosus. **B,** Atrial septectomy to avoid pulmonary venous hypertension. Patch closure of the distal main PA. Division and ligation of the ductus arteriosus. **C** and **D,** Construction of a "neoaorta" with use of the proximal main PA, diminutive ascending aorta, and vascular allograft. **E,** Pulmonary blood flow supplied by a right modified Blalock-Taussig shunt connecting the right subclavian artery to the right PA. *Ao,* Aorta; *LV,* left ventricle; *RV,* right ventricle.

associated with a primary Fontan procedure and to attempt to reduce the postoperative complications of effusions associated with it.[9] In the stage II procedure—hemi-Fontan—SVC blood flow is directed to the lungs and IVC blood flow continues to flow to the right ventricle. The third and final stage, the modified Fontan procedure, separates the systemic and pulmonary circulations.

Procedural considerations

Additional items for the open-heart setup include the following:

- Stage I: PTFE tube graft, 3.5 or 4 mm, and pulmonary homograft tissue.

- Stage II: Oscillating saw and pulmonary homograft tissue.
- Stage III: Oscillating saw and PTFE tube graft, 10 mm. A higher than usual supply of blood should be available.

Operative procedures

Stage I (Norwood Procedure) (Fig. 29-64)

1. A median sternotomy is performed. The aortic cannula is placed into the main pulmonary artery rather than the diminutive aorta, and the venous cannula is placed into the right atrium. CPB is instituted, and the right and left pulmonary arteries are immediately occluded with tourniquets to force

the blood through the ductus arteriosus to the systemic circulation.

2. When deep hypothermic circulatory arrest is about to be instituted, the innominate and left carotid arteries are occluded with tourniquets. The venous and aortic cannulas are removed.

3. The septum primum is excised through the venous cannulation site; occasionally a right atriotomy is necessary to facilitate the atrial septectomy.

4. The main pulmonary artery is transsected immediately before the takeoff of the right and left pulmonary arteries.

5. The distal pulmonary artery is closed with a small patch of homograft tissue.

6. The ductus arteriosus is then exposed and closed using a 2-0 Tevdek tie. The tie is left long to better expose the thoracic aorta. The ductus is transsected.

7. At the point where the ductus was attached to the aorta, the thoracic aorta is opened 1 to 2 cm, and the aortic arch and ascending aorta are opened to a point adjacent to the main pulmonary artery.

8. A gusset of homograft tissue is joined to the aorta starting at the thoracic end, and the pulmonary artery is incorporated at the proximal end of the ascending aorta. A continuous monofilament stitch is used. Occasionally interrupted sutures are used to attach the main pulmonary artery to the aorta.

9. To perform a right BT shunt, the innominate artery is cross-clamped and incised, and a 3.5 or 4 mm PTFE tube graft is interposed.

10. CPB is instituted, and the pulmonary end of the shunt is performed by incising the pulmonary artery and interposing the distal end of the tube graft.

11. Immediately after the shunt is completed, the shunt must be occluded with a bulldog clamp until termination of bypass.

Stage II (Hemi-Fontan Procedure) (Fig. 29-65)

1. Since these patients have had previous surgery, an oscillating saw is used for the median sternotomy.

2. The aorta, right atrium, and right BT shunt are exposed.

3. CPB is instituted, and the shunt is immediately occluded with a clip.

4. The branch pulmonary arteries are exposed.

5. Deep hypothermic circulatory arrest is instituted.

6. An incision is made in the confluence of the pulmonary arteries, extending to the pericardial reflections.

7. An incision is made in the dome of the right atrium, extending to the SVC.

8. The pulmonary artery is then anastomosed to the SVC–right atrial junction.

9. The pulmonary arteries are augmented with a gusset of homograft tissue, incorporating part of this tissue intraatrially as a dam between the common atrium and the vena cava–pulmonary artery anastomosis.

10. CPB is reinstituted until the patient is normothermic. CPB is discontinued, and chest closure is completed.

Stage III (Modified Fontan Procedure)
(Fig. 29-66)

1. Repeat step 1 of stage II (hemi-Fontan).

2. The aorta and right atrium are exposed.

3. CPB is instituted.

4. Deep hypothermic circulatory arrest is instituted.

5. A lateral incision is made in the right atrium.

6. A 10 mm PTFE tube graft is cut in half lengthwise and is placed intraatrially by suturing the inferior end of the graft around the orifice of the IVC and up the right lateral free wall of the right atrium to the superior dome of the right atrium. This creates a tunnel in which the inferior blood flow is directed to the pulmonary arteries. The superior vena cava blood flow was directed to the pulmonary arteries during the stage II repair. (One may perform variations on this procedure, such as excluding a hepatic vein or doing a fenestrated Fontan by making a series of small openings in the PTFE tube graft or a single 4 mm opening with an aortic punch in the graft material.)

7. The atria are closed, and CPB is reinstituted until the patient is normothermic. CPB is discontinued, and chest closure is completed.

Repair of Severely Diseased Aortic Valves

Discussion on impaired aortic valves and the surgical treatment of aortic valve replacement with a mechanical and biologic valve prosthesis is located in Chapter 27. An alternative to mechanical and allograft (homograft) replacement of aortic valves that cannot be repaired by valvuloplasty or annuloplasty involves using the patient's autologous pulmonary valve as a free-standing aortic root replacement and then replacing the patient's pulmonary outflow tract with pulmonary or aortic valve homograft tissue depending on size availability.

Ross Procedure

Experimental animal work from Lower and Shumway in 1960 showed that an excised pulmonary valve would function under systemic pressures. In 1967, Donald Ross performed the first surgical procedure replacing a patient's aortic valve with autologous pulmonary artery. Although the first procedures involved implanting the autograft in the subcoronary position, the autografts now are inserted as a free-standing root replacement to allow the valve to grow with the patient, prevent distortion and provide a competent mechanism. The autograft operation provides a permanent aortic valve replacement for patients and avoids the threat of embolism and anticoagulant hemorrhage from mechanical valves.[10]

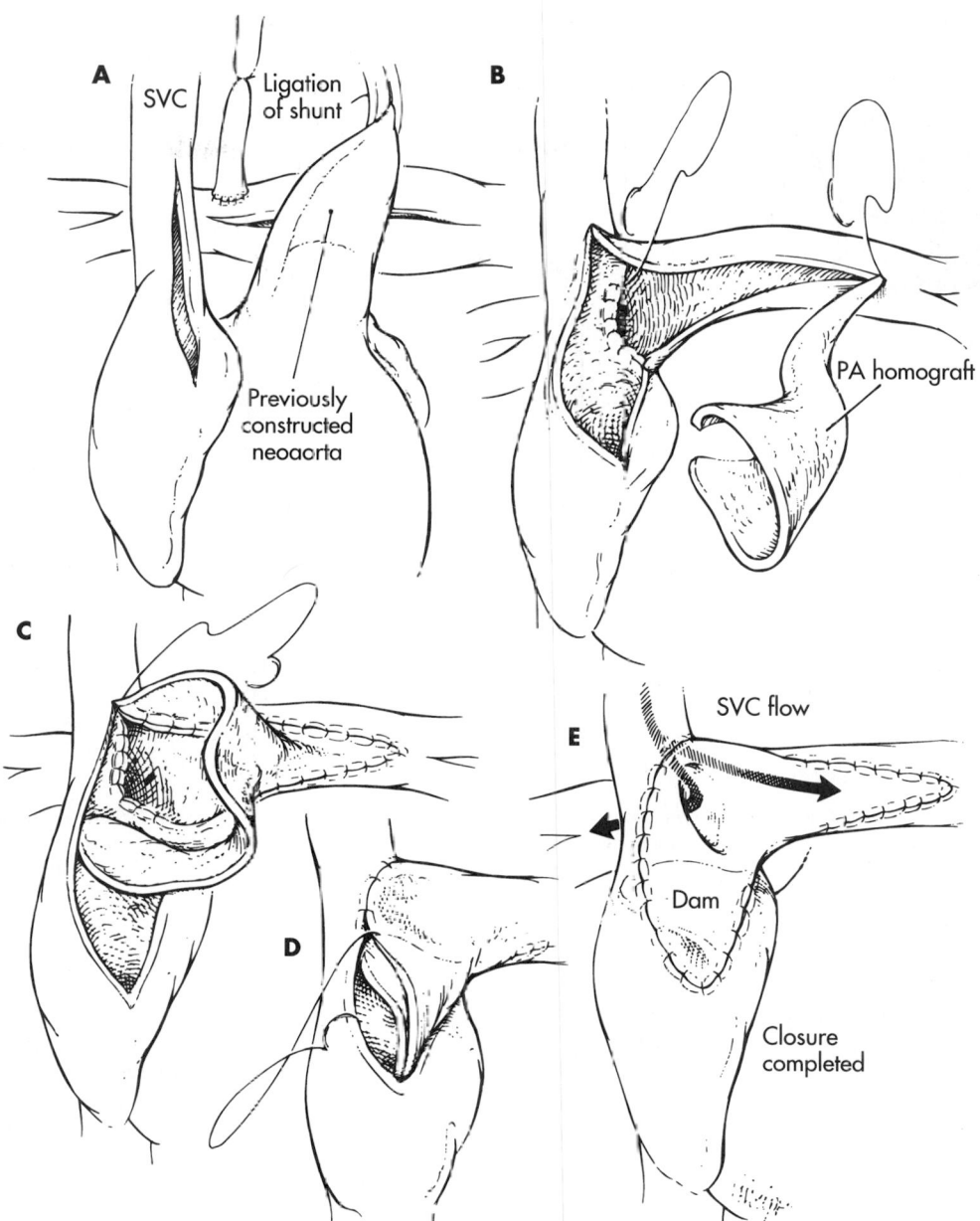

FIGURE 29-65 Hemi-Fontan procedure in a patient with hypoplastic left-sided heart syndrome. **A** and **B,** Ligation of the systemic–to–pulmonary artery shunt and side-to-side anastomosis of the superior vena cava *(SVC)* to the confluence of the pulmonary artery *(PA)* with allograft augmentation. **C** to **E,** Placement of a dam to close the junction of the atrium with the SVC so that saturated pulmonary venous blood mixes in the common atrium with desaturated blood draining from the inferior vena cava. Pulmonary blood flow is supplied exclusively through the SVC.

Procedural considerations

Additional items for the open-heart setup include the following: pulmonary valve homograft tissue, Spencer plegia cannula, appropriate solution and basins to rinse homograft, and felt.

Operative procedure

1. A median sternotomy is performed with a sternal saw if the patient has had no previous surgery or an oscillating saw if the patient has a former sternotomy incision.

2. The pericardium is opened, and the aorta, coronary arteries, pulmonary artery, and the superior and inferior venae cavae are exposed.

3. The aorta is cannulated close to the arch of the aorta. Superior and inferior venous cannulas are used.

4. Once on CPB the patient is cooled to 28° C, and the aorta is cross clamped. Cardioplegia is given retrograde through the ascending aorta if the aortic valve is stenotic. If the aorta valve is regurgitant, the aorta is opened, and the cardioplegia is given directly into the coronary ostium.

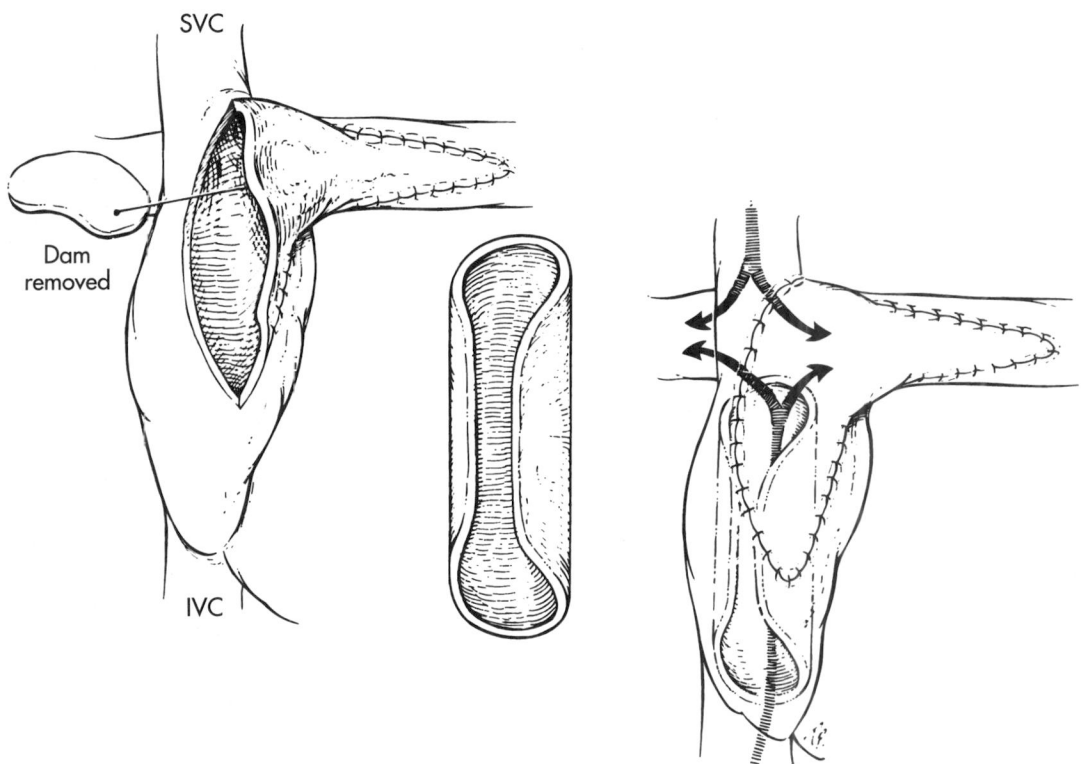

FIGURE 29-66 Conversion of hemi-Fontan to completion of Fontan. Excision of the dam between the right atrium and the superior vena cava–pulmonary artery anastomosis. Inferior vena cava flow is directed to the inlet of the superior vena cava–pulmonary artery anastomosis by a baffle. *IVC,* Inferior vena cava; *SVC,* superior vena cava.

5. The aorta is transsected (Fig. 29-67, *A*).

6. The pulmonary artery is transsected (Fig. 29-67, *B*).

7. The right ventricle is incised, and the pulmonary root is carefully dissected. Care is taken to avoid the first septal branch of the left anterior descending coronary artery (Fig. 29-67, *C*).

8. The pulmonary artery allograft is placed in saline for use later in the repair.

9. Cardioplegia is given intermittently before and during autograft implantation.

10. The orifice of the coronary arteries with a rim of adjacent coronary wall are excised (Fig. 29-67, *A*).

11. The edges of the aortic commissures are exposed with 2-0 silk suture.

12. The aortic valve is excised.

13. The pulmonary autograft is trimmed and implanted in the aortic root position with absorbable suture being used in younger patients and nonabsorbable suture in older patients. A felt ring may be needed to reinforce the suture (Fig. 29-67, *D*).

14. Sinuses are made in the pulmonary autograft, and the cuff and coronary artery are then sutured in place using continuous absorbable suture in younger patients and nonabsorbable suture in older patients (Fig. 29-67, *E*).

15. The distal pulmonary autograft is then anastomosed to the proximal aorta with continuous suture according to the patient's size and age.

16. The pulmonary homograft is trimmed, and the distal end is sewn to the bifurcation of the right and left pulmonary artery with a continuous nonabsorbable suture (Fig. 29-67, *F*).

17. The proximal end of the homograft is sewn to the right ventricle by means of a continuous nonabsorbable suture (Fig. 29-67, *G*).

18. Suture lines are inspected. When the patient is fully rewarmed and hemodynamically stable, CPB is discontinued. Chest closure is completed after transesophageal echocardiographic confirmation of satisfactory results.

Pulmonary Artery Banding

Pulmonary artery banding is the constriction of the pulmonary artery to reduce its diameter, thereby decreasing pulmonary blood flow (see Fig. 29-68, *B*).

An infant with an enlarged heart in intractable failure and a large left-to-right shunt may be treated effectively by a palliative pulmonary artery banding operation. This procedure is designed to reduce the flow of blood through the pulmonary artery to approximately one half to one

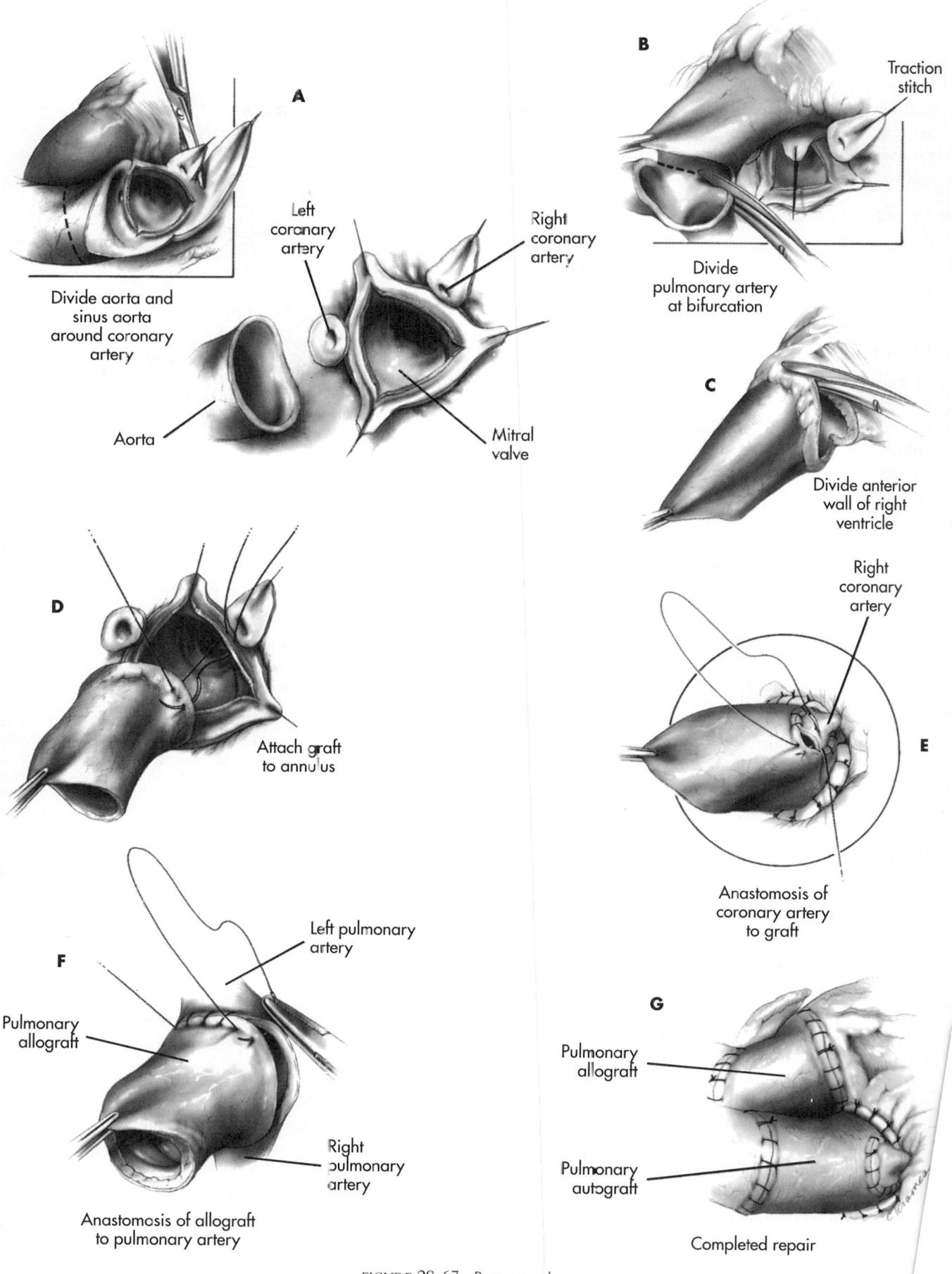

A Divide aorta and sinus aorta around coronary artery

Left coronary artery

Right coronary artery

Aorta

Mitral valve

B Traction stitch

Divide pulmonary artery at bifurcation

C Divide anterior wall of right ventricle

Right coronary artery

E Anastomosis of coronary artery to graft

D Attach graft to annulus

F Left pulmonary artery

Pulmonary allograft

Right pulmonary artery

Anastomosis of allograft to pulmonary artery

G Pulmonary allograft

Pulmonary autograft

Completed repair

FIGURE 29–67 Ross procedure.

third of the existing rate. A tape is looped about the artery and secured in place by a simple suture technique. Pressures are measured by direct needle puncture and before and after banding. A reduction of the distal pulmonary artery pressure by 50% to 70% is sought. Repair of the interventricular septal defect may be postponed until the child has been clinically stabilized and can withstand an open-heart procedure.

Procedural considerations

The child is placed in the left lateral position if an anterolateral incision is to be used or in the supine position if a median sternotomy is to be used. Silastic sheeting or polyester tape is cut by the surgeon to the appropriate size.

Shunt for Palliation

The shunt for palliation is one of several palliative procedures designed to divert poorly oxygenated blood from one of the major arteries back through one of the pulmonary arteries to the lungs for reoxygenation, thereby increasing the total blood flow in the pulmonary circulation.

Shunt procedures that increase pulmonary flow are described in Fig. 29-68, along with procedures to reduce pulmonary blood flow (pulmonary artery banding) and to increase intracardiac mixing of blood (Blalock-Hanlon ASD, as in Fig. 29-68, *C*, and Rashkind septostomy). The BT procedure consists in making an end-to-side anastomosis between the proximal end of the subclavian and the side of the pulmonary artery (Fig. 29-68, *A*). The procedure is performed on the side opposite the aortic arch. This shunt may be dismantled or ligated if a future operation for full correction is anticipated; however, the shunt has a tendency to decrease in size as the child grows. Currently the most commonly used form of shunt is a modification of the BT procedure in which a PTFE graft is used to connect pulmonary and systemic vasculature. It connects the subclavian artery to the ipsilateral pulmonary artery or the innominate artery to the right pulmonary artery. Occasionally one use a central shunt in which the PTFE graft connects the aorta and main pulmonary artery.

The Potts-Smith and Waterston procedures involve direct anastomosis of the aorta to the pulmonary arteries. These are rarely performed because of the potential for deformity of the pulmonary arteries, producing excessive pulmonary blood flow and CHF.[11]

The Glenn procedure consists in making an anastomosis of the SVC to the right pulmonary artery. This operation is employed infrequently in the treatment of tetralogy of Fallot (Fig. 29-68, *E*).

Procedural considerations

The child is placed in a position that is specific for each procedure (supine or right or left lateral position). Instruments are as previously described for open-heart surgery, plus the following, with appropriate sizes for

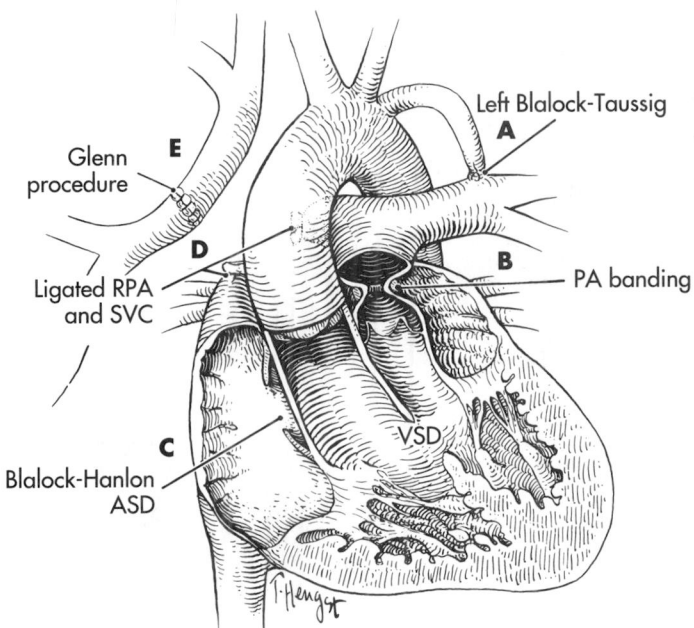

FIGURE 29-68 Palliative procedures for congenital cardiac anomalies. **A,** Left Blalock-Taussig subclavian-to-pulmonary artery shunt applicable for tetralogy of Fallot and also for other congenital anomalies associated with insufficient pulmonary arterial flow. (Modification of Blalock-Taussig procedure consists in interposing PTFE graft between the left subclavian artery and pulmonary artery, thereby preserving the subclavian artery.) **B,** Pulmonary artery banding used for anomalies associated with excessive pulmonary blood flow attributable to large intracardiac left-to-right shunt. These include ventricular septal defect, truncus arteriosus, and others. **C,** Blalock-Hanlon creation of interatrial septal defect used predominantly for transposition of great vessels but also for anomalies such as mitral or tricuspid atresia in which large opening is advantageous to reduce intraatrial pressure. Dilatation of patent foramen ovale may be done with balloon-tipped catheter (Rashkind technique). **D** and **E,** Glenn procedure is used primarily for tricuspid atresia but is also used for transposition of great vessels. In **D,** superior vena cava is anastomosed to right pulmonary artery to direct approximately 35% of systemic venous return to right lung for oxygenation. This technique cannot be used if pulmonary vascular resistance is elevated, as often occurs in transposition. Glenn procedure, **E,** is usually performed by implantation of distal end of pulmonary artery into side of superior vena cava. Cava is then ligated at atriocaval junction. Ligation of azygos vein may enhance flow through cavopulmonary anastomosis but may also increase pressure in veins draining upper half of body. Techniques of delayed azygos ligation have been described in infants and children.

infants and children: Potts-Smith aortic occlusion clamps, Johns Hopkins modified Potts clamps, Hendrin ductus clamps, and Cooley anastomosis clamps.

Operative procedures
Blalock-Taussig Procedure (Fig. 29-68, *A*)

1. An anterolateral incision is made from the sternal margin to the midaxillary line. The chest cavity is opened, and the lung is retracted, as described previously.
2. The mediastinal pleura is incised and retracted with a stay suture.

3. The pulmonary artery is dissected from the surrounding tissue, with vascular forceps, dry dissector sponges, and Metzenbaum scissors. As the artery and branches are mobilized, heavy ligatures, moistened umbilical tapes, or fine silicone tubing is placed about them.

4. Branches of the vagus nerve are protected and retracted.

5. The subclavian artery is dissected completely from its origin to where it produces the internal mammary and costocervical branches. Its distal end is marked with a silk suture.

6. The subclavian artery is occluded with a vascular clamp, a ligature is placed at the distal segment, and the vessel is divided.

7. The pulmonary artery is occluded temporarily with a curved vascular clamp.

8. An incision of sufficient size to accommodate the subclavian artery is made with a scalpel with a #11 knife blade and Potts scissors.

9. An end-to-side anastomosis is completed with cardiovascular suture.

10. The clamps are released, and the suture line is inspected for hemostasis.

11. The mediastinal pleura is closed.

12. Closed chest drainage is established, and the chest wound is closed.

Potts-Smith Procedure

1. A left posterolateral incision is made in the fourth intercostal space.

2. The pulmonary artery is dissected from its surrounding tissue, and the descending aorta is mobilized. Occluding tapes and Blalock or Potts-Smith clamps are applied.

3. A longitudinal incision is made in each artery, and a side-to-side anastomosis is completed with cardiovascular sutures.

4. The pulmonary artery is released, and the suture line is inspected for hemostasis.

5. The aortic clamps are then removed.

Waterston Procedure

1. A right anterolateral incision is made in the fourth interspace. The pericardium is opened, and the ascending aorta is exposed.

2. The right pulmonary artery is dissected as it passes beneath the ascending aorta.

3. A heavy suture is passed around the right pulmonary artery and is used to occlude the artery temporarily. A curved vascular clamp is placed so that one blade is behind the pulmonary artery and the other occludes a posterolateral portion of the ascending aorta.

4. On closure of the clamp, both the right pulmonary artery and a posterior portion of the ascending aorta are occluded.

5. Parallel incisions are made in the aorta and the right pulmonary artery.

6. An anastomosis is then made between the ascending aorta and the right pulmonary artery.

Extracorporeal Membrane Oxygenation (ECMO)

Extracorporeal membrane oxygenation (ECMO) is a therapy used on pediatric patients who have reversible pulmonary or cardiac disease. Many patients are neonates with respiratory disease syndrome (RDS), persistent pulmonary hypertension (PPH), meconium aspiration (MA), or congenital diaphragmatic hernia (CHD) requiring adequate tissue oxygenation and waste removal from the body. In the cardiac patient it may be used on a child after surgery with pulmonary hypertension or cardiogenic shock. It may also be used as a bridge to heart or lung transplantation until donor organs are available. To perform ECMO a program must be in place at the patient's hospital or the patient will need to be transferred to a facility with an established ECMO service.

Most of the time children are placed on ECMO in the intensive care unit (ICU). For venoarterial ECMO the surgical approach is usually through the right carotid artery and internal jugular vein. For the cardiac patient after surgical repair, cannulation of the carotid artery and jugular vein provide good venous drainage of the right atrium, and the incision site is remote from the sternotomy wound.[12] However, the surgeon may choose to reopen the sternum on the postoperative patients and cannulate the aorta and right atrium. In the operating room, for a patient who cannot be successfully weaned from bypass after surgery, the patient's bypass circuit may be switched to an ECMO circuit, and the patient may be transferred on ECMO to the ICU.

Procedural considerations

An area by the patient's bedside should be provided for the ECMO pump, surgical table and instrumentation, electrocautery machine, surgeon's headlight, and defibrillator with external and sterile internal paddles. A wall suction outlet should be available. Appropriate surgical attire should be provided for everyone involved with the procedure, and traffic should be limited.

Operative procedures
For Neck Cannulation

1. Place a shoulder roll under the patient and prep the neck and chest to the nipple line and drape. The ears should also be exposed and prepped for use as reference points.

2. Secure the suction tubing, electrocautery pencil, and ECMO tubing to the sterile field as indicated by the institution's protocol.

3. An incision is made in the neck, and the right common carotid artery and right internal jugular vein are exposed for venoarterial ECMO.

4. The surgeon may cannulate the vessels through a

purse-string suture and then reconstruct these vessels at the time of decannulation.

5. After insertion of the arterial and venous cannulas, the clamped cannulas are connected to the ECMO circuit. All the air is eliminated.

6. The cannulas are secured to the skin. The neck incision is closed and dressed. The surgical instruments are kept sterile until proper positioning of the venous and arterial cannulas is confirmed by x-ray examination.

For Median Sternotomy Cannulation

1. Prep the patient from neck to umbilicus and drape.

2. Repeat step 2 for neck cannulation.

3. The patient has usually had a prior sternotomy incision, and so the sternum is opened with wire cutters.

4. A chest retractor is inserted, and purse-string sutures for cannulation are placed in the aorta and right atrium.

5. The aorta and venous cannulas are inserted and clamped.

6. The clamped cannulas are connected to the ECMO circuit. All the air is eliminated.

7. The sternum is left open to prevent kinking of the cannulas and ECMO pump tubing. The wound is closed with a synthetic patch sutured to the skin. An antibiotic ointment may be applied and an "Open chest" sign placed on top of the outer dressing to serve as a warning related to potential chest compressions.

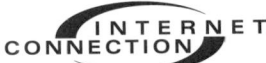

American Academy of Pediatrics: http://www.aap.org/

Association of Pediatric Oncology Nurses:
http://www.apon.org

National Association of Neonatal Nurses:
http://www.nann.org

National Association of Pediatric Nurse Associates and Practitioners: http://www.napnap.org

DRS4Kids: http://www.drs4kids.com

Pediatric Points of Interest:
http://www.med.jhu.edu/peds/neonatology/poi.html

The Johns Hopkins Hospital Virtual Children's Center:
http://www.med.jhu.edu/peds/pedspage.html

Pediatric Essentials Current Updates:
http://www.mosby.com/mosby/open/hcom_wong

Pediatric Radiology:
http://www.vh.org/Patients/IHB/PedsRad.html

Children's Eye Center:
http://www.ach.uams.edu:80/services/ophth/

The Virtual Hospital: http://indy.radiology.uiowa.edu

Resources for Nurses and Families:
http://pegasus.cc.ucf.edu/~wink/

Pediatric-Related List Serve:
e-mail listproc@u.washington.edu

REFERENCES

1. Cardona, V.D. (1994). *Trauma nursing* (ed. 2). Philadelphia: W.B. Saunders.

2. *Child health care.* (1993). AAP Research Update, a publication of the American Academy of Pediatrics, No. 9.

3. Cohn, L.H., Doty, D.B., & McElvein, R.B. (1993). *Decision-making in cardiothoracic surgery.* St. Louis: Mosby.

4. Holder, T.M., & Manning, P.B. (1991). Esophageal atresia with tracheoesophageal fistula. In Grosfeld, J.L. (Ed.). *Common problems in pediatric surgery.* St. Louis: Mosby.

5. Jacobs, M.L., & Norwood, W.I. (1992). *Pediatric cardiac surgery.* Boston: Butterworth Heinemann.

6. Johnson, D.G. (1991). Gastroesophageal reflux. In Grosfeld, J.L. (Ed.). *Common problems in pediatric surgery.* St. Louis: Mosby.

7. Lavoie, J., Burrows, F., & Hansen, D. (1996). Video-assisted thoracoscopic surgery for the treatment of congenital cardiac defects in the pediatric population. *Anesthesia and Analgesia, 82*(3), 563.

8. Merrill, W., Hoff, S., & Bender, H. (1994). Surgical treatment of atrioventricular septal defects. In Marroudis, C., & Backer, C. (Eds.). *Pediatric cardiac surgery.* St. Louis: Mosby.

9. Nicolson, S., Steven, J., & Jobes, D. (1995). Hypoplastic left heart syndrome. In Nichols, G., Cameron, D., Greeley, W., et al. (Eds.). *Critical heart disease in infants and children.* St. Louis: Mosby.

10. Ross, D. (1995). Pulmonary autografts. In Acar, J., & Bodnar, E. (Eds.). *Textbook of acquired heart valve disease.* London: ICR Publishers.

11. Sade, R.M. (1992). Surgical options in univentricular atrioventricular connection. In Jacobs, M.L., & Norwood, W.I. (Eds.). *Pediatric cardiac surgery.* Boston: Butterworth-Heinemann.

12. Spray, T.L. (1993). Extracorporeal membrane oxygenation for pediatric cardiac support. *Cardiac Surgery: State of the Art Reviews, 7*(2), 179.

13. Vegunta, R.K., Cooney, D.E., & Cooney, D.R. (1993). Surgical management of abdominal wall defects in infants. *AORN Journal, 58*(1), 53.

14. West, K.W. (1991). Intussusception. In Grosfeld, J.L. (Ed.). *Common problems in pediatric surgery.* St. Louis: Mosby.

15. Woolley, M.M. (1991). Type A esophageal atresia. In Grosfeld, J.L. (Ed.). *Common problems in pediatric surgery.* St. Louis: Mosby.

CHAPTER THIRTY

Geriatric Surgery

Patricia Felice Meckes

AS A BIOLOGIC process, aging has changed little in the last 300 years. In general, we age neither faster nor slower than we did in Colonial America, and our maximum life span has not changed substantially. The number of people living beyond their tenth decade has increased more recently. However, estimates of maximum survival potential remain between 85 and 115 years.[28] What has changed is our ability to age successfully and thereby forestall the negative effects of the aging process. Abrams et al.[1] compared "usual" with "successful" aging to explain the effects of intrinsic aging. "Successful aging refers to changes due solely to the aging process uncomplicated by damage from environment, lifestyle, or disease, whereas usual aging refers to changes due to the combined effects of the aging process, disease, adverse environment, and lifestyle factors." Essentially, we will enjoy a period of sustained but undramatic growth in the elderly population for the next 10 to 13 years. With the aging of the "Baby Boomers," the gerontology boom will emerge producing the most rapid increase in the older population somewhere between 2010 and 2030.

The older population, which includes those 65 and older, numbered 33.5 million in 1995 and represented 12.8% of the United States population. The number of older Americans increased by 2.3 million or 7% since 1990, compared with an increase of 5% for the under-65 population. By 2030 there will be about 70 million older persons, which represents more than twice their number in 1990. Persons over 65 years of age are expected to represent 13% of the population in the year 2000 and continue to increase to 20% by 2030. In 1995 persons reaching 65 years of age could expect to live an additional 17.4 years (19.0 years for women and 15.6 for men). Experts on aging agree that we should be able to add 3 or 4 years to life expectancy over the next 50 years.[19] If current fertility and immigration levels remain stable, the only age groups to experience significant growth in the next century will be those past 55 years of age. In 1995 the 65- to 74-year age group (18.8 million) was eight times larger than it was in 1900, the 75- to 84-year age group (11.1 million) was 14 times larger, and the over–85-year age group (3.6 million) was 29 times larger.[2]

Now surpassing the 80- to 85-year age group, the elderly over 100 years of age are the fastest-growing age group among the over-65 United States population. The U.S. Census Bureau, generally conservative in its estimates of the aged population thus far, now predicts an astonishing 1 million American centenarians by the year 2050 and close to 2 million of them by 2080. Advances in health care and the treatment and prevention of disease may mean that the average percentage of centenarians within each generation—currently about 1%—could increase to 2% or more in future years. Today even the 100-year-old elderly are expected to live an additional 2.5 years.[28]

Translating these demographics into health care trends produces even more startling implications for perioperative care. As a result of the "graying" of America, the health care business will never be the same. Most older persons have at least one chronic condition; many have multiple conditions. In 1994 the most frequently occurring conditions per 100 noninstitutionalized elderly were arthritis, 50%; hypertension, 36%; heart disease, 32%; hearing impairments, 29%; cataracts, 17%; orthopedic impairments, 16%; sinusitis, 15%; and diabetes, 10%. Of all hospital stays in 1994, older people accounted for 37% of them and 47% of all days of care in hospitals. The average length of hospital stay for older people was 7.4 days, as compared with 4.8 days for those under 65 years of age. However, the average length of stay for older adults decreased 6.8 days since 1968 and 3.3 days since 1980.[2]

This dramatic growth in elderly (over 65) and aged (over 85) surgical patients punctuates the necessity for perioperative nurses to recognize the special needs of these patients. Understanding how normal aging changes and chronic disease affect the successful outcome of any surgical procedure is of utmost importance and is therefore the emphasis of this chapter.

PERIOPERATIVE NURSING CONSIDERATIONS

Preliminary Evaluation

Before an elderly patient actually arrives in the operating room for surgery, many preliminary decisions are made by the physician to determine whether the benefit of surgery outweighs potential risks. In the past the elderly were not considered good candidates for surgery merely because of age. Surgeons tended to avoid surgery in geriatric patients until all nonsurgical modalities were exhausted. Research as far back as the early 1900s through the present chronicle the attitude of surgeons regarding the operative risks of elders.[28] Because surgical morbidity and mortality increase with age, the surgeon's reluctance is understandable (Research Highlight 30-1). Perioperative mortality in geriatric surgical patients includes three factors—presence of coexisting disease, emergency surgery, and site of surgery.[4]

1. *Presence of coexisting disease as quantified by the American Society of Anesthesiologists' Physical Status Classification.* The patients with statuses IV and V are consistently found to have greater mortality than those with physical statuses I and II.
2. *Emergency surgery.* Surgical risk in the elderly increases dramatically when the surgery is of an emergent nature.
3. *Site of surgery.* Major vascular, intrathoracic, and intraabdominal procedures have a higher surgical risk than other surgical procedures in the elderly.

Most surgeons agree that age alone is not a contraindication to surgery. In fact, studies confirm that even the very old can have successful positive surgical outcomes (Research Highlight 30-2). Buxbaum and Schwartz[4] further reported results of research studies that indicated patients over 65 years of age with no coexisting disease and undergoing an elective surgical procedure had mortality rates similar to those of patients under 65 years of age. More recently attitudes have changed toward a more aggressive approach and a belief that surgical risk can be substantially reduced by careful evaluation preoperatively.

30-1 RESEARCH HIGHLIGHT

Through a review of literature, Buxbaum and Schwartz reported the results of several research studies that substantiated the increase in mortality and morbidity in geriatric surgical patients. Their findings showed a mortality of 8.2% in patients over 81 years of age compared to overall mortality of 1.9% of surgical patients within 7 days of anesthesia.

From Buxbaum, J.L., & Schwartz, A.J. (1994). Perianesthetic considerations for the elderly patient. *Surgical Clinics of North America,* 74(1), 41-58.

Surgical decision making in the elderly can be a difficult task. A frequent mistake is to compare the risk in elderly patients with that of younger patients. What should be considered more often is the risk of not operating and the quality of life expected. The decision for surgery is within the purview of the physician, but nurses should be aware of its implications. Important factors that need to be evaluated are (1) life expectancy versus the natural course of the disease, (2) independence versus dependence, (3) motivation, and (4) risk of nonoperative management versus surgical risks.[8]

1. *Life expectancy versus natural course of disease.* If the patient has surpassed the expected norm for number of years of survival (persons reaching 65 years of age in 1995 had a further life expectancy of 19.0 years for women and 15.6 years for men), surgical intervention may not be appropriate if the course of the disease is poor. However, if the patient has several years of life expectancy left and is likely to outlive the condition with minimal morbidity, surgical treatment may be the treatment of choice.
2. *Independence versus dependence.* The patient's right to self-determination and making healthcare decisions should always be considered. The need for independence is of utmost importance to elderly persons, and they are far more interested in maintaining health and independence than longevity. Complications of surgery are not well tolerated by the elderly and can quickly develop into life-threatening situations. If surgical

---

30-2 RESEARCH HIGHLIGHT

Ackerman and colleagues studied the surgical outcomes of elderly patients 90 or more years of age. A total of 116 patients had 134 major operative procedures. The patients ranged in age from 90 to 103 years. Ninety-two patients were women, 75 were white, 63 were nursing home residents, and 77 had minimal impairment in functional status. The most common procedure was repair of fractured hip, second was gangrene of the lower extremity, and third was small bowel obstruction. The overall mortality was 19.8%, with the highest being in those who had abdominal procedures. Survival was significantly longer when patients came from a family residence (1.6 years) as compared to those from a nursing home (0.7 year). Eighty-four of the 97 survivors maintained their functional status. Once past the postoperative period the mortality of the very old is similar to that of the general population.

From Ackerman, R.J., et al. (1995). Surgery in nonogenarians: morbidity, mortality and functional outcomes, *Journal of Family Practice, 40,* 129-135.

intervention will further incapacitate an already debili-tated person, alternative treatment should be consid-ered. However, if surgery will help to alleviate debilitating conditions and improve or maintain inde-pendence, it should be considered an appropriate modality of care.

3. *Motivation.* Evaluation of the elderly patient's level of motivation must be considered when surgery is planned. Many elderly patients are reluctant to undergo surgery. They are concerned that the surgery will not improve their quality of life and that it will make them more dependent on others or destine them to a life in a care facility.[12] In addition, they do not want to withstand the pain, discomfort, and rigors of surgery and the recuperative period necessary to treat a condition that really doesn't bother them very much or that they have "learned to live with." This lack of motivation will have a negative influence on the results of the surgery. Patients who show a strong sense of determination in doing all that is necessary to get well and stay well are more likely candidates for surgery than those who believe illness is a prelude to death. Obviously the outcome of surgery is enhanced if the patient is motivated to have a positive result.

4. *Risk of nonoperative management versus surgical risks.* Making a decision between the risks of nonoperative management and surgical intervention is particularly difficult with elderly patients. Mortalities for emer-gency surgery in elderly patients are double that of elective surgery. Surgical and anesthetic risk increase in proportion to the emergent nature of the patient's condition. When an acute emergency condition taxes an already overburdened physiologic state, the chances of survival are less likely. The elderly patient's family does not find consolation in knowing that their loved one died as a result of a "successful" surgery. To increase the chances of survival from a surgical procedure, the elderly person must be in optimum condition, and adequate preoperative assessment and preparation must precede an elective procedure.

Another important consideration relates to the extent of surgical treatment. The decision for surgery relies heavily on the patient's physical status at the time of surgery and how extensively the disease has progressed. When treating patients who are nearing the end of life, there should be a shift from maximizing survival alone to maximizing the quality of life and dignity while minimiz-ing suffering. Early identification of problems with aggressive, preventive surgical treatment are considered more appropriate than waiting for problems to develop.[28]

Assessment

In elderly persons a preoperative medical assessment is conducted mainly to determine present physiologic func-tioning. Application of these findings identifies operative risk, minimizes postoperative complications, and estab-lishes the presence and status of any concomitant disease process that could negatively affect the outcome of the surgery. The preoperative nursing assessment is conducted to plan patient care throughout the perioperative period. In particular, assessment data are used to establish presurgi-cal baseline data so that health status changes, primarily during the intraoperative and postoperative periods, are more readily recognized.

Chronologic age as a valid predictor of a patient's response to surgery is not a reliable measurement. A person of 75 years of age can be in better physical and mental condition for surgery than a person 65 years of age or even younger. Biologic age as a measurement criterion is much more reliable. Establishing biologic age, however, becomes the greatest challenge. Chronic conditions may interfere with the elderly person's ability to distinguish between recent and long-standing ailments. Therefore the preop-erative interview, especially in elderly persons, should be conducted in a quiet, relaxed environment with as few distractions as possible. The elderly person should be allowed to respond to each question independently without prompting from a spouse or other family members unless absolutely necessary (Fig. 30-1). This helps to maintain the patient's dignity, independence, and control, which are extremely important to the older adult.

Normal age-related changes

In general, the aging process imposes a decline in organ functions, atypical responses to pain and temperature, alterations in pharmacokinetics, and atypical signs and symptoms of disease, all of which may vary from one

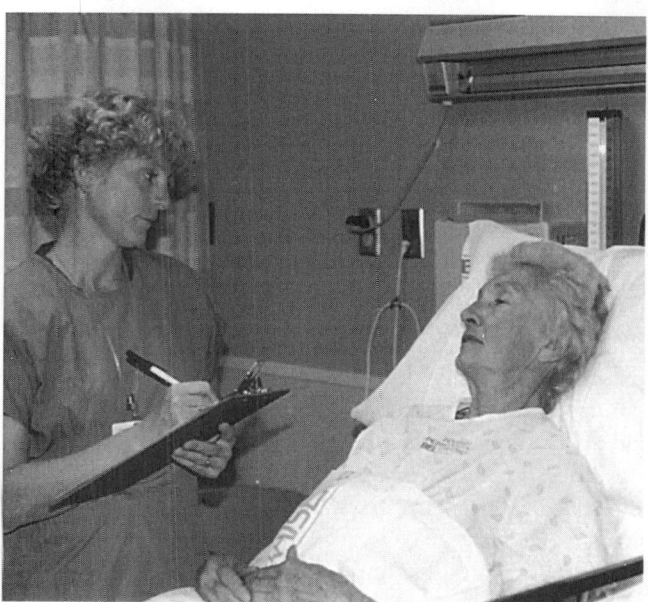

FIGURE 30-1 Allowing elderly person to respond to questions independently, without prompting from family members, helps main-tain patient's dignity and control.

elderly person to the next. Having a clear understanding of normal age changes helps to establish appropriate nursing diagnoses and care plan development. The following review of systems focuses on age-specific changes of particular importance to perioperative care planning.

Physiologic Changes

Integumentary system

The nails become thick and tough, and the circulation in the feet can be decreased. A nick or cut can lead to a serious infection. Hair color and texture changes and the loss of pigmentation results in greying of hair. Decrease in oil makes the hair dull and lifeless, and the amount of hair decreases. The skin loses elasticity and subcutaneous fat and becomes more prone to shear force and pressure injury. Because of the thinness of the skin and small vessel fragility, bruising is quite common. Dry skin develops because of decreased oils and sweat glands. Because of the thinness of the skin, hemorrhaging is quite common, and skin breakdown and pressure ulcers develop more easily. The vascular system of the skin has nutritional and protective roles. It is necessary for body heat regulation, provides defenses against microbial and physical damage, provides nutrient supply to the avascular epidermis, and promotes wound healing. All these roles are extremely important for a patient undergoing surgical intervention. However, papillary capillaries, responsible for epidermal nourishment and heat dissipation, degenerate with aging. What is left is only the horizontal arteriovenous plexus lying beneath the skin surface. This progressive impairment of vascular circulation and tissue nutrition and the loss of subcutaneous tissue predispose to a feeling of cold, especially in cool environments like the operating room. Therefore the ability to maintain thermoregulation is compromised in the elderly and must be controlled through external measures.

Respiratory system

Lungs lose elasticity, which contributes to an increase in functional residual capacity, residual volume, and dead space. Lungs increase in size and are lighter in weight than previously. Calcification of costal cartilages, dorsal kyphosis, and osteoporosis result in a rigid chest wall. Muscles responsible for inhalation and exhalation may be weakened, resulting in a diminished ability to increase and decrease the size of the thoracic cavity. All these changes contribute to a minimal tidal exchange, which makes the elderly patient more susceptible to pulmonary complications. The elderly person's lung changes are not usually obvious at rest. However, when the person becomes active, breathing may be more difficult. The ability to cough and clear the upper airway is lessened, and such reduction may increase the chance of respiratory infections and diseases. Some can be severe enough to threaten the elderly person's life.

Cardiovascular system

A 35% decrease in coronary artery blood flow is more likely in elderly persons.[16] Because of a shift in blood flow, there is a greater decrease in circulation to the kidneys and liver than to the brain and heart. Blood pressure rises as a result of increased arterial resistance. When the elderly person is at rest, the heart rate remains approximately the same as that of a younger person. However, the older heart requires a longer recovery time after each beat, which means that it reacts poorly to stress and anxiety-produced tachycardia. In general, the capacity of the cardiovascular system to tolerate and buffer insults is limited. Activity, exercise, excitement, and illness increase the body's need for oxygen and nutrients. The older heart may be unable to meet these needs. Arteries lose their elasticity and become narrow causing a weakened heart to work harder. As a result, less blood flows through the arteries, causing poor circulation in many parts of the body.

Digestive system

The secretion of digestive glands decreases, mucus becomes thicker causing dysphagia, and saliva becomes more alkaline. Loss of teeth and poorly fitted dentures make chewing difficult resulting in digestion problems. Foods that are difficult to eat are avoided, and such avoidance can affect overall nutrition. Decrease in peristalsis and a reduction of gastric motility—the results of muscle tone loss—cause a delay in stomach emptying. The absorption of drugs is affected because of a reduction of blood flow to abdominal viscera, hydrochloric acid, and delayed gastric emptying. Decrease of total body water and plasma volume results in a smaller volume of distribution for water-soluble drugs. Lean body mass decreases, and the percentage of body fat increases, a condition that increases the volume of distribution and storage of lipophilic drugs such as diazepam and lidocaine. These factors are of particular importance for assessing the patient's response to preoperative, anesthetic, and postoperative medications.

Urinary system

Nephrons decrease in function with age, so by 75 years of age a person has probably lost a third to a half of original nephron function. Elasticity and tone are lost in the ureters, bladder, and urethra, which leads to incomplete emptying of the bladder. Benign prostatic hypertrophy is almost universal; it is found in 70% of elderly male patients. Difficulty in voiding and retention are common with this condition. Total bladder capacity also declines, so elderly persons experience a more frequent and urgent need to urinate. Because blood flow to the kidneys is decreased, elimination of drugs through these organs is affected. The danger lies in the possible cumulative and adverse effects of drugs. Close observation and consideration of the effect of age-related changes on the kidneys are extremely important during the perioperative period. During this part of the patient's hospital stay the greatest number and variety of drugs are given, increasing the chances for adverse and consequential results.

Musculoskeletal system

A significant change in the elderly person's skeleton is the loss of bone mass, which contributes to skeletal instability and makes fractures of the hip and vertebrae very common. Curvature of the spine and arthritis of the joints are also commonplace. Back pain is related to dehydration and decreased flexibility of the vertebral disks. These changes result in a gradual loss of height, loss of strength, and decreased mobility. Poor posture tends to be proportional to the degree of back pain experienced and may greatly compromise internal organ function. Joint range of motion is impaired to varying degrees and may affect surgical positioning.

Nervous system

Although not functionally significant, a steady loss of neurons begins at about 25 years of age. An inappropriate or slow response to stimuli is primarily a result of a decrease in some organ systems' ability to send reliable messages to the brain and spinal cord. Nerve cells are particularly sensitive to lack of oxygen. Because elderly persons may have, in varying degrees, cerebral arteriosclerosis and atherosclerosis, decreased blood flow and nervous system deficits such as insomnia, irritability, visual motor deficits, and memory loss are not uncommon. Other neurologic changes significant to perioperative care include a loss of position sense in the toes, decreased tactile sense, and atypical response to pain. In addition, benign hypothermia (temperature below 98.6° F) is a common problem in the elderly. In the operating room maintaining balance between heat gain (metabolic production, muscular contraction, and hot ambient temperature) and heat loss (radiation, convection, evaporation, ventilation, cold fluid infusion, blood loss, antithermoregulatory drugs, and impaired heat production) is difficult at best in older surgical patients.

Sensory changes

Sensory changes in vision, hearing, taste, smell, and touch may have an influence on the patient's response to care. Farsightedness in the aging person, or presbyopia, is a result of the lens becoming more rigid and less pliable with age. Consequently visual acuity and accommodation are decreased. Color perception changes, as a result of a yellowing of the lens, make distinguishing blue, green, and purple more difficult for the elderly person. Of particular importance in the operating room is an awareness of the older person's difficulty in adapting to changes in light. Moving patients from a dimly lit holding area to the bright lights of the operating room can cause momentary "blindness."

Presbycusis, or loss of hearing sensitivity, is irreversible, bilateral, and primarily sensorineural, although metabolic and mechanical causes are also possible. It is the most frequent cause of hearing loss in the geriatric patient. Hearing loss, which appears to be greater in men than in women, is mostly within the higher frequencies (above 1000 Hz). In addition, cerumen thickens, and the eardrum becomes less pliable, and such changes also contribute to diminished hearing. Often geriatric patients are labeled "confused" or "senile" because they respond inappropriately to questions they did not hear or describe what they see inaccurately because of poor vision.

Significant changes in taste related to aging are unlikely to occur before 70 years of age. The number of tastebuds decreases, and half are basically nonfunctional. The taste buds at the front of the tongue, which are responsible for sweet and salty tastes, are usually the first to decrease in function. Those buds for bitter and sour taste continue to function longer. For this reason, many older adults may complain that their food tastes bitter or sour.

There is a close association between the sense of smell and human behavior. Smell can affect emotions when a person recalls a particular odor. Other functions include protection of the individual by warning of danger in the air, such as smoke or gas fumes; assistance in digestions; and helping a person to remember or recollect. In the elderly, the sense of smell is reduced as well as the ability to identify odors. Demented elderly in particular have a severe decrease in their ability to identify and discriminate food odors.

Changes in sensitivity to touch often accompany the aging process, but the degree of change varies among individuals. In some cases, losses can be related to neuropathy caused by disease, injury, or circulatory problems. Decreased ability in the sense of touch can affect the elderly person's ability to localize stimuli and can also reduce the speed of reaction to tactile stimulation. An example is an older person having difficulty differentiating between coins, fastening buttons, or grasping small items.

Psychologic Changes

Physiologic and psychologic stress may result in confusion in the geriatric patient, which is analogous to convulsions as a stress reaction in the pediatric patient. In the elderly, mental change can be a warning of some underlying problem. Confusion should therefore not be dismissed as an expected behavior of the geriatric patient who is, after all, "just senile." The most important assessment factor is determining whether the confusion is chronic or acute. Chronic conditions such as depression and Alzheimer's disease can make communication with the patient difficult. Depending on the stage of disease, patients may or may not be able to understand explanations. Family members are the best resource in determining the patient's ability to comprehend and respond to questions and instructions. Behavioral changes such as aggressiveness, agitation, and paranoia are not uncommon. Soft restraints may be necessary during local procedures in the operating room to ensure patient safety. Taking the time to talk slowly, being deliberate in movements, getting to know the patient, and developing a trusting relationship before surgery can help to lessen the patient's anxiety and control the combative outbursts that occur in some Alzheimer patients.

Acute confusional states in the elderly can be precipitated by any number of conditions. Some of the most common predisposing factors for confusion in hospitalized elders are increasing age, baseline brain damage, drug or alcohol addictions, fatigue, social and psychologic stressors, and sleep deprivation. Causes of confusion include drugs, alcohol withdrawal, infections, metabolic disorders, cardiac disorders, cancer, trauma, and cerebrovascular disorders.[11] Other conditions such as fecal impaction, urinary bladder distention, dehydration, and electrolyte imbalance can also affect cognition in the elderly. Even the disruption of relocation into the hospital, which brings the patient into an unfamiliar environment, can cause acute confusion, particularly during the postoperative period. Validation of the patient's previous mental state with a relative or significant other can help to determine if the onset occurred since hospitalization.

Routine laboratory and diagnostic tests

The physiologic changes of aging do not significantly alter the diagnostic values of complete blood count (CBC), differential cell count, platelets, urinalysis, and blood chemistry results; therefore abnormalities should be evaluated. A slight increase may be noted in potassium levels, fasting blood glucose, postprandial blood glucose, oral glucose tolerance, total cholesterol, and thyroid-stimulating hormone. A decrease in vitamin B_{12}, folic acid, magnesium, creatinine clearance, and albumin may also be noted.[11] The chest x-ray film may reveal increased anteroposterior diameter, osteopenia, and degenerative joint disease. The heart size should appear normal, even in the elderly. Cardiomegaly can contribute to postoperative complications and should be evaluated. The ECG may show P-wave notching, ST-segment depression, and T-wave flattening or inversion. An increase in bundle branch block, hemiblock, and first-degree block may also be noted, largely as a result of degenerative disease of the conduction system. Other diagnostic tests that are considered important for elderly surgical patients are hemoglobin or hematocrit, creatinine, BUN, glucose, and arterial blood gases. Serum electrolytes are evaluated because they demonstrate underlying disease and increased risk. In particular, they should be evaluated when patients are taking diuretics because muscle relaxants, mechanical ventilation, and IV fluids can exacerbate an electrolyte disturbance.[1]

Because many elderly patients take several medications, assessing their drug history is important. Digoxin and nitroglycerin may be stopped during the perioperative period, whereas diuretics and antihypertensives may be taken as needed but not used routinely during the postoperative period. Any patient who had been receiving steroids within the previous 12 months should receive parenteral steroids starting the evening before surgery and continuing through the initial postoperative course.

Control of diabetes is often difficult during the perioperative period. For patients taking oral hypoglycemics the medication is stopped, and serum glucose and urinary glucose are closely monitored. Long-acting parenteral insulin is discontinued, and regular insulin is given during the preoperative period. Patients who are fasting the morning of surgery should have an IV line inserted with 5% dextrose and water and receive half their usual morning dose of insulin. Thereafter, until the patient assumes a normal diet, serum glucose levels are covered as necessary with insulin.[4]

Additional assessment data

Another very important but often overlooked area of assessment is dental evaluation. The condition of the patient's temporomandibular joint and the presence of a mouth disorder including loose teeth and dentures can make the difference between a smooth and safe anesthetic and a disastrous outcome. Misconceptions about oral health in the elderly have changed in part because of research conducted in this area of elder care (Research Highlight 30-3). Tooth loss is not considered to be an inevitable consequence of aging. Currently in the United States only one third of those 65 years of age and over are completely edentulous, a situation that is a considerable change from 30 to 40 years ago.[10] A mouth disorder, like any number of physiologic, psychologic, or social factors, can affect the nutritional condition of the

30-3 RESEARCH HIGHLIGHT

Garcia (1995) reported the results of two major longitudinal studies of aging and oral health. The findings indicate that oral disease or dysfunction in the elderly appears to be related to the presence of comorbidity rather than to any normal age-related change. Additionally findings have shown that salivary gland function remains functionally unchanged with aging and dry mouth is more likely associated with certain systemic conditions or medications taken.

From García, R.I. (1995). Geriatric dentistry. In Reichel, W. (Ed.), *Care of the elderly: clinical aspects of aging* (ed. 4). Baltimore: Williams & Wilkins.

patient. Many elderly persons simply do not care to eat because of ill-fitting dentures or poor oral health.

Life changes can also affect the nutritional state. As previously mentioned, normal age changes in taste and smell may negatively affect nutritional status postoperatively. Of particular importance are the losses endured with aging such as the loss of one's spouse, family, or friends through death or relocation; loss of a prior standard of living through retirement; and loss of physical or mental well-being. These changes can affect older persons to the point that they either cannot afford to buy nutritious foods or lose the ability or interest to prepare food. The ultimate effect, among other things, is a nutritionally debilitated patient. Any nutritional deficits should be corrected before surgery because the success of the operative procedure, the rate of wound healing, and the length of hospital stay are directly related to the nutritional state.

Determination of operative risk

After assessment of the patient is completed, conditions that can add to the patient's operative risk may be identified. Surgical procedures, including cardiac, abdominal, thoracic, and multioperations performed on an emergency basis, significantly increase operative risk (Box 30-1). Whenever possible, medical conditions are treated before surgery. Sometimes correction is not possible, and the risk of forestalling surgery outweighs any other medical problem. The determination of operative risk for the patient is generally based on the physical status scale of the American Society of Anesthesiologists.[4] Although the actual classification of the patient is done by the anesthesia provider, noting the parameters from which a decision is made is important.

- Class I: Normal healthy patient
- Class II: Patient with mild to moderate systemic disease
- Class III: Patient with severe systemic disease that limits activity but is not incapacitating
- Class IV: Patient with incapacitating systemic disease that is a constant threat to life
- Class V: Moribund patient not expected to survive 24 hours with or without the operation
- Class E: Emergency procedure (applied to any classification above)

As previously mentioned, operative risk should not be based on age alone. More recently, the evaluation of operative risk, even for major surgical procedures, has focused more on clinical status than on chronologic age (Research Highlight 30-4).

Nursing Diagnoses

In evaluating, synthesizing, and prioritizing the data collected during the preoperative assessment, the perioperative nurse can formulate nursing diagnoses that will form the basis of the plan of care.

Nursing diagnoses related to the care of geriatric surgical patients might include the following:

- Risk for infection
- Risk for fluid volume deficit
- Ineffective thermoregulation
- Risk for impaired skin integrity
- Sensory or perceptual alterations (visual or auditory)

BOX 30-1	**Risk Factors for Surgery in Elderly Patients**

Surgical Risks

Emergency surgery
Site of surgery
  Vascular
  Aortic
  Intrathoracic
  Intraperitoneal
Duration of procedure (>3.5 hours)

Anesthetic Risks

ASA Classification as classes IV and V
Age >75
Preexisting medical disease

Disease-Related Risks

Cardiovascular
  Angina
  Previous myocardial infarction
  Congestive heart failure
Pulmonary
  Bronchitis
  Pneumonia
  Cigarette smoking
Digestive
  Poor nutritional status or malnutrition
  Protein deficiency
  Cirrhosis
  Active peptic ulcer
Endocrine
  Adrenal insufficiency
  Hypothyroidism

Cognitive Impairment

Dementia
Acute confusional state (delirium)

Other Conditions

Dehydration
Anemia
Recent stroke
Malignancy

Adapted from Barry, P.P. (1997). Perioperative care. In Ham, R.J., & Sloane, P.D. (Eds.), *Primary care geriatrics: a case based approach,* (ed. 3). St. Louis: Mosby.

30-4 RESEARCH HIGHLIGHT

A case-controlled study compared a group of 115 elderly patients 70+ years to a group of 115 younger patients for complications, mortality, and survival rates. The subjects were drawn from patients admitted over a 10-year period for treatment of head and neck cancers. Although disease extension was similar in both groups of subjects, a highly significant number of the elderly group were classified as operative risk III and IV. Results showed that local and systemic complications occurred at a similar rate in both groups; risk of recurrence was slightly reduced in the elderly group; and at the close of the study 30% of the elderly and 37% of the younger group were alive. The 5-year actuarial survival rate was 43% for patients older than 70 years versus 56% for the younger controls. The conclusions of this study indicated that elderly patients undergoing radical surgery had postoperative mortality and complication rates comparable to those of the younger patients. Although the elderly group had 1.4 times the risk of death than their younger controls, rates of cancer-related death were similar for the two groups.

Benedetti et al. reported the results of a study conducted to determine the outcomes of kidney transplants in patients older than 60. Subjects 18 to 59 years of age were compared to 60+ year olds to determine surgical outcomes including patient and graft survival, hospital length of stay, incidence of rejection and rehospitalization, and the causes of graft loss. Results of 2828 transplantation patients were reported for data collected over a 23-year period from 1970 to 1993. Recipients and graft-survival rates in the older group were similar to those in the younger group until 3 years after transplantation when the mortality increased for the older patients. Longer initial hospitalization was required for the elderly group, but they had fewer rejection episodes and fewer hospitalizations than the younger group had. Quality-of-life scores for surviving transplantation recipients from the 60+ years group were similar to the national norms. The researcher concluded that kidney transplantation is successful in patients 60 years or older and that the incidence of extrarenal disease at the time of transplantation was not a predictive factor of outcome and should not be used as an exclusion for transplantation in older patients.

From Kowalski, L.P., Alcantara, P.S., Magrin, J., & Parise, O. (1994). A case control study on complications and survival in elderly patients undergoing major head and neck surgery. *American Journal of Surgery, 168,* 485-490; and from Benedetti, E., Matas, A.J., Hakim, N., et al. (1994). Renal transplantation for patients 60 years of age or older: a single-institution experience. *Annals of Surgery, 220,* 445-460.

Outcome Identification

Outcomes identified for the selected nursing diagnoses could be stated as follows:

- The patient will be free from infection throughout the postoperative period.
- The patient will maintain adequate fluid-volume levels intraoperatively and postoperatively.
- The patient will maintain normothermia ±1° F throughout the perioperative period.
- The patient will maintain skin integrity intraoperatively.
- The patient will accurately perceive and interpret environmental and sensory stimuli throughout the perioperative period.

Planning

As a result of anatomic and physiologic effects of aging, geriatric patients have, in varying degrees, a general decline in organ function and an altered ability to recover from stressful events. In addition to normal age changes, many older adults suffer from one or more chronic conditions that influence the risk of surgery. Successful surgical outcomes in the geriatric patient depend on elective versus emergency surgical procedures, optimum physical condition of the patient, thorough preoperative assessment, close intraoperative and postoperative monitoring, and preventive measures to decrease the likelihood of complications.

A Sample Care Plan for a geriatric surgical patient is shown on p. 1291.

Implementation

Perioperative geriatric patient care is very similar to the care provided to younger adults. However, modifications that involve consideration of age-specific differences between the two groups are made. The perioperative nurse who recognizes the special needs of the elderly patient during what may be the most critical period of hospitalization helps to enhance the course of surgical intervention and postoperative recovery.

Preoperative preparation

The preoperative period is an opportune time to evaluate the patient's psychosocial status and educational needs. As previously mentioned, the motivation of the patient can have an effect on operative risk and successful surgical outcomes. Awareness of psychologic and emotional status is equally important as physiologic status. Often the patient's concerns are focused on spouse or other family members rather than on the impending

S A M P L E   C A R E   P L A N

Nursing Diagnosis: Risk for wound infection related to intraoperative procedures and length of surgery secondary to age-associated reduction in efficiency of the antigen-antibody reaction and endocrine function

Outcome: Patient will be free from infection throughout the postoperative period.

Interventions:

Monitor for breaks in aseptic technique throughout the procedure.

Take corrective action for breaks in techniques immediately.

Perform preoperative skin preparation using appropriate technique as defined by AORN recommended practices and hospital policy.

Restrict traffic within the operating room.

Keep doors closed during surgical procedures.

Check equipment and assemble all supplies before surgery to prevent intraoperative delays.

Confine and contain contaminants.

Ensure availability of antibiotics as needed.

Nursing Diagnosis: Risk for fluid volume deficit related to NPO status and intraoperative blood and body fluid losses secondary to age-associated decreases in total body water and plasma volume

Outcome: Patient will maintain adequate fluid volume levels intraoperatively and postoperatively.

Interventions:

Monitor and record intraoperative intake and output.

Provide visualization of sponges and suction canister.

Closely monitor blood versus irrigation fluid amounts in suction bottle.

Ensure visualization of the urine drainage bag.

Ensure availability of blood replacement as needed.

Ensure availability of IV fluids as needed.

Report intake and output to PACU nurse.

Nursing Diagnosis: Ineffective thermoregulation related to poikilothermy secondary to age-associated physiologic decompensation

Outcome: Patient will maintain normothermia ±1° F throughout the perioperative period.

Interventions:

Use warm blankets during transport to operating room and replenish as needed throughout the perioperative period.

Place warmed sheet on OR bed before patient transfer.

Use hyperthermia blanket beneath patient for lengthy procedures; begin warming before patient's arrival in operating room.

Maintain room temperature at comfortable levels.

Monitor patient for fluctuations in temperature.

Provide additional head covering (cloth, plastic, or reflective) during surgical procedure.

Prevent overexposure of patient.

Use warmed irrigation and prep (as recommended by manufacturer) solutions.

Administer warmed blood and blood products and IV fluids at room temperature.

Remove wet linens before transport to PACU.

Nursing Diagnosis: Risk for impaired skin integrity related to surgical positioning secondary to alterations in skin turgor, sensation, peripheral tissue perfusion, and skeletal prominence

Outcome: Patient will maintain skin integrity intraoperatively.

Interventions:

Assess potential pressure areas before anesthesia and positioning.

Avoid shearing forces by utilizing a four-person lift when transferring patient to or from the OR bed.

Place safety strap above the knees; prevent undue pressure on the popliteal space and heels.

Provide pillows and other padding devices during positioning to protect potential pressure areas.

Maintain body alignment within restrictions imposed by musculoskeletal age-related changes.

Prevent wrinkling of linen under the patient or positioning devices.

Place electrosurgical dispersive pad in the most appropriate area while avoiding bony prominences.

Avoid pooling of solutions under the patient.

Apply tape sparingly to prevent skin injury during removal.

Nursing Diagnosis: Sensory or perceptual alterations: visual or auditory related to removal of eyeglasses or hearing aid in the operating room secondary to age-associated changes in sensory organs

Outcome: Patient will accurately perceive and interpret environmental and sensory stimuli throughout the perioperative period.

Interventions:

Remove operating room mask to introduce self and explain procedures before surgery.

Ask the patient to state his or her name and continue to call the patient by stated name.

Attract the patient's attention before speaking.

Face the patient directly when speaking.

Speak slowly and distinctly in a low-pitched, clear voice.

Use gestures to supplement words.

Write instructions as needed to clarify information.

Allow ample time for patient to ask questions.

Prepare patient for changes in light intensity.

Assist patient with transfers and mobility.

Inform patient before positioning or procedures done before anesthesia.

surgery. An unexpected hospitalization can be very disruptive to an elderly patient who perhaps was the sole caretaker of an ill spouse, a parent, or even a pet. The worry of how that individual or pet will be cared for can have an effect on the surgical outcome. In addition, the concern for quality of life and the fear of institutionalization after surgery can be extremely upsetting. Utilizing the assistance of the discharge planner or case manager to arrange for resources may help to allay the patient's concerns.

Sensory deficits occurring either as a result of age-related changes or merely because eyeglasses and hearing aids are removed can make communication with geriatric patients more difficult. Unresponsive or uncooperative behavior may be inappropriately diagnosed as dementia and therefore expected as part of aging and ignored. As discussed earlier, acute confusion in the elderly is the most important indicator of possible underlying conditions that could seriously and adversely affect surgical intervention and outcomes. Knowing whether the patient's cognitive impairment is recent or chronic will provide direction for planning postoperative care.

The nurse should take advantage of the time spent in the presurgical care unit, preoperative holding, or the surgical corridor to introduce herself or himself and explain events to follow. Because a surgical mask is generally not required in these areas, this is the most opportune time for talking with the older adult and thus facilitating better communication. Once the patient is taken into the operating room, a reassuring touch and remaining close to the patient, particularly during anesthesia induction, can help to decrease anxiety (Fig. 30-2).

Anesthesia induction

Pertinent assessment data that may affect anesthesia is obtained by the perioperative nurse and shared with anesthesia personnel. A medical history of asthma, previous patient or family anesthesia problems, abnormal laboratory data, and physical limitations affecting induction or airway management are important findings.[13]

Geriatric patients frequently have changes in airway anatomy that make appropriate ventilation difficult. Changes in facial contour from sunken cheeks or lack of dentition result in an inadequately fitting anesthesia mask. Keeping dentures in place often offsets this problem; however, if intubation is planned, dentures are usually removed. The joints of the head and neck may exhibit limited range of motion, making intubation and airway management more difficult in the elderly. Assessment of these potential problems before anesthesia facilitates a smooth induction period.

The choice of anesthesia in the elderly patient depends on physiologic status, length of the operative procedure, and preference of the anesthesia provider. No evidence indicates that a specific inhaled or injected drug is preferable as an anesthetic for older adults. Regional

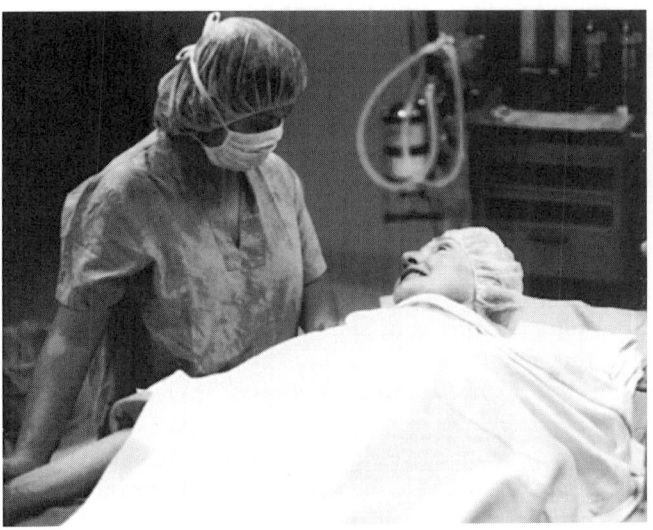

FIGURE 30-2 Perioperative nurse's presence and reassuring touch help to allay patient's anxiety before anesthesia induction.

anesthesia on an alert, cooperative patient is an acceptable alternative to general anesthesia.[18] Accurate predictions of how the elderly patient will respond to drugs or anesthesia are difficult to make because of a decrease in systems function. Older patients have both an altered pharmacodynamic (relation between plasma concentration and drug effect) and pharmacokinetic (distribution and elimination of drugs) response to drugs. This is important in understanding the increased incidence of side effects. The increasing age of the patient decreases the dose requirement of anesthesia. This includes agents that induce anesthesia (such as thiopental sodium, etomidate, propofol) and narcotics. The induction dose of a barbiturate required for a 70 year old is approximately 30% less than patients 20 to 30 years of age.[18] Minimal blood levels of a drug may produce undesired side effects before therapeutic levels are reached. Likewise reduced liver and kidney function, altered body composition, decreased albumin, and decreased cardiac output all modify the aged person's ability to eliminate drugs from the body. Age-related changes in homeostatic mechanisms affect the older adult's ability to deal with physiologic stresses of surgery such as fluid depletion, volume overload, or hypoxemia. The nurse should be prepared to respond quickly in assisting the anesthesia provider to stabilize the patient when adverse reactions occur.

Positioning

Protection of skin integrity is of utmost importance. Loss of subcutaneous fat, poor skin turgor, and tissue fragility can potentiate a postoperative skin problem. Aging changes in the skin accentuate bony prominences and a decrease in the range of motion make positioning one of the most important considerations of care. Elderly patients should be lifted into position, rather than slid or dragged, to prevent shearing injuries.

Often, because of musculoskeletal deformity, elderly patients cannot fully extend the spine, neck, or upper and lower extremities. Using pillows or padding devices to compensate for these skeletal changes not only makes the patient more comfortable during the procedure but also prevents residual pain or injury postoperatively (Fig. 30-3). Depending on the situation, positioning the patient before anesthesia induction may be best so that the patient can direct positioning efforts in regard to comfort.

Skin preparation and thermoregulation

Temperature fluctuations are common in the elderly as a result of impaired thermoregulation. Response to cold including vasoconstriction and shivering is diminished in the elderly and is triggered by a lower core temperature than that in younger adults. Increasing the operating room temperature will help to stabilize effects of heat loss. Devices such as warmed blankets or temperature-regulating blankets are highly recommended, particularly when a lengthy surgical procedure is expected. Prepping solutions should be carefully chosen to prevent skin irritation and warmed (if recommended by the manufacturer) to help decrease hypothermic effects. Ensuring that the patient is not lying in a prep solution or on wet linens also helps to reduce skin injury and inadvertent lowering of body temperature.

When the body is exposed to cold temperatures, blood is shunted away from peripheral body parts to the head. Because the head lacks fat depots and vasoconstriction capabilities, heat loss from the head can be as much as 25% to 60% of total body heat loss. Elderly patients should therefore have some form of head covering to prevent the ill effects of hypothermia.

Aseptic techniques and safety measures

Age-related decline in the immune system and some age-associated diseases have a detrimental effect on the aging body's ability to appropriately respond to infectious agents. In the lungs, the cough reflex and ciliary action weaken specialized defense mechanisms against foreign-body invasion. Incomplete emptying of the bladder can cause urinary tract infection. Immobility and drug therapy can alter flora in the intestines and make the body more vulnerable to infectious organisms. Because infection and delayed healing of wounds are poorly tolerated and often fatal in the debilitated elderly patient, strict adherence to aseptic technique is extremely important. Because length of surgical procedure is related to incidence of infection, ensuring that needed supplies and equipment are readily available is important. This practice prevents unnecessary delays and decreases surgical exposure and also the length of time the elderly patient is under anesthesia.

Fluctuations in fluid volume are common in the geriatric patient. Volume deficits occur as a natural course

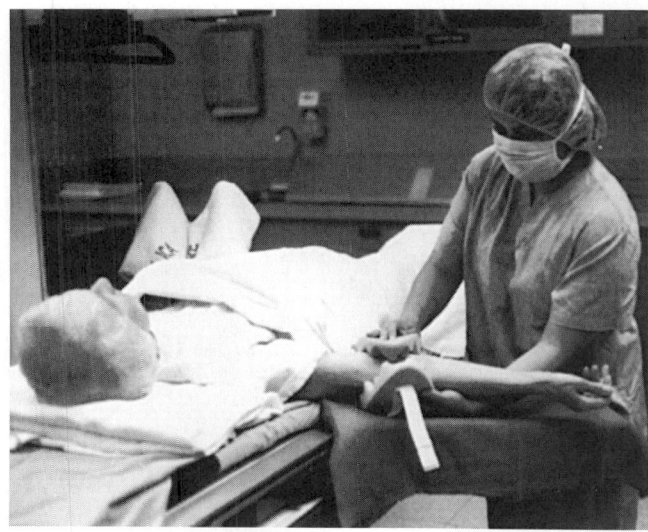

FIGURE 30-3 Pillows or padding devices aid patient comfort and prevent residual pain or injury postoperatively.

of aging, whereas volume excess can occur from intraoperative fluid replacement. Careful measurement of intake and output is essential. Closely monitoring sponges, suction bottle contents, and urinary drainage also helps to prevent potentially fatal complications.

Evaluation

Before transporting the patient to the PACU, the perioperative nurse should assess the care provided intraoperatively by evaluating expected versus actual outcomes. Specific outcome criteria established for each nursing diagnosis provide the basis for evaluation of care.

The skin is examined for signs of injury, particularly over bony prominences and under the electrosurgical dispersive pad. To prevent skin injury postoperatively, wet linens from beneath the patient are removed, and the patient is carefully lifted from the OR bed to the PACU stretcher. Anticipated frequency of dressing change, as in a draining wound, should govern the method used to secure the dressing. A minimal amount of tape should be used because its removal can cause additional skin trauma. Depending on the wound site, rolled gauze over the primary dressing may be the best choice so that tape is not applied directly to the skin. Another alternative is Montgomery straps. For smaller wounds the least possible amount of hypoallergenic tape should be used. Because infection is poorly tolerated, the choice of dressing should maximize wound protection while being the least irritating to the skin.

In collaboration with the anesthesia provider, an assessment of intake and output is completed and recorded. Because of the consequences of postoperative dehydration or fluid volume overload in the elderly patient, fluids are increased or decreased accordingly. Blood loss is carefully evaluated, recorded, and reported.

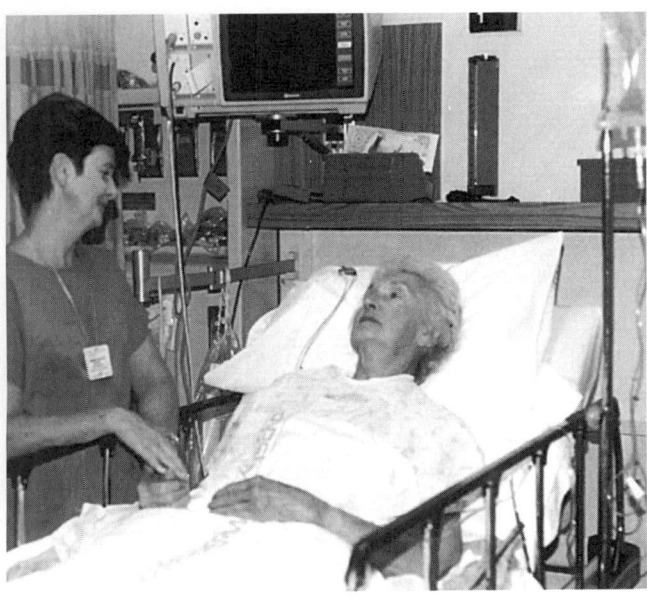

FIGURE 30-4 Explanations to elderly patient before any procedure enhance cooperation.

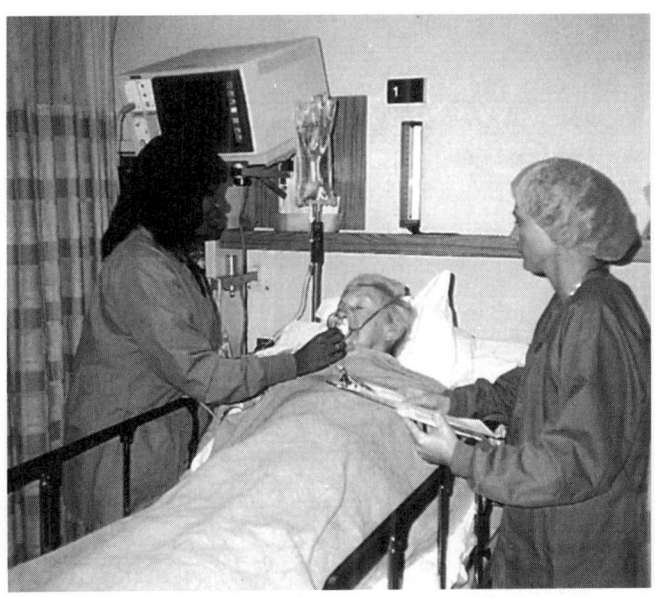

FIGURE 30-5 Pertinent information that could affect postoperative care outcomes is communicated to PACU nurse.

The wound is closely observed for bleeding before dressing application and postoperatively because the elderly person's ability to recover from hemorrhage and shock is extremely poor.

Evaluation of body temperature is particularly important in the elderly because postoperative hypothermia is quite common and can precipitate agitation and confusion. To prevent any adverse response, the patient should be covered with warmed blankets throughout the recovery period.

As previously discussed, the elderly patient responds poorly to infectious agents. Monitoring the patient frequently for potential sources of wound contamination is extremely important because physical reserves after surgery are greatly reduced. Special attention to sterile and clean procedures and frequent handwashing can make the difference between an uneventful surgical outcome and one fraught with complications.

Depending on the patient's level of consciousness, explanation should be given about the impending transfer to PACU as a form of reality orientation. As appropriate, the patient should be introduced to the PACU nurse and told what to expect in the unit. Explanations should always precede any procedure. Often the elderly person is reluctant to cooperate simply because no one has taken the time to explain what is going to happen (Fig. 30-4).

Because of the relatively fine line between stability and the development of postoperative complications, the elderly patient's response to surgery must be closely evaluated. Verbal communication between the perioperative and PACU nurses should include any pertinent preoperative and intraoperative information that could

affect postoperative care outcomes, including sensory limitations; intake and output; allergies; type and location of catheters, drains, packing, and implantable devices; anesthesia and medications received; and any unusual occurrences that could affect the patient's recovery (Fig. 30-5). The type and extent of surgery may affect postoperative pain. Elderly persons may not complain of pain, but it is not an indication that pain does not exist. There is some belief that pain sensitivity and perception decreases with aging; however, this belief is controversial. The consequences of this assumption may mean needless suffering and undertreatment of both the elderly person's pain and the underlying cause.[6]

Documentation of outcome evaluation can be phrased as follows:

- Skin integrity was maintained, free from redness, bruises, and abrasions; patient reports no pain or impairment of the skin or joint mobility.
- Fluid balance was maintained; urinary output was within normal limits; the patient's forehead skin was checked and had good turgor; and vital signs were stable.
- Temperature was ±1° F of normal range, skin was warm to touch, and patient verbalized comfort.
- Aseptic technique was maintained throughout the procedure; wound was dry and dressing intact; lab values and vital signs were within normal limits.
- The patient accurately perceived and interpreted environmental stimuli, expressed and demonstrated understanding of procedures, and responded appropriately to auditory and verbal stimuli.

Patient and Family Education and Discharge Planning

Education should be conducted at a time when the patient is at rest rather than during preoperative or postoperative procedures. Too much stimuli from outside sources can interfere with the patient's ability to concentrate and motivation to learn. Physical comfort should be assured. A patient who is uncomfortable or in pain will not be receptive to education. Age-related changes can affect the elderly patient's ability to learn new material; therefore modification of traditional teaching approaches should be used to enhance effectiveness.

Sensory changes in vision and hearing or cognitive impairment can interfere with the patient's ability to understand and retain information. Giving the patient postoperative instructions in written form helps with retention, and modification using large type on colored paper of warm tones (yellow, tan) makes them easier to read. Family members or significant others who are present should be included in the educational session so that they can provide assistance at home.

Content should be focused only on relevant information about surgical procedures or postoperative recoveries, and relating it to previous life experiences helps the patient to grasp the concepts more readily.[20]

Discharge planning begins during the preoperative assessment. Sufficient time is needed to make appropriate decisions about postdischarge care to prevent complications, reduce the risk of rehospitalization, and minimize stress to the patient and the caregivers.[7] The type of surgery and expected postoperative recovery period determines the extent of resources needed, such as durable medical equipment, home health and homemaker services, extended care, social and community services, or physical rehabilitation. The success of postdischarge outcomes in the elderly include the patient's self-assessment of health as good or excellent, the complexity of the patient's medical condition, history of being able to maintain responsibility for his or her own health, and family or social networks.[7] Discharge needs of the patient should be evaluated as early as possible so that appropriate education, referrals, and home preparation can be completed before the patient leaves the hospital or surgicenter.

SURGICAL INTERVENTIONS

Unlike that in the pediatric patient, surgery in the elderly does not include special instruments, equipment, or drapes that are made for the geriatric patient exclusively. Surgical procedures that can be considered classically geriatric are governed more by pathologic condition than by anatomy and are directly related to the common diseases affecting older adults.

Throughout the remainder of this chapter, surgical procedures that are commonly seen in geriatric patients are discussed briefly. Reference is made to other sections of the text for a more in-depth description of the technical aspects of the procedures.

COMMON SURGICAL PROCEDURES IN GERIATRIC PATIENTS

It is believed that the demographic structure of the population is a major influence on the numbers of surgical procedures performed on that population. Additionally however, it seems likely that a greater understanding and acceptance of the appropriateness of surgery in the old and the very old has affected the demand for and trending of surgical procedures in the elderly.

The frequency of surgical procedures correlates to the change in underlying patterns of disease in the elderly. A mnemonic used for remembering the most common diseases of aging is to think of the *i*'s: immobility, instability, incontinence, intellectual impairment, impaired homeostasis, impaired vision and hearing, insomnia, and iatrogenic disease.[22] The common primary discharge diagnoses for men in 1990 were heart disease, neoplasms, pneumonia, cerebrovascular disease, and hyperplasia of the prostate. In women the common discharge diagnoses were heart disease, neoplasms, cerebrovascular disease, fractures, and pneumonia.[22]

In comparing this information to the most common operative procedures in the elderly (65 years of age and over) as reported by McRae[22] and Hershey[14] it is not surprising that a close association exists between the two. In men the most common surgeries were reported as prostatectomy, cardiac catheterization, coronary bypass, pacemaker insertion or replacement, repair of inguinal hernia, digestive system biopsies, and extraction of lens.

For women, the common surgeries reported were cardiac catheterization, reduction of fracture (excluding head and facial), pacemaker insertion or replacement, digestive system biopsies, cholecystectomy, cataract extraction, and lens insertion.

These data, as compared to surgical procedures reported in 1989, show a dramatic increase in the number of cardiac procedures in the elderly for both males and females, whereas the incidence of other procedures remains similar over time.

ABDOMINAL SURGERY

Accurate diagnosis of abdominal disease is important in the elderly to plan timely and appropriate operations. However, clinical signs of abdominal disease such as tenderness, pain, muscle rigidity, and fever are frequently less obvious in elderly patients. The common use of nonsteroid antiinflammatory drugs (NSAIDs) may mask symptoms or even predispose elderly patients to acute abdominal disease.

GI surgery in the elderly is associated with a tripling of mortality and morbidity. Nearly 10% of surgery in the elderly is for gastrointestinal emergency surgery.[21]

Most often, operations are performed for complications of calculus disease and less often for malignant obstruction of the bile ducts. The incidence of gallstones increases with age with more than 50% in patients 70 years of age or over. In females the incidence rises from 5% at 20 years of age, to 25% at 60 years of age, and 35% at 80 years of age.

Research indicates that acute cholecystitis should be treated by cholecystectomy through open or endoscopic procedure, with use of general or local anesthesia even in the very oldest symptomatic patients. Because laparotomy is a stressor in older ill patients, laparoscopic cholecystectomy is considered the preferred surgical approach in elderly patients with symptomatic gallstone disease.[9] Asymptomatic stone patients should also be treated surgically because of the increased incidence of associated gallbladder carcinoma in about 1% of patients. Conservative treatment of an acute condition followed by interval cholecystectomy is not advisable because elderly men are prone to perforation of an acutely inflamed gallbladder, and the mortality rate is 15% to 25%. All biliary surgery in patients 70 years of age and older should be done with antibiotic prophylaxis. See Chapter 12 for an in-depth description of operations of the biliary tract.

Mortality for peptic ulcer disease complications can be 100 times higher in the elderly, with bleeding causing death most often. If bleeding necessitates hospitalization, 20% to 40% of patients with a gastric ulcer and 40% to 50% of patients with a duodenal ulcer require immediate surgical intervention.[21]

Perforation of gastroduodenal ulcer is second to bleeding as a cause of death in the elderly and accounts for one fourth of the ulcer-related deaths. After 50 years of age, the risk of perforation doubles. If surgical intervention does not occur within 12 to 18 hours after problem recognition, the mortality approaches 100%. Approximately 70% of peptic perforations are duodenal and 30% are gastric with similar mortality rates of 15% to 20%. The procedure chosen must consider the patient's overall condition, history of chronic versus acute ulcer symptoms, and ulcer location.[21] In poor-risk patients suture plication with vagotomy and pyloroplasty can lessen the operative risk. Elderly patients tolerate a surgical procedure better than prolonged or recurrent bleeding. See Chapter 11 for an in-depth description of ulcer surgery.

HERNIA

The elective repair of inguinal and femoral hernias is strongly advised because of the risk of incarceration with subsequent emergency operation. Approximately 20% of hernia repairs in elderly patients are emergency incarcerations and small bowel obstruction. As with other emergency procedures in the elderly, the mortality rate is 7.5% as compared with 1.37% for elective procedures. The operation can be performed as an ambulatory procedure, and local anesthesia provides a very satisfactory alternative to general or spinal anesthesia. General or spinal anesthesia is not believed to be necessary, may predispose the elderly patient to significant cardiopulmonary and urologic complications, and has been associated with significant perioperative hypotension.[26]

Laparoscopic techniques for hernia repair have gained popularity because of its associated shorter hospital stay, minimal pain postoperatively, and early recovery. However, the necessity for general anesthesia and unknown recurrence rates make this approach one that may not be advisable in the elderly. Decisions for local versus spinal or general anesthesia are made based on the patient's overall physiologic status and surgical risk.

In elderly men the coexistence of inguinal hernia and prostatism is fairly common. Depending on the size of the prostate, the hernioplasty should be postponed until after the prostate surgery.

Not unusual in the elderly are large neglected scrotal hernias. The repair of these hernias is not routine in that the abdominal wall defect may be so large that primary repair cannot take place without tension. Synthetic abdominal wall replacements are helpful in management of such large hernias. The repair of huge scrotal hernias can have a tremendous benefit on the personality of the geriatric patient, who is much relieved after removal of what can be considered an accessory appendage that is offensive, difficult to clean, and often an impedance to daily activities. See Chapter 13 for an in-depth description of herniorrhaphy.

GENITOURINARY SURGERY

The predominant reason for urologic surgery in elderly men is benign prostatic hypertrophy (BPH). The prevalence of the disease increases steadily with age involving more than half of prostates in men 51 to 60 years of age and 90% of men 81 to 90 years of age. BPH may be silent or have minimal symptoms in the presence of severe bladder decompensation. Prostate surgery, especially transurethral resection of the prostate (TURP), is relatively safe and generally well tolerated. The majority of the 400,000 or more BPH operations per year are performed to relieve symptoms, rather than for more serious problems such as retention, infections, bladder stones, hydronephrosis, and renal damage.[25] TURP is indicated if the surgeon believes that total resection can be accomplished in 1 hour and there is no bladder disease or impairment to urethral access.

A surgical alternative to TURP is transurethral incision of the prostate (TUIP). The resectoscope knife is used to make a full-thickness cut through the prostate from the bladder neck through the apex of the prostate with no tissue resection. Research to compare TUIP to TURP indicate that identical improvement in symptoms and urinary flows improved an average of 75% with TUIP versus 105% for TURP. TUIP complications are significantly less than TURP, especially bleeding, retrograde ejaculation, and impotence. It is a more desirable alternative to TURP for patients with prostates weighing less than 30 g.[25]

See Chapter 15 for an in-depth description of prostate surgery.

OPHTHALMIC SURGERY

Given a long life span, undergoing eye surgery (most commonly for cataracts) is more likely than other surgical procedures. Most ophthalmic procedures are minimally invasive and have a high success rate. Because elderly patients may have concurrent systemic disease, even a low-stress procedure should not be treated lightly. Elderly patients may be confused, be uncooperative, or have hearing problems that may make it impossible to follow directions. In addition, they may have significant musculoskeletal disease and be unable to lie still for long periods. Patients with chronic lung disease lying in the supine position may experience coughing, which can increase intraocular pressure and jeopardize the surgery.

Cataract surgery is among the most common and successful of all surgical procedures. The majority of these cases are performed in an ambulatory setting with patients returning home the day of surgery. Most eye surgery patients make the decision to have the procedure done after months of deliberation and slow, progressive loss of vision. The overall risk of death is low and doesn't change much whether local or general anesthesia is used. Nearly a million cataract operations are performed in the United States each year, and more than 90% of patients regain the potential for full visual acuity. Intraocular lenses can be safely implanted in the majority of patients. Microsurgical wound closure ensures a secure incision that allows immediate ambulation. The surgical stress is considered so low and visual rehabilitation so rapid that severe visual impairment is considered a reasonable indication to perform surgery even if the elderly patient is debilitated. See Chapter 18 for an in-depth description of cataract surgery.

ORTHOPEDIC SURGERY

Osteoporosis is the most obvious skeletal change that occurs with advancing age. It leads to susceptibility to fracture, which doubles every 5 years after 50 years of age.[24] An approximate loss of 40% of the mineral content of the bone must be present before detectable change is evident on x-ray films. To some degree osteoporosis is related to a lessening of physical activity, but it is also related to lessened hormonal secretion. Thus postmenopausal women are more prone to develop the condition and therefore more likely to sustain a hip fracture.

Age-related changes in bone increase the incidence of displaced femoral and intertrochanteric fractures of the upper femur. The incidence of hip fracture increases with advancing age, doubling for each decade beyond 50 years. Hip fracture is more common in women at a 2:1 ratio and higher in institutionalized patients, a level that is probably caused by dementia, comorbidity, and use of psychotropic drugs.[29] Because the usual cause of death in patients with upper femur fracture is pulmonary embolus, surgery is designed to relieve the severe pain, allow movement in and out of bed, and return the patient to his or her former environment as quickly as possible with minimal debilitation. Estimates of mortality within 1 year after hip fracture are 12% to 30%.[17]

A displaced femoral neck fracture must be surgically repaired or healing will not occur. In elderly patients, 70 and older, prosthetic replacement is usually done because it allows for early ambulation and will last throughout the remaining years of the patient's life. Intertrochanteric and subtrochanteric fractures are best treated with internal fixation. These methods also allow for early mobility.

Degenerative joint disease (osteoarthritis) and inflammatory polyarticular disease (rheumatoid arthritis) are the primary indications for total joint replacement in the hip and knee. In these patients pain that disrupts normal daily activities and interrupts sleep is the major reason for surgery regardless of the patient's age. Usually these procedures are elective, and patients have better functional status and a higher bone mass than those with hip fracture. These factors increase the success of the prosthesis.[24] See Chapter 22 for an in-depth description of hip and knee surgery.

CARDIOVASCULAR SURGERY

Cardiovascular disease remains the number one cause of death in the elderly with a prevalence of almost 50% and accounting for more than 40% of death in people over 65 years of age.[3] If it were successfully eliminated, approximately 14 years of additional life expectancy could be added at birth. In men 65 years of age it is estimated that 20% have ischemic heart disease, 10% have hypertensive heart disease, 7% have combined ischemic and hypertensive disease, and 4% have valvular disease. Elderly women have slightly different but very similar cardiovascular disease; 14% have hypertensive heart disease, 12% have ischemic disease, 7% have combined hypertensive and ischemic disease, and 6% have valvular disease.[27]

Coronary bypass surgery is performed in increasing numbers of patients over 65 with an operative mortality of 3% to 6%. Elective peripheral vascular reconstructive procedures are also encouraged in the geriatric patient. Patients older than 80 are reported to have had as little as

5.5% hospital mortality and a 13.8% complication rate in various vascular procedures, including cerebrovascular reconstruction, aortic aneurysms, grafts of upper and lower extremity vessels, and embolectomy in acute arterial occlusion. Newer intraoperative techniques introduced in the mid to late 1970s, including myocardial preservation, optical magnification, finer sutures, and membrane oxygenation, have greatly improved the outcome of surgery in older patients.[15]

In another group of 80 year olds undergoing elective aortic aneurysmectomy, the patients' mortality rate was reported to be only 4.7%, and 86% of the patients were reported to have quality of life equal to or better than their preoperative status. The facts that 25% of abdominal aortic aneurysms 4 to 7 cm in diameter do rupture and that the operative mortality for ruptured aneurysm is about 40% provide a strong argument for elective surgery in carefully screened and prepared elderly patients. See Chapters 26 and 27 for a more in-depth description of vascular and cardiac surgery.

ADDITIONAL CONSIDERATIONS

Every surgical procedure carries with it a certain amount of risk no matter what the age of the patient. As discussed previously, the physiologic deficits of aging increase surgical risk in the aged patient just as comorbidity and surgery done on an emergency basis do. Procedures that are performed in the thorax or the peritoneal cavity are considered of high risk of death. Procedures of moderate risk include vascular and hip procedures, and low-risk procedures include prostatectomy and mastectomy. However, any procedure, even those considered of low risk, can have poor outcomes, depending on the patient's overall condition.

Dodson and Seymour,[5] have proposed a code of practice for elderly surgical patients. Some of the points that they suggest should be used when consideration is made for surgical care of the elderly include the following:

- Age alone should not be a barrier to surgery in the elderly.
- Elderly persons with conditions treatable by surgery have as much right to benefit from modern surgery, anesthesia, and medical and intensive care techniques as younger patients have.
- Medical and surgical techniques that can enhance the older person's life should be equally available to the old and to the young.
- The majority of elderly patients are mentally competent and should therefore be involved in making decisions about their care or treatment plan.
- Elderly patients have special needs because of their atypical presentation of disease, multiple medical disorders or comorbidity, impaired homeostasis, and altered drug response.

- The perioperative nurse who approaches the care of the elderly with these points in mind will not only enhance the surgical outcome but will significantly affect the patient's overall quality of life.

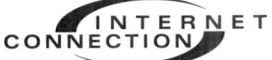

National Gerontological Nursing Association:
http://www.nursingcenter.com/people/nrsorgs/ngna/

Gerontological Society of America: http://www.geron.org/

National Institute on Aging: http://www.nih.gov/nia/

Geriatric Education: http://www.med.ufl.edu/medinfo/geri/

Topics in Geriatrics From the Mayo Clinic:
http://www.mayo.edu/geriatrics-rst/GeriArtcls.html

Geriatrics Care Pearls From the Mayo Clinic:
http://www.mayo.edu/geriatrics-rst/Pearls.html

Administration on Aging: http://www.aoa.dhhs.gov/

Geriatric Video Productions: http://geriatricvideo.com

REFERENCES

1. Abrams, W.B., Beers, M.H., Berkow, M.D., & Fletcher, A.J.. (1995). *The Merck manual of geriatrics* (ed. 2). Rahwah, N.J.: Merck Research Laboratories.
2. American Association of Retired Persons (AARP). (1996). *A profile of older Americans.* Washington, D.C.: AARP.
3. Aranki, S.F. (1994). Cardiovascular surgery in the elderly. In Homberger, F. (Ed.). *The rational use of advanced medical technology with the elderly.* New York: Springer Verlag.
4. Buxbaum, J.L., & Schwartz, A.J. (1994). Perianesthetic considerations for the elderly patient. *Surgical Clinics of North America, 74*(1), 41-58.
5. Dodson, M.E., & Seymour, G. (1992). Surgery and anaesthesia in old age. In Brocklehurst, J.C., et al. (Eds.). *Textbook of geriatric medicine and gerontology* (ed. 4). New York: Churchill Livingstone.
6. Ebersole, P., & Hess, P. (1994). *Toward healthy aging human needs and nursing response.* St. Louis: Mosby.
7. Eliopoulos, C. (1997). *Gerontological nursing* (ed. 4). Philadelphia: J.B. Lippincott.
8. Ferris, P. (1976). Surgical management of the elderly. *Hospital Practice, 11,* 65.
9. Fried, G.M., Clas, D., & Meakins, J.L. (1994). Minimally invasive surgery in the elderly patient. *Surgical Clinics of North America, 74*(2), 375-386.
10. Garcia, R.I. (1995). Geriatric dentistry. In Reichel, W. (Ed.). *Care of the elderly: clinical aspects of aging* (ed. 4). Baltimore: Williams & Wilkins.
11. Girard, N.J. (1997). Gerontological nursing in acute care settings. In Matteson, M.A., & McConnell, E.S. (Eds.). *Gerontological nursing: concepts and practice* (ed. 2). Philadelphia: W.B. Saunders.
12. Ham, R.J. (1997). Assessment. In Ham, R.J., & Sloane, P.D. (Eds.). *Primary care geriatrics a case based approach* (ed. 3). St. Louis: Mosby.
13. Hazen, S.E., Larsen, P.D., & Hoot Martin, J.L. (1997). General anesthesia and elderly surgical patients, *AORN Journal, 65*(4), 815-822.
14. Hershey, D.N. (1996). The aging patient. In Rothrock, J.C. (Ed.). *Perioperative nursing care planning* (ed. 2). St. Louis: Mosby.
15. Hochberg, M.S. (1990). Cardiac surgery in the elderly. In Katlic, M.R. (Ed.). *Geriatric surgery: comprehensive care of the elderly patient.* Baltimore: Urban & Schwarzenberg.

16. Jaffe, M. (1996). *Geriatric nursing care plans* (ed. 2). Englewood, Colo.: Skidmore-Roth.

17. Kane, R.L., Ouslander, J.G., & Abrass, I.B. (1994). *Essentials of clinical geriatrics* (ed. 3). New York: McGraw-Hill.

18. Kelly, M. (1995). Surgery, anesthesia, and the geriatric patient, *Geriatric Nursing, 16*(5), 213-216.

19. Kirkland, R.I. (1994). Why we will live longer. . . and what it will mean. *Fortune, Feb.:* 66-77.

20. Lusis, S.A. (1996). The challenges of nursing elderly surgical patients. *AORN Journal, 64*(6), 954-962.

21. McFadden, D.W., & Zinner, M.J. (1994). Gastroduodenal disease in the elderly patient, *Surgical Clinics of North America, 74*(1), 113-126.

22. McRae, T.D. (1995). Common complaints of the elderly. In Reichel, W. (Ed.). *Care of the elderly: clinical aspects of aging* (ed. 4). Baltimore: Williams & Wilkins.

23. Muravchick, S. (1997). Geriatric patients. In Longnecker, D.E., & Murphy, F.L. (Eds.). *Dripps-Eckenhoff-Vandam Introduction to anesthesia* (ed. 9). Philadelphia: W.B. Saunders.

24. Ochs, M. (1990). Surgical management of the hip in the elderly patient. *Clinics in Geriatric Medicine, 6*(3), 571-587.

25. Payne, C.K., Babiarz, J.W., & Raz, S. (1994). Genitourinary problems in the elderly patient. *Surgical Clinics of North America, 74*(2), 401-429.

26. Rosenthal, R.A. (1994). Small-bowel disorders and abdominal wall hernia in the elderly patient. *Surgical Clinics of North America, 74*(2), 261-291.

27. Weitz, H.H. (1990). Noncardiac surgery in the elderly patient with cardiovascular disease. *Clinics in Geriatric Medicine, 6*(3), 511-529.

28. Zenilman, M.E. (1994). Surgery in the nursing home patient. *Surgical Clinics of North America, 74*(1), 63-77.

29. Zuckerman, J.D., & Spivak, J.M. (1990). Orthopedic surgery in the elderly. In Katlic, M.R. (Ed.). *Geriatric surgery: comprehensive care of the elderly patient.* Baltimore: Urban & Schwarzenberg.

CHAPTER THIRTY ONE | # Trauma Surgery

Antoinette Frances Kanne

TRAUMA IS RANKED as the foremost health care problem in the United States today. It accounts for the cause of death for approximately 160,000 Americans per year.[5] Injury, resulting from trauma, is the leading cause of death for people 44 years or less, with men having a greater risk of death than women have. Whether the injury is a result of a motor vehicle collision, violence, crime, or work-related injury, trauma occurs unplanned and without warning. The unpredictable nature of trauma can pose a great challenge to the perioperative nurse.

The potential for injury has existed since the beginning of mankind. Most of the major advances in care of the critically injured have been accomplished through experience in the military. Clearly, the shorter the response time, the greater the survival rate for casualties. This was demonstrated by the success of the Mobile Army Surgical Hospitals (MASH) during the Korean conflict, which brought the necessary supplies, equipment, and personnel closer to the battlefields and consequently improved patient outcomes.

Eventually this concept was applied to the civilian population and is most commonly referred to as the "golden hour" of trauma care. More specifically, the golden hour refers to the time immediately after the injury when rapid and definitive interventions can be most effective in the reduction of morbidity and mortality.[7]

Traumatic death may occur in three phases.[9] The first phase occurs immediately after the injury. This accounts for about 50% of the deaths from trauma and is usually a result of lacerations to the heart or aorta or brainstem injury. These patients rarely survive to the hospital and die at the scene. The second phase of deaths occurs within the first 1 to 2 hours after the injury, representing about 30% of the total fatalities. These patients have injuries to the spleen, liver, lung, or other organs that result in significant blood loss. This is the group in which definitive trauma care (that is, appropriate and aggressive resuscitation with adequate volume replacement) may have the largest effect (the golden hour). The third phase of deaths occurs days to weeks after the injury, often during the intensive care phase, and is usually caused by complications or a failure of multiple organ systems[6] (Fig. 31-1). In other words, time is of the essence in providing definitive care to the critically injured.

A significant number of deaths can be prevented if there is provision for rapid transport from the accident scene to a facility equipped to provide resuscitation and treatment in an efficient and timely manner. This concept is reflected in the national development of the Emergency Medical Services (EMS) system. Facilities and resources are allocated and coordinated to provide specific interventions for a group of patients. For example, in the trauma system facilities that meet certain criteria to accommodate the specialized needs of the critically injured patient are designated as trauma centers. Transfer and triage protocols that allow for a trauma patient to reach the appropriate facility with the least out-of-hospital time possible are established. This may be accomplished by a helicopter with a specially trained flight crew or through the use of ground transport by means of an advances life support (ALS) ambulance team (Fig. 31-2).

Trauma centers are designated by four specific levels of care. A level I trauma center is committed to provision of qualified personnel and technologic equipment necessary for rapid diagnosis and treatment on a 24-hour basis. A level II center is able to treat the seriously injured but lacks some of the specialized clinicians and resources required for the level I designation. A level III trauma center may be a community hospital in an area that does not have a level I or level II facility. A level IV trauma center has the ability to provide advanced trauma life support before patient transfer. These facilities may be located in rural areas with limited access and may be a clinic or a hospital. Consequently the tiering of the trauma system allows injured patients to be stabilized and transferred according to preestablished protocols that allow for the most efficient access to definitive care.[3]

A level I trauma facility is the receiving institution for severely injured patients in the region. In rural areas there can be a long transport time in the absence of helicopter availability. Therefore time is of the essence. A level II facility may provide surgical intervention if resources match the patient need or if the critical nature of the injury dictates immediate intervention before transfer to a major trauma facility.

Trauma patients require immediate access to the operating room 24 hours a day, 365 days a year. A sudden influx of a large number of trauma patients to a trauma center may necessitate triage or classification of those less seriously injured as less urgent allowing immediate access to the critically injured. The elective surgery schedule may need to be interrupted to expedite care for the trauma patient. Such scheduling policies and procedures should be established collaboratively by the departments of surgery, trauma, anesthesia, and perioperative nursing services. Consequently the perioperative nurse should be familiar with supplies and equipment located in the operating room designated for trauma or in the operating rooms most frequently used for these patients.

PERIOPERATIVE NURSING CONSIDERATIONS

Preliminary Evaluation: Mechanism of Injury

Because of the unpredictable timing of trauma, it is often the on-call perioperative nursing team who cares for injured patients requiring surgical intervention. In contrast to the elective procedure, little information is known about these patients, and preparation time is often minutes at the most. A working knowledge of the mechanism of injury is essential to assist the perioperative nurse in rapid assessment of the patient soon to arrive.

Mechanism of injury (MOI), or kinematics, involves the action of forces on the human body and their effects. Knowing the forces applied provides invaluable information in evaluation of the patient and injuries that may be present. Upon initial evaluation of the trauma patient at the scene of the injury, careful observations are made by the first responding EMS team. For example, the position of the victim in a car, whether the person was the driver or a passenger seated in the back seat or front seat, estimated velocity of the vehicle, location of impact, and use of seat belt or air bag are all pieces of information to increase the index of suspicion about the probable causes of injuries of the patient (Fig. 31-3). After addressing the immediate

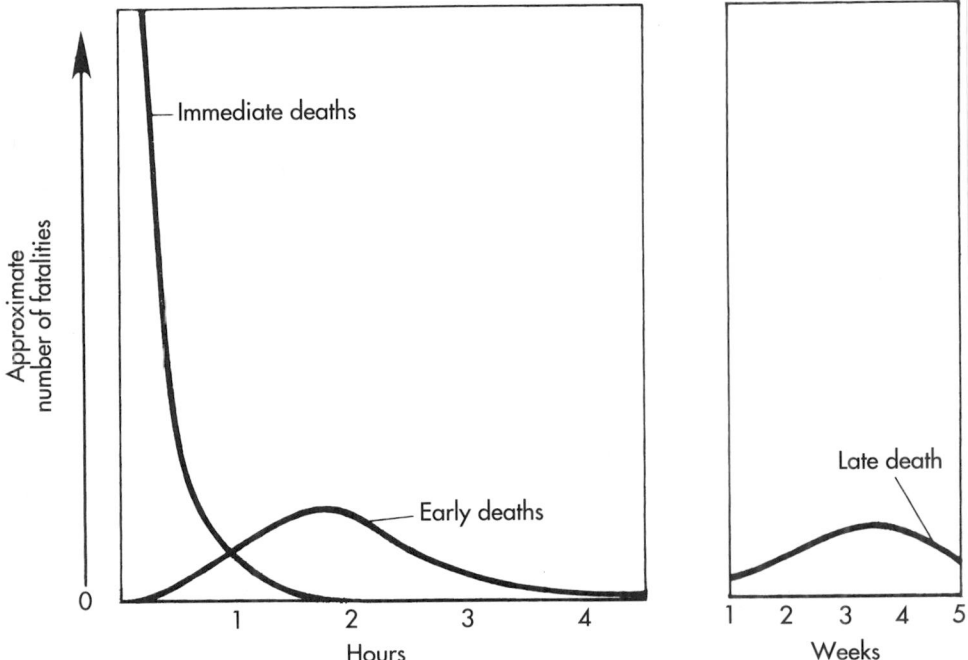

FIGURE 31-1   Distribution of fatalities caused by trauma as function of time after injury. Notice that trimodal distribution occurs: 50% of deaths occur in first phase (immediate deaths), 30% of deaths occur in second phase (early deaths), and 20% of deaths occur in third phase (late deaths).

threats to life, the MOI can provide valuable clues as to probable cause of injuries (Fig. 31-4). This systematic approach can reduce morbidity and mortality (Box 31-1).

The MOI is a product of the type of injuring force and the resulting tissue response. The velocity of the collision, shape of the object, and the tissue's flexibility are influential in the magnitude of the injury sustained. For example, long-bone tissue has little or no flexibility. A strong collision involving a long bone most often results in a fracture of some type (Fig. 31-5). This is a tissue stressor greater than the tissue's ability to recover. In contrast, soft-tissue injury from a colliding force may result in a contusion, a localized bruising, since this tissue has greater flexibility.

Blunt trauma is injury resulting from a combination of forces, such as acceleration, deceleration, shearing, and compression, that does not result in a break of the skin. Morbidity and mortality may be greater than with penetrating trauma because identification of injuries is more difficult when injuries are less obvious. Examples of blunt trauma include motor vehicle crashes (MVCs), falls, contact sports injuries, and aggravated assault. The spleen is the most common abdominal organ injured. Head, spinal, thoracic, and skeletal system injuries can also occur.

Acceleration and deceleration injuries occur most frequently in blunt trauma. A ruptured thoracic aorta is an example of an injury that occurs as a result of these types of forces (Research Highlight 31-1). In an MVC the large vessels are stopped or decelerated rapidly, resulting in vessel damage caused by stretching that exceeds its elastic ability. This affects the aorta at the ligamentum arteriosum, the anatomic point where it is affixed tightly to the chest wall, just below the origin of the subclavian artery. This shearing below the attachment site causes a rupture as the aorta continues to move in a forward motion after the chest wall motion has stopped.

MVCs account for approximately 50% of blunt trauma.[5] During an MVC, three collisions occur. The first collision is that of a car into another object. The second collision is that of the occupant's body impacting on the vehicle's interior. The third collision happens when an

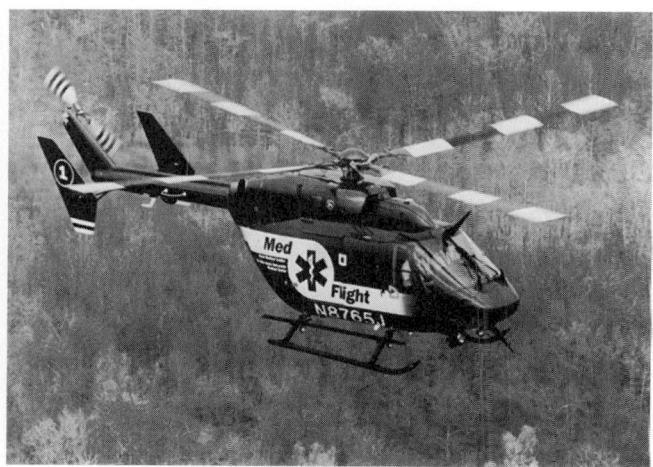

FIGURE 31-2 BK-117 rotary-wing craft.

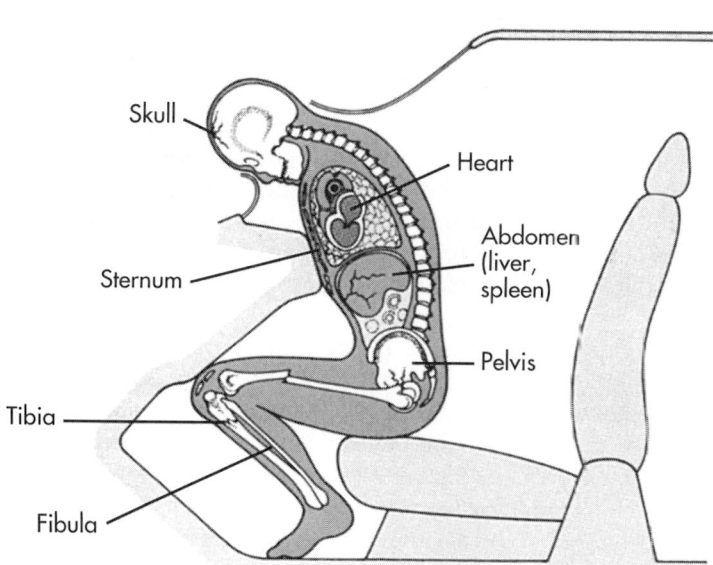

FIGURE 31-3 Potential injury sites of unrestrained passenger in front seat.

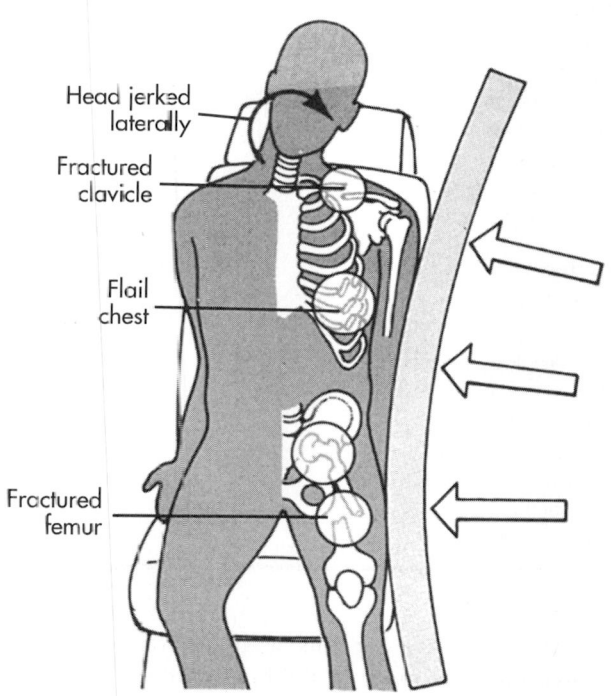

FIGURE 31-4 Potential injury sites in lateral-impact collision. Notice that injury is still possible in lateral crash, even with airbag inflation, because airbags were designed specifically for frontal crashes. However, injuries are usually fewer in lateral-impact crashes with airbag inflation than without.

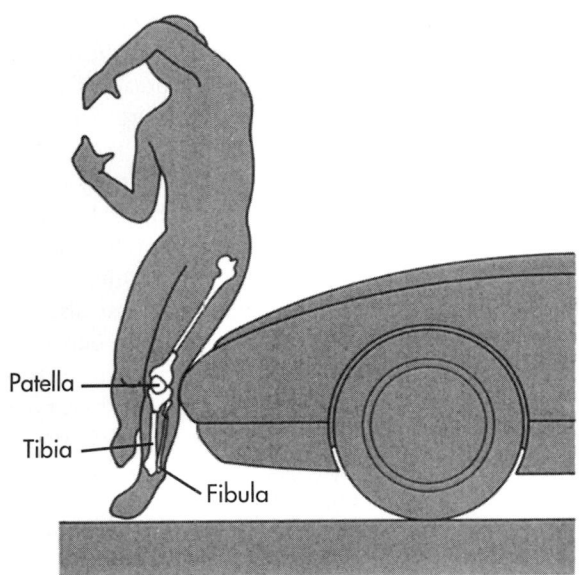

FIGURE 31-5 Potential primary injury sites of adult pedestrian.

BOX 31-1	**Predictable Injuries in Motor Vehicle Crashes**

Unrestrained Driver

Head injuries
Facial injuries
Neck injuries
Fractured larynx
Fractured sternum
Cardiac contusion
Pulmonary contusion
Lacerated liver or spleen
Lacerated great vessels
Fractured patella and femur
Fractured clavicle

Restrained Driver

Caused by lap restraint
   Pelvic injuries
   Spleen, liver, and pancreas injuries
Caused by shoulder restraint
   Cervical fractures
   Rupture of mitral valve or diaphragm
Caused by air bag deployment
   Nasal fracture
   Forearm fractures

---

internal body structure hits a rigid bony surface. A coup-contrecoup injury of the brain, for example, is the result of an acceleration force to one area of the brain and a deceleration force to an opposite area.

Falls also contribute highly to the cause of traumatic death in the United States.[1] Injuries are most commonly associated in children experiencing falls greater than twice

---

31-1 RESEARCH HIGHLIGHT

Katyal et al. conducted a study to examine the relationship between traumatic rupture of the thoracic aorta (TRA) and the direction of impact at the time of the motor vehicle crash. This was a retrospective review of patients with TRA conducted over a 4.5-year period from two different data sources, that is, the coroner's office and a trauma registry. Criteria for inclusion in the study included confirmation of vehicle impact by police reports and documented rupture of the thoracic aorta either at autopsy or time of surgical intervention. Ninety-seven patients met the study criteria. Forty-eight cases (49.5%) were involved in lateral impact crashes. Twenty-eight drivers and 20 passengers were victims of TRA also from lateral, or side, impact crashes. The authors concluded that lateral impact crashes have a strong correlation with TRA. The study recommended that traumatic rupture of the aorta should maintain a high index of suspicion with a mechanism of lateral impact.

From Katyal, D., McLellan, B.A., Brenneman, F.D., et al. (1997). Lateral impact motor vehicle collisions: significant cause of blunt traumatic rupture of the thoracic aorta. *The Journal of Trauma, 42*(5), 769-772.

---

their height. In adults, falls greater than 10 to 15 feet are usually accompanied by significant injury. Deceleration forces in falls produce forces of stretching, shearing, and compression. Consequently, aortic injuries are also suspect in this group of patients. Skeletal injuries occur as well, because of the compressive forces present.

Penetrating trauma is a result of the passage of a foreign object through tissue. The degree or extent of tissue injury is a function of the energy that is dissipated to the tissue and the surrounding areas. The anatomic structures most often injured include the liver, intestines, and vascular system. Extent of the injury includes the nature of the foreign object, such as bullet caliber, size of knife, distance from the weapon, structures penetrated, and amount of energy dissipated to the structures.

The velocity of a bullet is responsible for the degree of injury or cavitation to the tissue. A low-velocity bullet is one that travels at a lower speed (1000 feet per second or less) and disrupts only the bullet tract and its immediate surrounding area. A high-velocity, or military, weapon fires a bullet traveling at a greater speed (3000 feet per second or greater) and causes significantly more damage and tissue destruction, since the bullet tract involves more extensive surrounding tissue (Fig. 31-6). The distance from the weapon also influences the degree of injury because the velocity is greatest when the bullet leaves the weapon and decreases as it travels. Type of bullet (such as shotgun shells with multiple pellets and hollow-point

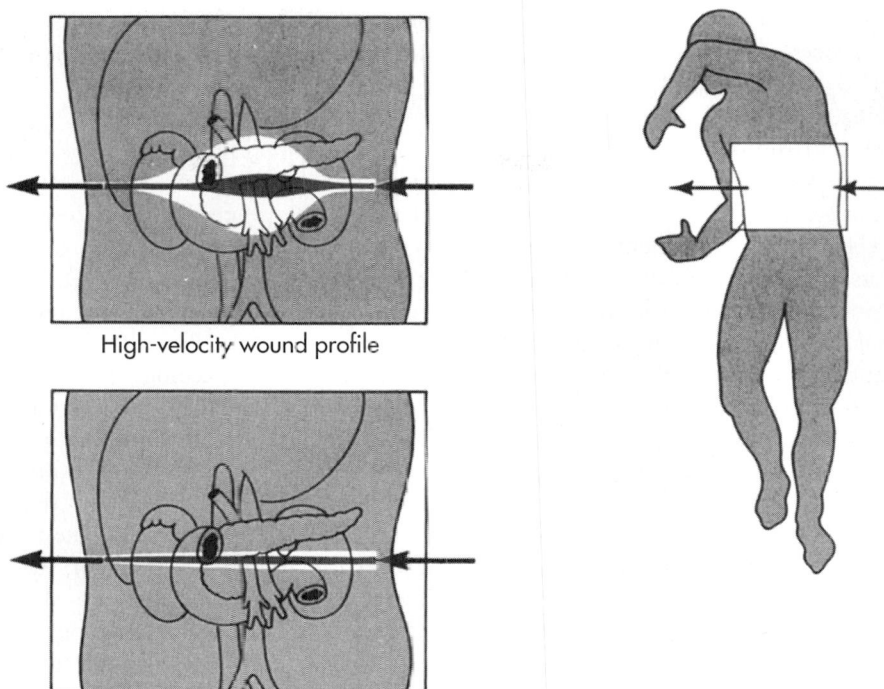

High-velocity wound profile

Low-velocity wound profile

FIGURE 31-5   Potential injury path of high- and low-velocity bullets.

bullets, which mushroom on impact) influences the degree of injury. Commonly the entrance wound is smaller than the exit wound because of the dissipation of energy, but an exit wound may not always be present. If the bullet completely fragments or is lodged in a structure internally, there will not be an exit wound. Depending on the position of the bullet and any resultant injury it may cause, bullets are not always removed.

Stab and impalement wounds are considered to be low-velocity wounds. The associated injuries usually correspond to the path of the penetrating object. Factors of the object, such as width and length, assist in identification of the possible occurrence of injuries. A single injury site may penetrate several different organs or cavities. Penetrating injuries located at or below the nipple line may cause both chest and abdominal injuries. This is attributable to the diaphragmatic excursion that occurs with inspiration and expiration.

Impaled objects should not be removed at the scene or in the emergency department (ED). The impaled object provides a tampon effect to injured blood vessels and is removed only when the ability to control potential bleeding from those vessels is present. Wound debridement may also be necessary. These objects are removed in an operating room where the needed supplies and instrumentation are present.

Injuries that result from explosions are related to the effects of the blast. Fragments may become high-velocity missiles, and shock waves can also produce tissue disruption. Traumatic amputations are also possible.

TABLE 31-1	Revised Trauma Score (Range 12 to 0)		
GLASGOW COMA SCALE	SYSTOLIC BLOOD PRESSURE	RESPIRATORY RATE	CODED VALUE
13-15	>89	10-29	= 4
9-12	76-89	7-29	= 3
6-8	50-75	6-9	= 2
4-5	1-49	1-5	= 1
3	0	0	= 0

From Champion, H.R., Sacco, W.J., Copes, W.S., et al. (1989). A revision of the trauma score. *Journal of Trauma, 29*(5), 623-629.

Thermal and electrical tissue damage and inhalation injuries may occur from an explosion or as a sole mechanism of injury. These patients are usually resuscitated and require operative intervention for debridement on a nonemergent basis, unless the injury is limb or life threatening.

Injuries can be scored objectively according to the severity. This scoring system assists medical personnel in more effective triage and provides a universal method of communication between facilities, departments, and nursing personnel. The revised trauma score (RTS)[2] incorporates physiologic criteria including head injury severity (Glasgow Coma Scale). The RTS scale ranges from 0 to 12. An RTS of 11 or less at initial triage is usually an indication for transfer to a trauma center (Table 31-1).

Assessment

The resuscitative process begins upon arrival of emergency personnel to the scene and ends when the patient has been stabilized, received definitive care, and undergone a complete and thorough physical exam for determination of all injuries sustained. Upon arrival at the ED, the trauma team initiates a primary assessment. This is a logical, orderly process of patient assessment for potential life threats. These assessment activities are based on established protocols outlined in the *Advanced Trauma Life Support* (ATLS) *Manual*.[3] Use of the acronym "ABCDE", representing assessment of *a*irway (with cervical spine precautions), *b*reathing, *c*irculation, *d*isability or brief neurologic exam, and *e*xposure (to reveal all life-threatening injuries), is accomplished. Airway interventions may include manual maneuvers (chin lift, jaw thrust), oral or nasopharyngeal airways, or intubation. Emergent procedures, such as tracheostomy or needle cricothyrotomy may also be utilized to obtain an airway. Pulse oximetry and capnography are also utilized.

During this time the trauma surgeon or ED physician and trauma team identify life threats that are present and correct life threats as they are identified before progressing to the next part of the exam.[3] For example, a patient may have a penetrating wound with evisceration of abdominal contents. However, the obvious, which is currently not life threatening, is ignored until the trauma team is assured of a patent airway, cervical spine precautions have been implemented, and an effective breathing pattern exists. An evisceration needs to be corrected, but an inadequate airway is an immediate life threat and assumes primary priority.

After completion of the primary assessment and correction of any immediate life threats, the secondary assessment is completed. The purpose of the secondary assessment is to identify all injuries present. Sometimes this second assessment may be completed by the perioperative nurse, the postanesthesia recovery nurse, or the critical care nurse. A patient requiring immediate surgery is transported to the operating room, undergoes surgical intervention, and then is transferred to the PACU or ICU, depending on his or her condition. This assessment is a more in-depth exam of the patient from head to toe, including a back exam. All vital signs, including a rectal or tympanic temperature unless contraindicated, are obtained. Inspection, palpation, percussion, and auscultation are used in the complete head-to-toe assessment to reveal any other sites of injury.

A brief history is obtained from his or her family or significant other when possible. This history is referred to as the "AMPLE" history and may be obtained even after the patient is transferred to the operating room by the ED personnel. The history includes *a*llergies, *m*edications, *p*ast medical history, *l*ast meal, *l*ast menstrual period (if appropriate), and *e*vents or *e*nvironment leading to the accident or injury.[3] If the history is obtained after the initiation of surgery, it is important to communicate it to the surgeon and the anesthesia team.

Routine Laboratory Tests

During the resuscitation phase two large-bore intravenous line (16 gauge or larger) are inserted, and blood is drawn. Appropriate laboratory tests include a minimum of a complete blood count (CBC), hemoglobin and hematocrit (H/H), blood alcohol level (BAL), and a type and screen. Other tests may be requested during evaluation, such as prothrombin time (PT), activated partial thromboplastin (APTT), toxicology screen, and a serum electrolyte panel (Box 31-2). The results of the laboratory studies, as applicable to the patient, should be reviewed and communicated as appropriate. Abnormal clotting studies are of obvious significance in this patient population. These results may be attributable to anticoagulant medication the patient is taking or the effects of profound hypothermia. H/H values are also important to note. Caution is advised in evaluating an H/H drawn in the ED. There can be a significant time delay between bleeding and a drop in H/H.[7] Frequently, abnormal values in the blunt trauma patient alert the team to the possibility of internal bleeding. BAL also assists the trauma team in their evaluation. If the level is significantly high, the physical exam and patient response may be unreliable. In addition, the neurologic status of these patients is very difficult to assess.

A blood type and screen allows the blood bank to decrease time in obtaining a crossmatch if needed later. Most trauma centers have several units of type O negative blood (universal donor) available in the event that a blood transfusion is required before a type and crossmatch (T&C) can be performed. Because of regional shortages of O-negative blood, O-positive blood can be used in male patients and adult female patients of nonchildbearing age. Initially, trauma patients are resuscitated with crystalloid solutions such as lactated Ringer's solution or normal saline solution. If a patient presents in a hypotensive state, 2 liters of warmed crystalloid may be given as a fluid challenge.[8] If the patient's blood pressure responds, the diagnostic examination continues. However, if the hypotension returns, blood may be initiated, and the patient may be transported immediately to the operating room for exploratory surgery.

If indicated by the injury, an arterial blood gas (ABG) measurement is also taken (Box 31-3). This test provides an accurate assessment of the ventilatory status of the patient and also evaluates resuscitative airway and breathing interventions. Metabolic acidosis or a large base deficit, with all other causes ruled out, may be indicative of internal bleeding.

Often during resuscitation a Foley catheter is inserted. After insertion, urine is obtained for a urinalysis and urine drug screen (Box 31-4). The identification of specific drugs in the urine may assist in further diagnosis and

BOX 31-2	Normal Laboratory Values: Blood and Serum Electrolytes

Red Blood Cells (RBCs, Erythrocytes)

RBC values vary, depending on age, sex, and geographic location (in relation to sea level) of the patient.

Normal values

Neonate (up to 2 months)	4.4-5.8 million/μl
Infant (over 2 months)	3-3.8 million/μl
Child (>1 year)	4.6-4.8 million/μl
Adult:	
Male	4.5-5.3 million/μl
Female	4.2-5.4 million/μl
Pregnant female	Elevated

Abnormal values   *Probable cause*

↑
↓

- Dehydration
- Hypovolemia
- Fluid overload (dilutional)

White Blood Cells (WBCs, Leukocytes)

A white blood cell count is obtained to identify the presence of an infection.

Normal values

4100-10,900/μl (elevated in pregnancy)

Abnormal values   *Probable cause*

>10,900/μl

- Infection/inflammation
- Tissue necrosis
- Immunocompromise

Hematocrit (HCT)

A hematocrit value is obtained to determine the percentage of red blood cells in whole blood.

Normal values

Neonate	55%-68%
7-day-old infant	47%-65%
1-month-old infant	37%-49%
3-month-old infant	30%-36%
1-year-old	29%-41%
10-year-old	36%-40%
Adult:	
Male	42%-54%
Female	35%-46%
Pregnant female	Elevated

Abnormal values in trauma

↓

- Hemodilution
  From compensated hypovolemia
  From excessive volume replacement

↑

- Hemoconcentration

Note: When blood is lost acutely, the amount of hematocrit lost is in the same ratio as that of whole blood. Therefore the percentage of hematocrit in a whole blood sample would remain normal. It is only after hemodilution occurs (from shock compensation or crystalloid replacement) that hematocrit drops.

Hemoglobin (HGB)

Hemoglobin value is obtained to measure the amount of hemoglobin in whole blood. The amount of hemoglobin determines the oxygen-carrying capacity of blood.

Normal values

Neonate	17-22 g/dl
1-week-old infant	15-20 g/dl
1-month-old infant	11-15 g/dl
Child	11-13 g/dl
Adult:	
Male	14-18 g/dl
Female	12.4-14.9 g/dl
Pregnant female	Elevated
Elderly female	11.7-13.8 g/dl

Continued

BOX 31-2	Normal Laboratory Values: Blood and Serum Electrolytes—cont'd

Abnormal values in trauma   *Possible cause*

↓   Hemorrhage

Note: When whole blood is lost acutely, the amount of hemoglobin that is lost is proportionate. It is only after hemodilution occurs (as a result of shock compensation or crystalloid volume replacement) that hemoglobin drops.

Platelets (Thrombocytes)

A platelet count is obtained to test the amount of platelet function. Platelets play an essential role in coagulation. Particularly in trauma, platelets are essential to hemostasis when vascular trauma occurs.

Normal values

130,000-370,000/mm^3

Abnormal values   *Probable causes*

↑
- Splenectomy
- Living at high altitude
- Hemorrhage

↓
- Disseminated intravascular coagulation

Coagulation Studies: Prothrombin Time (PT/Protime)

A prothrombin time is evaluated in trauma patients to measure clotting time (caused by factors V, VII, and X, fibrinogen, and prothrombin). This is important in determining the blood's ability to clot.

Normal values

Males   9.6-11.8 sec

Females   9.5-11.3 sec

Abnormal values   *Probable cause*

↑   Deficiency of factors V, VII, X, fibrin, or prothrombin; 2.5× normal values means that there is an abnormal bleeding tendency

Note: There may be prolonged clotting times in the presence of excessive alcohol ingestion or the use of anabolic steroids. Clotting times decrease with the use of antihistamines and diuretics.

Coagulation Studies: Activated Partial Thromboplastin Time (APTT)

An APTT is obtained to screen for problems with intrinsic clotting factors (except factors VII and XIII). It can also be used to monitor the effectiveness of anticoagulation with heparin. This laboratory test measures the amount of time it takes for fibrin to form a clot. In the trauma patient, it is used to determine the patient's tendency to bleed.

Normal values

25-36 seconds for the clot to form (after the clinical reagent is added)

Abnormal values   *Probable cause*

>36 seconds
- Intrinsic factor deficiency

Note: Be sure to fill the lab tube because the tube contains anticoagulant and the ratio of blood to anticoagulant may be altered, causing a false prolonged clotting time if the tube is not filled.

Serum Electrolytes: Sodium (Na)

Sodium is one of the two major extracellular cations. It is the major cause of osmotic pressure in extracellular fluid. Sodium also plays a major part in both acid-base balance and neuromuscular function.

Normal value

135-145 mEq/L

Abnormal values   *Possible causes*

>145 mEq/L (hypernatremia)
- ↓ Fluid intake/fluid loss
- ↑ Sodium intake

<135 mEq/L
- ↓ Sodium intake
- ↑ Sodium loss

Serum Electrolytes: Potassium (K$^+$)

Because potassium is one of the two major cellular cations, it is essential for the maintenance of cellular osmosis. It plays a major role in the electrical conductivity of both cardiac and skeletal muscle. In addition, potassium plays a major role in both acid-base balance and kidney function.

Normal value

3.8-5.5 mEq/L

BOX 31-2 | **Normal Laboratory Values: Blood and Serum Electrolytes—cont'd**

Abnormal values	*Possible causes*
>5.5 mEq/L (hyperkalemia)	• Major burns
	• Renal failure
	• Major crush injuries
<3.8 mEq/L (hypokalemia)	• Hypovolemia

Serum Electrolytes: Chlorides (Cl)

Measurement of serum chlorides is important for the assessment of acid-base status. Chloride is a major extracellular anion that plays a role in the maintenance of oncotic pressure and thus blood volume and arterial pressure.

Normal value
100-108 mEq/L

Abnormal values	*Possible causes*
>108 mEq/L (hyperchloremia)	• Dehydration
	• Renal failure
	• CNS trauma with central neurogenic breathing
<100 mEq/L (hypochloremia)	• Excess vomiting
	• Excess gastric suctioning

BOX 31-3 | **Normal Laboratory Values: Arterial Blood Gases**

Normal Values

Pao_2	Amount of oxygen in arterial blood	80-100 mm Hg
$Paco_2$	Pressure of carbon dioxide in arterial blood and a measurement of how well the lungs are getting rid of carbon dioxide (CO_2 is controlled by the lungs)	35-45 mm Hg
pH	Acidity or alkalinity of arterial blood; a measurement of hydrogen-ion concentration	7.35-7.45
HCO_3	Amount of bicarbonate in arterial blood; it s controlled by the kidneys	22-26 mEq/L
O_2 saturation	Percentage of hemoglobin that is carrying oxygen	94%-100%

Abnormal Values

		Possible Cause
Pao_2	<50 mm Hg	Hypoxia
pH	<7.35	Acidosis
	>7.45	Alkalosis
$Paco_2$	>45 mm Hg	Hypoventilation/CO_2 retention by lungs
HCO_3	<22 mEq/L	Renal excretion of too much bicarbonate
	>26 mEq/L	Renal retention of too much bicarbonate

---

treatment. The urine will also be tested to determine the presence of red blood cells. Depending on the amount of hematuria present, there may be a renal contusion or other renal injury.

The perioperative nurse may be asked to insert an indwelling urethral catheter in the operating room. The urinary meatus should be inspected for the presence of blood before insertion. If blood is noted, the surgeon should be notified and catheter not inserted. The patient may have a ruptured bladder or a urethral injury, either of which is commonly associated with a pelvis fracture. The surgeon at this point may wish to perform a retrograde urethrogram to examine the bladder and urethra for the presence of tears or disruption.

Diagnostic Procedures
Radiology

Depending on the trauma center protocol, a blunt trauma radiographic series is part of the resuscitative phase. This minimally includes a lateral view of the cervical spine and an anteroposterior (AP) view of the chest. In addition, lateral thoracic and lumbar spine films and an AP of the pelvis are taken. Any area with deformity, swelling, or pain may also be radiographed. Trauma patients are always treated as if they have a cervical spine injury until proved otherwise. Adequate spine films for clearance of the cervical spine from injury are imperative.

If the resources are available, trauma center protocol may also include computerized axial tomography (CAT

BOX 31-4 | **Normal Laboratory Values: Urinalysis (UA)**

A urinalysis is done to check for injury to the genitourinary system and for the presence of specific diseases.

Normal Values

Color	Yellow straw
Appearance	Clear
Specific gravity	1.005-1.020
pH	4.5-8.0
Protein	Negative
Glucose	Negative
Ketones	Negative
Microscopic findings:	
RBCs	0-3/hpf
WBCs	0-4/hpf
Epithelial cells	Few
Casts	0
Crystals	Few
Bacteria	0
Yeast	0
Parasites	0

Abnormal Values

		In Trauma, May Indicate
Color	Dark or red	• Presence of blood
Appearance	Dark or red	• Presence of blood
Specific gravity	>1.020	• Shock
pH	Alkaline >8.0	• Alkalosis
	Acidic <4.5	• Acidosis
Glucose	Present	• Diabetes
		• Increased intracranial pressure
Protein	Present	• Renal failure
Ketone	Present	• Diabetes
		• Diarrhea and vomiting
Microscopic findings:		
RBCs	3/hpf	• Kidney, ureteral, bladder trauma
WBCs	4/hpf	• Urinary tract infection
Epithelial cells	↑	• Renal tubular necrosis
Casts	↑	• Glomerular capsule trauma
Bacteria		• Abnormalities not usually seen in early trauma
Yeast		
Parasites		

Hpf, High-power field.

---

scan) as a diagnostic or screening tool. Depending on the MOI, such as a fall, a CAT scan of the head and abdomen may be performed. Since injuries in blunt trauma are very difficult to diagnose, the CAT scan is frequently done before patient transfer to the operating room. A high index of suspicion is maintained for other injuries until proved otherwise. Bowel injuries may be missed during initial scanning. A CAT scan of the brain revealing an injury incompatible with life may alter the course of definitive treatment for a patient.

An arteriogram may be indicated in diagnosis of vascular injuries. If the patient is hemodynamically stable, this test is of great value in determining the extent of the injury. It is particularly beneficial in the diagnosis of a ruptured thoracic aorta, in which extravasation of the dye at the area of aortic fixation to the chest wall is noted. Other uses include evaluation of penetrating wounds, especially in the extremity. Vessel injury can be noted and the need for surgical intervention accomplished.

Other diagnostic tests

Cardiac monitoring is also a component of the initial phase of trauma care and is particularly important in blunt trauma. Early detection of ventricular arrhythmias may be indicative of a myocardial contusion or bruising of the heart. An electrocardiogram (ECG) is obtained when indicated by the mechanism of injury or patient symptoms. Undiagnosed heart disease, as evidenced by an abnormal ECG, is noteworthy in a patient requiring operative intervention.

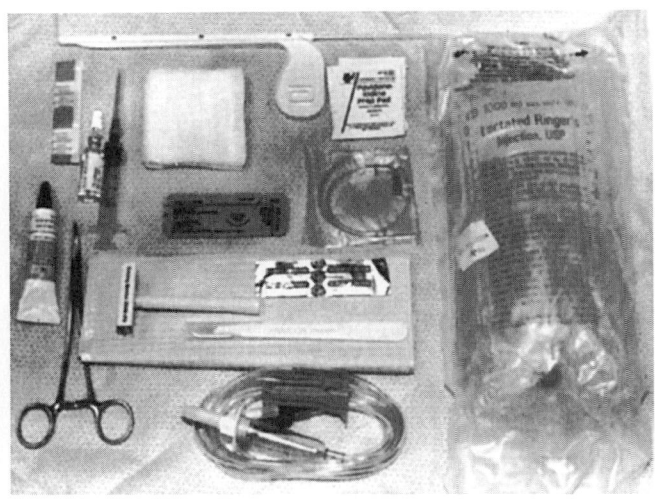

FIGURE 31-7   Basic equipment for peritoneal lavage.

Ultrasonic examination of the abdomen at the bedside is utilized in some facilities as an adjunct to diagnosis. Sonography can assist in detecting the presence of hemoperitoneum and visceral injury in the hands of the experienced operator. The abdominal exam is divided into four quadrants. Presence of blood in at least two of the four quadrants indicates a need for immediate abdominal exploration.

Diagnostic peritoneal lavage (DPL) can be performed to determine the presence of abdominal injury. This diagnostic tool is of particular benefit when evaluation of the abdomen is difficult, as when the patient is intoxicated, unconscious, or hemodynamically unstable. However, the presence of retroperitoneal blood may be missed. DPLs can be performed in the ED, operating room, postanesthesia recovery room, or the ICU (Fig. 31-7). It may be performed closed (Seldinger technique) or open (exposure of peritoneum), based on established protocols, except for the pregnant or obese patient and the patient with a pelvic fracture. If any of these factors are present, an open procedure is performed.[1] Before the DPL an indwelling urethral catheter and nasogastric tube are placed to decompress the bladder and stomach, respectively, to avoid injury. In the presence of facial fractures the nasogastric tube is placed orally. A local anesthetic is injected just below the umbilicus, and a long trocar needle or catheter over a stylette is inserted and syringe attached. If 10 ml of frank red blood are withdrawn, the tap is considered positive. Otherwise, 1 liter of warmed normal saline or lactated Ringer's solution is infused, with a pressure bag or by gravity drainage, into the abdomen. The liter bag is then inverted, the fluid is allowed to return by gravity, and a sample of the fluid is sent to the laboratory for analysis. The presence of food particles, greater than $100,000/mm^3$ red blood cells, greater than $500/mm^3$ white blood cells, or amylase greater than 175 U/dl is considered a positive result.[5] A positive result is indicative of an injury necessitating surgical intervention.

Internal compartment pressures may be measured in the patient with an injury to the extremity. Swelling of the muscles below the fascia covering may compromise circulation and result in the eventual loss of the extremity caused by tissue necrosis. This is known as the *compartment syndrome*. Compartment pressures are measured by the use of a manometer/stopcock/syringe (Fig. 31-8) or a commercial compartment-measuring device (Fig. 31-9). Normal compartmental pressures are less than 20 mm. Pressures greater than 30 mm require a fasciotomy. Symptoms include severe pain, paresthesias and a decrease in motor movement in the involved extremity, especially on passive movement (Table 31-2).

Admission Assessment

The perioperative nurse may not obtain information concerning the trauma patient until the patient arrives in the operating room area for surgical intervention. If the patient's condition permits, the perioperative nurse should obtain a precise but brief report from the ED nurse containing the following information: MOI, an AMPLE history (if available), condition upon arrival (level of consciousness), availability or prior administration of blood products, spine clearance, injuries present, and any other pertinent information (such as family present, completion of secondary assessment). If the injury is life or limb threatening, implied surgical consent is assumed (that is, if the patient were able, consent would be given).

Additional data are collected as the perioperative nurse accompanies the patient to the operating room. The status of the airway as well as breathing patterns and circulatory condition can be observed. The ED record also provides information concerning amount and type of IV fluid received, vital signs, core temperature, and laboratory and diagnostics performed. A quick visual survey of the patient when the perioperative nurse is preparing for the procedure enables the nurse to identify other sites of injury that might require attention.

The patient's psychologic status can also be assessed. If the patient is awake, the perioperative nurse is challenged to allay fear and anxiety. The trauma patient has endured a very frightening experience and is in need of support. The perioperative nurse is often the best member of the surgical team to communicate with the patient and explain the interventions occurring before anesthesia induction. A touch or handhold is an important aspect of this communication process.

Nursing Diagnosis

Nursing diagnoses related to the care of trauma patients undergoing operative intervention might include the following:

- Anxiety related to recent traumatic injury
- Fluid volume deficit related to the excessive blood loss or decreased plasma volume, or both
- Potential for infection related to presence of traumatized

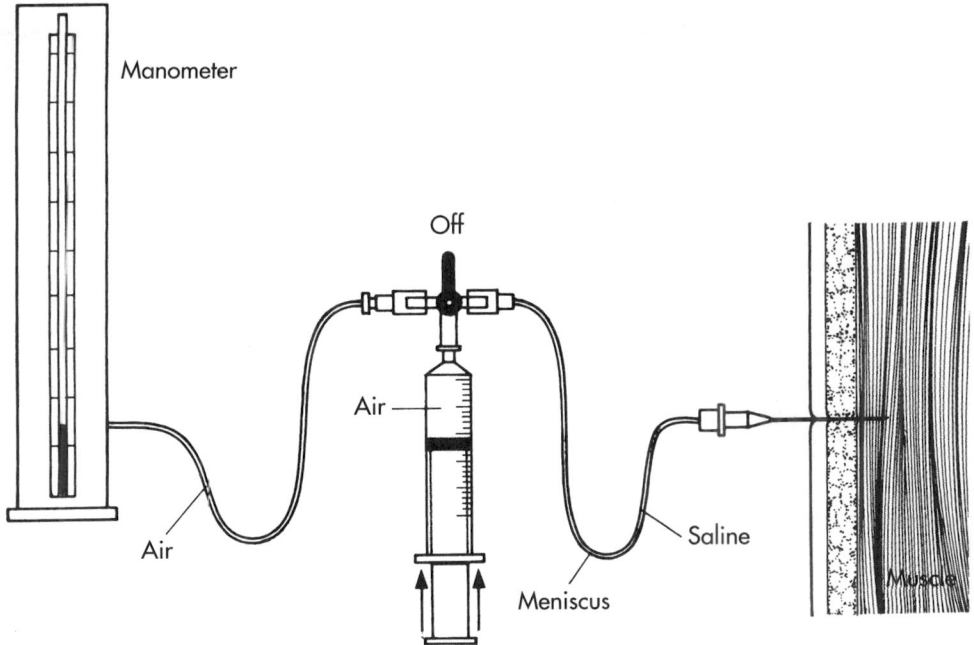

FIGURE 31-8 Whitesides technique of tissue pressure measurement. Tubing is fitted to mercury manometer tubing and side port. Needle is inserted into muscle through skin, subcutaneous tissue, and fascia.

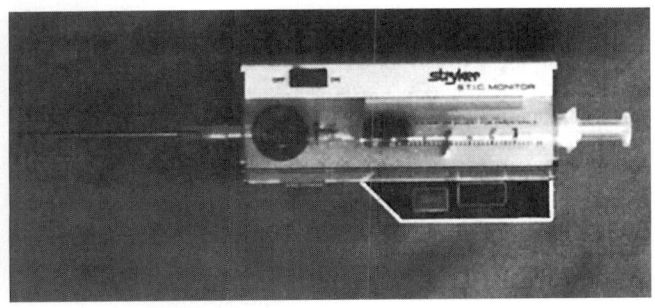

FIGURE 31-9 Stryker Solid-State Transducer Intra Compartmental (STIC) pressure monitor system.

tissue and increased environmental exposure and contamination
- Risk for aspiration related to reduced level of consciousness
- Acute pain related to traumatic injury

Outcome Identification

Outcomes identified for the selected nursing diagnoses could be stated as follows:

- The patient will demonstrate decreased level of anxiety as evidenced by less apprehension, ability to maintain eye contact, decreased quivering voice, and ability to follow directions even though anxiety persists.
- The patient will be afebrile with BP and pulse within normal limits for the patient, will have an H/H within

normal limits postoperatively, and will have a balanced intake and output.
- The patient will be free from signs and symptoms of infection postoperatively.
- The patient will be free from signs and symptoms of aspiration pneumonia.
- The patient reports reasonable relief from acute pain when analgesia is used.

Planning

Because of the unexpected nature of trauma, planning perioperative care is of the utmost importance. Utilizing a knowledge of kinematics, the perioperative nurse can optimize the minimal preparation time available. A high index of suspicion is maintained for potentially related injuries until the injury is ruled out. Consequently equipment, instruments, and supplies that have a high probability of use must be immediately available. Autotransfusion or cell-saving devices should also be considered during patient care preparation.

A Sample Care Plan for a trauma patient is shown on p. 1314.

Implementation
Multiple operative procedures

Depending on the severity of the injuries, the multiple trauma patient may require many surgical interventions. Some of these procedures may be performed simultaneously. This is determined through a collaborative effort among the trauma surgeon, anesthesiologist, specialty surgeons, and the perioperative nurse. If a patient has

TABLE 31-2 | **Signs and Symptoms Associated with Compartmental Syndromes**

COMPARTMENT	LOCATION OF SENSORY CHANGES	MOVEMENT WEAKENED	PAINFUL PASSIVE MOVEMENT	LOCATION OF PAIN OR TENSENESS
Lower Leg				
Anterior	First web space	Toe extension	Toe flexion	Along lateral side of anterior tibia
Lateral	Dorsum (top) of foot	Foot eversion	Foot inversion	Lateral lower leg
Superficial posterior	None	Foot plantar flexion	Foot corsiflexion	Calf
Deep posterior	Sole of foot	Toe flexion	Toe extension	Deep calf—palpable between Achilles' tendon and medial malleoli
Forearm				
Volar	Volar (palmar) aspect of fingers	Wrist and finger flexion	Wrist and finger extension	Volar forearm
Dorsal	None	Wrist and finger extension	Wrist and finger flexion	Dorsal forearm
Hand				
Intraosseous	None	Finger adduction and abduction	Finger adduction and abduction	Between metacarpals on dorsum of hand

Adapted from Matsen, F.A. (1975). Compartmental syndromes: a unified concept. *Clinical Orthopedics and Related Research, 113,* 10.

sustained severe head and abdominal trauma, the neurosurgeon will need to place an intracranial pressure–monitoring device into the head to monitor the intracranial pressure. However, the exploratory celiotomy is also emergently indicated. Consequently the severe condition of the patient may require performance of both these procedures at the same time.

Multiple procedures, either simultaneously or in succession, require a great deal of preparation by the perioperative nurse and the trauma team. The order of procedures is determined by the presence or absence of life threats. The usual order of priority is chest, abdomen, head, and extremities. However, this priority must be determined for each individual patient situation.

Performance of simultaneous procedures should be encouraged when physically possible. Anesthesia time is decreased for the critically ill patient, and definitive surgical interventions are accomplished more rapidly.

Increased risk of infection

Many trauma patients suffer wounds that are contaminated with roadside debris, dirt, grass, or automobile parts. Others perforate a full stomach and release food particles into the peritoneum, increasing the risk of peritonitis. Consequently these patients are at a very high risk for infection. Sterile technique may be compromised secondary only to immediate life threat. Pouring of povidone-iodine solution across the surgical site may be the only surgical skin preparation allowed when an immediate life threat exists.

Wounds may be grossly decontaminated before the surgical prep. Sterile scrub brushes or a mechanical irrigation-under-pressure device may be utilized preoperatively and intraoperatively. Care must be exercised to remove as much contamination as possible, without creating further damage to the wound or body part.

Traffic in the operating room should be limited to essential personnel. Often a broadcast on the radio or television will precipitate a parade of curious staff members. Increased traffic in the room increases chances for contamination to an already compromised patient as well as potentially interfering with expedient care.

Procedure preparation

Most level I trauma centers have a designated trauma operating room that contains all equipment and supplies potentially needed for trauma patients. Many hospitals maintain an emergency abdominal procedure set, craniotomy procedure set, and chest procedure set either within the operating-room-suite sterile supply area or immediately available in the central supply department. This streamlines preparation for the surgical procedure and allows for the possibility of rapid preparation in those instances where the patient bypasses the emergency room upon arrival and is transported directly to the operating room suite.

Once the perioperative nurse is notified of the surgical procedure, operating room determination is made in consultation with the anesthesia staff and surgeon. Considerations include the following:

- Equipment required by the surgeon or surgeons to perform the surgical procedure
- Room availability

SAMPLE CARE PLAN

Nursing Diagnosis: Anxiety related to recent trauma

Outcome: The patient will demonstrate decreased level of anxiety as evidenced by less apprehension, ability to maintain eye contact, decreased quivering voice, and ability to follow directions even though anxiety persists.

Interventions:

Monitor level of anxiety by assessing the patient's state of alertness, ability to comprehend, and ability to follow directions.

Help patient to focus on the present situation to assist in identifying coping mechanisms to decrease anxiety.

Reassure patient during interactions by touch and empathetic verbal and nonverbal exchanges.

Reduce excessive stimulation by maintaining a calm and safe environment.

Explain environment to the patient and what to expect to assist in reduction of anxiety.

Instruct patient to take slow, deep breaths and utilize deep breathing techniques as necessary.

Nursing Diagnosis: Fluid volume deficit related to excessive blood loss or decreased plasma volume.

Outcome: The patient will be afebrile with BP and pulse within normal limits for patient, will have an H/H within normal limits postoperatively, and will have a balanced intake and output.

Interventions:

Assist in accurate monitoring of intake and output during the surgical procedure.

Monitor and report blood loss intraoperatively.

Assist in monitoring fluid volume status by completion of intraoperative labwork: H/H, serum electrolytes, BUN, and creatinine.

Consider autotransfusion or cell-saving devices when patient injuries are suspected or excessive preoperative blood loss is present.

Assist with placement of invasive monitoring lines (arterial, CVP) and required fluid volume replacement therapy.

Nursing Diagnosis: Potential for infection related to presence of traumatized tissue and increased environmental exposure and contamination.

Outcome: The patient is free from signs and symptoms of infection postoperatively.

Interventions:

Preoperatively assess the wound and identify presence of risk factors or environmental contamination.

Determine and document the appropriate wound classification.

Consider utilization of pressurized wound irrigation for wounds contaminated with debris.

Maintain a sterile environment.

Administer antibiotics as ordered.

Nursing Diagnosis: Risk for aspiration related to reduced level of consciousness.

Outcome: The patient will be free from signs and symptoms of aspiration pneumonia.

Interventions:

Ensure operation of suction apparatus preoperatively.

Have suction canister and Yankauer suction tip available at bedside during anesthesia induction and postoperatively.

Provide cricoid pressure, under direction of the anesthesia team, during induction until correct intubation is confirmed and endotracheal tube cuff is inflated.

Assist with placement of nasogastric or orogastric tube.

Nursing Diagnosis: Acute pain related to trauma

Outcome: The patient reports reasonable relief from acute pain when analgesia is utilized.

Interventions:

Collaborate with anesthesia provider and surgeon on pain management to increase patient's level of comfort, if condition permits.

Assess nonverbal cues regarding level of pain and discomfort.

Provide care in a supportive manner.

Convey acceptance of patient's report of discomfort by a willingness to provide comfort measures.

Reassure patient in a quiet, calming manner.

Use a visual or numerical scale to assess change in discomfort.

- Room size (equipment, staff, and multiple procedures)
- Need for additional staff
- Capability for autotransfusion or cell-saver
- Availability of emergency procedure supplies (including power equipment)
- Selection of OR bed

Additional diagnostic procedures are often required during multiple trauma procedures. A fluoroscopic electric OR bed provides increased flexibility in patient management. The bed can be rotated on its base to facilitate two teams operating at once. The fluoroscopic capabilities allow for additional radiographs and arteriograms as needed. The bed should easily transform into different positions such as lithotomy or lateral rotation. Although this bed is not required for trauma surgery, it may be considered a necessary adjunct to surgical trauma care. If a fluoroscopic bed is not available, consideration for performance of radiologic diagnostic procedures intraoperatively must be considered.

Before transfer of the patient to the OR bed, the perioperative nurse must ascertain if the spinal column has been cleared by the trauma surgeon or attending physician as free from injury. If the spine has not been cleared, the surgeon must be consulted before removal of the patient from the backboard. Logrolling technique must be utilized in transfer of the patient from the cart to the OR bed. This necessitates a minimum of four people, positioned on either side and one each at the head and foot of the transfer cart. The person at the head of the patient is deemed in charge. This person maintains manual in-line cervical spine immobilization at all times and counts out loud before the rolling and transfer of the patient. The nose of the patient is kept in line with the umbilicus and feet as the patient is rolled as one unit, avoiding any twisting of the spinal column. Even if the spine is cleared, remember that initial radiographs are examined rapidly during initial evaluation, and a very subtle injury to the vertebrae may be overlooked. Therefore use of log-rolling technique during all patient transfers is advocated and should be documented as such.

Positioning of the patient is based on the surgical approach. This is of the greatest consequence concerning chest and orthopedic procedures. Ascertaining the location of the wound, anterior or posterior, and type of operative procedure dictates the patient position. For example, an aortic injury may be approached through a thoracotomy or a median sternotomy incision. The thoracotomy requires lateral positioning devices, and the sternotomy necessitates a supine position.

If several procedures are being performed, positioning may change intraoperatively. Changing the anesthetized patient's position is accomplished under the supervision of the anesthesia team. The patient is moved slowly, allowing for assessment of vital sign changes in response to the position movement. All precautions regarding positioning are reexecuted with special attention provided to the electrosurgical grounding pad. This pad may loosen during patient repositioning and may require replacement to ensure adequate pad contact.

Established sponge, instrument, and sharp count policies should address surgical procedures of an emergent nature within the institution. Every attempt is made to verify appropriate numbers of counted items, without compromising the timeliness of intervention in a life-threatening situation. If a preprocedural count is not performed, the perioperative nurse must document the occurrence and rationale used in accordance with established hospital policies and procedures. Some institutions require an x-ray exam postoperatively to examine the patient for the presence of a retained object.

In the presence of clotting difficulties or specific types of organ injuries with continuous oozing of blood, the surgeon may elect to pack the surgical site with laparotomy sponges and close the patient as a temporary measure. After a period of 24 to 48 hours, the patient returns to the operating room for removal of the laparotomy sponges and primary closure, if possible. In such instances the perioperative nurse must document and record accurately the number of sponges utilized for packing. When the sponges are removed, the exact number is verified, and the sponges are isolated and contained in accordance with established hospital policy and procedure.

Autotransfusion

In this era of blood-borne disease, and considering the high blood loss associated with traumatic injuries, autotransfusion has become a vital asset in trauma care. Preoperative blood loss that is associated with an isolated hemothorax is collected in a designated chest-drainage device for reinfusion within 4 hours to avoid bacterial contamination. Intraoperative blood loss is collected, filtered, and reinfused to the patient. This provides immediate volume replacement, decreases the amount of bank blood used, and negates the possibility of transfusion reactions or risk of the spread of infectious disease.

The autotransfusion device or cell-saver requires some specialized training for operation. Institutional policies vary regarding appropriate personnel designated for operation of the equipment. Capabilities for autotransfusion should be considered during procedure preparation, since additional qualified personnel may be required.

During cell-saver use the sterile scrub team member squeezes out additional blood and fluid from saturated sponges before discarding them from the surgical field. The cell-saver suction is used whenever possible to maximize the amount of blood salvaged. However, care must be taken to ensure that the blood collected in the cell-saver is free from contamination. For instance, if the abdomen is contaminated with free food particles or colonic perforation is present, the blood cannot be used. Similarly, once antibiotic irrigation is initiated, the cell-saver is not utilized.

Evidence preservation

If the injury to the patient is a result of a violent crime, attention must be given to preservation of evidence during the course of patient care. Physical evidence (bullets, bags of powder, weapons, pills, and other foreign objects), trace evidence (hair and fibers), biologic evidence (body fluids and blood), and clothing are considered types of evidence to be preserved. Specific procedures on handling of evidence may differ by institution and law-enforcement agencies.

Clothing must be handled properly. When clothing is removed from the patient, it should be cut along the seams or around the bullet or stab wound holes. The shape of the hole may help in identification of the weapon used. A clean white sheet may be placed on the floor and clothing is placed on it to collect potential evidence. The sheet is folded up and given to law-enforcement personnel. Clothing is placed in paper bags and labeled appropriately.

Plastic bags trap moisture and may facilitate growth of mold, which could destroy evidence. The transfer cart sheet should also be handled in a similar manner, since evidence may be present. Descriptions of wound appearances, body markings consistent with gang or cult activity, and statements from the patient must be accurately recorded.

The chain of custody for all evidence is followed, including clothing. This process allows for identification of all people handling the evidence. Documentation must verify that the evidence has been in secure possession at all times. All evidence discovered must be recorded as to site of origin and when and to whom it was given. A system of documentation using receipts or a specific form should be established to ensure appropriate compliance.

Gunpowder residues, tissue, hair, or other valuable information may be present on the hands of a trauma patient. This evidence can be preserved by placing the patient's hands in a paper bag and securing it with tape. Washing the hands should be avoided. If the patient survives the injury, such avoidance may not be feasible.

Bullets and retained implements offer valuable evidence as well in identifying the assailant. The weapon firing the bullet and the bullet itself can be linked together by the specific grooves and markings placed on the bullet by the gun barrel when fired. Most bullets are composed of soft lead, and handling with metal instruments can interfere with the markings. Therefore the use of metal instruments in the handling of bullets is avoided.[6] Once a bullet is removed, it should be placed in dry, clean gauze into a plastic specimen container and passed off the sterile field to the circulator. The container is labeled appropriately. After the chain of custody procedures, the circulator should dispose of the bullet according to established institutional policies. Some of the newer exploding types of bullets can offer a risk to perioperative team members during wound exploration. Care should be exercised to avoid sterile glove tears and personal injury, since these types of bullets are extremely sharp.

Deep vein thrombosis prophylaxis

Because of the prolonged immobilization anticipated for the trauma patient, prevention of deep vein thrombosis is an important concern. Placement of sequential compression devices preoperatively is ideal. These pneumatic compression devices are believed to decrease the possibility of deep vein thrombosis, and their effect is optimized when applied before surgical intervention. Preoperative placement is subject to the physician's preference; clinical research regarding similar devices and demonstrated product effectiveness is ongoing. Subsequent insertion of an inferior vena cava filter may be performed in high-risk patients to prevent pulmonary embolus (PE). Risk factors include prolonged immobility, multiple pelvis and lower extremity fractures, previous history of PE, or spinal cord injury with paralysis.

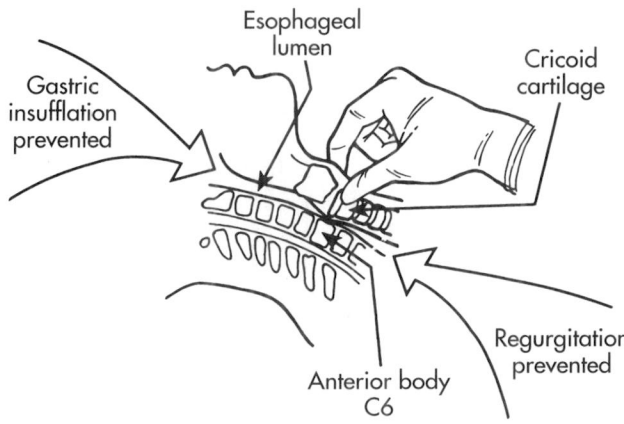

FIGURE 31-10 Application of cricoid pressure. Thumb and forefinger are used to depress cricoid cartilage, causing it to impinge on lumen of esophagus and sealing it closed against anterior body of C6. As a result, gastric insufflation secondary to positive-pressure ventilation (bag-valve-mask apparatus) from above, as well as regurgitation of stomach contents from below, is largely prevented.

Anesthesia implications

Depending on institutional protocol, the anesthesia team may be directly involved in resuscitation of the trauma patient immediately after arrival at the ED. The anesthesia member maintains the airway inclusive of intubation, if necessary. In addition, some interventions are performed in the ED of a trauma center. These interventions vary from insertion of an intracranial pressure monitor to an emergent exploratory thoracotomy.

However, if diagnostic evaluation can be accomplished without intubation and sedation, the patient may arrive at the operating room awake. A trauma patient is assumed to have a full stomach. Thus these patients are at high risk for aspiration and resultant pneumonia. Under the direction of the attending anesthesia team member, cricoid pressure (Sellick's maneuver) is provided by the perioperative nurse (Fig. 31-10). This pressure is maintained over the cricoid area until the cuff on the endotracheal tube is inflated and tube placement is verified. This type of intubation is often referred to as a crash induction and is used in the presence of a hiatal hernia or when NPO status is uncertain.

In addition, the patient may require intubation for protection of the airway before radiologic examination of the cervical spine. If the cervical spine is not cleared or if the radiographic screening exam is not performed before intubation, endotracheal intubation is done while cervical spine precautions (that is, in-line intubation) are maintained (Fig. 31-11). Hyperextension of the neck is avoided, since an injury to the cervical spine is always presumed until proved otherwise in the trauma setting. This type of intubation procedure requires a person to be positioned at the head of the patient, whose only responsibility is to maintain the head in midline position during the intubation procedure.

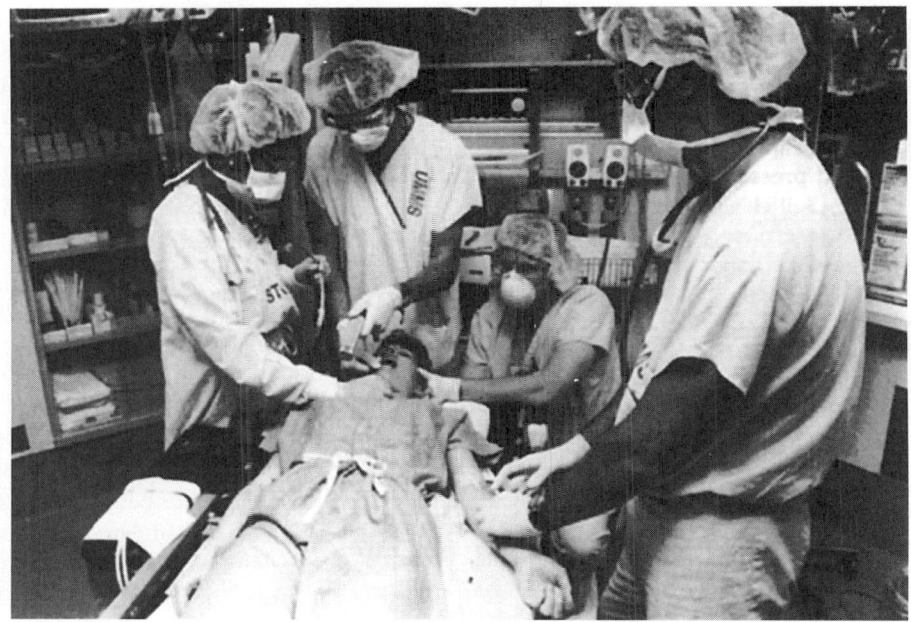

FIGURE 31-11 Technique of oral intubation performed by four-person team using laryngoscopy and "manual-in-line axial traction" in emergency trauma patient. Individual on left applies cricoid pressure (while also identifying landmarks for a cricothyroidotomy if it becomes necessary) and holds endotracheal tube ready. At center, intubator opens patient's mouth with right hand and holds laryngoscope with left hand. On right, assistant (ideally the neurosurgical consultant) uses both hands to stabilize head and neck. Notice that anterior portion of cervical collar has been removed. Fourth person is responsible for administering intravenous induction agents.

In injuries of the face, where midface fractures are present, nasal intubation and nasogastric tube placement are avoided. Documented tube placement in the brain through a fracture of the cribriform plate is a well-known complication. In these instances oral endotracheal intubation is the technique of choice. Stomach decompression will be achieved by placement of the gastric tube orally. An awake oral intubation is often necessitated because anesthesia and muscle relaxants can result in the loss of any remaining airway in the presence of facial trauma.

Large-bore IV tubing used with rapid fluid warmers may be employed in the ED. These fluid warmers can deliver high volumes of crystalloid solution at body temperature (Fig. 31-12). Use of the fluid warmer may continue during the intraoperative phase to facilitate volume replacement.

Hypothermia

The trauma patient may suffer from prolonged environmental exposure and be subject to a decrease in core temperature. Immersion victims or patients whose accident occurred several hours before discovery may be hypothermic despite the ambient temperature. The perioperative nurse needs to be aware of several effects on the body when hypothermia is present. For purposes of definition, generalized hypothermia is considered to be present when the core temperature is below 35° C. These patients are subject to prolonged bleeding and clotting times. Coagulopathies of this sort become clinically significant in a multiple trauma patient undergoing surgical intervention. Viscosity of the blood is also increased. Thrombocytopenia has been noted. Many facilities utilize a thermister Foley catheter to monitor core temperature. Additional information concerning hypothermia is discussed in a later section of this chapter.

Pregnancy

The normal physiologic changes that occur during pregnancy increase the challenge of evaluation and treatment when these individuals are victims of trauma. It is most important to remember that two patients are being treated. The key to resuscitation of the fetus is to resuscitate the mother. One of the first physiologic changes to note is that the pregnant trauma patient has a much larger circulatory volume. The cardiac output may be increased by as much as 40%. Oxygen requirements are increased. Heart rate increases over the prepregnant state (Table 31-3). It becomes obvious that the usual clinical indicators of hypovolemic shock are unreliable in the pregnant trauma patient (Table 31-4). It is imperative that the pregnant trauma victim be assumed to be in shock until proved otherwise. Early aggressive treatment is a must. The uterus is enlarged and no longer a pelvic organ, and it elevates the bladder out of the pelvis as well. Supine position for the pregnant patient can result in a decrease in cardiac output as a result of compression of the inferior vena cava. By term, there can be as much as 30% reduction of cardiac output as a result of compression on the inferior vena cava.[1] Consequently, patients who are 20 weeks or more into their pregnancy should be placed in the left lateral decubitus position to avoid a hypotensive episode. If this is not possible, manual displacement of the uterus by lateral abdominal pressure should be attempted.

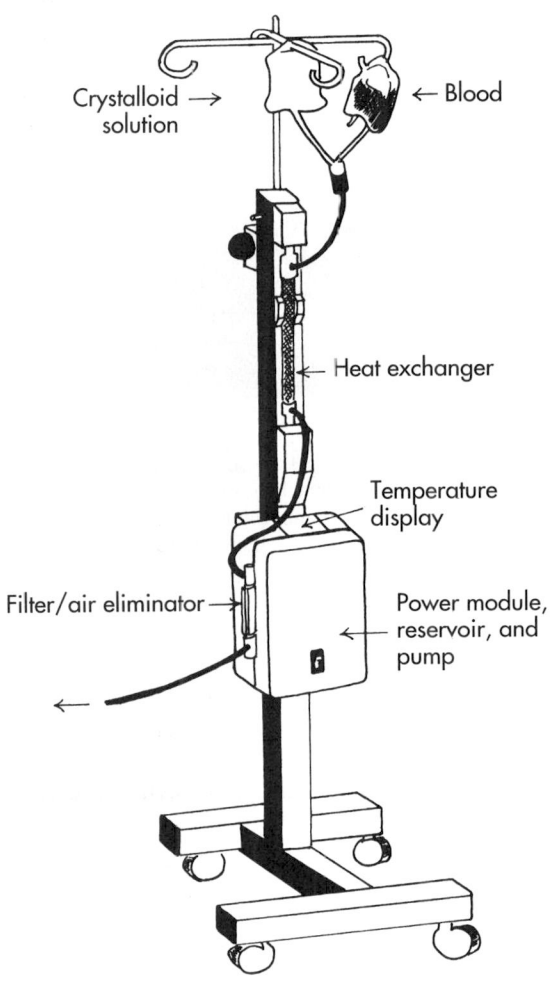

Crystalloid → solution

← Blood

→ Heat exchanger

Temperature display

Filter/air eliminator →

Power module, reservoir, and pump

FIGURE 31-12   Level I System 250 fluid warmer unit.

The pregnant trauma patient and fetus are treated as one during the resuscitative phase. The best chance of maintaining the viability of the fetus is in expedient treatment of the mother. Ultrasound studies are conducted to determine viability of the fetus when possible. In the event of a ruptured uterus, a cesarean section and hysterectomy may be required if the fetus is viable. Neonatal resuscitation is of the utmost importance immediately on delivery of the fetus.

Fetuses of pregnant patients requiring surgery require fetal assessment intraoperatively. Any fetal movement should be noted. In addition, fetal monitoring is continuous. This is inclusive of fetal heart rate and uterine contractions. Fetal monitoring provides information on the condition of the fetus and response to uterine contractions, if present. Fetal heart rate can usually be obtained after 10 weeks of gestation. Abnormalities in fetal heart rate can be an early sign of maternal compromise because the pregnant uterus is viewed as a nonessential peripheral organ in states of hypovolemic shock. Personnel qualified in the interpretation of fetal heart rate patterns must be present. This expertise may be provided by the obstetric nursing staff.

Perimortem (postmortem) cesarean section may be performed in the event of the sudden death of the mother and presence of a viable fetus. The fetus can survive approximately 10 minutes of anoxia without severe side effects.[6]

Pediatric trauma patients

Special considerations related to the care of infants and children who have sustained a trauma are described in Chapter 29.

Elderly trauma patients

As the number of adults over 65 years of age continues to grow, so does the number of elderly patients requiring surgical intervention related to trauma. The physiologic effects of aging combined with the preinjury health status

TABLE 31-3 | **Central Hemodynamic Changes During Pregnancy**

PARAMETER	NONPREGNANT	PREGNANT
Cardiac output (L/min)	4.3 ± 0.9	6.2 ± 1.0
Heart rate (beats/min)	70 ± 10.0	83 ± 10.0
Systemic vascular resistance (dyne $\times$ cm $\times$ sec^{-5})	1530 ± 520	1210 ± 266
Pulmonary vascular resistance (dyne $\times$ cm $\times$ sec^{-5})	119 ± 47.0	78 ± 22
Colloid oncotic pressure (mm Hg)	20.8 ± 1.0	18.0 ± 1.5
Colloid oncotic pressure/pulmonary capillary wedge pressure (mm Hg)	14.5 ± 2.5	10.5 ± 2.7
Mean arterial pressure (mm Hg)	86.4 ± 7.5	90.3 ± 5.8
Pulmonary capillary wedge pressure (mm Hg)	6.3 ± 2.1	7.5 ± 1.8
Central venous pressure (mm Hg)	3.7 ± 2.6	3.6 ± 2.5
Left ventricular stroke	41 ± 8	48 ± 6

From Clark, S., Cotton, O., Lee, W., et al. (1989). Central hemodynamic assessment of normal term pregnancy. *American Journal of Obstetrics and Gynecology, 161,* 1439-1442.

of many elderly patients significantly affect their ability to respond to initial treatment for traumatic injuries and subsequent surgical intervention. Consequently, the mortality rate for elderly trauma patients is significantly higher than that in younger patients with the same level of injury. Preexisting medical conditions, decreased physiologic reserves, and the physical and psychologic stress experienced during surgical interventions place elderly trauma victims at increased risk for perioperative complications.[4] See Chapter 30 for the physiologic and psychologic changes that occur in geriatric patients, affecting the outcomes of care associated with traumatic injuries.

Invasive emergency department interventions

If a patient has had very recent loss of vital signs, either en route to the hospital or upon arrival at the ED, the trauma surgeon may elect to perform an emergency thoracotomy in the ED. A left-sided approach is usually performed because this allows rapid access to the heart for external cardiac massage and exposure of the great vessels for clamping in the event of severe blood loss. The incision can be extended to the right side by cutting across the sternum. This procedure can be used to gain control in hemorrhage of the great vessels, to access the heart, or in a grave situation as a final effort to save a life (Fig. 31-13). The procedure is utilized more often in penetrating injuries where a laceration to a ventricle or other potentially treatable, life-threatening injury may be present.

Because of the knowledge of surgical instrumentation held by the perioperative nurse, assistance in this procedure in the ED is often required of the perioperative team.

TABLE 31-4 | **Signs of Hypovolemic Shock in Pregnancy**

CIRCULATING BLOOD VOLUME DEFICIT	EARLY (20%)	LATE (25%)
Pulse	<100 beats/min	>100 beats/minute
Respiratory rate	12-20/min	>20/minute
Blood pressure	Normal	Hypotensive
Skin perfusion	Warm, dry skin	Cool, ashen skin
Capillary refill	<2 seconds	>2 seconds
Level of consciousness	Alert	Agitated, lethargic
Urine output	>30-50 ml/hour	<30-50 ml/hour
Fetal heart rate (normally 120-160 beats/min)	High, low, with late decelerations	High, low, absent, late decelerations

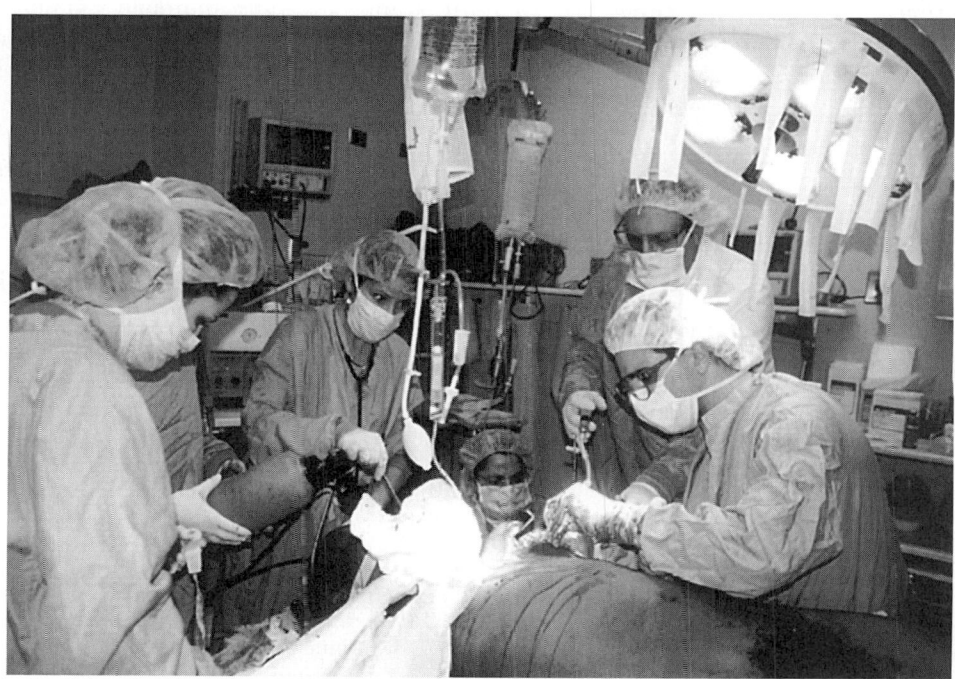

FIGURE 31-13   Patient undergoing emergency department exploratory thoracotomy.

Rapid access to the heart and great vessels is the goal. The patient is transported to the operating room suite for additional interventions once hemorrhage control is established.

In a similar fashion an exploratory laparotomy can be initiated in the ED to control abdominal hemorrhage, especially when a splenic rupture is suspected and the patient is severely compromised.

If all other techniques of airway access are unsuccessful, a cricothyrotomy is performed. A vertical incision is made through the skin, and the cricothyroid membrane is incised. An endotracheal or tracheostomy tube can be inserted through the membrane to create an airway. In the event a tube is not immediately available, a large-bore needle can be inserted into the membrane and the catheter left in place. This provides a temporary airway access measure but is inadequate to ventilate the patient without a jet oscillating ventilator.

Successive surgical interventions

Often the multiple trauma patient requires a multitude of surgical procedures, either specialty related or as a stepwise progression in the primary treatment of the initial injury. Acalculous cholecystitis is often a secondary complication of the trauma patient's postoperative course, which requires cholecystectomy. Secondary wound closures, debridements, and fixation of initially undiscovered fractures compose the majority of follow-up procedures. Initially the trauma patient is critically ill and requires intensive care facilities. When surgery is scheduled, the perioperative nurse may need additional assistance in transport of the patient, and transport monitoring of the ECG, arterial line, and blood pressure is performed. Oxygen and mechanical ventilation with Ambu Bag are necessary for the intubated patient.

Additional opportunities for intervention are afforded the perioperative nurse because the patient might undergo several surgical procedures during a week. Increased familiarity with the patient's needs as well as the ability to monitor the patient's recovery progress is possible.

Evaluation

The evaluation of the patient should reflect the effectiveness of the interventions. Did the patient remain free from untoward complications? Was there progress toward the expected outcomes as described in the perioperative care plan? The following are examples of evaluation statements in relation to the Sample Care Plan:

- The patient demonstrates decreased level of anxiety as evidenced by less apprehension, ability to maintain eye contact, decreased quivering voice, and ability to follow directions even though anxiety persists.
- The patient is afebrile with BP and pulse within normal limits for patient, has an H/H within normal limits postoperatively, and has a balanced intake and output postoperatively.

- The patient is free from signs and symptoms of infection postoperatively.
- The patient is free from signs and symptoms of aspiration pneumonia.
- The patient reports reasonable relief from acute pain when analgesia is utilized.

Upon completion of the procedure or procedures the perioperative nurse is afforded an opportunity to further assess the trauma patient as well as evaluate the plan of care implemented. If the patient has sustained numerous injuries and remains critically injured, the PACU may be bypassed, and the patient may be transferred directly to the ICU. The perioperative nurse should accompany the patient, along with the anesthesia team, to the ICU. Once the anesthesia report is given, the perioperative nurse can provide a wealth of information to the critical care nurse. At this point, family members may have been contacted or are present, allowing more specific medical history information to be obtained. However, the mechanism of injury and events surrounding the accident are still significant. A high index of suspicion remains during postoperative care of the patient sustaining multiple injuries. Attention can be diverted from a less-significant injury in the presence of a highly visible or obvious trauma. Once the obvious trauma undergoes intervention, pain or discomfort from other injuries becomes more apparent. In the care of a patient with neurologic deficit, physical assessment and continued evaluation are essential because patient self-report is nonexistent.

Status of progress in the secondary assessment should also be reported. Any additional laboratory work or interventions that have yet to be completed should be discussed. It is imperative in a thorough examination to view the back of the patient in an effort to locate all injuries.

Additional diagnostic procedures may be required after completion of the surgical procedure if the patient's condition is stable. The perioperative nurse may be requested to accompany the patient to diagnostics with the anesthesia team. In addition, respiratory care may assist in patient transport and maintenance of the airway.

Critical-Incident-Stress Debriefing

Unfortunately, some accidental injuries result in death. This can be particularly difficult for the perioperative team, since most surgical interventions are of a curative or restorative nature. In many emergency medical systems a critical-incident-stress debriefing team exists. It is composed of mental health professionals and specially trained volunteers who are also professionals and peers in the healthcare field. Police officers, firefighters, paramedics, ED nurses, and ICU nurses can also be on the team. In the event of a particularly tragic death of a patient, the team can be contacted and a meeting with that patient's care providers is arranged. The benefit of this team is enhanced when intervention is timely. Opportunity for the patient care members to discuss their feelings and emotions is provided and encouraged as each provider discusses feelings related to personal participation in care of the patient. Critical-incident-stress debriefing teams enhance coping mechanisms and are very successful and can provide a healthy professional growth from what is otherwise a tragedy.

Patient and Family Education and Discharge Planning

Traumatic injury to a family member or significant other occurs without warning. Patients may be traveling or visiting out of town or state at the time of injury. Families or friends involved in a motor vehicle collision may be triaged to several different facilities based on severity of injury or age. A family member or significant other may not be contacted until several hours or even days after the injury. Sometimes the patient's identity is either unknown or must be confidential to prevent further harm. Both the patient and family member are truly victims of traumatic injury. Consequently, patients and family members are in a time of crisis.

Some families may handle the crisis with utmost ease, whereas others become dysfunctional. Coping strategies may be inappropriate at times as the patient and family attempt to reestablish patterns of function. A family system already taxed before the event may be overwhelmed with the additional stress of a sudden traumatic event.

It is of vital importance for the perioperative nurse to be prepared for a variety of responses, both from the patient and the family or significant other. Interaction with the patient before surgical intervention may be brief or impossible because of the severity of the injury, such as prior intubation or hemodynamic instability. The perioperative nurse will need to offer brief, simple instructions and educational information when possible. This may include the following:

- Explanation of background noise as caregivers prepare for emergent intervention
- Perception of cold within the OR room
- Placement of safety straps, armboards, warming devices, pneumatic compression stockings, and so on.
- Invasive interventions such as additional intravenous access or arterial line monitoring.

A reassuring touch or hand hold may be the only communication possible.

In accordance with hospital policies and procedures, the perioperative nurse may call the surgical waiting room with periodic updates on the patient's condition. The information shared is subject to the trauma surgeon's discretion and is usually concise in nature, such as, "At this time the extent of injury is unknown; his condition is critical." When permitted, these contacts with the family are appreciated because frequently they are unable to contact the patient before the operation.

Many facilities have a chaplain or social worker available to assist family members during this time of crisis. These caregivers assist in the initial family contact and provide immediate support. The utilization of the chaplain or social worker's expertise can augment the intervention of the perioperative nurse.

All injuries and possible subsequent complications may not be known at the time of operative intervention. The multiply injured patient frequently requires rehabilitation or an extended stay in a skilled nursing facility before discharge. Continued therapy, such as neuropsychology (for cognitive impairment), or occupational and physical therapy may be on an outpatient basis. Consequently, information regarding recovery and rehabilitation is limited upon admission to the hospital. Many facilities have access to or provide support groups for patients and families related to the type of injury and its subsequent lifelong effects.

SURGICAL INTERVENTIONS
INJURIES OF THE HEAD
AND SPINAL COLUMN

Trauma to the head is responsible for half of all trauma deaths. Brain injury occurs either as a direct result of the trauma to the tissue or as a complication. Often forces of energy from the impact are tolerated by the rigid skull, but the soft tissue of the brain is traumatized. This results in formation of subdural, epidural, or intracerebral hematomas (Fig. 31-14). In addition, cerebral swelling

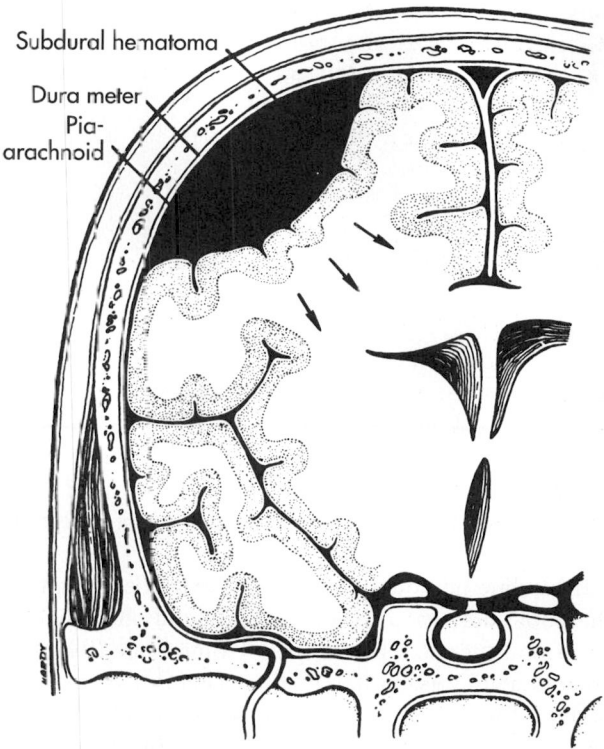

FIGURE 31-14 Subdural hematoma causing increased intracranial pressure with shifting of tissue.

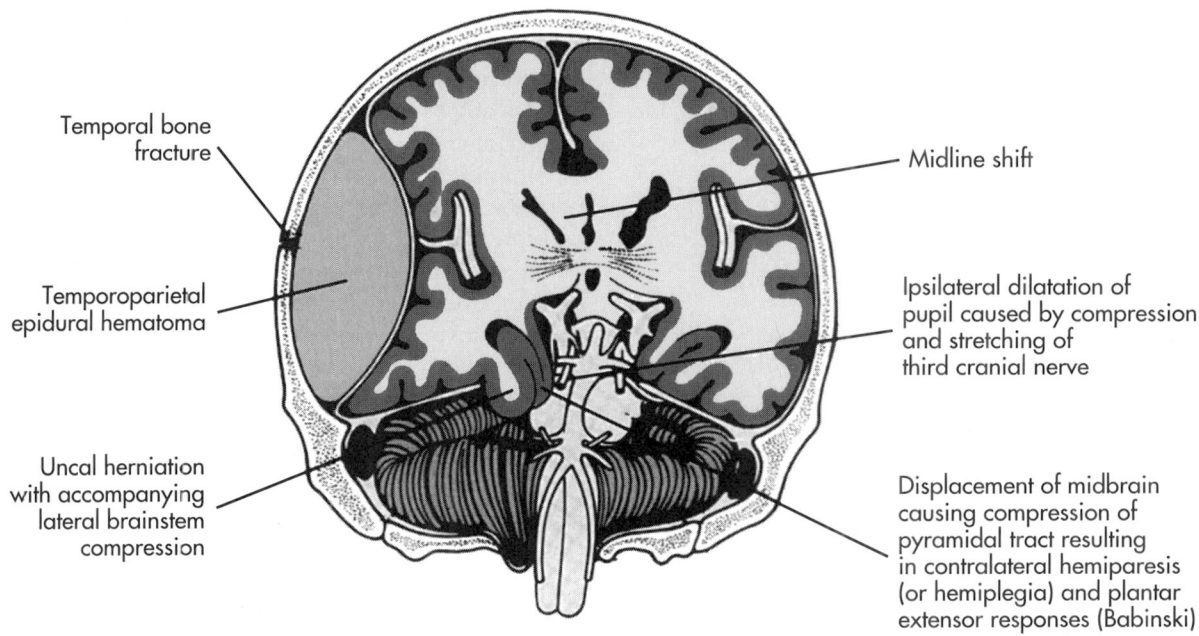

FIGURE 31-15   Cross section showing herniation of lower portion of temporal lobe (uncus) through tentorium caused by temporoparietal epidural hematoma. Herniation may occur also in cerebellum. Notice mass effect and midline shift.

BOX 31-5	The Glasgow Coma Scale (GCS)★	
Subscale	**Description**	**Score**
Eye opening	Spontaneously	4
	To speech	3
	To pain	2
	Do not open	1
Best verbal response	Oriented	5
	Confused	4
	Inappropriate speech	3
	Unintelligible speech	2
	No verbalization	1
Best motor response	Obeys command	6
	Localized pain	5
	Withdraws from pain	4
	Abnormal flexion	3
	Abnormal extension	2
	No motor response	1

★Best total score = 15: E4, V5, M6. Worst score = 3

can result in herniation of the brain despite treatment (Fig. 31-15).

A baseline neurologic exam is of extreme importance. The pupils are examined and the presence or absence of posturing is noted. The Glasgow Coma Scale (Box 31-5) provides a universally accepted mechanism to assess the baseline data for the trauma team. However, in the presence of alcohol or drug intoxication in chemical paralysis or in a pediatric patient the scale cannot be

used. For patients with a score of less than or equal to 8, intubation with hyperventilation is the immediate treatment of choice. In the highly combative patient, intubation may also be performed to allow adequate assessment of the extent of injury.

Hyperventilation may be utilized only for brief periods in the presence of acute neurologic deterioration to decrease intracranial pressure during initial management of the patient. An osmotic diuretic, such as mannitol, can be used if the patient is not severely hypotensive. The diuresis assists in lowering the intracranial pressure. Elevation of the head of the bed at 30 degrees and keeping the head midline (to promote venous drainage) can also be beneficial.

Skull fractures usually do not require operative intervention when there is no displacement and the fracture is linear. Depressed fractures or the presence of bone in the brain frequently requires elevation and debridement (Fig. 31-16). Hematoma evacuation is based on the location of the hematoma, size, and number present. Before a craniotomy or burr hole is performed, the CT scan, the neurologic status of the patient, morbidity or mortality associated with the procedure, other injuries present, and any underlying medical problems if known are evaluated. An intracranial pressure monitor may be placed in the patient who is at risk for increased intracranial pressure. At some institutions this procedure is performed in the trauma room of the ED or in the ICU. The perioperative team may be asked to assist with the procedure wherever it is done. Specific discussion of the neurosurgical procedures is found in Chapter 23.

In the trauma patient the spinal cord is always considered to be injured until proved otherwise. The

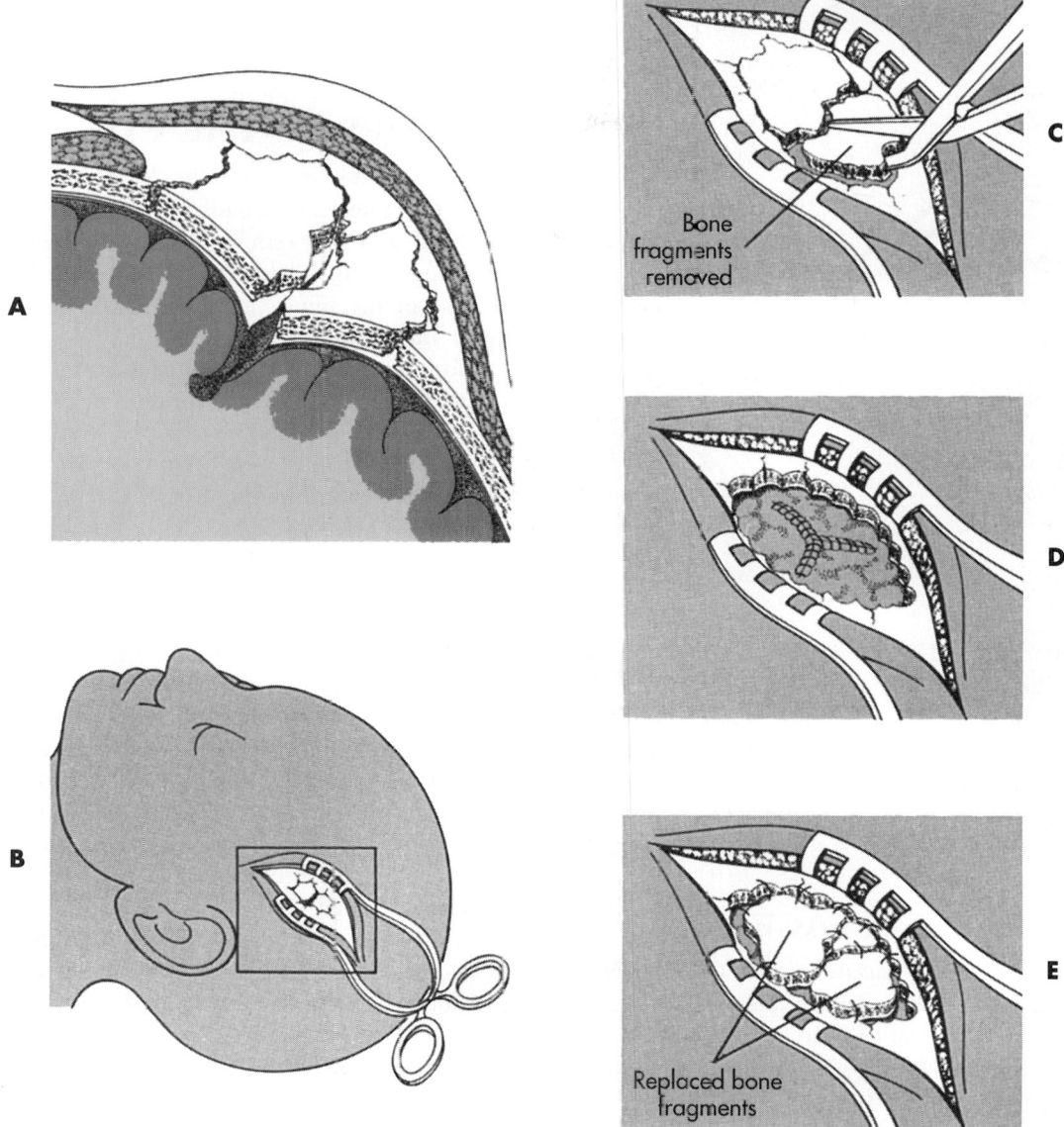

FIGURE 31-16   Treatment of compound depressed fracture of skull. **A**, Depressed skull fracture and scalp injury. **B**, Incision to expose fracture and remove devitalized scalp. **C**, Removal of impacted bone by burr hole to locate and identify normal dura, followed by resection of bone fragments. **D**, Watertight closure of dura after brain debridement. **E**, Replacement and fixation of bone fragments.

patient with a cervical spine injury at or near C3 to C5 is at great risk for respiratory difficulties because this is the area of diaphragmatic innervation. There is also the possibility of swelling above the area of injury, and the perioperative nurse should be alert for the potential of respiratory distress even if not initially present. A 24- to 48-hour dose of methylprednisolone (Solu-Medrol), calculated by body weight, is believed to decrease initial cord swelling.

The standard indicators of possible cord injury are absence of rectal tone and bradycardia in the presence of hypotension. The body's normal response is to increase heart rate in the presence of decreased blood flow or hypotension. These responses are not present in injury of the spinal cord, and vagal control results in bradycardia.

Injuries involving the spinal cord can range from complete transsection, without hope of recovery, to a contusion of the cord. Fractures or dislocation of the vertebra can result in the protrusion of small pieces into the spinal canal. This is known as a burst fracture. Several vertebrae may be fractured or have fractured components. Generally, in compression fractures, if the loss of vertebral height is greater than 20%, surgical treatment may be indicated. Bracing can be considered an option if the compression is less than 20%, and no neurologic symptoms are present.

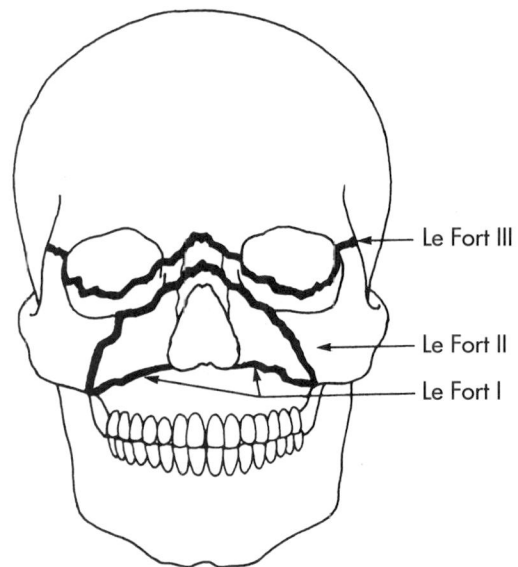

FIGURE 31-17   Le Fort's classification of maxillary fractures.

Treatment of spinal column fractures can involve surgery. Stabilization of the fracture may be necessary, depending on the severity of the injury. For cervical spine fractures traction may be used initially to reduce the fracture followed by surgical intervention as soon as patient condition permits. Internal fixation devices are discussed in Chapter 22.

INJURIES OF THE FACE

Motor vehicle crashes account for about 60% of maxillofacial injuries.[5] Mandibular fractures alone are highly associated with assault as the MOI. In the patient who presents with facial injury, the airway must be secured. This requires removing any items that pose the threat of aspiration in addition to ensuring patency. If a midface fracture is present, nasogastric tube placement and nasotracheal intubation are avoided. A tracheostomy may need to be performed before initiation of the operative procedure. Control of scalp or facial hemorrhage can be achieved through a pressure dressing until surgical intervention is possible, since exsanguination can occur. Treatment of the fracture may be delayed until the immediate life threats have been successfully managed. Goals of operative intervention are to reduce and immobilize the fracture, prevent infection, and restore facial cosmesis and function.

Facial fractures can be categorized into Le Fort I, II, or III (Fig. 31-17). A Le Fort I fracture is the most common maxillary fracture. It involves a horizontal interruption of the anterior and lateral wall of the maxillary sinus. Le Fort II is a pyramidal fracture along the maxilla and lacrimal bones and through the infraorbital rim. Le Fort III is otherwise known as *craniofacial disjunction*. The midface is completely disengaged from the cranial base, resulting from a fracture across the frontomaxillary sutures. Specific information regarding these injuries is located in Chapter 24.

INJURIES OF THE EYE

Injuries to the eye can result from blunt or penetrating types of trauma. Penetrating objects in the globe are stabilized and not removed until the patient is in the operating room. These injuries threaten loss of vision because of the injury itself, inflammation, or infection. Blunt injury to the eye can result in hematomas and accompanying fractures. A blowout fracture is the result of a blunt force to the eye that pushes soft tissue through the thin bony orbital floor. The patient has recession of the eye into the orbit and loses the ability to gaze upward. Surgical repair is often indicated. For further information see Chapter 18.

INJURIES OF THE NECK

Injury to the neck and soft-tissue structures is most commonly a result of penetrating trauma. The neck can be divided into three zones with respect to injury and consequence. Zone I is the base of the neck below the clavicles. Anatomic structures located in this region are the great vessels and aortic arch, the innominate veins, trachea, esophagus, and lungs. Zone II is the area in the middle of the neck between the clavicles and the mandible. Structures located in this area include the carotid artery, internal jugular vein, trachea, and esophagus. Zone III is located between the angle of the mandible and the base of the skull. The primary target of evaluation in these injuries is vascular structures.

Zone II injuries may necessitate an otolaryngology specialist. Penetrating injuries to the larynx and trachea can be primarily repaired. Blunt force to the larynx can result in a fracture and impose immediate airway obstruction. These patients require immediate tracheostomy followed by repair of the fracture when it is unstable or displaced. Specific information concerning these procedures is located in Chapter 21.

INJURIES OF THE CHEST AND HEART

Trauma to the chest area is the primary cause of death in 25% of trauma victims.[1] Blunt trauma is most often associated with high-speed motor vehicle accidents. Penetrating trauma is on the rise with an increase in violent crimes. Penetrating injuries at or immediately below the nipple line or level of the scapular tips is evaluated for both chest and abdominal involvement. Diaphragmatic injury is also a possibility.

Deceleration injury, such as that from a fall or striking the steering wheel in a motor vehicle accident, may cause

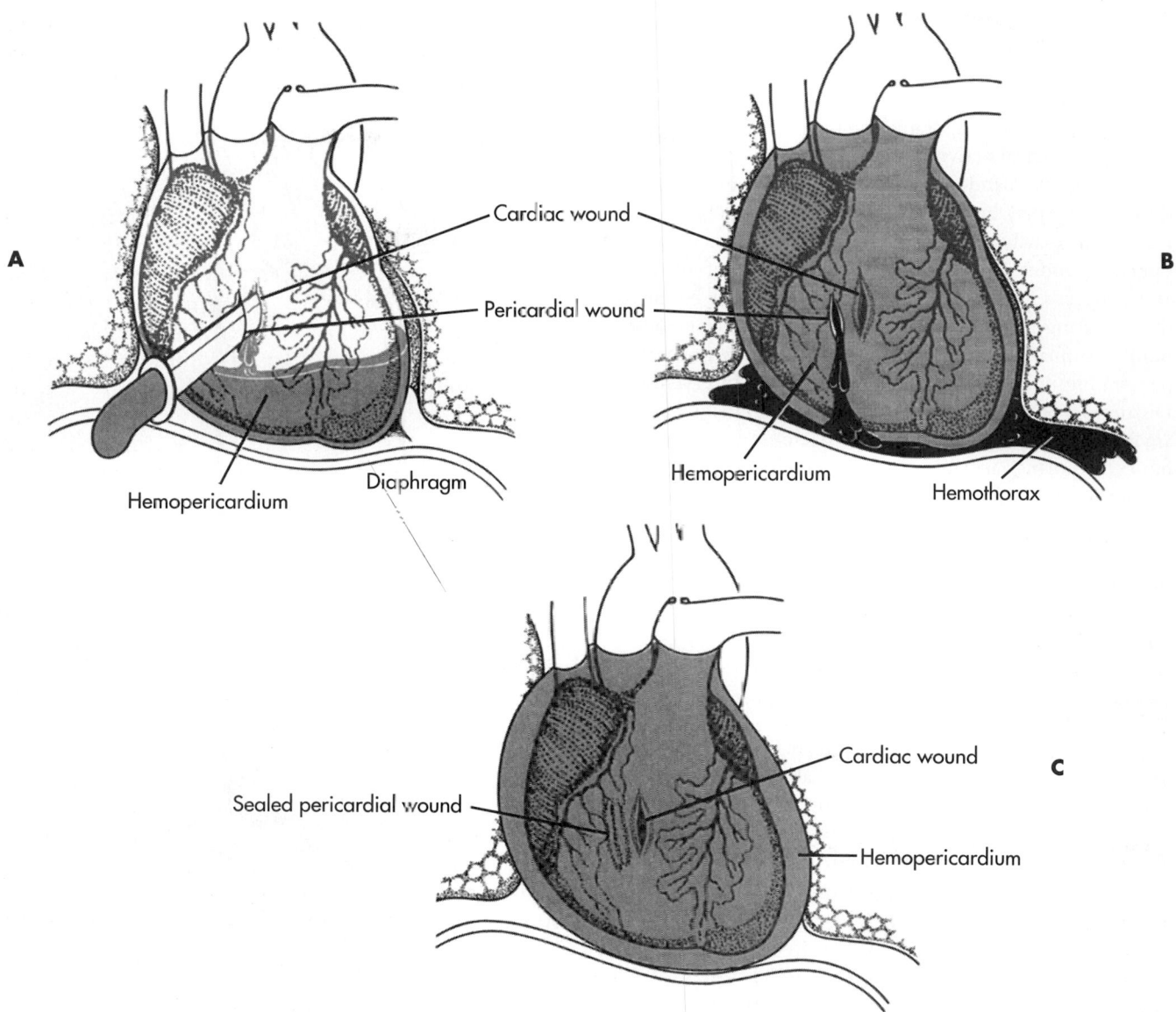

FIGURE 31-18   **A**, Cardiac injury with pericardial disruption. **B**, Bleeding from heart through pericardial tear into pleural space. **C**, Self-sealing of pericardial wound resulting in pericardial tamponade.

contusions of the chest wall, rib or sternal fractures, cardiac or pulmonary contusions, or rupture of the aorta and other major vessels. Rib fractures are also associated with a hemothorax or pneumothorax. A flail-chest segment may result when two or more adjacent ribs are broken in two or more places. This results in a paradoxical chest wall movement as a result of loss of bony support. The segment of chest wall will move in the opposite direction. If there is respiratory distress and diminished breath sounds, a chest tube is indicated immediately. An autotransfusion chest-drainage device should be considered. Chest tube output must be closely monitored intraoperatively because accumulation of 1000 to 1500 ml of blood is an indication for chest exploration. Penetrating wounds, either as a result of gunshot or stab injuries, may cause hemothoraces and pneumothoraces as well. Lacerations or perforation of the

lung, heart, great vessels, trachea, esophagus, and bronchus are possible.

Myocardial contusion usually involves the right ventricle and can be evidenced by dysrhythmias upon patient arrival or shortly thereafter. The patient is monitored on a telemetry unit, and surgical intervention is not required. Rupture of a heart valve can occur, depending on which part of the cardiac cycle the heart is in at the time of contusion. If valve rupture has occurred, surgical repair is necessary. Heart sounds should be evaluated during the secondary assessment to document the presence or absence of murmurs. Heart valve rupture can occur as a late complication of myocardial contusion. Pericardiocentesis is performed for signs and symptoms of pericardial tamponade (Fig 31-18). These include jugular venous distention, muffled heart sounds, and a narrowing pulse pressure. Patients may present to the operating room for a pericardial window either emergently or during the recovery phase.

An emergency thoracotomy may be indicated in the patient with penetrating trauma to the chest in full arrest or pulseless electrical activity on ECG. If a laceration to the heart is suspected and the patient is rapidly deteriorating, a thoracotomy may be performed in the ED. The laceration may be primarily repaired and the patient taken to the operating room for irrigation, debridement of wounds, and closure. Otherwise, surgical intervention is begun in the operating room. Wounds located across the mediastinum accompanied by hemodynamic instability or massive penetrating lung injuries require surgical intervention. Disruption of the trachea, bronchus, or esophagus is also an indication. Rupture of the thoracic aorta is another injury requiring an operation and includes the use of extracorporeal bypass. This injury is an obvious life threat but may be difficult to diagnose. An arch aortogram is indicated in patients with significant mechanism to cause such an injury. This injury is associated with first rib or sternal fractures. Chapters 25 and 27 provide additional information on associated surgical procedures.

INJURIES OF THE ABDOMEN

When the trauma patient is transferred to the operating room, the extent of injury is not always known. The perioperative nurse should prep from the suprasternal notch to the midthigh area. This allows for rapid access to the chest to clamp the aorta should massive hemorrhage control be indicated, as well as exposure of the femoral arteries for potential cannulation and access to the thigh for harvesting of a saphenous vein. The spleen is the most common organ injured in blunt trauma, and the liver, because of its large size, is the most common organ injured in penetrating trauma. Historically, initial efforts were aimed at performing splenectomy with splenic injury. However, research has shown the role of the spleen in the body's defense against infection. Therefore every effort is made to control hemorrhage in the spleen and avoid its removal. Injury to the spleen occurs with deceleration injuries resulting in fracture of the organ because of its multiple fixation points. Rupture of the spleen can be immediate or delayed. Splenic lacerations are treated nonoperatively by close monitoring and bed rest or may be treated operatively if necessary. Treatment is determined by the condition of the spleen and of the patient. A midline incision is used, which allows for exposure of all abdominal contents. Splenorrhaphy, because it is the placement of an absorbable polyglycolic acid mesh around the spleen, is utilized in capsular tears (Fig. 31-19). Topical hemostatic agents are also used with success as well as suturing and argon laser in some instances. A laceration involving the splenic hilum or complete shattering of the organ usually results in splenectomy.

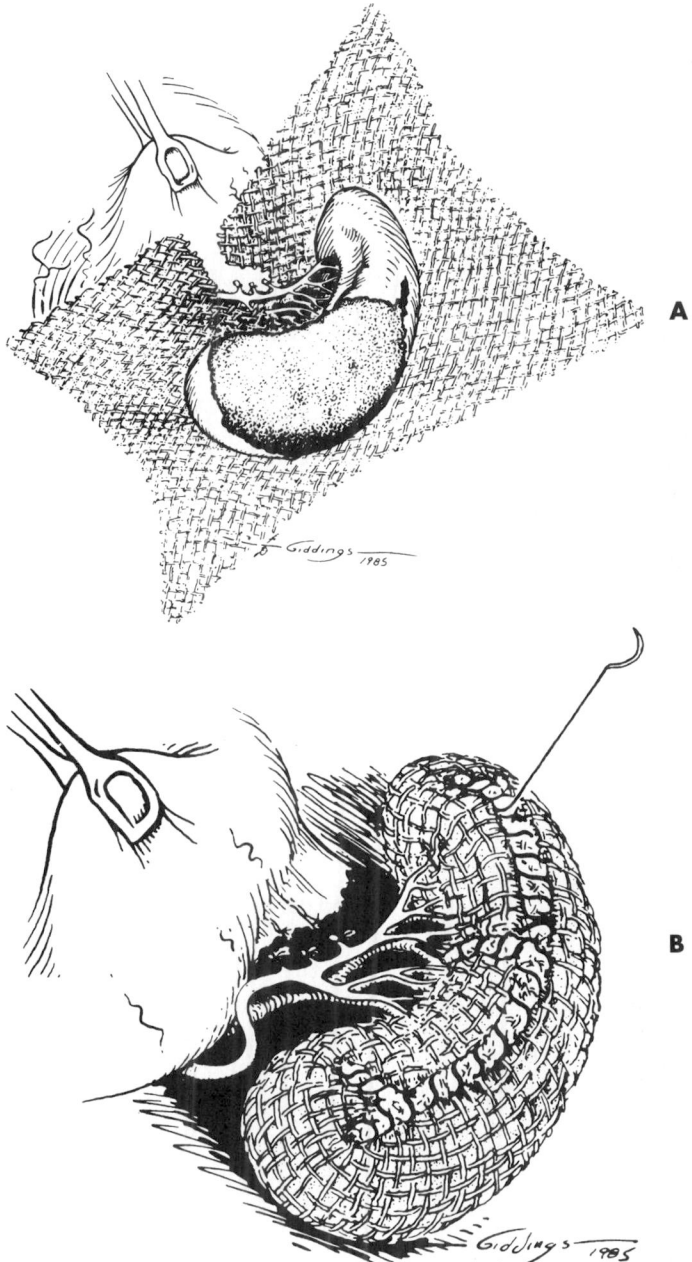

FIGURE 31-19 **A**, With capsular loss, the spleen may be encased in a woven polyglycolic acid mesh. **B**, The mesh is sutured along the anterior surface of the spleen.

Liver injury is managed in much the same way. Nonoperative treatment is indicated in minor capsular and subcapsular injuries. This can be accomplished with bed rest and close monitoring. Topical hemostatic agents and suturing are techniques of management in minor injuries. Fibrin glue is also used in some institutions as a topical hemostatic agent. More severe injuries with active expanding hematomas or lobe disruption may necessitate hepatic resection or ligation of associated vasculature. With massive hemorrhage, control of bleeding is the utmost

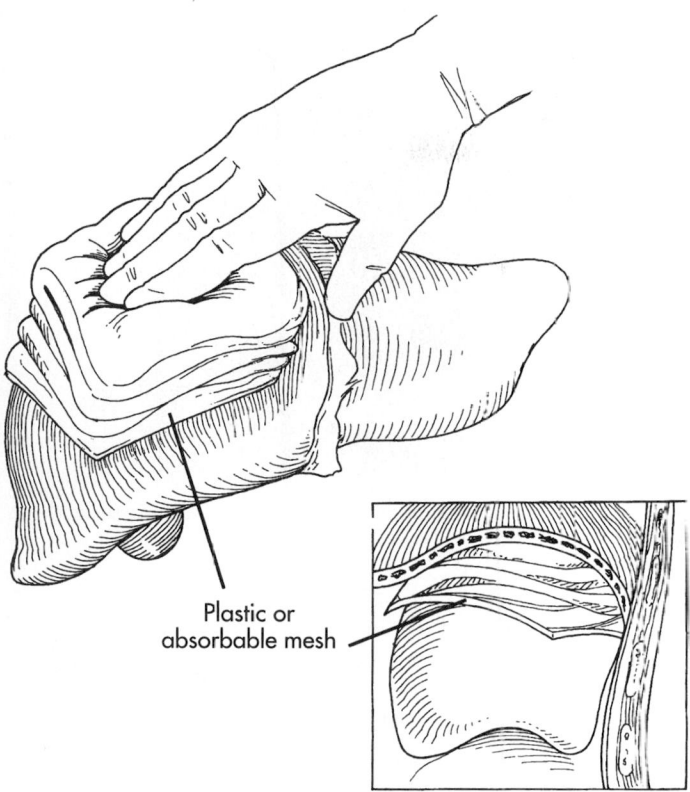

Plastic or
absorbable mesh

FIGURE 31-20   Perihepatic packing using a folded Steri-Drape and laparotomy pads.

concern. Packing with laparotomy sponges may be indicated along with manual compression of the organ if intraoperative hypotension become severe (Fig. 31-20). A pressure dressing of absorbable mesh laparotomy sponges may be applied and the wound closed temporarily until associated coagulopathies, hypothermia, and hemodynamic instability can be corrected. The patient is returned to the operating room usually within 24 to 72 hours postoperatively, or when the condition permits, for further exploration and removal of the sponges.

Injuries to the gastrointestinal system are also associated with abdominal trauma. Bowel injuries may be missed on abdominal CT scan during the initial diagnostic period. Any perforation of the gastrointestinal tract carries with it a chance for peritonitis and sepsis. In the event of a penetrating injury, the trajectory of the missile or the implement is examined and organs within the area are considered potentially injured. Exploration is indicated, and the components of the gastrointestinal system are thoroughly examined for any perforations, contusion, hemorrhage, or compromise of vasculature, such as a mesenteric hematoma. Once the injury is identified, suturing, stapling, or segmental excision may be indicated. Further information on these procedures is in Chapter 11.

Diagnostic laparoscopy is being used increasingly for

31-2   RESEARCH HIGHLIGHT

Murray et al. performed a study with two objectives: (1) examine the incidence of diaphragmatic injuries in penetrating left thoracoabdominal trauma and (2) review the role of laparoscopy in determining clinically occult diaphragmatic injuries. One-hundred-seven patients presenting to a large urban trauma center were fully evaluated for penetrating injuries to the left thoracoabdominal region over an 8-month period. These patients underwent either an exploratory celiotomy (those who were hemodynamically unstable or had peritonitis) or laparoscopy (those with no urgent indication for abdominal exploration). Fifty patients had a celiotomy on an emergent basis. Fifty-seven patients were candidates for laparoscopy. In the study population 42% of the patients had a diaphragmatic injury (59% gunshot wounds, 32% stab wounds). The 45 patients with diaphragmatic injury had some clinically occult preoperative findings; 31% had no abdominal tenderness; 40% normal chest roentgenogram; 49% associated hemopneumothorax. Twenty-six percent of the patients who underwent laparoscopy had occult diaphragmatic injuries. Diagnosis of diaphragmatic injuries can be difficult. The authors concluded that there is a high incidence of diaphragmatic injuries occurring with penetrating left thoracoabdominal trauma. Clinical examination and roentgenographic results are not reliable in the detection of these injuries. Laparoscopy has a role in detecting occult diaphragmatic injuries in patients not requiring initial celiotomy.

From Murray, J.A., Demetriades, D., Cornwell, E.E. III, et al. (1997). Penetrating left thoracoabdominal trauma: the incidence and clinical presentation of diaphragm injuries. *The Journal of Trauma, 43*(4), 624-626.

direct visualization of abdominal organs to diminish the need for a negative exploratory celiotomy. This procedure allows the surgeon to more effectively evaluate for the presence of injury and develop an appropriate plan of treatment in the stable patient. Some interventions may also be performed through the laparoscope, so that the more invasive celiotomy is avoided (Research Highlight 31-2). Laparoscopy can be assistive in evaluating patients with penetrating abdominal injuries. However, there is some concern that bowel injuries are not always identified. The increased intraabdominal pressure may also pose an adverse ventilatory effect. In the presence of abdominal vein injury with low pressures, CO_2 could leak into the vasculature and result in CO_2 emboli to the heart or lungs. Tension pneumothorax may be created in patients with a diaphragmatic injury. Indications for this procedure in the trauma setting continue to be evaluated.

INJURIES OF THE GENITOURINARY SYSTEM

Laceration of the kidney, a retroperitoneal structure, is closely associated with fracture of the ribs and transverse vertebral processes. Since the organ is retroperitoneal, the presence of bleeding may not be observed on diagnostic peritoneal lavage. Renal contusions often produce hematuria. Gross clots may also be seen in more serious injury, but it should be noted that hematuria is not present in a complete avulsion injury. Management of renal contusions can be nonoperative with monitoring of hematuria. Lacerations involving the collecting system, severe crush injuries, or pedicle injuries necessitate surgical intervention. Nephrectomy may be indicated with severe injury of the pedicle or massive hemorrhage.

Rupture of the bladder and urethral injury are most often associated with pelvic fractures. Both blunt and penetrating trauma are causative factors. The type of bladder injury is a direct result of the amount of urine present in the bladder at the time of injury. Blunt forces applied to a full bladder result in an intraperitoneal rupture. This type of rupture is closely associated with alcohol consumption because of alcohol's diuretic effect. Pelvic fracture is associated with an extraperitoneal bladder rupture. Most often these patients present with gross hematuria. A small extraperitoneal rupture may be managed by urinary catheter drainage. A large extraperitoneal rupture and intraperitoneal rupture require surgical intervention. A suprapubic cystostomy tube may be placed, and the bladder is repaired. Pelvic fracture reduction and fixation are also performed.

Urethral injuries require exploration and primary repair. These types of injuries are more common in the male. A fall or straddle type of injury is usually responsible. This injury is detected by the presence of blood at the urinary meatus. In these instances an indwelling urethral catheter should not be inserted. Blood at the urinary meatus may be indicative of a tear in the anterior urethra. A retrograde urethrogram may be performed to evaluate for extravasation of urine and potential injury. Chapter 15 provides additional information on urologic procedures.

SKELETAL INJURIES

Trauma to the skeletal system usually results in contusion or fracture. After stabilization of the patient, any body part that is distorted, edematous, painful, or highly suspicious for fracture or dislocation is radiographed. Treatment of fractures is aimed at restoring function with a minimum of complications. Immobilization of fractures can be accomplished by casting, bracing, splinting, and application of traction or hardware fixation. Femur fractures in particular can be associated with a high risk of hemorrhage and require traction before surgical repair. Closed and open reductions, application of internal and

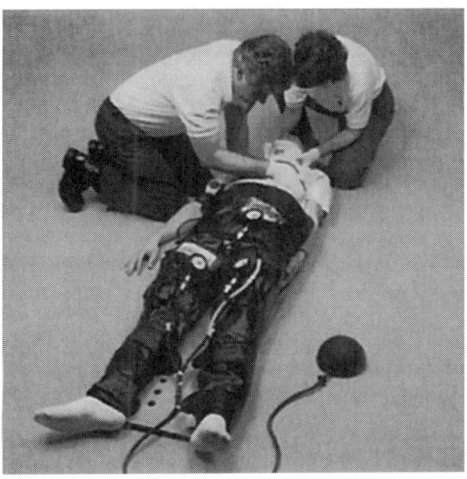

FIGURE 31-21   After PASG positioning, the Velcro straps are securely fastened.

external fixators, and some types of traction may be performed in the operating room. The perioperative nurse involved in care of the trauma patient must have a working knowledge of the orthopedic specialty. Fractures must be repaired in a timely manner to avoid untoward complications; however, immediate life threats are corrected first. Open fractures are at an increased risk of infection. Chapter 22 contains information on the surgical procedures utilized in fracture management.

Pelvic fractures may pose an additional challenge to the perioperative team. Fractures within the pelvic ring are associated with hemorrhage and shock. Systemic peripheral vascular resistance is increased. A tamponade effect may be provided to blood vessels that are disrupted because of the pelvic fracture. Pneumatic antishock garment (PASG) or PASG trousers provide stabilization of the fracture and also can reduce associated hemorrhage when applied to the patient before arrival at the hospital (Fig. 31-21). However, there is much controversy concerning their use and possible complications. Once applied, the patient may be transported to the operating room with the trousers still inflated. The perioperative nurse must be familiar with deflation procedures. The attending anesthesia member directs deflation in collaboration with the surgeon. Blood pressure and other vital signs are closely monitored. The abdominal compartment is deflated first. Deflation continues slowly while IV fluids are infused to maintain blood pressure. A 5 mm Hg drop in blood pressure requires fluid resuscitation of approximately 200 ml before deflation of the next compartment. If the patient remains stable, each leg compartment is deflated slowly, one at a time. Severe hemorrhage associated with the fracture may be controlled by arterial embolization performed in the radiology department if surgical intervention must be delayed. Fixation of the fracture ultimately provides hemorrhage control.

Soft-tissue injuries of an extremity are subject to

compartment syndrome. This is a result of swelling of the soft tissues and muscles encased in the fascia. With a significant amount of swelling, pain is increased, and the surrounding circulation may be compromised. The patient may experience a decrease in motor and sensory function. This injury must be treated surgically by performance of a fasciotomy. Incising the fascia allows space for tissue swelling. Several days later, the patient returns to the operating room for closure, which may require skin grafting for complete coverage.

HYPOTHERMIA

Hypothermia can be classified into three types. *Mild hypothermia* is a core temperature between 32° and 35° C. These patients may appear gray and are cool to the touch. Some alterations in level of consciousness can be present. Treatment is aimed at passive rewarming of the patient by means of warm fluids and blankets. *Moderate hypothermia* is characterized as core temperatures between 30° and 32° C. Warmed fluids are given IV and also by gastric or peritoneal lavage. A warming blanket may also be initiated. Immersion in a Hubbard tank filled with warm water has also been successful. An irritable myocardium may cause dysrhythmias to be present. Shivering may or may not be present. *Severe hypothermia* is diagnosed in the patient with a temperature below 30° C.[3] The heart rate and the respiratory rate are greatly decreased. This patient is comatose, often appears dead, and requires active rewarming processes. It is advisable to warm the core first to avoid complications associated with rewarming. This can best be accomplished by core heating by means of a cardiopulmonary bypass, which directly warms internal vital organs, including the heart. The patient should be handled gently during transfers to avoid further tissue injury and stimulation of an irritable myocardium.[1]

It should be noted that severe cases of hypothermia mimic death, and no patient can be pronounced dead until he or she is warm and dead. Resuscitation measures are ceased if the patient is rewarmed to at least 35° C and cardiac functions are still nonexistent.

THERMAL INJURIES

Heat and cold exposure injuries require prompt initial management in the ED setting. Some institutions transfer pediatric burn patients and severely burned adult patients to a burn center for treatment once the patient is stabilized. In addition to treatment of the site of injury to decrease further tissue damage, fluid management is of the utmost importance in these patients. After hemodynamic stabilization of the patient, burn and frostbite wounds usually require a series of debridement. These patients may have multiple surgical debridement procedures before skin grafting and cosmetic interventions. Restoration of function is important. Circumferential burns may restrict the neurovascular structures during eschar formation. Chest burns with eschar may restrict movement of the chest wall and ventilatory function. An escharotomy (incision of the eschar) may be performed to alleviate the constriction. If necessary, this procedure may be performed at the bedside, and the perioperative team may be asked to assist.

ORGAN AND TISSUE PROCUREMENT

As previously noted, trauma primarily affects young people. In the event that resuscitation efforts or surgical interventions are not successful, the patient may be declared dead. Depending on the cause of death and preexisting medical conditions, the patient may be an organ-donor candidate. Both federal and state laws mandate that local organ-procurement facilities are notified of potential donors and that families are informed that organ donation exists as an option. Organ-donation agencies can be contacted early and will assist in assessing the potential donor as well as providing a protocol for donor management once the patient is declared dead. Definition of brain death is not uniform throughout the country. The perioperative nurse should be familiar with the state's definition of brain death and the institution's criteria for the declaration. Once a patient is declared dead and becomes a potential organ donor, all financial costs acquired from that point are not incurred by the patient's family. The patient is not disfigured in any way that will interfere with bereavement rituals.

Patients up to 70 years of age may be considered potential organ donors. Exclusion criteria include the presence of IV drug abuse, preexisting untreated infection, malignancy (exclusive of brain tumor), and active tuberculosis.[1]

A transplantation coordinator assists in managing the organ donor patient in the ICU setting until the procurement teams arrive. The perioperative nurse must prepare for the organ-procurement procedure. The harvesting of organs and tissue may take several hours and additional members of the perioperative team. Different organ-procurement agencies will provide a surgical team, but require additional scrub and circulating personnel are needed. The transplantation coordinators actively seek tissue and organ recipients during the harvest procedure. Most organ-transplantation agencies contact the institution and provide follow-up information regarding the ultimate success of the transplantation procedures and information about the recipients.

The heart is removed first, followed by the lungs, pancreas, liver, and kidneys. Tissue dissection is performed in such a manner as to allow for optimal organ transplantation. Sterile technique remains important. In addition, traffic control is of concern during these procedures. Any nonessential personnel should be limited. Bone, skin, and corneas can also be removed. Some procurement agencies remove bone and corneas in the morgue, rather than in the operating room.

SUMMARY

Nowhere is the team concept more important than in the provision of definitive care to the multiple trauma patient. The perioperative nurse is a vital member of the trauma team. Through the application of principles of trauma care as outlined in this chapter, perioperative nurses can significantly contribute to positive outcomes for trauma patients.

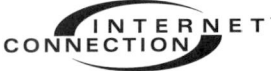

American Association of Critical Care Nurses (AACN):
http://aacn.org

Emergency Nurses Association (ENA): http://www.ena.org

American Association for the Surgery of Trauma:
http://www.aast.org/

University of Texas Health Sciences Center - San Antonio Trauma Page: http://rmstewart.uthsca.edu/

Federal Emergency Management Agency (FEMA):
http://www.fema.gov/

Journal of Emergency Medical Services:
http://wwwdotcom.com/jems/jems/jems1.html

Emergency Medicine:
http://www.medconnect.com/finalhtm/pedjclemclbhm.htm

REFERENCES

1. Cardona, V.D., Hurn, P.D., Bastnagel Mason, P.J., et al. (1994). *Trauma nursing* (ed. 2). Philadelphia: W.B. Saunders.
2. Champion, H.R., Sacco, W.J., Copes, W.S., et al. (1989). A revision of the Trauma Score. *The Journal of Trauma, 29*(5), 623–629.
3. Committee on Trauma (1997). *Advanced trauma life support program.* Chicago: American College of Surgeons.
4. Keough, V., & Letizia, M. (1996). Perioperative care of elderly trauma patients, *AORN Journal, 63*(5), 932–937.
5. Lopez–Viego, M.A. (Ed.). (1994). *The Parkland trauma handbook.* St. Louis: Mosby.
6. Neff, J.A., & Kidd, P.S. (1993). *Trauma nursing: the art and science.* St. Louis: Mosby.
7. Sheehy, S.B., & Jimmerson, C.L. (1994). *Manual of clinical trauma care* (ed. 2). St. Louis: Mosby.
8. State of Illinois Trauma Nurse Specialist Course Manual. (1990). Springfield, Ill: Illinois Department of Health.
9. Trunkey, D. (1983). Trauma. *Scientific American, 249,* 28–35.

CHAPTER THIRTY TWO | # Contemporary Issues

Donna S. Watson

THE CHANGES IN current health care management and practices are challenging many of nursing's fundamental principles. The area of greatest concern is the ability to deliver safe, quality patient care. The *American Journal of Nursing* Patient Care Survey[31] validates that nurses are taking on more responsibilities with less time for direct patient care. Downsizing, restructuring, and the substitution of unlicensed assistive personnel (UAP) in place of the registered nurse (RN) are common in the present healthcare system. The effects on perioperative nursing practice as a result of changes in the healthcare system are far reaching; these include a steady rise in outpatient surgery, rapid technologic advances, integration of managed care plans, higher patient acuity, and greater responsibilities and accountability. To be successful the perioperative nurse must recognize the importance of awareness and participation in contemporary issues that are the focus of this chapter. It is these issues that will shape and form the perioperative practice of tomorrow.

BEST PRACTICES

In 1996, a group of nursing organizations participated in a summit held by the American Nurses Association (ANA) and the American Association of Critical Care Nurses (AACN) to address the delivery of safe, high-quality, accessible, and cost-effective healthcare. The outcome is the best practices network, Creative Solutions, dedicated to creating a renaissance for healthcare innovation. The Association of Operating Room Nurses (AORN) is one of the participating founders and supporters of Creative Solutions. Presently, 21 professional nursing organizations have donated financial and clinical expertise in support of this new global network.

Creative Solutions is the publisher of the *Best Practice Directory* and sponsor of the international conference "Showcase for Innovative Practice," a conference dedicated to the best of best practices. Another initiative is the Best Practice Network (www.best4health.org), a forum of sharing ideas by various healthcare providers.

"Best Practice" is described as a better way or a new way of providing a particular healthcare service or program. Categories of best practices include internal, competitive, functional, or generic. Each represents an innovative healthcare practice, process, or service that has been successfully implemented and is viewed as a creative solution. For example, the best practice called *Skin Care Protocol*[16] describes a 220-bed community hospital's comprehensive effort to address the problem of pressure ulcers. The goal was to create a state-of-the-art skin-care protocol based on current research. The best practice discusses Agency for Health Care Policy and Research (AHCPR) Clinical Practice Guidelines, state legislation, and the Joint Commission for Accreditation of Healthcare Organizations (JCAHO) standards and requirements used in planning, setting objectives and performance measures, implementation, and evaluation of the best practice. For additional information contact the Best Practice Network at 1-800-809-2273.

Perioperative Nursing Implications

A Best Practice is a service or program that is recognized for its excellence. The program or service has met requirements that support significant benefits for the patient or community, has been tested with successful implementation in a clinical setting, demonstrates an improvement in current practices, and is an innovative approach to solving a problem. When one is looking at a specific problem or population, the Best Practice Network should be consulted to look for a better or new way for achieving a positive outcome. Those individuals or institutions with innovative solutions and approaches for perioperative programs or services should consider submission to the Best Practice Network.

BENCHMARKING

The term *benchmarking* is a misunderstood concept with different definitions for various organizations. A common definition is that benchmarking is the "process of identifying and learning from best practices anywhere in the world."[5] The process of benchmarking is becoming increasingly popular, as healthcare managers are forced into making tough decisions about reducing overall cost while maintaining quality of care. The benchmarking process allows for an organization to "compare data with other providers to target areas for quality improvement and reduction of resources utilization."[32]

Czarnecki[15] has identified the following steps for an organization participating in the benchmarking process:

- *Deciding what to benchmark.* The process for benchmarking begins with identifying what to benchmark. The focus may be on an administrative component such as determining the labor cost per surgical minute or on a clinical component such as decreasing the length of stay for a specific diagnosis related group.
- *Enlisting partners.* Groups of organizations are encouraged to work together as benchmarking partners.
- *Defining and mapping a process.* A team from the enlisting organizations defines the process that will be used for collecting and analyzing the data.
- *Conducting library research.* There is a variety of useful resources that may provide information on other organizations' best practices.
- *Developing surveys.* Most often some form of written survey is developed and utilized. The team will develop the tool and distribute it to participants for data collection. Perioperative data elements collected might include case length, turnaround time, supply cost, staffing, and so forth. There is a variety of external vendors that now supply benchmarking data specific to the perioperative environment (such as Healthcare Investment Analysts, Allegiance Healthcare Consulting Services, O.R. Benchmarks, Inc.).
- *Gathering performance-measurement data.* Data are collected for organizational comparison with other known best practices.
- *Measuring performance.* An organization's performance is compared with that of other organizations to identify existing performance gap or gaps.
- *Visiting the best practitioners.* A formal written survey often misses critical information that is gathered by direct observation of best practitioners.
- *Conducting best practice workshops.* When organizations are involved in studies together, a formal presentation of the results may be presented or written for publication.[24,32]

By utilizing benchmarking measures an organization's performance is compared with that of other organizations with known best practices. Areas for improvement in administrative and operational processes and clinical procedures are identified. Other industries have utilized the benchmarking process with great success. The use of benchmarking is proving to be an effective quality-improvement tool for healthcare managers looking for effective ways to lower costs while maintaining quality.

UNLICENSED ASSISTIVE PERSONNEL

The growing use of unlicensed assistive personnel (UAP) is a major concern for the nursing community. Legislation such as the Patient Safety Act is a direct result of public demand to know who is providing their care, staffing levels and mix, and patient outcomes. Many states are moving to regulating UAP, and this has created debate within the profession of nursing.

The 1995 AORN House of Delegates revised and ratified the "AORN Official Statement on Unlicensed Assistive Personnel"[7] (Box 32-1). The AORN monitors and participates as appropriate in state legislation related to unlicensed assistive personnel. Perioperative nurses must continue to take an active and aggressive role in keeping abreast of state legislation. It is one of nursing's responsibilities to monitor and participate in discussions related to regulatory decisions that affect the care and well-being of patients. For current legislative priorities related to perioperative nursing practice, refer to the AORN Government Affairs page on the Internet at http://www.aorn.org/GOVT/index.htm.

SURGICAL TECHNOLOGISTS

These are tumultuous times for nurses who practice in the perioperative setting. Because of healthcare reform and necessary reduction of costs in all areas, managers are forced to look at job classifications, education requirements, and implement strategies for work redesign. This has resulted in surgical technologists (STs) assuming some roles and responsibilities traditionally performed only by registered nurses.

STs work under the direction of either a physician or nurse; they are not independent practitioners. When selecting appropriate nursing activities that may delegated, the RN must conduct an assessment of the patient, identify nursing diagnoses, determine patient acuity level and appropriate nursing interventions, determine necessary equipment and supplies, identify expected patient outcomes, and assess the level of skills, education, experience, and competency of the ST to whom selected nursing activities may be appropriately delegated.

The current work-redesign efforts have perioperative nurses assuming additional roles and responsibilities for

| BOX 32–1 | AORN Official Statement on Unlicensed Assistive Personnel |

Preamble

Market forces and anticipation of health care reform compel perioperative registered nurses to reexamine their traditional practice roles and the nursing tasks delegated to unlicensed assistive personnel (UAP). These forces provide an opportunity for perioperative registered nurses to focus their leadership skills on coordinating patient care and directing the activities of the perioperative nursing team. The perioperative nursing team consists of multiskilled nursing care providers working in a collaborative partnership to achieve expected patient outcomes and satisfaction. Team members must perform patient care activities consistent with the needs of the patient and the provider's education, training, and skills to ensure patient safety.

The restructuring of traditional roles does not replace perioperative registered nurses with UAP but rather provides perioperative registered nurses with support for the delivery of nursing care. Perioperative registered nurses demonstrate leadership by selecting nursing activities that may be safely and legally delegated to competent UAP.

Position Statement

Perioperative registered nurses are accountable for patient outcomes resulting from the nursing care provided during the perioperative experience. A perioperative registered nurse must plan and direct the care of every patient undergoing operative and other invasive procedures. A 1:1 perioperative RN to patient ratio is required for each patient during operative and other invasive procedures.[1] To ensure that patients receive the highest quality and standard of care, the circulating nurse must always be a registered professional nurse.

The core activities of perioperative nursing care are assessment, diagnosis, outcome identification, planning, implementation, and evaluation. The perioperative registered nurse may not delegate assessment, diagnosis, outcome identification, planning, and evaluation; however, depending on the patient's potential for adverse outcomes and need for complex interventions and teaching, the perioperative registered nurse may delegate appropriate patient care activities. The perioperative registered nurse uses judgment to decide to whom and under what circumstances to delegate these activities.

Unlicensed assistive personnel, in a variety of job categories, may assist in the implementation of delegated patient care activities according to the unlicensed individual's level of education, training, and demonstrated competency in the required skill set. Unlicensed assistive personnel are accountable to and work under the direct or indirect supervision of perioperative registered nurses when performing delegated patient care activities.

Perioperative registered nurses must consider the following factors before delegating patient care activities to UAP:

- assessment of the patient's condition;
- complexity of the patient's condition;
- complexity of technology and surgery;
- predictability of patient outcome(s);
- level of preparation and education of UAP;
- competency of UAP;

- ratio of registered nurses to UAP based on patient need; and
- amount of supervision registered nurses will be able to provide.

Perioperative registered nurses define and supervise the training and utilization of UAP who provide direct and indirect patient care in the perioperative setting. Unlicensed assistive personnel must receive appropriate training and demonstrate competency before assuming new and expanded responsibilities within the perioperative setting. Educational preparation and training of UAP must be commensurate with the activities that will be delegated.

Perioperative nurses must participate in decisions regarding the appropriate position descriptions and job duties for all UAP. Perioperative registered nurses also validate the competencies of UAP on an ongoing basis to ensure that role expectations delineated in institutional performance descriptions are being met.

The facility must provide an appropriate number of perioperative registered nurses to perform the core activities of assessment, diagnosis, outcome identification, planning, implementation, and evaluation and to supervise and coordinate patient care delivery by UAP.

Definitions

The following are operational definitions of terms used in the statement.

Competency. The knowledge, skills, and abilities to fulfill patient care activities in the operating room. Competency is defined by the policies and procedures of the health care facility/unit.

Delegation. The transfer of responsibility for the performance of an activity from one individual to another while retaining accountability for the outcome. It is the registered nurse who uses judgment to determine the appropriate activities to delegate.[2] The term *assignment* is used in place of *delegation* in some states. Refer to state nurse practice acts for the appropriate application of the terms *delegation* and *assignment*.

Supervision. The active process of directing, guiding, and influencing the outcome of an individual's performance of an activity.[3]

On-site (direct). Physically present or immediately available while the activity is being performed.

Off-site (indirect). Direction provided through various means of written and verbal communications.

Assistive personnel. Individuals trained to assist registered nurses in providing patient care activities as delegated by registered nurses. Assistive personnel include, but are not limited to, nurses' aides/assistants, orderlies, technicians, and technologists.

Skill set. A designated group of activities required to perform specific functions.

Notes

1. "Statement on mandate for the registered nurse as circulator in the operating room," in *AORN Standards and Recommended Practices* (Denver: Association of Operating Room Nurses, Inc, 1994) 23; "Resolution on the necessity for the registered nurse in the operating room," in *AORN Standards and Recommended Practices* (Denver: Association of Operating Room Nurses, Inc, 1994) 31.

2. American Nurses Association, *Position Statement on Registered Nurse Utilization of Unlicensed Assistive Personnel, Attachment 1, Definition Related to ANA Position Statement on Unlicensed*

Continued

BOX 32-1 | **AORN Official Statement on Unlicensed Assistive Personnel—cont'd**

Assistive Personnel (Washington, DC: American Nurses Association, 1992).
   3. *Ibid.*

Suggested reading

Abbott, C. "Intraoperative nursing activities performed by surgical technologists." *AORN Journal* 60 (September 1994) 382-393.

Phippen, M.L.; Applegeet, C. "Unlicensed assistive personnel in the perioperative setting." (Clinical Issues) *AORN Journal* 60 (September 1994) 455-458.

Ponder, K.S. "The RN circulator." (Opinion) *AORN Journal* 60 (September 1994) 459-462.

Submitted: 3/95
Revised and ratified: 3/9/95
House of Delegates,
Atlanta, Georgia
Sunset review: 3/2000

From *AORN standards, recommended practices, and guidelines.* (1997). Denver, Colo.: Association of Operating Room Nurses, pp. 21-22.

---

management of the surgical patient. Because STs are skilled and competent in certain areas, the perioperative nurse delegates selected nursing activities that may be performed by STs. Abbott[1] (Research Highlight 32-1) identified frequently delegated nursing activities performed by STs to include the following:

1. *Counts*: counting instruments, sponges, sharps; communicating count results; and initiating corrective actions when incorrect.
2. *Sterile field*: gowning, gloving, surgical hand scrub, draping, inspecting items when opened, correcting breaks in aseptic technique; flash sterilization, soaking items for sterilization or disinfection.
3. *Equipment and supplies*: selection of appropriate equipment, assuring proper functioning, and processing of instrumentation.
4. *Patients' rights*: protection of patient privacy and maintenance of confidentiality.

Activities of assessing patient needs, determining appropriate interventions, prioritizing interventions, developing goals, and evaluation of the care are solely and legally within the scope of the professional registered nurse. Professional nursing care is based on assessment, diagnosis, outcome identification, planning, implementation, and evaluation. Those aspects of the nursing process that may be delegated are dependent on individual state nurse practice acts.

Because downsizing has occurred, many institutions have moved to a skill mix of one registered nurse to one ST for each surgical patient. Together the RN, ST, anesthesia provider, and surgeon compose the surgical team. Each group of providers bring specific education, training, skills, and competency that collectively contribute to delivery of quality patient care.

Recently, the Association of Surgical Technologists (AST) and AORN have begun to meet jointly to discuss issues of mutual interest between the two groups. Together, the two organizations represent over 61,000 members. Ongoing dialog between the two organizations is indicated because of the close working relationships between STs and RNs. The organizations agreed that working on issues of mutual concern will benefit the surgical patient and surgical environment.[12]

HEALTHCARE REPORT CARDS

Report cards for healthcare that include detailed information about local health plans can now be purchased by consumers.[20] The National Committee for Quality Assurance (NCQA) sponsored and collected data on six Denver healthcare plans. Areas surveyed included member satisfaction, women's health, heart disease, children's health, mental health, and prevention of complications from chronic disease. Other cities surveyed included Pittsburgh and Dallas. The NCQA uses 60 criteria in evaluating managed care plans. The comparative data between the different plans allows employers and employees to closely critique and select plans that will best meet their needs.

The ANA has also developed a prototype for nursing report cards that measures the effect of nursing on several patient outcomes.[4] The ANA has developed 21 measurable structure, process, and outcomes indicators for acute care settings.[3] As the need for database comparison increases, standardized computer-based record systems will emerge, allowing for easier generation of nursing, financial, and strategic operating indicator comparisons between various institutions.

HEALTHCARE REFORM

Nursing is involved daily with America's crisis in healthcare. The nurse can easily identify with the patient who is denied access to care and at the same time envision a better future that supports universal access. It was estimated that between 34 and 37 million Americans were uninsured in 1993, with more than a fourth of these being children. In addition, approximately 60 million were underinsured in the event of a serious illness.

Some financial policies that have influenced nursing practice include legislation in 1983 that changed Medicare

32-1 RESEARCH HIGHLIGHT

In this study, intraoperative nursing activities delegated to surgical technologists (STs) were identified. The AORN competency statements of intraoperative nursing were used as the conceptual framework for the development of the Abbott Intraoperative Nursing questionnaire (AINQ). The AINQ included 59 nursing activities that were identified as low-risk or high-risk patient care situations. Subjects were requested to rate each nursing activity on a five-point scale of the Likert type ranging from ST never performed to ST always performed. The sample $n = 343$ consisted of OR directors, perioperative nurses, and STs from rural and community hospitals and medical centers.

Intraoperative activities that the surgical technologists frequently performed included four categories: (1) surgical counts category: counting instruments, sponges, sharps; communicating count results; and initiating corrective actions when incorrect. (2) Sterile field category: gowning, gloving, surgical scrubbing, draping; inspection of sterile items; corrective actions for breaks in aseptic technique; cleaning, disinfection, and sterilization of instrumentation. (3) Equipment and supplies category: selecting equipment and supplies, checking function of equipment, and processing for sterilization. (4) Patients' rights category: protecting and maintaining patient privacy and confidentiality.

Intraoperative activities STs performed infrequently included: (1) patients' rights category: knowledge of spiritual and ethnic beliefs, contact of religious counselor; (2) sterile field category: specimens, cultures, forms for laboratory, hair removal, and skin preparation; (3) OR environment category: monitor traffic patterns, temperature, electrical safety, light and noise; (4) transportation category: transfer patient, determine method of transfer, confirm patient identity, arrange for patient transfer, support patients' emotional needs; (5) counts category: documentation; (6) teaching category: identification of needs, assessment of readiness to learn, instruction, and documentation; (7) equipment and supplies category: application and removal of electrosurgical-unit dispersive pad, evaluation of skin condition, documentation of implant information; charges; (8) patient monitoring category: assist anesthesia, evaluate laboratory results, perform physical examination and patient assessment, check for blood loss and physical status during procedure.

To successfully delegate nursing activities to the STs, the nurse must be aware of appropriate direct and indirect patient care activities that may be performed by the STs. These delegated activities should be appropriate to the STs, education, skills, competency, and training and be based on the complexity of patient care.

From Abbott, C. (1994). Intraoperative nursing activities performed by surgical technologists. *AORN Journal, 60*(3), 382-393.

---

reimbursement from a retrospective cost-based system to a prospective payment system. This system, based on diagnosis related groups (DRGs), established a payment system for Medicare inpatient hospital services before services are provided. It encourages decreased admissions and shorter lengths of stay for patients. Reimbursement is at a fixed rate. If the institution's costs are less than the DRG payment, the institution benefits fiscally.

In 1986 the Physician Payment Review Commission (PPRC) was established by Congress. It advises Congress on what to pay physicians for services rendered to Medicare patients. Nursing closely monitors the activities of the PPRC to determine how physician payment is reviewed and revised and how nursing payment may be developed in the future. The PPRC has recommended the Resource Based Relative Value Scale (RBRVS) for payment to nonphysician providers who render care to Medicare patients. This system does not pay nonphysician and physician providers equally for like services.

The present payment mechanisms are not effective. It is projected that the Medicare trust fund will be depleted by the year 2005. Private payer insurance companies are indirectly paying for medical care of uninsured people. Insurance rates continue to spiral upward, with no ceiling in sight. The private payer is paying increasingly more. Many businesses have increased copayments of insurance or completely dropped insurance as an employee benefit because the costs often exceed their profits. Most state-operated Medicaid programs are on the brink of financial disaster.

As the country attempts to overhaul the healthcare system for its 260 million citizens, nursing has been visible in making known that the profession of nursing is not being used to its fullest potential. Opportunities that allow for greater responsibilities and better use of nursing services include prescriptive authority, which is now in effect in some states, direct reimbursement for nursing services, education of the public in techniques that contribute to promotion of wellness and prevention of illness, and privileges to admit patients to the hospital when designated criteria are met. Nursing has the capability of delivering 60% to 80% of preventive and primary care services, currently provided by physicians, and at a lower cost.[14] New York's Columbia/Presbyterian

Medical Center and Connecticut-based Oxford Health Plans use nurse practitioners as primary care providers.[19] The Commonwealth of Massachusetts utilize advanced practice nurses for management of care for surgical patients.[18] Nursing will continue to emerge as a significant contributor and participant in the reformed healthcare system. As reform measures are phased in, nursing will keep some of its traditional roles and gain many nontraditional roles.

The roles and responsibilities of the perioperative nurse are certain to be affected by healthcare reform. No longer are the definitions of scrub nurse and circulator adequate to reflect the actual practices and responsibilities of perioperative nurses. Additional current roles for perioperative nurses include pain management, patient teaching, first assisting, case management, utilization review, discharge planning, information systems, environmental waste management, risk management, research, consulting, and policy making. In the future it might be the perioperative nurse who administers specific short-term therapeutic, screening, and diagnostic procedures. Perhaps the future perioperative nurse will routinely repair simple lacerations, administer intravenous conscious sedation throughout the institution, function as the first assistant on all surgical procedures, and accompany the patient home for postoperative care. Although it is uncertain what specific new roles and responsibilities will emerge with the reforming of healthcare, it is certain that the perioperative nurse of today is actively participating in shaping the perioperative challenges of tomorrow.

MANAGEMENT OF MEDICAL WASTE

Medical waste disposal is increasingly becoming a major issue of healthcare facilities. As technology has advanced, so has the packaging and use of disposable items. Many institutions prefer disposables to reusables because the product is ensured of sterility and function. In addition, potential exposure to bloodborne pathogens during cleaning is decreased, and overall productivity of the nurse is increased, allowing more time for patient care.[28] The operation of a single surgical suite generates a significant amount of medical waste. There are gloves, gowns, backtable covers, patient drapes, needles and other sharps, sponges, body fluids and secretions, and other items that must be disposed of. This does not include medical waste from the private offices of dentists and physicians. The cumulative effect of disposal is significant, and the effect on the environment is becoming more apparent.

Society has demanded accountability of healthcare facilities in proper disposal of medical waste. Reports of shoreline contamination with syringes, bloody vials, and needles from medical waste resulted in public outrage and began the quest for more efficient methods of medical waste disposal. Public attention was in part attributable to the fear and concern of exposure to the human immunodeficiency virus (HIV) and the hepatitis B virus (HBV). Management of medical waste quickly became a widespread public concern.

Tracking of medical waste is costly and time consuming. In addition to tracking facilities such as hospitals, private physicians' offices, ambulatory surgery centers, and blood banks, methods would have to be developed to track medical waste related to patient home care, IV drug users, and private clinics.

The 1994 AORN House of Delegates ratified the position statement on "Regulated Medical Waste Definition and Treatment: A Collaborative Document."[6] The collaborative document includes input from representatives of 13 organizations with each recognizing that there is little consensus on an accepted definition and management of regulated medical waste. However, it is generally agreed that medical waste "has the potential to transmit infectious disease."[6] In 1997, the ANA House of Delegates endorsed the "Regulated Medical Waste Definition and Treatment: A Collaborative Document"[8] (Box 32-2).

An institution defining medical waste should closely evaluate the type of pathogen, transmission, host, and appropriate safe disposal of the waste. Medical waste is disposed of by methods such as steam sterilization, thermal inactivation, chemical disinfection, grinding, microwaves, high-density lasers, and dumping into landfills. Some companies offer recycling options for their products. One reason for not having a universally accepted treatment requirement for management of medical waste, hospital waste, infectious waste, and regulated medical waste is attributable to the inconsistencies in definitions.

Applying the definition of infectious waste as medical waste that is considered infectious and may cause disease, one could interpret infectious waste as any material exposed to blood and body secretions. This could imply that all materials in contact with the patient are infectious waste. Such a misinterpretation would have a significant effect. Not only would the disposal and cost be insurmountable, but also the environmental effect would be significant. There are fewer landfills available, and other methods of disposal come with potential hazards to the environment.

Classification and standardization of waste management definitions would eliminate some confusion. Also, there is a lack of regulatory control on proper removal, storage, and disposal of hospital waste. Recommendations vary according to city, state, and federal sources, and there are inconsistencies. Institutions may be fined large amounts when disposal recommendations are not followed.

In the perioperative setting infectious waste will continue to be an issue well into the next decade. The AORN Statement on Protection of the Environment[9]

BOX 32-2	AORN Position Statement: Regulated Medical Waste Definition and Treatment: a Collaborative Document

In November 1992 in Atlanta, AORN convened a collaborative meeting. Representatives of 13 organizations participated in the discussion of the issues that resulted in this document.

Introduction

There are three types of regulated waste from health care facilities. The first two are radioactive waste, which is regulated by the Nuclear Regulatory Agency, and hazardous chemical waste, which is regulated by the US Environmental Protection Agency (EPA). The third type is potentially infective waste, which, for the purposes of this document, will be referred to as regulated medical waste. This document will focus primarily on the environmental issues arising from regulated medical waste. This document addresses what hospital waste should be considered as regulated medical waste and what should constitute acceptable treatment, on site or off site, to allow safe handling and disposal of such waste.

Two concerns arise when discussing the disposal of items that have been in contact with potentially infectious materials. The first of these concerns is the transmission of disease through occupational exposure (ie, contact that occurs from the point of contamination to final disposal). This concern is addressed by the proper adherence to the December 1991 Occupational Safety and Health Administration (OSHA) final rule on bloodborne pathogens.[1] The second concern is the environmental and public health implications of regulated medical waste.

Background

Considerable confusion and difference of opinion exist in what should be designated as regulated medical waste and how it should be managed. The importance of properly defining regulated medical waste is shown in a recent study by Rutala.[2] This study estimates that under the Centers for Disease Control and Prevention (CDC) definitions, about 6% of hospital waste would be considered regulated medical waste, whereas under the Medical Waste Tracking Act (MWTA) definitions from the EPA, as much as 45% of hospital waste could be considered regulated medical waste. On average, American hospitals designate approximately 15% of their waste as regulated medical waste. Regulated medical waste is 0.3% of the total municipal solid waste Americans produce annually.[2] In a 1990 report from the Agency for Toxic Substances and Disease Registry to Congress, the executive summary states that "the general public's health is not likely to be adversely affected by medical waste generated in the traditional healthcare setting."[4]

The 1991 OSHA rule on bloodborne pathogens designates certain types of medical waste as "regulated waste." If these designations are included in the definition of regulated medical waste, the amount of health care waste considered as regulated would be further increased.

The Department of Transportation (DOT) recently issued performance-oriented packaging standards specifying package requirements for transportation of regulated medical waste. The definition of regulated medical waste used in these standards matches that of the EPA.[5] In addition to multiple federal definitions, states, counties, and municipalities have developed their own requirements, leading to further confusion.

Medical waste contains a significantly lower content of microbes than household waste, and it is widely recognized that household waste poses no threat. According to the position paper on this issue by the Society for Hospital Epidemiology of America (SHEA).

> *Household waste contains more microorganisms with pathogenic potential for humans on average than medical waste. We can deduce from our daily exposure to household waste and the decades of sanitary landfill burial that the public health risks for the less microbially contaminated hospital waste are nominal.[6]*

While there are documented instances of occupational illness resulting from exposure to regulated medical waste, there are no known instances of public illness caused by such exposure.

The definition and treatment of regulated medical waste from health care facilities should be based on scientifically sound epidemiological and microbiological information.

Costs

Escalating health care costs are a growing concern to both the public and governmental officials. Regulated medical waste is only one component of these costs, but it is one that can be reduced by adopting the uniform definitions and treatment recommendations contained in this document.

As mandated by Congress in the MWTA, the EPA has conducted a demonstration project to regulate and track medical waste. As the result of this project, which terminated in June 1991, the EPA is to provide Congress with recommendations for managing medical waste. The definition of medical waste used in this program includes "any solid waste generated in the diagnosis, treatment, or immunization of human beings or animals" and specifies seven classes of regulated medical waste.

The EPA originally estimated that the average cost per hospital for complying with the MWTA would be $3,757 per year. Several studies have shown that the actual costs to hospitals are many times more than that. In one anecdotal example, a New York teaching/medical center reported an increase in the amount of regulated medical waste of 315% between 1984 (443,000 lb) to 1989 (1,837,000 lb). The cost increased 700% from $106,000 to $835,000 per year largely as a result of considering a larger portion of medical waste as regulated medical waste and the resultant higher cost of treatment and disposal.[7]

Another study conducted by the Voluntary Hospitals of America showed that when 10 sample hospitals went to MWTA requirements from the previous CDC guidelines, their increased costs of complying with the new rules ranged from $80,000 to $700,000 per year. Again, these higher costs were due to both increased amounts of regulated waste and higher costs of treatment and disposal.[8]

Such cost increases will be incurred by health care providers and passed directly on to the public. In an era of healthcare cost containment, it is critical that any new rules and regulations for managing regulated medical waste be based on scientific evidence of need and demonstrated benefit to public health and the environment.

Definition of Regulated Medical Waste

Although it is generally agreed that regulated medical waste refers to that portion of medical waste that has the potential to transmit infectious disease, no uniform definition of what constitutes regulated medical waste has been universally accepted. Any definition of

Continued

BOX 32-2 | **AORN Position Statement: Regulated Medical Waste Definition and Treatment: a Collaborative Document—cont'd**

waste capable of causing infectious disease must consider the factors related to induction of such disease in humans:

- There must be the presence of a pathogen. Pathogens are microorganisms that can cause infection. Many microorganisms are incapable of causing infection in humans.
- The pathogen must be of sufficient virulence. Virulence is the disease-evoking power of a microorganism. Not all pathogens are equally capable of causing infectious disease.
- The pathogen must be present in sufficient dose. There must be a sufficient number of microorganisms present for infection to occur. This number varies with several factors (eg, organism type, host susceptibility, portal of entry).
- The organisms must have a portal of entry or a way to get into the body (eg, puncture, cut, wound).
- There must be a susceptible host. All persons are not equally susceptible to infectious diseases.[9]

Because it is not practical or realistic to assay medical waste to determine the presence and number of suspected pathogens, the identification of regulated medical waste tends to focus on the potential presence of pathogens and possible portal of entry.

Based on these considerations, there are four categories of medical waste that should be included in the definition of regulated medical waste because of risk they represent to the public health and the environment.

Sharps (used and unused). Discarded medical devices that have been used in animal or human patient care, medical research, or industrial laboratories and that are capable of puncturing or cutting the skin, thereby creating a portal of entry, should be classified as regulated medical waste. This includes, but is not limited to, needles; syringes with needles attached; trocars; pipettes; scalpel blades; blood vials; and broken or unbroken glassware that has been in contact with infectious agents, including serum culture bottles, slides, and coverslips.

Rationale. Used sharps have been associated with injury and disease transmission in occupational settings and represent the greatest hazard for health care workers and trash handlers because of potential contamination with infectious agents and their ability to cause a portal of entry. Unused sharps are included since it may not be apparent whether discarded sharps have been used or not.

Cultures and stocks of infectious wastes. Discarded cultures and stocks of infectious agents and associated microbiologicals should be considered regulated medical waste. This category includes human and animal cell cultures from medical and pathological laboratories; cultures and stocks of infectious agents from research and industrial laboratories; wastes from the production of biologicals; discarded live and attenuated vaccines; and culture dishes and devices used to transfer, inoculate, and mix cultures of infectious agents.

Rationale. Cultures and stocks of infectious agents pose a potential risk for disease transmission because they have a higher number of microorganisms and therefore a higher potential for survival of sufficient numbers to produce disease. Also, they are usually in glass or plastic containers that, if broken, become contaminated sharps that can create a portal of entry.

Animal waste. Discarded material originating from animals inoculated with infectious agents during research or production of biological or pharmaceutical testing is regulated medical waste.

Examples are carcasses, body parts, blood, and bedding of animals known to have been in contact with infectious agents.

Rationale. These waste materials pose a potential risk because they can contain a sufficient number of viable infectious agents to cause disease provided an appropriate portal of entry is present in a susceptible host.

Selected isolation waste. Biological waste and discarded materials contaminated with blood, excretion, exudates, or secretions from humans who are isolated to protect others from certain highly virulent diseases (ie, Class 4 etiologic agents) or from isolated animals known to be infected with these diseases should be treated as regulated medical waste.

Rationale. Although very rarely seen in the United States, there are certain highly virulent diseases, such as Lassa fever, that deserve special mention. These diseases are caused by Class 4 etiologic agents as defined by the CDC, and waste from patients treated in isolation for these diseases should be considered regulated medical waste.[10]

The following two categories of waste are usually included in regulated medical waste, not because they pose any environmental or public health risks but because of aesthetic concerns of the public.

Pathological waste. Discarded pathological wastes (eg, human tissues, organs, body parts) removed during surgery, autopsy, or other medical procedures.

Human blood, blood products, body fluids. This category includes discarded free-flowing human blood and blood products (eg, plasma, serum), any free-flowing body secretion containing blood components (eg, pleural, peritoneal, amniotic fluid), and any other fluid visibly contaminated with blood. Human excretions (eg, urine, stool) are specifically excluded because they have accepted means of disposal.

Rationale. Although blood, blood products, and body fluids containing blood components may represent an occupational hazard, especially in the presence of sharps, they do not pose a risk to public health or the environment when disposed of properly. We recognize that these substances present a heightened concern to the public; however, scientific information and practical experience have demonstrated that they only need to be included from an aesthetic viewpoint.

Disposal, Treatment of Regulated Medical Waste

For the four categories that pose some public health risk, some treatment to reduce the microbiological content is recommended. Methods usually employed to decontaminate medical waste are divided into three general categories: heat treatment (eg, incineration, autoclaving, microwaving, pyrolysis), chemical treatment (eg, hypochlorite, chlorine dioxide), and, much less popular, radiation treatment (eg, gamma ray, electron beam).[11] Each method's efficacy and efficiency depends on factors such as contact time; bioload (ie, number of microorganisms in the material to be treated); and organic content, volume, and physical state of the waste (ie, liquid, solid). The presence of other waste products (eg, radioisotopes, hazardous chemicals) also must be taken into account when determining the proper method of waste treatment.

For the categories that represent aesthetic concerns, there are recognized standard practices for dealing with this waste. Pathological waste should be incinerated or interred. Free-flowing blood and body fluids should be discarded into a sanitary sewer system taking

---

BOX 32-2 | **AORN Position Statement: Regulated Medical Waste Definition and Treatment: a Collaborative Document—cont'd**

proper precautions to prevent exposure to those dispensing the fluid into the drain.

Although there are no known health risks associated with the current treatment technologies, further research of efficacy, cost, and environmental impact needs to be done to allow valid scientific comparisons.

Notes

1. "Occupational exposure to bloodborne pathogens; Final rule," *Federal Register* 56 (Dec 6, 1991) 64175.

2. W A Rutala, R I Odette, G P Samsa, "Management of infectious waste by US hospitals," *Journal of the American Medical Association* 262 (Sept 22, 1989) 1635-1640.

3. Agency for Toxic Substances and Disease Registry, *The Public Health Implications of Medical Waste: A Report to Congress* (Atlanta: US Department of Health & Human Services, 1990).

4. *Ibid.*

5. "Performance-oriented packaging standards," *Federal Register* 56 (Dec 20, 1991) 66144-66145.

6. W A Rutala, C G Mayhall, "SHEA position paper: Medical waste," *Infection Control and Hospital Epidemiology* 13 (January 1992) 43-44.

7. J T Marchese et al, "Regulated medical waste disposal at a university and university hospital: Future implications," paper presented at the Third International Conference on Nosocomial Infections, Atlanta, August, 1990.

8. *Modern Healthcare,* 4 Nov 1991, 19; *Medical Waste News,* 3:22, 31 Oct 1991, 169-170.

9. US Environmental Protection Agency, *Infectious Waste Management Guidelines* (Springfield, Va: National Technical Information Service, 1986).

10. American Hospital Association, *Shaping State and Local Regulation of Medical Waste and Hazardous Materials: A Report of the Ad Hoc Committee on Medical Waste and Hazardous Materials* (Chicago: American Hospital Association, 1990).

11. Agency for Toxic Substances and Disease Registry, *The Public Health Implications of Medical Waste: A Report to Congress.*

The following organizations participated in the Atlanta meeting. Participation does not imply endorsement. Some organizations have a nonendorsement policy or have individual position statements on this issue.

American Association of Critical-Care Nurses
American Association of Nurse Anesthetists
American College of Surgeons
American Hospital Association
American Society for Microbiology
American Society of Anesthesiologists
Association of Operating Room Nurses, Inc
Association of Practitioners in Infection Control
Centers for Disease Control and Prevention
Emergency Nurses Association
Medical Waste Institute
Society of Hospital Epidemiologists of America
University of North Carolina School of Medicine

The following organizations have reviewed and endorsed this document as of June 30, 1997:

Academy of Medical-Surgical Nurses
American Association of Critical-Care Nurses
American Association of Nurse Anesthetists
American Association of Occupational Health Nurses, Inc
American College of Surgeons
American Nephrology Nurses Association
American Nurses Association
Association of Operating Room Nurses, Inc
Emergency Nurses Association
Healthcare Resource Conservation Coalition
Oncology Nursing Society
ONE-California

Ratified by House of Delegates March 14, 1994

From *AORN standards, recommended practices, and guidelines.* (1997). Denver, Colo.: Association of Operating Room Nurses, pp. 33-36.

(Box 32-3) supports the ongoing examination of waste management and notes implications specific to perioperative practice and contributions that can be made by the nurse. The perioperative nurse advocating a cleaner environment should pursue the following:

1. Increase awareness of the problem and become intensely involved with both federal and state regulatory agencies regarding management of medical waste and infectious waste.
2. Become part of the solution by closely evaluating the products that are to be used in the operating room.
3. Consider using reusable items instead of disposables and evaluate options for reprocessing of single-use sterile items.

BOX 32-3 | **AORN Position Statement on Protection of the Environment**

AORN recognizes that aspects of perioperative practice result in the generation of medical waste that impacts the environment. The Association strongly supports efforts to improve and preserve the environment through judicious selection, management, and disposal of surgical supplies and through environmentally sound programs of waste management. The Association encourages individual members to participate in research, to promote education, and to dialogue with others for the purpose of developing effective means to reduce the environmental impact of surgical waste.

From *AORN standards, recommended practices, and guidelines.* (1998). Denver, Colo.: Association of Operating Room Nurses, p. 30.

4. Select and evaluate surgical products wisely to decrease unnecessary medical waste.
5. Educate colleagues and the general public. Become an advocate for the environment. Many are unaware of the acute problem of medical waste management both on a professional and personal level.

Every perioperative nurse must accept this challenge, examine what changes can be initiated, and implement these changes accordingly. Perioperative nurses must be proactive in preserving the environment not only for themselves, but also for future generations.

ETHICAL ISSUES

The nursing profession is involved with ethical decisions related to healthcare reform: the continuous surge of technology, how it is used, and who benefits from it; aggressive surgery for the terminally ill; and decisions of patients' access to needed services by managed care companies. The perioperative nurse is not immune to ethical dilemmas and the influence that ethical decision making has. Ethical decisions are especially critical for surgical patients who are sedated or unconscious and unable to provide decisions related to their care. As the patient's advocate, the perioperative nurse may have to intervene on behalf of the patient's rights and wishes.

Ethical situations specific to the perioperative setting may result from a technical error made by the surgeon, who then requests no documentation be made of the incident; performing surgery on a brain-dead child for the sake of the family; issues of mandatory HIV testing for both the patient and healthcare worker; having unauthorized persons present in the operating room during a procedure; suspected drug abuse by one of the team members; operating on the wrong patient or wrong side; rushing "do-not-resuscitate" patients to the postanesthesia care unit to expire; performing additional procedures not listed on surgical consent; and unclear criteria for confirming death in a patient.

Perioperative nurses dealing with what is ethically and morally right or wrong should base their decisions and actions in accordance with the ANA Code for Nurses with Interpretive Statement—Explications for Perioperative Nursing.[30] These professional codes of conduct establish expectations for the perioperative nurse, who is accountable for upholding them and being responsible to the public, healthcare team members, and the profession of nursing.

Many perioperative nurses are members of their institution's nursing ethics committee. Nursing ethics committees allows nurses to focus on ethical problems that might otherwise be avoided on a hospital-wide ethics committees (such as nurse-physician conflicts). Nursing ethics committees serve as a resource for evaluation of existing ethical standards of care such as organ procurement, do-not-resuscitate protocol, patient rights, informed consent, and patient confidentiality. Members of the nursing ethics committee assist staff by facilitating a better understanding of ethical principles and decision making.

Organ Procurement

Most perioperative nurses have participated in organ procurement. For many the most difficult time occurs when the organs are procured and the anesthesia machine is turned off. The procurement team departs quickly to implant the organs, anesthesia personnel are gone, and the perioperative nurse is left to prepare the patient for the family. This should not overshadow the opportunities offered to the recipients, but in reality it is a difficult time for the surgical team and especially the perioperative nurse.

Since the 1970s there has been widespread acceptance of guidelines for brain death and criteria that allow the patient to become a candidate as a heart-beating cadaver donor. More recently, because of the increasing need for organs, the University of Pittsburgh Medical Center and the Regional Organ Bank of Illinois have become pioneers in new criteria and protocols for organ donors that differ from the traditional method of using brain death as a determinant.

The University of Pittsburgh is using cardiopulmonary status as a determinant for non–heart beating cadaver donors, for which the timing and place of death are controlled.[34] The Pittsburgh protocol involves the family decision of forgoing all life-sustaining treatment. When this decision has been made, consent is obtained from the family. The patient is then transported to the operating room, and the organs are removed immediately after pronouncement of death. It is preferable that the surgical team is not present in the operating room until death has been declared. The certification of death is met when the following criteria have been determined: the patient who is apneic and unresponsive is weaned from the ventilator and may be administered sedatives and narcotics if pain is demonstrated; irreversible cessation of cardiac function must occur (2 minutes of pulselessness), and rigorous documentation accompanies the course of events.

The Regional Organ Bank of Illinois is using a protocol that includes infusing the kidneys with cold preservation solution at the time of uncontrolled death. Death is determined by cardiopulmonary criteria and usually involves patients who have undergone unsuccessful resuscitation or polytrauma. Initially, the center obtained permission before infusing the kidneys with preservation fluid. But because of the high incidence of family refusal, consent is no longer required. By proceeding with methods to preserve the kidneys, the families have more time for a final decision.

Both of these protocols present tremendously complex ethical dilemmas for the medical profession, nursing profession, and society. Although death is a natural occurrence of life, it rarely is easy. What seems to be overlooked with both protocols is the involvement of family at the time of death. With one protocol the patient, in essence, dies without the presence of loved ones. The other involves the intervention of preserving the kidneys without the family's permission. The definition of death and whether death is being hastened for the supply and demand of available organs can be made an issue. In addition, the surgical team may feel that they are participating in the termination of life.

As new opportunities arise to meet the endless list of recipients for donated organs, new ethical dilemmas emerge. The professionals, patients, and society will need to discuss these issues and come to a common understanding for application of new criteria and practices for procuring organs from non–heart-beating cadaver donors.

Do-Not-Resuscitate Orders

The do-not-resuscitate order "is deemed clinically, ethically, and legally appropriate when resuscitation would be futile and would prolong the patient's death."[22] It is common practice in the operating room to suspend do-not-resuscitate (DNR) orders when the patient is undergoing a surgical procedure, since surgery on a DNR patient may be performed for a variety of reasons. Most often it is related to an attempt to decrease patient suffering (such as decreasing pain related to an obstruction or pressure from a growing mass). Although surgery is not curative for the terminally ill patient, it may offer an opportunity for an increased level of comfort and may increase the quality of life. Ethically, DNR orders suspended in the operating room could be challenged, based on refusal or lack of recognition by the surgical team to implement a patient's legal right, even if the result is death.[22]

Institutions are increasingly becoming aware of the ethical inconsistencies that exist when DNR orders are suspended in the operating room. The AORN Position Statement on Perioperative Care of Patients with Do-Not-Resuscitate Orders[10] states that "automatically suspending a DNR order during surgery undermines a patient's right to self-determination" (Box 32-4).

Many institutions are developing interdisciplinary policies addressing DNR orders specific for the operating room. Developing a policy for patients with advance directives, such as a living will that includes the patient's desire not to be resuscitated, allows for staff input and discussion on the ethical issues and concerns. Do-not-resuscitate orders are honored throughout an institution's various units. Why should this standard of care be any different for the operating room? A DNR policy should include a clear chain of communication for resolving questions about DNR orders and protocols to assist the surgical team in the event of death of any patient.[17] Today patients and families are participants in their own care, demanding to be heard and to be the final decision makers.

Advance Directives

The 1990 Patient Self-Determination Act requires hospitals, skilled nursing facilities, home health agencies, and hospice agencies to ask patients if they have advance directives. The bill requires every patient to be given written information regarding their rights under state law to accept or refuse medical care and to write advance directives. Advance directives may be written instructions through a living will, which specifies the patient's present and future decisions for medical care in the event they become unable to participate in decisions regarding their care. A living will should address the patient's preference for life-sustaining treatment (such as resuscitation orders and ventilator use). All 50 states have living-will laws.[29]

Durable power of attorney is another option for the patient. In this document, the patient has designated a person to act on the patient's behalf in the event the patient is unable to do so. This document is also recognized by most states. If an institution fails to comply with the requirements of the Patient Self-Determination Act it could lose Medicare and Medicaid funding.

Unfortunately, only about 15% of adults have any type of signed advance directives.[25] Although living wills or durable power of attorney are recognized by all states, state law requirements vary and should be reviewed. The perioperative nurse should be aware of the state's requirements for advance directives, required documentation, and institution policy (Research Highlight 32-2). As an advocate for the patient, the nurse must monitor that the patient's wishes and intent are followed.

OPERATING ROOM RISK MANAGEMENT

The Association of Operating Room Nurses has developed Standards of Perioperative Nursing, which include Standards of Clinical Practice and Standards of Professional Performance.[11] These standards are developed from the American Nurses Association Standards of Clinical Nursing Practice. The standards, which are broad in scope, relevant, attainable, and definitive, serve as the foundation for the practice of perioperative nursing. In addition, AORN develops recommended practices that address technical areas of perioperative care and guidelines that are based on scientific evidence. The AORN Standards of Practice, Recommended Practices, and Guidelines delineate expected competencies for the perioperative nurse. Frequently, these are used in malpractice lawsuits to determine whether reasonable and prudent care was provided for the patient by the perioperative nurse and surgical team.

Nurses are responsible for maintaining competency through current knowledge and skills in their given specialty of practice. Knowledge and skills may be enhanced through a variety of educational activities. The nurse must be aware of national standards, guidelines,

BOX 32-4	AORN Position Statement: Perioperative Care of Patients with Do–Not–Resuscitate (DNR) Orders

Preamble

Nurses have a responsibility to uphold the rights of patients.[1] A patient with a do-not-resuscitate (DNR) order may require surgical procedures and anesthesia management. These procedures often are for palliative care, to relieve pain or distress, to facilitate care, or to improve the patient's quality of life. A DNR order should not mean that all treatment is stopped and the need for medical and nursing care is eliminated, but rather that the patient has made certain choices about end-of-life decisions.[2] A patient's rights do not stop at the entrance to the operating room.[3] Automatically suspending a DNR order during surgery undermines a patient's right to self-determination.[4] Development of a policy related to DNR orders in the operating room is supported by the Patient Self-Determination Act,[5] the Joint Commission on Accreditation of Healthcare Organizations (JCAHO), the "ANA code for nurses with interpretative statements—explications for perioperative nursing,"[6] and *A Patient's Bill of Rights.*[7]

Position Statement

Required reconsideration of DNR decisions with patients is an integral component of the care of patients undergoing surgery.[8] Required reconsideration of DNR decisions ensures that the risks and benefits of anesthesia and surgery are discussed by health care providers and patients or patients' surrogate decision makers before surgery.

Guidelines

Patient autonomy must be respected as the professional responsibility of the health care team.[9] The patient's physicians are responsible for discussing and documenting issues with the patient and/or family to determine whether the DNR order is to be maintained or completely or partially suspended during anesthesia and surgery. The discussion needs to describe potential resuscitation efforts during surgery and whether withholding resuscitation compromises the patient's basic objectives for surgery.[10] Discussion involved with the required reconsideration should include

- the goals of the surgical treatment,
- the possibility of resuscitative measures,
- a description of what these measures include, and
- possible outcomes with and without resuscitation.

If the patient has chosen to suspend the DNR order during the intraoperative period, it should be documented when the DNR order is to be reinstated.

Preoperatively, communication among the health care team, the patient, and the patient's family about DNR decisions must occur. Adequate information must be given so that the surgical team supports the patient's or the patient's surrogate's right to participate in the health care decision.[11] A method of communication needs to be developed so that all health care team members are informed of the patient's decision. Following the discussion, the decision and plan must be clearly documented and communicated to all health care providers potentially involved in the perioperative care of the patient. Throughout the process, the patient has the right to modify any decision, and this also must be communicated to all involved health care providers. Patient situations that may require further ethical deliberation before surgical intervention may benefit from consultation with the hospital's ethics advisory committee.

The perioperative nurse, as a patient advocate, has a moral responsibility to the patient.[12] If the perioperative nurse has a moral objection to the patient's decision, he or she should be allowed to make a reasonable effort to find another nurse willing to provide care to the patient. If another nurse is not available, the patient's decision will be upheld with recognition that there are times when a patient's wishes take precedence in a clinical situation.

Operational Definitions

The following are operational definitions of terms used in the statement.

Do-not-resuscitate (DNR) order. A specific directive, written by a physician, mandating that cardiopulmonary resuscitation should not be performed.[13]

Do-not-resuscitate (DNR) decision. The patient's or surrogate's directives regarding end-of-life choices.

Required reconsideration. An event that allows a patient or surrogate to participate in decisions about the use of cardiopulmonary resuscitation and that offers caregivers an opportunity to explain the significance of cardiac arrest and resuscitation in the perioperative setting.[14]

Health care team. Nurses, physicians, and all others involved in clinical disciplines.[15]

Notes

1. S Igoe, S Cascella, K Stockdale, "Ethics in the OR: DNR and patient autonomy," *Nursing Management* 24 (September 1993) 112A, 112D, 112H.

2. J M Reeder, "Do-not-resuscitate orders in the operating room," *AORN Journal* 57 (April 1993) 947-951.

3. S J Youngner, H F Cascorbi, J M Shuck, "DNR in the operating room: Not really a paradox," *Journal of the American Medical Association* 266 (November 1991) 2433-2434.

4. Igoe, Cascella, Stockdale, "Ethics in the OR: DNR and patient autonomy," 112A, 112D, 112H.

5. *Patient Self-Determination Act,* Public Law 101-508, *Federal Register* 57 (March 6, 1992).

6. "ANA code for nurses with interpretive statements—explications for perioperative nursing," in *AORN Standards and Recommended Practices* (Denver: Association of Operating Room Nurses, Inc, 1994) 39-56.

7. American Hospital Association, *A Patient's Bill of Rights,* second ed (Chicago: American Hospital Association, 1994).

8. C B Cohen, P J Cohen, "Required reconsideration of 'do-not-resuscitate' orders in the operating room and certain other treatment settings," *Law, Medicine & Health Care* 20 (Winter 1992) 354-363.

9. Igoe, Cascella, Stockdale, "Ethics in the OR: DNR and patient autonomy," 112A, 112D, 112H.

10. P Patterson, "Suspension of DNR orders in the OR being questioned," *OR Manager* 8 (February 1992) 1, 5-8.

11. Reeder, "Do-not-resuscitate orders in the operating room," 947-951.

12. M J Keffer, H L Keffer, "The do-not-resuscitate order: Moral responsibilities of the perioperative nurse," *AORN Journal* 54 (March 1994) 641-650.

| BOX 32-4 | **AORN Position Statement: Perioperative Care of Patients with Do-Not-Resuscitate (DNR) Orders—cont'd** |

13. Cohen, Cohen, "Required reconsideration of 'do-not-resuscitate' orders in the operating room and certain other treatment settings," 354-363.

14. *Ibid.*

15. J L Levenson, L Pettrey, "Controversial decisions regarding treatment and DNR: An algorithmic guide for the uncertain in decision-making ethics (GUIDE)," *American Journal of Critical Care* 3 (March 1994).

Suggested reading

American College of Surgeons. "Statement of the American College of Surgeons on Advance Directives by Patients: 'Do Not Resuscitate' in the Operating Room." *ACS Bulletin* 79 (September 1994) 29.

American Nurses Association Center for Human Rights Task Force. *Compendium of Position Statements on the Nurse's Role in End-of-Life Decisions.* Washington, DC: American Nurses Association, 1993.

American Society of Anesthesiologists. "Ethical guidelines for the anesthesia care of patients with do-not-resuscitate orders or

other directives that limit care." In *ASA Standards, Guidelines, and Statements.* Park Ridge, Ill: American Society of Anesthesiologists, 1993.

Keffer, M J; Keffer, H L. "Do-not-resuscitate in the operating room: Moral obligation of anesthesiologists." *Anesthesia and Analgesia* 74 (June 1992) 901-905.

Tomlinson, T; Brody, H. "Futility and the ethics of resuscitation." *Journal of the American Medical Association* 264 (September 1990) 1276-1280.

Walker, R M. "DNR in the OR: Resuscitation as an operative risk." *Journal of the American Medical Association* 266 (November 1991) 2407-2412.

Submitted: 3/95
Adopted: 3/6/95
House of Delegates,
Atlanta, Georgia
Sunset review: 3/2000

From *AORN standards, recommended practices, and guidelines.* (1997). Denver, Co o.: Association of Operating Room Nurses, pp. 18-19.

32-2 RESEARCH HIGHLIGHT

Weiler et al. conducted a study questionnaire on "Iowa Nurses Knowledge of Cancer Pain and Living Wills." The questionnaire was designed to answer the following questions: (1) Were Iowa nurses aware of the living-will statute? (2) What sources of information did nurses use to learn about this legislation? (3) What were nurses' perceptions of patients' rights? (4) What were nurses' perceptions of the nurses' role involving living wills? (5) Were living wills followed? (6) If not followed, which factors contributed to the failure to honor a living will? (7) Which communication mechanisms were used to alert nurses to a living will? The questionnaire was mailed to 10,000 registered nurses and licensed practical nurses throughout the state with a response rate of 27%. Seventy percent were aware of Iowa's living-will legislation; sources of information included professional journals, media, continuing education programs, colleagues, and their own advance directives. Overall the nurses supported the belief that the patient should have control over healthcare treatment decisions. Only 39% indicated that it was a nursing responsibility to give information to patients and families regarding advance directives; 56% indicated that living wills were honored; family opposition was cited as the most frequent reason for not following living-will terms; and the patient's medical record was cited as the most frequent source for identifying an existing living will. Recommendations from the study include the development of institution educational programs to update nurses on current legislation and skills for dealing with opposition from family members and other members of the healthcare team. It was also suggested that nurses should set an example by having their own living wills.

From Weiler, K., Eland, J., & Buckwalter, K.C. (1996). Iowa nurses' knowledge of living wills and perceptions of patient autonomy. *Journal of Professional Nursing, 12*(4), 245-252.

---

recommended practices, and the institution's standard of care. The nurse should follow them accordingly; failure could result in legal implications if patient harm occurs. When an incident occurs, an incident report is usually required to be completed by the nurse. Various types of incidents may occur related to an act of the patient, equipment and supplies, medications, patient or visitor complaint, treatment or procedure, act of a visitor or caregiver or significant other, a fall, or the actual surgical procedure. Documentation should include the outcome of the incident and actions taken after the incident. Only factual comments should be documented without speculation on the cause or blaming anyone for the incident. Incident reports are forwarded to the risk management department. In the event of a medical lawsuit, an incident report may or may not be admitted as evidence, dependent on state law.

All nurses must be familiar with the scope and limitations of nursing practice in their individual states' practice acts under which they are licensed. They should know the standards of nursing practice and implementation, attend education activities that will enhance or maintain nursing knowledge, and keep abreast of current issues by reading nursing literature. Standards of nursing practice are integrated into everyday practice and generally are documented as standards of care for an institution.

PEW HEALTH PROFESSIONS COMMISSION

Tracking state responses to the Pew Commission recommendations for healthcare work force regulation is one of the top-ranked legislative priorities for the AORN. In 1989, the Pew Health Professions Commission convened as a think tank to address issues to assist healthcare professionals, legislators, regulators, work-force policy makers, and institutions meet the needs of the future healthcare system. The initial intent of the commission was to develop a guide to aid in the survival and thriving of evolving healthcare forces. The outcome included recommendations for all healthcare professionals, allied health, medicine, nursing, and public health. These recommendations were based on predictions that indicate an alarming surplus of 200,000 to 300,000 nurses, 150,000 physicians, and 40,000 pharmacists.[26]

Later the commission convened a task force to address health professionals' education, governance, credentialing, and regulation. The task force released 10 recommendations and policy options for state consideration. The following summarizes the Pew Health Professions Commission Taskforce on Health Care Workforce Regulation report.

Recommendation One: Standardizing Regulatory Terms

This recommendation suggests that "states should use standardized and understandable language for health professions regulation and its functions to clearly describe them for consumers, provider organizations, businesses, and the professions."[28] Misuse of terms such as licensure, certification, and registration were cited. For example RNs are licensed, not registered; certified patient care technicians are certified by a hospital; and a CNOR certification is by a private accrediting body after successful completion of a standardized national examination. The inconsistent terminology creates confusion among the healthcare professionals, regulators, legislators, and consumers. The task force suggests that states' future use of the term "licensure" should be limited to any regulation of practice acts and title protection and the use of the term

"certification" should be reserved for use of private-sector credentialing bodies.

Recommendation Two: Standardizing Entry-to-Practice Requirements

"States should standardize entry-to-practice requirements and limit them to competence assessments for health professions to facilitate the physical and professional mobility of the health professions."[27] The task force suggested that policy options for states include adopting uniform professional entry-to-practice standards, adopting mutual recognition of licensure through endorsement legislation, partnering with private-sector bodies and states to develop standardized competency examinations to test competence, entry-to-practice requirements through alternatives such as experience, and eliminating entry-to-practice standards that do not contribute to competence, skills, training, or knowledge.

Nursing has been successful with the administration of a standardized national examination that is recognized by all states allowing for interstate mobility. Through endorsement the RN may obtain licensure in a state other than the original state of licensure. However this is not the case for many professionals (such as dentists). Today's integrated healthcare delivery systems, telemedicine, downsizing, and increasing population mobility necessitate standardization of entry-to-practice requirements for all professionals.

Recommendation Three: Removing Barriers to the Full Use of Competent Health Professionals

Recommendation three suggests that "states should base practice acts on demonstrated initial and continuing competence. This process must allow and expect different professions to share overlapping scopes of practice. States should explore pathways to allow all professionals to provide services to the full extent of their current knowledge, training, experience, and skills."[27] The task force suggests that states eliminate exclusive scopes of practice that unnecessarily restrict other professionals from providing care that is competent, effective, and accessible; allow for provision of same services by different professionals who can demonstrate knowledge, training, experience, and skills; grant title protection without accompanying scope of practice acts for some professions; and allow individual professionals to practice "overlapping" scopes of practice with the demonstration of appropriate competency.

Recommendation Four: Redesigning Board Structure and Function

"States should redesign health professional boards and their functions to reflect the interdisciplinary and public accountability demands of the changing healthcare delivery system."[27] A policy option for state consideration is the establishment of an interdisciplinary oversight board to ensure that the public's best interest is reflected. The board's composition should include healthcare representatives with a majority of representatives from the state's public urban, rural, ethnic, and cultural communities. The board would have authority to approve, amend, and reject any decision made by an individual state board. It is recommended that the board structure and function be consolidated around service areas (such as medical and nursing care, vision healthcare, and oral healthcare). The task force also suggests that "board membership include significant, meaningful and effective public representation to improve board credibility and accountability."[27] The boards should be staffed and financed to perform their missions efficiently and effectively.

Recommendation Five: Informing the Public

Recommendation five states that "boards should educate consumers to assist them in obtaining the information necessary to make decisions about practitioners and to improve the board's public accountability."[27] The public is entitled to information on their healthcare professionals, and the task force recommends that the state collect such information (that is, demographics, education, practice, employment, disciplinary actions, criminal convictions, and malpractice judgments). This information should be made accessible and understandable to the consumer unless forbidden by the state law.

Because many health professional regulatory boards do not disclose specific information on individual practitioners, it is perceived as inaccessible. Nursing has always been a strong supporter of the public's right to be informed about their health professional providers. In addition, nursing supports the disclosure of information regarding staffing levels, mix, and patient outcomes. Legislation will be reintroduced in the 105th Congress requiring these disclosures and whistleblower protection for those reporting unsafe patient conditions.[13,33]

Recommendation Six: Collecting Data on the Health Professional

"Boards should cooperate with other public and private organizations in collecting data on regulated health professions to support effective workforce planning."[27] Without current and reliable data, policy makers are limited on how to best guide decisions related to public policy. Data-set elements might include primary and secondary specialty, board or specialty certification, continuing education completed, hospital admitting privileges, ethnic origin, institutions attended for education and professional training, research and teaching activities, practice location, and licenses and certificates from other states. State boards are in key positions to collect essential information that is key in shaping work-force policy and planning.

Recommendation Seven: Assuring Practitioner Competence

Recommendation seven suggests that "states should require each board to develop, implement, and evaluate continuing competency requirements to assure the continuing competence of regulated health care professionals."[27] The task force recommends that states consider a policy that requires demonstration of competency for regulated health professionals through appropriate testing mechanisms. Testing mechanisms could include a variety of markers such as the number of disciplinary actions, lack of specialty or private certification, length of time in solo practice number of procedures performed, peer review (such as targeted or random), or others as determined. The issue is that the public is protected. Credentials required in the beginning of one's career change and practitioners must continually update their knowledge, skills, and clinical judgment.

Recommendation Eight: Reforming the Professional Disciplinary Process

"States should maintain a fair, cost-effective, and uniform disciplinary process to exclude incompetent practitioners to protect and promote the public's health."[27] There is concern regarding the present process of investigation, reporting, and disciplinary action of health professionals who have violated state statutes, rules, or regulations. The task force recommends that the process and oversight for investigating complaints, resolution, and disciplinary action should be assigned to an existing or newly established authoritative body to ensure that all professional boards are acting in the best interest of the public. States should establish a single process to assure that all complaints are handled in an objective manner. Involved parties should be regularly informed of investigation status, and this information should be accessible to the public.

Recommendation Nine: Evaluating Regulatory Effectiveness

"States should develop evaluation tools that assess the objectives, successes, and shortcomings of their regulatory systems and bodies to best protect and promote the public's health."[27] It is important to determine if regulatory boards are effective in doing what they are intended to, that is, protecting and promoting the public's health. The task force recommends policy options for states to include some type of external and internal evaluations such as legislative sunset audit and review and a comprehensive internal self-assessment.

Recommendation Ten: Understanding the Organizational Context of Health Professions Regulation

"States should understand the links, overlaps and conflicts among their health care workforce regulatory systems and other systems which affect the education, regulation, and practice of health care practitioners and work to develop partnerships to streamline regulatory structures and processes."[27] Health professions regulation systems are inconsistent from state-to-state and are complex. The task force recommends a comprehensive analysis of the different systems and streamlining when appropriate, with the goal being a "state health professional regulator system that is standardized, accountable, flexible, effective, and efficient in protecting and promoting the public's health, safety, and welfare."[27]

Nursing's Response

The American Nurses Association (ANA) and the National Council of State Boards of Nursing (NCSBN) have published responses to the Pew Taskforce on Health Care Workforce Regulation.[2,23] The Association of Operating Room Nurses (AORN) responded to each report integrating comments and feedback from the perioperative nursing community.

The Pew Health Professions Commission will establish two new task forces to address issues of medical education federal policies, use of foreign medical graduates, and location of graduate health professions training and state regulatory reforms. A follow-up report on the responses to the Pew report recommendations is expected. Nursing will continue to track the ramifications at both state and federal levels.

Perioperative Nursing Implications

The perioperative nurse should continuously monitor and become active in state legislation regarding unlicensed assistive personnel and healthcare profession regulation. Many states have proposed legislation or movement regarding state licensure or registration of STs, use of unlicensed assistive personnel, and other related health profession regulations. Perioperative nurses should pay close attention to the third Pew recommendation of "removing barriers to the full use of competent health professionals." If states implement this recommendation, STs may be permitted to circulate and first assist provided that they can demonstrate competence.

AGENCY FOR HEALTH CARE POLICY AND RESEARCH

The 1970s brought about drastic changes in the United States healthcare system. Cost containment was key. Doing business as usual in healthcare was no longer acceptable. An outgrowth of this philosophy included new payment mechanisms such as prospective payment systems, health maintenance organizations (HMOs), managed care plans, and peer review organizations. These mechanisms, however, offered no answers and seemed to create more problems than they were developed to solve. Many consider the present healthcare system as wasteful and inefficient.

In an effort to offset upward spiraling of healthcare costs and increase the quality, Congress mandated the establishment of the Agency for Health Care Policy and Research (AHCPR). This agency is a part of the U.S. Department of Health and Human Services Public Health Service and its purpose is to support research designed to improved the quality of a specific health service, reduce the cost, and increase access to services. These services are provided by many functional components of the agency.

Evidence-based research for the AHCPR falls under the Office of the Forum for Quality and Effectiveness in Health Care, which is responsible for the development of performance measures, standards of quality, and review criteria and for updating AHCPR clinical guidelines. The office investigates practice variations and develops guidelines that may reduce clinically significant variations among physicians. For example, if a diagnostic procedure does not contribute to a beneficial outcome, it may not be recommended for a certain condition. The practitioner may choose to use it anyway, however, if deemed appropriate for that patient. It is believed that significant healthcare expenditures can be saved by the reduction of variations in practice for a given condition.

The AHCPR definition for clinical guidelines is "systematically developed statements to assist practitioner and patient decisions for appropriate health care for specific clinical circumstances." Guidelines assist the practitioner in managing patient care while allowing both the practitioner and patient alternative choices. Current guideline development for clinical conditions is based on needs and priority areas determined by the Medicare and Medicaid programs.

The intent of the guidelines is to provide the practitioner and patient with what is considered appropriate care specific to prevention, diagnosis, treatment, and management of a given clinical condition. Clinical conditions are selected for guideline development based on how frequently the clinical condition occurs, evidence that variation in practice occurs, risk to the population, and cost of treatment.

Once a guideline is developed, the most effective plan of care is described, based on scientific evidence obtained by means of a comprehensive review of the literature and consensus of the panel's clinical experts and consumer representatives. Up to now the following guidelines have been developed:

- Prediction, prevention, and early treatment of pressure ulcers in adults
- Acute pain management

- Urinary incontinence in the adult, 1996 update (see Chapter 15)
- Diagnosis and treatment of depressed outpatients in primary care settings
- Management of functional impairment caused by cataract in the adult
- Diagnosis and treatment of benign prostatic hyperplasia
- Sickle cell disease
- Otitis media with effusion
- Diagnosis and treatment of heart failure secondary to coronary vascular disease
- Poststroke rehabilitation
- HIV-positive asymptomatic patient: evaluation and early intervention
- Management of cancer-related pain
- Treatment of stage II and greater pressure ulcers
- Acute low back problems in adults
- Recognition and initial assessment of Alzheimer's disease
- Quality determinants of mammography
- Smoking cessation
- Unstable angina

Perioperative nurses should be aware of the AHCPR guidelines and use them appropriately in daily practice. One example of perioperative application into clinical practice is for the AHCPR pressure ulcer guideline.[21] Every perioperative patient should be assessed for factors that place the patient at increased risk for the development of pressure ulcers. Such factors might include patients with immobility, limited activity levels, incontinence, inadequate nutrition, altered level of consciousness, and dry, flaky, or scaling skin.

Patients at risk for pressure ulcer development are identified by the nurse and appropriate preventive interventions are initiated. A systematic inspection of the skin should be conducted before the patient is positioned and interventions are taken to prevent adverse effects related to positioning and external forces such as pressure, friction, and shearing applied. Several nursing interventions intended to prevent or decrease the risk for development of a pressure ulcer include:

- Padding and positioning bony prominences to protect the skin
- Cleansing skin to eliminate sources of contamination from fecal or urinary incontinence and chemical sources such as pooling of prep solutions
- Minimizing exposure to cold operating room temperature
- Draping patient in a manner to optimize moisture resistance to avoid pooling of fluids
- Using appropriate personnel to position patient so as to avoid skin injury caused by pressure, friction, and shear forces
- Applying protective padding to decrease friction around all pressure areas (such as heels, elbows, occiput, sacrum); doughnut devices should not be used

- Avoiding placing bony prominences (such as ankles and knees) in direct contact with each other
- Avoiding direct pressure on the trochanter when patient is placed in a lateral position, as well as padding knees, feet, dependent ankle, and dependent knee
- Determining patient's risk of pressure ulcer development and utilizing foam, alternating air, gel, or water mattress as procedure permits
- Assessing every patient for postural alignment, distribution of weight, balance, stability, and pressure point relief

Educational programs for preventing pressure ulcers in adults should be structured, organized, and comprehensive. All perioperative staff who assist in transporting, transferring, and positioning the surgical patient should participate. The perioperative nurse makes a major contribution in reducing the incidence of pressure ulcers for the surgical patient.

The AORN is active in guideline development and translation specific for care of the perioperative patient. Future nursing guideline development might include multispecialty and multidisciplinary representation with a focus on patient care for a given patient problem, population, or technology. The developed guideline would be published with endorsement or recognition of appropriate nursing and medical organizations and associations. To gain support and recognition, guideline development must be based on scientific research and not consensus alone.

SUMMARY

With over 2.2 million in their ranks, nurses are the largest group of healthcare professionals. The resulting changes in the evolving healthcare system are creating many challenges; within these challenges are unique opportunities for the perioperative nurse to make a significant effect on the delivery of care to the patient. Contemporary issues related to the reform of health care include reimbursement for nursing services, medical waste management, ethical dilemmas, risk management, and appropriate utilization of unlicensed assistive personnel and STs. Nurses are a powerful driving force in healthcare and will chart their own course in shaping a preferred future by developing new roles and responsibilities necessary for practice in the twenty-first century.

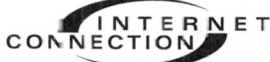

Virtual Medical Law Center:
http://www-sci.lib.uci.edu/HSGLegal.html

Merci Project (Cost Containment Issues):
http://www.med.Virginia.EDU/~hmf2e/merci.html

Agency for Health Care Policy and Research:
http://www.ahcpr.gov/

Medical Outcomes Trust: http://www.outcomes-trust.org

MCW Bioethics Online Service:
http://www.mcw.edu/bioethics/

MaClean Center for Clinical Medical Ethics:
http://ccme-mac4.bsd.uchicago.edu/CCMEHomePage.html

Advance Directives:
http://www.ama-assn.org/public/booklets/livgwill.htm

National Committee for Quality Assurance:
http:www.ncqa.org

Transcultural Nursing Society:
http://www.nursingcenter.com/people/nrsorgs/tcn/

AORN Governmental Affairs: http://www.aorn.org/GOVT/

FedWorld Information Network: http://www.fedworld.gov/

Legislative Information: http://thomas.loc.gov/

National Conference of State Legislatures:
http://www.ncsl.org/

Library of Congress:
http://lcweb.loc.gov/global/state/stategov.html#info

Hot Topics in Health Care: http://www.ahcpub.com/

AMSO Managed Care Forum: http://www.amso.com

Telemedicine Information Exchange: http://tie.telemed.org/

REFERENCES

1. Abbott, C. (1994). Intraoperative nursing activities performed by surgical technologists. *AORN Journal, 60*(3), 382-393.
2. American Nurses Association. (December 5, 1996a). *The American Nurses Association's response to the Pew report on health care workforce regulation.* Washington, D.C.: ANA.
3. American Nurses Association. (1996b). *Nursing quality indicators, definitions, and implications.* Washington, D.C.: ANA.
4. American Nurses Association. (1997). *Implementing nursing's report card: a study of RN staffing, length of stay and patient outcomes.* Washington, D.C.: ANA.
5. American Productivity and Quality Center. (1997). *The benchmarking code of conduct.* Houston, Texas: American Productivity and Quality Center.
6. Association of Operating Room Nurses. (1994). Business proceedings: regulated medical waste definition and treatment: a collaborative document. *AORN Journal, 59*(6), 1176-1183.
7. Association of Operating Room Nurses. (1998). AORN official position statement on unlicensed assistive personnel, 21-22. In *AORN standards, recommended practices, and guidelines.* Denver, Colo.: AORN.
8. Association of Operating Room Nurses. (1998). AORN official position statement on regulated medical waste definition and treatment: a collaborative document, 33-36. In *AORN standards, recommended practices, and guidelines.* Denver, Colo.: AORN.
9. Association of Operating Room Nurses. (1998). AORN official position statement on protection of the environment, 30. In *AORN standards, recommended practices, and guidelines.* Denver, Colo.: AORN.
10. Association of Operating Room Nurses. (1998). AORN official position statement on perioperative care of patients with do-not-resuscitate (DNR) orders, 18-19. In *AORN standards, recommended practices, and guidelines.* Denver, Colo.: AORN.
11. Association of Operating Room Nurses. (1998). *AORN standards, recommended practices, and guidelines.* Denver, Colo.: AORN.
12. AORN Policy Profile. (1996). *Regulation of surgical technologists.* Denver, Colo.: AORN.
13. Canavan, K. (July-August 1997). ANA, SNAs use legislation, grant programs to help nurses protect patients. *The American Nurse, 29*(4), 1-2.
14. Cassetta, R.A. (1993). Opening doors for advanced practice opportunities. *The American Nurse, 25*(6), 18-19.
15. Czarnecki, M.T. (1996). Benchmarking: a data-oriented look at improving health care performance. *Journal of Nursing Care Quality, 10*(3), 1-6.
16. Dahl B., & Beaman, C. (1997). *Skin care protocol: best practices.* Aliso Viejo, Calif.: The Best Practice Network.
17. Giordano, B. (1993). Symposium on the operating room environment. *AORN Journal, 58,* 340-344.
18. Hylka, S.C., & Beschle, J.C. (1997). The role of advanced practice nurses in surgical services. *AORN Journal, 66*(3), 481-485.
19. Keepnews, D. (1997). Does APRN:MD = UAP:RN? *The American Nurse, 29*(4), 7.
20. Krampf, L. (1996). Health care 'report cards' go on sale at newsstands. *OR Manager, 12*(3), 18.
21. Meeker, M., Carelock, H., Gregory, B., et al. *From guidelines to practice: interpreting the clinical practice guideline for pressure ulcers in adults for perioperative patient care.* AORN Pre-Congress, February 27, 1993, Anaheim, Calif.
22. Murphy, E. (1993). Do-not-resuscitate orders in the OR. *AORN Journal, 58*(2), 399-401.
23. National Council of State Boards of Nursing. (August 1996). *Response to the Pew taskforce on health care workforce regulation.* Chicago: National Council of State Boards of Nursing.
24. OR Manager. (1995). Hospital consortium collaborates on benchmarking. *OR Manager, 11*(5), 13.
25. Ott, B.B., & Hardie, T.L. (1997, First Quarter). Readability of advance directive documents. *Image Journal of Nursing Scholar, 29,* 53-57.
26. Pew Health Professions Commission. (1995a). *Critical challenges: revitalizing the health professions for the twenty-first century.* San Francisco, Calif.: UCSF Center for the Health Professions, p. i.
27. Pew Health Professions Commission. (1995b). *Reforming health care workforce regulation policy considerations for the twenty first century.* San Francisco, Calif.: UCSF Center for the Health Professions.
28. Reichert, M. (1993). Laparoscopic instruments. *AORN Journal, 57*(3), 637-655.
29. Rosen, L.F. (1996). Self-determination (part II). *Today's Surgical Nurse, 18*(5), 49-50.
30. Seifert, P.C., Killen, A.R., Bray, C.A., et al. (1993). ANA code for nurses with interpretive statements—explications for perioperative nursing. *AORN Journal, 58*(2), 369-388.
31. Shindul-Rothschild, J., Berry, D., & Long-Middleton, E. (1996). Where have all the nurses gone? final results of our patient care survey. *American Journal of Nursing, 96*(11), 25-39.
32. Tortorice, J., Martorella, C., Harlan, K., & Gertner, H. (1996). Clinical benchmarking carotid endarterectomy. *Surgical Services Management, 2*(11), 26-28.
33. Walker, J.F. (1996). Patient safety act of 1996 introduced. *AORN Journal, 60*(1), 119-121.
34. Youngener, S.J., & Arnold, R.M. (1993). Ethical, psychosocial, and public policy implications of procuring organs from non–heart beating cadaver donors. *Journal of the American Medical Association, 269*(21), 2769-2774.

Cover photo, Unit I photo, Courtesy Joseph T. Rothrock, III, Medical Photographer, Cooper Hospital/University Medical Center, Camden, New Jersey.

Chapter 1

1-1, Courtesy University of Pennsylvania School of Medicine, Philadelphia, Pennsylvania; **1-4,** Reprinted with permission from AORN *Clinical Path Template,* 1997, pp. 8-9. Copyright AORN, Inc., Denver, Colorado.

Chapter 2

2-1, Courtesy Valleylab, Inc., Pfizer Hospital Products Group, Boulder, Colorado; **2-2, 2-5,** Used with permission from Maine Medical Center, Brighton Campus, Portland, Maine; **2-3, 2-4,** From Beare, P.G., & Myers, J.L. (1998). *Principles and practices of adult health nursing* (ed. 3). St. Louis: Mosby.

Chapter 3

3-1, 3-38, 3-39, 3-44, Courtesy Olympus America, Inc., Melville, New York; **3-2,** From Bau, K.A. (1997) Endoscopic Surgery, St. Louis: Mosby; **3-3, 3-34, 3-35, 3-40, 3-43, 3-45,** Courtesy Circon ACMI, Santa Barbara, California; **3-5, 3-9, 3-10, 3-20,** Courtesy Karl Storz, Culver City, California; **3-6, 3-30,** Courtesy STERIS Corp., Mentor, Ohio; **3-7, 3-36, 3-37, 3-42, 3-46, 3-51,** Courtesy MP Video, Hopkinton, Massachussets; **3-11, 3-12, 3-13, 3-16, 3-22, 3-24, 3-58, 3-59, 3-61, 3-62, 3-64,** Courtesy Ethicon Endo-Surgery, Cincinnati, Ohio; **3-14, 3-18, 3-19, 3-21, 3-23, 3-25, 3-26, 3-27,** Copyright 1993 United States Surgical Corporation. All rights reserved. Reprinted with permission of United States Surgical Corporation; **3-17,** Courtesy Aesculap, Inc., South San Francisco, California; **3-28,** Courtesy Specialty Medical Systems, Shawnee Mission, Kansas; **3-29,** Courtesy API Airclean Systems, Raleigh, North Carolina; **3-41, A,** Courtesy O.R. Concepts, Inc., Burnsville, Minnesota; **3-41, B,** Courtesy Dexide, Inc., Fort Worth, Texas; **3-47,** Courtesy Computer Motion, Goleta, California; **3-48,** Courtesy United Medical Network, Dublin, Ohio; **3-49,** From Ponsky, J. (1992). *Atlas of surgical endoscopy,* St. Louis: Mosby; **3-52,** Courtesy Snowden-Pencer, Inc., Tucker, Georgia; **3-53, 3-54, 3-55, 3-56, 3-57,** From Ball, K. (1995). *Lasers: the perioperative challenge* (ed. 2). St. Louis: Mosby; **3-60, 3-63, 3-68,** Courtesy Valleylab, Inc., Boulder, Colorado; **3-65,** Courtesy Cabot Medical Corporation, Langhorne, Pennsylvania; **3-66,** Courtesy Sanese Medical Corporation, Columbus, Ohio; **3-67,** Courtesy Davol, Inc., Cranston, Rhode Island.

Chapter 4

4-1, Courtesy Charleston Area Medical Center; **4-2,** From Wong, D. (1995). *Whaley & Wong's nursing care of infants and children* (ed. 5). St. Louis: Mosby; **4-3, 4-5, 4-6,** Courtesy STERIS Corp., Mentor, Ohio.

Chapter 5

5-1, 5-2, Courtesy STERIS Corporation, Mentor, OH; **5-5,** From Atkinson, L.J., Fortunato, N.M. (1996) *Berry & Kohn's operating room technique* (ed. 8). St. Louis: Mosby.

Chapter 6

6-3, 6-6, 6-7, 6-8, 6-9, 6-10, 6-11, Davis & Geck (1992) surgical atlas and suture guide (ed. 2), 1992, American Cyanamid Co., Wayne, New Jersey; **6-4,** Courtesy 3M, St. Paul, Minnesota; **6-5,** From Atkinson, L.J., Fortunato, N.M. (1996) *Berry & Kohn's operating room technique* (ed. 8). St. Louis: Mosby; **6-14,** Courtesy Miltex Instrument Company; **6-21, 6-22, 6-23, 6-24, 6-25,** Brooks-Tighe, S.M. (1994). *Instrumentation for the operating room* (ed. 4). St. Louis: Mosby; **6-26, 6-27, 6-28, 6-29,** Copyright 1993 United States Surgical Corporation, Norwalk, Connecticut.

Chapter 7

7-1 From Atkinson, R.S., Rushman, G.B., & Lee, J.A. (1982). *A synopsis of anaesthesia.* London: John Wright & Sons, Ltd., Medical Publishers; **7-2, 7-3, 7-5, 7-7, 7-8, 7-9, 7-11, 7-13,** Courtesy Scott & White Memorial Hospital, Temple, Texas; **7-6,** Courtesy Brain Medical, Ltd.; **7-10,** Modified from Dripps, R.D., Eckenhoff, J.E., & Vandam, L.D. (1982). *Introduction to anesthesia: the principles of safe practice* (ed. 6). Philadelphia: W.B. Saunders.

Chapter 8

8-1, 8-2, From Litwack, K. (1995). *Post anesthesia care nursing* (ed. 2). St. Louis: Mosby; **8-3,** Courtesy Forrest General Hospital, Hattiesburg, Mississippi; **8-4, 8-5,** From Phipps, W.J., et al. (1995). *Medical-surgical nursing: concepts and clinical practice* (ed. 5). St. Louis: Mosby; **8-6,** Courtesy Augustine Medical, Minneapolis, Minnesota; **8-7, 8-8, ABC,** From Acute Pain Management Guideline Panel. (1992). Acute pain management in adults: operative procedures: quick reference guide for clinicians. *AHCPR* Pub. No. 92-0019. Rockville, Maryland: Agency for Health Care Policy and Research; **8-8, D,** From Wong, D.L. (1995). *Whaley & Wong's nursing care of infants and children* (ed. 5). St. Louis: Mosby; **8-9,** From Long, B.C., et al. (1993). *Medical-surgical nursing: a nursing process approach* (ed. 3). St. Louis: Mosby.

Chapter 9

9-1, From Bolton, L., & Rijswijk, L. (1991). Wound dressings: meeting clinical and biological needs. *Dermatology Nursing, 3*(3), 147; **9-2, 9-4, 9-7,** Courtesy Johnson and Johnson Patient Care, Inc., New Brunswick, New Jersey; **9-3,** From Gogia, P. (1992). The biology of wound healing. *Ostomy/Wound management, 38*(9), Nov/Dec 13; **9-5,** Courtesy Vanderbilt University Hospital, Nashville, Tennessee; **9-8,** Courtesy Zimmer, Inc., Warsaw, Indiana.

Chapter 10

10-1, 10-2, Courtesy Jenny Pierce, RN, MSN, CNS, Mother Francis Hospital, Tyler, Texas; **10-3,** From McHatton, M. (1985). A theory for timely teaching. *AJN, 85,* 799; **10-5, 10-6,** From Lorig, K. (1992). *Patient education: a practical approach,* (ed. 2). Thousand Oaks: Sage Publications.

Unit II photo, Courtesy Indiana University Medical Center, Indianapolis, Indiana. Used with permission from DePuy Orthopaedics, Inc., Warsaw, Indiana.

Chapter 11

11-2, From Thibodeau, G.A. (1990). *Anthony's textbook of anatomy and physiology* (ed. 13). St. Louis: Mosby; **11-10, 11-11, 11-12, 11-13, 11-15, 11-24, 11-26, 11-27, 11-28, 11-31, 11-32, 11-33,** Thompson, J.C. (1992). *Atlas of surgery of the stomach, duodenum, and small bowel.* St. Louis: Mosby; **11-17, 11-25, 11-34, 11-35, 11-36, 11-38, 11-39, 11-40, 11-41, 11-42,** From Bauer, J.J. (1993). *Colorectal surgery illustrated,* St. Louis: Mosby; **11-18, 11-19, 11-20, 11-21, 11-22,** *1, 2, 4,* **11-23,** Courtesy Codman & Shurtleff, Inc., Randolph, Massachusetts; **11-22,** *3,* Courtesy American V. Mueller, Deerfield, Illinois; **11-22,** *5,* Courtesy Edward Weck & Co., Research Triangle Park, North Carolina.

Chapter 12

12-1, 12-2, 12-12, 12-13, 12-16, 12-17, 12-19, 12-20, 12-21, 12-22, From Davis, J.H., & Sheldon, G.F. (1995). *Surgery: a problem-solving approach* (ed. 2). St Louis: Mosby; **12-4, 12-5,** From Cooperman, A.M., & Hoerr, S.O. (Eds.). (1978). *Surgery of the pancreas: a text and atlas.* St. Louis: Mosby; **12-6,** From Thibodeau, G.A., & Patton, K.T. (1996). *Anatomy and physiology* (ed. 3). St. Louis: Mosby; **12-7, 12-8, 12-9,** Courtesy Codman & Shurtleff, Inc., Randolph, Massachusetts; **12-10, 12-27, 12-35, 12-36,** From Daly, J.M., & Cady, B. (1993). *Atlas of surgical oncology.* St. Louis: Mosby; **12-14,** Reprinted with permission from AORN Clinical Path Template, 1997, pp. 10-13. Copyright AORN. Inc., Denver, Colorado; **12-15, 12-16,** From Quilici, P.J. (1992). New developments in laparoscopy. Norwalk, Conn.: U.S. Surgical Corporation; **12-23, 12-24,** From Cerilli, G.J. (1988). *Organ transplantation and replacement.* Philadelphia: J.B. Lippincott; **12-25,** From Davis, J.H., et al (1987) Clinical Surgery, Vol. 2. St. Louis: Mosby; **12-26, 12-28, 12-29,** **12-30, 12-31, 12-32, 12-33, 12-34,** Copyright 1990 Lahey Clinic, Burlington, Massachusetts; **12-37,** Courtesy Neoprobe Corp., Columbus, Ohio; **12-38,** From Anscher, N.L., et al. (1984). In Simmons R.L., et al. (Eds.). *Manual of vasuclar access, organ donation, and transplantation.* New York: Springer-Verlag.

Chapter 13

13-1, From Davis, J.H., & Sheldon, G.F. (1995). *Surgery: a problem-solving approach* (ed. 2). St Louis: Mosby; **13-2, 13-4, 13-15,** From Schumpelick, V. (1990). *Atlas of hernia surgery* Toronto: B.C. Decker; **13-12,** Courtesy Davol Inc. Subsidiary of C.R. Bard, Inc., Cranston, Rhode Island; **13-13,** From Zollinger, R.M., & Zollinger, R.M., Jr. (1993). *Atlas of surgical operations* (ed 7). New York: McGraw-Hill; **13-17,** From Liechty, R.D., & Soper, R.T. (1985). *Synopsis of surgery* (ed. 5). St. Louis: Mosby.

Chapter 14

14-1, 14-2, 14-3, 14-4, 14-5, 14-6, From Lowdermilk, D.L., et al. (1997). *Maternity and women's health care* (ed. 6). St. Louis: Mosby; **14-8, 14-9, 14-10, 14-11,** *1, 3, 4, 5,* **14-12, 14-13, 14-14,** Courtesy Codman & Shurtleff, Inc., Randolph, Massachusetts; **14-11,** *2,* Courtesy DISC Co., Inc., Malvern, Pennsylvania; **14-17,** Redrawn from Symmonds, R.E. (1984). Relaxation of pelvic supports. In Benson, R.C. (Ed.). *Current obstetric and gynecologic diagnosis and treatment* (ed. 5). Los Altos: Lange Medical Publications; **14-18, 14-19,** From Herbst, A.L., et al. (1992). *Comprehensive gynecology* (ed. 2). St. Louis: Mosby; **14-24, 14-30, 14-40, 14-44,** From Ball, T.L. (1963). *Gynecologic surgery and urology* (ed. 2). St. Louis: Mosby; **14-27,** From Schrock, T.R. (1994). *Handbook of surgery* (ed. 10). St. Louis: Mosby; **14-28, 14-29, 14-35, 14-36, 14-38, 14-41, 14-45, 14-46, 14-47,** From Nichols, D.H. (1993). *Gynecologic and obstetric surgery,* St. Louis: Mosby; **14-37,** From Marlow Surgical Technologies, Inc.; **14-39,** Courtesy Cooper Health Systems, Camden, New Jersey; **14-48,** Courtesy Ohio Medical Products, Madison, Wisconsin; **14-49,** Courtesy Edward Weck & Co., Research Triangle Park, North Carolina.

Chapter 15

15-1, 15-6, 15-7, Modified from Seidel, H.M., et al. (1995). *Mosby's guide to physical examination* (ed. 3). St. Louis: Mosby; **15-3, 15-33, 15-72,** From Nagle, G.M. (1997). *Genitourinary surgery.* St. Louis: Mosby; **15-9, 15-16, 15-17, 15-19, 15-21, 15-34, 15-35, 15-53, 15-54, 15-57, 15-71,** Courtesy Circon Corp., Santa Barbara, California; **15-11,** Courtesy Cook Urological, Spencer, Indiana; **15-18, 15-22, 15-40,** Courtesy Greenwald Surgical Co., Inc., Lake Station, Indiana; **15-23, 15-26, 15-27, 15-28, 15-30, 15-64,** *A,* Courtesy American Medical Systems, Minnetonka, Minnesota; **15-29, 15-43, 15-44, 15-45, 15-49, 15-50, 15-51, 15-62, 15-63, 15-64,** *B,* **15-74, 15-75,** From Droller,

M.J. (1992). *Surgical management of urologic disease.* St. Louis: Mosby; **15-31, 15-65, 15-66, 15-69, 15-70,** From Gillenwater, J.Y., et al. (1996). *Adult and pediatric urology* (ed. 3)., vol. 2, St. Louis: Mosby; **15-42, 15-48,** Courtesy Omni-Tract Surgical, a division of MN Scientific, Inc., St. Paul, Minnesota; **15-59,** Courtesy Pilling Company, Fort Washington, Pennsylvania; **15-60,** Courtesy Influence, Inc., San Francisco, California; **15-67,** From Gray, M. (1992). *Genitourinary disorders,* St. Louis: Mosby; **15-68,** From Brundage, D. (1992). *Renal disorders,* St. Louis: Mosby.

Chapter 16

16-2, 16-8, From Healy, J., & Hodge, J. (1990). *Surgical anatomy* (ed. 2). Philadelphia: B.C. Decker; **16-4,** Courtesy Tucson Medical Center, Tucson, Arizona; **16-6, 16-7,** From Clark, O.H. (1985). *Endocrine surgery of the thyroid and parathyroid glands.* St. Louis: Mosby.

Chapter 17

17-1, 17-2, 17-3, 17-9, From Isaacs, J.H. (1992). *Textbook of breast disease.* St. Louis: Mosby; **17-4, 17-5, 17-6,** Courtesy Wende W. Logan, MD, Rochester, New York and the Breast Clinic of Rochester; **17-7, 17-8,** Copyright 1997 United States Surgical Corporation. All rights reserved. Reprinted with the permission of United States Surgical Corporation. Trademark of United States Surgical Corporation; **17-10,** Courtesy Vanderbilt University Medical Center, Nashville, Tennessee; **17-11,** Redrawn from Zollinger, R.M. (1988). *Atlas of surgical operations* (ed. 6). New York: MacMillan.

Chapter 18

18-1, 18-2, 18-3, From Thompson, J.M., et al. (1997). *Mosby's clinical nursing* (ed. 4). St. Louis: Mosby; **18-4,** From Phipps, W.J., et al. (1995). *Medical-surgical nursing: concepts and clinical practice* (ed. 5). St. Louis: Mosby; **18-7, 18-55, 18-64, 18-65,** From Federman, J.L., et al. (1994). *Retina and vitreous.* London: Mosby; **18-10,** Modified from Thibodeau, G.A. (1990). *Anthony's textbook of anatomy and physiology* (ed. 13). St. Louis: Mosby; **18-13,** From Stein, H.A., Slatt, B.J., & Stein, R.M. (1994). *The ophthalmic assistant: a guide for ophthalmic medical personnel* (ed. 6.) St. Louis: Mosby; **18-15,** From Mawhinney, M.S. (1989). Operative stretchers: use in ophthalmologic procedures, *AORN Journal, 50,* 314; **18-20,** Courtesy Zeiss, Inc.; **18-24, 18-26, 18-27, 18-28,** From Tenzel, R.R. (1993). *Textbook of ophthalmology, vol. 4, orbit and oculoplastics.* London: Gower; **18-25, 18-30,** From Saunders, W.H., et al. (1979). *Nursing care in eye, ear, nose, and throat disorders* (ed. 4). St. Louis: Mosby; **18-33,** From Allen, J.H. (Ed.). (1963). *May's manual of the diseases of the eye* (ed. 23). Baltimore: Williams & Wilkins; **18-42, 18-43,** From Newell, F.W. (1992). *Ophthalmology: principles and concepts* (ed. 7). St. Louis: Mosby; **18-44,** From Rothrock, J.C. (1996). Perioperative Nursing Care Plans (ed. 2). St. Louis: Mosby; **18-46, 18-53, 18-58, 18-59, 18-60, 18-61,**

Courtesy Visual Communications, The Methodist Hospital, Houston, Texas; **18-47, 18-49, 18-50,** From Lindquist, T.D., & Lindstrom, R.L. (1990). *Ophthalmic surgery: looseleaf and update service,* St. Louis: Mosby; **18-54,** From Ryan, S.J., et al. (1995). *Retina* (ed. 2). St. Louis: Mosby.

Chapter 19

19-1, 19-2, 19-4, 19-5, From Seidel, H.M., et al. (1995). *Mosby's guide to physical examination* (ed. 3). St. Louis: Mosby; **19-3, 19-17, 19-23,** From DeWeese, D.D., et al. (1988). *Otolaryngology: head and neck surgery* (ed. 7). St. Louis: Mosby; **19-6, 19-7, 19-8,** Courtesy Marvin P. Fried, MD, Boston, Massachusetts; **19-9,** Courtesy XOMED, Jacksonville, Florida; **19-18,** From Saunders, W.H., et al. (1979). *Nursing care in eye, ear, nose, and throat disorders* (ed. 4). St. Louis: Mosby; **19-19,** Courtesy Vanderbilt University Hospital, Nashville, Tennessee; **19-21,** Courtesy Oto-Med, Inc., Lake Havasu, Arizona; **19-24,** From Cummings, C.W., et al. (1997). *Otolaryngology: head and neck surgery* (ed. 8). St. Louis: Mosby; **19-25,** From Tjellstrom, H., & Hakansson, B. (1995). The bone-anchored hearing aid, *Otolaryngologic Clinics of North America, 1*(1).

Chapter 20

20-2, From Saunders, W.H., et al. (1979). *Nursing care in eye, ear, nose, and throat disorders.* St. Louis: Mosby; **20-5, 20-6, 20-7, 20-8,** Courtesy Codman & Shurtleff, Inc., Randolph, Massachusetts; **20-9, 20-36,** From DeWeese, D.D., & Saunders, W.H. (1982). *Textbook of otolaryngology* (ed. 6). St. Louis: Mosby; **20-10,** Courtesy Ohio State University Medical Center, Columbus, Ohio; **20-12, 20-14,** From Schuller, D.E., & Schleuning, A.J. (1994). *Otolaryngology: head and neck surgery* (ed. 8). St. Louis: Mosby; **21-13,** From Cummings, C.W., et al. (1993). *Otolaryngology: head and neck surgery* (ed. 3). St. Louis: Mosby; **20-15, 20-16,** Courtesy Vanderbilt University Medical Center, Nashville, Tennessee; **20-17, 20-18, 10-19, 20-20, 20-21, 20-22, 20-23, 20-24, 20-25, 20-25, 20-27, 20-28, 20-29, 20-30, 20-31, 20-32, 20-33,** From Stammberger, H. (1991). *Functional endoscopic sinus surgery.* Philadelphia: B.C. Decker; **20-34,** From Thawley, S.E., & Garrett, H. (1988). Endoscopic sinus surgery; an outpatient procedure that minimizes tissue removal. *AORN Journal, 47,* 902. Copyright AORN, Inc. Denver, Colorado.

Chapter 21

21-1, 21-2, 21-3, From Marino, L.B. (1981). *Cancer nursing,* St. Louis: Mosby; **21-4, 21-11, 21-12, 21-13, 21-17, 21-18, 21-19, 21-20, B, 21-22, 21-23, 21-24,** From Cummings, C.W., et al. (1993). *Otolaryngology: head and neck surgery* (ed. 3). St. Louis: Mosby; **21-6, A, 21-14.** From DeWeese, D.D. (1982). *Textbook of otolaryngology* (ed. 6). St. Louis: Mosby; **21-6, B,** Courtesy Pilling Company, Philadelphia, Pennsylvania; **21-10,** From McCance, K.L.

(1998). *Pathophysiology: the biologic basis for disease in adults and children* (ed. 3). St. Louis: Mosby; **21-15,** Lewis, S.M., et al. (1996). *Medical-surgical nursing* (ed. 4). St. Louis: Mosby; **21-16,** From Luckmann, J. (1987). *Medical-surgical nursing* (ed. 3). Philadelphia: W.B. Saunders; **21-20,** *A,* From Sigler, B.A., et al. (1993). *Ear, nose and throat disorders.* St. Louis: Mosby; **21-21,** Courtesy Johns Hopkins Hospital, Baltimore, Maryland.

Chapter 22

22-1, From Gosling, J.A., et al. (1996). *Human anatomy* (ed. 3). London: Mosby; **22-2, 22-4, 22-5, 22-6, 22-7, A, 22-8, 22-9, 22-12, 22-126,** From Thibodeau, G.A., & Patton, K.T. (1996). *Anatomy and physiology* (ed. 3). St. Louis: Mosby; **22-3,** Redrawn from Lewis, R.C. (1988). *Primary care orthopedics.* New York: Churchill Livingstone; **22-11, 22-15, 22-19, 22-39, 22-43, 22-54, 22-71, 22-76, 22-93, 22-102, 22-105, 22-127,** Courtesy Zimmer, Inc., Warsaw, Indiana; **22-13,** Courtesy Franciscan Hospital, Mount Airy Campus, Cincinnati, Ohio; **22-14,** Courtesy McConnell Orthopaedic Manufacturing Company, Greenville, Texas; **22-16, 22-83, 22-119,** Courtesy Acufex Microsurgical, Inc., Mansfield, Massachusetts; **22-17,** Courtesy OSI, Hayward, California; **22-18, 22-37, 22-50, 22-52, 22-63, 22-79, 22-107, 22-109, 22-110,** From Gregory, B. (1994). *Orthopaedic surgery.* St. Louis: Mosby; **22-20, 22-21, 22-68,** Courtesy Zimmer Traction Handbook, 1989, Zimmer, Inc., Warsaw, Indiana; **22-23,** From Mourad, L.A. (1991). *Orthopedic disorders.* St. Louis: Mosby; **22-24,** Courtesy Span & Aids, McGaw Park, Illinois; **22-25, 22-80, 22-91, 22-94, 22-99,** From DePuy ACE Medical Company, El Segundo, California; **22-26, 22-74, 22-96, 22-98, 22-111, 22-113, 22-115, 22-116,** Courtesy Stryker Surgical, Kalamazoo, Michigan; **22-33,** Courtesy Hall Surgical Division, Carpinteria, California; **22-34,** Courtesy Osteotech, Shrewsbury, New Jersey; **22-35,** From Phipps, W.J., et al. (1995). *Medical-surgical nursing* (ed. 5). St. Louis: Mosby; **22-36,** Courtesy Orthopaedic Division of Telectronics Proprietary, Ltd., Englewood, Colorado; **22-38, 22-43, 22-65, 22-67,** From Gustilo, R.B., et al. (1993). *Fractures and dislocations, vol. 2.* St. Louis: Mosby; **22-40, 22-42, 22-57,** Courtesy Synthes U.S.A., Paoli, Pennsylvania; **22-41,** Courtesy Richards Medical Co., Memphis, Tennessee; **22-45,** Courtesy LTI Medica and the UpJohn Company. Illustration by Beverly Kessler, 1982, Learning Technology, Inc.; **22-46, 22-56, 22-59, 22-61,** From Crenshaw, A.H. (1992). *Campbell's operative orthopaedics* (ed. 8). St. Louis: Mosby; **22-47,** Courtesy Biomet, Inc., Warwaw, Indiana; **22-49,** Redrawn from Rockwood, C.A., Jr., et al. (1984). *Fractures in adults* (ed. 2). Philadelphia: J.B. Lippincott; **22-51,** Courtesy The Anspach Effort, Inc., Palm Beach Gardens, Florida, **22-53,** Redrawn from Neer, C.S., II. (1970). *Journal of Bone and Joint Surgery, 52-A:*1007; **22-60,** From Knight, R.A. (1957). *AAOS Inst Course Lecture, 14:*123; **22-62, 22-87,** From Muller, M.E., et al. (1990). *Manual of internal fixation: techniques recommended by AO-ASIF group* (ed. 3). Berlin: Springer-Verlag; **22-64,** Redrawn from Sprague, H.H., & Howard, F.M. (1988). *Contemporary Orthopedics, 16:*18; **22-68,** Courtesy Zimmer Technique Manual, Warsaw, Indiana; **22-69, 22-97, 22-125,** Courtesy Richards Medical Company, Memphis, Tennessee; **22-70, 22-86,** From Canale, S.T. (1998). *Campbell's Operative Orthopaedics,* (ed. 9). St. Louis: Mosby; **22-72, 22-73, 22-85, 22-95, 22-100, 22-101, 22-106,** Courtesy Howmedica, Inc., Rutherford, New Jersey; **22-75,** From Gustilo, R.B. (1991). *The Fracture Classification Manual.* St. Louis: Mosby; **22-77,** Redrawn from Muller, M.E., et al. (1990). *The comprehensive classification of fractures of long bones,* Berlin: Springer-Verlag; **22-78,** Redrawn from Schatzker, J., McBroom, R., & Bruce, D. (1979). *Clinical Orthopedics, 138,* 94; **22-81,** Courtesy 3M Health Care, St. Paul, Minnesota; **22-82,** Redrawn from Cox, J.S. (1976). *American Journal of Sports Medicine, 4,* 72; **22-84,** Courtesy Linvatec; **22-88,** From Richards, V. (1956). *Surgery for general practice.* St. Louis: Mosby; **22-90,** From Tile, M. (1988). *Journal of Bone and Joint Surgery, 70-B,* 3; **22-92,** From Cameron, H.U. (1992). *The technique of total hip arthroplasty.* St. Louis: Mosby; **22-103,** Courtesy 3M Orthopedic Products, St. Paul, Minnesota; **22-104,** Redrawn from Gristina, A.G., & Webb, L.X. (1983). *Proximal humeral and monospherical glenoid replacement: surgical technique.* Rutherford: Howmedica, Inc.; **22-108,** Courtesy Dow Corning Wright, Arlington, Texas; **22-112, 22-124,** Courtesy Smith + Nephew Dyonics, Andover, Massachussets; **22-114,** Courtesy Arthrex, Inc., Naples, Florida; **22-117, 22-118,** From Shahriaree, H. (1984). *O'Connor's textbook of arthroscopic surgery.* Philadelphia: J.B. Lippincott; **22-120,** Courtesy Johnson and Johnson; **22-122,** From Laurin, C.A., et al. (1992). *Atlas of orthopaedic surgery,* vol. 3, *lower extremity.* Masson; **22-128,** From Bradford, D.S., et al. (1987). *Moe's textbook of scoliosis and other spinal deformities* (ed. 2). Philadelphia: W.B. Saunders; **22-129,** Courtesy Danek, Memphis, Tennessee.

Chapter 23

23-1, 23-2, 23-3, 23-4, 23-19, From Thibodeau, G.A., & Patton, K.T. (1996). *Anatomy and physiology* (ed. 3). St. Louis: Mosby; **23-5, 23-7, 23-8, 23-9, 23-10, 23-21,** From Conway-Rutkowski, B.L. (1982). *Carini and Owens' neurological and neurosurgical nursing* (ed. 8). St. Louis: Mosby; **23-6, 23-12, 23-13, 23-14, 23-15,** From Anthony, C.P., & Thibodeau, G.A. (1983). *Textbook of anatomy and physiology* (ed. 11). St. Louis: Mosby; **23-11,** From Nolte, J. (1988). *The human brain: an introduction to its fundamental anatomy* (ed. 2). St. Louis: Mosby; **23-16,** Modified from Mettler, F.A. (1948). *Neuroanatomy* (ed. 2). St. Louis: Mosby. In Conway-Rutkowski, B.L. (1982). *Carini and Owens' neurological and neurosurgical nursing* (ed. 8). St. Louis: Mosby; **23-17, 23-18,** From Mettler, F.A. (1948). *Neuroatomy* (ed. 2). St. Louis: Mosby; **23-22, 23-23, 23-24, 23-28, A, 23-32, 23-43, A, 23-45, 23-47, 23-48, 23-49, 23-50, 23-51, 23-52, 23-53,**

23-54, 23-55, 23-56, 23-59, 23-60, 23-66, 23-67, 23-73, Courtesy Codman & Shurtleff, Inc., Randolph, Massachussets; **23-26, 23-43, C, 23-63,** Courtesy Omi Surgical Products, a division of Ohio Medical Instrument Company, Cincinnati, Ohio; **23-28, B,** Courtesy Valley-Lab, Inc., Boulder, Colorado; **23-29,** Courtesy Zimmer-Reed, Midlothian, Virginia; **23-30,** Courtesy Midas Rex Corp., Fort Worth, Texas; **23-35,** Courtesy HEALTH-SOUTH Medical Center, Richmond, Virginia; **23-36, 23-37,** From Richards, V. (1956). *Surgery for general practice.* St. Louis: Mosby; **23-38, 23-41,** From Kempe, L.G. (1968). *Operative neurosurgery,* vols. 1 and 2. New York: Springer-Verlag; **23-39,** From Barber, J., et al. (1977). *Adult and child care* (ed. 2). St. Louis: Mosby; **23-40, 23-42, 23-69, 23-70, 23-72,** From Carini, E., & Owens, G. (1974). *Neurological and neurosurgical nursing* (ed. 6). St. Louis: Mosby; **23-43, B,** Courtesy Holco Instrument Corp., New York, New York; **23-44,** Courtesy Aesculap, Burlingame, California; **23-57, 23-58,** From *Neurosurgery wound closure,* Ethicon, Inc., **23-61, 23-68, 23-76,** From Sachs, E. (1949). *Diagnosis and treatment of brain tumors and the care of the neurosurgical patient* (ed. 2). St. Louis: Mosby; **23-62, 23-65,** From Barker, E. (1994). *Neuroscience nursing.* St. Louis: Mosby; **23-64,** Courtesy Cordis Corporation, Miami, Florida; **23-71,** Courtesy K. Cramer Lewis, Department of Illustrations, Washington University School of Medicine, St. Louis, Missouri; **23-74,** Courtesy Vanderbilt University Medical Center Nashville, Tennessee.

Chapter 24

24-1, From Stuart, G.W., & Laraia, M.T. (1993). *Stuart & Sundeen's principles and practices of psychiatric nursing* (ed. 6). St. Louis: Mosby; **24-2,** Courtesy Vanderbilt University Medical Center, Nashville, Tennessee; **24-29,** From Neff, J.A., & Kidd, P.M. (1993). *Trauma nursing: the art and science.* St. Louis: Mosby; **24-30, 24-39,** From Thibodeau, G.A., & Patton, K.T. (1997). *The human body in health and disease* (ed. 2). St. Louis: Mosby; **24-36,** From Fortunato, N. (1998). *Plastic and reconstructive surgery.* St. Louis: Mosby; **24-40,** From Hollinshead, W.H. (1969). *Anatomy for surgeons,* vol 3, *the back and limb* (ed. 2). New York: Harper & Row.

Chapter 25

25-5, 25-6, From Schottelius, B.A., & Schottelius, D.D. (1978). *Textbook of physiology* (ed. 18). St. Louis: Mosby; **25-7, 25-8, 25-9, 25-11, 25-12, 25-15, 1, 5, 6, 10-18,** Courtesy Pilling Company, Fort Washington, Pennsylvania; **25-10** Courtesy Olympus, New Hyde Park, New York; **25-14, 1-7,** Courtesy Codman & Shurtleff, Inc., Randolph, Massachusetts; **25-14, 8, 25-15, 7,** Courtesy Zimmer, Inc., Warsaw, Indiana; **25-15, 2, 4, 8-9,** Courtesy Edward Weck & Co., Research Triangle Park, North Carolina; **25-16,** From Johnson, J., & Kirby, C.K. (1970). *Surgery of the chest* (ed. 4). Chicago: Year Book; **25-17,** From Thompson, J.M., et al. (1993). *Mosby's clinical*

nursing (ed. 4). St. Louis: Mosby; **25-20,** Courtesy Vanderbilt University Medical Center, Nashville, Tennessee; **25-24,** Redrawn from Dehnel, W. (1973). *AORN Journal, 18,* 296.

Chapter 26

26-1, B, 26-2, 26-3, 26-4, 26-11, From Thibodeau, G.A., & Patton, K.T. (1996). *Anatomy and physiology* (ed. 3). St. Louis: Mosby; **26-5,** From Dettenmeier, P.A. (1995). *Radiographic assessment for nurses.* St. Louis: Mosby; **26-8, 26-9, 26-15, 26-17,** From MacVittie, B.A. (1998). *Vascular surgery.* St. Louis: Mosby; **26-12,** From Haimovici, H. (1984). *Vascular surgery: principles and technique.* Norwalk: Appleton-Century-Crofts; **26-14, 26-18,** From Hershey, F.B., & Calman, C.H. (1973). *Atlas of vascular surgery* (ed. 3). St. Louis: Mosby; **26-16,** Reprinted with permission from AORN Clinical Path Template, 1997, pp. 14-17. Copyright AORN, Inc., Denver, Colorado; **26-22, 26-24, 26-25,** From Wilson, S.E. (1996). *Vascular access: principles and practice* (ed. 3). St. Louis: Mosby; **26-23** From Calne, R., & Pollard, S.G. (1992). *Operative surgery.* London: Gower; **26-26,** From Ballinger, P.W. (1995). *Merrill's atlas of radiographic positions and radiologic procedures,* vol. 2 (ed. 8). St. Louis: Mosby.

Unit III photo: Courtesy Joseph T. Rothrock, III. Medical Photographer, Cooper Hospital/University Medical Center, Camden, New Jersey.

Chapter 27

27-1, 27-2, 27-6, From Seifert, P.C. (1994). *Cardiac surgery.* St. Louis: Mosby. Drawings by Peter Stone; **27-4,** From Berne, R.N., & Levy, M.N. (1997). *Cardiovascular physiology* (ed. 7). St. Louis: Mosby; **27-5,** From Thompson, J.M., et al. (1997). *Mosby's clinical nursing* (ed. 4). St. Louis: Mosby; **27-8, 27-11,** From Canobbio, M. (1990). *Cardiovascular disorders.* St. Louis; Mosby; **27-9, 27-10,** Courtesy Edward A. Lefrak, MD, Annandale, Virginia. **27-12,** From Kinney, M., & Packa, D. (1995). *Andreoli's comprehensive cardiac care* (ed. 7). St. Louis: Mosby; **27-13,** From Brooks-Tighe, S. (1994). *Instrumentation for the operating room* (ed. 4). St. Louis: Mosby; **27-14,** Courtesy Scanlan International, St. Paul, Minnesota; **27-15,** Courtesy Rultract, Inc., Cleveland, Ohio; **27-16,** Courtesy Pilling Company, Fort Washington, Pennsylvania; **27-17, 27-50,** Courtesy United States Surgical Cororation, Cardiovascular Division, Holly Springs, North Carolina; **27-18,** Courtesy Hewlett-Packard Company, Medical Products Group, Andover, Massachusetts; **27-20, 27-21, 27-22,** Courtesy Meadox Medicals, a division of Boston Scientific Company; **27-23,** Courtesy of St. Jude Medical, Inc. St. Paul, Minnesota; **27-24,** Courtesy Sulzer Carbomedics, Inc., Austin, Texas; **27-25, 27-27, 27-28, 27-29, 27-33,** Courtesy Baxter Healthcare Corp., Edwards CVS division, Santa Ana, California. **27-26, 27-32, 27-73, 27-76, 27-78,** Courtesy Medtronic, Inc, Minneapolis, Minnesota; **27-30, 27-31,** Courtesy CryoLife, Inc.,

Marietta, Georgia; **27-35, 27-41,** Courtesy Bard Cardiopulmonary GTC, Haverhill, Massachusetts; **27-36, 27-37, 27-38, 27-40, 27-43, 27-44, 27-46, 27-47, 27-49, 27-51, 27-52. 28-56, 27-57, 27-58, 27-59, 27-60, 27-61, 27-62, 27-63, 27-64, 27-66, 27-67, 27-68, 27-69, 27-70, 27-71, 27-74, 27-75, 27-77, 27-79,** From Waldhausen, J.A., Pierce, W.S., & Campbell, D.B. (1996). *Johnson's surgery of the chest* (ed. 6). St. Louis: Mosby; **27-39, 27-55,** Courtesy Heartport, Inc., Redwood City, California; **27-42,** From Drinkwater, D.C., Laks, H., & Buckberg, G.D. (1990). A new simplified method of optimizing cardioplegic delivery without right heart isolation antegrade/retrograde blood cardioplegia. *Journal of Thoracic and Cardiovascular Surgery, 100,* 56; **27-45,** Courtesy Bev DeBold; **27-48,** From Lytle, B.W., et al. (1989). Coronary artery bypass grafting with the right gastroepiploic artery. *Journal of Thoracic and Cardiovascular Surgery,* 97(6), 826; **27-54,** Courtesy CardioThoracic Systems, Cupertino, California; **27-65, 27-72,** From Doty, D.B. (1997). *Cardiac surgery: operative technique.* St. Louis: Mosby.

Chapter 28

28-1 to 28-6 Courtesy Saint Francis Hospital, Tulsa, Oklahoma.

Chapter 29

29-1, 29-2, 29-3, 29-8, 29-11, 29-13, From Coran, A.G., et al. (1978). *Surgery of the neonate.* Boston: Little, Brown; **29-5,** From Randolph, J.G. (1985). *Annals of Surgery, 198,* 579; **29-6,** From Benson, C.D. (1969). *Infants' hypertrophic pyloric stenosis.* In Mustard, W.T., et al. *Pediatric surgery* (ed. 2). Chicago: Year Book; **29-7,** Modified from Gross, R.E. (1970). *An atlas of children's surgery.* Philadelphia: W.B. Saunders; **29-9, 29-14,** From Lewis, J.E. (1967). *Atlas of infant surgery.* St. Louis: Mosby; **29-10,** Modified from Boley, S.J. (1968). An endorectal pull-through operation with primary anastomosis for Hirschsprung's disease, *Surgery, Gynecology and Obstetrics,* 127:(2), 253; **29-12,** From DeVries, P.A. (1984). *Posterior sagittal anorectoplasty.* In Holmann von Kap, herr S. (Ed.). *Anorektale Fehlbildungen.* Stuttgart: Gustav Fischer-Verlag; **29-15,** Courtesy Karl Storz, Culver City, California; **29-17,** Modified from Gillenwater, J.Y. (1991). *Adult and pediatric urology.* St. Louis: Mosby; **29-18, 29-19, 29-23,** Modified from Droller, M.J. (1992). *Surgical management of urologic disease.* St. Louis: Mosby; **29-20,** From Devine, C.J., Jr. (1983). *Chordee and hypospadias.* In Glenn, J.F., & Boyce, W.H. (Eds.). *Urologic surgery* (ed. 3). Philadelphia: J.B. Lippincott; **29-24,** Modified from Culp, D.A., et al. (1985). *Surgical urology* (ed. 5). Chicago: Year Book; **29-25,** Modified from DeWeese, D.D., & Saunders, W.H. (1982). *Textbook of otolaryngology* (ed. 6). St. Louis: Mosby; **29-26,** From Saunders, W.H., et al. (1979). *Nursing care in eye, ear, nose and throat disorders* (ed. 4). St. Louis: Mosby; **29-27,** Courtesy Codman & Shurtleff, Inc., Randolph, Massachussetts; **29-28,** From Luckmann, J., & Sorenson, K.C.

(1987). *Medical-surgical nursing* (ed. 3). Philadelphia: W.B. Saunders; **29-29,** From *Neurosurgery wound closure,* Ethicon, Inc., **29-35, 29-36, 29-37,** Courtesy Emory University School of Medicine, Atlanta, Georgia; **29-39, A,** Redrawn from Chameides, L. (1988). *Pediatric advanced life support.* Dallas: American Heart Association; **29-39, B,** Barkin, R.M., & Rosen, P. (1990). *Emergency pediatrics: a guide to ambulatory care* (ed. 3). St. Louis: Mosby; **29-40, 29-43, 29-46, 29-49, 29-52, 29-56, 29-59, 29-64, 29-65, 29-66,** From Nichols, D.G., et al. (1994). *Critical heart disease in infants and children.* St. Louis: Mosby; **29-41, 29-45, 29-47, 29-48, 29-50, 29-51, 29-55, 29-58, 29-61, 29-63,** From Wong, D.L. (1995). *Whaley & Wong's nursing care of infants and children* (ed. 5). St. Louis: Mosby; **29-42,** Courtesy Vanderbilt University Medical Center, Nashville, Tennesee, **29-44,** From Cooley, D.A., & Norman, J.C. (1975). *Techniques in cardiac surgery.* Houston: Texas Medical Press; **29-53, 29-54, 29-62,** From Mavroudis, C., & Backer, C.L. (1994). *Pediatric cardiac surgery* (ed. 2) St. Louis: Mosby; **29-57,** From Effler, D.B. (1978). *Elades' surgical disease of the chest* (ed. 4). St. Louis: Mosby; **29-60,** From Burke, R.P., & Wernovsky, G. (1997). Thoracoscopic clipping of patent ductus arteriosus, *New England Journal of Medicine,* 336(3), 185; **29-67,** From Doty, D.B. (1997). *Cardiac surgery operative technique.* St. Louis: Mosby; **29-68,** From Cooley, D.A. (1984). *Techniques in cardiac surgery* (ed. 2). Philadelphia: W.B. Saunders.

Chapter 31

31-1, 31-3, 31-4, 31-5, 31-6, 31-12, 31-17, 31-18, From Neff, J.A., & Kidd, P.S. (1993). *Trauma nursing: the art and science.* St. Louis: Mosby; **31-2,** Courtesy MedFlight; **31-7,** From Sheehy, S.B., & Jimmerson, C.L. (1994). *Manual of clinical trauma care: the first hour* (ed. 2). St. Louis: Mosby; **31-8,** From Kuska, B.M. (1982). Acute onset of compartment syndrome, *Journal of Emergency Nursing,* 8(2), 78; **31-9,** Courtesy Stryker, Inc., Kalamazoo, Michigan; **31-10,** From Grande, C.M. (1993). *Textbook of trauma anesthesia and critical care.* St. Louis: Mosby; **31-11,** From Criswell, J.C., & Parr, M.J.A. (June 1992). *Emergency airway management in trauma patients with cervical spine injury;* presented at 5th Annual Trauma Anesthesia and Critical Care Symposium, Amsterdam; **31-14,** From Cosgriff, J.H., Jr., & Anderson, D.L. *The practice of emergency care* (ed. 2). Philadelphia: J.B. Lippincott; **31-15,** Redrawn from Kintzel, K.C. (1977). *Advanced concepts in clinical nursing* (ed. 2). Philadelphia: J.B. Lippincott; **31-16,** Redrawn from Becker, D.P., Gade, G.F., Young, H.F., & Fewerman, T.F. (1990). Diagnosis and treatment of head injury. In Youman, J.R. (Ed.). *Neurological surgery* (ed. 3). Philadelphia: W.B. Saunders; **31-19,** From Feliciano, D.V., Moore, E.E., & Mattox, K.L. (1996). *Trauma* (ed. 3). Stamford: Appelton & Lange; **31-20,** From Feliciano, D.V., et al. Packing for control of hepatic hemorrhage, *Journal of Trauma, 26,* 738-743; **31-21,** From Sanders, M.J. (1994). *Mosby's paramedic textbook.* St. Louis: Mosby.

Index